Colon and Other Gastrointestinal Cancers

Cancer

Principles & Practice of Oncology

10th edition

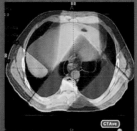
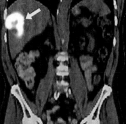
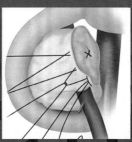
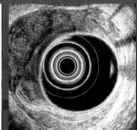

Vincent T. DeVita, Jr., MD

Amy & Joseph Perella Professor of Medicine
Yale Comprehensive Cancer Center and Smilow
   Cancer Hospital at Yale-New Haven
Professor of Epidemiology and Public Health
Yale University School of Public Health
New Haven, Connecticut

Theodore S. Lawrence, MD, PhD

Isadore Lampe Professor and Chair
Department of Radiation Oncology
University of Michigan
Ann Arbor, Michigan

Steven A. Rosenberg, MD, PhD

Chief, Surgery Branch, National Cancer Institute, National Institutes of Health
Professor of Surgery, Uniformed Services University of the Health Sciences
School of Medicine
Bethesda, Maryland
Professor of Surgery
George Washington University School of Medicine
Washington, District of Columbia

Acquisitions Editor: Julie Goolsby
Senior Product Development Editor: Emilie Moyer
Editorial Assistant: Brian Convery
Production Project Manager: David Orzechowski
Marketing Manager: Rachel Mante Leung
Senior Designer: Stephen Druding
Illustration Coordinator: Jennifer Clements
Illustrator: Jason McAlexander, Electronic Publishing Services, Inc.
Manufacturing Coordinator: Beth Welsh
Prepress Vendor: Absolute Service, Inc.
Prepress Vendor Project Manager: Harold Medina

Library of Congress Cataloging-in-Publication Data

Names: DeVita, Vincent T., Jr., 1935- , editor. | Lawrence, Theodore S.,
    editor. | Rosenberg, Steven A., editor.
Title: Cancer : principles & practice of oncology. Colon and other
    gastrointestinal cancers / [edited by] Vincent T. DeVita, Jr., Theodore S.
    Lawrence, Steven A. Rosenberg.
Other titles: Colon and other gastrointestinal cancers
Description: Philadelphia : Wolters Kluwer Health, [2016] | Contained in:
    Devita, Hellman, and Rosenberg's cancer. 10th edition. [2015]. | Includes
    bibliographical references and index.
Identifiers: LCCN 2016005138 | ISBN 9781496333964
Subjects: | MESH: Gastrointestinal Neoplasms
Classification: LCC RC261 | NLM WI 149 | DDC 616.99/4--dc23 LC record available at
http://lccn.loc.gov/2016005138

Ghassan Abou-Alfa, MD
Associate Attending
Department of Medicine
Memorial Sloan-Kettering Cancer Center
Associate Professor
Department of Medicine
Weill Cornell Medical College
New York, New York

Ross A. Abrams, MD
Chairman and Hendrickson Professor of
    Radiation Oncology
Rush University Medical Center
Chicago, Illinois

Gregory P. Adams, PhD
Associate Professor Developmental
    Therapeutics Program
Director of Biological Research and
    Therapeutics
Fox Chase Cancer Center
Philadelphia, Pennsylvania

Bharat B. Aggarwal, PhD
Professor of Cancer Research
Professor of Cancer Medicine
    (Biochemistry)
Chief, Cytokine Research Laboratory
Department of Experimental
    Therapeutics
The University of Texas MD Anderson
    Cancer Center
Houston, Texas

Shahab Ahmed, MD
Data Analyst, Department of
    Gastrointestinal Medical Oncology
The University of Texas MD Anderson
    Cancer Center
Houston, Texas

Shirin Arastu-Kapur, PhD
Associate Director
Biology at Onyx Pharmaceuticals
South San Francisco, California

Alan Ashworth, FRS
Professor and Chief Executive
The Institute of Cancer Research
London, United Kingdom

Itzhak Avital, MD, FACS
Professor of Surgery
Executive Medical Director
Bon Secours Cancer Institute
Richmond, Virginia

Jennifer E. Axilbund, MS, CGC
Cancer Risk Assessment Program
The Johns Hopkins Hospital
Baltimore, Maryland

Sharyn D. Baker, PharmD, PhD
Associate Member
Pharmaceutical Sciences Department
St. Jude Children's Research Hospital
Memphis, Tennessee

Alberto Bardelli, MD
Laboratory of Molecular Genetics
Institute for Cancer Research and
    Treatment
University of Torino Medical School
Candiolo, Italy

Susan E. Bates, MD
Head, Molecular Therapeutics Section
Developmental Therapeutics Branch
Center for Cancer Research
National Cancer Institute
Bethesda, Maryland

Stephen B. Baylin, MD
Professor of Oncology
Professor of Medicine
Johns Hopkins University School of
    Medicine
Deputy Director of the Cancer Center
Baltimore, Maryland

Andrew Berchuck, MD
Professor and Director
Gynecologic Oncology Program
Division of Gynecologic Oncology
Department of Obstetrics and
    Gynecology
Duke Cancer Institute
Duke University Medical Center
Durham, North Carolina

Leslie Bernstein, MS, PhD
Professor and Director
Division of Cancer Etiology
Department of Population Sciences
Beckman Research Institute
City of Hope Dean for Faculty Affairs
City of Hope National Medical Center
    and the Beckman Research Institute
Duarte, California

Bryan L. Betz, PhD
Assistant Professor
Department of Pathology
University of Michigan
Technical Director
Molecular Diagnostics Laboratory
University of Michigan Health System
Ann Arbor, Michigan

Lawrence H. Boise, PhD
Professor
Winship Cancer Institute of Emory
    University
Departments of Hematology/Medical
    Oncology and Cell Biology
Emory School of Medicine
Atlanta, Georgia

Danielle C. Bonadies, MS, CGC
Director, Cancer Genetics Division
Gene Counsel, LLC
New Haven, Connecticut

Mitesh J. Borad, MD
Assistant Professor
Department of Medicine
Director, Phase I Drug Development
Mayo Clinic
Scottsdale, Arizona

Hossein Borghaei, MS, DO
Associate Professor
Chief, Thoracic Medical Oncology
Fox Chase Cancer Center
Philadelphia, Pennsylvania

Otis W. Brawley, MD, FACP
Chief Medical Officer
American Cancer Society, Inc.
Atlanta, Georgia

Dean E. Brenner, MD
Kutsche Family Professor of Internal
    Medicine
Professor of Pharmacology
University of Michigan Comprehensive
    Cancer Center
Ann Arbor, Michigan

Jonathan R. Brody, PhD
Associate Professor
Director of Surgical Research
Department of Surgery
Jefferson Medical College of Thomas
    Jefferson University
Philadelphia, Pennsylvania

Christopher B. Buck, PhD
Investigator
Head, Tumor Virus Molecular Biology
    Section
Laboratory of Cellular Oncology
Center for Cancer Research
National Cancer Institute
Bethesda, Maryland

Tim E. Byers, MD, MPH
Associate Dean for Public Health Practice
Colorado School of Public Health
Associate Director for Cancer Prevention
    and Control
University of Colorado Cancer Center
Aurora, Colorado

A. Hilary Calvert
Professor
Gynecologic Oncology
University College Hospitals (UCLH)
London, United Kingdom

Paolo G. Casali, MD
Head
Adult Mesenchymal Tumor Medical
    Oncology Unit
Fondazione Instituto di Ricovero
    Carattere Scientifico
Instituto Nazionale dei Tumori
Milano, Italy

**Ronald S. Chamberlain, MD, MPA,
    FACS**
Chairman and Surgeon-in-Chief
Department of Surgery
Saint Barnabas Medical Center
Livingston, New Jersey

Cindy H. Chau, PharmD, PhD
Scientist
Medical Oncology Branch
Center for Cancer Research
National Cancer Institute
National Institutes of Health
Bethesda, Maryland

Edward Chu, MD
Professor of Medicine and Pharmacology
    & Chemical Biology
Chief, Division of Hematology-Oncology
Deputy Director, University of Pittsburgh
    Cancer Institute
University of Pittsburgh School of
    Medicine
Pittsburgh, Pennsylvania

Nicki Chun, MS, LCGC
Clinical Assistant Professor of Pediatrics/
    Genetics
Stanford Cancer Genetics Clinic
Stanford, California

Jessica Clague, PhD, MPH
Assistant Research Professor
Division of Cancer Etiology
Department of Population Sciences
Beckman Research Institute
City of Hope National Medical Center
Duarte, California

M. Sitki Copur, MD, FACP
Medical Director of Oncology
Saint Francis Cancer Treatment Center
Grand Island, Nebraska
Professor, Department of Medicine
Division of Hematology Oncology
Adjunct Faculty
University of Nebraska Medical Center
Omaha, Nebraska

Brian G. Czito, MD
Gary Hock and Lynn Proctor Associate
    Professor, Department of Radiation
    Oncology
Duke Cancer Institute
Duke University Medical Center
Durham, North Carolina

Angelo Paolo Dei Tos, MD
Director, Department of Oncology
Director of Anatomic Pathology
Scientific Director
Veneto Region Cancer Registry
General Hospital of Treviso
Treviso, Italy

Hari A. Deshpande, MD
Associate Professor of Medicine
Yale University School of Medicine
Section of Medical Oncology
Yale New Haven Hospital
New Haven, Connecticut

Khanh T. Do, MD
Senior Clinical Fellow
Division of Cancer Treatment and
    Diagnosis
National Cancer Institute
National Institutes of Health
Bethesda, Maryland

James H. Doroshow, MD
Director, Division of Cancer Treatment
    and Diagnosis
Deputy Director for Clinical and
    Translational Research
National Cancer Institute
National Institutes of Health
Bethesda, Maryland

Damian E. Dupuy, MD, FACR
Professor of Diagnostic Imaging
The Warren Alpert Medical School of
    Brown University
Director of Tumor Ablation
Rhode Island Hospital
Providence, Rhode Island

Cathy Eng, MD, FACP
Associate Professor
Associate Medical Director, Colorectal
    Center
Director, MD Anderson Cancer Center
    Clinical Trials Network
Gastrointestinal Medical Oncology
    Co-Chair
Southwest Oncology Group
Rectal Subcommittee
National Clinical Trials Network
    Institutional Grant
Lead Contact Principle Investigator
Department of Gastrointestinal Medical
    Oncology
The University of Texas MD Anderson
    Cancer Center
Houston, Texas

Charles Erlichman, MD
Professor, Department of Oncology
Deputy Director, Clinical Research
Peter and Frances Georgeson Professor of
    Gastroenterology Cancer Research
Mayo Clinic
Rochester, Minnesota

Steven A. Feldman, PhD
Staff Scientist
Director, Surgery Branch
Vector Production Facility
National Cancer Institute
Bethesda, Maryland

Mary Feng, MD
Associate Professor, Department of
    Radiation Oncology
University of Michigan Health System
Ann Arbor, Michigan

**William Douglas Figg, Sr., PharmD,
    MBA**
Senior Investigator and Head of the
    Clinical Pharmacology Program
Clinical Director, Center for Cancer
    Research
Head of the Molecular Pharmacology
    Section
Medical Oncology Branch
Center for Cancer Research
National Cancer Institute
National Institutes of Health
Bethesda, Maryland

Antonio Tito Fojo, MD, PhD
Medical Oncology Branch and Affiliates
Head, Experimental Therapeutics
    Section
Senior Investigator
Center for Cancer Research
National Cancer Institute
Bethesda, Maryland

Yuman Fong, MD
Chairman, Department of Surgery
Associate Director, International
  Relations
City of Hope Medical Center
Duarte, California

James M. Ford, MD
Associate Professor
Departments of Medicine, Pediatrics and
  Genetics
Divisions of Oncology and Medical
  Genetics
Director, Clinical Cancer Genomics
  Program
Stanford University School of Medicine
Stanford, California

Larissa V. Furtado, MD
Assistant Professor
Department of Pathology
Assistant Director
Division of Genomics and Molecular
  Pathology
University of Chicago
Chicago, Illinois

**Sheryl G. A. Gabram-Mendola, MD,
  MBA, FACS**
Surgeon-in-Chief
Grady Memorial Hospital
Emory University School of Medicine
Deputy Director
Georgia Cancer Center for Excellence
Director, AVON Comprehensive Breast
  Center at Grady
Director, High Risk Assessment Program
Winship Cancer Institute of Emory
  University
Georgia Cancer Coalition Distinguished
  Cancer Scholar
Atlanta, Georgia

Jared J. Gartner, DO
Biologist, National Cancer Institute
Surgery Branch
National Institute of Health
Bethesda, Maryland

Scott Nicholas Gettinger, MD
Associate Professor of Medicine
Thoracic Oncology Program
Developmental Therapeutics
Yale Cancer Center
New Haven, Connecticut

Matthew P. Goetz, MD
Associate Professor of Pharmacology
Associate Professor of Oncology
Mayo Clinic
Rochester, Minnesota

Sarah B. Goldberg, MD, MPH
Assistant Professor of Internal Medicine
Medical Oncology
Yale Cancer Center
Yale University School of Medicine
New Haven, Connecticut

Steven D. Gore, MD
Yale University School of Medicine
New Haven, Connecticut

Ellen R. Gritz, PhD
Professor and Chair
Department of Behavioral Science
The University of Texas MD Anderson
  Cancer Center
Houston, Texas

Alessandro Gronchi, MD
Surgical Oncologist, Department of
  Surgery
Chief, Sarcoma Service
Fondazione IRCCS
Istituto Nazionale dei Tumori
Milan, Italy

José G. Guillem, MD, MPH
Department of Surgery
Memorial Sloan-Kettering Cancer Center
New York, New York

Douglas Hanahan, PhD
Director
Swiss Institute for Experimental Cancer
  Research (ISREC)
Lausanne, Switzerland

Lyndsay N. Harris, MD, FRCP(C)
Diana Hyland Chair in Breast Cancer
Director, Breast Cancer Program
Seidman Cancer Center
University Hospitals Case Medical Center
Professor of Medicine
Division of Hematology and Oncology
Case Western Reserve University
Cleveland, Ohio

James G. Herman, MD
Johns Hopkins University
Baltimore, Maryland

Jay L. Hess, MD, PhD
Professor, Department of Pathology
Carl V. Weller Professor and Chair
Professor, Department of Internal
  Medicine
University of Michigan Health System
Ann Arbor, Michigan

Christopher J. Hoimes, DO
Assistant Professor
UH Case Medical Center
Department of Medicine-Hematology
  and Oncology
Cleveland, Ohio

Ralph H. Hruban, MD
Professor, Department of Pathology
Director, The Sol Goldman Pancreatic
  Cancer Research Center
Johns Hopkins University School of
  Medicine
Baltimore, Maryland

Vanessa W. Hui, MD
Department of Surgery
Memorial Sloan-Kettering Cancer Center
New York, New York

David H. Ilson, MD, PhD
Professor and Attending Physician
Department of Medicine
Memorial Sloan-Kettering Cancer Center
  and Weill Cornell Medical College
  Memorial Hospital
New York, New York

Kory W. Jasperson, MS, CGC
Genetic Counselor
Department of Internal Medicine
Huntsman Cancer Institute
University of Utah
Salt Lake City, Utah

Matthew Kalady, MD
Associate Professor of Surgery
Krause-Lieberman Chair in Colorectal
  Surgery
Department of Colorectal Surgery
Digestive Disease Institute
Cleveland Clinic
Cleveland, Ohio

David P. Kelsen, MD
Edward S Gordon Chair in Medical
  Oncology
Attending Physician, Department of
  Medicine
Memorial Sloan-Kettering Cancer Center
Professor of Medicine Weill Cornell
  Medical College
New York, New York

Scott E. Kern, MD
Everett and Marjorie Kovler Professor of
  Pancreas Cancer Research
Department of Oncology
Sidney Kimmel Comprehensive Cancer
  Center at Johns Hopkins
Baltimore, Maryland

Christopher J. Kirk, MD
Vice President of Research
Onyx Pharmaceuticals, Inc.
South San Francisco, California

James N. Kochenderfer, MD
Investigator, Experimental Transplantation
  and Immunology Branch
National Cancer Institute
National Institutes of Health
Bethesda, Maryland

Manish Kohli, MD
Associate Professor of Oncology
Department of Oncology
College of Medicine
Mayo Clinic
Joint Appointment, Department of
  Urology
Mayo Clinic
Rochester, Minnesota

Shivaani Kummar, MD, FACP
Head, Early Clinical Trials Development
Office of the Director
Division of Cancer Treatment and
    Diagnosis
National Cancer Institute
Bethesda, Maryland

Theodore S. Lawrence, MD, PhD
Isadore Lampe Professor and Chair
Department of Radiation Oncology
University of Michigan Health System
Ann Arbor, Michigan

Rebecca A. Levine, MD
Assistant Professor, Department of
    Surgery
Montefiore Medical Center
Albert Einstein College of Medicine
Bronx, New York

Nancy L. Lewis, MD
Associate Professor
Department of Medical Oncology
Clinical Director
Experimental Therapeutics
Thomas Jefferson University
Kimmel Cancer Center
Philadelphia, Pennsylvania

Steven K. Libutti, MD, FACS
Director, Montefiore-Einstein Center for
    Cancer Care
Vice Chairman, Department of Surgery
Montefiore-Einstein Center for Cancer
    Care
Bronx, New York

Scott M. Lippman, MD
Director, Senior Associate Dean, &
    Associate Vice Chancellor
Cancer Research and Care
Chugai Pharmaceutical Chair
Professor of Medicine
University of California, San Diego
Moores Cancer Center
La Jolla, California

Mats Ljungman, PhD
Professor, Departments of Radiation
Oncology and Environmental Health
    Sciences
Translational Oncology Program
University of Michigan Medical School
Ann Arbor, Michigan

Carlos López-Otín, PhD
Professor, Department of Biochemistry
    and Molecular Biology
Universidad de Oviedo
Principality of Asturias, Spain

Charles L. Loprinzi, MD
Regis Professor of Breast Cancer Research
Department of Oncology
Mayo Clinic
Rochester, Minnesota

Yani Lu, PhD
Assistant Research Professor
Division of Cancer Etiology
Department of Population Science
Beckman Research Institute of the City
    of Hope
Duarte, California

Xiaomei Ma, PhD
Associate Professor, Department of
    Chronic Disease Epidemiology
Yale University School of Public Health
New Haven, Connecticut

Krishnaraj Mahendraraj, MD
Resident, Department of Surgery
St. Barnabas Medical Center
Livingston, New Jersey

Jens U. Marquardt, MD
Resident Physician
Department of Medicine
University of Mainz
Mainz, Germany
Laboratory of Experimental
    Carcinogenesis
Center for Cancer Research
National Cancer Institute
National Institutes of Health
Bethesda, Maryland

Ellen T. Matloff, MS, CGC
President & CEO
Gene Counsel, LLC
New Haven, Connecticut

Susan T. Mayne, PhD
C.-E.A. Winslow Professor of Epidemiology
Chair, Department of Chronic Disease
    Epidemiology
Yale University School of Public Health
Associate Director for Population
    Sciences
Yale Cancer Center
New Haven, Connecticut

Howard L. McLeod, PharmD
Medical Director, DeBartolo Family
Personalized Medicine Institute
Senior Member, Division of Population
    Sciences
H. Lee Moffitt Cancer Center
Tampa, Florida

Karin B. Michels, ScD, PhD
Associate Professor
Obstetrician/Gynecologist
Epidemiology Center
Department of Obstetrics, Gynecology
    and Reproductive Biology
Brigham and Women's Hospital
Harvard Medical School
Boston, Massachusetts

Bruce D. Minsky, MD
Professor and Frank T. McGraw
    Memorial Chair
Deputy Head, Division of Radiation
    Oncology
The University of Texas MD Anderson
    Cancer Center
Houston, Texas

Jeffrey F. Moley, MD
Chief, Section of Endocrine and
    Oncologic Surgery
Professor of Surgery
Washington University School of
    Medicine
St. Louis, Missouri

Meredith A. Morgan, PhD
Research Assistant Professor
Department of Radiation Oncology
University of Michigan
Ann Arbor, Michigan

Jeffrey A. Norton, MD
Professor, Department of Surgery
Chief, Section of Surgical Oncology and
    Division of General Surgery
Department of Surgery
Stanford University Hospital
Stanford, California

Richard J. O'Connor, PhD
Associate Member, Department of Health
    Behavior
Division of Cancer Prevention and
    Population Sciences
Roswell Park Cancer Institute
Buffalo, New York

Peter J. O'Dwyer, MD
Professor of Medicine
Abramson Cancer Center
University of Pennsylvania
Philadelphia, Pennsylvania

Howard L. Parnes, MD
Chief
Prostate and Urologic Cancer Research
    Group
Division of Cancer Prevention
National Cancer Institute
Rockville, Maryland

Tushar Patel, MBChB
Professor of Medicine
Mayo Clinic
Jacksonville, Florida

Giao Q. Phan, MD, FACS
Associate Professor
Division of Surgical Oncology
Massey Cancer Center
Virginia Commonwealth University
Richmond, Virginia

Peter W. T. Pisters, MD, FACS
Professor, Department of Surgical Oncology
Division of Surgery
The University of Texas MD Anderson
Cancer Center
Houston, Texas

Yves Pommier, MD, PhD
Chief, Laboratory of Molecular
Pharmacology
Head, DNA Topoisomerase/Integrase
Group
Center for Cancer Research
National Cancer Institute
Bethesda, Maryland

Mitchell C. Posner, MD, FACS
Thomas D. Jones Professor of Surgery
and Vice-Chairman
Chief, Section of General Surgery and
Surgical Oncology
Professor, Radiation and Cellular Oncology
Medical Director, Clinical Cancer
Programs
The University of Chicago Medicine
Chicago, Illinois

Sahdeo Prasad, PhD
Cytokine Research Laboratory
Department of Experimental
Therapeutics
The University of Texas MD Anderson
Cancer Center
Houston, Texas

Lee Ratner, MD, PhD
Professor Departments of Medicine and
Molecular Microbiology
Co-Director, Medical & Molecular
Oncology
Washington University School of
Medicine
Barnes-Jewish Hospital
St. Louis, Missouri

Paul F. Robbins, PhD
National Institutes of Health
Bethesda, Maryland

Matthew K. Robinson, PhD
Assistant Professor, Developmental
Therapeutics Program
Fox Chase Cancer Center
Philadelphia, Pennsylvania

Steven A. Rosenberg, MD, PhD
Chief, Surgery Branch, National Cancer
Institute, National Institutes of Health
Professor of Surgery, Uniformed Services
University of the Health Sciences
School of Medicine
Bethesda, Maryland
Professor of Surgery
George Washington University School of
Medicine
Washington, District of Columbia

Anil K. Rustgi, MD
T. Grier Miller Professor of Medicine &
Genetics
Chief of Gastroenterology
University of Pennsylvania Perelman
School of Medicine
Philadelphia, Pennsylvania

M. Wasif Saif, MD, MBBS
Director, Gastrointestinal Oncology
Program
Leader, Experimental Therapeutics
Program
Tufts Medical Center
Tufts University School of Medicine
Boston, Massachusetts

Leonard B. Saltz, MD
Professor, Department of Medicine
Chief, Gastrointestinal Oncology Service
Memorial Sloan-Kettering Cancer Center
New York, New York

Yardena Samuels, PhD
Knell Family Professorial Chair
Department of Molecular Cell Biology
Weizmann Institute of Science
Rehovot, Israel

Charles L. Sawyers, MD
Investigator, Howard Hughes Medical
Institute
Chair, Human Oncology and
Pathogenesis Program
Memorial Sloan-Kettering Cancer Center
New York, New York

Leigha Senter-Jamieson, MS, CGC
Director of Clinical Supervison
Associate Professor
Division of Human Genetics
Department of Internal Medicine
The Ohio State University
Columbus, Ohio

Syed Ammer Shah, MD
Postgraduate Year Four
Surgical Resident
Saint Barnabas Medical Center
Caldwell, New Jersey

Peter G. Shields, MD
Deputy Director, Comprehensive Cancer
Center
Professor, College of Medicine
James Cancer Hospital
The Ohio State University
Columbus, Ohio

Ramesh A. Shivdasani, MD, PhD
Associate Professor, Department of
Medical Oncology
Dana-Farber Cancer Institute
Department of Medicine
Harvard Medical School
Boston, Massachusetts

Alex Sparreboom, PhD
Associate Member, Department of
Pharmaceutical Sciences
St. Jude Children's Research Hospital
Memphis, Tennessee

Alexander Stojadinovic, MD
Bon Secours Cancer Institute
Richmond, Virginia

Irene M. Tamí-Maury, DMD, DrPH, MSc
The University of Texas MD Anderson
Cancer Center
Houston, Texas

**Randall K. Ten Haken, PhD, FAAPM,
FInstP, FASTRO, FACR**
Professor, Associate Chair, and Physics
Division Director
Department of Radiation Oncology
University of Michigan Medical School
Ann Arbor, Michigan

Kenneth D. Tew, PhD, DSc
Chairman and John C. West Chair in
Cancer Research
Cell and Molecular Pharmacology
Medical University of South Carolina
Charleston, South Carolina

Snorri S. Thorgeirsson, MD, PhD
Head, Center of Excellence in Integrative
Cancer Biology and Genomics
Chief, Laboratory of Experimental
Carcinogenesis Center for Cancer
Research
National Cancer Institute
National Institutes of Health
Bethesda, Maryland

Benjamin A. Toll, PhD
Associate Professor of Psychiatry
Yale University School of Medicine
Yale Comprehensive Cancer Center
Program Director, Smoking Cessation
Service
Smilow Cancer Hospital at Yale-New
Haven
New Haven, Connecticut

Brian B. Tuch, PhD
Associate Director, Translational
Genomics
Onyx Pharmaceuticals
South San Francisco, California

Christine M. Walko, PharmD, BCOP
Clinical Pharmacogenetic Scientist
DeBartolo Family Personalized Medicine
Institute
Applied Clinical Scientist, Division of
Population Science
H. Lee Moffitt Cancer Center and
Research Institute
Tampa, Florida

Graham W. Warren, MD, PhD
Associate Professor
Vice Chair for Research in Radiation
    Oncology
Department of Radiation Oncology
Department of Cell and Molecular
    Pharmacology
Hollings Cancer Center
Medical University of South Carolina
Charleston, South Carolina

Robert A. Weinberg, PhD
Member, Whitehead Institute for
    Biomedical Research
Department of Biology
Massachusetts Institute of Technology
Director, Ludwig Center for Molecular
    Oncology
Whitehead Institute for Biomedical
    Research
Cambridge, Massachusetts

Louis M. Weiner, MD
Director, Lombardi Comprehensive
    Cancer Center
Professor and Chair, Department of
    Oncology
Francis L. and Charlotte G. Gragnani
    Chair
Georgetown University Medical Center
Washington, District of Columbia

Elizabeth L. Wiley, MD
Professor and Director, Division of
    Surgical Pathology
Department of Pathology
University of Illinois Hospital and Health
    Sciences System
University of Illinois College of Medicine
Chicago, Illinois

Christopher G. Willett, MD
Professor and Chairman, Department of
    Radiation Oncology
Duke University
Durham, North Carolina

Walter C. Willett, MD, DrPH
Professor and Chair, Department of
    Nutrition
Harvard School of Public Health
Boston, Massachusetts

Jordan M. Winter, MD
Assistant Professor, Department of Surgery
Thomas Jefferson University
Philadelphia, Pennsylvania

Charles J. Yeo, MD
Samuel D. Gross Professor and Chair
Department of Surgery
Jefferson Medical College
Philadelphia, Pennsylvania

Herbert Yu, MD, PhD
Professor and Director
Cancer Epidemiology Program
Associate Director for Population
Sciences and Cancer Control
University of Hawaii Cancer Center
Adjunct Professor, Department of
    Chronic Disease Epidemiology
Yale School of Public Health
Honolulu, Hawaii

Stuart H. Yuspa, MD
Chief, Laboratory of Cancer Biology and
    Genetics
Center for Cancer Research
National Cancer Institute
Bethesda, Maryland

CONTENTS

PART I

Principles
of Oncology

1 The Cancer Genome

Yardena Samuels, Alberto Bardelli, Jared J. Gartner, and Carlos López-Otín

INTRODUCTION

There is a broad consensus that cancer is, in essence, a genetic disease, and that accumulation of molecular alterations in the genome of somatic cells is the basis of cancer progression (Fig. 1.1).[1] In the past 10 years, the availability of the human genome sequence and progress in DNA sequencing technologies has dramatically improved knowledge of this disease. These new insights are transforming the field of oncology at multiple levels:

1. The genomic maps are redesigning the tumor taxonomy by moving it from a histologic- to a genetic-based level.
2. The success of cancer drugs designed to target the molecular alterations underlying tumorigenesis has proven that somatic genetic alterations are legitimate targets for therapy.
3. Tumor genotyping is helping clinicians individualize treatments by matching patients with the best treatment for their tumors.
4. Tumor-specific DNA alterations represent highly sensitive biomarkers for disease detection and monitoring.
5. Finally, the ongoing analyses of multiple cancer genomes will identify additional targets, whose pharmacologic exploitation will undoubtedly result in new therapeutic approaches.

This chapter will review the progress that has been made in understanding the genetic basis of sporadic cancers. An emphasis will be placed on an introduction to novel integrated genomic approaches that allow a comprehensive and systematic evaluation of genetic alterations that occur during the progression of cancer. Using these powerful tools, cancer research, diagnosis, and treatment are poised for a transformation in the next years.

CANCER GENES AND THEIR MUTATIONS

Cancer genes are broadly grouped into oncogenes and tumor suppressor genes. Using a classical analogy, oncogenes can be compared to a car accelerator, so that a mutation in an oncogene would be the equivalent of having the accelerator continuously pressed.[2] Tumor suppressor genes, in contrast, act as brakes,[2] so that when they are not mutated, they function to inhibit tumorigenesis. Oncogene and tumor suppressor genes may be classified by the nature of their somatic mutations in tumors. Mutations in oncogenes typically occur at specific hotspots, often affecting the same codon or clustered at neighboring codons in different tumors.[1] Furthermore, mutations in oncogenes are almost always missense, and the mutations usually affect only one allele, making them heterozygous. In contrast, tumor suppressor genes are usually mutated throughout the gene; a large number of the mutations may truncate the encoded protein and generally affect both alleles, causing loss of heterozygosity (LOH). Major types of somatic mutations present in malignant tumors include nucleotide substitutions, small insertions and deletions (*indels*), chromosomal rearrangements, and copy number alterations.

IDENTIFICATION OF CANCER GENES

The completion of the Human Genome Project marked a new era in biomedical sciences.[3] Knowledge of the sequence and organization of the human genome now allows for the systematic analysis of the genetic alterations underlying the origin and evolution of tumors. Before elucidation of the human genome, several cancer genes, such as *KRAS*, *TP53*, and *APC*, were successfully discovered using approaches based on an oncovirus analysis, linkage studies, LOH, and cytogenetics.[4,5] The first curated version of the Human Genome Project was released in 2004,[3] and provided a sequence-based map of the normal human genome. This information, together with the construction of the HapMap, which contains single nucleotide polymorphisms (SNP), and the underlying genomic structure of natural human genomic variation,[6,7] allowed an extraordinary throughput in cataloging somatic mutations in cancer. These projects now offer an unprecedented opportunity: the identification of all the genetic changes associated with a human cancer. For the first time, this ambitious goal is within reach of the scientific community. Already, a number of studies have demonstrated the usefulness of strategies aimed at the systematic identification of somatic mutations associated with cancer progression. Notably, the Human Genome Project, the HapMap project, as well as the candidate and family gene approaches (described in the following paragraphs), utilized capillary-based DNA sequencing (first-generation sequencing, also known as Sanger sequencing).[8] Figure 1.2 clearly illustrates the developments in the search of cancer genes, its increased pace, as well as the most relevant findings in this field.

Cancer Gene Discovery by Sequencing Candidate Gene Families

The availability of the human genome sequence provides new opportunities to comprehensively search for somatic mutations in cancer on a larger scale than previously possible. Progress in the field has been closely linked to improvements in the throughput of DNA analysis and in the continuous reduction in sequencing costs. What follows are some of the achievements in this research area, as well as how they affected knowledge of the cancer genome.

A seminal work in the field was the systematic mutational profiling of the genes involved in the RAS-RAF pathway in multiple tumors. This candidate gene approach led to the discovery that *BRAF* is frequently mutated in melanomas and is mutated at a lower frequency in other tumor types.[9] Follow-up studies quickly revealed that mutations in *BRAF* are mutually exclusive with alterations in *KRAS*,[9,10] genetically emphasizing that these genes function in the same pathway, a concept that had been previously demonstrated in lower organisms such as *Caenorhabditis elegans* and *Drosophila melanogaster*.[11,12]

In 2003, the identification of cancer genes shifted from a candidate gene approach to the mutational analyses of gene families. The first gene families to be completely sequenced were those that

A metastatic cancer genome requires decades to develop

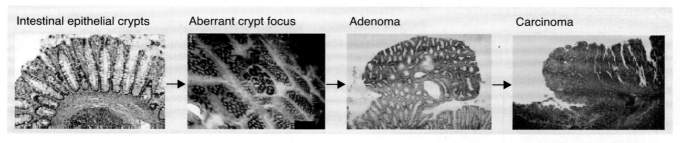

Intestinal epithelial crypts   Aberrant crypt focus   Adenoma   Carcinoma

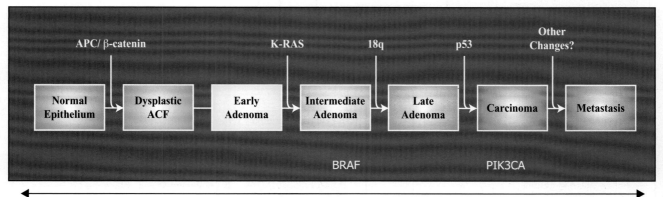

~10–30 Years

Figure 1.1 Schematic representation of the genomic and histopathologic steps associated with tumor progression: from the occurrence of the initiating mutation in the founder cell to metastasis formation. It has been convincingly shown that the genomic landscape of solid tumors such as that of pancreatic and colorectal tumors requires the accumulation of many genetic events, a process that requires decades to complete. This timeline offers an incredible window of opportunity for the early detection, which is often associated with an excellent prognosis, of this disease.

involved protein[13,14] and lipid phosphorylation.[15] The rationale for initially focusing on these gene families was threefold:

- The corresponding proteins were already known at that time to play a pivotal role in the signaling and proliferation of normal and cancerous cells.
- Multiple members of the protein kinases family had already been linked to tumorigenesis.
- Kinases are clearly amenable to pharmacologic inhibition, making them attractive drug targets.

The mutational analysis of all the tyrosine-kinase domains in colorectal cancers revealed that 30% of cases had a mutation in at least one tyrosine-kinase gene, and overall mutations were identified in eight different kinases, most of which had not previously been linked to cancer.[13] An additional mutational analysis of the coding exons of 518 protein kinase genes in 210 diverse human cancers, including breast, lung, gastric, ovarian, renal, and acute lymphoblastic leukemia, identified approximately 120 mutated genes that probably contribute to oncogenesis.[14] Because kinase activity is attenuated by enzymes that remove phosphate groups called phosphatases, the rational next step in these studies was to perform a mutation analysis of the protein tyrosine phosphatases. A mutational investigation of this family in colorectal cancer identified that 25% of cases had mutations in six different phosphatase genes (*PTPRF, PTPRG, PTPRT, PTPN3, PTPN13,* or *PTPN14*).[16] A combined analysis of the protein tyrosine kinases and the protein tyrosine phosphatases showed that 50% of colorectal cancers had mutations in a tyrosine-kinase gene, a protein tyrosine phosphatase gene, or both, further emphasizing the pivotal role of protein phosphorylation in neoplastic progression. Many of the identified genes had previously been linked to human cancer, thus validating

the unbiased comprehensive mutation profiling. These landmark studies led to additional gene family surveys.

The phosphatidylinositol 3-kinase (*PI3K*) gene family, which also plays a role in proliferation, adhesion, survival, and motility, was also comprehensively investigated.[17] Sequencing of the exons encoding the kinase domain of all 16 members belonging to this family pinpointed *PIK3CA* as the only gene to harbor somatic mutations. When the entire coding region was analyzed, *PIK3CA* was found to be somatically mutated in 32% of colorectal cancers. At that time, the *PIK3CA* gene was certainly not a newcomer in the cancer arena, because it had previously been shown to be involved in cell transformation and metastasis.[17] Strikingly, its staggeringly high mutation frequency was discovered only through systematic sequencing of the corresponding gene family.[15] Subsequent analysis of *PIK3CA* in other tumor types identified somatic mutations in this gene in additional cancer types, including 36% of hepatocellular carcinomas, 36% of endometrial carcinomas, 25% of breast carcinomas, 15% of anaplastic oligodendrogliomas, 5% of medulloblastomas and anaplastic astrocytomas, and 27% of glioblastomas.[18–22] It is known that *PIK3CA* is one of the two (the other being *KRAS*) most commonly mutated oncogenes in human cancers. Further investigation of the *PI3K* pathway in colorectal cancer showed that 40% of tumors had genetic alterations in one of the *PI3K* pathway genes, emphasizing the central role of this pathway in colorectal cancer pathogenesis.[23]

Although most cancer genome studies of large gene families have focused on the kinome, recent analyses have revealed that members of other families highly represented in the human genome are also a target of mutational events in cancer. This is the case of proteases, a complex group of enzymes consisting of at least 569 components that constitute the so-called human degradome.[24] Proteases exhibit an elaborate interplay with kinases and

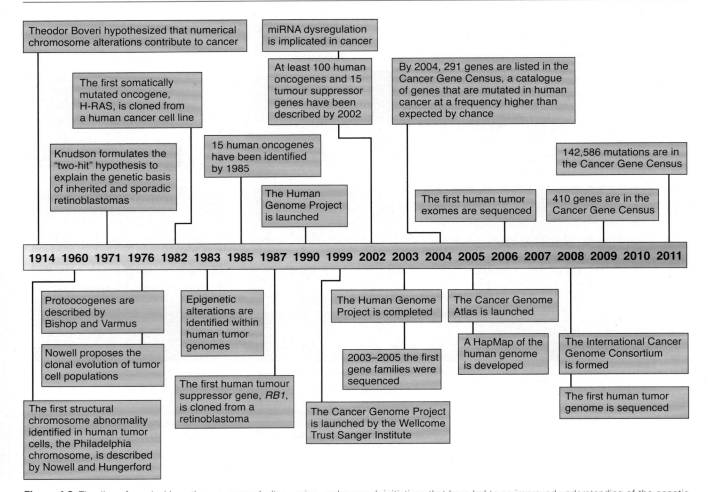

Figure 1.2 Timeline of seminal hypotheses, research discoveries, and research initiatives that have led to an improved understanding of the genetic etiology of human tumorigenesis within the past century. The consensus cancer gene data were obtained from the Wellcome Trust Sanger Institute Cancer Genome Project Web site (http://www.sanger.ac.uk/genetics/CGP). (Redrawn from Bell DW. Our changing view of the genomic landscape of cancer. *J Pathol* 2010;220:231–243.)

have traditionally been associated with cancer progression because of their ability to degrade extracellular matrices, thus facilitating tumor invasion and metastasis.[25,26] However, recent studies have shown that these enzymes hydrolyze a wide variety of substrates and influence many different steps of cancer, including early stages of tumor evolution.[27] These functional studies have also revealed that beyond their initial recognition as prometastatic enzymes, they play dual roles in cancer, as assessed by the identification of a growing number of tumor-suppressive proteases.[28]

These findings emphasized the possibility that mutational activation or inactivation of protease genes occurs in cancer. A systematic analysis of genetic alterations in breast and colorectal cancers revealed that proteases from different catalytic classes were somatically mutated in cancer.[29] These results prompted the mutational analysis of entire protease families such as matrix metalloproteinases (MMP), a disintegrin and metalloproteinase (ADAM), and ADAMs with thrombospondin domains (ADAMTS) in different tumors. These studies led to the identification of protease genes frequently mutated in cancer, such as *MMP8*, which is mutated and functionally inactivated in 6.3% of human melanomas.[30,31]

The mutational status of caspases has also been extensively analyzed in different tumors because these proteases play a fundamental role in the execution of apoptosis, one of the hallmarks of cancer.[32] These studies demonstrated that *CASP8* is deleted in neuroblastomas and inactivated by somatic mutations in a variety of human malignancies, including head and neck, colorectal, lung, and gastric carcinomas.[33–35] Other large protease families

whose components are often mutated in cancer are the deubiquitinating enzymes (DUB), which catalyze the removal of ubiquitin and ubiquitin-like modifiers of their target proteins.[36] Some DUBs were initially identified as oncogenic proteins, but further work has shown that other deubiquitinases, such as CYLD, A20, and BAP1, are tumor suppressors inactivated in cancer. *CYLD* is mutated in patients with familial cylindromatosis, a disease characterized by the formation of multiple tumors of skin appendages.[37] A20 is a DUB family member encoded by the *TNFAIP3* gene, which is mutated in a large number of Hodgkin lymphomas and primary mediastinal B-cell lymphomas.[38–41] Finally, the *BAP1* gene, encoding an ubiquitin C-terminal hydrolase, is frequently mutated in metastasizing uveal melanomas[42] and in other human malignancies, such as mesothelioma and renal cell carcinoma.[43]

Mutational Analysis of Exomes Using Sanger Sequencing

Although the gene family approach for the identification of cancer genes has proven extremely valuable, it still is a candidate approach and thus biased in its nature. The next step forward in the mutational profiling of cancer has been the sequencing of exomes, which is the entire coding portion of the human genome (18,000 protein-encoding genes). The exomes of many different tumors—including breast, colorectal, pancreatic, and ovarian clear cell carcinomas; glioblastoma multiforme; and medulloblastoma—have been analyzed using Sanger sequencing. For the first time, these large-scale analyses allowed researchers to describe and understand the genetic complexity of human cancers.[29,44-48] The declared goals of these exome studies were to provide methods for exomewide mutational analyses in human tumors, to characterize their spectrum and quantity of somatic mutations, and, finally, to discover new genes involved in tumorigenesis as well as novel pathways that have a role in these tumors. In these studies, sequencing data were complemented with gene expression and copy number analyses, thus providing a comprehensive view of the genetic complexity of human tumors.[45-48] A number of conclusions can be drawn from these analyses, including the following:

- Cancer genomes have an average of 30 to 100 somatic alterations per tumor in coding regions, which was a higher number than previously thought. Although the alterations included point mutations, small insertions, deletions, or amplifications, the great majority of the mutations observed were single-base substitutions.[45,46]
- Even within a single cancer type, there is a significant intertumor heterogeneity. This means that multiple mutational patterns (encompassing different mutant genes) are present in tumors that cannot be distinguished based on histologic analysis. The concept that individual tumors have a unique genetic milieu is highly relevant for personalized medicine, a concept that will be further discussed.
- The spectrum and nucleotide contexts of mutations differ between different tumor types. For example, over 50% of mutations in colorectal cancer were C:G to T:A transitions, and 10% were C:G to G:C transversions. In contrast, in breast cancers, only 35% of the mutations were C:G to T:A transitions, and 29% were C:G to G:C transversions. Knowledge of mutation spectra is vital because it allows insight into the mechanisms underlying mutagenesis and repair in the various cancers investigated.
- A considerably larger number of genes that had not been previously reported to be involved in cancer were found to play a role in the disease.
- Solid tumors arising in children, such as medulloblastomas, harbor on average 5 to 10 times less gene alterations compared to a typical adult solid tumor. These pediatric tumors also harbor fewer amplifications and homozygous deletions within coding genes compared to adult solid tumors.

Importantly, to deal with the large amount of data generated in these genomic projects, it was necessary to develop new statistical and bioinformatic tools. Furthermore, an examination of the overall distribution of the identified mutations allowed for the development of a novel view of cancer genome landscapes and a novel definition of cancer genes. These new concepts in the understanding of cancer genetics are further discussed in the following paragraphs. The compiled conclusions derived from these analyses have led to a paradigm shift in the understanding of cancer genetics.

A clear indication of the power of the unbiased nature of the whole exome surveys was revealed by the discovery of recurrent mutations in the active site of *IDH1*, a gene with no known link to gliomas, in 12% of tumors analyzed.[46] Because malignant gliomas are the most common and lethal tumors of the central nervous system, and because glioblastoma multiforme (GBM; World Health Organization grade IV astrocytoma) is the most biologically aggressive subtype, the unveiling of *IDH1* as a novel GBM gene is extremely significant. Importantly, mutations of *IDH1* predominantly occurred in younger patients and were associated with a better prognosis.[49] Follow-up studies showed that mutations of *IDH1* occur early in glioma progression; the R132 somatic mutation is harbored by the majority (greater than 70%) of grades II and III astrocytomas and oligodendrogliomas, as well as in secondary GBMs that develop from these lower grade lesions.[49-55] In contrast, less than 10% of primary GBMs harbor these alterations. Furthermore, analysis of the associated *IDH2* revealed recurrent somatic mutations in the R172 residue,

which is the exact analog of the frequently mutated R132 residue of *IDH1*. These mutations occur mostly in a mutually exclusive manner with *IDH1* mutations,[49,51] suggesting that they have equivalent phenotypic effects. Subsequently, *IDH1* mutations have been reported in additional cancer types, including hematologic neoplasias.[56-58]

Next-Generation Sequencing and Cancer Genome Analysis

In 1977, the introduction of the Sanger method for DNA sequencing with chain-terminating inhibitors transformed biomedical research.[8] Over the past 30 years, this first-generation technology has been universally used for elucidating the nucleotide sequence of DNA molecules. However, the launching of new large-scale projects, including those implicating whole-genome sequencing of cancer samples, has made necessary the development of new methods that are widely known as next-generation sequencing technologies.[59-61] These approaches have significantly lowered the cost and the time required to determine the sequence of the 3×10^9 nucleotides present in the human genome. Moreover, they have a series of advantages over Sanger sequencing, which are of special interest for the analysis of cancer genomes.[62] First, next-generation sequencing approaches are more sensitive than Sanger methods and can detect somatic mutations even when they are present in only a subset of tumor cells.[63] Moreover, these new sequencing strategies are quantitative and can be used to simultaneously determine both nucleotide sequence and copy number variations.[64] They can also be coupled to other procedures such as those involving paired-end reads, allowing for the identification of multiple structural alterations, such as insertions, deletions, and rearrangements, that commonly occur in cancer genomes.[63] Nonetheless, next-generation sequencing still presents some limitations that are mainly derived from the relatively high error rate in the short reads generated during the sequencing process. In addition, these short reads make the task of de novo assembly of the generated sequences and the mapping of the reads to a reference genome extremely complex. To overcome some of these current limitations, deep coverage of each analyzed genome is required and a careful validation of the identified variants must be performed, typically using Sanger sequencing. As a consequence, there is a substantial increase in both the cost of the process and in the time of analysis. Therefore, it can be concluded that whole-genome sequencing of cancer samples is already a feasible task, but not yet a routine process. Further technical improvements will be required before the task of decoding the entire genome of any malignant tumor of any cancer patient can be applied to clinical practice.

The number of next-generation sequencing platforms has substantially grown over the past few years and currently includes technologies from Roche/454, Illumina/Solexa, Life/APG's SOLiD3, Helicos BioSciences/HeliScope, and Pacific Biosciences/PacBio RS.[61] Noteworthy also are the recent introduction of the Polonator G.007 instrument, an open source platform with freely available software and protocols; the Ion Torrent's semiconductor sequencer; as well as those involving self-assembling DNA nanoballs or nanopore technologies.[65-67] These new machines are driving the field toward the era of third-generation sequencing, which brings enormous clinical interest because it can substantially increase the speed and accuracy of analyses at reduced costs and can facilitate the possibility of single-molecule sequencing of human genomes. A comparison of next-generation sequencing platforms is shown in Table 1.1. These various platforms differ in the method utilized for template preparation and in the nucleotide sequencing and imaging strategy, which finally result in their different performance. Ultimately, the most suitable approach depends on the specific genome sequencing projects.[61]

Current methods of template preparation first involve randomly shearing genomic DNA into smaller fragments, from which

TABLE 1.1

Comparative Analysis of Next-Generation Sequencing Platforms

Platform	Library/Template Preparation	Sequencing Method	Average Read-Length (Bases)	Run Time (Days)	Gb Per Run	Instrument Cost (U.S.$)	Comments
Roche 454 GS FLX	Fragment, mate-pair Emulsion PCR	Pyrosequencing	400	0.35	0.45	500,000	Fast run times High reagent cost
Illumina HiSeq 2000	Fragment, mate-pair Solid phase	Reversible terminator	100–125	8 (mate-pair run)	150–200	540,000	Most widely used platform Low multiplexing capability
Life/APG's SOLiD 5500xl	Fragment, mate-pair Emulsion PCR	Cleavable probe, sequencing by ligation	35–75	7 (mate-pair run)	180–300	595,000	Inherent error correction Long run times
Helicos BioSciences HeliScope	Fragment, mate-pair Single molecule	Reversible terminator	32	8 (fragment run)	37	999,000	Nonbias template representation Expensive, high error rates
Pacific Biosciences PacBio RS	Fragment Single molecule	Real-time sequencing	1,000	1	0.075	NA	Greatest potential for long reads Highest error rates
Polonator G.007	Mate pair Emulsion PCR	Noncleavable probe, sequencing by ligation	26	5 (mate-pair run)	12	170,000	Least expensive platform Shortest read lengths

NA, not available.
Data represent an update of information provided in Metzker ML. Sequencing technologies—the next generation. *Nat Rev Genet* 2010;11:31–46.

a library of either fragment templates or mate-pair templates are generated. Then, clonally amplified templates from single DNA molecules are prepared by either emulsion polymerase chain reaction (PCR) or solid-phase amplification.[68,69] Alternatively, it is possible to prepare single-molecule templates through methods that require less starting material and that do not involve PCR amplification reactions, which can be the source of artifactual mutations.[70] Once prepared, templates are attached to a solid surface in spatially separated sites, allowing thousands to billions of nucleotide sequencing reactions to be performed simultaneously.

The sequencing methods currently used by the different next-generation sequencing platforms are diverse and have been classified into four groups: cyclic reversible termination, single-nucleotide addition, real-time sequencing, and sequencing by ligation (Fig. 1.3).[61,71] These sequencing strategies are coupled with different imaging methods, including those based on measuring bioluminescent signals or involving four-color imaging of single molecular events. Finally, the extraordinary amount of data released from these nucleotide sequencing platforms is stored, assembled, and analyzed using powerful bioinformatic tools that have been developed in parallel with next-generation sequencing technologies.[72]

Next-generation sequencing approaches represent the newest entry into the cancer genome decoding arena and have already been applied to cancer analyses. The first research group to apply these methodologies to whole cancer genomes was that of Ley et al.,[73] who reported in 2008 the sequencing of the entire genome of a patient with acute myeloid leukemia (AML) and its comparison with the normal tissue from the same patient, using the Illumina/Solexa platform. As further described, this work allowed for the identification of point mutations and structural alterations of putative oncogenic relevance in AML and represented proof

of principle of the relevance of next-generation sequencing for cancer research.

Whole-Genome Analysis Utilizing Second-Generation Sequencing

The sequence of the first whole cancer genome was reported in 2008, where AML and normal skin from the same patient were described.[73] Numerous additional whole genomes, together with the corresponding normal genomes of patients with a variety of malignant tumors, have been reported since then.[56,63,74–86]

The first available whole genome of a cytogenetically normal AML subtype M1 (AML-M1) revealed eight genes with novel mutations along with another 500 to 1,000 additional mutations found in noncoding regions of the genome. Most of the identified genes had not been previously associated with cancer. However, validation of the detected mutations did not identify novel recurring mutations in AML.[73] Concomitantly, with the expansion in the use of next-generation sequencers, many other whole genomes from a number of cancer types started to be evaluated in a similar manner (Fig. 1.4).[87]

In contrast to the first AML whole genome, the second did observe a recurrent mutation in *IDH1*, encoding isocitrate dehydrogenase.[56] Follow-up studies extended this finding and reported that mutations in *IDH1* and the related gene *IDH2* occur at a 20% to 30% frequency in AML patients and are associated with a poor prognosis in some subgroups of patients.[79,80,88] A good example illustrating the high pace at which second-generation technologies and their accompanying analytical tools are found is demonstrated by the following finding derived from a reanalysis of the first AML whole genome. Thus, when improvements in sequencing

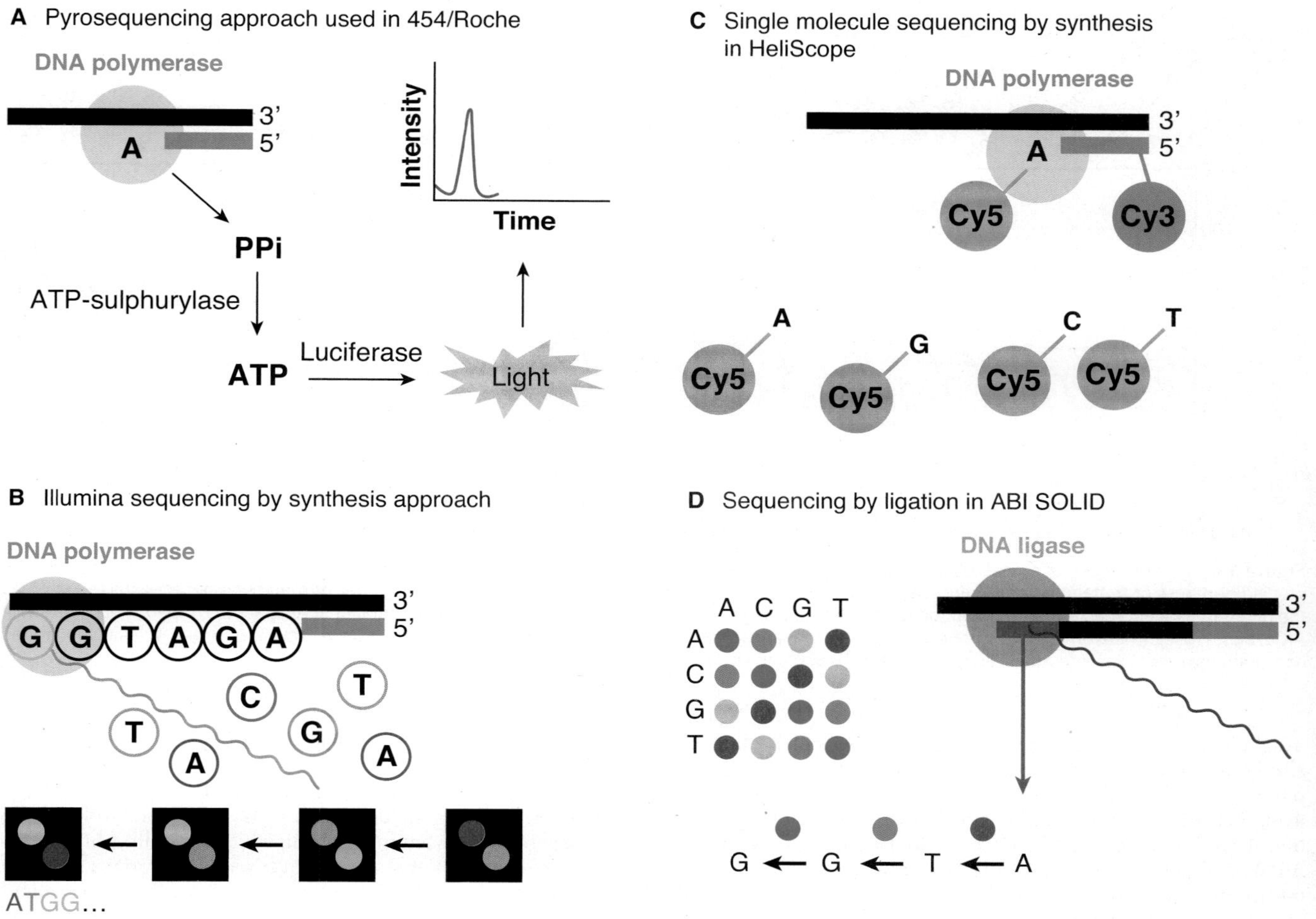

A Pyrosequencing approach used in 454/Roche

C Single molecule sequencing by synthesis in HeliScope

B Illumina sequencing by synthesis approach

D Sequencing by ligation in ABI SOLID

Figure 1.3 Advances in sequencing chemistry implemented in next-generation sequencers. **(A)** The pyrosequencing approach implemented in 454/Roche sequencing technology detects incorporated nucleotides by chemiluminescence resulting from PPi release. **(B)** The Illumina method utilizes sequencing by synthesis in the presence of fluorescently labeled nucleotide analogs that serve as reversible reaction terminators. **(C)** The single-molecule sequencing by synthesis approach detects template extension using Cy3 and Cy5 labels attached to the sequencing primer and the incoming nucleotides, respectively. **(D)** The SOLiD method sequences templates by sequential ligation of labeled degenerate probes. Two-base encoding implemented in the SOLiD instrument allows for probing each nucleotide position twice. (From Morozova O, Hirst M, Marra MA. Applications of new sequencing technologies for transcriptome analysis. *Annu Rev Genomics Hum Genet* 2009;10:135–151.)

techniques were available, the first AML whole genome (described previously), which identified no recurring mutations and had a 91.2% diploid coverage, was reevaluated by deeper sequence coverage, yielding 99.6% diploid coverage of the genome. This improvement, together with more advanced mutation calling algorithms, allowed for the discovery of several nonsynonymous mutations that had not been identified in the initial sequencing. This included a frameshift mutation in the DNA methyltransferase gene *DNMT3A*. Validation of *DNMT3A* in 280 additional de novo AML patients to define recurring mutations led to the significant discovery that a total of 22.1% of AML cases had mutations in *DNMT3A* that were predicted to affect translation. The median overall survival among patients with *DNMT3A* mutations was significantly shorter than that among patients without such mutations (12.3 months versus 41.1 months; p <0.001).

Shortly after this study, complete sequences of a series of cancer genomes, together with matched normal genomes of the same patients, were reported.[56,78,83,84] These works opened the way to more ambitious initiatives, including those involving large international consortia, aimed at decoding the genome of malignant tumors from thousands of cancer patients. Thus, over the last 2 years, many whole genomes of different human malignancies have been made available.[74–76]

In addition to direct applications of next-generation sequencing technologies for the mutational analysis of cancer genomes, these methods have an additional range of applications in cancer research. Thus, genome sequencing efforts have begun to elucidate the genomic changes that accompany metastasis evolution through a comparative analysis of primary and metastatic lesions from breast and pancreatic cancer patients.[77,81,82,85] Likewise, massively parallel sequencing has been used to analyze the evolution of a tongue adenocarcinoma in response to selection by targeted kinase inhibitors.[89] Detailed information of several of these whole genome projects is found in the following paragraph.

The first solid cancer to undergo whole-genome sequencing was a malignant melanoma that was compared to a lymphoblastoid cell line from the same individual.[83] Impressively, a total of 33,345 somatic base substitutions were identified, with 187 nonsynonymous substitutions in protein-coding sequences, at least one order of magnitude higher than any other cancer type. Most somatic base substitutions were C:G > T:A transitions, and of the 510 dinucleotide substitutions, 360 were CC.TT/GG.AA changes, which is consistent with ultraviolet light exposure mutation signatures previously reported in melanoma.[14] Such results from the most comprehensive catalog of somatic mutations not only provide

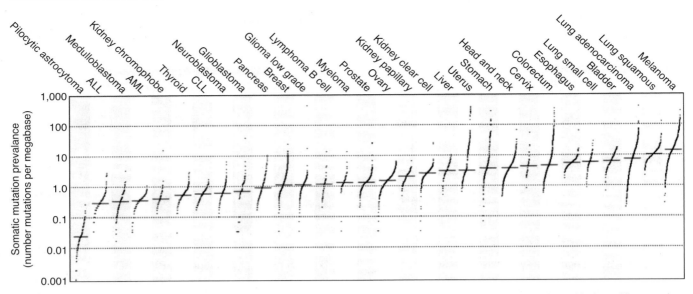

Figure 1.4 The prevalence of somatic mutations across human cancer types. Every *dot* represents a sample, whereas the *red horizontal lines* are the median numbers of mutations in the respective cancer types. The vertical axis (log scaled) shows the number of mutations per megabase, whereas the different cancer types are ordered on the horizontal axis based on their median numbers of somatic mutations. ALL, acute lymphoblastic leukemia; AML, acute myeloid leukemia; CLL, chronic lymphocytic leukemia. (Used with permission from Alexandrov LB, Nik-Zainal S, Wedge DC, et al. Signatures of mutational processes in human cancer. *Nature* 2013;500:415–421.)

insight into the DNA damage signature in this cancer type, but can also be useful in determining the relative order of some acquired mutations. Indeed, this study shows that a significant correlation exists between the presence of a higher proportion of C.A/G.T transitions in early (82%) compared to late mutations (53%). Another important aspect that the comprehensive nature of this melanoma study provided was that cancer mutations are spread out unevenly throughout the genome, with a lower prevalence in regions of transcribed genes, suggesting that DNA repair occurs mainly in these areas.

An interesting and pioneering example of the power of whole-genome sequencing in deciphering the mutation evolution in carcinogenesis was seen in a study in which a basallike breast cancer tumor, a brain metastasis, a tumor xenograft derived from the primary tumor, and the peripheral blood from the same patient were compared (Fig. 1.5).[85] This analysis showed a wide range of

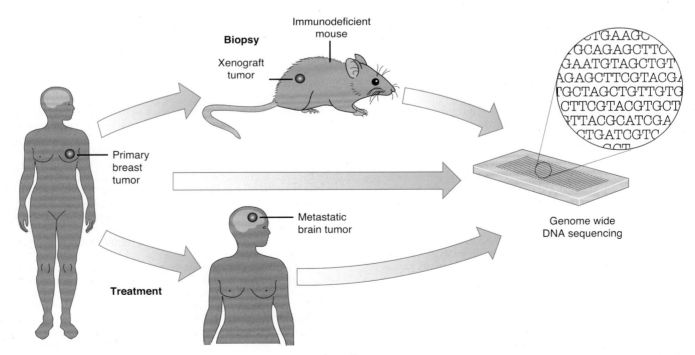

Figure 1.5 Covering all the bases in metastatic assessment. Ding et al.[85] performed a genomewide analysis on three tumor samples: a patient's primary breast tumor; her metastatic brain tumor, which formed despite therapy; and a xenograft tumor in a mouse, originating from the patient's breast tumor. They find that the primary tumor differs from the metastatic and xenograft tumors mainly in the prevalence of genomic mutations. (With permission from Gray J. Cancer: genomics of metastasis. *Nature* 2010;464:989–990.)

mutant allele frequencies in the primary tumor, which was narrowed in the metastasis and xenograft samples. This suggested that the primary tumor was significantly more heterogeneous in its cell populations compared to its matched metastasis and xenograft samples because these underwent selection processes whether during metastasis or transplantation. The clear overlap in mutation incidence between the metastatic and xenograft cases suggests that xenografts undergo similar selection as metastatic lesions and, therefore, are a reliable source for genomic analyses. The main conclusion of this whole-genome study was that, although metastatic tumors harbor an increased number of genetic alterations, the majority of the alterations found in the primary tumor are preserved. Interestingly, single-cell genome sequencing of a breast primary tumour and its liver metastasis indicated that a single clonal expansion formed the primary tumor and seeded the metastasis.[90] Further studies have confirmed and extended these findings to metastatic tumors from different types, including renal and pancreatic carcinomas.[91]

The importance of performing whole-genome sequencing has also been emphasized by the recent identification of somatic mutations in regulatory regions, which can also elicit tumorigenesis. In a study reviewing the noncoding mutations in 19 melanoma whole-genome samples, two recurrent mutations in 17 of the 19 cases studied within the *telomerase reverse transcriptase (TERT)* promoter region were revealed.[92] When these two mutations were investigated in an extension of 51 additional tumors and their matched normal tissues, it was observed that 33 tumors harbored one of the mutations and that the mutations occurred in a mutually exclusive manner. These two mutations generate an identical 11 bp nucleotide stretch that contains the consensus binding site for E-twenty-six (ETS) transcription factors. When cloned into a luciferase reporter assay system, it was shown that these mutations conferred a two- to fourfold increase in transcriptional activity of this promoter in five melanoma cell lines. Although this alteration is much more frequent in melanoma, it is also present in other cancer types because 16% of the cancers listed in the Cancer Cell Line Encyclopedia harbor one of the two *TERT* mutations. In combination, these *TERT* mutations are seen in a greater frequency than *BRAF*- and *NRAS*-activating mutations. They occur in a mutually exclusive manner and in regions that do not show a large background mutation rate, all suggesting that these mutations are important driver events contributing to oncogenesis. Further supporting this was another recent study that identified these same two mutations in the germ line of familial melanoma patients.[93]

As the *TERT* promoter mutation discovery shows, regions of the genome that do not code for proteins are just as vital in our understanding of the biology behind tumor development and progression. Another class of non–protein-coding regions in the genome are the noncoding RNAs. One class of noncoding RNAs are microRNAs (miRNA). Discovered 20 years ago, miRNAs are known to be expressed in a tissue or developmentally specific manner and their expression can influence cellular growth and differentiation along with cancer-related pathways such as apoptosis or stress response. miRNAs do this through either overexpression, leading to the targeting and downregulation of tumor suppressor genes, or inversely through their own downregulation, leading to increased expression of their target oncogene. miRNAs have been extensively studied in cancer and their functional effects have been noted in a wide variety of cancers like glioma[94] and breast cancer,[95] to name just a few.

Another class of noncoding RNAs (ncRNA) are the long noncoding RNAs (lncRNA). These RNAs are typically greater than 200 bp and can range up to 100 kb in size. They are transcribed by RNA polymerase II and can undergo splicing and polyadenylation. Although much less extensively studied when compared to miRNAs for their role in cancer, lncRNAs are beginning to come under much more scrutiny. A recent study of the steroid receptor RNA activator (SRA) revealed two transcripts, a lncRNA (SRA) and a translated transcript (steroid receptor RNA activator protein [SRAP]), that coexist within breast cancer cells. However, their expression varies within breast cancer cell lines with·different phenotypes. It was shown that in a more invasive breast cancer line, higher relative levels of the noncoding transcript were seen.[96] Because this ncRNA acts as part of a ribonucleoprotein complex that is recruited to the promoter region of regulatory genes, it has been hypothesized that this shift in balance between both noncoding and coding transcripts may be associated with growth advantages. When this balance was shifted in vitro, it led to a large increase in transcripts associated with invasion and migration. The results of this study highlight the importance of the investigation into the roles of ncRNA in tumor development or progression and confirm again that the study of coding variants is not sufficient in determining the full genomic spectrum of cancer.

It must be also noted that the recent analysis of whole genomes of many different human tumors has provided additional insights into cancer evolution. Thus, it has been demonstrated that multiple mutational processes are operative during cancer development and progression, each of which has the capacity to leave its particular mutational signature on the genome. A remarkable and innovative study in this regard was aimed at the generation of the entire catalog of somatic mutations in 21 breast carcinomas and the identification of the mutational signatures of the underlying processes. This analysis revealed the occurrence of multiple, distinct single- and double-nucleotide substitution signatures. Moreover, it was reported that breast carcinomas harboring *BRCA1* or *BRCA2* mutations showed a characteristic combination of substitution mutation signatures and a particular profile of genomic deletions. An additional contribution of this analysis was the identification of a distinctive phenomenon of localized hypermutation, which has been termed *kataegis*, and which has also subsequently been observed in other malignancies distinct from breast carcinomas.[87]

Whole-genome sequencing of human carcinomas has also allowed for the ability to characterize other massive genomic alterations, termed *chromothripsis* and *chromoplexy*, occurring across different cancer subtypes.[97] Chromothripsis implies a massive genomic rearrangement acquired in a one-step catastrophic event during cancer development and has been detected in about 2% to 3% of all tumors, but is present at high frequency in some particular cases, such as bone cancers.[98] Chromoplexy has been originally described in prostate cancer and involves many DNA translocations and deletions that arise in a highly interdependent manner and result in the coordinate disruption of multiple cancer genes.[99] These newly described phenomena represent powerful strategies of rapid genome evolution, which may play essential roles during carcinogenesis.

Whole-Exome Analysis Utilizing Second-Generation Sequencing

Another application of second-generation sequencing involves utilizing nucleic acid "baits" to capture regions of interest in the total pool of nucleic acids. These could either be DNA, as described previously,[100,101] or RNA.[102] Indeed, most areas of interest in the genome can be targeted, including exons and ncRNAs. Despite inefficiencies in the exome-targeting process—including the uneven capture efficiency across exons, which results in not all exons being sequenced, and the occurrence of some off-target hybridization events—the higher coverage of the exome makes it highly suitable for mutation discovery in cancer samples.

Over the last few years, thousands of cancer samples have been subjected to whole-exome sequencing. These studies, combined with data from whole-genome sequencing, have provided an unprecedented level of information about the mutational landscape of the most frequent human malignancies.[74–76] In addition, whole-exome sequencing has been used to identify the somatic mutations characteristic of both rare tumors and those that are prevalent in certain geographical regions.[76]

Overall, these studies have provided very valuable information about mutation rates and spectra across cancer types and subtypes.[87,103,104] Remarkably, the variation in mutational frequency between different tumors is extraordinary, with hematologic and pediatric cancers showing the lowest mutation rates (0.001 per Mb of DNA), and melanoma and lung cancers presenting the highest mutational burden (more than 400 per Mb). Whole-exome sequencing has also contributed to the identification of novel cancer genes that had not been previously described to be causally implicated in the carcinogenesis process. These genes belong to different functional categories, including signal transduction, RNA maturation, metabolic regulation, epigenetics, chromatin remodeling, and protein homeostasis.[74] Finally, a combination of data from whole-exome and whole-genome sequencing has allowed for the identification of the signatures of mutational processes operating in different cancer types.[87] Thus, an analysis of a dataset of about 5 million mutations from over 7,000 cancers from 30 different types has allowed for the extraction of more than 20 distinct mutational signatures. Some of them, such as those derived from the activity of APOBEC cytidine deaminases, are present in most cancer types, whereas others are characteristic of specific tumors. Known signatures associated with age, smoking, ultraviolet (UV) light exposure, and DNA repair defects have been also identified in this work, but many of the detected mutational signatures are of cryptic origin. These findings demonstrate the impressive diversity of mutational processes underlying cancer development and may have enormous implications for the future understanding of cancer biology, prevention, and treatment.

SOMATIC ALTERATION CLASSES DETECTED BY CANCER GENOME ANALYSIS

Whole-genome sequencing of cancer genomes has an enormous potential to detect all major types of somatic mutations present in malignant tumors. This large repertoire of genomic abnormalities includes single nucleotide changes, small insertions and deletions, large chromosomal reorganizations, and copy number variations (Fig. 1.6).

Nucleotide substitutions are the most frequent somatic mutations detected in malignant tumors, although there is a substantial variability in the mutational frequency among different cancers.[60] On average, human malignancies have one nucleotide change per million bases, but melanomas reach mutational rates 10-fold higher, and tumors with mutator phenotype caused by DNA mismatch repair deficiencies may accumulate tens of mutations per million nucleotides. By contrast, tumors of hematopoietic origin have less than one base substitution per million. Several bioinformatic tools and pipelines have been developed to efficiently detect somatic nucleotide substitutions through comparison of the genomic information obtained from paired normal and tumor samples from the same patient. Likewise, there are a number of publicly available computational methods to predict the functional relevance of the identified mutations in cancer specimens.[60] Most of these bioinformatic tools exclusively deal with nucleotide changes in protein coding regions and evaluate the putative structural or functional effect of an amino acid substitution in a determined protein, thus obviating changes in other genomic regions, which can also be of crucial interest in cancer. In any case, current computational methods used in this regard are far from being optimal, and experimental validation is finally required to assess the functional relevance of nucleotide substitutions found in cancer genomes.

For years, the main focus of cancer genome analyses has been on identifying coding mutations that cause a change in the amino acid sequence of a gene. The rationale behind this is quite sound because any mutation that creates a novel protein or truncates an essential protein has the potential to drastically change the cellular environment. Examples of this have been shown earlier in the chapter with BRAF and KRAS along with many others. With the advancements in next-generation sequencing, larger studies are able to be conducted. These studies give the power to detect mutations occurring in the cancer genome at a lower frequency. Interesting to note is that these studies are leading to the discovery that recurrent synonymous mutations occur in cancer. Previously believed to be merely neutral mutations that maintain no functional role in tumorigenesis, these mutations were largely ignored, but a recent study shows[105] that simply dismissing these mutations as silent may be premature.

In a review of only 29 melanoma exomes and genomes, 16 recurring synonymous mutations were discovered. When these mutations were screened in additional samples, a synonymous mutation in the gene BCL2L12 was discovered in 12 out of 285 total samples. The observed frequency of this recurrent mutation is greater than expected by chance, suggesting that it has undergone some type of selective pressure during tumor development.[105] Noting that BCL2L12 had previously been linked to tumorigenesis, the mutation was further evaluated for its functional effect, with the finding that it led to an abrogation of the effect of a miRNA, leading to the deregulated expression of BCL2L12. BCL2L12 is a negative regulator of the gene p53, which functions by binding and inhibiting apoptosis in glioma.[106] Accordingly, the dysregulation observed in BCL2L12 led to a reduction in p53 target gene expression.

Small insertions and deletions (indels) represent a second category of somatic mutations that can be discovered by whole-genome sequencing of cancer specimens. These mutations are about 10-fold less frequent than nucleotide substitutions, but may also have an obvious impact in cancer progression. Accordingly, specific bioinformatic tools have been created to detect these indels in the context of the large amount of information generated by whole-genome sequencing projects.[107]

The systematic identification of large chromosomal rearrangements in cancer genomes represents one of the most successful applications of next-generation sequencing methodologies. Previous strategies in this regard had mainly been based on the utilization of cytogenetic methods for the identification of recurrent translocations in hematopoietic tumors. More recently, a combination of bioinformatics and functional methods has allowed for the finding of recurrent translocations in solid epithelial tumors such as TMPRSS2–ERG in prostate cancer and EML4–ALK in non–small-cell lung cancer.[108,109] Now, by using a next-generation sequencing analysis of genomes and transcriptomes, it is possible to systematically search for both intrachromosomal and interchromosomal rearrangements occurring in cancer specimens. These studies have already proven their usefulness for cancer research through the discovery of recurrent translocations involving genes of the RAF kinase pathway in prostate and gastric cancers and in melanomas.[110] Likewise, massively parallel paired-end genome and transcriptome sequencing has already been used to detect new gene fusions in cancer and to catalog all major structural rearrangements present in some tumors and cancer cell lines.[63,111–113] The ongoing cancer genome projects involving thousands of tumor samples will likely lead to the detection of many other chromosomal rearrangements of relevance in specific subsets of cancers. It is also remarkable that whole-genome sequencing may also facilitate the identification of other types of genomic alterations, including rearrangements of repetitive elements, such as active retrotransposons, or insertions of foreign gene sequences, such as viral genomes, which can contribute to cancer development. Indeed, a next-generation sequencing analysis of the transcriptome of Merkel cell carcinoma samples has revealed the clonal integration within the tumor genome of a previously unknown polyomavirus likely implicated in the pathogenesis of this rare but aggressive skin cancer.[114]

Finally, next-generation sequencing approaches have also demonstrated their feasibility to analyze the pattern of copy number

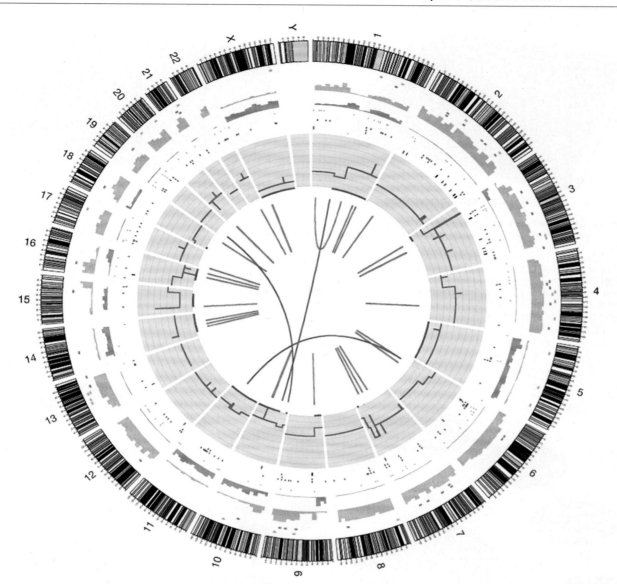

Figure 1.6 The catalog of somatic mutations in COLO-829. Chromosome ideograms are shown around the *outer ring* and are oriented pter–qter in a clockwise direction with centromeres indicated in *red*. Other tracks contain somatic alterations (*from outside to inside*): validated insertions *(light green rectangles)*; validated deletions *(dark green rectangles)*; heterozygous *(light orange bars)*, and homozygous *(dark orange bars)* substitutions shown by density per 10 megabases; coding substitutions *(colored squares: silent in gray, missense in purple, nonsense in red, and splice site in black)*; copy number *(blue lines)*; regions of loss of heterozygosity (LOH) *(red lines)*; validated intrachromosomal rearrangements *(green lines)*; validated interchromosomal rearrangements *(purple lines)*. (From Pleasance ED, Cheetham RK, Stephens PJ, et al. A comprehensive catalogue of somatic mutations from a human cancer genome. *Nature* 2010;463:191–196.)

alterations in cancer, because they allow researchers to count the number of reads in both tumor and normal samples at any given genomic region and then to evaluate the tumor-to-normal copy number ratio at this particular region. These new methods offer some advantages when compared with those based on microarrays, including much better resolution, precise definition of the involved breakpoints, and absence of saturation, which facilitates the accurate estimation of high copy number levels occurring in some genomic loci of malignant tumors.[60]

PATHWAY-ORIENTED MODELS OF CANCER GENOME ANALYSIS

Genomewide mutational analyses suggest that the mutational landscape of cancer is made up of a handful of genes that are mutated in a high fraction of tumors, otherwise known as *mountains*, and most mutated genes are altered at relatively low frequencies, otherwise known as *hills* (Fig. 1.7).[29] The mountains probably give a high selective advantage to the mutated cell, and the hills might provide a lower advantage, making it hard to distinguish them from passenger mutations. Because the hills differ between cancer types, it seems that the cancer genome is more complex and heterogeneous than anticipated. Although highly heterogeneous, bioinformatic studies suggest that the mountains and hills can be grouped into sets of pathways and biologic processes. Some of these pathways are affected by mutations in a few pathway members and others by numerous members. For example, pathway analyses have allowed for the stratification of mutated genes in pancreatic adenocarcinomas to 12 core pathways that have at least one member mutated in 67% to 100% of the tumors analyzed (Fig. 1.8).[45] These core pathways deviated to some that harbored one single highly mutated gene,

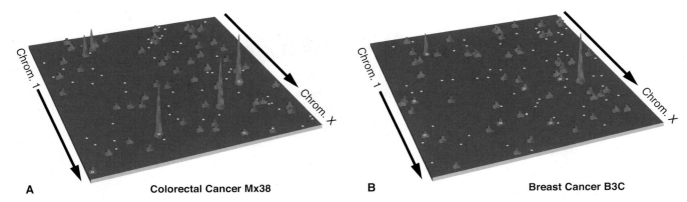

Figure 1.7 Cancer genome landscapes. Nonsilent somatic mutations are plotted in a two-dimensional space representing chromosomal positions of RefSeq genes. The telomere of the short arm of chromosome 1 is represented in the rear left corner of the *green plane* and ascending chromosomal positions continue in the direction of the arrow. Chromosomal positions that follow the front edge of the plane are continued at the back edge of the plane of the adjacent row, and chromosomes are appended end to end. Peaks indicate the 60 highest ranking CAN genes for each tumor type, with peak heights reflecting CaMP scores. The *dots* represent genes that were somatically mutated in the individual colorectal (Mx38) **(A)** or breast tumor (B3C) **(B)**. The *dots* corresponding to mutated genes that coincided with hills or mountains are black with white rims; the remaining *dots* are white with red rims. The mountain on the right of both landscapes represents *TP53* (chromosome 17), and the other mountain shared by both breast and colorectal cancers is *PIK3CA* (upper left, chromosome 3). (Redrawn from Wood LD, Parsons DW, Jones S, et al. The genomic landscapes of human breast and colorectal cancers. *Science* 2007;318:1108–1113. Reprinted with permission from the American Association for the Advancement of Science).

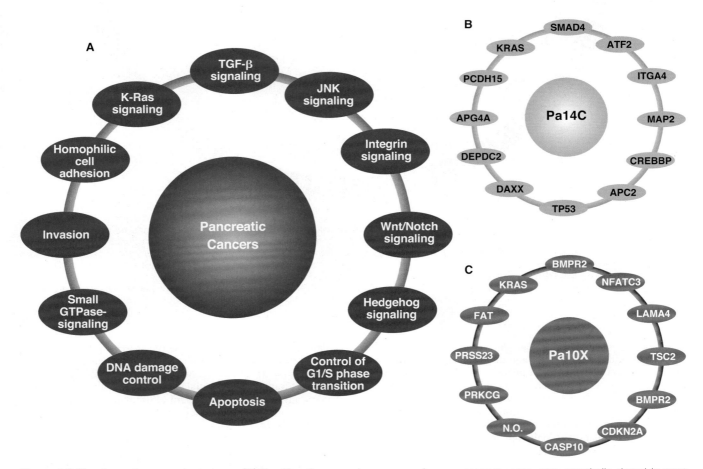

Figure 1.8 Signaling pathways and processes. **(A)** The 12 pathways and processes whose component genes were genetically altered in most pancreatic cancers. **(B,C)** Two pancreatic cancers (Pa14C and Pa10X) and the specific genes that are mutated in them. The positions around the circles in **(B)** and **(C)** correspond to the pathways and processes in **(A)**. Several pathway components overlapped, as illustrated by the BMPR2 mutation that presumably disrupted both the SMAD4 and Hedgehog signaling pathways in Pa10X. Additionally, not all 12 processes and pathways were altered in every pancreatic cancer, as exemplified by the fact that no mutations known to affect DNA damage control were observed in Pa10X. NO, not observed. (Redrawn from Jones S, Zhang X, Parsons DW, et al. Core signaling pathways in human pancreatic cancers revealed by global genomic analyses. *Science* 2008;321:1801–1806. Reprinted with permission from the American Association for the Advancement of Science).

such as in *KRAS* in the G1/S cell cycle transition pathway and pathways where a few mutated genes were found, such as the transforming growth factor (TGF-β) signaling pathway. Finally, there were pathways in which many different genes were mutated, such as invasion regulation molecules, cell adhesion molecules, and integrin signaling. Importantly, independent of how many genes in the same pathway are affected, if they are found to occur in a mutually exclusive fashion in a single tumor, they most likely give the same selective pressure for clonal expansion.

The idea of genetically analyzing pathways rather than individual genes has been applied previously, revealing the concept of mutual exclusivity. Mutual exclusivity has been shown elegantly in the case of *KRAS* and *BRAF*, where a *KRAS*-mutated cancer generally does not also harbor a *BRAF* mutation, because *KRAS* is upstream of *BRAF* in the same pathway.[9] A similar concept was applied for *PIK3CA* and *PTEN*, where both mutations do not usually occur in the same tumor.[23]

With the ever expanding amounts of genetic information being gathered, the ability to search for common pathways being affected in cancer is increasing. One new pathway that is beginning to emerge is the glutamate-signaling pathway. Glutamate dysregulation has been implicated in a number of cancers. In a study of pancreatic duct adenocarcinoma (PDAC), it was seen that glutamate levels were significantly higher in the tissue of individuals with chronic pancreatitis (CP) and PDAC when compared to normal pancreas tissue.[115] It was also observed that the increased glutamate levels led to proinvasion and antiapoptotic signaling through the activation of AMPA receptors.

Also in this regard, and through the use of whole-exome sequencing, it has been recently shown that the glutamate receptor gene *GRIN2A* is highly mutated in melanoma. The finding that many of these mutations are nonsense has suggested that *GRIN2A* is a novel tumor suppressor. Additional genes in the glutamate pathway have also found mutated in melanomas.[116] Pathway analyses and statistical testing on the whole-exome data have also revealed the glutamate signaling pathway to be dysregulated. These results have been further corroborated in another study reporting mutations in the metabotropic glutamate receptor GRM3[117,118] in melanoma. A functional analysis of mutations found in *GRM3* in melanoma tumor samples has shown an increased activation of MEK1/2 kinase, increased migration, and anchorage-independent growth.[117]

Passenger and Driver Mutations

By the time a cancer is diagnosed, it is comprised of billions of cells carrying DNA abnormalities, some of which have a functional role in malignant proliferation; however, many genetic lesions acquired along the way have no functional role in tumorigenesis.[14] The emerging landscapes of cancer genomes include thousands of genes that were not previously linked to tumorigenesis but are found to be somatically mutated. Many of these changes are likely to be *passengers*, or neutral, in that they have no functional effects on the growth of the tumor.[14] Only a small fraction of the genetic alterations are expected to drive cancer evolution by giving cells a selective advantage over their neighbors. Passenger mutations occur incidentally in a cell that later or in parallel develops a *driver* mutation, but are not ultimately pathogenic.[119] Although neutral, cataloging passengers mutations is important because they incorporate the signatures of the previous exposures the cancer cell underwent as well as DNA repair defects the cancer cell has. In many cases, the passenger and driver mutations occur at similar frequencies and the identification of drivers versus the passenger is of utmost relevance and remains a pressing challenge in cancer genetics.[120–122] This goal will eventually be achieved through a combination of genetic and functional approaches, some of which are listed as follows.

The most reliable indicator that a gene was selected for and therefore is highly likely to be pathogenic is the identification of recurrent mutations, whether at the same exact amino acid position

or in neighboring amino acid positions in different patients. More than that, if somatic alterations in the same gene occur very frequently (mountains in the tumor genome landscape), these can be confidently classified as drivers. For example, cancer alleles that are identified in multiple patients and different tumors types, such as those found in *KRAS*, *TP53*, *PTEN*, and *PIK3CA*, are clearly selected for during tumorigenesis.

However, most genes discovered thus far are mutated in a relatively small fraction of tumors (hills), and it has been clearly shown that genes that are mutated in less than 1% of patients can still act as *drivers*.[123] The systematic sequencing of newly identified putative cancer genes in the vast number of specimens from cancer patients will help in this regard. However, even if examining large numbers of samples can provide helpful information to classify drivers versus passengers, this approach alone is limited by the marked variation in mutation frequency among individual tumors and individual genes. The statistical test utilized in this case calculates the probability that the number of mutations in a given gene reflects a mutation frequency that is greater than expected from the nonfunctional background mutation rate,[29,124] which is different between different cancer types. These analyses incorporate the number of somatic alterations observed, the number of tumors studied, and the number of nucleotides that were successfully sequenced and analyzed.

Another approach often used to distinguish driver from passenger mutations exploits the statistical analysis of synonymous versus nonsynonymous changes.[125] In contrast to nonsynonymous mutations, synonymous mutations do not alter the protein sequence. Therefore, they do not usually apply a growth advantage and would not be expected to be selected during tumorigenesis. This strategy works by comparing the observed-to-expected ratio of synonymous with that of nonsynonymous mutation. An increased proportion of nonsynonymous mutations from the expected 2:1 ratio implies selection pressure during tumorigenesis.

Other approaches are based on the concept that driver mutations may have characteristics similar to those causing Mendelian disease when inherited in the germ line and may be identifiable by constraints on tolerated amino acid residues at the mutated positions. In contrast, passenger mutations may have characteristics more similar to those of nonsynonymous SNPs with high minor allele frequencies. Based on these premises, supervised machine learning methods have been used to predict which missense mutations are drivers.[126] Additional approaches to decipher drivers from passengers include the identification of mutations that affect locations that have previously been shown to be cancer causing in protein members of the same gene family. Enrichment for mutations in evolutionarily conserved residues are analyzed by algorithms, such as SIFT (sorting intolerant from tolerant (SIFT),[127] which estimates the effects of the different mutations identified.

Probably the most conclusive methods to identify driver mutations will be rigorous functional studies using biochemical assays as well as model organisms or cultured cells, using knockout and knockin of individual cancer alleles.[128] Unfortunately, these methods are not well suited to the analysis of the hundreds of gene candidates that arise from every large-scale cancer genome project. In conclusion, it is fair to say that sequencing cancer genomes is only the beginning of a journey that will ultimately be completed when the thousands of the newly discovered alleles are annotated as being the drivers of this disease. A summary of the various next-generation applications and approaches for their analysis is summarized in Figure 1.9 and Table 1.2.

NETWORKS OF CANCER GENOME PROJECTS

The repertoire of oncogenic mutations is extremely heterogeneous, suggesting that it would be difficult for independent cancer genome initiatives to address the generation of comprehensive

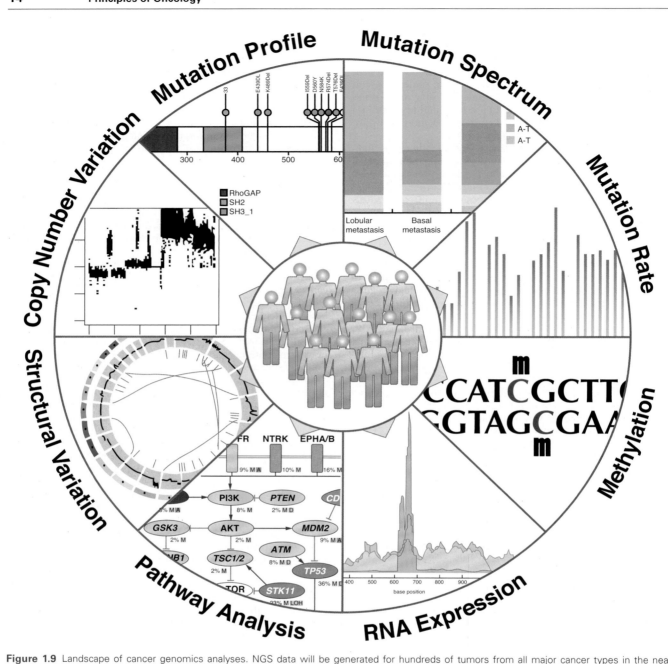

Figure 1.9 Landscape of cancer genomics analyses. NGS data will be generated for hundreds of tumors from all major cancer types in the near future. The integrated analysis of DNA, RNA, and methylation sequencing data will help elucidate all relevant genetic changes in cancers. (Used with permission from Ding L, Wendl MC, Koboldt DC, et al. Analysis of next-generation genomic data in cancer: accomplishments and challenges. *Hum Mol Genet* 2010;19:R188–R196.)

catalogs of mutations in the wide spectrum of human malignancies. Accordingly, there have been different efforts to coordinate the cancer genome sequencing projects being carried out around the world, including The Cancer Genome Atlas (TCGA) and the International Cancer Genome Consortium (ICGC). Moreover, there are other initiatives that are more focused on specific tumors, such as that led by scientists at St. Jude Children's Research Hospital in Memphis, and Washington University, which aims at sequencing multiple pediatric cancer genomes.[129]

TCGA began in 2006 in the United States as a comprehensive program in cancer genomics supported by the U.S. National Institutes of Health (NIH). The initial project focused on three tumors: GBM, serous cystadenocarcinoma of the ovary, and lung squamous carcinoma. These studies have already generated novel

and interesting information regarding genes mutated in these malignancies.[134] On the basis of these positive results, the NIH announced an expansion of the TCGA program with the aim to produce genomic data sets for at least 20 to 25 cancers during the next few years.

The ICGC was formed in 2008 to coordinate the generation of comprehensive catalogs of genomic abnormalities in tumors from 50 different cancer types or subtypes that are of clinical and societal importance across the world.[130] The project aims to perform systematic studies of over 25,000 cancer genomes at the genomic level and integrate this information with epigenomic and transcriptomic studies of the same cases as well as with clinical features of patients. At present, there are a total of 69 committed projects involving at least 16 different countries coordinated by

TABLE 1.2

Computational Tools and Databases Useful for Cancer Genome Analyses

Category	Tool/Database	URL
Alignment	Maq[a]	http://maq.sourceforge.net
	Burrows-Wheeler Aligner (BWA)[b]	http://bio-bwa.sourceforge.net
Mutation calling	SNVMix[c]	http://www.bcgsc.ca/platform/bioinfo/software/SNVMix
	SAMtools[d]	http://samtools.sourceforge.net
	VarScan[e]	http://varscan.sourceforge.net
	MuTect[f]	http://www.broadinstitute.org/cancer/cga/mutect
Indel calling	Pindel[g]	http://gmt.genome.wustl.edu/pindel/current/
Copy number analysis	CBS[h]	http://www.bioconductor.org
	SegSeq[i]	http://www.broadinstitute.org/cgi-bin/cancer/publications/pub_paper.cgi?mode=view&paper_id=182
Functional effect	SIFT[j]	http://sift.jcvi.org/
	PolyPhen-2[k]	http://genetics.bwh.harvard.edu/pph2
Visualization	CIRCOS[l]	http://mkweb.bcgsc.ca/circos
	Integrative Genomics Viewer (IGV)[m]	http://www.broadinstitute.org/igv
Repository	Catalogue of Somatic Mutations in Cancer (COSMIC)[n]	http://www.sanger.ac.uk/genetics/CGP/cosmic
	Cancer Genome Project (CGP)[o]	http://www.sanger.ac.uk/genetics/CGP
	dbSNP[p]	http://www.ncbi.nlm.nih.gov/SNP
	Gene Ranker[q]	http://cbio.mskcc.org/tcga-generanker/

[a] Li H, Durbin R. Fast and accurate short read alignment with Burrows–Wheeler transform. *Bioinformatics* 2009;25:1754–1760.
[b] Li H, Durbin R. Fast and accurate long-read alignment with Burrows–Wheeler transform. *Bioinformatics* 2010;26:589–595.
[c] Goya R, Sun MG, Morin RD, et al. SNVMix: predicting single nucleotide variants from next-generation sequencing of tumors. *Bioinformatics* 2010;26:730–736.
[d] Li H, Handsaker B, Wysoker A, et al. The Sequence Alignment/Map format and SAMtools. *Bioinformatics* 2009;25:2078–2079.
[e] Koboldt DC, Chen K, Wylie T, et al. VarScan: variant detection in massively parallel sequencing of individual and pooled samples. *Bioinformatics* 2009;25:2283–2285.
[f] Cibulskis K, Lawrence MS, Carter SL, et al. Sensitive detection of somatic point mutations in impure and heterogeneous cancer samples. *Nat Biotechnol* 2013;31:213–219.
[g] Ye K, Schulz MH, Long Q, et al. Pindel: a pattern growth approach to detect break points of large deletions and medium sized insertions from paired-end short reads. *Bioinformatics* 2009;25:2865–2871.
[h] Venkatraman ES, Olshen AB. A faster circular binary segmentation algorithm for the analysis of array CGH data. *Bioinformatics* 2007;23:657–663.
[i] Chiang DY, Getz G, Jaffe DB, et al. High-resolution mapping of copy-number alterations with massively parallel sequencing. *Nature Methods* 2009;6:99–103.
[j] Ng PC, Henikoff S. Predicting deleterious amino acid substitutions. *Genome Res* 2001;11:863–874.
[k] Idzhubei IA, Schmidt S, Peshkin L, et al. A method and server for predicting damaging missense mutations. *Nature Methods* 2010;7:248–249.
[l] Krzywinski M, Schein J, Birol I, et al. Circos: an information aesthetic for comparative genomics. *Genome Res* 2009;19:1639–1645.
[m] Robinson JT, Thorvaldsdóttir H, Winckler W, et al. Integrative Genomics Viewer. *Nat Biotechnol* 2011;29:24–26.
[n] Forbes SA, Bhamra S, Dawson E, et al. The catalogue of somatic mutations in cancer (COSMIC). *Curr Protoc Hum Genet* 2008;Chapter 10:Unit 10.11.
[o] Futreal PA, Coin L, Marshall M, et al. A census of human cancer genes. *Nat Rev Cancer* 2004;4:177–183.
[p] Sherry ST, Ward MH, Kholodov M, et al. dbSNP: The NCBI Database of genetic variation. *Nucleic Acids Res* 2001;29:308–311.
[q] The Cancer Genome Atlas Research Network. Comprehensive genomic characterization defines human glioblastoma genes and core pathways. *Nature* 2008;455:1061–1068.
Based on Meyerson M, Stacey G, Getz G. Advances in understanding cancer genomes through second generation sequencing. *Nature Rev Genet* 2010;11:685–696, Table 2.

the ICGC. All of these projects deal with at least 500 samples per cancer type from cancers affecting a variety of human organs and tissues, including blood, the brain, the breast, the esophagus, the kidneys, the liver, the oral cavity, the ovaries, the pancreas, the prostate, the skin, and the stomach.[130]

All of these coordinated projects have already provided new insights into the catalog of genes mutated in cancer and have unveiled specific signatures of the mutagenic mechanisms, including carcinogen exposures or DNA-repair defects, implicated in the development of different malignant tumors.[83,84,87,131] Furthermore, these cancer genome studies have also contributed to define clinically relevant subtypes of tumors for prognosis and therapeutic management, and in some cases have identified new targets and strategies for cancer treatment.[74–76] The rapid technological advances in DNA sequencing will likely drop the costs of sequencing cancer genomes to a small fraction of

the current price and will allow researchers to overcome some of the current limitations of these global sequencing efforts. Hopefully, worldwide coordination of cancer genome projects, including Pan-Cancer initiative, with those involving large-scale, functional analyses of genes in both cellular and animal models will likely provide us with the most comprehensive collection of information generated to date about the causes and molecular mechanisms of cancer.

THE GENOMIC LANDSCAPE OF CANCERS

Examining the overall distribution of the identified mutations redefined the cancer genome landscapes whereby the *mountains* are the handful of commonly mutated genes and the *hills* represent the vast majority of genes that are infrequently mutated.

One of the most striking features of the tumor genomic landscape is that it involves different sets of cancer genes that are mutated in a tissue-specific fashion.[132,133] To continue with the analogy, the scenery is very different if we observe a colorectal, a lung, or a breast tumor. This indicates that mutations in specific genes cause tumors at specific sites, or are associated with specific stages of development, cell differentiation, or tumorigenesis, despite many of those genes being expressed in various fetal and adult tissues. Moreover, different types of tumors follow specific genetic pathways in terms of the combination of genetic alterations that it must acquire. For example, no cancer outside the bowel has been shown to follow the classic genetic pathway of colorectal tumorigenesis. Additionally, *KRAS* mutations are almost always present in pancreatic cancers but are very rare or absent in breast cancers. Similarly, *BRAF* mutations are present in 60% of melanomas, but are very infrequent in lung cancers.[1] Another intriguing feature is that alterations in ubiquitous housekeeping genes, such as those involved in DNA repair or energy production, occur only in particular types of tumors.

In addition to tissue specificity, the genomic landscape of tumors can also be associated with gender and hormonal status. For example, *HER2* amplification and *PIK3C2A* mutations, two genetic alterations associated with breast cancer development, are correlated with the estrogen-receptor hormonal status.[134] The molecular basis for the occurrence of cancer mutations in tissue- and gender-specific profiles is still largely unknown. Organ-specific expression profiles and cell-specific neoplastic transformation requirements are often mentioned as possible causes for this phenomenon. Identifying tissue and gender cancer mutations patterns is relevant because it may allow for the definition of individualized therapeutic avenues.

INTEGRATIVE ANALYSIS OF CANCER GENOMICS

The implementation of novel high-throughput technologies is generating an extraordinary amount of information on cancer samples in many different ways other than those derived from whole-exome or whole-genome sequencing. Accordingly, there is a growing need to integrate genomic, epigenomic, transcriptomic, and proteomic landscapes from tumor samples, and then linking this integrated information with clinical outcomes of cancer patients. There are some examples of human malignancies in which this integrative approach has been already performed, such as for AML, glioblastoma, medulloblastoma, and renal cell, colorectal, ovarian, endometrial, prostate, and breast carcinomas.[135–142] In these cases, the integration of whole-exome and whole-genome sequencing with studies involving genomic DNA copy number arrays, DNA methylation, transcriptomic arrays, miRNA sequencing, and proteomic profiling has contributed to improving the molecular classification of complex and heterogeneous tumors. These integrative molecular analyses have also provided new insights into the mechanisms disrupted in each particular cancer type or subtype and have facilitated the association of genomic information with distinct clinical parameters of cancer patients and the discovery of novel therapeutic targets.[143] Also in this regard, there has been significant progress in the definition of the mechanisms by which the cancer genome and epigenome influence each other and cooperate to facilitate malignant transformation.[144,145] Thus, many tumor-suppressor genes are inactivated by either mutation or epigenetic silencing, and in some cases such as colorectal carcinomas, both mechanisms work coordinately to create a permissive environment for oncogenic transformation.[146] Moreover, mutations in epigenetic regulators such as DNA methyl transferases, chromatin remodelers, histones, and histone modifiers, are very frequent events in many tumors,

including hepatocellular carcinomas, renal carcinomas leukemias, lymphomas, glioblastomas, and medulloblastomas. These genetic alterations of epigenetic modulators cause widespread transcriptomic changes, thereby amplifying the initial effect of the mutational event at the cancer genome level.[145]

The recent availability of different platforms for integrative cancer genome analyses will be very helpful in enabling the classification, biologic characterization, and personalized clinical management of human cancers (Table 1.3).[144,147]

THE CANCER GENOME AND THE NEW TAXONOMY OF TUMORS

Deciphering the cancer genome has already impacted clinical practice at multiple levels. On the one hand, it allowed for the identification of new cancer genes such as *IDH1*, a gene involved in glioma, which was discovered recently (see previous), and on the other hand, it is redesigning the taxonomy of tumors.

Until the genomic revolution, tumors had been classified based on two criteria: their localization (site of occurrence) and their appearance (histology). These criteria are also currently used as primary determinants of prognosis and to establish the best treatments. For many decades, it has been known that patients with histologically similar tumors have different clinical outcomes. Furthermore, tumors that cannot be distinguished based on an histologic analysis can respond very differently to identical therapies.[148]

It is becoming increasingly clear that the frequency and distribution of mutations affecting cancer genes can be used to redefine the histology-based taxonomy of a given tumor type. Lung and colorectal tumors represent paradigmatic examples. Genomic analyses led to the identification of activating mutations in the receptor tyrosine kinase *EGFR* in lung adenocarcinomas.[149] The occurrence of *EGFR* mutations molecularly defines a subtype of non–small-cell lung cancers (NSCLC) that occur mainly in non-smoking women, that tend to have a distinctly enhanced prognosis, and that typically respond to epidermal growth factor receptor (EGFR)-targeted therapies.[150–152] Similarly, the recent discovery of the *EML4-ALK* fusion identifies yet another subset of NSCLC that is clearly distinct from those that harbor *EGFR* mutations, that have distinct epidemiologic and biologic features, and that respond to ALK inhibitors.[109,153]

The second example is colorectal cancers (CRC), the tumor type for which the genomic landscape has been refined with the highest accuracy. CRCs can be clearly categorized according to the mutational profile of the genes involved in the *KRAS* pathway (Fig. 1.10). It is now known that *KRAS* mutations occur in approximately 40% of CRCs. Another subtype of CRC (approximately 10%) harbors mutations in *BRAF*, the immediate downstream effectors of *KRAS*.[10]

In CRCs and other tumor types, *KRAS* and *BRAF* mutations are known to be mutually exclusive. The mutual exclusivity pattern indicates that these genes operate in the same signaling pathway. Large epidemiologic studies have shown that the prognosis of tumors harboring wild-type *KRAS/BRAF* genes is distinct, and typically more favorable, than that of the mutated ones.[154,155] Of note, *KRAS* and *BRAF* mutations have been recently shown to impair responsiveness to the anti-EGFR monoclonal antibodies therapies in CRC patients.[156–158] Clearly distinct subgroups can be genetically identified in both NSCLCs and CRCs with respect to prognosis and response to therapy. It is likely that as soon as the genomic landscapes of other tumor types are defined, molecular subgroups like those described previously will also become defined.

Genotyping tumor tissue in search of somatic genetic alterations for *actionable* information has become routine practice in clinical oncology. The genetic profile of solid tumors is currently obtained from surgical or biopsy specimens. As the techniques

TABLE 1.3

Useful Information for the Description and Management of Cancer

Bioinformatic Tool or Webservices	Database Used	Webservice or Tool	Upload of Data Possible	Gene Search	Chromosomal Region Search	mRNA Expression	SNV	CNV	Methylation	miRNA Expression	Protein	Pathways
cBioPortal for Cancer Genomics	TCGA	Webservice	—	✓	—	✓	✓	✓	—	—	✓	✓
PARADIGM, Broad GDAC Firehose	TCGA	Webservice	✓	✓	—	✓	✓	✓	✓	—	—	✓
WashU Epigenome Browser	ENCODE	Webservice	✓	✓	✓	✓	✓	✓	✓	—	—	✓
UCSC Cancer Genomics Browser	UCSC	Webservice	✓	✓	✓	✓	✓	✓	✓	✓	—	—
The Cancer Genome Workbench	TCGA	Webservice	—	✓	✓	✓	✓	✓	✓	—	—	—
EpiExplorer	ENCODE and ROADMAP	Webservice	✓	✓	✓	✓	✓	✓	✓	—	—	—
EpiGRAPH	ENCODE	Webservice	✓	✓	✓	✓	✓	✓	✓	—	—	—
Catalogue of Somatic Mutations in Cancer (COSMIC)	TCGA and ICGC	Webservice	—	✓	—	—	✓	✓	—	—	—	—
PCmtl, MAGIA, miRvar, CoMeTa, etc.*	GEO and TCGA	Webservice	✓	✓	—	✓	—	—	—	✓	—	✓
ICGC	ICGC	Webservice	—	✓	—	✓	✓	✓	—	—	—	—
Genomatix	User defined	Tool	—	✓	✓	✓	✓	✓	✓	—	—	✓
Caleydo	TCGA	Tool	—	✓	✓	✓	✓	✓	✓	✓	—	✓
Integrative Genomics Viewer (IGV)	ENCODE	Tool	—	✓	✓	✓	—	✓	✓	—	—	—
iCluster and iCluster Plus	User defined	Tool	—	✓	—	✓	—	✓	—	—	—	—

* Web Site with links for integrated analysis of microRNA and mRNA expression.
CNV, copy-number variation; ENCODE, Encyclopedia of DNA Elements; ICGC, the International Cancer Genome Consortium; GDAC, Genomic Data Analysis Center; GEO, Gene Expression Omnibus; miRNA, microRNA; SNV, single-nucleotide variation; TCGA, The Cancer Genome Atlas; UCSS, University of California, Santa Cruz;
Based on Plass C, Pfister SM, Lindroth AM, et al. Mutations in regulators of the epigenome and their connections to global chromatin patterns in cancer. *Nat Rev Genet* 2013;14:765–780, Table 1.

PRINCIPLES OF ONCOLOGY

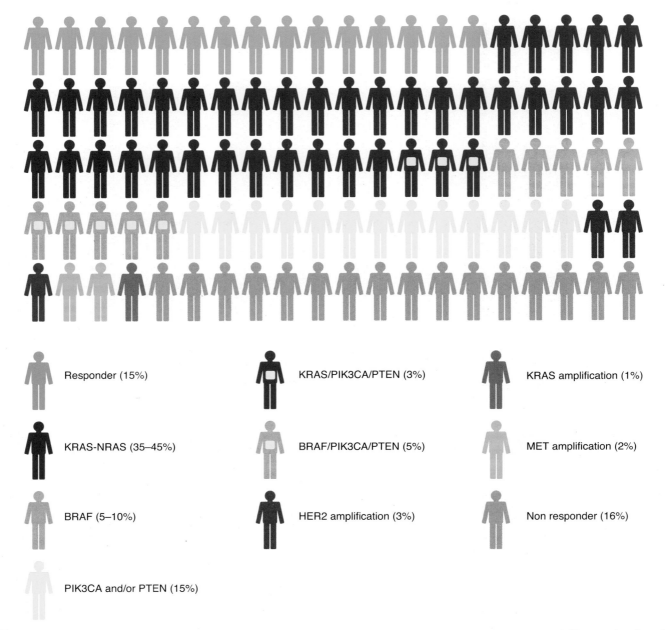

Figure 1.10 Graphic representation of a cohort of 100 patients with colorectal cancer treated with cetuximab or panitumumab. The genetic milieu of individual tumors and their impacts on the clinical response are listed. *KRAS, BRAF,* and *PIK3CA* somatic mutations as well as loss of PTEN protein expression are indicated according to different color codes. Molecular alterations mutually exclusive or coexisting in individual tumors are indicated using different color variants. The relative frequencies at which the molecular alterations occur in colorectal cancers are described. (Redrawn from Bardelli A, Siena S. Molecular mechanisms of resistance to cetuximab and panitumumab in colorectal cancer. *J Clin Oncol* 2010;28:1254–1261.)

that have enabled us to analyze tumor tissues become ever more sophisticated, we have realized the limitations of this approach. As previously discussed, cancers are heterogeneous, with different areas of the same tumor showing different genetic profiles (i.e., intratumoral heterogeneity); likewise, heterogeneity exists between metastases within the same patient (i.e., intermetastatic heterogeneity).[159] A tissue section (or a biopsy) from one part of a solitary tumor will miss the molecular intratumoral as well as intermetastatic heterogeneity. To capture tumor heterogeneity, techniques that are capable of interrogating the genetic landscapes of the overall disease in a single patient are needed.

In 1948, the publication of a manuscript describing the presence of cell-free circulating DNA (cfDNA) in the blood of humans

offered—probably without realizing it—unprecedented opportunities in this area.[160] Only recently, the full potential of this seminal discovery has been appreciated. Several groups have reported that the analysis of circulating tumor DNA can, in principle, provide the same genetic information obtained from tumor tissue.[161] The levels of cfDNA are typically higher in cancer patients than healthy individuals, indicating that it is possible to screen for the presence of disease through a simple blood test. Furthermore, the specific detection of tumor-derived cfDNA has been shown to correlate with tumor burden, which changes in response to treatment or surgery.[162–164]

Although the detection of ctDNA has remarkable potential, it is also challenging for several reasons. The first is the need to discriminate DNA released from tumor cells (ctDNA) from circulating *normal* DNA. Discerning ctDNA from normal cfDNA is aided by the fact that tumor DNA is defined by the presence of mutations. These somatic mutations, commonly single base pair substitutions, are present only in the genomes of cancer cells or precancerous cells and are present in the DNA of normal cells of the same individual. Accordingly, ctDNA offers exquisite specificity as a biomarker. Unfortunately, cfDNA derived from tumor cells often represents a very small fraction (<1%) of the total cfDNA, thus limiting the applicability of the approach. The development and refinement of next-generation sequencing strategies as well as recently developed digital PCR techniques have made it possible to define rare mutant variants in complex mixtures of DNA. Using these approaches, it is possible to detect point mutations, rearrangements, and gene copy number changes in individual genes starting from a few milliliters of plasma.[165] Very recently, several groups have opened a new frontier by showing that exome analyses can also be performed from circulating DNA extracted from the blood of cancer patients.[166]

The detection of tumor-specific genetic alterations in patients' blood (often referred to as *liquid biopsies*) has several applications in the field of oncology, which are summarized as follows. Analyses of cfDNA can be used to genotype tumors when a tissue sample is not available or is difficult to obtain. Circulating tumor DNA fragments contain the identical genetic defects as the tumor themselves, thus the blood can reveal tumor point mutations (*EGFR*, *KRAS*, *BRAF*, *PIK3CA*), rearrangements (e.g., *EML4-ALK*), as well as tumor amplifications (*MET*).[167–169] *Liquid biopsies* may also be useful in monitoring tumor burden—a central aspect in the management of patients with cancer that is typically assessed with imaging. In this regard, several investigational studies have shown that ctDNA can be a surrogate for tumor burden and that, much like viral load changes (e.g., HIV viral load), levels of ctDNA correspond with clinical course. Another application of ctDNA is the detection of minimal residual disease following surgery or therapy with curative intent.[163] Finally, *liquid biopsies* can be used to monitor the genomic drift (clonal evolution) of tumors upon treatment.[166] In this setting, the analysis of ctDNA in plasma samples obtained pretreatment, during, and posttreatment can lead to an understanding of the mechanisms of primary and, especially, acquired resistance to therapies.[170,171]

Importantly, the advances in sequencing technologies have made the idea of personalized treatment of cancer a reality, which is most evident in the field of adoptive cell therapy (ACT). Although already a treatment in use, the ability to use a patient's autologous tumor-infiltrating lymphocytes (TIL) is in position to benefit greatly from advances in sequencing technologies. A recent study demonstrated this when whole-exome data, along with a major histocompatibility complex (MHC)-binding algorithm, were utilized to identify candidate tumor epitopes that are recognized by the patients' TILs.[172] This study should allow for future work in which the information obtained from the direct sequencing of a patient's tumor can quickly be used to generate tumor-reactive T cells that can then be used for a personalized treatment.

In conclusion, the taxonomy of tumors is being rewritten using the presence of genetic lesions as major criteria. Genome-based information will improve the diagnosis and will be used to determine personalized therapeutic regimens based on the genetic landscape of individual tumors.

CANCER GENOMICS AND DRUG RESISTANCE

Cancer genomics has dramatically impacted disease management, because its application is helping researchers determine which patients are likely to benefit from which drug. As discussed in great detail in Chapter 22, good examples for such treatment include targeted therapy using imatinib for chronic myeloid leukemia (CML) patients and the use of gefitinib and erlotinib for NSCLC patients.

The key to the successful development and application of anticancer agents is a better understanding of the effect of the therapeutic regimens and of resistance mechanisms that may develop. In most tumor types, a fraction of patients' tumors are refractory to therapies (intrinsic resistance). Even if an initial response to therapies is obtained, the vast majority of tumors subsequently become refractory (i.e., acquired resistance), and patients eventually succumb to disease progression. Therefore, secondary resistance should be regarded as a key obstacle to treatment progress. The analysis of the cancer genome represents a powerful tool both for the identification of chemotherapeutic signatures as well as to understand resistance mechanisms to therapeutic agents. Examples for each of these are described as follows.

An important application of systematic sequencing experiments is the identification of the effects of chemotherapy on the cancer genome. For example, gliomas that recur after temozolomide treatment have been shown to harbor large numbers of mutations with a signature typical of a DNA alkylating agent.[173,174] Because these alterations were detected using Sanger sequencing, which as described previously has limited sensitivity, the data suggested that the detected alterations were clonal. The model that unfolds from this study indicates that although temozolomide has limited efficacy, almost all of the cells in a glioma respond to the drug. However, a single cell that was resistant to the chemotherapy proliferated and formed a cell clone. Later genomic analyses of the cell clone allowed for the identification of the underlying mutated resistance genes.[173,174]

Single-molecule–targeted therapy is almost always followed by acquired drug resistance.[175–177] Genomic analyses can be successfully exploited to decipher resistance mechanisms to such inhibitors. A few paradigmatic examples are presented as follows, which will be discussed extensively in other chapters. Despite the effectiveness of gefitinib and erlotinib in EGFR mutant cases of NSCLC,[178] drug resistance develops within 6 to 12 months after the initiation of therapy. The underlying reason for this resistance was identified as a secondary mutation in *EGFR* exon 20, T790M, which is detectable in 50% of patients who relapse.[179–181] Importantly, some studies have shown the mutation to be present before the patient was treated with the drug,[182,183] suggesting that exposure to the drug selected for these cells.[184] Because the drug-resistant *EGFR* mutation is structurally analogous to the mutated gatekeeper residue T315I in BCR-ABL, T670I in c-Kit, and L1196M in EML4-ALK, which have been shown previously to confer resistance to imatinib and other kinase inhibitors,[176,185,186] this mechanism of resistance represents a general problem that needs to be overcome.

A recent elegant study, which also represents the use of genomics in understanding drug-resistance mechanisms, focused on the inhibition of activating *BRAF* (V600E) mutations, which occur in 7% of human malignancies and in 60% of melanomas.[9] Clinical trials using PLX4032, a novel class I RAF-selective inhibitor, showed an 80% antitumor response rate in melanoma patients with *BRAF* (V600E) mutations; however, cases of drug resistance were observed.[187] The use of microarray and sequencing technologies showed that, in this case, the resistance was not due to secondary mutations in *BRAF*, but due rather to either upregulation of *PDGFRB* or *NRAS* mutations.[188]

It was, however, the introduction of two anti-EGFR monoclonal antibodies, cetuximab and panitumumab, for the treatment of metastatic colorectal cancer, that provided the largest body of knowledge on the relationship between tumors' genotypes and the response to targeted therapies. The initial clinical analysis pointed out that only a fraction of metastatic CRC patients benefited from this novel treatment. Different from the NSCLC paradigm, it was found that EGFR mutations do not play a major role in the response. On the contrary, from the initial retrospective analysis, it became clear that somatic *KRAS* mutations, thought to be present in 35% to 45% of metastatic colorectal cancers, are important negative predictors of efficacy in patients who are given panitumumab or cetuximab.[156-158] Among tumors carrying wild-type *KRAS*, mutations of *BRAF* or *PIK3CA*, or a loss of phosphatase and tensin homolog (PTEN) expression may also predict resistance to EGFR-targeted monoclonal antibodies, although the latter biomarkers require further validation before they can be incorporated into clinical practice. From these few examples, it is clear that a future, deeper genomic understanding of targeted drug resistance is crucial to the effective development of additional as well as alternative therapies to overcome this resistance.

PERSPECTIVES OF CANCER GENOME ANALYSIS

The completion of the human genome project has marked a new beginning in biomedical sciences. Because human cancer is a genetic disease, the field of oncology has been one of the first to be impacted by this historic revolution. Knowledge of the sequence and organization of the human genome allows for the systematic analysis of the genetic alterations underlying the origin and evolution of tumors. High-throughput mutational profiling of common tumors, including lung, skin, breast, and colorectal cancers, and the application of next-generation sequencing to whole genome, whole exome, and whole transcriptome of cancer samples has allowed substantial advances in the understanding of this disease by facilitating the detection of all main types of somatic cancer genome alterations. These have also led to historical results, such as the identification of genetic alterations that are likely to be the major drivers of these diseases.

However, the genetic landscape of cancers is by no means complete, and what has been learned so far has raised new and exciting questions that must be addressed. There are still important technical challenges for the detection of somatic mutations.[60] Clinical tumor samples often contain large amounts of nonmalignant cells, which makes the identification of mutations in cancer genomes more challenging when compared with similar analyses of peripheral blood samples for germ-line genome studies. Moreover, the genomic instability inherent to cancer development and progression largely increases the complexity and diversity of genomic alterations of malignant tumors, making it necessary to distinguish between driver and passenger mutations. Likewise, the fact that malignant tumors are genetically heterogeneous and contain several clones simultaneously growing within the same tumor mass raises additional questions regarding the quality of the information currently derived from cancer genomes. Hopefully, in the near future, advances in third-generation sequencing technologies will make it feasible to obtain high-quality sequence data of a genome isolated from a single cell, an aspect of crucial relevance for cancer research.

One of the next imperatives is the definition of the oncogenomic profile of all tumor types. In particular, the less common—although not less lethal—ones are still largely mysterious to scientists and untreatable to clinicians. For some of these diseases, few new therapeutically amenable molecular targets have been discovered in the past years. For example, the identification of drugable genetic lesions associated with pancreatic and ovarian cancers could help define new therapeutic strategies for these aggressive diseases. To achieve this, detailed oncogenomic maps of the corresponding tumors must be drafted. The latter will hopefully be completed in the coming years, thanks to the systematic cancer genome projects that are presently being performed.

Even in the case of common cancers, a lot of genomic profiling efforts still lay ahead. For example, in a significant fraction of breast and lung tumors, the mutations that are likely to be drivers have not yet been found. This is not surprising considering that even in these tumor types only a limited number of samples have been systematically analyzed so far. Therefore, low incidence mutations that could represent potentially key therapeutic targets in a subset of tumors might have escaped detection. Consequently, the scaling up of the mutational profiling to large numbers of specimens for each tumor type is warranted.

Finally, understanding the cellular properties imparted by the hundreds of recently discovered cancer alleles is another area that must be developed. As a matter of fact, compared to the genomic discovery stage, the functional validation of putative novel cancer alleles, despite their potential clinical relevance, is substantially lagging behind. To achieve this, high-throughput functional studies in model systems that accurately recapitulate the genetic alterations found in human cancer must be developed.

To conclude, the eventual goal of profiling the cancer genome is not only to further understand the molecular basis of the disease, but also to discover novel diagnostic and drug targets. One might anticipate that the most immediate application of these new technologies will be noninvasive strategies for early cancer detection. Considering that oncogenic mutations are present only in cancer cells, screening for tumor-derived mutant DNA in patients' blood holds great potential and will progressively substitute current biomarkers, which have poor sensitivity and lack specificity.[171] Further improvements in next-generation sequencing technologies are likely to reduce their cost as well as make these analyses more facile in the future. Once this happens, most cancer patients will undergo in-depth genomic analyses as part of their initial evaluation and throughout their treatment. This will offer more precise diagnostic and prognostic information, which will affect treatment decisions. Although many challenges remain, the information gained from next-generation sequencing platforms is laying a foundation for personalized medicine, in which patients are managed with therapies that are tailored to the specific gene mutations found in their tumors. Ultimately, these should lead to therapeutic successes similar to the ones attained for CML patients with imatinib,[189,190] melanoma patients with PLX4032,[187] and NSCLC patients with gefitinib and erlotinib.[178] Clearly, this is the absolute goal for all of this work.

ACKNOWLEDGMENTS

This work was supported by the Intramural Research Programs of the National Human Genome Research Institute, National Institutes of Health, USA, YS is supported by the Henry Chanoch Krenter Institute for Biomedical Imaging and Genomics, Louis and Fannie Tolz Collaborative Research Project, Dukler Fund for Cancer Research, De Benedetti Foundation-Cherasco 1547, Peter and Patricia Gruber Awards, Gideon Hamburger, Israel, Estate of Alice Schwarz-Gardos, Estate of John Hunter and the Knell Family. YS is supported by the Israel Science Foundation grant numbers 1604/13 and 877/13 and the ERC (StG-335377). A.B. is supported by the European Communityís Seventh Framework Programme under grant agreement no. 259015 COLTHERES, Associazione Italiana per la Ricerca sul Cancro (AIRC) IG grant no. 12812 and Fondazione Piemontese per la Ricerca sul Cancro–ONLUS. C.L-O. is an Investigator of the Botin Foundation supported by grants from Ministerio de Economía y Competitividad-Spain and Instituto de Salud Carlos III (RTICC), Spain.

REFERENCES

1. Vogelstein B, Kinzler KW. Cancer genes and the pathways they control. *Nat Med* 2004;10:789–799.
2. Kinzler KW, Vogelstein B. Lessons from hereditary colon cancer. *Cell* 1996; 87:159–170.
3. International Human Genome Sequencing Consortium. Finishing the euchromatic sequence of the human genome. *Nature* 2004;431:931–945.
4. Stehelin D, Varmus HE, Bishop JM, et al. DNA related to the transforming gene(s) of avian sarcoma viruses is present in normal avian DNA. *Nature* 1976;260:170–173.
5. Rous P. Transmission of a malignant new growth by means of a cell-free filtrate. *J Am Med Assoc* 1911;56:198.
6. International HapMap Consortium. The International HapMap Project. *Nature* 2003;426:89–96.
7. International HapMap Consortium. A haplotype map of the human genome. *Nature* 2005;437:1299–1320.
8. Sanger F, Nicklen S, Coulson AR. DNA sequencing with chain-terminating inhibitors. *Proc Natl Acad Sci U S A* 1977;74:5463–5467.
9. Davies H, Bignell GR, Cox C, et al. Mutations of the BRAF gene in human cancer. *Nature* 2002;417:949–954.
10. Rajagopalan H, Bardelli A, Lengauer C, et al. Tumorigenesis: RAF/RAS oncogenes and mismatch-repair status. *Nature* 2002;418:934.
11. Moodie SA, Wolfman A. The 3Rs of life: Ras, Raf and growth regulation. *Trends Genet* 1994;10:44–48.
12. Hafen E, Dickson B, Brunner D, et al. Genetic dissection of signal transduction mediated by the sevenless receptor tyrosine kinase in Drosophila. *Prog Neurobiol* 1994;42:287–292.
13. Bardelli A, Parsons DW, Silliman N, et al. Mutational analysis of the tyrosine kinome in colorectal cancers. *Science* 2003;300:949.
14. Greenman C, Stephens P, Smith R, et al. Patterns of somatic mutation in human cancer genomes. *Nature* 2007;446:153–158.
15. Samuels Y, Wang Z, Bardelli A, et al. High frequency of mutations of the PIK3CA gene in human cancers. *Science* 2004;304:554.
16. Wang Z, Shen D, Parsons DW, et al. Mutational analysis of the tyrosine phosphatome in colorectal cancers. *Science* 2004;304:1164–1166.
17. Vivanco I, Sawyers CL. The phosphatidylinositol 3-Kinase AKT pathway in human cancer. *Nat Rev Cancer* 2002;2:489–501.
18. Broderick DK, Di C, Parrett TJ, et al. Mutations of PIK3CA in anaplastic oligodendrogliomas, high-grade astrocytomas, and medulloblastomas. *Cancer Res* 2004;64:5048–5050.
19. Lee JW, Soung YH, Kim SY, et al. PIK3CA gene is frequently mutated in breast carcinomas and hepatocellular carcinomas. *Oncogene* 2005;24:1477–1480.
20. Bachman KE, Argani P, Samuels Y, et al. The PIK3CA gene is mutated with high frequency in human breast cancers. *Cancer Biol Ther* 2004;3: 772–775.
21. Oda K, Stokoe D, Taketani Y, et al. High frequency of coexistent mutations of PIK3CA and PTEN genes in endometrial carcinoma. *Cancer Res* 2005;65:10669–10673.
22. Samuels Y, Waldman T. Oncogenic mutations of PIK3CA in human cancers. *Curr Top Microbiol Immunol* 2010;2:21–42.
23. Parsons DW, Wang TL, Samuels Y, et al. Colorectal cancer: mutations in a signalling pathway. *Nature* 2005;436:792.
24. Lopez-Otin C, Overall CM. Protease degradomics: a new challenge for proteomics. *Nat Rev Mol Cell Biol* 2002;3:509–519.
25. Liotta LA, Tryggvason K, Garbisa S, et al. Metastatic potential correlates with enzymatic degradation of basement membrane collagen. *Nature* 1980;284: 67–68.
26. Lopez-Otin C, Hunter T. The regulatory crosstalk between kinases and proteases in cancer. *Nat Rev Cancer* 2010;10:278–292.
27. Egeblad M, Werb Z. New functions for the matrix metalloproteinases in cancer progression. *Nat Rev Cancer* 2002;2:161–174.
28. Lopez-Otin C, Matrisian LM. Emerging roles of proteases in tumour suppression. *Nat Rev Cancer* 2007;7:800–808.
29. Wood LD, Parsons DW, Jones S, et al. The genomic landscapes of human breast and colorectal cancers. *Science* 2007;318:1108–1113.
30. Palavalli LH, Prickett TD, Wunderluch JR, et al. Analysis of the matrix metalloproteinase family reveals that MMP8 is often mutated in melanoma. *Nat Genet* 2009;41:518–520.
31. Lopez-Otin C, Palavalli LH, Samuels Y. Protective roles of matrix metalloproteinases: from mouse models to human cancer. *Cell Cycle* 2009;8:3657–3662.
32. Hanahan D, Weinberg RA. The hallmarks of cancer. *Cell* 2000;100:57–70.
33. Teitz T, Wei T, Valentine MB, et al. Caspase 8 is deleted or silenced preferentially in childhood neuroblastomas with amplification of MYCN. *Nat Med* 2000;6:529–535.
34. Mandruzzato S, Brasseur F, Andry G, et al. A CASP-8 mutation recognized by cytolytic T lymphocytes on a human head and neck carcinoma. *J Exp Med* 1997;186:785–793.
35. Soung YH, Lee JW, Kim SY, et al. CASPASE-8 gene is inactivated by somatic mutations in gastric carcinomas. *Cancer Res* 2005;65:815–821.
36. Fraile JM, Quesada V, Rodríguez D, et al. Deubiquitinases in cancer: new functions and therapeutic options. *Oncogene* 2012;31:2373–2388.
37. Bignell GR, Warren W, Seal S, et al. Identification of the familial cylindromatosis tumour-suppressor gene. *Nat Genet* 2000;25:160–165.
38. Schmitz R, Hansmann ML, Bohle V, et al. TNFAIP3 (A20) is a tumor suppressor gene in Hodgkin lymphoma and primary mediastinal B cell lymphoma. *J Exp Med* 2009;206:981–989.
39. Compagno M, Lim WK, Grunn A, et al. Mutations of multiple genes cause deregulation of NF-kappaB in diffuse large B-cell lymphoma. *Nature* 2009;459:717–721.
40. Kato M, Sanada M, Kato I, et al. Frequent inactivation of A20 in B-cell lymphomas. *Nature* 2009;459:712–716.
41. Novak U, Rinaldi A, Kwee I, et al. The NF-kappa B negative regulator TNFAIP3 (A20) is inactivated by somatic mutations and genomic deletions in marginal zone lymphomas. *Blood* 2009;113: 4918–4921.
42. Harbour JW, Onken MD, Roberson ED, et al. Frequent mutation of BAP1 in metastasizing uveal melanomas. *Science* 2010;330:1410–1413.
43. Carbone M, Yang H, Pass HI, et al. BAP1 and cancer. *Nat Rev Cancer* 2013; 13:153–159.
44. Sjöblom T, Jones S, Wood LD, et al. The consensus coding sequences of human breast and colorectal cancers. *Science* 2006;314:268–274.
45. Jones S, Zhang X, Parsons DW, et al. Core signaling pathways in human pancreatic cancers revealed by global genomic analyses. *Science* 2008;321:1801–1806.
46. Parsons DW, Jones S, Zhang X, et al. An integrated genomic analysis of human glioblastoma multiforme. *Science* 2008;321:1807–1812.
47. Jones S, Wang TL, Shih IeM, et al. Frequent mutations of chromatin remodeling gene ARID1A in ovarian clear cell carcinoma. *Science* 2010;330:228–231.
48. Parsons DW, Li M, Zhang X, et al. The genetic landscape of the childhood cancer medulloblastoma. *Science* 2011;331:435–439.
49. Yan H, Parsons DW, Jin G, et al. IDH1 and IDH2 mutations in gliomas. *N Engl J Med* 2009;360:765–773.
50. Bleeker FE, Lamba S, Leenstra S, et al. IDH1 mutations at residue p.R132 (IDH1(R132)) occur frequently in high-grade gliomas but not in other solid tumors. *Hum Mutat* 2009;30:7–11.
51. Hartmann C, Meyer J, Balss J, et al. Type and frequency of IDH1 and IDH2 mutations are related to astrocytic and oligodendroglial differentiation and age: a study of 1,010 diffuse gliomas. *Acta Neuropathol* 2009;118:469–474.
52. Hayden JT, Frühwald MC, Hasselblatt M, et al. Frequent IDH1 mutations in supratentorial primitive neuroectodermal tumors (sPNET) of adults but not children. *Cell Cycle* 2009;8:1806–1807.
53. Ichimura K, Pearson DM, Kocialkowski S, et al. IDH1 mutations are present in the majority of common adult gliomas but rare in primary glioblastomas. *Neuro Oncol* 2009;11:341–347.
54. Kang MR, Kim MS, Oh JE, et al. Mutational analysis of IDH1 codon 132 in glioblastomas and other common cancers. *Int J Cancer* 2009;125:353–355.
55. Watanabe T, Nobusawa S, Kleihues P, et al. IDH1 mutations are early events in the development of astrocytomas and oligodendrogliomas. *Am J Pathol* 2009;174:1149–1153.
56. Mardis ER, Ding L, Dooling DJ, et al. Recurring mutations found by sequencing an acute myeloid leukemia genome. *N Engl J Med* 2009;361:1058–1066.
57. Green A, Beer P. Somatic mutations of IDH1 and IDH2 in the leukemic transformation of myeloproliferative neoplasms. *N Engl J Med* 2010;362:369–370.
58. Gross S, Cairns RA, Minden Md, et al. Cancer-associated metabolite 2-hydroxyglutarate accumulates in acute myelogenous leukemia with isocitrate dehydrogenase 1 and 2 mutations. *J Exp Med* 2010;207:339–344.
59. Mardis ER, Wilson RK. Cancer genome sequencing: a review. *Hum Mol Genet* 2009;18:R163–R168.
60. Meyerson M, Gabriel S, Getz G. Advances in understanding cancer genomes through second-generation sequencing. *Nat Rev Genet* 2010;11:685–696.
61. Metzker ML. Sequencing technologies - the next generation. *Nat Rev Genet* 2010;11:31–46.
62. Bell DW. Our changing view of the genomic landscape of cancer. *J Pathol* 2010;220:231–243.
63. Campbell PJ, Pleasance ED, Stephens PJ, et al. Subclonal phylogenetic structures in cancer revealed by ultra-deep sequencing. *Proc Natl Acad Sci U S A* 2008;105:13081–13086.
64. Kidd JM, Cooper GM, Donahue WF, et al. Mapping and sequencing of structural variation from eight human genomes. *Nature* 2008;453:56–64.
65. Drmanac R, Sparks AB, Callow MJ, et al. Human genome sequencing using unchained base reads on self-assembling DNA nanoarrays. *Science* 2010; 327:78–81.
66. Clarke J, Wu HC, Jayasinghe L, et al. Continuous base identification for single-molecule nanopore DNA sequencing. *Nat Nanotechnol* 2009;4:265–270.
67. Schadt EE, Turner S, Kasarskis A. A window into third-generation sequencing. *Hum Mol Genet* 2010;19:R227–R240.
68. Dressman D, Yan H, Traverso G, et al. Transforming single DNA molecules into fluorescent magnetic particles for detection and enumeration of genetic variations. *Proc Natl Acad Sci U S A* 2003;100:8817–8822.
69. Fedurco M, Romieu A, Williams S, et al. BTA, a novel reagent for DNA attachment on glass and efficient generation of solid-phase amplified DNA colonies. *Nucleic Acids Res* 2006;34:e22.
70. Harris TD, Buzby PR, Babcock H, et al. Single-molecule DNA sequencing of a viral genome. *Science* 2008;320:106–109.
71. Morozova O, Hirst M, Marra MA. Applications of new sequencing technologies for transcriptome analysis. *Annu Rev Genomics Hum Genet* 2009;10: 135–151.

PRINCIPLES OF ONCOLOGY

72. Pop M, Salzberg SL. Bioinformatics challenges of new sequencing technology. *Trends Genet* 2008;24:142–149.

73. Ley TJ, Mardis ER, Ding L, et al. DNA sequencing of a cytogenetically normal acute myeloid leukaemia genome. *Nature* 2008;456:66–72.

74. Garraway LA, Lander ES. Lessons from the cancer genome. *Cell* 2013;15:17–37.

75. Vogelstein B, Papadopoulos N, Velculescu VE, et al. Cancer genome landscapes. *Science* 2013;339:1546–1558.

76. Watson IR, Takahashi K, Futreal PA, et al. Emerging patterns of somatic mutations in cancer. *Nat Rev Genet* 2013;14:703–718.

77. Campbell PJ, Yachida S, Mudie LJ, et al. The patterns and dynamics of genomic instability in metastatic pancreatic cancer. *Nature* 2010;467:1109–1113.

78. Lee W, Jiang Z, Liu J, et al. The mutation spectrum revealed by paired genome sequences from a lung cancer patient. *Nature* 2010;465:473–477.

79. Marcucci G, Maharry K, Wu YZ, et al. IDH1 and IDH2 gene mutations identify novel molecular subsets within de novo cytogenetically normal acute myeloid leukemia: a Cancer and Leukemia Group B study. *J Clin Oncol* 2010;28:2348–2355.

80. Paschka P, Schlenk RF, Gaidzik VI, et al. IDH1 and IDH2 mutations are frequent genetic alterations in acute myeloid leukemia and confer adverse prognosis in cytogenetically normal acute myeloid leukemia with NPM1 mutation without FLT3 internal tandem duplication. *J Clin Oncol* 2010;28:3636–3643.

81. Shah SP, Morin Rd, Khattra J, et al. Mutational evolution in a lobular breast tumour profiled at single nucleotide resolution. *Nature* 2009;461:809–813.

82. Yachida S, Jones S, Bozic I, et al. Distant metastasis occurs late during the genetic evolution of pancreatic cancer. *Nature* 2010;467:1114–1117.

83. Pleasance ED, Cheetham RK, Stephens PJ, et al. A comprehensive catalogue of somatic mutations from a human cancer genome. *Nature* 2010;463:191–196.

84. Pleasance ED, Stephens PJ, O'Meara S, et al. A small-cell lung cancer genome with complex signatures of tobacco exposure. *Nature* 2010;463:184–190.

85. Ding L, Ellis MJ, Li S, et al. Genome remodelling in a basal-like breast cancer metastasis and xenograft. *Nature* 2010;464:999–1005.

86. Ley TJ, Ding L, Walter MJ, et al. DNMT3A mutations in acute myeloid leukemia. *N Engl J Med* 2010;363:2424–2433.

87. Alexandrov LB, Nik-Zainal S, Wedge DC, et al. Signatures of mutational processes in human cancer. *Nature* 2013;500:415–421.

88. Ward PS, Patel J, Wise DR, et al. The common feature of leukemia-associated IDH1 and IDH2 mutations is a neomorphic enzyme activity converting alpha-ketoglutarate to 2-hydroxyglutarate. *Cancer Cell* 2010;17:225–234.

89. Jones SJ, Laskin J, Lu YY, et al. Evolution of an adenocarcinoma in response to selection by targeted kinase inhibitors. *Genome Biol* 2010;11:R82.

90. Navin N, Kendall J, Troge J, et al. Tumour evolution inferred by single-cell sequencing. *Nature* 2011;472:90–94.

91. Vanharanta S, Massague J. Origins of metastatic traits. *Cancer Cell* 2013;24:410–421.

92. Huang FW, Hodis E, Xu MJ, et al. Highly recurrent TERT promoter mutations in human melanoma. *Science* 2013;339:957–959.

93. Horn S, Figl A, Rachakonda PS, et al. TERT promoter mutations in familial and sporadic melanoma. *Science* 2013;339:959–961.

94. Ying Z, Li Y, Wu J, et al. Loss of miR-204 expression enhances glioma migration and stem cell-like phenotype. *Cancer Res* 2013;73:990–999.

95. Liang YJ, Wang QY, Zhou CX, et al. MiR-124 targets Slug to regulate epithelial-mesenchymal transition and metastasis of breast cancer. *Carcinogenesis* 2013;34:713–722.

96. Cooper C, Guo J, Yan Y, et al. Increasing the relative expression of endogenous non-coding Steroid Receptor RNA Activator (SRA) in human breast cancer cells using modified oligonucleotides. *Nucleic Acids Res* 2009;37:4518–4531.

97. Stephens PJ, Greenman CD, Fu B, et al. Massive genomic rearrangement acquired in a single catastrophic event during cancer development. *Cell* 2011;144:27–40.

98. Korbel JO, Campbell PJ. Criteria for inference of chromothripsis in cancer genomes. *Cell* 2013;152:1226–1236.

99. Baca SC, Prandi D, Lawrence MS, et al. Punctuated evolution of prostate cancer genomes. *Cell* 2013;153:666–677.

100. Turner EH, Lee C, Ng SB, et al. Massively parallel exon capture and library-free resequencing across 16 genomes. *Nat Methods* 2009;6:315–316.

101. Gnirke A, Melnikov A, Maguire J, et al. Solution hybrid selection with ultra-long oligonucleotides for massively parallel targeted sequencing. *Nat Biotechnol* 2009;27:182–189.

102. Levin JZ, Berger MF, Adiconis X, et al. Targeted next-generation sequencing of a cancer transcriptome enhances detection of sequence variants and novel fusion transcripts. *Genome Biol* 2009;10:R115.

103. Lawrence MS, Stojanov P, Polak P, et al. Mutational heterogeneity in cancer and the search for new cancer-associated genes. *Nature* 2013;499:214–218.

104. Kandoth C, McLellan MD, Vandin F, et al. Mutational landscape and significance across 12 major cancer types. *Nature* 2013;502:333–339.

105. Gartner JJ, Parker SC, Prickett TD, et al. Whole-genome sequencing identifies a recurrent functional synonymous mutation in melanoma. *Proc Natl Acad Sci U S A* 2013;110:13481–13486.

106. Stegh AH, Brennan C, Mahoney JA, et al. Glioma oncoprotein Bcl2L12 inhibits the p53 tumor suppressor. *Genes Dev* 2010;24:2194–2204.

107. Mullaney JM, Mills RE, Pittard WS, et al. Small insertions and deletions (INDELs) in human genomes. *Hum Mol Genet* 2010;19:R131–R136.

108. Tomlins SA, Rhodes DR, Perner S, et al. Recurrent fusion of TMPRSS2 and ETS transcription factor genes in prostate cancer. *Science* 2005;310:644–648.

109. Soda M, Choi YL, Enomoto M, et al. Identification of the transforming EML4-ALK fusion gene in non-small-cell lung cancer. *Nature* 2007;448:561–566.

110. Palanisamy N, Ateeq B, Kalyana-Sundaram S, et al. Rearrangements of the RAF kinase pathway in prostate cancer, gastric cancer and melanoma. *Nat Med* 2010;16:793–798.

111. Leary RJ, Kinde I, Diehl F, et al. Development of personalized tumor biomarkers using massively parallel sequencing. *Sci Transl Med* 2010;2:20ra14.

112. Maher CA, Kumar-Sinha C, Cao X, et al. Transcriptome sequencing to detect gene fusions in cancer. *Nature* 2009;458:97–101.

113. Stephens PJ, McBride DJ, Lin ML, et al. Complex landscapes of somatic rearrangement in human breast cancer genomes. *Nature* 2009;462:1005–1010.

114. Feng H, Shuda M, Chang Y, et al. Clonal integration of a polyomavirus in human Merkel cell carcinoma. *Science* 2008;319:1096–1100.

115. Herner A, Sauliunaite D, Michalski CW, et al. Glutamate increases pancreatic cancer cell invasion and migration via AMPA receptor activation and Kras-MAPK signaling. *Int J Cancer* 2011;129:2349–2359.

116. Wei X, Walia V, Lin JC, et al. Exome sequencing identifies GRIN2A as frequently mutated in melanoma. *Nat Genet* 2011;43:442–446.

117. Prickett TD, Wei X, Cardenas-Navia I, et al. Exon capture analysis of G protein-coupled receptors identifies activating mutations in GRM3 in melanoma. *Nat Genet* 2011;43:1119–1126.

118. Krauthammer M, Kong Y, Ha BH, et al. Exome sequencing identifies recurrent somatic RAC1 mutations in melanoma. *Nat Genet* 2012;44:1006–1014.

119. Davies H, Hunter C, Smith R, et al. Somatic mutations of the protein kinase gene family in human lung cancer. *Cancer Res* 2005;65:7591–7595.

120. Bozic I, Antal T, Ohtsuki H, et al. Accumulation of driver and passenger mutations during tumor progression. *Proc Natl Acad Sci U S A* 2010;107:18545–18550.

121. Parmigiani G, Boca S, Lin J, et al. Design and analysis issues in genome-wide somatic mutation studies of cancer. *Genomics* 2009;93:17–21.

122. Kaminker JS, Zhang Y, Waugh A, et al. Distinguishing cancer-associated missense mutations from common polymorphisms. *Cancer Res* 2007;67:465–473.

123. Futreal PA. Backseat drivers take the wheel. *Cancer Cell* 2007;12:493–494.

124. Greenman C, Wooster R, Futreal PA, et al. Statistical analysis of pathogenicity of somatic mutations in cancer. *Genetics* 2006;173:2187–2198.

125. Baudot A, Real FX, Izarzugaza JM, et al. From cancer genomes to cancer models: bridging the gaps. *EMBO Rep* 2009;10:359–366.

126. Carter H, Chen S, Isik L, et al. Cancer-specific high-throughput annotation of somatic mutations: computational prediction of driver missense mutations. *Cancer Res* 2009;69:6660–6667.

127. Ng PC, Henikoff S. SIFT: Predicting amino acid changes that affect protein function. *Nucleic Acids Res* 2003;31:3812–3814.

128. Kohli M, Rago C, Lengauer C, et al. Facile methods for generating human somatic cell gene knockouts using recombinant adeno-associated viruses. *Nucleic Acids Res* 2004;32:e3.

129. Downing JR, Wilson RK, Zhang J, et al. The Pediatric Cancer Genome Project. *Nat Genet* 2012;44:619–622.

130. Hudson TJ, Anderson W, Artez A, et al. International network of cancer genome projects. *Nature* 2010;464:993–998.

131. Bignell GR, Greenman CD, Davies H, et al. Signatures of mutation and selection in the cancer genome. *Nature* 2010;463:893–898.

132. Sieber OM, Tomlinson SR, Tomlinson IP. Tissue, cell and stage specificity of (epi)mutations in cancers. *Nat Rev Cancer* 2005;5:649–655.

133. Benvenuti S, Frattini M, Arena S, et al. PIK3CA cancer mutations display gender and tissue specificity patterns. *Hum Mutat* 2008;29:284–288.

134. Karakas B, Bachman KE, Park BH. Mutation of the PIK3CA oncogene in human cancers. *Br J Cancer* 2006;94:455–459.

135. Brennan CW, Werhaak RG, McKenna A, et al. The somatic genomic landscape of glioblastoma. *Cell* 2013;155:462–477.

136. Cancer Genome Atlas Network. Comprehensive molecular characterization of human colon and rectal cancer. *Nature* 2012;487:330–337.

137. Cancer Genome Atlas Network. Comprehensive molecular portraits of human breast tumours. *Nature* 2012;490:61–70.

138. Cancer Genome Atlas Research Network. Integrated genomic analyses of ovarian carcinoma. *Nature* 2011;474:609–615.

139. Cancer Genome Atlas Research Network. Comprehensive molecular characterization of clear cell renal cell carcinoma. *Nature* 2013;499:43–49.

140. Cancer Genome Atlas Research Network. Integrated genomic characterization of endometrial carcinoma. *Nature* 2013;497:67–73.

141. Weischenfeldt J, Simon R, Feuerbach L, et al. Integrative genomic analyses reveal an androgen-driven somatic alteration landscape in early-onset prostate cancer. *Cancer Cell* 2013;23:159–170.

142. Cancer Genome Atlas Research Network. Genomic and epigenomic landscapes of adult de novo acute myeloid leukemia. *N Engl J Med* 2013;368:2059–2074.

143. Dawson SJ, Rueda OM, Aparicio S, et al. A new genome-driven integrated classification of breast cancer and its implications. *EMBO J* 2013;32:617–628.

144. Plass C, Pfister SM, Lindroth AM, et al. Mutations in regulators of the epigenome and their connections to global chromatin patterns in cancer. *Nat Rev Genet* 2013;14:765–780.

145. Shen H, Laird PW. Interplay between the cancer genome and epigenome. *Cell* 2013;153:38–55.

146. Yamamoto E, Suzuki H, Yamano HO, et al. Molecular dissection of premalignant colorectal lesions reveals early onset of the CpG island methylator phenotype. *Am J Pathol* 2012;181:1847–1861.

147. Gao J, Aksoy BA, Dogrusoz U, et al. Integrative analysis of complex cancer genomics and clinical profiles using the cBioPortal. *Sci Signal* 2013;6:pl1.

148. Bleeker FE, Bardelli A. Genomic landscapes of cancers: prospects for targeted therapies. *Pharmacogenomics* 2007;8:1629–1633.

149. Paez JG, Jänne PA, Lee JC, et al. EGFR mutations in lung cancer: correlation with clinical response to gefitinib therapy. *Science* 2004;304:1497–1500.

150. Ciardiello F, Tortora G. EGFR antagonists in cancer treatment. *N Engl J Med* 2008;358:1160–1174.

151. Janku F, Stewart DJ, Kurzrock R. Targeted therapy in non-small-cell lung cancer—is it becoming a reality? *Nat Rev Clin Oncol* 2010;7:401–414.

152. Pao W, Chmielecki J. Rational, biologically based treatment of EGFR-mutant non-small-cell lung cancer. *Nat Rev Cancer* 2010;10:760–774.

153. Gerber DE, Minna JD. ALK inhibition for non-small cell lung cancer: from discovery to therapy in record time. *Cancer Cell* 2010;18:548–551.

154. Andreyev HJ, Norman AR, Cunningham D, et al. Kirsten ras mutations in patients with colorectal cancer: the multicenter "RASCAL" study. *J Natl Cancer Inst* 1998;90:675–684.

155. Roth AD, Tejpar S, Delorenzi M, et al. Prognostic role of KRAS and BRAF in stage II and III resected colon cancer: results of the translational study on the PETACC-3, EORTC 40993, SAKK 60-00 trial. *J Clin Oncol* 2010;28:466–474.

156. Bardelli A, Siena S. Molecular mechanisms of resistance to cetuximab and panitumumab in colorectal cancer. *J Clin Oncol* 2010;28:1254–1261.

157. Siena S, Sartore-Bianchi A, Di Nicolantonio F, et al. Biomarkers predicting clinical outcome of epidermal growth factor receptor-targeted therapy in metastatic colorectal cancer. *J Natl Cancer Inst* 2009;101:1308–1324.

158. Tejpar S, Bertagnolli M, Bosman F, et al. Prognostic and predictive biomarkers in resected colon cancer: current status and future perspectives for integrating genomics into biomarker discovery. *Oncologist* 2010;15:390–404.

159. Gerlinger M, Rowan AJ, Horswell S, et al. Intratumor heterogeneity and branched evolution revealed by multiregion sequencing. *N Engl J Med* 2012;366:883–892.

160. Mandel P, Metais P. [Not Available]. *C R Seances Soc Biol Fil* 1948;142:241–243.

161. Crowley E, Di Nicolantonio F, Loupakis F, et al. Liquid biopsy: monitoring cancer-genetics in the blood. *Nat Rev Clin Oncol* 2013;10:472–484.

162. Diehl F, Li M, Dressman D, et al. Detection and quantification of mutations in the plasma of patients with colorectal tumors. *Proc Natl Acad Sci U S A* 2005;102:16368–16373.

163. Diehl F, Schmidt K, Choti MA, et al. Circulating mutant DNA to assess tumor dynamics. *Nat Med* 2008;14:985–990.

164. Frattini M, Gallino G, Signoroni S, et al. Quantitative and qualitative characterization of plasma DNA identifies primary and recurrent colorectal cancer. *Cancer Lett* 2008;263:170–181.

165. Chan KC, Jiang P, Zheng YW, et al. Cancer genome scanning in plasma: detection of tumor-associated copy number aberrations, single-nucleotide variants, and tumoral heterogeneity by massively parallel sequencing. *Clin Chem* 2013;59:211–224.

166. Murtaza M, Dawson SJ, Tsui DW, et al. Non-invasive analysis of acquired resistance to cancer therapy by sequencing of plasma DNA. *Nature* 2013;497:108–112.

167. Bardelli A, Corso S, Bertotti A, et al. Amplification of the MET receptor drives resistance to anti-EGFR therapies in colorectal cancer. *Cancer Discov* 2013;3:658–673.

168. Higgins MJ, Jelovac D, Barnathan E, et al. Detection of tumor PIK3CA status in metastatic breast cancer using peripheral blood. *Clin Cancer Res* 2012;18:3462–3469.

169. Leary RJ, Sausen M, Kinde I, et al. Detection of chromosomal alterations in the circulation of cancer patients with whole-genome sequencing. *Sci Transl Med* 2012;4:162ra154.

170. Misale S, Yaeger R, Hobor S, et al. Emergence of KRAS mutations and acquired resistance to anti-EGFR therapy in colorectal cancer. *Nature* 2012;486:532–536.

171. Diaz LA Jr, Williams RT, Wu J, et al. The molecular evolution of acquired resistance to targeted EGFR blockade in colorectal cancers. *Nature* 2012;486:537–540.

172. Robbins PF, Lu YC, El-Gamil M, et al. Mining exomic sequencing data to identify mutated antigens recognized by adoptively transferred tumor-reactive T cells. *Nat Med* 2013;19:747–752.

173. Hunter C, Smith R, Cahill DP, et al. A hypermutation phenotype and somatic MSH6 mutations in recurrent human malignant gliomas after alkylator chemotherapy. *Cancer Res* 2006;66:3987–3991.

174. Cahill DP, Levine KK, Betensky RA, et al. Loss of the mismatch repair protein MSH6 in human glioblastomas is associated with tumor progression during temozolomide treatment. *Clin Cancer Res* 2007;13:2038–2045.

175. Engelman JA, Zejnullahu K, Mitsudomi T, et al. MET amplification leads to gefitinib resistance in lung cancer by activating ERBB3 signaling. *Science* 2007;316:1039–1043.

176. Gorre ME, Mohmmed M, Ellwood K, et al. Clinical resistance to STI-571 cancer therapy caused by BCR-ABL gene mutation or amplification. *Science* 2001;293:876–880.

177. Heinrich MC, Corless CL, Blanke CD, et al. Molecular correlates of imatinib resistance in gastrointestinal stromal tumors. *J Clin Oncol* 2006;24:4764–4774.

178. Shepherd FA, Rodrigues Pereira J, Ciuleanu T, et al. Erlotinib in previously treated non-small-cell lung cancer. *N Engl J Med* 2005;353:123–132.

179. Kobayashi S, Boggon TJ, Dayaram T, et al. EGFR mutation and resistance of non-small-cell lung cancer to gefitinib. *N Engl J Med* 2005;352:786–792.

180. Kwak EL, Sordella R, Bell DW, et al. Irreversible inhibitors of the EGF receptor may circumvent acquired resistance to gefitinib. *Proc Natl Acad Sci U S A* 2005;102:7665–7670.

181. Pao W, Miller VA, Politi KA, et al. Acquired resistance of lung adenocarcinomas to gefitinib or erlotinib is associated with a second mutation in the EGFR kinase domain. *PLoS Med* 2005;2:e73.

182. Shih JY, Gow CH, Yang PC. EGFR mutation conferring primary resistance to gefitinib in non-small-cell lung cancer. *N Engl J Med* 2005;353:207–208.

183. Bell DW, Gore I, Okimoto Ra, et al. Inherited susceptibility to lung cancer may be associated with the T790M drug resistance mutation in EGFR. *Nat Genet* 2005;37:1315–1316.

184. Inukai M, Toyooka S, Ito S, et al. Presence of epidermal growth factor receptor gene T790M mutation as a minor clone in non-small cell lung cancer. *Cancer Res* 2006;66:7854–7858.

185. Daub H, Specht K, Ullrich A. Strategies to overcome resistance to targeted protein kinase inhibitors. *Nat Rev Drug Discov* 2004;3:1001–1010.

186. Choi YL, Soda M, Yamashita Y, et al. EML4-ALK mutations in lung cancer that confer resistance to ALK inhibitors. *N Engl J Med* 2010;363:1734–1739.

187. Flaherty KT, Puzanov I, Kim KB, et al. Inhibition of mutated, activated BRAF in metastatic melanoma. *N Engl J Med* 2010;363:809–819.

188. Nazarian R, Shi H, Wang Q, et al. Melanomas acquire resistance to B-RAF(V600E) inhibition by RTK or N-RAS upregulation. *Nature* 2010;468:973–977.

189. Pompetti F, Spadano A, Sau A, et al. Long-term remission in BCR/ABL-positive AML-M6 patient treated with Imatinib Mesylate. *Leuk Res* 2007;31:563–567.

190. Druker BJ, Builhot F, O'Brien SG, et al. Five-year follow-up of patients receiving imatinib for chronic myeloid leukemia. *N Engl J Med* 2006;355:2408–2417.

2 Hallmarks of Cancer: An Organizing Principle for Cancer Medicine

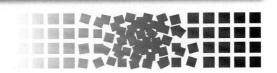

Douglas Hanahan and Robert A. Weinberg

INTRODUCTION

The hallmarks of cancer comprise eight biologic capabilities acquired by incipient cancer cells during the multistep development of human tumors. The hallmarks constitute an organizing principle for rationalizing the complexities of neoplastic disease. They include sustaining proliferative signaling, evading growth suppressors, resisting cell death, enabling replicative immortality, inducing angiogenesis, activating invasion and metastasis, reprogramming energy metabolism, and evading immune destruction. Facilitating the acquisition of these hallmark capabilities are genome instability, which enables mutational alteration of hallmark-enabling genes, and immune inflammation, which fosters the acquisition of multiple hallmark functions. In addition to cancer cells, tumors exhibit another dimension of complexity: They contain a repertoire of recruited, ostensibly normal cells that contribute to the acquisition of hallmark traits by creating the *tumor microenvironment*. Recognition of the widespread applicability of these concepts will increasingly influence the development of new means to treat human cancer.

At the beginning of the new millennium, we proposed that six *hallmarks of cancer* embody an organizing principle that provides a logical framework for understanding the remarkable diversity of neoplastic diseases.[1] Implicit in our discussion was the notion that, as normal cells evolve progressively to a neoplastic state, they acquire a succession of these hallmark capabilities, and that the multistep process of human tumor pathogenesis can be rationalized by the need of incipient cancer cells to acquire the diverse traits that in aggregate enable them to become tumorigenic and, ultimately, malignant.

We noted as an ancillary proposition that tumors are more than insular masses of proliferating cancer cells. Instead, they are complex tissues composed of multiple distinct types of neoplastic and normal cells that participate in heterotypic interactions with one another. We depicted the recruited normal cells, which form tumor-associated stroma, as active participants in tumorigenesis rather than passive bystanders; as such, these stromal cells contribute to the development and expression of certain hallmark capabilities. This notion has been solidified and extended during the intervening period, and it is now clear that the biology of tumors can no longer be understood simply by enumerating the traits of the cancer cells, but instead must encompass the contributions of the *tumor microenvironment* to tumorigenesis. In 2011, we revisited the original hallmarks, adding two new ones to the roster, and expanded on the functional roles and contributions made by recruited stromal cells to tumor biology.[2] Herein we reiterate and further refine the hallmarks-of-cancer perspectives we presented in 2000 and 2011, with the goal of informing students of cancer medicine about the concept and its potential utility for understanding the pathogenesis of human cancer, and the potential relevance of this concept to the development of more effective treatments for this disease.

HALLMARK CAPABILITIES, IN ESSENCE

The eight hallmarks of cancer—distinct and complementary capabilities that enable tumor growth and metastatic dissemination—continue to provide a solid foundation for understanding the biology of cancer (Fig. 2.1). The sections that follow summarize the essence of each hallmark, providing insights into their regulation and functional manifestations.

Sustaining Proliferative Signaling

Arguably, the most fundamental trait of cancer cells involves their ability to sustain chronic proliferation. Normal tissues carefully control the production and release of growth-promoting signals that instruct entry of cells into and progression through the growth-and-division cycle, thereby ensuring proper control of cell number and thus maintenance of normal tissue architecture and function. Cancer cells, by deregulating these signals, become masters of their own destinies. The enabling signals are conveyed in large part by growth factors that bind cell-surface receptors, typically containing intracellular tyrosine kinase domains. The latter proceed to emit signals via branched intracellular signaling pathways that regulate progression through the cell cycle as well as cell growth (that is, increase in cell size); often, these signals influence yet other cell-biologic properties, such as cell survival and energy metabolism.

Remarkably, the precise identities and sources of the proliferative signals operating within normal tissues remain poorly understood. Moreover, we still know relatively little about the mechanisms controlling the release of these mitogenic signals. In part, the study of these mechanisms is complicated by the fact that the growth factor signals controlling cell number and position within normal tissues are thought to be transmitted in a temporally and spatially regulated fashion from one cell to its neighbors; such paracrine signaling is difficult to access experimentally. In addition, the bioavailability of growth factors is regulated by their sequestration in the pericellular space and associated extracellular matrix. Moreover, the actions of these extracellular mitogenic proteins is further controlled by a complex network of proteases, sulfatases, and possibly other enzymes that liberate and activate these factors, apparently in a highly specific and localized fashion.

The mitogenic signaling operating in cancer cells is, in contrast, far better understood.[3–6] Cancer cells can acquire the capability to sustain proliferative signaling in a number of alternative ways: They may produce growth factor ligands themselves, to which they can then respond via the coexpression of cognate receptors, resulting in autocrine proliferative stimulation. Alternatively, cancer cells may send signals to stimulate normal cells within the supporting tumor-associated stroma; the stromal cells then reciprocate by supplying the cancer cells with various growth factors.[7,8] Mitogenic signaling can also be deregulated by elevating the levels of receptor proteins displayed at the cancer cell

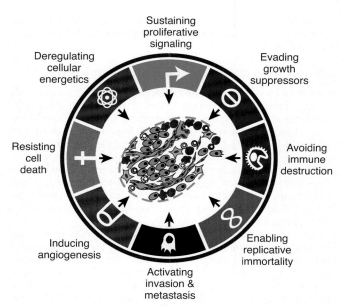

Figure 2.1 The hallmarks of cancer. Eight functional capabilities—the hallmarks of cancer—are thought to be acquired by developing cancers in the course of the multistep carcinogenesis that leads to most forms of human cancer. The order in which these hallmark capabilities are acquired and the relative balance and importance of their contributions to malignant disease appears to vary across the spectrum of human cancers. (Adapted from Hanahan D, Weinberg R. The hallmarks of cancer. *Cell* 2000;100:57–70; Hanahan D, Weinberg RA. Hallmarks of cancer: the next generation. *Cell* 2011;144:646–674.)

surface, rendering such cells hyperresponsive to otherwise limiting amounts of growth factor ligands; the same outcome can result from structural alterations in the receptor molecules that facilitate ligand-independent firing.

Independence from externally supplied growth factors may also derive from the constitutive activation of components of intracellular signaling cascades operating downstream of these receptors within cancer cells. These intracellular alterations obviate the need to stimulate cell proliferation pathways by ligand-mediated activation of cell-surface receptors. Of note, because a number of distinct downstream signaling pathways radiate from ligand-stimulated receptors, the activation of one or another of these downstream branches (e.g., the pathway responding to the Ras signal transducer) may only provide a subset of the regulatory instructions transmitted by a ligand-activated receptor.

Somatic Mutations Activate Additional Downstream Pathways

DNA sequencing analyses of cancer cell genomes have revealed somatic mutations in certain human tumors that predict constitutive activation of the signaling circuits, cited previously, that are normally triggered by activated growth factor receptors. The past 3 decades have witnessed the identification in tens of thousands of human tumors of mutant, oncogenic alleles of the *RAS* proto-oncogenes, most of which have sustained point mutations in the 12th codon, which results in RAS proteins that are constitutively active in downstream signaling. Thus, more than 90% of pancreatic adenocarcinomas carry mutant K-*RAS* alleles. More recently, the repertoire of frequently mutated genes has been expanded to include those encoding the downstream effectors of the RAS proteins. For example, we now know that ~40% of human melanomas contain activating mutations affecting the structure of the B-RAF protein, resulting in constitutive signaling through the RAF to the mitogen-activated protein (MAP)–kinase pathway.[9] Similarly, mutations in the catalytic subunit of phosphoinositide 3-kinase (PI3K)

isoforms are being detected in an array of tumor types; these mutations typically serve to hyperactivate the PI3K signaling pathway, causing in turn, excess signaling through the crucial Akt/PKB signal transducer.[10,11] The advantages to tumor cells of activating upstream (receptor) versus downstream (transducer) signaling remain obscure, as does the functional impact of cross-talk between the multiple branched pathways radiating from individual growth factor receptors.

Disruptions of Negative-Feedback Mechanisms that Attenuate Proliferative Signaling

Recent observations have also highlighted the importance of negative-feedback loops that normally operate to dampen various types of signaling and thereby ensure homeostatic regulation of the flux of signals coursing through the intracellular circuitry.[12–15] Defects in these negative-feedback mechanisms are capable of enhancing proliferative signaling. The prototype of this type of regulation involves the RAS oncoprotein. The oncogenic effects of mutant RAS proteins do not result from a hyperactivation of its downstream signaling powers; instead, the oncogenic mutations affecting *RAS* genes impair the intrinsic GTPase activity of RAS that normally serves to turn its activity off, ensuring that active signal transmission (e.g., from upstream growth factor receptors) is transient; as such, oncogenic RAS mutations disrupt an autoregulatory negative-feedback mechanism, without which RAS generates chronic proliferative signals.

Analogous negative-feedback mechanisms operate at multiple nodes within the proliferative signaling circuitry. A prominent example involves phosphatase and tensin homolog (PTEN), which counteracts PI3K by degrading its product, phosphatidylinositol 3,4,5-phosphate (PIP₃). Loss-of-function mutations in PTEN amplify PI3K signaling and promote tumorigenesis in a variety of experimental models of cancer; in human tumors, PTEN expression is often lost by the methylation of DNA at specific sites associated with the promoter of the *PTEN* gene, resulting in the shutdown of its transcription.[10,11]

Yet another example involves the mammalian target of rapamycin (mTOR) kinase, a key coordinator of cell growth and metabolism that lies both upstream and downstream of the PI3K pathway. In the circuitry of some cancer cells, mTOR activation results, via negative feedback, in the inhibition of PI3K signaling. Accordingly, when mTOR is pharmacologically inhibited in such cancer cells (e.g., by the drug rapamycin), the associated loss of negative feedback results in increased activity of PI3K and its effector, the Akt/PKB kinase, thereby blunting the antiproliferative effects of mTOR inhibition.[16,17] It is likely that compromised negative feedback loops in this and other signaling pathways will prove to be widespread among human cancer cells, serving as important means by which cancer cells acquire the capability of signaling chronically through these pathways. Moreover, disruption of such normally self-attenuating signaling can contribute to the development of adaptive resistance toward therapeutic drugs targeting mitogenic signaling.

Excessive Proliferative Signaling Can Trigger Cell Senescence

Early studies of oncogene action encouraged the notion that ever-increasing expression of such genes and the signals released by their protein products would result in proportionately increased cancer cell proliferation and, thus, tumor growth. More recent research has undermined this notion, in that it is now apparent that excessively elevated signaling by oncoproteins, such as RAS, MYC, and RAF, can provoke counteracting (protective) responses from cells, such as induction of cell death; alternatively, cancer cells expressing high levels of these oncoproteins may be forced to enter into the nonproliferative but viable state called senescence. These responses contrast with those seen in cells expressing lower levels of these proteins, which permit cells to avoid senescence or cell death and, thus, proliferate.[18–21]

Cells with morphologic features of senescence, including enlarged cytoplasm, the absence of proliferation markers, and the expression of the senescence-induced β-galactosidase enzyme, are abundant in the tissues of mice whose genomes have been reengineered to cause overexpression of certain oncogenes[19,20]; such senescent cells are also prevalent in some cases of human melanoma.[22]

These ostensibly paradoxical responses seem to reflect intrinsic cellular defense mechanisms designed to eliminate cells experiencing excessive levels of certain types of mitogenic signaling. Accordingly, the intensity of oncogenic signaling observed in naturally arising cancer cells may represent compromises between maximal mitogenic stimulation and avoidance of these anti-proliferative defenses. Alternatively, some cancer cells may adapt to high levels of oncogenic signaling by disabling their senescence- or apoptosis-inducing circuitry.

Evading Growth Suppressors

In addition to the hallmark capability of inducing and sustaining positively acting growth-stimulatory signals, cancer cells must also circumvent powerful programs that negatively regulate cell proliferation; many of these programs depend on the actions of tumor suppressor genes. Dozens of tumor suppressors that operate in various ways to limit cell proliferation or survival have been discovered through their inactivation in one or another form of animal or human cancer; many of these genes have been validated as bona fide tumor suppressors through gain- or loss-of-function experiments in mice. The two prototypical tumor suppressor genes encode the retinoblastoma (RB)-associated and TP53 proteins; they operate as central control nodes within two key, complementary cellular regulatory circuits that govern the decisions of cells to proliferate, or alternatively, to activate growth arrest, senescence, or the cell-suicide program known as apoptosis.

The RB protein integrates signals from diverse extracellular and intracellular sources and, in response, decides whether or not a cell should proceed through its growth-and-division cycle.[23–25] Cancer cells with defects in the RB pathway function are thus missing the services of a critical gatekeeper of cell-cycle progression whose absence permits persistent cell proliferation. Whereas RB transduces growth-inhibitory signals that largely originate outside of the cell, TP53 receives inputs from stress and abnormality sensors that function within the cell's intracellular operating systems. For example, if the degree of damage to a cell's genome is excessive, or if the levels of nucleotide pools, growth-promoting signals, glucose, or oxygenation are insufficient, TP53 can call a halt to further cell-cycle progression until these conditions have been normalized. Alternatively, in the face of alarm signals indicating overwhelming or irreparable damage to such cellular systems, TP53 can trigger apoptosis. Of note, the alternative effects of activated TP53 are complex and highly context dependent, varying by cell type as well as by the severity and persistence of conditions of cell-physiologic stress and genomic damage.

Although the two canonical suppressors of proliferation—TP53 and RB—have preeminent importance in regulating cell proliferation, various lines of evidence indicate that each operates as part of a larger network that is wired for functional redundancy. For example, chimeric mice populated throughout their bodies with individual cells lacking a functional *Rb* gene are surprisingly free of proliferative abnormalities, despite the expectation that a loss of RB function should result in unimpeded advance through the cell division cycle by these cells and their lineal descendants; some of the resulting clusters of *Rb*-null cells should, by all rights, progress to neoplasia. Instead, the *Rb*-null cells in such chimeric mice have been found to participate in relatively normal tissue morphogenesis throughout the body; the only neoplasia observed is of pituitary tumors developing late in life.[26] Similarly, *TP53*-null mice develop

normally, show largely normal cell and tissue homeostasis, and again develop abnormalities only later in life in the form of leukemias and sarcomas.[27]

Mechanisms of Contact Inhibition and Its Evasion

Four decades of research have demonstrated that the cell-to-cell contacts formed by dense populations of normal cells growing in 2-dimensional culture operate to suppress further cell proliferation, yielding confluent cell monolayers. Importantly, such *contact inhibition* is abolished in various types of cancer cells in culture, suggesting that contact inhibition is an in vitro surrogate of a mechanism that operates in vivo to ensure normal tissue homeostasis that is abrogated during the course of tumorigenesis. Until recently, the mechanistic basis for this mode of growth control remained obscure. Now, however, mechanisms of contact inhibition are beginning to emerge.[28]

One mechanism involves the product of the *NF2* gene, long implicated as a tumor suppressor because its loss triggers a form of human neurofibromatosis. Merlin, the cytoplasmic *NF2* gene product, orchestrates contact inhibition by coupling cell-surface adhesion molecules (e.g., E-cadherin) to transmembrane receptor tyrosine kinases (e.g., the EGF receptor). In so doing, Merlin strengthens the adhesiveness of cadherin-mediated cell-to-cell attachments. Additionally, by sequestering such growth factor receptors, Merlin limits their ability to efficiently emit mitogenic signals.[28–31]

Corruption of the TGF-β Pathway Promotes Malignancy

Transforming growth factor beta (TGF-β) is best known for its antiproliferative effects on epithelial cells. The responses of carcinoma cells to TGF-β's proliferation–suppressive effects is now appreciated to be far more elaborate than a simple shutdown of its signaling circuitry.[32–35] In normal cells, exposure to TGF-β blocks their progression through the G1 phase of the cell cycle. In many late-stage tumors, however, TGF-β signaling is redirected away from suppressing cell proliferation and is found instead to activate a cellular program, termed the epithelial-to-mesenchymal transition (EMT), which confers on cancer cells multiple traits associated with high-grade malignancy, as will be discussed in further detail.

Resisting Cell Death

The ability to activate the normally latent apoptotic cell-death program appears to be associated with most types of normal cells throughout the body. Its actions in many if not all multicellular organisms seems to reflect the need to eliminate aberrant cells whose continued presence would otherwise threaten organismic integrity. This rationale explains why cancer cells often, if not invariably, inactivate or attenuate this program during their development.[21,36–38]

Elucidation of the detailed design of the signaling circuitry governing the apoptotic program has revealed how apoptosis is triggered in response to various physiologic stresses that cancer cells experience either during the course of tumorigenesis or as a result of anticancer therapy. Notable among the apoptosis-inducing stresses are signaling imbalances resulting from elevated levels of oncogene signaling and from DNA damage. The regulators of the apoptotic response are divided into two major circuits, one receiving and processing extracellular death-inducing signals (the extrinsic apoptotic program, involving for example the Fas ligand/Fas receptor), and the other sensing and integrating a variety of signals of intracellular origin (the intrinsic program). Each of these circuits culminates in the activation of a normally latent protease (caspase 8 or 9, respectively), which proceeds to initiate a cascade of proteolysis involving effector caspases that are responsible for the execution phase of apoptosis. During this final phase, an apoptotic cell is progressively disassembled and then consumed, both by its neighbors and by professional phagocytic cells. Currently, the intrinsic apoptotic program is more widely implicated as a barrier to cancer pathogenesis.

The molecular machinery that conveys signals between the apoptotic regulators and effectors is controlled by counterbalancing pro- and antiapoptotic members of the Bcl-2 family of regulatory proteins.[36,37] The archetype, Bcl-2, along with its closest relatives (Bcl-XL, Bcl-W, Mcl-1, A1) are inhibitors of apoptosis, acting in large part by binding to and thereby suppressing two proapoptotic triggering proteins (Bax and Bak); the latter are embedded in the mitochondrial outer membrane. When relieved of inhibition by their antiapoptotic relatives, Bax and Bax disrupt the integrity of the outer mitochondrial membrane, causing the release into the cytosol of proapoptotic signaling proteins, the most important of which is cytochrome C. When the normally sequestered cytochrome C is released, it activates a cascade of cytosolic caspase proteases that proceed to fragment multiple cellular structures, thereby executing the apoptotic death program.[37,39]

Several abnormality sensors have been identified that play key roles in triggering apoptosis.[21,37] Most notable is a DNA damage sensor that acts through the TP53 tumor suppressor[40]; TP53 induces apoptosis by upregulating expression of the proapoptotic, Bcl-2-related Noxa and Puma proteins, doing so in response to substantial levels of DNA breaks and other chromosomal abnormalities. Alternatively, insufficient survival factor signaling (e.g., inadequate levels of interleukin (IL)-3 in lymphocytes or of insulinlike growth factors 1/2 [IGF1/2] in epithelial cells) can elicit apoptosis through another proapoptotic Bcl-2-related protein called Bim. Yet another condition triggering apoptosis involves hyperactive signaling by certain oncoproteins, such as Myc, which acts in part via Bim and other Bcl-2-related proteins.[18,21,40]

Tumor cells evolve a variety of strategies to limit or circumvent apoptosis. Most common is the loss of TP53 tumor suppressor function, which eliminates this critical damage sensor from the apoptosis-inducing circuitry. Alternatively, tumors may achieve similar ends by increasing the expression of antiapoptotic regulators (Bcl-2, Bcl-XL) or of survival signals (IGF1/2), by downregulating proapoptotic Bcl-2-related factors (Bax, Bim, Puma), or by short-circuiting the extrinsic ligand-induced death pathway. The multiplicity of apoptosis-avoiding mechanisms presumably reflects the diversity of apoptosis-inducing signals that cancer cell populations encounter during their evolution from the normal to the neoplastic state.

Autophagy Mediates Both Tumor Cell Survival and Death

Autophagy represents an important cell-physiologic response that, like apoptosis, normally operates at low, basal levels in cells but can be strongly induced in certain states of cellular stress, the most obvious of which is nutrient deficiency.[41–43] The autophagic program enables cells to break down cellular organelles, such as ribosomes and mitochondria, allowing the resulting catabolites to be recycled and thus used for biosynthesis and energy metabolism. As part of this program, intracellular vesicles (termed autophagosomes) envelope the cellular organelles destined for degradation; the resulting vesicles then fuse with lysosomes in which degradation occurs. In this fashion, low-molecular-weight metabolites are generated that support survival in the stressed, nutrient-limited environments experienced by many cancer cells. When acting in this fashion, autophagy favors cancer cell survival.

However, the autophagy program intersects in more complex ways with the life and death of cancer cells. Like apoptosis, the autophagy machinery has both regulatory and effector components.[41–43] Among the latter are proteins that mediate autophagosome formation and delivery to lysosomes. Of note, recent research has revealed intersections between the regulatory circuits governing autophagy, apoptosis, and cellular homeostasis. For example, the signaling pathway involving PI3K, AKT, and mTOR, which is stimulated by survival signals to block apoptosis, similarly inhibits autophagy; when survival signals are insufficient, the PI3K signaling pathway is downregulated, with the result that autophagy and/or apoptosis may be induced.[41,42,44,45]

Another interconnection between these two programs resides in the Beclin-1 protein, which has been shown by genetic studies to be necessary for the induction of autophagy.[41–44] Beclin-1 is a member of the Bcl-2 family of apoptotic regulatory proteins, and its BH3 domain allows it to bind the Bcl-2/Bcl-XL proteins. Stress sensor–coupled BH3-containing proteins (e.g. Bim, Noxa) can displace Beclin-1 from its association with Bcl-2/Bcl-XL, enabling the liberated Beclin-1 to trigger autophagy, much as they can release proapoptotic Bax and Bak to trigger apoptosis. Hence, stress-transducing Bcl-2–related proteins can induce apoptosis and/or autophagy depending on the physiologic state of the cell.

Genetically altered mice bearing inactivated alleles of the *Beclin-1* gene or of certain other components of the autophagy machinery exhibit increased susceptibility to cancer.[42,46] These results suggest that the induction of autophagy can serve as a barrier to tumorigenesis that may operate independently of or in concert with apoptosis. For example, excessive activation of the autophagy program may cause cells to devour too many of their own critical organelles, such that cell growth and division are crippled. Accordingly, autophagy may represent yet another barrier that needs to be circumvented by incipient cancer cells during multistep tumor development.[41,46]

Perhaps paradoxically, nutrient starvation, radiotherapy, and certain cytotoxic drugs can induce elevated levels of autophagy that apparently protect cancer cells.[45–48] Moreover, severely stressed cancer cells have been shown to shrink via autophagy to a state of reversible dormancy.[46,49] This particular survival response may enable the persistence and eventual regrowth of some late-stage tumors following treatment with potent anticancer agents. Together, observations like these indicate that autophagy can have dichotomous effects on tumor cells and, thus, tumor progression.[46,47] An important agenda for future research will involve clarifying the genetic and cell-physiologic conditions that determine when and how autophagy enables cancer cells to survive or, alternatively, causes them to die.

Necrosis Has Proinflammatory and Tumor-Promoting Potential

In contrast to apoptosis, in which a dying cell contracts into an almost invisible corpse that is soon consumed by its neighbors, necrotic cells become bloated and explode, releasing their contents into the local tissue microenvironment. A body of evidence has shown that cell death by necrosis, like apoptosis, is an organized process under genetic control, rather than being a random and undirected process.[50–52]

Importantly, necrotic cell death releases proinflammatory signals into the surrounding tissue microenvironment, in contrast to apoptosis, which does not. As a consequence, necrotic cells can recruit inflammatory cells of the immune system,[51,53,54] whose dedicated function is to survey the extent of tissue damage and remove associated necrotic debris. In the context of neoplasia, however, multiple lines of evidence indicate that immune inflammatory cells can be actively tumor-promoting by fostering angiogenesis, cancer cell proliferation, and invasiveness (discussed in subsequent sections). Additionally, necrotic cells can release bioactive regulatory factors, such as IL1α, which can directly stimulate neighboring viable cells to proliferate, with the potential, once again, to facilitate neoplastic progression.[53] Consequently, necrotic cell death, while seemingly beneficial in counterbalancing cancer-associated hyperproliferation, may ultimately do more damage to the patient than good.

Enabling Replicative Immortality

Cancer cells require unlimited replicative potential in order to generate macroscopic tumors. This capability stands in marked contrast to the behavior of the cells in most normal cell lineages in the body, which are only able to pass through a limited number of successive cell growth-and-division cycles. This limitation has been associated with two distinct barriers to proliferation: *replicative senescence*, a typically irreversible entrance into a nonproliferative but viable state, and *crisis*, which involves cell death. Accordingly, when cells are propagated in culture, repeated cycles of cell division lead first to induction of replicative senescence and then, for those cells that succeed in circumventing this barrier, to the crisis phase, in which the great majority of cells in the population die. On rare occasion, cells emerge from a population in crisis and exhibit unlimited replicative potential. This transition has been termed immortalization, a trait that most established cell lines possess by virtue of their ability to proliferate in culture without evidence of either senescence or crisis.

Multiple lines of evidence indicate that telomeres protecting the ends of chromosomes are centrally involved in the capability for unlimited proliferation.[55–58] The telomere-associated DNA, composed of multiple tandem hexanucleotide repeats, shortens progressively in the chromosomes of nonimmortalized cells propagated in culture, eventually losing the ability to protect the ends of chromosomal DNA from end-to-end fusions; such aberrant fusions generate unstable dicentric chromosomes, whose resolution during the anaphase of mitosis results in a scrambling of karyotype and entrance into crisis that threatens cell viability. Accordingly, the length of telomeric DNA in a cell dictates how many successive cell generations its progeny can pass through before telomeres are largely eroded and have consequently lost their protective functions.

Telomerase, the specialized DNA polymerase that adds telomere repeat segments to the ends of telomeric DNA, is almost absent in nonimmortalized cells but is expressed at functionally significant levels in the great majority (~90%) of spontaneously immortalized cells, including human cancer cells. By extending telomeric DNA, telomerase is able to counter the progressive telomere erosion that would otherwise occur in its absence. The presence of telomerase activity, either in spontaneously immortalized cells or in the context of cells engineered to express the enzyme, is correlated with a resistance to induction of both senescence and crisis/apoptosis; conversely, the suppression of telomerase activity leads to telomere shortening and to activation of one or the other of these proliferative barriers.

The two barriers to proliferation—replicative senescence and crisis/apoptosis—have been rationalized as crucial anticancer defenses that are hardwired into our cells and are deployed to impede the outgrowth of clones of preneoplastic and, frankly, neoplastic cells. According to this thinking, most incipient neoplasias exhaust their endowment of replicative doublings and are stopped in their tracks by either of these barriers. The eventual immortalization of rare variant cells that proceed to form tumors has been attributed to their ability to maintain telomeric DNA at lengths sufficient to avoid triggering either senescence or apoptosis, which is achieved most commonly by upregulating the expression of telomerase or, less frequently, via an alternative recombination-based (ALT) telomere maintenance mechanism.[59] Hence, telomere shortening has come to be viewed as a clocking device that determines the limited replicative potential of normal cells and, thus, one that must be overcome by cancer cells.

Reassessing Replicative Senescence

The senescent state induced by oncogenes, as described previously, is remarkably similar to that induced when cells are explanted from living tissue and introduced into culture, the latter being the replicative senescence just discussed. Importantly, the concept of replication-induced senescence as a general barrier requires refinement and reformulation. Recent experiments have revealed that the induction of senescence in certain cultured cells can be delayed and possibly eliminated by the use of improved cell culture conditions, suggesting that recently explanted primary cells may be intrinsically able to proliferate unimpeded in culture up the point of crisis and the associated induction of apoptosis triggered by critically shortened telomeres.[60–63] This result indicates that telomere shortening does not necessarily induce senescence prior to crisis. Additional insight comes from experiments in mice engineered to lack telomerase; this work has revealed that shortening telomeres can shunt premalignant cells into a senescent state that contributes (along with apoptosis) to attenuated tumorigenesis in mice genetically destined to develop particular forms of cancer.[58] Such telomerase-null mice with highly eroded telomeres exhibit multiorgan dysfunction and abnormalities that provide evidence of both senescence and apoptosis, perhaps similar to the senescence and apoptosis observed in cell culture.[58,64] Thus, depending on the cellular context, the proliferative barrier of telomere shortening can be manifested by the induction of senescence and/or apoptosis.

Delayed Activation of Telomerase May Both Limit and Foster Neoplastic Progression

There is now evidence that clones of incipient cancer cells in spontaneously arising tumors experience telomere loss-induced crisis relatively early during the course of multistep tumor progression due to their inability to express significant levels of telomerase. Thus, extensively eroded telomeres have been documented in premalignant growths through the use of fluorescence in situ hybridization (FISH), which has also revealed the end-to-end chromosomal fusions that signal telomere failure and crisis.[65,66] These results suggest that such incipient cancer cells have passed through a substantial number of successive telomere-shortening cell divisions during their evolution from fully normal cells of origin. Accordingly, the development of some human neoplasias may be aborted by telomere-induced crisis long before they have progressed to become macroscopic, frankly neoplastic growths.

A quite different situation is observed in cells that have lost the TP53-mediated surveillance of genomic integrity and, thereafter, experience critically eroded telomeres. The loss of the TP53 DNA damage sensor can enable such cells to avoid apoptosis that would otherwise be triggered by the DNA damage resulting from dysfunctional telomeres. Instead, such cells lacking TP53 continue to divide, suffering repeated cycles of interchromosomal fusion and subsequent breakage at mitosis. Such breakage-fusion-bridge (BFB) cycles result in deletions and amplifications of chromosomal segments, evidently serving to mutagenize the genome, thereby facilitating the generation and subsequent clonal selection of cancer cells that have acquired mutant oncogenes and tumor suppressor genes.[58,67] One infers, however, that the clones of cancer cells that survive this telomere collapse must eventually acquire the ability to stabilize and thus protect their telomeres via the activation of telomerase or the ALT mechanism noted previously.

These considerations present an interesting dichotomy: Although dysfunctional telomeres are an evident barrier to chronic proliferation, they can also facilitate the genomic instability that generates hallmark-enabling mutations, as will be discussed further. Both mechanisms may be at play in certain forms of carcinogenesis in the form of transitory telomere deficiency prior to telomere stabilization. Circumstantial support for this concept of transient telomere deficiency in facilitating malignant progression has come from comparative analyses of premalignant and malignant lesions in the human breast.[68,69] The premalignant lesions did not express significant levels of telomerase and were marked by telomere shortening and chromosomal aberrations. In contrast, overt carcinomas exhibited telomerase expression concordantly with the reconstruction of longer telomeres and the fixation of the aberrant karyotypes that would seem to have been acquired after telomere failure but before the acquisition of telomerase activity. When portrayed in this way, the delayed acquisition of telomerase function serves to generate tumor-promoting mutations, whereas its subsequent expression stabilizes the mutant genome and confers the unlimited replicative capacity that cancer cells require in order to generate clinically apparent tumors.

Inducing Angiogenesis

Like normal tissues, tumors require sustenance in the form of nutrients and oxygen as well as an ability to evacuate metabolic wastes and carbon dioxide. The tumor-associated neovasculature, generated by the process of angiogenesis, addresses these needs. During embryogenesis, the development of the vasculature involves the birth of new endothelial cells and their assembly into tubes (vasculogenesis) in addition to the sprouting (angiogenesis) of new vessels from existing ones. Following this morphogenesis, the normal vasculature becomes largely quiescent. In the adult, as part of physiologic processes such as wound healing and female reproductive cycling, angiogenesis is turned on, but only transiently. In contrast, during tumor progression, an *angiogenic switch* is almost always activated and remains on, causing normally quiescent vasculature to continually sprout new vessels that help sustain expanding neoplastic growths.[70]

A compelling body of evidence indicates that the angiogenic switch is governed by countervailing factors that either induce or oppose angiogenesis.[71,72] Some of these angiogenic regulators are signaling proteins that bind to stimulatory or inhibitory cell-surface receptors displayed by vascular endothelial cells. The well-known prototypes of angiogenesis inducers and inhibitors are vascular endothelial growth factor-A (VEGF-A) and thrombospondin-1 (Tsp-1), respectively.

The VEGF-A gene encodes ligands that are involved in orchestrating new blood vessel growth during embryonic and postnatal development, in the survival of endothelial cells in already-formed vessels, and in certain physiologic and pathologic situations in the adult. VEGF signaling via three receptor tyrosine kinases (VEGFR1–3) is regulated at multiple levels, reflecting this complexity of purpose. VEGF gene expression can be upregulated both by hypoxia and by oncogene signaling.[73–75] Additionally, VEGF ligands can be sequestered in the extracellular matrix in latent forms that are subject to release and activation by extracellular matrix-degrading proteases (e.g., matrix metallopeptidase 9 [MMP-9]).[76] In addition, other proangiogenic proteins, such as members of the fibroblast growth factor (FGF) family, have been implicated in sustaining tumor angiogenesis.[71] TSP-1, a key counterbalance in the angiogenic switch, also binds transmembrane receptors displayed by endothelial cells and thereby triggers suppressive signals that can counteract proangiogenic stimuli.[77]

The blood vessels produced within tumors by an unbalanced mix of proangiogenic signals are typically aberrant: Tumor neovasculature is marked by precocious capillary sprouting, convoluted and excessive vessel branching, distorted and enlarged vessels, erratic blood flow, microhemorrhaging, leaking of plasma into the tissue parenchyma, and abnormal levels of endothelial cell proliferation and apoptosis.[78,79]

Angiogenesis is induced surprisingly early during the multistage development of invasive cancers both in animal models and in humans. Histologic analyses of premalignant, noninvasive lesions, including dysplasias and in situ carcinomas arising in a variety of organs, have revealed the early tripping of the angiogenic switch.[70,80] Historically, angiogenesis was envisioned to be important only when rapidly growing macroscopic tumors had formed, but more recent data indicate that angiogenesis also contributes to the microscopic premalignant phase of neoplastic progression, further cementing its status as an integral hallmark of cancer.

Gradations of the Angiogenic Switch

Once angiogenesis has been activated, tumors exhibit diverse patterns of neovascularization. Some tumors, including highly aggressive types such as pancreatic ductal adenocarcinomas, are hypovascularized and replete with stromal deserts that are largely avascular and indeed may even be actively antiangiogenic.[81] In contrast, many other tumors, including human renal and pancreatic neuroendocrine carcinomas, are highly angiogenic and, consequently, densely vascularized.[82,83]

Collectively, such observations suggest an initial tripping of the angiogenic switch during tumor development, which is followed by a variable intensity of ongoing neovascularization, the latter being controlled by a complex biologic rheostat that involves both the cancer cells and the associated stromal microenvironment.[71,72] Of note, the switching mechanisms can vary, even though the net result is a common inductive signal (e.g., VEGF). In some tumors, dominant oncogenes operating within tumor cells, such as *Ras* and *Myc*, can upregulate the expression of angiogenic factors, whereas in others, such inductive signals are produced indirectly by immune inflammatory cells, as will be discussed.

Endogenous Angiogenesis Inhibitors Present Natural Barriers to Tumor Angiogenesis

A variety of secreted proteins have been reported to have the capability to help shut off normally transitory angiogenesis, including thrombospondin-1 (TSP-1), fragments of plasmin (angiostatin) and type 18 collagen (endostatin), along with another dozen candidate antiangiogenic proteins.[77,84–88] Most are proteins, and many are derived by proteolytic cleavage of structural proteins that are not themselves angiogenic regulators.

A number of these endogenous inhibitors of angiogenesis can be detected in the circulation of normal mice and humans. Genes that encode several endogenous angiogenesis inhibitors have been deleted from the mouse germ line without untoward developmental or physiologic effects; however, the growth of autochthonous and implanted tumors is enhanced as a consequence.[84,85,88] By contrast, if the circulating levels of an endogenous inhibitor are genetically increased (e.g., via overexpression in transgenic mice or in xenotransplanted tumors), tumor growth is impaired.[85,88] Interestingly, wound healing and fat deposition are impaired or accelerated by elevated or ablated expression of such genes.[89,90] The data suggest that, under normal conditions, endogenous angiogenesis inhibitors serve as physiologic regulators modulating the transitory angiogenesis that occurs during tissue remodeling and wound healing; they may also act as intrinsic barriers to the induction and/or persistence of angiogenesis by incipient neoplasias.

Pericytes Are Important Components of the Tumor Neovasculature

Pericytes have long been known as supporting cells that are closely apposed to the outer surfaces of the endothelial tubes in normal tissue vasculature, where they provide important mechanical and physiologic support to the endothelial cells. Microscopic studies conducted in recent years have revealed that pericytes are associated, albeit loosely, with the neovasculature of most, if not all, tumors.[91–93] More importantly, mechanistic studies (discussed subsequently) have revealed that pericyte coverage is important for the maintenance of a functional tumor neovasculature.

A Variety of Bone Marrow-Derived Cells Contribute to Tumor Angiogenesis

It is now clear that a repertoire of cell types originating in the bone marrow play crucial roles in pathologic angiogenesis.[94–97] These include cells of the innate immune system—notably, macrophages, neutrophils, mast cells, and myeloid progenitors—that assemble at the margins of such lesions or infiltrate deeply within them; the tumor-associated inflammatory cells can help to trip the angiogenic switch in quiescent tissue and sustain ongoing angiogenesis associated with tumor growth. In addition, they can help protect the vasculature from the effects of drugs targeting endothelial cell signaling.[98] Moreover, several types of bone marrow–derived *vascular progenitor cells* have been observed to have migrated into neoplastic lesions and become intercalated into the existing neovasculature, where they assumed the roles of either pericytes or endothelial cells.[92,99,100]

Activating Invasion and Metastasis

The multistep process of invasion and metastasis has been schematized as a sequence of discrete steps, often termed the invasion–metastasis cascade.[101,102] This depiction portrays a succession of cell-biologic changes, beginning with local invasion, then intravasation by cancer cells into nearby blood and lymphatic vessels, transit of cancer cells through the lymphatic and hematogenous systems, followed by the escape of cancer cells from the lumina of such vessels into the parenchyma of distant tissues (extravasation), the formation of small nests of cancer cells (micrometastases), and finally, the growth of micrometastatic lesions into macroscopic tumors, this last step being termed *colonization*. These steps have largely been studied in the context of carcinoma pathogenesis. Indeed, when viewed through the prism of the invasion–metastasis cascade, the diverse tumors of this class appear to behave in similar ways.

During the malignant progression of carcinomas, the neoplastic cells typically develop alterations in their shape as well as their attachment to other cells and to the extracellular matrix (ECM). The best-characterized alteration involves the loss by carcinoma cells of E-cadherin, a key epithelial cell-to-cell adhesion molecule. By forming adherens junctions between adjacent epithelial cells, E-cadherin helps to assemble epithelial cell sheets and to maintain the quiescence of the cells within these sheets. Moreover, increased expression of E-cadherin has been well established as an antagonist of invasion and metastasis, whereas a reduction of its expression is known to potentiate these behaviors. The frequently observed downregulation and occasional mutational inactivation of the E-cadherin–encoding gene, *CDH1*, in human carcinomas provides strong support for its role as a key suppressor of the invasion–metastasis hallmark capability.[103,104]

Notably, the expression of genes encoding other cell-to-cell and cell-to-ECM adhesion molecules is also significantly altered in the cells of many highly aggressive carcinomas, with those favoring cytostasis typically being downregulated. Conversely, adhesion molecules normally associated with the cell migrations that occur during embryogenesis and inflammation are often upregulated. For example, N-cadherin, which is normally expressed in migrating neurons and mesenchymal cells during organogenesis, is upregulated in many invasive carcinoma cells, replacing the previously expressed E-cadherin.[104]

Research into the capability for invasion and metastasis has accelerated dramatically over the past decade as powerful new research tools, and refined experimental models have become available. Although still an emerging field replete with major unanswered questions, significant progress has been made in delineating important features of this complex hallmark capability. An admittedly incomplete representation of these advances is highlighted as follows.

The Epithelial-to-Mesenchymal Transition Program Broadly Regulates Invasion and Metastasis

A developmental regulatory program, termed the EMT, has become implicated as a prominent means by which neoplastic epithelial cells can acquire the abilities to invade, resist apoptosis, and disseminate.[105–110] By co-opting a process involved in various steps of embryonic morphogenesis and wound healing, carcinoma cells can concomitantly acquire multiple attributes that enable invasion and metastasis. This multifaceted EMT program can be activated transiently or stably, and to differing degrees, by carcinoma cells during the course of invasion and metastasis.

A set of pleiotropically acting transcriptional factors (TF), including Snail, Slug, Twist, and Zeb1/2, orchestrate the EMT and related migratory processes during embryogenesis; most were initially identified by developmental genetics. These transcriptional regulators are expressed in various combinations in a number of malignant tumor types. Some of these EMT-TFs have been shown in experimental models of carcinoma formation to be causally important for programming invasion; others have been found to elicit metastasis when experimentally expressed in primary tumor cells.[105,111–114] Included among the cell-biologic traits evoked by these EMT-TFs are loss of adherens junctions and associated conversion from a polygonal/epithelial to a spindly/fibroblastic morphology, concomitant with expression of secreted matrix-degrading enzymes, increased motility, and heightened resistance to apoptosis, which are implicated in the processes of invasion and metastasis. Several of these transcription factors can directly repress E-cadherin gene expression, thereby releasing neoplastic epithelial cells from this key suppressor of motility and invasiveness.[115]

The available data suggest that EMT-TFs regulate one another as well as overlapping sets of target genes. Results from developmental genetics indicate that contextual signals received from neighboring cells in the embryo are involved in triggering expression of these transcription factors in cells that are destined to pass through an EMT[111]; in an analogous fashion, heterotypic interactions of cancer cells with adjacent tumor-associated stromal cells have been shown to induce expression of the malignant cell phenotypes that are known to be choreographed by one or more of these EMT-TFs.[116,117] Moreover, cancer cells at the invasive margins of certain carcinomas can be seen to have undergone an EMT, suggesting that these cancer cells are subject to microenvironmental stimuli distinct from those received by cancer cells located in the cores of these lesions.[118] Although the evidence is still incomplete, it would appear that EMT-TFs are able to orchestrate most steps of the invasion–metastasis cascade, except perhaps the final step of colonization, which involves adaptation of cells originating in one tissue to the microenvironment of a foreign, potentially inhospitable tissue.

We still know rather little about the various manifestations and temporal stability of the mesenchymal state produced by an EMT. Indeed, it seems increasingly likely that many human carcinoma cells only experience a *partial EMT*, in which they acquire mesenchymal markers while retaining many preexisting epithelial ones. Although the expression of EMT-TFs has been observed in certain nonepithelial tumor types, such as sarcomas and neuroectodermal tumors, their roles in programming malignant traits in these tumors are presently poorly documented. Additionally, it remains to be determined whether aggressive carcinoma cells invariably acquire their malignant capabilities through activation of components of the EMT program, or whether alternative regulatory programs can also enable expression of these traits.

Heterotypic Contributions of Stromal Cells to Invasion and Metastasis

As mentioned previously, cross-talk between cancer cells and cell types of the neoplastic stroma is involved in the acquired capabilities of invasiveness and metastasis.[94,119–121] For example, mesenchymal stem cells (MSC) present in the tumor stroma have been found to secrete CCL5/RANTES in response to signals released by cancer cells; CCL5 then acts reciprocally on the cancer cells to stimulate invasive behavior.[122] In other work, carcinoma cells secreting IL-1 have been shown to induce MSCs to synthesize a spectrum of other cytokines that proceed thereafter to promote activation of the EMT program in the carcinoma cells; these effectors include IL-6, IL-8, growth-regulated oncogene alpha (GRO-α), and prostaglandin E2.[123]

Macrophages at the tumor periphery can foster local invasion by supplying matrix-degrading enzymes such as metalloproteinases and cysteine cathepsin proteases[76,120,124,125]; in one model system, the invasion-promoting macrophages are activated by IL-4 produced by the cancer cells.[126] And in an experimental model of metastatic breast cancer, tumor-associated macrophages (TAM) supply epidermal growth factor (EGF) to breast cancer cells, while the cancer cells reciprocally stimulate the macrophages with colony stimulating factor 1 (CSF-1). Their concerted interactions facilitate intravasation into the circulatory system and metastatic dissemination of the cancer cells.[94,127]

Observations like these indicate that the phenotypes of high-grade malignancy do not arise in a strictly cell-autonomous manner, and that their manifestation cannot be understood solely through analyses of signaling occurring within tumor cells. One important implication of the EMT model, still untested, is that the ability of carcinoma cells in primary tumors to negotiate most of the steps of the invasion–metastasis cascade may be acquired in certain tumors without the requirement that these cells undergo additional mutations beyond those that were needed for primary tumor formation.

Plasticity in the Invasive Growth Program

The role of contextual signals in inducing an invasive growth capability (often via an EMT) implies the possibility of reversibility, in that cancer cells that have disseminated from a primary tumor to more distant tissue sites may no longer benefit from the activated stroma and the EMT-inducing signals that they experienced while residing in the primary tumor. In the absence of ongoing exposure to these signals, carcinoma cells may revert in their new tissue environment to a noninvasive state. Thus, carcinoma cells that underwent an EMT during initial invasion and metastatic dissemination may reverse this metamorphosis, doing so via a mesenchymal-to-epithelial transition (MET). This plasticity may result in the formation of new tumor colonies of carcinoma cells exhibiting an organization and histopathology similar to those created by carcinoma cells in the primary tumor that never experienced an EMT.[128]

Distinct Forms of Invasion May Underlie Different Cancer Types

The EMT program regulates a particular type of invasiveness that has been termed *mesenchymal*. In addition, two other distinct modes of invasion have been identified and implicated in cancer cell invasion.[129,130] *Collective invasion* involves phalanxes of cancer cells advancing en masse into adjacent tissues and is characteristic of, for example, squamous cell carcinomas. Interestingly, such cancers are rarely metastatic, suggesting that this form of invasion lacks certain functional attributes that facilitate metastasis. Less clear is the prevalence of an *amoeboid* form of invasion,[131,132] in which individual cancer cells show morphologic plasticity, enabling them to slither through existing interstices in the ECM rather than clearing a path for themselves, as occurs in both the mesenchymal and collective forms of invasion. It is presently unresolved whether cancer cells participating in the collective and amoeboid forms of invasion employ components of the EMT program, or whether entirely different cell-biologic programs are responsible for choreographing these alternative invasion programs.

Another emerging concept, noted previously, involves the facilitation of cancer cell invasion by inflammatory cells that assemble at the boundaries of tumors, producing the ECM-degrading enzymes and other factors that enable invasive growth.[76,94,120,133] These functions may obviate the need of invading cancer cells to produce these proteins through activation of EMT programs. Thus, rather than synthesizing these proteases themselves, cancer cells may secrete chemoattractants that recruit proinvasive inflammatory cells; the latter then proceed to produce matrix-degrading enzymes that enable invasive growth.

The Daunting Complexity of Metastatic Colonization

Metastasis can be broken down into two major phases: the physical dissemination of cancer cells from the primary tumor to distant tissues, and the adaptation of these cells to foreign tissue microenvironments that results in successful colonization (i.e., the growth of micrometastases into macroscopic tumors). The multiple steps of dissemination would seem to lie within the purview of the EMT and similarly acting migratory programs. Colonization, however, is not strictly coupled with physical dissemination, as evidenced by the presence in many patients of myriad micrometastases that have disseminated but never progress to form macroscopic metastatic tumors.[101,102,134–136]

In some types of cancer, the primary tumor may release systemic suppressor factors that render such micrometastases dormant, as revealed clinically by explosive metastatic growth soon after resection of the primary growth.[87,137] In others, however, such as breast cancer and melanoma, macroscopic metastases may erupt decades after a primary tumor has been surgically removed or pharmacologically destroyed. These metastatic tumor growths evidently reflect dormant micrometastases that have solved, after much trial and error, the complex problem of adaptation to foreign tissue microenvironments, allowing subsequent tissue colonization.[135,136,138] Implicit here is the notion that most disseminated cancer cells are likely to be poorly adapted, at least initially, to the microenvironment of the tissue in which they have landed. Accordingly, each type of disseminated cancer cell may need to develop its own set of ad hoc solutions to the problem of thriving in the microenvironment of one or another foreign tissue.[139]

One can infer from such natural histories that micrometastases may lack certain hallmark capabilities necessary for vigorous growth, such as the ability to activate angiogenesis. Indeed, the inability of certain experimentally generated dormant micrometastases to form macroscopic tumors has been ascribed to their failure to activate tumor angiogenesis.[135,140] Additionally, recent experiments have shown that nutrient starvation can induce intense autophagy that causes cancer cells to shrink and adopt a state of reversible dormancy. Such cells may exit this state and resume active growth and proliferation when permitted by changes in tissue microenvironment, such as increased availability of nutrients, inflammation from causes such as infection or wound healing, or other local abnormalities.[49,141] Other mechanisms of micrometastatic dormancy may involve antigrowth signals embedded in normal tissue ECM[138] and tumor-suppressing actions of the immune system.[135,142]

Metastatic dissemination has long been depicted as the last step in multistep primary tumor progression; indeed, for many tumors, that is likely the case, as illustrated by recent genome sequencing studies that provide genetic evidence for clonal evolution of pancreatic ductal adenocarcinoma to a metastatic stage.[143–145] Importantly, however, recent results have revealed that some cancer cells can disseminate remarkably early, dispersing from apparently noninvasive premalignant lesions in both mice and humans.[146,147] Additionally, micrometastases can be spawned from primary tumors that are not obviously invasive but possess a neovasculature lacking in luminal integrity.[148] Although cancer cells can clearly disseminate from such preneoplastic lesions and seed the bone marrow and other tissues, their capability to colonize these sites and develop into pathologically significant macrometastases remains unproven. At present, we view this early metastatic dissemination as a demonstrable phenomenon in mice and humans, the clinical significance of which is yet to be established.

Having developed such a tissue-specific colonizing ability, the cells in metastatic colonies may proceed to disseminate further, not only to new sites in the body, but also back to the primary tumors in which their ancestors arose. Accordingly, tissue-specific colonization programs that are evident among certain cells within a primary tumor may originate not from classical tumor progression occurring entirely within the primary lesion, but instead from immigrants that have returned home.[149] Such reseeding is consistent with the aforementioned studies of human pancreatic cancer metastasis.[143–145] Stated differently, the phenotypes and underlying gene expression programs in focal subpopulations of cancer cells within primary tumors may reflect, in part, the reverse migration of their distant metastatic progeny.

Implicit in this *self-seeding* process is another notion: The supportive stroma that arises in a primary tumor and contributes to its acquisition of malignant traits provides a hospitable site for reseeding and colonization by circulating cancer cells released from metastatic lesions.

Clarifying the regulatory programs that enable metastatic colonization represents an important agenda for future research. Substantial progress is being made, for example, in defining sets of genes (*metastatic signatures*) that correlate with and appear to facilitate the establishment of macroscopic metastases in specific tissues.[139,146,150–152] Importantly, metastatic colonization almost certainly requires the establishment of a permissive tumor microenvironment composed of critical stromal support cells. For these reasons, the process of colonization is likely to encompass a large number of cell-biologic programs that are, in aggregate, considerably more complex and diverse than the preceding steps of metastatic dissemination that allow carcinoma cells to depart from primary tumors to sites of lodging and extravasation throughout the body.

Reprogramming Energy Metabolism

The chronic and often uncontrolled cell proliferation that represents the essence of neoplastic disease involves not only deregulated control of cell proliferation but also corresponding adjustments of energy metabolism in order to fuel cell growth and division. Under aerobic conditions, normal cells process glucose, first to pyruvate via glycolysis in the cytosol and thereafter via oxidative phosphorylation to carbon dioxide in the mitochondria. Under anaerobic conditions, glycolysis is favored and relatively little pyruvate is dispatched to the oxygen-consuming mitochondria. Otto Warburg first observed an anomalous characteristic of cancer cell energy metabolism[153–155]: Even in the presence of oxygen, cancer cells can reprogram their glucose metabolism, and thus their energy production, leading to a state that has been termed *aerobic glycolysis.*

The existence of this metabolic specialization operating in cancer cells has been substantiated in the ensuing decades. A key signature of aerobic glycolysis is upregulation of glucose transporters, notably GLUT1, which substantially increases glucose import into the cytoplasm.[156–158] Indeed, markedly increased uptake and utilization of glucose has been documented in many human tumor types, most readily by noninvasively visualizing glucose uptake using positron-emission tomography (PET) with a radiolabeled analog of glucose (^{18}F-fluorodeoxyglucose [FDG]) as a reporter.

Glycolytic fueling has been shown to be associated with activated oncogenes (e.g., *RAS, MYC*) and mutant tumor suppressors (e.g., *TP53*),[18,156,157,159] whose alterations in tumor cells have been selected primarily for their benefits in conferring the hallmark capabilities of cell proliferation, subversion of cytostatic controls, and attenuation of apoptosis. This reliance on glycolysis can be further accentuated under the hypoxic conditions that operate within many tumors: The hypoxia response system acts pleiotropically to upregulate glucose transporters and multiple enzymes of the glycolytic pathway.[156,157,160] Thus, both the Ras oncoprotein and hypoxia can independently increase the levels of the HIF1α and HIF2α hypoxia-response transcription factors, which in turn upregulate glycolysis.[160–162]

The reprogramming of energy metabolism is seemingly counterintuitive, in that cancer cells must compensate for the ~18-fold lower efficiency of ATP production afforded by glycolysis relative to mitochondrial oxidative phosphorylation. According to one long-forgotten[163] and a recently revived and refined hypothesis,[164] increased glycolysis allows the diversion of glycolytic intermediates into various biosynthetic pathways, including those generating nucleosides and amino acids. In turn, this facilitates the biosynthesis of the macromolecules and organelles required for assembling new cells. Moreover, Warburg-like metabolism seems to be present in many rapidly dividing embryonic tissues, once again suggesting a role in supporting the large-scale biosynthetic programs that are required for active cell proliferation.

Interestingly, some tumors have been found to contain two subpopulations of cancer cells that differ in their energy-generating pathways. One subpopulation consists of glucose-dependent (Warburg-effect) cells that secrete lactate, whereas cells of the second subpopulation preferentially import and utilize the lactate produced by their neighbors as their main energy source, employing part of the citric acid cycle to do so.[165–168] These two populations evidently function symbiotically: The hypoxic cancer cells depend on glucose for fuel and secrete lactate as waste, which is imported and preferentially used as fuel by their better oxygenated brethren. Although this provocative mode of intratumoral symbiosis has yet to be generalized, the cooperation between lactate-secreting and lactate-utilizing cells to fuel tumor growth is in fact not an invention of tumors, but rather again reflects the co-opting of a normal physiologic mechanism, in this case one operative in muscle[165,167,168] and the brain.[169] Additionally, it is becoming apparent that oxygenation, ranging from normoxia to hypoxia, is not necessarily static in tumors, but instead fluctuates temporally and regionally,[170] likely as a result of the instability and chaotic organization of the tumor-associated neovasculature.

Finally, the notion of the Warburg effect needs to be refined for most if not all tumors exhibiting aerobic glycolysis. The effect does not involve a switching off oxidative phosphorylation concurrent with activation of glycolysis, the latter then serving as the sole source of energy. Rather, cancer cells become highly adaptive, utilizing both mitochondrial oxidative phosphorylation and glycolysis in varying proportions to generate fuel (ATP) and biosynthetic precursors needed for chronic cell proliferation. Finally, this capability for reprograming energy metabolism, dubbed to be an *emerging hallmark* in 2011,[2] is clearly intertwined with the hallmarks conveying deregulated proliferative signals and evasion of growth suppressors, as discussed earlier. As such, its status as a discrete, independently acquired hallmark remains unclear, despite growing appreciation of its importance as a crucial component of the neoplastic growth state.

Evading Immune Destruction

The eighth hallmark reflects the role played by the immune system in antagonizing the formation and progression of tumors. A longstanding theory of immune surveillance posited that cells and tissues are constantly monitored by an ever alert immune system, and that such immune surveillance is responsible for recognizing and eliminating the vast majority of incipient cancer cells and, thus, nascent tumors.[171,172] According to this logic, clinical detectable cancers have somehow managed to avoid detection by the various arms of the immune system, or have been able to limit the extent of immunologic killing, thereby evading eradication.

The role of defective immunologic monitoring of tumors would seem to be validated by the striking increases of certain cancers in immune-compromised individuals.[173] However, the great majority of these are virus-induced cancers, suggesting that much of the control of this class of cancers normally depends on reducing viral burden in infected individuals, in part through eliminating virus-infected cells. These observations, therefore, shed little light on the possible role of the immune system in limiting formation of the >80% of tumors of nonviral etiology. In recent years, however, an increasing body of evidence, both from genetically engineered mice and from clinical epidemiology, suggests that the immune system operates as a significant barrier to tumor formation and progression, at least in some forms of non–virus-induced cancer.[174–177]

When mice genetically engineered to be deficient for various components of the immune system were assessed for the development of carcinogen-induced tumors, it was observed that tumors arose more frequently and/or grew more rapidly in the immunodeficient mice relative to immune-competent controls. In particular, deficiencies in the development or function of either CD8+ cytotoxic T lymphocytes (CTL), CD4+ T_H1 helper T cells, or natural killer (NK) cells, each led to demonstrable increases in tumor incidence. Moreover, mice with combined immunodeficiencies in both T cells and NK cells were even more susceptible to cancer development. The results indicated that, at least in certain experimental models, both the innate and adaptive cellular arms of the immune system are able to contribute significantly to immune surveillance and, thus, tumor eradication.[142,178]

In addition, transplantation experiments have shown that cancer cells that originally arose in immunodeficient mice are often inefficient at initiating secondary tumors in syngeneic immunocompetent hosts, whereas cancer cells from tumors arising in immunocompetent mice are equally efficient at initiating transplanted tumors in both types of hosts.[142,178] Such behavior has been interpreted as follows: Highly immunogenic cancer cell clones are routinely eliminated in immunocompetent hosts—a process that has been referred to as *immunoediting*—leaving behind only weakly immunogenic variants to grow and generate solid tumors. Such weakly immunogenic cells can thereafter successfully colonize both immunodeficient and immunocompetent hosts. Conversely, when arising in immunodeficient hosts, the immunogenic cancer cells are not selectively depleted and can, instead, prosper along with their weakly immunogenic counterparts. When cells from such nonedited tumors are serially transplanted into syngeneic recipients, the immunogenic cancer cells are rejected when they confront, for the first time, the competent immune systems of their secondary hosts.[179] (Unanswered in these particular experiments is the question of whether the chemical carcinogens used to induce such tumors are prone to generate cancer cells that are especially immunogenic.)

Clinical epidemiology also increasingly supports the existence of antitumoral immune responses in some forms of human cancer.[180–182] For example, patients with colon and ovarian tumors that are heavily infiltrated with CTLs and NK cells have a better prognosis than those who lack such abundant killer lymphocytes.[176,177,182,183] The case for other cancers is suggestive but less compelling and is the subject of ongoing investigation. Additionally, some immunosuppressed organ transplant recipients have been observed to develop donor-derived cancers, suggesting that in ostensibly tumor-free organ donors, the cancer cells were held in check in a dormant state by a functional immune system,[184] only to launch into proliferative expansion once these *passenger cells* in the transplanted organ found themselves in immunocompromised patients who lack the physiologically important capabilities to mount immune responses that would otherwise hold latent cancer cells in check or eradicate them.

Still, the epidemiology of chronically immunosuppressed patients does not indicate significantly increased incidences of the major forms of nonviral human cancers, as noted previously. This might be taken as an argument against the importance of immune surveillance as an effective barrier to tumorigenesis and tumor progression. We note, however, that HIV and pharmacologically immunosuppressed patients are predominantly immunodeficient in the T- and B-cell compartments and thus do not present with the multicomponent immunologic deficiencies that have been produced in the genetically engineered mutant mice lacking both NK cells and CTLs. This leaves open the possibility that such

patients still have residual capability for mounting an anticancer immunologic defense that is mediated by NK and other innate immune cells.

In truth, the previous discussions of cancer immunology simplify tumor–host immunologic interactions, because highly immunogenic cancer cells may well succeed in evading immune destruction by disabling components of the immune system that have been dispatched to eliminate them. For example, cancer cells may paralyze infiltrating CTLs and NK cells by secreting TGF-β or other immunosuppressive factors.[32,185,186] Alternatively, cancer cells may express immunosuppressive cell-surface ligands, such as PD-L1, that prevent activation of the cytotoxic mechanisms of the CTLs. These PD-L1 molecules serve as ligands for the PD-1 receptors displayed by the CTLs, together exemplifying a system of *checkpoint* ligands and receptors that serve to constrain immune responses in order to avoid autoimmunity.[187–189] Yet other localized immunosuppressive mechanisms operate through the recruitment of inflammatory cells that can actively suppress CTL activity, including regulatory T cells (Tregs) and myeloid-derived suppressor cells (MDSC).[174,190–193]

In summary, these eight hallmarks each contribute qualitatively distinct capabilities that seem integral to most lethal forms of human cancer. Certainly, the balance and relative importance of their respective contributions to disease pathogenesis will vary among cancer types, and some hallmarks may be absent or of minor importance in some cases. Still, there is reason to postulate their generality and, thus, their applicability to understanding the biology of human cancer. Next, we turn to the question of how these capabilities are acquired during the multistep pathways through which cancers develop, focusing on two facilitators that are commonly involved.

TWO UBIQUITOUS CHARACTERISTICS FACILITATE THE ACQUISITION OF HALLMARK CAPABILITIES

We have defined the hallmarks of cancer as acquired functional capabilities that allow cancer cells to survive, proliferate, and disseminate. Their acquisition is made possible by two *enabling characteristics* (Fig. 2.2). Most prominent is the development of genomic instability in cancer cells, which generates random mutations, including chromosomal rearrangements, among which are rare genetic changes that can orchestrate individual hallmark capabilities. A second enabling characteristic involves the inflammatory state of premalignant and frankly malignant lesions. A variety of cells of the innate and adaptive immune system infiltrate neoplasias, some of which serve to promote tumor progression through various means.

An Enabling Characteristic: Genome Instability and Mutation

Acquisition of the multiple hallmarks enumerated previously depends in large part on a succession of alterations in the genomes of neoplastic cells. Basically, certain mutant genotypes can confer selective advantage to particular subclones among proliferating nests of incipient cancer cells, enabling their outgrowth and eventual dominance in a local tissue environment. Accordingly, multistep tumor progression can be portrayed as a succession of clonal expansions, most of which are triggered by the chance acquisition of an enabling mutation.

Indeed, it is apparent that virtually every human cancer cell genome carries mutant alleles of one or several growth-regulating genes, underscoring the central importance of these genetic alterations in driving malignant progression.[194] Still, we note that many heritable phenotypes—including, notably, inactivation of tumor suppressor genes—can be acquired through epigenetic

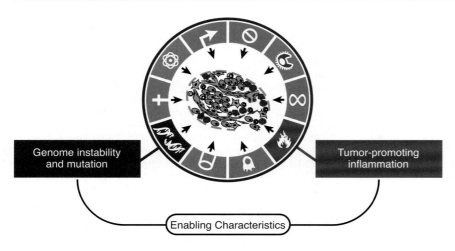

Figure 2.2 Enabling characteristics. Two ostensibly generic characteristics of cancer cells and the neoplasias they create are involved in the acquisition of the hallmark capabilities. First and foremost, the impairment of genome maintenance systems in aberrantly proliferating cancer cells enables the generation of mutations in genes that contribute to multiple hallmarks. Secondarily, neoplasias invariably attract cells of the innate immune system that are programmed to heal wounds and fight infections; these cells, including macrophages, neutrophils, and partially differentiated myeloid cells, can contribute functionally to acquisition of many of the hallmark capabilities. (Adapted from Hanahan D, Weinberg RA. Hallmarks of cancer: the next generation. *Cell* 2011;144:646–674.)

mechanisms, such as DNA methylation and histone modifications.[195–198] Thus, many clonal expansions may also be triggered by heritable nonmutational changes affecting the regulation of gene expression. At present, the relative importance of genetic versus heritable epigenetic alterations to the various clonal expansions remains unclear, and likely, varies broadly amongst the catalog of human cancer types.

The extraordinary ability of genome maintenance systems to detect and resolve defects in the DNA ensures that rates of spontaneous mutation in normal cells of the body are typically very low, both in quiescent cells and during cell division. The genomes of most cancer cells, by contrast, are replete with these alterations, reflecting loss of genomic integrity with concomitantly increased rates of mutation. This heightened mutability appears to accelerate the generation of variant cells, facilitating the selection of those cells whose advantageous phenotypes enable their clonal expansion.[199,200] This mutability is achieved through increased sensitivity to mutagenic agents, through a breakdown in one or several components of the genomic maintenance machinery, or both. In addition, the accumulation of mutations can be accelerated by aberrations that compromise the surveillance systems that normally monitor genomic integrity and force such genetically damaged cells into either quiescence, senescence, or apoptosis.[201–203] The role of TP53 is central here, leading to its being called the *guardian of the genome*.[204]

A diverse array of defects affecting various components of the DNA-maintenance machinery, referred to as the *caretakers* of the genome,[205] have been documented. The catalog of defects in these caretaker genes includes those whose products are involved in (1) detecting DNA damage and activating the repair machinery, (2) directly repairing damaged DNA, and (3) inactivating or intercepting mutagenic molecules before they have damaged the DNA.[199,201,202,206–208] From a genetic perspective, these caretaker genes behave much like tumor suppressor genes, in that their functions are often lost during the course of tumor progression, with such losses being achieved either through inactivating mutations or via epigenetic repression. Mutant copies of many of these caretaker genes have been introduced into the mouse germ line, resulting, not unexpectedly, in increased cancer incidence, thus supporting their involvement in human cancer development.[209]

In addition, research over the past decade has revealed another major source of tumor-associated genomic instability. As described earlier, the loss of telomeric DNA in many tumors generates karyotypic instability and associated amplification and deletion of chromosomal segments.[58] When viewed in this light, telomerase is more than an enabler of the hallmark capability for unlimited replicative potential. It must also be added to the list of critical caretakers responsible for maintaining genome integrity.

Advances in the molecular–genetic analysis of cancer cell genomes have provided the most compelling demonstrations of function-altering mutations and of ongoing genomic instability during tumor progression. One type of analysis—comparative genomic hybridization (CGH)—documents the gains and losses of gene copy number across the cell genome. In many tumors, the pervasive genomic aberrations revealed by CGH provide clear evidence for loss of control of genome integrity. Importantly, the recurrence of specific aberrations (both amplifications and deletions) at particular locations in the genome indicates that such sites are likely to harbor genes whose alteration favors neoplastic progression.[210]

More recently, with the advent of efficient and economical DNA sequencing technologies, higher resolution analyses of cancer cell genomes have become possible. Early studies are revealing distinctive patterns of DNA mutations in different tumor types (see: http://cancergenome.nih.gov/). In the not-too-distant future, the sequencing of entire cancer cell genomes promises to clarify the importance of ostensibly random mutations scattered across cancer cell genomes.[194] Thus, the use of whole genome resequencing offers the prospect of revealing recurrent genetic alterations (i.e., those found in multiple independently arising tumors) that in aggregate represent only minor proportions of the tumors of a given type. The recurrence of such mutations, despite their infrequency, may provide clues about the regulatory pathways playing causal roles in the pathogenesis of the tumors under study.

These surveys of cancer cell genomes have shown that the specifics of genome alteration vary dramatically between different tumor types. Nonetheless, the large number of already documented genome maintenance and repair defects, together with abundant evidence of widespread destabilization of gene copy number and nucleotide sequence, persuade us that instability of the genome is inherent to the cancer cells forming virtually all types of human tumors. This leads, in turn, to the conclusion that the defects in genome maintenance and repair are selectively advantageous and, therefore, instrumental for tumor progression, if only because they accelerate the rate at which evolving premalignant cells can accumulate favorable genotypes. As such, genome instability is clearly an *enabling characteristic* that is causally associated with the acquisition of hallmark capabilities.

An Enabling Characteristic: Tumor-Promoting Inflammation

Among the cells recruited to the stroma of carcinomas are a variety of cell types of the immune system that mediate various inflammatory functions. Pathologists have long recognized that some (but not all) tumors are densely infiltrated by cells of both the innate and adaptive arms of the immune system, thereby mirroring inflammatory conditions arising in nonneoplastic tissues.[211] With the advent of better markers for accurately identifying the distinct cell types of the immune system, it is now clear that virtually every neoplastic lesion contains immune cells present at densities ranging from subtle infiltrations detectable only with cell type–specific antibodies to gross inflammations that are apparent even by standard histochemical staining techniques.[183] Historically, such immune responses were largely thought to reflect an attempt by the immune system to eradicate tumors, and indeed, there is increasing evidence for antitumoral responses to many tumor types with an attendant pressure on the tumor to evade immune destruction,[174,176,177,183] as discussed earlier.

By 2000, however, there were also clues that tumor-associated inflammatory responses can have the unanticipated effect of facilitating multiple steps of tumor progression, thereby helping incipient neoplasias to acquire hallmark capabilities. In the ensuing years, research on the intersections between inflammation and cancer pathogenesis has blossomed, producing abundant and compelling demonstrations of the functionally important tumor-promoting effects that immune cells—largely of the innate immune system—have on neoplastic progression.[19,53,94,174,212,213] Inflammatory cells can contribute to multiple hallmark capabilities by supplying signaling molecules to the tumor microenvironment, including growth factors that sustain proliferative signaling; survival factors that limit cell death; proangiogenic factors; extracellular matrix-modifying enzymes that facilitate angiogenesis, invasion, and metastasis; and inductive signals that lead to activation of EMT and other hallmark-promoting programs.[53,94,116,212,213]

Importantly, localized inflammation is often apparent at the earliest stages of neoplastic progression and is demonstrably capable of fostering the development of incipient neoplasias into full-blown cancers.[94,214] Additionally, inflammatory cells can release chemicals—notably, reactive oxygen species—that are actively mutagenic for nearby cancer cells, thus accelerating their genetic evolution toward states of heightened malignancy.[53] As such, inflammation by selective cell types of the immune system is demonstrably an *enabling characteristic* for its contributions to the acquisition of hallmark capabilities. The cells responsible for this enabling characteristic are described in the following section.

THE CONSTITUENT CELL TYPES OF THE TUMOR MICROENVIRONMENT

Over the past 2 decades, tumors have increasingly been recognized as tissues whose complexity approaches and may even exceed that of normal healthy tissues. This realization contrasts starkly with the earlier, reductionist view of a tumor as nothing more than a collection of relatively homogeneous cancer cells, whose entire biology could be understood by elucidating the cell-autonomous properties of these cells (Fig. 2.3A). Rather, assemblages of diverse cell types associated with malignant lesions are increasingly documented to be functionally important for the manifestation of symptomatic disease (Fig. 2.3B). When viewed from this perspective, the biology of a tumor can only be fully understood by studying the individual specialized cell types within it. We enumerate as follows a set of accessory cell types recruited directly or indirectly by neoplastic cells into tumors, where they contribute in important ways to the biology of many tumors, and we discuss the regulatory mechanisms that control their individual and collective functions. Most of these observations stem from the study of carcinomas, in which the neoplastic epithelial cells constitute a compartment (the parenchyma) that is clearly distinct from the mesenchymal cells forming the tumor-associated stroma.

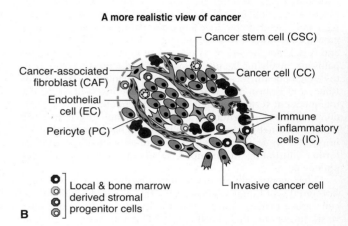

Figure 2.3 Tumors as outlaw organs. Research aimed at understanding the biology of tumors has historically focused on the cancer cells, which constitute the drivers of neoplastic disease. This view of tumors as nothing more than masses of cancer cells **(A)** ignores an important reality, that cancer cells recruit and corrupt a variety of normal cell types that form the tumor-associated stroma. Once formed, the stroma acts reciprocally on the cancer cells, affecting almost all of the traits that define the neoplastic behavior of the tumor as a whole **(B).** The assemblage of heterogeneous populations of cancer cells and stromal cells is often referred to as the tumor microenvironment (TME). (Adapted from Hanahan D, Weinberg R. The hallmarks of cancer. *Cell* 2000;100:57–70; Hanahan D, Weinberg RA. Hallmarks of cancer: the next generation. *Cell* 2011;144:646–674.)

Cancer-Associated Fibroblasts

Fibroblasts are found in various proportions across the spectrum of carcinomas, in many cases constituting the preponderant cell population of the tumor stroma. The term *cancer-associated fibroblasts* (CAFs) subsumes at least two distinct cell types: (1) cells with similarities to the fibroblasts that create the structural foundation supporting most normal epithelial tissues, and (2) myofibroblasts, whose biologic roles and properties differ markedly from those of the widely distributed tissue-derived fibroblasts. Myofibroblasts are identifiable by their expression of α-smooth muscle actin (αSMA). They are rare in most healthy epithelial tissues, although certain tissues, such as the liver and pancreas, contain appreciable numbers of αSMA-expressing cells. Myofibroblasts transiently increase in abundance in wounds and are also found in sites of chronic inflammation. Although beneficial to tissue repair, myofibroblasts are problematic in chronic inflammation, in that they contribute to the pathologic fibrosis observed in tissues such as the lung, kidney, and liver.

Recruited myofibroblasts and variants of normal tissue-derived fibroblastic cells have been demonstrated to enhance tumor phenotypes, notably cancer cell proliferation, angiogenesis, invasion, and metastasis. Their tumor-promoting activities have largely been defined by transplantation of cancer-associated fibroblasts admixed with cancer cells into mice, and more recently by genetic and pharmacologic perturbation of their functions in tumor-prone mice.[8,121,133,215–219] Because they secrete a variety of ECM components, cancer-associated fibroblasts are implicated in the formation of the desmoplastic stroma that characterizes many advanced carcinomas. The full spectrum of functions contributed by both subtypes of cancer-associated fibroblasts to tumor pathogenesis remains to be elucidated.

Endothelial Cells

Prominent among the stromal constituents of the TME are the endothelial cells forming the tumor-associated vasculature. Quiescent tissue capillary endothelial cells are activated by *angiogenic* regulatory factors to produce a neovasculature that sustains tumor growth concomitant with continuing endothelial cell proliferation and vessel morphogenesis. A network of interconnected signaling pathways involving ligands of signal-transducing receptors (e.g., the Angiopoeitin-1/2, Notch ligands, Semaphorin, Neuropilin, Robo, and Ephrin-A/B) is now known to be involved in regulating quiescent versus activated angiogenic endothelial cells, in addition to the aforementioned counterbalancing VEGF and TSP signals. This network of signaling pathways has been functionally implicated in developmental and tumor-associated angiogenesis, further illustrating the complex regulation of endothelial cell phenotypes.[220–224]

Other avenues of research are revealing distinctive gene expression profiles of tumor-associated endothelial cells and identifying cell-surface markers displayed on the luminal surfaces of normal versus tumor endothelial cells.[78,225,226] Differences in signaling, in transcriptome profiles, and in vascular *ZIP codes* will likely prove to be important for understanding the conversion of normal endothelial cells into tumor-associated endothelial cells. Such knowledge may lead, in turn, to opportunities to develop novel therapies that exploit these differences in order to selectively target tumor-associated endothelial cells. Additionally, the activated (*angiogenic*) tumor vasculature has been revealed as a barrier to efficient intravasation and a functional suppressor of cytotoxic T cells,[227] and thus, tumor endothelial cells can contribute to the hallmark capability for evading immune destruction. As such, another emerging concept is to normalize rather than ablate them, so as to improve immunotherapy[190] as well as delivery of chemotherapy.[228]

Closely related to the endothelial cells of the circulatory system are those forming lymphatic vessels.[229] Their role in the tumor-associated stroma, specifically in supporting tumor growth, is poorly understood. Indeed, because of high interstitial pressure within solid tumors, intratumoral lymphatic vessels are typically collapsed and nonfunctional; in contrast, however, there are often functional, actively growing (*lymphangiogenic*) lymphatic vessels at the periphery of tumors and in the adjacent normal tissues that cancer cells invade. These associated lymphatics likely serve as channels for the seeding of metastatic cells in the draining lymph nodes that are commonly observed in a number of cancer types. Recent results that are yet to be generalized suggest an alternative role for the activated (i.e., lymphangiogenic) lymphatic endothelial cells associated with tumors, not in supporting tumor growth like the blood vessels, but in inducing (via VEGF-C–mediated signaling) a lymphatic tissue microenvironment that suppresses immune responses ordinarily marshaled from the draining lymph nodes.[230] As such, the real value to a tumor from activating the signaling circuit involving the ligand VEGF-C and its receptor VEGFR3 may be to facilitate the evasion of antitumor immunity by abrogating the otherwise immunostimulatory functions of draining lymphatic vessels and lymph nodes, with the collateral effect of inducing lymphatic endothelial cells to form the new lymphatic vessels that are commonly detected in association with tumors.

Pericytes

Pericytes represent a specialized mesenchymal cell type that are closely related to smooth muscle cells, with fingerlike projections that wrap around the endothelial tubing of blood vessels. In normal tissues, pericytes are known to provide paracrine support signals to the quiescent endothelium. For example, Ang-1 secreted by pericytes conveys antiproliferative stabilizing signals that are received by the Tie2 receptors expressed on the surface of endothelial cells. Some pericytes also produce low levels of VEGF that serve a trophic function in endothelial homeostasis.[93,231] Pericytes also collaborate with the endothelial cells to synthesize the vascular basement membrane that anchors both pericytes and endothelial cells and helps vessel walls to withstand the hydrostatic pressure created by the blood.

Genetic and pharmacologic perturbation of the recruitment and association of pericytes has demonstrated the functional importance of these cells in supporting the tumor endothelium.[93,217,231] For example, the pharmacologic inhibition of signaling through the platelet-derived growth factor (PDGF) receptor expressed by tumor pericytes and bone marrow–derived pericyte progenitors results in reduced pericyte coverage of tumor vessels, which in turn destabilizes vascular integrity and function.[91,217,231] Interestingly, and in contrast, the pericytes of normal vessels are not prone to such pharmacologic disruption, providing another example of the differences in the regulation of normal quiescent and tumor vasculature. An intriguing hypothesis, still to be fully substantiated, is that tumors with poor pericyte coverage of their vasculature may be more prone to permit cancer cell intravasation into the circulatory system, thereby enabling subsequent hematogenous dissemination.[91,148]

Immune Inflammatory Cells

Infiltrating cells of the immune system are increasingly accepted to be generic constituents of tumors. These inflammatory cells operate in conflicting ways: Both tumor-antagonizing and tumor-promoting leukocytes can be found in various proportions in most, if not all, neoplastic lesions. Evidence began to accumulate in the late 1990s that the infiltration of neoplastic tissues by cells of the immune system serves, perhaps counterintuitively, to promote tumor progression. Such work traced its conceptual roots back to the observed association of tumor formation with sites of chronic inflammation. Indeed, this led some to liken tumors to "wounds that do not heal."[211,232] In the course of normal wound healing and the resolution of infections, immune inflammatory cells appear transiently and then disappear, in contrast to their persistence in sites of chronic inflammation, where their presence has been associated with a variety of tissue pathologies, including fibrosis, aberrant angiogenesis, and as mentioned, neoplasia.[53,233]

We now know that immune cells play diverse and critical roles in fostering tumorigenesis. The roster of tumor-promoting inflammatory cells includes macrophage subtypes, mast cells, and neutrophils, as well as T and B lymphocytes.[96,97,119,133,212,234,235] Studies of these cells are yielding a growing list of tumor-promoting signaling molecules that they release, which include the tumor growth factor EGF, the angiogenic growth factors VEGF-A/C, other proangiogenic factors such as FGF2, plus chemokines and cytokines that amplify the inflammatory state. In addition, these cells may produce proangiogenic and/or proinvasive matrix-degrading enzymes, including MMP-9 and other MMPs, cysteine cathepsin proteases, and heparanase.[94,96] Consistent with the expression of these diverse signals, tumor-infiltrating inflammatory cells have been shown to induce and help sustain tumor angiogenesis, to stimulate cancer cell proliferation, to facilitate tissue invasion, and to support the metastatic dissemination and seeding of cancer cells.[94,96,97,119,120,234–237]

In addition to fully differentiated immune cells present in tumor stroma, a variety of partially differentiated myeloid progenitors have been identified in tumors.[96] Such cells represent intermediaries between circulating cells of bone marrow origin and the differentiated immune cells typically found in normal and inflamed tissues. Importantly, these progenitors, like their more differentiated derivatives, have demonstrable tumor-promoting activity. Of particular interest, a class of tumor-infiltrating myeloid cells has been shown to suppress CTL and NK cell activity, having been identified as MDSCs that function to block the attack on tumors by the adaptive (i.e., CTL) and innate (i.e., NK) arms of the immune system.[94,133,193] Hence, recruitment of certain myeloid cells may be doubly beneficial for the developing tumor, by directly promoting angiogenesis and tumor progression, while at the same time affording a means of evading immune destruction.

These conflicting roles of the immune system in confronting tumors would seem to reflect similar situations that arise routinely in normal tissues. Thus, the immune system detects and targets infectious agents through cells of the adaptive immune response. Cells of the innate immune system, in contrast, are involved in wound healing and in clearing dead cells and cellular debris. The balance between the conflicting immune responses within particular tumor types (and indeed in individual patients' tumors) is likely to prove critical in determining the characteristics of tumor growth and the stepwise progression to stages of heightened aggressiveness (i.e., invasion and metastasis). Moreover, there is increasing evidence supporting the proposition that this balance can be modulated for therapeutic purposes in order to redirect or reprogram the immune response to focus its functional capabilities on destroying tumors.[133,238,239]

Stem and Progenitor Cells of the Tumor Stroma

The various stromal cell types that constitute the tumor microenvironment may be recruited from adjacent normal tissue—the most obvious reservoir of such cell types. However, in recent years, bone marrow (BM) has increasingly been implicated as a key source of tumor-associated stromal cells.[99,100,240–243] Thus, mesenchymal stem and progenitor cells can be recruited into tumors from BM, where they may subsequently differentiate into the various well-characterized stromal cell types. Some of these recent arrivals may also persist in an undifferentiated or partially differentiated state, exhibiting functions that their more differentiated progeny lack.

The BM origins of stromal cell types have been demonstrated using tumor-bearing mice in which the BM cells (and thus their disseminated progeny) have been selectively labeled with reporters such as green fluorescent protein (GFP). Although immune inflammatory cells have been long known to derive from BM, more recently progenitors of endothelial cells, pericytes, and several subtypes of cancer-associated fibroblasts have also been shown to originate from BM in various mouse models of cancer.[100,240–243] The prevalence and functional importance of endothelial progenitors for tumor angiogenesis is, however, currently unresolved.[99,242] Taken together, these various lines of evidence indicate that tumor-associated stromal cells may be supplied to growing tumors by the proliferation of preexisting stromal cells or via recruitment of BM-derived stem/progenitor cells.

In summary, it is evident that virtually all cancers, including even the *liquid tumors* of hematopoietic malignancies, depend not only on neoplastic cells for their pathogenic effects, but also on diverse cell types recruited from local and distant tissue sources to assemble specialized, supporting tumor microenvironments. Importantly, the composition of stromal cell types supporting a particular cancer evidently varies considerably from one tumor type to another; even within a particular type, the patterns and abundance can be informative about malignant grade and prognosis. The inescapable conclusion is that cancer cells are not fully autonomous, and rather depend to various degrees on stromal cells of the tumor microenvironment, which can contribute functionally to seven of the eight hallmarks of cancer (Fig. 2.4).

Heterotypic Signaling Orchestrates the Cells of the Tumor Microenvironment

Every cell in our bodies is governed by an elaborate intracellular signaling circuit—in effect, its own microcomputer. In cancer cells, key subcircuits in this integrated circuit are reprogrammed so as to activate and sustain hallmark capabilities. These changes are induced by mutations in the cells' genomes, by epigenetic alterations affecting gene expression, and by the receipt of a diverse array of signals from the tumor microenvironment. Figure 2.5A illustrates some of the circuits that are reprogrammed to enable cancer cells to proliferate chronically, to avoid proliferative brakes and cell death, and to become invasive and metastatic. Similarly, the intracellular integrated circuits that regulate the actions of stromal cells are also evidently reprogrammed. Current evidence suggests that stromal cell reprogramming is primarily affected by extracellular cues and epigenetic alterations in gene expression, rather than gene mutation.

Given the alterations in the signaling within both neoplastic cells and their stromal neighbors, a tumor can be depicted as a network of interconnected (cellular) microcomputers. This dictates that a complete elucidation of a particular tumor's biology will require far more than an elucidation of the aberrantly functioning integrated circuits within its neoplastic cells. Accordingly, the rapidly growing catalog of the function-enabling genetic mutations within cancer cell genomes[194] provides only one dimension to this problem. A reasonably complete, graphical depiction of the network of microenvironmental signaling interactions remains far beyond our reach, because the great majority of signaling molecules and their circuitry are still to be identified. Instead, we provide a hint of such interactions in Figure 2.5B. These few well-established examples are intended to exemplify a signaling network of remarkable complexity that is of critical importance to tumor pathogenesis.

Coevolution of the Tumor Microenvironment During Carcinogenesis

The tumor microenvironment described previously is not static during multistage tumor development and progression, thus creating another dimension of complexity. Rather, the abundance and functional contributions of the stromal cells populating neoplastic lesions will likely vary during progression in two respects. First, as the neoplastic cells evolve, there will be a parallel coevolution occurring in the stroma, as indicated by the shifting composition of stroma-associated cell types. Second, as cancer cells enter into different locations, they encounter distinct stromal microenvironments. Thus, the microenvironment in the interior of a primary tumor will likely be distinct both from locally invasive breakout lesions and from the one encountered by disseminated cells in distant organs (Fig. 2.6A). This dictates that the observed histopathologic progression of a tumor reflects underlying changes in heterotypic signaling between tumor parenchyma and stroma.

We envision back-and-forth reciprocal interactions between the neoplastic cells and the supporting stromal cells that change during the course of multistep tumor development and progression, as depicted in Figure 2.6B. Thus, incipient neoplasias begin the interplay by recruiting and activating stromal cell types that assemble into an initial preneoplastic stroma, which in turn responds reciprocally by enhancing the neoplastic phenotypes of the nearby cancer cells. The cancer cells, in response, may then undergo further genetic evolution, causing them to feed signals back to the stroma. Ultimately, signals originating in the stroma of primary tumors enable cancer cells to invade normal adjacent tissues and disseminate, seeding distant tissues and, with low efficiency, metastatic colonies (see Fig. 2.6B).

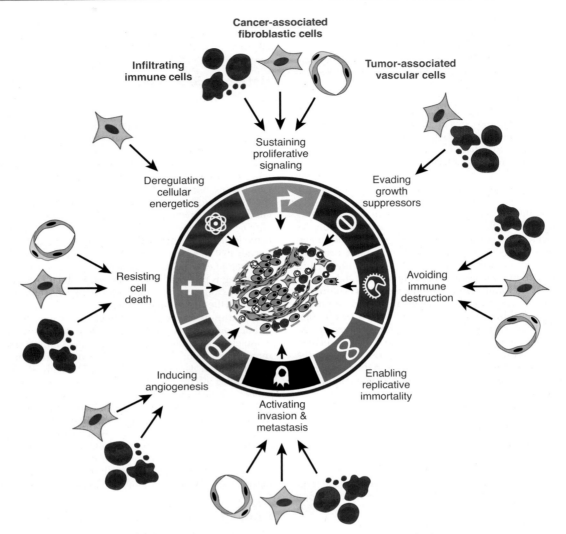

Figure 2.4 Diverse contributions of stromal cells to the hallmarks of cancer. Of the eight hallmark capabilities acquired by cancer cells, seven depend on contributions by stromal cells forming the tumor microenvironment.[2,213] The stromal cells can be divided into three general classes: infiltrating immune cells, cancer-associated fibroblastic cells, and tumor-associated vascular cells. The association of these corrupted cell types with the acquisition of individual hallmark capabilities has been documented through a variety of experimental approaches that are often supported by descriptive studies in human cancers. The relative importance of each of these stromal cell classes to a particular hallmark varies according to tumor type and stage of progression. (Adapted from Hanahan D, Coussens LM. Accessories to the crime: functions of cells recruited to the tumor microenvironment. *Cancer Cell* 2012;21:309–322.)

The circulating cancer cells that are released from primary tumors leave a microenvironment supported by this coevolved stroma. Upon landing in a distant organ, however, disseminated cancer cells must find a means to grow in a quite different tissue microenvironment. In some cases, newly seeded cancer cells must survive and expand in naïve, fully normal tissue microenvironments. In other cases, the newly encountered tissue microenvironments may already be supportive of such disseminated cancer cells, having been preconditioned prior to their arrival. Such permissive sites have been referred to as *premetastatic niches*.[146,244,245] These supportive niches may already preexist in distant tissues for various physiologic reasons,[101] including the actions of circulating factors dispatched systemically by primary tumors.[245]

The fact that signaling interactions between cancer cells and their supporting stroma are likely to evolve during the course of multistage primary tumor development and metastatic colonization clearly complicates the goal of fully elucidating the mechanisms of cancer pathogenesis. For example, this complexity poses challenges to systems biologists seeking to chart the crucial regulatory networks that orchestrate malignant progression, because much of the critical signaling is not intrinsic to cancer cells and instead operates through the interactions that these cells establish with their neighbors.

Cancer Cells, Cancer Stem Cells, and Intratumoral Heterogeneity

Cancer cells are the foundation of the disease. They initiate neoplastic development and drive tumor progression forward, having acquired the oncogenic and tumor suppressor mutations that define cancer as a genetic disease. Traditionally, the cancer cells within tumors have been portrayed as reasonably homogeneous cell populations until relatively late in the course of tumor progression, when hyperproliferation combined with increased genetic instability spawn genetically distinct clonal subpopulations. Reflecting such clonal heterogeneity, many human tumors are histopathologically diverse, containing regions demarcated by various

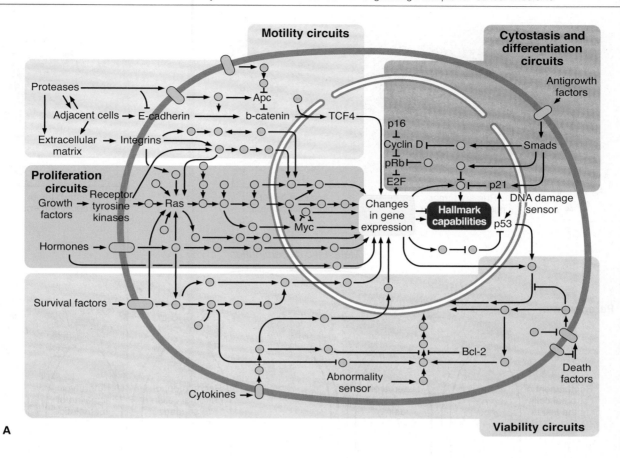

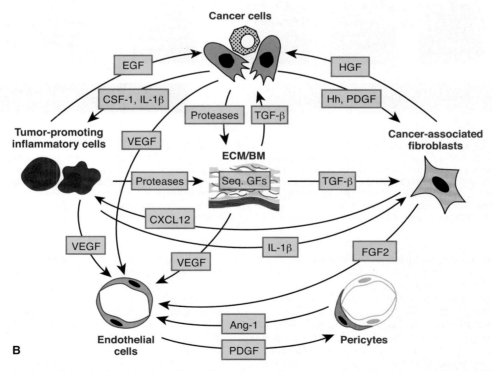

Figure 2.5 Reprogramming intracellular circuits and cell-to-cell signaling pathways dictates tumor inception and progression. An elaborate integrated circuit operating within normal cells is reprogrammed to regulate the hallmark capabilities acquired by cancer cells **(A)** and by associated stromal cells. Separate subcircuits, depicted here in differently colored fields, are specialized to orchestrate distinct capabilities. At one level, this depiction is simplistic, because there is considerable cross-talk between such subcircuits. More broadly, the integrated circuits operating inside cancer cells and stromal cells are interconnected via a complex network of signals transmitted by the various cells in the tumor microenvironment (in some cases via the extracellular matrix *[ECM]* and basement membranes *[BM]* they synthesize), of which a few signals are exemplified **(B)**. HGF, hepatocyte growth factor for the cMet receptor; Hh, hedgehog ligand for the Patched (PTCH) receptor; Seq. GF, growth factors sequestered in the ECM/BM. (Adapted from Hanahan D, Weinberg RA. Hallmarks of cancer: the next generation. *Cell* 2011;144:646–674.)

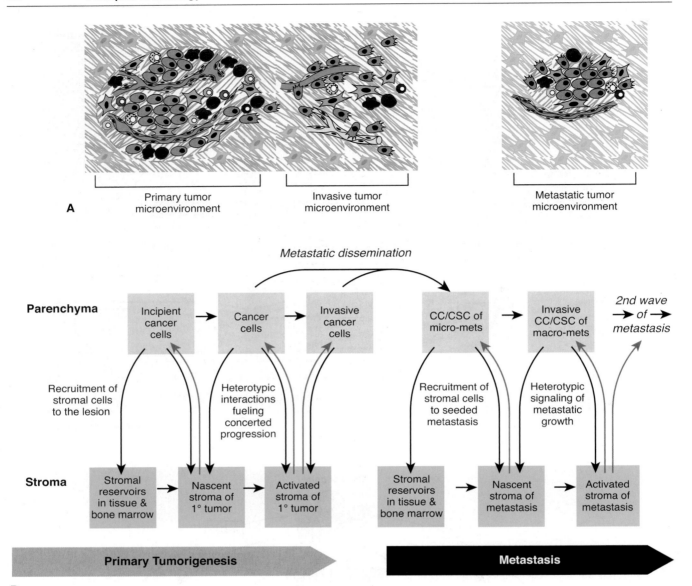

Figure 2.6 The dynamic variation and coevolution of the tumor microenvironment during the lesional progression of cancer. **(A)** Interactions between multiple stromal cell types and heterogeneously evolving mutant cancer cells create a succession of tumor microenvironments that change dynamically as tumors are initiated, invade normal tissues, and thereafter seed and colonize distant tissues. The abundance, histologic organization, and characteristics of the stromal cell types and associated extracellular matrix (hatched background) evolves during progression, thereby enabling primary, invasive, and then metastatic growth. **(B)** Importantly, the signaling networks depicted in Figure 2.5 involving cancer cells and their stromal collaborators change during tumor progression as a result of reciprocal signaling interactions between these various cells. CC, cancer cell; CSC, cancer stem cell; mets, metastases. (Adapted from Hanahan D, Weinberg RA. Hallmarks of cancer: the next generation. *Cell* 2011;144:646–674.)

degrees of differentiation, proliferation, vascularity, and invasiveness. In recent years, however, evidence has accumulated pointing to the existence of a new dimension of intratumor heterogeneity and a hitherto unappreciated subclass of neoplastic cells within tumors, termed cancer stem cells (CSC).

CSCs were initially implicated in the pathogenesis of hematopoietic malignancies,[246,247] and years later, were identified in solid tumors, in particular breast carcinomas and neuroectodermal tumors.[248,249] The fractionation of cancer cells on the basis of cell-surface markers has yielded subpopulations of neoplastic cells with a greatly enhanced ability, relative to the corresponding majority populations of non-CSCs, to seed new tumors upon implantation in immunodeficient mice. These, often rare, tumor-initiating cells have proven to share transcriptional profiles with certain normal tissue stem cells, thus justifying their designation as stemlike.

Although the evidence is still fragmentary, CSCs may prove to be a constituent of many, if not most tumors, albeit being present with highly variable abundance. CSCs are defined operationally through their ability to efficiently seed new tumors upon implantation into recipient host mice.[250–253] This functional definition is often complemented by profiling the expression of certain CSC-associated markers that are typically expressed by the normal stem cells in the corresponding normal tissues of origin.[249] Importantly, recent in vivo lineage-tracing experiments have provided an additional functional test of CSCs by demonstrating their ability to spawn large numbers of progeny, including non-CSCs within tumors.[250] At the same time, these experiments have provided the most compelling evidence to date that CSCs exist, and that they can be defined functionally through tests that do not depend on the implantation of tumor cells into appropriate mouse hosts.

The origins of CSCs within a solid tumor have not been clarified and, indeed, may well vary from one tumor type to another.[250,251,254] In some tumors, normal tissue stem cells may serve as the cells of origin that undergo oncogenic transformation to yield CSCs; in others, partially differentiated transit-amplifying cells, also termed progenitor cells, may suffer the initial oncogenic transformation, thereafter assuming more stemlike characters. Once primary tumors have formed, the CSCs, like their normal counterparts, may self-renew as well as spawn more differentiated derivatives. In the case of neoplastic CSCs, these descendant cells form the great bulk of many tumors and thus are responsible for creating many tumor-associated phenotypes. It remains to be established whether multiple distinct classes of increasingly neoplastic stem cells form during the inception and subsequent multistep progression of tumors, ultimately yielding the CSCs that have been described in fully developed cancers.

Recent research has interrelated the acquisition of CSC traits with the EMT transdifferentiation program discussed previously.[250,255] The induction of this program in certain model systems can induce many of the defining features of stem cells, including self-renewal ability and the antigenic phenotypes associated with both normal and cancer stem cells. This concordance suggests that the EMT program may not only enable cancer cells to physically disseminate from primary tumors, but can also confer on such cells the self-renewal capability that is crucial to their subsequent role as founders of new neoplastic colonies at sites of dissemination.[256] If generalized, this connection raises an important corollary hypothesis: The heterotypic signals that trigger an EMT, such as those released by an activated, inflammatory stroma, may also be important in creating and maintaining CSCs.

An increasing number of human tumors are reported to contain subpopulations with the properties of CSCs, as defined operationally through their efficient tumor-initiating capabilities upon xenotransplantation into mice. Nevertheless, the importance of CSCs as a distinct phenotypic subclass of neoplastic cells remains a matter of debate, as does their oft cited rarity within tumors.[254,257–259] Indeed, it is plausible that the phenotypic plasticity operating within tumors may produce bidirectional interconversion between CSCs and non-CSCs, resulting in dynamic variation in the relative abundance of CSCs.[250,260] Such plasticity could complicate a definitive measurement of their characteristic abundance. Analogous plasticity is already implicated in the EMT program, which can be engaged reversibly.[261]

These complexities notwithstanding, it is already evident that this new dimension of tumor heterogeneity holds important implications for successful cancer therapies. Increasing evidence in a variety of tumor types suggests that cells exhibiting the properties of CSCs are more resistant to various commonly used chemotherapeutic treatments.[255,262,263] Their persistence following initial treatment may help to explain the almost inevitable disease recurrence occurring after apparently successful debulking of human solid tumors by radiation and various forms of chemotherapy. Moreover, CSCs may well prove to underlie certain forms of tumor dormancy, whereby latent cancer cells persist for years or even decades after initial surgical resection or radio/chemotherapy, only to suddenly erupt and generate life-threatening disease. Hence, CSCs represent a double threat in that they are more resistant to therapeutic killing, and at the same time, are endowed with the ability to regenerate a tumor once therapy has been halted.

This phenotypic plasticity implicit in the CSC state may also enable the formation of functionally distinct subpopulations within a tumor that support overall tumor growth in various ways. Thus, an EMT can convert epithelial carcinoma cells into mesenchymal, fibroblast-like cancer cells that may well assume the duties of CAFs in some tumors (e.g., pancreatic ductal adenocarcinoma).[264] Intriguingly, several recent reports that have yet to be thoroughly validated in terms of generality, functional importance, or prevalence have documented the ability of glioblastoma cells (or possibly their associated CSC subpopulations) to transdifferentiate into endothelial-like cells that can substitute for bona fide host-derived endothelial cells in forming a tumor-associated neovasculature.[265–267] These examples suggest that certain tumors may induce some of their own cancer cells to undergo various types of metamorphoses in order to generate stromal cell types needed to support tumor growth and progression, rather than relying on recruited host cells to provide the requisite hallmark-enabling functions.

Another form of phenotypic variability resides in the genetic heterogeneity of cancer cells within a tumor. Genomewide sequencing of cancer cells microdissected from different sectors of the same tumor[145] has revealed striking intratumoral genetic heterogeneity. Some of this genetic diversity may be reflected in the long recognized histologic heterogeneity within individual human tumors. Thus, genetic diversification may produce subpopulations of cancer cells that contribute distinct and complementary capabilities, which then accrue to the common benefit of overall tumor growth, progression, and resistance to therapy, as described earlier. Alternatively, such heterogeneity may simply reflect the genetic chaos that arises as tumor cell genomes become increasingly destabilized.

THERAPEUTIC TARGETING OF THE HALLMARKS OF CANCER

We do not attempt here to enumerate the myriad therapies that are currently under development or have been introduced of late into the clinic. Instead, we consider how the description of hallmark principles is likely to inform therapeutic development at present and may increasingly do so in the future. Thus, the rapidly growing armamentarium of therapeutics directed against specific molecular targets can be categorized according to their respective effects on one or more hallmark capabilities, as illustrated in the examples presented in Figure 2.7. Indeed, the observed efficacy of these drugs represents, in each case, a validation of a particular capability: If a capability is truly critical to the biology of tumors, then its inhibition should impair tumor growth and progression.

Unfortunately, however, the clinical responses elicited by these targeted therapies have generally been transitory, being followed all too often by relapse. One interpretation, which is supported by growing experimental evidence, is that each of the core hallmark capabilities is regulated by a set of partially redundant signaling pathways. Consequently, a targeted therapeutic agent inhibiting one key pathway in a tumor may not completely eliminate a hallmark capability, allowing some cancer cells to survive with residual function until they or their progeny eventually adapt to the selective pressure imposed by the initially applied therapy. Such adaptation can reestablish the expression of the functional capability, permitting renewed tumor growth and clinical relapse. Because the number of parallel signaling pathways supporting a given hallmark must be limited, it may become possible to therapeutically cotarget all of these supporting pathways, thereby preventing the development of adaptive resistance.

Another dimension of the plasticity of tumors under therapeutic attack is illustrated by the unanticipated responses to antiangiogenic therapy, in which cancer cells reduce their dependence on this hallmark capability by increasing their dependence on another. Thus, many observers anticipated that potent inhibition of angiogenesis would starve tumors of vital nutrients and oxygen, forcing them into dormancy and possibly leading to their dissolution.[86,87,268] Instead, the clinical responses to antiangiogenic therapies have been found to be transitory, followed by relapse, implicating adaptive or evasive resistance mechanisms.[220,269–271] One such mechanism of evasive resistance, observed in certain preclinical models of antiangiogenic therapy, involves reduced dependence on continuing angiogenesis by increasing the activity of two other capabilities: invasiveness and metastasis.[269–271] By invading nearby and distant tissues, initially hypoxic cancer cells gain access to normal,

PRINCIPLES OF ONCOLOGY

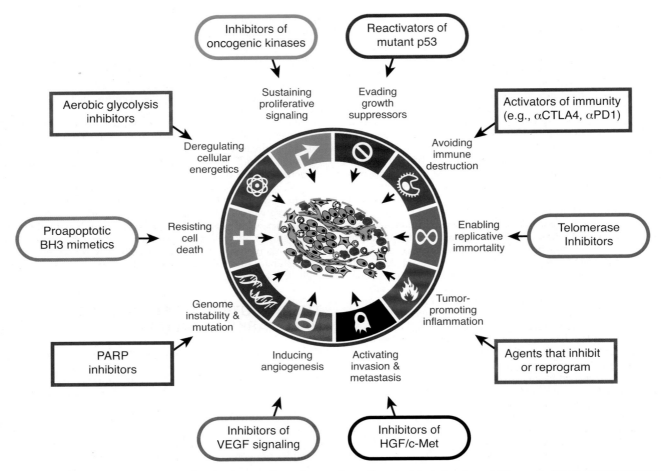

Figure 2.7 Therapeutic targeting of the hallmarks of cancer. Drugs that interfere with each of the hallmark capabilities and hallmark-enabling processes have been developed and are in preclinical and/or clinical testing, and in some cases, approved for use in treating certain forms of human cancer. A focus on antagonizing specific hallmark capabilities is likely to yield insights into developing novel, highly effective therapeutic strategies. PARP, poly ADP ribose polymerase. (Adapted from Hanahan D, Weinberg RA. Hallmarks of cancer: the next generation. *Cell* 2011;144:646–674.)

preexisting tissue vasculature. The initial clinical validation of this adaptive/evasive resistance is apparent in the increased invasion and local metastasis seen when human glioblastomas are treated with antiangiogenic therapies.[272–274] The applicability of this lesson to other human cancers has yet to be established.

Analogous adaptive shifts in dependence on other hallmark traits may also limit the efficacy of analogous hallmark-targeting therapies. For example, the deployment of apoptosis-inducing drugs may induce cancer cells to hyperactivate mitogenic signaling, enabling them to compensate for the initial attrition triggered by such treatments. Such considerations suggest that drug development and the design of treatment protocols will benefit from incorporating the concepts of functionally discrete hallmark capabilities and of the multiple biochemical pathways involved in supporting each of them. For these reasons, we envisage that attacking multiple hallmark capabilities with hallmark-targeting drugs (see Fig. 2.7), in carefully considered combinations, sequences, and temporal regimens,[275] will result in increasingly effective therapies that produce more durable clinical responses.

CONCLUSION AND A VISION FOR THE FUTURE

Looking ahead, we envision significant advances in our understanding of invasion and metastasis during the coming decade. Similarly, the role of altered energy metabolism in malignant growth will be

elucidated, including a resolution of whether this metabolic reprogramming is a discrete capability separable from the core hallmark of chronically sustained proliferation. We are excited about the new frontier of immunotherapy, which will be empowered to leverage detailed knowledge about the regulation of immune responses in order to develop pharmacologic tools that can modulate them therapeutically for the purpose of effectively and sustainably attacking tumors and, most importantly, their metastases.

Other areas are currently in rapid flux. In recent years, elaborate molecular mechanisms controlling transcription through chromatin modifications have been uncovered, and there are clues that specific shifts in chromatin configuration occur during the acquisition of certain hallmark capabilities.[195,196] Functionally significant epigenetic alterations seem likely to be factors not only in the cancer cells, but also in the altered cells of the tumor-associated stroma. At present, it is unclear whether an elucidation of these epigenetic mechanisms will materially change our overall understanding of the means by which hallmark capabilities are acquired, or simply add additional detail to the regulatory circuitry that is already known to govern them.

Similarly, the discovery of hundreds of distinct regulatory microRNAs has already led to profound changes in our understanding of the molecular control mechanisms that operate in health and disease. By now, dozens of microRNAs have been implicated in various tumor phenotypes.[276,277] Still, these only scratch the surface of the true complexity, because the functions of hundreds of microRNAs known to be present in our cells and to be altered in expression levels in different forms of cancer remain total mysteries. Here again, we are unclear whether future progress will cause fundamental shifts in our understanding of the pathogenic mechanisms of cancer, or only add detail to the elaborate regulatory circuits that have already been mapped out.

Finally, the existing diagrams of heterotypic interactions between the multiple distinct cell types that collaborate to produce malignant tumors are still rudimentary. We anticipate that, in another decade, the signaling pathways describing the intercommunication between these various cell types within tumors will be charted in far greater detail and clarity, eclipsing our current knowledge. And, as before,[1,2] we continue to foresee cancer research as an increasingly logical science, in which myriad phenotypic complexities are manifestations of an underlying organizing principle.

ACKNOWLEDGMENT

This chapter is modified from Hanahan D, Weinberg RA. Hallmarks of cancer: the next generation. *Cell* 2011;144(5):646–674.

REFERENCES

1. Hanahan D, Weinberg R. The hallmarks of cancer. *Cell* 2000;100:57–70.
2. Hanahan D, Weinberg RA. Hallmarks of cancer: the next generation. *Cell* 2011;144:646–674.
3. Lemmon MA, Schlessinger J. Cell signaling by receptor tyrosine kinases. *Cell* 2010;141:1117–1134.
4. Witsch E, Sela M, Yarden Y. Roles for growth factors in cancer progression. *Physiology* 2010;25:85–101.
5. Hynes NE, MacDonald G. ErbB receptors and signaling pathways in cancer. *Curr Opin Cell Biol* 2009;21:177–184.
6. Perona T. Cell signalling: growth factors and tyrosine kinase receptors. *Clin Transl Oncol* 2006;8:77–82.
7. Franco OE, Shaw AK, Strand DW, et al. Cancer associated fibroblasts in cancer pathogenesis. *Semin Cell Dev Biol* 2010;21:33–39.
8. Bhowmick NA, Neilson EG, Moses HL. Stromal fibroblasts in cancer initiation and progression. *Nature* 2004;432:332–337.
9. Davies MA, Samuels Y. Analysis of the genome to personalize therapy for melanoma. *Oncogene* 2010;29:5545–5555.
10. Jiang BH, Liu LZ. PI3K/PTEN signaling in angiogenesis and tumorigenesis. *Adv Cancer Res* 2009;102:19–65.
11. Yuan TL, Cantley LC. PI3K pathway alterations in cancer: variations on a theme. *Oncogene* 2008;27:5497–5510.
12. Wertz IE, Dixit VM. Regulation of death receptor signaling by the ubiquitin system. *Cell Death Differ* 2010;17:14–24.
13. Cabrita MA, Christofori G. Sprouty proteins, masterminds of receptor tyrosine kinase signaling. *Angiogenesis* 2008;11:53–62.
14. Amit I, Citri A, Shay T, et al. A module of negative feedback regulators defines growth factor signaling. *Nature Genet* 2007;39:503–512.
15. Mosesson Y, Mills GB, Yarden Y. Derailed endocytosis: an emerging feature of cancer. *Nat Rev Cancer* 2008;8:835–850.
16. Sudarsanam S, Johnson DE. Functional consequences of mTOR inhibition. *Curr Opin Drug Discov Devel* 2010;13:31–40.
17. O'Reilly KE, Rojo F, She QB, et al. mTOR inhibition induces upstream receptor tyrosine kinase signaling and activates Akt. *Cancer Res* 2006;66:1500–1508.
18. Dang CV. MYC on the path to cancer. *Cell* 2012;149:22–35.
19. Collado M, Serrano M. Senescence in tumours: evidence from mice and humans. *Nat Rev Cancer* 2010;10:51–57.
20. Evan GI, d'Adda di Fagagna F. Cellular senescence: hot or what? *Curr Opin Genet Dev* 2009;19:25–31.
21. Lowe SW, Cepero E, Evan G. Intrinsic tumour suppression. *Nature* 2004;432:307–315.
22. Mooi WJ, Peeper DS. Oncogene-induced cell senescence—halting on the road to cancer. *N Engl J Med* 2006;355:1037–1046.
23. Burkhart DL, Sage J. Cellular mechanisms of tumour suppression by the retinoblastoma gene. *Nat Rev Cancer* 2008;8:671–682.
24. Deshpande A, Sicinski P, Hinds PW. Cyclins and cdks in development and cancer: a perspective. *Oncogene* 2005;24:2909–2915.
25. Sherr CJ, McCormick F. The RB and p53 pathways in cancer. *Cancer Cell* 2002;2:103–112.
26. Lipinski MM, Jacks T. The retinoblastoma gene family in differentiation and development. *Oncogene* 1999;18:7873–7882.
27. Ghebranious N, Donehower LA. Mouse models in tumor suppression. *Oncogene* 1998;17: 3385–3400.
28. McClatchey AI, Yap AS. Contact inhibition (of proliferation) redux. *Curr Opin Cell Biol* 2012;24:685–694.
29. Curto M, Cole BK, Lallemand D, et al. Contact-dependent inhibition of EGFR signaling by Nf2/Merlin. *J Cell Biol* 2007;177:893–903.
30. Okada T, Lopez-Lago M, Giancotti FG. Merlin/NF-2 mediates contact inhibition of growth by suppressing recruitment of Rac to the plasma membrane. *J Cell Biol* 2005;171:361–371.
31. Stamenkovic I, Yu Q. Merlin, a "magic" linker between the extracellular cues and intracellular signaling pathways that regulate cell motility, proliferation, and survival. *Curr Protein Pept Sci* 2010;11:471–484.
32. Pickup M, Novitskiy S, Moses HL. The roles of TGFβ in the tumour microenvironment. *Nat Rev Cancer* 2013;13:788–799.
33. Ikushima H, Miyazono K. TGFbeta signalling: a complex web in cancer progression. *Nat Rev Cancer* 2010;10:415–424.
34. Massagué J. TGF-beta in cancer. *Cell* 2008;134:215–230.
35. Bierie B, Moses HL. Tumour microenvironment: TGF-beta: the molecular Jekyll and Hyde of cancer. *Nat Rev Cancer* 2006;6:506–520.
36. Strasser A, Cory S, Adams JM. Deciphering the rules of programmed cell death to improve therapy of cancer and other diseases. *EMBO J* 2011;30:3667–3683.
37. Adams JM, Cory S. The Bcl-2 apoptotic switch in cancer development and therapy. *Oncogene* 2007;26:1324–1337.
38. Evan G, Littlewood T. A matter of life and cell death. *Science* 2004;281:1317–1322.
39. Willis SN, Adams JM. Life in the balance: how BH3-only proteins induce apoptosis. *Curr Opin Cell Biol* 2005;17:617–625.
40. Junttila MR, Evan GI. p53 — a jack of all trades but master of none. *Nat Rev Cancer* 2009;9:821–829.
41. White E. Deconvoluting the context-dependent role for autophagy in cancer. *Nat Rev Cancer* 2012;12:401–410.
42. Levine B, Kroemer G. Autophagy in the pathogenesis of disease. *Cell* 2008;132:27–42.
43. Mizushima N. Autophagy: process and function. *Genes Dev* 2007;21:2861–2873.
44. Sinha S, Levine B. The autophagy effector Beclin 1: a novel BH3-only protein. *Oncogene* 2008;27:S137–S148.
45. Mathew R, Karantza-Wadsworth V, White E. Role of autophagy in cancer. *Nat Rev Cancer* 2007;7:961–967.
46. White E, DiPaola RS. The double-edged sword of autophagy modulation in cancer. *Clin Cancer Res* 2009;15:5308–5316.
47. Apel A, Zentgraf H, Büchler MW, et al. Autophagy—A double-edged sword in oncology. *Int J Cancer* 2009;125:991–995.
48. Amaravadi RK, Thompson CB. The roles of therapy-induced autophagy and necrosis in cancer treatment. *Clin Cancer Res* 2007;13:7271–7279.
49. Lu Z, Luo RZ, Lu Y, et al. The tumor suppressor gene ARHI regulates autophagy and tumor dormancy in human ovarian cancer cells. *J Clin Invest* 2008;118:3917–3929.
50. Vanden Berghe T, Linkermann A, Jouan-Lanhouet S, et al. Regulated necrosis: the expanding network of non-apoptotic cell death pathways. *Nat Rev Mol Cell Biol* 2014;15:135–147.
51. Galluzzi L, Kroemer G. Necroptosis: a specialized pathway of programmed necrosis. *Cell* 2008;135:1161–1163.
52. Zong WX, Thompson CB. Necrotic death as a cell fate. *Genes Dev* 2006;20:1–15.
53. Grivennikov SI, Greten FR, Karin M. Immunity, inflammation, and cancer. *Cell* 2010;140:883–899.
54. White E, Karp C, Strohecker AM, et al. Role of autophagy in suppression of inflammation and cancer. *Curr Opin Cell Biol* 2010;22:212–217.
55. Blasco MA. Telomeres and human disease: ageing, cancer and beyond. *Nat Rev Genet* 2005;6:611–622.
56. Shay JW, Wright WE. Hayflick, his limit, and cellular ageing. *Nat Rev Mol Cell Biol* 2000;1:72–76.
57. Shay JW, Wright WE. Telomeres and telomerase in cancer. *Sem Cancer Biol* 2011;21:349–353.
58. Artandi SE, DePinho RA. Telomeres and telomerase in cancer. *Carcinogenesis* 2010;31:9–18.
59. Cesare AJ, Reddel RR. Alternative lengthening of telomeres: models, mechanisms and implications. *Nat Rev Genet* 2010;11:319–330.
60. Ince TA, Richardson AL, Bell GW, et al. Transformation of different human breast epithelial cell types leads to distinct tumor phenotypes. *Cancer Cell* 2007;12:160–170.
61. Passos JF, Saretzki G, von Zglinicki T. DNA damage in telomeres and mitochondria during cellular senescence: is there a connection? *Nucleic Acids Res* 2007;35:7505–7513.
62. Zhang H, Herbert BS, Pan KH, et al. Disparate effects of telomere attrition on gene expression during replicative senescence of human mammary epithelial cells cultured under different conditions. *Oncogene* 2004;23:6193–6198.
63. Sherr CJ, DePinho RA. Cellular senescence: mitotic clock or culture shock? *Cell* 2000;102:407–410.
64. Feldser DM, Greider CW. Short telomeres limit tumor progression in vivo by inducing senescence. *Cancer Cell* 2007;11:461–469.
65. Kawai T, Hiroi S, Nakanishi K, et al. Telomere length and telomerase expression in atypical adenomatous hyperplasia and small bronchioloalveolar carcinoma of the lung. *Am J Clin Pathol* 2007;127:254–262.

66. Hansel DE, Meeker AK, Hicks J. Telomere length variation in biliary tract metaplasia, dysplasia, and carcinoma. *Mod Pathol* 2006;19:772–779.

67. Artandi SE, DePinho RA. Mice without telomerase: what can they teach us about human cancer? *Nature Med* 2000;6:852–855.

68. Raynaud CM, Hernandez J, Llorca FP, et al. DNA damage repair and telomere length in normal breast, preoplastic lesions, and invasive cancer. *Am J Clin Oncol* 2010;33:341–345.

69. Chin K, de Solorzano CO, Knowles D, et al. In situ analyses of genome instability in breast cancer. *Nature Genet* 2004;36:984–988.

70. Hanahan D, Folkman J. Patterns and emerging mechanisms of the angiogenic switch during tumorigenesis. *Cell* 1996;86:353–364.

71. Baeriswyl V, Christofori G. The angiogenic switch in carcinogenesis. *Semin Cancer Biol* 2009;19:329–337.

72. Bergers G, Benjamin LE. Tumorigenesis and the angiogenic switch. *Nat Rev Cancer* 2003;3:401–410.

73. Ferrara N. Vascular endothelial growth factor. *Arterioscler Thromb Vasc Biol* 2009;29:789–791.

74. Mac Gabhann F, Popel AS. Systems biology of vascular endothelial growth factors. *Microcirculation* 2008;15:715–738.

75. Carmeliet P. VEGF as a key mediator of angiogenesis in cancer. *Oncology* 2005;69:4–10.

76. Kessenbrock K, Plaks V, Werb Z. Matrix metalloproteinases: regulators of the tumor microenvironment. *Cell* 2010;141:52–67.

77. Kazerounian S, Yee KO, Lawler J. Thrombospondins in cancer. *Cell Mol Life Sci* 2008;65:700–712.

78. Nagy JA, Chang SH, Shih SC, et al. Heterogeneity of the tumor vasculature. *Semin Thromb Hemost* 2010;36:321–331.

79. Baluk P, Hashizume H, McDonald DM. Cellular abnormalities of blood vessels as targets in cancer. *Curr Opin Genet Dev* 2005;15:102–111.

80. Raica M, Cimpean AM, Ribatti D. Angiogenesis in pre-malignant conditions. *Eur J Cancer* 2009;45:1924–1934.

81. Olive KP, Jacobetz MA, Davidson CJ, et al. Inhibition of Hedgehog signaling enhances delivery of chemotherapy in a mouse model of pancreatic cancer. *Science* 2009;324:1457–1461.

82. Zee YK, O'Connor JP, Parker GJ, et al. Imaging angiogenesis of genitourinary tumors. *Nat Rev Urol* 2010;7:69–82.

83. Turner HE, Harris AL, Melmed S, et al. Angiogenesis in endocrine tumors. *Endocr Rev* 2003;24:600–632.

84. Xie L, Duncan MB, Pahler J, et al. Counterbalancing angiogenic regulatory factors control the rate of cancer progression and survival in a stage-specific manner. *Proc Natl Acad Sci U S A* 2011;108:9939–9944.

85. Ribatti D. Endogenous inhibitors of angiogenesis: a historical review. *Leuk Res* 2009;33:638–644.

86. Folkman J. Angiogenesis. *Annu Rev Med* 2006;57:1–18.

87. Folkman J. Role of angiogenesis in tumor growth and metastasis. *Semin Oncol* 2002;29:15–18.

88. Nyberg P, Xie L, Kalluri R. Endogenous inhibitors of angiogenesis. *Cancer Res* 2005;65:3967–3979.

89. Cao Y. Adipose tissue angiogenesis as a therapeutic target for obesity and metabolic diseases. *Nat Rev Drug Discov* 2010;9:107–115.

90. Seppinen L, Sormunen R, Soini Y, et al. Lack of collagen XVIII accelerates cutaneous wound healing, while overexpression of its endostatin domain leads to delayed healing. *Matrix Biol* 2008;27:535–546.

91. Raza A, Franklin MJ, Dudek AZ. Pericytes and vessel maturation during tumor angiogenesis and metastasis. *Am J Hematol* 2010;85:593–598.

92. Kovacic JC, Boehm M. Resident vascular progenitor cells: an emerging role for non-terminally differentiated vessel-resident cells in vascular biology. *Stem Cell Res* 2009;2:2–15.

93. Bergers G, Song S. The role of pericytes in blood-vessel formation and maintenance. *Neuro Oncol* 2005;7:452–464.

94. Qian BZ, Pollard JW. Macrophage diversity enhances tumor progression and metastasis. *Cell* 2010;141:39–51.

95. Zumsteg A, Christofori G. Corrupt policemen: inflammatory cells promote tumor angiogenesis. *Curr Opin Oncol* 2009;21:60–70.

96. Murdoch C, Muthana M, Coffelt SB, et al. The role of myeloid cells in the promotion of tumour angiogenesis. *Nat Rev Cancer* 2008;8:618–631.

97. De Palma M, Murdoch C, Venneri MA, et al. Tie2-expressing monocytes: regulation of tumor angiogenesis and therapeutic implications. *Trends Immunol* 2007;28:519–524.

98. Ferrara N. Pathways mediating VEGF-independent tumor angiogenesis. *Cytokine Growth Factor Rev* 2010;21:21–26.

99. Patenaude A, Parker J, Karsan A. Involvement of endothelial progenitor cells in tumor vascularization. *Microvasc Res* 2010;79:217–223.

100. Lamagna C, Bergers G. The bone marrow constitutes a reservoir of pericyte progenitors. *J Leukoc Biol* 2006;80:677–681.

101. Talmadge JE, Fidler IJ. AACR centennial series: the biology of cancer metastasis: historical perspective. *Cancer Res* 2010;70:5649–5669.

102. Fidler IJ. The pathogenesis of cancer metastasis: the "seed and soil" hypothesis revisited. *Nat Rev Cancer* 2003;3:453–458.

103. Berx G, van Roy F. Involvement of members of the cadherin superfamily in cancer. *Cold Spring Harb Perspect Biol* 2009;1:a003129.

104. Cavallaro U, Christofori G. Cell adhesion and signaling by cadherins and Ig-CAMs in cancer. *Nat Rev Cancer* 2004;4:118–132.

105. De Craene B, Berx G. Regulatory networks defining EMT during cancer initiation and progression. *Nat Rev Cancer* 2013;13:97–110.

106. Klymkowsky MW, Savagner P. Epithelial-mesenchymal transition: a cancer researcher's conceptual friend and foe. *Am J Pathol* 2009;174:1588–1592.

107. Polyak K, Weinberg RA. Transitions between epithelial and mesenchymal states: acquisition of malignant and stem cell traits. *Nat Rev Cancer* 2009;9:265–273.

108. Thiery JP, Acloque H, Huang RY, et al. Epithelial-mesenchymal transitions in development and disease. *Cell* 2009;139:871–890.

109. Yilmaz M, Christofori G. EMT, the cytoskeleton, and cancer cell invasion. *Cancer Metastasis Rev* 2009;28:15–33.

110. Barrallo-Gimeno A, Nieto MA. The Snail genes as inducers of cell movement and survival: implications in development and cancer. *Development* 2005;132:3151–3161.

111. Micalizzi DS, Farabaugh SM, Ford HL. Epithelial-mesenchymal transition in cancer: parallels between normal development and tumor progression. *J Mammary Gland Biol Neoplasia* 2010;15:117–134.

112. Taube JH, Herschkowitz JI, Komurov K, et al. Core epithelial-to-mesenchymal transition interactome gene-expression signature is associated with claudin-low and metaplastic breast cancer subtypes. *Proc Natl Acad Sci U S A* 2010;107:15449–15454.

113. Schmalhofer O, Brabletz S, Brabletz T. E-cadherin, beta-catenin, and ZEB1 in malignant progression of cancer. *Cancer Metastasis Rev* 2009;28:151–166.

114. Yang J, Weinberg RA. Epithelial-mesenchymal transition: at the crossroads of development and tumor metastasis. *Develop Cell* 2008;14:818–829.

115. Peinado H, Marin F, Cubillo E, et al. Snail and E47 repressors of E-cadherin induce distinct invasive and angiogenic properties in vivo. *J Cell Sci* 2004;117:2827–2839.

116. Karnoub AE, Weinberg RA. Chemokine networks and breast cancer metastasis. *Breast Dis* 2006;26:75–85.

117. Brabletz T, Jung A, Reu S, et al. Variable beta-catenin expression in colorectal cancers indicates tumor progression driven by the tumor environment. *Proc Natl Acad Sci U S A* 2001;98:10356–10361.

118. Hlubek F, Brabletz T, Budczies J, et al. Heterogeneous expression of Wnt/beta-catenin target genes within colorectal cancer. *Int J Cancer* 2007;121:1941–1948.

119. Egeblad M, Nakasone ES, Werb Z. Tumors as organs: complex tissues that interface with the entire organism. *Dev Cell* 2010;18:884–901.

120. Joyce JA, Pollard JW. Microenvironmental regulation of metastasis. *Nat Rev Cancer* 2009;9:239–252.

121. Kalluri R, Zeisberg M. Fibroblasts in cancer. *Nat Rev Cancer* 2006;6:392–401.

122. Karnoub AE, Dash AB, Vo AP, et al. Mesenchymal stem cells within tumour stroma promote breast cancer metastasis. *Nature* 2007;449:557–563.

123. Li HJ, Reinhart F, Herschman HR, et al. Cancer-stimulated mesenchymal stem cells create a carcinoma stem cell niche via prostaglandin E2 signaling. *Cancer Discov* 2012;2:840–855.

124. Palermo C, Joyce JA. Cysteine cathepsin proteases as pharmacological targets in cancer. *Trends Pharmacol Sci* 2008;29:22–28.

125. Mohamed MM, Sloane BF. Cysteine cathepsins: multifunctional enzymes in cancer. *Nat Rev Cancer* 2006;6:764–775.

126. Gocheva V, Wang HW, Gadea BB, et al. IL-4 induces cathepsin protease activity in tumor-associated macrophages to promote cancer growth and invasion. *Genes Dev* 2010;24:241–255.

127. Wyckoff JB, Wang Y, Lin EY, et al. Direct visualization of macrophage-assisted tumor cell intravasation in mammary tumors. *Cancer Res* 2007;67:2649–2656.

128. Hugo H, Ackland ML, Blick T, et al. Epithelial-mesenchymal and mesenchymal-epithelial transitions in carcinoma progression. *J Cell Physiol* 2007;213:374–383.

129. Friedl P, Wolf K. Plasticity of cell migration: a multiscale tuning model. *J Cell Biol* 2009;188:11–19.

130. Friedl P, Wolf K. Tube travel: the role of proteases in individual and collective cancer cell invasion. *Cancer Res* 2008;68:7247–7249.

131. Madsen CD, Sahai E. Cancer dissemination—lessons from leukocytes. *Dev Cell* 2010;19:13–26.

132. Sabeh F, Shimizu-Hirota R, Weiss SJ. Protease-dependent versus-independent cancer cell invasion programs: three-dimensional amoeboid movement revisited. *J Cell Biol* 2009;185:11–19.

133. Quail DF, Joyce JA. Microenvironmental regulation of tumor progression and metastasis. *Nat Med* 2013;19:1423–1437.

134. McGowan PM, Kirstein JM, Chambers AF. Micrometastatic disease and metastatic outgrowth: clinical issues and experimental approaches. *Future Oncol* 2009;5:1083–1098.

135. Aguirre-Ghiso JA. Models, mechanisms and clinical evidence for cancer dormancy. *Nat Rev Cancer* 2007;7:834–846.

136. Townson JL, Chambers AF. Dormancy of solitary metastatic cells. *Cell Cycle* 2006;5:1744–1750.

137. Demicheli R, Retsky MW, Hrushesky WJ, et al. The effects of surgery on tumor growth: a century of investigations. *Ann Oncol* 2008;19:1821–1828.

138. Barkan D, Green JE, Chambers AF. Extracellular matrix: a gatekeeper in the transition from dormancy to metastatic growth. *Eur J Cancer* 2010;46:1181–1188.

139. Gupta GP, Minn AJ, Kang,Y, et al. Identifying site-specific metastasis genes and functions. *Cold Spring Harb Symp Quant Biol* 2005;70:149–158.

140. Naumov GN, Folkman J, Straume O, et al. Tumor-vascular interactions and tumor dormancy. *APMIS* 2008;116:569–585.

141. Kenific CM, Thorburn A, Debnath J. Autophagy and metastasis: another double-edged sword. *Curr Opin Cell Biol* 2010;22:241–245.

142. Teng MW, Swann JB, Koebel CM, et al. Immune-mediated dormancy: an equilibrium with cancer. *J Leukoc Biol* 2008;84:988–993.

143. Campbell PJ, Yachida S, Mudie LJ, et al. The patterns and dynamics of genomic instability in metastatic pancreatic cancer. *Nature* 2010;467:1109–1113.

144. Luebeck EG. Cancer: genomic evolution of metastasis. *Nature* 2010;467:1053–1055.

145. Yachida S, Jones S, Bozic I, et al. Distant metastasis occurs late during the genetic evolution of pancreatic cancer. *Nature* 2010;467:1114–1117.

146. Coghlin C, Murray GI. Current and emerging concepts in tumour metastasis. *J Pathol* 2010;222:1–15.

147. Klein CA. Parallel progression of primary tumours and metastases. *Nat Rev Cancer* 2009;9:302–312.

148. Gerhardt H, Semb H. Pericytes: gatekeepers in tumour cell metastasis? *J Mol Med* 2008;86:135–144.

149. Kim MY, Oskarsson T, Acharyya S, et al. Tumor self-seeding by circulating cancer cells. *Cell* 2009;139:1315–1326.

150. Bos PD, Zhang XH, Nadal C, et al. Genes that mediate breast cancer metastasis to the brain. *Nature* 2009;459:1005–1009.

151. Olson P, Lu J, Zhang H, et al. MicroRNA dynamics in the stages of tumorigenesis correlate with hallmark capabilities of cancer. *Genes Dev* 2009;23:2152–2165.

152. Nguyen DX, Bos PD, Massagué J. Metastasis: from dissemination to organ-specific colonization. *Nat Rev Cancer* 2009;9:274–284.

153. Warburg OH. *The Metabolism of Tumours: Investigations from the Kaiser Wilhelm Institute for Biology, Berlin-Dahlem.* London, UK: Arnold Constable; 1930.

154. Warburg O. On the origin of cancer cells. *Science* 1956;123:309–314.

155. Warburg O. On respiratory impairment in cancer cells. *Science* 1956;124:269–270.

156. Jones RG, Thompson CB. Tumor suppressors and cell metabolism: a recipe for cancer growth. *Genes Dev* 2009;23:537–548.

157. DeBerardinis RJ, Lum JJ, Hatzivassiliou G, et al. The biology of cancer: metabolic reprogramming fuels cell growth and proliferation. *Cell Metab* 2008;7:11–20.

158. Hsu PP, Sabatini DM. Cancer cell metabolism: Warburg and beyond. *Cell* 2008;134:703–707.

159. Ward PS, Thompson CB. Metabolic reprogramming: a cancer hallmark even warburg did not anticipate. *Cancer Cell* 2012;21:297–308.

160. Semenza GL. HIF-1: upstream and downstream of cancer metabolism. *Curr Opin Genet Dev* 2010;20:51–56.

161. Semenza GL. Defining the role of hypoxia-inducible factor 1 in cancer biology and therapeutics. *Oncogene* 2010;29:625–634.

162. Kroemer G, Pouyssegur J. Tumor cell metabolism: cancer's Achilles' heel. *Cancer Cell* 2008;13:472–482.

163. Potter V. The biochemical approach to the cancer problem. *Fed Proc* 1958;17:691–697.

164. Vander Heiden MG, Cantley LC, Thompson CB. Understanding the Warburg effect: the metabolic requirements of cell proliferation. *Science* 2009;324:1029–1033.

165. Semenza GL. Tumor metabolism: cancer cells give and take lactate. *J Clin Invest* 2008;118:3835–3837.

166. Nakajima EC, Van Houten B. Metabolic symbiosis in cancer: refocusing the Warburg lens. *Mol Carcinog* 2013;52:329–337.

167. Kennedy KM, Dewhirst MW. Tumor metabolism of lactate: the influence and therapeutic potential for MCT and CD147 regulation. *Future Oncol* 2010;6:127–148.

168. Feron O. Pyruvate into lactate and back: from the Warburg effect to symbiotic energy fuel exchange in cancer cells. *Radiother Oncol* 2009;92:329–333.

169. Magistretti PJ. Neuron-glia metabolic coupling and plasticity. *J Exp Biol* 2006;209:2304–2311.

170. Hardee ME, Dewhirst MW, Agarwal N, et al. Novel imaging provides new insights into mechanisms of oxygen transport in tumors. *Curr Mol Med* 2009;9:435–441.

171. Burnet FM. The concept of immunological surveillance. *Prog Exp Tumor Res* 1970;13:1–27.

172. Thomas L. On immuosurveillance in human cancer. *Yale J Biol Med* 1982;55:329–333.

173. Vajdic CM, van Leeuwen MT. Cancer incidence and risk factors after solid organ transplantation. *Int J Cancer* 2009;125:1747–1754.

174. Elinav E, Nowarski R, Thaiss CA, et al. Inflammation-induced cancer: crosstalk between tumours, immune cells and microorganisms. *Nat Rev Cancer* 2013;13:759–771.

175. Swann JB, Smyth MJ. Immune surveillance of tumors. *J Clin Invest* 2007;117:1137–1146.

176. Fridman WH, Mlecnik B, Bindea G, et al. Immunosurveillance in human non-viral cancers. *Curr Opin Immunol* 2011;23:272–278.

177. Galon J, Angell HK, Bedognetti D, et al. The continuum of cancer immunosurveillance: prognostic, predictive, and mechanistic signatures. *Immunity* 2013;39:11–26.

178. Kim R, Emi M, Tanabe K. Cancer immunoediting from immune surveillance to immune escape. *Immunology* 2007;121:1–14.

179. Smyth MJ, Dunn GP, Schreiber RD. Cancer immunosurveillance and immune-editing: the roles of immunity in suppressing tumor development and shaping tumor immunogenicity. *Adv Immunol* 2006;90:1–50.

180. Bindea G, Mlecnik B, Fridman WH, et al. Natural immunity to cancer in humans. *Curr Opin Immunol* 2010;22:215–222.

181. Ferrone C, Dranoff G. Dual roles for immunity in gastrointestinal cancers. *J Clin Oncol* 2010;28:4045–4051.

182. Nelson BH. The impact of T-cell immunity on ovarian cancer outcomes. *Immunol Rev* 2008;222:101–116.

183. Pagès F, Galon J, Dieu-Nosjean MC, et al. Immune infiltration in human tumors: a prognostic factor that should not be ignored. *Oncogene* 2010;29:1093–1102.

184. Strauss DC, Thomas JM. Transmission of donor melanoma by organ transplantation. *Lancet Oncol* 2010;11:790–796.

185. Yang L, Pang Y, Moses HL. TGF-beta and immune cells: an important regulatory axis in the tumor microenvironment and progression. *Trends Immunol* 2010;31:220–227.

186. Shields JD, Kourtis IC, Tomei AA, et al. Induction of lymphoidlike stroma and immune escape by tumors that express the chemokine CCL21. *Science* 2010;328:749–752.

187. Korman AJ, Peggs KS, Allison J. Checkpoint blockade in cancer immunotherapy. *Adv Immunol* 2006;90:297–339.

188. Fife BT, Pauken KE, Eagar TN, et al. Interactions between programmed death-1 and programmed death ligand-1 promote tolerance by blocking the T cell receptor-induced stop signal. *Nat Immunol* 2009;10:1185–1192.

189. Pardoll DM. The blockade of immune checkpoints in cancer immunotherapy. *Nat Rev Cancer* 2012;12:252–264.

190. Motz GT, Coukos G. Deciphering and reversing tumor immune suppression. *Immunity* 2013;39:61–73.

191. Gabrilovich DI, Nagaraj S. Myeloid-derived suppressor cells as regulators of the immune system. *Nat Rev Immunol* 2009;9:162–174.

192. Mougiakakos D, Choudhury A, Lladser A, et al. Regulatory T cells in cancer. *Adv Cancer Res* 2010;107:57–117.

193. Ostrand-Rosenberg S, Sinha P. Myeloid-derived suppressor cells: linking inflammation and cancer. *J Immunol* 2009;182:4499–4506.

194. Garraway LA, Lander ES. Lessons from the cancer genome. *Cell* 2013;153:17–37.

195. You JS, Jones PA. Cancer genetics and epigenetics: two sides of the same coin? *Cancer Cell* 2012;22:9–20.

196. Berdasco M, Esteller M. Aberrant epigenetic landscape in cancer: how cellular identity goes awry. *Dev Cell* 2010;19:698–711.

197. Esteller M. Cancer epigenomics: DNA methylomes and histone-modification maps. *Nat Rev Genet* 2007;8:286–298.

198. Jones PA, Baylin SB. The epigenomics of cancer. *Cell* 2007;128:683–692.

199. Negrini S, Gorgoulis VG, Halazoneitis TD. Genomic instability—an evolving hallmark of cancer. *Nat Rev Mol Cell Bio* 2010;11:220–228.

200. Loeb LA. A mutator phenotype in cancer. *Cancer Res* 2001;61:3230–3239.

201. Jackson SP, Bartek J. The DNA-damage response in human biology and disease. *Nature* 2009;461:1071–1078.

202. Kastan MB. DNA damage responses: mechanisms and roles in human disease. *Mol Cancer Res* 2008;6:517–524.

203. Sigal A, Rotter V. Oncogenic mutations of the p53 tumor suppressor: the demons of the guardian of the genome. *Cancer Res* 2000;60:6788–6793.

204. Lane DP. Cancer. p53, guardian of the genome. *Nature* 1992;358:15–16.

205. Kinzler KW, Vogelstein B. Cancer-susceptibility genes. Gatekeepers and caretakers. *Nature* 1997;386:761–763.

206. Ciccia A, Elledge SJ. The DNA damage response: making it safe to play with knives. *Mol Cell* 2010;40:179–204.

207. Harper JW, Elledge SJ. The DNA damage response: ten years after. *Mol Cell* 2007;28:739–745.

208. Friedberg EC, Aguilera A, Gellert M, et al. DNA repair: from molecular mechanism to human disease. *DNA Repair (Amst)* 2006;5:986–996.

209. Barnes DE, Lindahl T. Repair and genetic consequences of endogenous DNA base damage in mammalian cells. *Annu Rev Genet* 2004;38:445–476.

210. Korkola J, Gray JW. Breast cancer genomes—form and function. *Curr Opin Genet Dev* 2010;20:4–14.

211. Dvorak HF. Tumors: wounds that do not heal. Similarities between tumor stroma generation and wound healing. *N Engl J Med* 1986;315:1650–1659.

212. De Nardo DG, Andreu P, Coussens LM. Interactions between lymphocytes and myeloid cells regulate pro- versus anti-tumor immunity. *Cancer Metastasis Rev* 2010;29:309–316.

213. Hanahan D, Coussens LM. Accessories to the crime: functions of cells recruited to the tumor microenvironment. *Cancer Cell* 2012;21:309–322.

214. de Visser KE, Eichten A, Coussens LM. Paradoxical roles of the immune system during cancer development. *Nat Rev Cancer* 2006;6:24–37.

215. Servais C, Erez N. From sentinel cells to inflammatory culprits: cancer-associated fibroblasts in tumour-related inflammation. *J Pathol* 2013;229:198–207.

216. Dirat B, Bochet L, Escourrou G, et al. Unraveling the obesity and breast cancer links: a role for cancer-associated adipocytes? *Endocr Dev* 2010;19:45–52.

217. Pietras K, Ostman A. Hallmarks of cancer: interactions with the tumor stroma. *Exp Cell Res* 2010;316:1324–1331.

218. Räsänen K, Vaheri A. Activation of fibroblasts in cancer stroma. *Exp Cell Res* 2010;316:2713–2722.

219. Shimoda M, Mellody KT, Orimo A. Carcinoma-associated fibroblasts are a rate-limiting determinant for tumour progression. *Sem Cell Dev Biol* 2010;21:19–25.

220. Welti J, Loges S, Dimmeler S, et al. Recent molecular discoveries in angiogenesis and antiangiogenic therapies in cancer. *J Clin Invest* 2013;123:3190–3200.

PRINCIPLES OF ONCOLOGY

221. Pasquale EB. Eph receptors and ephrins in cancer: bidirectional signalling and beyond. *Nat Rev Cancer* 2010;10:165–180.

222. Ahmed Z, Bicknell R. Angiogenic signalling pathways. *Methods Mol Biol* 2009;467:3–24.

223. Dejana E, Orsenigo F, Molendini C, et al. Organization and signaling of endothelial cell-to-cell junctions in various regions of the blood and lymphatic vascular trees. *Cell Tissue Res* 2009;335:17–25.

224. Carmeliet P, Jain RK. Angiogenesis in cancer and other diseases. *Nature* 2000;407:249–257.

225. Ruoslahti E, Bhatia SN, Sailor MJ. Targeting of drugs and nanoparticles to tumors. *J Cell Biol* 2010;188:759–768.

226. Ruoslahti E. Specialization of tumour vasculature. *Nat Rev Cancer* 2002;2:83–90.

227. Motz GT, Coukos G. The parallel lives of angiogenesis and immunosuppression: cancer and other tales. *Nat Rev Immunol* 2011;11:702–711.

228. Carmeliet P, Jain RK. Principles and mechanisms of vessel normalization for cancer and other angiogenic diseases. *Nat Rev Drug Discov* 2011;10:417–427.

229. Tammela T, Alitalo K. Lymphangiogenesis: Molecular mechanisms and future promise. *Cell* 2010;140:460–476.

230. Card CM, Yu SS, Swartz MA. Emerging roles of lymphatic endothelium in regulating adaptive immunity. *J Clin Invest* 2014;124:943–952.

231. Gaengel K, Genové G, Armulik A, et al. Endothelial-mural cell signaling in vascular development and angiogenesis. *Arterioscler Thromb Vasc Biol* 2009;29:630–638.

232. Schäfer M, Werner S. Cancer as an overhealing wound: an old hypothesis revisited. *Nat Rev Mol Cell Biol* 2008;9:628–638.

233. Karin M, Lawrence T, Nizet V. Innate immunity gone awry: linking microbial infections to chronic inflammation and cancer. *Cell* 2006;124:823–835.

234. Coffeldt SB, Lewis CE, Naldini L, et al. Elusive identities and overlapping phenotypes of proangiogenic myeloid cells in tumors. *Am J Pathol* 2010;176:1564–1576.

235. Johansson M, Denardo DG, Coussens LM. Polarized immune responses differentially regulate cancer development. *Immunol Rev* 2008;222:145–154.

236. Mantovani A. Molecular pathways linking inflammation and cancer. *Curr Mol Med* 2010;10:369–373.

237. Mantovani A, Allavena P, Sica A, et al. Cancer-related inflammation. *Nature* 2008;454:436–444

238. DeNardo DG, Brennan DJ, Rexhepaj E, et al. Leukocyte complexity predicts breast cancer survival and functionally regulates response to chemotherapy. *Cancer Discov* 2011;1:54–67.

239. De Palma M, Coukos G, Hanahan D. A new twist on radiation oncology: low-dose irradiation elicits immunostimulatory macrophages that unlock barriers to tumor immunotherapy. *Cancer Cell* 2013;24:559–561.

240. Koh BI, Kang Y. The pro-metastatic role of bone marrow-derived cells: a focus on MSCs and regulatory T cells. *EMBO Rep* 2012;13:412–422.

241. Bergfeld SA, DeClerck YA. Bone marrow-derived mesenchymal stem cells and the tumor microenvironment. *Cancer Metastasis Rev* 2010;29:249–261.

242. Fang S, Salven P. Stem cells in tumor angiogenesis. *J Mol Cell Cardiol* 2011;50:290–295.

243. Giaccia AJ, Schipani E. Role of carcinoma-associated fibroblasts and hypoxia in tumor progression. *Curr Top Microbiol Immunol* 2010;345:31–45.

244. Labelle M, Hynes RO. The initial hours of metastasis: the importance of cooperative host-tumor cell interactions during hematogenous dissemination. *Cancer Discov* 2012;2:1091–1099.

245. Peinado H, Lavothskin S, Lyden D. The secreted factors responsible for premetastatic niche formation: old sayings and new thoughts. *Semin Cancer Biol* 2011;21:139–146.

246. Reya T, Morrison SJ, Clarke MF, et al. Stem cells, cancer, and cancer stem cells. *Nature* 2001;414:105–111.

247. Bonnet D, Dick JE. Human acute myeloid leukemia is organized as a hierarchy that originates from a primitive hematopoietic cell. *Nature Med* 1997;3:730–737.

248. Gilbertson RJ, Rich JN. Making a tumour's bed: glioblastoma stem cells and the vascular niche. *Nat Rev Cancer* 2007;7:733–736.

249. al-Hajj M, Wicha M, Benito-Hernandez A, et al. Prospective identification of tumorigenic breast cancer cells. *Proc Natl Acad Sci U S A* 2003;100:3983–3988.

250. Beck B, Blanpain C. Unravelling cancer stem cell potential. *Nat Rev Cancer* 2013;13:727–738.

251. Magee JA, Piskounova E, Morrison SJ. Cancer stem cells: impact, heterogeneity, and uncertainty. *Cancer Cell* 2012;21:283–296.

252. Cho RW, Clarke MF. Recent advances in cancer stem cells. *Curr Opin Genet Devel* 2008;18:1–6.

253. Lobo NA, Shimono Y, Qian D, et al. The biology of cancer stem cells. *Annu Rev Cell Dev Biol* 2007;23:675–699.

254. Meacham CE, Morrison SJ. Tumour heterogeneity and cancer cell plasticity. *Nature* 2013;501:328–337.

255. Singh A, Settleman J. EMT, cancer stem cells and drug resistance: an emerging axis of evil in the war on cancer. *Oncogene* 2010;29:4741–4751.

256. Brabletz T, Jung A, Spaderna S, et al. Opinion: migrating cancer stem cells – an integrated concept of malignant tumor progression. *Nat Rev Cancer* 2005;5:744–749.

257. Boiko AD, Razorenova OV, van de Rijn M, et al. Human melanoma-initiating cells express neural crest nerve growth factor receptor CD271. *Nature* 2010;466:133–137.

258. Gupta P, Chaffer CL, Weinberg RA. Cancer stem cells: mirage or reality? *Nature Med* 2009;15:1010–1012.

259. Quintana E, Shackleton M, Sabel MS, et al. Efficient tumour formation by single human melanoma cells. *Nature* 2008;456:593–598.

260. Chaffer CL, Brueckmann I, Scheel C, et al. Normal and neoplastic nonstem cells can spontaneously convert to stem-like state. *Proc Natl Acad Sci U S A* 2011;108:7950–7955.

261. Thiery JP, Sleeman JR. Complex networks orchestrate epithelial-mesenchymal transitions. *Nat Rev Mol Cell Biol* 2006;7:131–142.

262. Creighton CJ, Li X, Landis M, et al. Residual breast cancers after conventional therapy display mesenchymal as well as tumor-initiating features. *Proc Natl Acad Sci U S A* 2009;106:13820–13825.

263. Buck E, Eyzaguirre A, Barr S, et al. Loss of homotypic cell adhesion by epithelial-mesenchymal transition or mutation limits sensitivity to epidermal growth factor receptor inhibition. *Mol Cancer Therap* 2007;6:532–541.

264. Rhim AD, Mirek ET, Aiello NM, et al. EMT and dissemination precede pancreatic tumor formation. *Cell* 2012;148:349–361.

265. Soda Y, Marumoto T, Friedmann-Morvinski D, et al. Transdifferentiation of glioblastoma cells into vascular endothelial cells. *Proc Natl Acad Sci U S A* 2011;108:4274–4280.

266. El Hallani S, Boisselier B, Peglion F, et al. A new alternative mechanism in glioblastoma vascularization: tubular vasculogenic mimicry. *Brain* 2010;133:973–982.

267. Wang R, Chadalavada K, Wilshire J, et al. Glioblastoma stem-like cells give rise to tumour endothelium. *Nature* 2010;468:829–833.

268. Folkman J, Kalluri R. Cancer without disease. *Nature* 2004;427:787.

269. Azam F, Mehta S, Harris AL. Mechanisms of resistance to antiangiogenesis therapy. *Eur J Cancer* 2010;46:1323–1332.

270. Ebos JM, Lee CR, Kerbel RS. Tumor and host-mediated pathways of resistance and disease progression in response to antiangiogenic therapy. *Clin Cancer Res* 2009;15:5020–5025.

271. Bergers G, Hanahan D. Modes of resistance to anti-angiogenic therapy. *Nat Rev Cancer* 2008;8:592–603.

272. Ellis LM, Reardon DA. Cancer: the nuances of therapy. *Nature* 2009;458:290–292.

273. Norden AD, Drappatz J, Wen PY. Antiangiogenic therapies for high-grade glioma. *Nat Rev Neurol* 2009;5:610–620.

274. Verhoeff JJ, van Tellingen O, Claes A, et al. Concerns about anti-angiogenic treatment in patients with glioblastoma multiforme. *BMC Cancer* 2009;9:444.

275. Hanahan D. Rethinking the war on cancer. *Lancet* 2014;383:558–563.

276. Pencheva N, Tavazoie SF. Control of metastatic progression by microRNA regulatory networks. *Nat Cell Biol* 2013;15:546–554.

277. Garzon R, Marcucci G, Croce CM. Targeting microRNAs in cancer: rationale, strategies and challenges. *Nat Rev Drug Discov* 2010;9:775–789.

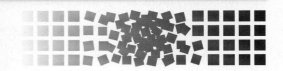

3 Molecular Methods in Cancer

Larissa V. Furtado, Jay L. Hess, and Bryan L. Betz

APPLICATIONS OF MOLECULAR DIAGNOSTICS IN ONCOLOGY

Molecular diagnostics is increasingly impacting a number of areas of cancer care delivery including diagnosis, prognosis, in predicting response to particular therapies, and in minimal residual disease monitoring. Each of these depends on detection or measurement of one or more disease-specific molecular biomarkers representing abnormalities in genetic or epigenetic pathways controlling cellular proliferation, differentiation, or cell death (Table 3.1). In addition, molecular diagnostics is beginning to play a role in predicting host metabolism of drugs—for example, in predicting fast versus slow thiopurine metabolizers using polymorphisms in the thiopurine methyltransferase (TPMT) allele and in use in dosing patients with thiopurine drugs.[1] Molecular diagnostics has also had a major impact on assessing an engraftment after bone marrow transplantation and in tissue typing for bone marrow and solid organ transplantation.

The ideal cancer biomarker is only associated with the disease and not the normal state. The utility of the biomarker largely depends on what the clinical effect the biomarker predicts for, how large the effect is, and how strong the evidence is for the effect. For clinical application, biomarkers need a high level of *analytic validity*, *clinical validity*, and *clinical utility*. Analytic validity refers to the ability of the overall testing process to accurately detect and, in many cases, measure the biomarker. Clinical validity is the ability of a biomarker to predict a particular disease behavior or response to therapy. Clinical utility, arguably the most difficult to assess, addresses whether the information available from the biomarker is actually beneficial for patient care.

Biomarkers can take many forms including *chromosomal translocations* and *other chromosomal rearrangements*, *gene amplification*, *copy number variation*, *point mutations*, *single nucleotide polymorphisms*, *changes in gene expression* (including micro RNAs), and *epigenetic alterations*. Most biomarkers in widespread use represent either gain of function or loss of function alterations in key signaling pathways. Those that occur early and at a high frequency in tumors tend to be *driver mutations*, whose function is important for the cancer cell's proliferation and/or survival. These are particularly useful as biomarkers because they often represent important therapeutic targets. However, cancer cells accumulate many genetic alterations, called *passenger mutations*, which tend to occur at a lower frequency overall and in a subset of a heterogeneous population of tumor cells that may contribute to the cancer phenotype but are not absolutely essential.[2] Distinguishing passenger from driver mutations using various functional assays has become a major focus of translational research in cancer. The same biomarker may have utility in a variety of settings. For example, the detection of the *BCR-ABL1* translocation, pathognomonic for chronic myelogenous leukemia (CML), is used for establishing the diagnosis, for the selection of therapy, and for monitoring for minimal residual disease during and after therapy.

Some of the most heavily used genetic biomarkers in cancer, particularly in hematologic malignancies, are *chromosomal translocations*. For certain diseases such as CML, detection of the *BCR-ABL1* translocation or in Burkitt lymphoma the immunoglobulin gene-*MYC* translocation is required, according to current World Health Organization (WHO) guidelines, to make the diagnosis. Identification of translocations is important in the diagnosis and subtyping of acute leukemias (e.g., detection of *PML-RARA* and variant translocations in acute promyelocytic leukemia) and is also extremely important for the diagnosis of sarcomas such as Ewing sarcoma. The discovery of chromosomal translocations, such as the *TMPRSS-ETS* in prostate cancer and *ALK* translocations in non–small-cell lung cancer, portends an importance of detecting translocations in solid tumors.[3] Chromosomal translocations, especially for hematologic malignancies, have been traditionally detected by classical karyotyping. This approach has limitations; in particular, it requires viable, dividing cells, which are often not readily available from solid tumor biopsies. In addition, a significant proportion of chromosomal translocations are not detectable by conventional karyotyping. For example, 5% to 10% of CML cases lack detectable t(9;22) by G banding. Such "cryptic" translocations require other approaches for detection, which are to be discussed, including *fluorescent in situ hybridization (FISH)*, *polymerase chain reaction (PCR)*, as well as *nucleic acid sequencing-based methods*.

In certain settings, it can be helpful to detect if a population of cells is clonal. For example, in some lymphoid infiltrates, the cells are well differentiated and it can be difficult to determine whether these represent a reactive or neoplastic infiltrate. If dispersed, cells are available and these could be analyzed by flow cytometer to detect whether a monotypic population expressing either immunoglobulin kappa or lambda light chains is present. In theory, immunohistochemical staining (IHC) for immunoglobulin light chains could be used to assess clonality; however, in practice this is done with more sensitivity using RNA in situ hybridization for immunoglobulin kappa and lambda light chain transcripts. The most sensitive way to detect clonality in a B-cell population is to analyze the size of the break point cluster region that arises as a result of VDJ recombination by *PCR*. Reactive B cells will show a distribution in the size of the VDJ recombination for the *IGH* or *IGK* or *IGL*, whereas clonal cells will show a predominant band that represents the size of the VDJ region of the dominant clone. Similarly, sometimes it can be difficult to distinguish neoplastic from reactive T-cell infiltrates. Given the large number of T-cell antigen receptors, it is not as simple to detect clonality by IHC or flow cytometry in T-cell proliferations. One approach is to use aberrant loss of T-cell antigen expression to aid in the diagnosis of T-cell neoplasms. Another is to detect clonal rearrangement of the VDJ region of the T-cell receptor gamma (*TCRγ*) gene, which can be done by PCR on both fresh and formalin-fixed paraffin-embedded (FFPE) tissue.

Gene amplification is another important mechanism in cancer that has been found to have high utility in a subset of cancers. *MYCN* amplification occurs in approximately 40% of undifferentiated or poorly differentiated neuroblastoma subtypes,[4,5] either appearing as double minute chromosomes or homogeneously

TABLE 3.1

Genomic Alterations as Putative Predictive Biomarkers for Cancer Therapy

Genes	Pathways	Aberration Type	Disease Examples	Putative or Proven Drugs
PIK3CA,[51,52] *PIK3R1*,[53] *PIK3R2, AKT1, AKT2*, and *AKT3*[54,55]	Phosphoinositide 3-kinase (PI3K)	Mutation or amplification	Breast, colorectal, and endometrial cancer	■ PI3K inhibitors ■ AKT inhibitors
PTEN[56]	PI3K	Deletion	Numerous cancers	■ PI3K inhibitors
MTOR,[57] *TSC1*,[58] and *TSC2*[59]	mTOR	Mutation	Tuberous sclerosis and bladder cancer	■ mTOR inhibitors
RAS family (*HRAS, NRAS, KRAS*), *BRAF*,[60] and *MEK1*	RAS–MEK	Mutation, rearrangement, or amplification	Numerous cancers, including melanoma and prostate cancers	■ RAF inhibitors ■ MEK inhibitors ■ PI3K inhibitors
Fibroblast growth factor receptor 1 (*FGFR1*), *FGFR2, FGFR3, FGFR4*[36]	FGFR	Mutation, amplification, or rearrangement	Myeloma, sarcoma, and bladder, breast, ovarian, lung, endometrial, and myeloid cancers	■ FGFR inhibitors ■ FGFR antibodies
Epidermal growth factor receptor (*EGFR*)	EGFR	Mutation, deletion, or amplification	Lung and gastrointestinal cancer	■ EGFR inhibitors ■ EGFR antibodies
ERBB2[61]	ERBB2	Amplification or mutation	Breast, bladder, gastric, and lung cancers	■ ERBB2 inhibitors ■ ERBB2 antibodies
SMO[62,63] and *PTCH1*[64]	Hedgehog	Mutation	Basal cell carcinoma	■ Hedgehog inhibitor
MET[65]	MET	Amplification or mutation	Bladder, gastric, and renal cancers	■ MET inhibitors ■ MET antibodies
JAK1, JAK2, JAK3,[66] *STAT1, STAT3*	JAK–STAT	Mutation or rearrangement	Leukemia and lymphoma	■ JAK–STAT inhibitors ■ STAT decoys
Discoidin domain-containing receptor 2 (*DDR2*)	RTK	Mutation	Lung cancer	■ Some tyrosine kinase inhibitors
Erythropoietin receptor (*EPOR*)	JAK–STAT	Rearrangement	Leukemia	■ JAK–STAT inhibitors
Interleukin-7 receptor (*IL-7R*)	JAK–STAT	Mutation	Leukemia	■ JAK–STAT inhibitors
Cyclin-dependent kinases (*CDKs*[67]; *CDK4, CDK6, CDK8*), *CDKN2A*, and cyclin D1 (*CCND1*)	CDK	Amplification, mutation, deletion, or rearrangement	Sarcoma, colorectal cancer, melanoma, and lymphoma	■ CDK inhibitors
ABL1	ABL	Rearrangement	Leukemia	■ ABL inhibitors
Retinoic acid receptor-α (*RARA*)	RARα	Rearrangement	Leukemia	■ All-trans retinoic acid
Aurora kinase A (*AURKA*)[68]	Aurora kinases	Amplification	Prostate and breast cancers	■ Aurora kinase inhibitors
Androgen receptor (*AR*)[69]	Androgen	Mutation, amplification, or splice variant	Prostate cancer	■ Androgen synthesis inhibitors ■ Androgen receptor inhibitors
FLT3[70]	FLT3	Mutation or deletion	Leukemia	■ FLT3 inhibitors
MET	MET–HGF	Mutation or amplification	Lung and gastric cancers	■ MET inhibitors
Myeloproliferative leukemia (*MPL*)	THPO, JAK–STAT	Mutation	Myeloproliferative neoplasms	■ JAK–STAT inhibitors
MDM2[71]	MDM2	Amplification	Sarcoma and adrenal carcinomas	■ MDM2 antagonist
KIT[72]	KIT	Mutation	GIST, mastocytosis, and leukemia	■ KIT inhibitors
PDGFRA and *PDGFRB*	PDGFR	Deletion, rearrangement, or amplification	Hematologic cancer, GIST, sarcoma, and brain cancer	■ PDGFR inhibitors
Anaplastic lymphoma kinase (*ALK*)[9,37,73,74]	ALK	Rearrangement or mutation	Lung cancer and neuroblastoma	■ ALK inhibitors

(continued)

TABLE 3.1

Genomic Alterations as Putative Predictive Biomarkers for Cancer Therapy *(continued)*

Genes	Pathways	Aberration Type	Disease Examples	Putative or Proven Drugs
RET	RET	Rearrangement or mutation	Lung and thyroid cancers	▪ RET inhibitors
ROS1[75]	ROS1	Rearrangement	Lung cancer and cholangiocarcinoma	▪ ROS1 inhibitors
NOTCH1 and *NOTCH2*	Notch	Rearrangement or mutation	Leukemia and breast cancer	▪ Notch signalling pathway inhibitors

PIK3CA, PI3K catalytic subunit-α; *PIK3R1*, PI3K regulatory subunit 1; *PI3K*, phosphoinositide 3-kinase; *AKT*, v-akt murine thymoma viral oncogene homolog; *PTEN*, phosphatase and tensin homolog; mTOR, mechanistic target of rapamycin; *TSC1*, tuberous sclerosis 1 protein; RAS–MEK, rat sarcoma; *MEK*, MAPK/ERK (mitogen-activated protein kinase/extracellular signal-regulated kinase) kinase; RAF, v-raf murine sarcoma viral oncogene homolog; *ERBB2*, also known as HER2; *SMO*, smoothened homolog; *PTCH1*, patched homolog; *MET*, hepatocyte growth factor receptor; *JAK*, Janus kinase; *THPO*, thrombopoietin; *STAT*, signal transducer and activator of transcription; RTK, receptor tyrosine kinase; *CDKN2A*, cyclin-dependent kinase inhibitor 2A; ABL, Abelson murine leukemia viral oncogene homolog 1; *FLT3*, FMS-like tyrosine kinase 3; *HGF*, hepatocyte growth factor; *MDM2*, mouse double minute 2; *KIT*, v-kit Hardy-Zuckerman 4 feline sarcoma viral oncogene homolog; GIST, gastrointestinal stromal tumor; PDGFR, platelet-derived growth factor receptor; *ROS1*, v-ros avian UR2 sarcoma virus oncogene homolog.
Reprinted by permission from Macmillan Publishers Limited: Nature Reviews Drug Discovery, Simon, R. and Rowchodhury, S. 12:358–369, 2013, ©2013.

staining regions. *MYCN* amplification is a very strong predictor of poor outcomes, particularly in patients with localized (stage 1 or stage 2) disease or in infants with stage 4S metastatic disease, where fewer than half of patients survive beyond 5 years.[6]

Use of *other chromosome abnormalities* has been largely limited to the diagnosis and prognostication of hematologic disorders. Roughly half of all myelodysplastic disorders show cytogenetically detectable chromosomal abnormalities, such as monosomy 5 or 7, partial chromosomal loss (5q-, 7q-), or complex chromosomal abnormalities. Certain abnormalities in isolation (e.g., 5q-) have a favorable prognosis, whereas many others (e.g., "complex" karyotypes with three or more abnormalities) carry a worse prognosis. Differences in ploidy have proven to be useful predictors in pediatric acute lymphocytic leukemia (ALL), with hyperdiploid cases (>50 chromosomes) showing a distinctly more favorable course compared with hypodiploid or near diploid cases.[7] Overall, DNA ploidy can be assessed by flow cytometry. Specific chromosomal copy number alterations can be detected by *conventional karyotyping*, *array hybridization methods*, or *FISH*.

Copy number variation (CNV) represents the most common type of structural chromosomal alteration. Regions affected by CNVs range from approximately 1 kilobase to several megabases that are either amplified or deleted. It is estimated that about 0.4% of the genomes of healthy individuals differ in copy number.[8] CNVs resulting in deletion of genes such as *BRCA1, BRCA2, APC*, mismatch repair genes, and *TP53* have been implicated in a wide range of highly penetrant cancers.[9,10] CNVs can be detected by a variety of means including *FISH, comparative or array genomic hybridization*, or *virtual karyotyping* using *single nucleotide polymorphism (SNP) arrays*. Increasingly, CNV is detected using *next-generation sequencing*.

Large-scale sequencing of tumors has identified many *mutations* that are of potential prognostic and therapeutic significance. As will be discussed further, a wide range of strategies is available for the detection of point mutations (Fig. 3.1). It is important to

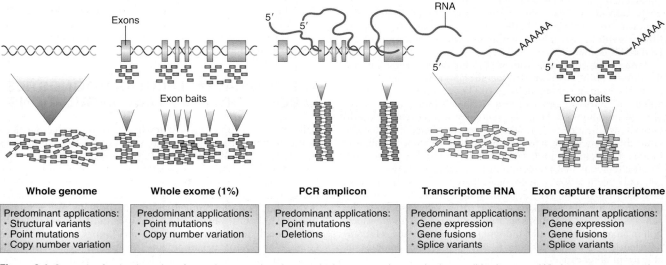

Whole genome	Whole exome (1%)	PCR amplicon	Transcriptome RNA	Exon capture transcriptome
Predominant applications: • Structural variants • Point mutations • Copy number variation	Predominant applications: • Point mutations • Copy number variation	Predominant applications: • Point mutations • Deletions	Predominant applications: • Gene expression • Gene fusions • Splice variants	Predominant applications: • Gene expression • Gene fusions • Splice variants

Figure 3.1 Strategies for the detection of mutations, translocations, and other structural genomic abnormalities in cancer. Whole genome sequencing, which involves determining the entire sequence of both introns and exons, is not only the most comprehensive, but also the most laborious and expensive approach. Exome sequencing uses *baits* to capture either the entire exome (roughly 20,000 genes [about 1% of the genome]) or else a subset of genes of interest. Amplicon-based sequencing uses PCR or other amplification techniques to amplify targets of interest for sequencing. Transcriptome sequencing, also known as RNAseq, is based on sequencing expressed RNA and can be used to detect not only mutations, but also translocations, other structural abnormalities, as well as differences in expression levels. This can be combined with exome capture techniques for a higher sensitivity analysis of genes of particular interest. (Reprinted by permission from Macmillan Publishers Limited: Nature Reviews Drug Discovery, Simon, R. and Rowchodhury, S. 12:358–369, 2013, ©2013.)

recognize that many nucleotide variations occur at any given allele in populations. Formally, the term *polymorphism* is used to describe genetic differences present in ≥1% of the human population, whereas *mutation* describes less frequent differences. However, in practice, *polymorphism* is often used to describe a nonpathogenic genetic change, and mutation a deleterious change, regardless of their frequencies.

Mutations can be classified according to their effect in the structure of a gene. The most common of these disease-associated alterations are single nucleotide substitutions (point mutations); however, many deletions, insertions, gene rearrangements, gene amplification, and copy number variations have been identified that have clinical significance. Point mutations may affect promoters, splicing sites, or coding regions. Coding region mutations can be classified into three kinds, depending on the impact on the codon: *missense mutation*, a nucleotide change leads to the substitution of an amino acid to another; *nonsense mutation*, a nucleotide substitution causes premature termination of codons with protein truncation; and *silent mutation*, a nucleotide change does not change the coded amino acid.

Loss of function mutations, either through point mutations or deletions in tumor suppression genes such as *APC* and *TP53*, are the most common mutations in cancers. Tumor suppression genes require two-hit (biallelic) mutations that inactivate both copies of the gene in order to allow tumorigenesis to occur. The first hit is usually an inherited or somatic point mutation, and the second hit is assumed to be an acquired deletion mutation that deletes the second copy of the tumor suppression gene. Promoter methylation of tumor suppressor genes is an alternative route to tumorigenesis that, to date, has not been commonly employed for molecular diagnostics.

Oncogenes originate from the deregulation of genes that normally encode for proteins associated with cell growth, differentiation, apoptosis, and signal transduction (proto-oncogenes, [e.g., *BRAF* and *KRAS*]). Proto-oncogenes generally require only one gain of function or activating mutation to become oncogenic. Common mutation types that result in proto-oncogene activation include point mutations, gene amplifications, and chromosomal translocations. One example is mutations in the epidermal growth factor receptor (*EGFR*) that occur in lung cancer, which are almost exclusively seen in nonmucinous bronchoalveolar carcinomas. Somatic mutations of *EGFR* constitutively activate the receptor tyrosine kinase (TK). Importantly, responsiveness of tumors harboring these mutations to the inhibitor gefitinib is highly coordinated with a mutation of the EGFR TK domain.[11,12]

One of the challenges with using mutations as biomarkers is that there can be many nucleotide alterations that affect a given gene. For example, there are over 100 known different point mutations in *EGFR* reported in non–small-cell lung cancer. Many of these mutations occur at low frequency and have an unknown clinical significance.[13,14] Another important concept is that the same driver oncogene may be mutated in a variety of different tumors. For example, lung cancers harbor a number of other different alterations that are common in other solid tumors, which generally occur at lower frequencies than *EGFR* mutations such as *KRAS*, *BRAF*, and *HER2*. Some lung cancers have translocations involving the *ALK* kinase gene. *ALK*, interestingly, is also activated by point mutations in a neuroblastoma as by translocation in anaplastic large cell lymphoma (Fig. 3.2). Hence, a therapy targeted to a genetic alteration in one cancer may demonstrate efficacy in other cancers.

The detection of mutations is also important in the evaluation of chemotherapy resistance. Roughly a third of CML patients are resistant to the frontline ABL1 kinase inhibitor imatinib, either at the time of initial treatment or, more commonly, secondarily. In cases of primary failure or secondary failure, over 100 different *ABL1* mutations have been identified, including particularly common ones such as T315I and P loop mutations. While some

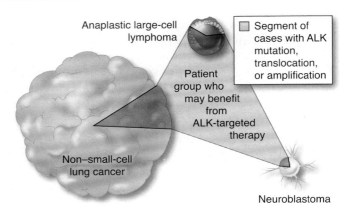

Figure 3.2 Activating genomic alterations occur in a variety of tumor types. *ALK* translocations, mutations, and amplifications occur in non–small-cell lung cancer, neuroblastomas, and in anaplastic large cell lymphomas. Such recurrent alterations in cancer, together with effective inhibitors of these pathways, are transforming oncologic therapies from organ-specific to pathway-specific interventions and are driving the use of molecular diagnostics in a wider range of tumor types. (Modified from McDermott, U. and Settleman, J. *J Clin Oncol* 2009;27:5650–5659.)

mutations, such as Y253H, respond to second generation TK inhibitors (TKI), others, such as the T315I mutation, are noteworthy because they confer resistance not only to imatinib, but also to nilotinib and dasatinib.

Mutations are also used as important predictive biomarkers (Table 3.1). Two of the most notable examples are the use of the *BRCA1* and *BRCA2* mutation analysis for women with a strong family history of breast cancer. Over 200 mutations (loss of function point mutations, small deletions, or insertions) occur in *BRCA* genes, which are distributed across the genes necessitating full sequencing for their detection. The overall prevalence of these occur in about 0.1% of the general population.[15,16] The lifetime risk of breast cancer for women carrying *BRCA1* mutations is in the range of 47% to 66%, whereas for *BRCA2* mutations, it is in the range of 40% to 57%.[17,18] In addition, the risk of other tumors including ovarian, fallopian, and pancreatic cancer is also increased. Detection of *BRCA1* and *BRCA2* mutations is, therefore, important for cancer prevention and risk reduction.

THE CLINICAL MOLECULAR DIAGNOSTICS LABORATORY: RULES AND REGULATIONS

Laboratories in the United States that perform molecular diagnostic testing are categorized as high-complexity laboratories under the Clinical Laboratory Improvement Amendments of 1988 (CLIA).[19] The CLIA program sets the minimum administrative and technical standards that must be met in order to ensure quality laboratory testing. Most laboratories in the United States that perform clinical testing in humans are regulated under CLIA. CLIA-certified laboratories must be accredited by professional organizations such as the Joint Commission, the College of American Pathologists, or another agency officially approved by the Centers for Medicare & Medicaid Services (CMS), and must comply with CLIA standards and guidelines for quality assurance. Although the regulation of laboratory services is in the U.S. Food and Drug Administration's (FDA) jurisdiction, the FDA has historically exercised enforcement discretion. Therefore, FDA approval is not currently required for clinical implementation of molecular tests as long as other regulations are met.[20,21]

SPECIMEN REQUIREMENTS FOR MOLECULAR DIAGNOSTICS

Samples typically received for molecular oncology testing include blood, bone marrow aspirates and biopsies, fluids, organ-specific fresh tissues in saline or tissue culture media such as Roswell Park Memorial Institute (RPMI), FFPE tissues, and cytology cell blocks. Molecular tests can be ordered electronically or through written requisition forms, but never through verbal requests only. All samples submitted for molecular testing need to be appropriately identified. Sample type, quantity, and specimen handling and transport requirements should conform to the laboratory's stated requirements in order to ensure valid test results.

Blood and bone marrow samples should be drawn into anticoagulated tubes. The preferred anticoagulant for most molecular assays is ethylenediaminetetraacetic acid (EDTA; lavender). Other acceptable collection tubes include ACD (yellow) solutions A and B. Heparinized tubes are not preferred for most molecular tests because heparin inhibits the polymerase enzyme utilized in PCR, which may lead to assay failure. Blood and bone marrow samples can be transported at ambient temperature. Blood samples should never be frozen prior to separation of cellular elements because this causes hemolysis, which interferes with DNA amplification. Fluids should be transported on ice. Tissues should be frozen (preferred method) as soon as possible and sent on dry ice to minimize degradation. Fresh tissues in RPMI should be sent on ice or cold packs. Cells should be kept frozen and sent on dry ice; DNA samples can be sent at ambient temperature or on ice.

For FFPE tissue blocks, typical collection and handling procedures include cutting 4 to 6 microtome sections of 10-micron thickness each on uncoated slides, air-drying unstained sections at room temperature, and staining one of the slides with hematoxylin and eosin (H&E). A board-certified pathologist reviews the H&E slides to ensure the tissue block contains a sufficient quantity of neoplastic tumor cells, and circles an area on the H&E slide that will be used as a template to guide macrodissection or microdissection of the adjacent, unstained slides. The pathologist also provides an estimate of the percentage of neoplastic cells in the area that will be tested, which should exceed the established limit of detection (LOD) of the assay.

MOLECULAR DIAGNOSTICS TESTING PROCESS

The workflow of a molecular test begins with receipt and accessioning of the specimen in the clinical molecular diagnostics laboratory followed by extraction of the nucleic acid (DNA or RNA), test setup, detection of analyte (e.g., PCR products), data analysis, and result reporting to the patient medical record (Fig. 3.3).

An extraction of intact, moderately high-quality DNA is essential for molecular assays. For DNA extraction, the preferred age for blood, bone marrow, and fluid samples is less than 5 days; for frozen or fixed tissue, it is indefinite; and for fresh tissue, it is overnight. Although there is no age limit for the use of a fixed and embedded tissue specimen for analysis, older specimens may yield a lower quantity and quality of DNA. Because RNA is significantly more labile than DNA, the preferred age for blood and bone marrow is less than 48 hours (from time of collection). Tissue samples intended for an RNA analysis should be promptly processed in fresh state, snap frozen, or preserved with RNA stabilizing agents for transport.

Dedicated areas, equipment, and materials are designated for various stages of DNA and RNA extraction procedures. DNA and RNA isolation can be done by manual or automated methods. Currently, most clinical laboratories employ commercial protocols based on liquid- or solid-phase extractions. Nucleated cells are isolated from biological samples prior to nucleic acid extraction.

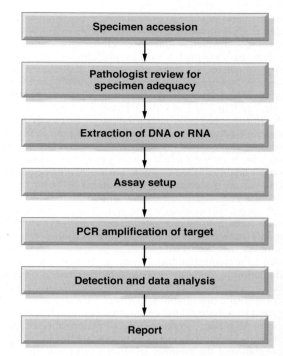

Figure 3.3 Simplified workflow of clinical molecular diagnostic testing.

White blood cells (WBC) can be isolated from blood and bone marrow samples by different methods. One method involves lysing the red blood cells with an ammonium chloride solution, which yields the total WBC population and other nucleated cells present. Another method involves a gradient preparation with a Ficoll solution, which yields the mononuclear cell population only. Sections of FFPE tissue blocks are prepared for DNA extraction by first removing the paraffin and disrupting the cell membranes with proteinase K digestion. Fresh and frozen tissues also undergo proteinase K digestion prior to nucleic acid extraction. DNA isolation protocols consist of several steps, including cell lysis, DNA purification by salting out the proteins and other debris (nonorganic method), or by solvent extractions of the proteins with phenol and chloroform solutions (organic method). The DNA is then precipitated out of the solution with isopropanol or ethanol. The pellet is washed with 70% to 80% ethanol and then solubilized in buffer, such as Tris-EDTA solution. Proteinase K can be added to assist in the disruption and to prevent nonspecific degradation of the DNA. RNase is sometimes added to eliminate contaminating RNA. The DNA yield is quantitated spectrophotometrically, and the DNA sample integrity is visually checked, if necessary, on an agarose gel followed by ethidium bromide staining. Intact DNA appears as a high–molecular-weight single band, whereas degraded DNA is identified as a smear of variably sized fragments. After extraction, the DNA is stored at 4°C prior to use in a PCR assay, and is then stored at −70°C after completion of the assay. Because the DNA extracted from formalin-fixed tissue is degraded to a variable extent, an analysis of the extraction product by gel electrophoresis is not informative. Yield and integrity of the extracted DNA is best assessed by an amplification control to ensure that the quality and quantity of input DNA is adequate to yield a valid result.

RNA isolation steps are similar to the ones described previously for DNA extraction. However, RNA is inherently less stable than DNA due to its single-strand conformation and susceptibility to degradation by RNase, which is ubiquitous in the environment. To ensure preservation of target RNA, special precautions are required, including the use of diethylpyrocarbonate (DEPC) water in all reagents used in RNA procedures, and special decontamination of work area and pipettes to prevent RNase contamination. The extracted RNA is usually degraded to a variable extent so that the analysis of the extraction product by gel electrophoresis is not informative. The quality of the RNA and its suitability for use in a reverse transcriptase polymerase chain reaction (RT-PCR)–based assay is assessed most appropriately by the demonstration of a positive result in an assay designed to detect the RNA transcripts for a "housekeeping gene," such as *ABL1* or *GAPDH*. Any RNA sample in which the 260/280-nm absorption ratio is below 1.9 or greater than 2.0 may contain contaminants and must be cleaned prior to analysis.

Following nucleic acid extraction, the assay is set up according to written procedures established during validation/verification of the assay by qualified laboratory staff. Dedicated areas, equipment, and materials are designated for various stages of the test (e.g., extraction, pre-PCR and post-PCR for amplification-based assays). For each molecular oncology test, appropriated positive and negative control specimens are included to each run as a matter of routine quality assessment. A no template (blank) control, containing the complete reaction mixture except for nucleic acids, is also included in amplification-based assays to evaluate for amplicon contamination in the assay reagents that may lead to inaccurate results. The controls are processed in the same manner as patient samples to ensure that established performance characteristics are being met for each step of the assay (extraction, amplification, and detection). All assay controls and overall performance of the run must be examined prior to interpretation of sample results. Following acceptance of the controls, results are electronically entered into reports. The final report is reviewed and signed by the laboratory director or a qualified designee who meets the same qualifications as the director, as defined by CLIA (see previous).

TECHNOLOGIES

Several traditional and emerging techniques are currently available for mutation detection in cancer (Table 3.2). In the era of personalized medicine, molecular oncology assays are rapidly moving from a mutational analysis of single genes toward a multigene panel analysis. As the number of "actionable" mutations such as *ALK*, *EGFR*, *BRAF*, and others increase, the use of next-generation sequencing platforms is expected to become much more widespread. Both traditional and emerging testing approaches have advantages and disadvantages that need to be balanced before a test platform is implemented into practice.

An important consideration when adding a new oncology test in the clinical laboratory menu is to define the intended use of the assay (e.g., diagnosis, prognosis, prediction of therapy response). The clinical utility of the assay, appropriate types of specimens, the spectrum of possible mutations that can be found in the genomic region of interest, and available methods for testing should also be determined. The laboratory director and ordering physicians should also discuss the estimated test volume, optimal reporting format, and required turnaround time for the proposed new test.[21–23]

Polymerase Chain Reaction

Polymerase chain reaction (PCR)[24,25] is widely used in all molecular diagnostics laboratories for the rapid amplification of targeted DNA sequences. The reaction includes the specimen template DNA, forward and reverse primers (18 to 24 oligonucleotides long), Taq DNA polymerase, and each of the four nucleotides bases (dATP, dTTP, dCTP, dGTP). During PCR, selected genomic sequences undergo repetitive temperature cycling (sequential heat and cooling) that allows for *denaturation* of double-stranded DNA template, *annealing* of the primers to the targeted complementary sequences on the template, and *extension* of new strands of DNA by Taq polymerase from nucleotides, using the primers as the starting point. Each cycle doubles the copy number of PCR

templates for the next round of polymerase activity, resulting in an exponential amplification of the selected target sequence. The PCR products (amplicons) are detected by electrophoresis or in real-time systems simultaneously to the amplification reaction (see real-time PCR, which follows).

PCR is specifically designed to work on DNA templates because the Taq polymerase does not recognize RNA as a starting material. Nonetheless, PCR can be adapted to RNA testing by including a reverse transcription step to convert a RNA sequence into its cognate cDNA sequence before the PCR reaction is performed (see reverse-transcription PCR, which follows). Multiplex PCR reactions can also be designed with multiple primers for simultaneous amplification of multiple genomic targets. PCR is a highly sensitive and specific technique that can be employed in different capacities for the detection of point mutations, small deletions, insertions and duplications, as well as gene rearrangements and clonality assessment. Limits of detection can reach 0.1% mutant allele or lower, which is important for the detection of somatic mutations in oncology because tumor specimens are usually composed of a mixture of tumor and normal cells. Reverse transcription PCR can also be used for the relative quantification of target RNA in minimal residual disease testing, such as *BCR-ABL1* transcripts in CML. Another advantage of PCR is its ability to amplify small amounts of low quality FFPE-derived DNA. However, applications of PCR can be limited because it cannot amplify across large or highly repetitive genomic regions. Also, the PCR reaction can be inhibited by heparin or melanin if present in the extracted DNA, which may lead to assay failure. Finally, the risk of false positives due to specimen or amplicon contamination is an important issue when using PCR-based techniques; therefore, stringent laboratory procedures, as described previously, are used to minimize contamination. With the exception of hybridization assays, such as fluorescence in situ hybridization and genomic microarrays, PCR is the necessary initial step in all current molecular oncology assays.

Targeted Mutation Analysis Methods

Real-Time PCR (q-PCR)

In real-time PCR (q-PCR), the polymerase chain reaction is performed with a PCR reporter that is usually a fluorescent double-stranded DNA binding dye or a fluorescent reporter probe. The intensity of the fluorescence produced at each amplification cycle is monitored in real time, and both quantification and detection of targeted sequences is accomplished in the reaction tube as the PCR amplification proceeds.

The intensity of the fluorescent signal for a given DNA fragment (wild type or mutant) is correlated with its quantity, based on the PCR cycle in which the fluorescence rises above the background (crossing threshold [Ct] or crossing point [Cp]).[26] The Ct value can be used for qualitative or quantitative analysis. Qualitative assays use the Ct as a cutoff for determining "presence" or "absence" of a given target in the reaction. A qualitative analysis by q-PCR is particularly useful for a targeted detection of point mutations that are located in mutational hotspots. Examples include the *JAK2* V617F mutation, which is located within exon 14, and is found in several myeloproliferative neoplasms (polycythemia vera, essential thrombocythemia, and primary myelofibrosis),[27] and the *BRAF* V600E,[28] which is located within exon 15, and is found in various cancer types including melanomas and thyroid and lung cancers.

For a quantitative analysis, the Ct of standards with known template concentration is used to generate a standard curve to which Ct values of unknown samples are compared. The concentration of the unknown samples is then extrapolated from values from the standard curve. The quantity of amplicons produced in a PCR reaction is proportional to the prevalence of the targeted sequence;

TABLE 3.2

Molecular Methods in Oncology

Method	Advantages	Disadvantages	Analytic Sensitivity	Examples of Applications in Oncology
Real-time PCR (q-PCR) Allele-specific PCR (AS-PCR) Reverse transcriptase PCR (RT-PCR)	Flexible platforms that permit detection of a variety of conserved hotspot mutations including nucleotide substitutions, small length mutations (deletions, insertions), and translocations High sensitivity is beneficial for residual disease testing and specimens with limited tumor content Adaptable to quantitative assays	Detects only specific targeted mutations/ chromosomal translocations Not suitable for variable mutations May not determine the exact change in nucleotide sequence	Very high	*KRAS, BRAF,* and *EGFR* mutations in solid tumors *JAK2* V617F and *MPL* mutations in myeloproliferative neoplasms *KIT* D816V mutation in systemic mastocytosis and AML Quantitation of *BCR-ABL1* and *PML-RARA* transcripts for residual disease monitoring in CML and APL, respectively
Fragment analysis	Detects small to medium insertions and deletions Detects variable insertions and deletions regardless of specific alteration Provides semiquantitative information regarding mutation level	Does not determine the exact change in nucleotide sequence Does not detect single nucleotide substitution mutations Limited multiplex capability	High	*NPM1* insertion mutations in AML *FLT3* internal tandem duplications in AML *JAK2* exon 12 insertions and deletions in PV *EGFR* exon 19 deletions in NSCLC
FISH	Detects chromosomal translocation, gene amplification, and deletion Morphology of tumor is preserved, allowing for a more accurate interpretation of heterogeneous samples	High cost Unable to detect small insertions and deletions Limited multiplex capability Does not determine the exact breakpoint and change in nucleotide sequence	High	*IGH/BCL2* translocation detection in follicular lymphoma and in a subset of diffuse large B-cell lymphoma *ALK* translocation in NSCLC *EWSR1* translocation in soft tissue tumors *HER2* amplification in breast cancer 1p/19q deletion in oligodendroglioma
High-resolution melting (HRM) curve analysis	Qualitative detection of variable single nucleotide substitutions and small insertions and deletions	Does not determine the exact mutation Result interpretation may require testing via an alternate technology Limited multiplex capability	Medium	*KRAS* and *BRAF* mutations in solid tumors *JAK2* exon 12 mutations in PV
Sanger sequencing	Detects variable single nucleotide substitutions and small insertions and deletions Provides semiquantitative information about mutation level Current gold standard for mutation detection	Low throughput Low analytic sensitivity limits application in specimens with low tumor burden Does not detect copy number changes or large (>500 bp) insertions and deletions	Low	*KIT* mutations in GIST and melanoma *CEBPA* mutations in AML *EGFR* mutations in NSCLC
Pyrosequencing	Higher analytical sensitivity than Sanger sequencing Detects variable single nucleotide substitutions and small insertions and deletions Provides quantitative information about mutation level	Short read lengths limit analysis to mutational hotspots Low throughput	Medium	*KRAS* and *BRAF* mutations in solid tumors
Single nucleotide extension assay (SNaPshot)	Simultaneous detection of targeted nucleotide substitution mutations Multiplex capability	Detects only targeted mutations	High	Small gene panels (3–10) for melanoma, NSCLC, breast cancer, and metastatic colorectal cancer

(continued)

PRINCIPLES OF ONCOLOGY

TABLE 3.2

Molecular Methods in Oncology *(continued)*

Method	Advantages	Disadvantages	Analytic Sensitivity	Examples of Applications in Oncology
Next-generation sequencing (NGS)	Quantitative detection of variable single nucleotide substitutions, small insertions and deletions, chromosomal translocations, and gene copy number variations Highly multiplexed High throughput	Requires costly investment in instrumentation and bioinformatics Technology is rapidly evolving Higher error rates for insertion and deletion mutations Limited ability to sequence GC-rich regions	High	Small to large gene panels (3–500) for solid tumor and hematologic malignancies
Genomic microarray	Simultaneous detection of copy number variation and LOH (SNP array)	Limited application to FFPE tissue Does not detect balanced translocations May not detect low-level mutant allele burden	Medium	Analysis of recurrent copy number variation and LOH in chronic lymphocytic leukemia and myeloproliferative neoplasms

AML, acute myelogenous leukemia; CML, chronic myelogenous leukemia; APL, acute promyelocytic leukemia; PV, polycythemia vera; NSCLC, non–small-cell lung carcinoma; GIST, gastrointestinal stromal tumor; GC, guanine-cytosine; LOH, loss of heterozygosity; FFPE, formalin-fixed paraffin-embedded.

therefore, samples with a higher template concentration reaches the Ct at earlier PCR cycles than one with a low concentration of the amplified target. Quantitative q-PCR has high analytical sensitivity for the detection of low mutant allele burden. For that reason, this method has been widely utilized for monitoring minimal residual disease.

Allele-Specific PCR

Allele-specific PCR (AS-PCR) is a variant of conventional PCR. The method is based on the principle that Taq polymerase is incapable of catalyzing chain elongation in the presence of a mismatch between the 3′ end of the primer and the template DNA. Selective amplification by AS-PCR is achieved by designing a forward primer that matches the mutant sequence at the 3′ end primer. A second mismatch within the primer can be introduced at the adjacent -1 or -2 position to decrease the efficiency of mismatched amplification products. This will minimize the chance of amplifying and, therefore, detecting the wild-type target. AS-PCR is usually performed as two PCR reactions: one employing a forward primer specific for the mutant sequence, the other using a forward primer specific for the correspondent wild-type sequence. In this case, a common reverse primer is used for both reactions. Following amplification, the PCR products are detected by electrophoresis (capillary or agarose gel) or in q-PCR systems. The detection of adequate PCR product in the wild-type amplification reaction is important to control for adequate specimen quality and quantity, particularly when the specimen is negative in the mutation-specific PCR reaction.

AS-PCR is particularly useful for the detection of targeted point mutations. Multiplex AS-PCR reactions can be designed for the simultaneous detection of multiple mutations by including several mutation-specific primers. The method has high analytical sensitivity and specificity and can be easily deployed in most clinical laboratories. However, an important limitation is that this approach will not detect mutations other than those for which specific primers are designed. Therefore, it is utilized for highly recurrent mutations that occur at specific locations within genes, rather than for the detection of variable mutations that may occur throughout a gene.

Examples of AS-PCR applications in oncology include the detection of *JAK2* V617F and *MPL* mutations in myeloprolifera-

tive neoplasms (primary myelofibrosis, essential thrombocythemia, and/or polycythemia vera),[29] the *BRAF* V600E mutation,[30] and *KIT* D816V mutations in cases of systemic mastocytosis and in acute myelogenous leukemia (AML).

Reverse Transcriptase PCR

RT-PCR is utilized for the detection and quantification of RNA transcripts. The first step for all amplification-based assays that use RNA as a starting material is reverse transcription of RNA into cDNA, because RNA is not a suitable substrate for Taq polymerase. In RT-PCR, RNA is isolated and reverse transcribed into cDNA by using a reverse transcriptase enzyme and one of the following: (1) random hexamer primers, which anneal randomly to RNA and reverse transcribe all RNA in the cell; (2) oligo dT primers, which anneal to the polyA tail of mRNA and reverse transcribe only mRNA; or (3) gene-specific primers that reverse transcribe only the target of interest. PCR is subsequently performed on the cDNA with forward and reverse primers specific to the gene(s) of interest. The RT-PCR products may then be analyzed by capillary electrophoresis or in real-time systems as in a standard PCR reaction.

RT-PCR is commonly used for detecting gene fusions during translocation analysis because breakpoints frequently occur within the intron of each partner gene and the precise intronic breakpoint locations may be variable. This variability complicates the design of primers used in DNA-based PCR assays. RT-PCR tests are advantageous because mature mRNA has intronic sequence spliced out, allowing for simplified primer design within the affected exon of each partner gene. In this setting, RT-PCR is useful in tests where both translocation partners are recurrent and only one or a few exons are involved in each partner gene. For instance, 95% of acute promyelocytic leukemia (APL) cases harbor the reciprocal t(15;17) chromosomal translocation and these breakpoints always occur within intron 2 of the *RARA* gene. By contrast, three distinct chromosome 15 breakpoints are involved, all occurring within the *PML* gene: intron 6, exon 6, and intron 3. Because the breakpoints in the two genes are recurrent, most of the reported *PML-RARA* fusions can be detected by targeting these three transcript isoforms.

RT-PCR is the method of choice when high sensitivity is required to detect gene translocations. For example, *PML-RARA*

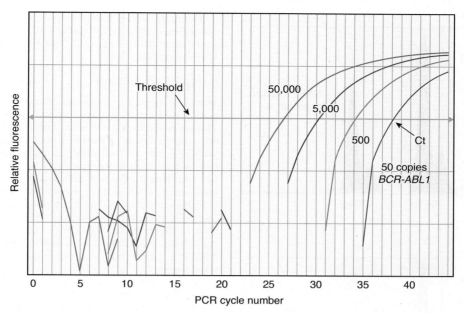

Figure 3.4 Reverse transcriptase PCR (RT-PCR) is a sensitive means to detect *BCR-ABL1* fusion transcripts in CML. RT-PCR can be combined with real-time PCR (q-PCR) to quantitate *BCR-ABL1* transcripts across four to six log range levels. Amplification products are detected during each PCR cycle using a fluorescent probe specific to the PCR product. The accumulated fluorescence in log(10) value is plotted against the number of PCR cycles. For a given specimen, the PCR cycle number is measured when the increase in fluorescence is exponential and exceeds a threshold. This point is called the Ct, which is inversely proportional to the amount of PCR target in the specimen (i.e., lower Ct values indicate a greater amount of target). Calibration standards of known quantity are used in standard curves to calculate the amount of target in a tested specimen. These are shown in the chart as different colored plots. Note that PCR increases the amount of amplification product by a factor of two with each PCR cycle. Therefore, specimens that produce a Ct value that is one cycle lower are expected to have a twofold higher concentration of target. Specimens that differ in target concentration by a factor of 10 (as shown) are expected to have a Ct value 3.3 cycles apart ($2^{3.3} = 10$).

transcript detection by RT-PCR can detect this fusion transcript down to 1 tumor cell in the background of 100,000 normal cells. Detecting low levels of fusion transcript can reveal relapse after consolidation and guide further treatment.[31] RT-PCR can also be used to quantitate the amount of expression of a gene. One major application of RT-PCR in this setting includes quantitative detection of *BCR-ABL1* fusion transcript for prognostication and minimal residual disease testing in CML (Fig. 3.4). In this setting, a three log decrease in *BCR-ABL1* levels is associated with an improved outcome.[32,33]

Fragment Analysis

A fragment analysis is a PCR amplicon-sizing technique that is relevant for the detection of small- to medium-length–affecting mutations (deletions, insertions, and duplications). This is typically performed by capillary electrophoresis, which is capable of resolving length mutations from approximately 1 to 500 base pairs in size.

Fragment analysis represents a practical strategy because it enables comprehensive detection of a wide variety of possible length mutations and has high analytic sensitivity. Further, it can provide semiquantitative information regarding the relative amount of mutated alleles. Limitations of this approach include the inability to objectively quantitate mutant allele burdens, the inability to determine the exact change in nucleotide sequence, and the inability to detect non–length-affecting mutations such as substitution mutations.

Examples of fragment analysis applications in oncology include the detection of *NPM1* insertion mutations (Fig. 3.5),[34] *EGFR* exon 19 deletions, *FLT3* internal tandem duplications, and *JAK2* exon 12 mutations.[35]

High-Resolution Melting Curve Analysis

A high-resolution melting (HRM) curve analysis is a mutation screening method that allows for the detection of DNA sequence variations based on specific sequence-related melting profiles of PCR products.[36] Because the melting property of DNA duplexes is dependent on the biophysical and chemical properties of the nucleotide sequences, mutant and wild-type DNA sequences can be differentiated from one another based on their melting characteristics.

An HRM analysis is preceded by a PCR. The reaction employs a pair of gene-specific forward and reverse primers, template DNA, and a reporter that can either be a double-stranded DNA binding dye or a fluorescent reporter probe. Following the last cycle of the PCR, the amplification products undergo a cooling step that generates homoduplexes (double-stranded molecules with perfect complementarity between alleles) and heteroduplexes (double-stranded molecules with sequence mismatch between alleles) followed by a heating step that denatures (i.e., melts) the double-stranded products. Heteroduplexes (mutant DNA) produce a melting profile different from that of wild-type samples (homoduplexes). In most cases, the reaction is performed in a q-PCR system that allows for an analysis of amplification and

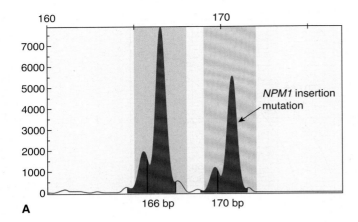

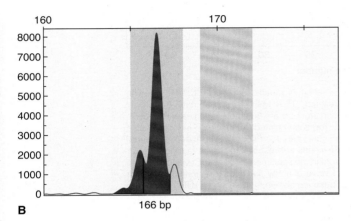

Figure 3.5 Fragment analysis. *NPM1* mutations are important prognostic markers in acute myeloid leukemia. Virtually all *NPM1* mutations result in a four nucleotide insertion within exon 12. Detection of these mutations can be accomplished by PCR utilizing primers that flank the mutation region. The amplification products are sized using capillary electrophoresis. A mutation is indicated by a PCR fragment that is 4 bp larger than the wild-type fragment. Mutation positive **(A)** and negative **(B)** cases are shown.

melting data in a close-tube format, thereby minimizing the risk of amplicon contamination.

An HRM analysis is useful for the qualitative detection of variable point mutations and small length-affecting mutations that occur within mutational hotspot regions. This method has high analytical sensitivity and can detect mutations even in a small fraction of alleles in a background of wild-type DNA. However, this assay does not characterize the specific sequence alteration in the mutant allele and may be challenging to interpret, especially for cases with mutation levels that approach the detection limit of the assay. Samples with a lower abundance of mutant alleles, and consequently a decreased fraction of heteroduplexes that produced fluorescence decay during the melting analysis, usually produce a melting curve that may not differ significantly from that of wild-type samples. Likewise, the detection of duplication mutations may be hampered by the similarity between the mutant and the duplicated wild-type genome sequences, which may produce only subtle differences in the melting behavior of the DNA duplexes, especially for samples with low mutant allele burden. Therefore, both the mutant sequence and the allelic burden play in the ability of an HRM analysis to detect mutations.[37] Poor quality and impurity of genomic DNA may also lower the sensitivity of an HRM analysis.[38] In instances of patients with a low mutant allelic burden, equivocal mutations identified by this approach may not be confirmable by an alternate method such as Sanger sequencing.

Examples of HRM applications in oncology include a mutational analysis of *KRAS* codons 12, 13, and 61[39]; a mutation screening of *BRAF* codon 600[39]; and the detection of *JAK2* exon 12 mutations (Fig. 3.6).[40]

Sanger Sequencing

Mutations in single gene assays are commonly analyzed by targeted nucleic acid sequencing, most commonly by Sanger sequencing.[41] This method, also known as dideoxy sequencing, is based on random incorporation of modified nucleotides (dideoxynucleotides [ddNTP]) into a DNA sequence during rounds of template extension that result in termination of the chain reaction at various fragment lengths. Because dideoxynucleotides lack a 3' hydroxyl group on the DNA pentose ring, which is required for the addition of further nucleotides during extension of the new DNA strand, the chain reaction is terminated at different lengths with the random incorporation of ddNTPs to the sequence. In addition to the dideoxy modification, each ddNTP (ddATP, ddTTP, ddCTP, ddGTP) is labeled with fluorescent tags of different fluorescence wavelengths.

In this method, repetitive cycles of primer extension are performed using denatured PCR products (amplicons) as templates. Unlike PCR, in which both forward and reverse primers are added to the same reaction, in Sanger sequencing, the forward and reverse reactions are performed separately. Bidirectional sequencing is performed to ensure that the entire region of interest

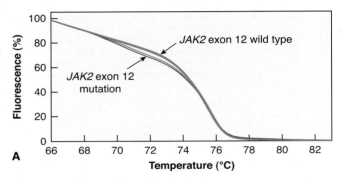

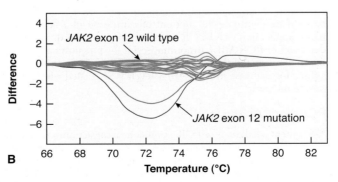

Figure 3.6 High resolution melting (HRM) curve analysis. An HRM analysis can be an efficient screening method for detecting a variety of mutations that may cluster in one or more hotspot regions, such as occurs with *JAK2* exon 12 mutations in polycythemia vera. PCR is utilized to amplify the target region in the presence of a fluorescent double-stranded DNA-binding dye. Following PCR, the product is gradually melted, and the emitted fluorescence is measured. **(A)** Plotting fluorescence versus temperature generates a melt curve characteristic of each amplicon. The presence of a mutation alters the melt profile due to mismatched double-stranded heteroduplexes of mutant and wild-type fragments. **(B)** A difference plot in which sample curves are subtracted from a wild-type control can accentuate the different melt profiles.

for each analysis is visualized adequately to produce unequivocal sequence readout. The sequencing products of increasing size are resolved by capillary electrophoresis, and the DNA sequence is determined by detection of the fluorescently labeled nucleotide sequences.

Sanger sequencing has the ability to detect a wide variety of nucleotide alterations in the DNA, including point mutations, deletions, insertions, and duplications. This technique is especially useful when mutations are scattered across the entire gene, when genes have not been sufficiently studied to determine mutational hot spots, or when it is relevant to determine the exact change in DNA sequence. Sanger sequencing can also provide semiquantitative information about mutation levels in a sample based on the evaluation of average peak drop values from forward and reverse mutant peaks on sequence chromatograms. Limitations of this approach include low throughput and limited diagnostic sensitivity. In general, heterozygous mutations at allelic levels lower than 20% may be difficult to detect by Sanger sequencing. This may be particularly problematic when testing for somatic mutations in oncogenes, such as *JAK2* exon 12 in polycythemia vera, which may occur at low levels.[35]

Examples of Sanger sequencing applications in oncology include the detection of *KIT* mutations for gastrointestinal stromal tumors (GIST) and melanomas that arise from mucosal membranes and acral skin, *EGFR* mutations for non–small-cell lung cancers, and *KRAS* mutations for colorectal and lung carcinomas (Fig. 3.7).

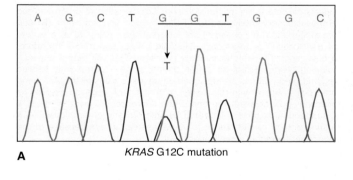

A   *KRAS* G12C mutation

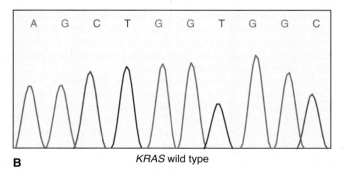

B   *KRAS* wild type

Figure 3.7 Sanger sequencing. *KRAS* mutation testing requires a technology like Sanger sequencing, which can detect the diverse variety of mutations that span multiple nucleotide sites. Overlapping peaks in the DNA sequence chromatogram indicate the presence of a mutation. The top panel **(A)** displays a G to T nucleotide substitution in codon 12. This results in a GGT to TGT codon change, leading to a glycine to cysteine (G12C) amino acid substitution. Activating mutations in *KRAS* such as G12C are associated with resistance to epidermal growth factor receptor (EGFR) targeted therapies in colon cancer. The bottom panel **(B)** displays a wild-type *KRAS* sequence.

Pyrosequencing

Pyrosequencing, also known as *sequencing by synthesis*, is based on the real-time detection of pyrophosphate release by nucleotide incorporation during DNA synthesis.[42] In the pyrosequencing reaction, as nucleotides are added to the nucleic acid chain by polymerase, pyrophosphate molecules are released and subsequently converted to ATP by ATP sulfurylase. Light is produced by an ATP-driven luciferase reaction via oxidation of a luciferin molecule. The amount of light produced is proportional to the number of incorporated nucleotides in the sequence. When a nucleotide is not incorporated into the reaction, no pyrophosphate is released and the unused nucleotide is degraded by apyrase. Light is converted into peaks in a charge-coupled device (CCD) camera. Individual dNTP nucleotides are sequentially added to the reaction, and the sequence of nucleotides that produce chemiluminescent signals allow the template sequence to be determined. Mutations appear as new peaks in the pyrogram sequence or variations of the expected peak heights.[43]

Pyrosequencing is particularly useful for the detection of point mutations and insertion/deletion mutations that occur at short stretches in mutational hotspots. This method has higher analytical sensitivity than Sanger sequencing and can provide quantitative information about mutation levels in a sample. Pyrosequencing can also be used for the detection and quantification of gene-specific DNA methylation and gene copy number assessments. A microfluidic pyrosequencing platform is available for massive parallel sequencing. However, this method is not well suited for detecting mutations that are scattered across the entire gene because pyrosequencing read lengths are limited to ~100 to 250 base pairs.[43]

Examples of pyrosequencing applications in oncology include the mutational analysis of *BRAF* (codon 600),[44,45] *KRAS* (codons 12, 13, 61),[45] *NRAS* (codon 61),[45] and the methylation analysis of *MGMT* in glioblastoma multiforme.[46,47]

Single Nucleotide Extension Assay (SNaPshot®)

The single nucleotide extension assay is a variant of dideoxy sequencing. This method consists of a single base extension of an unlabeled primer that anneals one base upstream to the relevant mutation with fluorophore-labeled dideoxynucleotides (ddNTP). Multiplexed reactions can be designed with multiple primers of differing lengths for simultaneous amplification of multiple genomic targets.[48] Mutations are identified based on amplicon size and fluorophore color via capillary electrophoresis. When a mutation is present, an alternative dideoxynucleotide triphosphate is incorporated, resulting in a different colored peak with a different amplicon length than the expected wild-type one.

The single nucleotide extension assay is particularly useful for the simultaneous detection of recurrent point mutations. Clinically, it has been employed for analyses of mutational hotspots in multiple genes involved in melanomas, non–small-cell lung cancers, breast cancers, and metastatic colorectal cancers.[49] The assay has higher analytical sensitivity than Sanger sequencing and can detect low-level mutations in FFPE-derived DNA, making it advantageous for biopsy specimens with limited tumor involvement. This assay, however, can only detect mutations that are immediately adjacent to the 3′ to the end of the primer.

Fluorescence In Situ Hybridization

FISH allows for the visualization of specific chromosome nucleic acid sequences within a cellular preparation. This method involves the annealing of a large single-stranded fluorophore-labeled oligonucleotide probe to complementary DNA target sequences within a tissue or cell preparation. The hybridization of the probe at the specific DNA region within a nucleus is visible by direct detection using fluorescence microscopy.

FISH can be used for the quantitative assessment of gene amplification or deletion and for the qualitative evaluation of gene rearrangements. Many oncologic FISH assays employ two probe types: *locus specific probes*, which are complementary to the gene of interest, and *centromeric probes*, which hybridize to the alpha-satellite regions near the centromere of a specific chromosome and help in the enumeration of the number of copies of that chromosome.

For the quantitative assessment of gene amplification, a locus-specific probe and a centromeric probe are labeled with two different fluorophores. The signals generated by each of these probes are counted and a ratio of the targeted gene to the chromosome copy number is calculated. The amount of signal produced by the locus-specific probe is proportional to the number of copies of the targeted gene in a cell. This type of gene amplification assay can be used for the detection of *HER2* gene amplification as an adjunct to existing clinical and pathologic information as an aid in the assessment of stage II, node-positive breast cancer patients for whom Herceptin treatment is being considered. It can also be used for an assessment of *MYCN* amplification in neuroblastoma.

For the detection of deletion mutations, dual-probe hybridization is usually performed using locus-specific probes. For instance, for the detection of 1p/19q codeletion in oligodendrogliomas, locus-specific probe sets for 1p36 and 19q13, and 1q25 and 19p13 (control) are used. The frequencies of signal patterns for each of these loci are evaluated. A signal pattern with 1p and 19q signals that are less than control signals is consistent with deletion of these loci.

Gene rearrangements/chromosomal translocations in hematologic or solid malignancies can be tested using locus-specific dual-fusion or break-apart probes. Dual-color, dual-fusion translocation assays employ two probes that are located in two separate genes involved in a specific rearrangement. Each gene probe is labeled in a different color. This design detects translocations by the juxtaposition of both probe signals. Dual-color, dual-fusion translocation assays are very specific for detecting a selected translocation. But, it can only be used for detecting translocations that involve consistent partners, where both partners are known. Alternate translocations with different fusion partners are not detected by this approach. Examples of application of dual-fusion probes in oncology include for the detection of the *IGH-BCL2* translocation that occurs in most follicular lymphomas and a subset of diffuse large B-cell lymphomas (Fig. 3.8) and for the detection of *IGH-CCND1* rearrangements in mantle cell lymphomas.

In break-apart FISH assays, both dual-colored probes flank the breakpoint region in a single gene that represents the constant partner in the translocation. By this approach, rearranged alleles show two split signals, whereas normal alleles show fusion signals. This design is particularly useful for genes that fuse with multiple translocation partners (e.g., *EWSR1* gene, which may undergo rearrangement with multiple partner genes, including *FLI1*, *ERG*, *ETV1*, *FEV*, and *E1AF* in Ewing sarcoma/primitive neuroectodermal tumor [PNET]; *WT1* in desmoplastic small round cell tumors; *CHN* in extraskeletal myxoid chondrosarcoma; and *ATF1* in clear cell sarcoma and angiomatoid fibrous histiocytoma).[50] The disadvantage of this approach is that break-apart FISH does not allow for the identification of the "unknown" partner in the translocation.

FISH has the advantage of being applicable to a variety of specimen types, including FFPE tissue. Because probes are hybridized to tissue in situ, the tumor morphology is preserved, which allows for an interpretation of the assay even in the context of heterogeneous samples. However, FISH is a targeted approach that will only detect specific alterations. Because most probes are large (e.g., >100 kb), small deletions or insertions will not be detected. In addition, poor tissue fixation, fixation artifacts, nuclear truncation on tissue slides, and nuclear overlaps are potential pitfalls of this technique that may hamper interpretation. Some intrachromosomal rearrangements (e.g., *RET-PTC* and *EML4-ALK*) may be challenging to interpret by FISH due to subtle rearrangements of the probe signals on the same chromosome arm.

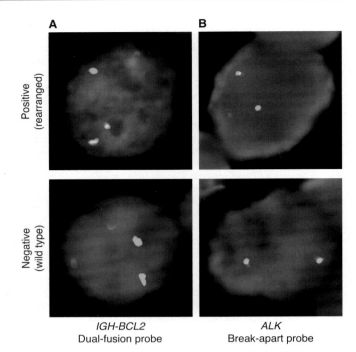

Figure 3.8 Fluorescence in situ hybridization (FISH). **(A)** Recurrent chromosomal translocations such as *IGH-BCL2* (occurring in B-cell lymphomas) can be effectively detected with a dual-fusion probe strategy. This design utilizes a green probe specific to the *IGH* locus and a red probe specific to the *BCL2* gene, with each probe spanning their respective breakpoint region. Individual green and red probe signals indicate a lack of translocation. Colocalization of green and red probes is observed when an *IGH-BCL2* translocation is present. **(B)** *ALK* rearrangements in non–small-cell lung cancers may involve a variety of translocation partners, including *EML4*, *TFG*, and *KIF5B*. Therefore, a break-apart FISH probe strategy is utilized that will detect any *ALK* rearrangement, regardless of the partner gene. Fluorescently labeled red and green probes are designed on opposite sides of the *ALK* gene breakpoint region. With this design, a normal *ALK* gene is observed as overlapping or adjacent red and green fluorescent signals, whereas a rearranged *ALK* gene is indicated by split red and green signals. *ALK* testing in lung cancer has become widespread in use because of the significant therapeutic implications.

Methylation Analysis

Changes in the methylation status of cytosine in DNA regions enriched for the sequence CpG (also known as CpG islands) are early events in many cancers and permanent changes found in many tumors. The detection of aberrant methylation of cancer-related genes may aid in the diagnosis, prognosis, and/or determination of the metastatic potential of tumors.

The most common approaches for the detection of methylation are based on the conversion of unmethylated cytosine bases into uracil after sodium bisulfite treatment, which is then converted to thymidine during PCR. By this approach, bisulfite-treated methylated alleles have different DNA sequences as compared with their corresponding unmethylated alleles. The differences between methylated and unmethylated DNA sequences can be evaluated by several methods, including methylation-sensitive restriction enzyme analysis, methylation-specific PCR, semiquantitative q-PCR, Sanger sequencing, pyrosequencing, and next-generation sequencing.

The methylation status of oncogenic genes can also be assessed by methylation-sensitive multiplex ligation-dependent probe amplification (MS-MLPA) assay.[51,52] MS-MLPA is a variant of multiplex PCR in which oligonucleotide probes hybridized to the targeted DNA samples are directly amplified using one pair of universal primers. This method is not based on bisulfite conversion of unmethylated cytosine bases into uracil. Instead, the target sequences detected by MS-MLPA probes contain a restriction site recognized by methylation-sensitive endonucleases. A probe amplification product will only be obtained if the CpG site is methylated because digested probes cannot be amplified during PCR. The level of methylation is determined by resolving PCR products by capillary electrophoresis and calculating the normalized ratio of each target probe peak area in both digested and undigested specimens. The ratio corresponds to the percentage of methylation present in the specimen.

Examples of applications of methylation analysis in oncology include an analysis of *MLH1* promoter hypermethylation in microsatellite unstable sporadic colorectal carcinomas, an analysis of *MGMT* promoter methylation status in glioblastoma multiforme patients treated with alkylating chemotherapy, and *SEPT9* promoter methylation in DNA derived from blood plasma in colorectal cancer patients.[53]

Microsatellite Instability Analysis

Microsatellites are short, tandem-repeated DNA sequences with repeating units of one to six base pairs in length. Microsatellites are distributed throughout the human genome, and individual repeat loci often vary in length from one individual to another. Microsatellite instability (MSI) is the change in length of a microsatellite allele due to either insertion or deletion of repeating units and a failure of the DNA mismatch repair (MMR) system to repair these replication errors. This genomic instability arises in a variety of human neoplasms where tumor cells have a decreased ability to faithfully replicate DNA. MSI is particularly associated with colorectal cancer, where 15% to 20% of sporadic tumors show MSI, in contrast to the more common chromosomal instability (CIN) phenotype, with MSI status being an independent prognostic indicator. MSI analysis is also clinically useful in identifying patients at increased risk of hereditary nonpolyposis colorectal cancer (HNPCC)/Lynch syndrome, where a germline mutation of an MMR gene causes a familial predisposition to colorectal cancer. MSI analysis alone is not sufficient to make a diagnosis of a germline MMR mutation given the high rate of sporadic MSI-positive colorectal tumors, but a positive result is an indication for follow-up genetic testing and counseling.

In an MSI analysis, DNA is extracted from tumor tissue and the corresponding adjacent normal mucosa. The DNA is subjected to multiplex PCR using fluorescent-labeled primers for coamplification of five mononucleotide repeat markers for MSI determination and two pentanucleotide markers for confirming tumor/normal sample identity. The resulting PCR fragments are separated and detected using capillary electrophoresis. Allelic profiles of normal versus tumor tissues are compared, and MSI is scored as the presence of novel microsatellite lengths in tumor DNA compared to normal DNA. Instability in two or more out of five mononucleotide microsatellite markers in tumor DNA compared to normal DNA is defined as MSI-H (high). MSI-L (low) is defined as instability in one out of five mononucleotide markers in tumor DNA compared to normal DNA. Tumors with no instability (zero out of five altered mononucleotide markers) are defined as microsatellite stable (MSS).[54,55]

Loss of Heterozygosity Analysis

Loss of heterozygosity (LOH) is a common event in cancer that usually occurs due to deletion of a chromosome segment and results in a loss of one copy of an allele. LOH is a common occurrence in tumor suppressor genes and may contribute to tumorigenesis when the second allele is subsequently inactivated by a second "hit" due to mutation or deletion.

LOH studies are used to identify genomic imbalance in tumors, indicating possible sites of tumor suppressor gene (TSG) deletion. LOH studies can be done by multiplex PCR analysis of microsatellites (short tandem repeats [STRs]), FISH, and genomic

microarrays). By PCR, microsatellites located in the vicinity of a tumor suppressor gene are used as surrogate markers for the presence of the gene of interest. DNA is extracted from tumor tissue and corresponding adjacent normal mucosa. The DNA is subjected to multiplex PCR using fluorescent-labeled STR primers. Peak height ratio of informative (nonhomozygous) alleles at each locus is calculated from both normal and tumor tissues. LOH is defined as the decrease in peak height of one of the two alleles, relative to the allele peak heights of the normal sample.

An example of applications of LOH studies in oncology include an analysis of 1p/19q loss in oligodendrogliomas, and an analysis of 1p loss in parathyroid carcinomas.

Whole Genome Analysis Methods

Next-Generation Sequencing

Next-generation sequencing (NGS), also known as massive parallel sequencing or deep sequencing, is an emerging technology that has revolutionized the speed, throughput, and cost of sequencing and has facilitated the discovery of clinically relevant genetic biomarkers for diagnosis, prognosis, and personalized therapeutics. By way of this technology, multiple genes or the entire exome or genome can be interrogated simultaneously in multiple parallel reactions instead of a single-gene basis as in Sanger sequencing or pyrosequencing. Currently, the most common NGS approach for cancer testing in the clinical setting employs targeted sequencing of specific genes and mutation hotspot regions. This targeted approach increases sensitivity for the detection of low-level mutations by increasing the depth of sequence coverage.

Presently, there are numerous NGS platforms that employ different sequencing technologies. A comprehensive review and comparison of NGS platforms is beyond the scope of this chapter and has been reviewed elsewhere.[56,57] A generalized clinical workflow is shown (Fig. 3.9). Frequently, multiple DNA samples are individually barcoded and pooled together to leverage platform throughput. Pooled libraries are prepared and enriched, and single DNA molecules are arrayed in solid surfaces, glass slides, or beads and sequenced in situ using reversible DNA chain terminators or iterative cycles of oligonucleotide ligation. NGS signal outputs are based on luminescence, fluorescence, or changes in ion concentration. Robust bioinformatics pipelines are required for an alignment of reads to a reference genome sequence, variant calling, variant annotation, and to assist with result reporting.[58]

NGS can be used for the detection of single nucleotide variants, small insertions and deletions, translocations, inversions, alternative splicing, and copy number variations given sufficient depth of genomic DNA sequence (Fig. 3.10). Technical limitations of this technique include difficulty in sequencing guanine-cytosine (GC)–rich genomic regions, and erroneous sequencing of homologous DNA regions (e.g., pseudogenes) that may confound interpretation.

Examples of applications of NGS in oncology include small targeted panels (3 to 50 genes) for non–small-cell lung cancers, melanomas, colon cancers, and acute myeloid leukemias.[57,59–62] Larger panels (50 to 500 genes) are increasingly being utilized, particularly in both clinical trials and research.

Massively parallel sequencing of RNA (RNA-Seq) can be used for determining sequence variants, alternative splicing, gene rearrangements, and allelic expression of mutant transcripts. To date, this technique has been used primarily for discovery rather than clinical applications, but it is likely to play an increasing role in clinical diagnostics as the technology improves. For transcriptome sequencing, the RNA must first be converted to cDNA, which is then fragmented and entered into library construction. After sequencing, reads are aligned to a reference genome, compared with known transcript sequences, or assembled de novo

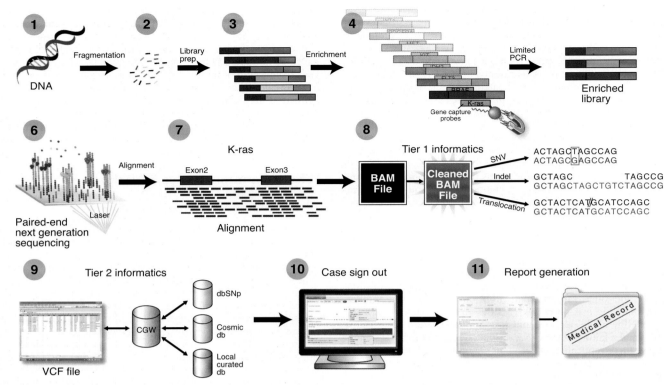

Figure 3.9 Next-generation sequencing (NGS) workflow in a clinical laboratory. Targeted-panel sequencing offers tremendous promise for cancer diagnostics due to the massive improvement in throughput, speed, and cost. NGS is a complex, multiday process that requires significant infrastructure and expertise to deploy in a clinical setting. The process begins with genomic DNA extraction, which is fragmented and to which linkers are ligated. In this targeted gene panel–based example, the sequencing libraries are enriched for the target genes, which are subjected to a limited PCR prior to sequencing. Sequence reads are mapped to a reference genome and subjected to several bioinformatics tools to provide variant calling results and variant annotation. Clinical interpretation and case sign out is performed by a physician with expertise in molecular pathology. BAM, Binary Sequence Alignment/Map; SNV, Single Nucleotide Variant; VCF, Variant Call Format; CGW, Clinical Genomicist Workstation; dbSNP, The Single Nucleotide Polymorphism Database. (Used with permission from Shashikant Kulkarni PhD and Eric Duncavage MD.)

to construct a genome-scale transcription map. Expression levels are determined from the total number of sequence reads that map to the exons of a particular gene, normalized by the length of exons that can be uniquely mapped.[56] Compared with genomic microarrays, RNA-Seq has a greater ability to distinguish RNA isoforms, determine allelic expression, and reveal sequence variants.

Chromatin immunoprecipitation with sequencing (ChIP-Seq) can be used to determine the genome-wide location of chromatin-binding transcription factors or specific epigenetic modifications of histones. This has proved to be a very powerful research tool, which to date has not been used for clinical diagnostics. Proteins in contact with genomic DNA are chemically cross-linked (usually with formaldehyde treatment) to their binding sites, the DNA is fragmented, and the proteins cross-linked with DNA are then immunoprecipitated with antibodies specific for the proteins (or specific epigenetic histone modification) of interest. The DNA harvested from the immunoprecipitate is converted into a library for NGS. The obtained reads are mapped to the reference genome of interest to generate a genome-wide protein binding map.[63,64] ChIP-Seq is rapidly replacing chromatin immunoprecipitation and microarray hybridization (ChIP-on-chip) technology[65] because of its higher sensitivity and resolution.[66]

Genomic Microarrays

High-density genomic microarrays are widely used for whole genome assessment of copy number changes, LOH, and geno-

typing. In array comparative genomic hybridization (aCGH), cloned genomic probes are arrayed onto glass slides and serves as targets for the competitive hybridization of normal and tumor DNA. In the aCGH reaction, tumor DNA and DNA from a normal control sample are labeled with different fluorophores. These samples are denatured and hybridized together to the arrayed single-strand probes. Digital imaging systems are used to quantify the relative fluorescence intensities of the labeled DNA probes that have hybridized to each target probe. The fluorescence ratio of the tumor and control hybridization signals is determined at different positions along the genome, which provides information on the relative copy number of sequences in the tumor genome as compared to the normal genome.[67] This method is able to detect copy number variation, such as deletions, duplications, and gene amplification, but it cannot detect polymorphic allele changes.

An SNP array has the ability to detect LOH profiles in addition to high-resolution detection of copy number aberrations, such as amplifications and deletions. This method employs thousands of unique fluorescent-labeled nucleotide probe sequences arrayed on a chip to which a fragmented single-stranded specimen DNA binds to their complementary partners. Each SNP site is interrogated by complementary sets of probes containing perfect matches and mismatches to each SNP site. Each probe is associated with one of the two alleles of an SNP (also known as A and B). Relative fluorescence intensity depends on both the amount of target DNA in the sample, as well as the affinity between target and probe. An analysis of the raw fluorescence intensity is done by computational

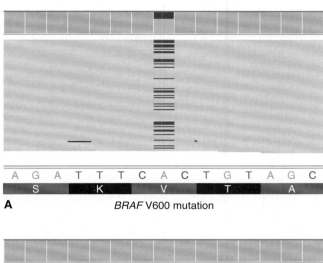

A   *BRAF* V600 mutation

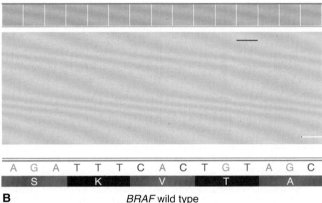

B   *BRAF* wild type

Figure 3.10 Next-generation sequencing (NGS). Hundreds to thousands of sequence reads are mapped and horizontally aligned to specific targeted regions in the reference genome (sequence shown on *bottom* of each panel). A software-assisted analysis assists in the detection of mutations, displayed as colored bars in each read above the mutation site. A wild-type sequence within each read is displayed in *gray*. Mutation frequency correlates to the number of times the mutant sequence is detected compared to the total number of reads at that nucleotide position. Shown are sequencing results from *BRAF* V600E mutation positive **(A)** and negative **(B)** melanomas. The A to T base substitution that leads to the V600E mutation is displayed in red. Patients with metastatic melanoma that harbors the *BRAF* V600E mutation are candidates for targeted therapy.

algorithms that convert the set of probe intensities into genotypes. Deleted genomic regions are identified as having an LOH associated with copy number reduction. A copy-neutral LOH is detected when SNPs expected to be heterozygous in the normal sample are detected as homozygous in the tumor sample without copy number variation. A copy neutral LOH may arise from somatic homologous recombination of a mutated tumor suppressor allele and its surrounding DNA that replaces the other allele (uniparental disomy [UPD]). SNP microarrays are the only genomic microarrays that are able to identify UPD. Array technologies cannot detect true balanced chromosome abnormalities and low-level mosaicism.

Examples of genomic microarrays applications in oncology include the detection of copy number variations and LOH in chronic lymphocytic leukemia[68] and recurrent cytogenetic abnormalities in MDS (e.g., 5q-, -7 or 7q-, +8, 20q-).[69]

Expression Panels

Gene expression signatures of multiple cancer biomarkers are starting to be incorporated into clinical practice as an adjunct to clinical and pathologic information in diverse cancer management settings. An example of a multigene expression–based test in current use includes Oncotype DX, which is a quantitative RT-PCR–based assay that measures the expression of 21 genes in FFPE breast tumors. The test is designed to predict the potential benefit of chemotherapy and the likelihood of distant breast cancer recurrence in women with node negative or node positive, estrogen receptor (ER)-positive, and *HER2*-negative invasive breast cancer. This test has been in-corporated into current American Society of Clinical Oncology (ASCO) and National Comprehensive Cancer Network (NCCN) for breast cancer management.[70] Prospective trials are in progress to evaluate other multigene tests for early stage breast cancer.

With the rapid advances in molecular diagnostic technologies, it is likely that many mutation- and expression-based panels analyzing hundreds if not thousands of genes, or even the complete genome or transcriptome, will enter widespread use. Some of the many challenges to address will be to provide evidence-based, actionable reports that guide the oncologist to more effective therapies, to learn from the results of such testing to improve the algorithms guiding therapy, to handle the incidental findings in such testing in an ethically responsible way, and ultimately, with the drugs available, to provide sufficient improvements in outcomes so that society will be willing to bear the costs.

PRINCIPLES OF ONCOLOGY

REFERENCES

1. Lennard L, Cartwright CS, Wade R, et al. Thiopurine methyltransferase genotype-phenotype discordance and thiopurine active metabolite formation in childhood acute lymphoblastic leukaemia. *Br J Clin Pharmacol* 2013;76(1):125–136.
2. Haber DA, Settleman J. Cancer: drivers and passengers. *Nature* 2007; 446(7132):145–146.
3. Hayashi T, Sudo J. Relieving effect of saline on cephaloridine nephrotoxicity in rats. *Chem Pharm Bull (Tokyo)* 1989;37(3):785–790.
4. Brodeur GM, Seeger RC, Schwab M, et al. Amplification of N-myc in untreated human neuroblastomas correlates with advanced disease stage. *Science* 1984;224(4653):1121–1124.
5. Seeger RC, Brodeur GM, Sather H, et al. Association of multiple copies of the N-myc oncogene with rapid progression of neuroblastomas. *N Engl J Med* 1985;313(18):1111–1116.
6. Weinstein JL, Katzenstein HM, Cohn SL. Advances in the diagnosis and treatment of neuroblastoma. *Oncologist* 2003;8(3):278–292.
7. Pui CH, Crist WM, Look AT. Biology and clinical significance of cytogenetic abnormalities in childhood acute lymphoblastic leukemia. *Blood* 1990;76(8):1449–1463.
8. Lee JA, Lupski JR. Genomic rearrangements and gene copy-number alterations as a cause of nervous system disorders. *Neuron* 2006;52(1):103–121.
9. Kuiper RP, Ligtenberg MJ, Hoogerbrugge N, et al. Germline copy number variation and cancer risk. *Curr Opin Genet Dev* 2010;20(3):282–289.
10. Shlien A, Malkin D. Copy number variations and cancer. *Genome Med* 2009;1(6):62.
11. Lynch TJ, Bell DW, Sordella R, et al. Activating mutations in the epidermal growth factor receptor underlying responsiveness of non–small-cell lung cancer to gefitinib. *N Engl J Med* 2004;350(21):2129–2139.
12. Paez JG, Janne PA, Lee JC, et al. EGFR mutations in lung cancer: correlation with clinical response to gefitinib therapy. *Science* 2004;304(5676): 1497–1500.
13. Forbes SA, Bindal N, Bamford S, et al. COSMIC: mining complete cancer genomes in the Catalogue of Somatic Mutations in Cancer. *Nucleic Acids Res* 2011;39(Database issue):D945–950.
14. Van Allen EM, Wagle N, Levy MA. Clinical analysis and interpretation of cancer genome data. *J Clin Oncol* 2013;31(15):1825–1833.
15. Newman B, Mu H, Butler LM, et al. Frequency of breast cancer attributable to BRCA1 in a population-based series of American women. *JAMA* 1998;279(12):915–921.
16. Ford D, Easton DF, Stratton M, et al. Genetic heterogeneity and penetrance analysis of the BRCA1 and BRCA2 genes in breast cancer families. The Breast Cancer Linkage Consortium. *Am J Hum Genet* 1998;62(3): 676–689.
17. Antoniou A, Pharoah PD, Narod S, et al. Average risks of breast and ovarian cancer associated with BRCA1 or BRCA2 mutations detected in case series unselected for family history: a combined analysis of 22 studies. *Am J Hum Genet* 2003;72(5):1117–1130.
18. Chen S, Iversen ES, Friebel T, et al. Characterization of BRCA1 and BRCA2 mutations in a large United States sample. *J Clin Oncol* 2006;24(6):863–871.

19. Bachner P, Hamlin W. Federal regulation of clinical laboratories and the Clinical Laboratory Improvement Amendments of 1988—Part II. *Clin Lab Med* 1993;13(4):987–994.

20. Halling KC, Schrijver I, Persons DL. Test verification and validation for molecular diagnostic assays. *Arch Pathol Lab Med* 2012;136(1):11–13.

21. Jennings L, Van Deerlin VM, Gulley ML, College of American Pathologists Molecular Pathology Resource C. Recommended principles and practices for validating clinical molecular pathology tests. *Arch Pathol Lab Med* 2009;133(5):743–755.

22. Jennings LJ, Smith FA, Halling KC, et al. Design and analytic validation of BCR-ABL1 quantitative reverse transcription polymerase chain reaction assay for monitoring minimal residual disease. *Arch Pathol Lab Med* 2012;136(1):33–40.

23. Pont-Kingdon G, Gedge F, Wooderchak-Donahue W, et al. Design and analytical validation of clinical DNA sequencing assays. *Arch Pathol Lab Med* 2012;136(1):41–46.

24. Saiki RK, Gelfand DH, Stoffel S, et al. Primer-directed enzymatic amplification of DNA with a thermostable DNA polymerase. *Science* 1988;239(4839):487–491.

25. Mullis KB. The unusual origin of the polymerase chain reaction. *Sci Am* 1990;262(4):56–61, 64–65.

26. Bernard PS, Wittwer CT. Real-time PCR technology for cancer diagnostics. *Clin Chem* 2002;48(8):1178–1185.

27. Bench AJ, Baxter EJ, Green AR. Methods for detecting mutations in the human JAK2 gene. *Methods Mol Biol* 2013;967:115–131.

28. Halait H, Demartin K, Shah S, et al. Analytical performance of a real-time PCR-based assay for V600 mutations in the BRAF gene, used as the companion diagnostic test for the novel BRAF inhibitor vemurafenib in metastatic melanoma. *Diagn Mol Pathol* 2012;21(1):1–8.

29. Furtado LV, Weigelin HC, Elenitoba-Johnson KS, et al. Detection of MPL mutations by a novel allele-specific PCR-based strategy. *J Mol Diagn* 2013;15(6):810–818.

30. Lang AH, Drexel H, Geller-Rhomberg S, et al. Optimized allele-specific real-time PCR assays for the detection of common mutations in KRAS and BRAF. *J Mol Diagn* 2011;13(1):23–28.

31. Wang ZY, Chen Z. Acute promyelocytic leukemia: from highly fatal to highly curable. *Blood* 2008;111(5):2505–2515.

32. O'Brien SG, Guilhot F, Larson RA, et al. Imatinib compared with interferon and low-dose cytarabine for newly diagnosed chronic-phase chronic myeloid leukemia. *N Engl J Med* 2003;348(11):994–1004.

33. Hughes TP, Kaeda J, Branford S, et al. Frequency of major molecular responses to imatinib or interferon alfa plus cytarabine in newly diagnosed chronic myeloid leukemia. *N Engl J Med* 2003;349(15):1423–1432.

34. Szankasi P, Jama M, Bahler DW. A new DNA-based test for detection of nucleophosmin exon 12 mutations by capillary electrophoresis. *J Mol Diagn* 2008;10(3):236–241.

35. Furtado LV, Weigelin HC, Elenitoba-Johnson KS, et al. A multiplexed fragment analysis-based assay for detection of JAK2 exon 12 mutations. *J Mol Diagn* 2013;15(5):592–599.

36. Reed GH, Kent JO, Wittwer CT. High-resolution DNA melting analysis for simple and efficient molecular diagnostics. *Pharmacogenomics* 2007;8(6):597–608.

37. Palais RA, Liew MA, Wittwer CT. Quantitative heteroduplex analysis for single nucleotide polymorphism genotyping. *Anal Biochem* 2005;346(1):167–175.

38. Carillo S, Henry L, Lippert E, et al. Nested high-resolution melting curve analysis a highly sensitive, reliable, and simple method for detection of JAK2 exon 12 mutations—clinical relevance in the monitoring of polycythemia. *J Mol Diagn* 2011;13(3):263–270.

39. Ney JT, Froehner S, Roesler A, et al. High-resolution melting analysis as a sensitive prescreening diagnostic tool to detect KRAS, BRAF, PIK3CA, and AKT1 mutations in formalin-fixed, paraffin-embedded tissues. *Arch Pathol Lab Med* 2012;136(9):983–992.

40. Jones AV, Cross NC, White HE, et al. Rapid identification of JAK2 exon 12 mutations using high resolution melting analysis. *Haematologica* Oct 2008;93(10):1560–1564.

41. Sanger F, Nicklen S, Coulson AR. DNA sequencing with chain-terminating inhibitors. *Proc Natl Acad Sci U S A* 1977;74(12):5463–5467.

42. Ronaghi M, Uhlén M, Nyrén P. A sequencing method based on real-time pyrophosphate. *Science* 1998;281(5375):363, 365.

43. Ronaghi M, Shokralla S, Gharizadeh B. Pyrosequencing for discovery and analysis of DNA sequence variations. *Pharmacogenomics* 2007;8(10):1437–1441.

44. Shigaki H, Baba Y, Watanabe M, et al. KRAS and BRAF mutations in 203 esophageal squamous cell carcinomas: pyrosequencing technology and literature review. *Ann Surg Oncol* 2013;20:485–491.

45. Vaughn CP, Zobell SD, Furtado LV, et al. Frequency of KRAS, BRAF, and NRAS mutations in colorectal cancer. *Genes Chromosomes Cancer* 2011;50(5):307–312.

46. Everhard S, Tost J, El Abdalaoui H, et al. Identification of regions correlating MGMT promoter methylation and gene expression in glioblastomas. *Neuro Oncol* 2009;11(4):348–356.

47. Mikeska T, Bock C, El-Maarri O, et al. Optimization of quantitative MGMT promoter methylation analysis using pyrosequencing and combined bisulfite restriction analysis. *J Mol Diagn* 2007;9(3):368–381.

48. Dias-Santagata D, Akhavanfard S, David SS, et al. Rapid targeted mutational analysis of human tumours: a clinical platform to guide personalized cancer medicine. *EMBO Mol Med* 2010;2(5):146–158.

49. Su Z, Dias-Santagata D, Duke M, et al. A platform for rapid detection of multiple oncogenic mutations with relevance to targeted therapy in non–small-cell lung cancer. *J Mol Diagn* 2011;13(1):74–84.

50. Lazar A, Abruzzo LV, Pollock RE, et al. Molecular diagnosis of sarcomas: chromosomal translocations in sarcomas. *Arch Pathol Lab Med* 2006;130(8):1199–1207.

51. Nygren AO, Ameziane N, Duarte HM, et al. Methylation-specific MLPA (MS-MLPA): simultaneous detection of CpG methylation and copy number changes of up to 40 sequences. *Nucleic Acids Res* 2005;33(14):e128.

52. Hömig-Hölzel C, Savola S. Multiplex ligation-dependent probe amplification (MLPA) in tumor diagnostics and prognostics. *Diagn Mol Pathol* 2012;21(4):189–206.

53. Warren JD, Xiong W, Bunker AM, et al. Septin 9 methylated DNA is a sensitive and specific blood test for colorectal cancer. *BMC Med* 2011;9:133.

54. Boland CR, Thibodeau SN, Hamilton SR, et al. A National Cancer Institute Workshop on Microsatellite Instability for cancer detection and familial predisposition: development of international criteria for the determination of microsatellite instability in colorectal cancer. *Cancer Res* 1998;58(22):5248–5257.

55. Umar A, Boland CR, Terdiman JP, et al. Revised Bethesda Guidelines for hereditary nonpolyposis colorectal cancer (Lynch syndrome) and microsatellite instability. *J Natl Cancer Inst* 2004;96(4):261–268.

56. Voelkerding KV, Dames SA, Durtschi JD. Next-generation sequencing: from basic research to diagnostics. *Clin Chem* 2009;55(4):641–658.

57. Cronin M, Ross JS. Comprehensive next-generation cancer genome sequencing in the era of targeted therapy and personalized oncology. *Biomarker Med* 2011;5(3):293–305.

58. Coonrod EM, Durtschi JD, Margraf RL, et al. Developing genome and exome sequencing for candidate gene identification in inherited disorders: an integrated technical and bioinformatics approach. *Arch Pathol Lab Med* 2013;137(3):415–433.

59. Grossmann V, Kohlmann A, Klein HU, et al. Targeted next-generation sequencing detects point mutations, insertions, deletions and balanced chromosomal rearrangements as well as identifies novel leukemia-specific fusion genes in a single procedure. *Leukemia* 2011;25(4):671–680.

60. Marchetti A, Del Grammastro M, Filice G, et al. Complex mutations & subpopulations of deletions at exon 19 of EGFR in NSCLC revealed by next generation sequencing: potential clinical implications. *PloS One* 2012;7(7):e42164.

61. McCourt CM, McArt DG, Mills K, et al. Validation of next generation sequencing technologies in comparison to current diagnostic gold standards for BRAF, EGFR and KRAS mutational analysis. *PloS One* 2013;8(7):e69604.

62. Thol F, Kölking B, Damm F, et al. Next-generation sequencing for minimal residual disease monitoring in acute myeloid leukemia patients with FLT3-ITD or NPM1 mutations. *Genes Chromosomes Cancer* 2012;51(7):689–695.

63. Barski A, Cuddapah S, Cui K, et al. High-resolution profiling of histone methylations in the human genome. *Cell* 2007;129(4):823–837.

64. Schones DE, Zhao K. Genome-wide approaches to studying chromatin modifications. *Nat Rev Genet* 2008;9(3):179–191.

65. Ren B, Robert F, Wyrick JJ, et al. Genome-wide location and function of DNA binding proteins. *Science* 2000;290(5500):2306–2309.

66. Robertson G, Hirst M, Bainbridge M, et al. Genome-wide profiles of STAT1 DNA association using chromatin immunoprecipitation and massively parallel sequencing. *Nat Methods* 2007;4(8):651–657.

67. Shinawi M, Cheung SW. The array CGH and its clinical applications. *Drug Discov Today* 2008;13(17–18):760–770.

68. Iacobucci I, Lonetti A, Papayannidis C, Martinelli G. Use of single nucleotide polymorphism array technology to improve the identification of chromosomal lesions in leukemia. *Curr Cancer Drug Targets* 2013;13(7):791–810.

69. Ahmad A, Iqbal MA. Significance of genome-wide analysis of copy number alterations and UPD in myelodysplastic syndromes using combined CGH - SNP arrays. *Curr Med Chem* 2012;19(22):3739–3747.

70. Goncalves R, Bose R. Using multigene tests to select treatment for early-stage breast cancer. *J Natl Compr Canc Netw* 2013;11(2):174–182.

PART II

Etiology and Epidemiology of Cancer

Section 1 Etiology of Cancer

4 Tobacco

Richard J. O'Connor

INTRODUCTION

Regrettably, tobacco use remains one of the leading causes of death worldwide. It is projected to leave over 1 billion dead in the 21st century, after killing nearly 100 million during the course of the 20th century.[1] Data from the Global Adult Tobacco Survey (GATS), which conducted representative household surveys in 14 low- and middle-income countries (Bangladesh, Brazil, China, Egypt, India, Mexico, Philippines, Poland, Russia, Thailand, Turkey, Ukraine, Uruguay, and Vietnam), suggest 41% of men and 5% of women across these countries currently smoke.[2] Compare this to approximately 24% of men and 16% of women in the United States.[3] A preponderance of the death and disease associated with tobacco use is associated with its combusted forms, particularly the cigarette. However, all forms of tobacco use have negative health consequences, the severity of which can vary among products. From the introduction of the mass-manufactured, mass-marketed cigarette (e.g., Camel in 1913), smoking rates grew, first among men then among women, and peaked in Western countries in the 1960s to 1970s, before beginning a steady decline.[4] The smoking rate among US adults has dropped from its peak in 1965 of 42% to 19% in 2011.[3] Per capita consumption has been dropping almost continuously since the 1960s, although the rate of decline has slowed since the early 2000s.[5] Among youth, smoking rates have been in decline since the 1990s,[6,7] although there is some evidence of growth in use of other forms of tobacco (e.g., cigars, water pipes, electronic cigarettes) in 2011 to 2012 that may be displacing cigarette use.[8]

Tobacco control policy interventions can impact both smoking prevalence and lung cancer incidence.[9] For example, a recent analysis suggests that implementation of graphic health warnings in Canada in 1999 resulted in a significant reduction (up to 4.5 percentage points) in smoking prevalence over a decade.[10] Increases in tobacco taxes have long been shown to reduce youth smoking initiation and to prompt more attempts to quit smoking.[11] Evidence from state comparisons in the United States suggests that comprehensive tobacco control measures effectively implemented (such as in California and Massachusetts) can reduce lung cancer incidence.[12] Indeed, Holford and colleagues[13] have shown that since the seminal 1964 Report of the Surgeon General, an estimated 157 million years of life (approximately 20 years per person) have been saved by tobacco control activities in the United States over 50 years. That is, tobacco control activities are estimated to have averted 8 million premature deaths and extended mean life span by 19 to 20 years.[13] However, the marketing of cigarettes has since shifted focus to the developing world, where smoking rates are on the increase. In an attempt to head off an epidemic of smoking and associated diseases, the World Health Organization initiated a public health treaty, the Framework Convention on Tobacco Control (FCTC), to coordinate international efforts to reduce tobacco use.[14] The FCTC binds parties to enact measures to control the labeling and marketing of tobacco products,

create a framework for testing and regulating product contents and emissions, combat smuggling and counterfeiting, and protect nonsmokers from secondhand smoke.[15] To date, the FCTC has been ratified by more than 150 countries. The FCTC provides governments the opportunity to regulate the marketing, labeling, and contents/emissions of tobacco products, as well as control the global trade in tobacco products. In the United States, which is currently not a party to FCTC, the U.S. Food and Drug Administration (FDA) has, since 2009, had authority to regulate tobacco products and their marketing along similar lines.[16]

EPIDEMIOLOGY OF TOBACCO AND CANCER

Linkages between tobacco use and cancers at various sites had been noted for several decades. In the late 1800s, it was believed that excessive cigar use created irritation that led to oral cancers.[17] In the 1930s, German scientists began to establish links between cigarette smoking and lung cancers.[18] However, it was not until the Doll and Hill[19] and Wynder and Graham[20] studies were published that the association was demonstrated in large samples and well-designed studies. Table 4.1 lists the cancers currently recognized by the U.S. Surgeon General as caused by smoking, along with their corresponding estimated mortality statistics.[21–23] Of these, the most well-publicized link is between smoking and lung cancer. In a recent examination of National Health and Nutrition Examination Survey (NHANES) data, Jha[24] showed a hazard ratio for lung cancer in smokers versus nonsmokers of 17.8 in women and 14.6 in men. However, smoking contributes substantially to overall cancer burden across multiple sites, including the oropharynx, cervix, and pancreas. Hazard ratios of 1.7 for women and 2.2 for men are seen for cancers other than in the lung in smokers versus nonsmokers.[24] Emerging evidence also links smoking with breast cancer, although the data are as yet insufficient to make causal conclusions.[23,25] Cancer risks associated with smoking, as well as outcomes and survival, depend on a number of factors. A common index of cancer risk is pack-years, or the number of packs of cigarettes smoked per day multiplied by the number of years smoked in the lifetime. In general, the higher the number of pack-years, the greater the cancer risk. Risks for lung cancer decline with smoking cessation, and the longer a former smoker remains off of cigarettes, the more the risk declines.[26] However, excepting those smokers who quit with relatively few pack years accumulated (typically before age 40), cancer risk rarely approaches that of a never smoker.[24,27]

A recent study using several large cohort studies examined death rates and the relative risks associated with smoking and smoking cessation for 3 epochs (1959 to 1965, 1982 to 1988, and 2000 to 2010).[27] Of most interest here is death from lung cancer. For men, the age-adjusted death rate from lung cancer increased from 1959 through 1965 to 1982 through1988, but then fell for 2000

TABLE 4.1

Level of Evidence for Smoking-Attributable Cancers According to the United States Office of the Surgeon General by Cancer Site and Yearly Smoking-Attributable Mortality at Sites with Available Estimates, United States, 2004

	Cancer Site	Yearly Smoking-Attributable Mortality
Evidence Sufficient to Infer Causal Relationship	Bladder	4,983
	Cervix	447
	Colon and rectum	N/A
	Esophagus	8,592
	Kidney	3,043
	Larynx	3,009
	Leukemia (AML)	1,192
	Liver	N/A
	Lung	125,522
	Oral cavity and pharynx	4,893
	Pancreas	6,683
	Stomach	2,484
Evidence Suggestive but Not Sufficient to Infer Causal Relationship	Breast	
Inadequate to Infer Presence or Absence of Causal Relationship	Ovary	
Evidence Sufficient to Infer No Causal Relationship	Prostate	

N/A, not available; AML, acute myeloid leukemia.

through 2010; for women, the age-adjusted death rate continued to rise over time, with the biggest increase between 1982 through 1988 to 2000 through 2010.[27] In relative risk terms, the likelihood of dying from lung cancer given current smoking has increased from 2.73 to 12.65 to 25.66 among women, and 12.22 to 23.81 to 24.97 for men. Equivalent risks for former smokers increased from 1.3 to 3.85 to 6.7 among women, versus 3.48 to 7.41 to 6.75 for men. These and other analyses suggest that the cancer risks from smoking may have increased with time.[27,28] The histologic subtypes of lung cancer seen in the US population have also shifted with time. Into the early 1980s, squamous cell carcinomas (SCC) were the most common manifestations of lung cancer. However, a rapid rise in adenocarcinomas has been noted, and by the 1990s, had overtaken SCC as the leading type of lung cancer.[23]

Tobacco Use Behaviors

The level of tobacco exposure is ultimately driven by use behaviors, including the number of cigarettes smoked, the patterns of smoking on individual cigarettes, and the number of years smoked. The primary driver of smoking behavior is nicotine—the major addictive substance and primary reinforcer of continued smoking.[29–31] Over time, smokers learn an *acceptable* level of nicotine intake that attains the beneficial effects they seek while avoiding negative withdrawal symptoms. Smokers can affect the amount of nicotine (and accompanying toxicants) they draw from a cigarette by altering the number of puffs taken, puff size,

frequency, duration, and velocity (collectively referred to as smoking topography).[32] Smokers tend to consume a relatively stable number of cigarettes per day and to smoke those cigarettes in a relatively consistent manner in order to maintain an acceptable level of nicotine in their system across the day.[33] The number of cigarettes smoked per day and the smoking pattern of an individual may be influenced by the rate of nicotine metabolism.[30] Nicotine is metabolized primarily to cotinine, which is further metabolized to trans-3'-hydroxycotinine (3HC), catalyzed by the liver cytochrome P450 2A6 enzyme.[34] Functional polymorphisms in the genes coding for these enzymes allow for the identification of *fast* metabolizers, who have more rapid nicotine clearance and show greater cigarette intake and more intensive smoking topography profiles relative to *normal* or *slow* metabolizers.[35–37] The ratio of 3HC to cotinine in plasma or saliva can be used as a reliable noninvasive phenotypic marker for CYP2A6 activity.[38,39] CYP2A6 activity is known to vary across racial/ethnic groups, with those of African or Asian descent showing slower metabolism than those of Caucasian descent.[40–42] Clinical trial data clearly show that the metabolite ratio can be used to predict success in quitting, and that the likelihood of quitting decreases as the ratio increases, such that slower metabolizers are more successful at achieving abstinence.[37,41,43] Despite their addiction to nicotine, most smokers in Western countries report that they regret ever starting to smoke and want to quit smoking, and there is evidence for similar regret in developing countries as well.[44–46] However, most smokers are unsuccessful in their attempts to quit smoking; the most effective evidence-based treatments increase the odds of quitting by 3 times, with 12-month cessation rates of approximately 40% relative to placebo.[47]

Evolution of Tobacco Products

Historically, tar was believed to be the main contributor to smoking-caused disease.[48] It is important to note that *tar* is not a specific substance, but simply the collected particulate matter from cigarette smoke, less water and nicotine (in technical reports, it is often referred to as nicotine-free dry particulate matter). Soon after the first studies were done showing that painting mice with cigarette tar caused cancerous tumors, it was theorized that reducing tar yields of cigarettes might also reduce the disease burden of smoking.[48] Concurrently, cigarette manufacturers were seeking to reassure their customers that their products were safe, that if hazardous compounds were identified they would be removed, and that product modifications could help to reduce risks.[4,49–51] Indeed, in the United States and United Kingdom, average tar levels of cigarettes dropped dramatically from the 1960s through the 1990s, and have since leveled off.[52,53] The European Union took the tar reduction mentality to heart in crafting maximum levels of tar in cigarettes that could be sold in member countries, beginning at 15 mg in 1992, then dropping to 12 mg in 1998, and 10 mg in 2005.[54] Unfortunately, these reductions in tar yields have not translated into changes in disease risks among smokers.[55] Despite initial optimism about these products, both laboratory-based and epidemiologic studies indicate neither an individual, nor a public health benefit from *low-tar* cigarettes as compared to *full-flavor* varieties.[56–58] The health consequences of mistakenly accepting the purported benefits of lower tar and nicotine products have been significant. The increases in adenocarcinoma of the lung observed in the United States over recent decades may reflect changes made to the cigarette, such as filters, filter ventilation, and tobacco-specific nitrosamines (TSNA) in smoke produced by the relatively high amount of burley tobacco used in the typical US cigarette blend.[23,59] Tobacco manufacturers engineered cigarettes be *elastic*; that is, cigarettes allow smokers to adjust their puffing patterns to regulate their intake of nicotine, regardless of how the cigarette might perform under the standard testing conditions that drove the labeling and advertising of the products.[55] Researchers have since come to determine that filter vents are the main design feature the industry relied on in creating elastic products.[54,55,60,61] Vents facilitate taking larger puffs and also contribute to sensory perceptions, because they dilute the smoke with air.[62] So, even with a larger puff, the same mass of toxins can seem less harsh and irritating because it is diluted by a proportionate amount of air, which may in turn underscore smokers' beliefs that they are smoking safer cigarettes.[62–64] Other smoke components (e.g., acetaldehyde, ammonia, minor tobacco alkaloids) and aspects of cigarette engineering (e.g., menthol, flavor additives) may further contribute to the addictiveness of cigarettes.[65]

Since the 1980s, manufacturers have introduced products that make more explicit claims about reduced health risks. Examples of modified cigarettelike products include Premier (RJ Reynolds), Eclipse (RJ Reynolds), Accord/Heatbar (Philip Morris), Omni (Vector Tobacco), and Advance (Brown and Williamson).[66] In the 2000s, as evidence of reduced lung cancer incidence and coincident increases in snus use in Sweden appeared,[67,68] manufacturers began to promote smokeless tobacco products as reduced harm alternatives. Most recently, electronic cigarettes, which vaporize a nicotine solution, have gained increasing popularity and generated concern among public health practitioners, particularly with regard to effects on youth.[8,69,70] In the United States, the FDA has authority to authorize marketing claims about reduced risk, which an Institute of Medicine panel concluded should be based on extensive testing of abuse liability, likely health effects, and effects on the whole population.[71]

CARCINOGENS IN TOBACCO PRODUCTS AND PROCESSES OF CANCER DEVELOPMENT

Cigarette smoke has been identified as carcinogenic since the 1950s, and efforts have continued to identify specific carcinogens in smoke and smokeless tobacco products. The International Agency for Research on Cancer (IARC) has classified both cigarette smoke and smokeless tobacco as Group 1 carcinogens.[72,73] IARC has also identified 72 measurable carcinogens in cigarette smoke where evidence is sufficient to classify them as Group 1 (carcinogenic to humans), 2A (probably carcinogenic to humans), or 2B (possibly carcinogenic to humans).[72] The IARC list, in addition to data from the U.S. Environmental Protection Agency (EPA), the National Toxicology Program, and the National Institute for Occupational Safety and Health (NIOSH), informed the FDA's development of a list of Harmful and Potentially Harmful Constituents (HPHC) in tobacco and tobacco smoke, which manufacturers will be required to report.[74] Table 4.2 illustrates the carcinogens listed as HPHC alongside their carcinogenicity classifications by IARC or the EPA.

Compounds of Particular Concern

Research groups have listed components of cigarette smoke theorized to impact health risk, often relying on carcinogenic potency indices and relative concentrations in smoke.[75,76] In these analyses, the N-nitrosamines, benzene, 1,3-butadiene, aromatic amines, and cadmium often rank highly. Polycyclic aromatic hydrocarbons (PAH), many of which are carcinogenic, consist of three or more fused aromatic rings resulting from incomplete combustion of organic (carbonaceous) materials, and are often found in coal tar, soot, broiled foods, and automobile engine exhaust.[77] A compound of particular concern in cigarette smoke historically has been benzo(a)pyrene (BaP), which has substantial carcinogenic activity and is considered carcinogenic to humans by the IARC.[77] In addition to PAH, other hydrocarbons found in significant quantities in cigarette smoke include benzene (a long-established cause

of leukemia), 1,3-butadiene (a potent multiorgan carcinogen), naphthalene, and styrene. Carbonyl compounds, such as formaldehyde and acetaldehyde, are found in copious amounts in cigarette smoke, primarily coming from the combustion of sugars and cellulose.[78] However, there are numerous other noncigarette exposures to these compounds, including endogenous formation during metabolism. Smoke contains a number of aromatic amines, such as known bladder carcinogens 2-aminonaphthalene and 4-aminobiphenyl, heterocyclic amines, and furans. Toxic metals, including beryllium, cadmium, lead, and polonium-210, are also present in cigarette smoke in measurable quantities,[79,80] levels of which may depend in part on the region of the world where the tobacco was grown.[81] Much attention has been focused on the N-nitrosamines, primarily because they are well-established carcinogens.[82–85] Nitrosamines form through reactions of nitrite with amino groups. In tobacco, two compounds of concern are 4-(methylnitrosamino)-1-(3-pyridyl)-1-butanone (NNK), which is derived from nitrosation of nicotine, and N′-nitrosonornicotine (NNN), which is derived from nitrosation of nornicotine. Both of these compounds are tobacco specific. NNN and NNK primarily form during the curing process for tobacco, where the leaves are dried through contact with combustion gases from heat (flue) curing or microbial activity in air curing.[78] NNK is known to be a potent lung carcinogen, but also shows tumor induction activity in the nasal cavity, the pancreas, and the liver, whereas NNN has been shown to induce tumors along the respiratory tract and esophagus in various animal models. Because they are produced in the curing process and transfer into smoke, rather than being formed by combustion, it is possible to reduce nitrosamines by changing curing and storage practices.[78,86,87]

Smokeless tobacco products, although they are not burned, nonetheless contain substantial levels of carcinogens, most prominently the N-nitrosamines.[73] Here, product type and composition has an enormous effect on nitrosamine levels. For example, US moist snuff has substantially higher levels than that sold in Sweden (snus), whereas smokeless products available in India are often far higher in nitrosamines.[88] US smokeless products also can contain PAH and carbonyl compounds, likely derived from fire curing the constituent tobacco.[89] Similar to cigarettes, smokeless products would also contain toxic metals.[79,80]

Although tobacco is an exceedingly complex mixture, it is possible to use animal model and epidemiologic evidence to postulate relationships between specific components and known tobacco-induced cancers.[90–92] There is strong evidence from multiple studies to suggest that PAH and N-nitrosamines are involved in lung carcinogenesis. For example, PAH–DNA adducts are observed in lung tissues, and p53 tumor suppressor mutations in lung tumors resemble the damage created by PAH diol epoxide metabolites in vitro.[93–96] NNK appears to preferentially induce lung tumors in the rat, regardless of the route of administration, and DNA–nitrosamine adducts are detectable in lung tissues.[97,98] Most importantly, nitrosamine metabolite levels measured in smokers were prospectively related to the risk of lung cancer in cohort studies, even adjusting for other indices of smoking exposure (e.g., cotinine, pack-years).[98–102] PAH and nitrosamines are also likely to be implicated in cancers along the respiratory tract and the cervix.[103,104] Considerable evidence exist that aromatic amines such as 4-aminobiphenyl and 2-naphthylamine are potent bladder carcinogens, and smokers are known to be at an elevated risk of bladder cancer, so these are presumed to be the primary causative agents.[105–107] Similarly, as benzene is a known cause of leukemia, it is presumed that this is the link to leukemia observed in smokers.

Important to examining the role of various smoke components in cancer is the ability to measure the exposure of smokers to these components. Biomarkers of exposure may also be crucial for examining products for their potential to reduce health risks associated with tobacco use.[71,108,109] Validation of tobacco exposure biomarkers is threefold: method validation, validation with respect to product use, and validation with respect to disease risk.[71]

TABLE 4.2

Carcinogens in Tobacco and Tobacco Smoke Identified as Harmful and Potentially Harmful by the U.S. Food and Drug Administration, with International Agency for Research on Cancer Carcinogenecity (IARC) Classifications as of 2013

Compound	CAS No.	IARC Group	IARC Volume	Year
1,3-Butadiene	106-99-0	1	100F	2012
2-Aminonaphthalene	91-59-8	1	100F	2012
4-(Methylnitrosamino)-1-(3-pyridyl)-1-butanone (NNK)	64091-91-4	1	100E	2012
4-Aminobiphenyl	92-67-1	1	100F	2012
Aflatoxin B1	1162-65-8	1	100F	2012
Arsenic	7440-38-2	1	100C	2012
Benzene	71-43-2	1	100F	2012
Benzo[a]pyrene	50-32-8	1	100F	2012
Beryllium	7440-41-7	1	100C	2012
Cadmium	7440-43-9	1	100C	2012
Chromium (Hexavalent compounds)	18540-29-9	1	100C	2012
Ethylene oxide	75-21-8	1	100F	2012
Formaldehyde	50-00-0	1	100F	2012
N-Nitrosonornicotine (NNN)	16543-55-8	1	100E	2012
Nickel (compounds)		1	100C	2012
o-Toluidine	95-53-4	1	100F	2012
Polonium-210	7440-08-6	1	100D	2012
Uranium (235, 238 Isotopes)	7440-61-1	1	100D	2012
Vinyl chloride	75-01-4	1	100F	2012
Acrylamide	79-06-1	2A	60	1994
Cyclopenta[c,d]pyrene	27208-37-3	2A	92	2010
Dibenz[a,h]anthracene	53-70-3	2A	92	2010
Dibenzo[a,l]pyrene	191-30-0	2A	92	2010
Ethyl carbamate (urethane)	51-79-6	2A	96	2010
IQ (2-Amino-3-methylimidazo[4,5-f]quinoline)	76180-96-6	2A	56	1993
N-Nitrosodiethylamine	55-18-5	2A	SUP 7	1987
N-Nitrosodimethylamine (NDMA)	62-75-9	2A	SUP 7	1987
2-Nitropropane	79-46-9	2B	71	1999
2,6-Dimethylaniline	87-62-7	2B	57	1993
5-Methylchrysene	3697-24-3	2B	92	2010
A-α-C (2-Amino-9H-pyrido[2,3-b]indole)	26148-68-5	2B	SUP 7	1987
Acetaldehyde	75-07-0	2B	71	1999
Acetamide	60-35-5	2B	71	1999
Acrylonitrile	107-13-1	2B	71	1999
Benz[a]anthracene	56-55-3	2B	92	2010
Benz[j]aceanthrylene	202-33-5	2B	92	2012
Benzo[b]fluoranthene	205-99-2	2B	92	2010
Benzo[b]furan	271-89-6	2B	63	1995
Benzo[c]phenanthrene	195-19-7	2B	92	2010
Benzo[k]fluoranthene	207-08-9	2B	92	2010
Caffeic acid	331-39-5	2B	56	1993
Catechol	120-80-9	2B	71	1999
Chrysene	218-01-9	2B	92	2010
Cobalt	7440-48-4	2B	52	1991

(continued)

TABLE 4.2

Carcinogens in Tobacco and Tobacco Smoke Identified as Harmful and Potentially Harmful by the U.S. Food and Drug Administration, with International Agency for Research on Cancer Carcinogenecity (IARC) Classifications as of 2013 (continued)

Compound	CAS No.	IARC Group	IARC Volume	Year
Dibenzo[a,h]pyrene	189-64-0	2B	92	2010
Dibenzo[a,i]pyrene	189-55-9	2B	92	2010
Ethylbenzene	100-41-4	2B	77	2000
Furan	110-00-9	2B	63	1995
Glu-P-1 (2-Amino-6-methyldipyrido[1,2-a:3′,2′-d]imidazole)	67730-11-4	2B	SUP 7	1987
Glu-P-2 (2-Aminodipyrido[1,2-a:3′,2′-d]imidazole)	67730-10-3	2B	SUP 7	1987
Hydrazine	302-01-2	2B	71	1999
Indeno[1,2,3-cd]pyrene	193-39-5	2B	92	2010
Isoprene	78-79-5	2B	71	1999
Lead	7439-92-1	2B	SUP 7	1987
MeA-α-C (2-Amino-3-methyl)-9H-pyrido[2,3-b]indole)	68006-83-7	2B	SUP 7	1987
N-Nitrosodiethanolamine (NDELA)	1116-54-7	2B	77	2000
N-Nitrosomethylethylamine	10595-95-6	2B	SUP 7	1987
N-Nitrosomorpholine (NMOR)	59-89-2	2B	SUP 7	1987
N-Nitrosopiperidine (NPIP)	100-75-4	2B	SUP 7	1987
N-Nitrosopyrrolidine (NPYR)	930-55-2	2B	SUP 7	1987
N-Nitrososarcosine (NSAR)	13256-22-9	2B	SUP 7	1987
Naphthalene	91-20-3	2B	82	2002
Nickel	7440-02-0	2B	49	1990
Nitrobenzene	98-95-3	2B	65	1996
Nitromethane	75-52-5	2B	77	2000
o-Anisidine	90-04-0	2B	73	1999
PhIP (2-Amino-1-methyl-6-phenylimidazo[4,5-b]pyridine)	105650-23-5	2B	56	1993
Propylene oxide	75-56-9	2B	60	1994
Styrene	100-42-5	2B	82	2002
Trp-P-1 (3-Amino-1,4-dimethyl-5H-pyrido[4,3-b]indole)	62450-06-0	2B	SUP 7	1987
Trp-P-2 (3-Amino-1-Methyl-5H-pyrido[4,3-b]indole)	62450-07-1	2B	SUP 7	1987
Vinyl acetate	108-05-4	2B	63	1995
1-Aminonaphthalene	134-32-7	3	SUP 7	1987
Chromium	7440-47-3	3	49	1990
Crotonaldehyde	4170-30-3	3	63	1995
Dibenzo[a,e]pyrene	192-65-4	3	92	2010
Mercury	7439-97-6	3	58	1993
Quinoline	91-22-5	EPA Group B2		
Cresols (o-, m-, and p-cresol)	1319-77-3	EPA Group C		

Notes: Most recently published IARC monograph for each compound is listed.
Quinoline and cresols have not been evaluated by IARC, but have been evaluated by U.S. Environmental Protection Agency.
IARC Groups: 1, Carcinogenic to humans; 2A, Probably carcinogenic to humans; 2B, Possibly carcinogenic to humans; 3, Not classifiable as to its carcinogenicity to humans; http://monographs.iarc.fr/ENG/Classification/ClassificationsAlphaOrder.pdf
EPA Groups: B2, Likely to be carcinogenic in humans; C, Possible human carcinogen.
CAS No., Chemical Abstracts Service registry number. *CAS Registry Number is a Registered Trademark of the American Chemical Society.* EPA, Environmental Protection Agency.
Quinoline: http://www.epa.gov/iris/subst/1004.htm
Cresols: http://www.epa.gov/iris/subst/0300.htm; http://www.epa.gov/iris/subst/0301.htm; http://www.epa.gov/iris/subst/0302.htm

TABLE 4.3

Commonly Used Biomarkers of Exposure to Carcinogens in Tobacco Smoke

Biomarker	Tobacco Smoke Source	Matrices
Monohydroxy-30butenyl mercapturic acid (MHBMA)	1,3-butadiene	Urine
4-Aminobiphenyl-globin	4-aminobiphenyl	Blood
N-(2-hydroxypropyl)methacrylamide (HPMA)	Acrolein	Urine
Carbamoylethylvaline	Acrylamide	Blood
Cyanoethylvaline	Acrylonitrile	Blood
S-phenylmercapturic acid (SPMA)	Benzene	Urine
Cd	Cadmium	Urine
3-hydroxypropyl mercapturic acid (HBMA)	Crotonaldehyde	Urine
2-hydroxyethyl mercapturic acid (HEMA)	Ethylene oxide	Urine
Nicotine equivalents (nicotine, cotinine, trans-3'-hydroxycotinine, and their respective glucuronides)	Nicotine	Urine
Total 4-(methylnitrosamino)-1-(3-pyridyl)-1-butanol (NNAL) (NNAL + NNAL glucuronide)	NNK	Urine
Total NNN (NNN + NNN glucuronide)	NNN	Urine
1-Hydroxypyrene	Pyrene (representative of other PAH)	Urine

Adapted from Hecht SS, Yuan JM, Hatsukami D. Applying tobacco carcinogen and toxicant biomarkers in product regulation and cancer prevention. *Chem Res Toxicol* 2010;23:1001–1008.

ETIOLOGY AND EPIDEMIOLOGY OF CANCER

Validation with respect to product use means that levels of a given biomarker differ substantially between users and nonusers, and that biomarker levels decrease substantially when product use is stopped. Validation with respect to disease risk implies that variation in biomarker levels in product users are predictive of variations in disease outcomes. Over the last decade, the development of modern high-throughput, high-resolution mass spectrometry has allowed for the measurement of multiple metabolites of tobacco carcinogens.[110–113] Commonly used biomarkers of tobacco exposure are listed in Table 4.3.

How Tobacco Use Leads to Cancer

A recent U.S. Surgeon General's report provides extensive detail on the current state of knowledge of how smoking causes cancer.[65] Therefore, only a brief overview is provided here. Hecht[101,113–116] has argued for a major pathway by which tobacco use leads to cancer: carcinogen exposure leads to the formation of carcinogen–DNA adducts, which then cause mutations that, if not repaired or removed by apoptosis, will eventually give rise to cancer. It is important to keep perspective that, whereas each cigarette may contain seemingly low levels of a given carcinogen, smoking is, for most people, a long-term addiction. Thus, a mixture of numerous carcinogens is administered multiple times per day over the course of decades. Further, compounds taken in during smokers can be metabolically activated, thus increasing their activity. Cigarette smoke compounds appear to induce the cytochrome P450 system, which facilitates the metabolic activation of carcinogens to electrophilic entities that are able to covalently bind DNA.[117,118] DNA adducts appear to be crucial to the cancer process, and numerous studies show that smoker tissues contain higher levels of DNA adducts than nonsmokers, and that DNA adduct levels are associated with cancer risk.[119,120] At the same time, other systems are involved in the detoxification and deactivation of smoke constituents, typically catalyzed by UDP-glucuronosyltransferases and glutathione-S-transferases, resulting in excretion of inactive compounds.[121,122] An individual's balance of activation and deactivation of toxicants

may be an important predictor of cancer risk, although evidence for this is mixed in the literature.[123,124] Similarly, DNA repair capacity is an important consideration, because, even if adducts are formed, processes exist to remove such perturbations to normalize DNA structure. Enzymatic processes of DNA repair include alkytransferases, nucleotide excision, and mismatch repair. Polymorphisms in genes coding for these enzymes may relate to individual cancer susceptibility. Table 4.4 outlines the metabolic activation/detoxification, DNA-adduct formation, and repair processes believed to be involved for four tobacco carcinogens (nitrosamines, PAH, benzene, 4-aminobiphenyl).[65,120]

Those DNA adducts that persist can cause miscoding during DNA replication. Smoke carcinogens are known to cause G:A and G:T mutations, and mutations in the *KRAS* oncogene and the *P53* tumor suppressor gene are strongly associated with tobacco-caused cancers.[95,114,125–127] Inactivation of *P53*, together with the activation of *KRAS*, appear to reduce survival in non–small-cell lung cancer.[65] Gene mutations that do not result in apoptosis may go on to influence a number of downstream processes, which may lead to genomic instability, proliferation, and eventually, malignancy.[128–130] Some smoke constituents may also act in ways that indirectly support the development of cancer. Nicotine, although not a carcinogen in itself, is known to reduce apoptosis and increase angiogenesis and transformation processes via nuclear factor kappa B (NF-κB).[65,131] Activation of nicotinic acetylcholine receptors (nAChR) in lung epithelium by nicotine or NNK is associated with survival and proliferation of malignant cells.[65] Nitrosamines also appear to have similar activities via the activation of protein kinases A and B.[132] NNK may bind β-adrenergic receptors to stimulate the release of arachidonic acid, which is converted to prostaglandin E2 by cyclooxygenase (COX)-2. Smoke compounds appear to activate epidermal growth factor receptor (EGFR) and COX-2, both of which are found to be elevated in many cancers.[133] Ciliatoxic, inflammatory, and oxidizing compounds, such as acrolein and ethylene oxide in smoke, may also impact the likelihood of cancer development. Epigenetic changes such as hypermethylation, particularly at P16, may also play a role in lung cancer development.[65]

TABLE 4.4

Key Pathways and Processes Where Selected Smoke Constituents Are Activated and Detoxified

	NNN, NNK	PAH	Benzene	4-ABP
Metabolic Activation	Alpha hydroxylation	Diol epoxide formation	Epoxide/oxepin formation	N-oxidation
Cytochrome P450 Enzymes Involved	2A6, 2A13, 2E1	1A1, 1B1	2E1	1A2
Enzymes Involved in Detoxification/ Activation	UGT	MEH, GST, UGT	MEH, GST	UGT, NAT
DNA Adduct Formation Sites				
Lung	O6-POB-deoxyguanosine	BPDE-N2-deoxyguanosine		
Bladder				C-8 deoxyguanosine
DNA Repair Pathways	AGT, BER	NER, MMR	BER, NER, NIR	NER

UGT, uridine-5′-diphosphate-glucuronosyltransferases; MEH, microsomal epoxide hydrolases; NAT, N-Acetyltransferases; GST, glutathione-S-transferases; AGT, O6-alkylguanine–DNA alkyltransferase; BER, base excision repair; NER, nucleotide excision repair; MMR, mismatch repair; NIR, nucleotide incision repair.

REFERENCES

1. World Health Organization, Research for International Tobacco Control. *WHO Report on the Global Tobacco Epidemic, 2008: the MPOWER Package*. Geneva: World Health Organization; 2008.
2. Giovino GA, Mirza SA, Samet JM, et al. Tobacco use in 3 billion individuals from 16 countries: an analysis of nationally representative cross-sectional household surveys. *Lancet* 2012;380:668–679.
3. Centers for Disease Control and Prevention (CDC). Current cigarette smoking among adults—United States, 2011. *MMWR Morb Mortal Wkly Rep* 2012;61:889–894.
4. Proctor R. *Golden Holocaust: Origins of the Cigarette Catastrophe and the Case for Abolition*. Berkeley: University of California Press; 2011.
5. Centers for Disease Control and Prevention (CDC). Consumption of cigarettes and combustible tobacco—United States, 2000-2011. *MMWR Morb Mortal Wkly Rep* 2012;61:565–569.
6. Centers for Disease Control and Prevention (CDC). Cigarette use among high school students—United States, 1991–2009. *MMWR Morb Mortal Wkly Rep* 2010;59:797–801.
7. Centers for Disease Control and Prevention (CDC). Tobacco use among middle and high school students—United States, 2000–2009. *MMWR Morb Mortal Wkly Rep* 2010;59:1063–1068.
8. Centers for Disease Control and Prevention (CDC). Tobacco product use among middle and high school students—United States, 2011 and 2012. *MMWR Morb Mortal Wkly Rep* 2013;62:893–897.
9. Cummings KM, Fong GT, Borland R. Environmental influences on tobacco use: evidence from societal and community influences on tobacco use and dependence. *Annu Rev Clin Psychol* 2009;5:433–458.
10. Huang J, Chaloupka FJ, Fong GT. Cigarette graphic warning labels and smoking prevalence in Canada: a critical examination and reformulation of the FDA regulatory impact analysis. *Tob Control* 2014;1:i7–i12.
11. Chaloupka FJ, Yurekli A, Fong GT. Tobacco taxes as a tobacco control strategy. *Tob Control* 2012;21:172–180.
12. Centers for Disease Control and Prevention (CDC). State-specific trends in lung cancer incidence and smoking—United States, 1999-2008. *MMWR Morb Mortal Wkly Rep* 2011;60:1243–1247.
13. Holford TR, Meza R, Warner KE, et al. Tobacco control and the reduction in smoking-related premature deaths in the United States, 1964–2012. *JAMA* 2014;311:164–171.
14. Slama K. The FCTC enters into effect in 2005. *Int J Tuberc Lung Dis* 2005;9:119.
15. Liberman J. Four COPs and counting: achievements, underachievements and looming challenges in the early life of the WHO FCTC Conference of the Parties. *Tob Control* 2012;21:215–220.
16. Deyton LR. FDA tobacco product regulations: a powerful tool for tobacco control. *Public Health Rep* 2011;126:167–169.
17. Patterson JT. *The Dread Disease: Cancer and Modern American Culture*. Cambridge, MA: Harvard University Press; 1987.
18. Proctor R. *The Nazi War on Cancer*. Princeton: Princeton University Press; 1999.
19. Doll R, Hill AB. Smoking and carcinoma of the lung: a preliminary report. *BMJ* 1950;2:739–748.
20. Wynder EL, Graham EA. Tobacco smoking as a possible etiologic factor in bronchiogenic carcinoma: a study of six hundred and eighty-four proved cases. *JAMA* 1950;143:329–336.
21. US Department of Health and Human Services. *The Health Consequences of Smoking: A Report of the Surgeon General*. Atlanta: Department of Health and Human Services, Centers for Disease Control and Prevention, National Center for Chronic Disease Prevention and Health Promotion, Office on Smoking and Health; 2004.
22. Centers for Disease Control and Prevention (CDC). Smoking-attributable mortality, years of potential life lost, and productivity losses—United States, 2000-2004. *MMWR Morb Mortal Wkly Rep* 2008;57:1226–1228.
23. US Department of Health and Human Services. *The Health Consequences of Smoking—50 Years of Progress. A Report of the Surgeon General*. Atlanta: U.S. Department of Health and Human Services, Centers for Disease Control and Prevention, National Center for Chronic Disease Prevention and Health Promotion, Office on Smoking and Health; 2014.
24. Jha P, Ramasundarahettige C, Landsman V, et al. 21st-century hazards of smoking and benefits of cessation in the United States. *N Engl J Med* 2013;368:341–350.
25. Gaudet MM, Gapstur SM, Sun J, et al. Active smoking and breast cancer risk: original cohort data and meta-analysis. *J Natl Cancer Inst* 2013;105:515–525.
26. Peto R, Darby S, Deo H, et al. Smoking, smoking cessation, and lung cancer in the UK since 1950: combination of national statistics with two case-control studies. *BMJ* 2000;321:323–329.
27. Thun MJ, Carter BD, Feskanich D, et al. 50-year trends in smoking-related mortality in the United States. *N Engl J Med* 2013;368:351–364.
28. Burns DM, Anderson CM, Gray N. Has the lung cancer risk from smoking increased over the last fifty years? *Cancer Causes Control* 2011;22:389–397.
29. Benowitz NL. Clinical pharmacology of nicotine: implications for understanding, preventing, and treating tobacco addiction. *Clin Pharmacol Ther* 2008;83:531–541.
30. Benowitz NL. Pharmacology of nicotine: addiction, smoking-induced disease, and therapeutics. *Annu Rev Pharmacol Toxicol* 2009;49:57–71.
31. Benowitz NL. Nicotine addiction. *N Engl J Med* 2010;362:2295–2303.
32. Scherer G. Smoking behaviour and compensation: a review of the literature. *Psychopharmacology (Berl)* 1999;145:1–20.
33. Hammond D, Fong GT, Cummings KM, et al. Smoking topography, brand switching, and nicotine delivery: results from an in vivo study. *Cancer Epidemiol Biomarkers Prev* 2005;14:1370–1375.
34. Benowitz NL, Hukkanen J, Jacob P. Nicotine chemistry, metabolism, kinetics and biomarkers. *Handb Exp Pharmacol* 2009:29–60.
35. Benowitz NL, Swan GE, Jacob P, et al. CYP2A6 genotype and the metabolism and disposition kinetics of nicotine. *Clin Pharmacol Ther* 2006;80:457–467.
36. Johnstone E, Benowitz N, Cargill A, et al. Determinants of the rate of nicotine metabolism and effects on smoking behavior. *Clin Pharmacol Ther* 2006;80:319–330.
37. Malaiyandi V, Lerman C, Benowitz NL, et al. Impact of CYP2A6 genotype on pretreatment smoking behaviour and nicotine levels from and usage of nicotine replacement therapy. *Mol Psychiatry* 2006;11:400–409.
38. Lea RA, Dickson S, Benowitz NL. Within-subject variation of the salivary 3HC/COT ratio in regular daily smokers: prospects for estimating CYP2A6 enzyme activity in large-scale surveys of nicotine metabolic rate. *J Anal Toxicol* 2006;30:386–389.
39. St Helen G, Novalen M, Heitjan DF, et al. Reproducibility of the nicotine metabolite ratio in cigarette smokers. *Cancer Epidemiol Biomarkers Prev* 2012;21:1105–1114.

40. Benowitz NL, Dains KM, Dempsey D, et al. Racial differences in the relationship between number of cigarettes smoked and nicotine and carcinogen exposure. *Nicotine Tob Res* 2011;13:772–783.

41. Dempsey DA, St Helen G, Jacob P, et al. Genetic and pharmacokinetic determinants of response to transdermal nicotine in white, black, and asian nonsmokers. *Clin Pharmacol Ther* 2013;94:687–694.

42. Zhu AZ, Renner CC, Hatsukami DK, et al. The ability of plasma cotinine to predict nicotine and carcinogen exposure is altered by differences in CYP2A6: the influence of genetics, race, and sex. *Cancer Epidemiol Biomarkers Prev* 2013;22:708–718.

43. Schnoll RA, Patterson F, Wileyto EP, et al. Nicotine metabolic rate predicts successful smoking cessation with transdermal nicotine: a validation study. *Pharmacol Biochem Behav* 2009;92:6–11.

44. Fong GT, Hammond D, Laux FL, et al. The near-universal experience of regret among smokers in four countries: findings from the International Tobacco Control Policy Evaluation Survey. *Nicotine Tob Res* 2004;6:S341–S351.

45. Lee WB, Fong GT, Zanna MP, et al. Regret and rationalization among smokers in Thailand and Malaysia: findings from the International Tobacco Control Southeast Asia Survey. *Health Psychol* 2009;28:457–464.

46. Sansone N, Fong GT, Lee WB, et al. Comparing the experience of regret and its predictors among smokers in four Asian countries: findings from the ITC surveys in Thailand, South Korea, Malaysia, and China. *Nicotine Tob Res* 2013;15:1663–1672.

47. Tobacco Use and Dependence Guideline Panel. *Treating Tobacco Use and Dependence: 2008 Update.* Rockville, MD: U.S. Department of Health and Human Services; 2008.

48. Wynder EL, Hoffmann D. *Tobacco and Tobacco Smoke.* New York: Academic Press; 1967.

49. Cummings KM, Morley CP, Hyland A. Failed promises of the cigarette industry and its effect on consumer misperceptions about the health risks of smoking. *Tob Control* 2002;11:I110–I117.

50. Pollay RW, Dewhirst T. The dark side of marketing seemingly "Light" cigarettes: successful images and failed fact. *Tob Control* 2002;11:I18–I31.

51. Fairchild A, Colgrove J. Out of the ashes: the life, death, and rebirth of the "safer" cigarette in the United States. *Am J Public Health* 2004;94:192–204.

52. Hoffmann D, Hoffmann I. The changing cigarette, 1950–1995. *J Toxicol Environ Health.* 1997;50:307–364.

53. Jarvis MJ. Trends in sales weighted tar, nicotine, and carbon monoxide yields of UK cigarettes. *Thorax* 2001;56:960–963.

54. O'Connor RJ, Cummings KM, Giovino GA, et al. How did UK cigarette makers reduce tar to 10 mg or less? *BMJ.* 2006;332:302.

55. National Cancer Institute. *Risks Associated with Smoking Cigarettes with Low Machine-Measured Yields of Tar and Nicotine.* Bethesda, MD: The Institute; 2001.

56. Harris JE, Thun MJ, Mondul AM, et al. Cigarette tar yields in relation to mortality from lung cancer in the cancer prevention study II prospective cohort, 1982-8. *BMJ* 2004;328:72.

57. Thun MJ, Burns DM. Health impact of "reduced yield" cigarettes: a critical assessment of the epidemiological evidence. *Tob Control* 2001;10:i4–i11.

58. Benowitz NL, Jacob P, Bernert JT, et al. Carcinogen exposure during short-term switching from regular to "light" cigarettes. *Cancer Epidemiol Biomarkers Prev* 2005;14:1376–1383.

59. Burns DM, Anderson CM, Gray N. Do changes in cigarette design influence the rise in adenocarcinoma of the lung? *Cancer Causes Control* 2011;22:13–22.

60. Kozlowski LT, Mehta NY, Sweeney CT, et al. Filter ventilation and nicotine content of tobacco in cigarettes from Canada, the United Kingdom, and the United States. *Tob Control* 1998;7:369–375.

61. Kozlowski LT, O'Connor RJ, Giovino GA, et al. Maximum yields might improve public health—if filter vents were banned: a lesson from the history of vented filters. *Tob Control* 2006;15:262–266.

62. Kozlowski LT, O'Connor RJ. Cigarette filter ventilation is a defective design because of misleading taste, bigger puffs, and blocked vents. *Tob Control* 2002;11:I40–I50.

63. Kozlowski LT, Goldberg ME, Yost BA, et al. Smokers are unaware of the filter vents now on most cigarettes: results of a national survey. *Tob Control* 1996;5:265–270.

64. O'Connor RJ, Caruso RV, Borland R, et al. Relationship of cigarette-related perceptions to cigarette design features: findings from the 2009 ITC U.S. Survey. *Nicotine Tob Res* 2013;15:1943–1947.

65. Centers for Disease Control and Prevention, National Center for Chronic Disease Prevention and Health Promotion, Office on Smoking and Health. *How Tobacco Smoke Causes Disease: The Biology and Behavioral Basis for Smoking-Attributable Disease: A Report of the Surgeon General.* Rockville, MD: Centers for Disease Control and Prevetion; 2010.

66. Stratton KR. *Clearing the Smoke: Assessing the Science Base for Tobacco Harm Reduction.* Washington, DC: Institute of Medicine, National Academy Press; 2001.

67. Foulds J, Ramstrom L, Burke M, et al. Effect of smokeless tobacco (snus) on smoking and public health in Sweden. *Tob Control* 2003;12:349–359.

68. Henningfield JE, Fagerstrom KO. Swedish Match Company, Swedish snus and public health: a harm reduction experiment in progress? *Tob Control* 2001;10:253–257.

69. Pepper JK, Brewer NT. Electronic nicotine delivery system (electronic cigarette) awareness, use, reactions and beliefs: a systematic review. *Tob Control* 2013 [Epub ahead of print].

70. Schaller K, Ruppert L, Kahnert S, et al. *Electronic Cigarettes—An Overview.* Heidelberg: German Cancer Research Center (DKFZ); 2013. http://www.dkfz.de/en/presse/download/RS-Vol19-E-Cigarettes-EN.pdf

71. Institute of Medicine. *Scientific Standards for Studies on Modified Risk Tobacco Products.* Washington, DC: National Academies Press; 2012.

72. International Agency for Research on Cancer. *Tobacco Smoke and Involuntary Smoking.* Vol 83. Lyon: International Agency for Research on Cancer, World Health Organization; 2004.

73. International Agency for Research on Cancer. *Smokeless Tobacco and Tobacco-Specific Nitrosamines.* Vol 89. Lyon: International Agency for Research on Cancer, World Health Organization; 2007.

74. Center for Tobacco Products. *Reporting Harmful and Potentially Harmful Constituents in Tobacco Products and Tobacco Smoke Under Section 904(a)(3) of the Federal Food, Drug, and Cosmetic Act.* Rockville, MD: Department of Health and Human Services; 2012.

75. Fowles J, Dybing E. Application of toxicological risk assessment principles to the chemical constituents of cigarette smoke. *Tob Control* 2003;12:424–430.

76. Burns DM, Dybing E, Gray N, et al. Mandated lowering of toxicants in cigarette smoke: a description of the World Health Organization tobacco regulation proposal. *Tob Control* 2008;17:132–141.

77. Straif K, Baan R, Gosse Y, et al. Carcinogenicity of polycyclic aromatic hydrocarbons. *Lancet Oncol* 2005;6:931–932.

78. O'Connor RJ, Hurley PJ. Existing technologies to reduce specific toxicant emissions in cigarette smoke. *Tob Control* 2008;17:i39–i48.

79. Pappas RS. Toxic elements in tobacco and in cigarette smoke: inflammation and sensitization. *Metallomics* 2011;3:1181–1198.

80. Marano KM, Naufal ZS, Kathman SJ, et al. Cadmium exposure and tobacco consumption: biomarkers and risk assessment. *Regul Toxicol Pharmacol* 2012;64:243–252.

81. Stephens WE, Calder A, Newton J. Source and health implications of high toxic metal concentrations in illicit tobacco products. *Environ Sci Technol* 2005;39:479–488.

82. Hecht SS, Hoffmann D. Tobacco-specific nitrosamines, an important group of carcinogens in tobacco and tobacco smoke. *Carcinogenesis* 1988;9:875–884.

83. Hecht SS. Biochemistry, biology, and carcinogenicity of tobacco-specific N-nitrosamines. *Chem Res Toxicol* 1998;11:559–603.

84. Hoffmann D, Rivenson A, Hecht SS. The biological significance of tobacco-specific N-nitrosamines: smoking and adenocarcinoma of the lung. *Crit Rev Toxicol* 1996;26:199–211.

85. Nilsson R. The molecular basis for induction of human cancers by tobacco specific nitrosamines. *Regul Toxicol Pharmacol* 2011;60:268–280.

86. Hecht SS, Stepanov I, Hatsukami DK. Major tobacco companies have technology to reduce carcinogen levels but do not apply it to popular smokeless tobacco products. *Tob Control* 2011;20:443.

87. Stepanov I, Knezevich A, Zhang L, et al. Carcinogenic tobacco-specific N-nitrosamines in US cigarettes: three decades of remarkable neglect by the tobacco industry. *Tob Control* 2012;21:44–48.

88. Stanfill SB, Connolly GN, Zhang L, et al. Global surveillance of oral tobacco products: total nicotine, unionised nicotine and tobacco-specific N-nitrosamines. *Tob Control* 2011;20:e2.

89. Stepanov I, Villalta PW, Knezevich A, et al. Analysis of 23 polycyclic aromatic hydrocarbons in smokeless tobacco by gas chromatography-mass spectrometry. *Chem Res Toxicol* 2010;23:66–73.

90. Stanton MF, Miller E, Wrench C, et al. Experimental induction of epidermoid carcinoma in the lungs of rats by cigarette smoke condensate. *J Natl Cancer Inst* 1972;49:867–877.

91. Hoffmann D, Stepanov I, Hecht SS, et al. *Tobacco Carcinogenesis.* New York: Academic Press; 1978.

92. Deutsch-Wenzel R, Brune H, Grimmer G. Experimental studies in rat lungs on the carcinogenicity and dose-response relationships of eight frequently occurring environmental polycyclic aromatic hydrocarbons. *J Natl Cancer Inst* 1983;71:539–544.

93. Pfeiffer GP, Denissenko MF, Olivier M, et al. Tobacco smoke carcinogens, DNA damage and p53 mutations in smoking-associated cancers. *Oncogene* 2002;21:7435–7451.

94. Boysen G, Hecht SS. Analysis of DNA and protein adducts of benzo[a]pyrene in human tissues using structure-specific methods. *Mutat Res* 2003;543:17–30.

95. Phillips DH. Smoking-related DNA and protein adducts in human tissues. *Carcinogenesis* 2002;23:1979–2004.

96. Liu Z, Muehlbauer KR, Schmeiser HH, et al. p53 Mutations in benzo[a]pyrene-exposed human p53 knock-in murine fibroblasts correlate with p53 mutations in human lung tumors. *Cancer Res* 2005;65:2583–2587.

97. Belinsky SA, Foley JF, White CM, et al. Dose-response relationship between O6-methylguanine formation in Clara cells and induction of pulmonary neoplasia in the rat by 4-(methylnitrosamino)-1-(3-pyridyl)-1-butanone. *Cancer Res* 1990;50:3772–3780.

98. Stepanov I, Sebero E, Wang R, et al. Tobacco-specific N-nitrosamine exposures and cancer risk in the Shanghai cohort study: remarkable coherence with rat tumor sites. *Int J Cancer* 2014;134:2278–2283.

99. Yuan JM, Koh WP, Murphy SE, et al. Urinary levels of tobacco-specific nitrosamine metabolites in relation to lung cancer development in two prospective cohorts of cigarette smokers. *Cancer Res* 2009;69:2990–2995.

ETIOLOGY AND EPIDEMIOLOGY OF CANCER

100. Church TR, Anderson SE, Caporaso NE, et al. A prospectively measured serum biomarker for a tobacco-specific carcinogen and lung cancer in smokers. *Cancer Epidemiol Biomarkers Prev* 2009;18:260–266.

101. Hecht SS, Murphy SE, Stepanov I, et al. Tobacco smoke biomarkers and cancer risk among male smokers in the Shanghai Cohort Study. *Cancer Lett* 2012 [Epub ahead of print].

102. Yuan JM, Butler LM, Gao YT, et al. Urinary metabolites of a polycyclic aromatic hydrocarbon and volatile organic compounds in relation to lung cancer development in lifelong never smokers in the Shanghai Cohort Study. *Carcinogenesis* 2014;35:339–345.

103. Melikian AA, Sun P, Prokopczyk B, et al. Identification of benzo[a]pyrene metabolites in cervical mucus and DNA adducts in cervical tissues in humans by gas chromatography-mass spectrometry. *Cancer Lett* 1999;146: 127–134.

104. Prokopczyk B, Trushin N, Leszczynska J, et al. Human cervical tissue metabolizes the tobacco-specific nitrosamine, 4-(methylnitrosamino)-1-(3-pyridyl)-1-butanone, via alpha-hydroxylation and carbonyl reduction pathways. *Carcinogenesis* 2001;22:107–114.

105. Castelao JE, Yuan JM, Skipper PL, et al. Gender- and smoking-related bladder cancer risk. *J Natl Cancer Inst* 2001;93:538–545.

106. Sugimura T. History, present and future, of heterocyclic amines, cooked food mutagens. *Princess Takamatsu Symp* 1995;23:214–231.

107. Turesky RJ. Heterocyclic aromatic amine metabolism, DNA adduct formation, mutagenesis, and carcinogenesis. *Drug Metab Rev* 2002; 34:625–650.

108. Ashley DL, O'Connor RJ, Bernert JT, et al. Effect of differing levels of tobacco-specific nitrosamines in cigarette smoke on the levels of biomarkers in smokers. *Cancer Epidemiol Biomarkers Prev* 2010;19:1389–1398.

109. Hatsukami DK, Benowitz NL, Rennard SI, et al. Biomarkers to assess the utility of potential reduced exposure tobacco products. *Nicotine Tob Res* 2008;8: 169–191.

110. Carmella SG, Chen M, Han S, et al. Effects of smoking cessation on eight urinary tobacco carcinogen and toxicant biomarkers. *Chem Res Toxicol* 2009;22:734–741.

111. Carmella SG, Ming X, Olvera N, et al. High throughput liquid and gas chromatography-tandem mass spectrometry assays for tobacco-specific nitrosamine and polycyclic aromatic hydrocarbon metabolites associated with lung cancer in smokers. *Chem Res Toxicol* 2013;26:1209–1217.

112. Church TR, Anderson KE, Le C, et al. Temporal stability of urinary and plasma biomarkers of tobacco smoke exposure among cigarette smokers. *Biomarkers* 2010;15:345–352.

113. Hecht SS, Yuan JM, Hatsukami D. Applying tobacco carcinogen and toxicant biomarkers in product regulation and cancer prevention. *Chem Res Toxicol* 2010;23:1001–1008.

114. Hecht SS. Tobacco smoke carcinogens and lung cancer. *J Natl Cancer Inst* 1999;91:1194–1210.

115. Hecht SS. Tobacco carcinogens, their biomarkers, and tobacco-induced cancer. *Nature Rev Cancer* 2003;3:733–744.

116. Hecht SS. Lung carcinogenesis by tobacco smoke. *Int J Cancer* 2012;131: 2724–2732.

117. Guengerich FP. Common and uncommon cytochrome P450 reactions related to metabolism and chemical toxicity. *Chem Res Toxicol* 2001; 14:611–650.

118. Jalas J, Hecht SS, Murphy SE. Cytochrome P450 2A enzymes as catalysts of metabolism of 4-(methylnitrosamino)-1-(3-pyridyl)-1-butanone (NNK), a tobacco-specific carcinogen. *Chem Res Toxicol* 2005;18:95–110.

119. Nebert DW, Dalton TP, Okey AB, et al. Role of aryl hydrocarbon receptor-mediated induction of the CYP1 enzymes in environmental toxicity and cancer. *J Biol Chem* 2004;279:23847–23850.

120. Hang B. Formation and repair of tobacco carcinogen-derived bulky DNA adducts. *J Nucleic Acids* 2010;2010:709521.

121. Burchell B, McGurk K, Brierley CH, et al. *UDP-Glucuronosyltransferases.* Vol 3. New York: Elsevier Science; 1997.

122. Armstrong RN. *Glutathione-S-Transferases.* Vol 3. New York: Elsevier Science; 1997.

123. Vineis P, Veglia F, Benhamou S, et al. CYP1A1 T3801 C polymorphism and lung cancer: a pooled analysis of 2451 cases and 3358 controls. *Int J Cancer* 2003;104:650–657.

124. Carlsten C, Sagoo GS, Frodsham AJ, et al. Glutathione S-transferase M1 (GSTM1) polymorphisms and lung cancer: a literature-based systematic HuGE review and meta-analysis. *Am J Epidemiol* 2008;167:759–774.

125. Ahrendt SA, Decker PA, Alawi EA, et al. Cigarette smoking is strongly associated with mutation of the K-ras gene in patients with primary adenocarcinoma of the lung. *Cancer* 2001;92:1525–1530.

126. Ding L, Getz G, Wheeler DA, et al. Somatic mutations affect key pathways in lung adenocarcinoma. *Nature* 2008;455:1069–1075.

127. Johnson L, Mercer K, Greenbaum D, et al. Somatic activation of the K-ras oncogene causes early onset lung cancer in mice. *Nature* 2001;410:1111–1116.

128. Sekido Y, Fong KW, Minna JD. Progress in understanding the molecular pathogenesis of human lung cancer. *Biochim Biophys Acta* 1998;1378:F21–F59.

129. Bode AM, Dong A. Signal transduction pathways in cancer development and as targets for cancer prevention. *Prog Nucleic Acid Res Mol Biol* 2005;79:237–297.

130. Schuller HM. Mechanisms of smoking-related lung and pancreatic adenocarcinoma development. *Nat Rev Cancer* 2002;2:455–463.

131. Heeschen C, Jang JJ, Weis M, et al. Nicotine stimulates angiogenesis and promotes tumor growth and atherosclerosis. *Nat Med* 2001;7:833–839.

132. West KA, Brognard J, Clark AS, et al. Rapid Akt activation by nicotine and a tobacco carcinogen modulates the phenotype of normal human airway epithelial cells. *J Clin Invest* 2003;111:81–90.

133. Moraitis D, Du B, De Lorenzo MS, et al. Levels of cyclooxygenase-2 are increased in the oral mucosa of smokers: evidence for the role of epidermal growth factor receptor and its ligands. *Cancer Res* 2005;65:664–670.

5 Oncogenic Viruses

Christopher B. Buck and Lee Ratner

PRINCIPLES OF TUMOR VIROLOGY

Viral infections are estimated to play a causal role in at least 11% of all new cancer diagnoses worldwide.[1] A vast majority of cases (>85%) occur in developing countries, where poor sanitation, high rates of cocarcinogenic factors such as HIV/AIDS, and lack of access to vaccines and cancer screening all contribute to increased rates of virally induced cancers. Even in developed countries, where effective countermeasures are widely available, cancers attributable to viral infection account for at least 4% of new cases.[2,3]

Viruses thought to cause various forms of human cancer come from six distinct viral families with a range of physical characteristics (Table 5.1). All known human cancer viruses are capable of establishing durable, long-term infections and cause cancer only in a minority of persistently infected individuals. The low penetrance of cancer induction is consistent with the idea that a virus capable of establishing a durable productive infection would not benefit from inducing a disease that kills the host.[4] The slow course of cancer induction (typically over a course of many years after the initial infection) suggests that viral infection alone is rarely sufficient to cause human malignancy and that virally induced cancers arise only after additional oncogenic "hits" have had time to accumulate stochastically.

In broad terms, viruses can cause cancer through either (or both) of two broad mechanisms: direct or indirect. Direct mechanisms, in which the virus-infected cell ultimately becomes malignant, are typically driven by the effects of viral oncogene expression or through direct genotoxic effects of viral gene products. In most established examples of direct viral oncogenesis, the cancerous cell remains "addicted" to viral oncogene expression for ongoing growth and viability.

A common feature of DNA viruses that depend on host cell DNA polymerases for replication (e.g., papillomaviruses, herpesviruses, and polyomaviruses) is the expression of viral gene products that promote progression into the cell cycle. A typical mechanism of direct oncogenic effects is through the inactivation of tumor suppressor proteins, such as the guardian of the genome, p53, and retinoblastoma protein (pRB). This effectively primes the cell to express the host machinery necessary for replicating the viral DNA. The study of tumor viruses has been instrumental in uncovering the existence and function of key tumor suppressor proteins, as well as key cellular proto-oncogenes, such as Src and Myc.

In theory, viruses could cause cancer via direct hit-and-run effects. In this model, viral gene products may serve to preserve cellular viability and promote cell growth in the face of otherwise proapoptotic genetic damage during the early phases of tumor development. In principle, the precancerous cell might eventually accumulate enough additional genetic hits to allow for cell growth and survival independent of viral oncogene expression. This would allow for stochastic loss of viral nucleic acids from the nascent tumor, perhaps giving a growth advantage due to the loss of "foreign" viral antigens that might otherwise serve as targets for immune-mediated clearance of the nascent tumor. Although hit-and-run effects have been observed in animal models of virally

induced cancer,[5] these effects are extremely difficult to address in humans. Currently, there are no clearly established examples of hit-and-run effects in human cancer.

In indirect oncogenic mechanisms, the cells that give rise to the malignant tumor have never been infected by the virus. Instead, the viral infection is thought to lead to cancer by attracting inflammatory immune responses that, in turn, lead to accelerated cycles of tissue damage and regeneration of noninfected cells. In some instances, virally infected cells may secrete paracrine signals that drive the proliferation of uninfected cells. At a theoretical level, it may be difficult to distinguish between indirect carcinogenesis and hit-and-run direct carcinogenesis, because, in both cases, the metastatic tumor may not contain any viral nucleic acids.

A variety of hunting approaches have been used to uncover etiologic roles for viruses in human cancer. The first clues that high-risk human papillomaviruses (HPVs), Epstein-Barr virus (EBV), Kaposi's sarcoma–associated herpesvirus (KSHV), and Merkel cell polyomavirus (MCPyV) might be carcinogenic were based on the detection of virions, viral DNA, or viral RNA in the tumors these viruses cause. A common feature of known virally induced cancers is that they are more prevalent in immunosuppressed individuals, such as individuals suffering from HIV/AIDS or patients on immunosuppressive therapy after organ transplantation. This is thought to reflect the lack of immunologic control over the cancer-causing virus. Studies focused on AIDS-associated cancers provided the first evidence for the carcinogenic potential of KSHV and MCPyV. A theoretical limitation of this approach is that some virally induced cancers may not occur at dramatically elevated rates in all types of immunosuppressed subjects, particularly if the virus causes only a fraction of cases (e.g., HPV-induced head and neck cancers). Fortunately, the unbiased analysis of nucleic acid sequences found in tumors has become substantially more tractable as deep-sequencing methods have continued to fall in price. In the coming years, it should be increasingly possible to search for viral sequences without making the starting assumption that all virally induced tumors are associated with immunosuppression.[6]

One limitation of tumor sequencing approaches is that they might miss undiscovered divergent viral species within viral families known to have extensive sequence diversity[7] and could miss viral families that have not yet been discovered.[8] Tumor-sequencing approaches might also miss viruses that cause cancer by hit-and-run or indirect mechanisms. It is conceivable that this caveat could be addressed by focusing on sequencing early precancerous lesions thought to ultimately give rise to metastatic cancer.

An additional successful approach to hunting cancer viruses involves showing that individuals who are infected with a particular virus have an increased long-term risk of developing particular forms of cancer. This approach was successful for identifying and validating the carcinogenic roles of high-risk HPV types, hepatitis B virus (HBV), hepatitis C virus (HCV), KSHV, and human T-lymphotropic virus 1 (HTLV-1). Although viruses that are extremely prevalent, such as EBV and MCPyV, are not amenable to this approach per se, it may still be possible to draw connections

TABLE 5.1
Oncogenic Viruses

Virus	Taxon	Viral Genome	Virion	Infection Rate	Site of Persistance	Diseases in Normal Hosts	Diseases in Immunocompromised Hosts	Associated Cancers
High-risk human papillomavirus types (e.g., HPV16)	*Alphapapillomavirus*	8 kb circular dsDNA	Nonenveloped	>70%	Anogential mucosa, oral mucosa	Carcinomas of the cervix, penis, anus, vagina, vulva, tonsils, base of tongue	Increased incidence of same diseases	610,000
Hepatitis B virus (HBV)	*Hepadnaviridae*	3 kb ss/dsDNA	Enveloped	2%–8%	Hepatocytes	Cirrhosis, hepatocellular carcinoma	Same diseases, increased incidence with AIDS	380,000
Hepatitis C virus (HCV)	*Flaviviridae*	10 kb +RNA	Enveloped	~3%	Hepatocytes	Cirrhosis, hepatocellular carcinoma, splenic marginal zone lymphoma	Same diseases, increased incidence with AIDS	220,000
Epstein-Barr virus (EBV, HHV-4)	*Gammaherpesvirinae*	170 kb linear DNA	Enveloped	90%	B cells, pharyngeal mucosa	Mononucleosis, Burkitt lymphoma, other non-Hodgkin lymphoma, nasopharyngeal carcinoma	Increased incidence of same diseases, lymphoproliferative disease, other lymphomas, oral hairy leukoplakia, leiomyosarcoma	110,000
Kaposi's sarcoma herpesvirus (KSHV, HHV-8)	*Gammaherpesvirinae*	170 kb linear DNA	Enveloped	2%–60%	Oral mucosa, endothelium, B cells	Kaposi's sarcoma (KS), multicentric Castleman disease (MCD)	Increased KS, MCD incidence, primary effusion lymphoma	43,000
Merkel cell polyomavirus (MCPyV, MCV)	*Orthopolyomavirus*	5 kb circular dsDNA	Nonenveloped	75%	Skin (lymphocytes?)	Merkel cell carcinoma (MCC)	Increased MCC incidence	1,500 (US)
Human T-cell leukemia virus (HTLV-1)	*Deltaretrovirus*	9 kb +RNA (RT)	Enveloped	0.01%–6%	T and B cells	Adult T-cell leukemia/lymphoma, tropical spastic paraparesis, myelopathy, uveitis, dermatitis	Unknown	2,100

Note: Ranges for infection rates imply major variations in prevalence among populations in different world regions. *Associated cancers* indicates the annual number of new cases clearly attributable to viral infection. An estimate for the worldwide incidence of Merkel cell carcinoma is not currently available and an estimate of the annual new cases in the United States alone is given instead.
ds, double-stranded; ss, single-stranded; HHV, human herpesvirus; RT, reverse transcriptase.
Adapted from de Martel C, Ferlay J, Franceschi S, et al. Global burden of cancers attributable to infections in 2008: a review and synthetic analysis. *Lancet Oncol* 2012;13(6):607–615; Schiller JT, Lowy DR. Virus infection and human cancer: an overview. *Recent Results Cancer Res* 2014;193:1–10; Chen CJ, Hsu WL, Yang HI, et al. Epidemiology of virus infection and human cancer. *Recent Results Cancer Res* 2014;193:11–32; and Virgin HW, Wherry EJ, Ahmed R. Redefining chronic viral infection. *Cell* 2009;138(1):30–50.

between cancer risk and either unusually high serum antibody titers against viral antigens or unusually high viral load. Relatively high serologic titers reflect either comparatively poor control of the viral infection in at-risk individuals or expression of viral antigens in tumors or tumor precursor cells.[9,10]

The finding that a virus causes cancer is good news, in the sense that it can suggest possible paths to clinical intervention. These can include the development of vaccines or antiviral agents that prevent, attenuate, or eradicate the viral infection and thereby prevent cancer; the development of methods for early detection or diagnosis of cancer based on assays for viral nucleic acids or gene products; or the development of drugs or immunotherapeutics that treat cancer by targeting viral gene products. Unfortunately, establishing the carcinogenicity of a given viral species is an arduous process that must inevitably integrate multiple lines of evidence.[11] The demonstration that the virus can transform cells in culture and/or cause cancer in animal models provides circumstantial evidence of the oncogenic potential of a virus. All known human cancer viruses meet this criterion. However, it is important to recognize that viruses can theoretically coevolve to be noncarcinogenic in their native host (e.g., humans) and cause cancer only in the dysregulated environment of a nonnative host animal. This caveat may apply to human adenoviruses.

Finding that viral DNA is clonally integrated in a primary tumor and its metastatic lesions helps address the caveat that the virus might merely be a hitchhiker that finds the tumor cell a conducive environment in which to replicate (as opposed to playing a causal carcinogenic role). This caveat is also addressed by the observation that, in most instances, viruses found in tumors have lost the ability to exit viral latency and are functionally unable to produce new progeny virions. An unfortunate consequence of this is that vaccines or antiviral agents that target virion proteins (e.g., vaccines against high-risk HPVs or HBV) or gene products expressed late in the viral life cycle (e.g., herpesvirus thymidine kinase, which is the target of drugs such as ganciclovir) are rarely effective for treating existing virally induced tumors.

Demonstrating that a vaccine or antiviral agent targeting the virus either prevents or treats human cancer is by far the strongest form of evidence that a given virus causes human cancer. This type of proof has fully validated the causal role of HBV in human liver cancer. Compelling clinical trial data also show that antiherpesvirus therapeutics can prevent KSHV- or EBV-associated lymphoproliferative disorders, and that vaccination against HPV can prevent the development of precancerous lesions on the uterine cervix.

PAPILLOMAVIRUSES

History

The idea that cancer of the uterine cervix might be linked to sexual behavior was first proposed in the mid 19th century by Dominico Rigoni-Stern, who observed that nuns rarely contracted cervical cancer, whereas prostitutes suffered from cervical cancer more often than the general populace.[12] Another major milestone in cervical cancer research was Georgios Papanikolaou's development of the so-called Pap smear for early cytologic diagnosis of precancerous cervical lesions.[13] This form of screening, which allows for surgical intervention to remove precancerous lesions, has saved many millions of lives in developed countries, where public health campaigns have made testing widely available.

Although observations in the early 1980s suggested the possibility of a hit-and-run carcinogenic role for herpes simplex viruses in cervical cancer,[14] this hypothesis was abandoned in light of studies led by Harald zur Hausen. Low-stringency hybridization approaches revealed the presence of two previously unknown papillomavirus types, HPV16 and HPV18, in various cervical cancer cell lines, including the famous HeLa cell line.[15,16] There is now

overwhelming evidence that a group of more than a dozen sexually transmitted HPV types, including HPV16 and HPV18, play a causal role in essentially all cases of cervical cancer. HPVs associated with a high risk of cancer also cause about half of all penile cancers, 88% of anal cancers, 43% of vulvar cancers, 70% of vaginal cancers,[2] and an increasing fraction of head and neck cancers (see the following). In 2008, zur Hausen was awarded the Nobel Prize for his groundbreaking work establishing the link between HPVs and human cancer.

The viral family *Papillomaviridae* is named for the benign skin warts (papillomas) that some members of the family cause. In the early 1930s, Richard Edwin Shope and colleagues demonstrated viral transmission of papillomas in a rabbit model system.[17] Using this system, Peyton Rous and others showed that cottontail rabbit papillomavirus-induced lesions can progress to malignant skin cancer.[18,19] This was the first demonstration of a cancer-causing virus in mammals, building on Rous' prior work demonstrating a virus capable of causing cancer in chickens (the Rous sarcoma retrovirus).

Tissue Tropism and Gene Functions

Although papillomaviruses can achieve infectious entry into a wide variety of cell types in vitro and in vivo, the late phase of the viral life cycle, during which the viral genome undergoes vegetative replication and the L1 and L2 capsid proteins are expressed, is strictly dependent on host cell factors found only in differentiating keratinocytes near the surface of the skin or mucosa. Interestingly, a majority of HPV-induced cancers appear to arise primarily at zones of transition between stratified squamous epithelia and the single-layer (columnar) epithelia of the endocervix, the inner surface of the anus, and tonsillar crypts. It is thought that the mixed phenotypic milieu in cells at squamocolumnar transition zones may cause dysregulation of the normal coupling of the HPV life cycle to keratinocyte differentiation.

There are nearly 200 known HPV types.[20] In general, each papillomavirus type is a functionally distinct serotype, meaning that serum antibodies that neutralize one HPV type do not robustly neutralize other HPV types. Various HPV types preferentially infect different skin or mucosal surfaces. Different types tend to establish either transient infections that may be cleared over the course of months, or stable infections where virions are chronically shed from the infected skin surface for the lifetime of the host. HPV infections may or may not be associated with the formation of visible warts or other lesions. High-risk HPV types, with clearly established causal links to human cancer, are preferentially tropic for the anogenital mucosa and the oral mucosa, are usually transmitted by sexual contact, rarely cause visible warts, and usually establish only transient infections in a great majority of exposed individuals. The lifetime risk of sexual exposure to a high-risk HPV type has been estimated to be >70%. Individuals who fail to clear their infection with a high-risk HPV type and remain persistently infected are at much greater risk of developing cancer. Polymerase chain reaction (PCR)-based screening for the presence of high-risk HPV types thus serves as a useful adjunct to, or even a replacement for, the traditional Pap test.[21]

A consequence of the strict tissue-differentiation specificity of the papillomavirus life cycle is that HPVs do not replicate in standard monolayer cell cultures. Papillomaviruses also seem to be highly species restricted, and there are no known examples of an HPV type capable of infecting animals.[22] Thus, the investigation of key details of papillomavirus biology has relied almost entirely on modern recombinant DNA and molecular biologic analyses.

Papillomavirus genomes are roughly 8 kb, double-stranded, closed-circular DNA molecules (essentially reminiscent of a plasmid). During the normal viral life cycle, the genome does not adopt a linear form, does not integrate into the host cell chromosome, and remains as an extrachromosomal episome or minichromosome.

All the viral protein-coding sequences are arranged on one strand of the genome. The expression of various proteins is regulated by differential transcription and polyadenylation, as well as effects at the level of RNA splicing, export from the nucleus, and translation. In addition to the late half of the viral genome, which encodes the L1 and L2 capsid proteins, all papillomaviruses encode six key early region genes: E1, E2, E4, E5, E6, and E7.

The master transcriptional regulator E2 serves as a transcriptional repressor, and loss of E2 expression (typically through integration of the viral episome into the host cell DNA) results in the upregulation of early gene expression. The most extensively studied early region proteins are the E6 and E7 oncogenes of HPV16 and HPV18. The E6 protein of high-risk HPV types triggers the destruction of p53 by recruiting a host cell ubiquitin–protein ligase, E6AP.[23–25] Another important oncogenic function of E6 is the activation of cellular telomerase.[26] A wide variety of additional high-risk E6 activities that do not involve p53 have been identified.[27]

Most E7 proteins, including those of many low-risk HPV types, contain a conserved LXCXE motif that mediates interaction with pRB and the related "pocket" proteins p107 and p130.[28] Interestingly, the LXCXE motif is present in a wide variety of other oncogenes, most notably the T antigens of polyomaviruses and the E1A oncogenes of adenoviruses. The interaction of E7 with pRB disrupts the formation of a complex between pRB and E2F transcription factors, thereby blocking the ability of pRB to trigger cell cycle arrest.[29] The E7 proteins of high-risk HPVs can also contribute to chromosomal mis-segregation and aneuploidy, which may in turn contribute to malignant progression.[30] Like E6, E7 interacts with a wide variety of additional cellular targets, the spectrum of which seems to vary with different HPV types.[27]

Some papillomavirus types express an E5 oncogene, which functions as an agonist for cell surface growth factor receptors such as platelet-derived growth factor beta (PDGF-β) and epidermal growth factor (EGF) receptor.[31] Because E5 expression is uncommon in cervical tumors, it is uncertain whether the protein plays a key role in human cancer.

Human Papilloma Virus Vaccines

Two preventive vaccines against cancer-causing HPVs, trade named Gardasil (Merck) and Cervarix (GSK), are currently marketed worldwide for the prevention of cervical cancer. Both vaccines contain recombinant L1 capsid proteins based on HPV16 and HPV18 that are assembled in vitro into virus-like particles (VLPs). Together, HPV16 and HPV18 cause about 70% of all cases of cervical cancer worldwide. Gardasil also includes VLPs based on HPV types 6 and 11, which rarely cause cervical cancer but together cause about 90% of all genital warts. The VLPs contained in the vaccines are highly immunogenic in humans, eliciting high-titer serum antibody responses against L1 that are capable of neutralizing the infectivity of the cognate HPV types represented in the vaccine. It appears that the current HPV vaccines may confer lifelong immunity against new infection with the HPV types represented in the vaccine.[32] The vaccines elicit lower titer cross-neutralizing responses against a subset of cancer-causing HPV types that are closely related to HPV16 and HPV18.[33] Although these cross-neutralizing responses can at least partially protect vaccinees against a new infection with additional high-risk types, such as HPV31 and HPV45, it remains unclear how durable the lower level cross-protection will be.[33]

Because L1 is not expressed in latently infected keratinocyte stem cells residing on the epithelial basement membrane, current HPV vaccines are very unlikely to eradicate existing infections.[34,35] Like keratinocyte stem cells, cervical cancers and precursor lesions rarely or never express L1. Thus, the existing L1-based vaccines seem unlikely to serve as therapeutic agents for treating cervical cancer.

Three types of next-generation HPV vaccines are currently in human clinical trials. Merck has recently announced that a newer version of Gardasil, which contains VLPs based on a total of nine different HPV types, remained highly effective against HPV16 and HPV18 and also prevented 97% of precancerous cervical lesions caused by a wider variety of high-risk HPV types.[36] Another class of second-generation vaccines targets the papillomavirus minor capsid protein L2. An N-terminal portion of L2 appears to represent a highly conserved "Achilles' heel", which contains conserved protein motifs required for key steps of the infectious entry process.[37] Anti-L2 antibodies can neutralize a broad range of different human and animal HPV types, and thus, L2 vaccines are hoped to offer protection against all HPVs that cause cervical cancer, all low-risk HPV types that cause abnormal Pap smear results, as well as the full range of HPV types that cause skin warts. Finally, a wide variety of vaccines that seek to elicit cell-mediated immune responses against the E6 and E7 oncoproteins are aimed at a therapeutic intervention for the treatment of cervical cancer.[38]

Oropharyngeal Cancer

It is well established that tobacco products and alcohol cause head and neck cancer. In the late 1990s, Maura Gillison and colleagues noted a surprising number of new cases of tonsillar cancer in nonsmokers.[39] Many of the tumors found in nonsmokers were found to have wild-type p53 genes, raising the possibility that the tumor might be dependent on a p53-suppressing viral oncogene (as seen in cervical cancer). Gillison and colleagues went on to show that nearly half of all tonsillar cancers contain HPV DNA, most commonly HPV16. Interestingly, HPV-positive oropharyngeal cancers tend to be less lethal than tobacco-associated HPV-negative tumors. This finding has important implications for treatment of HPV-positive head and neck cancers.[40]

Although the incidence of tobacco-associated head and neck cancer has been declining in recent decades due to decreased tobacco use, recent studies suggest an ongoing increase in the incidence of HPV-associated cancers of the tonsils and the base of the tongue. By 2025, the number of new HPV-induced head and neck cancer cases in the United States is expected to roughly equal the number of new cervical cancer cases.[39] Based in part on these observations, the U.S. Centers for Disease Control and Prevention recommends that boys, in addition to girls, should be vaccinated against high-risk HPVs.

Nonmelanoma Skin Cancer

Epidermodysplasia verruciformis (EV) is a rare immunodeficiency that is characterized by the appearance of numerous flat, wartlike lesions across wide areas of skin. The lesions typically contain genus betapapillomaviruses, such as HPV5 or HPV8. EV patients frequently develop squamous cell carcinomas (SCC) in sun-exposed skin areas (suggesting that ultraviolet [UV] light exposure is a cofactor). It is also well established that other immunosuppressed individuals, such as organ transplant recipients and HIV-infected individuals, are at increased risk of developing SCC.[41,42] Although the E6 and E7 proteins of betapapillomaviruses appear to exert a different spectrum of effects than the E6 and E7 proteins of HPV types associated with cervical cancer,[43–45] Betapapillomavirus oncogenes can transform cells in vitro.[46] Although these circumstantial lines of evidence suggest that infectious agents, such as Betapapillomaviruses, might play a causal role in SCC, recent deep sequencing studies have observed few or no viral sequences in SCC tumors.[47] Although the results argue against durable direct oncogenic effects of any known viral species in SCC, an animal model system using bovine papillomavirus type 4 strongly suggests that papillomaviruses can cause cancer by hit and run mechanisms.[5] Thus, the question of whether hit-and-run or indirect oncogenic effects of HPVs may be at play in human SCC remains open.

POLYOMAVIRUSES

History

In the early 1950s, Ludwik Gross showed that a filterable infectious agent could cause salivary gland cancer in laboratory mice.[48] Later work by Bernice Eddy and Sarah Stewart showed that the murine polyoma (Greek for "many tumors") virus caused many different types of cancer in experimentally infected mice.[49] The discovery that murine polyomavirus could be grown in cell culture helped rekindle research interest in tumor virology and interest in the question of whether viruses might cause human cancer.

Like papillomaviruses, polyomaviruses have a nonenveloped capsid assembled from 72 pentamers of a single major capsid protein (VP1). Both viral families also carry circular dsDNA genomes. These physical similarities initially led to the classification of both groups into a single family, *Papovaviridae*. When sequencing studies ultimately revealed that polyomaviruses have a unique genome organization (with early and late genes being arranged on opposing strands of the genome) and almost no sequence homology to papillomaviruses, the two groups of viruses were divided into separate families.

In the early 1960s, Bernice Eddy, Maurice Hilleman, and Benjamin Sweet reported the discovery of simian vacuolating virus 40 (SV40), a previously unknown polyomavirus that was found as a contaminant in vaccines against poliovirus.[50,51] SV40 was derived from the rhesus monkey kidney cells used to amplify poliovirus virions in culture.[52] SV40 rapidly became an important model polyomavirus, and studies of its major and minor tumor antigens (large T [LT] and small t [ST], respectively) have played an important role in understanding various aspects of carcinogenesis. Despite significant alarm about the possible risk SV40 might pose to exposed individuals, a comprehensive, decades long series of studies have failed to uncover compelling evidence that SV40 exposure is causally associated with human cancer.[53]

Two naturally human-tropic polyomaviruses, BK virus (BKV) and John Cunningham virus (JCV), were first reported in back-to-back publications in 1971.[54,55] BKV and JCV are known to cause kidney disease and a lethal brain disease called progressive multifocal leukoencephalopathy, respectively, in immunosuppressed individuals. Although both viruses can cause cancer in experimentally exposed animals, it remains unclear whether either virus plays a causal role in human cancer. Although BKV LT expression can frequently be observed in the inflammatory precursor lesions that

are thought to give rise to prostate cancer,[56] there is no evidence for the persistence of BKV DNA in malignant prostate tumors.[57] There have been case studies finding BKV T-antigen expression in bladder cancer,[58] and some reports have indicated the presence of JCV DNA in colorectal tumors. The long history of conflicting evidence concerning possible roles for BKV or JCV in human cancer is reviewed elsewhere.[59,60]

Merkel Cell Polyomavirus

In 2008, Yuan Chang and Patrick Moore reported their lab's discovery of the fifth known human polyomavirus species, which they named Merkel cell polyomavirus (MCV or MCPyV) based on its presence in Merkel cell carcinoma (MCC).[61] The discovery used an RNA deep sequencing approach called digital transcriptome subtraction. Using classic Southern blotting, this report demonstrated the clonal integration of MCPyV in an MCC tumor and its distant metastases. Many other labs worldwide have independently confirmed the presence of MCPyV DNA in about 80% of MCC tumors.[11]

MCC is a rare but highly lethal form of cancer that typically presents as a fast-growing lesion on sun-exposed skin surfaces (Fig. 5.1).[62] The risk of MCC is dramatically higher in HIV/AIDS patients, offering an initial clue that MCC might be a virally induced cancer.[63] Although MCC tumors express neuroendocrine markers associated with sensory Merkel cells of the epidermis, one recent report has shown that some MCC tumors also express B-cell markers, including rearranged antibody loci.[64] Currently, there is no clear evidence for the involvement of MCPyV in other tumors with neuroendocrine features.

In 2012, the International Agency for Research on Cancer (IARC) concluded that MCPyV is a class 2A carcinogen (probably carcinogenic to humans).[10,53] It should be noted that IARC evaluations rely heavily on animal carcinogenicity studies, and the 2A designation was assigned prior to a recent report showing that MCV-positive MCC lines are tumorigenic in a mouse model system.[65]

A great majority of healthy adults have serum antibodies specific for the MCPyV major capsid protein VP1. A majority also shed MCPyV virions from apparently healthy skin surfaces, and there is a strong correlation between individual subjects' serologic titer against VP1 and the amount of MCPyV DNA they shed.[66–68] Interestingly, MCC patients tend to have exceptionally strong serologic titers against VP1.[69] MCC tumors do not express detectable amounts of VP1, so this is unlikely to reflect direct exposure to

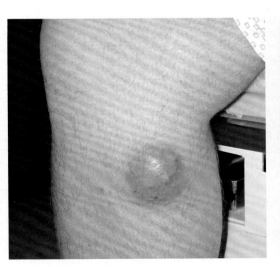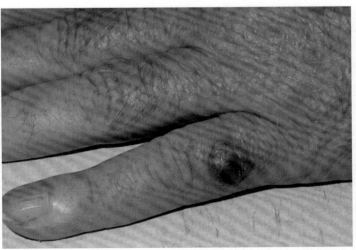

Figure 5.1 Merkel cell carcinoma (MCC). The *left panel* shows an MCC tumor on the calf. The *right panel* shows an MCC tumor on the finger. Photographs provided with permission by Dr. Paul Nghiem (University of Washington, www.merkelcell.org).

the tumor and instead likely represents a history of a high MCPyV load in MCC patients. A recent study of archived serum samples shows that unusually high serologic titers against MCPyV VP1 often precede the development of MCC by many years.[70]

Like the LT protein of SV40 (and the E7 proteins of high-risk HPVs), an N-terminal portion of the MCPyV LT protein contains an LXCXE motif that mediates inactivation of pRB function. In contrast to SV40 LT, which carries a p53-inactivation domain that overlaps the C-terminal helicase domain, MCPyV LT does not appear to inactivate p53 function.[71] Instead, the MCPyV LT helicase domain activates DNA damage responses and induces cell cycle arrest in cultured cell lines.[72] This may explain why the LT genes found in MCC tumors essentially always carry mutations that truncate LT upstream of the helicase domain. siRNA experiments indicate that most (although possibly not all) MCC tumors are "addicted" to the expression of MCPyV T antigens.[73–75] Interestingly, patients with higher levels of MCPyV DNA in their tumors, stronger T-antigen expression, and tumors that have been infiltrated by CD8+ T cells appear to have better prognoses.[76] This is consistent with the idea that cell-mediated immunity can help clear MCC tumors that express MCPyV antigens.

Recent work has shown that the pRB interacting domain of LT mediates increased expression of the cellular gene survivin. The knockdown of survivin using siRNAs results in MCC tumor cell death and YM155, a small molecule inhibitor of survivin expression, protects mice from MCC tumors in a xenograft challenge system.[77,78]

In contrast to SV40, where LT appears to be the dominant oncogene, the MCPyV ST protein appears to play a key role in cell transformation. In addition to modifying the signaling functions of the cellular proto-oncogene PP2A, ST triggers the phosphorylation of eukaryotic translation initiation factor 4E binding protein 1.[79] This results in dysregulation of cap-dependent translation and cellular transformation.

Although there is an intriguing epidemiologic correlation between MCC and chronic lymphocytic leukemia (CLL),[80] there are conflicting reports concerning the presence of MCPyV in CLL and other lymphocytic cancers.[81–83]

Other Human Polyomaviruses

In recent years, the number of known human polyomaviruses has expanded dramatically. Of the 12 currently known HPyV species, only MCPyV has been clearly linked to human cancer. One new HPyV, trichodysplasia spinulosa polyomavirus (TSV or TSPyV) has been found in association with abnormal spiny growths on the facial skin of a small number of immunocompromised individuals.

EPSTEIN-BARR VIRUS

History

In 1958, Denis Burkitt provided the first clear clinical description of an unusual B-cell–derived tumor that frequently affects the jawbones of children in equatorial Africa.[84] After hearing Burkitt give a 1961 lecture entitled "The Commonest Children's Cancer in Tropical Africa – A Hitherto Unrecognized Syndrome," Michael Epstein became interested in the idea that an insect vector-borne infection might account for the high incidence of Burkitt lymphoma in tropical Africa. Epstein, together with then PhD candidate Yvonne Barr, began examining tumor samples sent to them by Burkitt. Electron micrographs of lymphoid cells that grew out of the tumors in culture revealed viral particles with a morphology strikingly similar to herpes simplex viruses.[85] It was soon shown that Epstein-Barr herpesvirus (EBV, later designated human herpesvirus 4 [HHV-4]) can transform cultured B cells and is the agent responsible for infectious mononucleosis.[86–88]

Although the initial conjecture that tropically endemic Burkitt lymphoma depends on a geographically restricted infectious agent ultimately proved correct, it was quickly established that the EBV infection is not restricted to the tropics. It instead appears likely that the malaria parasite *Plasmodium falciparum* is a key geographically restricted cocarcinogen responsible for endemic Burkitt lymphoma.[53] In areas where children suffer repeated malaria infections, it appears that the parasite triggers abnormal B-cell responses, as well as weakened cell-mediated immune function, and these effects of recurring malaria infection in turn promote or allow the development of EBV-induced Burkitt tumors.[11]

Epstein-Barr Virus Life Cycle

EBV chronically infects nearly all humans. In a great majority of individuals, the infection is initially established in early childhood and is never associated with any noticeable symptoms. The infection is typically transmitted when virions, shed in the saliva of a chronically infected individual, come in contact with the oropharyngeal epithelium of a naïve individual. Although infected epithelial cells, such as keratinocytes, might serve to amplify the virus in some circumstances,[89] the establishment of chronic infection is ultimately dependent on mature B cells, as subjects with X-linked agammaglobulinemia (who lack mature B cells) appear to be immune to stable EBV infection.[90] Individuals who escape infection during childhood and instead first become infected during adolescence or adulthood often develop mononucleosis, which is associated with fevers and extreme fatigue lasting for weeks or sometimes months. Interestingly, late-infected individuals who experience mononucleosis and high EBV viral load are at increased risk of developing EBV-positive Hodgkin lymphoma.[91]

EBV-infected B cells can either go on to produce new virions, which are typically associated with cell lysis, or the virus can enter a nonproductive state known as latency. Viral latency is defined as a condition in which the virus expresses few (or possibly no) gene products but can, under some conditions, "reawaken" to express the full range of viral gene products and produce new progeny virions. Latently infected cells are highly resistant to immune clearance.

There are three recognized forms of EBV latency. In latency I, EBV nuclear antigen-1 (EBNA1), which is required for the stable maintenance of the circularized viral DNA minichromosome, is the only viral protein expressed. EBV-derived microRNAs (miRs) may also be expressed. At the other end of the spectrum, latency III is characterized by the expression of EBNA1–6, several latent membrane proteins (LMP1, 2A, and 2B), two noncoding RNAs (EBER1 and 2), the BCL-2 homolog BHRF1, BARF0, and multiple miRs. Although the initial discovery of EBV involved the visualization of virions, indicating that the virus had exited latency and entered the productive lytic phase of the life cycle, viral gene expression in EBV-induced cancers generally follows one of the three latent patterns. The oncogenic activities of various EBV gene products have recently been reviewed.[87,88]

In a great majority of healthy individuals, EBV exists almost exclusively in a latent state, with the occasional asymptomatic shedding of virions in the saliva. The infection is controlled, at least in part, by CD8+ T cells specific for various latency proteins. EBV, like other herpesviruses, expresses a variety of proteins that interfere with cell-mediated immune responses. Intriguingly, results from mouse model systems suggest that the chronic immunostimulatory effects of persistent gammaherpesvirus emergence (or abortive emergence) from latency in healthy hosts can nonspecifically boost immunity to other infections.[92]

Lymphomas

In addition to endemic Burkitt lymphoma, EBV is often present in sporadic cases of Burkitt lymphoma in individuals who have not been exposed to malaria. Although nearly all cases of endemic

Burkitt's lymphoma contain EBV DNA in the tumor (typically in a latency I–like state), only about 20% of sporadic cases arising in immunocompetent individuals contain EBV. Rates of Burkitt lymphoma are elevated in HIV-infected individuals, and HIV-associated Burkitt lymphomas contain EBV in about 30% of cases.

A common hallmark of all types of Burkitt's lymphomas is deregulation of the cellular Myc proto-oncogene. A classic mutation involves chromosomal translocation of the Myc gene to the antibody heavy chain locus. Burkitt's lymphoma tumors that lack detectable EBV DNA tend to carry multiple additional mutations in host cell genes, raising the possibility that an originally EBV-positive precursor cell ultimately accumulated mutations that rendered it independent of viral genes.[88,93]

In addition to Burkitt lymphoma, EBV is associated, to varying extents, with a histologically diverse range of other lymphoid cancers, including Hodgkin lymphoma, natural killer (NK)/T-cell lymphoma, primary central nervous system (CNS) lymphoma, and diffuse large B-cell lymphoma. The incidence of these various forms of lymphoma is significantly increased both in AIDS patients as well as in iatrogenically and congenitally immunosuppressed individuals.[88] In particular, the essentially universal presence of EBV in CNS lymphomas in AIDS patients makes it possible to diagnose the disease with a PCR test for EBV that, together with radiologic findings, can obviate the need for a brain biopsy.

EBV is almost invariably associated with lymphoproliferative disorders, such as plasmacytic hyperplasia and polymorphic B cell hyperplasia, which are often observed in organ transplant recipients. These polyclonal lymphoproliferative responses can, in some instances, progress to oligoclonal or monoclonal lymphomas of various types. The occurrence of EBV-associated lymphoproliferative disease in immunosuppressed patients is generally heralded by the increased detection of EBV DNA in the peripheral blood and the oral cavity. This presumably reflects the failure of cellular immune responses to drive the virus into full latency and perhaps also a failure of cell-mediated immune responses targeting latency-associated EBV gene products present in the nascent tumor.

Carcinomas

In Southern China, NPC affects 25 out of 100,000 people, accounting for 18% of all cancers in China as a whole.[94] Most other world regions have a 25- to 100-fold lower rate of NPC. EBV is present in nearly all cases of NPC, both in endemic and nonendemic regions. Although there is support for the idea that dietary intake of salted fish and other preserved foods is a factor in endemic NPC, it remains possible that genetic traits or as yet unidentified environmental cocarcinogenic factors may play a role as well. Individuals with rising or relatively high IgA antibody responses to EBNA1, DNase, and/or EBV capsid antigens have a dramatically increased risk of developing NPC, offering an early detection method for at-risk individuals.[87]

EBV is also present in a small percentage (5% to 15%) of gastric adenocarcinomas and over 90% of gastric lymphoepithelioma-like carcinomas. In contrast to NPC, the prevalence of EBV-associated gastric cancer is similar in all world regions. As with NPC, elevated antibody responsiveness to EBV antigens may offer a method for identifying individuals at greater risk of gastric cancer.

Prevention and Treatment

The reduction of immunosuppression in response to increasing EBV loads is a standard approach to preventing EBV diseases in T-cell immunosuppressed individuals. Another approach to the prevention of EBV disease relies on ganciclovir (or related antiherpesvirus drugs), which can trigger the death of cells that express the EBV thymidine kinase gene. Pretreating at-risk individuals, such as organ transplant recipients, with ganciclovir has been shown to effectively prevent the development of EBV-induced

lymphoproliferative disorders.[95] However, it is important to note that thymidine kinase is only expressed in the lytic phase of the viral life cycle, and drugs of this class are not generally effective for treating existing tumors, presumably due to the fact that EBV gene expression in tumors is typically of a latent type.

Although a recently developed vaccine targeting the EBV gp350 virion surface antigen did not provide sterilizing immunity to EBV infection, vaccinees did experience lower peak EBV viral loads upon infection.[96] Given the strong correlation between high EBV loads and the development of EBV diseases, it is hoped that the vaccine's ability to merely blunt the acute infection may offer significant protection against disease.

Most forms of EBV-associated lymphoid cancers express the B-cell marker CD20, making rituximab (an anti-CD20 mAb) a potentially effective adjunct therapy.[97,98] An emerging treatment approach that has recently entered clinical trials involves stimulating T cells ex vivo against peptides based on EBV antigens or against autologous EBV-transformed B cells.

KAPOSI'S SARCOMA HERPESVIRUS

History and Epidemiology

In the late 19th century, Hungarian dermatologist Moritz Kaposi's described a relatively rare type of indolent pigmented skin sarcoma affecting older men.[99] Kaposi's sarcoma (KS) was later found to be more prevalent in the Mediterranean region and in eastern portions of sub-Saharan Africa.[100] An early clue to the emergence of the HIV/AIDS pandemic in the early 1980s was a dramatic increase in the incidence of highly aggressive forms of KS, particularly in gay men who were much younger than typical KS patients. After the discovery of HIV, it was briefly hypothesized that HIV might be a direct cause of KS. However, this hypothesis failed to explain the existence of KS long prior to the HIV pandemic and the low incidence of KS in individuals who became infected with HIV via blood products. This latter observation was more easily explained by the existence of a sexually transmitted cofactor other than HIV.[101]

Using a subtractive DNA hybridization approach known as representational difference analysis, Yuan Chang, Patrick Moore, and colleagues discovered the presence of a previously unknown herpesvirus in KS tumors.[102] The newly founded field of research rapidly established key lines of evidence supporting the conclusion that KSHV (later designated human herpesvirus-8 [HHV-8]) is a causal factor in KS.[11]

It is now clear that the rate of KSHV infection varies greatly in different world regions.[11,103] In North America and Western Europe, KSHV seroprevalence in the general population ranges from 1% to 7%. Seroprevalence among gay men in these regions is substantially higher (25% to 60%), suggesting a possible link to sexual transmission. KSHV infection is much more prevalent in the general population in central and eastern Africa, where seroprevalence ranges from 23% to 70%. In endemic areas, up to 15% of children are seropositive, suggesting either vertical transmission or transmission via nonsexual casual contact (presumably via saliva). In endemic regions, KS is estimated to be the third most common cancer among adults.[104]

Kaposi's Sarcoma-Associated Herpesvirus in Kaposi's Sarcoma

KS tumors are complex on a number of levels. In contrast to most other forms of cancer, where it is often clear that a single cell type has proliferated out of control, KS tumors are composed of cells from multiple lineages (Fig. 5.2). KSHV-infected cells in the tumor often have a spindle-shaped morphology. Interestingly,

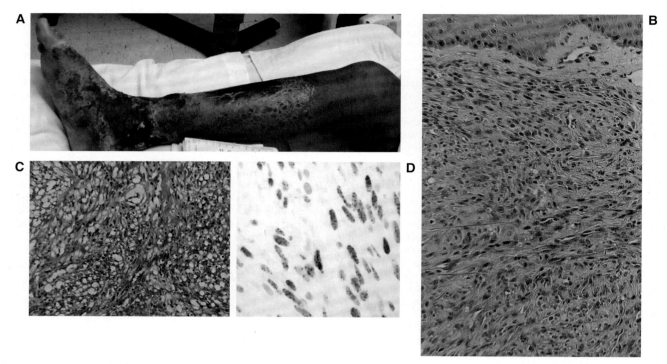

Figure 5.2 Kaposi's sarcoma (KS). **(A)** Photograph of the lower leg of an individual with severe, diffuse KS involving the lower leg. **(B)** Histology of the skin. **(C)** Lung shows a mixture of spindle to epithelioid cells, with slitlike vascular spaces intermixed with red blood cells and red blood cell fragments. **(D)** Immunohistochemical detection of KSHV LANA in the cutaneous tumor. Photographs provided with permission by Drs. Odey Ukpo and Ethel Cesarman.

spindle cells do not exhibit a highly transformed phenotype and tend to show relatively little chromosomal instability. In a culture, the cells are highly dependent on exogenous cytokines and other factors present in the tumor microenvironment in vivo. Although spindle cells express a number of markers of the endothelial lineage, it is uncertain whether they are derived from mature endothelial cells, the early precursor cells that give rise to smooth muscle and vascular endothelial cells, or cells of the lymphatic endothelial lineage. KS tumors also contain infiltrating lymphocytes and monocytes, as well as aberrant neovascular spaces lined with infected and uninfected endothelial cells. The aberrant blood vessels in KS lesion vessels rupture easily and leak red blood cells, giving KS tumors their classic dark red, brown, or purple color.

The latency status of KSHV in KS tumors is also complex, with the expression of gene products typical of latency (e.g., LANA) as well as lytic-phase genes (e.g., RTA/ORF50). Some of these gene products, such as the viral interleukin (IL)-6 homolog (vIL-6), trigger proliferation and secondary cytokine signaling in noninfected cells within the tumor. The tumorigenic effects of individual KSHV gene products have recently been reviewed.[88,103] In contrast to EBV, where tumorigenesis is driven by latency gene expression, it appears that KS pathogenesis is often dependent on lytic phase gene expression. This may explain why ganciclovir, which is not a particularly effective treatment for EBV tumors, was found to prevent the formation of new KS lesions in HIV-positive patients.[105] However, it should be noted that this outcome has more recently proven difficult to reproduce.[106] At present, there are no recommended preventive therapies for individuals at risk of KS, but this is an area of active investigation.

There are a variety of possible explanations for the need for lytic-phase KSHV gene expression during tumor development. For example, infected spindle cells may lose the viral DNA during cell division and require reinfection for ongoing tumorigenicity. Alternatively, factors secreted by a small fraction of tumor cells that enter the lytic phase may be required for tumorigenesis. An important area of current research focus is the role of KSHV gene products in the regulation of angiogenesis in KS lesions[107] and several current trials are investigating inhibitors of angiogenic pathways for the treatment of KS.

Lymphoproliferative Disorders

KSHV causes two forms of B-cell proliferative disorder: multicentric Castleman disease (MCD) and primary effusion lymphoma (PEL). Both diseases are most commonly found in association with HIV infection. In HIV-infected individuals, MCD tumors contain KSHV in nearly all cases, whereas in HIV-negative individuals, the tumor contains KSHV in only about 50% of cases.[108] KSHV in MCD tumors exhibits periodic activation of lytic replication and the expression of lytic phase genes.[109] The expression of vIL-6 during disease flare-ups appears to play a role in MCD pathogenesis, raising the possibility that tocilizumab (a mAb therapeutic that targets the IL-6 receptor) may be of therapeutic benefit.

PEL comprises about 4% of all HIV-associated non-Hodgkin lymphomas.[110] Typically, PEL tumors express markers of both plasma cells (akin to multiple myeloma tumors) and immunoblasts (similar to some EBV-induced tumors). In AIDS patients, essentially all PEL tumors are infected with KSHV and a great majority are also coinfected with EBV.[88] Although PEL is rare in HIV-negative individuals, PEL tumors in such individuals contain KSHV in about 50% of cases.

A common approach to the treatment of all KSHV-associated diseases is the restoration of immune function, either through antiretroviral therapy of HIV/AIDS or through a reduction of immunosuppressive therapy. The general success of immune reconstitution in many KSHV-associated diseases presumably involves an immune-mediated attack of cells expressing KSHV gene products, particularly the many lytic-phase gene products the virus can produce in various disease states.

ANIMAL AND HUMAN RETROVIRUSES

The first oncogenic retroviruses were discovered by Ellerman and Bang in 1908 and by Rous in 1911, but it was many years before the significance of these findings was appreciated.[111] One reason the field was stymied was the failure to identify RNA forms of the viral genome in infected cells. This led to the discovery of the reverse transcriptase independently by Baltimore and Temin in 1970. Another major development was the finding in 1976 of viral oncogenes derived from cellular genes, with the identification by Varmus and Bishop of the first dominant oncogene, *src*. With the discovery of IL-2 by Gallo in 1976, it became possible to culture the first human retrovirus, HTLV-1, from a form of adult T-cell leukemia/lymphoma (ATLL) that was first recognized by Takatsuki and coworkers.[112] These advances opened the door for Montagnier and colleagues' isolation of HIV-1 in 1983, a discovery confirmed independently by Gallo and Levy. This breakthrough led to the first licensed HIV test in 1985.

Retroviruses are positive single-strand RNA viruses that utilize transcription of their RNA genome into a DNA intermediate during virus replication.[111] This accounts for their name, retroviruses, because this is opposite to the normal flow of eukaryotic genetic information. They infect a wide range of vertebrate animal species and are distantly related to repetitive elements in the human genome, known as retrotransposons. Retroviruses are also related to hepadnaviruses, double-stranded DNA viruses, such as hepatitis B virus, which also undergo a reverse transcription step in their replication.

Retroviruses may be classified as *endogenous* or *exogenous* depending on whether they appear in the genome of the host species. There are approximately 100,000 endogenous retroviral elements in the human genome, making up nearly 8% of the genetic information, but their potential roles in disease are unclear.[113] Retroviruses may also be classified as *ecotropic*, *xenotropic*, or *polytropic* depending on whether they infect cells of the same animal species from which they are derived, infect cells of a different species, or both. *Amphotropic* retroviruses infect cells of the species of origin without producing disease, but infect cells of other species and may produce disease.

Retroviruses that produce disease after a long incubation period are termed *lentiviruses* and include human, simian, feline, ovine, caprine, and bovine immunodeficiency viruses. Another group of retroviruses that are not clearly associated with disease are known as *spumaviruses* and include human and simian foamy viruses. HTLV-1, which is classified in the genus Delta, is the only retrovirus known to be oncogenic in humans. A member of the retroviral genus Gamma identified in 2008, designated xenotropic murine leukemia virus-related virus (XMRV), was thought to be associated with human prostate cancer; however, more recent studies showed XMRV to be a lab-derived artifact.[114] A genus betaretrovirus related to the mouse mammary tumor virus has been suggested to be associated with biliary cirrhosis, but this finding requires independent validation.[115]

Retroviruses producing tumors in animals or birds are designated transforming viruses and may be classified as acute or chronic transforming retroviruses. Acute transforming retroviruses have acquired a mutated cellular gene, termed *oncogene*, and induce cancer in an animal within a few weeks. Many dominant acting proto-oncogenes in humans (e.g., *ras*, *myc*, and *erbB*), were first identified as retroviral oncogenes.

Chronic transforming retroviruses integrate almost randomly in the genome, but when integrated in the vicinity of specific genes disrupt their regulation and induce cell proliferation or resistance to apoptosis. Chronic transforming retroviruses induce malignancy only after many weeks to months of infection. The use of a murine leukemia virus vector for gene therapy in children with a form of severe combined immune deficiency syndrome characterized by defective expression of the common gamma chain of the IL-2 receptor resulted in T-cell acute lymphoblastic leukemia.

This was found to be the result of persistent expression of the LIM domain only 2 (LMO2) gene triggered by the nearby integration of the retroviral vector.[116]

In addition to acute or chronic transformation mechanisms, retroviruses can transform cells through direct effects on cell physiology mediated by structural or nonstructural viral proteins. Transforming genes of HTLV-1 are nonstructural viral proteins that activate host cell signaling pathways.[117] Because the oncogenic effects of HTLV-1 transforming genes generally take many years to cause cancer, the virus does not fit the precise definition of having either an acute or a chronic oncogenic mechanism.

HIV-1 infection is also associated with a variety of malignancies, but only by indirect effects of suppressing immunity to oncogenic virus infections, such as gammaherpesviruses, high-risk human papillomaviruses, and hepatitis viruses.

Human T-Cell Leukemia Virus Epidemiology

Four species of human T-cell leukemia virus have been identified. HTLV-1 was identified in 1980 as the first human retrovirus associated with cancer, and it is the focus of the remainder of this section.[118] HTLV-2 was discovered in 1982 and shares 70% genomic homology with HTLV-1.[119] HTLV-3 and -4 were sporadically isolated from individuals who had contact with monkeys.[120] HTLV-2, -3, and -4 do not appear to be associated with disease in humans.

HTLV-1 is present in 15 to 20 million individuals worldwide, most commonly in the Caribbean Islands, South America, southern Japan, and parts of Australia, Melanesia, Africa, and Iran.[121] In the United States, Canada, and Europe, 0.01% to 0.03% of blood donors are infected with HTLV-1. It is most commonly found in individuals who emigrated from endemic regions or among African Americans. HTLV-1 is transmitted sexually, by contaminated cell-associated blood products, or by breast-feeding.[122] Only 2% to 5% of HTLV-1–infected individuals develop disease, and ATLL only occurs in individuals who acquired HTLV-1 by breast-feeding.

Human T-Cell Leukemia Virus Molecular Biology

HTLV-1, like other retroviruses, encodes Gag, Protease, Pol, and Envelope proteins.[123] Gag proteins compose the inner nucleocapsid core of the virus. The Pol proteins include the reverse transcriptase and integrase. The reverse transcriptase copies the single-stranded viral RNA into double-stranded DNA, and it is inhibited by several nucleoside analogs, but not by the nonnucleoside reverse transcriptase inhibitors approved for HIV-1.[124] The integrase is responsible for inserting the linear double-stranded DNA product of reverse transcription into the host chromosomal DNA. At least one integrase inhibitor, raltegravir, now approved for HIV-1, is active against HTLV-1.[125] Integration occurs throughout the human genome, but there is preference for integration into transcriptionally active genomic regions.[126] The viral protease proteolytically processes Gag, Protease, and Pol precursor proteins to the mature individual proteins, but it is not affected by inhibitors of HIV-1 protease. The envelope proteins include the transmembrane protein, which anchors the surface envelope protein on the virion, which mediates binding to the viral receptor.[127]

The viral genome also encodes regulatory proteins, including Tax and HTLV-1 bZIP factor (HBZ).[117] Tax is a transcriptional transactivator protein that functions as a coactivator to induce members of the cAMP response element-binding protein/activating transcription factor (CREB/ATF) family, nuclear factor kappa B (NF-κB), and serum response factor (SRF) pathways. Tax activation of the CREB/ATF pathway is responsible for upregulation of the viral promoter. Tax induction of NF-κB promotes cell proliferation and resistance to apoptosis. Tax also binds and activates cyclin-dependent kinases and inhibits cell cycle checkpoint proteins. Tax is important for tumor initiation, whereas HBZ may be important in tumor maintenance.[128]

HTLV-1 preferentially immortalizes CD4+ T lymphocytes and induces tumors in mice.[129] Tax also promotes the leukemia-initiating activity of ATLL cells in mouse models.[130] In immunodeficient mice reconstituted with human hematopoietic cells, HTLV-1 causes CD4+ lymphomas.[131]

Clinical Characteristics and Treatment of HTLV-Associated Malignancies

The diagnosis of HTLV-1 is based on serologic assays.[132] HTLV-1 is associated with various inflammatory disorders, including uveitis, polymyositits, pneumonitis, Sjögren syndrome, and myelopathy. Infected patients are susceptible to certain infectious disorders (e.g. staphylococcal dermatitis) and opportunistic infections such as pneumocystis pneumonia, disseminated cryptococcosis, strongyloidiasis, or toxoplasmosis.[133] Vaccines have not been developed for HTLV infections.

T-lymphocyte proliferative disorders develop in 1% to 5% of infected individuals and are generally CD2+, CD3+, CD4+, CD5+, CD25+, CD29+, CD45RO+, CD52+, HLA-DR+, T-cell receptor αβ+, and variably CD30+, and lack CD7, CD8, and CD26 expression. The virus is clonally integrated in the malignant cells. Complex karyotypes are often found, and cytogenetic analysis is rarely useful. The histologic features of lymph nodes in ATLL may be indistinguishable from those of other peripheral T-cell lymphomas.[134] Circulating tumor "flower cells" are helpful in the diagnosis (Fig. 5.3).

ATLL is categorized in four subtypes.[135] (1) Smoldering ATLL is defined as 5% or more abnormal T lymphocytes and lactate dehydrogenase (LDH) levels up to 1.5× the upper limit of normal, with normal lymphocyte count, calcium, and no lymph node or visceral disease other than skin or pulmonary disease. (2) Chronic ATLL is characterized by lymphocytosis, LDH up to 2× the upper limit of normal, no hypercalcemia, and no CNS, bone, pleural, peritoneal, or gastrointestinal involvement, although the lymph nodes, liver, spleen, skin, or lungs may be involved. The mean survival of these forms of ATLL is 2 to 5 years.[136] No intervention in these subtypes of ATLL has been defined that prevents progression to the more aggressive forms of ATLL. Although chronic or smoldering ATLL may respond to zidovudine and interferon, randomized studies have not been conducted.[137] (3) Lymphoma-type ATLL is characterized by ≤1% abnormal T lymphocytes and features of non-Hodgkin lymphoma. (4) Acute-type ATLL includes the remaining patients. Even with optimal therapy, the median survival of lymphoma and acute-type ATLL is less than 1 year.[138] Lymphoma and acute types of ATLL are the most common presenting subtypes. Other major prognostic factors include performance status, age, the presence of more than three involved lesions, and hypercalcemia.[139]

Combination chemotherapy for lymphoma or acute-type ATLL with the infusional etoposide, prednisone, vincristine, and doxorubicin (EPOCH) regimen or the LSG-15 regimen results in complete remission rates of 15% to 40%.[140,141] However, responses are short lived, with <10% of patients free of disease at 4 years. The addition of anti-CCR4 antibody, mogamulizumab, may improve response rates, but studies are still underway.[142]

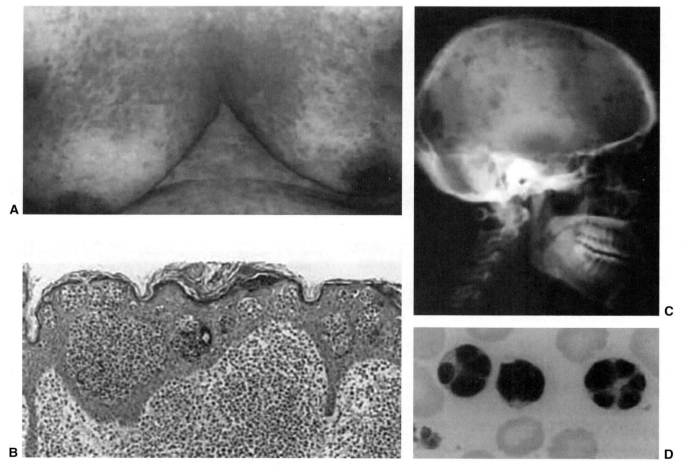

Figure 5.3 Clinical manifestation of adult T-cell leukemia/lymphoma. **(A–B)** Infiltration of malignant T lymphocytes into the skin. **(C)** Lytic bone lesions seen on lateral skull x-ray. **(D)** "Flower cells" in the blood.

The combination of interferon and zidovudine with or without arsenic may result in the remission of acute, but not lymphoma subtypes.[143] Allogenic transplantation may result in long-term, disease-free survival for patients with complete or near complete remission of disease, although infectious complications have been notable in these studies.[144]

HEPATITIS VIRUSES

The earliest record of an epidemic caused by a hepatitis virus was in 1885, occurring in individuals vaccinated for smallpox with lymph from other people.[145] The cause of the epidemic, HBV, was not identified until 1966, when Blumberg discovered the *Australian antigen* now known to be the hepatitis B surface antigen (HBsAg). This was followed by the discovery of the virus particle by Dane in 1970. In the early 1980s, the HBV genome was sequenced and the first vaccines were tested. In the mid 1970s, Alter described cases of hepatitis not due to hepatitis A or B viruses, and the suspected agent was designated non-A, non-B hepatitis virus, now known as HCV.[146] In 1987, Houghton used molecular cloning to identify the HCV genome and develop a diagnostic test, which was licensed in 1990.

Approximately 240 million people are chronically infected with HBV and 150 to 200 million people are infected with HCV worldwide, according to the World Health Organization (WHO). About 1 million deaths per year are attributed to the chronic diseases such as liver cirrhosis and hepatocellular carcinoma (HCC) that result from viral hepatitis infections. HBV and HCV are the leading cause of liver cancer in the world, accounting for almost 80% of the cases. In the United States, Europe, Egypt, and Japan, more than 60% of HCC cases are associated with HCV, and 20% are related to HBV and chronic alcoholism.[147] In Africa and Asia, 60% of HCC is associated with HBV, 20% related to HCV, and the remainder related to other risk factors, such as alcohol and aflatoxin. HCC is the sixth most common cancer worldwide and is the third most common cause of cancer death.[148]

In Asia and Africa, up to 70% of individuals have serologic evidence of current or prior HBV infection, and 8% to 15% of these subjects have a chronic active infection. Rates of HCV infection of >3.5% occur in Central and East Asia, North Africa, and the Middle East. In the United States, 0.8 to 1.4 million individuals are infected with HBV, and 3.2 million with HCV. The incidence of HCC in the United States tripled between 1975 and 2005, particularly in African American and Hispanic males.[149]

HBV is transmitted primarily through exposure to infected blood, semen, and other body fluids, whereas HCV is transmitted primarily by contact with contaminated blood. Acute HCV infection causes mild and vague symptoms in about 15% of individuals and resolves spontaneously in 10% to 50% of cases.[150] Liver enzymes are normal in 5% to 50% of individuals with chronic HCV infection.[151] After 20 years of an HCV infection, the likelihood of cirrhosis is 10% to 15% for men, and 1.5% for women.[152] Cofactors that increase the likelihood of cirrhosis are coinfection with both hepatitis viruses, persistently high levels of HBV or HCV viremia, HBeAg, certain viral genotypes, schistosoma, HIV, alcoholism, male gender, advanced age at the time of infection, diabetes, and obesity.[153,154]

Hepatitis B Virus

HBV is an enveloped DNA virus that is a member of the *Hepadnaviridae* family.[155] HBV has a strong preference for infecting hepatocytes, but small amounts of viral DNA can also be found in kidney, pancreas, and mononuclear cells, although it is not linked to extrahepatic disease. The viral genome is a relaxed circular, partially double-stranded (ds) DNA of 3.2 kb. The genome exists as an episomal covalently closed circular dsDNA (cccDNA)

molecule in the nucleus of infected cells, although chromosomal integration of viral genomic sequences can occur during cycles of hepatocyte regeneration and proliferation. In addition to 40 to 42 nm virions, HBV-infected cells also produce noninfectious 20-nm spherical and filamentous particles. The viral genome encodes four open reading frames. The presurface–surface (preS-S) region encodes three proteins from different translational initiation sites; these include the S (HBsAg), M (or pre-S2), and L (or pre-S1) proteins. The L protein is responsible for receptor binding and virion assembly. The precore–core (preC-C) region encodes the HBcAg and HBeAg. The P region encodes the viral polymerase, and the X (HBx) protein modulates host-signal transduction.

After infection, the viral genome is transcribed by host RNA polymerase II, and viral proteins are translated. Nucleocapsids assemble in the cytosol, incorporating a molecule of pregenomic RNA into the viral core, where reverse transcription occurs to produce the dsDNA viral genome. Viral cores are enveloped with intracellular membranes and viral L, M, and S surface antigens, which are exported from the cells.

HBV replication is not cytotoxic. Instead, liver injury is due to the host immune response, primarily T-cell and proinflammatory cytokine responses. Chronic HBV carriers exhibit an attenuated virus-specific T-cells response, although a vigorous humoral response is still evident. About 5% of infections in adults and up to 90% of infections in neonates result in a persistent infection, which may or may not be associated with symptoms and elevated serum aminotransferase levels. About 20% of such individuals develop cirrhosis. Immunosuppressed individuals also have a higher likelihood of a persistent infection.

With acute infection, viral titers of 10^9 to 10^{10} virions per mililiter are present, whereas levels of 10^7 to 10^9 virions per mililiter and HBsAg, and in some cases, HBeAg are present in the blood of individuals with a persistent infection. The resolution of infection, which is associated with declining viral DNA titers, is observed at a rate of 5% to 10% per year in persistently infected individuals. However, even subjects who have resolved the infection continue to have very low levels of viral DNA (10^3 to 10^5 copies per mililiter) for most of their lives.

HBV infection can be managed with alpha interferon or nucleos(t)ide analogs that inhibit the viral polymerase, such as lamivudine, telbivudine, entecavir, adefovir, and tenofovir.[156] Entecavir and tenofovir are both effective at inducing viral suppression, and may be used in combination in patients with high HBV DNA load or multidrug resistance. Because these agents are all associated with some toxicity, current guidelines recommend therapy only when liver disease is clinically apparent, with continued treatment for 6 to 12 months after clearance of HBeAg or HBsAg. Although these drugs effectively control HBV, they typically fail to cure the infection due to the long-term persistence of the cccDNA form of the viral genome. Other nucleos(t)ide analogs are currently in clinical trials, as well as a novel form of interferon (IFN-λ) and an inhibitor of virus release.[157]

Hepatitis D virus (HDV) occurs only in individuals coinfected with HBV. HDV is composed a single-stranded circular viral RNA genome of 1,679 nucleotides, a central core of HDAg, and an outer coat with all three HBV envelope proteins. HDV infection results in more severe complications than infection with HBV alone, with a higher likelihood and more rapid progression to cirrhosis and HCC.

Hepatits C Virus

HCV is an enveloped RNA virus associated with cancer, primarily HCC and, rarely, splenic marginal zone lymphoma.[158] HCV is a positive-sense, single-stranded RNA virus of the *Flaviviridae* family.[159] There are seven genotypes of HCV; in the United States, about 70% of infections are caused by genotype 1.[160] HCV replicates in the cytoplasm and does not integrate into the host cell genome. The viral RNA is 9.6 kb and encodes a single polyprotein of 3,010 amino acids that is proteolytically processed into structural and nonstructural proteins. In addition to the structural roles of the core (C) protein, it has also been reported to affect various host cell functions. The envelope glycoproteins E1 and E2 mediate infectious entry through tetraspanin CD81 and other receptors on hepatocytes and B lymphocytes.

HCV non structural proteins NS2, NS3, NS4A, NS4B, NS5A, NS5B, and p7 are required for virus replication and assembly. NS2 is a membrane-associated cysteine protease. NS3 is a helicase and NTPase that unwinds RNA and DNA substrates. The complex of NS3 with NS4A forms a serine protease. NS4B induces the formation of a membranous web associated with the viral RNA replicase. NS5A is an RNA-binding phosphoprotein, whereas NS5B is the RNA-dependent RNA polymerase. The p7 protein forms a cation channel in infected cells that has a role in particle maturation and release.

Treating an HCV infection typically utilizes 24 to 48 weeks of pegylated IFN-α and ribavirin.[161] Treatment with IFN and ribavirin alone produces sustained virologic responses in 70% to 80% of subjects with genotype 2 or 3 infections. Recently approved inhibitors of the NS3-4A protease (e.g., telaprevir, boceprevir, or simeprevir) may be included in IFN-based regimens, particularly if the patient has failed prior therapy. Protease inhibitors are currently approved for use in IFN/ribavirin combination therapy for HCV genotype 1 or 4 infection. Sofosbuvir, a nucleoside analog inhibitor of the viral NS5B polymerase, has recently been approved for use in combination with ribavirin alone for genotypes 2 or 3, or in triple therapy for genotypes 1 and 4. Recently, IFN-free regimens have also been approved. Additional protease and polymerase inhibitors are currently in development. A recent meta-analysis of eight randomized controlled trials comparing antiviral therapy with placebo suggested that antiviral therapy resulted in a 50% reduced risk of HCC.[162]

Hepatitis Virus Pathogenesis

HBV and HCV depress innate immune responses by inhibiting Toll-like receptor signaling through effects of HBx and NS3-4A.[147] In addition, HCV C inhibits the Janus kinase (JAK)-signal transducer and activator of transcription (STAT) signaling, and NS5A and E2 inhibit IFN signaling. Through an undefined mechanism, HBV can inhibit JAK-STAT signaling as well.

HBV and HCV induce HCC by direct and indirect mechanisms.[147] Both HBV and HCV encode proteins that have pro- and antiapoptotic properties. High levels of HBx block activation of the NF-κB pathway, whereas HCV C and NS5A block apoptosis by the activation of AKT and NF-κB, respectively. The C and NS5A proteins may also induce epithelial–mesenchymal transition (EMT), which is important for liver fibrosis, through effects on transforming growth factor β and Src signaling. Mice transgenic for NS5A develop steatosis and HCC.

HBx and HCV C are associated with mitochondria, where they trigger oxidative stress that induces apoptosis. In addition, HBs and HBx and NS3-4A alter calcium signaling and increase reactive oxygen species, which trigger endoplasmic reticulum (ER) stress, an unfolded protein response, and the production of proinflammatory cytokines that induce collagen synthesis, which drives the development of fibrosis. Autophagy is triggered by both viruses to restore ER integrity, which promotes cell survival and viral persistence.

HBV and HCV also disrupt tumor suppressor proteins. HCV NS5B recruits an ubiquitin ligase protein to modify pRB and induce its degradation, whereas HBx and HCV C proteins both inhibit p16INK4a and p21 cell cycle inhibitors, which leads to the inactivating phosphorylation of pRB. The HBx and HCV C, NS3, and NS5A proteins deregulate p53 tumor suppressor activity, by compromising p53-mediated DNA repair. HBV and HCV also induce alterations in micro-RNAs that are partially responsible for cell cycle effects.

Although not part of the normal virus replication cycle, the tendency of HBV genomic DNA sequences to integrate within the host cell chromosomes also contributes to the pathogenesis of HBV-associated HCC. In most hepatoma cells, HBV replication is extinguished, and integration at certain sites provides a growth or survival advantage, leading to tumors that are clonal with respect to viral integration. Whole-genome sequencing studies have identified a number of cellular loci, including *TERT* and *MLL*, where HBV integration is associated with HCC.[163,164]

Both HBV and HCV promote characteristics of cancer stem cells. HBx promotes the expression of Nanog, Kruppel-like factor 4, octamer-binding transcription factor 4, and Myc. These markers are also induced by HBV and HCV-induced hypoxia and hypoxia-induced factors.

Clinical Characteristics and Treatment of Hepatitis Virus-Associated Malignancies

HBV and HCV infections are diagnosed by serologic assays, and/or antigen assays in the case of HBV.[153] Quantitative HBV DNA and HCV RNA polymerase chain reactions are utilized to measure virus load. No vaccine has been identified that protects against HCV because infections consist of a genetically heterogenous "swarm" of virus particles, some of which escape neutralization. However, a vaccine, which now utilizes a recombinant HBsAg produced in yeast cells, has been available for HBV prevention for more than 30 years. The HBV vaccine reduces the risk of infection by more than 70%.[157] Factors associated with HBV vaccination failure in adults include increased age, obesity, smoking, diabetes, end-stage renal disease, HIV infection, alcoholism, or recipients of liver or kidney transplantation. There have been recent suggestions that emerging HBV strains may be evolving to escape neutralizing antibodies elicited by the current vaccine.[165] Novel vaccine adjuvants are currently in clinical trials, as well as studies of a therapeutic HBV vaccine.

Because an early diagnosis of HCC is key to a successful treatment, there has been extensive research on surveillance techniques in HBV- and HCV-infected individuals.[166] The U.S. Centers for Disease Control and Prevention has recently recommended that all individuals born between 1945 and 1965 be tested for HCV infection. The American Association for the Study of Liver Diseases, as well as the European and Asian Pacific Associations for the Study of the Liver, endorse surveillance in HCV-infected individuals with cirrhosis using ultrasound every 6 months. Viral eradication does not fully eliminate the risk of HCC, and thus, continued surveillance is still recommended in cirrhotic patients.

Therapeutic options for HCC are determined not only by the number and size of HCC nodules as well as the presence or absence of vascular invasion and metastases, but also by liver function and the presence or absence of portal hypertension.[167] HCC amenable to liver transplantation is usually defined as either one tumor measuring ≤50 mm in diameter or two to three tumors measuring ≤30 mm in diameter without vascular extension or metastasis (Milan criteria).[168] Up to 30% of all cases of HCC present with multiple nodules of HCC, suggesting a field carcinogenesis effect of HBV and HCV.[169] HBV- and HCV-infected patients may have a lower survival than noninfected patients after liver transplantation.[170] Hepatitis B immune globulin and nucleos(t)ide analogs are recommended for reinfection prophylaxis in the posttransplant period for HBV-infected individuals.[171] Studies are underway to examine the appropriate use of antiviral therapy for HCV-infected patients undergoing liver transplantation.

Reactivation of HCV can occur with chemotherapy or monoclonal antibody-based immunosuppressive therapies, but is less frequent as compared to HBV infection.[172] Individuals who appear to have cleared an HBV infection and who have an undetectable viral load can experience HBV reactivation on rituximab therapy. Monitoring hepatic function and virus load is indicated during chemoimmunotherapy of HBV- or HCV-positive patients.[173] Although there is controversy regarding the role of virus screening for patients undergoing chemotherapy, antiviral therapy is recommended for high-risk HBV-infected patients undergoing chemoimmunotherapy, such as rituximab-based chemotherapy regimens.[174]

An association between HCV and B-cell non-Hodgkin lymphoma (NHL) has also been demonstrated in highly endemic geographic areas.[175] Lymphoproliferation has been linked to type II mixed cryoglobulinemia in many of these individuals. In addition to diffuse large B-cell lymphoma, marginal zone lymphoma and lymphoplasmacytic lymphomas are the histologic subtypes most frequently associated with HCV infection. Antiviral treatment with IFNα with or without ribavirin has been effective in the treatment of HCV-infected patients with indolent lymphoma, but rarely in individuals with aggressive lymphomas.

CONCLUSION

Oncogenic viruses are important causes of cancer, especially in less industrialized countries and in immunosuppressed individuals. They are common causes of anogenital cancers, lymphomas, oral and hepatocellular carcinomas and are associated with a variety of other malignancies. Vaccines and antiviral agents play an important role in the prevention of virus-induced cancers. Studies of virus pathogenesis will continue to establish paradigms that are critical to our understanding of cancer etiology in general.

REFERENCES

1. de Martel C, Ferlay J, Franceschi S, et al. Global burden of cancers attributable to infections in 2008: a review and synthetic analysis. *Lancet Oncol* 2012;13(6):607–615.
2. Schiller JT, Lowy DR. Virus infection and human cancer: an overview. *Recent Results Cancer Res* 2014;193:1–10.
3. Chen CJ, Hsu WL, Yang HI, et al. Epidemiology of virus infection and human cancer. *Recent Results Cancer Res* 2014;193:11–32.
4. Virgin HW, Wherry EJ, Ahmed R. Redefining chronic viral infection. *Cell* 2009;138(1):30–50.
5. Campo MS, O'Neil BW, Barron RJ, et al. Experimental reproduction of the papilloma-carcinoma complex of the alimentary canal in cattle. *Carcinogenesis* 1994;15(8):1597–1601.
6. Khoury JD, Tannir NM, Williams MD, et al. Landscape of DNA virus associations across human malignant cancers: analysis of 3,775 cases using RNA-Seq. *J Virol* 2013;87(16):8916–8926.
7. zur Hausen H, de Villiers EM. TT viruses: oncogenic or tumor-suppressive properties? *Curr Top Microbiol Immunol* 2009;331:109–116.
8. Mizutani T, Sayama Y, Nakanishi A, et al. Novel DNA virus isolated from samples showing endothelial cell necrosis in the Japanese eel, Anguilla japonica. *Virology* 2011;412(1):179–187.
9. Paulson KG, Carter JJ, Johnson LG, et al. Antibodies to merkel cell polyomavirus T antigen oncoproteins reflect tumor burden in merkel cell carcinoma patients. *Cancer Res* 2010;70:8388–8397.
10. International Agency for Research on Cancer (IARC) Working Group. *IARC Monographs on the Evaluation of Carcinogenic Risks to Humans. Malaria and Some Polyomaviruses (SV40, BK, JC, and Merkel Cell Viruses)*, Vol. 104. Lyon, France: IARC; 2013.
11. Moore PS, Chang Y. The conundrum of causality in tumor virology: the cases of KSHV and MCV. *Semin Cancer Biol* 2013;26C:4–12.
12. Rigoni-Stern D. Fatti statistici relativi alle malattie cancrose. *Giornale Service Progr Pathol Terap Ser* 1842;2:507–517.
13. Lowy DR. History of papillomavirus research. In: Garcea RL, DiMaio D, eds. *The Papillomaviruses.* New York, NY: Springer; 2007:13–28.
14. zur Hausen H. Herpes simplex virus in human genital cancer. *Int Rev Exp Pathol* 1983;25:307–326.
15. Durst M, Gissmann L, Ikenberg H, et al. A papillomavirus DNA from a cervical carcinoma and its prevalence in cancer biopsy samples from different geographic regions. *Proc Natl Acad Sci U S A* 1983;80(12):3812–3815.
16. Boshart M, Gissmann L, Ikenberg H, et al. A new type of papillomavirus DNA, its presence in genital cancer biopsies and in cell lines derived from cervical cancer. *Embo J* 1984;3(5):1151–1157.
17. Christensen ND. Cottontail rabbit papillomavirus (CRPV) model system to test antiviral and immunotherapeutic strategies. *Antivir Chem Chemother* 2005;16(6):355–362.
18. Rous P, Beard J. The progression to carcinoma of virus induced rabbit papillomas (Shope). *J Exp Med* 1935;62:523–545.
19. Syverton JT, Berry GP. Carcinoma in the cottontail rabbit following spontaneous virus papilloma (Shope). *Proc Soc Exp Biol Med* 1935;33:399–400.
20. de Villiers EM. Cross-roads in the classification of papillomaviruses. *Virology* 2013;445(1-2):2–10.
21. Bosch FX, Broker TR, Forman D, et al. Comprehensive control of human papillomavirus infections and related diseases. *Vaccine* 2013;31 Suppl 8:I1–I31.
22. Van Doorslaer K. Evolution of the papillomaviridae. *Virology* 2013;445(1–2):11–20.
23. Scheffner M, Werness BA, Huibregtse JM, et al. The E6 oncoprotein encoded by human papillomavirus types 16 and 18 promotes the degradation of p53. *Cell* 1990;63(6):1129–1136.
24. Scheffner M, Huibregtse JM, Vierstra RD, Howley PM. The HPV-16 E6 and E6–AP complex functions as a ubiquitin-protein ligase in the ubiquitination of p53. *Cell* 1993;75(3):495–505.
25. Huibregtse JM, Scheffner M, Howley PM. Cloning and expression of the cDNA for E6-AP, a protein that mediates the interaction of the human papillomavirus E6 oncoprotein with p53. *Mol Cell Biol* 1993;13(2):775–784.
26. Klingelhutz AJ, Foster SA, McDougall JK. Telomerase activation by the E6 gene product of human papillomavirus type 16. *Nature* 1996;380(6569):79–82.
27. White EA, Howley PM. Proteomic approaches to the study of papillomavirus-host interactions. *Virology* 2013;435(1):57–69.
28. Dyson N, Howley PM, Munger K, et al. The human papilloma virus-16 E7 oncoprotein is able to bind to the retinoblastoma gene product. *Science* 1989;243(4893):934–937.
29. Munger K, Howley PM. Human papillomavirus immortalization and transformation functions. *Virus Res* 2002;89(2):213–228.
30. Duensing S, Lee LY, Duensing A, et al. The human papillomavirus type 16 E6 and E7 oncoproteins cooperate to induce mitotic defects and genomic instability by uncoupling centrosome duplication from the cell division cycle. *Proc Natl Acad Sci U S A* 2000;97(18):10002–10007.
31. DiMaio D, Petti LM. The E5 proteins. *Virology* 2013;445(1–2):99–114.
32. Schiller JT, Lowy DR. Understanding and learning from the success of prophylactic human papillomavirus vaccines. *Nat Rev Microbiol* 2012;10(10):681–692.
33. Kemp TJ, Safaeian M, Hildesheim A, et al. Kinetic and HPV infection effects on cross-type neutralizing antibody and avidity responses induced by Cervarix((R)). *Vaccine* 2012;31(1):165–170.
34. Haupt RM, Wheeler CM, Brown DR, et al. Impact of an HPV6/11/16/18 L1 virus-like particle vaccine on progression to cervical intraepithelial neoplasia in seropositive women with HPV16/18 infection. *Int J Cancer* 2011;129(11):2632–2642.
35. Kreuter A, Wieland U. Lack of efficacy in treating condyloma acuminata and preventing recurrences with the recombinant quadrivalent human papillomavirus vaccine in a case series of immunocompetent patients. *J Am Acad Dermatol* 2013;68(1):179–180.
36. Joura E, Team V-S, eds. Abstract SS 8–4: Efficacy and immunogenicity of a novel 9-valent HPV L1 virus-like particle vaccine in 16- to 26-year-old women. Paper presented at: Eurogin 2013 International Multidisciplinary Congress; 2013; Florence, Italy.
37. Wang JW, Roden RB. L2, the minor capsid protein of papillomavirus. *Virology* 2013;445(1–2):175–186.
38. Ma B, Maraj B, Tran NP, et al. Emerging human papillomavirus vaccines. *Expert Opin Emerg Drugs* 2012;17(4):469–492.
39. Scudellari M. HPV: sex, cancer and a virus. *Nature* 2013;503(7476):330–332.
40. Gillison ML, Alemany L, Snijders PJ, et al. Human papillomavirus and diseases of the upper airway: head and neck cancer and respiratory papillomatosis. *Vaccine* 2012;30 Suppl 5:F34–54.
41. Silverberg MJ, Leyden W, Warton EM, et al. HIV infection status, immunodeficiency, and the incidence of non-melanoma skin cancer. *J Natl Cancer Inst* 2013;105(5):350–360.
42. Kempf W, Mertz KD, Hofbauer GF, et al. Skin cancer in organ transplant recipients. *Pathobiology* 2013;80(6):302–309.
43. Wallace NA, Gasior SL, Faber ZJ, et al. HPV 5 and 8 E6 expression reduces ATM protein levels and attenuates LINE-1 retrotransposition. *Virology* 2013;443(1):69–79.
44. White EA, Kramer RE, Tan MJ, et al. Comprehensive analysis of host cellular interactions with human papillomavirus E6 proteins identifies new E6 binding partners and reflects viral diversity. *J Virol* 2012;86(24):13174–13186.
45. White EA, Sowa ME, Tan MJ, et al. Systematic identification of interactions between host cell proteins and E6 and E7 oncoproteins from diverse human papillomaviruses. *Proc Natl Acad Sci U S A* 2012;109(5):E260–267.
46. Caldeira S, Zehbe I, Accardi R, et al. The E6 and E7 proteins of the cutaneous human papillomavirus type 38 display transforming properties. *J Virol* 2003;77(3):2195–2206.
47. Arron ST, Ruby JG, Dybbro E, et al. Transcriptome sequencing demonstrates that human papillomavirus is not active in cutaneous squamous cell carcinoma. *J Invest Dermatol* 2011;131(8):1745–1753.
48. Gross L. A filterable agent, recovered from Ak leukemic extracts, causing salivary gland carcinomas in C3H mice. *Proc Soc Exp Biol Med* 1953;83(2):414–421.

49. Eddy BE, Stewart SE. Characteristics of the SE polyoma virus. *Am J Public Health Nations Health* 1959;49:1486–1492.

50. Sweet BH, Hilleman MR. The vacuolating virus, S.V. 40. *Proc Soc Exp Biol Med* 1960;105:420–427.

51. Eddy BE, Borman GS, Grubbs GE, et al. Identification of the oncogenic substance in rhesus monkey kidney cell culture as simian virus 40. *Virology* 1962;17:65–75.

52. Dang-Tan T, Mahmud SM, Puntoni R, et al. Polio vaccines, simian virus 40, and human cancer: the epidemiologic evidence for a causal association. *Oncogene* 2004;23(38):6535–6540.

53. Bouvard V, Baan RA, Grosse Y, et al. Carcinogenicity of malaria and of some polyomaviruses. *Lancet Oncol* 2012;13(4):339–340.

54. Gardner SD, Field AM, Coleman DV, et al. New human papovavirus (B.K.) isolated from urine after renal transplantation. *Lancet*. 1971;1(7712): 1253–1257.

55. Padgett BL, Walker DL, ZuRhein GM, et al. Cultivation of papova-like virus from human brain with progressive multifocal leucoencephalopathy. *Lancet* 1971;1(7712):1257–1260.

56. Das D, Wojno K, Imperiale MJ. BK virus as a cofactor in the etiology of prostate cancer in its early stages. *J Virol* 2008;82(6):2705–2714.

57. Akgul B, Pfister D, Knuchel R, et al. No evidence for a role of xenotropic murine leukaemia virus-related virus and BK virus in prostate cancer of German patients. *Med Microbiol Immunol* 2012;201(2):245–248.

58. Alexiev BA, Randhawa P, Vazquez Martul E, et al. BK virus-associated urinary bladder carcinoma in transplant recipients: report of 2 cases, review of the literature, and proposed pathogenetic model. *Human Pathol* 2013;44(5):908–917.

59. Abend JR, Jiang M, Imperiale MJ. BK virus and human cancer: innocent until proven guilty. *Semin Cancer Biol* 2009;19(4):252–260.

60. Maginnis MS, Atwood WJ. JC virus: an oncogenic virus in animals and humans? *Semin Cancer Biol* 2009;19(4):261–269.

61. Feng H, Shuda M, Chang Y, et al. Clonal integration of a polyomavirus in human Merkel cell carcinoma. *Science* 2008;319(5866):1096–1100.

62. Hodgson NC. Merkel cell carcinoma: changing incidence trends. *J Surg Oncol* 2005;89(1):1–4.

63. Engels EA, Frisch M, Goedert JJ, et al. Merkel cell carcinoma and HIV infection. *Lancet* 2002;359(9305):497–498.

64. Zur Hausen A, Rennspiess D, Winnepenninckx V, et al. Early B-cell differentiation in Merkel cell carcinomas: clues to cellular ancestry. *Cancer Res* 2013;73(16):4982–4987.

65. Guastafierro A, Feng H, Thant M, et al. Characterization of an early passage Merkel cell polyomavirus-positive Merkel cell carcinoma cell line, MS-1, and its growth in NOD scid gamma mice. *J Virol Methods* 2013;187(1):6–14.

66. Schowalter RM, Pastrana DV, Pumphrey KA, et al. Merkel cell polyomavirus and two previously unknown polyomaviruses are chronically shed from human skin. *Cell Host Microbe* 2010;7(6):509–515.

67. Faust H, Pastrana DV, Buck CB, et al. Antibodies to Merkel cell polyomavirus correlate to presence of viral DNA in the skin. *J Infect Dis* 2011;203(8):1096–1100.

68. Pastrana DV, Wieland U, Silling S, et al. Positive correlation between Merkel cell polyomavirus viral load and capsid-specific antibody titer. *Med Microbiol Immunol* 2011;201(1):17–23.

69. Pastrana DV, Tolstov YL, Becker JC, et al. Quantitation of human serorresponsiveness to Merkel cell polyomavirus. *PLoS Pathog* 2009;5(9):e1000578.

70. Faust H, Andersson K, Ekstrom J, et al. Prospective study of Merkel cell polyomavirus and risk of Merkel cell carcinoma. *Int J Cancer* 2014;134(4):844–848.

71. Cheng J, Rozenblatt-Rosen O, Paulson KG, et al. Merkel cell polyomavirus large T antigen has growth-promoting and inhibitory activities. *J Virol* 2013;87(11):6118–6126.

72. Li J, Wang X, Diaz J, et al. Merkel cell polyomavirus large T antigen disrupts host genomic integrity and inhibits cellular proliferation. *J Virol* 2013;87(16):9173–9188.

73. Houben R, Shuda M, Weinkam R, et al. Merkel cell polyomavirus-infected Merkel cell carcinoma cells require expression of viral T antigens. *J Virol* 2010;84(14):7064–7072.

74. Houben R, Grimm J, Willmes C, et al. Merkel cell carcinoma and Merkel cell carcinoma polyomavirus: evidence for hit-and-run oncogenesis. *J Invest Dermatol* 2012;132(1):254–256.

75. Shuda M, Chang Y, Moore PS. Merkel cell polyomavirus positive Merkel cell carcinoma requires viral small T antigen for cell proliferation. *J Invest Dermatol* 2013 [Epub ahead of print].

76. Paulson KG, Iyer JG, Tegeder AR, et al. Transcriptome-wide studies of merkel cell carcinoma and validation of intratumoral CD8+ lymphocyte invasion as an independent predictor of survival. *J Clin Oncol* 2011;29(12):1539–1546.

77. Arora R, Shuda M, Guastafierro A, et al. Survivin is a therapeutic target in Merkel cell carcinoma. *Sci Transl Med* 2012;4(133):133ra56.

78. Dresang LR, Guastafierro A, Arora R, et al. Response of merkel cell polyomavirus-positive merkel cell carcinoma xenografts to a survivin inhibitor. *PloS One* 2013;8(11):e80543.

79. Shuda M, Kwun HJ, Feng H, et al. Human Merkel cell polyomavirus small T antigen is an oncoprotein targeting the 4E-BP1 translation regulator. *J Clin Invest* 2011;121(9):3623–3634.

80. Howard RA, Dores GM, Curtis RE, et al. Merkel cell carcinoma and multiple primary cancers. *Cancer Epidemiol Biomarkers Prev* 2006;15(8):1545–1549.

81. Pantulu ND, Pallasch CP, Kurz AK, et al. Detection of a novel truncating Merkel cell polyomavirus large T antigen deletion in chronic lymphocytic leukemia cells. *Blood* 2010;116(24):5280–5284.

82. Tolstov YL, Arora R, Scudiere SC, et al. Lack of evidence for direct involvement of Merkel cell polyomavirus (MCV) in chronic lymphocytic leukemia (CLL). *Blood* 2010;115(23):4973–4974.

83. Cimino PJ, Jr., Bahler DW, Duncavage EJ. Detection of Merkel cell polyomavirus in chronic lymphocytic leukemia T-cells. *Exp Mol Pathol* 2013;94(1):40–44.

84. Burkitt D. A sarcoma involving the jaws in African children. *Br J Surg* 1958;46(197):218–223.

85. Epstein MA, Achong BG, Barr YM. Virus particles in cultured lymphoblasts from Burkitt's lymphoma. *Lancet* 1964;1(7335):702–703.

86. Henle G, Henle W, Diehl V. Relation of Burkitt's tumor-associated herpesytpe virus to infectious mononucleosis. *Proc Natl Acad Sci U S A* 1968;59(1): 94–101.

87. Longnecker RM, Kieff E, Cohen JI. Epstein-Barr virus. In: Knipe DM, Howley PM, eds. *Fields Virology*. 6th ed. Philadelphia, PA: Lippincott Williams & Wilkins; 2013.

88. Cesarman E. Gammaherpesviruses and lymphoproliferative disorders. *Annu Rev Pathol* 2014;9:349–372.

89. Shannon-Lowe C, Rowe M. Epstein-Barr virus infection of polarized epithelial cells via the basolateral surface by memory B cell-mediated transfer infection. *PLoS Pathog* 2011;7(5):e1001338.

90. Faulkner GC, Burrows SR, Khanna R, et al. X-Linked agammaglobulinemia patients are not infected with Epstein-Barr virus: implications for the biology of the virus. *J Virol* 1999;73(2):1555–1564.

91. Hjalgrim H, Smedby KE, Rostgaard K, et al. Infectious mononucleosis, childhood social environment, and risk of Hodgkin lymphoma. *Cancer Res* 2007;67(5):2382–2388.

92. Barton ES, White DW, Cathelyn JS, et al. Herpesvirus latency confers symbiotic protection from bacterial infection. *Nature* 2007;447(7142):326–329.

93. Giulino-Roth L, Cesarman E. Molecular biology of Burkitt lymphoma. In: Robertson E, ed. *Burkitt's Lymphoma*. New York, NY: Springer; 2013: 211–226.

94. Chang ET, Adami HO. The enigmatic epidemiology of nasopharyngeal carcinoma. *Cancer Epidemiol Biomarkers Prev* 2006;15(10):1765–1777.

95. Murukesan V, Mukherjee S. Managing post-transplant lymphoproliferative disorders in solid-organ transplant recipients: a review of immunosuppressant regimens. *Drugs* 2012;72(12):1631–1643.

96. Cohen JI, Mocarski ES, Raab-Traub N, et al. The need and challenges for development of an Epstein-Barr virus vaccine. *Vaccine* 2013;31(Suppl 2): B194–196.

97. Choquet S, Leblond V, Herbrecht R, et al. Efficacy and safety of rituximab in B-cell post-transplantation lymphoproliferative disorders: results of a prospective multicenter phase 2 study. *Blood* 2006;107(8):3053–3057.

98. Barnes JA, Lacasce AS, Feng Y, et al. Evaluation of the addition of rituximab to CODOX-M/IVAC for Burkitt's lymphoma: a retrospective analysis. *Ann Oncol* 2011;22(8):1859–1864.

99. Kaposi M. Idiopathisches multiples Pigmentsarkom der Haut. *Archiv für Dermatologie und Syphilis* 1872;4(2):265–273.

100. Antman K, Chang Y. Kaposi's sarcoma. *N Engl J Med* 2000;342(14):1027–1038.

101. Beral V, Peterman TA, Berkelman RL, et al. Kaposi's sarcoma among persons with AIDS: a sexually transmitted infection? *Lancet* 1990;335(8682):123–128.

102. Chang Y, Cesarman E, Pessin MS, et al. Identification of herpesvirus-like DNA sequences in AIDS-associated Kaposi's sarcoma. *Science* 1994;266(5192): 1865–1869.

103. Damania BA, Cesarman E. Kaposi's sarcoma-associated herpesvirus. In: Knipe DM, Howley PM, eds. *Fields Virology*. 6th ed. Philadelphia, PA: Lippincott Williams & Wilkins; 2013.

104. Cook-Mozaffari P, Newton R, Beral V, et al. The geographical distribution of Kaposi's sarcoma and of lymphomas in Africa before the AIDS epidemic. *Br J Cancer* 1998;78(11):1521–1528.

105. Martin DF, Kuppermann BD, Wolitz RA, et al. Oral ganciclovir for patients with cytomegalovirus retinitis treated with a ganciclovir implant. Roche Ganciclovir Study Group. *N Engl J Med* 1999;340(14):1063–1070.

106. Krown SE, Dittmer DP, Cesarman E. Pilot study of oral valganciclovir therapy in patients with classic Kaposi sarcoma. *J Infect Dis* 2011;203(8):1082–1086.

107. Sakakibara S, Tosato G. Regulation of angiogenesis in malignancies associated with Epstein-Barr virus and Kaposi's sarcoma-associated herpes virus. *Future Microbiol* 2009;4(7):903–917.

108. Soulier J, Grollet L, Oksenhendler E, et al. Kaposi's sarcoma-associated herpesvirus-like DNA sequences in multicentric Castleman's disease. *Blood* 1995;86(4):1276–1280.

109. Polizzotto MN, Uldrick TS, Wang V, et al. Human and viral interleukin-6 and other cytokines in Kaposi sarcoma herpesvirus-associated multicentric Castleman disease. *Blood* 2013;122(26):4189–4198.

110. Simonelli C, Spina M, Cinelli R, et al. Clinical features and outcome of primary effusion lymphoma in HIV-infected patients: a single-institution study. *J Clin Oncol* 2003;21(21):3948–3954.

111. Coffin JM, Hughes SH, Varmus HE, eds. The interactions of retroviruses and their hosts. *Retroviruses*. Cold Spring Harbor, NY: Cold Spring Harbor Laboratory Press; 1997.

112. Gallo RC. History of the discovery of the first human retroviruses: HTLV-1 and HTLV-2. *Oncogene* 2005;24:5926–5930.

113. Smit AF, Riggs AD. Tiggers and DNA transposon fossils in the human genome. *Proc Natl Acad Sci U S A* 1996;93:1443–1448.

114. Delviks-Frankenberry K, Paprotka T, Cingöz O, et al. Generation of multiple replication-competent retroviruses through recombination between PreXMRV-1 and PreXMRV-2. *J Virol* 2013;87:11525–11537.

115. Mason AL, Zhang G. Linking human beta retrovirus infection with primary biliary cirrhosis. *Gastroenterol Clin Biol* 2010;34:359–366.

116. Hacein-Bey-Abina S, VonKalle C, Schmidt M, et al. LMO2-associated clonal T cell proliferation in two patients after gene therapy for SCID-X1. *Science* 2003;302:415–419.

117. Matsuoka M, Jeang K-T. Human T-cell leukaemia virus type 1 (HTLV-1) infectivity and cellular transformation. *Nat Rev Cancer* 2007;7:270–280.

118. Poiesz BJ, Ruscetti FW, Mier JW, et al. T-cell lines established from human T-lymphocytic neoplasias by direct response to T-cell growth factor. *Proc Natl Acad Sci U S A* 1980;77:6815–6819.

119. Kalyanaraman VS, Sarngadharan MG, Robert-Guroff M, et al. A new subtype of human T-cell leukemia virus (HTLV-II) associated with a T-cell variant of hairy cell leukemia. *Science* 1982;218:571–573.

120. Wolfe ND, Heneine W, Carr JK, et al. Emergence of unique primate T-lymphotropic viruses among central African bushmeat hunters. *Proc Natl Acad Sci U S A* 2005;102:7994–7999.

121. Goncalves DU, Prioietti FA, Ribas JGR, et al. Epidemiology, treatment, and prevention of human T-cell leukemia virus type 1-associated diseases. *Clin Microbiol Rev* 2010;23:577–589.

122. Hino S, Sugiyama H, Doi H, et al. Breaking the cycle of HTLV-1 transmission via carrier mothers' milk. *Lancet Oncol* 1987;2:158–159.

123. Kannian P, Green PL. Human T lymphotropic virus type 1 (HTLV-1): molecular biology and oncogenesis. *Viruses* 2010;2:2037–2077.

124. Hill SA, Lloyd PA, McDonald S, et al. Susceptibility of human T cell leukemia virus type I to nucleoside reverse transcriptase inhibitors. *J Infec Dis* 2003;188:424–427.

125. Seegulam ME, Ratner L. Integrase inhibitors effective against human T-cell leukemia virus type 1. *Antimicrob Agents Chemother* 2011;55:2011–2017.

126. Derse D, Crise B, Li Y, et al. Human T-cell leukemia virus type 1 integration target sites in the human genome: comparison with those of other retroviruses. *J Virol* 2007;81:6731–6741.

127. Jones KS, Lambert S, Bouttier M, et al. Molecular aspects of HTLV-1 entry: functional domains of the HTLV-1 surface subunit (SU) and their relationships to the entry receptors. *Viruses* 2011;3:794–810.

128. Matsuoka M, Green PL. The HBZ gene, a key player in HTLV-1 pathogenesis. *Retrovirology* 2009;6:71.

129. Grossman WJ, Kimata JT, Wong FH, et al. Development of leukemia in mice transgenic for the tax gene of human T-cell leukemia virus type I. *Proc Natl Acad Sci U S A* 1995;92:1057–1061.

130. El Hajj H, El-Sabban M, Hasegawa H, et al. Therapy-induced selective loss of leukemia-initiating activity in murine adult T cell leukemia. *J Exp Med* 2010;207:2785–2792.

131. Villaudy J, Wencker M, Gadot N, et al. HTLV-1 propels thymic human T cell development in "human immune system" Rag2-/-IL-2Rgammac-/- mice. *PLoS Pathog* 2011;7:e1002231.

132. Costa EAS, Magri MC, Caterino-de-Arujo A. The best algorithm to confirm the diagnosis of HTLV-1 and HTLV-2 in at-risk individuals from Sao Paulo, Brazil. *J Virol Methods* 2011;173:280–286.

133. Barros N, Wolf F, Watanabe L, et al. Are increased Foxp3+ regulatory T cells responsible for immunosuppression during HTLV-1 infection? Case reports and review of the literature. *BMJ Case Rep* 2012;bcr2012006574.

134. Cook LB, Rowan AG, Melamed A, et al. HTLV-1-infected T cells contain a single integrated provirus in natural infection. *Blood* 2012;120:3488–3490.

135. Shimoyama M. Diagnostic criteria and classification of clinical subtypes of adult T-cell leukemia-lymphoma: a report from the Lymphoma Study Group. *Br J Hematol* 1991;79:426–437.

136. Takasaki Y, Iwanaga M, Imaizumi Y, et al. Long-term study of indolent adult T-cell leukemia-lymphoma. *Blood* 2010;115:4337–4343.

137. Bazarbachi A, Plumelle Y, Ramos JC, et al. Meta-analysis on the use of zidovudine and interferon-alfa in adult T-cell leukemia/lymphoma showing improved survival in the leukemic subtypes. *J Clin Oncol* 2010;28:4177–4183.

138. Katsuya H, Yamanka T, Ishitsuka K, et al. Prognostic index for acute- and lymphoma-type adult T-cell leukemia/lymphoma. *J Clin Oncol* 2012;30:1635–1640.

139. Tsukasaki K, Hermine O, Bazarbachi A, et al. Definition, prognostic factors, treatment, and reponse criteria of adult T-cell leukemia-lymphoma: a proposal from an international consensus meeting. *J Clin Oncol* 2009;27:453–459.

140. Yamada Y, Tomonaga M, Fukuda H, et al. A new G-CSF supported combination chemotherapy, LSG15, for adult T-cell leukemia-lymphoma: Japan Clinical Oncology Group Study 9303. *Br J Hematol* 2001;113:375–382.

141. Ratner L, Harrington W, Feng X, et al. Human T cell leukemia virus reactivation with progression of adult T-cell leukemia-lymphoma. AIDS Malignancy Consortium. *PLoS One* 2009;4:e4420.

142. Tatsuro J, Ishida T, Takemoto S, et al., eds. Randomized phase II study of mogamulizumab (KW-0761) plus VCAP-AMP-VECP (mLSG15) versus mLSG15 alone for newly diagnosed aggressive adult T-cell leukemia-lymphoma (ATL). Paper presented at: 2013 ASCO Annual Meeting; 2013; Chicago, IL.

143. Bazarbachi A, Suarez F, Fields P, et al. How I treat adult T-cell leukemia/lymphoma. *Blood* 2011;118:1736–1745.

144. Utsonomiya A, Miyazaki Y, Takasuka Y, et al. Improved outcome of adult T cell leukemia/lymphoma with allogeneic hematopoietic stem cell transplanation. *Bone Marrow Transplant* 2001;27:15–20.

145. Blumberg BS. The discovery of the hepatitis B virus and the intervention of the vaccine: a scientific memoir. *J Gastroenterol Hepatol* 2002;17(Supplement s4):S502–S503.

146. Houghton M. Discovery of the hepatitis C virus. *Liver Int* 2009;29(Supplement 1):82–88.

147. Arzumanyan A, Reis HM, Feitelson MA. Pathogenic mechanisms in HBV- and HCV-associated hepatocellular carcinoma. *Nat Rev Cancer* 2013;13:123–135.

148. Soerjomataram I, Lortet-Tieulent J, Parkin DM, et al. Global burden of cancer in 2008: a systematic analysis of disability-adjusted life-years in 12 world regions. *Lancet* 2012;380:1840–1850.

149. Altekruse SF, McGlynn KA, Reichman ME. Hepatocellular carcinoma incidence, mortality, and survival trends in the United States from 1975 to 2005. *J Clin Oncol* 2009;27:1485–1491.

150. Shiffman ML, ed. *Chronic Hepatitis C Virus: Advances in Treatment, Promise for the Future.* New York: Springer Verlag; 2011.

151. Nicot F, Nassim K, Lionel R, et al. Occult hepatitis C virus infection: Where are we now? *Liver Biopsy in Modern Med* 2004;307–334.

152. Freeman AJ, Dore GJ, Law MG, et al. Estimating progression to cirrhosis in chronic hepatitis C virus infection. *Hepatology* 2001;34:809–816.

153. Wilkins T, Malcom JK, Raina D, et al. Hepatitis C: diagnosis and treatment. *Am Fam Physician* 2010;81:1351–1357.

154. Fallot G, Neuveut C, Buendia M-A. Diverse roles of hepatitis B virus in liver cancer. *Curr Opin Virol* 2012;2:467–473.

155. Ganem D, Prince AM. Hepatitis B virus infection - natural history and clinical consequences. *N Engl J Med* 2004;350:1118–1129.

156. Tujios SR, Lee WM. Update in the management of chronic hepatitis B. *Curr Opin Gastroenterol* 2013;29:250–256.

157. Seto W-K, Fung J, Yuen M-F, et al. Future prevention and treatment of chronic hepatitis B infection. *J Clin Gastroenterol* 2012;46:725–734.

158. Wang WK, Levy S. Hepatitis C virus (HCV) and lymphomagenesis. *Leuk Lymphoma* 2003;44:1113–1120.

159. Fernandez-Garcia M-D, Mazzon M, Jacobs M, et al. Pathogenesis of flavivirus infections: using and abusing the host cell. *Cell Host Microbe* 2009;318:318–328.

160. Moradpour D, Penin F, Rice CM. Replication of hepatitis c virus. *Nat Rev Microbiol* 2007;5:453–463.

161. Liang TJ, Ghany MG. Current and future therapies for hepatitis C virus infection. *N Engl J Med* 2013;368:1907–1917.

162. Kimer N, Dahl EK, Gluud LL, et al. Antiviral therapy for prevention of hepatocellular carcinoma in chronic hepatitis C: systematic review and meta-analysis of randomised controlled trials. *BMJ Open* 2012;2:e001313.

163. Fujimoto A, Totoki Y, Abe T, et al. Whole-genome sequencing of liver cancers identifies etiological influences on mutation patterns and recurrent mutations in chromatin regulators. *Nat Genet* 2012;44:760–764.

164. Sung WK, Zheng H, Li S, et al. Genome-wide survey of recurrent HBV integration in hepatocellular carcinoma. *Nat Genet* 2012;44:765–769.

165. Devi U, Locarnini S. Hepatitis B antivirals and resistance. *Curr Opin Virol* 2013;3:495–500.

166. Aghemo A, Colombo M. Hepatocellular carcinoma in chronic hepatitis C: from bench to bedside. *Semin Immunopathol* 2013;35:111–120.

167. Bruix J, Sherman M. Management of hepatocellular carcinoma: an update. *Hepatology* 2011;53:1020–1022.

168. Mazzaferro V, Regalia E, Doci R, et al. Liver transplantation for the treatment of small hepatocellular carcinomas in patients with cirrhosis. *N Engl J Med* 1996;334:693–699.

169. Mino M, Lauwers GY. Pathologic spectrum and prognostic significance of underlying liver disease in hepatocellular carcinoma. *Surg Oncol Clin N Am* 2003;12:13–24.

170. Burton JR, Everson GT. Management of the transplant recipient with chronic hepatitis C. *Clin Liver Dis* 2013;17:73–91.

171. Beckebaum S, Kabar I, Cicinnati VR. Hepatitis B and C in liver transplantation: new strategies to combat the enemies. *Rev Med Virol* 2012;23:172–193.

172. Torres HA, Davila M. Reactivation of hepatitis B virus and hepatitis C virus in patients with cancer. *Nat Rev Clin Oncol* 2012;9:156–166.

173. Huang Y-H, Hsaio L-T, Hong Y-C, et al. Randomized controlled trial of entecavir prophylaxis for rituximab-associated hepatitis B virus reactivation in patients with lymphoma and resolved hepatitis. *J Clin Oncol* 2013;31:2765–2772.

174. Artz AS, Somerfield MR, Feld JJ, et al. American Society of Clinical Oncology provisional clinical opinion: chronic hepatitis B virus infection screening in patients receiving cytotoxic chemotherapy for treatment of malignant diseases. *J Clin Oncol* 2010;28:3199–3202.

175. Forghieri F, Luppi M, Barozzi P, et al. Pathogenetic mechanisms of hepatitits C virus-induced B-cell lymphomagenesis. *Clin Dev Immunol* 2012;2012:807351.

ETIOLOGY AND EPIDEMIOLOGY OF CANCER

6 Inflammation

Sahdeo Prasad and Bharat B. Aggarwal

INTRODUCTION

Extensive research over the last half a century indicates that inflammation plays an important role in cancer. Although acute inflammation can play a therapeutic role, low-level chronic inflammation can promote cancer. Different inflammatory cells, the various cell signaling pathways that lead to inflammation, and biomarkers of inflammation have now been well defined. These inflammatory pathways, which are primarily mediated through the transcription factors nuclear factor kappa B (NF-κB) and signal transducer and activator of transcription 3 (STAT3), have been linked to cellular transformation, tumor survival, proliferation, invasion, angiogenesis, and metastasis of cancer. These pathways have also now been linked with chemoresistance and radioresistance. This chapter considers the role of inflammation in cancer and its potential for cancer prevention and treatment.

Inflammation is the complex biologic responses of the body to irritation, injury, or infection. The recognition of inflammation dates back to antiquity. As documented by Aulus Cornelius Celsus, a Roman of the 1st century AD, inflammation is characterized by the tissue response to injury that results in *rubor* (redness, due to hyperemia), *tumor* (swelling, caused by increased permeability of the microvasculature and leakage of protein into the interstitial space), *calor* (heat, associated with increased blood flow and the metabolic activity of the cellular mediators of inflammation), and *dolor* (pain, in part due to changes in the perivasculature and associated nerve endings). Rudolf Virchow subsequently added *functio laesa* (dysfunction of the organs involved) in the 1850s. The process includes increased blood flow with an influx of white blood cells and other chemical substances that facilitate healing. Inflammation is also considered the body's self-protective attempt to remove harmful stimuli, including damaged cells, irritants, or pathogens, and to begin the healing process.

The word inflammation is derived from the Latin *inflammo* (meaning "I set alight, I ignite"). Because inflammation is a stereotyped response, it is considered a mechanism of innate immunity, as compared with adaptive immunity. On the basis of longevity, inflammation is classified as acute or chronic. When inflammation is short term, usually appearing within a few minutes or hours and ceasing upon the removal of the injurious stimulus, it is called acute. However, if it persists longer, it is called chronic inflammation, which leads to simultaneous destruction from the inflammatory process. Inflammation is beneficial when it is acute; however, chronic inflammation leads to several diseases, including cancer. Cancer is primarily a disease of lifestyle, with 30% of all cancers having been linked to smoking, 35% to diet, 14% to 20% to obesity, 18% to infection, and 7% to environmental pollution and radiation (Fig. 6.1).[1] Smoking, obesity, infections, pollution, and radiation are all known to activate proinflammatory pathways.[2] Therefore, understanding how inflammation contributes to cancer etiology is important for both cancer prevention and treatment.[3]

MOLECULAR BASIS OF INFLAMMATION

Although it is clear that inflammation and cancer are closely related, the mechanisms underlying persistent and chronic inflammation in chronic diseases remain unclear. Numerous cytokines have been linked with inflammation, including tumor necrosis factor (TNF), interleukin (IL)-1, IL-6, IL-8, IL-17, and vascular endothelial growth factor (VEGF). Among various cytokines that have been linked with inflammation, TNF is a primary mediator of inflammation linked to cancer.[4] However, it has been shown that proinflammatory transcriptional factors (activator protein [AP]-1, STAT3, NF-κB, hypoxia-inducible factor [HIF]-1, and β-catenin/Wnt) are ubiquitously expressed and control numerous physiologic processes, including development, differentiation, immunity, and metabolism in chronic diseases. Although these transcription factors are regulated by completely different signaling mechanisms, they are activated in response to various stimuli, including stresses and cytokines, and are involved in inflammation-induced tumor development and its metastasis.[5] Interestingly, inflammation plays a role at all stages of tumor development: initiation, progression, and metastasis.[2] In initiation, inflammation induces the release of a variety of cytokines and chemokines that promote the release of inflammatory cells and associated factors. This further causes oxidative damage, DNA mutations, and other changes in the tissue microenvironment, making it more conducive to cell transformation, increased survival, and proliferation. Inflammation also contributes to tissue injury, remodeling of the extracellular matrix, angiogenesis, and fibrosis in diverse target tissues. Among all the inflammatory cell signaling pathways, NF-κB has been shown to play a major role in cancer,[6,7] and TNF is one of the most potent activators of NF-κB.[8,9]

ROLE OF INFLAMMATION IN TRANSFORMATION

Transformation is the process by which the cellular and molecular makeup of a cell is altered as it becomes malignant. Numerous factors are involved in the process of cell transformation, including inflammation. A clinical study has shown that chronic inflammation due to heavy metal deposition in lymph nodes leads to malignant transformation and, finally, to patient death.[10] More recently, chronic exposure to cigarette smoke extract[11] and arsenite[12] has been shown to induce inflammation followed by epithelial–mesenchymal transition and transformation of human bronchial epithelial (HBE) cells. Furthermore, activation of NF-κB and HIF-2α increased the levels of the proinflammatory IL-6, IL-8, and IL-1β, which are essential for the malignant progression of transformed HBE cells. Sox2, another important molecular factor, cooperates with inflammation-mediated STAT3 activation, which precedes the malignant transformation of foregut basal progenitor cells.[13] A clinical study reported that the p53 mutation is a critical event for the malignant transformation of sinonasal inverted papilloma. This p53 mutation resulted in cyclooxygenase (COX)-2–mediated inflammatory signals that contribute to the proliferation

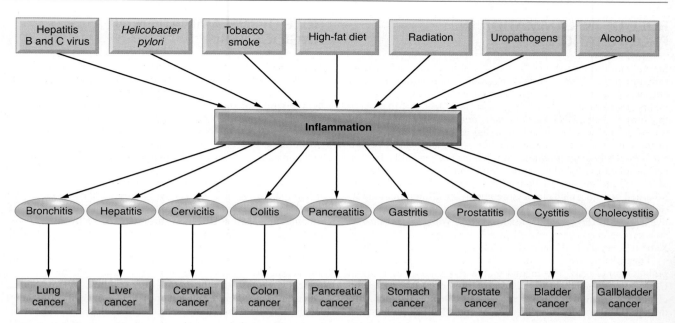

Figure 6.1 Origin of inflammation and its role in various cancers.

of advanced sinonasal inverted papilloma.[14] In another study in patients, the YKL-40 protein was found to be involved in chronic inflammation and oncogenic transformation of human breast tissues.[15] Inflammation-mediated transformation was also found to be regulated by MyD88 in a mouse model through Ras signaling.[16] In addition, inflammation contributed to the activation of the epidermal growth factor receptor (EGFR) and its subsequent interaction with PKCδ, which leads to the transformation of normal esophageal epithelia to squamous cell carcinoma.[17] Activation of Src oncoprotein triggers an inflammatory response mediated by NF-κB that directly activates Lin28 transcription and rapidly reduces let-7 microRNA levels. The inflammatory cytokine IL-6 mediates the activation of STAT3 transcription factor, which results in the transformation of cells.[18]

ROLE OF INFLAMMATION IN SURVIVAL

Numerous findings across different cancer populations have suggested that inflammation has an important role in carcinogenesis and disease progression.[19,20] The important markers of systemic inflammatory response in both in vitro findings and clinical outcomes include plasma C-reactive protein (CRP) concentration,[21,22] hypoalbuminemia,[23] and the Glasgow Prognostic Score (GPS), which combines CRP and albumin.[24,25] In addition to these, hematologic markers of systemic inflammatory response such as absolute white-cell count or its components (neutrophils, neutrophil-to-lymphocyte ratio [NLR]),[26–28] platelets, and a platelet-to-lymphocyte ratio[29,30] are also prognostic indicators for cancer clinical outcomes. Whether these inflammatory biomarkers influence the survival of cancer patients is discussed in this section.

In a study of 416 patients with renal cell carcinoma, with 362 patients included in the analysis, elevated neutrophil count, elevated platelet counts, and a high NLR were found. This inflammatory response was predictive for shorter overall patient survival.[31] Another study in unresectable malignant biliary obstruction (UMBO) found that patients with low GPS (0 and 1) had better postoperative survivals than did patients with a higher GPS. The 6-month and 1-year survival rates were 58.1% to 27.3%, respectively, for patients with low GPS and 25% to 6.2%, respectively, for patients with a higher GPS.[32] It has been also shown that prostate

cancer patients with aggressive, clinically significant disease and an elevated GPS[2] had a higher risk of death overall as well as high-grade disease.[33] Other than GPS, age and gastrectomy have also been shown to independently influence the disease-specific and progression-free survival of gastric cancer patients.[34] A biomarker of systemic inflammation, the blood NLR, predicted patient survival with hepatocellular carcinoma (HCC) after transarterial chemoembolization. Patients in whom the NLR remained stable or became normalized after transarterial chemoembolization showed improved overall survival compared with patients showing a persistently abnormal index of NLR.[35]

A further study found that inflammatory transcription factors and cytokines contribute to the overall survival of patients. One study found that 97% of patients with epithelial tumors of malignant pleural mesothelioma and 95% of patients with nonepithelial tumors expressed IL-4Rα protein, and this strong IL-4Rα expression was correlated with a worse survival. In response to IL-4, human malignant pleural mesothelioma cells showed increased STAT6 phosphorylation and increased production of IL-6, IL-8, and VEGF without any effect on proliferation or apoptosis. This finding indicates that high expression of STAT6 as well as STAT3 and cytokines is inversely correlated with survival in patients.[36,37] NF-κB, along with IL-6, contributes to the survival of mammospheres in culture, because NF-κB and IL-6 were hyperactive in breast cancer–derived mammospheres.[38] In addition, elevated CRP and serum amyloid A (SAA) were associated with reduced disease-free survival of breast cancer patients.[39] In gastroesophageal cancer, proinflammatory cytokines IL-1β, IL-6, IL-8, and TNF-α and acute phase protein concentrations (CRP) were found to be elevated, and these levels were associated with reduced survival of patients.[40] Additionally, the Bcl-2 family protein COX-2, which is regulated by inflammatory transcription factors, is also involved in the survival of cancer cells.[41,42] Thus, we conclude that inflammation in general contributes to poor survival of patients.

In contrast to these findings, an in vivo study of dogs with osteosarcoma showed that survival improvement was apparent with inflammation or lymphocyte-infiltration scores >1, as well as in dogs that had apoptosis scores in the top 50th percentile.[43] Also, in patients with epithelioid malignant pleural mesothelioma, a high degree of chronic inflammatory cell infiltration in the stromal component was associated with improved overall survival.[44]

ROLE OF INFLAMMATION IN PROLIFERATION

Several studies have shown that cell proliferation is affected by inflammation.[45] More significantly, proliferation in the setting of chronic inflammation predisposes humans to carcinoma in the esophagus, stomach, colon, liver, and urinary bladder.[46] In postgastrectomy patients, *Helicobacter pylori* induced inflammation and was associated with increased epithelial cell proliferation.[47] Even in the mouse model, chronic infection with *Helicobacter hepaticus* induced hepatic inflammation, which further led to hepatic cell proliferation.[48] Other reports found an increased expression of the cell proliferative markers PCNA and Ki-67 in the linings of inflamed odontogenic keratocysts compared with noninflamed lesions.[49,50] These findings suggest the existence of greater proliferative activity in the cells with inflammation. Wang et al.[51] showed an increased expression of cell proliferative markers PCNA and Ki-67 in a sample of 45 patients with benign prostatic hyperplasia.

The inflammatory biomarker COX-2 was also associated with the proliferation of cells. The highest proliferation index was found in COX-2–positive epithelium.[51] The association of COX-2 and proliferation was also reported in a rat model. The carcinogen dimethylhydrazine (DMH) induces an increase in epithelial cell proliferation and in the expression of COX-2 in the colon of rats.[52] Erbb2, a kinase, regulates inflammation through the induction of NF-κB, Comp1, IL-1β, COX-2, and multiple chemokines in the skin by ultraviolet (UV) exposure. This inflammation has been shown to increase the proliferation of skin tissue after UV irradiation.[53]

ROLE OF INFLAMMATION IN INVASION

A characteristic of invasive cancer cells is survival and growth under nonadhesive conditions. This invasion of cancer cells causes the disease to spread, which results in poor patient survival.[54] A strong relationship has been documented between inflammation and cancer cell invasion.[55,56] In a study of 150 patients with HCC, a high GPS score was associated with a high vascular invasion of cancer cells.[57] Another study of colorectal cancer also supports the links between inflammation and the invasion of cancer cells, with a finding that a high GPS increased the invasion of colorectal cancer cells.[58] In patients with esophageal squamous cell carcinoma, a high GPS score also showed a close relationship with lymphatic and venous invasion.[59]

At the molecular level, various proteins are known to be involved in tumor cell invasion. MMP-9, a gelatinase that degrades type IV collagen—the major structural protein component in the extracellular matrix and basement membrane—is thought to play an important role in facilitating tumor invasion, as it is highly expressed in various malignant tumors.[60,61] Additionally, the high expression of HIF-1α has been proposed as being associated with a greater incidence of vascular invasion of HCC. This expression of HIF-1α was further correlated with high expression of the inflammatory molecule COX-2.[62]

Breast cancer invasion has been linked to proteolytic activity at the tumor cell surface. In inflammatory breast cancer (IBC) cells, high expression of cathepsin B, a cell surface proteolytic enzyme, has been shown to be associated with invasiveness of IBC. In addition, a high coexpression of cathepsin B and caveolin-1 was found in IBC patient biopsies. Thus, proteolytic activity of cathepsin B and its coexpression with caveolin-1 contributes to the invasiveness of IBC.[63] In IBC, RhoC GTPase is also responsible for the invasive phenotype.[64] In addition, the PI3K/Akt signaling pathway is crucial in IBC invasion. The molecules involved in cell motility are specifically upregulated in IBC patients compared with stage-matched and cell-type-of-origin–matched non-IBCs patients. Distinctively, RhoC GTPase is a substrate for Akt1, and its phosphorylation is absolutely essential for IBC cell invasion.[65]

ROLE OF INFLAMMATION IN ANGIOGENESIS

Angiogenesis—the formation of new blood vessels from existing vessels—is tightly linked to chronic inflammation and cancer. Angiogenesis is one of the molecular events that bridges the gap between inflammation and cancer. Angiogenesis results from multiple signals acting on endothelial cells. Mature vessels control exchanges of hematopoietic cells and solutes between blood and surrounding tissues by responding to microenvironmental cues, including inflammation. Although inflammation is essential to defend the body against pathogens, it has adverse effects on the surrounding tissue, and some of these effects induce angiogenesis. Inflammation and angiogenesis are thereby linked processes, but exactly how they are related has not been well understood. Both inflammation and angiogenesis are exacerbated by an increased production of chemokines/cytokines, growth factors, proteolytic enzymes, proteoglycans, lipid mediators, and prostaglandins.

A close relationship has been reported between inflammation and angiogenesis in breast cancer. Tissue section staining showed increased vascularity with the intensity of diffuse inflammation.[66] Offersen et al.[67] found that inflammation was significantly correlated in bladder carcinoma with microvessel density, which is a marker of angiogenesis. Leukocytes have been described as mediators of inflammation-associated angiogenesis. In addition, the stable expression of TNF-α in endothelial cells increased angiogenic sprout formation independently of angiogenic growth factors. Furthermore, in work using the Matrigel plug assay in vivo, increased angiogenesis was observed in endothelial TNF-α–expressing mice. Thus, chronic inflammatory changes mediated by TNF-α can induce angiogenesis in vitro and in vivo, suggesting a direct link between inflammation and angiogenesis.[68] TNF-α–induced inhibitor of nuclear factor kappa kinase (IKK)-β activation also activates the angiogenic process. IKK-β activates the mammalian target of rapamycin (mTOR) pathway and enhances angiogenesis through VEGF production.[66] In addition to TNF-α, proinflammatory cytokines IL-1 (mainly IL-1β) and IL-8 were also found to be major proangiogenic stimuli of both physiologic and pathologic angiogenesis.[69,70] Recently, another cytokine macrophage migration inhibitory factor (MIF) was found to play a role in neoangiogenesis/vasculogenesis by endothelial cell activation along with inflammation.[71]

Benest et al.[72] found that a well-known regulator of angiogenesis, angiopoietin-2 (Ang-2), can upregulate inflammatory responses, indicating a common signaling pathway for inflammation and angiogenesis. TGF-β induction was also reported in head and neck epithelia and human head and neck squamous cell carcinomas (HNSCC), with severe inflammation that leads to angiogenesis.[73] The tumor-derived cytokine endothelial monocyte-activating polypeptide II (EMAP-II) has been shown to have profound effects on inflammation as well as on the processes involved in angiogenesis.[74] NF-κB plays an important role in inflammation as well as in angiogenesis, because the suppression of NF-κB and IkB-2A blocks basic fibroblast growth factor–induced angiogenesis in vivo. NF-κB regulates the angiogenic protein VEGF promoted by α5β1 integrin, which coordinately regulates angiogenesis and inflammation.[75] It has been also reported that a coculture of cancer cells with macrophages synergistically increased the production of various angiogenesis-related factors when stimulated by the inflammatory cytokine. This inflammatory angiogenesis was mediated by the activation of NF-κB and activator protein 1 (Jun/Fos), because the administration of either NF-κB–targeting drugs or COX-2 inhibitors or the depletion of macrophages blocked inflammatory angiogenesis.[76]

In a mouse model, cigarette smoke induced the inflammatory protein 5-lipoxygenase (5-LOX), and this induction activated matrix metalloproteinase 2 (MMP-2) and VEGF to induce the angiogenic process.[77] A cellular enzyme, Tank-binding kinase 1

(TBK-1), has been proposed as a putative mediator in tumor angiogenesis. TBK-1 mediates angiogenesis through the upregulation of VEGF and exerts proinflammatory effects via the induction of inflammatory cytokines. Thus, these pathways, including TBK-1, are an important cross-link between angiogenesis and inflammation.[78]

ROLE OF INFLAMMATION IN METASTASIS

Inflammation plays a regulatory role in cancer progression and metastasis. Chronic or tumor-derived inflammation and inflammation-related stimuli within the tumor microenvironment promote blood and lymphatic vessel formation and aid in invasion and metastasis.[79,80] The association of inflammation and metastasis has been observed in several cancer types. In an immunohistochemical analysis of lung cancer tissues, a remarkably high level of metastasis was observed with severe inflammation.[81] A mouse model of breast cancer found that mammary tumors increased the frequency of lung metastases, and this effect was associated with the recruitment of inflammatory cells to the lung as well as elevated levels of IL-6 in the lung airways.[82] In another murine model, implanting human ovarian tumor cells into the ovaries of severe combined immunodeficient mice resulted in peritoneal inflammation and tumor cell dissemination from the ovaries. In addition, enhancement of the inflammatory response with thioglycolate accelerated the development of ascites and metastases, and its suppression with acetylsalicylic acid delayed metastasis.[83] Thus, it can be concluded that inflammation facilitates ovarian tumor metastasis by a mechanism largely mediated by cytokines.

It has been shown that metastatic tumor cells entering a distant organ such as the liver trigger a proinflammatory response involving the Kupffer cell–mediated release of TNF-α and the upregulation of vascular endothelial cell adhesion receptors, such as E-selectin.[84] The physiologic expression of the selectins is tightly controlled to limit the inflammatory response, but dysregulated expression of selectins contributes to inflammatory and thrombotic disorders as well as tumor metastases.[85] Using P-selectin knockout mice, the importance of P-selectin–mediated cell adhesive interactions in the pathogenesis of inflammation and metastasis of cancers has been clearly demonstrated.[86]

Tumor-associated inflammatory monocytes and macrophages are essential promoters of tumor cell migration, invasion, and metastasis.[87] Macrophages and their mediators affect the multistep process of invasion and metastasis, from interaction with the extracellular matrix to the construction of a premetastatic niche. Monocytes are attracted by cytokines and chemokines (e.g., CSF-1, GM-CSF, and MCP-1), which are released by tumor cells or cells of the tumor microenvironment. These monocytes are then induced to express proangiogenic and metastatic factors, including VEGF, fibroblast growth factor (FGF)-2, platelet-derived growth factor (PDGF), intercellular adhesion molecule (ICAM)-1, vascular cell adhesion molecule (VCAM)-1, E-selectin, P- selectin, and MMP-9.[88] Versican, a large extracellular matrix proteoglycan, has been shown to activate tumor-infiltrating myeloid cells through Toll-like receptor (TLR) 2 and its coreceptors TLR6 and CD14 and to elicit the production of proinflammatory cytokines (including TNF-α), which enhance tumor metastasis. TLR2 increases the secretion of IL-8, which potentiates metastatic growth. Ligation of TLR2 by versican induces inflammatory cytokine secretion, providing a link between inflammation and cancer metastasis.[89]

IKK-α has been shown to be important in the inflammation-associated metastasis of cancer cells. Luo et al.[90] demonstrated that activation and nuclear localization of IKK-α by tumor-infiltrating immune cells in prostatic epithelial tumor cells leads to malignant prostatic epithelial cells with a metastatic fate. Src family kinases, when inappropriately activated, promote pathologic inflammatory processes and tumor metastasis, in part through their effects on the regulation of endothelial monolayer permeability.[91] Platelet-activating factor (PAF), an inflammatory biolipid, has also been shown to increase metastasis. In particular, Melnikova et al.[92] demonstrated that PAF receptor antagonists can effectively inhibit the metastatic potential of human melanoma cells in nude mice. Mesenchymal stem cells promote HCC metastasis under the influence of inflammation through TGF-β.[93]

EPIGENETIC CHANGES AND INFLAMMATION

Epigenetics considers the heritable changes in the activity of gene expression without the alteration of DNA sequences, and such changes have been linked to many human diseases, including cancer.[94] DNA methylation and histone modification are well-known epigenetic changes that can lead to gene activation or inactivation.[94–96] DNA methylation occurs primarily at cytosine-phosphate-guanine (CpG) dinucleotides as well as at transcriptional regulatory sites on the gene promoter.[96–98] Epigenetic abnormalities result in dysregulated gene expression and function, which can further lead to cancer. Inflammation and epigenetic abnormalities in cancer are highly associated. Inflammation induces aberrant epigenetic alterations in a tissue early in the process of carcinogenesis, and accumulation of such alterations forms an epigenetic field for cancer. Yara et al.[99] have shown that increased inflammation, as evidenced by the activation of NF-κB, production of IL-6 and COX-2, as well as the decrease of IκB, leads to the promoter's methylation. However, preincubation of cells with a demethylating agent prevented inflammation.

Infectious agents also contribute to inflammation-induced epigenetic changes. Infectious agents such as *H. pylori* and hepatitis C virus as well as intrinsic mediators of inflammatory responses, including proinflammatory cytokines, induce genetic and epigenetic changes, including point mutations, deletions, duplications, recombinations, and methylation of various tumor-related genes. Interestingly, disturbances in cytokine and chemokine signals and the induction of cell proliferation are important ways that inflammation induces aberrant DNA methylation. A study has shown that infection of human gastric mucosae with *H. pylori* induces chronic inflammation and further gastric cancers.[100] This inflammation is associated with high methylation levels or high incidences of methylation.[101–103]

Furthermore, numerous reports have documented the fact that inflammation is linked with epigenetic changes in carcinogenesis. Recently, Achyut[104] reported that inflammation in stromal fibroblasts caused epigenetic silencing of p21 and further tumor progression. Chronic inflammation also led to epigenetic regulation of p16 and activation of DNA damage in a lung carcinogenesis model.[105]

A transient inflammatory signal has been shown to initiate an epigenetic switch from nontransformed cells to cancer cells via a positive feedback loop involving NF-κB, Lin28, let-7, and IL-6. This IL-6 induced STAT3, directly activated miR-21 and miR-181b-1, and further induced the epigenetic switch. Thus, STAT3 underlies the epigenetic switch of mir-21 and mir-181b-1 that links inflammation to cancer.[106] Another report also showed that transient activation of Src oncoprotein mediates an epigenetic switch from immortalized breast cells to a stably transformed line that contained cancer stem cells. Thus, inflammation activates a positive feedback loop that maintains the epigenetic transformed state for many generations in the absence of the inducing signal.[18]

DNA hypermethylation at promoter CpG islands is an important mechanism by which carcinogenesis occurs through the inactivation of tumor-suppressor genes. Aberrant CpG island hypermethylation is also frequently observed in chronic inflammation and precancerous lesions, which again suggests links between inflammation and epigenetic change.[107] In addition, inflammation induced the halogenation of cytosine nucleotide. Damage products of this inflammation-mediated halogenated cytosine interfere with normal epigenetic control by altering DNA-protein interactions that are critical for gene regulation and the heritable transmission of methylation patterns. These inflammation-mediated cytosine damage products also provide a mechanistic link between inflammation and cancer.[108]

ROLE OF INFLAMMATION IN CANCER DIAGNOSIS

Chronic inflammation plays an important role in the etiology and progression of chronic diseases, including cancer. Hence, chronic inflammation may have an important diagnostic role in cancer. Inflammation induced by inflammatory cells such as infiltrating cells and mesothelial cells is mediated via the release of various mediators and proteins, including PDGF, IL-8, monocyte chemotactic peptide (MCP-1), nitric oxide (NO), collagen, antioxidant enzymes, and the plasminogen activation inhibitor (PAI). Furthermore, several inflammatory mediators have been shown to be detected at increased concentrations, thereby aiding in the disease diagnosis.[109]

In one study, numerous inflammatory disorders were detected based on inflammation measured in gastric biopsies of patients by Fourier transform infrared spectroscopy (FT-IR). Using endoscopic samples, gastritis and gastric cancer were diagnosed.[110] Furthermore, the degree of prostate inflammation has been used to determine the level of incidental prostatitis.[111] An assessment of the expression of cytokines and other immune stimulatory molecules that drive B-cell activation provides insight into the etiology of cancers. It has been shown that the dysregulation of cytokine production precedes the diagnosis of non-Hodgkin lymphoma.[112]

Inflammation parameters have been used to diagnose cancer in patients. Inflammation parameters, including CRP, were found to differ in patients with cancer and in those without. In clinical practice, however, such parameters are considered to have modest diagnostic value for cancer.[113] In a study with 1,275 patients, granulomatous inflammation was identified in 154 patients (12.1%), of whom 12 out of 154 (7.8%) had a concurrent diagnosis of cancer.[114] In another study with 173 patients, 52% had lung adenocarcinoma. Patients with high systemic inflammation were more likely to have more than two sites of metastatic disease and to have poor performance status and less likely to receive any chemotherapy. Systemic inflammation at diagnosis is considered to be an independent marker of poor outcome in patients with advanced non-small cell lung cancer (NSCLC).[115]

INFLAMMATION AND GENOMICS

Recently, the genomic landscape of the most common forms of human cancer have been examined.[116] Almost 140 genes and 12 cell signaling pathways have been linked with most cancers. Several of these genes and pathways are directly or indirectly linked with inflammation. A cytokine pattern in patients with cancer has been identified.[117]

INFLAMMATION AND TARGETED THERAPIES

That inflammation can be used as a target for cancer prevention and treatment is indicated by the fact that several drugs approved by the U.S. Food and Drug Administration (FDA) actually modulate proinflammatory pathways. For instance, EGFR, HER2, VEGF, CXCR4, and proteasome have been shown to activate NF-κB–mediated proinflammatory pathways, and their inhibitors have been approved by the FDA for the treatment of various cancers. Similarly, steroids such as dexamethasone, nonsteroidal anti-inflammatory drugs (NSAIDs), and statins that are currently used for prevention or treatment have also been found to suppress the NF-κB pathway. Thus, these observations indicate that inflammatory pathways are excellent targets for cancer.

CONCLUSIONS

According to Colditz et al.,[118] almost 50% of all cancers can be prevented based on what we know today. All the studies summarized previously suggest that inflammation is closely linked to cancer, and the incidence of most cancers can be reduced by controlling inflammation. Proinflammatory conditions such as colitis, bronchitis, hepatitis, and gastritis can all eventually lead to cancer. Thus, one must find ways to treat these conditions before the appearance of cancer. All these studies indicate that an anti-inflammatory lifestyle could play an important role in both the prevention and treatment of cancer.

REFERENCES

1. Anand P, Kunnumakkara AB, Sundaram C, et al. Cancer is a preventable disease that requires major lifestyle changes. *Pharm Res* 2008;25:2097–2116.
2. Aggarwal BB, Gehlot P. Inflammation and cancer: how friendly is the relationship for cancer patients? *Curr Opin Pharmacol* 2009;9:351–369.
3. Coussens LM, Zitvogel L, Palucka AK. Neutralizing tumor-promoting chronic inflammation: a magic bullet? *Science* 2013;339:286–291.
4. Sethi G, Sung B, Aggarwal BB. TNF: a master switch for inflammation to cancer. *Front Biosci* 2008;13:5094–5107.
5. Karin M. Nuclear factor-kappaB in cancer development and progression. *Nature* 2006;441:431–436.
6. Aggarwal BB. Nuclear factor-kappaB: the enemy within. *Cancer Cell* 2004; 6:203–208.
7. Chaturvedi MM, Sung B, Yadav VR, et al. NF-kappaB addiction and its role in cancer: 'one size does not fit all'. *Oncogene* 2011;30:1615–1630.
8. Aggarwal BB. Signalling pathways of the TNF superfamily: a double-edged sword. *Nat Rev Immunol* 2003;3:745–756.
9. Aggarwal BB, Gupta SC, Kim JH. Historical perspectives on tumor necrosis factor and its superfamily: 25 years later, a golden journey. *Blood* 2012; 119:651–665.
10. Iannitti T, Capone S, Gatti A, et al. Intracellular heavy metal nanoparticle storage: progressive accumulation within lymph nodes with transformation from chronic inflammation to malignancy. *Int J Nanomed* 2010;5:955–960.
11. Zhao Y, Xu Y, Li Y, et al. NF-kappaB-mediated inflammation leading to EMT via miR-200c is involved in cell transformation induced by cigarette smoke extract. *Toxicol Sci* 2013;135:265–276.
12. Xu Y, Zhao Y, Xu W, et al. Involvement of HIF-2alpha-mediated inflammation in arsenite-induced transformation of human bronchial epithelial cells. *Toxicol Appl Pharmacol* 2013;272:542–550.

13. Liu K, Jiang M, Lu Y, et al. Sox2 cooperates with inflammation-mediated Stat3 activation in the malignant transformation of foregut basal progenitor cells. *Cell Stem Cell* 2013;12:304–315.
14. Yoon BN, Chon KM, Hong SL, et al. Inflammation and apoptosis in malignant transformation of sinonasal inverted papilloma: the role of the bridge molecules, cyclooxygenase-2, and nuclear factor kappaB. *Am J Otolaryngol* 2013;34:22–30.
15. Roslind A, Johansen JS. YKL-40: a novel marker shared by chronic inflammation and oncogenic transformation. *Methods Mol Biol* 2009;511:159–184.
16. Coste I, Le Corf K, Kfoury A, et al. Dual function of MyD88 in RAS signaling and inflammation, leading to mouse and human cell transformation. *J Clin Invest* 2010;120:3663–3667.
17. Parthasarathy S, Dhayaparan D, Jayanthi V, et al. Aberrant expression of epidermal growth factor receptor and its interaction with protein kinase C delta in inflammation associated neoplastic transformation of human esophageal epithelium in high risk populations. *J Gastroenterol Hepatol* 2011;26:382–390.
18. Iliopoulos D, Hirsch HA, Struhl K. An epigenetic switch involving NF-kappaB, Lin28, Let-7 MicroRNA, and IL6 links inflammation to cell transformation. *Cell* 2009;139:693–706.
19. Colotta F, Allavena P, Sica A, et al. Cancer-related inflammation, the seventh hallmark of cancer: links to genetic instability. *Carcinogenesis* 2009;30: 1073–1081.
20. Hanahan D, Weinberg RA. Hallmarks of cancer: the next generation. *Cell* 2011;144:646–674.
21. Canna K, McMillan DC, McKee RF, et al. Evaluation of a cumulative prognostic score based on the systemic inflammatory response in patients undergoing potentially curative surgery for colorectal cancer. *Br J Cancer* 2004;90: 1707–1709.

22. Hilmy M, Bartlett JM, Underwood MA, et al. The relationship between the systemic inflammatory response and survival in patients with transitional cell carcinoma of the urinary bladder. *Br J Cancer* 2005;92:625–627.

23. Forrest LM, McMillan DC, McArdle CS, et al. Evaluation of cumulative prognostic scores based on the systemic inflammatory response in patients with inoperable non-small-cell lung cancer. *Br J Cancer* 2003;89:1028–1030.

24. Ramsey S, Lamb GW, Aitchison M, et al. Evaluation of an inflammation-based prognostic score in patients with metastatic renal cancer. *Cancer* 2007;109:205–212.

25. Crumley AB, Stuart RC, McKernan M, et al. Comparison of an inflammation-based prognostic score (GPS) with performance status (ECOG-ps) in patients receiving palliative chemotherapy for gastroesophageal cancer. *J Gastroenterol Hepatol* 2008;23:e325–329.

26. Yamanaka T, Matsumoto S, Teramukai S, et al. The baseline ratio of neutrophils to lymphocytes is associated with patient prognosis in advanced gastric cancer. *Oncology* 2007;73:215–220.

27. Halazun KJ, Aldoori A, Malik HZ, et al. Elevated preoperative neutrophil to lymphocyte ratio predicts survival following hepatic resection for colorectal liver metastases. *Eur J Surg Oncol* 2008;34:55–60.

28. Huang ZL, Luo J, Chen MS, et al. Blood neutrophil-to-lymphocyte ratio predicts survival in patients with unresectable hepatocellular carcinoma undergoing transarterial chemoembolization. *J Vasc Interv Radiol* 2011;22:702–709.

29. Heng DY, Xie W, Regan MM, et al. Prognostic factors for overall survival in patients with metastatic renal cell carcinoma treated with vascular endothelial growth factor-targeted agents: results from a large, multicenter study. *J Clin Oncol* 2009;27:5794–5799.

30. Smith RA, Bosonnet L, Raraty M, et al. Preoperative platelet-lymphocyte ratio is an independent significant prognostic marker in resected pancreatic ductal adenocarcinoma. *Am J Surg* 2009;197:466–472.

31. Fox P, Hudson M, Brown C, et al. Markers of systemic inflammation predict survival in patients with advanced renal cell cancer. *Br J Cancer* 2013; 109:147–153.

32. Iwasaki Y, Ishizuka M, Kato M, et al. Usefulness of an inflammation-based prognostic score (mGPS) for predicting survival in patients with unresectable malignant biliary obstruction. *World J Surg* 2013;37:2222–2228.

33. Shafique K, Proctor MJ, McMillan DC, et al. Systemic inflammation and survival of patients with prostate cancer: evidence from the Glasgow Inflammation Outcome Study. *Prostate Cancer Prostatic Dis* 2012;15:195–201.

34. Kunisaki C, Takahashi M, Ono HA, et al. Inflammation-based prognostic score predicts survival in patients with advanced gastric cancer receiving biweekly docetaxel and s-1 combination chemotherapy. *Oncology* 2012;83:183–191.

35. Pinato DJ, Sharma R. An inflammation-based prognostic index predicts survival advantage after transarterial chemoembolization in hepatocellular carcinoma. *Transl Res* 2012;160:146–152.

36. Burt BM, Bader A, Winter D, et al. Expression of interleukin-4 receptor alpha in human pleural mesothelioma is associated with poor survival and promotion of tumor inflammation. *Clin Cancer Res* 2012;18:1568–1577.

37. Sethi G, Shanmugam MK, Ramachandran L, et al. Multifaceted link between cancer and inflammation. *Biosci Rep* 2012;32:1–15.

38. Papi A, Guarnieri T, Storci G, et al. Nuclear receptors agonists exert opposing effects on the inflammation dependent survival of breast cancer stem cells. *Cell Death Differ* 2012;19:1208–1219.

39. Pierce BL, Ballard-Barbash R, Bernstein L, et al. Elevated biomarkers of inflammation are associated with reduced survival among breast cancer patients. *J Clin Oncol* 2009;27:3437–3444.

40. Deans DA, Wigmore SJ, Gilmour H, et al. Elevated tumour interleukin-1beta is associated with systemic inflammation: a marker of reduced survival in gastro-oesophageal cancer. *Br J Cancer* 2006;95:1568–1575.

41. Chen LS, Balakrishnan K, Gandhi V. Inflammation and survival pathways: chronic lymphocytic leukemia as a model system. *Biochem Pharmacol* 2010;80:1936–1945.

42. Sharma-Walia N, Paul AG, Bottero V, et al. Kaposi's sarcoma associated herpes virus (KSHV) induced COX-2: a key factor in latency, inflammation, angiogenesis, cell survival and invasion. *PLoS Pathog* 2010;6:e1000777.

43. Modiano JF, Bellgrau D, Cutter GR, et al. Inflammation, apoptosis, and necrosis induced by neoadjuvant fas ligand gene therapy improves survival of dogs with spontaneous bone cancer. *Mol Ther* 2012;20:2234–2243.

44. Suzuki K, Kadota K, Sima CS, et al. Chronic inflammation in tumor stroma is an independent predictor of prolonged survival in epithelioid malignant pleural mesothelioma patients. *Cancer Immunol Immunother* 2011;60:1721–1728.

45. Hu B, Elinav E, Flavell RA. Inflammasome-mediated suppression of inflammation-induced colorectal cancer progression is mediated by direct regulation of epithelial cell proliferation. *Cell Cycle* 2011;10:1936–1939.

46. Sugar LM. Inflammation and prostate cancer. *Can J Urol* 2006;13(Suppl 1):46–47.

47. Safatle-Ribeiro AV, Ribeiro U, Jr., Clarke MR, et al. Relationship between persistence of *Helicobacter pylori* and dysplasia, intestinal metaplasia, atrophy, inflammation, and cell proliferation following partial gastrectomy. *Dig Dis Sci* 1999;44:243–252.

48. Ihrig M, Schrenzel MD, Fox JG. Differential susceptibility to hepatic inflammation and proliferation in AXB recombinant inbred mice chronically infected with *Helicobacter hepaticus*. *Am J Pathol* 1999;155:571–582.

49. de Paula AM, Carvalhais JN, Domingues MG, et al. Cell proliferation markers in the odontogenic keratocyst: effect of inflammation. *J Oral Pathol Med* 2000;29:477–482.

50. Kaplan I, Hirshberg A. The correlation between epithelial cell proliferation and inflammation in odontogenic keratocyst. *Oral Oncol* 2004;40:985–991.

51. Wang W, Bergh A, Damber JE. Chronic inflammation in benign prostate hyperplasia is associated with focal upregulation of cyclooxygenase-2, Bcl-2, and cell proliferation in the glandular epithelium. *Prostate* 2004;61:60–72.

52. Demarzo MM, Martins LV, Fernandes CR, et al. Exercise reduces inflammation and cell proliferation in rat colon carcinogenesis. *Med Sci Sports Exerc* 2008;40:618–621.

53. Madson JG, Lynch DT, Tinkum KL, et al. Erbb2 regulates inflammation and proliferation in the skin after ultraviolet irradiation. *Am J Pathol* 2006; 169:1402–1414.

54. Bondong S, Kiefel H, Hielscher T, et al. Prognostic significance of L1CAM in ovarian cancer and its role in constitutive NF-kappaB activation. *Ann Oncol* 2012;23:1795–1802.

55. Wu Y, Zhou BP. Inflammation: a driving force speeds cancer metastasis. *Cell Cycle* 2009;8:3267–3273.

56. Aggarwal BB, Vijayalekshmi RV, Sung B. Targeting inflammatory pathways for prevention and therapy of cancer: short-term friend, long-term foe. *Clin Cancer Res* 2009;15:425–430.

57. Kinoshita A, Onoda H, Imai N, et al. The Glasgow Prognostic Score, an inflammation based prognostic score, predicts survival in patients with hepatocellular carcinoma. *BMC Cancer* 2013;13:52.

58. Toiyama Y, Miki C, Inoue Y, et al. Evaluation of an inflammation-based prognostic score for the identification of patients requiring postoperative adjuvant chemotherapy for stage II colorectal cancer. *Exp Ther Med* 2011;2:95–101.

59. Kobayashi T, Teruya M, Kishiki T, et al. Inflammation-based prognostic score, prior to neoadjuvant chemoradiotherapy, predicts postoperative outcome in patients with esophageal squamous cell carcinoma. *Surgery* 2008;144:729–735.

60. Nelson AR, Fingleton B, Rothenberg ML, et al. Matrix metalloproteinases: biologic activity and clinical implications. *J Clin Oncol* 2000;18:1135–1149.

61. Clark ES, Weaver AM. A new role for cortactin in invadopodia: regulation of protease secretion. *Eur J Cell Biol* 2008;87:581–590.

62. Dai CX, Gao Q, Qiu SJ, et al. Hypoxia-inducible factor-1 alpha, in association with inflammation, angiogenesis and MYC, is a critical prognostic factor in patients with HCC after surgery. *BMC Cancer* 2009;9:418.

63. Victor BC, Anbalagan A, Mohamed MM, et al. Inhibition of cathepsin B activity attenuates extracellular matrix degradation and inflammatory breast cancer invasion. *Breast Cancer Res* 2011;13:R115.

64. van Golen KL, Bao LW, Pan Q, et al. Mitogen activated protein kinase pathway is involved in RhoC GTPase induced motility, invasion and angiogenesis in inflammatory breast cancer. *Clin Exp Metastasis* 2002;19:301–311.

65. Lehman HL, Van Laere SJ, van Golen CM, et al. Regulation of inflammatory breast cancer cell invasion through Akt1/PKBalpha phosphorylation of RhoC GTPase. *Mol Cancer Res* 2012;10:1306–1318.

66. Lee DF, Kuo HP, Chen CT, et al. IKK beta suppression of TSC1 links inflammation and tumor angiogenesis via the mTOR pathway. *Cell* 2007;130: 440–455.

67. Offersen BV, Knap MM, Marcussen N, et al. Intense inflammation in bladder carcinoma is associated with angiogenesis and indicates good prognosis. *Br J Cancer* 2002;87:1422–1430.

68. Rajashekhar G, Willuweit A, Patterson CE, et al. Continuous endothelial cell activation increases angiogenesis: evidence for the direct role of endothelium linking angiogenesis and inflammation. *J Vasc Res* 2006;43:193–204.

69. Voronov E, Carmi Y, Apte RN. Role of IL-1-mediated inflammation in tumor angiogenesis. *Adv Exp Med Biol* 2007;601:265–270.

70. Qazi BS, Tang K, Qazi A. Recent advances in underlying pathologies provide insight into interleukin-8 expression-mediated inflammation and angiogenesis. *Int J Inflam* 2011;2011:908468.

71. Asare Y, Schmitt M, Bernhagen J. The vascular biology of macrophage migration inhibitory factor (MIF). Expression and effects in inflammation, atherogenesis and angiogenesis. *Thromb Haemost* 2013;109:391–398.

72. Benest AV, Kruse K, Savant S, et al. Angiopoietin-2 is critical for cytokine-induced vascular leakage. *PLoS One* 2013;8: e70459.

73. Lu SL, Reh D, Li AG, et al. Overexpression of transforming growth factor beta1 in head and neck epithelia results in inflammation, angiogenesis, and epithelial hyperproliferation. *Cancer Res* 2004;64:4405–4410.

74. Berger AC, Tang G, Alexander HR, et al. Endothelial monocyte-activating polypeptide II, a tumor-derived cytokine that plays an important role in inflammation, apoptosis, and angiogenesis. *J Immunother* 2000;23:519–527.

75. Klein S, de Fougerolles AR, Blaikie P, et al. Alpha 5 beta 1 integrin activates an NF-kappa B-dependent program of gene expression important for angiogenesis and inflammation. *Mol Cell Biol* 2002;22:5912–5922.

76. Ono M. Molecular links between tumor angiogenesis and inflammation: inflammatory stimuli of macrophages and cancer cells as targets for therapeutic strategy. *Cancer Sci* 2008;99:1501–1506.

77. Ye YN, Liu ES, Shin VY, et al. Contributory role of 5-lipoxygenase and its association with angiogenesis in the promotion of inflammation-associated colonic tumorigenesis by cigarette smoking. *Toxicology* 2004;203:179–188.

78. Czabanka M, Korherr C, Brinkmann U, et al. Influence of TBK-1 on tumor angiogenesis and microvascular inflammation. *Front Biosci* 2008;13: 7243–7249.

79. Solinas G, Marchesi F, Garlanda C, et al. Inflammation-mediated promotion of invasion and metastasis. *Cancer Metastasis Rev* 2010;29:243–248.

80. Affara NI, Coussens LM. IKKalpha at the crossroads of inflammation and metastasis. *Cell* 2007;129:25–26.

81. Kayser K, Bulzebruck H, Ebert W, et al. Local tumor inflammation, lymph node metastasis, and survival of operated bronchus carcinoma patients. *J Natl Cancer Inst* 1986;77:77–81.

ETIOLOGY AND EPIDEMIOLOGY OF CANCER

82. Hobson J, Gummadidala P, Silverstrim B, et al. Acute inflammation induced by the biopsy of mouse mammary tumors promotes the development of metastasis. *Breast Cancer Res Treat* 2013;139:391–401.

83. Robinson-Smith TM, Isaacsohn I, Mercer CA, et al. Macrophages mediate inflammation-enhanced metastasis of ovarian tumors in mice. *Cancer Res* 2007;67:5708–5716.

84. Khatib AM, Auguste P, Fallavollita L, et al. Characterization of the host proinflammatory response to tumor cells during the initial stages of liver metastasis. *Am J Pathol* 2005;167:749–759.

85. McEver RP. Selectin-carbohydrate interactions during inflammation and metastasis. *Glycoconj J* 1997;14:585–591.

86. Geng JG, Chen M, Chou KC. P-selectin cell adhesion molecule in inflammation, thrombosis, cancer growth and metastasis. *Curr Med Chem* 2004; 11:2153–2160.

87. Condeelis J, Pollard JW. Macrophages: obligate partners for tumor cell migration, invasion, and metastasis. *Cell* 2006;124:263–266.

88. Siegel G, Malmsten M. The role of the endothelium in inflammation and tumor metastasis. *Int J Microcirc Clin Exp* 1997;17:257–272.

89. Wang W, Xu GL, Jia WD, et al. Ligation of TLR2 by versican: a link between inflammation and metastasis. *Arch Med Res* 2009;40:321–323.

90. Luo JL, Tan W, Ricono JM, et al. Nuclear cytokine-activated IKKalpha controls prostate cancer metastasis by repressing Maspin. *Nature* 2007;446:690–694.

91. Kim MP, Park SI, Kopetz S, et al. Src family kinases as mediators of endothelial permeability: effects on inflammation and metastasis. *Cell Tissue Res* 2009;335:249–259.

92. Melnikova V, Bar-Eli M. Inflammation and melanoma growth and metastasis: the role of platelet-activating factor (PAF) and its receptor. *Cancer Metastasis Rev* 2007;26:359–371.

93. Jing Y, Han Z, Liu Y, et al. Mesenchymal stem cells in inflammation microenvironment accelerates hepatocellular carcinoma metastasis by inducing epithelial-mesenchymal transition. *PLoS One* 2012;7:e43272.

94. Jones PA, Baylin SB. The epigenomics of cancer. *Cell* 2007;128:683–692.

95. Esteller M. Aberrant DNA methylation as a cancer-inducing mechanism. *Annu Rev Pharmacol Toxicol* 2005;45:629–656.

96. Thiagalingam S, Cheng KH, Lee HJ, et al. Histone deacetylases: unique players in shaping the epigenetic histone code. *Ann N Y Acad Sci* 2003; 983:84–100.

97. Li E, Beard C, Jaenisch R. Role for DNA methylation in genomic imprinting. *Nature* 1993;366:362–365.

98. Antequera F, Bird A. Number of CpG islands and genes in human and mouse. *Proc Natl Acad Sci U S A* 1993;90:11995–11999.

99. Yara S, Lavoie JC, Beaulieu JF, et al. Iron-ascorbate-mediated lipid peroxidation causes epigenetic changes in the antioxidant defense in intestinal epithelial cells: impact on inflammation. *PLoS One* 2013;8:e63456.

100. Uemura N, Okamoto S, Yamamoto S, et al. Helicobacter pylori infection and the development of gastric cancer. *N Engl J Med* 2001;345:784–789.

101. Maekita T, Nakazawa K, Mihara M, et al. High levels of aberrant DNA methylation in Helicobacter pylori-infected gastric mucosae and its possible association with gastric cancer risk. *Clin Cancer Res* 2006;12:989–995.

102. Nakajima T, Maekita T, Oda I, et al. Higher methylation levels in gastric mucosae significantly correlate with higher risk of gastric cancers. *Cancer Epidemiol Biomarkers Prev* 2006;15:2317–2321.

103. Perri F, Cotugno R, Piepoli A, et al. Aberrant DNA methylation in non-neoplastic gastric mucosa of H. Pylori infected patients and effect of eradication. *Am J Gastroenterol* 2007;102:1361–1371.

104. Achyut BR, Bader DA, Robles AI, et al. Inflammation-mediated genetic and epigenetic alterations drive cancer development in the neighboring epithelium upon stromal abrogation of TGF-beta signaling. *PLoS Genet* 2013;9:e1003251.

105. Blanco D, Vicent S, Fraga MF, et al. Molecular analysis of a multistep lung cancer model induced by chronic inflammation reveals epigenetic regulation of p16 and activation of the DNA damage response pathway. *Neoplasia* 2007;9:840–852.

106. Iliopoulos D, Jaeger SA, Hirsch HA, et al. STAT3 activation of miR-21 and miR-181b-1 via PTEN and CYLD are part of the epigenetic switch linking inflammation to cancer. *Mol Cell* 2010;39:493–506.

107. Suzuki H, Toyota M, Kondo Y, et al. Inflammation-related aberrant patterns of DNA methylation: detection and role in epigenetic deregulation of cancer cell transcriptome. *Methods Mol Biol* 2009;512:55–69.

108. Valinluck V, Sowers LC. Inflammation-mediated cytosine damage: a mechanistic link between inflammation and the epigenetic alterations in human cancers. *Cancer Res* 2007;67:5583–5586.

109. Kroegel C, Antony VB. Immunobiology of pleural inflammation: potential implications for pathogenesis, diagnosis and therapy. *Eur Respir J* 1997; 10:2411–2418.

110. Li QB, Sun XJ, Xu YZ, et al. Use of Fourier-transform infrared spectroscopy to rapidly diagnose gastric endoscopic biopsies. *World J Gastroenterol* 2005;11:3842–3845.

111. Difuccia B, Keith I, Teunissen B, et al. Diagnosis of prostatic inflammation: efficacy of needle biopsies versus tissue blocks. *Urology* 2005;65:445–448.

112. Vendrame E, Martinez-Maza O. Assessment of pre-diagnosis biomarkers of immune activation and inflammation: insights on the etiology of lymphoma. *J Proteome Res* 2011;10:113–119.

113. Baicus C, Caraiola S, Rimbas M, et al. Utility of routine hematological and inflammation parameters for the diagnosis of cancer in involuntary weight loss. *J Investig Med* 2011;59:951–955.

114. DePew ZS, Gonsalves WI, Roden AC, et al. Granulomatous inflammation detected by endobronchial ultrasound-guided transbronchial needle aspiration in patients with a concurrent diagnosis of cancer: a clinical conundrum. *J Bronchology Interv Pulmonol* 2012;19:176–181.

115. Jafri SH, Shi R, Mills G. Advance lung cancer inflammation index (ALI) at diagnosis is a prognostic marker in patients with metastatic non-small cell lung cancer (NSCLC): a retrospective review. *BMC Cancer* 2013;13:158.

116. Vogelstein B, Papadopoulos N, Velculescu VE, et al. Cancer genome landscapes. *Science* 2013;339:1546–1558.

117. Lippitz BE. Cytokine patterns in patients with cancer: a systematic review. *Lancet Oncol* 2013;14:e218–228.

118. Colditz GA, Wolin KY, Gehlert S. Applying what we know to accelerate cancer prevention. *Sci Transl Med* 2012;4(127):127rv4.

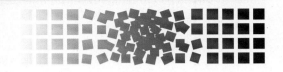

7 Chemical Factors

Stuart H. Yuspa and Peter G. Shields

ETIOLOGY AND EPIDEMIOLOGY OF CANCER

INTRODUCTION

As early as the 1800s, initial observations of unusual cancer incidences in occupational groups provided the first indications that chemicals were a cause of human cancer, which was then confirmed in experimental animal studies during the early and mid 1900s. However, the extent to which chemical exposures contribute to cancer incidence was not fully appreciated until population-based studies documented differing organ-specific cancer rates in geographically distinct populations and in cohort studies such as those that linked smoking to lung cancer.[1] The most commonly occurring chemical exposures that increase cancer risk are tobacco, alcoholic beverages, diet, and reproductive factors (e.g., hormones). Today, it is recognized that cancer results not solely from chemical exposure (e.g., in the workplace or at home), but that a variety of biologic, social, and physical factors contribute to cancer pathogenesis.[2,3] For some common cancers, it also has been recognized that heritable factors also contribute to cancer risk from chemical exposure (e.g., genes involved in carcinogen metabolism, DNA repair, a variety of cancer pathways).[4] Twin studies show that for common cancers, nongenetic risk factors are dominant, and the best associations for genetic risks of sporadic cancers indicate that the risks for specific genetic traits are typically less than 1.5-fold.[5–7] The role of the tumor microenvironment, the cancer stem cells, and feedback signaling to and from the tumor also have been recently recognized as important contributors to carcinogenesis, although how chemicals affect these have yet been clearly demonstrated.[8–10]

The experimental induction of tumors in animals, the neoplastic transformation of cultured cells by chemicals, and the molecular analysis of human tumors have revealed important concepts regarding the pathogenesis of cancer and how laboratory studies can be used to better understand human cancer pathogenesis.[7,11,12] Chemical carcinogens usually affect specific organs, targeting the epithelial cells (or other susceptible cells within an organ) and causing genetic damage (genotoxic) or epigenetic effects regulating DNA transcription and translation. Chemically related DNA damage and consequent somatic mutations relevant to human cancer can occur either directly from exogenous exposures or indirectly by activation of endogenous mutagenic pathways (e.g., nitric oxide, oxyradicals).[13,14] The risk of developing a chemically induced tumor may be modified by nongenotoxic exogenous and endogenous exposures and factors (e.g., hormones, immunosuppression triggered by the tumor), and by accumulated exposure to the same or different genotoxic carcinogens.[7,15]

Analyses of how chemicals induce cancer in animal models and human populations has had a major impact on human health. Experimental studies have been instrumental in replicating hypotheses generated from human studies and identifying pathobiologic mechanisms. For example, animal experiments confirmed the carcinogenic and cocarcinogenic properties of cigarette smoke and identified bioactive chemical and gaseous components.[1] The transplacental carcinogenicity of diethylstilbestrol and the hazards of specific occupational carcinogens such as vinyl chloride,

benzene, aromatic amines, and bis(chloromethyl)ether led to a reduction in allowable exposures of suspected human carcinogens from the workplace and a reduction in cancer rates. Dietary factors that enhance or inhibit cancer development and the contribution of obesity to specific organ sites have been identified in models of chemical carcinogenesis, and alterations in diet and obesity are expected to result in reduced cancer risk. Experimental animal studies are the mainstay of risk assessment as a screening tool to identify potential carcinogens in the workplace and the environment, although these studies do not prove specific chemical etiologies as a cause of human cancer because of interspecies differences and the use of maximally tolerated doses that do not replicate human exposure.

THE NATURE OF CHEMICAL CARCINOGENS: CHEMISTRY AND METABOLISM

The National Toxicology Program, based mostly on experimental animal studies and supported by epidemiology studies when available, lists 45 chemical, physical, and infectious agents as known human carcinogens and about 175 that are reasonably anticipated to be human carcinogens (http://ntp.niehs.nih.gov/?objectid=035E57E7-BDD9-2D9B-AFB9D1CADC8D09C1), whereas the International Agency for Research on Cancer (IARC) lists 113 agents as carcinogenic to humans and 66 that are probably carcinogenic to humans (http://monographs.iarc.fr/ENG/Classification/index.php). Table 7.1 provides a selected list of known human carcinogens, as indicated by the IARC, which are continuously updated.[16] Most chemical carcinogens first undergo metabolic activation by cytochrome P450s or other metabolic pathways so that they react with DNA and/or alter epigenetic mechanisms.[11,17] This process, evolutionarily presumed to have been developed to rid the body of foreign chemicals for excretion, inadvertently generates reactive carcinogenic intermediates that can bind cellular molecules, including DNA, and cause mutations or other alterations.[18] Recent data indicate that metabolizing enzymes also have the ability to cross-talk with transcription factors involved in the regulation of other metabolizing and antioxidant enzymes.[19] DNA is considered the ultimate target for most carcinogens to cause either mutations or gross chromosomal changes, but epigenetic effects, such as altered DNA methylation and gene transcription, also promote carcinogenesis.[20] The formation of DNA adducts, where chemicals bind directly to DNA to promote mutations, is likely necessary but not sufficient to cause cancer.

Genotoxic carcinogens may transfer simple alkyl or complexed (aryl) alkyl groups to specific sites on DNA bases.[18,21] These alkylating and aryl-alkylating agents include, but are not limited to, N-nitroso compounds, aliphatic epoxides, aflatoxins, mustards, polycyclic aromatic hydrocarbons, and other combustion products of fossil fuels and vegetable matter. Others transfer arylamine residues to DNA, as exemplified by aryl aromatic

TABLE 7.1

Known Chemical Carcinogens in Humans[a]

Target Organ	Agents	Industries	Tumor Type
Lung	Tobacco smoke, arsenic, asbestos, crystalline silica, benzo(a)pyrene, beryllium, bis(chloro)methyl ether, 1,3-butadiene, chromium VI compounds, coal tar and pitch, diesel exhaust, nickel compounds, soot, mustard gas, cobalt-tungsten carbide powders	Aluminum production, coal gasification, coke production, painting, hematite mining, painting, grinding in oil and gas	Squamous, large cell, and small cell cancer and adenocarcinoma
Pleura	Asbestos, erionite, painting	Insulation, mining	Mesothelioma
Oral cavity	Tobacco smoke, alcoholic beverages, nickel compounds, betel quid	–	Squamous cell cancer
Esophagus	Tobacco smoke, alcoholic beverages, betel quid	–	Squamous cell cancer
Gastric	Tobacco smoking	Rubber industry	Adenocarcinoma
Colon	Alcohol, tobacco smoking	–	Adenocarcinoma
Liver	Aflatoxin, vinyl chloride, tobacco smoke, alcoholic beverages	–	Hepatocellular carcinoma, hemangiosarcoma
Kidney	Tobacco smoke, trichloroethylene	–	Renal cell cancer
Bladder	Tobacco smoke, 4-aminobiphenyl, benzidine, 2-napthylamine, cyclophosphamide, phenacetin	Magenta manufacturing, auramine manufacturing, painting, rubber production	Transitional cell cancer
Prostate	Cadmium	–	Adenocarcinoma
Skin	Arsenic, benzo(a)pyrene, coal tar and pitch, mineral oils, soot, cyclosporin A, azathioprine, shale oils	–	Squamous cell cancer, basal cell cancer
Bone marrow	Benzene, tobacco smoke, ethylene oxide, antineoplastic agents, cyclosporin A, formaldehyde	Rubber workers	Leukemia, lymphoma

[a]The carcinogen designations are determined by the International Agency for Research on Cancer (http://monographs.iarc.fr/index.php). They do not imply proof of carcinogenicity in individuals. This table is not all inclusive. For additional information, the reader is referred to agency documents and publications.

amines, aminoazo dyes, and heterocyclic aromatic amines. For genotoxic carcinogens, the interaction with DNA is not random, and each class of agents reacts selectively with purine and pyrimidine targets.[7,18,21] Furthermore, targeting carcinogens to particular sites in DNA is determined by nucleotide sequence, by host cell, and by selective DNA repair processes (see later discussion), making some genetic material at risk over others. As expected from this chemistry, genotoxic carcinogens can be potent mutagens and particularly adept at causing nucleotide base mispairing or small deletions, leading to missense or nonsense mutations. Others may cause macrogenetic damage, such as chromosome breaks and large deletions. In some cases, such genotoxic damage may result in changes in transcription and translation that affect protein levels or function, which in turn alter the behavior of the specific host cell type. For example, there may be effects on cell proliferation, programmed cell death, or DNA repair. This is best typified by the signature mutations detected in the p53 gene caused by ingested aflatoxin in human liver cancer[22] and by polycyclic aromatic hydrocarbons human lung cancer caused by the inhalation of cigarette smoke.[15,23,24] Similarly, a distinct pattern of mutations is detected in pancreatic cancers from smokers when compared with pancreatic cancers from nonsmokers.[25]

Some chemicals that cause cancers in laboratory rodents are not demonstrably genotoxic. In general, these agents are carcinogenic in laboratory animals at high doses and require prolonged exposure. Synthetic pesticides and herbicides fall within this group, as do a number of natural products that are ingested. The mechanism of action by nongenotoxic carcinogens is not well understood, and may be related in some cases to toxic cell death and regenerative hyperplasia. They may also induce endogenous mutagenic mechanisms through the production of free radicals, increasing

rates of depurination, and the deamination of 5-methylcytosine. In other cases, nongenotoxic carcinogens may have hormonal effects on hormone-dependent tissues. For example, some pesticides, herbicides, and fungicides have endocrine-disrupting properties in experimental models, although the relation to human cancer risk is unknown.

ANIMAL MODEL SYSTEMS AND CHEMICAL CARCINOGENESIS

Most human chemical carcinogens can induce tumors in experimental animals; however, the tumors may not be in the same organ, the exposure pathways may differ from human exposure, and the causative mechanisms may not exist in humans. In many cases, however, the cell of origin, morphogenesis, phenotypic markers, and genetic alterations are qualitatively identical to corresponding human cancers. Furthermore, animal models have revealed the constancy of carcinogen–host interaction among mammalian species by reproducing organ-specific cancers in animals with chemicals identified as human carcinogens, such as coal tar and squamous cell carcinomas, vinyl chloride and hepatic angiosarcomas, aflatoxin and hepatocellular carcinoma, and aromatic amines and bladder cancer. The introduction of genetically modified mice designed to reproduce specific human cancer syndromes and precancer models has accelerated both the understanding of the contributions of chemicals to cancer causation and the identification of potential exogenous carcinogens.[26,27] Furthermore, construction of mouse strains genetically altered to express human drug–metabolizing enzymes has added both to the relevance of mouse studies for understanding human carcinogen metabolism and the prediction of genotoxicity from suspected human carcinogens and other chemical exposures.[28] Together, these studies have indicated that carcinogenic agents can directly activate oncogenes, inactivate tumor suppressor genes, and cause the genomic changes that are associated with autonomous growth, enhanced survival, and modified gene expression profiles that are required for the malignant phenotype.[29]

Genetic Susceptibility to Chemical Carcinogenesis in Experimental Animal Models

The use of inbred strains of rodents and spontaneous or genetically modified mutant strains have led to the identification and characterization of genes that modify risks for cancer development.[30–32] For a variety of tissue sites, including the lungs, the liver, the breast, and the skin, pairs of inbred mice can differ by 100-fold in the risk for tumor development after carcinogen exposure. Genetically determined differences in the affinity for the aryl hydrocarbon hydroxylase (Ah) receptor or other differences in metabolic processing of carcinogens is one modifier that has a major impact on experimental and presumed human cancer risk.[33–35] The development of mice reconstituted with components of the human carcinogen–metabolizing genome should facilitate the extrapolation of metabolic activity by human enzymes and cancer risk.[27,28,36] Such mice also show that other loci regulate the growth of premalignant foci, the response to tumor promoters, the immune response to metastatic cells, and the basal proliferation rate of target cells.[30] In mice susceptible to colon cancer due to a carcinogen-induced constitutive mutation in the APC gene, a locus on mouse chromosome 4 confers resistance to colon cancer.[31] The identification of the phospholipase A2 gene at this locus and subsequent functional testing in transgenic mice revealed an interesting paracrine protective influence on tumor development.[31] This gene, and several other genes mapped for susceptibility to chemically induced mouse tumors (PTPRJ, a receptor type tyrosine phosphatase, and STK6/STK15, an aurora kinase), have now been shown to influence susceptibility to organ-specific cancer induction in humans.[30,31]

MOLECULAR EPIDEMIOLOGY, CHEMICAL CARCINOGENESIS, AND CANCER RISK IN HUMAN POPULATIONS

Molecular epidemiology is the application of biologically based hypotheses using molecular and epidemiologic methods and measures. New technologies continue to allow epidemiologic studies to improve the testing of biologically based hypotheses and to develop large datasets for hypothesis generation, most notably the application of various –omics technologies via next-generation sequencing (e.g., genomics, epigenomics, transcriptomics), proteomics, and metabolomics. The greatest challenge now is to develop methods that allow for analysis cutting across various technologies.[37–43] Recent advances now include the role of microRNA and long noncoding RNAs in tumor development and progression because of their impact on the regulation of gene expression.[44,45] Chemical effects on microRNAs and the resultant gene expression is currently being identified.[46] Using such technologies, emerging evidence is noting the importance of the microbiome and associated infections as a risk of human cancer.[47–50] The complexity of environmental exposure and how it interacts with humans to affect numerous biologic pathways has been characterized as the exposome, also expressed as a multidimensional complex dataset.[51] Therefore, the important goal remains: to characterize cancer risk based on gene–environment interactions. However, we remain challenged because cancer is a complex disease of diverse etiologies by multiple exposures causing damage in different genes; for example, $gene^n$–$environment^n$ interactions, for which the variable n is not known.

Two fundamental principles underlie current studies of molecular epidemiology. First, carcinogenesis is a multistage process, and behind each stage are numerous genetic events that occur either due to an exogenous insult such as a chemical exposure or an endogenous insult, such as from free radicals generated via cellular processes or errors in DNA replication. Therefore, identifying a cancer risk factor can be challenging because of the multifactorial nature of carcinogenesis, given that any one risk factor occurs within a background of many risk factors. Second, wide interindividual variation in response to carcinogen exposure and other carcinogenic processes indicate that the human response is not homogeneous, so that experimental models and epidemiology (e.g., the use of a single cell clone to study a gene's effect experimentally or the assumption that the population responds similarly to the mean in epidemiology studies), might not be representative of susceptible and resistant groups within a population.

Genetic Susceptibility

In humans, the determination of genetic susceptibility can be assessed by phenotyping or genotyping methods. Phenotypes generally represent complex genotypes. Examples of phenotypes include the assessment of DNA repair capacity in cultured blood cells, mammographic breast density, or the quantitation of carcinogen-DNA adducts in a target organ. Phenotypes now also include profiles of methylation that affect gene expression, a so-called epigenetic effect, for example, identified though next-generation sequencing or other methods.[52] The contribution of genetics to cancer risk from chemical carcinogens can range from small to large, depending on its penetrance.[4] Highly penetrant cancer-susceptibility genes cause familial cancers, but account for less than 5% of all cancers. Low-penetrant genes cause common sporadic cancers, which have large public health consequences.

A genetic polymorphism (e.g., single nucleotide polymorphisms) is defined as a genetic variant present in at least 1% of the population. Because of the advent of improved genotyping methods that have reduced cost and increased high throughput, haplotyping and whole genomewide association studies are ongoing. Although haplotyping studies, facilitated through the International HapMap Project (www.hapmap.org), have not proven useful for predicting human cancers; high-density, whole genomewide, single nucleotide polymorphism association studies have shown remarkable consistency for many gene loci, although the risk estimates are only 1.0 to 1.4, which are not useful in the clinic for individual risk assessment.[6] For example, the contribution of genetic polymorphisms to cancer risk, at least for breast cancer, appears to improve risk modeling by only a few percent; known breast cancer risk factors account for about 58% of risk, and adding 10 genetic variants increases the risk prediction only to 62%.[53] Genes under study are from pathways that affect behavior, activate and detoxify carcinogens, affect DNA repair, govern cell-cycle control, trigger apoptosis, effect cell signaling, and so forth.

Biomarkers of Cancer Risk

The evaluation of dose and risk estimates in epidemiologic studies can include four components: namely, external exposure measurements, internal exposure measurements, biomarkers estimating the biologically effective dose, and biomarkers of effect or harm. The latter three measurements are biomarkers that improve on the first by quantifying exposure inside the individual and at the cellular level to characterize low-dose exposures in low-risk populations, providing a relative contribution of individual chemical carcinogens from complex mixtures, and/or estimating total burden of a particular exposure where there are many sources.[54]

Chemicals cause genetic damage in different ways, namely in the formation of carcinogen-DNA adducts leading to base mutations or gross chromosomal changes. Adducts are formed when a mutagen, or part of it, irreversibly binds to DNA so that it can cause a base substitution, insertion, or deletion during DNA replication. Gross chromosomal mutations are chromosome breaks, gaps, or translocations. The level of DNA damage is the biologically effective dose in a target organ, and reflects the net result of carcinogen exposure, activation, lack of detoxification, lack of effective DNA repair, and lack of programmed cell death. A variety of assays have been used for determining carcinogen-macromolecular adducts in human tissues; for example, for assessing risk from tobacco smoking for lung cancer and aflatoxin and liver cancer.[55,56] Important considerations for the assessment of biomarkers include sensitivity, specificity, reproducibility, accessibility for human use, and whether it represents a risk measured in a target organ or surrogate tissue. No single biomarker has been considered to be sufficiently validated for use as a cancer risk marker in an individual as it relates to chemical carcinogenesis.[57] However, there is some evidence that DNA adducts are cancer risk factors in both cohort and case-control studies.[58]

People are commonly exposed to N-nitrosamine and other N-nitroso compounds from dietary and tobacco exposures, which are associated with DNA adduct formation and cancer. Exposure can occur through endogenous formation of N-nitrosamines from nitrates in food or directly from dietary sources, cosmetics, drugs, household commodities, and tobacco smoke. Endogenous formation occurs in the stomach from the reaction of nitrosatable amines and nitrate (used as a preservative), which is converted to nitrites by bacteria. The N-nitrosamines undergo metabolic activation by cytochrome P450s (CYP2E1, CYP2A6, and CYP2D6) and form DNA adducts. Biomarkers are available to assess N-nitrosamine exposure from tobacco smoke (e.g., urinary tobacco-specific nitrosamine levels) or DNA, including in target organs such as the lungs. Recent data indicate that increasing levels of tobacco-specific nitrosamine metabolites are associated with increased lung cancer risk.[55]

Heterocyclic amines are formed from the overheating of food with creatine, such as meat, chicken, and fish.[59] Heterocyclic amines, estimated based on consumption of well-done meat, have been associated with breast and colon cancer, presumably through metabolic activation mechanisms and DNA damage.[59] Aflatoxins, another food contaminant, are considered to be a major contributor to liver cancer in China and parts of Africa, especially interacting with hepatitis viruses, and urinary aflatoxin adduct levels are predictors of liver cancer risk.[56]

Aromatic amines are another class of human carcinogens. Aryl aromatic amines have been implicated in bladder carcinogenesis, especially in occupationally exposed cohorts (e.g., dye workers) and tobacco smokers.[60] These compounds are activated by cytochrome P4501A2 and excreted via the N-acetyltransferase 2 gene. They are genotoxic, and the quantitative assessment using biomarkers has been more difficult, but some persons have studied DNA adducts as well.[61]

Polycyclic aromatic hydrocarbons (PAH) are large, aromatic (three or more fused benzene rings) compounds that are a class of more than 200 chemicals. These compounds are ubiquitous in the environment and present in the ambient air. They are formed from overcooking foods, fireplaces, charcoal barbeques, burning of coal and crude oil, tobacco smoke, and can be found in various occupational settings. In order for PAHs to exert their toxic effect, they must undergo metabolic activation via cytochromes P4501A1 and P4503A4 to form DNA adducts, or are excreted via pathways involving the glutathione-S-transferase genes. PAHs are associated with an increased risk of lung and skin cancer in the occupational setting, although risk varies by type of industry and the individual being

exposed.[62,63] Benzo(a)pyrene (BaP), the most frequently studied PAH, serves as a model for chemical carcinogens. The bay region diol epoxide binds to DNA, mostly as the N2-deoxyguanosine adduct. The evidence linking BaP-deoxyguanosine adducts with a carcinogenic effect in lung cancer is very strong, including site-specific hotspot mutations in the p53 tumor suppressor gene.[64–68] Various biomarkers of exposure have been developed for assessing PAH exposure. These include measuring DNA adducts, protein adducts, and urinary 1-hydroxypyrene; only the latter is a validated biomarker of exposure and no adducts have been validated as biomarkers of cancer risk. However, recent data indicate that PAH metabolites might be risk factors for lung cancer.[58]

Air pollution has been recently classified by the IARC as a known human lung carcinogen.[69] Studies that support the conclusion include cohort studies that use biomarkers of exposure.[70] Such markers include measurements of 1-hydroxypyrene, DNA adducts, chromosomal aberrations, micronuclei, oxidative damage to nucleobases, and methylation changes.[71]

Epidemiologic and experimental studies have linked benzene to hematologic toxicity, including aplastic anemia, myelodysplastic syndrome, and acute myeloid leukemia.[72–74] Benzene is metabolized by hepatic P4502E1 (CYP2E1), yielding benzene oxide and hydroquinone, among other reactive metabolites. Circulating hydroquinones may be further metabolized to reactive benzoquinones by myeloperoxidase in bone marrow white blood cell precursors and stroma. Benzene metabolites are reported to have a variety of biologic consequences on bone marrow cells, including covalent binding to DNA and protein, alterations in gene expression, cytokine and chemokine abnormalities, and chromosomal aberrations.[75] There are well-established biomarkers of exposure to benzene, but to date, biomarkers of toxicity have not been validated (except for high-level exposure workplaces and effects of peripheral blood counts).

ARISTOLOCHIC ACID AND UROTHELIAL CANCERS AS A MODEL FOR IDENTIFYING HUMAN CARCINOGENS

Aristolochic acids come from the Aristolochia genus of plants, which have been used for herbal remedies (e.g., birthwort, Dutchman's pipe). The case of the carcinogen aristolochic acid, which is identified as a Class 1 human carcinogen by the IARC (http://monographs.iarc.fr/ENG/Monographs/vol100A/mono100A-23.pdf), presents a powerful example of how the forces of epidemiology, classical chemical carcinogenesis, and genomics collaborate to unravel the pathogenesis and prevention of a specific human cancer.[76] In the 1990s, epidemiologists independently reported on three distinct unrelated population groups that developed nephrotoxicity (interstitial fibrosis) and an extraordinary high incidence of urothelial cancer of the upper urinary track after exposure for different reasons and in different parts of the world (Belgium, the Balkans, and China). In Belgian women ingesting an extract from plants of the Aristolochia species for weight reduction, which was provided to them in a weight loss clinic, nearly 50% developed this unusual syndrome. A similar clinical picture (so-called Balkan endemic nephropathy) was reported for residents farming around the Danube River and eating home-baked bread from wheat contaminated with seeds from Aristolochia weeds grown in the same fields. In China, the Aristolochia herbs have been used for centuries in Chinese medicine and are prominently prescribed in Taiwan, a nation with the highest incidence of urothelial cancer in the world, as remedies for ailments of the heart, liver, snake bites, arthritis, gout, childbirth, and others.

Common to all Aristolochia species are one of two major nitrophenanthrene carboxylic acid toxicants, namely, aristolochic acid I and II (http://monographs.iarc.fr/ENG/Monographs/vol100A/

mono100A-23.pdf).[77,78] The oral administration of aristolochic acid to rodents is highly carcinogenic, producing predominantly forestomach cancers and lymphomas, along with cancers of the lung, kidney, and urothelium (http://monographs.iarc.fr/ENG/Monographs/vol100A/mono100A-23.pdf). The major route of excretion of aristolochic acid is through the kidneys. These clinical and experimental observations inspired further analyses of the mechanism of action of these potent human carcinogens. Studies in intact mice and mice reconstituted with humanized P450 revealed that CYP1a and CYP2a were responsible for both the activation and the detoxification of aristolochic acid I and II, and that NAD(P)H:quinone oxidoreductase produced the ultimate reactive aristolactam I nitrenium species.[78] The molecular action of the ultimate carcinogen is remarkably specific, targeting purine nucleotides in DNA to form DNA adducts and binding at the exocyclic amino group of deoxyadenosine and deoxyguanosine with a far greater affinity for dA over dG (Fig. 7.1). DNA adducts from aristolochic acids have been found in both experimental animals and humans. Furthermore, unlike any other human carcinogen, the predominant mutagenic outcome is an A:T transversion with a marked preference for the nontranscribed strand of DNA, notably in the p53 gene.[77,79] The A:T to T:A transversions

are extremely uncommon among the mutation spectrum in all eukaryotes. These unique properties of aristolochic acid DNA adducts appear to elude DNA repair mechanisms that commonly focus on transcribing DNA, resulting in persistent carcinogen-DNA adducts in human tissues and surgical tumor specimens, thus confirming the association of exposure with a biologic effect.[80] In experimental models in mice where human p53 is substituted for the mouse gene, multiple sites on p53 are mutated, almost all of which are those unusual A:T transversions.[81] Modern genomic techniques have unraveled other selective properties of this unusual but potent human chemical carcinogen. Whole genome and exome sequencing of multiple aristolochic-associated kidney cancers from patients confirmed the high frequency of the unusual A:T to T:A transversion mutations. Furthermore, an unusual pattern emerges where there is selectivity for mutations at splice sites with a preferable consensus sequence of T/CAG. Among the many mutations detected, certain targets stand out, particularly in p53, MLL2, and other genes the products of which function in regulating gene expression through higher chromosome order.[82,83] This cancer story covers the gamut of all elements of chemical carcinogenesis, and its illumination has opened a door for cancer prevention.

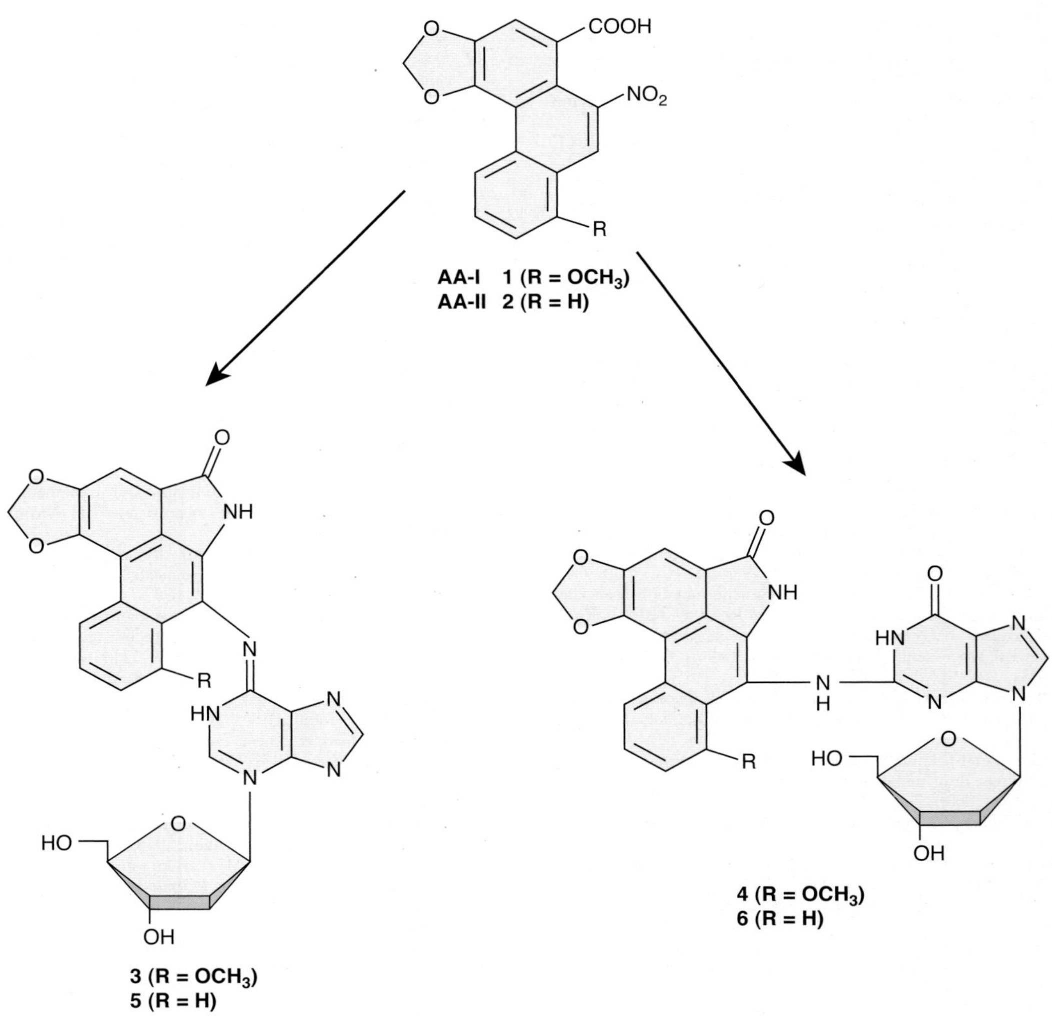

Figure 7.1 Aristolochic acid I and II form DNA adducts through the exocyclic amino group of deoxyadenosine and deoxyguanosine. The deoxyadenosine adduct is highly favored. For more detailed analysis of the complete metabolic profile, see Attaluri et al.[79]

REFERENCES

1. U.S. Department of Health and Human Services. *The Health Consequences of Smoking: 50 Years of Progress. A Report of the Surgeon General.* Atlanta: Author; 2014.
2. Colditz GA, Wei EK. Preventability of cancer: the relative contributions of biologic and social and physical environmental determinants of cancer mortality. *Annu Rev Public Health* 2012;33:137–156.
3. Lynch SM, Rebbeck TR. Bridging the gap between biologic, individual, and macroenvironmental factors in cancer: a multilevel approach. *Cancer Epidemiol Biomarkers Prev* 2013;22:485–495.
4. Rahman N. Realizing the promise of cancer predisposition genes. *Nature* 2014;505:302–308.
5. Lichtenstein P, Holm NV, Verkasalo PK, et al. Environmental and heritable factors in the causation of cancer—analyses of cohorts of twins from Sweden, Denmark, and Finland. *N Engl J Med* 2000;343:78–85.
6. Hunter DJ, Chanock SJ. Genome-wide association studies and "the art of the soluble." *J Natl Cancer Inst* 2010;102:836–837.
7. Luch A. Nature and nurture - lessons from chemical carcinogenesis. *Nat Rev Cancer* 2005;5:113–125.
8. Taddei ML, Giannoni E, Comito G, et al. Microenvironment and tumor cell plasticity: an easy way out. *Cancer Lett* 2013;341:80–96.
9. Fessler E, Dijkgraaf FE, De Sousa E Melo, et al. Cancer stem cell dynamics in tumor progression and metastasis: is the microenvironment to blame? *Cancer Lett* 2013;341:97–104.
10. Hanahan D, Coussens LM. Accessories to the crime: functions of cells recruited to the tumor microenvironment. *Cancer Cell* 2012;21:309–322.
11. Irigaray P, Belpomme D. Basic properties and molecular mechanisms of exogenous chemical carcinogens. *Carcinogenesis* 2010;31:135–148.
12. Xia HJ, Chen CS. Progress on non-human primate animal models of cancers. *Dongwuxue Yanjiu* 2011;32:70–80.
13. Yi C, He C. DNA repair by reversal of DNA damage. *Cold Spring Harb Perspect Biol* 2013;5:a012575.
14. Dizdaroglu M. Oxidatively induced DNA damage: mechanisms, repair and disease. *Cancer Lett* 2012;327:26–47.
15. Wogan GN, Hecht SS, Felton JS, et al. Environmental and chemical carcinogenesis. *Semin Cancer Biol* 2004;14:473–486.
16. Baan R, Grosse Y, Straif K, et al. A review of human carcinogens—Part F: chemical agents and related occupations. *Lancet Oncol* 2009;10:1143–1144.
17. Rendic S, Guengerich FP. Contributions of human enzymes in carcinogen metabolism. *Chem Res Toxicol* 2012;25:1316–1383.
18. Luch A. The mode of action of organic carcinogens on cellular structures. *EXS* 2006;65–95.
19. Anttila S, Raunio H, Hakkola J. Cytochrome P450-mediated pulmonary metabolism of carcinogens: regulation and cross-talk in lung carcinogenesis. *Am J Respir Cell Mol Biol* 2011;44:583–590.
20. Pogribny IP, Beland FA. DNA methylome alterations in chemical carcinogenesis. *Cancer Lett* 2012 [Epub ahead of print].
21. Shrivastav N, Li D, Essigmann JM. Chemical biology of mutagenesis and DNA repair: cellular responses to DNA alkylation. *Carcinogenesis* 2010;31:59–70.
22. Kew MC. Aflatoxins as a cause of hepatocellular carcinoma. *J Gastrointestin Liver Dis* 2013;22:305–310.
23. Feng Z, Hu W, Hu Y, et al. Acrolein is a major cigarette-related lung cancer agent: preferential binding at p53 mutational hotspots and inhibition of DNA repair. *Proc Natl Acad Sci U S A* 2006;103:15404–15409.
24. Porta M, Crous-Bou M, Wark PA, et al. Cigarette smoking and K-ras mutations in pancreas, lung and colorectal adenocarcinomas: etiopathogenic similarities, differences and paradoxes. *Mutat Res* 2009;682:83–93.
25. Blackford A, Parmigiani G, Kensler TW, et al. Genetic mutations associated with cigarette smoking in pancreatic cancer. *Cancer Res* 2009;69:3681–3688.
26. Eastmond DA, Vulimiri SV, French JE, et al. The use of genetically modified mice in cancer risk assessment: challenges and limitations. *Crit Rev Toxicol* 2013;43:611–631.
27. Boverhof DR, Chamberlain MP, Elcombe CR, et al. Transgenic animal models in toxicology: historical perspectives and future outlook. *Toxicol Sci* 2011;121:207–233.
28. Cheung C, Gonzalez FJ. Humanized mouse lines and their application for prediction of human drug metabolism and toxicological risk assessment. *J Pharmacol Exp Ther* 2008;327:288–299.
29. Hanahan D, Weinberg RA. Hallmarks of cancer: the next generation. *Cell* 2011;144:646–674.
30. Demant P. Cancer susceptibility in the mouse: genetics, biology and implications for human cancer. *Nat Rev Genet* 2003;4:721–734.
31. Klatt P, Serrano M. Engineering cancer resistance in mice. *Carcinogenesis* 2003;24:817–826.
32. Lynch D, Svoboda J, Putta S, et al. Mouse skin models for carcinogenic hazard identification: utilities and challenges. *Toxicol Pathol* 2007;35:853–864.
33. Lash LH, Hines RN, Gonzalez FJ, et al. Genetics and susceptibility to toxic chemicals: do you (or should you) know your genetic profile? *J Pharmacol Exp Ther* 2003;305:403–409.
34. Di PG, Magno LA, Rios-Santos F. Glutathione S-transferases: an overview in cancer research. *Expert Opin Drug Metab Toxicol* 2010;6:153–170.
35. Feng S, Cao Z, Wang X. Role of aryl hydrocarbon receptor in cancer. *Biochim Biophys Acta* 2013;1836:197–210.
36. Jiang XL, Gonzalez FJ, Yu AM. Drug-metabolizing enzyme, transporter, and nuclear receptor genetically modified mouse models. *Drug Metab Rev* 2011;43:27–40.
37. Tuna M, Amos CI. Genomic sequencing in cancer. *Cancer Lett* 2013;340:161–170.
38. MacConaill LE. Existing and emerging technologies for tumor genomic profiling. *J Clin Oncol* 2013;31:1815–1824.
39. Watson IR, Takahashi K, Futreal PA, et al. Emerging patterns of somatic mutations in cancer. *Nat Rev Genet* 2013;14:703–718.
40. Dumas ME. Metabolome 2.0: quantitative genetics and network biology of metabolic phenotypes. *Mol Biosyst* 2012;8:2494–2502.
41. Adamski J, Suhre K. Metabolomics platforms for genome wide association studies—linking the genome to the metabolome. *Curr Opin Biotechnol* 2013;24:39–47.
42. Verma M, Khoury MJ, Ioannidis JP. Opportunities and challenges for selected emerging technologies in cancer epidemiology: mitochondrial, epigenomic, metabolomic, and telomerase profiling. *Cancer Epidemiol Biomarkers Prev* 2013;22:189–200.
43. Edwards SL, Beesley J, French JD, et al. Beyond GWASs: illuminating the dark road from association to function. *Am J Hum Genet* 2013;93:779–797.
44. Di LG, Garofalo M, Croce CM. MicroRNAs in cancer. *Annu Rev Pathol* 2014;9:287–314.
45. Cheetham SW, Gruhl F, Mattick JS, et al. Long noncoding RNAs and the genetics of cancer. *Br J Cancer* 2013;108:2419–2425.
46. Izzotti A, Pulliero A. The effects of environmental chemical carcinogens on the microRNA machinery. *Int J Hyg Environ Health* 2014 [Epub ahead of print].
47. Kostic AD, Gevers D, Pedamallu CS, et al. Genomic analysis identifies association of Fusobacterium with colorectal carcinoma. *Genome Res* 2012;22:292–298.
48. Compare D, Nardone G. Contribution of gut microbiota to colonic and extracolonic cancer development. *Dig Dis* 2011;29:554–561.
49. Ahn J, Chen CY, Hayes RB. Oral microbiome and oral and gastrointestinal cancer risk. *Cancer Causes Control* 2012;23:399–404.
50. Schwabe RF, Jobin C. The microbiome and cancer. *Nat Rev Cancer* 2013;13:800–812.
51. Wild CP, Scalbert A, Herceg Z. Measuring the exposome: a powerful basis for evaluating environmental exposures and cancer risk. *Environ Mol Mutagen* 2013;54:480–499.
52. Brennan K, Flanagan JM. Epigenetic epidemiology for cancer risk: harnessing germline epigenetic variation. *Methods Mol Biol* 2012;863:439–465.
53. Wacholder S, Hartge P, Prentice R, et al. Performance of common genetic variants in breast-cancer risk models. *N Engl J Med* 2010;362:986–993.
54. Boffetta P, van der Hel O, Norppa H, et al. Chromosomal aberrations and cancer risk: results of a cohort study from Central Europe. *Am J Epidemiol* 2007;165:36–43.
55. Yuan JM, Gao YT, Wang R, et al. Urinary levels of volatile organic carcinogen and toxicant biomarkers in relation to lung cancer development in smokers. *Carcinogenesis* 2012;33:804–809.
56. Wogan GN, Kensler TW, Groopman JD. Present and future directions of translational research on aflatoxin and hepatocellular carcinoma. A review. *Food Addit Contam Part A Chem Anal Control Expo Risk Assess* 2012;29:249–257.
57. Hatsukami DK, Benowitz NL, Rennard SI, et al. Biomarkers to assess the utility of potential reduced exposure tobacco products. *Nicotine Tob Res* 2006;8:599–622.
58. Yuan JM, Gao YT, Murphy SE, et al. Urinary levels of cigarette smoke constituent metabolites are prospectively associated with lung cancer development in smokers. *Cancer Res* 2011;71:6749–6757.
59. Turesky RJ, Le ML. Metabolism and biomarkers of heterocyclic aromatic amines in molecular epidemiology studies: lessons learned from aromatic amines. *Chem Res Toxicol* 2011;24:1169–1214.
60. Burger M, Catto JW, Dalbagni G, et al. Epidemiology and risk factors of urothelial bladder cancer. *Eur Urol* 2013;63:234–241.
61. Besaratinia A, Tommasi S. Genotoxicity of tobacco smoke-derived aromatic amines and bladder cancer: current state of knowledge and future research directions. *FASEB J* 2013;27:2090–2100.
62. International Agency for Research on Cancer. *IARC Monographs on the Evaluation of Carcinogenic Risks to Humans: Some Non-Heterocyclic Polycyclic Aromatic Hydrocarbons and Some Related Exposures.* Volume 92. Lyon, France: World Health Organization; 2010.
63. Boffetta P, Autier P, Boniol M, et al. An estimate of cancers attributable to occupational exposures in France. *J Occup Environ Med* 2010;52:399–406.
64. Mordukhovich I, Rossner P Jr, Terry MB, et al. Associations between polycyclic aromatic hydrocarbon-related exposures and p53 mutations in breast tumors. *Environ Health Perspect* 2010;118:511–518.
65. Pfeifer GP, Denissenko MF, Olivier M, et al. Tobacco smoke carcinogens, DNA damage and p53 mutations in smoking-associated cancers. *Oncogene* 2002;21:7435–7451.
66. Pfeifer GP, Hainaut P. On the origin of G → T transversions in lung cancer. *Mutat Res* 2003;526:39–43.
67. Sjaastad AK, Jorgensen RB, Svendsen K. Exposure to polycyclic aromatic hydrocarbons (PAHs), mutagenic aldehydes and particulate matter during pan frying of beefsteak. *Occup Environ Med* 2010;67:228–232.

68. Hussain SP, Amstad P, Raja K, et al. Mutability of p53 hotspot codons to benzo(a)pyrene diol epoxide (BPDE) and the frequency of p53 mutations in nontumorous human lung. *Cancer Res* 2001;61:6350–6355.

69. Loomis D, Grosse Y, Lauby-Secretan B, et al. The carcinogenicity of outdoor air pollution. *Lancet Oncol* 2013;14:1262–1263.

70. Raaschou-Nielsen O, Andersen ZJ, Beelen R, et al. Air pollution and lung cancer incidence in 17 European cohorts: prospective analyses from the European Study of Cohorts for Air Pollution Effects (ESCAPE). *Lancet Oncol* 2013;14:813–822.

71. Demetriou CA, Raaschou-Nielsen O, Loft S, et al. Biomarkers of ambient air pollution and lung cancer: a systematic review. *Occup Environ Med* 2012;69:619–627.

72. Galbraith D, Gross SA, Paustenbach D. Benzene and human health: A historical review and appraisal of associations with various diseases. *Crit Rev Toxicol* 2010;40:1–46.

73. Vlaanderen J, Portengen L, Rothman N, et al. Flexible meta-regression to assess the shape of the benzene-leukemia exposure-response curve. *Environ Health Perspect* 2010;118:526–532.

74. Vlaanderen J, Lan Q, Kromhout H, et al. Occupational benzene exposure and the risk of chronic myeloid leukemia: a meta-analysis of cohort studies incorporating study quality dimensions. *Am J Ind Med* 2012;55:779–785.

75. Snyder R. Leukemia and benzene. *Int J Environ Res Public Health* 2012;9:2875–2893.

76. Grollman AP. Aristolochic acid nephropathy: harbinger of a global iatrogenic disease. *Environ Mol Mutagen* 2013;54:1–7.

77. Hollstein M, Moriya M, Grollman AP, et al. Analysis of TP53 mutation spectra reveals the fingerprint of the potent environmental carcinogen, aristolochic acid. *Mutat Res* 2013;753:41–49.

78. Stiborova M, Martinek V, Frei E, et al. Enzymes metabolizing aristolochic acid and their contribution to the development of aristolochic acid nephropathy and urothelial cancer. *Curr Drug Metab* 2013;14:695–705.

79. Attaluri S, Bonala RR, Yang IY, et al. DNA adducts of aristolochic acid II: total synthesis and site-specific mutagenesis studies in mammalian cells. *Nucleic Acids Res* 2010;38:339–352.

80. Sidorenko VS, Yeo JE, Bonala RR, et al. Lack of recognition by global-genome nucleotide excision repair accounts for the high mutagenicity and persistence of aristolactam-DNA adducts. *Nucleic Acids Res* 2012;40:2494–2505.

81. Nedelko T, Arlt VM, Phillips DH, et al. TP53 mutation signature supports involvement of aristolochic acid in the aetiology of endemic nephropathy-associated tumours. *Int J Cancer* 2009;124:987–990.

82. Hoang ML, Chen CH, Sidorenko VS, et al. Mutational signature of aristolochic acid exposure as revealed by whole-exome sequencing. *Sci Transl Med* 2013;5:197ra102.

83. Poon SL, Pang ST, McPherson JR, et al. Genome-wide mutational signatures of aristolochic acid and its application as a screening tool. *Sci Transl Med* 2013;5:197ra101.

ETIOLOGY AND EPIDEMIOLOGY OF CANCER

8

Physical Factors

Mats Ljungman

INTRODUCTION

Ionizing radiation (IR) and ultraviolet (UV) light have challenged the genetic integrity of all living organisms throughout time. By inducing DNA damage and subsequent mutations, these physical agents have promoted diversity through natural selection, and, as a result, organisms from all kingdoms of life carry genes that encode proteins that repair damaged DNA. In higher, multicellular organisms, many additional mechanisms of genome preservation have evolved, such as cell cycle checkpoints and apoptosis. Despite the many sophisticated mechanisms to safeguard the human genome from the mutagenic actions of DNA-damaging agents, not all exposed cells successfully restore the integrity of their DNA and some cells may subsequently progress into malignant cancer cells. Furthermore, through manmade activities, we are now exposed to many new physical agents, such as radiofrequency and microwave radiation, electromagnetic fields, asbestos, and nanoparticles, for which evolution has not yet had time to deliver genome-preserving response mechanisms. This chapter will highlight the molecular mechanisms by which these physical agents affect cells and how human exposure may lead to cancer.

IONIZING RADIATION

IR is defined as radiation that has sufficient energy to ionize molecules by displacing electrons from atoms. IR can be electromagnetic, such as x-rays and gamma rays, or can consist of particles, such as electrons, protons, neutrons, alpha particles, or carbon ions. Natural sources of IR make up about 80% of human exposure and medical sources make up about 20%.[1] The increased medical use of diagnostic x-rays and computed tomography (CT) scanning procedures likely translates into higher incidences of cancer. Of the natural sources, radon exposure is the most significant exposure risk to humans. Importantly, with better and more comprehensive screening techniques, the human exposure to radon could be dramatically lowered.

Mechanisms of Damage Induction

Linear Energy Transfer

The biologic effects of IR are unique in that the induced damage is clustered due to the local deposition of energy in radiation tracks. The distance between the depositions of energy is biologically very relevant and unique to the energy and the type of radiation. The term *linear energy transfer (LET)* denotes the energy transferred per unit length of a track of radiation. Electromagnetic radiation, such as x-rays or gamma rays, are sparsely ionizing and therefore classified as low LET radiation, whereas particulate radiation, such as neutrons, protons, and alpha particles, are examples of high LET radiation.[1]

Radiation Biochemistry

Radiation-induced damage to cellular target molecules, such as DNA, proteins, and lipids, can be either direct or indirect

(Fig. 8.1). The *direct action* of radiation, which is the dominant mode of action of high LET radiation, is due to the deposition of energy directly to the target molecule, resulting in one or more ionization events. The *indirect action* of radiation is due to the radiolysis of water molecules, which, after initial absorption of radiation energy, become excited and generate different types of radiolysis products where the reactive hydroxyl radical ($\bullet$OH), can damage both DNA and proteins. About two-thirds of the damage induced by low LET radiation is due to the indirect action of radiation. Since the hydroxyl radical is very reactive (half-life is 10^{-9} seconds), it does not diffuse more than a few nanometers after it is formed before it reacts with other molecules, and, thus, only radicals formed in close proximity to the target molecule will contribute to the damage of that target.[2] However, by chemical recombination of the primary radiolysis products, hydrogen peroxide (H_2O_2) is formed, which in turn can produce hydroxyl radicals at a later time through the Fenton reaction, involving free metals. Because H_2O_2 is not very reactive, it can diffuse long distances away from the initial site of energy deposition.

Radical scavengers normally present in cells, such as glutathione, can protect target molecules by reacting with the hydroxyl radical (see Fig. 8.1). Even after the target molecule has been hit and ionized, glutathione can contribute to cell protection by donating a hydrogen atom to the radical, allowing the unpaired electron present in the radical to pair up with the electron from the hydrogen atom. This is considered the simplest of all types of repair and is called *chemical repair*.[3] However, if oxygen molecules are present, they will compete with scavenger molecules for the ionized molecule, and if oxygen reacts with the ionized target molecule before the hydrogen donation occurs, the damage will be solidified as a peroxide, which is not amendable to chemical repair. Instead, this lesion will require enzymatic repair for the restoration of DNA. This augmenting biologic effect of oxygen is called the *oxygen effect* and is considered an important factor for the effectiveness of radiation therapy.[1]

Damage to DNA

The direct and indirect effects of radiation induce more or less identical types of lesions in DNA. However, the density of lesions induced in a stretch of DNA is higher for high LET radiation, and this increased complexity is thought to complicate the repair of these lesions. Radiation-induced lesions consist of more than 100 chemically distinct base lesions, such as the mutagenic lesions thymine glycol and 8-hydroxyguanine.[2,4,5] Furthermore, damage to the sugar moiety in the backbone of DNA and some types of base damage can result in single-strand breaks (SSB). Because the energy deposition of radiation is clustered even for low LET radiation, it is possible that two individual strand breaks are formed in close proximity on opposite strands, resulting in the formation of a double-strand break (DSB). It has been estimated that 1 Gy of ionizing radiation gives rise to about 40 DSBs, 1,000 SSBs, 1,000 base lesions, and 150 DNA-protein cross-links per cell.[2] For a similarly lethal dose of UV light, about 400,000 lesions are required, demonstrating that the lesions induced by IR are much more toxic

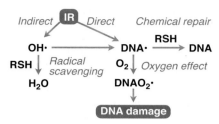

Figure 8.1 Factors affecting the induction of DNA damage by ionizing radiation (IR). Ionizing radiation can ionize DNA either by direct action or by indirect action, in which radiation energy is absorbed by neighboring molecules, such as water, leading to the generation of hydroxyl radicals that attack DNA. Sulfur-containing cellular molecules (RSH), such as glutathione, can scavenge hydroxyl radicals by hydrogen atom donations and thereby protect the DNA from the indirect action of radiation. Glutathione can also donate hydrogen atoms to ionized DNA, thereby restoring the integrity of DNA in a process termed *chemical repair*. Oxygen can compete with chemical repair in a process termed the *oxygen effect*, resulting in the enhancement of the biologic effect of ionizing radiation by the fixation of the initial DNA damage into DNA peroxides ($DNAO_2\bullet$).

than lesions induced by UV light. It is believed that DSBs are the critical lesions that lead to cell lethality following exposure to ionizing radiation.[6]

Damage to Proteins

Although proteins and lipids are subject to damage following exposure to IR, the common belief is that DNA is the critical target for the biologic effects of radiation. Indeed, abrogation of DNA damage surveillance or repair processes in cells results in the enhanced induction of mutations and decreased cell survival following radiation.[5] However, studies of radiation-sensitive and radiation-resistant bacteria imply that mechanisms that suppress protein damage may also play important roles in radiation resistance.[7] *Deinococcus radiodurans* is a bacterium that can survive radiation exposures of up to 17,000 Gy, and its extreme radioresistance has been linked to high intracellular levels of manganese, which protect proteins from oxidation. The thought is that if a cell can limit protein oxidation, then its enzymes will remain active, and cellular functions such as DNA repair will be able to restore the integrity of DNA even after severe DNA damage.[8] It would be interesting to explore whether the concentration of manganese can be manipulated to sensitize tumor cells to radiation therapy. Furthermore, because protein damage due to reactive oxygen species (ROS) accumulate during the aging process, could supplements of manganese turn back the clock on aging?

Cellular Responses

DNA Repair

Ever since organisms started to utilize atmospheric oxygen for metabolic respiration many millions of years ago, they have been forced to deal with the cellular damage induced by ROS. Base excision repair (BER) evolved to remove many of the different types of oxidative base lesions and DNA SSBs induced by ROS. However, ROS seldom induce DSBs unless the generation of hydroxyl radicals is clustered near the DNA molecule. A more important source of intracellular generation of DSBs may instead be the process of DNA replication, and it is possible that homologous recombination (HR) repair primarily evolved to overcome DSBs sporadically induced during the replication process. The other major pathway of DSB repair is the nonhomologous end-joining (NHEJ) pathway, which is utilized by immune cells in the process of antibody generation. Although the HR pathway has high fidelity due to the utilization of homologous sister chromatids to ensure that correct DNA ends are joined, the NHEJ pathway lacks this

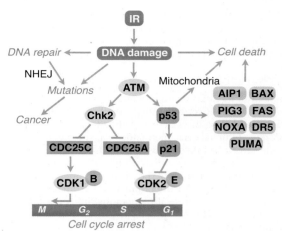

Figure 8.2 Cellular responses to ionizing radiation. Ionizing radiation induces predominantly base lesions and single- and double-strand breaks. Base lesions and single-strand breaks are repaired by base excision repair (BER), whereas double-strand breaks are repaired by nonhomologous end joining (NHEJ) and homologous recombination (HR). If DNA lesions are misrepaired by NHEJ or not repaired at all before cells enter S phase or mitosis, genomic instability is manifested as mutations or chromosome aberrations that promote carcinogenesis. In order for cells to assist DNA repair and safeguard against genetic instability and cancer, cells can induce cell cycle arrest or apoptosis. The ATM kinase is an early responder to DNA damage induced by ionizing radiation that activates the cell cycle checkpoint kinase Chk2 and the tumor suppressor p53. Chk2 inactivates the CDC25A and CDC25C phosphatases that are critical in promoting cell cycle progression by activating the cyclin-dependent kinases CDK2 or CDK1 and thereby arresting the cells at the G_1/S or G_2/M checkpoints. In addition, p53 can arrest cells at the G_1/S checkpoint by inducing the CDK inhibitor p21. p53 also plays a role in promoting apoptosis by inducing a number of proapoptotic proteins as well as translocating to mitochondria where it inhibits the actions of antiapoptotic factors. AIP1, actin interacting protein 1; BAX, bcl-2-like protein; PIG3, p53-inducible gene 3.

control mechanism and therefore occasionally rejoins ends incorrectly. Thus, the NHEJ pathway may contribute to the generation of mutations following radiation (Fig. 8.2). However, NHEJ is the only mechanism available for DSB repair in postmitotic cells and cells in the G_1 phase of the cell cycle because no sister chromatids are available in these cells to support HR repair.

Ataxia-Telangiectasia Mutated and Cell Cycle Checkpoints

Due to the enormous task of replicating the whole genome during the S phase and segregating the chromosomes during mitosis, proliferating cells are generally much more vulnerable to radiation than stationary cells. To prevent cells with damaged DNA from entering into these critical stages of the cell cycle, cells can activate cell cycle checkpoints (see Fig. 8.2). The major sensor of radiation-induced damage in cells is the ataxia-telangiectasia mutated (ATM) kinase, which, following activation, can phosphorylate more than 700 proteins in cells.[9] Two ATM substrates, p53 and Chk2, are critical for the activation of cell cycle arrests at multiple sites in the cell cycle.[10,11] The kinase p53 regulates the gene expression of specific genes such as *p21*, which inhibits cyclin-dependent kinase (CDK)2- and CDK4-mediated phosphorylation of the retinoblastoma protein, resulting in a block in the progression from the G_1 phase to the S phase of the cell cycle.[12,13] The Chk2 kinase promotes checkpoint activation in G_1 by targeting the cell division cycle 25 homolog A (CDC25A) phosphatase[14] and, in G_2/M, by targeting the CDC25C phosphatase.[15] The activation of a cell cycle arrest following DNA damage provides the cell with additional time to repair the DNA before entering critical cell cycle stages, which promotes genetic stability. Loss or defects in the *ATM* or *p53* genes result in abrogation of radiation-induced cell cycle checkpoints, which manifests itself as the highly cancer-prone human syndromes ataxia telangiectasia[16] or Li-Fraumeni,[17] respectively.

Radiation-Induced Cell Death

Terminally differentiated and stationary cells, such as kidney, lung, brain, muscle, and liver cells, are generally more resistant to radiation-induced killing than are cells with a high turnover rate, such as different epithelial cells, spermatogonia, and hair follicles. However, the spleen and thymus, which consist of mostly nondividing cells, are among the most radiosensitive tissues, implying that the rate of cell proliferation is not the sole determiner of the radiation sensitivity of a tissue. An important factor regulating the induction of programmed cell death (apoptosis) in tissues is the tumor suppressor p53.[18] The p53 protein is activated in cells following exposure to IR by the ATM kinase (see Fig. 8.2). When activated, it regulates the expression of multiple genes that have roles in DNA repair, cell cycle arrest, and apoptosis. p53 can also localize to mitochondria following irradiation, where it triggers apoptosis through the inactivation of antiapoptotic regulatory proteins.[19] Not all tissues induce the p53 response to the same degree after similar doses of IR, nor do they activate downstream pathways, such as DNA repair, cell cycle arrest, and apoptosis, in a similar way. For example, thymocytes have an intrinsic setting that favors apoptosis over cell cycle arrest following IR, whereas fibroblasts rarely induce apoptosis, but instead activate a strong and lasting cell cycle arrest.[18]

IR can induce cell death in tissues by many different mechanisms. Apoptosis can occur rapidly in a p53-dependent manner or later in a p53-independent manner. This later wave of radiation-induced apoptosis is often initiated by mitotic catastrophe, which occurs as a result of complications during chromosome segregation. Cell death induced by IR may in some cases be associated with autophagy, also called autophagocytosis, in which cells degrade cellular components via the lysosomal machinery. Whether autophagy is a programmed cell death or occurs in parallel with cell death is not clear. Interestingly, for some cell types, autophagy has been shown to actually protect the cells from radiation-induced death. Finally, tissue can undergo necrotic cell death following exposure to IR. Necrosis is a clinical problem following radiation therapy that can occur in normal tissues many months after treatment and can contribute to the inflammatory response.

Cancer Risks

It is clear from epidemiologic studies of radiation workers and atomic bomb and Chernobyl victims that IR can induce cancer.[20] Twenty years after the atomic bomb explosions in Japan during World War II, significant increases in the incidence of thyroid cancer and leukemia were observed. However, it took almost 50 years before solid tumors appeared in the population as a result of radiation exposure from the atomic bombs.[21] The incidences of solid tumors, such as breast, ovary, bladder, lung, and colon cancers, were estimated to have increased by a factor of 2 in the exposed group during this time period. The epidemiology studies following the nuclear power plant disaster in Chernobyl showed a clear increase in thyroid cancer as early as 4 years after the accident.[22] Young children were the most vulnerable to radiation exposure, with 1-year-old children being 237-fold more susceptible to thyroid cancer than the control group, while 10-year-old children were found to be sixfold more susceptible to thyroid cancer. Many of the thyroid cancers that developed following the Chernobyl disaster could have been prevented if the population had not consumed locally produced milk that was contaminated with radioactive iodine.

The molecular signatures of radiation-induced tumors are complex but involve point mutations that could lead to the activation of the *RAS* oncogene or inactivation of the tumor suppressor

gene *p53*. Furthermore, IR induces DNA DSBs that may be unfaithfully repaired by the NHEJ pathway, leading to chromosome rearrangements. One such rearrangement found in 50% to 90% of the thyroid cancers examined following the Chernobyl accident involved the receptor tyrosine kinase c-RET, which promotes cell growth when activated.[22] Furthermore, a great majority of the thyroid cancers found in the exposed children harbored kinase fusion oncogenes affecting the mitogen-activated protein kinase (MAPK) signaling pathway.[23]

The correlation between high exposure to IR and cancer following the atomic bomb explosions and the Chernobyl accident is clear. What about the cancer risk following lower radiation exposures occurring in daily life? There are four theoretical risk models of radiation-induced cancer to consider. First, the *linear, no threshold* (LNT) *model* suggests that the induction of cancer is directly proportional to the dose of radiation, even at low doses of exposure. Second, the *sublinear* or *threshold model* suggests that below a certain threshold dose the risk of radiation-induced cancers is negligible. At these lower doses of radiation exposure, the DNA damage surveillance and repair mechanisms are thought to be fully capable of safeguarding the DNA to avoid the induction of mutations and cancer. Third, the *supralinear* or *stealth model* suggests that doses below a certain threshold or radiation with sufficiently low dose rates may not trigger the activation of DNA damage surveillance and repair mechanisms, resulting in suboptimal activation of cell cycle checkpoints and repair. This would be expected to lead to a higher rate of mutations and cancers than predicted by the LNT model, but may be balanced by a higher incident of cell death. Fourth, the *linear-quadratic model* suggest that radiation effects at low doses are due to a single track of radiation hitting multiple targets, resulting in a linear induction rate, whereas at higher doses, multiple radiation tracks hit multiple cellular targets, resulting in a quadratic induction rate.

The Biological Effects of Ionizing Radiation (BEIR) VII report, released by the Committee on Biological Effects of Ionizing Radiation of the National Academy of Sciences and commissioned by the US Environmental Protection Agency (EPA), is a review of published data regarding human health and cancer risks from exposure to low levels of IR. Although this topic is controversial and not fully settled, the BIER VII report favored the LNT model.[24] Thus, the "official" view is that no level of radiation is safe; therefore, a careful consideration of risks versus benefits is necessary to ensure that the general population only receives radiation doses as low as reasonably achievable. Furthermore, the BIER VII committee concluded that the heritable effects of radiation were not evident in the published data, indicating that an individual is not likely to develop cancer due to radiation exposure of his or her parents.

The largest source of radiation exposure to the population is radon, which is a natural radioactive gas formed as a decay product of radium in the decay chain of uranium. Radon gas can accumulate to high levels in poorly ventilated basements in houses built on rock containing uranium. The major risk with radon is that some of its radioactive decay products can attach to dust particles that accumulate in the lungs, leading to a continuous exposure of the lung tissues to high LET alpha particles. Due to this radiation exposure, the EPA claims that radon is the second leading cause of lung cancer in the United States. Another important source of human exposure to IR is medical x-ray devices, and there is a growing concern about the dramatically increased use of whole body CT scans for diagnostic purposes. For a typical CT scan, a patient will receive about 100-fold more radiation than from a typical mammogram.[24] It is recommended that the use of whole body CT scans for children be very restricted due to the elevated risk of developing radiation-induced cancer for this age group.

Cancer patients who receive radiation therapy are at risk of developing secondary tumors induced by the radiation therapy treatment.[1] This is particularly a concern for young patients since (1) children are more prone to radiation-induced cancer,

(2) children have a relatively good chance of surviving the primary cancer and would have long life expectancies so a secondary tumor would have plenty of time to develop, and (3) many childhood cancers are promoted by genetic defects in DNA damage response pathways, making these patients highly prone to the genotoxic effects of radiation and subsequent secondary cancers. The most sensitive tissues for the development of secondary cancer have been found to be bone marrow (leukemia), the thyroid, breast, and lung.[1]

ULTRAVIOLET LIGHT

Depending on the wavelength, UV light is categorized into UVA (320 to 400 nm), UVB (290 to 320 nm), and UVC (240 to 290 nm) radiation. Most of the UVC light emitted from the sun is absorbed by the ozone layer in the atmosphere, and, thus, living organisms are mostly exposed to UVA and UVB irradiation.

Mechanisms of Damage Induction

UVC light is more damaging to DNA than UVA and UVB because the absorption maximum of DNA is around 260 nm. UVB and UVC induce predominantly pyrimidine dimers and 6-4 photoproducts, which consist of covalent ring structures that link two adjacent pyrimidines on the same DNA strand.[5] The formation of these lesions results in the bending of the DNA helix, resulting in the interference with both DNA and RNA synthesis. UVA light does not induce pyrimidine dimers or 6-4 photoproducts but can induce ROS, which in turn can form SSBs and base lesions in DNA of exposed cells.

Cellular Responses

DNA Repair

The nucleotide excision repair (NER) pathway removes pyrimidine dimers and 6-4 photoproducts from cellular DNA.[5] This pathway involves proteins that recognize the DNA lesions, nucleases that excise the DNA strand that contains the lesion, a DNA polymerase that synthesizes new DNA to fill the gap, and a DNA ligase that joins the backbone in the newly synthesized strand. Genetic defects in the NER pathway result in the human syndrome xeroderma pigmentosum, with individuals more than 1,000-fold more prone to sun-induced skin cancer than normal individuals. In addition, human polymorphisms in certain NER genes are thought to predispose individuals to cancers such as lung cancer, nonmelanoma skin cancer, head and neck cancer, and bladder cancer, indicating that NER is responsible for safeguarding the genome against many types of DNA adducts in addition to UV-induced lesions.[5]

UV-induced lesions formed in the transcribed strand of active genes block the elongation of RNA polymerase II, and if a cell does not restore transcription within a certain time frame, it may undergo apoptosis (Fig. 8.3).[25,26] To rapidly restore RNA synthesis and avoid cell death, NER enzymes are recruited to the sites of blocked RNA polymerase II and the lesions are removed in a process called transcription-coupled repair (TCR).[27] Individuals with Cockayne syndrome (CS), trichothiodystrophy, or the UV-sensitive syndrome, are unable to utilize the TCR pathway following UV irradiation.[5] Cells from these individuals do not recover RNA synthesis following UV irradiation and are therefore very prone to UV-induced apoptosis. Interestingly, despite a clear DNA repair defect, these individuals are not predisposed to UV-induced skin cancer. It is thought that the inability of CS cells to remove the toxic lesions that block transcription following UV irradiation results in the suppression of tumorigenesis by the elimination of damaged cells by apoptosis. However, while protecting against

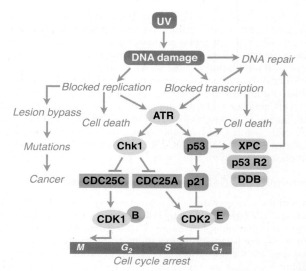

Figure 8.3 Cellular responses to ultraviolet (UV) light–induced DNA damage. UV light predominantly induces bulky DNA lesions that interfere with the processes of DNA replication and transcription. These lesions are removed from the global genome by global genomic nucleotide excision repair (GG-NER) and from transcribed DNA strands by transcription-coupled NER (TC-NER). Lesions blocking replication can be bypassed by exchanging processive DNA polymerases with less processive translesion DNA polymerases. While these polymerases allow cells to continue DNA synthesis and progress through the cell cycle, they have low fidelity, resulting in the potential induction of mutations promoting UV-induced carcinogenesis. To suppress mutations and support DNA repair efforts, the ataxia-telangiectasia and Rad3-related (ATR) kinase is activated in response to blocked replication or transcription. ATR activates the cell cycle checkpoint kinase Chk1, which, similar to Chk2, arrests cells in the G_1/S and G_2/M checkpoints by inhibiting CDC25A and CDC25C. ATR also activates p53, promoting G_1/S checkpoint activation via the induction of the Cdk-inhibitor p21. p53 also stimulates GG-NER by the transactivation of various NER genes and can promote apoptosis by the induction of proapoptotic factors and translocation to mitochondria. Finally, apoptosis is induced if cells do not recover transcription in a certain time frame, potentially due to the loss of survival factors or complications in the S phase when replication encounters stall the transcription complexes.

tumorigenesis, the elevated level of apoptosis in these cells leads to increased cell loss, which in turn may lead to neurologic degeneration.[25,28] Persistent transcription-blocking lesions in the genome have also been linked to aging.[29–31]

Translesion DNA Synthesis

Proliferating skin cells are very vulnerable to UV light because UV lesions block DNA replication (see Fig. 8.3). Cells that have entered the S phase and have initiated DNA synthesis have no choice but to finish replicating the whole genome or they will die. If DNA repair enzymes are not able to remove the blocking lesions from the template, the processive DNA polymerases may be exchanged for other, less processive DNA polymerases that can bypass the lesions. This is part of a "tolerance" mechanism, which allows cells to complete replication and eventually divide.[5] However, the translesion DNA polymerases do not have the same fidelity as the processive DNA polymerases; thus, mutations may occur. This is thought to be a major pathway by which UV light induces mutagenesis and, subsequently, cancer (see Fig. 8.3).

ATM and Rad3-Related Mediated Cell Cycle Checkpoints

In addition to utilizing the NER and BER pathways to repair UV-induced DNA damage, proliferating cells activate cell cycle checkpoints to allow more time for repair before entering critical parts of the cell cycle, such as the S phase and mitosis. The ATM and Rad3-related (ATR) kinase is activated following UV irradiation by blocked replication or transcription (see Fig. 8.3).[32] ATR phosphorylates a large number of proteins, many of which are the same as those phosphorylated by ATM after exposure to ionizing radiation.[9] Two important substrates of ATR are p53 and Chk1, which are critical in promoting cell cycle arrest. When induced by ATR, p53 transactivates the gene that encodes the cell cycle inhibitor p21, leading to the arrest of cells in the G_1 phase of the cell cycle, while Chk1 phosphorylates the CDK-activating phosphatases CDC25A and CDC25C, which targets them for degradation, resulting in an S-phase or G_2-phase arrest (see Fig. 8.3).[33]

Activation of Cell Membrane Receptors

In addition to triggering cellular stress responses by inducing DNA damage, UV light can directly induce membrane receptor signaling by receptor phosphorylation. This is thought to be due to the direct UV-mediated inhibition of protein-tyrosine phosphatases that regulate the phosphorylation levels of various membrane receptors.[34] In addition, membrane receptors may physically aggregate following UV irradiation, leading to the activation of signal transduction pathways that regulate cell growth[35] or apoptosis.[36]

Cell Death

UV light effectively induces apoptosis in skin cells. The mechanism by which UV light induces cell death is not fully understood, but failure to adequately resume RNA synthesis following UV light exposure is strongly linked to apoptosis (see Fig. 8.3).[25] Many potential mechanisms of how blocked transcription results in apoptosis have been suggested, such as a physical clash during the S phase between elongating replication machineries and transcription complexes stalled at UV lesions. Another possible mechanism involves the preferential loss of survival factors coded by highly unstable mRNAs.[37] The induction of p53 may also contribute to UV-induced apoptosis,[38] although p53 appears to protect human fibroblasts[39] and keratinocytes[40] from UV-induced apoptosis. Although complications induced by DNA damage may be the predominant mechanism by which cells die following UV irradiation, UV light may induce apoptosis in certain cell types by directly promoting the physical aggregation of the death receptor Fas/APO1.[36]

Cancer Risks

The incidence of sun-induced skin cancer, especially melanoma, is on the increase due to higher rates of sun exposure in the general population. The link between UV light exposure and skin cancer is very strong, but the role of UV light in the etiology of nonmelanoma and melanoma skin cancer differs. Although the risk of nonmelanoma cancer relates to the cumulative lifetime exposure to UV light, the risk of contracting melanoma appears to be linked to high sunlight exposure during childhood.[41] What makes UV light such a potent carcinogen is that it can initiate carcinogenesis by inducing DNA lesions as well as suppressing the immune system, resulting in a greater probability that initiated cells will survive and grow into tumors.[42,43]

Nonmelanoma Skin Cancer

Basal cell carcinoma (BCC) and squamous cell carcinoma (SCC) are the two most common skin cancer types. BCC and SCC occur predominantly in sun-exposed areas of the skin, but there are examples of these cancers forming in nonexposed areas as well. The tumor suppressor genes *p53* and *p16* are frequently inactivated in BCC and SCC, while the hedgehog-signaling pathway is activated primarily by mutations to the patched gene (percutaneous transhepatic cholangiography [*PTCH*]). This

scenario promotes proliferation without the opposition of the cell cycle inhibitors p53 and p16.

Melanoma

Melanoma arises from mutations in epidermal melanocytes and is the most dangerous form of skin cancer because it has the highest propensity to metastasize. It is formed in both sun-exposed and shielded areas of the skin; therefore, the role of UV light as the major carcinogen in melanoma has been controversial.[41] Defects in the NER pathway do not seem to predispose the development of melanoma, suggesting that pyrimidine dimers or 6-4 photoproducts induced by UVB are not the initiators of melanoma carcinogenesis. Instead, ROS induced by UVA may be responsible for the development of melanoma.[41] However, a study using next-generation sequencing techniques to catalog all mutations in a melanoma cell line found a mutational spectrum of the over 33,000 mutations detected that strongly indicated that pyrimidine dimers and 6-4 photoproducts are the major mutagenic lesions in melanoma, whereas a subset of mutations may be induced by ROS.[44] The incidence of mutations in the *p16* and *ARF* genes is high, whereas *p53* and *RAS* mutations are fairly uncommon in melanoma.

Photoimmunosuppression

Studies of transplantation of mouse skin cancers into syngeneic mice revealed that prior UVB irradiation of recipient mice promoted tumor growth, whereas transplantation into naïve nonirradiated mice led to rejection.[43] These studies established that UV light has local immunosuppressing ability, and subsequent studies found that UV light preferentially depletes Langerhans cells from irradiated skin.[42] Langerhans cells play an important role in the immune response by presenting antigens to the immune cells, and, thus, depletion of these cells leads to local immunosuppression. In addition to local immunosuppression, UV light has been shown to promote systemic immunosuppression.[45] This response is complex, but it is known that UV-induced DNA lesions in skin cells contribute to the systemic immunosuppression response.[46] The secretion of the immunosuppressing cytokine interleukin (IL)-10 from irradiated keratinocytes as well as UV-induced structural alteration of the epidermal chromophore urocanic acid may mediate the long-range immunosuppressive effects of UV light.[42,45]

RADIOFREQUENCY AND MICROWAVE RADIATION

Radiofrequency radiation (RFR) is electromagnetic radiation in the frequency range 3 kHz to 300 MHz, whereas microwave radiation (MR) is in the frequency range between 300 MHz to 300 GHz. RFR and MR do not have sufficient energies to cause ionizations in target tissues. Rather, the radiation energy is converted into heat as the radiation energy is absorbed. Sources of radiofrequency and microwave radiation include mobile phones, radio transmitters of wireless communication, radars, medical devices, and kitchen appliances.

Mechanism of Damage Induction

Because human exposure to RFR has increased dramatically in recent years, it is important to know whether this type of radiation gives rise to genotoxic damage. Although there are many studies showing that RFR can induce ROS, leading to genetic damage in cell culture systems, other studies have generated conflicting results.[47] One confounding factor when assessing the genotoxic effect of RFR, and especially MR, is the heating effect that occurs in the tissue when the radiation energy is absorbed. A recent study controlling for the potential heating effect of exposure found that RFR induces ROS and DNA damage in human spermatozoa in vitro, which is an alarming finding considering the potential hereditary implications.[48] It has been suggested that MR may affect the folding of proteins in cells that promote new protein synthesis.[49] Furthermore, exposure of cells to MR has been shown to lead to the phosphorylation of numerous cellular proteins largely through the activation of the p38/MAPK stress response pathway.[50] However, the biologic consequences of these cellular changes are not clear. Epidemiology studies that monitored the genetic effects in individuals exposed to high levels of RF have revealed evidence of increased induction of chromosome aberrations in lymphocytes.[51] However, there is a level of uncertainty in these studies about exposure levels, making it difficult to come to meaningful conclusions.

Cancer Risks

Because the population's exposure to RFR and MR has dramatically increased in recent years, it is of great importance to assess the potential cancer risks of these types of radiation so that appropriate exposure limits can be implemented. A number of studies have focused on the potential cancer risks from mobile phone usage, and some of these studies indicate that long-term mobile phone usage may be associated with increased risks of developing brain tumors (see the following). Other epidemiologic studies of cancer incidences in populations living near radio towers or mobile phone base stations are inconclusive. Some studies have shown a connection between proximity to mobile phone base stations and increased cancer incidence,[52] whereas another study found no association between exposure to RFR from mobile phone base stations and early childhood cancers.[53]

ELECTROMAGNETIC FIELDS

An electromagnetic field (EMF) is a physical field produced by electrically charged objects that can affect other charged objects in the field. Typical sources of EMFs are electric power lines, electrical devices, and magnetic resonance imaging (MRI) machines.

Mechanisms of Damage Induction

A low frequency EMF does not transmit energy high enough to break chemical bonds; therefore, it is not thought to directly damage DNA or proteins in cells. The data obtained from studies to assess the potential genotoxic effects of EMF do not provide a clear conclusion. Some of the results obtained in cell culture studies suggest a harmful effect of EMFs, but the concerns are that these effects may be related to heat production induced by EMFs rather than from the magnetic field itself. A recent in vitro study detected DNA strand breaks in cells exposed to EMFs, but this induction was thought to not be the result of ROS production, but rather due to indirect effects through interference with DNA replication and induction of apoptosis in a subset of cells.[54] A study using an MRI found no evidence of an induced formation of DNA DSBs in cell cultures.[55] EMFs have been shown to induce nongenotoxic effects in cells, such as interference with cellular signaling pathways,[56] which could contribute to neurodegeneration.[57]

Cancer Risks

Studies with rodents have largely failed to detect an association between exposure to EMFs and cancer. This is also true for numerous epidemiology studies, with the only exception being the association between EMF exposure and childhood leukemia where children exposed to doses of 0.4 mcT or above may have about a twofold increased risk of developing leukemia.[58,59] There is no strong link between EMF exposure and increased risks of contracting adult leukemia, brain tumors, or breast cancer.[60,61] Furthermore, a study investigating whether EMF exposure was associated with heritable effects found no correlation between parental exposure and childhood cancer.[62]

Potential Cancer Risks from Mobile Phone Usage

Mobile phones emit RFR and generate EMFs. The biggest health concern with mobile phone usage is its potential role in the development of brain tumors. During mobile phone use, the brain tissue is exposed to doses, giving peak specific absorption rates (SAR) of 4 to 8 W/kg. At these intensities, the induction of DNA damage has been detected in laboratory studies.[63] The current epidemiologic data are largely inconclusive on the association between mobile phone usage and brain tumor incidence. Meta-analysis studies of populations who had used mobile phones for more than 10 years concluded that mobile phone usage was associated with an elevated risk for brain tumors, such as acoustic neuroma and glioma cancer.[64–66] In contrast, other large prospective studies did not observe a correlation between mobile phone usage and incidences of glioma, meningioma, or non–central nervous system (CNS) cancers.[67,68] It is important to point out that, generally, it takes 30 to 40 years for brain tumors to develop, and because mobile phones have only been in general use for about 15 years, there has not been sufficient time to fully evaluate the brain cancer risks of mobile phone usage.

ASBESTOS

Asbestos is a class of naturally occurring silicate minerals that have been widely used in building materials for its heat, sound, and electrical insulating qualities. Asbestos becomes a serious health hazard if the fibers are inhaled over a long period of time, and these health effects are increased dramatically if the exposed individual is a smoker. It was first reported in 1935 that asbestos might be an occupational health hazard that could induce cancer.[69,70] However, it was not until 1986 that the International Labor Organization recommended banning asbestos.[71] The use of asbestos products peaked in the 1970s, yet remains a major health hazard in many places around the world today.

Mechanisms of Damage Induction

Asbestos fibers can enter cells and induce ROS, especially if they contain high levels of iron.[72] In addition, ROS can be generated by "frustrated" phagocytosis, and this in turn can lead to the release of proinflammatory cytokines with subsequent inflammation of the tissue. ROS have been implicated to originate from affected mitochondria leading to induction of SSBs and base damage, such as 8-hydroxyguanine in DNA.[73] Furthermore, if not successfully repaired, asbestos-induced DNA damage has been shown to result in chromosome aberrations, micronuclei formation, and increased rates of sister chromatid exchanges.[74]

Cellular and Tissue Responses

Asbestos-induced ROS cause base lesions and DNA strand breaks, which require base excision repair for the restoration of DNA and for minimizing mutagenesis. In addition to DNA repair, a number of cellular signaling pathways are activated by asbestos. These include the epidermal growth factor receptor (EGFR) and the MAPK pathway, leading to the activation of nuclear factor kappa B

ETIOLOGY AND EPIDEMIOLOGY OF CANCER

(NF-κB) and transcription factor AP-1.[72,74] Activation of the NF-κB pathway leads to the induction of proinflammatory genes such as tumor necrosis factor (TNF), *IL-6*, *IL-8*, and proliferation-promoting genes such as *c-Myc*, leading to inflammation and increased cell proliferation. Asbestos exposure also stimulates the expression of the transforming growth factor beta (TGF-β), which, in turn, stimulates fibrogenesis in exposed tissues.[74]

Cancer Risks

Lung Cancer

Epidemiologic studies have found a strong link between asbestos exposure and lung cancer.[74] It has been estimated that about 5% to 7% of all lung cancers are attributable to asbestos exposure, and asbestos and tobacco smoking act in synergy to induce lung cancer. Mutational spectra due to 8-hydroxyguanine lesions formed by ROS can be linked to asbestos exposure, and point mutations in the tumor suppressor genes *p53* and *p16/INK4A* and in the *KRAS* oncogene have been found in tumors from asbestos-exposed individuals.

Mesothelioma

After being taken up by lung tissues, asbestos fibers can translocate into the pleura, the body cavity that surrounds the lungs. The pleura are covered with a protective lining, the mesothelium, which consists of squamouslike epithelial cells. Mesothelial cells can internalize asbestos fibers, resulting in the induction of ROS and inflammatory responses, subsequently leading to the initiation and progression of malignant mesothelioma.[75] Asbestos is considered one of the major causes of malignant mesothelioma, and frequent mutations are found in the *p16/INK4A* and *NF2* genes, whereas *p53* mutations are fairly rare.

NANOPARTICLES

Nanoparticles are defined as ultrafine particles of the size range 1 to 100 nm in diameter. Nanoparticle chemistry of a certain compound is different from bulk chemistry of that compound because of the high percentage of atoms at the surface of the particle. The production of nanoparticles has increased dramatically in recent years, and they are found in many industrial and consumer products such as paint, cosmetics, and sunscreens. They also have many potential medical applications, such as delivery vehicles for specific drugs to specific target tissues or tumors.

Mechanisms of DNA Damage Induction

Many of the cellular effects of nanoparticles are similar to the effects exerted by asbestos, such as the generation of ROS and inflammation.[72] Nanoparticles have been shown to induce oxidative DNA damage, such as DNA strand breaks and 8-hydroxyguanine lesions both in cell culture[76, 77] and in vivo.[78] Nanoparticle-induced DNA lesions are manifested as histone γ-H2AX nuclear foci, chromosome deletions, and micronuclei.

Cellular Responses

Nanoparticles induce ROS either directly or indirectly, resulting in DNA lesions, such as 8-hydroxyguanine–base damage and DNA strand breaks. These lesions are repaired by the base excision repair. The phosphorylation of histone H2AX has been shown to occur following exposure of cells to nanoparticles, suggesting that the DNA lesions trigger the activation of ATM or ATR stress kinases.[79] Nanoparticles have also been found to affect the immune system[80] and can induce the release of the proinflammatory cytokine TNF-α from cells.

Cancer Risks

Some nanoparticles, such as titanium dioxide, which is used as pigments in paint, have been classified by the International Agency for Research on Cancer (IARC) as a group 2B carcinogen, "possible carcinogenic to humans." However, rigorous epidemiologic data is lacking to fully evaluate the cancer-inducing potential of nanoparticles.[81]

REFERENCES

1. Hall E, Giaccia A. *Radiobiology for the Radiologist.* Philadelphia: Lippincott Williams & Wilkins; 2012.
2. Ward JF. DNA damage produced by ionizing radiation in mammalian cells: identities, mechanisms of formation, and repairability. *Prog Nucleic Acid Res Mol Biol* 1988;35:95–125.
3. Prutz WA. 'Chemical repair' in irradiated DNA solutions containing thiols and/or disulphides. Further evidence for disulphide radical anions acting as electron donors. *Int J Radiat Biol* 1989;56:21–33.
4. Hutchinson F. Chemical changes induced in DNA by ionizing radiation. *Prog Nucleic Acid Res Mol Biol* 1985;32:115–154.
5. Friedberg E, Walker G, Siede W, et al. DNA *Repair and Mutagenesis.* 2nd ed. Washington, D.C.: ASM Press; 2006.
6. Radford IR. The level of induced DNA double-strand breakage correlates with cell killing after X-irradiation. *Int J Radiat Biol Relat Stud Phys Chem Med* 1985;48:45–54.
7. Daly MJ. A new perspective on radiation resistance based on *Deinococcus radiodurans. Nat Rev Microbiol* 2009;7:237–245.
8. Krisko A, Radman M. Biology of extreme radiation resistance: the way of *Deinococcus radiodurans. Cold Spring Harb Perspect Biol* 2013;5.
9. Matsuoka S, Ballif BA, Smogorzewska A, et al. ATM and ATR substrate analysis reveals extensive protein networks responsive to DNA damage. *Science* 2007;316:1160–1166.
10. Kastan M, Onyekwere O, Sidransky D, et al. Participation of p53 protein in the cellular response to DNA damage. *Cancer Res* 1991;51:6304–6311.
11. Matsuoka S, Huang M, Elledge SJ. Linkage of ATM to cell cycle regulation by the Chk2 protein kinase. *Science* 1998;282:1893–1897.
12. Harper J, Adami G, Wei N, et al. The p21 cdk-interacting protein Cip1 is a potent inhibitor of G1 cyclin-dependent kinases. *Cell* 1993;75:805–816.
13. El-Deiry W, Tokino T, Velculescu V, et al. WAF1, a potential mediator of p53 tumor suppression. *Cell* 1993;75:817–825.
14. Falck J, Mailand N, Syljuasen RG, et al. The ATM-Chk2-Cdc25A checkpoint pathway guards against radioresistant DNA synthesis. *Nature* 2001;410:842–847.
15. Bartek J, Falck J, Lukas J. Chk2 kinase—a busy messenger [Review]. *Nat Rev Mol Cell Biol* 2001;2:877–886.
16. Savitsky K, Bar-Shira A, Gilad S, et al. A single ataxia telangiectasia gene with a product similar to PI-3 kinase. *Science* 1995;268:1749–1753.
17. Srivastava S, Zou ZQ, Pirollo K, et al. Germ-line transmission of a mutated p53 gene in a cancer-prone family with Li-Fraumeni syndrome. *Nature.* 1990;348:747–749.
18. Gudkov AV, Komarova EA. The role of p53 in determining sensitivity to radiotherapy. *Nat Rev Cancer* 2003;3:117–129.
19. Mihara M, Erster S, Zaika A, et al. p53 has a direct apoptogenic role at the mitochondria. *Mol Cell* 2003;11:577–590.
20. Williams D, Baverstock K. Chernobyl and the future: too soon for a final diagnosis. *Nature* 2006;440:993–994.
21. Thompson DE, Mabuchi K, Ron E, et al. Cancer incidence in atomic bomb survivors. Part II: Solid tumors, 1958–1987. *Radiat Res* 1994;137:S17–67.
22. Williams D. Cancer after nuclear fallout: lessons from the Chernobyl accident. *Nat Rev Cancer* 2002;2:543–549.
23. Ricarte-Filho JC, Li S, Garcia-Rendueles ME, et al. Identification of kinase fusion oncogenes in post-Chernobyl radiation-induced thyroid cancers. *J Clin Invest* 2013;123:4935–4944.
24. National Research Council. *Health Risks from Exposure to Low Levels of Ionizing Radiation: BEIR VII Phase 2.* Washington, D.C.: National Academy Press; 2006.
25. Ljungman M, Zhang F. Blockage of RNA polymerase as a possible trigger for u.v. light-induced apoptosis. *Oncogene.* 1996;13:823–831.
26. Brash DE, Wikonkal NM, Remenyik E, et al. The DNA damage signal for Mdm2 regulation, Trp53 induction, and sunburn cell formation in vivo originates from actively transcribed genes. *J Invest Derm* 2001;117:1234–1240.

27. Hanawalt PC, Spivak G. Transcription-coupled DNA repair: two decades of progress and surprises. *Nat Rev Mol Cell Biol* 2008;9:958–970.

28. Lehmann AR. DNA repair-deficient diseases, xeroderma pigmentosum, Cockayne syndrome and trichothiodystrophy. *Biochimie* 2003;85:1101–1111.

29. Andressoo JO, Hoeijmakers JH. Transcription-coupled repair and premature ageing. *Mutat Res* 2005;577:179–194.

30. de Boer J, Andressoo JO, de Wit J, et al. Premature aging in mice deficient in DNA repair and transcription. *Science* 2002;296:1276–1279.

31. Garinis GA, Uittenboogaard LM, Stachelscheid H, et al. Persistent transcription-blocking DNA lesions trigger somatic growth attenuation associated with longevity. *Nat Cell Biol* 2009;11:604–615.

32. Derheimer FA, O'Hagan HM, Krueger HM, et al. RPA and ATR link transcriptional stress to p53. *Proc Natl Acad Sci U S A* 2007;104:12778–12783.

33. Kastan MB, Bartek J. Cell-cycle checkpoints and cancer. *Nature* 2004;432:316–323.

34. Gross S, Knebel A, Tenev T, et al. Inactivation of protein-tyrosine phosphatases as mechanism of UV-induced signal transduction. *J Biol Chem* 1999;274:26378–26386.

35. Sachsenmaier C, Radlerpohl A, Zinck R, et al. Involvement of growth factor receptors in the mammalian UVC response. *Cell* 1994;78:963–972.

36. Rehemtulla A, Hamilton CA, Chinnaiyan AM, et al. Ultraviolet radiation-induced apoptosis is mediated by activation of CD-95 (Fas/APO-1). *J Biol Chem* 1997;272:25783–25786.

37. Ljungman M, Lane DP. Transcription - guarding the genome by sensing DNA damage. *Nat Rev Cancer* 2004;4:727–737.

38. Ziegler A, Jonason AS, Leffell DJ, et al. Sunburn and p53 in the onset of skin cancer. *Nature* 1994;372:773–776.

39. McKay B, Ljungman M. Role for p53 in the recovery of transcription and protection against apoptosis induced by ultraviolet light. *Neoplasia* 1999;1:276–284.

40. Chaturvedi V, Sitailo LA, Qin JZ, et al. Knockdown of p53 levels in human keratinocytes accelerates Mcl-1 and Bcl-x(L) reduction thereby enhancing UV-light induced apoptosis. *Oncogene* 2005;24:5299–5312.

41. Maddodi N, Setaluri V. Role of UV in cutaneous melanoma. *Photochem Photobiol* 2008;84:528–536.

42. Murphy GM. Ultraviolet radiation and immunosuppression. *Br J Dermatol* 2009;161(Suppl 3):90–95.

43. Fisher MS, Kripke ML. Systemic alteration induced in mice by ultraviolet light irradiation and its relationship to ultraviolet carcinogenesis. *Proc Natl Acad Sci U S A* 1977;74:1688–1692.

44. Pleasance ED, Cheetham RK, Stephens PJ, et al. A comprehensive catalogue of somatic mutations from a human cancer genome. *Nature* 2010;463:191–196.

45. Schwarz T. Photoimmunosuppression. *Photodermatol Photoimmunol Photomed* 2002;18:141–145.

46. Kripke ML, Cox PA, Alas LG, et al. Pyrimidine dimers in DNA initiate systemic immunosuppression in UV-irradiated mice. *Proc Natl Acad Sci U S A* 1992;89:7516–7520.

47. Vijayalaxmi, Prihoda TJ. Genetic damage in mammalian somatic cells exposed to radiofrequency radiation: a meta-analysis of data from 63 publications (1990–2005). *Radiat Res* 2008;169:561–574.

48. De Iuliis GN, Newey RJ, King BV, et al. Mobile phone radiation induces reactive oxygen species production and DNA damage in human spermatozoa in vitro. *PLoS One* 2009;4:e6446.

49. Gerner C, Haudek V, Schandl U, et al. Increased protein synthesis by cells exposed to a 1,800-MHz radio-frequency mobile phone electromagnetic field, detected by proteome profiling. *Int Arch Occup Environ Health* 2010;83:691–702.

50. Leszczynski D, Joenvaara S, Reivinen J, et al. Non-thermal activation of the hsp27/p38MAPK stress pathway by mobile phone radiation in human endothelial cells: molecular mechanism for cancer- and blood-brain barrier-related effects. *Differentiation* 2002;70:120–129.

51. Verschaeve L. Genetic damage in subjects exposed to radiofrequency radiation. *Mutat Res* 2009;681:259–270.

52. Khurana VG, Hardell L, Everaert J, et al. Epidemiological evidence for a health risk from mobile phone base stations. *Int J Occup Environ Health* 2010;16:263–267.

53. Elliott P, Toledano MB, Bennett J, et al. Mobile phone base stations and early childhood cancers: case-control study. *BMJ* 2010;340:c3077.

54. Focke F, Schuermann D, Kuster N, et al. DNA fragmentation in human fibroblasts under extremely low frequency electromagnetic field exposure. *Mutat Res* 2010;683:74–83.

55. Schwenzer NF, Bantleon R, Maurer B, et al. Detection of DNA double-strand breaks using gammaH2AX after MRI exposure at 3 Tesla: an in vitro study. *J Magn Reson Imaging* 2007;26:1308–1314.

56. Girgert R, Hanf V, Emons G, et al. Signal transduction of the melatonin receptor MT1 is disrupted in breast cancer cells by electromagnetic fields. *Bioelectromagnetics* 2010;31:237–245.

57. Consales C, Merla C, Marino C, et al. Electromagnetic fields, oxidative stress, and neurodegeneration. *Int J Cell Biol* 2012;2012:683897.

58. Ahlbom A, Day N, Feychting M, et al. A pooled analysis of magnetic fields and childhood leukaemia. *Br J Cancer* 2000;83:692–698.

59. Malagoli C, Fabbi S, Teggi S, et al. Risk of hematological malignancies associated with magnetic fields exposure from power lines: a case-control study in two municipalities of northern Italy. *Environ Health* 2010;9:16.

60. Kheifets L, Monroe J, Vergara X, et al. Occupational electromagnetic fields and leukemia and brain cancer: an update to two meta-analyses. *J Occup Environ Med* 2008;50:677–688.

61. Chen C, Ma X, Zhong M, et al. Extremely low-frequency electromagnetic fields exposure and female breast cancer risk: a meta-analysis based on 24,338 cases and 60,628 controls. *Breast Cancer Res Treat* 2010;123:569–576.

62. Hug K, Grize L, Seidler A, et al. Parental occupational exposure to extremely low frequency magnetic fields and childhood cancer: a German case-control study. *Am J Epidemiol* 2010;171:27–35.

63. Hardell L, Sage C. Biological effects from electromagnetic field exposure and public exposure standards. *Biomed Pharmacother* 2008;62:104–109.

64. Hardell L, Carlberg M, Hansson Mild K. Mobile phone use and the risk for malignant brain tumors: a case-control study on deceased cases and controls. *Neuroepidemiology* 2010;35:109–114.

65. Hardell L, Carlberg M, Soderqvist F, et al. Meta-analysis of long-term mobile phone use and the association with brain tumours. *Int J Oncol* 2008;32:1097–1103.

66. Myung SK, Ju W, McDonnell DD, et al. Mobile phone use and risk of tumors: a meta-analysis. *J Clin Oncol* 2009;27:5565–5572.

67. Benson VS, Pirie K, Schuz J, et al. Mobile phone use and risk of brain neoplasms and other cancers: prospective study. *Int J Epidemiol* 2013;42:792–802.

68. Poulsen AH, Friis S, Johansen C, et al. Mobile phone use and the risk of skin cancer: a nationwide cohort study in Denmark. *Am J Epidemiol* 2013;178:190–197.

69. Lynch K, Smith W. Pulmonary asbestosis. III. Carcinoma of lung in asbestos-silicosis. *Am J Cancer* 1935;24:56–64.

70. Gloyne S. Two cases of squamous carcinoma of the lung occuring in asbestosis. *Tubercele* 1935;17:5–10.

71. LaDou J. The asbestos cancer epidemic. *Environ Health Perspect* 2004;112:285–290.

72. Pacurari M, Castranova V, Vallyathan V. Single- and multi-wall carbon nanotubes versus asbestos: are the carbon nanotubes a new health risk to humans? *J Toxicol Environ Health A* 2010;73:378–395.

73. Liu G, Cheresh P, Kamp DW. Molecular basis of asbestos-induced lung disease. *Annu Rev Pathol* 2013;8:161–187.

74. Nymark P, Wikman H, Hienonen-Kempas T, et al. Molecular and genetic changes in asbestos-related lung cancer. *Cancer Lett* 2008;265:1–15.

75. Jaurand MC, Renier A, Daubriac J. Mesothelioma: do asbestos and carbon nanotubes pose the same health risk? *Part Fibre Toxicol* 2009;6:16.

76. Shukla RK, Kumar A, Gurbani D, et al. TiO(2) nanoparticles induce oxidative DNA damage and apoptosis in human liver cells. *Nanotoxicology* 2013;7:48–60.

77. Horie M, Nishio K, Endoh S, et al. Chromium(III) oxide nanoparticles induced remarkable oxidative stress and apoptosis on culture cells. *Environ Toxicol* 2013;28:61–75.

78. Trouiller B, Reliene R, Westbrook A, et al. Titanium dioxide nanoparticles induce DNA damage and genetic instability in vivo in mice. *Cancer Res* 2009;69:8784–8789.

79. Prasad RY, Chastain PD, Nikolaishvili-Feinberg N, et al. Titanium dioxide nanoparticles activate the ATM-Chk2 DNA damage response in human dermal fibroblasts. *Nanotoxicology* 2013;7:1111–1119.

80. Zolnik BS, Gonzalez-Fernandez A, Sadrieh N, et al. Nanoparticles and the immune system. *Endocrinology* 2010;151:458–465.

81. Shi H, Magaye R, Castranova V, et al. Titanium dioxide nanoparticles: a review of current toxicological data. *Part Fibre Toxicol* 2013;10:15.

ETIOLOGY AND EPIDEMIOLOGY OF CANCER

9 Dietary Factors

Karin B. Michels and Walter C. Willett

INTRODUCTION

Over two decades ago, Doll and Peto[1] speculated that 35% (range: 10% to 70%) of all cancer deaths in the United States may be preventable by alterations in diet. The magnitude of the estimate for dietary factors exceeded that for tobacco (30%) and infections (10%).

Studies of cancer incidence among populations migrating to countries with different lifestyle factors have indicated that most cancers have a large environmental etiology. Although the contribution of environmental influences differs by cancer type, the incidence of many cancers changes by as much as five- to tenfold among migrants over time, approaching that of the host country. The age at migration affects the degree of adaptation among first-generation migrants for some cancers, suggesting that the susceptibility to environmental carcinogenic influences varies with age by cancer type. Identifying the specific environmental and lifestyle factors most important to cancer etiology, however, has proven difficult.

Environmental factors such as diet may influence the incidence of cancer through many different mechanisms and at different stages in the cancer process. Simple mutagens in foods, such as those produced by the heating of proteins, can cause damage to DNA, but dietary factors can also influence this process by inducing enzymes that activate or inactivate these mutagens, or by blocking the action of the mutagen. Dietary factors can also affect every pathway hypothesized to mediate cancer risk–for example, the rate of cell cycling through hormonal or antihormonal effects, aiding or inhibiting DNA repair, promoting or inhibiting apoptosis, and DNA methylation. Because of the complexity of these mechanisms, knowledge of dietary influences on risk of cancer will require an empirical basis with human cancer as the outcome.

METHODOLOGIC CHALLENGES

Study Types and Biases

The association between diet and the risk of cancer has been the subject of a number of epidemiologic studies. The most prevalent designs are the case-control study, the cohort study, and the randomized clinical trial. When the results from epidemiologic studies are interpreted, the potential for confounding must be considered. Individuals who maintain a healthy diet are likely to exhibit other indicators of a healthy lifestyle, including regular physical activity, lower body weight, use of multivitamin supplements, lower smoking rates, and lower alcohol consumption. Even if the influence of these confounding variables is analytically controlled, residual confounding remains possible.

Ecologic Studies

In ecologic studies or international correlation studies, variation in food disappearance data and the prevalence of a certain disease are correlated, generally across different countries. A linear association may provide preliminary data to inform future research but, due to the high probability of confounding, cannot provide strong evidence for a causal link. Food disappearance data also may not provide a good estimate for human consumption. The gross national product is correlated with many dietary factors such as fat intake.[2] Many other differences besides dietary fat exist between the countries with low fat consumption (less affluent) and high fat consumption (more affluent); reproductive behaviors, physical activity level, and body fatness are particularly notable and are strongly associated with specific cancers.

Migrant Studies

Studies of populations migrating from areas with low incidence of disease to areas with high incidence of disease (or vice versa) can help sort out the role of environmental factors versus genetics in the etiology of a cancer, depending on whether the migrating group adopts the cancer rates of the new environment. Specific dietary components linked to disease are difficult to identify in a migrant study.

Case-Control Studies

Case-control studies of diet may be affected by recall bias, control selection bias, and confounding. In a case-control study, participants affected by the disease under study (cases) and healthy controls are asked to recall their past dietary habits. Cases may overestimate their consumption of foods that are commonly considered "unhealthy" and underestimate their consumption of foods considered "healthy." Giovannucci et al.[3] have documented differential reporting of fat intake before and after disease occurrence. Thus, the possibility of recall bias in a case-control study poses a real threat to the validity of the observed associations. Even more importantly, in contemporary case-control studies using a population sample of controls, the participation rate of controls is usually far from complete, often 50% to 70%. Unfortunately, health-conscious individuals may be more likely to participate as controls and will thus be less overweight, will consume fruits and vegetables more frequently, and will consume less fat and red meat, which can substantially distort associations observed.

Cohort Studies

Prospective cohort studies of the effects of diet are likely to have a much higher validity than retrospective case-control studies because diet is recorded by participants before disease occurrence. Cohort studies are still affected by measurement error because diet consists of a large number of foods eaten in complex combinations. Confounding by other unmeasured or imperfectly measured lifestyle factors can remain a problem in cohort studies.

Now that the results of a substantial number of cohort studies have become available, their findings can be compared with those of case-control studies that have examined the same relations. In many cases, the findings of the case-control studies have not been confirmed; for example, the consistent finding of lower risk of many cancers with higher intake of fruits and vegetables in case-control studies has generally not been seen in cohort studies.[4] These findings suggest that the concerns about biases in case-control studies of diet, and probably many other lifestyle factors, are justified, and findings from such studies must be interpreted cautiously.

Randomized Clinical Trials

The gold standard in medical research is the randomized clinical trial (RCT). In an RCT on nutrition, participants are randomly assigned to one of two or more diets; hence, the association between diet and the cancer of interest should not be confounded by other factors. The problem with RCTs of diet is that maintaining the assigned diet strictly over many years, as would be necessary for diet to have an impact on cancer incidence, is difficult. For example, in the dietary fat reduction trial of the Women's Health Initiative (WHI), participants randomized to the intervention arm reduced their fat intake much less than planned.[5] The remaining limited contrast between the two groups left the lack of difference in disease outcomes difficult to interpret. Furthermore, the relevant time window for intervention and the necessary duration of intervention are unclear, especially with cancer outcomes. Hence, randomized trials are rarely used to examine the effect of diet on cancer but have better promise for the study of diet and outcomes that require a considerably shorter follow-up time (e.g., adenoma recurrence). Also, the randomized design may lend itself better to the study of the effects of dietary supplements such as multivitamin or fiber supplements, although the control group may adopt the intervention behavior because nutritional supplements are widely available. For example, in the WHI trial of calcium and vitamin D supplementation, two-thirds of the study population used vitamin D or calcium supplements that they obtained outside of the trial, again rendering the lack of effect in the trial uninterpretable.

Diet Assessment Instruments

Observational studies depend on a reasonably valid assessment of dietary intake. Although, for some nutrients, biochemical measurements can be used to assess intake, for most dietary constituents, a useful biochemical indicator does not exist. In population-based studies, diet is generally assessed with a self-administered instrument. Since 1980, considerable effort has been directed at the development of standardized questionnaires for measuring diet, and numerous studies have been conducted to assess the validity of these methods. The most widely used diet assessment instruments are the food frequency questionnaire, the 7-day diet record, and the 24-hour recall. Although the 7-day diet record may provide the most accurate documentation of intake during the week the participant keeps a diet diary, the burden of computerizing the information and extracting foods and nutrients has prohibited the use of the 7-day diet record in most large-scale studies. The 24-hour recall provides only a snapshot of diet on one day, which may or may not be representative of the participant's usual diet and is thus affected by both personal variation and seasonal variation. The food frequency questionnaire, the most widely used instrument in large population-based studies, asks participants to report their average intake of a large number of foods during the previous year. Participants tend to substantially overreport their fruit and vegetable consumption on the food frequency questionnaire.[6] This tendency may reflect social desirability bias, which leads to overreporting healthy foods and underreporting less healthy foods. Studies of validity using biomarkers or detailed measurements of diet as comparisons have suggested that carefully designed questionnaires can have sufficient validity to detect moderate to strong associations. Validity can be enhanced by using the average of repeated assessments over time.[7]

THE ROLE OF INDIVIDUAL FOOD AND NUTRIENTS IN CANCER ETIOLOGY

Energy

The most important impact of diet on the risk of cancer is mediated through body weight. Overweight, obesity, and inactivity are major contributors to cancer risk. (A more detailed discussion is provided in Chapter 10.) In the large American Cancer Society Cohort, obese individuals had substantially higher mortality from all cancers and, in particular, from colorectal cancer, postmenopausal breast cancer, uterine cancer, cervical cancer, pancreatic cancer, and gallbladder cancer than their normal-weight counterparts.[8] Adiposity and, in particular, waist circumference are predictors of colon cancer incidence among women and men.[9,10] A weight gain of 10 kg or more is associated with a significant increase in postmenopausal breast cancer incidence among women who never used hormone replacement therapy, whereas a weight loss of comparable magnitude after menopause substantially decreases breast cancer risk.[11] Regular physical activity contributes to a lower prevalence of being overweight and obesity and consequently reduces the burden of cancer through this pathway.

The mechanisms whereby adiposity increases the risk of various cancers are probably multiple. Being overweight is strongly associated with endogenous estrogen levels, which likely contribute to the excess risks of endometrial and postmenopausal breast cancers. The reasons for the association with other cancers are less clear, but excess body fat is also related to higher circulating levels of insulin, insulin-like growth factor (IGF)-1, and C-peptide (a marker of insulin secretion), lower levels of binding proteins for sex hormones and IGF-1, and higher levels of various inflammatory factors, all of which have been hypothesized to be related to risks of various cancers.

Energy restriction is one of the most effective measures to prevent cancer in the animal model. While energy restriction is more difficult to study in humans, voluntary starvation among anorectics and situations of food rationing during famines provide related models. Breast cancer rates were substantially reduced among women with a history of severe anorexia.[12] Although breast cancer incidence was higher among women exposed to the Dutch famine during childhood or adolescence, such short-term involuntary food rationing for 9 months or less was often followed by overnutrition.[13] A more prolonged deficit in food availability during World War II in Norway was associated with a reduction in adult risk of breast cancer if it occurred during early adolescence.[14]

Alcohol

Aside from body weight, alcohol consumption is the best established dietary risk factor for cancer. Alcohol is classified as a carcinogen by the International Agency for Research on Cancer. The consumption of alcohol increases the risk of numerous cancers, including those of the liver, esophagus, pharynx, oral cavity, larynx, breast, and colorectum in a dose-dependent fashion.[15] Evidence is convincing that excessive alcohol consumption increases the risk of primary liver cancer, probably through cirrhosis and alcoholic hepatitis. At least in the developed world, about 75% of cancers of the esophagus, pharynx, oral cavity, and larynx are attributable to alcohol and tobacco, with a marked increase in risk among drinkers who also smoke, suggesting a multiplicative effect. Mechanisms may include direct damage to the cells in the upper gastrointestinal tract; modulation of DNA methylation, which affects susceptibility to DNA mutations; and an increase in acetaldehyde, the main metabolite of alcohol, which enhances the proliferation of epithelial cells, forms DNA adducts, and is a recognized carcinogen. The association between alcohol consumption and breast cancer is notable because a small but significant risk has been found even with one drink per day. Mechanisms may include an interaction with folate, an increase in endogenous estrogen levels, and an elevation of acetaldehyde. Some evidence suggests that the excess risk is mitigated by adequate folate intake possibly through an effect on DNA methylation.[16] Notably, for most cancer sites, no important difference in associations was found with the type of alcoholic beverage, suggesting a critical role of ethanol in carcinogenesis.

Dietary Fat

In recent years, reducing dietary fat has been at the center of cancer prevention efforts. In the landmark 1982 National Academy of Sciences review of diet, nutrition, and cancer, a reduction in fat intake to 30% of calories was the primary recommendation.

Interest in dietary fat as a cause of cancer began in the first half of the 20th century, when studies by Tannenbaum[17] indicated that diets high in fat could promote tumor growth in animal models. Dietary fat has a clear effect on tumor incidence in many models, although not in all; however, a central issue has been whether this is independent of the effect of energy intake. In the 1970s, the possible relation of dietary fat intake to cancer incidence gained greater attention as the large international differences in rates of many cancers were noted to be strongly correlated with apparent per capita fat consumption in ecologic studies.[2] Particularly strong associations were seen with cancers of the breast, colon, prostate, and endometrium, which include the most important cancers not due to smoking in affluent countries. These correlations were observed to be limited to animal, not vegetable, fat.

Dietary Fat and Breast Cancer

Breast cancer is the most common malignancy among women, and incidence has been increasing for decades, although a decline has been noted starting with the new millennium. Rates in most parts of Asia, South America, and Africa have been only approximately one-fifth that of the United States, but in almost all these areas rates of breast cancer are also increasing. Populations that migrate from low- to high-incidence countries develop breast cancer rates that approximate those of the new host country. However, rates do not approach those of the general US population until the second or third generation.[18] This slower rate of change for immigrants may indicate delayed acculturation; although because a similar delay in rate increase is not observed for colon cancer, it may suggest an origin of breast cancer earlier in the life course.

The results from 12 smaller case-control studies that included 4,312 cases and 5,978 controls have been summarized in a meta-analysis.[19] The pooled relative risk (RR) was 1.35 ($P < .0001$) for a 100-g increase in daily total fat intake, although the risk was somewhat stronger for postmenopausal women (RR, 1.48; $P < .001$). This magnitude of association, however, could be compatible with biases due to recall of diet or the selection of controls.

Because of the prospective design of cohort studies, most of the methodologic biases of case-control studies are avoided. In an analysis of the Nurses' Health Study that included 121,700 US female registered nurses, no association with total fat intake was observed, and there was no suggestion of any reduction in risk at intakes below 25% of energy.[20] Because repeated assessments of diet were obtained at 2- to 4-year intervals, this analysis provided a particularly detailed evaluation of fat intake over an extended period in relation to breast cancer risk. Similar observations were made in the National Institutes of Health (NIH)–American Association of Retired Persons (AARP) Diet and Health Study including 188,736 postmenopausal women[21] and in the European Prospective Investigation into Cancer and Nutrition (EPIC), which included 7,119 incident cases.[22] In a pooled analysis of seven prospective studies, which included 337,000 women who developed 4,980 incident cases of breast cancer, no overall association was seen for fat intake over the range of less than 20% to more than 45% energy (reflecting the current range observed

internationally).[23] A similar lack of association was seen for specific types of fat. This lack of association with total fat intake was confirmed in a subsequent analysis of the pooled prospective studies of diet and breast cancer, which included over 7,000 cases.[24] Therefore, these cohort findings do not support the hypothesis that dietary fat is an important contributor to breast cancer incidence.

Endogenous estrogen levels have now been established as a risk factor for breast cancer. Thus, the effects of fat and other dietary factors on estrogen levels are of potential interest. Vegetarian women, who consume higher amounts of fiber and lower amounts of fat, have lower blood levels and reduced urinary excretion of estrogens, apparently due to increased fecal excretion. A meta-analysis has suggested that a reduction in dietary fat reduces plasma estrogen levels,[25] but the studies included were plagued by the lack of concurrent controls, the short duration, and the negative energy balance. In a large, randomized trial among postmenopausal women with a previous diagnosis of breast cancer, a reduction in dietary fat did not affect estradiol levels when the data were appropriately analyzed.[26]

The WHI Randomized Controlled Dietary Modification Trial similarly suggested no association between fat intake and breast cancer incidence,[5] but these results are difficult to interpret.[27] The data on biomarkers that reflect fat intake suggest little if any difference in fat intake between the intervention and control groups.[28] Even if dietary fat does truly have an effect on cancer incidence and other outcomes, this lack of adherence to the dietary intervention could explain the absence of an observed effect on total cancer incidence and total mortality. In another randomized trial in Canada that tested an intervention target of 15% of calories from fat, a small but significant difference in high-density lipoprotein (HDL) levels was observed after 8 to 9 years of follow-up suggesting a difference in fat intake in the two groups.[29] The incidence of breast cancer in the intervention and the control group did not differ significantly.

Some prospective cohort studies suggest an inverse association between monounsaturated fat and breast cancer. This is an intriguing observation because of the relatively low rates of breast cancer in southern European countries with high intakes of monounsaturated fats due to the use of olive oil as the primary fat. In case-control studies in Spain, Greece, and Italy, women who used more olive oil had reduced risks of breast cancer.

In a report of findings from the Nurses' Health Study II cohort of premenopausal women, a higher intake of animal fat was associated with an approximately 50% greater risk of breast cancer, but no association was seen with intake of vegetable fat.[30] This suggests that factors in foods containing animal fats, rather than fat per se, may account for the findings. In the same cohort, an intake of red meat and total fat during adolescence was also associated with the risk of premenopausal breast cancer.[31,32]

Dietary Fat and Colon Cancer

In comparisons among countries, rates of colon cancer are strongly correlated with a national per capita disappearance of animal fat and meat, with correlation coefficients ranging between 0.8 and 0.9.[2] Rates of colon cancer rose sharply in Japan after World War II, paralleling a 2.5-fold increase in fat intake. Based on these epidemiologic investigations and on animal studies, a hypothesis has developed that higher dietary fat increases the excretion of bile acids, which can be converted to carcinogens or act as promoters. However, evidence from many studies on obesity and low levels of physical activity increasing the risk of colon cancer suggests that at least part of the high rates in affluent countries previously attributed to fat intake is probably due to a sedentary lifestyle.

The Nurses' Health Study suggested an approximately twofold higher risk of colon cancer among women in the highest quintile of animal fat intake than in those in the lowest quintile.[33] In a multivariate analysis of these data, which included red meat intake and animal fat intake in the same model, red meat intake remained significantly predictive of colon cancer risk, whereas the association with animal fat was eliminated. Other cohort studies have supported associations of colon cancer and the consumption of red meat and processed meats but not other sources of fat or total fat.[34-36] Similar associations were also observed for colorectal adenomas. In a meta-analysis of prospective studies, red meat consumption was associated with a risk of colon cancer (RR = 1.24; 95% confidence interval [CI], 1.09 to 1.41 for an increment of 120 g per day).[37] The association with the consumption of processed meats was particularly strong (RR = 1.36; 95% CI, 1.15 to 1.61 for an increment of 30 g per day).

The apparently stronger association with red meat consumption than with fat intake in most large cohort studies needs further confirmation, but such an association could result if the fatty acids or nonfat components of meat (e.g., the heme iron or carcinogens created by cooking) were the primary etiologic factors. This issue has major practical implications because current dietary recommendations support the daily consumption of red meat as long as it is lean.[38]

Dietary Fat and Prostate Cancer

Although further data are desirable, the evidence from international correlations, case-control[39] and cohort studies[40-44] provides some support for an association between the consumption of fat-containing animal products and prostate cancer incidence. This evidence does not generally support a relation with intake of vegetable fat, which suggests that either the type of fat or other components of animal products are responsible. Some evidence also indicates that animal fat consumption may be most strongly associated with the incidence of aggressive prostate cancer, which suggests an influence on the transition from the widespread indolent form to the more lethal form of this malignancy. Data are limited on the relation of fat intake to the probability of survival after the diagnosis of prostate cancer.

Dietary Fat and Other Cancers

Rates of other cancers that are common in affluent countries, including those of the endometrium and ovary, are also correlated with fat intake internationally. In prospective studies between Iowa and Canadian women, no evidence of a relation between fat intake and risk of endometrial cancer was found. Positive associations between dietary fat and lung cancer have been observed in many case-control studies. However, in a pooled analysis of large prospective studies that included over 3,000 incident cases, no association was observed.[45] These findings provide further evidence that the results of case-control studies of diet and cancer are likely to be misleading.

Summary

Largely on the basis of the results of animal studies, international correlations, and a few case-control studies, great enthusiasm developed in the 1980s that modest reductions in total fat intake would have a major impact on breast cancer incidence. As the findings from large prospective studies have become available, however, support for this relation has greatly weakened. Although evidence suggests that a high intake of animal fat early in adult life may increase the risk of premenopausal breast cancer, this is not likely to be due to fat per se because vegetable fat intake was not related to risk. For colon cancer, the associations seen with animal fat intake internationally have been supported in numerous case-control and cohort studies, but this also appears to be explained by factors in red meat other than simply its fat content. Further, the importance of physical activity and leanness as protective factors against colon cancer indicates that international correlations probably overstate the contribution of diet to differences in colon cancer incidence. At present, the available evidence most strongly suggests an association between animal fat consumption and risk of prostate cancer, particularly the aggressive form of this disease.

As with colon cancer, the possibility remains that other factors in animal products contribute to risk.

Despite the large body of data on dietary fat and cancer that has accumulated since 1985, any conclusions should be regarded as tentative, because these are disease processes that are poorly understood and are likely to take many decades to develop. Because most of the reported literature from prospective studies is based on fewer than 20 years' follow-up, further evaluations of the effects of diet earlier in life and at longer intervals of observation are needed to fully understand these complex relations. Nevertheless, persons interested in reducing their risk of cancer could be advised, as a prudent measure, to minimize their intake of foods high in animal fat, particularly red meat. Such a dietary pattern is also likely to be beneficial for the risk of cardiovascular disease. On the other hand, unsaturated fats (with the exception of *transfatty* acids) reduce blood low-density lipoprotein cholesterol levels and the risk of cardiovascular disease, and little evidence suggests that they adversely affect cancer risk. Thus, efforts to reduce unsaturated fat intake are not warranted at this time and are likely to have adverse effects on cardiovascular disease risk. Because excess adiposity increases the risk of several cancers and cardiovascular disease, balancing calories from any source with adequate physical activity is extremely important.

Fruits and Vegetables

General Properties

Fruits and vegetables have been hypothesized to be major dietary contributors to cancer prevention because they are rich in potential anticarcinogenic substances. Fruits and vegetables contain antioxidants and minerals and are good sources of fiber, potassium, carotenoids, vitamin C, folate, and other vitamins. Although fruits and vegetables supply less than 5% of total energy intake in most countries worldwide on a population basis, the concentration of micronutrients in these foods is greater than in most others.

The comprehensive report of the World Cancer Research Fund and the American Institute for Cancer Research, published in 2007 and titled *Food, Nutrition, Physical Activity, and the Prevention of Cancer: A Global Perspective*, reached the consensus based on the available evidence: "findings from cohort studies conducted since the mid-1990s have made the overall evidence, that vegetables or fruits protect against cancers, somewhat less impressive. In no case now is the evidence of protection judged to be convincing."[15]

Fruit and Vegetable Consumption and Colorectal Cancer

The association between fruit and vegetable consumption and the incidence of colon or rectal cancer has been examined prospectively in at least six studies. In some of these prospective cohorts, inverse associations were observed for individual foods or particular subgroups of fruits or vegetables, but no consistent pattern emerged and many comparisons revealed no such links. The results from the largest studies, the Nurses' Health Study and the Health Professionals' Follow-Up Study, suggested no important association between the consumption of fruits and vegetables and the incidence of cancers of the colon or rectum during 1,743,645 person-years of follow-up.[46] In these two large cohorts, diet was assessed repeatedly during follow-up with a detailed food frequency questionnaire. Similarly, in the Pooling Project of Prospective Studies of Diet and Cancer, including 14 studies, 756,217 participants, and 5,838 cases of colon cancer, no association with overall colon cancer risk was found.[47]

Fruit and Vegetable Consumption and Stomach Cancer

At least 12 prospective cohort studies have examined the consumption of some fruits and vegetables and the incidence of stomach cancer.[15] Seven of these studies considered total vegetable intake. Three found significant protection from stomach cancer, whereas three did not. All other comparisons were made for subgroups of vegetables and produced inconsistent results. Nine prospective cohort studies investigated the association between fruit consumption and stomach cancer risk. Four studies found an inverse association of borderline statistical significance.

Fruit and Vegetable Consumption and Breast Cancer

The most comprehensive evaluation of fruit and vegetable consumption and the incidence of breast cancer was provided by a pooled analysis of all cohort studies.[48] Data were pooled from eight prospective studies that included 351,825 women, 7,377 of whom developed incident invasive breast cancer during follow-up. The pooled relative risk adjusted for potential confounding variables was 0.93 (95% CI, 0.86 to 1.0; P for trend, .08) for the highest versus the lowest quartile of fruit consumption, 0.96 (95% CI, 0.89 to 1.04; P for trend, .54) for vegetable intake, and 0.93 (95% CI, 0.86 to 1.0; P for trend, .12) for total consumption of fruits and vegetables combined. The EPIC study confirmed this lack of association.[49] In a recent analysis within the Nurses' Health Study, an inverse association was seen between vegetable intake and the risk of estrogen receptor–negative breast cancer.[50] This observation was confirmed in the pooling project of prospective studies: The pooled relative risk for the highest vs. the lowest quintile of total vegetable consumption was 0.82 (95% CI 0.74 to 0.90) for estrogen-receptor negative breast cancer.[51]

Fruit and Vegetable Consumption and Lung Cancer

The relation between fruit and vegetable consumption and the incidence of lung cancer was examined in the pooled analysis of cohort studies.[52] Overall, no association was observed, although a modest increase in lung cancer incidence was evident among participants with the lowest fruit and vegetable consumption.

Fruit and Vegetable Consumption and Total Cancer

An analysis of the Nurses' Health Study and the Health Professionals' Follow-Up Study, including over 9,000 incident cases of cancer, did not reveal a benefit of fruit and vegetable consumption for total cancer incidence.[53] Observations from the EPIC cohort were essentially consistent with these findings.[54] Although there may be no or only a very weak protection conferred for cancer from consuming an abundance of fruits and vegetables, there is a substantial benefit for protection from cardiovascular disease.

Summary

The consumption of fruits and vegetables and some of their main micronutrients appear to be less important in cancer prevention than previously assumed. With an accumulation of data from prospective cohort studies and randomized trials, a lack of association of these foods and nutrients with cancer outcomes has become apparent. A modest association cannot be excluded because of an imperfect measurement of diet, and it remains possible that a high consumption of fruits and vegetables during childhood and adolescence is more effective at reducing cancer risk than consumption in adult life due to the long latency of cancer manifestation.

Conversely, it is possible that, with the fortification of breakfast cereal, flour, and other staple foods, the frequent consumption of fruits and vegetables has become less essential for cancer prevention. Nevertheless, an abundance of fruits and vegetables as part of a healthy diet is recommended, because evidence consistently suggests that it lowers the incidence of hypertension, heart disease, and stroke.

Fiber

General Properties

Dietary fiber was defined in 1976 as "all plant polysaccharides and lignin which are resistant to hydrolysis by the digestive enzymes of men."[55] Fiber, both soluble and insoluble, is fermented by the luminal bacteria of the colon. Among the properties of fiber that make it a candidate for cancer prevention are its "bulking" effect, which reduces colonic transit time, and the binding of potentially carcinogenic luminal chemicals. Fiber may also aid in producing short-chain fatty acids that may be directly anticarcinogenic. Fiber may also induce apoptosis.

Dietary Fiber and Colorectal Cancer

In 1969, Dennis Burkitt hypothesized that dietary fiber is involved in colon carcinogenesis.[56] While working as a physician in Africa, Burkitt noticed the low incidence of colon cancer among African populations whose diets were high in fiber. Burkitt concluded that a link might exist between the fiber-rich diet and the low incidence of colon cancer. Burkitt's observations were followed by numerous case-control studies that seemed to confirm his theories. A combined analysis of 13 case-control studies[57] as well as a meta-analysis of 16 case-control studies[58] suggested an inverse association between fiber intake and the risk of colorectal cancer. The inclusion of studies was selective, however, and effect estimates unadjusted for potential confounders were used for most studies. Moreover, recall bias is a severe threat to the validity of retrospective case-control studies of fiber intake and any disease outcome.

Data from prospective cohort studies have largely failed to support an inverse association between dietary fiber and colorectal cancer incidence. Initial analyses from the Nurses' Health Study and the Health Professionals' Follow-Up Study[36] found no important association between dietary fiber and colorectal cancer. A significant inverse association between fiber intake and incidence of colorectal cancer was reported from the EPIC study. The analysis presented on dietary fiber and colorectal cancer encompassed 434,209 women and men from eight European countries.[59] The analytic model used by the EPIC investigators included adjustments for age, height, weight, total caloric intake, sex, and center assessed at baseline and identified[60] a significant inverse association between fiber intake and colorectal cancer. Applying the same analytic model used in EPIC to data from the Nurses' Health Study and the Health Professionals' Follow-Up Study encompassing 1.8 million person-years of follow-up and 1,572 cases of colorectal cancer revealed associations similar to those found in the EPIC study.[61] After a more complete adjustment for confounding variables, however, the association vanished.[61] Results from the pooled analysis of 13 prospective cohort studies, including 8,081 colorectal cancer cases diagnosed during over 7 million person-years of follow-up, suggested an inverse relation between dietary fiber and colorectal cancer incidence in age-adjusted analyses, but this association disappeared after appropriate adjustment for confounding variables, particularly other dietary factors.[62] The NIH–AARP study, which included 2,974 cases of colorectal cancer, confirmed the lack of association between total dietary fiber and colorectal cancer risk.[63]

The association between dietary fiber and colorectal cancer appears to be confounded by a number of other dietary and nondietary factors. These methodologic considerations must be taken into account when interpreting the evidence. It is possible that other dietary factors such as folate intake are more important for colorectal cancer pathogenesis than dietary fiber.

Dietary Fiber and Colorectal Adenomas

In a few prospective cohort studies, the primary occurrence of colorectal polyps was investigated, but no consistent relation was found.

The study of fiber intake and colorectal adenoma recurrence lends itself to a randomized clinical trial design because of the relatively short follow-up necessary and because fiber can be provided as a supplement. A number of RCTs have explored the effect of fiber supplementation on colorectal adenoma recurrence. Evidence has fairly consistently indicated no effect of fiber intake.[64–68] In one RCT, an increase in adenoma recurrence was observed among participants randomly assigned to use a fiber supplement, which was stronger among those with high dietary calcium.[69]

Dietary Fiber and Breast Cancer

Investigators have speculated that dietary fiber may reduce the risk of breast cancer through a reduction in intestinal absorption of estrogens excreted via the biliary system.

Relatively few epidemiologic studies have examined the association between fiber intake and breast cancer. In a meta-analysis of 10 case-control studies, a significant inverse association was observed. However, these retrospective studies were likely affected by the aforementioned biases—selection and recall bias, in particular. Results from at least six prospective cohort studies consistently suggested no association between fiber intake and breast cancer incidence.[70–75]

Dietary Fiber and Stomach Cancer

The results from retrospective case-control studies of fiber intake and gastric cancer risk are inconsistent. In the Netherlands Cohort Study, dietary fiber was not associated with an incidence of gastric carcinoma.[76] Further investigations through prospective cohort studies must be completed before conclusions about the relation between fiber intake and stomach cancer incidence can be drawn.

Summary

The observational data presently available do not indicate an important role for dietary fiber in the prevention of cancer, although small effects cannot be excluded. The long-held perception that a high intake of fiber conveys protection originated largely from retrospectively conducted studies, which are affected by a number of biases, in particular, the potential for differential recall of diet, and from studies that were not well controlled for potential confounding variables.

OTHER FOODS AND NUTRIENTS

Red Meat

The regular consumption of red meat has been associated with an increased risk of colorectal cancer. In a recent meta-analysis, the increase in risk associated with an increase in intake of 120 g per day was 24% (95% CI, 9% to 41%).[37] The association was strongest for processed meat; the relative risk of colorectal cancer was 1.36 (95% CI, 1.15 to 1.61) for a consumption of 30 g per day.[37] No overall association has been observed between red meat consumption and breast cancer in a pooled analysis of prospective cohorts.[77] However, among premenopausal women in the Nurses' Health Study II, the risk for estrogen-receptor–positive and progesterone-receptor–positive breast cancer doubled with 1.5 servings of red meat per day compared to three or fewer servings per week.[78] No associations have been found in studies on poultry or fish.[15] Mechanisms through which red meat may increase cancer risk include anabolic hormones routinely used in meat production in the United States, heterocyclic amines, and polycyclic aromatic hydrocarbons formed during cooking at high temperatures, the high amounts of heme iron, and nitrates and related compounds in smoked, salted, and some processed meats that can convert to carcinogenic nitrosamines in the colon.

Milk, Dairy Products, and Calcium

Regular milk consumption has been associated with a modest reduction in colorectal cancer in both a pooling project[79] and a meta-analysis of cohort studies,[80] possibly due to its calcium content. In the pooling project of prospective studies of diet and cancer, a modest inverse association was also seen for calcium intake.[79] This finding is consistent with the results of a randomized trial in which calcium supplements reduced the risk of colorectal adenomas.[81] Associations with cheese and other dairy products have been less consistent.[79,80]

Conversely, in multiple studies, a high intake of calcium or dairy products has been associated with an increased risk of prostate cancer,[80,82–86] specifically fatal prostate cancer.[87,88] Similar observations were made in the NIH–AARP study, although the increase in risk there did not reach statistical significance.[89] While the Multiethnic Cohort[90] and the Prostate, Lung, Colorectal, and Ovarian Cancer Screening Trial[91] did not find an important association between dairy consumption and prostate cancer, these cohort studies did not specifically include fatal prostate cancer cases. A meta-analysis of prospective studies generated an overall relative risk of advanced prostate cancer of 1.33 (95% CI, 1.00 to 1.78) for the highest versus the lowest intake categories of dairy products.[92] In another meta-analysis, no significant association was found for cohort studies on dairy or milk consumption, but relative risk estimates suggested a positive association.[93] Thus, although the findings are not entirely consistent and are complicated by the widespread use of prostate-specific antigen (PSA) screening in the United States, the global evidence suggests a positive association between the regular consumption of dairy products and the risk of fatal prostate cancer. Consuming three or more servings of dairy products per day has been associated with endometrial cancer among postmenopausal women not using hormonal therapy.[94] A high intake of lactose from dairy products has also been associated with a modestly higher risk of ovarian cancer.[95]

These observations are particularly important in the context of national dietary recommendations to drink three glasses of milk per day.[38] Possible mechanisms include an increase in endogenous IGF-1 levels[96] and steroid hormones contained in cows' milk.[97]

Vitamin D

In 1980, Garland and Garland[98] hypothesized that sunlight and vitamin D may reduce the risk of colon cancer. Since then, substantial research has been conducted in this area supporting an inverse association between circulating 25-hydroxyvitamin D (25[OH]D) levels and colorectal cancer risk.[99–103] A meta-analysis, including five nested case-control studies with prediagnostic serum, suggested a reduction of colorectal cancer risk by about half among individuals with serum 25(OH)D levels of more than 82 nmol/L compared to individuals with less than 30 nmol/L.[104] A subsequent meta-analysis including eight studies confirmed these associations.[105] These observations are supported by similar findings for colorectal adenomas.[106] Vitamin D levels may particularly affect colorectal cancer prognosis; colorectal cancer mortality was 72% lower among individuals with 25(OH)D concentrations of 80 nmol/L or higher.[107]

The evidence for other cancers has been less consistent. High plasma levels of vitamin D have been associated with a decreased risk of several other cancers, including cancer of the breast[108–111]; prostate, especially fatal prostate cancer[112]; and ovary.[113,114] Whether vitamin D plays a role in pancreatic cancerogenesis remains to be determined with one pooling project, suggesting a positive association,[115] whereas other prospective studies[116] and a pooling project of cohort studies found inverse associations.[117]

The activation of vitamin D receptors by 1,25(OH)^{2}D induces cell differentiation and inhibits proliferation and angiogenesis.[118] Solar ultraviolet B radiation is the major source of plasma vitamin D, and dietary vitamin D without supplementation has a minor effect on plasma vitamin D. To achieve sufficient plasma levels through sun exposure, at least 15 minutes of full-body exposure to bright sunlight is necessary. Physical activity has to be considered as possible confounder of studies on plasma levels of vitamin D and cancer. Sunscreen effectively blocks vitamin D production. Populations who live in geographic areas with limited or seasonal sun exposure may benefit from a vitamin D supplementation of 1,000 IU per day.

Folate

Folate is a micronutrient commonly found in fruits and vegetables, particularly oranges, orange juice, asparagus, beets, and peas. Folate may affect carcinogenesis through various mechanisms: DNA methylation, DNA synthesis, and DNA repair. In the animal model, folate deficiency enhances intestinal carcinogenesis.[119] Folate deficiency is related to the incorporation of uracil into human DNA and to an increased frequency of chromosomal breaks. A number of epidemiologic studies suggest that a diet rich in folate lowers the risk of colorectal adenomas and colorectal cancer.[15] Because the folate content in foods is generally relatively low, is susceptible to oxidative destruction by cooking and food processing, and is not well absorbed, folic acid from supplements and fortification plays an important role. Pooled results from 13 prospective studies suggests that intake of 400 to 500 μg per day is required to minimize risk.[120]

Potential interactions among alcohol consumption, folic acid intake, and methionine intake have been described. Although alcohol consumption has been fairly consistently related to an increase in breast cancer incidence, the potential detrimental effect of alcohol seems to be eliminated in women with high folic acid intake.[16] A similar folic acid or methionine–alcohol interaction has been observed for colorectal cancer risk.[119]

Genetic susceptibility may also modify the relation between folate intake and cancer risk. A polymorphism of the *methylenetetrahydrofolate reductase (MTHFR)* gene (cytosine to thymine transition at position 677) may result in a relative deficiency of methionine. Individuals with the common C677T mutation appear to experience the greatest protection from high folic acid or methionine intake and low alcohol consumption.[121] Although the interaction between this polymorphism and dietary factors needs to be investigated further, the consistently observed association between this polymorphism and the risk of colorectal cancer supports a role of folate in the etiology of colorectal cancer.

Folate levels also affect the availability of methyl groups via S-adenosylmethionine in the one-carbon metabolism.[122] Low red blood cell folate levels are associated with low DNA methylation status among homozygous *MTHFR* 677T/T mutation carriers, whereas at high red blood cell folate levels, the amount of methylated cytosine in DNA is similar to that of the heterozygote *MTHFR* C677T genotype.[123]

Conversely, evidence from animal and human studies suggests that a high folate status may promote the progression of existing neoplasias.[122,124,125] The randomization of folic acid supplements among individuals with a history of colorectal adenoma resulted in either no effect on recurrent adenoma recurrence[126] or an increase in recurrence with over 6 to 8 years of follow-up.[127] The high proliferation rate of neoplastic cells requiring increased DNA synthesis is likely supported by folate, which is necessary for thymidine synthesis.[122,125] The effects of folate on de novo methylation and subsequent gene silencing have been insufficiently studied. An increase in colorectal cancer rates has been observed in the United States and Canada concurrent with the introduction of the folic acid fortification program, but this could be an artifact due to increased use of colonoscopies.[128] The lack of increase in mortality, but an acceleration in a long-term downward trend suggests the latter explanation (http://progressreport.cancer.gov/).

Carotenoids

Carotenoids, antioxidants prevalent in fruits and vegetables, enhance cell-to-cell communication, promote cell differentiation, and modulate immune response. In 1981, Doll and Peto[1] speculated that beta-carotene may be a major player in cancer prevention and encouraged testing its anticarcinogenic properties. Indeed, subsequent observational studies, mostly case-control investigations, suggested a reduced cancer risk—especially of lung cancer—with a high intake of carotenoids. In contrast, clinical trials randomizing the intake of beta-carotene supplements have not revealed the evidence of a protective effect of beta-carotene. In fact, beta-carotene was found to increase the risk of lung cancer and total mortality among smokers in the Finnish Alpha-Tocopherol, Beta-Carotene Cancer Prevention Study.[129] However, these adverse affects disappeared during longer periods of follow-up.[130] In a detailed analysis of prospective studies, no association was seen between the intake of beta-carotene and the risk of lung cancer.[131]

The pooled analysis of 18 cohort studies including more than 33,000 breast cancer cases suggested inverse associations between the intake of several carotenoids (beta-carotene, alpha-carotene, luteine/zeaxanthin) and estrogen-receptor–negative breast cancer incidence, whereas no association was found for estrogen-receptor–positive tumors.[132] Similarly, in a pooled analysis of data from eight prospective studies including about 3,055 breast cancer cases, blood levels of carotenoids were inversely related to estrogen-receptor–negative mammary tumor incidence.[133] Women in the highest quintile of beta-carotene levels had about half the risk of developing estrogen-receptor–negative breast cancer than women in the lowest quintile (hazard ratio [HR] = 0.52; 95% CI, 0.36 to 0.77).

The particularly pronounced antioxidant properties of lycopene, a carotenoid mainly found in tomatoes, may explain the inverse associations with some cancers. The frequent consumption of tomato-based products has been associated with a decreased risk of prostate, lung, and stomach cancers.[134] The bioavailability of lycopene from cooked tomatoes is higher than from fresh tomatoes, making tomato soup and sauce excellent sources of the carotenoid.

Selenium

Selenium has long been of interest in cancer prevention due to its antioxidative properties. Its intake is difficult to estimate because food content depends on the selenium content of the soil it is grown in. Selenium enriches in toenails, which provide an integrative measure of intake during the previous year and therefore are popular biomarkers in epidemiologic studies. Inverse associations with toenail selenium levels have been found in several prospective studies, especially for fatal protate cancer.[135–137] In a recent meta-analysis, plasma/serum selenium was also inversely correlated with prostate cancer.[138] In the Selenium and Vitamin E Cancer Prevention Trial (SELECT), no protective effect of selenium was found for prostate cancer. However, the trial was terminated prematurely after 4 years, which is a short period in which to expect a reduction in cancer.[139]

Soy Products

The role of soy products has been considered for breast carcinogenesis. In Asian countries, which traditionally have a high consumption of soy foods, breast cancer rates have been low until recently. In Western countries, soy consumption is generally low, and between-person variation may be insufficient to allow meaningful comparisons. Soybeans contain isoflavones, which are phytoestrogens that compete with estrogen for the estrogen receptor. Hence, soy consumption may affect estrogen concentrations differently depending on the endogenous baseline level. This mechanism may also contribute to the equivocal results of studies on soy foods and breast cancer risk. In a recent meta-analysis of 18 epidemiologic studies, including over 9,000 breast cancer cases, frequent soy intake was associated with a modest decrease in risk (odds ratio = 0.86; 95% CI, 0.75 to 0.99).[140] Wu et al.[141] observed that childhood intake of soy was more relevant to breast cancer prevention than adult consumption.

Carbohydrates

The Warburg hypothesis postulated in 1924 that tumor cells mainly generate energy by the nonoxidative breakdown of glucose (glucolysis) instead of pyrovate.[142] Carbohydrates with a high glycemic load increase blood glucose levels after consumption, which results in insulin spikes increasing the risk for type 2 diabetes. Several cancers, including colorectal cancer[143] and breast cancer,[144] have been associated with type 2 diabetes. The evidence on the consumption of sucrose and refined, processed flour and cancer incidence is heterogeneous.[145] Whereas in some prospective cohort studies an increase in colon cancer incidence was observed,[146] this was not found in other studies.[147] In large cohort studies, associations have been observed for pancreatic[148] and endometrial[145] cancer risk, but not for postmenopausal breast cancer.[149] Especially in obese, sedentary individuals, abnormal glucose and insulin metabolism may contribute to tumorigenesis.

DIETARY PATTERNS

Foods and nutrients are not consumed in isolation, and, when evaluating the role of diet in disease prevention and causation, it is sensible to consider the entire dietary pattern of individuals. Public health messages may be better framed in the context of a global diet than individual constituents.

The role of vegetarian diets for cancer incidence has been examined in a few studies. In the Adventist Health Study-2, vegetarians had an 8% lower incidence of cancer than nonvegetarians (95% CI, 1 to 15%).[150] The protective association was strongest for cancers of the gastrointestinal tract with 24% (95% CI, 10 to 37%). Vegans had a 16% (95%, 1 to 28%) lower incidence of cancer, with a particular protection conferred to female cancers of 34% (95% CI, 8 to 53%). A combined analysis of data from the Oxford Vegetarian Study and EPIC similarly suggest a 12% (95% CI, 4 to 19%) reduction in cancer incidence among vegetarians compared to meat eaters.[151]

During the past decade, dietary pattern analyses have gained popularity in observational studies. The most commonly employed methods are factor analyses and cluster analyses, which are largely data-driven methods, and investigator-determined methods such as dietary indices and scores. The search for associations between distinct patterns such as the "Western pattern," which is characterized by a high consumption of red and processed meats; high fat dairy products, including butter and eggs; and refined carbohydrates, such as sweets, desserts, and refined grains, and the "prudent pattern," which is defined by the frequent consumption of a variety of fruits and vegetables, whole grains, legumes, fish, and poultry, and the risk of cancer has been largely disappointing. Notable exceptions were the link between a Western dietary pattern and colon cancer incidence and an inverse relation between a prudent diet[152] and estrogen-receptor–negative breast cancer.[153] These findings were subsequently in the California Teachers Study.[154] The general lack of association between global dietary patterns and cancer supports a more modest role of nutrition during adult life in carcinogenesis than previously assumed.

DIET DURING THE EARLY PHASES OF LIFE

Some cancers may originate early in the course of life. A high birth weight is associated with an increase in the risk of childhood leukemia,[155] premenopausal breast cancer,[156] and testicular cancer.[157] Tall height is an indicator of the risk of many cancers and is in part determined by nutrition during childhood.[15] Until recently, most studies focused on the role of diet during adult life. However, the critical exposure period for nutrition to affect cancer risk may be earlier, and because the latent period for cancer may span several decades, diet during childhood and adolescence may be important. However, relating dietary information during early life and cancer outcomes prospectively is difficult because nutrition records from the remote past are not available. Studies in which recalled diet during youth is used have to be interpreted cautiously due to misclassification, although recall has been found reasonably reproducible and consistent with recalls provided by participants' mothers.[158,159] The role of early life diet has been explored in only a few studies in relation to breast cancer risk. In a study nested in the Nurses' Health Study cohorts that used data recalled by mothers, frequent consumption of french fries was associated with an increased risk of breast cancer, whereas whole milk consumption was inversely related to risk.[160] Similarly, an inverse association with milk consumption during childhood was found among younger women (30 to 39 years), but not among older premenopausal women (40 to 49 years) in a Norwegian cohort.[161] Dietary habits during high school recalled by adult participants of the Nurses' Health Study II (but before the diagnosis of breast cancer) suggested a positive association of total fat and red meat consumption.[31,32] More data are needed in this promising area of research.[162]

DIET AFTER A DIAGNOSIS OF CANCER

The role of diet in the secondary prevention of cancer recurrence and survival is generally of great interest to cancer patients because they are highly motivated to make lifestyle changes to optimize their prognosis. The compliance of cancer patients makes the RCTs a more feasible design to evaluate the role of diet than among healthy individuals. However, concurrent cancer treatments may make any effect of diet more difficult to isolate.

Most evidence is available for breast cancer, colorectal, and prostate cancer. Observational data suggest a limited role of diet in the prevention of breast cancer recurrence and survival. The Life After Cancer Epidemiology (LACE) Cohort supported a beneficial role for vitamin C and E supplement use but the effect of other health-seeking behaviors is difficult to exclude.[163] In a pooled analysis, alcohol consumption after a diagnosis did not affect survival.[164] Several randomized trials have addressed the role of diet in breast cancer prognosis. In the Women's Intervention Nutrition Study (WINS), 2,437 women with early stage breast cancer were randomized to a dietary goal of 15% of calories from fat or maintenance of their usual dietary habits.[165] The intervention group received dietary counseling by registered dieticians and, according to self-reports, a difference of 19 g in daily fat intake was maintained between the intervention and the control group after 60 months of follow-up. However, at that time, women in the intervention group were also 6 pounds lighter, making it difficult to separate an effect of dietary fat from a nonspecific effect of intensive dietary intervention, which quite consistently produces weight loss. Breast cancer recurrence was 29% lower in the intervention group (95% CI, 6% to 47%), whereas overall survival was not affected. In the Women's Healthy Eating and Living (WHEL) RCT, 3,088 early stage breast cancer patients were randomly assigned to a target of five vegetable servings, three fruit servings, 30 g fiber per day, and 15% to 20% of calories from fat.[166] After 72 months, the intervention versus control group reports were 5.8 versus 3.6 servings of vegetables, 3.4 versus 2.6 servings of fruit, 24.2 versus 18.9 g fiber per day, and 28.9% versus 32.4% of calories from fat. The total plasma carotenoid concentration, a biomarker of vegetable and fruit intake, was 43% higher in the intervention group than the comparison group after 4 years (p<0.001). Neither recurrence rates nor mortality were affected by the intervention after the 7.3-year follow-up. Overall, diet is unlikely a major factor influencing breast cancer prognosis. However, because the prognosis for breast cancer is relatively good, women diagnosed with breast cancer remain at risk for cardiovascular disease and other causes of death that affect those without breast cancer. Thus, among women in the Nurses' Health Study diagnosed with breast cancer, a higher diet quality, which was assessed by the Alternative Healthy Eating Index, was not associated with mortality due to breast cancer but was associated with substantially lower mortality due to other causes.[167] Similarly, among over 4,000 women with breast cancer, intakes of saturated and trans fat, but not of total fat, were associated with significantly greater total mortality but not specifically breast cancer mortality. Thus, there is good reason for women with breast cancer to adopt a healthy diet even if it does not affect the prognosis of breast cancer.

In a systematic review, no consistent association between individual dietary components and colorectal cancer prognosis outcome was found.[168] However, in an observational study including 1,009 patients with stage III colon cancer, a Western dietary pattern was associated with lower rates of disease-free survival, recurrence-free survival, and overall survivals.[169] In the same patient population, higher dietary glycemic load and total carbohydrate intake were significantly associated with an increased risk of recurrence and mortality.[170] These findings support a possible role of glycemic load in colon cancer progression.

In the Physician's Health Study, whole milk consumption among men with incident prostate cancer was associated with double the risk of progression to fatal disease.[171] Among men with nonmetastatic prostate cancer in the Health Professionals' Follow-up Study, replacing 10% of energy intake from carbohydrates with vegetable fat was associated with a lower risk of lethal prostate cancer.[172] A marginally increased risk of progression of localized to lethal prostate cancer among these men was also associated with postdiagnostic poultry and processed red meat consumption,[173] whereas postdiagnostic consumption of fish and tomato sauce were inversely related with a risk of progression.[174] In an intervention study, 93 patients with early stage prostate cancer (PSA = 4 to 10 ng per mililiter and Gleason score <7) were randomized to comprehensive lifestyle changes, including a vegan diet based on 10% of calories from fat and consisting predominantly of vegetables, fruit, whole grains, legumes, and soy protein.[175] Other interventions included moderate exercise, stress management, and relaxation. After 1 year, PSA values decreased 4% in the intervention group, but increased 6% in the control group. Six patients in the control group, but none in the experimental group, underwent conventional prostate cancer treatment. Although the impact of the different intervention components are difficult to separate in this study, further data on diet and the prognosis for patients with localized prostate cancer are needed.

SUMMARY

A considerable proportion of cancers are potentially preventable through lifestyle changes. Besides a curtailment of smoking, the most important strategies are maintaining a healthy body weight and regular physical activity, which contribute to a lower prevalence of being overweight and obesity. The avoidance of a positive energy balance and becoming overweight are the most important nutritional factors in cancer prevention.

Although dietary patterns, including frequent fruit and vegetable consumption, appear to play a modest role in cancer prevention, knowledge gained about some specific foods and nutrients might inform a targeted approach. Vitamin D is a strong candidate to counter carcinogenesis, thus supplementation could be a feasible and safe route to avoid several types of cancer. Although the data on vitamin D and cancer incidence are not conclusive, the

prevention of bone fractures is a sufficient reason to maintain good vitamin D status.

Limiting or avoiding red meat, processed meat, and alcohol reduces the risk of breast, colorectal, stomach, esophageal, and other cancers. Although the role of dairy products and milk remains to be more fully elucidated, current evidence suggests a probable increase in the risk of prostate cancer with frequent milk consumption, and possibly endometrial cancer, which raises concern regarding current dietary recommendations of three glasses of milk per day. The relation of calcium and dairy intake to cancer is complex, as the evidence for a reduction in the risk of colorectal cancer is strong, but high intakes appear likely to increase the risk of fatal prostate cancer. The consumption of tomato-based products may contribute to the prevention of prostate cancer. Finally, diet may influence the prognosis of colorectal and prostate cancer, but more data are needed in this area. Because most people with cancer remain at risk of cardiovascular disease and other common conditions related to unhealthy diets, an overall healthy diet can be recommended while further research on diet and cancer survival is ongoing.

LIMITATIONS

Studying the role of diet in health and disease requires overcoming a number of hurdles. Because biomarkers reflecting nutrient intake with sufficient accuracy are largely lacking, assessing nutrition in a population-based study has to rely on self-reports by individuals, which inevitably leads to imprecision or error in the diet assessment. Such misclassification may produce spurious associations in case-control studies or may lead to an underestimation of true associations in prospective cohort studies. Ideally, hypotheses relating dietary factors to cancer risks would be tested in large randomized trials. Besides being extremely expensive, maintaining adherence to assigned diets has been challenging; for example, in the WHI trial that focused on dietary fat reduction, there were no differences between intervention and control groups in blood lipid fractions that are known to change with a reduction in fat intake, indicating a failure to test the hypothesis.[28]

Most observational studies are conducted within populations or countries. Although reasonable variations in nutritional habits exist within populations, allowing for the detection of substantial dietary risk factors for cardiovascular disease and diabetes, these contrasts may be too limited to detect small relative risks as they may exist for cancer. The pooled analysis of large prospective cohort studies across countries and continents attempts to overcome this limitation. Studies taking advantage of the large between-population variation in diets across developed and developing countries would appear to be advantageous, but would be plagued by confounding by other differences in lifestyle factors that might be difficult to assess and control adequately.

Few epidemiologic studies repeatedly capture dietary habits over time and thus account for potential changes in diet over time. Furthermore, the length of follow-up in prospective studies may not be sufficient to capture the impact of diets assessed at baseline. In case-control studies, a recall of dietary habits prior to the disease onset may be influenced by current disease status; moreover, the relevant time for nutrition to act may be decades earlier, which is more difficult to remember.

Most epidemiologic studies of diet and cancer have assessed intake among adults. Due to greater susceptibility to genotoxic influences earlier in life, it is possible that data on diet during childhood or early adolescence are more relevant for carcinogenesis and cancer prevention. Studies that have collected dietary data during childhood and followed the subjects for cancer incidence would be most informative but are virtually nonexistent and will be challenging to conduct.

Finally, data on special diets including organic foods, whole foods, raw foods, and a vegan diet are limited.

FUTURE DIRECTIONS

Some of the most promising research at present is in the areas of vitamin D, milk consumption, and the effect of diet early in life on cancer incidence. Recent nutrition changes in countries previously maintaining a more traditional diet such as Japan and some developing countries have already been followed by increased rates of some cancers (but declines in stomach cancer), providing a setting to study the effect of change over time. Additional insight may come from studies on gene–nutrient interaction and epigenetic changes induced by the diet. To improve observational research methods, refined dietary assessment methods, including the identification of new biomarkers, will be advantageous.

RECOMMENDATIONS

A wealth of data are available from observational studies on diet and cancer, and the current evidence supports suggestions made by Doll and Peto[1] that approximately 30% to 40% of cancers may be avoidable with changes in nutrition; however, much of this risk of cancer is related to being overweight and to inactivity. Excessive energy intake and lack of physical activity, marked by rapid growth in childhood and being overweight, have become growing threats to population health and are important contributors to risks of many cancers. Nevertheless, the cumulative incidence for many cancers has decreased over the past decade, in part due to the decreasing prevalence of smoking and use of hormone therapy.

Dietary recommendations must integrate the goal of overall avoidance of disease and maintenance of health and, thus, should not focus singularly on cancer prevention. The strength of the evidence and magnitude of the expected benefit should also be considered in recommendations. With these considerations in mind, the following recommendations are outlined, which are largely in agreement with the guidelines put forth by the American Cancer Society in 2012:[176]

1. *Engage in regular physical activity.* Physical activity is a primary method of weight control and it also reduces risk of several cancers, especially colon cancer, through independent mechanisms. Moderate to vigorous exercise for at least 30 minutes on most days is a minimum and more will provide additional benefits.

2. *Avoid being overweight and weight gain in adulthood.* A positive energy balance that results in excess body fat is one of the most important contributors to cancer risk. Staying within 10 pounds of body weight at age 20 may be a simple guide, assuming no adolescent obesity.

3. *Limit alcohol consumption.* Alcohol consumption contributes to the risk of many cancers and increases the risk of accidents and addiction, but low to moderate consumption has benefits for coronary heart disease risk. The individual family history of disease as well as personal preferences should be considered.

4. *Consume lots of fruits and vegetables.* Frequent consumption of fruits and vegetables during adult life is not likely to have a major effect on cancer incidence, but will reduce the risk of cardiovascular disease.

5. *Consume whole grains and avoid refined carbohydrates and sugars.* A regular consumption of whole grain products instead of refined flour and a low consumption of refined sugars lower the risk of cardiovascular disease and diabetes. The effect on cancer risk is less clear.

6. *Replace red meat and dairy products with fish, nuts, and legumes.* Red meat consumption increases the risk of colorectal cancer, diabetes, and coronary heart disease and should be largely avoided. Frequent dairy consumption may increase the risk of prostate cancer. Fish, nuts, and legumes are excellent sources of valuable mono- and polyunsaturated fats and vegetable proteins and may contribute to lower rates of cardiovascular disease and diabetes.

7. *Consider taking a vitamin D supplement.* A substantial proportion of the population, especially those living at higher latitudes, are vitamin D deficient. Most adults may benefit from taking 1,000 IU of vitamin D^3 per day during months of low sunlight intensity. Vitamin D supplementation will, at a minimum, reduce bone fracture rates, probably colorectal cancer incidence, and possibly other cancers.

ETIOLOGY AND EPIDEMIOLOGY OF CANCER

REFERENCES

1. Doll R, Peto R. The causes of cancer: quantitative estimates of avoidable risks of cancer in the United States today. *J Natl Cancer Inst* 1981;66:1191–1308.
2. Armstrong B, Doll R. Environmental factors and cancer incidence and mortality in different countries, with special reference to dietary practices. *Int J Cancer* 1975;15:617–631.
3. Giovannucci E, Stampfer MJ, Colditz GA, et al. A comparison of prospective and retrospective assessments of diet in the study of breast cancer. *Am J Epidemiol* 1993;137:502–511.
4. Riboli E, Norat T. Epidemiologic evidence of the protective effect of fruit and vegetables on cancer risk. *Am J Clin Nutr* 2003;78:559S–569S.
5. Prentice RL, Caan B, Chlebowski RT, et al. Low-fat dietary pattern and risk of invasive breast cancer: the Women's Health Initiative Randomized Controlled Dietary Modification Trial. *JAMA* 2006;295:629–642.
6. Michels KB, Bingham SA, Luben R, et al. The effect of correlated measurement error in multivariate models of diet. *Am J Epidemiol* 2004;160:59–67.
7. Willett W. *Nutritional Epidemiology.* 3rd ed. New York: Oxford University Press; 2013.
8. Calle EE, Rodriguez C, Walker-Thurmond K, et al. Overweight, obesity, and mortality from cancer in a prospectively studied cohort of U.S. adults. *N Engl J Med* 2003;348:1625–1638.
9. Giovannucci E, Ascherio A, Rimm EB, et al. Physical activity, obesity, and risk for colon cancer and adenoma in men. *Ann Intern Med* 1995;122:327–334.
10. Martinez ME, Giovannucci E, Spiegelman D, et al. Leisure-time physical activity, body size, and colon cancer in women. Nurses' Health Study Research Group. *J Natl Cancer Inst* 1997;89:948–955.
11. Eliassen AH, Colditz GA, Rosner B, et al. Adult weight change and risk of postmenopausal breast cancer. *JAMA* 2006;296:193–201.
12. Michels KB, Ekbom A. Caloric restriction and incidence of breast cancer. *JAMA* 2004;291:1226–1230.
13. Elias SG, Peeters PH, Grobbee DE, et al. Breast cancer risk after caloric restriction during the 1944–1945 Dutch famine. *J Natl Cancer Inst* 2004;96:539–546.
14. Tretli S, Gaard M. Lifestyle changes during adolescence and risk of breast cancer: an ecologic study of the effect of World War II in Norway. *Cancer Causes Control* 1996;7:507–512.
15. World Cancer Research Fund/American Institute for Cancer Research. *Food, Nutrition, Physical Activity, and the Prevention of Cancer: A Global Perspective.* Washington, D.C.: AICR; 2007.
16. Zhang S, Hunter DJ, Hankinson SE, et al. A prospective study of folate intake and the risk of breast cancer. *JAMA* 1999;281:1632–1637.
17. Tannenbaum A. The genesis and growth of tumors. III. Effects of a high-fat diet. *Cancer Res* 1942;2:468–475.
18. Kolonel L, Hinds M, Hankin J. *Cancer Patterns Among Migrant and Native-Born Japanese in Hawaii in Relation to Smoking, Drinking, and Dietary Habits.* Tokyo: Japan Scientific Societies Press; 1980.
19. Howe GR, Hirohata T, Hislop TG, et al. Dietary factors and risk of breast cancer: combined analysis of 12 case-control studies. *J Natl Cancer Inst* 1990;82:561–569.
20. Kim EH, Willett WC, Colditz GA, et al. Dietary fat and risk of postmenopausal breast cancer in a 20-year follow-up. *Am J Epidemiol* 2006;164:990–997.
21. Thiebaut AC, Kipnis V, Chang SC, et al. Dietary fat and postmenopausal invasive breast cancer in the National Institutes of Health-AARP Diet and Health Study cohort. *J Natl Cancer Inst* 2007;99:451–462.
22. Sieri S, Krogh V, Ferrari P, et al. Dietary fat and breast cancer risk in the European Prospective Investigation into Cancer and Nutrition. *Am J Clin Nutr* 2008;88:1304–1312.
23. Hunter DJ, Spiegelman D, Adami HO, et al. Cohort studies of fat intake and the risk of breast cancer—a pooled analysis. *N Engl J Med* 1996;334:356–361.
24. Smith-Warner SA, Spiegelman D, Adami HO, et al. Types of dietary fat and breast cancer: a pooled analysis of cohort studies. *Int J Cancer* 2001;92:767–774.
25. Wu AH, Pike MC, Stram DO. Meta-analysis: dietary fat intake, serum estrogen levels, and the risk of breast cancer. *J Natl Cancer Inst* 1999;91:529–534.

26. Rose DP, Connolly JM, Chlebowski RT, et al. The effects of a low-fat dietary intervention and tamoxifen adjuvant therapy on the serum estrogen and sex hormone-binding globulin concentrations of postmenopausal breast cancer patients. *Breast Cancer Res Treat* 1993;27:253–262.

27. Michels KB. The women's health initiative—curse or blessing? *Int J Epidemiol* 2006;35:814–816.

28. Michels KB, Willett WC. The Women's Health Initiative Randomized Controlled Dietary Modification Trial: a post-mortem. *Breast Cancer Res Treat* 2009;114:1–6.

29. Martin LJ, Li Q, Melnichouk O, et al. A randomized trial of dietary intervention for breast cancer prevention. *Cancer Res* 2011;71:123–133.

30. Cho E, Spiegelman D, Hunter DJ, et al. Premenopausal fat intake and risk of breast cancer. *J Natl Cancer Inst* 2003;95:1079–1085.

31. Linos E, Willett WC, Cho E, et al. Red meat consumption during adolescence among premenopausal women and risk of breast cancer. *Cancer Epidemiol Biomarkers Prev* 2008;17:2146–2151.

32. Linos E, Willett WC, Cho E, et al. Adolescent diet in relation to breast cancer risk among premenopausal women. *Cancer Epidemiol Biomarkers Prev* 2010;19:689–696.

33. Willett WC, Stampfer MJ, Colditz GA, et al. Relation of meat, fat, and fiber intake to the risk of colon cancer in a prospective study among women. *N Engl J Med* 1990;323:1664–1672.

34. Bostick RM, Potter JD, Kushi LH, et al. Sugar, meat, and fat intake, and non-dietary risk factors for colon cancer incidence in Iowa women (United States). *Cancer Causes Control* 1994;5:38–52.

35. Goldbohm RA, van den Brandt PA, van't Veer P, et al. A prospective cohort study on the relation between meat consumption and the risk of colon cancer. *Cancer Res* 1994;54:718–723.

36. Giovannucci E, Rimm EB, Stampfer MJ, et al. Intake of fat, meat, and fiber in relation to risk of colon cancer in men. *Cancer Res* 1994;54:2390–2397.

37. Norat T, Lukanova A, Ferrari P, et al. Meat consumption and colorectal cancer risk: dose-response meta-analysis of epidemiological studies. *Int J Cancer* 2002;98:241–256.

38. Dietary Guidelines for Americans. DietaryGuidelines.gov Web site. http://www.health.gov/dietaryguidelines/.

39. Whittemore AS, Kolonel LN, Wu AH, et al. Prostate cancer in relation to diet, physical activity, and body size in blacks, whites, and Asians in the United States and Canada. *J Natl Cancer Inst* 1995;87:652–661.

40. Crowe FL, Key TJ, Appleby PN, et al. Dietary fat intake and risk of prostate cancer in the European Prospective Investigation into Cancer and Nutrition. *Am J Clin Nutr* 2008;87:1405–1413.

41. Giovannucci E, Rimm EB, Colditz GA, et al. A prospective study of dietary fat and risk of prostate cancer. *J Natl Cancer Inst* 1993;85:1571–1579.

42. Mills PK, Beeson WL, Phillips RL, et al. Cohort study of diet, lifestyle, and prostate cancer in Adventist men. *Cancer* 1989;64:598–604.

43. Park S-Y, Murphy SP, Wilkens LR, et al. Fat and meat intake and prostate cancer risk: The multiethnic cohort study. *Int J Cancer* 2007;121:1339–1345.

44. Schuurman AG, van den Brandt PA, Dorant E, et al. Association of energy and fat intake with prostate carcinoma risk: results from The Netherlands Cohort Study. *Cancer* 1999;86:1019–1027.

45. Smith-Warner SA, Ritz J, Hunter DJ, et al. Dietary fat and risk of lung cancer in a pooled analysis of prospective studies. *Cancer Epidemiol Biomarkers Prev* 2002;11:987–992.

46. Michels KB, Edward G, Joshipura KJ, et al. Prospective study of fruit and vegetable consumption and incidence of colon and rectal cancers. *J Natl Cancer Inst* 2000;92:1740–1752.

47. Koushik A, Hunter DJ, Spiegelman D, et al. Fruits, vegetables, and colon cancer risk in a pooled analysis of 14 cohort studies. *J Natl Cancer Inst* 2007;99:1471–1483.

48. Smith-Warner SA, Spiegelman D, Yaun SS, et al. Intake of fruits and vegetables and risk of breast cancer: a pooled analysis of cohort studies. *JAMA* 2001;285:769–776.

49. van Gils CH, Peeters PH, Bueno-de-Mesquita HB, et al. Consumption of vegetables and fruits and risk of breast cancer. *JAMA* 2005;293:183–193.

50. Fung TT, Hu FB, McCullough ML, et al. Diet quality is associated with the risk of estrogen receptor-negative breast cancer in postmenopausal women. *J Nutr* 2006;136:466–472.

51. Jung S, Spiegelman D, Baglietto L, et al. Fruit and vegetable intake and risk of breast cancer by hormone receptor status. *J Natl Cancer Inst* 2013;105:219–236.

52. Smith-Warner SA, Spiegelman D, Yaun SS, et al. Fruits, vegetables and lung cancer: a pooled analysis of cohort studies. *Int J Cancer* 2003;107:1001–1011.

53. Hung HC, Joshipura KJ, Jiang R, et al. Fruit and vegetable intake and risk of major chronic disease. *J Natl Cancer Inst* 2004;96:1577–1584.

54. Boffetta P, Couto E, Wichmann J, et al. Fruit and vegetable intake and overall cancer risk in the European Prospective Investigation into Cancer and Nutrition (EPIC). *J Natl Cancer Inst* 2010;102:529–537.

55. Trowell H, Southgate DA, Waolever TM, et al. Letter: Dietary fibre redefined. *Lancet* 1976;1:967.

56. Burkitt DP. Related disease—related cause? *Lancet* 1969;2:1229–1231.

57. Howe GR, Benito E, Castelleto R, et al. Dietary intake of fiber and decreased risk of cancers of the colon and rectum: evidence from the combined analysis of 13 case-control studies. *J Natl Cancer Inst* 1992;84:1887–1896.

58. Trock B, Lanza E, Greenwald P. Dietary fiber, vegetables, and colon cancer: critical review and meta-analyses of the epidemiologic evidence. *J Natl Cancer Inst* 1990;82:650–661.

59. Bingham SA, Day NE, Luben R, et al. Dietary fibre in food and protection against colorectal cancer in the European Prospective Investigation into Cancer and Nutrition (EPIC): an observational study. *Lancet* 2003;361:1496–1501.

60. Fuchs CS, Giovannucci EL, Colditz GA, et al. Dietary fiber and the risk of colorectal cancer and adenoma in women. *N Engl J Med* 1999;340:169–176.

61. Michels KB, Fuchs CS, Giovannucci E, et al. Fiber intake and incidence of colorectal cancer among 76,947 women and 47,279 men. *Cancer Epidemiol Biomarkers Prev* 2005;14:842–849.

62. Park Y, Hunter DJ, Spiegelman D, et al. Dietary fiber intake and risk of colorectal cancer: a pooled analysis of prospective cohort studies. *JAMA* 2005;294:2849–2857.

63. Schatzkin A, Mouw T, Park Y, et al. Dietary fiber and whole-grain consumption in relation to colorectal cancer in the NIH-AARP Diet and Health Study. *Am J Clin Nutr* 2007;85:1353–1360.

64. Alberts DS, Martinez ME, Roe DJ, et al. Lack of effect of a high-fiber cereal supplement on the recurrence of colorectal adenomas. Phoenix Colon Cancer Prevention Physicians' Network. *N Engl J Med* 2000;342:1156–1162.

65. Jacobs ET, Giuliano AR, Roe DJ, et al. Intake of supplemental and total fiber and risk of colorectal adenoma recurrence in the wheat bran fiber trial. *Cancer Epidemiol Biomarkers Prev* 2002;11:906–914.

66. MacLennan R, Macrae F, Bain C, et al. Randomized trial of intake of fat, fiber, and beta carotene to prevent colorectal adenomas. The Australian Polyp Prevention Project. *J Natl Cancer Inst* 1995;87:1760–1766.

67. McKeown-Eyssen GE, Bright-See E, Bruce WR, et al. A randomized trial of a low fat high fibre diet in the recurrence of colorectal polyps. Toronto Polyp Prevention Group. *J Clin Epidemiol* 1994;47:525–536.

68. Schatzkin A, Lanza E, Corle D, et al. Lack of effect of a low-fat, high-fiber diet on the recurrence of colorectal adenomas. Polyp Prevention Trial Study Group. *N Engl J Med* 2000;342:1149–1155.

69. Bonithon-Kopp C, Kronborg O, Giacosa A, et al. Calcium and fibre supplementation in prevention of colorectal adenoma recurrence: a randomised intervention trial. European Cancer Prevention Organisation Study Group. *Lancet* 2000;356:1300–1306.

70. Graham S, Zielezny M, Marshall J, et al. Diet in the epidemiology of postmenopausal breast cancer in the New York State Cohort. *Am J Epidemiol* 1992;136:1327–1337.

71. Horn-Ross PL, Hoggatt KJ, West DW, et al. Recent diet and breast cancer risk: the California Teachers Study (USA). *Cancer Causes Control* 2002;13:407–415.

72. Jarvinen R, Knekt P, Seppanen R, et al. Diet and breast cancer risk in a cohort of Finnish women. *Cancer Lett* 1997;114:251–253.

73. Terry P, Jain M, Miller AB, et al. No association among total dietary fiber, fiber fractions, and risk of breast cancer. *Cancer Epidemiol Biomarkers Prev* 2002;11:1507–1508.

74. Verhoeven DT, Assen N, Goldbohm RA, et al. Vitamins C and E, retinol, beta-carotene and dietary fibre in relation to breast cancer risk: a prospective cohort study. *Br J Cancer* 1997;75:149–155.

75. Willett WC, Hunter DJ, Stampfer MJ, et al. Dietary fat and fiber in relation to risk of breast cancer. An 8-year follow-up. *JAMA* 1992;268:2037–2044.

76. Botterweck AA, van den Brandt PA, Goldbohm RA. Vitamins, carotenoids, dietary fiber, and the risk of gastric carcinoma: results from a prospective study after 6.3 years of follow-up. *Cancer* 2000;88:737–748.

77. Missmer SA, Smith-Warner SA, Spiegelman D, et al. Meat and dairy food consumption and breast cancer: a pooled analysis of cohort studies. *Int J Epidemiol* 2002;31:78–85.

78. Cho E, Chen WY, Hunter DJ, et al. Red meat intake and risk of breast cancer among premenopausal women. *Arch Intern Med* 2006;166:2253–2259.

79. Cho E, Smith-Warner SA, Spiegelman D, et al. Dairy foods, calcium, and colorectal cancer: a pooled analysis of 10 cohort studies. *J Natl Cancer Inst* 2004;96:1015–1022.

80. Aune D, Lau R, Chan DS, et al. Dairy products and colorectal cancer risk: a systematic review and meta-analysis of cohort studies. *Ann Oncol* 2012;23:37–45.

81. Baron JA, Beach M, Mandel JS, et al. Calcium supplements for the prevention of colorectal adenomas. Calcium Polyp Prevention Study Group. *N Engl J Med* 1999;340:101–107.

82. Allen NE, Key TJ, Appleby PN, et al. Animal foods, protein, calcium and prostate cancer risk: the European Prospective Investigation into Cancer and Nutrition. *Br J Cancer* 2008;98:1574–1581.

83. Kurahashi N, Inoue M, Iwasaki M, et al. Dairy product, saturated fatty acid, and calcium intake and prostate cancer in a prospective cohort of Japanese men. *Cancer Epidemiol Biomarkers Prev* 2008;17:930–937.

84. Chan JM, Stampfer MJ, Ma J, et al. Dairy products, calcium, and prostate cancer risk in the Physicians' Health Study. *Am J Clin Nut* 2001;74:549–554.

85. Mitrou PN, Albanes D, Weinstein SJ, et al. A prospective study of dietary calcium, dairy products and prostate cancer risk (Finland). *Int J Cancer* 2007;120:2466–2473.

86. Tseng M, Breslow RA, Graubard BI, et al. Dairy, calcium, and vitamin D intakes and prostate cancer risk in the National Health and Nutrition Examination Epidemiologic Follow-up Study cohort. *Am J Clin Nutr* 2005;81:1147–1154.

87. Giovannucci E, Liu Y, Stampfer MJ, et al. A prospective study of calcium intake and incident and fatal prostate cancer. *Cancer Epidemiol Biomarkers Prev* 2006;15:203–210.

88. Snowdon DA, Phillips RL, Choi W. Diet, obesity, and risk of fatal prostate cancer. *Am J Epidemiol* 1984;120:244–250.

89. Park Y, Mitrou PN, Kipnis V, et al. Calcium, dairy foods, and risk of incident and fatal prostate cancer: the NIH-AARP Diet and Health Study. *Am J Epidemiol* 2007;166:1270–1279.

90. Park SY, Murphy SP, Wilkens LR, et al. Calcium, vitamin D, and dairy product intake and prostate cancer risk: the Multiethnic Cohort Study. *Am J Epidemiol* 2007;166:1259–1269.

91. Ahn J, Albanes D, Peters U, et al. Dairy products, calcium intake, and risk of prostate cancer in the prostate, lung, colorectal, and ovarian cancer screening trial. *Cancer Epidemiol Biomarkers Prev* 2007;16:2623–2630.

92. Gao X, LaValley MP, Tucker KL. Prospective studies of dairy product and calcium intakes and prostate cancer risk: a meta-analysis. *J Natl Cancer Inst* 2005;97:1768–1777.

93. Huncharek M, Muscat J, Kupelnick B. Dairy products, dietary calcium and vitamin D intake as risk factors for prostate cancer: a meta-analysis of 26,769 cases from 45 observational studies. *Nutr Cancer* 2008;60:421–441.

94. Ganmaa D, Cui X, Feskanich D, et al. Milk, dairy intake and risk of endometrial cancer: a 26-year follow-up. *Int J Cancer* 2012;130:2664–2671.

95. Genkinger JM, Hunter DJ, Spiegelman D, et al. Dairy products and ovarian cancer: a pooled analysis of 12 cohort studies. *Cancer Epidemiol Biomarkers Prev* 2006;15:364–372.

96. Hoppe C, Molgaard C, Juul A, et al. High intakes of skimmed milk, but not meat, increase serum IGF-I and IGFBP-3 in eight-year-old boys. *Eur J Clin Nutr* 2004;58:1211–1216.

97. Ganmaa D, Wang PY, Qin LQ, et al. Is milk responsible for male reproductive disorders? *Med Hypotheses* 2001;57:510–514.

98. Garland CF, Garland FC. Do sunlight and vitamin D reduce the likelihood of colon cancer? *Int J Epidemiol* 1980;9:227–231.

99. Feskanich D, Ma J, Fuchs CS, et al. Plasma vitamin D metabolites and risk of colorectal cancer in women. *Cancer Epidemiol Biomarkers Prev* 2004; 13:1502–1508.

100. Woolcott CG, Wilkens LR, Nomura AM, et al. Plasma 25-hydroxyvitamin D levels and the risk of colorectal cancer: the multiethnic cohort study. *Cancer Epidemiol Biomarkers Prev* 2010;19:130–134.

101. Jenab M, Bueno-de-Mesquita HB, Ferrari P, et al. Association between pre-diagnostic circulating vitamin D concentration and risk of colorectal cancer in European populations: a nested case-control study. *BMJ* 2010; 340:b5500.

102. Wactawski-Wende J, Kotchen JM, Anderson GL, et al. Calcium plus vitamin D supplementation and the risk of colorectal cancer. *N Engl J Med* 2006;354:684–696.

103. Park SY, Murphy SP, Wilkens LR, et al. Calcium and vitamin D intake and risk of colorectal cancer: the Multiethnic Cohort Study. *Am J Epidemiol* 2007;165:784–793.

104. Gorham ED, Garland CF, Garland FC, et al. Optimal vitamin D status for colorectal cancer prevention: a quantitative meta analysis. *Am J Prev Med* 2007;32:210–216.

105. Yin L, Grandi N, Raum E, et al. Meta-analysis: longitudinal studies of serum vitamin D and colorectal cancer risk. *Aliment Pharmacol Ther* 2009;30: 113–125.

106. Wei MY, Garland CF, Gorham ED, et al. Vitamin D and prevention of colorectal adenoma: a meta-analysis. *Cancer Epidemiol Biomarkers Prev* 2008; 17:2958–2969.

107. Freedman DM, Looker AC, Chang SC, et al. Prospective study of serum vitamin D and cancer mortality in the United States. *J Natl Cancer Inst* 2007;99:1594–1602.

108. Bertone-Johnson ER, Chen WY, Holick MF, et al. Plasma 25-hydroxyvitamin D and 1,25-dihydroxyvitamin D and risk of breast cancer. *Cancer Epidemiol Biomarkers Prev* 2005;14:1991–1997.

109. McCullough ML, Rodriguez C, Diver WR, et al. Dairy, calcium, and vitamin D intake and postmenopausal breast cancer risk in the Cancer Prevention Study II Nutrition Cohort. *Cancer Epidemiol Biomarkers Prev* 2005;14: 2898–2904.

110. Chen P, Hu P, Xie D, et al. Meta-analysis of vitamin D, calcium and the prevention of breast cancer. *Breast Cancer Res Treat* 2010;121:469–477.

111. Platz EA, Leitzmann MF, Hollis BW, et al. Plasma 1,25-dihydroxy- and 25-hydroxyvitamin D and subsequent risk of prostate cancer. *Cancer Causes Control* 2004;15:255–265.

112. Shui IM, Mucci LA, Kraft P, et al. Vitamin D-related genetic variation, plasma vitamin D, and risk of lethal prostate cancer: a prospective nested case-control study. *J Natl Cancer Inst* 2012;104:690–699.

113. Tworoger SS, Lee IM, Buring JE, et al. Plasma 25-hydroxyvitamin D and 1,25-dihydroxyvitamin D and risk of incident ovarian cancer. *Cancer Epidemiol Biomarkers Prev* 2007;16:783–788.

114. Toriola AT, Surcel HM, Agborsangaya C, et al. Serum 25-hydroxyvitamin D and the risk of ovarian cancer. *Eur J Cancer* 2010;46:364–369.

115. Stolzenberg-Solomon RZ, Jacobs EJ, Arslan AA, et al. Circulating 25-hydroxyvitamin D and risk of pancreatic cancer: Cohort Consortium Vitamin D Pooling Project of Rarer Cancers. *Am J Epidemiol* 2010; 172:81–93.

116. Skinner HG, Michaud DS, Giovannucci E, et al. Vitamin D intake and the risk for pancreatic cancer in two cohort studies. *Cancer Epidemiol Biomarkers Prev* 2006;15:1688–1695.

117. Wolpin BM, Ng K, Bao Y, et al. Plasma 25-hydroxyvitamin D and risk of pancreatic cancer. *Cancer Epidemiol Biomarkers Prev* 2012;21:82–91.

118. Giovannucci E. Epidemiology of vitamin D and colorectal cancer: casual or causal link? *J Steroid Biochem Mol Biol* 2010;121(1–2):349–354.

119. Giovannucci E. Epidemiologic studies of folate and colorectal neoplasia: a review. *J Nutr* 2002;132:2350S–2355S.

120. Kim D, Smith-Warner S, Spiegelman D, et al. Pooled analysis of 13 prospective cohort studies on folate and colon cancer. *Cancer Causes Control* 2010;21:1919-1930.

121. Chen J, Giovannucci E, Kelsey K, et al. A methylenetetrahydrofolate reductase polymorphism and the risk of colorectal cancer. *Cancer Res* 1996;56:4862–4864.

122. Osterhues A, Holzgreve W, Michels KB. Shall we put the world on folate? *Lancet* 2009;374:959–961.

123. Friso S, Choi SW, Girelli D, et al. A common mutation in the 5,10-methylene-tetrahydrofolate reductase gene affects genomic DNA methylation through an interaction with folate status. *Proc Natl Acad Sci U S A* 2002;99:5606–5611.

124. Kim YI. Folate: a magic bullet or a double edged sword for colorectal cancer prevention? *Gut* 2006;55:1387–1389.

125. Mason JB. Folate, cancer risk, and the Greek god, Proteus: a tale of two chameleons. *Nutr Rev* 2009;67:206–212.

126. Wu K, Platz EA, Willett W, et al. A randomized trial on folic acid supplementation and risk of recurrent colorectal adenoma. *Am J Clin Nutr* 2009; 90:1623–1631.

127. Cole BF, Baron JA, Sandler RS, et al. Folic acid for the prevention of colorectal adenomas: a randomized clinical trial. *JAMA* 2007;297:2351–2359.

128. Mason JB, Dickstein A, Jacques PF, et al. A temporal association between folic acid fortification and an increase in colorectal cancer rates may be illuminating important biological principles: a hypothesis. *Cancer Epidemiol Biomarkers Prev* 2007;16:1325–1329.

129. The effect of vitamin E and beta carotene on the incidence of lung cancer and other cancers in male smokers. The Alpha-Tocopherol, Beta Carotene Cancer Prevention Study Group. *N Engl J Med* 1994;330:1029–1035.

130. Virtamo J, Pietinen P, Huttunen JK, et al. Incidence of cancer and mortality following alpha-tocopherol and beta-carotene supplementation: a postintervention follow-up. *JAMA* 2003;290:476–485.

131. Mannisto S, Smith-Warner SA, Spiegelman D, et al. Dietary carotenoids and risk of lung cancer in a pooled analysis of seven cohort studies. *Cancer Epidemiol Biomarkers Prev* 2004;13:40–48.

132. Zhang X, Spiegelman D, Baglietto L, et al. Carotenoid intakes and risk of breast cancer defined by estrogen receptor and progesterone receptor status: a pooled analysis of 18 prospective cohort studies. *Am J Clin Nutr* 2012;95:713–725.

133. Eliassen AH, Hendrickson SJ, Brinton LA, et al. Circulating carotenoids and risk of breast cancer: pooled analysis of eight prospective studies. *J Natl Cancer Inst* 2012;104:1905–1916.

134. Giovannucci E. Tomatoes, tomato-based products, lycopene, and cancer: review of the epidemiologic literature. *J Natl Cancer Inst* 1999;91:317–331.

135. Yoshizawa K, Willett WC, Morris SJ, et al. Study of prediagnostic selenium level in toenails and the risk of advanced prostate cancer. *J Natl Cancer Inst* 1998;90:1219–1224.

136. Amaral AF, Cantor KP, Silverman DT, et al. Selenium and bladder cancer risk: a meta-analysis. *Cancer Epidemiol Biomarkers Prev* 2010;19:2407–2415.

137. Geybels MS, Verhage BA, van Schooten FJ, et al. Advanced prostate cancer risk in relation to toenail selenium levels. *J Natl Cancer Inst* 2013;105:1394–1401.

138. Hurst R, Hooper L, Norat T, et al. Selenium and prostate cancer: systematic review and meta-analysis. *Am J Clinical Nutr* 2012;96:111–122.

139. Lippman SM, Klein EA, Goodman PJ, et al. Effect of selenium and vitamin E on risk of prostate cancer and other cancers: the Selenium and Vitamin E Cancer Prevention Trial (SELECT). *JAMA* 2009;301:39–51.

140. Trock BJ, Hilakivi-Clarke L, Clarke R. Meta-analysis of soy intake and breast cancer risk. *J Natl Cancer Inst* 2006;98:459–471.

141. Wu AH, Wan P, Hankin J, et al. Adolescent and adult soy intake and risk of breast cancer in Asian-Americans. *Carcinogenesis* 2002;23:1491–1496.

142. Warburg O, Posener K, Negelein E. Ueber den Stoffwechsel der Tumoren. *Biochemische Zeitschrift* 1924;152:319.

143. Hu FB, Manson JE, Liu S, et al. Prospective study of adult onset diabetes mellitus (type 2) and risk of colorectal cancer in women. *J Natl Cancer Inst* 1999;91:542–547.

144. Michels KB, Solomon CG, Hu FB, et al. Type 2 diabetes and subsequent incidence of breast cancer in the Nurses' Health Study. *Diabetes Care* 2003;26:1752–1758.

145. Gnagnarella P, Gandini S, La Vecchia C, et al. Glycemic index, glycemic load, and cancer risk: a meta-analysis. *Am J Clinical Nutr* 2008;87:1793–1801.

146. Slattery ML, Benson J, Berry TD, et al. Dietary sugar and colon cancer. *Cancer Epidemiol Biomarkers Prev* 1997;6:677–685.

147. Terry PD, Jain M, Miller AB, et al. Glycemic load, carbohydrate intake, and risk of colorectal cancer in women: a prospective cohort study. *J Natl Cancer Inst* 2003;95:914–916.

148. Michaud DS, Liu S, Giovannucci E, et al. Dietary sugar, glycemic load, and pancreatic cancer risk in a prospective study. *J Natl Cancer Inst* 2002; 94:1293–1300.

149. Jonas CR, McCullough ML, Teras LR, et al. Dietary glycemic index, glycemic load, and risk of incident breast cancer in postmenopausal women. *Cancer Epidemiol Biomarkers Prev* 2003;12:573–577.

150. Tantamango-Bartley Y, Jaceldo-Siegl K, Fan J, et al. Vegetarian diets and the incidence of cancer in a low-risk population. *Cancer Epidemiol Biomarkers Prev* 2013;22:286–294.

151. Key TJ, Appleby PN, Spencer EA, et al. Cancer incidence in British vegetarians. *Br J Cancer* 2009;101:192–197.

ETIOLOGY AND EPIDEMIOLOGY OF CANCER

152. Fung T, Hu FB, Fuchs C, et al. Major dietary patterns and the risk of colorectal cancer in women. *Arch Intern Med* 2003;163:309–314.

153. Fung TT, Hu FB, Holmes MD, et al. Dietary patterns and the risk of postmenopausal breast cancer. *Int J Cancer* 2005;116:116–121.

154. Link LB, Canchola AJ, Bernstein L, et al. Dietary patterns and breast cancer risk in the California Teachers Study cohort. *Am J Clin Nutr* 2013;98:1524–1532.

155. Caughey RW, Michels KB. Birth weight and childhood leukemia: a meta-analysis and review of the current evidence. *Int J Cancer* 2009;124:2658–2670.

156. Michels KB, Xue F. Role of birthweight in the etiology of breast cancer. *Int J Cancer* 2006;119:2007–2025.

157. Michos A, Xue F, Michels KB. Birth weight and the risk of testicular cancer: a meta-analysis. *Int J Cancer* 2007;121:1123–1131.

158. Chavarro JE, Rosner BA, Sampson L, et al. Validity of adolescent diet recall 48 years later. *Am J Epidemiol* 2009;170:1563–1570.

159. Maruti SS, Feskanich D, Colditz GA, et al. Adult recall of adolescent diet: reproducibility and comparison with maternal reporting. *Am J Epidemiol* 2005;161:89–97.

160. Michels KB, Rosner BA, Chumlea WC, et al. Preschool diet and adult risk of breast cancer. *Int J Cancer* 2006;118:749–754.

161. Hjartaker A, Laake P, Lund E. Childhood and adult milk consumption and risk of premenopausal breast cancer in a cohort of 48,844 women - the Norwegian women and cancer study. *Int J Cancer* 2001;93:888–893.

162. Michels KB, Mohllajee AP, Roset-Bahmanyar E, et al. Diet and breast cancer: a review of the prospective observational studies. *Cancer* 2007;109:2712–2749.

163. Greenlee H, Kwan ML, Kushi LH, et al. Antioxidant supplement use after breast cancer diagnosis and mortality in the Life After Cancer Epidemiology (LACE) cohort. *Cancer* 2012;118:2048–2058.

164. Kwan ML, Chen WY, Flatt SW, et al. Postdiagnosis alcohol consumption and breast cancer prognosis in the after breast cancer pooling project. *Cancer Epidemiol Biomarkers Prev* 2013;22:32–41.

165. Chlebowski RT, Blackburn GL, Thomson CA, et al. Dietary fat reduction and breast cancer outcome: interim efficacy results from the Women's Intervention Nutrition Study. *J Natl Cancer Inst* 2006;98:1767–1776.

166. Pierce JP, Natarajan L, Caan BJ, et al. Influence of a diet very high in vegetables, fruit, and fiber and low in fat on prognosis following treatment for breast cancer: the Women's Healthy Eating and Living (WHEL) randomized trial. *JAMA* 2007;298:289–298.

167. Izano MA, Fung TT, Chiuve SS, et al. Are diet quality scores after breast cancer diagnosis associated with improved breast cancer survival? *Nutr Cancer* 2013;65:820–826.

168. van Meer S, Leufkens AM, Bueno-de-Mesquita HB, et al. Role of dietary factors in survival and mortality in colorectal cancer: a systematic review. *Nutrition Rev* 2013;71:631–641.

169. Meyerhardt JA, Niedzwiecki D, Hollis D, et al. Association of dietary patterns with cancer recurrence and survival in patients with stage III colon cancer. *JAMA* 2007;298:754–764.

170. Meyerhardt JA, Sato K, Niedzwiecki D, et al. Dietary glycemic load and cancer recurrence and survival in patients with stage III colon cancer: findings from CALGB 89803. *J Natl Cancer Inst* 2012;104:1702–1711.

171. Song Y, Chavarro JE, Cao Y, et al. Whole milk intake is associated with prostate cancer-specific mortality among U.S. male physicians. *J Nutr* 2013;143:189–196.

172. Richman EL, Kenfield SA, Chavarro JE, et al. Fat intake after diagnosis and risk of lethal prostate cancer and all-cause mortality. *JAMA Intern Med* 2013;173:1318–1326.

173. Richman EL, Kenfield SA, Stampfer MJ, et al. Egg, red meat, and poultry intake and risk of lethal prostate cancer in the prostate-specific antigen-era: incidence and survival. *Cancer Prev Res (Phila)* 2011;4:2110–2121.

174. Chan JM, Holick CN, Leitzmann MF, et al. Diet after diagnosis and the risk of prostate cancer progression, recurrence, and death (United States). *Cancer Causes Control* 2006;17:199–208.

175. Ornish D, Weidner G, Fair WR, et al. Intensive lifestyle changes may affect the progression of prostate cancer. *J Urol* 2005;174:1065–1070.

176. Kushi LH, Doyle C, McCullough M, et al. American Cancer Society Guidelines on nutrition and physical activity for cancer prevention: reducing the risk of cancer with healthy food choices and physical activity. *CA Cancer J Clin* 2012;62:30–67.

10 Obesity and Physical Activity

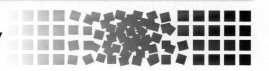

Yani Lu, Jessica Clague, and Leslie Bernstein

INTRODUCTION

Evidence showing that physical activity is associated with decreased cancer risk and that obesity is associated with increased cancer risk at certain sites is rapidly accumulating. It is not yet known whether these two factors are interrelated or independent. Physical activity may act to decrease cancer risk primarily by preventing weight gain and obesity. However, physical activity may also have independent effects on cancer risk. In this chapter, we present a summary of the current epidemiologic literature on the possible associations between physical activity and obesity and risk of cancer at several organ sites.

Physical activity is defined as any movement of the body that results in energy expenditure. In this chapter, we focus on recreational physical activity, also called leisure-time physical activity or exercise, and occupational physical activity, including household activity.[1] Occupational physical activity typically occurs over a longer period of time and generally requires less energy expenditure per hour than bouts of strenuous or moderate recreational physical activity. The distinction between recreational and occupational activity is important because increasing mechanization and technologic advances have led to decreased occupational physical activity in developed areas of the world, perhaps contributing to a decrease in overall physical activity.

Obesity is defined as the condition of being extremely overweight. In epidemiologic studies, the usual, but not necessarily the best, measure of body mass in adults is Quetelet's Index, or body mass index (BMI), which is measured as weight in kilograms (kg) divided by the square of height in meters (m^2). In the year spanning 2009 to 2010, the prevalence of obesity, defined by having a BMI of 30 kg/m^2 or greater, in the US population was 35.5% for adult men and 35.8% for adult women.[2] Physical inactivity has likely contributed to the high prevalence of obesity in the United States; data from the 2003 to 2004 National Health and Nutritional Examination Survey, a cross-sectional study of a sample of the civilian, noninstitutionalized population of the United States, has indicated that less than 5% of US adults achieve 30 minutes per day of physical activity, and that men are more physically active than women.[3]

Epidemiologic evidence on the associations of physical activity and obesity with cancer come from observational studies, including cohort studies, which follow populations forward in time after collecting exposure information, and case-control studies, which optimally identify a population-based series of newly diagnosed cases and healthy control subjects, collecting information retrospectively on exposures. In both study designs, physical activity information is usually self-reported and measures vary substantially with respect to timing and level of detail. Studies have measured lifetime or long-term physical activity, activity at defined ages or time points in life, and/or current or recent activity. Ideally, a study would capture activity by type (recreational, occupational, or other, such as an activity related to transportation), duration (minutes per session), frequency (sessions per day), and intensity (low, moderate, or strenuous as defined by examples of activity types) across the lifetime. These studies have often measured height and weight by self-report at one time point, such as at the time of study entry. Some studies have collected other or more detailed anthropometric information, such as waist circumference, hip circumference, or weight at an additional time point like age 18. Anthropometrics are directly measured by trained study personnel in only a few studies.

Epidemiologic evidence for a role of physical activity or obesity in relation to cancer risk exists for cancers of the breast, colon, endometrium, esophagus, kidney, and pancreatic cancer. Evidence is accumulating to link at least one of these "exposures" to the incidence of gallbladder cancer, non-Hodgkin lymphoma (NHL), and advanced prostate cancer. The evidence for an association between either physical activity or obesity and lung and ovarian cancer is inconclusive.

In addition to specific biologic mechanisms pertinent to physical activity or to obesity at each specific organ site, several global mechanisms have been implicated in both relationships across a number of these organ sites. The steroid hormone and insulin/insulinlike growth factor (IGF) pathways are two such global mechanisms hypothesized to be involved in the links between physical activity or obesity and cancer.[4] The role of steroid hormones as a mediator in these relationships is perhaps best understood in the context of breast cancer and endometrial cancer, and will be discussed in those sections. The roles of the insulin and IGF pathways have been discussed in depth with respect to colon cancer and, thus, will be presented in that context. Other global mechanisms have been proposed that have more generalized anticancer impacts and may explain associations between physical activity and several cancer sites; these include heightening immune surveillance, reducing inflammation, increasing insulin sensitivity, controlling growth factor production and activation, decreasing obesity and central adiposity, optimizing DNA repair capacity, and reducing oxidative stress.[5,6] Further, obesity has been shown to produce a proinflammatory state and, thus, inflammation may mediate the relationship between obesity and cancer risk.[7] It is highly plausible that several of these mechanisms act simultaneously and that they interact synergistically to mediate the associations between physical activity, obesity, and cancer.

BREAST CANCER

Low level of physical activity is an established breast cancer risk factor among postmenopausal women and, to a lesser extent, premenopausal women.[4,8,9] The evidence for an association between physical activity and breast cancer has been classified as convincing, with a 20% to 40% reduced risk among physically active women.[10] Obesity appears to have a paradoxical relationship with breast cancer risk in that it is an established breast cancer risk factor among postmenopausal women, but may offer some protection for breast cancer among premenopausal women.[4]

The epidemiologic literature has shown with relative consistency that breast cancer risk is reduced by increasing one's amount of physical activity.[4,8,9,11–13] One of the earliest studies, a case-control study of women age 40 years or younger, showed a dramatic reduction in risk of approximately 50% among women who averaged about 4 hours of activity per week during their reproductive years.[14] Similarly, among postmenopausal women, those with higher levels of recreational physical activity during their lifetimes have been shown to have lower breast cancer risk.[15] A meta-analysis of 29 case-control studies and 19 cohort studies published between 1994 and 2006 provided strong evidence for an inverse association between physical activity and risk of breast cancer, citing that the evidence for an association between physical activity and premenopausal breast cancer was not as strong as that for postmenopausal breast cancer.[8] The conclusion of the meta-analysis was that each additional hour of physical activity per week decreases breast cancer by approximately 6%.

Epidemiologists require that a risk factor demonstrate consistency across populations before considering it as accepted. Recently, studies have been published on the association between physical activity and breast cancer risk among Japanese,[16] Chinese,[17] Mexican,[18] Tunisian,[19] and African American women.[20] All studies showed a decreased risk of breast cancer with increasing physical activity. Interestingly, both Suzuki et al.[17] and Pronk et al.[21] observed the strongest associations among "heavier" women (BMI $\geq$25 kg/m^2 and 23.73 kg/m^2, respectively). In the California Teachers Study (CTS), a prospective cohort study of over 133,000 female public school professionals, a variable combining strenuous and moderate long-term recreational physical activity was associated with a reduced risk of estrogen receptor (ER)-negative but not ER-positive invasive breast cancer.[11] On the contrary, the Women's Health Initiative (WHI) observed decreases in breast cancer risk associated with recreational physical activity among postmenopausal women with ER-positive breast cancer and triple negative breast cancer, with only results for ER-positive breast cancer demonstrating a 15% statistically significant reduced risk (when comparing the highest versus lowest tertile of moderate-intensity physical activity).[22] Similar but not statistically significant results were observed for strenuous recreational physical activity.[22] A major limitation to this and previous studies stratifying by hormone receptor status is the inability to comprehensively classify triple negative breast cancer due to missing HER2 status (unknown in 40% of cases in the WHI study). The use of hormone therapy did not alter the inverse association between recreational physical activity and invasive breast cancer in the Women's Contraceptive and Reproductive Experiences (CARE) Study.[23] Most recently, in the American Cancer Society Cancer Prevention Study II Nutrition Cohort, it was observed that postmenopausal women who engage in at least 7 hours of walking over the course of a week had a modest decreased risk of breast cancer, even in the absence of more vigorous exercise.[24] Further, this association did not differ by ER status, BMI, adult weight gain, postmenopausal hormone therapy use, or time spent sitting.[24]

Lastly, whether physical activity reduces breast cancer risk by impacting preinvasive disease has been studied by assessing the associations with in situ breast cancer and benign breast disease. In the CTS cohort, increasing levels of long-term strenuous recreational physical activity were associated with a decreasing risk of in situ breast cancer.[11] Furthermore, a report from the Nurses' Health Study II cohort showed that lifetime recreational physical activity was associated with a decreased risk of benign breast disease and columnar cell lesions, which may be precursors to breast cancer.[25]

In summary, epidemiologic studies investigating the association between physical activity and breast cancer risk have produced relatively consistent results showing a reduction in breast cancer risk with increasing level of physical activity. Results to date suggest that moderate-to-strenuous activity may be required for the effect between physical activity and breast cancer risk to be clear; however, clarification of other key details, such as the importance of timing and intensity of activity or variation in effects by tumor characteristics, is pending.

Adult obesity and adult weight gain have both been associated with increased breast cancer risk among postmenopausal women, especially among women who were not current users of menopausal hormone therapy.[4,26,27] Most studies among postmenopausal women show a 1.5- to 2-fold increase in risk of invasive breast cancer when comparing the most obese women or those with the largest weight gain to normal-weight women (BMI: 18.5 to 24.9 kg/m^2) or those with the least weight gain.[4] Paradoxically, overweight or obese premenopausal women have a slightly decreased risk of breast cancer compared with normal-weight or thinner women. Whether larger waist circumference is more important than BMI has been studied in order to separate overall weight gain from abdominal obesity (i.e., visceral fat, which is one element of metabolic syndrome); however, most studies have reported a null association between waist circumference, used as a surrogate for visceral fat, and risk of postmenopausal breast cancer after adjustment for BMI.[26] In contrast to the results for postmenopausal women, waist circumference and a positive association with premenopausal breast cancer was found after adjustment for BMI.[26] A recent analysis of the Nurses' Health Study suggests that self-rated body fatness during youth and BMI at age 18 years are both inversely associated with breast cancer risk, with similar results for premenopausal and postmenopausal breast cancer.[28]

Hormones are central to the discussion of biologic mechanisms linking both physical activity and obesity with breast cancer risk. Physical activity can alter menstrual cycle patterns in premenopausal women, and hormone profiles in both premenopausal and postmenopausal women. Physical activity may lower body fat among children,[29] which in turn may delay age at menarche.[30] Later age at menarche has been associated with reduced breast cancer risk.[31] Physical activity may reduce the frequency of ovulatory cycles.[32] Having less frequent and therefore fewer cumulative ovulatory cycles is likely to reduce the lifetime exposure of the breast to endogenous ovarian hormones,[31] which are proven proliferative agents.[33] Physical activity also can have a direct impact on circulating estrogen levels among postmenopausal women.[34]

In the postmenopausal period, adipose tissue is the primary source of endogenous hormones via aromatization of androstenedione to estrone.[35] Thus, heavier postmenopausal women have higher levels of circulating estrogen than women with less adipose tissue. The involvement of estrogen in the relationship between obesity and breast cancer risk is supported by the observation that obesity does not independently increase breast cancer risk among menopausal hormone therapy users[27]; the obesity-related increase in estrogen over that provided by exogenous estrogens is negligible. The breast tissue of overweight or obese perimenopausal and postmenopausal women with relatively high risk of breast cancer has been shown to have cytologic abnormalities and higher epithelial cell counts than that of normal-weight women.[36] In contrast, obese premenopausal women experience menstrual cycle disturbances, including anovulatory cycles and secondary amenorrhea, thereby lowering their cumulative exposure to estradiol and progesterone.[31] A possible explanation for the inverse association between youth body fatness and breast cancer risk is that youth body size is inversely associated with adult IGF-1 levels.[28]

Other likely mechanisms that may link physical activity[37,38] and obesity[39,40] with breast cancer risk include aspects of immune function, inflammatory mechanisms, oxidative stress and DNA repair capability, metabolic hormones, and growth factors.

COLON AND RECTAL CANCER

An inverse association between physical activity and colon cancer risk has been consistently observed among epidemiologic studies; however, the evidence for rectal cancer remains inconclusive. Historically, comprehensive reviews have estimated that physical activity may reduce colon cancer risk by 20% to 25% when comparing individuals with the highest levels to those with the lowest levels of activity.[41] Risk reductions are greater for case-control studies (24%) than for cohort studies (17%), and risk reductions for occupational activity (22%) and recreational activity (23%) are similar.[41] In cohort studies, colon cancer risk reduction associated with physical activity is greater for men than for women, which may be due to the influence of hormone therapy on colon cancer risk,[42] although case-control studies suggest similar benefits for men and women.[43]

Whether physical activity preferentially protects against proximal or distal colon cancer is of interest. A meta-analysis including 21 cohort and case-control studies that examined associations between physical activity and the risks of proximal colon and distal colon cancers produced results suggesting that physical activity is associated with a reduced risk of both proximal colon and distal colon cancers, and that the magnitude of the association does not differ by subsite.[44]

Although the majority of previous studies have not found an association between physical activity and rectal cancer,[41] the National Institutes of Health (NIH)–AARP Diet and Health Study observed a modest reduction in rectal cancer risk for men but not for women after 6.9 years of follow-up.[45] Further, in a case-control study conducted in Australia, rectal cancer risk was reduced among men but not among women who participated in vigorous recreational physical activity averaging at least 6 metabolic equivalent task (MET)-hours per week during their adult years.[46]

An emphasis has been made on trying to identify risk factors for colon adenomas, which are considered precursor lesions for colon cancer; these are detected and removed during colonoscopy or sigmoidoscopy. Wolin et al. conducted a meta-analysis of 20 studies published through April 2010 that investigated the association between recreational physical activity and colon adenomas.[47] Adenoma risk was reduced by 19% among men and by 13% among women and, when combining men and women, the inverse association with physical activity was strongest for large/advanced polyps.

Obesity is an established risk factor for colon cancer in both men and women, although the relative risks for men have been higher than those for women.[4,26] The adverse impact of being overweight or obese on colon cancer risk is stronger for distal than for proximal colon cancers. In addition, visceral adiposity appears to confer greater risk than general adiposity.[26] In the European Prospective Investigation into Cancer and Nutrition (EPIC) study, abdominal obesity as well as adult weight gain were strongly associated with colon cancer risk in both men and women.[48,49] No association between these adiposity measures and colon cancer risk was evident among postmenopausal women who had used menopausal hormone therapy, and no association was observed between any measure of adiposity and rectal cancer risk.[48] The positive association between obesity and risk of colon cancer was further supported by the findings that both general obesity and abdominal obesity increase the risk of colon adenomas[47] with one study of women indicating that the distal colon is the main target site.[50]

Given that a higher BMI and lack of physical activity are both risk factors for colon cancer, several statistical approaches have been employed to tease apart their joint and independent effects on colon cancer risk. In the Netherlands Cohort Study,[51] colorectal cancer risk was increased at each subsite among larger women in the lowest recreational activity category (<30 minutes per day) than in smaller women in the highest recreational activity category (>90 minutes per day); however, the interaction between physical activity and body size was statistically significant only for proximal tumors. Using different fatness measures for men, the only similar finding was that men with low levels of physical activity whose trouser size was below the median of that for the cohort had an increased risk of distal colon cancer; no differences in risk were noted for other subsites or for men with larger trouser sizes.[51]

The mechanisms explaining the relationship between physical activity and colon cancer are not clearly established, but include the impact on insulin sensitivity and IGF profiles, and inflammation, as well as some colon-specific mechanisms. Physical activity may stimulate stool transit in the colon, thereby decreasing the exposure of colonic mucosa to carcinogens in the stool.[6] Alternatively, physical activity–induced decreases in prostaglandin E_2 may decrease colonic cell proliferation rates and increase colonic motility.[6] In addition to steroid hormones, which have been clearly implicated as biologic modifiers of the effect of physical activity and obesity on colon cancer risk, the insulin and IGF pathways may mediate the associations between these exposures and colon cancer risk. For obesity in particular, the link can be inferred because obesity can lead to insulin resistance,[52] a syndrome characterized by high circulating insulin levels. High insulin levels appear to promote cell proliferation and tumor growth in the colon[7] and may also suppress the expression of IGF-binding proteins 1 and 2, leading to increased bioavailable IGF-1 levels.[53] Another possible mechanism is obesity-enhanced inflammation in which increases in adipose tissue macrophages lead to the secretion of inflammatory cytokines associated with colon cancer risk (e.g., tumor necrosis factor [TNF]-α, monocyte chemoattractant protein [MCP]-1, and interleukin [IL]-6).

ENDOMETRIAL CANCER

The evidence for an association between physical activity and endometrial cancer risk is accumulating[4,54–58] but is not definitive. A meta-analysis of prospective cohort studies results published through 2009 indicates that recreational physical activity lowers endometrial cancer risk by 27%, and occupational activity lowers risk by 21%.[59] Adjustments for BMI minimally change relative risk estimates, suggesting that physical activity is independently associated with endometrial cancer. Although physical activity is associated with a decreased risk of endometrial cancer in both normal-weight and obese women, two recent studies have suggested that this association is more pronounced for obese women.[54,58]

Two meta-analyses of the association between physical activity and endometrial cancer have identified some inconsistencies in dose-response relationships, indicating the importance of differences in activity type and intensity.[55,56] Little evidence exists on how long-term or lifetime physical activity and activity patterns during different life periods might influence endometrial cancer risk; it has been suggested that recent or long-term activity might be more important than activity at early ages.[56] In the CTS, higher levels of recent (at cohort formation) strenuous recreational physical activity was associated with lower levels of endometrial cancer risk; among women exercising >3 hours per week per year, risk was approximately 25% lower than that of women exercising <0.5 hour per week per year.[60] This inverse association was limited to overweight and obese women (BMI ≥25 kg/m^2). Finally, sitting time has been independently associated with increased endometrial cancer risk.[59]

Epidemiologic studies have established a strong association between obesity and endometrial cancer risk.[26] Recent studies have suggested a linear trend between increasing body weight or BMI and increasing endometrial cancer risk among postmenopausal women, whereas among premenopausal women, no trend is observed, but rather, only obese women have an increased risk.[26] Furthermore, the strong association among postmenopausal women is only observed among those who are not using hormone therapy.[26] Finally, BMI appears to exert an effect on the risk of endometrial cancer that is independent of physical activity.[55]

Physical activity and obesity are likely to influence endometrial cancer risk by altering endogenous hormone profiles.[31,53] Heavier postmenopausal women have higher circulating levels of estrogen than do lighter postmenopausal women because of the aromatization of androstenedione to estrone in adipose tissue. This is pertinent to endometrial cancer risk because this aromatization occurs in the absence of progesterone, which opposes the proliferative effects of estrogen on endometrial tissue. Physical activity may counter the proliferative effects of estrogen either directly or by restricting weight gain. Some evidence also links elevated insulin levels and diabetes to endometrial cancer risk.[61] Physical inactivity and obesity play a role in the development of insulin insensitivity and diabetes, providing another mechanism by which they may influence endometrial cancer risk.

ETIOLOGY AND EPIDEMIOLOGY OF CANCER

ADENOCARCINOMA OF THE ESOPHAGUS

Several case-control studies[62–64] and one cohort study[65] have examined the association between physical activity and risk of adenocarcinoma of the esophagus. Zhang et al.[62] reported a modest association between participation in recreational physical activity more than once per week and a decreased risk of all esophageal cancer (adenocarcinomas and squamous cell tumors), although the result was not statistically significant. Lagergren et al.[63] reported no association between total, usual recreational and occupational physical activity and esophageal adenocarcinoma. Vigen et al.[64] showed that lifetime occupational physical activity was modestly associated with a lower risk of adenocarcinoma of the esophagus: the average annual level of occupational physical activity before age 65 years was associated with an approximately 40% reduction in risk of esophageal adenocarcinoma when the highest was compared with the lowest occupational physical activity category. Results from the NIH–AARP Diet and Health Study also support the hypothesis that physical activity lowers the risk of esophageal adenocarcinoma, but no association between physical activity and the risk of squamous cell esophageal cancer was found.[65]

Obesity is strongly associated with an increased risk of esophageal adenocarcinoma.[66,67] A pooled analysis of existing data showed that individuals with severe obesity (BMI $\geq$40 kg/m^2) had a 4.8-fold greater risk than individuals who were not overweight (BMI <25 kg/m^2), with similar risk estimates for men and women.[68] Several studies have examined the effect of abdominal adiposity, which have suggested that the risk associated with obesity is driven primarily by abdominal fatness.[26]

It is likely that obesity impacts esophageal adenocarcinoma risk because it is associated with the risk of gastroesophageal reflux disease (GERD). GERD may cause changes in the esophageal epithelium, leading to Barrett esophagus, a well-established precancerous condition for esophageal adenocarcinoma. On the other hand, obesity is associated with a systemic inflammatory state, which includes the exposure to adipocytokines and procoagulant factors released by adipocytes in central fat, which may also contribute to the development of esophageal adenocarcinoma.[67] Physical activity may influence the risk of esophageal adenocarcinoma by increasing digestive track transit time, thus reducing exposure of the esophagus to putative cancer-causing agents.

KIDNEY/RENAL CELL CANCER

Physical activity has been studied in relation to renal cell carcinoma in part because of the known deleterious effects of high BMI and hypertension on the risk of renal cell cancer; however, no association has been firmly established. A review of physical activity and risk of genitourinary cancers noted significant protective effects in 8 of 15 studies of physical activity in relation to renal cell carcinoma, with an average 8% reduction in risk when comparing individuals with the highest level of physical activity to those with the lowest level of activity.[69] Reductions in risk were greater for recreational than for other forms of activity and for activity performed later in life.

Obesity, in addition to high blood pressure and diabetes, is an established risk factor for kidney cancer.[26] It is still uncertain whether a gender difference exists, however. A meta-analysis has suggested a similar impact of BMI on kidney cancer risk among women and men, with an approximate 7% increase in risk per unit increase in BMI.[26] The effect of obesity may differ by histology; a recent study reported an increased risk observed for clear cell and chromophobe cancers, but not papillary renal cell cancer.[70]

PANCREATIC CANCER

Pancreatic cancer is generally diagnosed at an advanced stage and is associated with high mortality rates. A meta-analysis of 28 studies of pancreatic cancer showed that higher total lifetime physical activity and occupational activity were associated with a lower risk.[71] Nonsignificant reductions in risk were observed for recreational physical activity and transportation (walking and cycling as a form of commuting). Significant heterogeneity was present across the studies, making it difficult to find a definitive answer.

Evidence indicating that obesity is a risk factor for pancreatic cancer is convincing. Three large pooled analyses and three of four meta-analyses that encompass a range of well-designed, independent observational epidemiologic studies have demonstrated a positive association between obesity and pancreatic cancer risk.[72,73] Effects were relatively consistent across studies, with an approximate 10% or greater increase in risk for every 5 kg/m^2 increase in BMI. Two of the pooled analyses and one of the meta-analyses assessed measures of adiposity such as waist circumference or waist-to-hip ratio (WHR); each of the results suggested positive associations with pancreatic cancer risk.[72,74,75] The pooled analyses reported at least a 35% greater risk when the fourth quartile of WHR was compared to the first quartile. The meta-analysis study reported an 11% increase in risk associated with each 10-cm increase in waist circumference and a 19% increase in risk for each 0.1-unit increment in WHR.

GALLBLADDER CANCER

Gallbladder cancer occurs more frequently in women than in men, and the major risk factor is a history of gallstones,[10] which has been associated with the use of exogenous estrogens.[76] To date, we have found no epidemiologic literature investigating the possible association of physical activity and gallbladder cancer, although several studies have suggested a positive association between obesity and gallbladder cancer. In a meta-analysis comprised of 3,288 cases derived from eight cohort studies and three case-control studies, obesity was associated with a 66% increased risk of gallbladder cancer, and the increase in risk was larger for women than for men.[77] Further, two studies found that WHR was positively associated with gallbladder cancer risk among men and women with and without a history of gallstones, suggesting that abdominal obesity may be important in the etiology of this disease.[78,79]

NON-HODGKIN LYMPHOMA

Studies addressing physical inactivity and obesity as potential risk factors for NHL have been mixed, in part because they have not had a sufficient number of cases to assess risk by NHL subtype. Generally, studies have shown no overall association between physical activity and NHL risk.[4] The results of four cohort studies, the CTS,[80] WHI,[81] EPIC,[82] and the American Cancer Society Prevention Study-II[83] have been unconvincing, with WHI showing a nonstatistically significant positive association, whereas the other studies showed no association.

In 2008, the International Lymphoma Epidemiology Consortium (InterLymph) published a pooled analysis of 18 case-control studies with more than 10,000 cases reporting no association between BMI around the time of diagnosis and NHL risk overall, but an increased risk of diffuse NHL for severe obesity (BMI $\geq$40 kg/m^2).[84] The results from meta-analyses of cohort studies suggested a weak positive association overall and for diffuse NHL.[85,86] An analysis of two cohort studies has suggested that body size in early adulthood may be more predictive of NHL risk than that later in life for all NHL and for the diffuse and follicular subtypes.[87]

PROSTATE CANCER

More than 20 studies have assessed the potential association between physical activity and prostate cancer.[4,88,89] Regardless of the different approaches used, the populations studied, or the sample sizes of the studies, the majority of studies have suggested a modest reduction in risk with an increased level of physical activity.[4] In a review of the literature, Friedenreich and Orenstein[88] concluded that prostate cancer risk is reduced 10% to 30% when comparing the most active with the least active men and suggested that it may be high levels of physical activity earlier in life that are most relevant to this disease. An update to this review, based on 22 additional studies, indicates that the majority of recent research studies observed protective effects.[90] Leitzmann and Rohrmann[91] added that the associations with reduced risk may be most apparent for fatal prostate cancer. A current systematic review and meta-analysis, including 19 cohort and 24 case-control studies, agrees.[92] A pooled 19% reduction in risk was observed for occupational physical activity, and a 5% reduction was observed for recreational physical activity comparing the most physically active men to the least active.[92] An issue that somewhat reduces our confidence in these estimates is that considerable heterogeneity between studies was observed. Further, it is not yet clear whether these results reflect a true causal association or whether they are due to confounding by prostate-specific antigen testing, which may be more common among physically active men.

The early epidemiologic literature on the potential association between obesity and prostate cancer provided no consistent evidence of any relationship.[4] Recent studies have suggested that obesity may have a dual effect on prostate cancer risk. One meta-analysis reported that the risk of early-stage prostate cancer decreased by 6%, whereas the risk of advanced prostate cancer increased 9% per 5-kg/m^2 increase in BMI.[93] Another possibility is that obesity may decrease the likelihood of diagnosis of less aggressive prostate cancer. Proposed mechanisms include the paradoxical effects of testosterone on low-grade versus more advanced prostate cancer and alterations in insulin and circulating IGF-1.[94]

LUNG CANCER

Physical activity may reduce lung cancer risk by 30% to 40%,[88] but no definitive conclusion can be drawn because one cannot ignore potential residual confounding or effect modification due to smoking as an explanation for any observed association. Recent studies have attempted to address this issue by estimating risk within subgroups defined by smoking status. A recent review suggests an inverse relationship between heavy lifetime physical activity and lung cancer in former and current smokers that is consistent across all histologies, but is not observed among never smokers.[5] A small case-control study of current and former smokers enrolled in the Cologne Smoking Study came to a similar conclusion, observing a lower risk of lung cancer among participants who were physically active compared to those who were not.[95] In the large NIH–AARP Diet and Health Study, no associations were observed between occupational or recreation physical activity and lung cancer risk among those who never smoked.[96]

Due to sex differences in lung cancer pathology, risk factors, and prognosis, current research has also begun to investigate the association for men and women separately.[97] The recent literature consists of small case-control studies,[98] which lack statistical power to examine risks in subgroups defined by histology, smoking status, or sex, and which may be affected by survival bias in that rapidly fatal cases or those who are too ill to be interviewed are excluded from the study population.

Several studies have suggested the existence of an inverse association between increasing BMI and lung cancer risk.[99–102] Nevertheless, this inverse effect may have been due to residual confounding by smoking because the inverse association was restricted to ever smokers. One meta-analysis showed an inverse association between BMI and lung cancer in nonsmokers[103]; however, caution should be exercised when interpreting the results due to concerns about heterogeneity of risk estimates across studies, the quality of the original studies, and confounding by smoking.[104]

OVARIAN CANCER

The literature on ovarian cancer risk in relation to physical activity and obesity has been inconclusive. More than 18 studies have assessed the impact of physical activity on ovarian cancer risk. A meta-analysis of 12 studies found an approximate 20% decrease in ovarian cancer risk associated with physical activity when the highest category of exercise was compared to the lowest.[105] Four[106–109] of five[110] additional studies found no association; the fifth study found a nonsignificant 10% to 20% reduction in ovarian cancer risk for women who participated in at least 1 hour per week of recreational aerobic activity.

The evidence for an association between obesity and increased ovarian cancer risk is weak, with few studies showing a statistically significant result.[4,111] A meta-analysis of 16 studies indicated that adult obesity increases the risk for ovarian cancer; the overall pooled effect estimate was a 30% increase in ovarian cancer risk associated with adult obesity with a possible dose-response effect, but no variation in risk estimates across histologic subtypes.[111] In contrast, the results from the Ovarian Cancer Association Consortium, based on original data from 15 case-control studies, suggest that obesity only increases the risk of the less common histologic subtypes of ovarian cancer; obesity does not increase risk of high-grade invasive serous cancers, the most common subtype.[112] A pooled analysis of 12 cohort studies reported that BMI was not associated with ovarian cancer risk in postmenopausal women, but was positively associated with risk in premenopausal women.[113] Another meta-analysis, using 47 studies, showed that the positive association between BMI and ovarian cancer was restricted to women who had never used hormone therapy; among these women, risk increased by 10% with every 5 kg/m^2 increase in BMI.[114]

CONCLUSIONS

Table 10.1 illustrates the strength of evidence regarding increased physical activity as a protective factor and obesity as a risk factor

TABLE 10.1

Summary of the Strength of the Observational Epidemiologic Evidence for Physical Activity as a Protective Factor and Obesity as a Risk Factor for Cancer, By Type of Cancer

	Physical Activity	Overweight/Obesity
Breast, postmenopausal	+++	+++
Breast, premenopausal	++	++ (protection)
Colon	+++	+++
Endometrium	+	+++
Esophagus, adenocarcinoma	?	+++
Kidney/renal cell	?	+++
Gallbladder	?	++
Pancreas	?	+++
Non-Hodgkin lymphoma	?	+
Prostate, aggressive	+	+
Lung	+	?
Ovary	?	?

+++, evidence is convincing; ++, evidence is probable; +, evidence is possible; ?, evidence remains insufficient/inconclusive.

for cancer. The strength of evidence for each exposure is classified as convincing (+++), probable (++), possible (+), or insufficient and inconclusive (?). Overall, for physical activity, convincing evidence exists for an association with postmenopausal breast cancer and colon cancer; for obesity, the evidence is convincing for breast, colon, endometrial, esophageal, and kidney/renal cell cancer. Evidence for associations between these exposures and several other cancer sites is accumulating. Despite some convincing evidence of the effects of physical activity and obesity on the risk of certain cancers, it is difficult to make recommendations as to appropriate changes in lifestyle that will reduce a person's chances of developing cancer. We have no physical activity prescriptions to give at this time. Many questions remain to be answered: What are the ages at which physical activity will provide the most benefit? What types of activity should one do and at what intensity, frequency (times per week), and duration (hours per week)? Similarly, for BMI, is there some threshold below which the individual will not have excess cancer risk? Does purposeful weight loss during the adult years lower the risk associated with being overweight or obese? Finally, necessary research is ongoing to identify the biologic mechanisms that account for these effects and to determine whether all persons are affected equally. For instance, it is possible that genetically defined subgroups of the population respond to physical activity or obesity differently. Understanding mechanisms and population variation in these effects will illuminate appropriate prescriptions for lifestyle change.

REFERENCES

1. Caspersen CJ, Powell KE, Christenson GM. Physical activity, exercise, and physical fitness: definitions and distinctions for health-related research. *Public Health Rep* 1985;100(2):126–131.
2. Flegal KM, Carroll MD, Kit BK, et al. Prevalence of obesity and trends in the distribution of body mass index among US adults, 1999-2010. *JAMA* 2012;307(5):491–497.
3. Troiano RP, Berrigan D, Dodd KW, et al. Physical activity in the United States measured by accelerometer. *Med Sci Sports Exerc* 2008;40(1):181–188.
4. Vainio H, Bianchini F, eds. *IARC Handbooks of Cancer Prevention Volume 6: Weight Control and Physical Activity*. Lyon, France: IARC Press; 2000.
5. Anzuini F, Battistella A, Izzotti A. Physical activity and cancer prevention: a review of current evidence and biological mechanisms. *J Prev Med Hyg* 2011;52(4):174–180.
6. Hardman AE. Physical activity and cancer risk. *Proc Nutr Soc* 2001;60(1):107–113.
7. Gunter MJ, Leitzmann MF. Obesity and colorectal cancer: epidemiology, mechanisms and candidate genes. *J Nutr Biochem* 2006;17(3):145–156.
8. Monninkhof EM, Elias SG, Vlems FA, et al. Physical activity and breast cancer: a systematic review. *Epidemiol* 2007;18(1):137–157.
9. World Cancer Research Fund/American Institute for Cancer Research. *Food, Nutrition, Physical Activity, and the Prevention of Cancer: A Global Perspective.* Washington, D.C.: World Cancer Research Fund/American Institute for Cancer Research; 2007.
10. Ishiguro S, Inoue M, Kurahashi N, et al. Risk factors of biliary tract cancer in a large-scale population-based cohort study in Japan (JPHC study); with special focus on cholelithiasis, body mass index, and their effect modification. *Cancer Causes Control* 2008;19(1):33–41.
11. Dallal CM, Sullivan-Halley J, Ross RK, et al. Long-term recreational physical activity and risk of invasive and in situ breast cancer: The California Teachers Study. *Arch Intern Med* 2007;167(4):408–415.
12. Lahmann P, Friedenreich C, Schuit A, et al. Physical activity and breast cancer risk: The European Prospective Investigation into Cancer and Nutrition. *Cancer Epidemiol Biomarkers Prev* 2007;16(1):36–42.
13. Maruti SS, Willett WC, Feskanich D, et al. A prospective study of age-specific physical activity and premenopausal breast cancer. *J Natl Cancer Inst* 2008;100(10):728–737.
14. Bernstein L, Henderson BE, Hanisch R, et al. Physical exercise and reduced risk of breast cancer in young women. *J Natl Cancer Inst* 1994;86(18):1403–1408.
15. Carpenter CL, Ross RK, Paganini-Hill A, et al. Effect of family history, obesity and exercise on breast cancer risk among postmenopausal women. *Int J Cancer* 2003;106(1):96–102.
16. Iwasaki M, Tsugane S. Risk factors for breast cancer: epidemiological evidence from Japanese studies. *Cancer Sci* 2011;102(9):1607–1614.
17. Pronk A, Ji BT, Shu XO, et al. Physical activity and breast cancer risk in Chinese women. *Br J Cancer* 2011;105(9):1443–1450.
18. Sanchez-Zamorano LM, Flores-Luna L, Angeles-Llerenas A, et al. Healthy lifestyle on the risk of breast cancer. *Cancer Epidemiol Biomarkers Prev* 2011;20(5):912–922.
19. Awatef M, Olfa G, Rim C, et al. Physical activity reduces breast cancer risk: a case-control study in Tunisia. *Cancer Epidemiol* 2011;35(6):540–544.
20. Sheppard VB, Makambi K, Taylor T, et al. Physical activity reduces breast cancer risk in African American women. *Ethn Dis* 2011;21(4):406–411.
21. Suzuki R, Iwasaki M, Yamamoto S, et al. Leisure-time physical activity and breast cancer risk defined by estrogen and progesterone receptor status—the Japan Public Health Center-based Prospective Study. *Prev Med* 2011;52(3-4):227–233.
22. Phipps AI, Chlebowski RT, Prentice R, et al. Body size, physical activity, and risk of triple-negative and estrogen receptor-positive breast cancer. *Cancer Epidemiol Biomarkers Prev* 2011;20(3):454–463.
23. Dieli-Conwright CM, Sullivan-Halley J, Patel A, et al. Does hormone therapy counter the beneficial effects of physical activity on breast cancer risk in postmenopausal women? *Cancer Causes Control* 2011;22(3):515–522.
24. Hildebrand JS, Gapstur SM, Campbell PT, et al. Recreational physical activity and leisure-time sitting in relation to postmenopausal breast cancer risk. *Cancer Epidemiol Biomarkers Prev* 2013;22(10):1906–1912.
25. Jung MM, Colditz GA, Collins LC, et al. Lifetime physical activity and the incidence of proliferative benign breast disease. *Cancer Causes Control* 2011;22(9):1297–1305.
26. Boeing H. Obesity and cancer—the update 2013. *Best Pract Res Clin Endocrinol Metab* 2013;27(2):219–227.
27. Lahmann PH, Schulz M, Hoffmann K, et al. Long-term weight change and breast cancer risk: The European Prospective Investigation into Cancer and Nutrition (EPIC). *Br J Cancer* 2005;93(5):582–589.
28. Harris HR, Tamimi RM, Willett WC, et al. Body size across the life course, mammographic density, and risk of breast cancer. *Am J Epidemiol* 2011;174(8):909–918.
29. Goran MI. Energy metabolism and obesity. *Med Clin North Am* 2000;84(2):347–362.
30. Frisch R, McArthur J. Menstrual cycles: fatness as a determinant of minimum weight for height necessary for their maintenance or onset. *Science* 1974;185:949–951.
31. Bernstein L. Epidemiology of endocrine-related risk factors for breast cancer. *J Mammary Gland Biol Neoplasia* 2002;7(1):3–15.
32. Bernstein L, Ross RK, Lobo RA, et al. The effects of moderate physical activity on menstrual cycle patterns in adolescence: implications for breast cancer prevention. *Br J Cancer* 1987;55(6):681–685.
33. Anderson E, Clarke RB, Howell A. Estrogen responsiveness and control of normal human breast proliferation. *J Mammary Gland Biol Neoplasia* 1998;3(1):23–35.
34. Cauley JA, Gutai JP, Kuller LH, et al. The epidemiology of serum sex hormones in postmenopausal women. *Am J Epidemiol* 1989;129(6):1120–1131.
35. MacDonald PC, Edman CD, Hemsell DL, et al. Effect of obesity on conversion of plasma androstenedione to estrone in postmenopausal women with and without endometrial cancer. *Am J Obstet Gynecol* 1978;130(4):448–455.
36. Seewaldt FL, Goldenberg V, Jones LW, et al. Overweight and obese perimenopausal and postmenopausal women exhibit increased abnormal mammary epithelial cytology. *Cancer Epidemiol Biomarkers Prev* 2007;16:613–616.
37. Bernstein L. Exercise and breast cancer prevention. *Curr Oncol Reports* 2009;11(6):490–496.
38. Neilson HK, Friedenreich CM, Brockton NT, et al. Physical activity and postmenopausal breast cancer: proposed biologic mechanisms and areas for future research. *Cancer Epidemiol Biomarkers Prev* 2009;18(1):11–27.
39. Cleary MP, Grossmann ME. Obesity and breast cancer: the estrogen connection. *Endocrinol* 2009;150(6):2537–2542.
40. Brown KA, Simpson ER. Obesity and breast cancer: progress to understanding the relationship. *Cancer Res* 2010;70(1):4–7.
41. Friedenreich CM, Neilson HK, Lynch BM. State of the epidemiological evidence on physical activity and cancer prevention. *Eur J Cancer* 2010;46(14):2593–2604.
42. Mai PL, Sullivan-Halley J, Ursin G, et al. Physical activity and colon cancer risk among women in the California Teachers Study. *Cancer Epidemiol Biomarkers Prev* 2007;16(3):517–525.
43. Wolin KY, Yan Y, Colditz GA, et al. Physical activity and colon cancer prevention: a meta-analysis. *Br J Cancer* 2009;100(4):611–616.
44. Boyle T, Keegel T, Bull F, et al. Physical activity and risks of proximal and distal colon cancers: a systematic review and meta-analysis. *J Natl Cancer Inst* 2012;104(20):1548–1561.
45. Howard RA, Freedman DM, Park Y, et al. Physical activity, sedentary behavior, and the risk of colon and rectal cancer in the NIH-AARP Diet and Health Study. *Cancer Causes Control* 2008;19(9):939–953.
46. Boyle T, Heyworth J, Bull F, et al. Timing and intensity of recreational physical activity and the risk of subsite-specific colorectal cancer. *Cancer Causes Control* 2011;22(12):1647–1658.
47. Wolin KY, Yan Y, Colditz GA. Physical activity and risk of colon adenoma: a meta-analysis. *Br J Cancer* 2011;104(5):882–885.
48. Pischon T, Lahmann PH, Boeing H, et al. Body size and risk of colon and rectal cancer in the European Prospective Investigation Into Cancer and Nutrition (EPIC). *J Natl Cancer Inst* 2006;98(13):920–931.
49. Aleksandrova K, Pischon T, Buijsse B, et al. Adult weight change and risk of colorectal cancer in the European Prospective Investigation into Cancer and Nutrition. *Eur J Cancer* 2013;49(16):3526–3536.
50. Nimptsch K, Giovannucci E, Willett WC, et al. Body fatness during childhood and adolescence, adult height, and risk of colorectal adenoma in women. *Cancer Prev Res* 2011;4(10):1710–1718.

51. Hughes LA, Simons CC, van den Brandt PA, et al. Body size and colorectal cancer risk after 16.3 years of follow-up: an analysis from the Netherlands Cohort Study. *Am J Epidemiol* 2011;174(10):1127–1139.
52. Abate N. Insulin resistance and obesity. The role of fat distribution pattern. *Diabetes Care* 1996;19(3):292–294.
53. Calle EE, Kaaks R. Overweight, obesity and cancer: epidemiological evidence and proposed mechanisms. *Nat Rev Cancer* 2004;4(8):579–591.
54. Gierach GL, Chang SC, Brinton LA, et al. Physical activity, sedentary behavior, and endometrial cancer risk in the NIH-AARP Diet and Health Study. *Int J Cancer* 2009;124(9):2139–2147.
55. Voskuil DW, Monninkhof EM, Elias SG, et al. Physical activity and endometrial cancer risk, a systematic review of current evidence. *Cancer Epidemiol Biomarkers Prev* 2007;16(4):639–648.
56. Cust AE, Armstrong BK, Friedenreich CM, et al. Physical activity and endometrial cancer risk: a review of the current evidence, biologic mechanisms and the quality of physical activity assessment methods. *Cancer Causes Control* 2007;18(3):243–258.
57. Friedenreich C, Cust A, Lahmann PH, et al. Physical activity and risk of endometrial cancer: The European Prospective Investigation into Cancer and Nutrition. *Int J Cancer* 2007;121(2):347–355.
58. Patel AV, Feigelson HS, Talbot JT, et al. The role of body weight in the relationship between physical activity and endometrial cancer: results from a large cohort of US women. *Int J Cancer* 2008;123(8):1877–1882.
59. Moore SC, Gierach GL, Schatzkin A, et al. Physical activity, sedentary behaviours, and the prevention of endometrial cancer. *Br J Cancer* 2010;103(7):933–938.
60. Dieli-Conwright CM, Ma H, Lacey JV, Jr., et al. Long-term and baseline recreational physical activity and risk of endometrial cancer: The California Teachers Study. *Br J Cancer* 2013;109(3):761–768.
61. Kaaks R, Lukanova A, Kurzer MS. Obesity, endogenous hormones, and endometrial cancer risk: a synthetic review. *Cancer Epidemiol Biomarkers Prev* 2002;11(12):1531–1543.
62. Zhang ZF, Kurtz RC, Sun M, et al. Adenocarcinomas of the esophagus and gastric cardia: medical conditions, tobacco, alcohol, and socioeconomic factors. *Cancer Epidemiol Biomarkers Prev* 1996;5(10):761–768.
63. Lagergren J, Bergstrom R, Nyren O. Association between body mass and adenocarcinoma of the esophagus and gastric cardia. *Ann Intern Med* 1999;130(11):883–890.
64. Vigen C, Bernstein L, Wu AH. Occupational physical activity and risk of adenocarcinomas of the esophagus and stomach. *Int J Cancer* 2006;118(4):1004–1009.
65. Leitzmann MF, Koebnick C, Freedman ND, et al. Physical activity and esophageal and gastric carcinoma in a large prospective study. *Am J Prev Med* 2009;36(2):112–119.
66. Lepage C, Drouillard A, Jouve JL, et al. Epidemiology and risk factors for oesophageal adenocarcinoma. *Dig Liver Dis* 2013;45(8):625–629.
67. Ryan AM, Duong M, Healy L, et al. Obesity, metabolic syndrome and esophageal adenocarcinoma: epidemiology, etiology and new targets. *Cancer Epidemiol* 2011;35(4):309–319.
68. Hoyo C, Cook MB, Kamangar F, et al. Body mass index in relation to oesophageal and oesophagogastric junction adenocarcinomas: a pooled analysis from the International BEACON Consortium. *Int J Epidemiol* 2012;41(6):1706–1718.
69. Leitzmann MF. Physical activity and genitourinary cancer prevention. *Recent Results Cancer Res* 2011;186:43–71.
70. Purdue MP, Moore LE, Merino MJ, et al. An investigation of risk factors for renal cell carcinoma by histologic subtype in two case-control studies. *Int J Cancer* 2013;132(11):2640–2647.
71. O'Rorke MA, Cantwell MM, Cardwell CR, et al. Can physical activity modulate pancreatic cancer risk? A systematic review and meta-analysis. *Int J Cancer* 2010;126(12):2957–2968.
72. Aune D, Greenwood DC, Chan DS, et al. Body mass index, abdominal fatness and pancreatic cancer risk: a systematic review and non-linear dose-response meta-analysis of prospective studies. *Ann Oncol* 2012;23(4):843–852.
73. Bracci PM. Obesity and pancreatic cancer: overview of epidemiologic evidence and biologic mechanisms. *Mol Carcinog* 2012;51(1):53–63.
74. Arslan AA, Helzlsouer KJ, Kooperberg C, et al. Anthropometric measures, body mass index, and pancreatic cancer: a pooled analysis from the Pancreatic Cancer Cohort Consortium (PanScan). *Arch Intern Med* 2010;170(9):791–802.
75. Genkinger JM, Spiegelman D, Anderson KE, et al. A pooled analysis of 14 cohort studies of anthropometric factors and pancreatic cancer risk. *Int J Cancer* 2010;129(7):1708–1717.
76. Uhler ML, Marks JW, Judd HL. Estrogen replacement therapy and gallbladder disease in postmenopausal women. *Menopause* 2000;7(3):162–167.
77. Larsson SC, Wolk A. Obesity and the risk of gallbladder cancer: a meta-analysis. *Br J Cancer* 2007;96(9):1457–1461.
78. Hsing AW, Sakoda LC, Rashid A, et al. Body size and the risk of biliary tract cancer: a population-based study in China. *Br J Cancer* 2008;99(5):811–815.
79. Schlesinger S, Aleksandrova K, Pischon T, et al. Abdominal obesity, weight gain during adulthood and risk of liver and biliary tract cancer in a European cohort. *Int J Cancer* 2013;132(3):645–657.
80. Lu Y, Prescott J, Sullivan-Halley J, et al. Body size, recreational physical activity, and B-cell non-Hodgkin lymphoma risk among women in the California Teachers Study. *Am J Epidemiol* 2009;170(10):1231–1240.
81. Kabat GC, Kim MY, Jean Wactawski W, et al. Anthropometric factors, physical activity, and risk of non-Hodgkin's lymphoma in the Women's Health Initiative. *Cancer Epidemiol* 2012;36(1):52–59.
82. van Veldhoven CM, Khan AE, Teucher B, et al. Physical activity and lymphoid neoplasms in the European Prospective Investigation into Cancer and Nutrition (EPIC). *Eur J Cancer* 2011;47(5):748–760.
83. Teras LR, Gapstur SM, Diver WR, et al. Recreational physical activity, leisure sitting time and risk of non-Hodgkin lymphoid neoplasms in the American Cancer Society Cancer Prevention Study II Cohort. *Int J Cancer* 2012;131(8):1912–1920.
84. Willett EV, Morton LM, Hartge P, et al. Non-Hodgkin lymphoma and obesity: a pooled analysis from the InterLymph Consortium. *Int J Cancer* 2008;122(9):2062–2070.
85. Larsson SC, Wolk A. Body mass index and risk of non-Hodgkin's and Hodgkin's lymphoma: a meta-analysis of prospective studies. *Eur J Cancer* 2011;47(16):2422–2430.
86. Larsson SC, Wolk A. Obesity and risk of non-Hodgkin's lymphoma: a meta-analysis. *Int J Cancer* 2007;121(7):1564–1570.
87. Bertrand KA, Giovannucci E, Zhang SM, et al. A prospective analysis of body size during childhood, adolescence, and adulthood and risk of non-Hodgkin lymphoma. *Cancer Prev Res* 2013;6(8):864–873.
88. Friedenreich CM, Orenstein MR. Physical activity and cancer prevention: Etiologic evidence and biological mechanisms. *J Nutr* 2002;132(11 Suppl):3456S–3464S.
89. Friedenreich CM, McGregor SE, Courneya KS, et al. Case-control study of lifetime total physical activity and prostate cancer risk. *Am J Epidemiol* 2004;159(8):740–749.
90. Young-McCaughan S. Potential for prostate cancer prevention through physical activity. *World J Urol* 2012;30(2):167–179.
91. Leitzmann MF, Rohrmann S. Risk factors for the onset of prostatic cancer: age, location, and behavioral correlates. *Clin Epidemiol* 2012;4:1–11.
92. Liu Y, Hu F, Li D, et al. Does physical activity reduce the risk of prostate cancer? A systematic review and meta-analysis. *Eur Urol* 2011;60(5):1029–1044.
93. Discacciati A, Orsini N, Wolk A. Body mass index and incidence of localized and advanced prostate cancer—a dose-response meta-analysis of prospective studies. *Ann Oncol* 2012;23(7):1665–1671.
94. Rodriguez C, Freedland SJ, Deka A, et al. Body mass index, weight change, and risk of prostate cancer in the Cancer Prevention Study II Nutrition Cohort. *Cancer Epidemiol Biomarkers Prev* 2007;16(1):63–69.
95. Schmidt A, Jung J, Ernstmann N, et al. The association between active participation in a sports club, physical activity and social network on the development of lung cancer in smokers: A case-control study. *BMC Res Notes* 2012;5:2.
96. Lam TK, Moore SC, Brinton LA, et al. Anthropometric measures and physical activity and the risk of lung cancer in never-smokers: a prospective cohort study. *PLoS One* 2013;8(8):e70672.
97. Tardon A, Lee WJ, Delgado-Rodriguez M, et al. Leisure-time physical activity and lung cancer: a meta-analysis. *Cancer Causes Control* 2005;16(4):389–397.
98. Lin Y, Cai L. Environmental and dietary factors and lung cancer risk among Chinese women: a case-control study in Southeast China. *Nutr Cancer* 2012;64(4):508–514.
99. Bethea TN, Rosenberg L, Charlot M, et al. Obesity in relation to lung cancer incidence in African American women. *Cancer Causes Control* 2013;24(9):1695–1703.
100. Smith L, Brinton LA, Spitz MR, et al. Body mass index and risk of lung cancer among never, former, and current smokers. *J Natl Cancer Inst* 2012;104(10):778–789.
101. Andreotti G, Hou L, Beane Freeman LE, et al. Body mass index, agricultural pesticide use, and cancer incidence in the Agricultural Health Study cohort. *Cancer Causes Control* 2010;21(11):1759–1775.
102. Tarnaud C, Guida F, Papadopoulos A, et al. Body mass index and lung cancer risk: results from the ICARE Study, a large, population-based case-control study. *Cancer Causes Control* 2012;23(7):1113–1126.
103. Yang Y, Dong J, Sun K, et al. Obesity and incidence of lung cancer: a meta-analysis. *Int J Cancer* 2013;132(5):1162–1169.
104. El-Zein M, Parent ME, Rousseau MC. Comments on a recent meta-analysis: obesity and lung cancer. *Int J Cancer* 2012;132(8):1962–1963.
105. Olsen CM, Bain CJ, Jordan SJ, et al. Recreational physical activity and epithelial ovarian cancer: A case-control study, systematic review, and meta-analysis. *Cancer Epidemiol Biomarkers Prev* 2007;16(11):2321–2330.
106. Weiderpass E, Margolis KL, Sandin S, et al. Prospective study of physical activity in different periods of life and the risk of ovarian cancer. *Int J Cancer* 2006;118(12):3153–3160.
107. Lahmann PH, Friedenreich C, Schulz M, et al. Physical activity and ovarian cancer risk: The European Prospective Investigation into Cancer and Nutrition. *Cancer Epidemiol Biomarkers Prev* 2009;18(1):351–354.
108. Leitzmann MF, Koebnick C, Moore SC, et al. Prospective study of physical activity and the risk of ovarian cancer. *Cancer Causes Control* 2009;20(5):765–773.
109. Xiao Q, Yang HP, Wentzensen N, et al. Physical activity in different periods of life, sedentary behavior, and the risk of ovarian cancer in the NIH-AARP Diet and Health Study. *Cancer Epidemiol Biomarkers Prev* 2013;22(11):2000–2008.
110. Moorman PG, Jones LW, Akushevich L, et al. Recreational physical activity and ovarian cancer risk and survival. *Ann Epidemiol* 2011;21(3):178–187.
111. Olsen CM, Green AC, Whiteman DC, et al. Obesity and the risk of epithelial ovarian cancer: a systematic review and meta-analysis. *Eur J Cancer* 2007;43(4):690–709.
112. Olsen CM, Nagle CM, Whiteman DC, et al. Obesity and risk of ovarian cancer subtypes: evidence from the Ovarian Cancer Association Consortium. *Endocr Relat Cancer* 2013;20(2):251–262.
113. Schouten LJ, Rivera C, Hunter DJ, et al. Height, body mass index, and ovarian cancer: a pooled analysis of 12 cohort studies. *Cancer Epidemiol Biomarkers Prev* 2008;17(4):902–912.
114. Collaborative Group on Epidemiological Studies of Ovarian Cancer. Ovarian cancer and body size: individual participant meta-analysis including 25,157 women with ovarian cancer from 47 epidemiological studies. *PLoS Med* 2012;9(4):e1001200.

ETIOLOGY AND EPIDEMIOLOGY OF CANCER

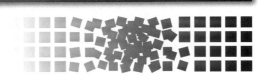

11 Epidemiologic Methods

Xiaomei Ma and Herbert Yu

INTRODUCTION

Epidemiology is the study of the distribution and determinants of health-related states or events in specified populations and the application of this study to control health problems.[1] Epidemiologic principles and methods have long been applied to cancer research, with the assumptions that cancer does not occur at random and the nonrandomness of carcinogenesis can be elucidated through systematic research. An example of such applications is the lung cancer study conducted by Doll and Hill in the early 1950s, which linked tobacco smoking to an increased mortality of lung cancer in over 40,000 medical professionals in the United Kingdom.[2] The observation from this study and many other studies, in conjunction with laboratory findings regarding the underlying biologic mechanisms for the effect of tobacco smoking, helped establish the role of tobacco smoking in the etiology of lung cancer. Epidemiologic methods are also used in clinical settings, where trials are conducted to evaluate the efficacy of new treatment protocols or preventive measures and where observational studies of prognostic factors are done.

Epidemiologic studies can take different forms, but generally they can be classified into two broad categories, observational studies and experimental studies (Fig. 11.1). In experimental studies, an investigator allocates different study regimens to the subjects, usually with randomization (experimental studies without randomization are sometimes referred to as "quasi-experiments").[3] Experimental studies can be individual based or community based. An experimental study most closely resembles laboratory experiments in that the investigator has control over the study condition. Experimental studies can be used to evaluate the efficacy of a treatment protocol (e.g., low-dose compared with standard-dose chemotherapy for non-Hodgkin's lymphoma)[4] or preventive measures (e.g., tamoxifen for women at an increased risk of breast cancer).[5] Although experimental studies are often considered the "gold standard" because of well-controlled study situations, they are only suitable for the evaluation of effects that are beneficial or at least not harmful due to ethical concerns. Experimental studies are discussed in detail in other chapters of this book. This section will focus on observational studies.

Observational studies do not involve the artificial manipulation of study regimens. In an observational study, an investigator stands by to observe what happens or happened to the subjects, in terms of exposure and outcome. Observational studies can be further divided into descriptive and analytical studies (see Fig. 11.1). Descriptive studies focus on the *distribution* of diseases with respect to person, place, and time (i.e., who, where, and when), whereas analytical studies focus on the *determinants* of diseases. Descriptive studies are often used to *generate* hypotheses, whereas analytical studies are often used to *test* hypotheses. However, the two types of studies should not be considered mutually exclusive entities; rather, they are the opposite ends of a continuum. Descriptive studies are discussed in detail in other chapters of this book.

ANALYTICAL STUDIES

Ecologic Studies

As in experimental studies, the unit of analysis can be individuals or groups of people in observational studies. Studies that use groups of people as the unit of analysis are called ecologic studies, which are relatively easy to carry out when group level measures are available. However, a relationship observed between variables on a group level does not necessarily reflect the relationship that exists at an individual level. For example, the fraction of energy supply from animal products was found to be positively correlated with breast cancer mortality in a recent ecologic study, which used preexisting data on both dietary supply and breast cancer mortality rates from 35 countries.[6] Because the data were country based, no reliable inference can be made at an individual level. Within each country, it could be that the people who had a low fraction of energy supply from animal products were actually dying from breast cancer. Results from ecologic studies are useful for inference at an individual level only when the within-group variability of the exposure is low so that a group-level measure can reasonably reflect exposure at an individual level. Alternatively, if the implications for prevention or intervention are at a group level (e.g., taxation of cigarettes to reduce smoking), results from ecologic studies are very useful.

Cross-Sectional Studies

There are three main types of analytical studies in which the unit of analysis is individuals: cross-sectional, cohort, and case-control studies. In a cross-sectional study, the information on various factors is collected from the study population at a given point in time. From a public health perspective, data collected in cross-sectional studies can be of great value in assessing the general health status of a population and allocating resources. For example, the National Health and Nutrition Examination Survey has provided valuable national estimates of health and nutritional status of the US civilian, noninstitutionalized population.[7] Findings from cross-sectional studies can also help generate hypotheses that may be tested later in other types of studies. However, it should be noted that cross-sectional studies have serious methodologic limitations if the research purpose is etiologic inference. Because exposures and disease status are evaluated simultaneously, it is usually not possible to know the temporality of events unless the exposure cannot change over time (e.g., blood type, skin color, race, country of birth). If one observes that more brain cancer patients are depressed than people without brain cancer in a cross-sectional study, the correlation does not necessarily mean that depression causes brain cancer. Depression may simply have resulted from the pathogenesis and diagnosis of brain cancer, or depression may

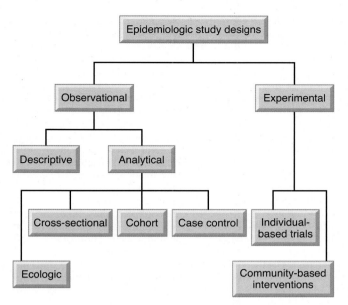

Figure 11.1 Classification of epidemiologic study designs.

have caused brain cancer in some patients and resulted from brain cancer in other patients. Without additional information on the timing of events, no conclusions can be made. Another concern in cross-sectional studies is the enrollment of prevalent cases, who survived different lengths of time after the incidence of disease. Factors that affect survival may also influence incidence. Prevalent cases may not be representative of incident cases, which makes etiologic inferences based on cross-sectional studies suspect at best.

Cohort Studies

In a cohort study, a study population free of a specific disease (or any other health-related condition) is grouped based on their exposure status and followed up for a certain period of time. Then the exposed and unexposed subjects are compared with respect to disease status at the end of the follow-up. The objective of a cohort study is usually to evaluate whether the incidence of a disease is associated with an exposure. The cohort design is fundamental in observational epidemiology and is considered "ideal" in that, if unbiased, cohort data reflect the real-life cause/effect sequence of disease.[8] Subjects in cohort studies may be a sample of the general population in a geographic area, a group of workers who are exposed to certain occupational hazards in a specific industry, or people who are considered at a high risk for a specific disease. A cohort study is considered prospective or concurrent if the investigator starts following up the cohort from the present time into the future, and retrospective or historical if the cohort is established in the past based on existing records (e.g., an occupational cohort based on employment records) and the follow-up ends before or at the time of the study. Alternatively, a cohort study can be ambidirectional in that data collection goes both directions.[9] Whether a cohort study is prospective, retrospective, or ambidirectional, the key feature is that all the subjects were free of the disease at the beginning of the follow-up and the study tracks the subjects from exposure to disease. Follow-up time, ranging from days to decades, is an essential element in cohort studies.

In a cohort study, the incidence of disease in the exposed group and the unexposed group is compared. The incidence measure can be cumulative incidence or incidence density, depending on the availability of data. When comparing the incidence in the two groups, both relative differences and absolute differences can be assessed. In cohort studies, the relative risk of developing

the disease is expressed as the ratio of the cumulative incidence in the exposed group to that in the unexposed group, which is also called cumulative incidence ratio or risk ratio. If we have data on the exact person-time of follow-up for every subject, we can also calculate an incidence density ratio (also called rate ratio) in a similar way. The numeric value of the risk or rate ratio reflects the magnitude of the association between an exposure and a disease. For example, a risk ratio of 2 would be interpreted as exposed individuals have a doubled risk of developing a disease than unexposed individuals, whereas a risk ratio of 5 indicates that exposed individuals have 5 times the risk of developing a disease compared with unexposed individuals. To put in another way, a factor with a risk ratio of 5 has a stronger effect than another factor with a risk ratio of 2. In addition to risk ratio and rate ratio, another relative measure called probability odds ratio can be calculated in cohort studies. The probability odds of disease is the number of subjects who developed a disease divided by the number of subjects who did not develop the disease, and the probability odds ratio is the probability odds in the exposed group divided by the probability odds in the unexposed group. Many investigators prefer risk ratio or rate ratio to probability odds ratio in cohort studies, because the ability to directly measure the risk of developing a disease is one of the most significant advantages in cohort studies. In practice, however, a probability odds ratio is often used as an approximation for risk or rate ratio, especially when multivariate logistic regression models are employed to adjust for the effect of other factors that may influence the relationship between an exposure and a disease.

As for absolute differences, a commonly used measure is called attributable risk in the exposed, which is the incidence in the exposed group minus the incidence in the unexposed group. Attributable risk reflects the disease incidence that could be attributed to the exposure in exposed individuals and the reduction in incidence that we would expect if the exposure can be removed from the exposed individuals, provided that there is a causal relationship between the exposure and the disease. Another absolute measure called population attributable risk extends this concept to the general population; it estimates the disease incidence that could be attributed to an exposure in the general population. Because both relative and absolute differences can be assessed in cohort studies, a natural question to ask is what measures to choose. In general, the relative differences are used more often if the main research objective is etiologic inference, and they can be used for the judgment of causality. Once causality is established, or at least assumed, measures of absolute differences are more important from a public health perspective. This point can be illustrated using the following hypothetical example. Assume the following: toxin X in the environment triples the risk of bladder cancer and toxin Y doubles the risk of bladder cancer, the effects of X and Y are entirely independent of each other, the prevalence of exposure to toxin Y in the general population is 20 times higher than the prevalence of exposure to toxin X, and there are only resources available to reduce the exposure to one toxin. It would be more effective to use the resources to reduce the exposure to toxin Y instead of toxin X. This is because the population attributable risk due to Y is higher than that due to X, although the risk ratio associated with toxin Y is smaller than that associated with toxin X.

Cohort studies have many advantages. A cohort design is the best way to study the natural history of a disease.[9] There is usually a clear temporal relationship between an exposure and a disease because all the subjects are free of the disease at the beginning of the follow-up (it can be a problem if a subject has a subclinical disease such as undetected prostate cancer). Furthermore, multiple diseases can be studied with respect to the same exposure. On the other hand, cohort studies, especially prospective cohort studies, are costly in terms of both time and money. A cohort design requires the follow-up of a large number of study participants over a sometimes extremely lengthy period of time and usually extensive data collection through questionnaires, physical measurements, and/or biologic specimens at regular intervals. Participants may be "lost" during the follow-up because they became tired of the study, moved away from the study area, or died from some causes other than the disease under study. If the subjects who were lost during the follow-up are different from those who remained under observation with respect to exposure, disease, or other factors that may influence the relationship between the exposure and the disease, results from the study may be biased. To date, cohort studies have been used to study the etiology of a wide spectrum of diseases, including different types of cancer. If a cohort study is conducted to evaluate the etiology of cancer, usually the study sample size would need to be very large (such as the National Institutes of Health-AARP Diet and Health Study, which included more than half million subjects[10]) and the follow-up time would need to be long, unless the cohort selected is a high-risk population.

For simplicity, we have discussed cohort studies in which the outcome of interest is the incidence of a specific disease and there are only two exposure groups. In practice, any health-related event can be the outcome of interest, and multiple exposure groups can be compared.

Case-Control Studies

Case-control design is an alternative to cohort design for the evaluation of the relationship between an exposure and a disease (or any other health condition). A case-control approach compares the odds of past exposure between cases and noncases (controls) and uses the exposure odds ratio as an estimate for relative risk. A primary goal in a case-control study is to reach the same conclusions as what would have been obtained from a cohort study, if one had been done.[11] If appropriately designed and conducted, a case-control study can optimize speed and efficiency as the need for follow-up is avoided.[8] The starting point of a case-control study is a source population from which the cases arise. Instead of obtaining the denominators for the calculation of risks or rates in a cohort study, a control group is sampled from the entire source population. After selecting control subjects, who ideally would have become cases had they developed the disease, an investigator collects data on past exposures from both the cases and the controls and then calculates an odds ratio, which is the odds of exposure in the cases divided by the odds of exposure in the controls.

There are two main types of case-control studies: case-based case-control studies and case-control studies within defined cohorts.[8] Some variations of the case-control design also exist. For instance, if the effect of an exposure is transient, sometimes a case can be used as his/her own control (case cross-over design). In case-based case-control studies, cases and controls are selected at a given point in time from a hypothetical cohort (e.g., at the end of follow-up). A cross-sectional ascertainment of cases will result in a case group that mostly contains prevalent cases who may have survived for different lengths of time after disease incidence. Cases who died before an investigator began subject ascertainment would not be eligible to be included in the study. As a result, the cases finally included in the study may not be representative of all the cases from the entire hypothetical cohort. Another disadvantage of enrolling prevalent cases is that cases that were diagnosed a long time ago will likely have difficulties recalling exposures that occurred before the disease incidence. In case-control studies, it is preferable to ascertain incident cases as soon as they are diagnosed and to select controls as soon as cases are identified. Case-control studies that enroll only incident cases are sometimes called *prospective* case-control studies because the investigators need to wait for the incident cases to develop and get diagnosed. For cancer studies, the cases can be ascertained from population-based cancer registries or hospitals. A major advantage of using a cancer registry is the completeness of case ascertainment; however, the reporting of cancer cases to registries is usually not instantaneous. There could be a lag time of several months or even over a year, and some cases could have died during the lag time. If the cancer

under study has a poor survival rate and/or clinical specimens need to be obtained in a timely manner, it may be preferable to identify cases directly from hospitals using a rapid ascertainment protocol. As for the selection of controls, the key issue is that controls should be representative of the source population from which the cases arise and, theoretically, the controls would have been ascertained as cases had they developed the disease. The most common types of controls include population-based controls (often selected through random digit dialing in case-control studies of cancer etiology), hospital controls, and friend controls. The advantages and disadvantages of different types of controls have been nicely summarized by Wacholder et al.[12] Because no follow-up is involved in case-based case-control studies, the incidence risk or rate cannot be calculated directly for case and control groups. The odds ratio will be a good estimate of relative risk if the disease is uncommon.

In addition to case-based case-control studies, there are also case-control studies within defined cohorts (also known as hybrid or ambidirectional designs), including case-cohort studies and nested case-control studies. In case-cohort studies, cases are identified from a well-defined cohort after some follow-up time, and controls are selected from the baseline cohort. In nested case-control studies, cases are also identified from a cohort, but controls are selected from the individuals at risk at the time each case occurs (i.e., incidence density sampling).[8] In these types of designs, controls are a sample of the cohort and the controls selected can theoretically become cases at some point. The possibility of selection bias in case-control studies within defined cohorts is lower than that in case-based case-control studies because the cases and the controls are selected from the same source population. Because of an increased awareness of the methodological issues inherent in the design of case-based case-control studies and the availability of a growing number of large cohorts, case-control studies within defined cohorts have become more common in recent years. The advantage of case-control studies within cohorts over traditional cohort studies is mainly the efficiency in additional data collection. For instance, a recent nested case-control study evaluated the relationship between endogenous sex hormones and prostate cancer risk.[13] Instead of measuring the serum hormones levels of the entire cohort (over 12,000 subjects), investigators chose to measure 300 cases and 300 controls selected from the cohort. Doing so not only significantly reduced the cost of measurements and the time it took to address the research question, but also helped preserve valuable serum samples for possible analyses in the future. In a case-cohort design, an odds ratio estimates risk ratio; in a nested case-control design, an odds ratio estimates rate ratio. In both designs, the disease under study does not have to be rare for the odds ratio to be a good estimate of the risk ratio or rate ratio.[8,14]

The biggest advantage of a case-control design is the speed and efficiency of obtaining data. It is claimed that investigators implement case-control studies more frequently than any other analytical epidemiologic study.[15] Because most types of cancer are uncommon and take a long time to develop, to date, most epidemiologic studies of cancer have been case-control instead of cohort in design. A case-control study can be conducted to evaluate the relationship between many different exposures and a specific disease, but the study will have limited statistical power if the exposure is rare. In general, a case-control design tends to be more susceptible to biases than a cohort design. Such biases include, but are not limited to, selection bias when choosing and enrolling subjects (especially controls) and recall bias when obtaining data from the subjects. The status of the subjects—that is, case or control—may affect how they recall and report previous exposures, some of which occurred years or even decades ago. It is important for investigators to explicitly define the diagnostic and eligibility criteria for cases, to select controls from the same population as the cases independent of the exposures of interest, to blind data collection staff to the case or control status of subjects and/or the main hypotheses of the study, to ascertain exposure in a similar manner from cases and controls, and to take into account other factors that may influence the relationship between an exposure and a disease.[15]

INTERPRETATION OF EPIDEMIOLOGIC FINDINGS

We have discussed measures of effects in various study designs. However, a risk ratio of 3 from a cohort study or an odds ratio of 2.5 from a case-control study does not necessarily mean that there is an association between an exposure and a disease. Several alternative explanations need to be assessed, including chance (random error), bias (systematic error), and confounding. Potential interaction also needs be evaluated.

Statistical methods are required to evaluate the role of chance. A usual way is to calculate the upper and lower limits of a 95% confidence interval around a point estimate for relative risk (risk ratio, rate ratio, or odds ratio). If the confidence interval does not include one, one would say that the observed association is statistically significant; if the confidence interval includes one, one would say that the observed relationship is not statistically significant. The width of a confidence interval is directly related to the number of participants in a study, which is called sample size. A larger sample size leads to less variability in the data, a tighter confidence interval, and a higher possibility in finding a statistically significant association if one truly exists. A 95% confidence interval means that if the data collection and analysis could be replicated many times, the confidence interval should include the correct value of the measure 95% of the time.[16] It is better to consider a confidence interval to be a general guide to the amount of random error in the data but not necessarily a literal measure of statistical variability.[16]

Bias can be defined as any systematic error in an epidemiologic study that results in an incorrect estimate of the association between exposure and disease, and it can occur in every type of epidemiologic study design. There are two main types of bias: selection bias and information bias. Selection bias is present when individuals included in a study are systematically different from the target population. For example, a selection bias would occur if a study aimed to generate a sample representing all women in the United States, but of the women contacted, more with a family history of breast cancer agreed to participate. This sample would be at a higher risk for breast cancer than the target population. Refusal to participate poses a constant challenge in epidemiologic studies. As individuals have become more concerned about privacy issues and as studies have become more demanding of time, biologic specimens, and other impositions, participation rates have dropped substantially in recent years. If nonparticipants are different from the participants with respect to study-related characteristics, the validity of the study is threatened. Information bias occurs when the data collected from the study subjects are erroneous. Information bias is also known as misclassification if the variable is measured on a categorical scale and the error causes a subject to be placed in a wrong category. Misclassification can happen to both exposure and disease. For example, in a case-control study of previous reproductive history and ovarian cancer, a woman who had an extremely early pregnancy loss might not even realize that she was ever pregnant and would mistakenly report no pregnancy, and another woman who has only subclinical presentations of ovarian cancer might be mistakenly selected as a control. Misclassification can be differential or nondifferential. An exposure misclassification is considered differential if it is related to disease status and nondifferential if not related to disease status. Similarly, a disease misclassification is considered differential if it is related to exposure status and nondifferential if not related to exposure status. If a binary exposure variable and a binary disease variable are analyzed, a nondifferential misclassification will result in an underestimate of the true association. Differential misclassification can either exaggerate or underestimate a true effect. Usually not much can be done to control or correct bias at the data analysis stage; therefore,

it is important to establish research protocols that are not prone to bias. The evaluation of potential bias is critical to the interpretation of study results. An invalid estimate is worse than no estimate.

Confounding refers to a situation in which the association between an exposure and a disease (or any health-related condition) is influenced by a third variable. This third variable is considered a confounding variable or confounder. A confounder must fulfill three criteria: (1) be associated with the exposure, (2) be associated with the disease independent of the exposure, and (3) not be an intermediate step between the exposure and the disease (i.e., not on the causal pathway). Unlike bias, which is primarily introduced by the investigator or study participants, confounding is a function of the complex interrelationship between various exposures and disease.[17] In a hypothetical case-control study of the effect of alcohol drinking on lung cancer, we may observe an odds ratio of 2.5 (usually called a "crude" odds ratio in the sense that no other variables were taken into account), which indicates that alcohol drinking increases the risk of lung cancer by 1.5-fold. However, if we classify all study subjects into two strata based on a history of cigarette smoking and then calculate the odds ratio in the two strata (smokers and nonsmokers) separately, we may have two stratum-specific odds ratios both equal to one, indicating that alcohol drinking is not associated with lung cancer risk. In this example, the crude odds ratio calculated to estimate the association between alcohol drinking and lung cancer without considering smoking is simply misleading. Being associated with both the exposure (i.e., alcohol drinking) and the disease (i.e., lung cancer), smoking acted as a confounder in this example. A stratified analysis is needed to evaluate the potential confounding effect of a third variable, whether it is done with pencil and paper or statistical modeling. Usually data are stratified based on the level of a third variable. If the stratum-specific effect measures are similar to each other but different from the crude effect measure, confounding is said to be present. In this section, we have illustrated basic epidemiologic principles using an overly simplified scenario and only considered a single exposure. In practice, most if not all diseases, cancer included, have a multifactorial etiology. Consequently, it is usually necessary to assess the potential confounding effect of a group of variables simultaneously using multivariate statistical models. The effect measure derived from a multivariate model will then be called an "adjusted" one in the sense that the effect of other factors was also adjusted for. Without controlling for the potential effect of other variables, an investigator cannot really judge whether an observed association between a given exposure and a specific disease is spurious.

If the effect of an exposure on the risk of a disease is not homogeneous in strata formed by a third variable, the third variable is considered an effect modifier, and the situation is called interaction or effect modification. Put in other words, interaction exists when the stratum-specific effect measures are different from each other. In the lung cancer example given previously, if the odds ratio for alcohol drinking is 1 in smokers but 3 in nonsmokers, then there is interaction and smoking is an effect modifier. The evaluation of interaction is essentially a stratified analysis, which is similar to the evaluation of confounding. Confounding and interaction can be both present in a given study. However, when interaction occurs, the stratum-specific effect measures should be reported. It is no longer appropriate to report a summary measure in the presence of interaction. Unlike confounding, which is a nuisance that an investigator hopes to remove, interaction is a more detailed description of the true relationship between an exposure and a disease.

CANCER OUTCOMES RESEARCH

The discussion of epidemiologic methods in this section focuses primarily on etiological research, which aims at identifying the risk factors of cancer. However, similar principles and methods are applicable to cancer outcomes research, which aims at studying a variety of factors related to the early identification, treatment, prognosis, health related quality of life, and cost of care. Cancer outcomes research can be experimental or observational in nature. For example, randomized clinical trials have been conducted to assess the impact of screening on prostate cancer mortality[18] and to compare the effect of radical prostatectomy versus observation in patients with localized prostate cancer.[19] Observational studies of cancer outcomes, especially those that build upon preexisting resources,[20,21] can be carried out in a large group of patients with relatively little cost to capture the patterns and cost of care and to address many other research questions that have important clinical implications. Although the findings of such observation studies are subject to bias and confounding inherent in an observational design, these studies are complementary to experimental studies and have their unique value. Given an increasing interest in improving the effectiveness and value of cancer care, more cancer outcomes research is to be expected in the future.

MOLECULAR EPIDEMIOLOGY

Molecular epidemiology involves multidisciplinary and transdisciplinary research that entails not only traditional epidemiology and biostatistics, but also genetics, molecular biology, biochemistry, cellular biology, analytical chemistry, toxicology, pharmacology, and laboratory medicine. Unlike traditional epidemiology research of cancer, which focuses on exposures or risk factors ascertained through questionnaire-based interviews or surveys, molecular epidemiology studies expand the assessment of exposure to a much broader scope that includes an analysis of biomarkers underlying internal exposure of exogenous and endogenous carcinogenic agents or risk factors, molecular alterations in response to exposure, and genetic susceptibility to cancer. The biomarkers often measured in molecular epidemiology research include DNA, RNA, proteins, chromosomes, compound molecules (e.g., DNA and protein adducts), and various metabolites as well as other endogenous and exogenous substances (e.g., steroids, nutrients, chemical or biologic toxins, and phytochemicals). Molecular markers can reflect different aspects of the tumorigenic process, which include biomarkers of internal exposure, biomarkers of molecular or cellular changes in response to exposure, and biomarkers of precursor lesions or early diseases.[22,23] Depending on the source of molecules and location of diseases, surrogates are often used in epidemiologic studies. When using a surrogate marker or tissue, the relevance of a proxy to its underlying target needs to be established or justified.[23] This justification is especially important when conducting population-based epidemiologic studies that focus on organ-specific cancers, because assessing biomarkers in target tissue is difficult for controls; molecular markers from blood samples are often used as substitutes. If a biomarker in the blood does not travel to or act on the tissue or organ of interest, an association between the circulating marker and the cancer may not be relevant. Thus, establishing a close link between a surrogate and its target is crucial in molecular epidemiology research.

Gene-environment interaction plays an essential role in cancer development.[24] Common genetic variations are considered an important determinant of host susceptibility and are a major focus of molecular epidemiology research. Depending on the biologic mechanism involved, genetic variations can influence every aspect of the carcinogenic process, ranging from external and internal exposure to carcinogens or risk factors to molecular and cellular damage, alteration, and response.[22,23] Currently, single nucleotide polymorphisms (SNPs) are the most studied genetic variations. It is believed that even if SNPs confer a small risk, they may still be important at the population level because these variations are common in the general population. It is also important that the impacts of SNPs on cancer are considered under the context of gene–gene and gene–environment interactions. As genotyping technology has advanced substantially with respect to its analytic

quality, capacity, and cost, research of genetic polymorphisms has evolved rapidly from investigations of a single SNP to studies of haplotypes and tag SNPs, and from a pathway-based candidate gene approach to genome-wide association studies (GWAS).[25] A GWAS analyzes hundreds of thousands of SNPs simultaneously for hundreds or even thousands of study subjects. When these data are further combined with questionnaire information such as environmental exposures, lifestyle factors, dietary habits, and medical history, enormous information is generated, which requires a huge sample size to allow for a reliable and complete assessment of these variables individually and jointly. A single epidemiologic study can no longer provide sufficient power for this type of investigation. Multicenter investigations or study consortia that pool study information and specimens together are developed to address the sample size issue.[26] False-positive findings resulting from multiple comparisons constitute a major challenge in epidemiologic studies of genetic associations with cancer.[27] A meta-analysis or pooled analysis can be used to address this problem if sufficient studies are already published and available for evaluation. To address this issue at the time of study design, one may adopt a two- or multiphase study design in which study subjects are divided into two or multiple groups for genotyping and data analysis. Selected or genomewide SNPs are first screened in one group of the study subjects (discovery phase), and then the significant findings determined by stringent statistical criteria (usually p values less than 1×10^{-5} or 1×10^{-7}) are reanalyzed in one or several other groups of subjects for verification (validation phase). This study design also lowers the cost of genotyping. False-positive findings can also be addressed with various statistical methods, such as bootstrap, permutation test, estimate of false positive report probability, prediction of false discovery rate, and the use of a much more stringent p value to accommodate multiple comparisons. For epidemiologic studies that are not population based or not conducted strictly following epidemiology principles, population stratification is a potential source of bias that may distort genetic associations.[28]

A large number of GWAS have been completed in search for SNPs that influence host susceptibility to cancer. Considering that more than 5 million SNPs are present in the human genome, the numbers of SNPs that are found to be associated with cancer risk after rigorous validation are much fewer than what one would have anticipated. In addition, the risk associations detected are quite weak, with most of the odds ratios ranging from 1.1 to 1.5, and the functional relevance or biologic implications are unclear for most of the SNPs. Furthermore, not many SNPs associated with cancer risk are located in protein-coding regions, and even fewer are in the loci of candidate genes suspected to be involved in tumorigenesis, such as oncogenes, tumor suppressor genes, DNA repair genes, and xenobiotic metabolizing or detoxification genes. Genes where SNPs are found to be linked to cancer by GWAS include *FGFR2, MAP3K1, MRPS30, LSP1, TNRC9, TOX3, STXBP1,* and *RAD51L1* for breast cancer[29–31]; *JAZF1, HNF1B, MSMB, CTBP2,* and *KLK2/KLK3* for prostate cancer[29,32]; *SMAD7, CRAC1, EIF3H, BMP4, CDH1,* and *RHPN2* for colorectal cancer[29,33]; *CHRNA3* and *CHRNA5* for lung cancer[34,35]; *ABO* for pancreatic cancer[36]; *TACC3* and *PSCA* for bladder cancer[37,38]; and *KRT5* for basal cell carcinoma.[39] Among these genes identified by GWAS, two findings are considered especially interesting. One is the association of lung cancer with *CHRNA3* and *CHRNA5,* which encode neuronal nicotinic acetylcholine receptor subunits. Different genotypes of these receptor subunits appear to influence individual's addiction to tobacco, which further leads to different smoking exposure and lung cancer risk.[40,41] Another is the link of the *ABO* gene to pancreatic cancer. The association between pancreatic cancer risk and ABO blood type was observed 50 years ago. The GWAS finding not only confirms the relationship, but also provides new clues for understanding the underlying biologic mechanism.

Besides intragenic SNPs, GWAS also found many intergenic SNPs in association to cancer risk, which include those in the regions of 8q24, 5p15, 1p11, 1p36, 1q42, 2p15, 2q35, 3p12, 3p24,

3q28, 6p21, 6q25, 7q21, 7q32, 9p21, 9p22, 9p24, 9q22, 10p14, 11q13, 11q23, 14q13, 18q23, and 20p12.[29–31,33,39,42–48] Of these loci, SNPs in 8q24 are associated with several cancer sites, including prostate, breast, colon, and bladder.[29,31–33,47–49] Further analysis of 8q24 indicates that there are nine SNPs in five regions and each region is independently related to different types of cancer, with SNPs in regions 1, 4, and 5 associated exclusively with prostate cancer, a SNP in region 2 related to breast cancer, and SNPs in region 3 linked to prostate, colon, and ovarian cancers.[50] No known genes are located within the region of 8q24, but an oncogene c-MYC resides about 330 kb downstream of the region.[51] An initial investigation found no evidence of the SNPs' influence on c-MYC expression,[47] but a later study suggests that the SNPs in 8q24 may be distal enhancers of c-MYC, interacting with its promoter through a chromatin loop.[52] Another genomic region that is associated with the risk of multiple cancer sites is 5p15, a region involving telomerase reverse transcriptase (TERT) cleft lip and palate transmembrane protein 1–like protein (CLPTM1L). Five types of cancer are found to be linked to this region, including basal cell carcinoma, lung, bladder, prostate, and cervical cancers.[53] TERT extends the length of telomere and is associated with cell proliferation and abnormal telomere maintenance.[54] The risk alleles of TERT are associated with shorter telomere length among the elderly and with higher DNA adduct in the lungs.[53,55]

GWAS has demonstrated its value in identifying disease-related SNPs in unknown regions of the genome, which provides new clues for investigators to interrogate and understand different regions of the human genome, especially in the gene-desert areas. Despite the strength, the low yield of significant findings from the GWAS has raised concerns in several areas, including the SNP coverage in the genome (rare SNPs and SNP representativeness in unknown regions), associations with low statistical significance (p value between 0.01 and 1×10^{-5}, the GWAS cutoff), other forms of genetic variations (copy number variation and other structural variations), cancer subtypes, and genetic interplay with environmental factors (gene–environment interaction).[56,57] To address these issues, investigators propose to perform fine-mapping and resequencing of genetic regions more specifically and meticulously. Epidemiologists suggest that detailed environmental exposure and lifestyle factors should be included in the next wave of GWAS. Furthermore, to make the study more reliable and compelling, DNA specimens, instead of convenient samples, should come from well-designed and well-executed epidemiologic studies that pay close attention to the selection of study subjects and the measurement of environmental and lifestyle factors to eliminate or minimize selection bias and measurement errors.

As described earlier, analytical epidemiology has two major study designs: the case-control study and the cohort study. It is important that investigators choose an appropriate study design to investigate molecular markers in epidemiologic studies. Two types of molecular markers, genotypic and phenotypic markers, can be considered. Genotypic markers refer to nucleotide sequences of genomic DNA, and all other molecules are considered phenotypic markers, including most of the chemical modifications on DNA, such as cytosine methylation. The distinction between the two is a marker's status in relation to an outcome variable, usually a disease. Genotypic markers generally do not change over time and are not affected by the development of a disease, whereas phenotypic markers are likely to change over time or be influenced by the presence of a disease, either itself or the treatment associated with it. If measurements of a phenotypic marker are made from the specimens that are collected after or at the time of cancer diagnosis, investigators will have difficulties determining the status of the phenotypic marker before the cancer was diagnosed. A disease condition, however, does not affect genotypic markers such as SNPs; therefore, a temporal relationship can be easily established even if the samples are collected after the disease is diagnosed. Based on this distinction, one can evaluate genotypic markers either in case-control or cohort studies, but a case-control study would be the design of choice because of efficiency and cost-effectiveness. A prospective cohort study design is ideal for phenotypic markers. Investigators, however, may use other study designs if they can demonstrate that the disease status does not influence the phenotypic markers of interest. To reduce study cost, investigators usually use nested case-control or case-cohort designs to avoid analyzing specimens from the entire cohort. The main purpose in choosing a cohort study design for a molecular epidemiology investigation is to ensure that biospecimens are collected before the development of a disease so that a temporal relationship between a marker and disease development can be established.

The differences between molecular epidemiology and genetic epidemiology are the scope of the molecular analysis and the emphasis on heredity. Sometimes molecular and genetic epidemiology both investigate genetic factors in association with cancer risk, but each has its own emphasis. The former assesses genetic involvement, but not necessarily inheritance, whereas the latter focuses mainly on heredity. Because of the difference in focus, study populations are different between the two types of investigation. Molecular epidemiology studies unrelated individuals, whereas genetic epidemiology investigates family members in the format of pedigrees, parent–child trios, or sibling pairs. Given the different research focus between genetic and molecular epidemiology, these investigations evaluate different genetic markers. Genetic epidemiology research is designed to identify genetic markers with high penetrance (strong association with an underlying disease) but low prevalence in the general populations, whereas a molecular epidemiology investigation targets low penetrance markers that are commonly present in the general population. Given the difference in study design, the analysis of genetic marker's link to cancer is also different between the studies. Relative risks or odds ratios are calculated in molecular epidemiology studies because study participants are unrelated individuals, whereas linkage analysis is used in genetic epidemiology because individuals in the study are genetically related family members. Recently, both genetic and molecular epidemiology study designs have been considered in GWAS to improve study validity and to minimize false positive findings. Another difference between genetic and molecular epidemiology research is that molecular epidemiology also studies nongenetic molecules. Thus, the scope of molecular analysis is much broader in molecular epidemiology research than in genetic epidemiology studies.

A laboratory analysis of molecular markers is another integral part of molecular epidemiology research, which has unique features that are different from basic science research. Collecting biologic specimens is difficult and expensive in population-based epidemiologic studies. It not only increases the study cost, but also imposes constraints to multiple areas of epidemiology research. Specimen collection may adversely influence the response rate of study participants, potentially compromising study validity. For organ-specific cancer research, investigating molecular markers in target tissue is difficult. Blood is the most common and versatile specimen used in molecular epidemiology research; other specimens used include urine, stool, nail, hair, sputum, buccal cells, and saliva. Tissue samples, either fresh frozen or chemically fixed, are also used, but the availability of these samples is highly limited to patients or selected subgroups of a general study population. Comparability and generalizability are always problems in epidemiologic studies involving tissue specimens, except for those investigations that focus on cancer prognosis or treatment in which only cancer patients are involved. Attempts have been made to use special body fluids for epidemiologic research, such as nipple aspirate and breast or pulmonary lavage, but the difficulty in specimen collection and preparation makes these samples impractical in large population-based studies.

Given the research value of biologic specimens and the difficulty in collecting them for population-based studies, technical issues related to specimen collection, processing, and storage become especially important in molecular epidemiology research.

These include time and conditions for specimen transportation and processing, a sample aliquot and labeling system, a sample special treatment for storage and analysis, a sample storage and tracking system, as well as backup plans and equipment for unexpected adverse events during long-term storage (e.g., power failure, earthquake, flooding). Laboratory methods used to analyze biomarkers are also important in molecular epidemiology. Because large numbers of specimens are involved, laboratory methods are required to be robust, reproducible, high throughput, low cost, and easy to use. These requirements are often met in the analysis of nucleotide sequences that serve as genotypic markers. However, for phenotypic markers, many methods do not readily meet these requirements. Moreover, many phenotypic markers, such as proteins, require both qualitative and quantitative assessments. An ideal laboratory method should be quantitative (able to measure a wide range of values), sensitive (able to detect a small amount of analyte), specific (able to detect only the molecule of interest, no other molecules), reproducible (high precision and low variation), and versatile (easy to use). In addition, investigators need to implement appropriate quality assurance procedures during sample processing and testing as well as include appropriate quality control samples in specimen analysis.

Host–environment interaction is believed to play a key role in the etiology of most types of cancer. Genetic factors, including mutations and polymorphisms, are initially considered important host factors, but recent developments in cancer research has indicated that epigenetic factors may also play a critical role in cancer as a host factor involved in host–environment interaction. Epigenetic factors, which regulate the function of human genome without altering the physical sequences of nucleotides, include pretranscription regulation through nucleotide modification (e.g., cytosine methylation at CpG sites), chromosome modification (e.g., histone acetylation), and posttranscription regulation by noncoding small RNA (e.g., microRNAs). These epigenetic factors have two unique features that have captured the attention of cancer researchers, especially cancer epidemiologists who are interested in the gene–environment interaction. It is known that epigenetic factors are heritable, but these inherited features are readily modifiable by environmental and lifestyle factors. Monozygotic twins have an identical genome as well as epigenome at birth, but the latter undergoes substantial changes over time, resulting in distinct epigenetic profiles that depend heavily on their environmental exposures.[58] Animal studies also indicated that the maternal intake of dietary nutrients involving one-carbon metabolism could influence offsprings' growth phenotypes, which are regulated by DNA methylation.[59] As evidence mounts on epigenetic involvement in cancer, molecular epidemiologists will start to look for clues in human populations that can link epigenetic factors to both lifestyle factors and cancer risk. Given that epigenetic regulation is tissue specific and time dependent, investigators face challenges in accurately assessing these phenotypic markers in etiologic studies. However, progress in the analysis of circulating methylation markers and microRNAs may provide an alternative to study epigenetic regulation in human cancer. Furthermore, methods for a genome-wide analysis of DNA methylation have been developed and applied in epidemiologic studies, which can substantially accelerate the search for cancer-related DNA methylation. Together with the high-throughput, high-dimensional analysis of DNA methylation, two other evolving fields that will have significant impacts on molecular epidemiology of cancer research are metagenomics and metabolomics. The former focuses on environmental genomics of the microbiome that resides in our body and influences one's biologic functions and health status. The latter refers to the analysis of hundreds or thousands of metabolites in a biologic specimen, including tissue, blood, urine, body fluids, and fecal samples. These new analyses will add tremendous value to epidemiologic studies.

REFERENCES

1. Last J. *A Dictionary of Epidemiology*. 3rd ed. New York: Oxford University Press; 1995.
2. Doll R, Hill AB. Lung cancer and other causes of death in relation to smoking: a second report on the mortality of British doctors. *Br Med J* 1956;12:1071–1081.
3. Kleinbaum D, Kupper L, Morgenstern H. *Epidemiologic Research*. New York: Van Nostrand Reinhold; 1982.
4. Kaplan LD, Straus DJ, Testa MA, et al. Low-dose compared with standard-dose m-BACOD chemotherapy for non-Hodgkin's lymphoma associated with human immunodeficiency virus infection. National Institute of Allergy and Infectious Diseases AIDS Clinical Trials Group. *N Engl J Med* 1997;336:1641–1648.
5. Dunn BK, Kramer BS, Ford LG. Phase III, large-scale chemoprevention trials. Approach to chemoprevention clinical trials and phase III clinical trial of tamoxifen as a chemopreventive for breast cancer—the US National Cancer Institute experience. *Hematol Oncol Clin North Am* 1998;12:1019–1036, vii.
6. Grant WB. An ecologic study of dietary and solar ultraviolet-B links to breast carcinoma mortality rates. *Cancer* 2002;94:272–281.
7. National Center for Health Statistics. Third National Health and Nutrition Examination Survey, 1988-1994, Plan and Operations Procedures Manuals (CD-ROM). Hyattsville, MD: U.S. Department of Health and Human Services (DHHS), Centers for Disease Control and Prevention; 1996.
8. Szklo M, Nieto F. *Epidemiology: Beyond the Basics*. Gaithersburg, MD: Aspen Publishers; 2000.
9. Grimes DA, Schulz KF. Cohort studies: marching towards outcomes. *Lancet* 2002;359:341–345.
10. Schatzkin A, Subar AF, Thompson FE, et al. Design and serendipity in establishing a large cohort with wide dietary intake distributions: the National Institutes of Health-American Association of Retired Persons Diet and Health Study. *Am J Epidemiol* 2001;154:1119–1125.
11. Mantel N, Haenszel W. Statistical aspects of the analysis of data from retrospective studies of disease. *J Natl Cancer Inst* 1959;22:719–748.
12. Wacholder S, Silverman DT, McLaughlin JK, et al. Selection of controls in case-control studies. II. Types of controls. *Am J Epidemiol* 1992;135:1029–1041.
13. Chen C, Weiss NS, Stanczyk FZ, et al. Endogenous sex hormones and prostate cancer risk: a case-control study nested within the Carotene and Retinol Efficacy Trial. *Cancer Epidemiol Biomarkers Prev* 2003;12:1410–1416.
14. Pearce N. What does the odds ratio estimate in a case-control study? *Int J Epidemiol* 1993;22:1189–1192.
15. Schulz KF, Grimes DA. Case-control studies: research in reverse. *Lancet* 2002;359:431–434.
16. Rothman K. *Epidemiology: An Introduction*. New York: Oxford University Press; 2002.
17. Hennekens C, Buring J. *Epidemiology in Medicine*. Boston: Little, Brown and Company; 1987.
18. Andriole GL, Crawford ED, Grubb RL 3rd, et al. Mortality results from a randomized prostate-cancer screening trial. *N Engl J Med* 2009;360:1310–1319.
19. Wilt TJ, Brawer MK, Jones KM, et al. Radical prostatectomy versus observation for localized prostate cancer. *N Engl J Med* 2012;367:203–213.
20. Yu JB, Soulos PR, Herrin J, et al. Proton versus intensity-modulated radiotherapy for prostate cancer: patterns of care and early toxicity. *J Natl Cancer Inst* 2013;105:25–32.
21. Ma X, Wang R, Long JB, et al. The cost implications of prostate cancer screening in the Medicare population. *Cancer* 2014;120(1):96–102.
22. Rundle A, Schwartz S. Issues in the epidemiological analysis and interpretation of intermediate biomarkers. *Cancer Epidemiol Biomarkers Prev* 2003;12:491–496.
23. Shields PG. Tobacco smoking, harm reduction, and biomarkers. *J Natl Cancer Inst* 2002;94:1435–1444.
24. Hunter DJ. Gene-environment interactions in human diseases. *Nat Rev Genet* 2005;6:287–298.
25. Hirschhorn JN, Daly MJ. Genome-wide association studies for common diseases and complex traits. *Nat Rev Genet* 2005;6:95–108.
26. Breast Cancer Association Consortium. Commonly studied single-nucleotide polymorphisms and breast cancer: results from the Breast Cancer Association Consortium. *J Natl Cancer Inst* 2006;98:1382–1396.
27. Wacholder S, Chanock S, Garcia-Closas M, et al. Assessing the probability that a positive report is false: an approach for molecular epidemiology studies. *J Natl Cancer Inst* 2004;96:434–442.
28. Clayton DG, Walker NM, Smyth DJ, et al. Population structure, differential bias and genomic control in a large-scale, case-control association study. *Nat Genet* 2005;37:1243–1246.
29. Easton DF, Eeles RA. Genome-wide association studies in cancer. *Hum Mol Genet* 2008;17:R109–115.
30. Ahmed S, Thomas G, Ghoussaini M, et al. Newly discovered breast cancer susceptibility loci on 3p24 and 17q23.2. *Nat Genet* 2009;41:585–590.
31. Thomas G, Jacobs KB, Kraft P, et al. A multistage genome-wide association study in breast cancer identifies two new risk alleles at 1p11.2 and 14q24.1 (RAD51L1). *Nat Genet* 2009;41:579–584.
32. Thomas G, Jacobs KB, Yeager M, et al. Multiple loci identified in a genome-wide association study of prostate cancer. *Nat Genet* 2008;40:310–315.

33. Le Marchand L. Genome-wide association studies and colorectal cancer. *Surg Oncol Clin N Am* 2009;18:663–668.

34. Hung RJ, McKay JD, Gaborieau V, et al. A susceptibility locus for lung cancer maps to nicotinic acetylcholine receptor subunit genes on 15q25. *Nature* 2008;452:633–637.

35. Amos CI, Wu X, Broderick P, et al. Genome-wide association scan of tag SNPs identifies a susceptibility locus for lung cancer at 15q25.1. *Nat Genet* 2008;40:616–622.

36. Amundadottir L, Kraft P, Stolzenberg-Solomon RZ, et al. Genome-wide association study identifies variants in the ABO locus associated with susceptibility to pancreatic cancer. *Nat Genet* 2009;41:986–990.

37. Kiemeney LA, Sulem P, Besenbacher S, et al. A sequence variant at 4p16.3 confers susceptibility to urinary bladder cancer. *Nat Genet* 2010;42(5):415–419.

38. Wu X, Ye Y, Kiemeney LA, et al. Genetic variation in the prostate stem cell antigen gene PSCA confers susceptibility to urinary bladder cancer. *Nat Genet* 2009;41:991–995.

39. Stacey SN, Sulem P, Masson G, et al. New common variants affecting susceptibility to basal cell carcinoma. *Nat Genet* 2009;41:909–914.

40. Thorgeirsson TE, Geller F, Sulem P, et al. A variant associated with nicotine dependence, lung cancer and peripheral arterial disease. *Nature* 2008;452:638–642.

41. Spitz MR, Amos CI, Dong Q, et al. The CHRNA5-A3 region on chromosome 15q24-25.1 is a risk factor both for nicotine dependence and for lung cancer. *J Natl Cancer Inst* 2008;100:1552–1556.

42. Zheng W, Long J, Gao YT, et al. Genome-wide association study identifies a new breast cancer susceptibility locus at 6q25.1. *Nat Genet* 2009;41:324–328.

43. Gudmundsson J, Sulem P, Gudbjartsson DF, et al. Common variants on 9q22.33 and 14q13.3 predispose to thyroid cancer in European populations. *Nat Genet* 2009;41:460–464.

44. Gudmundsson J, Sulem P, Gudbjartsson DF, et al. Genome-wide association and replication studies identify four variants associated with prostate cancer susceptibility. *Nat Genet* 2009;41:1122–1126.

45. Song H, Ramus SJ, Tyrer J, et al. A genome-wide association study identifies a new ovarian cancer susceptibility locus on 9p22.2. *Nat Genet* 2009;41:996–1000.

46. Stacey SN, Gudbjartsson DF, Sulem P, et al. Common variants on 1p36 and 1q42 are associated with cutaneous basal cell carcinoma but not with melanoma or pigmentation traits. *Nat Genet* 2008;40:1313–1318.

47. Zanke BW, Greenwood CM, Rangrej J, et al. Genome-wide association scan identifies a colorectal cancer susceptibility locus on chromosome 8q24. *Nat Genet* 2007;39:989–994.

48. Haiman CA, Patterson N, Freedman ML, et al. Multiple regions within 8q24 independently affect risk for prostate cancer. *Nat Genet* 2007;39:638–644.

49. Kiemeney LA, Thorlacius S, Sulem P, et al. Sequence variant on 8q24 confers susceptibility to urinary bladder cancer. *Nat Genet* 2008;40:1307–1312.

50. Ghoussaini M, Song H, Koessler T, et al. Multiple loci with different cancer specificities within the 8q24 gene desert. *J Natl Cancer Inst* 2008;100:962–966.

51. Harismendy O, Frazer KA. Elucidating the role of 8q24 in colorectal cancer. *Nat Genet* 2009;41:868–869.

52. Wright JB, Brown SJ, Cole MD. Upregulation of c-MYC in cis through a large chromatin loop linked to a cancer risk-associated single-nucleotide polymorphism in colorectal cancer cells. *Mol Cell Biol* 2010;30:1411–1420.

53. Rafnar T, Sulem P, Stacey SN, et al. Sequence variants at the TERT-CLPTM1L locus associate with many cancer types. *Nat Genet* 2009;41:221–227.

54. Fernandez-Garcia I, Ortiz-de-Solorzano C, Montuenga LM. Telomeres and telomerase in lung cancer. *J Thorac Oncol* 2008;3:1085–1088.

55. Zienolddiny S, Skaug V, Landvik NE, et al. The TERT-CLPTM1L lung cancer susceptibility variant associates with higher DNA adduct formation in the lung. *Carcinogenesis* 2009;30:1368–1371.

56. Ioannidis JP, Thomas G, Daly MJ. Validating, augmenting and refining genome-wide association signals. *Nat Rev Genet* 2009;10:318–329.

57. Chung CC, Magalhaes WC, Gonzalez-Bosquet J, et al. Genome-wide association studies in cancer—current and future directions. *Carcinogenesis* 2010;31:111–120.

58. Fraga MF, Ballestar E, Paz MF, et al. Epigenetic differences arise during the lifetime of monozygotic twins. *Proc Natl Acad Sci U S A* 2005;102:10604–10609.

59. Dolinoy DC, Weidman JR, Waterland RA, et al. Maternal genistein alters coat color and protects Avy mouse offspring from obesity by modifying the fetal epigenome. *Environ Health Perspect* 2006;114:567–572.

ETIOLOGY AND EPIDEMIOLOGY OF CANCER

Trends in United States Cancer Mortality

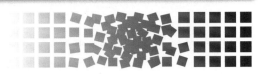

Tim E. Byers

INTRODUCTION

Cancer incidence registries now cover nearly all of the US population. State-based vital records systems and aggregate national systems regularly report trends in both cancer incidence and mortality, and national surveys routinely monitor cancer-related risk factors in the population. These surveillance systems have documented substantial changes in both risk factors for cancer and in cancer incidence and mortality rates in the United States over the past 3 decades. In 1996, the American Cancer Society (ACS) set an ambitious challenge for the United States: to reduce cancer mortality rates from their apparent peak in 1990 by 50% in the 25-year period ending in 2015.[1] In 1998, the ACS then challenged the United States to also reduce cancer incidence rates from their peak in 1992 by 25% by the year 2015.[2] In this chapter, we will examine trends in cancer risk factors as well as trends in cancer incidence and mortality rates in the United States over the 25-year period between 1990 and 2015.

CANCER SURVEILLANCE SYSTEMS

Collecting cancer incidence rates is largely a state-based activity in the United States, because cancer is a reportable disease in all states. The Centers for Disease Control and Prevention (CDC) organizes all state-based cancer registries within the National Program of Cancer Registries, which now reports collective data on cancer incidence from over 40 different state-based registries, providing data that meets strict quality standards.[3] The National Cancer Institute has supported high-quality cancer incidence and outcomes registration in selected states and cities since 1973 within the Surveillance, Epidemiology, and End Results (SEER) Program.[4] The most precise measures of long-term trends in cancer incidence come from SEER-9, a set of nine SEER registries that together include about 10% of the US population. The populations included in the SEER-9 registries document the most detailed history of cancer trends beginning in the 1970s based on highly standardized cancer case ascertainment, staging, treatment, and outcomes. Deaths from cancer are well ascertained in all states via state-based vital records, which are aggregated into annual national mortality reports by the CDC's National Center for Health Statistics.[5] Each year, the ACS, the National Cancer Institute, and the CDC publish a *Report to the Nation* on trends in cancer incidence and mortality in the United States.[6] Trends in the prevalence of behavioral factors that affect cancer risk are tracked by the Health Interview Survey, an ongoing, in-person interview of a nationally representative sample of adults, and in annual reports by the Behavioral Risk Factor Surveillance System, a continuously operating telephone-based survey operated by state departments of health and organized by the CDC.[7]

MAKING SENSE OF CANCER TRENDS

Understanding the reasons for cancer trends requires understanding trends in cancer-related risk factors. For factors like tobacco,

relating trends in exposure to trends in rates is easy, because those effects are large and single. However, for many other cancer risk factors, because effects are much smaller and multifactorial, simple correlations over time are less apparent. In most situations, all that maybe possible are crude qualitative relationships between temporal trends in cancer risk factors and subsequent trends in cancer rates. Statistical methods such as linear regression joinpoint analysis can tell us when inflections in cancer trends occur, but accounting for the precise reasons for changing rates is often impaired by our incomplete knowledge about the interacting impacts of variations in cancer screening, diagnosis, and treatment, and by uncertainties about latencies between interventions and outcomes.[8]

TRENDS IN CANCER RISK FACTORS AND SCREENING

Trends in major cancer risk factors have been mixed (Table 12.1). Although the downward trends in tobacco smoking among adults that began in the 1960s slowed after 1990, there has been a continuing downward trend in the number of cigarettes smoked per day by continuing smokers.[9] Obesity trends have been adverse among both men and women since the 1970s, with more than a doubling of the prevalence of obesity between 1990 and 2010. Long-term trends in the use of hormone replacement therapy (HRT) are not routinely monitored in the Behavioral Risk Factor Surveillance System (BRFSS), but HRT use increased substantially in the last 2 decades of the 20th century. Then, following the 2002 publication of the Women's Health Initiative trial, which showed clear adverse effects of HRT, there was a rapid and substantial drop in HRT use.[10,11] The use of endoscopic screening for colorectal cancer (sigmoidoscopy or colonoscopy) has increased substantially in recent years, approximately doubling since the mid 1990s, so that, as of 2010, about two-thirds of Americans age 50 and older reported ever having had an endoscopic examination. Mammography use increased progressively through the 1990s, but mammogram rates then leveled off after 2000.[12] Widespread prostate-specific antigen (PSA) testing began in the mid to late 1980s, then increased substantially during the 1990s. By 2002, a majority of US men age 50 and older reported having been tested.

CANCER INCIDENCE AND MORTALITY

In this chapter, we describe and discuss cancer trends for the time period 1990 through 2010 using cancer incidence data from the SEER-9 registry (Table 12.2 and Fig. 12.1) and US cancer mortality data from the National Center for Health Statistics (Table 12.3).[4,5] All rates were age-adjusted to the US 2000 standard population by the direct method, using 10-year age intervals.

Lung Cancer

The lung is the second leading site for cancer incidence and the leading site for cancer death among both men and women in the

TABLE 12.1

Trends in Risk Factors and Cancer Screening Practices in the United States, 1990–2010[a]

	Men		Women		Both Genders	
	Smoking	**PSA Screening**	**Smoking**	**Mammography**	**Obesity**	**CRC Screening**
1990	24.9	—	21.3	58.3	11.6	—
1991	25.1	—	21.3	62.2	12.6	—
1992	24.2	—	21.0	63.1	12.6	—
1993	24.0	—	21.1	66.5	13.7	—
1994	23.9	—	21.6	66.6	14.4	—
1995	24.8	—	20.9	68.6	15.8	29.4
1996	25.5	—	21.9	69.2	16.8	—
1997	25.4	—	21.1	70.3	16.6	32.4
1998	25.3	—	20.9	72.3	18.3	—
1999	24.2	—	20.8	72.8	19.7	43.7
2000	24.4	—	21.2	76.1	20.1	—
2001	25.4	—	21.2	—	21.0	—
2002	25.7	53.9	20.8	75.9	22.1	48.1
2003	24.8	—	20.2	—	—	—
2004	23.0	52.1	19.0	74.7	23.2	53.0
2005	22.1	—	19.2	—	24.4	—
2006	22.2	53.8	18.4	76.5	25.1	57.1
2007	21.2	—	18.4	—	26.3	—
2008	20.3	54.8	16.7	76.0	26.6	61.8
2009	19.5	—	16.7	—	27.1	—
2010	18.5	53.2	15.8	75.2	27.5	65.2

CRC, colorectal cancer; PSA, prostate-specific antigen.
[a] Median percent of the population across all states in the Behavioral Risk Factor Surveillance System. The survey covered such areas as body mass index and was based on self-reported height and weight. Questions included: Are you a regular cigarette smoker? Have you ever had a sigmoidoscopy or proctoscopic examination? For women age 40 and older, the following question was included: Have you had a mammogram in the past 2 years? For men aged 50 and older, the following question was included: Have you had a PSA test in the last 2 years? (From Centers for Disease Control and Prevention. Behavioral Risk Factor Surveillance System Web site. http://cdc.gov/brfss.)

United States.[6] There are now more deaths from lung cancer in the United States than from the sum of colorectal, breast, and prostate cancers. Trends in lung cancer incidence and mortality have been nearly identical because there are few effective treatments for lung cancer, and survival time remains short. Lung cancer trends follow historic declines in tobacco use, lagged by about 20 years.[13] Between 1965 and 1985, tobacco use among US adults dropped substantially, and more in men than in women. Lung cancer mortality rates began to decline among men in 1990, but rates increased among women throughout the 1990s. The stabilization of lung cancer incidence trends among women from 2000 to 2005 and the beginning of a decline in the period 2005 to 2010 foretells a coming persistent decline in lung cancer mortality among women in the United States.

The effectiveness of annual examinations by use of chest radiographs in reducing lung cancer mortality was studied as part of the Prostate, Lung, Colorectal, Ovary (PLCO) trial, and the effectiveness of annual screening by low-dose computed tomography (LDCT) of the lung fields was studied in the National Lung Screening Trial (NLST).[14,15] In brief, screening with standard chest radiography finds more cancers earlier but does not affect mortality, whereas screening with LDCT reduces the risk of death from lung cancer by at least 20%.[14,15] Therefore, both the ACS and the US Preventive Services Task Force have issued recommendations that favor informed decision making for lung cancer screening using LDCT.[16,17]

The major factor that will determine lung cancer incidence in the coming decade is the past history of tobacco use, but future screening will also reduce future mortality rates. Considering all factors, it is likely that over the coming decade the downward trends in mortality from lung cancer will continue at about the same rate among men, and soon will become more apparent among women.

Colorectal Cancer

The colorectum is the third leading site for cancer incidence and the second leading site for cancer death in the United States.[6] Colorectal cancer incidence rates increased until 1985, when they began to decline. The reasons for this decline are not clear, but could be related to downward trends in cigarette smoking and the increasing use of both nonsteroidal anti-inflammatory drugs (NSAIDs) and HRT.[18] The rapid decline in HRT use following the publication of the Women's Health Initiative trial results in 2002 may adversely affect colorectal trends among women in the coming years, because HRT reduces the risk for colorectal cancer among women.[11] Recent trials have demonstrated the potential for NSAIDs to reduce colorectal neoplasia, but adverse effects from these agents will limit their widespread use for that explicit purpose. Nonetheless, even the common sporadic use of NSAIDs for other indications will contribute to continuing declines in colorectal cancer incidence in the coming years.

Screening with either sigmoidoscopy or colonoscopy leads to the identification and removal of adenomas, thus preventing the development of colorectal cancer.[19,20] Medicare included

TABLE 12.2

Trends in Age-Adjusted Cancer Incidence Rates in the United States by Cancer Site, 1990–2010[a]

	Men		Women		Both Genders	
	Lung	**Prostate**	**Lung**	**Breast**	**Colorectal**	**All Sites**
1990	96.9	171.0	47.8	131.8	60.7	482.0
1991	97.2	214.8	49.6	133.9	59.5	503.0
1992	97.2	237.4	49.9	132.1	58.0	510.6
1993	94.0	209.5	49.2	129.2	56.8	493.4
1994	90.9	180.3	50.5	131.0	55.6	483.5
1995	89.8	169.3	50.4	132.6	54.0	476.9
1996	88.0	169.5	50.2	133.7	54.8	479.1
1997	86.3	173.5	52.6	138.0	56.4	486.4
1998	88.0	171.0	53.0	141.4	56.8	488.2
1999	84.6	183.4	52.4	141.5	55.5	490.4
2000	82.1	183.0	51.2	136.4	54.1	486.0
2001	81.4	184.8	51.7	138.7	53.6	489.7
2002	80.4	182.2	52.5	135.6	53.1	487.5
2003	81.0	169.6	53.0	126.8	50.8	475.2
2004	76.2	165.7	52.0	128.0	50.0	476.1
2005	75.8	156.5	53.7	126.4	47.8	471.9
2006	74.2	171.5	53.4	126.0	46.8	475.0
2007	73.5	174.3	53.4	127.9	46.3	480.5
2008	72.0	157.0	51.6	128.0	45.2	473.4
2009	70.2	153.7	51.8	130.3	43.0	470.5
2010	66.8	145.1	49.2	126.0	40.6	457.5
Average annual % change 1990–2010	−1.8	−0.5	+0.2	−0.2	−2.0	−0.2

[a] Data source is the Surveillance, Epidemiology, and End Results-9 populations for cancer incidence. Rates are age-adjusted to the year 2000 population standard. The annual percent change is the mean percent change per year across the 20-year period, 1990 to 2010. (From National Cancer Institute. Surveillance, Epidemiology, and End Results Program Web site. http://seer.cancer.gov.)

coverage for all recommended colorectal screening methods in 2001, and national publicity has substantially increased public interest in screening.[21] Colorectal screening rates have increased over time, now with about two-thirds of adults over age 50 reporting having ever been screened by lower gastrointestinal endoscopy (see Table 12.1).

Decreasing rates of colorectal cancer incidence are occurring in spite of the obesity epidemic, which is an adverse force on colorectal cancer risk, because obesity may account for as much as 20% of colorectal cancer in the United States.[22] Recently, however, obesity trends have stabilized in the United States.[23] As a result of the increased use of lower gastrointestinal endoscopy for colorectal screening and this stabilization of obesity trends, the incidence of colorectal cancer may exceed the ACS goal for 2015 of a 25% reduction, and there is a high likelihood that the rate of decline in deaths from colorectal cancer will be steep enough to reach the 2015 ACS mortality reduction goal of 50%.

Breast Cancer

The breast is the leading site of cancer incidence and the second leading site for cancer death among women in the United States.[6] Over the period 1990 to 2001, no substantial changes in incidence

rates were observed, but after 2000, breast cancer incidence began to decline. The decline in breast cancer incidence observed after 2002 seems to have been the result of the sudden decline in the use of HRT following the 2002 publication of the Women's Health Initiative results.[10,11] It is likely that persisting lower rates of HRT use will cause a continued decline in breast cancer incidence in the coming years. Countering this favorable trend, however, are the adverse effects of the obesity epidemic. Obesity, a major risk factor for postmenopausal breast cancer, increased substantially between 1990 and 2005, now with over 25% of US women being obese. However, the slowing of the obesity epidemic since 2005 may have substantial beneficial effects on the future trends in breast cancer incidence.

After persistent increases in the use of mammography over a 20-year period, mammography rates declined modestly between 2000 and 2004, and then leveled off. The downgrading of the evidence recommendations by the US Preventive Services Task Force for mammography for women age 40 to 49 and recommendations for every other year mammographies for women age 50 and older have resulted in lower mammogram utilization, which is likely to continue into the coming decade.[17] This trend will have an adverse effect on breast cancer mortality, but will tend to reduce breast cancer incidence somewhat because of a lack of detection of very early stage cancers.

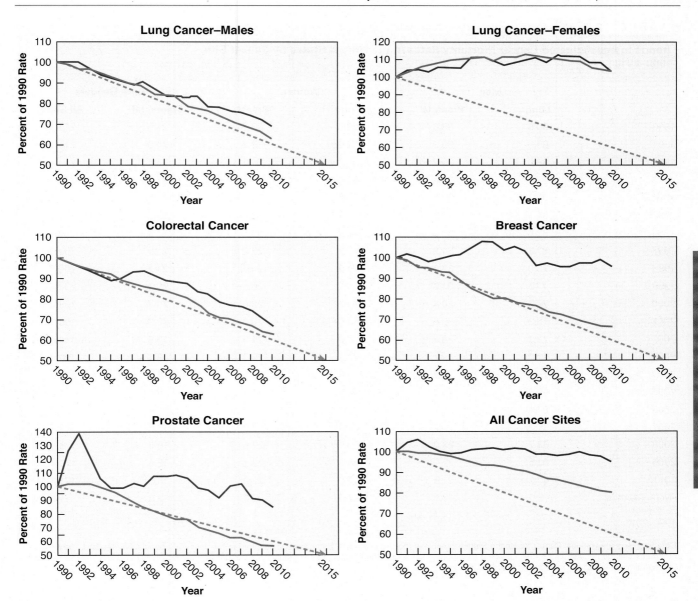

Figure 12.1 (A–F) Trends in cancer incidence and mortality between 1990 and 2010. Incidence rates are for the populations in the Surveillance, Epidemiology, and End Results Program; registries and mortality rates are for the entire United States. Rates are age-adjusted to the year 2000 standard. The y-axis rates are expressed as a percentage of the 1990 incidence and mortality rates. The *red lines* represent incidence rates, and the *blue lines* represent mortality rates. The *straight dotted green lines* represent the linear trend that would need to be followed to achieve a 50% mortality reduction between 1990 and 2015. (Data from National Cancer Institute. Surveillance, Epidemiology, and End Results Program Web site. http://seer .cancer.gov, and Centers for Disease Control and Prevention. U.S. mortality data. http://wonder.cdc.gov/ucd-icd10.html)

ETIOLOGY AND EPIDEMIOLOGY OF CANCER

The antiestrogens tamoxifen and raloxifene have both been shown to reduce the risk of incident breast cancer.[24] The safety profile for tamoxifen discourages its widespread use, but there is a more favorable risk/benefit balance of raloxifene. Nonetheless, neither of these drugs is commonly used for breast cancer prevention among postmenopausal women in the United States.

The average decline in breast cancer death rates of 2% per year since 1990 is the combined result of earlier diagnosis and better treatment.[25] Progress in breast cancer treatment is continuing, especially in the development and application of hormone-targeted therapies. Aromatase inhibitors have largely replaced tamoxifen therapy for breast cancer treatment for postmenopausal women. Because all antiestrogens substantially reduce the incidence of second primary cancers in the contralateral breast, they impact both therapy and prevention. In the coming decade, the longer term effects of decreased HRT use, increased antiestrogen use, reversal

of the obesity trends, and continued improvements in therapies will likely lead to continued decreases in both the incidence and mortality rates from breast cancer.

Prostate Cancer

The prostate is the leading site for cancer incidence and the second leading site for cancer death among men in the United States.[6] The incidence of prostate cancer has been extremely variable over the period 1990 to 2010. The incidence spike observed in the early 1990s actually began in the late 1980s, coincident with the advent of PSA testing. The reasons for the 2.8% annual downward trend in prostate cancer mortality since 1990 are uncertain, however, because the ongoing PSA screening trials have not yet demonstrated a mortality benefit from screening anywhere as large as the downward mortality

TABLE 12.3

Trends in Age-Adjusted Cancer Mortality Rates in the United States by Cancer Site, 1990–2010[a]

	Men		Women		Both Genders	
	Lung	**Prostate**	**Lung**	**Breast**	**Colorectal**	**All Sites**
1990	90.6	38.6	36.8	33.1	24.6	214.9
1991	89.9	39.3	37.6	32.7	24.0	215.1
1992	88.0	39.2	38.7	31.6	23.6	213.5
1993	87.6	39.3	39.3	31.4	23.3	213.4
1994	85.7	38.5	39.6	30.9	22.9	211.7
1995	84.4	37.3	40.3	30.6	22.6	210.0
1996	82.8	36.0	40.4	29.5	21.9	207.0
1997	81.3	34.2	40.8	28.2	21.5	203.6
1998	79.9	32.6	41.0	27.5	21.2	200.8
1999	77.0	31.6	40.2	26.6	20.9	200.7
2000	76.5	30.4	41.1	26.6	20.7	198.8
2001	75.3	29.5	41.0	26.0	20.2	196.3
2002	73.7	28.7	41.6	25.6	19.8	194.4
2003	72.0	27.2	41.3	25.3	19.1	190.9
2004	70.4	26.2	41.0	24.5	18.1	186.8
2005	69.5	25.4	40.7	24.1	17.6	185.2
2006	67.4	24.2	40.3	23.6	17.3	182.0
2007	65.2	24.2	40.1	23.0	16.9	179.3
2008	63.7	23.0	39.1	22.6	16.5	176.3
2009	61.5	22.1	38.6	22.2	15.8	173.4
2010	60.1	21.8	38.0	22.0	15.5	171.8
Average annual % change 1990–2010	−2.0	−2.8	+0.2	−2.0	−2.3	−1.1

[a] Data source is the National Center for Health Statistics national mortality data set. Rates are age-adjusted to the year 2000 population standard. The average percentage change per year is the mean percent change per year across the 20-year period, 1990 to 2010. (From Centers for Disease Control and Prevention. U.S. mortality data. http://wonder.cdc.gov/ucd-icd10.html)

decline observed since 1990.[26,27] In fact, the US trial findings suggest that there was virtually no mortality benefit within the first decade following the initiation of screening.[28] Therefore, it is not possible to know how much of this favorable trend was related to early diagnosis, how much was related to improvements in treatment, or how much might have been related to other factors, such as changes in the way cause of death has been listed on death certificates.

The Prostate Cancer Prevention Trial provided an important proof of principle that antiandrogen therapies can reduce prostate cancer risk.[29] Although the net benefits of finasteride for prevention are not clearly demonstrated from this trial, other agents that interfere with androgen effects on prostate cancer growth could prove to be useful for prostate cancer chemoprevention in the future. Prostate cancer incidence trends will likely continue to be largely driven by rates of PSA screening in the coming decade. Longer term results of a clearer benefit to mortality from either the PLCO trial in the United States or the European PSA trial would help to better specify screening recommendations.

Other Cancers

Even though mortality rates have been declining by about 2% per year from the four most common causes of cancer death (lung,

colorectal, breast, and prostate), very little progress has been made in reducing death rates from the other half of all adult cancers in the United States. Continuing progress in tobacco control will have beneficial effects on many other types of cancer linked to tobacco, and stopping the obesity epidemic will have favorable effects on many obesity-related cancers that have been increasing in recent years, such as adenocarcinoma of the esophagus and renal cancer.[30] Melanoma incidence rates have been increasing substantially in recent years, likely the result of the combined effects of previous sun exposure and increased awareness and surveillance for pigmented skin lesions, but recent advances in therapy for metastatic melanoma may foretell future declines in melanoma morality. Declining rates of stomach cancer incidence and mortality over several decades may be related to the combined effects of historic improvements in nutrition and the declining prevalence of chronic infection with *Helicobacter pylori*. Liver cancer incidence has been substantially increasing in recent years, likely resulting from historic trends in chronic infection with hepatitis B and C viruses. As a result, liver cancer will likely continue to rise in the United States over the coming decade.

The incidence of thyroid cancer has been increasing in the United States for the past several decades, but thyroid cancer mortality rates have been stable, a pattern most likely due to increased detection from improved diagnostic techniques. Invasive cervical cancer is uncommon in the United States because of widespread screening using Pap smears. Although the vaccination for human papillomavirus (HPV) has been shown to be highly effective in protecting against the serotypes that together account for 70% of cervical cancer cases, so far, HPV vaccine coverage has been low among young women in the United States.[6] For many of the other cancers, such as cancers of the pancreas, brain, ovary, and the hematopoietic malignancies, risk factors are poorly understood, and there are no effective early detection methods. For these cancers, the current hope for improvement resides in the development of better methods for early cancer detection and treatment.

PREDICTING FUTURE CANCER TRENDS

In the United States, cancer is now the leading cause of death under age 85 years. Over the first half of the ACS 25-year challenge period, overall cancer incidence rates have declined by about 0.2% per year, and mortality rates have declined by about 1% per year. The trends in both incidence and mortality from the four leading cancer sites are summarized in Figure 12.1. Using simple linear extrapolation, it therefore seems that the ACS challenge goals of reducing cancer incidence by 25% and mortality by 50% over 25 years may be only half achieved.[31,32] Clearly, though, estimating future trends only by linear extrapolation is a crude way to foretell future events. Projecting cancer trends into the more distant future using complex modeling is possible, however, as knowledge about changes in major cancer risk factors can lead to reasonable predictions about the direction and approximate slope of future trends. One method to incorporate knowledge about trends in risk factors into estimates of future cancer trends is to estimate the impact of changes in the attributable risk (also called the *preventable fraction*) in the population for each risk factor. By making assumptions about latency period, then tying changes in factors to changes in cancer incidence and mortality, cancer trends resulting from risk factor changes can be predicted. For example, if there were a factor that explained 30% of a particular cancer, then cutting that exposure in half would eventually lead to a projected 15% reduction in rates (50% of 30%). This method was used to project cancer mortality trends to 2015 and seems to have projected trends that are quite similar to those observed in recent years.[33]

Progress in cancer prevention, early detection, and treatment since 1990 has been persistent, and there are many reasons to be optimistic about the future. Just how much steeper the future downward slope in cancer death rates can be driven will depend on the extent to which we can discover new factors causing cancer, and effectively deploy ways to better act on our current knowledge about how to prevent and control cancer. Especially important will be progress in reversing the epidemics of tobacco use and obesity, and ensuring that the coming improvements to health care access will lead to access to state-of-the-art cancer screening and therapy for all.

REFERENCES

1. American Cancer Society Board of Directors. ACS Challenge goals for U.S. Cancer Mortality for the Year 2015. *Proceedings of the Board of Directors.* Atlanta, GA: American Cancer Society, 1996.
2. American Cancer Society Board of Directors. ACS Challenge goals for U.S. Cancer Incidence for the Year 2015. *Proceedings of the Board of Directors.* Atlanta, GA: American Cancer Society, 1998.
3. Centers for Disease Control and Prevention. National Program of Cancer Registries (NPCR) Web site. http://cdc.gov/cancer/npcr.
4. National Cancer Institute. Surveillance, Epidemiology, and End Results Program Web site. http://seer.cancer.gov.
5. Centers for Disease Control and Prevention. U.S. mortality data. http://wonder.cdc.gov/ucd-icd10.html.
6. Jemal A, Simard E, Dorell C, et al. Annual report to the nation on the status of cancer, 1975–2009, featuring the burden and trends in human papillomavirus (HPV)–associated cancers and HPV vaccination coverage levels. *J Natl Cancer Inst* 2013;105:175–201.
7. Centers for Disease Control and Prevention. Behavioral Risk Factor Surveillance System Web site. http://cdc.gov/brfss.
8. Ward E, Thun M, Hannan L, et al. Interpreting cancer trends. *Ann N Y Acad Sci* 2006;1076:29–53.
9. Centers for Disease Control and Prevention. Smoking & Tobacco Use Web site. http://cdc.gov/tobacco.
10. Rossouw JE, Anderson GL, Prentice RL, et al. Risks and benefits of estrogen plus progestin in healthy postmenopausal women: principal results from the Women's Health Initiative randomized controlled trial. *JAMA* 2002; 288:321–333.
11. Hersh A, Stefanick M, Stafford R. National use of postmenopausal hormone therapy: annual trends and response to recent evidence. *JAMA* 2004;291:47–53.
12. Ryerson AB, Miller J, Eheman CR, et al. Use of mammograms among women aged ≥40 years—United States, 2000–2005. *MMWR* 2007;56:49–51.
13. Giovino GA. Epidemiology of tobacco use in the United States. *Oncogene* 2002;21:7326–7340.
14. Oken M, Hocking W, Kvale P, et al. Screening by chest radiograph and lung cancer mortality. *JAMA* 2011;306:1865–1873.
15. The National Lung Screening Trial Research Team. Reduced lung-cancer mortality with low-dose computed tomographic screening. *N Engl J Med* 2011; 365:395–409.
16. Smith R, Brooks D, Cokkinides V, et al. Cancer screening in the United States, 2013: a review of current American Cancer Society guidelines, current issues in cancer screening, and new guidance on cervical cancer screening and lung cancer screening. *CA Cancer J Clin* 2013;63:88–105.
17. U.S. Preventive Services Task Force. U.S. Preventive Services Task Force Web site. http://uspreventiveservicestaskforce.org.
18. Martinez ME. Primary prevention of colorectal cancer: lifestyle, nutrition, exercise. *Recent Results Cancer Res* 2005;166:177–211.
19. Atkin W, Edwards R, Kralj-Hans I, et al. Once-only flexible sigmoidoscopy screening in prevention of colorectal cancer: a multicentre randomized controlled trial. *Lancet* 2010;375:1624–1633.
20. Schoen RE, Pinsky PF, Weissfeld JL, et al. Colorectal-cancer incidence and mortality with screening flexible sigmoidoscopy. *N Engl J Med* 2012; 366:2345–2357.
21. Cram P, Fendrick A, Inadomi J, et al. The impact of celebrity promotional campaign on the use of colon cancer screening: the Katie Couric effect. *Arch Intern Med* 2003;163(13):1601–1605.
22. World Cancer Research Fund/American Institute for Cancer Prevention. *Policy and Action for Cancer Prevention. Food, Nutrition, and Physical Activity: A Global Perspective.* Washington, DC: AICR; 2009.
23. Ogden CL, Carroll MD, Curtin LR, et al. Prevalence of overweight and obesity in the United States, 1999–2004. *JAMA* 2006;295:1549–1555.
24. Vogel V, Constantino J, Wickerham D, et al. Effects of tamoxifen vs raloxifene on the risks of developing invasive breast cancer and other disease outcomes: the NSABP Study of Tamoxifen and Raloxifene (STAR) P-2 trial. *JAMA* 2006;295:2727–2741.
25. Berry D, Cronin K, Plevritis S, et al. Effect of screening and adjuvant therapy on mortality from breast cancer. *N Engl J Med* 2005;353:1784–1792.
26. Andriole GL, Crawford ED, Grubb RL 3rd, et al. Mortality results from a randomized prostate-cancer screening trial. *N Engl J Med* 2009;360(13):1310–1319.
27. Schröder FH, Hugosson J, Roobol MJ, et al. Screening and prostate-cancer mortality in a randomized European study. *N Engl J Med* 2009;360(13):1320–1328.
28. Andriole G, Crawford D, Grubb R, et al. Prostate cancer screening in the randomized Prostate, Lung, Colorectal, and Ovarian Cancer Screening Trial: mortality results after 13 years of follow-up. *J Natl Cancer Inst* 2012;104: 125–132.
29. Thompson I, Goodman P, Tangen C, et al. Long-term survival of participants in the prostate cancer prevention trial. *N Engl J Med* 2013;369:603–610.
30. International Agency for Cancer Research. *Weight Control and Physical Activity. Handbook 6.* Lyon, France: IARC Press; 2002.
31. Sedjo R, Byers T, Barrera E, et al. A midpoint assessment of the American Cancer Society challenge goal to decrease cancer incidence by 25% between 1992 and 2015. *CA Cancer J Clin* 2007;57:326–340.
32. Byers T, Barrera E, Fontham E, et al. A midpoint assessment of the American Cancer Society challenge goal to halve the U.S. cancer mortality rates between the years 1990 and 2015. *Cancer* 2006;107:396–405.
33. Byers T, Mouchawar J, Marks J, et al. The American Cancer Society challenge goals. How far can cancer rates decline in the U.S. by the year 2015? *Cancer* 1999;86:715–727.

ETIOLOGY AND EPIDEMIOLOGY OF CANCER

PART III

Cancer Therapeutics

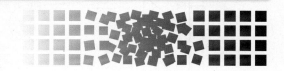

13 Essentials of Radiation Therapy

Meredith A. Morgan, Randall K. Ten Haken, and Theodore S. Lawrence

INTRODUCTION

The beneficial use of radiation was launched by the experiments of Wilhelm Roentgen, who, in 1895, found that x-rays could pass through materials that were impenetrable to light. Emil Grubbe provided one of the early examples of the therapeutic use of radiation by treating an advanced ulcerated breast cancer with x-rays in January 1896. We have made great progress since these early days, which has been strongly influenced by research in radiation chemistry, biology, and physics.

BIOLOGIC ASPECTS OF RADIATION ONCOLOGY

Radiation-Induced DNA Damage

Radiation is administered to cells either in the form of photons (x-rays and gamma rays) or particles (protons, neutrons, and electrons). When photons or particles interact with biologic material, they cause ionizations that can either directly interact with subcellular structures or they can interact with water, the major constituent of cells, and generate free radicals that can then interact with subcellular structures (Fig. 13.1).

The direct effects of radiation are the consequence of the DNA in chromosomes absorbing energy that leads to ionizations. This is the major mechanism of DNA damage induced by charged nuclei (such as a carbon nucleus) and neutrons and is termed *high linear energy transfer* (Fig. 13.2). In contrast, the interaction of photons with other molecules, such as water, results in the production of free radicals, some of which possess a lifetime long enough to be able to diffuse to the nucleus and interact with DNA in the chromosomes. This is the major mechanism of DNA damage induced by x-rays and has been termed *low linear energy transfer*.[1]

A free radical generated through the interaction of photons with other molecules that possess an unpaired electron in their outermost shell (e.g., hydroxyl radicals) can abstract a hydrogen molecule from a macromolecule such as DNA to generate damage. Cells that have increased levels of free radical scavengers, such as glutathione, would have less DNA damage induced by x-rays, but would have similar levels of DNA damage induced by a carbon nucleus that is directly absorbed by chromosomal DNA. Furthermore, a low oxygen environment would also protect cells from x-ray–induced damage because there would be fewer radicals available to induce DNA damage in the absence of oxygen, but this environment would have little impact on DNA damage induced by carbon nuclei.[2]

Cellular Responses to Radiation-Induced DNA Damage

Checkpoint Pathways

The cell cycle must progress in a specific order; checkpoint genes ensure that the initiation of late events is delayed until earlier events are complete. There are three principal places in the cell cycle at which checkpoints induced by DNA damage function: the border between G1 phase and S phase, intra-S phase, and the border between G2 phase and mitosis (Fig. 13.3). Cells with an intact checkpoint function that have sustained DNA damage stop progressing through the cycle and become arrested at the next checkpoint in the cell cycle. For example, cells with damaged DNA in G1 phase avoid replicating that damage by arresting at the G1/S interface. If irradiated cells have already passed the restriction point, a position in G1 phase that is regulated by the phosphorylation of the retinoblastoma tumor suppressor gene (*Rb*) and its dissociation from the E2F family of transcription factors, they will transiently arrest in S phase. The G1/S and intra-S phase checkpoints inhibit the replication of damaged DNA and work in a coordinated manner with the DNA repair machinery to permit the restitution of DNA integrity, thereby increasing cell survival.

The earliest response to radiation is the activation of ataxia-telangiectasia mutated (ATM), which involves a conformational change that results in the activation of its kinase domain and phosphorylation of serine 1981 (see Fig. 13.3).[3] This phosphorylation causes the ATM homodimer to dissociate into active monomers that phosphorylate a wide range of proteins such as 53BP1, the histone variant H2AX, Nbs1 (Nijmegen breakage syndrome; a member of the *MRN complex*, composed of Mre11, Rad50, and Nbs1), BRCA1, and SMC1 (structural maintenance of chromosomes), and these proteins coordinate repair with the cell cycle.[4] In response to DNA damage, H2AX is rapidly phosphorylated by ATM and localizes to sites of DNA double-strand breaks in multiprotein complexes described as foci (Fig. 13.4). Phosphorylation of H2AX by ATM results in the direct recruitment of Mdc1 and forms a complex with H2AX to recruit additional ATM molecules, forming a positive feedback loop.

The G1/S phase checkpoint is the best understood. In response to DNA damage, activated ATM can directly phosphorylate p53 and mdm2, the ubiquitin ligase that targets p53 for degradation. These phosphorylations are important for increasing the stability of the p53 protein. In addition to ATM, checkpoint kinase 2 (Chk2) also phosphorylates p53 and can enhance p53 stability. Activated p53 transcriptionally increases the expression of the *p21*[WAF1/CIP1] gene, which results in a sustained inhibition of G1 cyclin/Cdk, and prevents phosphorylation of pRb and progression from G1 into S.[5] Mutations in p53 that are commonly found in solid tumors result in loss of transcriptional activity and compromised checkpoint function.

Control of the S-phase checkpoint is mediated in part by the Cdc25A phosphatase inhibiting Cdk2 activity and the loading of Cdc45 onto chromatin. If Cdc45 fails to bind to chromatin, DNA polymerase α is not recruited to replication origins and replicon initiation fails to occur.[6] A more prominent mechanism for S-phase arrest is signaled through the MRN complex and the cohesin protein SMC1 by ATM.[7] Loss of ATM, MRN components, or SMC1 leads to the loss of the intra-S phase checkpoint function and increased radiosensitivity. Both the CDC45 and ATM pathways represent parallel, but seemingly independent, pathways to protect replication forks from trying to replicate through DNA strand

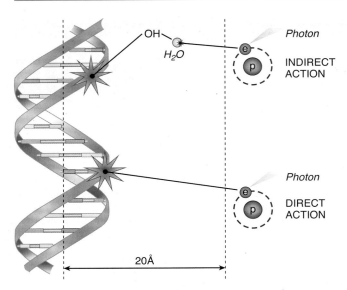

Figure 13.1 The direct and indirect effects of ionizing radiation on DNA. Incident photons transfer part of their energy to free electrons (Compton scattering). These electrons can directly interact with DNA to induce DNA damage, or they can first interact with water to produce hydroxyl radicals that can then induce damage.

breaks. Although ATM has received the lion's share of attention in signaling checkpoint activation in response to ionizing radiation, its family member ATR (ataxia telangiectasia and rad3-related) also plays a role in S-phase checkpoint responses.[8] ATM kinase activity is inducible by radiation, whereas ATR kinase activity is constitutive and does not significantly change with irradiation. (ATR is described in more detail in Chapter 19.) In contrast to Cdc45 and ATM, ATR is probably more important in monitoring

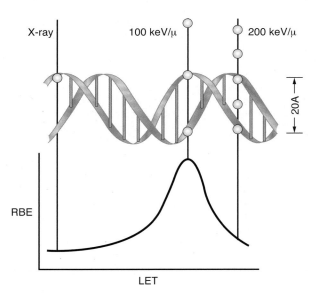

Figure 13.2 Linear energy transfer and DNA damage. Ionizing radiation deposits energy along the track (linear energy transfer [LET]), which causes DNA damage and cell killing. The most biologically potent (highest relative biologic effectiveness [RBE]) LET is 100 keV per μm because the separation between ionizing events is the same as the diameter of the DNA double helix (2 nm). (From Hall EJ, Giaccia AJ. *Radiobiology for the Radiologist.* Philadelphia: Lippincott Williams & Williams; 2012, with permission.)

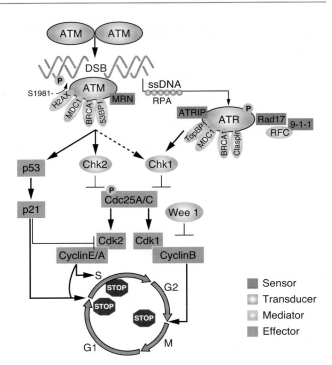

Figure 13.3 In response to DNA damage, the MRN complex—composed of MRE11, Rad50, and NBS1—together with ataxia-telangiectasia mutation (ATM) and H2AX are the earliest proteins recruited to the site of the break. ATM is released from its homodimer complex, activated by transautophosphorylation and, in turn, phosphorylates H2AX. Other members are recruited to the complex such as BRCA1 and 53BP1. As the DNA at the double-strand break (DSB) is resected, single-stranded DNA is formed and bound by replication protein A (RPA), resulting in the activation of the ataxia-telangiectasia and Rad3-related (ATR) pathway. The net result of ATM/ATR activation is the downstream activation of p53, leading to the transcription of the Cdk inhibitor, p21, and the activation of Chk1/Chk2, resulting in the degradation of Cdc25 phosphatases, Cdk-cyclin complex inactivation, and cell cycle arrest at phase G1, intra S, or G2. Note that ATM is also partially activated by changes in chromatin structure induced by DNA double-strand breaks.

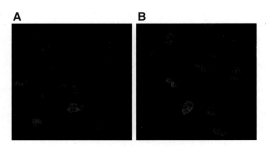

Figure 13.4 Phosphorylated histone variant H2AX as a marker of DNA damage. Phosphorylated histone variant H2AX (also called gamma H2AX) localizes to sites of DNA double-strand breaks, so that its appearance and disappearance correspond with induction and repair of breaks. The cells in panels **A** and **B** have been stained with DAPI (4',6-diamidino-2-phenylindole) (*blue*) in order to visualize cell nuclei and stained with an antibody, which recognizes *gamma* H2AX (*red*). The cells in **A** are untreated and exhibit little to no gamma H2AX staining, whereas the cells in **B** are treated with 7.5 Gy radiation and exhibit strong gamma H2AX staining at punctate foci in the nuclei, which are thought to correlate with sites of DNA double-strand breaks. (Image provided by Dr. Leslie Parsels, University of Michigan.)

perturbations in replication that are the result of stalled replication forks to prevent the formation of DNA double-strand breaks.

The arrest of cells in the G2 phase following DNA damage is one of the most conserved evolutionary responses to ionizing radiation. It makes sense to have a final checkpoint in the G2 phase to prevent cells from entering into mitosis with damaged DNA that could be transmitted to their progeny. It follows that cells lacking the G2 checkpoint are radiosensitive because they try to divide with damaged chromosomes that cannot be aligned at metaphase to be properly apportioned to daughter cells. At the biochemical level, the regulation of the mitosis-promoting factor cyclin B/Cdk1 is the critical step in the activation of this checkpoint. At the molecular level, ATM and Chk1/2 are activated by DNA damage in the G2 phase and inhibit the activation of Cdc25A and C phosphatases, which are essential for the activation of cyclin B/Cdk1.[9, 10] The pololike kinase family (Plk1 and Plk3) also responds to DNA damage and can inhibit Cdc25C activation.[11] A great deal of effort has been focused on the development of small molecules to inhibit checkpoint response proteins, such as Chk1, with the idea that they would inhibit radiation-induced G2 arrest and perhaps repair and thus be used as radiation sensitizers.[12]

DNA Repair

Ionizing radiation causes base damage, single-strand breaks, double-strand breaks, and sugar damage, as well as DNA–DNA, and DNA–protein cross-links. The critical target for ionizing radiation-induced cell inactivation and cell killing is the DNA double-strand break.[13,14] In eukaryotic cells, DNA double-strand breaks can be repaired by two processes: homologous recombination repair (HRR), which requires an undamaged DNA strand as a participant in the repair, and nonhomologous end joining (NHEJ), which mediates end-to-end joining.[15] In lower eukaryotes, such as yeast, HRR is the predominant pathway used for repairing DNA double-strand breaks, whereas mammalian cells use both HHR and non-HHR to repair their DNA. In mammalian cells, the choice of repair is biased by the phase of

the cell cycle and by the abundance of repetitive DNA. HRR is used primarily in the late S phase/G2 phases of the cell-cycle, and NHEJ predominates in the G1-phase of the cell cycle (Fig. 13.5). NHEJ and HRR are not mutually exclusive, and both have been found to be active in the late S/G2 phase of the cell cycle, indicating that factors in addition to the cell-cycle phase are important in determining which mechanism will be used to repair DNA strand breaks.

Nonhomologous End Joining. In the G1-phase of the cell cycle, the ligation of DNA double-strand breaks is primarily through NHEJ because a sister chromatid does not exist to provide a template for HRR. The damaged ends of DNA double-strand breaks must first be modified before rejoining. The process of NHEJ can be divided into at least four steps: synapsis, end processing, fill-in synthesis, and ligation (Fig. 13.6).[16] Synapsis is the critical initial step where the Ku heterodimer and the DNA-dependent protein kinase catalytic subunit (DNA-PKcs) bind to the ends of the DNA double-strand break. Ku recruits not only DNA-PKcs to

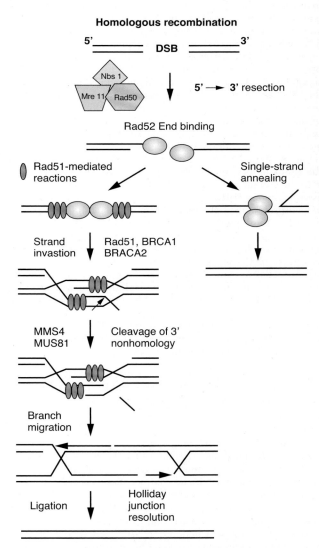

Figure 13.6 Schematic of the critical steps and proteins involved in homologous recombination repair (HRR). The process of HRR can be divided into the following steps: double-strand break (DSB) targeting by H2AX and the MRN complex, recruitment of the ataxia-telangiectasia mutation (ATM) kinase, end processing and protection, strand exchange, single-strand gap filling, and resolution into unique double-stranded molecules.

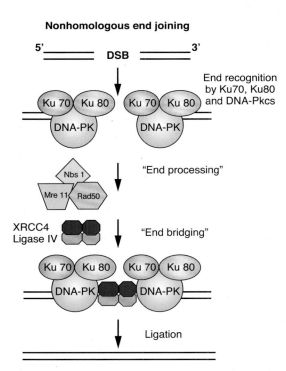

Figure 13.5 Schematic of the critical steps and proteins involved in nonhomologous end joining (NHEJ). The process of NHEJ can be divided into at least four steps: synapsis, end processing, fill-in synthesis, and ligation. DSB, double-strand break.

the DNA ends, but also artemis, a protein that possesses endonuclease activity for 5′ and 3′ overhangs as well as hairpins.[17] DNA-PKcs that is bound to the broken DNA ends phosphorylates artemis and activates its endonuclease activity for end processing. This role of artemis' endonuclease activity in NHEJ may not necessarily be required for the ligation of blunt ends or ends with compatible termini. DNA polymerase μ is associated with the Ku/DNA/XRCC4/DNA ligase IV complex, and is probably the polymerase that is used in the fill-in reaction. The actual rejoining of DNA ends is mediated by a XRCC4/DNA ligase IV complex, which is also probably recruited by the Ku heterodimer.[18,19] Although NHEJ is effective at rejoining DNA double-strand breaks, it is highly error prone. In fact, the main physiologic role of NHEJ is to generate antibodies through V(D)J rejoining, and the error-prone nature of NHEJ is essential for generating antibody diversity.

Homologous Recombination.   HRR provides the mammalian genome a high-fidelity pathway of repairing DNA double-strand breaks. In contrast to NHEJ, HRR requires physical contact with an undamaged DNA template, such as a sister chromatid, for repair to occur. In response to a double-strand break, ATM as well as the complex of Mre11, Rad50, and Nbs1 proteins (MRN complex), are recruited to sites of DNA double-strand breaks (Fig. 13.6).[20] The MRN complex is also involved in the recruitment of the breast cancer tumor suppressor gene, *BRCA1*, to the site of the break.[21] In addition to recruiting *BRCA1* to the site of the DNA strand break, Mre11 and as yet unidentified endonucleases resect the DNA, resulting in a 3′ single-strand DNA that serves as a binding site for Rad51. *BRCA2*, which is recruited to the double-strand break by BRCA1, facilitates the loading of the Rad51 protein onto replication protein A (RPA)-coated single-strand overhangs that are produced by endonuclease resection.[22] The Rad51 protein is a homolog of the *Escherichia coli* recombinase RecA, and possesses the ability to form nucleofilaments and catalyze strand exchange with the complementary strand of the undamaged chromatid, an essential step in HRR. Five additional paralogs of Rad51 also bind to the RPA-coated single-stranded region and recruit Rad52, which binds DNA and protects against exonucleolytic degradation.[23] To facilitate repair, the Rad54 protein uses its ATPase activity to unwind the double-stranded molecule. The two invading ends serve as primers for DNA synthesis, resulting in structures known as Holliday junctions. These Holliday junctions are resolved either by noncrossing over, in which case the Holliday junctions disengage and the DNA strands align followed by gap filling, or by crossing over of the Holliday junctions and gap filling. Because inactivation of most of the HRR genes discussed previously results in radiosensitivity and genomic instability, these genes provide a critical link between HRR and chromosome stability.

Chromosome Aberrations Result from Faulty DNA Double-Strand Break Repair

Unfaithful restitution of DNA strand breaks can lead to chromosome aberrations such as acentric fragments (no centromeres) or terminal deletions (uncapped chromosome ends). Radiation-induced DNA double-strand breaks also induce exchange-type aberrations that are the consequence of symmetric translocations between two DNA double-strand breaks in two different chromosomes (Fig. 13.7). Symmetrical chromosome translocations often do not lead to lethality, because genetic information is not lost in subsequent cell divisions. In contrast, when two DNA double-strand breaks in two different chromosomes recombine to form one chromosome with two centromeres and two fragments of chromosomes without centromeres or telomeres, cell death is inevitable. These types of chromosome aberrations are the consequence of asymmetrical chromosome translocations where the genetic material is recombined in what has been termed an *illegitimate* manner (e.g., a chromosome containing an extra centromere).

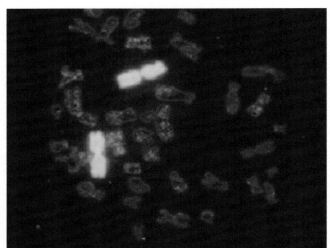

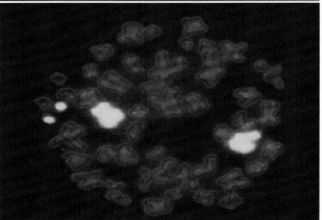

Figure 13.7 Fluorescent in situ hybridization of DNA probes that specifically recognize chromosome 4. In unirradiated cells **(top)**, two chromosome 4s are visualized. In irradiated cells **(bottom)**, one chromosome 4 illegitimately recombined with another chromosome to produce an asymmetrical chromosome aberration, with resulting acentric fragments that will be lost in subsequent cell divisions.

During mitosis, when a cell divides, aberrant chromosomes that have two centromeres, lack a centromere, or are in the shape of a ring have difficulty in separating, resulting in daughter cells with unequal or asymmetric distribution of the parental genetic material. The quantification of asymmetric chromosome aberrations induced by radiation is difficult and has to be performed by the first cell division because these aberrations will be lost during subsequent cell divisions. For this reason, symmetrical chromosome aberrations have been used to assess radiation-induced damage many generations after exposure because they are not lost from the population of exposed cells. In fact, symmetrical chromosome aberrations can be detected in the descendants of survivors of Hiroshima and Nagasaki, indicating that they are stable biomarkers of radiation exposure.[24]

Membrane Signaling

Apart from the direct of effects on DNA, radiation also affects cellular membranes. As part of the cellular stress response, radiation activates membrane receptor signaling pathways such those initiated via epidermal growth factor receptor (EGFR) and transforming growth factor β (TGF-β).[25,26] Activation of these pathways promotes overall survival in response to radiation by promoting DNA damage repair and/or cellular proliferation. In addition,

Cellular Response to Genotoxic Stress

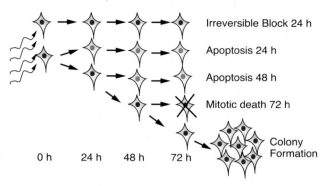

Irreversible Block 24 h

Apoptosis 24 h

Apoptosis 48 h

Mitotic death 72 h

Colony Formation

0 h   24 h   48 h   72 h

Figure 13.8 Consequences of exposure to ionizing radiation at the cellular level. Cells exposed to ionizing radiation can enter a state of senescence where they are unable to divide, but are still able to secrete growth factors. Alternatively, cells can die through apoptosis, mitotic linked cell death, or they can repair their DNA damage and produce viable progeny.

radiation also induces ceramide production at the membrane via activation of sphingomyelinases, which hydrolyze sphingomyelin to form ceramide. Ceramide production is linked to radiation-induced apoptosis.[27]

The Effect of Radiation on Cell Survival

The major potential consequences of cells exposed to ionizing radiation are normal cell division, DNA damage–induced senescence (reproductively inactive but metabolically active), apoptosis, or mitotic-linked cell death (Fig. 13.8). These manifestations of DNA damage can occur within one or two cell divisions or can manifest at later times after many cell divisions.[28] Effects that occur at later times have been termed *delayed reproductive cell death* and may also be influenced by secreted factors that are induced in response to radiation.[29]

The ability to culture cells derived from both normal and tumor tissues has allowed us to gain insight into how radiosensitivity varies between tissues by analyzing the shape of survival curves. Survival curves of tumor cells often possess a shouldered region at low doses that becomes shallower as the dose increases and eventually becomes exponential. A shoulder on a survival means that these low doses of radiation are less efficient in cell killing, presumably because cells are efficient at repairing DNA strand breaks.[13,14] Killing at low doses of radiation can be described in the form of a linear quadratic equation: $S = e^{-\alpha D - \beta D2}$ (Fig. 13.9).[30] In this equation, S is the fraction of cells that survive a dose (D) of radiation, whereas α and β are constants. Cell killing by the linear and quadratic components are equal when $\alpha D = \beta D^2$ or $D = \alpha/\beta$. Over a larger dose range, the relationship between cell killing and dose is more complex and is described by three different components: an initial slope (D_1), a final slope (D_o), and the width of the shoulder (n, the extrapolation number) or D_q, the quasi-threshold dose (Fig. 13.10). The extrapolation number, n, defines the place where the shoulder intersects the ordinate when the dose is extrapolated to zero, and the quasithreshold dose, D_q, defines the width of the shoulder by cutting the dose axis when there is a survival fraction of unity. In contrast to photons, the shoulder on the survival curve disappears when cells are exposed to densely ionizing radiation from particles, indicating that this form of radiation is highly effective at killing cells at both low and high doses.

In Vivo Survival Determination of Normal Tissue Response to Radiation

Although much of our knowledge on the effects of radiation on cell survival has come from cell culture studies, investigators have also devised experimental approaches to assess the clonogenic survival of normal tissues. The earliest example came from McCulloch and Till,[31] who developed an assay to measure the

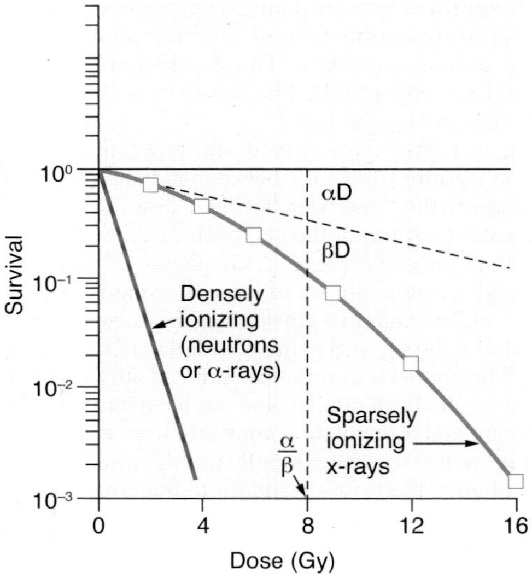

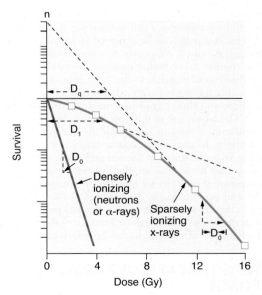

Figure 13.9 An analysis of survival curves for mammalian cells exposed to radiation by the linear quadratic model. The probability of hitting a critical target is proportional to dose (aD): the alpha component. The probability of hitting two critical targets will be the product of those probabilities; therefore, it will be proportional to dose² (βD²): the beta component. The dose at which killing by both the alpha and beta components is equal is defined as D = α/β. (From Hall EJ, Giaccia AJ. *Radiobiology for the Radiologist*. Philadelphia: Lippincott Williams & Williams; 2012, with permission.)

Figure 13.10 An analysis of survival curves for mammalian cells exposed to radiation by the multitarget model. This survival is described by an initial slope (D₁; dose to decreased survival to 37% on initial portion of the curve), a final slope (D₀; dose to decrease survival from starting point to 37% of that point on straight line portion of the curve), an extrapolation number (n; an estimate of the width of the shoulder), and a quasithreshold (D_q; a type of threshold dose below which radiation has no effect). (From Hall EJ, Giaccia AJ. *Radiobiology for the Radiologist*. Philadelphia: Lippincott Williams & Williams; 2012, with permission.)

clonogenic survival of bone marrow–derived cells in response to radiation by injecting them into a recipient mouse and quantifying the number of colonies that developed in the spleen. An analysis of these in vivo spleen assays indicated that bone marrow cells are highly radiosensitive (perhaps the most radiosensitive of all mammalian cells) in that their cell survival curve lacked a shoulder. These experiments represent two important firsts in the radiation sciences: They described the first development of an in vivo assay to assess normal tissue survival to radiation, and they demonstrated the first existence of normal tissue stem cells. Soon after, Withers and colleagues[32] developed an assay to assess the survival of skin stem cells, and Withers and Elkind[33] developed an assay to quantify the viability of small intestinal clonogens.

Because these ingenious approaches cannot be applied to all normal tissues, loss of tissue function instead of clonogenic survival has been used as an end point to assess radiation effects. Effects on tissue function can be grouped into the acute or late variety. Desquamation of skin by radiation is an example of an acute loss of function, whereas loss of spinal cord function is an example of a late functional effect. Acutely sensitive tissues such as skin, bone marrow, and intestinal mucosa possess a significant component of tissue cell division, whereas delayed sensitive tissues, such as spinal cord, breast, and bone, do not possess a significant amount of cell division or turnover and manifest radiation effects at later times.

In Vivo Determination of Tumor Response to Radiation

Assays have also been developed to assess the clonogenic survival of tumor cells in animals. Perhaps the most relevant of these assays is the tumor control dose 50% (TCD_{50}) assay,[34] in which the dose of radiation needed to control the growth of 50% of the tumors is determined in large cohorts of tumor-bearing animals. The TCD_{50} assay in animals most closely approximates the clinical situation because tumors are irradiated in animals and the ability to kill all viable tumor cells is assessed. Unlike assays in which tumor cells are irradiated ex vivo, the TCD_{50} assay takes into account the effects of the tumor microenvironment on tumor response. In contrast to the TCD_{50} assay, the tumor growth delay assay reflects the time after irradiation that a transplanted tumor reaches a fixed multiple of the pretreatment volume compared to an unirradiated control. This end point can be achieved by measuring tumor volume through the use of calipers or by a noninvasive measurement of tumor volume using bioluminescent molecules such as luciferase or fluorescent proteins. In the latter approach, all the tumor cells are stably transfected with a bioluminescent marker before implantation, and tumor growth is measured by bioluminescent activity.[35] The advantage of this approach is that tumor cells can be assessed even if they are orthotopically transplanted into their tissue of origin. In another approach, tumors or cells are first irradiated in vivo, the tumor is excised and made into a single-cell suspension, and these cells are then injected into a non–tumor-bearing animal. If the cells are injected subcutaneously under the skin, the end point is tumor formation.[36] If the tumor cells are injected in the tail vein of the mouse, the end point is colony formation in the lungs.[37] The major advantage of these assays is that the actual number of viable cells can be determined.

FACTORS THAT AFFECT RADIATION RESPONSE

The Fundamental Principles of Radiobiology

Studies on split-dose repair (SDR) by Elkind et al.[38] uncovered three of what we now recognize as the most fundamental principles of fractionated radiotherapy: repair, reassortment, and repopulation (Fig. 13.11). (Reoxygenation, described in the following paragraphs, is the fourth). SDR describes the increased survival

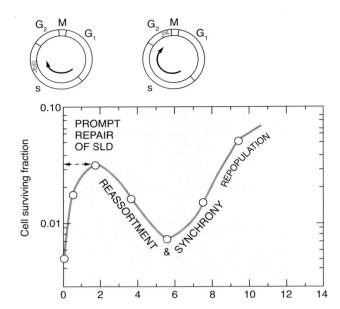

Figure 13.11 Idealized survival curve of rodent cells exposed to two fractions of x-rays. This figure illustrates how the time interval between doses alters the sensitivity of cells when exposed to multiple fractions. In this case, cells move from a resistant phase of the cell cycle (late S phase) to a sensitive phase of the cell cycle (G2 phase). This is known as *reassortment*. If longer periods of time occur between fractions of radiation, cells will undergo division. This latter process is called *repopulation*. SLD, sublethal damage. (From Hall EJ, Giaccia AJ. *Radiobiology for the Radiologist*. Philadelphia: Lippincott Williams & Williams; 2012, with permission.)

or tumor growth delay found if a dose of radiation is split into two fractions compared to the same dose administered in one fraction. This repair is likely due to DNA double-strand break rejoining. Elkind et al. found that the survival of cells increased with an increase in time between doses for up to a maximum of about 6 hours. This finding is consistent with the clinical observation that a separation of radiation treatments by 6 hours produces similar normal tissue injury as a 24-hour separation. The shoulder of a survival curve is strongly influenced by SDR: The broader the shoulder, the more SDR and the smaller α/β ratio.

Similar to repair, reassortment and repopulation are also dependent on the interval of time between radiation fractions. If cells are given short time intervals between doses, they can progress from a resistant portion of the cell cycle (e.g., S phase) to a sensitive portion of the cell cycle (e.g., G2 phase). This transit between resistant and sensitive phases of the cell cycle is termed *reassortment*. If irradiated cells are provided even longer intervals of time between doses, the survival of the population of irradiated cells will increase. This increase in split-dose survival after longer periods of time is the result of cell division and has been termed *repopulation*. Reassortment and repopulation appear to have more protracted kinetics in normal tissues than rapidly proliferating tumor cells, and thereby enhance the tumor response to fractionated radiotherapy compared to normal tissues.

Dose-Rate Effects

For sparsely ionizing radiation, dose rate plays a critical factor in cell killing. Lowering the dose rate, and thereby increasing exposure time, reduces the effectiveness of killing by x-rays because of increased SDR. A further reduction in dose rate results in more SDR and reduces the shoulder of the survival curve. Thus, if one plots the survival for individual doses in a multifraction experiment so that there is sufficient time for SDR to occur, the resulting survival curve would have little shoulder and appear almost linear.[39]

In some cell types, there is a threshold to the lowering of dose rate, and in fact, one paradoxically finds an increase, instead of a decrease, in cell killing. This increase in cell killing under these conditions of protracted dose rate is due to the accumulation of cells in a radiosensitive portion of the cell cycle. In summary, the magnitude of the dose rate effect varies between cell types because of SDR, the redistribution of cells through the cell cycle, and the time for cell division to occur.

Cell Cycle

The phase of the cell cycle at the time of radiation influences the cell's inherent sensitivity to radiation. Cells synchronized in late G1/early S and G2/M phases are most sensitive, whereas cells in G1 and mid to late S phase are more resistant to radiation.[1] These differences in sensitivity during the cell cycle are exploited by the concept of reassortment during fractioned radiotherapy as well by the use of chemotherapeutic agents, which reassort cells into more sensitive phases of the cell cycle in combination with radiation.

Tumor Oxygenation

The major microenvironmental influence on tumor response to radiation is molecular oxygen.[40] Decreased levels of oxygen (hypoxia) in tissue culture result in decreased killing after radiation, which can be expressed as an *oxygen enhancement ratio* (OER). Operationally, OER is defined as the ratio of doses to give the same killing under hypoxic and normoxic conditions. At high doses of radiation, the OER is approximately 3, whereas at low doses, it is closer to 2.[41] Oxygen must be present within 10 μs of irradiation to achieve its radiosensitizing effect. Under hypoxic conditions, damage to DNA can be repaired more readily than under oxic conditions, where damage to DNA is "fixed" because of the interaction of oxygen with free radicals generated by radiation. These changes in radiation sensitivity are detectable at oxygen ranges below 30 mm Hg. Most tumor cells exhibit a survival difference halfway between fully aerobic and fully anoxic cells when exposed to a partial pressure of oxygen between 3 and 10 mm Hg.[1] The presence of hypoxia has greater significance for single-dose fractions used in the treatment of certain primary tumors and metastases and is less important for fractionated radiotherapy, where reoxygenation occurs between fractions. Furthermore, most hypoxic cells are not actively undergoing cell division, thus impeding the efficacy of conventional chemotherapeutic agents that are targeted to actively dividing cells.

Although normal tissue and tumors vary in their oxygen concentrations, only tumors possess levels of oxygen low enough to influence the effectiveness of radiation killing. Although the variations in normal tissue oxygenation are in large part due to physiology governing acute changes in oxygen consumption, the variations in tumor oxygen can be directly attributed to abnormal vasculature that results in a more chronic condition. Thomlinson and Gray[42] observed that variations in tumor oxygen occur because there is insufficient vasculature to provide oxygen to all tumor cells. They hypothesized that oxygen is unable to reach tumor cells beyond 10 to 12 cell diameters from the lumen of a tumor blood vessel because of metabolic consumption by respiring tumor cells. This form of hypoxia caused by metabolic consumption of oxygen has been termed *chronic* or *diffusion-mediated hypoxia*. In contrast, changes in blood flow due either to interstitial pressure changes in tumor blood vessels that lack a smooth muscle component or red blood cell fluxes can cause transient occlusion of blood vessels resulting in *acute* or *transient hypoxia*. Chronically, hypoxic cells will only become reoxygenated when their distance from the lumen of a blood vessel decreases, such as during fractionated radiotherapy when tumor cords shrink. In contrast, tumor cells that are acutely hypoxic because of changes in blood flow or interstitial pressure often cycle in an unpredictable manner between oxic and hypoxic states as blood flow changes.

Based on studies demonstrating that hypoxia can alter radiation sensitivity and decrease tumor control by radiotherapy, strategies have been developed to increase tumor oxygenation. Most importantly, it appears that tumor oxygen levels increase during a course of fractionated radiation. This may be one of the most important benefits of fractionated radiation and is termed *reoxygenation* (the fourth of the four Rs of radiobiology). Tumor reoxygenation during a course of fractionated radiation may also offer an explanation for the general lack of clinical efficacy of hypoxic cell sensitizers despite the clear evidence that hypoxia causes radioresistance.

Aside from using fractionated radiation, the most direct approach to increasing tumor oxygenation is to expose patients receiving radiotherapy to hyperbaric oxygen therapy. The underlying concept is that increasing the amount of oxygen in the bloodstream should result in more oxygen being available for diffusion to the hypoxic regions of tumors. Experimentally, hyperbaric oxygen therapy increases the sensitivity of transplanted tumors to radiation. The results of clinical studies with hyperbaric oxygen therapy, when combined with radiotherapy, showed improvement for two sites—head and neck cancers, and cervix cancers—but failed to show an improvement with other sites, thus calling into question its general usefulness in radiotherapy.[43] In a related approach, erythropoietin (EPO), a hormone released by the kidney that increases red blood cell production, should also increase tumor oxygenation by increasing the delivery of hemoglobin-bound oxygen molecules. EPO has been effective at correcting anemia, but has not been successful in combination with radiation to control head and neck cancer and may, in fact, stimulate tumor growth.[44, 45]

Another strategy to increase tumor oxygenation has been the combined use of nicotinamide, which increases tissue perfusion and carbogen (95% O_2 and 5% CO_2) breathing (accelerated radiotherapy with carbogen and nicotinamide [ARCON] therapy). Recently, a randomized phase III clinical trial demonstrated improved regional but not local tumor control in larynx cancer patients treated with nicotinamide, carbogen, and radiation versus radiation alone.[46] Biologics such as antivascular endothelial growth factor (anti-VEGF) therapy have also been demonstrated to increase tumor oxygenation.[47] Anti-VEGF therapy may increase tumor oxygenation by eliminating abnormal vessels that are inadequate in perfusing tumor cells—the so-called *vascular normalization hypothesis*. Although there is solid experimental evidence to support this hypothesis, there appears to be only a short window of time in which it could be effectively combined with radiotherapy.

Because the presence of hypoxia has both prognostic and potential therapeutic implications, a substantial effort has been invested in trying to image hypoxia.[48] The goal of using imaging to "paint" radiation doses to different regions of tumors, although technically possible (as described in the next section, Radiation Physics), faces the problem that changes in oxygenation are dynamic.[49] In the future, hypoxia-directed treatment may evolve from the use of hypoxic cell cytotoxins to targeted drugs that exploit cellular signaling changes induced by hypoxia such as hypoxia-inducible factor 1α (HIF-1α). However, despite the strong rationale supporting their use, at this time, there are no agents used in the clinic that target hypoxia.

Immune Response

The abscopal effects of radiation (i.e., tumor cell killing outside of the radiation field) have been attributed to the activation of antigen and cytokine release by radiation, which subsequently activates a systemic immune response against tumor cells.[50,51] This response begins with the transfer of tumor cell antigens to dendritic cells and, subsequently, the activation of tumor-specific T cells and *immunogenic tumor cell death*. It is likely that radiation dose and fractionation influence the optimal immune response with higher doses and fewer fractions of radiation than those used in conventional fractionation schemes appearing superior in experimental models. Unfortunately, abscopal effects are uncommon because immune system evasion is an inherent characteristic of cancer cells that often dominates, even in the presence of a radiation-induced immune response. Strategies to amplify radiation-induced immune responses, and thus to overcome tumor cell evasion of the immune system, are under investigation. The combination of radiation with immune *checkpoint* modulators such as ipilimumab, an antibody against cytotoxic T-lymphocyte antigen 4 (CTLA-4), have shown promising, albeit anecdotal, clinical effects.

DRUGS THAT AFFECT RADIATION SENSITIVITY

For over 30 years now, chemotherapy and radiotherapy have been administered concurrently. In order to maximize the efficacy of radiochemotherapy, it is necessary to understand the biologic mechanisms underlying radiosensitization by chemotherapeutic agents. The several classes of standard chemotherapeutic agents as well as novel molecularly targeted agents that possess radiosensitizing properties will be discussed in this section.

Antimetabolites

5-fluorouracil is among the most commonly used chemotherapeutic radiation sensitizers. Given in combination with radiation, it has led to clinical improvements in a variety of cancers, including those of the head and neck, the esophagus, the stomach, the pancreas, the rectum, the anus, and the cervix. The combination of 5-fluorouracil with radiation is now a standard therapy for cancers of the stomach (adjuvant), the pancreas (unresectable), and the rectum. For other cancers such as head and neck, esophagus, or anal, 5-fluorouracil and radiation are combined with cisplatin or mitomycin C, respectively. Being an analog of uracil, 5-flourouracil is misincorporated into RNA and DNA. However, the ability of 5-fluorouracil to radiosensitize is related to its ability to inhibit thymidylate synthase, which leads to the depletion of thymidine triphosphate (dTTP) and the inhibition of DNA synthesis. This slowed, inappropriate progression through S phase in response to 5-fluorouracil is thought to be the mechanism underlying radiosensitization.[52] Similar to 5-fluorouracil, the oral thymidylate synthase inhibitor, capecitabine, is also being increasingly used in combination with radiation.

Gemcitabine (2', 2'-deoxyfluorocytidine [dFdCyd]) is another potent antimetabolite radiosensitizer. Preclinical studies have demonstrated that radiosensitization by gemcitabine involves the depletion of deoxyadenosine triphosphate (dATP) (related to the ability of gemcitabine diphosphate (dFdCDP) to inhibit ribonucleotide reductase) as well as the redistribution of cells into the early S phase of the cell cycle.[53] The combination of gemcitabine with radiation in clinical trials has suggested improved clinical outcomes for patients with cancers of the lung, pancreas, and bladder. Gemcitabine-based chemoradiation has developed into a standard therapy for locally advanced pancreatic cancer. However, in some clinical trials, such as those in lung and head and neck cancers, the combination of gemcitabine with radiation has led to increased mucositis and esophagitis.[54] Thus, it should be emphasized that in the presence of gemcitabine, radiation fields must be defined with great caution. Such is the case with pancreatic cancer, where the combination of full-dose gemcitabine with radiation to the gross tumor can be safely administered if clinically uninvolved lymph nodes are excluded.[55] Conversely, the inclusion of the regional lymphatics in the treatment field in combination with full-dose gemcitabine produces unacceptable toxicities.[56]

Platinums and Temozolomide

Cisplatin is likely the most commonly used chemotherapeutic agent in combination with radiation. Although cisplatin was the prototype for several other platinum analogs, carboplatin is also frequently used in combination with radiation. Cisplatin, in combination with radiation, and sometimes in conjunction with a second chemotherapeutic agent, is indicated for cancers of the head and neck, esophagus (with 5-fluorouracil), the lung, the cervix, and the anus. Radiosensitization by cisplatin is related to its ability to cause inter- and intra-strand DNA cross-links. Removal of these cross-links during the repair process results in DNA strand breaks. Although there are multiple theories to explain the mechanism(s) of radiosensitization by cisplatin, two plausible explanations are that cisplatin inhibits the repair (both homologous and nonhomologous) of radiation-induced DNA double-strand breaks and/or increases the number of lethal radiation-induced double-strand breaks.[57]

Temozolomide in combination with radiation is standard therapy for glioblastoma. Temozolomide is an alkylating agent, which forms methyl adducts at the O^6 position of guanine (as well as at N^7 and N^3-guanine) that are subsequently improperly repaired by the mismatch repair pathway. Radiosensitization by temozolomide involves the inhibition of DNA repair and/or an increase in radiation-induced DNA double-strand breaks due to radiation-induced single-strand breaks in proximity to O^6 methyl adducts. Like cisplatin, temozolomide-mediated radiosensitization does not seem to require cell cycle redistribution.

Taxanes

The taxanes, paclitaxel and docetaxel, act to stabilize microtubules resulting in the accumulation of cells in G2/M, the most radiation-sensitive phase of the cell cycle. The radiosensitizing properties of the taxanes are thought to be attributable to the redistribution of cells into G2/M. Paclitaxel, in combination with radiation (and carboplatin), has demonstrated a clinical benefit in the treatment of resectable lung carcinoma.[58]

Molecularly Targeted Agents

Molecularly targeted agents are especially appealing in the context of radiosensitization because they are generally less toxic than standard chemotherapeutic agents and need to be given in multimodality regimens (given their often inadequate efficacy as single agents). The EGFR has been intensely pursued as a target; both antibody and small molecule EGFR inhibitors, such as cetuximab and erlotinib, respectively, have been developed. The head and neck seem to be the most promising tumor sites for the combination of EGFR inhibitors with radiation therapy. Preclinical data have demonstrated that the schedule of administration of EGFR inhibitors with radiation is important; EGFR inhibition before chemoradiation may produce antagonism.[59] In a randomized phase III trial, cetuximab plus radiation produced a significant survival advantage over radiation alone in patients with locally advanced head and neck cancer.[60] In a subsequent trial, however, cetuximab in combination with concurrent, cisplatin-based chemoradiation failed to produce a survival benefit in head and neck cancer patients.[61] The combination of EGFR inhibitor with cisplatin-radiation requires further preclinical investigation.

Although EGFR inhibition, concurrent with radiation, is by far the best established combination of a molecularly targeted agent with radiation, other exciting molecularly targeted agents are being developed as radiation sensitizers. Targeting DNA damage response pathways is one approach to radiosensitization. Recently, agents that abrogate radiation-induced cell cycle checkpoints, such as Wee1 and Chk1 inhibitors, have been shown to radiosensitize tumor cells and are currently in clinical development in combination with chemotherapy, with clinical trials planned in combination with radiation.[62,63] In addition, poly(ADP-ribose) polymerase (PARP) inhibitors have been demonstrated to preclinically induce radiosensitization, and several clinical trials combining PARP inhibitors with radiation therapy are underway.[64]

Other Agents

Although the most common clinically used agents in combination with radiation have been shown to produce significant clinical benefit, as described previously, other agents with different mechanisms of action have been used as radiation sensitizers as well as radiation protectors. The vinca alkaloids, such as vincristine, possess radiosensitizing properties due to their ability to block mitotic spindle assembly and, thus, arrest cells in M phase. Although vincristine is used in combination with radiation to treat medulloblastoma, rhabdomyosarcoma, and brain stem glioma, its use is principally based on its lack of myelosuppressive side effects, which are dose limiting for radiation in these types of tumors, rather than its potential radiosensitizing properties.

Also worth mention in a discussion of modulators of radiation sensitivity are agents designed to radioprotect normal tissues. One such type of drug, amifostine, is a free radical scavenger with some selectivity toward normal tissues that express more alkaline phosphatase than tumor cells, the enzyme of which converts amifostine to a free thiol metabolite. Clinical trials in head and neck as well as lung cancers have shown a reduction in radiation-related toxicities such as xerostomia, mucositis, esophagitis, and pneumonitis, respectively.[65,66] However, further clinical investigations are necessary to conclusively demonstrate a lack of tumor protection and safety in combination with chemoradiotherapy regimens.

RADIATION PHYSICS

Physics of Photon Interactions

Tumors requiring radiation can be found at depths ranging from zero to 10s of centimeters below the skin. The goal of treatment is to deliver sufficient ionizing radiation to the tumor site, which can result in an absorbed dose. This involves both the availability of treatment beams and delivery techniques, and the methods to plan the treatments and ensure their safe delivery. This section will establish the general physical basis for the use of ionizing radiation in the treatment of tumors, briefly describe some of the treatment equipment, indicate physical qualities of the treatment beams themselves, and summarize the treatment planning process. Those who desire more in-depth details are referred to textbooks and other resources dedicated to medical physics and the technologic aspects of radiation oncology.[67] Most patients who are treated with radiation receive high-energy, external-beam photon therapy. Here, *external* indicates that the treatment beam is generated and delivered from outside of the body. High-energy (6 to 20 MV) photon beams (electromagnetic radiation) penetrate tissue, enabling the treatment of deep-seated tumors. Modern equipment generates these beams with sufficient fluence to ensure delivery of therapeutic fractions of dose in short treatment sessions. Other types of particles and beams also exist for use in treating tumors both externally and internally. They are mentioned briefly later. However, as external photon beams dominate the practice (and as common basic physics principles related to delivered dose exist among the modalities), the focus here will be on photon beam generation and interactions in tissue.

As mentioned earlier, ionizing radiation kills cells via both direct and indirect mechanisms. Radiation therapy aims to instigate those ionizations and events in the tumor cells. Photons are massless, uncharged packets of energy that primarily interact with matter via electromagnetic processes. As a consequence of those interactions, an incident photon can become either entirely absorbed (giving up its energy to the ejection of an atomic electron [photoelectric effect]), or create an energetic electron-positron pair (pair production), or scatter off an electron with a reduction in energy and a change in direction and subsequent transfer of parts of its energy to the free electron (Compton scattering). The secondary electrons generated as a consequence of these interactions have residual energy, mass, and, most importantly, electric charge. They slow down in matter through multiple interactions with (primarily) the electrons of atoms, leading to excitation and ionization of those atoms. These ionizations (hence the term *ionizing radiation*) lead to a local absorption of energy (i.e., dose = energy absorbed per unit mass) and the direct and indirect cell killing effects necessary to treat tumors.

Thus, the use of external photon beams for cancer therapy involves a two-step process: interaction (scattering) of the photons, with subsequent dose deposition via the secondary electrons. The probability of photon interactions is energy dependent. Photoelectric interactions dominate at lower photon energies. Whereas these beams are ideal for diagnostic procedures (for their preferential absorption by tissues of differing atomic number, leading to good subject contrast), they are attenuated too quickly in tissues to supply enough interactions to be useful for therapy for any but the most superficial tumors. Pair production interactions dominate at higher photon energies; however, the probability of interacting in tissues for those high-energy photons is so low as to preclude them from general use as well. In the 10s to 100s of kiloelectron volt (keV) to the few megaelectron volt (MeV) photon energy range, Compton scattering dominates. As will be shown, these beams have sufficient penetration and can be generated with sufficient intensity to be useful for tumor treatments, especially when combined in treatment plans that comprise multiple beams entering the patient from different directions but overlapping at the tumor.

It is useful to point out physical scales of reference for external photon beam therapy. A typical megavoltage photon beam may have an average photon energy near 2 MeV. Those photons primarily undergo Compton scattering with a mean free path in tissue of approximately 20 cm. An average Compton interaction results in a secondary electron with a mean energy near 0.5 MeV (and a Compton scattered photon near 1.5 MeV, which likely escapes or scatters elsewhere in the patient). A typical secondary electron of approximately 0.5 MeV will cause excitations and ionizations of atoms as it dissipates its energy over a path length of approximately 2 mm. This could be expected to lead to approximately 10,000 ionizations, or about 5 ionizations per micron of tissue. As can be seen, therapeutic damage to the DNA of cancer cells (2 nm; see Fig. 13.2) will require very many Compton scatterings with statistical interaction among the ionizations resulting from the slowing down of the secondary electrons.

Photon Beam Generation and Treatment Delivery

As previously mentioned, effective external-beam photon treatments require higher energy beams capable of reaching deep-seated tumors with sufficient fluence to make it likely that the dose deposition will kill the tumor cells. To spare normal tissues and maximize targeting, beams are arranged to enter the patient from several directions and to intersect at the center of the tumor (treatment isocenter). Although machines containing collimated beams from high-intensity radioactive sources (primarily cobalt 60 [^{60}Co]) are still in use, today's modern treatment machine accelerates electrons to high (MeV) energy and impinges them onto an x-ray production target, leading to the generation of intense beams of Bremsstrahlung x-rays. A typical photon beam treatment machine[68,69] (Fig. 13.12) consists of a high-energy (6 to 20 MeV) linear electron accelerator, electromagnetic beam steering and

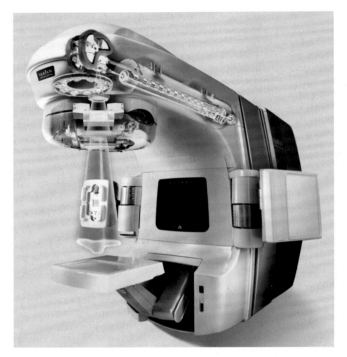

Figure 13.12 A shadow view of a C-arm linear accelerator. The electron beam (originating at upper right) is accelerated through a linear accelerator wave guide, selected for correct energy in a bending magnet, and then impinges on an x-ray production target. The x-ray beam (originating at target upper left) is flattened and collimated before leaving the treatment head. Also illustrated (downstream from the beam) is an electric portal imager that is used to measure (image) the beam exiting a patient. (From Varian Medical Systems, Palo Alto, CA, with permission.)

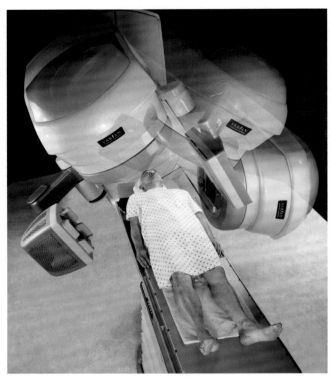

Figure 13.13 Model in treatment position on the patient support table. The treatment delivery head on the gantry's C-arm rotates about the patient, enabling the delivery of beams throughout 360 degrees of rotation. (From Varian Medical Systems, Palo Alto, CA, with permission.)

monitoring systems, x-ray generation targets, high-density treatment field-shaping devices (collimators), and up to a ton of radiation shielding on a mechanical C-arm gantry that can rotate precisely around a treatment couch (Fig. 13.13). These treatment-delivery machines routinely maintain mechanical isocenters for patient treatments to within a sphere of 1 mm radius. The development of *stereotactic radiotherapy*, which will be described in the section titled Clinical Application of Types of Radiation, depends on this level of machine precision.

X-ray production by monoenergetic high-energy electrons results in an x-ray (photon) beam that contains a continuous spectrum of energies with maximum photon energy near that of the incident electron beam. Lower energy photons appear with a much greater probability than do the highest energy ones, but they also become preferentially filtered out of the beam through the absorption in the target and the attenuation in the flattening filter. This generally results in a treatment beam energy spectrum with a mean photon energy of approximately one-third of the initial electron beam energy. In this energy range, the resulting photon beam exits the production target with a narrow angular spread focused primarily in the forward direction. These forward-peaked intensity distributions generally need to be modulated (flattened) to produce a large (up to 40 cm diameter at the patient) photon beam with uniform intensity across the beam. All modern treatment units take advantage of extensive computer control, monitoring, and feedback to produce highly stable and reproducible treatment beams.

The resulting photon beam requires beam shaping for conformal dose delivery. Some combination of primary, high-density field blocks (collimators) together with additional edge blocks generally provide the required shaping and shielding. Modern machines use computer-controlled multileaf collimators (Fig. 13.14)

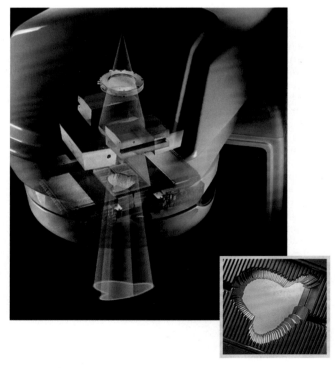

Figure 13.14 Multileaf collimator shaping of an x-ray treatment beam from a linear accelerator. *Inset* shows a view of the multileaf collimator. (From Varian Medical Systems, Palo Alto, CA, with permission.)

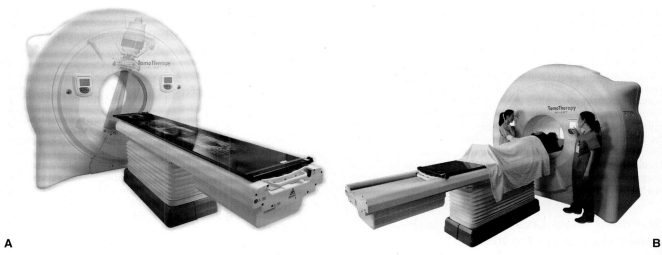

A

B

Figure 13.15 (A) A shadow view of linear accelerator, x-ray beam production system, and x-ray fan beam for helical tomotherapy treatment delivery. The beam production system rotates within its enclosed gantry. **(B)** The model patient on treatment table slides into the treatment unit. During treatment, the table moves as the collimated fan beam rotates about the patient, creating a modulated helical dose delivery pattern. (From TomoTherapy, Inc., Madison, WI, with permission.)

for the edge sculpting subsequent to setting the primary collimators for maximal shielding. This computer control provides high precision and reproducibility in the definition of field edges. Additionally, automation allows for a precise reshaping of the treatment beam for each angle of incidence, allowing not only conformation of irradiation to target volumes, but also modulation of the beam intensity patterns across the field (intensity-modulated radiation therapy [IMRT]).

Variations on the standard linear accelerator (linac) plus C-arm scenario that are being used for external-beam radiation treatments throughout the body include helical tomotherapy and nonisocentric miniature linac robotic delivery systems.[70] In helical tomotherapy, the accelerator, photon-production target, and collimation system are mounted on a ring gantry (similar to those found on diagnostic computed tomography [CT] scanners) (Fig. 13.15). It produces a fan beam of photons, and the intensity of each part of the fan being modulated by a binary collimator. As the gantry rotates, the patient simultaneously slides through the bore of the machine (again analogous to modern x-ray/CT imagers), which allows for the continuous delivery of intensity-modulated radiation in a helical pattern from all angles around a patient. Another delivery system uses an industrial robot to hold a miniature accelerator plus photon beam-production system (Fig. 13.16). The bulk of the system is reduced by keeping the field sizes small (spotlike). However, computer control of the robot provides flexibility in irradiating tumors from nearly any position external to the patient. The same control allows for the selection and use of many differing beam angles to build up the dose at the tumor location.

To take advantage of the precision of modern beam delivery, it is crucial to localize the patient's tumor and normal tissue.[71] This process can be divided into patient immobilization (i.e., limiting the motion of the patient) and localization (i.e., knowing the tumor and normal tissue location precisely in space). Although these concepts of immobilization and localization are related, they are not identical. Patients can be held reasonably comfortable in their treatment pose with the aid of foam molds and meshes (i.e., immobilization devices). Traditionally, localization has been achieved by indexing the immobilization device to the computer-controlled treatment couch and by using low-power laser beams aligned to skin marks. These techniques make it possible to reproducibly couple the surface of each patient with the treatment machine isocenter.

However, what is truly needed is to localize the tumor and normal tissues. The development of in-room, online x-ray, ultrasound, and infrared imaging equipment can now be used to ensure that the intended portions of each patient's internal anatomy are correctly positioned at the time of treatment. In particular, the development of rugged, low-profile, active matrix, flat-panel imaging devices, either attached to the treatment gantry or placed in the vicinity of the treatment couch, together with diagnostic x-ray generators or the patient treatment beam (see Fig. 13.13), allows the digital capture of projection x-ray images of patient anatomy with respect to the isocenter and treatment field borders. These digitized electronic images are immediately available for analysis. Software tools allow for a comparison to reference images and the generation of correction coordinates, which are in turn available for downloading to the treatment couch for automated fine adjustment of the patient's treatment position. Other precise localization systems rely on the identification of the positions of small, implanted radiopaque markers or other types of *smart* position-reporting devices. Careful use of these image-guided radiation

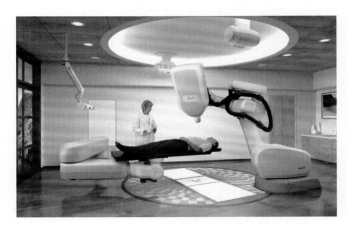

Figure 13.16 A miniature accelerator plus x-ray production system on a robotic delivery arm. Both the treatment table and the treatment head is set by a computer for multiple arbitrary angles of incidence. (From Accuray, Sunnyvale, CA, with permission.)

therapy (IGRT) systems[71, 72] can result in the repeated reducibility of patient position to within a few millimeters over a 5- to 8-week course of treatment.

The final part of external-beam patient treatment is dose delivery. All modern treatment units have computer monitoring (and often control) of all mechanical and dose-delivery components. Treatment-planning information (treatment machine parameters, treatment field configurations, dose per treatment field segment) is downloaded to a work station at the treatment unit that first assists with and then records treatment. This information, together with the readbacks from the treatment machine, are used to reproducibly set up and then verify each patient's treatment parameters, which prevents many of the variations that used to occur when all treatment was performed simply by following instructions written in a treatment chart.

Treatment Beam Characteristics and Dose-Calculation Algorithms

Beyond a basic understanding of the interactions of ionizing radiation with matter lies the requirement of being able to characterize the treatment beams for purposes of planning and verifying treatments. By virtue of a few underlying principles, this generally can be accomplished via a two-step process of absolute calibration of the dose at some reference point in a phantom (i.e., measurement media representative of a patient's tissues), with relative scaling of dose values in other parts of the beam or phantom with respect to that point.

As mentioned earlier, the predominant mode of interaction for therapeutic energy photon beams in tissuelike materials is through Compton scattering. The probability of Compton scattering events is primarily proportional to the relative electron density of the media with which they interact. Because many body tissues are waterlike in composition, it has been possible to make photon beam dosimetric measurements in phantoms consisting mostly of water (water tanks) or tissue-equivalent plastic and to then scale the interactions via relative electron density values (for example, as can be derived from computed x-ray/CT) to other waterlike materials. Thus, the relative fluence of photons in a therapeutic treatment beam is attenuated as it passes through a phantom, primarily via Compton scattering.

It was stated earlier that the photon beam is generated at a small region in the head of the machine. That fluence of photons spreads out through the collimating system before reaching the patient. Thus, without any interactions (e.g., if the beam were in a vacuum), the number of photons crossing any plane perpendicular to the beam direction would remain constant. However, the cross-sectional area of the plane gets larger the farther it is located from the source point. In fact, both the width and length of the cross-sectional area increase in proportion to the distance from the source, and thus the area increases in proportion to the square of the distance. This means that the primary photon fluence per unit area in a plane perpendicular to the beam direction of a pointlike source also decreases as one over the square of the distance, the so-called $1/r^2$ reduction in fluence as a function of distance, r, from the source.

Thus, we have two processes, attenuation and $1/r^2$ reduction, which reduce the photon fluence from an external therapeutic beam as a function of depth in a patient. There is also a process that can increase the photon fluence at a point downstream. Recall that Compton scattering interactions lead not only to secondary electrons (which are responsible for deposition of dose), but also to Compton scattered photons. These photons are scattered from the interaction sites in multiple, predominantly forward-looking directions. Thus, Compton-scattered photons originating from many other places can add to the photon fluence at another point. As the irradiated area (field size) increases, the amount of scattered radiation also increases.

As mentioned earlier, dose *deposition* is a two-step process of photon interaction (proportional to the local fluence of photons) and energy transfer to the medium via the slowing down of secondary electrons. Thus, the point where a photon interacts is not the place where the dose is actually deposited, which happens over the track of the secondary electron. Dose has a very strict definition of energy *absorbed* per unit mass (i.e., due to the slowing down charged particles) and should be distinguished from the energy released at a point, defined as kerma (e.g., energy transfer from the scattering incident photon). Thus, although the photon beam fluence will always be greatest at the entrance to a patient or phantom, the actual *absorbed dose* for a megavoltage photon beam builds up over the first couple of centimeters, reaching a maximum (d-max) at a depth corresponding to the range of the higher energy Compton electrons set in motion. This turns out to be a second desirable characteristic of these beams (beyond their ability to treat deep-seated lesions), because the dose to the skin (a primary dose-limiting structure in earlier times) is greatly reduced.

The relative distributions of dose, normalized to an absolute dose measurement (using a small thimblelike air ionization chamber at a standard depth and for a standard field size according to nationally and internationally accepted protocols), are the major inputs into treatment-planning systems. The major features of these distributions are (1) the initial dose buildup up to a depth of d-max, with a more gradual drop off in dose as a function of depth into the phantom due to the attenuation and $1/r^2$ factors at deeper depths (relative depth dose), and (2) the shape of the dose in the plane perpendicular to the direction of the beams; both as a function of field size. Central axis depth dose curves for typical external photon beams are shown in Figure 13.17 for two beam energies and for both a large and smaller field size. Notice both the expected increase in penetration with increasing beam energy and the increase in dose at a particular depth with increasing field size; the latter effect due to increased numbers of secondary Compton-scattered photons for larger irradiated areas. The change in dose perpendicular to the central axis is less remarkable, because the beams are designed to be uniform across a field as a function of depth.

It is useful to also point out the depth dose characteristics of clinical external treatment beams produced using ionizing

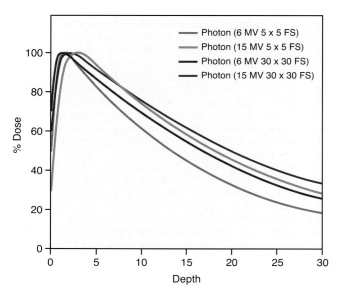

Figure 13.17 Sample depth-dose curves (change in delivered dose as a function of depth) along the central axis of some typical photon treatment beams for low (6 MV) and intermediate (15 MV) energy beams, and large (30 × 30 cm²) and smaller (5 × 5 cm²) field sizes (FS).

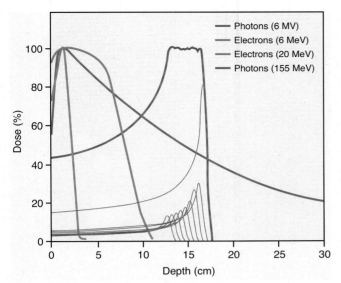

Figure 13.18 Sample depth-dose curves along the central axis of some typical charged particle treatment beams compared with that of a 6-MV proton beam. The spread out Bragg peak at the end of the 155-MeV proton beam (*thick pink curve*) is a composite dose deposition pattern from the addition of the multiple range-shifted proton curves (*thinner pink curves*).

radiations other than photons, primarily through the direct use of charged particles. Those beams (Fig. 13.18) illustrate interesting characteristics, which, when added to the options available for treatment planning (or used by themselves), can produce advantageous results. Relative to the photon beam, the direct use of electron beams leads to deposition of dose over a more localized range, but at the expense of a relative lack of penetration. Thus, electron beams are most widely used for treating, or boosting the treatment of, more superficial tumors and regions (see the section titled Clinical Application of Types of Radiation). The heavier charged particle beams (protons and carbon ions) appear to exhibit even more interesting *depth-dose* characteristics, with the advantage of both (when necessary) being highly penetrating and also lacking a significant dose beyond a certain depth (a depth that can be controlled and purposefully placed, for example, at the distal edge of a target volume).

The results of measurements such as these have been modeled so as to develop dose-calculation algorithms used in treatment-planning systems. These models all use measured beam data to set or adjust parameters used by those algorithms in their dose-distribution computations. Because most of the input data used for beam fitting come from measurements in water phantoms (or waterlike plastic phantoms), patient-specific adjustments are needed for the water phantom data to account for both geometry and tissue properties. It is the task of the dose-calculation algorithms to take those changes into account. The accuracy and precision actually realized for all dose-calculation algorithms generally need to be traded off against the time required to complete the calculation. Although the availability of ever more powerful computers has made calculation time less of a concern for broad, open-beam treatment planning, issues still remain for more specialized planning exercises that use many small beams or parts of beams such as IMRT (discussed later). Typically, relative dose distributions can be computed within patients on the scale of a few millimeters with a precision of better than a few percentage points.

An important area of research is the development of treatment-planning systems that calculate dose based on the principles of how radiation interacts with tissues, rather than simply by fitting data. These approaches use Monte Carlo techniques,[71,73] which

build a dose distribution by summing the calculated paths of thousands of photons and scattered electrons. This approach is more accurate than beam-fitting algorithms in regions of differing tissue densities, such as the lung, and therefore, will ultimately replace the current generation of treatment-planning systems, particularly for complex conditions. However, the time to perform these calculations is still prohibitive for a clinic, and it is anticipated that Monte Carlo calculations will be introduced over a period of years by balancing the need for accuracy in a particular clinical situation with the need to initiate patient treatment.

TREATMENT PLANNING

As discussed in the previous section, single-treatment beams usually deposit more of the dose closer to where they enter the patient than they do at depths corresponding to where a deep-seated tumor might be located. The use of multiple beams entering the patient from different directions that overlap at the target produces more dose per unit volume throughout the tumor volume than is received by normal tissues. In fact, as noted earlier, the treatment-delivery machines are designed to make this easy to accomplish. Planning patient treatments under these circumstances should be a somewhat trivial matter of first selecting a sufficient number of beam angles to realize the desired buildup of the dose in the overlap region relative to the doses in the upstream parts of each beam, and then second, designing beam apertures that shape the edges of the beams to match the target. However, dose-limiting normal tissues often also lie in the paths of one or more of the beams. These normal tissues are often more sensitive to radiation damage than the tumor, and regardless, it is best practice to minimize the dose in any case as a general principle. Computerized treatment-planning systems function to develop patient-specific anatomic or geometric models and then use these models together with the beam-specific dose deposition properties (derived from phantom measurements, as previously described) to select beam angles, shapes, and intensities that meet an overall prescribed objective. That is, modern radiation oncology dose prescriptions contain both tumor and normal tissue objectives, and the modern computerized treatment-planning systems make it possible to design treatments that meet these objectives.

The development and use of three-dimensional (3D) models of each patient's anatomy, treatment geometry, and dose distribution led to a paradigm shift in radiation therapy treatment planning. Computerized radiation treatment planning began in the 1980s as a mainly x-ray/CT–based reconstruction of 3D geometries from information manually contoured on multiple two-dimensional (2D) transverse CT images. Today, these models often incorporate imaging data from multiple sources. Geometrically accurate anatomic information from an x-ray/CT scan still anchors these studies (as well as provides tissue density information necessary for dose calculations). However, it is now quite common to also register the CT data set with other studies such as magnetic resonance imaging (MRI), which may add anatomic detail for soft tissues, or functional MRI or positron emission tomography (PET) studies,[74,75] which provide physiologic or molecular information about tumors and normal tissues. Once registered with each other, the unique or complementary information from each data set can be fused for inspection and incorporated into the design of each patient's target and normal tissue volumes (Fig. 13.19). Beyond the ability to more fully define the extent of the primary target volume (for instance, as the encompassing envelope of disease appreciated on all the imaging studies) lies the ability to define subvolumes of the tumor volume that might be appropriate for simultaneous treatment to higher dose. For example, it should soon become possible to define different biologic components of the tumor that could potentially be targeted and then monitored for response using these same imaging techniques.[76]

Current treatment planning makes the tacit assumption that the planning image yields "the truth" about the location and condition

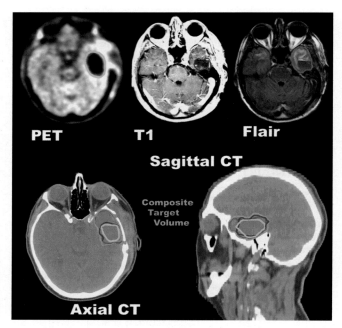

Figure 13.19 An illustration of the brain tumor target volume delineated on coregistered nuclear medicine and magnetic resonance imaging studies fused with computed tomography (CT) data for treatment planning. PET, positron emission tomography.

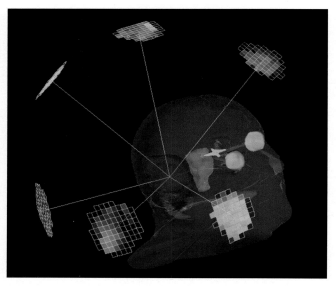

Figure 13.20 Six intensity-modulated treatment ports planned for treatment of a brain tumor (*large object in red*). Differing intensities of the 5 × 5 mm *beamlets* in each port illustrated by gray scale (brighter beamlet = higher intensity). The computer optimization of the beamlet intensities is designed to generate a delivered dose distribution that will conform to the tumor region, yet avoid critical normal tissues such as the brain stem (*dark pink*), optic chiasm (*green*), and optic nerves (*red tubular structures*).

of tumors and normal tissues throughout the course of treatment. However, this ignores the complexity inherent in attempting to build accurate 3D models from multimodality imaging for purposes of planning patient treatments. First, patients breathe and undergo other physiologic processes during a single treatment, changes that require dynamic modeling or other methods of accounting for the changes. Furthermore, the patient's condition may change over time (and hence their model). Thus, a complete design and assessment of a patient undergoing high-precision treatment requires the construction of four-dimensional (4D) patient models. Indeed, the recent ready availability of multidetector CT scanners with subsecond gantry rotations, and even more recently, the availability of cone-beam CT capabilities on the radiation therapy treatment simulators and treatment machines themselves, now makes it possible to construct 4D patient models. A very active area of physics research[72,75] deals with IGRT, including the formation of 4D patient models (including distortions and changes in anatomy) of the motion over time and the determination of the accumulated dose received by a moving tumor as well as the surrounding normal tissues such as uninvolved lung.

Complementary to the availability of these patient and dose models has come a much better understanding of the doses safely tolerated by normal tissues adjacent to a tumor volume (e.g., spinal cord) or surrounding it (e.g., brain, lung, liver).[77] Indeed, not only has knowledge of whole organ tolerances to irradiation been obtained, but it has also become possible to characterize in some detail the complex dependence of the probability of incurring a complication with respect to the highly (intentionally) inhomogeneous dose distributions these normal tissues receive as part of the planning process designed to avoid treating them. Modeling partial organ tolerances to irradiation is of great use in planning patient treatments because it enables[78] integration and manipulation of variable dose and volume distributions with respect to possible clinical outcomes.

Making the vast amount of tumor and normal tissue information useful for planning treatments requires equally sophisticated new ways of planning and delivering dose, potentially preferentially targeting subvolumes of the tumor regions or specifically avoiding selected portions of adjacent organs at risk. As mentioned earlier, modern treatment machines are capable of either varying the intensity of the radiation across each treatment port or projecting many small beams at a targeted region. This modulation of beam intensities (IMRT) from a given beam direction, together with the use of multiple beams (or parts of beams) from different directions, gives many degrees of freedom to create highly sculpted dose distributions, given that a system for designing the intensity modulation is available. Much computer programming and computational analysis has gone into the design of treatment-planning optimization systems to perform these functions.[79,80]

In IMRT, as most often applied, each treatment beam portal is broken down into simple basic components called beamlets, typically 0.5 to 1 cm × 1 cm in size, evenly distributed on a grid over the cross-section of each beam. Optimization begins with precomputation of the relative dose contribution that each of these beamlets gives to every subportion of tumor and normal tissue that the beamlet traverses as it goes through the patient model. Sophisticated optimization engines and search routines then iteratively alter the relative intensities of each beamlet in all the beams to minimize a cost function associated with target and normal tissue treatment goals. These, often hundreds of beamlets (each with its own intensity) (Fig. 13.20), provide the necessary flexibility and degrees of freedom to create dose distributions that can preferentially irradiate subportions of targets and also produce sharp dose gradients to avoid nearby organs at risk (Fig. 13.21). The cost-function approach also facilitates the ability to include factors such as the normal tissue and tumor-response models, mentioned previously in the optimization process, thus integrating the overall effects of the complex dose distributions across whole organ systems or target volumes within the planning process.

OTHER TREATMENT MODALITIES

Other types of external-beam radiation treatments use atomic or nuclear particles rather than photons. Beams of fast neutrons have been used for some cancers,[81] primarily because of the

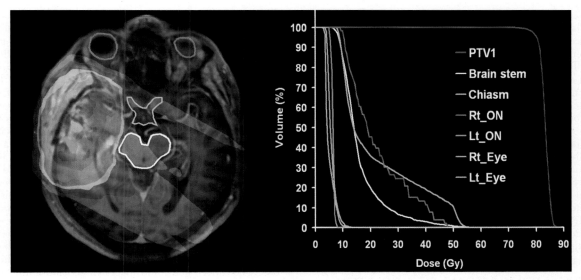

Figure 13.21 Resulting isodose distribution for an optimized intensity-modulated brain treatment. Dose-intensity pattern in the *left panel* is overlaid on the patient's magnetic resonance images used in planning. Also contoured are the optic chiasm (*green*), the brain stem (*white*), and the eyes (*orange*). In the *right panel*, the dose distribution throughout all slices of the patient's anatomy is summarized via cumulative dose-volume histograms for the various tissues and volumes that have been previously segmented. Each location on each curve represents the fraction of the volume of that tissue (%) that receives greater than or the same as the corresponding dose level.

dense ionization patterns they produce as they slow down in tissue (making cell killing less dependent on the indirect effect previously discussed). Being uncharged particles, neutron beams of therapeutic energy penetrate in tissue (have depth-dose characteristics) similar to photon beams, but with denser dose deposition in the cellular scale. Most other external-beam treatments use charged particles, primarily either electrons[82] (produced on the same machines used for photon beam treatments) or protons or heavier particles such as carbon ions.[83,84] The latter beams have desirable dose-deposition properties (see Fig. 13.18), because they can spare tissues downstream from the target volume and generally give less overall dose to normal tissue. There can also be some radiobiologic advantage to the heavier charged particle beams, similar to neutrons. The generation and delivery of proton beams and heavier charged particle beams generally requires an accelerator (in its own vault) plus a beam transport system and some sort of treatment nozzle, often located on an isocentric gantry. The cost of the accelerator is generally leveraged by having it supply beams to multiple treatment rooms, but these units still cost many times that of a standard linear accelerator.

Brachytherapy[85] is a form of treatment that uses direct placement of radioactive sources or materials within tumors (interstitial brachytherapy) or within body or surgical cavities (intracavitary brachytherapy), either permanently (allowing for full decay of short-lived radioactive materials) or temporarily (either in one extended application or over several shorter term applications). The ability to irradiate tumors from close range (even from the inside out) can lead to conformal treatments with low normal tissue doses. The radioactive isotopes most generally used for these treatments are contained within small tubelike or seedlike sealed source enclosures (which prevents direct contamination). They emit photons (gamma and x-rays) during their decay, which penetrate the source cover and interact with tissue via the same physical processes as described for external-beam treatments. The treatments have the advantage of providing a high fluence (and dose) very near each source that drops in intensity as 1 over the square of the distance from the source ($1/r^2$). Radioactive sources decay in an exponential fashion characterized by their individual half-lives. After each half-life ($T_{1/2}$) the strength of each source decreases by half. Brachytherapy treatments are further generally classified into the two broad categories of low–dose-rate and

high–dose-rate treatments. Low–dose-rate treatments attempt to deliver tumoricidal doses via continuous irradiation from implanted sources over a period of several days. High–dose-rate treatments use one or more higher activity sources (stored external to the patient) together with a remote applicator or source transfer system to give one or more higher dose treatments on time scales and schedules more like external-beam treatments.

Isotopes for brachytherapy treatments are selected on the basis of a combination of specific activity (i.e., how much activity can be achieved per unit mass [i.e., to keep the source sizes small]), the penetrating ability of the decay photons (together with the $1/r^2$ fall off determines how many sources or source location will be required for treatment), and the half-life of the radioactive material (which must be accounted for in computation of dose, but also determines how often reusable sources will need to be replaced). Table 13.1 lists those isotopes most commonly used, along with some of their primary applications.

The dose-deposition patterns surrounding each type of source can be measured or computed. These data (or the parameterization

TABLE 13.1

Common Isotopes for Brachytherapy Treatment

Isotope	Form	Primary Applications
^{125}I	Implantable sealed seed	LDR: Permanent prostate implants, brain implants, tumor bed implants, eye plaques
^{192}Ir	Implantable sealed seed	LDR: Interstitial solid tumor treatments
^{192}Ir	High activity sealed source on a remote transfer wire	HDR: Intracavitary GYN treatments, intraluminal irradiations
^{137}Cs	Sealed source tubes	LDR: Intracavitary GYN treatments

LDR, low-dose rate; HDR, high-dose rate; GYN, gynecologic; ^{137}Cs, caesium-137.

of same) can be stored within a computerized treatment-planning system. Planning a brachytherapy treatment-delivery scheme (desirable source strengths and arrangements) proceeds within the planning system by distributing the sources throughout the treatment area and having the computer add up the contributions of each source to designated tumor and normal tissue locations (e.g., obtained from a CT scan). Source strengths or spacing can be adjusted until an acceptable result is obtained. Indeed, optimization systems are now routinely used to fine tune this process.

Other types of therapeutic treatments with internal sources of ionizing radiation, generally classified as systemic targeted radionuclide therapy (STaRT), use antibodies or other conjugates or carriers such as microspheres to selectively deliver radionuclides to cancer cells.[86] Computing the effective dose to tumors and normal tissues via these techniques requires information on how much of the injected activity reaches the targets (biodistribution) as well as the energy and decay properties of the radionuclide being delivered. Imaging techniques and computer models are aiding in these computations.

CLINICAL APPLICATIONS OF RADIATION THERAPY

In contrast to surgical oncology and medical oncology, which focus on early- or late-stage disease, respectively, the field of radiation oncology encompasses the 1p8.49 entire spectrum of oncology. Board certification requires 5 years of postdoctoral training, typically beginning with an internship in internal medicine or surgery, followed by 4 years of radiation oncology residency. Education, as defined by leaders in the field,[87] begins with a thorough knowledge of the biology, physics, and clinical applications of radiation. It also includes training in the theoretical and practical aspects of the administration of radiation protectors and anticancer agents used as radiation sensitizers and the management of toxicities resulting from those treatments. In addition, residents receive education in palliative care, supportive care, and symptom and pain management. This training is in preparation for a practice that, in a given week, might include patients with a 2-mm vocal cord lesion or a 20-cm soft tissue sarcoma, both of whom can be treated with curative intent, as well as a patient with widely metastatic disease who needs palliative radiation, medical care for pain and depression, and discussion of end-of-life issues. More than 50% of (nonskin) cancer patients receive radiation therapy during the course of their illness.[88]

Clinical Application of Types of Radiation

Electrons are now the most widely used form of radiation for superficial treatments. Because the depth of penetration can be well controlled by the energy of the beam, it is possible to treat, for instance, skin cancer, a small part of the breast while sparing the underlying lung, or the cervical lymph nodes but not the spinal cord, which lies several centimeters more deeply. Superficial tumors, such as of skin cancers, can also be treated very effectively with low-energy (kilovoltage) photons, but their use has decreased because a separate machine is required for their production.

The main form of treatment for deep tumors is photons. As described in the Radiation Physics section, photons spare the skin and deposit dose along their entire path until the beam leaves the body. The use of multiple beams that intersect on the tumor permit high doses to be delivered to the tumor with a relative sparing of normal tissue. The pinnacle of this concept is IMRT, which uses hundreds of beams and can treat concave shapes with relative sparing of the central region (see Figs. 13.20 and 13.21). However, as each beam continues on its path beyond the tumor, this use of multiple beams means that a significant volume of normal tissue receives a low dose. There has been considerable debate concerning the magnitude of the risk of second cancers produced by radiating large volumes with low doses of radiation.[89] Charged particle beams (proton and carbon, in this discussion) differ from photons in that they interact only modestly with tissue until they reach the end of their path, where they then deposit the majority of their energy and stop (the Bragg peak; see Fig. 13.18). This ability to stop at a chosen depth decreases the region of low dose. The chief form of charged particle used today is the proton. In the decade from 1980 to 1990, proton therapy could deliver higher doses of radiation to the target than photon therapy because protons could produce a more rapid fall off of dose between the target and the critical normal tissue (e.g., tumor and brain stem). Therefore, initially, their main application was in the treatment uveal melanomas, base-of-skull chondrosarcomas, and chordomas. In contrast, today's IMRT photons are more conformal in the high-dose region than protons due to the range uncertainty of the latter.[90] Thus, it seems unlikely that protons will permit a higher target dose to be delivered than photons. In contrast, protons have the potential to decrease regions of low dose. This would be of particular advantage in the treatment of pediatric malignancies, where low doses of radiation would tend to increase the chance of second cancers and could affect neurocognitive function in the treatment of brain tumors.

A carbon ion beam has an additional potential biologic advantage over protons. As discussed in the section Biologic Aspects of Radiation Oncology, hypoxic cells, which are found in many tumors, are up to 3 times more resistant to photon or proton radiation than well-oxygenated cells. In contrast, hypoxia does not cause resistance to a carbon beam. Whether hypoxia is a cause of clinical resistance to fractionated radiation is still debated.[91] A carbon beam is available at a few sites in Europe and Japan.

Two major issues have affected the widespread acceptance of protons. The most widely recognized is cost. Proton (approximately $120 million) and carbon beam facilities (in excess of $200 million) are substantially more expensive than a similar-sized photon facility (approximately $25 million). The operating costs appear to be significantly higher as well. Although the majority of patients who have received proton therapy have prostate cancer, there is no evidence that protons produce superior results to those obtained with IMRT planned photons.[92,93] The lack of solid evidence that protons are superior to photons for any disease site and the magnitude of these costs are of societal importance.[94] Although less expensive single gantry proton units are under construction, there are no functioning units at the time of this writing. A second, less well-appreciated issue concerns the need to develop full integration of charged particle beams with IGRT, as has already been accomplished with photons, although this feature is being incorporated into second-generation proton units.

Neutron therapy attracted significant interest in the 1980s, based on the principle that it would be more effective than photons against hypoxic cells that some have thought are responsible for radiation resistance of tumors. The effectiveness of neutron therapy has been limited by initial difficulties with collimation and targeting, although there is evidence that they have a role in the treatment of refractory parotid gland tumors.[95]

Brachytherapy refers to the placement of radioactive sources next to or inside the tumor. The chief sites where brachytherapy plays a role are in prostate and cervical cancer, although it has applications in head and neck cancers, soft tissue sarcomas, and other sites. In the case of prostate cancer, most experience is with low–dose-rate permanent implants using iodine-125 (^{125}I) or, more recently, palladium-103 (^{103}Pd). Over the last 5 years, there has been an increasing emphasis on improving the accuracy of seed placement, guided by ultrasound and confirmed by CT or MRI, and in skilled hands, outstanding results can be achieved.[96] In the case of cervical cancer, high–dose-rate treatment, which can be performed in an outpatient setting, has essentially replaced low–dose-rate treatment, which typically requires general anesthesia and a 2-day hospital stay. The results from both techniques appear to be approximately equivalent.

Yttrium microspheres represent a distinct form of brachytherapy. These spheres carry yttrium-90 (^{90}Y), a pure beta emitter with a range of about 1 cm. These have been used to treat both primary hepatocellular cancer and colorectal cancer metastatic to the liver (hepatic arterial or systemic chemotherapy) by administration through the hepatic artery.

TREATMENT INTENT

Radiation doses are chosen so as to maximize the chance of tumor control without producing unacceptable toxicity. The dose of radiation required depends on the tumor type, the volume of disease (number of tumor cells), and the use of radiation-modifying agents (such as chemotherapeutic drugs used as radiation sensitizers). Except for a subset of tumors that are exquisitely sensitive to radiation (e.g., seminoma, lymphoma), doses that are required are often close to the tolerance of the normal tissue. A key fact driving the choice of dose is that a 1-cm^3 tumor contains approximately 1 billion cells. It follows that the reduction of a tumor that is 3 cm in diameter to 3 mm, which would be called a complete response by CT scan, would still leave 1 million tumor cells. Because each radiation fraction appears to kill a fixed fraction of the tumor, the dose to cure occult disease needs to be more similar to the dose for gross disease than one might otherwise expect. Thus, radiation doses (using the standard fractionation) of 45 to 54 Gy are typically used in the adjuvant setting when there is moderate suspicion for occult disease, 60 to 65 Gy for positive margins or when there is a high suspicion for occult disease, and 70 Gy or more for gross disease.

It is common during the course of radiation to give higher doses of radiation to regions that have a higher tumor burden. For example, regions that are suspected of harboring occult disease may be targeted to receive (in once daily 2-Gy fractions) 54 Gy, whereas, to control the gross tumor, the goal may be to administer a total dose of 70 Gy. Because the gross tumor will invariably reside within the region at risk for occult disease, it has become standard practice to deliver 50 Gy to the entire region, and then an additional *boost* dose of 20 Gy to the tumor. This sequence is called the *shrinking field technique*. With the development of IMRT, it has become possible to treat both regions with a different dose each day and achieve both goals simultaneously. For example, on each of the 35 days of treatment, the gross tumor might receive 2 Gy, and the region of occult disease 1.7 Gy, for a total dose of 59.5 Gy, which is of approximately equal biologic effectiveness to 54 Gy in 1.8-Gy fractions because of the lower dose per fraction (see the section Biologic Aspects of Radiation Oncology).

Radiation therapy alone is often used with curative intent for localized tumors. The decision to use surgery or radiation therapy involves factors determined by the tumor (e.g., is it resectable without a serious compromise in function?) and the patient (e.g., is the patient a good operative candidate?). The most common tumor in this group is prostate cancer, but patients with early-stage larynx cancer often receive radiation for voice preservation, and there are many patients with early-stage lung cancer who are not operative candidates. Control rates for these early-stage lesions are in excess of 70% (and as high as 90% for early-stage larynx cancer) and are usually a function of tumor size.

Stereotactic body radiation therapy (SBRT; sometimes called *stereotactic ablative radiation*) uses many (typically more than eight) cross-firing beams and provides an improved method of curing early-stage lung cancer[97] and liver metastases.[98] This approach uses precise localization and image guidance to deliver a small number (less than five) of high doses of radiation, with the concept of ablating the tumor, rather than using fractionation to achieve a therapeutic index (see the section title Fractionation). SBRT can provide long-term, local control rates of >90% for tumors less than 4 to 5 cm with minimal side effects.

Locally advanced or aggressive cancers can be cured with radiation alone or with a combination of radiation and chemotherapy or a molecularly targeted therapy. The most common examples here are locally advanced lung cancer, head and neck, esophageal, and cervix cancers, with cure rates in the 15% to 40% range, and are discussed in detail in their own chapters. A general principle that has emerged during the last decade is that combination chemoradiation has increased the cure rates of locally advanced cancers by 5% to 10% at the cost of increased toxicity.

An important consideration in the use of radiation (with or without chemotherapy) with curative intent is the concept of organ preservation. Perhaps the best example of achieving organ preservation in the face of gross disease involves the use of chemotherapy and radiation to replace laryngectomy in the treatment of advanced larynx cancer. Combined radiation and chemotherapy does not improve overall survival compared with radical surgery; however, the organ-conservation approach permits voice preservation in approximately two-thirds of patients with advanced larynx cancer.[99] The treatment of anal cancer with chemoradiation can also be viewed in this light, with chemoradiotherapy producing organ conservation and cure rates superior to radical surgery used decades ago.[100] Multiple randomized trials have demonstrated that lumpectomy plus radiation for breast cancer produces survival rates equal to that of modified radical mastectomy, while allowing for the preservation of the breast.

In the last decade, it has become clear that some patients with metastatic disease can be cured with radiation (with or without chemotherapy). The concept underlying this approach was established by the surgical practice of resecting a limited number of liver or lung metastases. A significant fraction of patients have a limited number of liver metastases that cannot be resected because of location, but are able to undergo high-dose radiation (often combined with chemotherapy). This radical approach to *oligometastases*[101] can produce 5-year survivals in the range of 20% in selected patients.[102] Patients with a limited number of lung metastases from colorectal cancer or soft tissue sarcomas are now being approached with stereotactic body radiation with a similar concept as has been used to justify surgical resection.[102] In addition to the direct effect of radiation on metastatic tumor, there is now anecdotal but provocative evidence that radiation can stimulate the immune system so that tumors distant from the irradiated tumor can respond. Distant (abscopal) responses have been reported in patients who receive immune checkpoint inhibitors such as ipilimumab.[103]

Radiation therapy can also contribute to the cure of patients when used in an adjuvant setting. If the risk of recurrence after surgery is low or if a recurrence could be easily addressed by a second resection, adjuvant radiation therapy is not usually given. However, when a gross total resection of the tumor is still associated with a high risk of residual occult disease or if local recurrence is morbid, adjuvant treatment is often recommended. A general finding across many disease sites is that adjuvant radiation can reduce local failure rates to below 10%, even in high-risk patients, if a gross total resection is achieved. If gross disease or positive margins remain, higher doses and/or larger volumes may be required, which may be less well tolerated and are less successful in achieving tumor control.

Adjuvant therapy can be delivered before or after definitive surgery. There are some advantages to giving radiation therapy after surgery. The details of the tumor location are known and, with the surgeon's cooperation, clips can be placed in the tumor bed, permitting increased treatment accuracy. In addition, compared with preoperative therapy, postoperative therapy is associated with fewer wound complications. However, in some cases, it is preferable to deliver preoperative radiation. Radiation can shrink the tumor, diminishing the extent of the resection, or making an unresectable tumor resectable. In the case of rectal cancer, the response to treatment may carry more prognostic information than the initial TNM staging.[104] In patients who will undergo significant surgeries (particularly a Whipple procedure or an esophageal resection), preoperative (sometimes called neoadjuvant) therapy can be more reliably administered than postoperative therapy. Most importantly, after resection of abdominal or pelvic tumors (such as rectal cancers or retroperitoneal sarcomas), the small bowel may become fixed by adhesions in the region requiring treatment, thus increasing the morbidity of postoperative treatment. A randomized trial has shown that preoperative therapy produces fewer gastrointestinal side effects and has at least as good efficacy as postoperative adjuvant therapy for locally advanced rectal cancer.[105] Taken together, there appears to be a trend toward preoperative or neoadjuvant therapy in cancers of the gastrointestinal track (esophagus, stomach, pancreas, rectum), postoperative radiation seems to be favored in head and neck, lung, and breast cancer, and soft tissue sarcoma seems equally split.

The effectiveness of adjuvant therapy in decreasing local recurrence has been demonstrated in randomized trials in lung, rectal, and breast cancers. More recently, randomized trials have shown that postmastectomy radiation improved the survival for women with breast cancer and four or more positive lymph nodes, all of whom also received adjuvant chemotherapy. A fascinating analysis has revealed that, across many treatment conditions, each 4% increase in 5-year local control is associated with a 1% increase in 5-year survival.[106] It has been proposed that the long-term survival benefit of radiation in these more recent studies was revealed by the introduction of effective chemotherapy, which prevented such a high fraction of women from dying early with metastatic disease.[107] This concept has been developed into a hypothesis that the effect of adjuvant radiation on survival will depend on the effectiveness of adjuvant chemotherapy. If chemotherapy is either ineffective or very effective, adjuvant radiation may have little influence on the survival in a disease in which systemic relapse dominates survival. Radiation will have its greatest impact on survival when chemotherapy is moderately effective.[108]

In addition to these curative roles, radiation plays an important part in palliative treatment. Perhaps most importantly, emergency irradiation can begin to reverse the devastating effects of spinal cord compression and of superior vena cava syndrome. A single 8-Gy fraction is highly effective for many patients with bone pain from a metastatic lesion. There is increasing evidence of the effectiveness of body stereotactic radiation to treat vertebral body metastases in patients who have a long projected survival or who need retreatment after previous radiation.[109] Stereotactic treatment can relieve symptoms from a small number of brain metastasis, and fractionated whole-brain radiation can mitigate the effects of multiple metastases. Bronchial obstruction can often be relieved by a brief course of treatment as can duodenal obstruction from pancreatic cancer. Palliative treatment is usually delivered in a smaller number of larger radiation fractions (see the section titled Fractionation) because the desire to simplify the treatment for a patient with limited life expectancy outweighs the somewhat increased potential for late side effects.

FRACTIONATION

Two crucial features that influence the effectiveness of a physical dose of radiation are the dose given in each radiation treatment (i.e., the fraction) and the total amount of time required to complete the course of radiation. Standard fractionation for radiation therapy is defined as the delivery of one treatment of 1.8 to 2.25 Gy per day. This approach produces a fairly well-understood chance of tumor control and risk of normal tissue damage (as a function of volume). By altering the fractionation schemes, one may be able to improve the outcome for patients undergoing curative treatment or to simplify the treatment for patients receiving palliative therapy.

Two forms of altered fractionation have been tested for patients undergoing curative treatment: accelerated fractionation and hyperfractionation. Accelerated fractionation emerged from analyses of the control of head and neck cancer as a function of dose administered and total treatment time. It was found that with an increasing dose there was increasing local control, but that protraction of treatment was associated with a loss of local control that

was equivalent to about 0.75 Gy per day.[110] The data were best modeled by assuming that, approximately 2 weeks into treatment, tumor cells began to proliferate more rapidly than they were proliferating early in treatment (called *accelerated repopulation*).[111] In accelerated fractionation, the goal is to complete radiation before the accelerated tumor cell proliferation occurs. The most common method of achieving accelerated fractionation is to give a standard fraction to the entire field in the morning and to give a second treatment to the boost field in the afternoon (called *concomitant boost*). As in standard radiation, the boost would be given by extending the length of the treatment course; this concomitant boost approach can shorten treatment from 7 weeks to 5 weeks in head and neck cancer.

The second approach to altering fractionation is called *hyperfractionation*. Hyperfractionation is defined as the use of more than one fraction per day separated by more than 6 hours (see the section titled Biologic Aspects of Radiation Oncology), with a dose per fraction that is less than standard. Hyperfractionation is expected to produce fewer late complications for the same acute effects against both rapidly dividing normal tissues and tumors. Pure hyperfractionation might give 1 Gy twice a day, so that the total dose per day would be 2 Gy, and thus be equal to standard fractionation. In practice, hyperfractionated treatments are usually in the range of 1.2 Gy, which means that, compared with a standard fractionation, a somewhat higher dose is administered during the same period of time (so that most hyperfractionation also includes modest acceleration). The overall effect is to increase the acute toxicity (which resolves) and tumor response, while not increasing the (dose-limiting) late toxicity, which can improve cure rate. Both accelerated fractionation and hyperfractionation have been demonstrated in a meta-analysis to be superior to standard fractionation in the treatment of head and neck cancer with radiation alone.[112] However, a recent randomized trial has shown that there is no increase in control or survival, but there is an increase toxicity using chemotherapy with hyperfractionation compared to standard chemoradiation; therefore, the use of altered fractionation schemes has decreased dramatically during the last few years.[113]

Hypofractionation refers to the administration of a smaller number of larger fractions than is standard. Hypofractionation might be expected to cause more late toxicity for the same antitumor effect than standard or hyperfractionation. In the past, this approach was reserved for palliative cases, with the sense that a modest potential for increased late toxicity was not a major concern in patients with limited life expectancy. However, more recently, it has been proposed that the ability to better exclude normal tissue by using IGRT may permit hypofractionation to be used safely and that, in the specific case of prostate cancer, hypofractionation may have beneficial effects.[114]

ADVERSE EFFECTS

Radiation produces adverse effects in normal tissues. Although these are discussed in detail in later chapters as part of comprehensive discussions of organ toxicity, it is worth making some general comments here from the perspective of how radiation biology relates to the clinical toxicities. The term *radiation toxicity* is used to describe the adverse effects caused by radiation alone and radiation plus chemotherapy. Although this latter toxicity would be better labeled as *combined modality toxicity*, the pattern typically resembles a more severe form of the toxicity produced by radiation alone. Adverse effects from radiation can be divided into acute, subacute, and chronic (or late) effects. Acute effects are common, rarely serious, and usually self-limiting. Acute effects tend to occur in organs that depend on rapid self-renewal, most commonly the skin or mucosal surfaces (oropharynx, esophagus, small intestine, rectum, and bladder). This is due to radiation-induced cell death that occurs during mitosis, so that cells that divide rapidly show the most rapid cell loss. In the treatment of head and neck cancer, mucositis becomes worse during the first 3 to 4 weeks of therapy, but then will often stabilize as the normal mucosa cell proliferation increases in response to mucosal cell loss. It seems likely that normal tissue stem cells are relatively resistant to radiation compared with the more differentiated cells, because these stem cells survive to permit the normal mucosa to reepithelialize. Acute side effects typically resolve within 1 to 2 weeks of treatment completion, although occasionally these effects are so severe that they lead to consequential late effects, as described later.

Because lymphocytes are exquisitely sensitive to radiation, there has been considerable investigation into the effects of radiation on immune function. In contrast to mucosal cell killing, which requires mitosis, radiation kills lymphocytes in all phases of the cell cycle by apoptosis, so that lymphocyte counts decrease within days of initiating treatment. These effects do not tend to put patients at risk for infection, because granulocytes, which are chiefly responsible for combating infections, are relatively unaffected.

Two acute side effects of radiation do not fit neatly into these models relating to cell kill: nausea[115,116] and fatigue.[117,118] The origin of radiation-induced nausea is not related to acute cell loss, because it can occur within hours of the first treatment. Nausea is usually associated with radiation of the stomach, but it can sometimes occur during brain irradiation or from large-volume irradiation that involves neither the brain nor the stomach. Irradiation typically produces fatigue, even if relatively small volumes are irradiated. It seems likely that the origins of both of these *abscopal* effects of radiation (i.e., effects that occur systemically or at a distance for the site of irradiation) are related to the release of cytokines, but little is known.

Radiation can also produce subacute toxicities in the form of radiation pneumonitis and radiation-induced liver disease. These typically occur 2 weeks to 3 months after radiation is completed. The risk of radiation pneumonitis and radiation-induced liver disease is proportional to the mean dose delivered.[119,120] Thus, the 3D tools that permit the calculation of dose-volume histograms (described in the physics section) are currently used to determine the maximum safe treatment that can be delivered in terms of dose and volume. These toxicities appear to be initiated subclinically during the course of radiation as a cascade of cytokines in which TGF-β, tumor necrosis factor α, interleukin 6, and other cytokines play a role.[121] High TGF-β plasma levels during a course of treatment have been found to be associated with a greater risk of radiation pneumonitis.[122] Thus, in the future, we might look toward a combination of physical dose delivery, measured by the dose-volume histogram, the functional imaging of normal tissue damage, and the detection of biomarkers of toxicity, such as TGF-β, to improve the ability to individualize therapy. Attempts to determine the genomic basis of radiation sensitivity, beyond the known rare genetic defects such as ataxia telangiectasia, have not yet been successful.[123]

Late effects, which are typically seen 6 or more months after a course of radiation, include fibrosis, fistula formation, or long-term organ damage. Two theories for the origin of late effects have been put forth: late damage to the microvasculature and direct damage to the parenchyma. Although the vascular damage theory is attractive, it does not account for the differing sensitivities of organs to radiation. Perhaps the microvasculature is unique in each organ.[124] Regardless of the mechanism of toxicity, the tolerance of whole-organ radiation is now fairly well established (Table 13.2). Late complications can also be divided into two categories: consequential and true late effects. The best example of a consequential late effect is fibrosis and dysphagia after high-dose chemoradiation for head and neck cancer. Here, late fibrosis or ulceration appears to be the result of the mucosa becoming denuded for a prolonged time period. Late consequential effects are distinct from true late effects, which can follow a normal treatment course of self-limited toxicity and a 6-month or more symptom-free period. Examples of true late effects are radiation myelitis, radiation brain necrosis, and radiation-induced bowel obstruction. In the past, radiation fibrosis was thought to be an irreversible condition. Therefore, an exciting recent development is that severe radiation-induced breast fibrosis is an active process that can be reversed by drug therapy (pentoxifylline and vitamin E).[125]

CANCER THERAPEUTICS

TABLE 13.2

Radiation Tolerance Doses for Normal Tissues

Site	TD 5/5 (Gy)[a] Portion of Organ Irradiated			TD 50/5 (Gy)[b] Portion of Organ Irradiated			Complication End Point(s)
	$^1/_3$	$^2/_3$	$^3/_3$	$^1/_3$	$^2/_3$	$^3/_3$	
Kidney	50	30	23	—	40	28	Nephritis
Rain	60	50	45	75	65	60	Necrosis, infarct
Brain stem	60	53	50	—	—	65	Necrosis, infarct
Spinal cord	50 (5–10 cm)	—	47 (20 cm)	70 (5–10 cm)	—	—	Myelitis, necrosis
Lung	45	30	17.5	65	40	24.5	Radiation pneumonitis
Heart	60	45	40	70	55	50	Pericarditis
Esophagus	60	58	55	72	70	68	Stricture, perforation
Stomach	60	55	50	70	67	65	Ulceration, perforation
Small intestine	50	—	40	60	—	55	Obstruction, perforation, fistula
Colon	55	—	45	65	—	55	Obstruction, perforation, fistula, ulceration
Rectum	(100 cm³ volume)		60	(100 cm³ volume)		80	Severe proctitis, necrosis, fistula
Liver	50	35	30	55	45	40	Liver failure

[a] TD 5/5, the average dose that results in a 5% complication risk within 5 years.
[b] TD 50/5, the average dose that results in a 50% complication risk within 5 years.
Adapted from Emami B, Lyman J, Brown A, et al. Tolerance of normal tissue to therapeutic irradiation. *Int J Radiat Oncol Biol Phys* 1991;21:109–122.

PRINCIPLES OF COMBINING ANTICANCER AGENTS WITH RADIATION THERAPY

Combining chemotherapy with radiation therapy has produced important improvements in treatment outcome. Randomized clinical trials show improved local control and survival through the use of concurrent chemotherapy and radiation therapy for patients with high-grade gliomas and locally advanced cancers of the head and neck, lung, esophagus, stomach, rectum, prostate, and anus. There are least two proposed reasons why chemoradiotherapy might be successful. The first is radiosensitization. In the laboratory, radiosensitization is defined as a synergistic relationship, using mathematical approaches such as isobologram or median effect analysis.[126,127] The underlying concept is that the observed effect of using chemotherapy and radiation concurrently is greater than simply adding the two together. A second proposed reason to combine radiation and chemotherapy is to realize the benefit of improved local control radiation along with the systemic effect of chemotherapy, a concept called *spatial additivity*.[128]

Clinical results show that both radiosensitization and spatial additivity contribute to varying extents in different clinical settings. In the case of head and neck cancer, radiosensitization predominates. This conclusion is supported by the meta-analysis of head and neck cancer: sequential chemotherapy and radiotherapy produces little if any improvement in survival, whereas concurrent chemoradiation produces a significant increase in survival.[129] Furthermore, in the early positive studies using concurrent chemoradiation, systemic metastases were unaffected even though survival was improved. Radiosensitization may also predominate in the success of chemoradiotherapy for locally advanced lung cancer. For instance, although initial studies indicated that sequential chemotherapy and radiation had some benefit for lung cancer,[130] more recent work indicates that concurrent therapy is superior, and it is now the standard treatment.[131] However, there are also examples of spatial additivity. For example, both radiosensitization and spatial additivity is provided by the use of chemoradiation for locally advanced cervical cancer in that both local and systemic relapses are decreased by combined therapy.[132]

By targeting the aberrant growth factor or proangiogenic pathways that are specific to cancer cells rather than all rapidly proliferating cells, molecularly targeted therapies offer the potential to improve outcome without increasing toxicity. Even a selective cytostatic effect against the tumor would be predicted to act synergistically with radiation (Fig. 13.22). Although preclinical studies (summarized in the previous biology section) have highlighted the potential therapeutic gains that could be achieved by adding EGFR inhibitors to radiation, the best validation of this combination has been from the results of clinical trials in head and neck cancer. A phase III clinical trial demonstrated that, in a cohort of 424 patients with local–regionally advanced squamous cell carcinoma of the head and neck, the addition of cetuximab nearly doubled the median survival of patients (compared to radiotherapy alone), from 28 to 54 months. This study represents the first major success

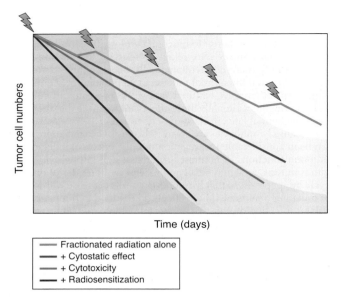

Figure 13.22 Potential mechanisms of synergy between epidermal growth factor receptor (EGFR) inhibitors and radiation. Although each daily radiation treatment kills a fraction of the cells, some cells grow back by the next day, which attenuates the effectiveness of radiation. If an EGFR inhibitor has only a selective cytostatic effect and blocks regrowth between fractions, the result would be a dramatic increase in radiation efficacy. The benefit of the inhibitor would be even greater if it caused tumor cell cytotoxicity or radiosensitization.

achieved by the addition of an EGFR antagonist to radiotherapy. This improvement was achieved without enhanced toxicity. Notably, the rates of pharyngitis and weight loss were identical in the two arms.[60] Local control was improved rather than the development of metastases, suggesting synergy rather than spatial additivity. Thus, the principle that can be derived from this study is that in tumors expressing high EGFR levels and that are likely to depend on aberrant EGF signaling, combining a true cytotoxic agent such as radiation with a cytostatic agent such as cetuximab has considerable promise.

Because of the success of chemoradiotherapy, the natural tendency has not been to substitute molecularly targeted agents such as cetuximab for chemotherapy, but to add cetuximab to chemoradiotherapy. Thus, the combination of cisplatin, cetuximab, and radiation was recently found to have the same control rate as cisplatin and radiation for patients with locally advanced head and neck cancer, but the cetuximab arm had greater toxicity. Unfortunately, the triple therapy was never evaluated preclinically, and it has been shown preclinically that when EGFR inhibitors are given prior to chemotherapy, they can produce antagonism.[133] The principles of adding molecularly targeted therapy to chemoradiation are still evolving.[63]

REFERENCES

1. Hall EJ, Giaccia AJ. *Radiobiology for the Radiologist*. Philadelphia: Lippincott Williams & Williams; 2012.
2. Fowler JF. Developing aspects of radiation oncology. *Med Phys* 1981;8:427–434.
3. Lavin MF. Ataxia-telangiectasia: from a rare disorder to a paradigm for cell signalling and cancer. *Nat Rev Mol Cell Biol* 2008;9:759–769.
4. Thompson LH. Recognition, signaling, and repair of DNA double-strand breaks produced by ionizing radiation in mammalian cells: the molecular choreography. *Mutat Res* 2012;751:158–246.
5. Sherr CJ, McCormick F. The RB and p53 pathways in cancer. *Cancer Cell* 2002;2:103–112.
6. Bartek J, Lukas J. Chk1 and Chk2 kinases in checkpoint control and cancer. *Cancer Cell* 2003;3:421–429.

7. Kitagawa R, Bakkenist CJ, McKinnon PJ, et al. Phosphorylation of SMC1 is a critical downstream event in the ATM-NBS1-BRCA1 pathway. *Genes Dev* 2004;18:1423–1438.
8. Abraham RT. Cell cycle checkpoint signaling through the ATM and ATR kinases. *Genes Dev* 2001;15:2177–2196.
9. Mailand N, Podtelejnikov AV, Groth A, et al. Regulation of G(2)/M events by Cdc25A through phosphorylation-dependent modulation of its stability. *EMBO J* 2002;21:5911–5920.
10. Donzelli M, Draetta GF. Regulating mammalian checkpoints through Cdc25 inactivation. *EMBO Rep* 2003;4:671–677.
11. Tsvetkov L. Polo-like kinases and Chk2 at the interface of DNA damage checkpoint pathways and mitotic regulation. *IUBMB Life* 2004;56:449–456.

12. Dai Y, Grant S. New insights into checkpoint kinase 1 in the DNA damage response signaling network. *Clin Cancer Res* 2010;16:376–383.

13. Giaccia A, Weinstein R, Hu J, et al. Cell cycle-dependent repair of double-strand DNA breaks in a gamma-ray-sensitive Chinese hamster cell. *Somat Cell Mol Genet* 1985;11:485–491.

14. Kemp LM, Sedgwick SG, Jeggo PA. X-ray sensitive mutants of Chinese hamster ovary cells defective in double-strand break rejoining. *Mutat Res* 1984;132:189–196.

15. Helleday T, Lo J, van Gent DC, et al. DNA double-strand break repair: from mechanistic understanding to cancer treatment. *DNA Repair (Amst)* 2007;6:923–935.

16. Hefferin ML, Tomkinson AE. Mechanism of DNA double-strand break repair by non-homologous end joining. *DNA Repair (Amst)* 2005;4:639–648.

17. Ma Y, Pannicke U, Schwarz K, et al. Hairpin opening and overhang processing by an Artemis/DNA-dependent protein kinase complex in nonhomologous end joining and V(D)J recombination. *Cell* 2002;108:781–794.

18. Grawunder U, Wilm M, Wu X, et al. Activity of DNA ligase IV stimulated by complex formation with XRCC4 protein in mammalian cells. *Nature* 1997;388:492–495.

19. Chen L, Trujillo K, Sung P, et al. Interactions of the DNA ligase IV-XRCC4 complex with DNA ends and the DNA-dependent protein kinase. *J Biol Chem* 2000;275:26196–26205.

20. Tsukuda T, Fleming AB, Nickoloff JA, et al. Chromatin remodelling at a DNA double-strand break site in Saccharomyces cerevisiae. *Nature* 2005;438:379–383.

21. Yang YG, Saidi A, Frappart PO, et al. Conditional deletion of Nbs1 in murine cells reveals its role in branching repair pathways of DNA double-strand breaks. *EMBO J* 2006;25:5527–5538.

22. Esashi F, Galkin VE, Yu X, et al. Stabilization of RAD51 nucleoprotein filaments by the C-terminal region of BRCA2. *Nat Struct Mol Biol* 2007;14:468–474.

23. Sleeth KM, Sorensen CS, Issaeva N, et al. RPA mediates recombination repair during replication stress and is displaced from DNA by checkpoint signalling in human cells. *J Mol Biol* 2007;373:38–47.

24. Littlefield LG, Kleinerman RA, Sayer AM, et al. Chromosome aberrations in lymphocytes—biomonitors of radiation exposure. *Prog Clin Biol Res* 1991;372:387–397.

25. Toulany M, Rodemann HP. Membrane receptor signaling and control of DNA repair after exposure to ionizing radiation. *Nuklearmedizin* 2010;49:S26–S30.

26. Barcellos-Hoff MH, Akhurst RJ. Transforming growth factor-beta in breast cancer: too much, too late. *Breast Cancer Res* 2009;11:202.

27. Deng X, Yin X, Allan R, et al. Ceramide biogenesis is required for radiation-induced apoptosis in the germ line of C. elegans. *Science* 2008;322:110–115.

28. Thompson LH, Suit HD. Proliferation kinetics of x-irradiated mouse L cells studied WITH TIME-lapse photography. II. *Int J Radiat Biol Relat Stud Phys Chem Med* 1969;15:347–362.

29. Sowa Resat MB, Morgan WF. Radiation-induced genomic instability: a role for secreted soluble factors in communicating the radiation response to non-irradiated cells. *J Cell Biochem* 2004;92:1013–1019.

30. Elkind MM. The initial part of the survival curve: does it predict the outcome of fractionated radiotherapy? *Radiat Res* 1988;114:425–436.

31. McCulloch EA, Till JE. The sensitivity of cells from normal mouse bone marrow to gamma radiation in vitro and in vivo. *Radiat Res* 1962;16:822–832.

32. Withers HR. Recovery and repopulation in vivo by mouse skin epithelial cells during fractionated irradiation. *Radiat Res* 1967;32:227–239.

33. Withers HR, Elkind MM. Microcolony survival assay for cells of mouse intestinal mucosa exposed to radiation. *Int J Radiat Biol Relat Stud Phys Chem Med* 1970;17:261–267.

34. Suit H, Wette R. Radiation dose fractionation and tumor control probability. *Radiat Res* 1966;29:267–281.

35. O'Neill K, Lyons SK, Gallagher WM, et al. Bioluminescent imaging: a critical tool in pre-clinical oncology research. *J Pathol* 2010;220:317–327.

36. Hewitt HB, Wilson CW. Survival curves for tumor cells irradiated in vivo. *Ann N Y Acad Sci* 1961;95:818–827.

37. Hill RP, Bush RS. A lung-colony assay to determine the radiosensitivity of cells of a solid tumour. *Int J Radiat Biol Relat Stud Phys Chem Med* 1969;15:435–444.

38. Elkind MM, Sutton-Gilbert H, Moses WB, et al. Radiation response of mammalian cells grown in culture. V. Temperature dependence of the repair of x-ray damage in surviving cells (aerobic and hypoxic). *Radiat Res* 1965;25:359–376.

39. Elkind MM, Whitmore GF. *Radiobiology of Cultured Mammalian Cells*. New York: Gordon and Breach; 1967.

40. Mottram JC. Factors of importance in radiosensitivity of tumors. *Br J Radiol* 1936;9:606.

41. Palcic B, Skarsgard LD. Reduced oxygen enhancement ratio at low doses of ionizing radiation. *Radiat Res* 1984;100:328–339.

42. Thomlinson RH, Gray LH. The histological structure of some human lung cancers and the possible implications for radiotherapy. *Br J Cancer* 1955;9:539–549.

43. Overgaard J, Horsman MR. Modification of hypoxia-induced radioresistance in tumors by the use of oxygen and sensitizers. *Semin Radiat Oncol* 1996;6:10–21.

44. Machtay M, Pajak TF, Suntharalingam M, et al. Radiotherapy with or without erythropoietin for anemic patients with head and neck cancer: a randomized trial of the Radiation Therapy Oncology Group (RTOG 99-03). *Int J Radiat Oncol Biol Phys* 2007;69:1008–1017.

45. Henke M, Laszig R, Rube C, et al. Erythropoietin to treat head and neck cancer patients with anaemia undergoing radiotherapy: randomised, double-blind, placebo-controlled trial. *Lancet* 2003;362:1255–1260.

46. Janssens GO, Rademakers SE, Terhaard CH, et al. Accelerated radiotherapy with carbogen and nicotinamide for laryngeal cancer: results of a phase III randomized trial. *J Clin Oncol* 2012;30:1777–1783.

47. Willett CG, Boucher Y, di Tomaso E, et al. Direct evidence that the VEGF-specific antibody bevacizumab has antivascular effects in human rectal cancer. *Nat Med* 2004;10:145–147.

48. Lapi SE, Voller TF, Welch MJ. Positron emission tomography imaging of hypoxia. *PET Clin* 2009;4:39–47.

49. Lee NY, Mechalakos JG, Nehmeh S, et al. Fluorine-18-labeled fluoromisonidazole positron emission and computed tomography-guided intensity-modulated radiotherapy for head and neck cancer: a feasibility study. *Int J Radiat Oncol Biol Phys* 2008;70:2–13.

50. Schaue D, Xie MW, Ratikan JA, et al. Regulatory T cells in radiotherapeutic responses. *Front Oncol* 2012;2:90.

51. Formenti SC, Demaria S. Combining radiotherapy and cancer immunotherapy: a paradigm shift. *J Natl Cancer Inst* 2013;105:256–265.

52. Lawrence TS, Davis MA, Tang HY, et al. Fluorodeoxyuridine-mediated cytotoxicity and radiosensitization require S phase progression. *Int J Radiat Biol* 1996;70:273–280.

53. Lawrence TS, Chang EY, Hahn TM, et al. Radiosensitization of pancreatic cancer cells by 2′,2′-difluoro-2′-deoxycytidine. *Int J Radiat Oncol Biol Phys* 1996;34:867–872.

54. Eisbruch A, Shewach DS, Bradford CR, et al. Radiation concurrent with gemcitabine for locally advanced head and neck cancer: a phase I trial and intracellular drug incorporation study. *J Clin Oncol* 2001;19:792–799.

55. Ben-Josef E, Schipper M, Francis IR, et al. A phase I/II trial of intensity modulated radiation (IMRT) dose escalation with concurrent fixed-dose rate gemcitabine (FDR-G) in patients with unresectable pancreatic cancer. *Int J Radiat Oncol Biol Phys* 2012;84:1166–1171.

56. Wolff RA, Evans DB, Gravel DM, et al. Phase I trial of gemcitabine combined with radiation for the treatment of locally advanced pancreatic adenocarcinoma. *Clin Cancer Res* 2001;7:2246–2253.

57. Wilson GD, Bentzen SM, Harari PM. Biologic basis for combining drugs with radiation. *Semin Radiat Oncol* 2006;16:2–9.

58. Bradley JD, Paulus R, Graham MV, et al. Phase II trial of postoperative adjuvant paclitaxel/carboplatin and thoracic radiotherapy in resected stage II and IIIA non-small-cell lung cancer: promising long-term results of the Radiation Therapy Oncology Group—RTOG 9705. *J Clin Oncol* 2005;23:3480–3487.

59. Nyati MK, Morgan MA, Feng FY, et al. Integration of EGFR inhibitors with radiochemotherapy. *Nat Rev Cancer* 2006;6:876–885.

60. Bonner JA, Harari PM, Giralt J, et al. Radiotherapy plus cetuximab for locoregionally advanced head and neck cancer: 5-year survival data from a phase 3 randomised trial, and relation between cetuximab-induced rash and survival. *Lancet Oncol* 2010;11:21–28.

61. Ang KK, Zhang QE, Rosenthal DI, et al. A randomized phase III trial (RTOG 0522) of concurrent accelerated radiation plus cisplatin with or without cetuximab for stage III-IV head and neck squamous cell carcinomas (HNC). *J Clin Oncol* 2011;29.

62. Engelke CG, Parsels LA, Qian Y, et al. Sensitization of pancreatic cancer to chemoradiation by the Chk1 inhibitor MK8776. *Clin Cancer Res* 2013;19:4412–4421.

63. Morgan MA, Parsels LA, Maybaum J, et al. Improving the efficacy of chemoradiation with targeted agents. *Cancer Discov* 2014;4:280–291.

64. Chalmers AJ, Lakshman M, Chan N, et al. Poly(ADP-ribose) polymerase inhibition as a model for synthetic lethality in developing radiation oncology targets. *Semin Radiat Oncol* 2010;20:274–281.

65. Brizel DM, Wasserman TH, Henke M, et al. Phase III randomized trial of amifostine as a radioprotector in head and neck cancer. *J Clin Oncol* 2000;18:3339–3345.

66. Winczura P, Jassem J. Combined treatment with cytoprotective agents and radiotherapy. *Cancer Treat Rev* 2010;36:268–275.

67. Van Dyk J, ed. Radiation oncology medical physics resources for working, teaching, and learning. In: *The Modern Technology of Radiation Oncology*. Volume 3. Medical Physics Publishing Web site. http://www.medicalphysics.org/vandykch16.pdf. Madison, WI: Medical Physics Publishing; 2013.

68. Karzmark C, Nunan C, Tanabe E. *Medical Electron Accelerators*. New York: McGraw-Hill Ryerson; 1993.

69. Greene D, Williams P. *Linear Accelerators for Radiation Therapy*. 2nd ed. New York: Taylor and Francis Group; 1997.

70. Fenwick JD, Tome WA, Soisson ET, et al. Tomotherapy and other innovative IMRT delivery systems. *Semin Radiat Oncol* 2006;16:199–208.

71. Curran B, Balter J, Chetty I, eds. *Integrating New Technologies into the Clinic: Monte Carlo and Image-Guided Radiation Therapy*. Madison, WI: Medical Physics Publishing; 2006.

72. Bourland J, ed. *Image-Guided Radiation Therapy*. Boca Raton, FL: Taylor & Francis; 2012.

73. Seco J, Verhaegen F, eds. *Monte Carlo Techniques in Radiation Therapy*. Boca Raton, FL: Taylor & Francis; 2013.

74. Kessler ML. Image registration and data fusion in radiation therapy. *Br J Radiol* 2006;79:S99–S108.

75. Brock K, ed. *Image Processing in Radiation Therapy*. Boca Raton, FL: Taylor & Francis Group; 2014.

76. Sovik A, Malinen E, Olsen DR. Strategies for biologic image-guided dose escalation: a review. *Int J Radiat Oncol Biol Phys* 2009;73:650–658.

77. Marks LB, Ten Haken RK, Martel MK. Guest editor's introduction to QUANTEC: a users guide. *Int J Radiat Oncol Biol Phys* 2010;76:S1–S2.

CANCER THERAPEUTICS

78. Li A, Alber M, Deasy JO, et al. The use and QA of biologically related models for treatment planning: short report of the TG-166 of the therapy physics committee of the AAPM. *Med Phys* 2012;39:1386–1409.

79. Bortfeld T. IMRT: a review and preview. *Phys Med Biol* 2006;51:R363–R379.

80. Webb S. *Contemporary IMRT Developing Physics and Clinical Implementation.* London: IOP Publishing; 2005.

81. Maughan R, Yudelev M. Neutron therapy. In: Van Dyk J, ed. *The Modern Technology of Radiation Oncology.* Madison, WI: Medical Physics Publishing; 1999.

82. Hogstrom KR, Almond PR. Review of electron beam therapy physics. *Phys Med Biol* 2006;51:R455–R489.

83. Schlegel W, Bortfeld T, Grosu A, eds. *New Technologies in Radiation Oncology.* Heidelberg: Springer-Verlag; 2006.

84. Ma C-MC, Lomax T, eds. *Proton and Carbon Ion Therapy.* Boca Raton, FL: Taylor & Francis Group; 2012.

85. Venselaar J, Meigooni A, Baltas D, et al., eds. *Comprehensive Brachytherapy: Physical and Clinical Aspects.* Boca Raton, FL: Taylor & Francis Group; 2012.

86. Meredith RF. Systemic targeted radionuclide therapy symposium introduction. *Int J Radiat Oncol Biol Phys* 2006;66:S7.

87. Tripuraneni P, Watson RL, Ang KK, et al. Intersociety Radiation Oncology Summit-SCOPE II. *Int J Radiat Oncol Biol Phys* 2008;72:323–326.

88. Delaney G, Jacob S, Featherstone C, et al. The role of radiotherapy in cancer treatment: estimating optimal utilization from a review of evidence-based clinical guidelines. *Cancer* 2005;104:1129–1137.

89. Zelefsky MJ, Housman DM, Pei X, et al. Incidence of secondary cancer development after high-dose intensity-modulated radiotherapy and image-guided brachytherapy for the treatment of localized prostate cancer. *Int J Radiat Oncol Biol Phys* 2012;83:953–959.

90. Combs SE, Laperriere N, Brada M. Clinical controversies: proton radiation therapy for brain and skull base tumors. *Semin Radiat Oncol* 2013;23:120–126.

91. Overgaard J. Hypoxic radiosensitization: adored and ignored. *J Clin Oncol* 2007;25:4066–4074.

92. Mouw KW, Trofimov A, Zietman AL, et al. Clinical controversies: proton therapy for prostate cancer. *Semin Radiat Oncol* 2013;23:109–114.

93. Yu JB, Soulos PR, Herrin J, et al. Proton versus intensity-modulated radiotherapy for prostate cancer: patterns of care and early toxicity. *J Natl Cancer Inst* 2013;105:25–32.

94. Brada M, Pijls-Johannesma M, De Ruysscher D. Proton therapy in clinical practice: current clinical evidence. *J Clin Oncol* 2007;25:965–970.

95. Douglas JG, Koh WJ, Austin-Seymour M, et al. Treatment of salivary gland neoplasms with fast neutron radiotherapy. *Arch Otolaryngol Head Neck Surg* 2003;129:944–948.

96. Shilkrut M, Merrick GS, McLaughlin PW, et al. The addition of low-dose-rate brachytherapy and androgen-deprivation therapy decreases biochemical failure and prostate cancer death compared with dose-escalated external-beam radiation therapy for high-risk prostate cancer. *Cancer* 2013;119:681–690.

97. Iyengar P, Timmerman R. Stereotactic ablative radiotherapy for non-small cell lung cancer: rationale and outcomes. *J Natl Compr Canc Netw* 2012;10:1514–1520.

98. Lo SS, Moffatt-Bruce SD, Dawson LA, et al. The role of local therapy in the management of lung and liver oligometastases. *Nat Rev Clin Oncol* 2011;8:405–416.

99. Forastiere AA, Zhang Q, Weber RS, et al. Long-term results of RTOG 91-11: a comparison of three nonsurgical treatment strategies to preserve the larynx in patients with locally advanced larynx cancer. *J Clin Oncol* 2013;31:845–852.

100. Gunderson LL, Winter KA, Ajani JA, et al. Long-term update of US GI intergroup RTOG 98-11 phase III trial for anal carcinoma: survival, relapse, and colostomy failure with concurrent chemoradiation involving fluorouracil/mitomycin versus fluorouracil/cisplatin. *J Clin Oncol* 2012;30:4344–4351.

101. Hellman S, Weichselbaum RR. Oligometastases. *J Clin Oncol* 1995;13:8–10.

102. Hortobagyi GN. Can we cure limited metastatic breast cancer? *J Clin Oncol* 2002;20:620–623.

103. Stamell EF, Wolchok JD, Gnjatic S, et al. The abscopal effect associated with a systemic anti-melanoma immune response. *Int J Radiat Oncol Biol Phys* 2013;85:293–295.

104. Nagtegaal ID, Gosens MJ, Marijnen CA, et al. Combinations of tumor and treatment parameters are more discriminative for prognosis than the present TNM system in rectal cancer. *J Clin Oncol* 2007;25:1647–1650.

105. Sauer R, Becker H, Hohenberger W, et al. Preoperative versus postoperative chemoradiotherapy for rectal cancer. *N Engl J Med* 2004;351:1731–1740.

106. Clarke M, Collins R, Darby S, et al. Effects of radiotherapy and of differences in the extent of surgery for early breast cancer on local recurrence and 15-year survival: an overview of the randomised trials. *Lancet* 2005;366:2087–2106.

107. Hellman S. Stopping metastases at their source. *N Engl J Med* 1997;337:996–997.

108. Marks LB, Prosnitz LR. Postoperative radiotherapy for lung cancer: the breast cancer story all over again? *Int J Radiat Oncol Biol Phys* 2000;48:625–627.

109. Wang XS, Rhines LD, Shiu AS, et al. Stereotactic body radiation therapy for management of spinal metastases in patients without spinal cord compression: a phase 1-2 trial. *Lancet Oncol* 2012;13:395–402.

110. Tarnawski R, Fowler J, Skladowski K, et al. How fast is repopulation of tumor cells during the treatment gap? *Int J Radiat Oncol Biol Phys* 2002;54:229–236.

111. Peters LJ, Withers HR. Applying radiobiological principles to combined modality treatment of head and neck cancer—the time factor. *Int J Radiat Oncol Biol Phys* 1997;39:831–836.

112. Bourhis J, Overgaard J, Audry H, et al. Hyperfractionated or accelerated radiotherapy in head and neck cancer: a meta-analysis. *Lancet* 2006;368:843–854.

113. Bourhis J, Sire C, Graff P, et al. Concomitant chemoradiotherapy versus acceleration of radiotherapy with or without concomitant chemotherapy in locally advanced head and neck carcinoma (GORTEC 99-02): an open-label phase 3 randomised trial. *Lancet Oncol* 2012;13:145–153.

114. Adkison JB, McHaffie DR, Bentzen SM, et al. Phase I trial of pelvic nodal dose escalation with hypofractionated IMRT for high-risk prostate cancer. *Int J Radiat Oncol Biol Phys* 2012;82:184–190.

115. Feyer P, Maranzano E, Molassiotis A, et al. Radiotherapy-induced nausea and vomiting (RINV): antiemetic guidelines. *Support Care Cancer* 2005;13:122–128.

116. Horiot JC. Prophylaxis versus treatment: is there a better way to manage radiotherapy-induced nausea and vomiting? *Int J Radiat Oncol Biol Phys* 2004;60:1018–1025.

117. Hickok JT, Roscoe JA, Morrow GR, et al. Frequency, severity, clinical course, and correlates of fatigue in 372 patients during 5 weeks of radiotherapy for cancer. *Cancer* 2005;104:1772–1778.

118. Schwartz AL, Nail LM, Chen S, et al. Fatigue patterns observed in patients receiving chemotherapy and radiotherapy. *Cancer Invest* 2000;18:11–19.

119. Dawson LA, Ten Haken RK. Partial volume tolerance of the liver to radiation. *Semin Radiat Oncol* 2005;15:279–283.

120. Kong FM, Hayman JA, Griffith KA, et al. Final toxicity results of a radiation-dose escalation study in patients with non-small-cell lung cancer (NSCLC): predictors for radiation pneumonitis and fibrosis. *Int J Radiat Oncol Biol Phys* 2006;65:1075–1086.

121. Fleckenstein K, Gauter-Fleckenstein B, Jackson IL, et al. Using biological markers to predict risk of radiation injury. *Semin Radiat Oncol* 2007;17:89–98.

122. Hart JP, Broadwater G, Rabbani Z, et al. Cytokine profiling for prediction of symptomatic radiation-induced lung injury. *Int J Radiat Oncol Biol Phys* 2005;63:1448–1454.

123. Barnett GC, Coles CE, Elliott RM, et al. Independent validation of genes and polymorphisms reported to be associated with radiation toxicity: a prospective analysis study. *Lancet Oncol* 2012;13:65–77.

124. Fajardo LF. Is the pathology of radiation injury different in small vs large blood vessels? *Cardiovasc Radiat Med* 1999;1:108–110.

125. Delanian S, Porcher R, Rudant J, et al. Kinetics of response to long-term treatment combining pentoxifylline and tocopherol in patients with superficial radiation-induced fibrosis. *J Clin Oncol* 2005;23:8570–8579.

126. Chou TC, Talalay P. Quantitative analysis of dose-effect relationships: the combined effects of multiple drugs or enzyme inhibitors. *Adv Enzyme Regul* 1984;22:27–55.

127. Steel GG, Peckham MJ. Exploitable mechanisms in combined radiotherapy-chemotherapy: the concept of additivity. *Int J Radiat Oncol Biol Phys* 1979;5:85–91.

128. Tannock IF. Treatment of cancer with radiation and drugs. *J Clin Oncol* 1996;14:3156–3174.

129. Blanchard P, Baujat B, Holostenco V, et al. Meta-analysis of chemotherapy in head and neck cancer (MACH-NC): a comprehensive analysis by tumour site. *Radiother Oncol* 2011;100:33–40.

130. Dillman RO, Herndon J, Seagren SL, et al. Improved survival in stage III non-small-cell lung cancer: seven-year follow-up of cancer and leukemia group B (CALGB) 8433 trial. *J Natl Cancer Inst* 1996;88:1210–1215.

131. De Ruysscher D, Belderbos J, Reymen B, et al. State of the art radiation therapy for lung cancer 2012: a glimpse of the future. *Clin Lung Cancer* 2013;14:89–95.

132. Klopp AH, Eifel PJ. Chemoradiotherapy for cervical cancer in 2010. *Curr Oncol Rep* 2011;13:77–85.

133. Chun PY, Feng FY, Scheurer AM, et al. Synergistic effects of gemcitabine and gefitinib in the treatment of head and neck carcinoma. *Cancer Res* 2006;66:981–988.

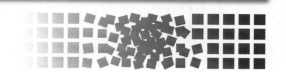

14   Cancer Immunotherapy

Steven A. Rosenberg, Paul F. Robbins, Giao Q. Phan,
Steven A. Feldman, and James N. Kochenderfer

INTRODUCTION

Progress in understanding basic aspects of cellular immunology and tumor–host immune interactions have led to the development of immune-based therapies capable of mediating the rejection of metastatic cancer in humans. Early studies of allografts and transplanted syngeneic tumors in mice demonstrated that it was the cellular arm of the immune response rather than the action of antibodies (humoral immunity) that was responsible for tissue rejection. Thus, studies of immunotherapy have focused on enhancing antitumor immune responses of T cells that recognize cancer antigens. Antibodies that recognize growth factors on the surface of tumors can contribute to tumor regression, primarily by interfering with growth signals rather than by the direct destruction of tumor cells. The use of monoclonal antibodies in cancer treatment will be considered in Chapter 29.

Evidence for specific tumor recognition by cells of the immune system was obtained in experiments first conducted in the 1940s using murine tumors generated or induced by the mutagen methylcholanthrene (MCA). Mice that received a surgical resection of previously inoculated tumors could be protected against a subsequent tumor challenge with the immunizing tumor but not generally protected against challenge with additional MCA tumors. The observation that CD8+ cytotoxic T cells were primarily responsible for mediating the rejection of MCA-induced tumors in mice led to the identification of genes that encoded tumor rejection antigens expressed on murine tumors as well as the subsequent identification of antigens recognized by human tumor-reactive T cells. The identification of widely shared nonmutated tumor antigens led to the expectation that effective vaccine therapies could be developed for the treatment of cancer patients; however, the response rates in clinical cancer vaccine trials targeting these antigens have, to this point, been disappointingly low. Vaccination with viruslike particles expressing human papilloma virus (HPV) proteins are successful in preventing the establishment of cervical cancer and immunization with peptides derived from the oncogenic HPV E6 and E7 proteins can mediate tumor regression in woman with high vulvar neoplasia.[1] Immune-based therapies have, however, been identified that mediate the regression of large, established tumor metastases. Nonspecific immune stimulation with interleukin-2 (IL-2) administration can lead to objective clinical responses in patients with melanoma and renal cancer,[2] and inhibition of regulatory pathways mediated by CTLA-4[3] or PD-1[4] can lead to tumor regression in patients with metastatic melanoma and lung cancer. The adoptive transfer of melanoma reactive T cells can mediate objective clinical responses in 50% to 70% of patients with melanoma,[5] and the ability to genetically modify antitumor lymphocytes is expanding this cell transfer therapy approach to the treatment of patients with other cancer histologies.[6] Studies aimed at identifying potent tumor rejection antigens, as well as mechanisms that regulate immune responses to cancer, are being actively pursued.

HUMAN TUMOR ANTIGENS

To be recognized by immune lymphocytes, intracellular proteins must be digested and the resulting peptides transported to the cell surface and bound to Class I or II main histocompatibility molecules (Fig. 14.1). A variety of approaches have been used to identify the antigens that are naturally processed and presented on tumor cells. These include evaluating the ability of cells transfected with tumor cDNA library pools along with genes encoding autologous major histocompatibility complex (MHC) molecules, as well as the ability of target cells pulsed with peptides eluted from tumor cell surface MHC molecules for their ability to stimulate tumor reactive T cells. Reverse immunology approaches that involve either repeated in vitro T cell sensitization or in vivo immunization with candidate peptides or proteins have also lead to the identification of tumor antigens. Candidate epitopes identified on the basis of their ability to bind to a particular MHC molecule, however, may not necessarily be naturally processed and presented on the tumor cell surface, and there are conflicting reports on the ability of T cells generated using some candidate epitopes to recognize unmanipulated tumor targets, as discussed further.

Additional tumor antigens have been identified using antisera from cancer patients to screen tumor cell cDNA libraries, a method that has been termed serological analysis of recombinant cDNA expression (SEREX).[7] Although some of the proteins identified using this technique are expressed in a tumor-specific manner, many of these antigens are simply expressed at higher levels in tumor cells than in normal cells. This may occur due to the release of normal self-proteins from necrotic and apoptotic tumor cells leading to the generation of antibodies against intracellular proteins that are normally sequestered from the immune system.

Finally, the use of recently described approaches involving whole exomic sequencing of tumor cells has led to the identification of mutated tumor antigens. These studies will be discussed further in the section devoted to mutated tumor antigens

Cancer/Germ-Line Antigens

The first antigen identified as a target of human tumor reactive T cells was isolated by screening a melanoma genomic DNA library with an autologous cytotoxic T lymphocyte (CTL) clone.[8] The gene that was isolated, termed *MAGE-1*, was found to be a nonmutated gene that was a member of a large, previously unidentified gene family, many of whose members encode antigens recognized by tumor reactive T cells.[9] Members of this family of antigens are expressed in the testes and placenta, both of which lack an expression of MHC molecules, but often not in other normal tissues, which has led to their designation as cancer germ-line (CG) antigens. Members of the MAGE gene family are expressed in a variety of tumor types, including melanoma, breast, prostate, and esophageal cancers. The expression patterns of three

167

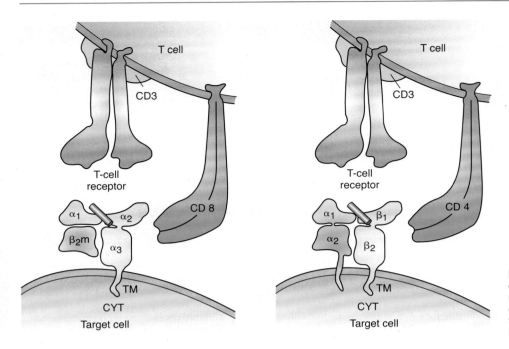

Figure 14.1 CD8 and CD4 cells use different molecules that interact with major histocompatibility complex (MHC) class I and II molecules respectively on the cell surface and serve to potentiate immune reactions.

different cancer/testes antigens in multiple tumor types is shown in Figure 14.2. The NY-ESO-1 antigen—a CG antigen that is unrelated to the MAGE family of genes—is expressed in approximately 30% of breast, prostate, and melanoma tumors, as well as between 70% and 80% of synovial cell sarcomas.[10]

Clinical adoptive immunotherapy trials targeting CG antigens have now been conducted in patients with melanoma as well as other tumor types. In a recent trial, objective clinical responses were seen in approximately 50% of patients with melanoma and 80% of patients with synovial cell sarcoma receiving autologous peripheral blood mononuclear cell (PBMC) transduced with a T-cell receptor directed against an HLA-A*02:01 restricted NY-ESO-1 epitope.[6] A trial targeting a MAGEA3

epitopes was recently carried out using a T-cell receptor (TCR) isolated from an HLA-A*02:01+ transgenic mouse immunized with the MAGEA3:112–120 peptide.[11] Objective clinical responses were observed in five of nine melanoma patients receiving the adoptively transferred PBMC that were transduced with the MAGEA3-reactive TCR.[12] Unexpectedly, neural toxicity was observed in three of the patients treated in this trial, two of whom lapsed into a coma and subsequently died. Autopsy samples of patients' brains revealed that *MAGEA12*, which encodes a cross-reactive epitope recognized by the MAGEA3 TCR, was expressed at low levels in patients' brains, which may have been responsible for the observed neurologic toxicities. In a recent trial carried out using an affinity-enhanced human TCR directed against the

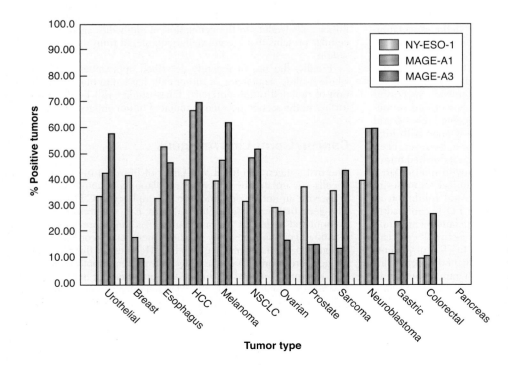

Figure 14.2 Expression of three different cancer/testes antigens in many different tumor types is shown. These data reflect reverse transcription–polymerase chain reaction measurements and is more sensitive than results obtained by immunohistochemistry. NSCLC, non–small-cell lung cancer. (Data compiled by Dr. J. Wargo. Massachusetts General Hospital.)

HLA-A*01:01-restricted, MAGEA3:168-176 epitope, the first two patients receiving TCR-transduced autologous PBMC died of cardiac arrest 4 to 5 days following infusion, which was attributed to cross-reactivity with titin, a protein expressed at high levels in cardimyocytes.[13] Taken together, these findings demonstrate the need for caution in evaluating cross-reactivity of high affinity TCRs recognizing tumor antigens.

Melanocyte Differentiation Antigens

Melanoma-reactive T cells have been frequently found to recognize gene products, termed melanocyte differentiation antigens (MDA), that are expressed in melanomas as well as in normal melanocytes present in the skin, eye, and ear but not in other normal tissues or tumor types. These include epitopes derived from gp100,[14,15] tyrosinase,[16] TRP-1,[17] and TRP-2,[18] proteins that had previously been found to play important roles in melanin synthesis. The screening of melanoma cDNA libraries with an HLA-A2–restricted tumor reactive T cells lead to the isolation of a previously unidentified gene, termed MART-1[19] or Melan-A.[20] The MART-1 antigen, which is expressed in 80% to 90% of fresh melanomas and cultured melanoma cell lines as well as normal melanocytes, represents an MDA of unknown function. The majority of melanoma reactive, HLA-A2–restricted tumor-infiltrating lymphocytes (TIL) recognize a single MART-1 epitope.[21] Studies carried out using a variety of approaches have also resulted in the identification of human leukocyte antigen (HLA) class II restricted epitopes of tyrosinase, TRP-1, TRP-2, and gp100.[9]

Overexpressed Gene Products

Gene products that are expressed at low levels in a variety of normal tissues but are overexpressed in a variety of tumor types have also been shown to be recognized by T cells. Screening of an autologous renal carcinoma cDNA library with a tumor reactive, HLA-A3–restricted T-cell clone resulted in the isolation of FGF5,[22] a protein that was expressed only at low levels in normal tissues but upregulated in multiple renal carcinomas as well as prostate and breast carcinomas. The peptide epitope recognized by FGF5-reactive T cells was generated by protein splicing, a process in which distant protein regions are joined together in the proteasome that had previously only been described in plants[23] and unicellular organisms.[24] Subsequent studies have led to the identification of multiple epitopes that result from protein splicing, suggesting that this represents a general mechanism for generating T-cell epitopes.[25–28] Screening of an autologous cDNA library led to the identification of a previously unknown gene that was termed *PRAME*.[29] This gene product was expressed in relatively high levels in melanomas as well as in additional tumor types but was also expressed at lower levels in a variety of normal tissues that included the testis, endometrium, ovary, and adrenals. The HLA-A24–restricted PRAME reactive T-cell clone, however, expressed the natural killer (NK) inhibitory receptor p58.2, and tumor cell recognition was dependent on the loss of expression of the HLA C*07 allele that represented the ligand for the inhibitory receptor, which may explain the lack of recognition of normal tissues that express relatively high levels of this HLA gene product.

Attempts have also been made to generate T cells directed against overexpressed candidate antigens by repeatedly stimulating PBMC in vitro with peptides that were identified as high binders for particular MHC molecules either using direct binding assays or *in silico* analysis carried out using peptide/MHC binding algorithms.[30,31] Using this approach, candidate epitopes have been identified from a variety of proteins that include prostate-specific antigen (PSA)[32] and prostate-specific membrane antigen (PSMA),[33] as well as Her-2/neu, a protein that is frequently overexpressed in a variety of tumor types, including breast carcinomas. Initial studies indicated that T cells derived by in vitro stimulation

with a peptide that was predicted to bind with high affinity to HLA-A*02:01, Her-2/neu:369–377, recognized the appropriate natural tumor targets.[34] In one study, T cells generated following two in vitro stimulations of postvaccination PBMC from three of the four patients who were tested efficiently recognized peptide-pulsed targets but failed to recognize appropriate tumor targets.[35] Similarly, although stimulation with a peptide corresponding to amino acids 540 through 548 of the human telomerase reverse transcriptase (hTERT) catalytic subunit was initially reported to generate tumor-reactive T cells,[36] additional observations indicated that T cells generated using this peptide failed to recognize tumor targets.[37] These factors responsible for these discrepancies remain unresolved, although the in vitro stimulation of T cells with target cells pulsed with relatively high peptide concentrations could have led to the generation of low-avidity T cells that were incapable of recognizing naturally processed antigens.

Alternative screening approaches employed for tumor antigen discovery that may help to address these issues include the use of tandem mass spectrometry to sequence peptides that have been eluted from tumor cell surface MHC molecules. Use of this technique, coupled with microarray gene expression profiling, resulted in the identification of peptides derived from proteins that appeared to be overexpressed in tumor cells.[38] Peptides identified using this approach may, in many cases, not be immunogenic due to the fact that their expression in normal tissues, although lower than in tumor cells, may be high enough to lead to central or peripheral tolerance. Nevertheless, one of the peptides that were identified in this study also appeared to be recognized by human tumor reactive T cells. Recently, a similar approach was used to identify candidate peptides presented on cell surface MHC molecules that appeared to be derived from proteins that were overexpressed on glioblastomas.[39] In a clinical trial involving vaccination of patients with pools of the identified peptides, overall survival was associated with the number of peptides in the vaccine pool that elicited immune response[40]; however, this may simply reflect the fact that T cells from healthier patients can more readily generate peptide-specific responses.

Transgenic mice that express human HLA molecules have also been immunized with candidate antigens in an attempt to identify high avidity tumor-reactive T cells. Immunization of transgenic mice expressing HLA-A*0201 with the native human p53:264–272 peptide that differed from the corresponding murine p53 sequence at a single position lead to the generation of T cells that recognized tumor cells expressing high levels of p53.[41] Human T cells transduced with a murine p53 TCR isolated from an immunized mouse recognized a variety of human tumor cells; however, transduced T cells also recognized normal cells expressing lower p53 levels, indicating the dangers of targeting a normal self-protein whose expression is not strictly limited to tumor cells.[42] Similarly, a TCR that was highly reactive with HLA-A*02:01+ tumor cells expressing the human carcinoembryonic antigen (CEA), a protein that is overexpressed in colon and breast carcinomas, was isolated by immunizing HLA-A*02:01+ transgenic mice with the CEA:691–699 peptide.[43] The adoptive transfer of human PBMC transduced with the CEA-reactive TCR lead to an objective clinical response in one of the three treated patients; however, severe colitis was observed in all three of the treated patients.[44] In general, immunotherapies that target antigens present even in small amounts on normal tissues have led to normal tissue destruction and must be applied with caution.

Mutated Gene Products Recognized by CD8+ and CD4+ T Cells

A variety of mutated antigens have also been identified as targets of tumor reactive T cells. The majority of mutated antigens identified using these approaches appear to be unique or only expressed in a relatively small percentage of cancers, and so do not represent targets that are broadly applicable to the treatment of multiple patients. Nevertheless, these studies have in some cases provided insights into mechanisms involved with tumor development, as the mutations may represent drivers of the transformed phenotype. The CDK4 gene product that was cloned using a CTL clone contained a point mutation that enhanced the binding to the HLA-A2 restriction element.[45] This mutation, which was identified in 1 of an additional 28 melanomas that were analyzed, led to the inhibition of binding to the cell cycle inhibitory protein p16^{INK4a} and may have played a role in the loss of growth control in this tumor cell. A point-mutated product of the β-catenin gene, containing a substitution of phenylalanine for serine at position 37, was isolated by screening a cDNA library with an HLA-24–restricted, melanoma reactive TIL.[46] This mutation was found to stabilize the β-catenin gene product by altering a critical serine phosphorylation site, and 2 of 24 additional melanoma cell lines were found to express transcripts with identical mutations.[47]

The observation that immunization against individual murine tumors did not generally cross-protect against challenge with additional syngeneic murine tumors has provided support for the hypothesis that mutant T-cell epitopes represent the predominant antigens responsible for tumor rejection.[48] Mutated epitopes also represent a foreign antigen, which may render them more immunogenic than the majority of normal self-antigens. Although many of the mutations are specific for individual tumors, T cells have been generated by carrying out in vitro sensitization with peptides encoded at mutational hot spots present in *driver* genes.[49]

Recently, novel approaches have been developed that involve the sequencing of tumor cell DNA to identify potential mutated epitopes. In one study, whole exome sequencing of the murine B16 melanoma led to the identification of mutated epitopes that elicited a T cell that appeared to specifically recognize the mutated but not the corresponding wild-type peptides.[50] In a second study, a mutated antigen was identified by screening candidate epitopes that were expressed by tumors derived from immunodeficient mice that regressed in immune-competent mice.[51] More recently, melanomas from three patients who responded to adoptive immunotherapy were subjected to whole exome sequencing, followed by *in silico* analysis using peptide/MHC binding algorithms to identify candidate epitopes that were predicted to bind to the patients' MHC molecules.[52] Using this approach, a total of seven peptides were identified as targets of the TIL that were administered to these patients. Two mutated epitopes were recently identified by whole exome sequencing of a melanoma from a patient who demonstrated a partial response to treatment with the anti–CTLA-4 antibody ipilimumab, followed by a screening of a panel of mutated candidate peptide/MHC tetramers that were predicted to bind to the patient's HLA-A and B alleles.[53] In addition, a mutated epitope expressed by a bile duct cancer was identified by screening tandem minigenes encoding all mutated epitopes that were identified by whole exome sequencing.[54] The adoptive transfer of T cells directed against this mutation-mediated regression of the patient's cancer. Mutations unique to each cancer represent ideal targets for immunotherapy and can potentially lead to the development of personalized therapies directed against these unique targets.

Antigens Identified in Viral-Associated Cancers

Viruses do not appear to play a role in the development of the majority of human cancers; however, an infection with HPV, a group of double-stranded DNA viruses that infect squamous epithelium, is highly associated with the development of a variety of genital lesions that range from warts to carcinomas, as well as the majority of oropharyngeal carcinomas. Recombinant vaccines have been produced by the generation of viruslike particles (VLP),

self-assembling particles that form following the expression of the HPV L1 protein in recombinant viral and yeast systems that were initially found to be protective in animal models. The results of a phase II trial in which 2,392 women between 16 and 23 years of age were immunized with HPV-16 VLPs indicated that 100% of those who were vaccinated were protected against infection with HPV-16.[55,56] Although vaccination with VLP does not lead to the regression of established disease, some success has been seen in therapeutic vaccination trials that target the oncogenic viral proteins E6 and E7. In a trial involving the vaccination of women with HPV-16–positive high-grade vulvar intraepithelial neoplasia with synthetic long peptides that encompass both HLA class I and class II restricted epitopes from the oncogenic HPV proteins E6 and E, clinical responses were observed in 15 of the 19 vaccinated patients, and complete regression of all lesions were seen in 9 of the 19 patients in this trial.[1]

Targeting foreign antigens thus may represent a strategy that can lead to more effective immunotherapies. These include viral epitopes as well as mutated epitopes that are also foreign to the host and therefore may represent more effective targets for these therapies than normal self-antigen.

HUMAN CANCER IMMUNOTHERAPIES

A wide variety of therapies have been evaluated in model systems and are now being developed for the treatment of patients with cancer. These include nonspecific approaches, those that involve direct immunization of patients with a variety of immunogens and approaches that involve the adoptive transfer of activated effector cells (Table 14.1). Much confusion related to the effectiveness of cancer immunotherapy has resulted from the lack of proper evaluation of the results of therapy using standard, accepted oncologic criteria such as the World Health Organization or the Response Evaluation Criteria in Solid Tumors (RECIST). Many clinical trials reported a positive use of *soft* criteria such as lymphoid infiltration or tumor necrosis that can occur in the natural course of cancer growth. Because of the delayed responses seen with some immunotherapy approaches, including tumor regression after initial tumor growth, guidelines have been published suggesting the use of an alternate set of immune-related response criteria for the evaluation of immune-based cancer treatments.[57,58] Other confusion has arisen from the use of inappropriate animal models. Although animal model systems have provided important clues that may lead to improved therapies, model systems that employ artificially introduced foreign antigens or that evaluate protection from tumor challenge do not appear to be relevant to the treatment of patients with bulky metastases. Short-term lung metastasis models involve the treatment of relatively small, nonvascularized tumors and also may not be directly relevant to the majority of tumors that are the targets of current clinical trials.

TABLE 14.1

Three Main Approaches to Cancer Immunotherapy

1. Nonspecific stimulation of immune reactions
   a) Stimulate effector cells
      IL-2 (melanoma and renal cancer)
   b) Inhibit regulatory factors
      Anti-CTLA4 (melanoma)
      Anti–PD-1 (melanoma, lung cancer)
2. Active immunization to enhance antitumor reactions (cancer vaccines)
3. Passively transfer activated immune cells with antitumor activity (adoptive immunotherapy)

Nonspecific Approaches to Cancer Immunotherapy

Progress has surged in the past 10 years in the understanding and utilization of nonspecific immune stimulation for the treatment of metastatic cancers. These agents aim to activate quiescent tumor-reactive immune cells or to remove inhibitory mechanisms to allow immunosuppressed cells to function to their full capacity. Although IL-2 and ipilimumab are currently the only immune stimulants approved by the U.S. Food and Drug Administration (FDA) for the treatment of metastatic renal cell carcinoma (IL-2) and melanoma (IL-2 and ipilimumab), new immune checkpoint inhibitors such as anti–programmed cell death 1 (anti–PD-1) have shown impressive results in recent clinical trials for patients with melanoma, renal cell cancer, and also non–small-cell lung cancer (NSCLC), and will likely be approved in the near future. As expected with nonspecific immunostimulation, systemic and bystander immune-related adverse events such as colitis has been reported with all agents in varying degrees, although most side effects are controllable and reversible if addressed aggressively and promptly by experienced clinicians. Importantly, antitumor responses seen with these immune-based modalities appear to be durable for some patients and may even be potentially curative. As with many therapies for metastatic solid tumors, preliminary trials using combination therapies have suggested better than expected response rates and survival, and confirmatory trials are in process to validate and ensure that toxicities from combining agents would not be prohibitive. Overall, patients with metastatic solid tumors may soon have wider armamentarium of off-the-shelf immunotherapy options.

Interleukin-2

Morgan et al.[59] showed that a *factor* produced in the medium from stimulated normal human blood lymphocytes can allow ex vivo growth and expansion of human T lymphocytes. The identification of this soluble T-cell growth factor (IL-2)[60,61] allowed the ability to culture T cells in vitro. IL-2 is a 15-kd glycoprotein produced in minute amounts by activated peripheral blood lymphocytes, and even with using T-cell hybridomas, minimal quantities could be purified; thus, research using IL-2 was impeded by the limited amounts of purified IL-2 available. The isolation of the cDNA clone in 1983[62] enabled the development in 1984 of recombinant IL-2,[63] which permitted the ability to mass manufacture IL-2. Although murine studies demonstrated the ability of IL-2 to mediate tumor regression,[64] early phase I clinical trials did not show any antitumor response,[65] but was instructive in showing pharmacokinetics and toxicities, which led to more effective regimens. Subsequently, IL-2 was given in higher doses (up to 720,000 IU/kg intravenously every 8 hours) in a landmark trial involving 25 patients, along with nonspecific lymphokine-activated natural killer (LAK) cells, which are non-T and non-B lymphocytes.[66] This report was the first to document the regression of advanced solid cancers (melanoma, renal cell, lung, and colon) using immunotherapy in humans.[66] A follow-up trial randomizing 181 patients to either high-dose IL-2 alone (720,000 IU/kg intravenously every 8 hours) or high-dose IL-2 and LAK cells showed that the tumor response was due to IL-2 alone and not to the nonspecific LAK cells.[67] This study also narrowed the IL-2–sensitive histologies to melanoma and renal cell cancer, which had more consistent responses.

IL-2 Therapy for Metastatic Renal Cell Cancer

Subsequent to the studies discussed previously, high-dose IL-2 was tested by additional centers and in combination with other agents for renal cell cancer. A randomized phase II trial involving 99 kidney cancer patients showed no increase in antitumor responses with the addition of interferon alfa-2b (IFNα-2b). Responses were seen for 12 (17%) of 71 patients who received high-dose IL-2 alone, with 4 complete regressions.[68] A summary report of 227 patients

with metastatic renal cell cancer treated with high-dose IL-2 (defined as 600,000 IU/kg or 720,000 IU/kg given intravenously every 8 hours as tolerated up to 15 doses) from 1985 to 1996 at the Surgery Branch of the National Cancer Institute (NCI) documented a total response rate of 19%, with 10% partial and 9% complete; the longest duration of a complete response was over 10 years ongoing (134+ months).[69] Another summary report from seven phase II clinical trials from multiple institutions involving 255 patients with metastatic renal cell cancer receiving high-dose IL-2 showed the overall response rate was 14%, with 9% partial and 5% complete, and responses occurred in all sites of disease, including primary kidney tumors, bone metastases, and bulking visceral tumor burdens.[70] Although the response rates were modest, the durability of the responses was remarkable, with many responses lasting over 5 years ongoing (see Fig. 14.2). Because of the striking durability of the antitumor responses, IL-2 received FDA approval for the treatment of metastatic renal cell cancer in 1992. A follow-up report in 2000 showing the response rates of the 255 renal cell patients in the seven phase II studies to be the same, with complete responses lasting over 10 years ongoing (131+ months for the longest responder), suggesting a potential cure.[71]

To ascertain whether lower doses and/or different administration routes, which would decrease toxicity and obviate the need for inpatient hospitalization for IL-2 therapy, a trial randomizing 400 patients with metastatic renal cell cancer to either standard high-dose intravenous IL-2, low-dose intravenous IL-2 (at 72,000 IU/kg), or low-dose subcutaneous IL-2 (250,000 U/kg per dose daily Monday through Friday in the first week and then 125,000 U/kg per dose daily during the next 5 weeks).[72] Although responses were seen with all three regimens, including complete responses in the low-dose subcutaneous regimen, standard high-dose IL-2 had higher overall response rates (21%) versus low-dose intravenous IL-2 (13%; p = 0.048) and low-dose subcutaneous IL-2 (10%; p = 0.033), suggesting the superiority of the high-dose intravenous regimen.[72]

The administration of IL-2 represents the only known curative treatment for patients with metastatic renal cell cancer and should be considered as front-line therapy for suitable patients.

IL-2 Therapy for Metastatic Melanoma

Between 1985 and 1993, 270 patients with metastatic melanoma enrolled into eight clinical trials in multiple centers using high-dose IL-2 (defined as 600,000 IU/kg or 720,000 IU/kg given intravenously every 8 hours as tolerated up to 15 doses). Atkins et al.[73] reported overall response rates of 16% (43 patients), with 10% partial and 6% complete; responses occurred at all tumor sites and regardless of initial tumor burden. With median follow-up at that time of 62 months, 20 responders (47%) were still alive, with 15 surviving over 5 years.[73] A follow-up report on those patients in 2000 showed that the response rates were unchanged; with the longest response duration of >12 years ongoing, disease progression was not observed in any patient responding greater than 30 months.[74] As with renal cell cancer, the flat *tail* of the Kaplan-Meier response duration and overall survival curves (Fig. 14.3), showing the potential curative nature of the antitumor responses, was the main compelling reason the FDA approved IL-2 for the treatment of metastatic melanoma in 1998.

Research in subsequent years aimed to increase the response rates of IL-2, led by increasing interests in tumor vaccinations as melanoma-associated antigens were being characterized.[75] Pilot studies suggested that vaccinations using modified melanoma differentiation antigens such as gp100:209–217(210M) could elicit immunologic responses in nearly all patients, and when combined with high-dose IL-2, could elicit potentially higher than expected clinical antitumor responses.[75] A follow-up phase III study[76] randomized 185 patients with HLA*A0201 from 21 centers to either high-dose IL-2 or high-dose IL-2 plus gp100:209–217(210M) concurrent immunization. Although the response rates for the

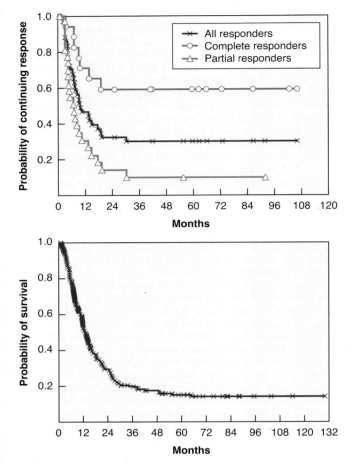

Figure 14.3 Kaplain-Meier plots of response duration (*top*) and overall survival (*bottom*) for 270 patients with metastatic melanoma who were treated with high-dose bolus IL-2 from 1985 to 1993 in eight clinical trials.[73]

IL-2 plus vaccine arm was statistically improved compared to IL-2 alone (16% versus 6%; p = 0.03), the IL-2 alone arm was notable for being much lower than in all prior studies.[76] In addition, a pilot trial of 36 melanoma patients treated high-dose IL-2 concurrently with ipilimumab (an antibody against cytotoxic T lymphocyte–associated antigen 4 discussed in the following section) gave a 25% OR rate, with 17% achieving complete response[77]; however, these data have not been further tested.

Correlative studies suggest that the total doses of IL-2 received during the first treatment course was significantly higher in patients achieving a complete response[69]; however, when limited to patients who were able to complete both cycles of the course, there was no statistical significance, suggesting that patients whose tumors progressed significantly after one cycle (and was not able to complete the second cycle of the course) accounted for some of the difference seen.[78] Responders did have a higher maximal lymphocyte count[69,78] immediately posttherapy and were more likely to develop vitiligo and thyroid dysfunction.[78] There has not been a consistent pretherapy factor that is predictive of response, although one retrospective correlative study involving 374 patients showed that patients with M1a (subcutaneous- and/or cutaneous-only disease) have a response rate of 54% compared with 12% for those with visceral M1b/c (P$_2$ <0.0001).[78]

Toxicities and Safe Administration of IL-2

High-dose IL-2 has been shown to be associated with adverse events that impact multiple organ systems.[73,79,80] The main component of the toxicities is due to an inflammatory response mediated by the release of cytokines such as IFNγ and tumor necrosis factor alpha (TNF-α)[81] resulting in a capillary-leak syndrome[82] and decreased systemic vascular resistance, which can lead to fever, hypotension, cardiac arrhythmia, lethargy, renal insufficiency, hepatic dysfunction, body edema, pulmonary edema, and confusion; other side effects can also include nausea, diarrhea, rash, anemia, thrombocytopenia, lymphocytosis, and neutrophil chemotactic defect[83] that predispose patients to gram-positive line infections. Since the first clinical trials with IL-2 in 1984, however, much has been learned to permit its safe dosing for appropriately screened patients[82,84,85]; importantly, if patients are appropriately supported, side effects are quickly reversible once IL-2 dosing ceases.[85] Kammula et al.[86] compared the incidences of grade 3/4 toxicities between the 155 patients treated from 1985 to 1986 to 156 patients treated from 1993 through 1997 at the NCI Surgery Branch: grade 3/4 hypotension decreased from 81% to 31%, intubations from 12% to 3%, neuropsychiatric toxicities from 19% to 8%, diarrhea from 92% to 12%, line sepsis from 18% to 4%, cardiac ischemia from 3% to 0%, and mortality from 3% to 0%. In fact, no fatality occurred strictly due to IL-2 therapy since 1989.[86] Overall strategies for the safe administration of high-dose IL-2 include careful screening for appropriately selected patients with adequate cardiopulmonary reserve, having an experienced team of physicians and nurses who are cognizant of the expected toxicities of IL-2, having routine preemptive measures such as prophylactic antibiotics to prevent line infections, and aggressive and prompt management of toxicities.

Checkpoint Modulators

Anti–Cytotoxic T Lymphocyte Antigen 4

CTLA-4 is an immunosuppressive *costimulatory* receptor found on newly activated T cells (and on regulatory T cells) that binds with costimulatory ligands B7-1 and B7-2 on antigen-presenting cells.[87,88] When CTLA-4 is engaged by B7-1 or B7-2, the T cells becomes inhibited,[89,90] suggesting that CTLA-4 likely evolved as a self-protective mechanism to prevent autoimmunity (Fig. 14.4). Thus, overcoming this *checkpoint* molecule was an aim of cancer immunotherapy. After CTLA-4 blockade in murine models led to antitumor immunity,[91,92] anti–CTLA-4 antibodies were tested in clinical trials starting in 2002.

The combination of anti–CTLA-4 blocking antibodies and vaccination worked well in murine models and led to one of the early phase II studies using ipilimumab (a fully human immunoglobulin [IgG$_1$] monoclonal antibody previously called MDX-010) with two gp100 vaccines, gp100:209–217(210M) and gp100:280–288(288V), in patients with metastatic melanoma.[93] Antitumor regressions were seen (from 11% to 22% overall response rates, with up to 8% complete response rates), along with severe autoimmune toxicities such as colitis, dermatitis, and even hypophysitis,[93–95] as would be expected based on the mechanism of CTLA-4 blockade. In fact, autoimmunity adverse events appeared to correlate with response to ipilimumab.[3] The experience with these early studies led to management strategies to screen aggressively for immune-related adverse events (IRAE), such as routine screening of endocrinopathies, and to treat IRAEs promptly, including high-dose steroids if needed for severe colitis.[96,97] Overall, ipilimumab was in some ways easier to manage for the patients than IL-2 because it was an outpatient infusion given every 3 weeks; IRAEs were unpredictable, however, and can appear suddenly many weeks after receiving a dose.

In 2010, results from a landmark phase III randomized trial comparing three treatment strategies (ipilimumab alone, gp100 peptide vaccine alone, or ipilimumab plus gp100 peptide vaccine) in 676 patients with metastatic melanoma were published showing improvement in median survival in the two arms that received ipilimumab (10 months) compared to the gp100 alone arm (6 months, p <0.001), despite showing a low response rate of 7% (among 540 patients who received ipilimumab).[98] Another

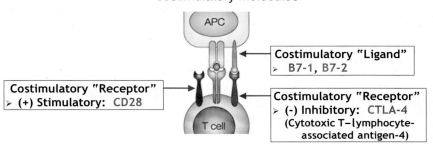

"Second Signal"

Additional signal(s) via costimulatory molecules

Figure 14.4 Mechanism of action of cytotoxic T-lymphocyte–associated antigen 4 (CTLA-4). When CD28 is engaged on the T cell, reactivity of the T cell is enhanced. When CTLA-4 is engaged on the T cell, reactivity of the T cell is inhibited. Blocking of CTLA-4 with a monoclonal antibody can elicit antitumor immunity but also autoimmunity.

phase III randomized trial comparing dacarbazine plus ipilimumab versus dacarbazine alone again showed improved survival in that arm containing dacarbazine (11.2 months versus 9.1 months; p <0.001).[99] These studies showing survival benefit led to FDA approval of ipilimumab for advanced melanoma in 2011.

The responses seen with ipilimumab appear to be durable.[100] A follow-up study of 177 patients with metastatic melanoma treated on the earliest trials at the NCI Surgery Branch using ipilimumab showed that response duration could last 99+ months ongoing.[77] In fact, 14 out of the 15 complete responders remain disease free 54+ to 99+ months ongoing, suggesting a potential cure for some patients. Interestingly, several patients who were deemed partial responders converted to complete responders several years later, because it look an average of 30 months to have all visible tumor marks on imaging scans to disappear.[77]

Ipilimumab was also tested on other solid tumors, and renal cell cancer again appears to be the only other type beside melanoma that had significant responses. Sixty-one patients with metastatic renal cell cancer were treated, and six developed a response (10%); however, 33% developed grade 3/4 IRAEs.[101] Subsequently, the availability of agents with lower toxicity profiles such as sunitinib and sorafenib prevented further enthusiasm to pursue this drug for renal cell cancer.

Another anti–CTLA-4 antibody, tremelimumab (previously called CP-675,206), has also demonstrated durable responses in melanoma patients.[102,103] A phase III randomized trial randomizing 655 patients with metastatic melanoma to either tremelimumab or physician's choice chemotherapy, however, failed to show a survival difference (despite a significantly different response duration favoring tremelimumab, 35.8 months versus 13.7 months; p = 0.0011), possibly due to crossover of chemotherapy patients enrolling into ipilimumab trials and expanded access programs.[103]

Anti–Programmed Death 1 and Anti–Programmed Death Ligand 1

PD-1 is another checkpoint modulator expressed on activated T cells. Although CTLA-4 appears to be involved in the early activation of T cells, PD-1 is involved in the later effector phase of T-cell activation and can function to prevent excessive damage to self by activated T cells in the periphery.[104,105] Interaction with its corresponding ligand, PD-L1 (B7-H1) and PD-L2 (B7-H2) leads to suppressed T-effector function. PD-L1 is expressed on hematopoietic and epithelial cells and is upregulated by cytokines such as IFNγ,[106] whereas PD-L1 is mainly on antigen-presenting cells. Given the clinical results with inhibiting the CTLA-4 checkpoint, recent efforts have focused on inhibiting the PD-1/PD-L1 and PD-1/PD-L2 interactions.

Nivolumab (previously known as BMS-936558, MDX-1106, and ONO-4538) is a fully human anti–PD-1 IgG4 monoclonal antibody that was initially tested in a phase I trial published in 2010 in which 39 patients with advanced solid cancers were treated in escalating doses.[107] Responses were seen in one patient with colon cancer, one with melanoma, and one with renal cell cancer; one patient developed colitis.[108] These hopeful results lead to a larger study in which 236 patients with either NSCLC (74 patients), melanoma (94 patients), or renal cell cancer (33 patients).[4] Objective responses were seen in 18% of patients with NSCLC, 28% with melanoma, and 27% with renal cell cancer.[4] Grade 3/4 adverse events occurred in 14% of patients, including those previously seen with ipilimumab (dermatitis, colitis, hepatitis, thyroiditis, hypophysitis, and pneumonitis). Nine patients developed pneumonitis, six of whom was reversible, and three (1%) with grade 3/4 died despite steroids and infliximab therapy.[4] An update on the status of 107 melanoma patients treated from 2008 to 2012 shows a 31% tumor response rate, with a median response duration of 2 years and a median overall survival of 16.8 months.[109]

Nivolumab was also tested in combination with ipilimumab in melanoma in either concurrent (53 patients) or sequenced (33 patients) regimens. The concurrent group experienced an overall response rate of 40%, whereas the sequenced group had a 20% response rate.[110] The concurrent group also experienced a higher rate of grade 3/4 adverse events (53%), compared to 18% in the sequenced group. Interestingly, 16 of 21 responders in the concurrent group experienced tumor reduction of 80% or greater by 12 weeks,[110] a tempo that is faster than was seen with ipilimumab.

Another anti–PD-1 developed independently, lambrolizumab (previously known as MK-3475, a humanized IgG4κ monoclonal antibody), was tested on 135 patients with metastatic melanoma.[111] The response rate was found to be 38% and was similar between those who had received ipilimumab and those who were ipilimumab naïve,[111] confirming that the antitumor response from lambrolizumab occurs via a different mechanism. Similar to nivolumab, 13% of patients developed grade 3/4 adverse events, with 4% developing pneumonitis, although none developed grade 3/4 pneumonitis.[111]

BMS-936559 is a fully human IgG4 monoclonal antibody that blocks PD-L1 ligation to both PD-1 and CD80. A phase I study was tested in 207 patients (75 with NSCLC, 55 with melanoma, 18 with colon cancer, and 17 with renal cell cancer, 17 with ovarian cancer, 14 with pancreatic cancer, 7 with gastric cancer, and 4 with breast cancer).[112] Among patients who were evaluated for response, objective responses were seen in 16% of melanoma patients, 17% of renal cell cancer patients, 10% of NSCLC patients, and 1 out of 17 ovarian cancer patients. Grade 3/4 toxicities were seen in 9% of patients.[112]

The advent of these checkpoint inhibitors brings additional treatment options to patients with selected advanced cancers, particularly those with histologies deemed previously to be outside the realm of immunotherapy such as NSCLC.[108,113] In addition, a new anti–PD-L1 (MPDL3280A) in clinical trials has also shown some efficacy in melanoma, renal cell cancer, and NSCLC in early reports.

Active Immunization Approaches to Cancer Therapy (Cancer Vaccines)

The molecular characterization of multiple cancer antigens led to a large number of clinical trials that attempted to actively immunize against these antigens with the expectation that cellular immune reactions would be generated capable of inhibiting the growth of established cancers. The results of these efforts have yet to produce significant vaccine efforts of value in the treatment of human cancer. There is a paucity of murine tumor models that suggests that active vaccine approaches can mediate the regression of established vascularized tumors; therefore, it is not surprising that these approaches have, with a few exceptions, shown little efficacy in humans. Enthusiasm about the effectiveness of cancer vaccines has often been grounded in surrogate and subjective end points, rather than reliable objective cancer regressions using standard oncologic criteria. In a review of the world literature, including 107 published cancer vaccine trials involving 2,242 patients, a 3.4% overall objective response rate was observed (Table 14.2).[114,115] In many cases, relatively soft criteria such as stable disease or the regression of individual metastases in the presence of progressive disease at other sites have been reported. A variety of immunizing vectors have been used, including tumor-derived peptides, proteins, whole tumor cells, recombinant viruses, dendritic cells, and heat-shock proteins.[116–122] Although many of these approaches can lead to the development of circulating T cells that can recognize the immunizing tumor antigen, these T cells rarely cause the inhibition of established tumors, a point that has led to much confusion in the field of tumor immunology. The generation of antitumor T cells in vivo is likely a necessary, but certainly not a sufficient criteria for the development of a clinically active immunotherapy. Often, T cells with weak avidity for tumor recognition are generated, and the tolerizing and inhibitory influences that exist in vivo must be overcome for an effective immune response to cause tumor destruction.

A prospective randomized trial of immunization with antigen-presenting cells was carried out by the Dendreon Corporation (Seattle, Washington). This trial used an antigen-presenting cell vaccine loaded with prostatic acid phosphatase linked to GM-CSF compared to placebo in men with hormone-refractory prostate cancer.[123] Of 330 patients who received the vaccine treatment,

TABLE 14.2

Experience with Therapeutic Cancer Vaccines

	Number of Trials	Number of Patients	Objective Responses
Surgery Branch, National Cancer Institute	25	541	14 (2.6%)
Published before 2005[114]	33	765	29 (4.0%)
Published 2005–2010[115]	49	936	34 (3.7%)
Total	107	2,242	77 (3.4%)

Note: Vaccines include: peptide, protein, dendritic cell, virus, plasmid DNA, and whole tumor cells.

1 objective partial response was seen. Only 8 patients experienced a PSA drop of at least 50%. There was no difference in the time to disease progression; however, the vaccine group had a median survival of 25.8 months compared to 21.7 months in the placebo group, and based on this statistically significant survival improvement, this treatment was approved by the FDA (Fig. 14.5).

Adoptive Cell Transfer Immunotherapy

Adoptive cellular immunotherapy refers to the transfer to the tumor-bearing host of immune lymphocytes with anticancer activity. The first successful administration of adoptive cell therapy (ACT) involving TIL, in combination with high-dose IL-2 was carried out at the National Cancer Institute Surgery Branch in 1988.[124] Studies that used cell transfer therapy in patients with metastatic melanoma have provided the clearest evidence of the power of the immune system to mediate the regression of advanced metastatic cancers in humans. Adoptive cell therapy has several theoretical as well as practical advantages.[125] Lymphocytes with antitumor activity can be expanded to very large numbers ex vivo for infusion into cancer patients. These cells can be tested in vitro for antitumor activity, and cells with appropriate properties such as high avidity for tumor recognition and a high proliferative potential

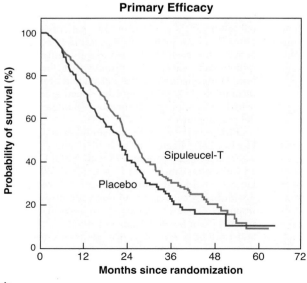

Primary Efficacy

Number at risk

Sipuleucel-T	341	274	129	49	14	1
Placebo	171	123	55	19	4	1

Figure 14.5 Kaplan-Meier estimate of the overall survival in patients with metastatic castration-resistant prostate cancer treated with Sipuleucel-T antigen–presenting cell immunotherapy. A modest but statistically significant improvement in survival was seen (*P* = 0.03).

Adoptive Transfer of Tumor Infiltrating Lymphocytes (TIL)

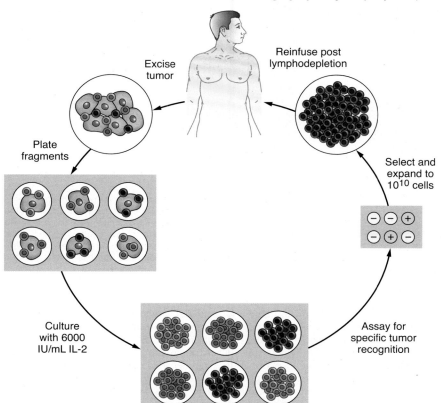

Figure 14.6 Diagram of the adoptive cell therapy of patients with metastatic melanoma. Tumors are resected and individual cultures are grown and tested for antitumor reactivity. Optimal cultures are expanded in vitro and reinfused into the autologous patient who had received a preparative lymphodepleting chemotherapy.

can be identified and selectively expanded for treatment. These cells can be activated in vitro and thus are not subjected to the tolerizing influences that exist in vivo. Perhaps, most important, the host can be manipulated prior to the transfer of the anticancer cells to provide an optimal tumor microenvironment free of in vivo suppressive factors.[125] Studies have shown that the transfer of cultured lymphocytes with antiviral activity can prevent Epstein-Barr virus (EBV) infections as well as the subsequent development of posttransplant lymphoproliferative diseases. Cultured lymphocytes have been used for the treatment of patients with established EBV-induced lymphomas.[126]

The best evidence for the ability of adoptive cell transfer to successfully treat patients with solid tumors comes from the treatment of patients with metastatic melanoma. A diagram that describes the nature of this treatment is shown in Figure 14.6. In patients with

metastatic melanoma, TILs can be obtained from resected tumor deposits and individual cultures tested to identify those with optimal anticancer activity.[124,127] These cells are then expanded ex vivo and reinfused along with IL-2, which is the requisite growth factor required for the survival and persistence of these cells. The administration of a preparative lymphodepleting chemotherapy regimen, consisting of cyclophosphamide and fludarabine with or without 2 or 12 Gy total body irradiation, could substantially enhance the survival and persistence of the transferred cells and increase their in vivo antitumor effectiveness.[128,129] In a series of three pilot trials with 93 patients, objective responses were seen in 49% to 72% of patients.[5,130] Of the 93 patients, 20 (22%) experienced a complete regression of all metastatic melanoma. Only 1 of these 20 patients has recurred, and the remaining patients have ongoing complete regressions from 80 to over 104 months (Table 14.3, Fig. 14.7).

TABLE 14.3				
Cell Transfer Therapy				
Treatment	Total	PR	CR	OR
		Number of Patients (Percentage) (Duration in Months)		
No TBI	43	16 (37%) (84, 36, 29, 28, 14, 12, 11, 7, 7, 7, 7, 4, 4, 2, 2, 2)	5 (12%) (114+, 112+, 111+, 97+, 86+)	21 (49%)
200 TBI	25	8 (32%) (14, 9, 6, 6, 5, 4, 3, 3)	5 (20%) (101+, 98+, 93+, 90+, 70+)	13 (52%)
1,200 TBI	25	8 (32%) (21, 13, 7, 6, 6, 5, 3, 2)	10 (40%) (81+, 78+, 77+, 72+, 72+, 71+, 71+, 70+, 70+, 19)	18 (72%)

Note: 20 complete responses: 19 ongoing at 70 to 114 months.

CANCER THERAPEUTICS

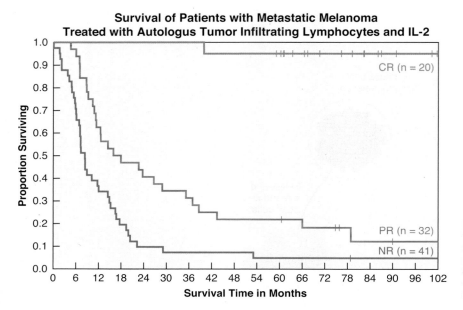

Survival of Patients with Metastatic Melanoma Treated with Autologus Tumor Infiltrating Lymphocytes and IL-2

Figure 14.7 Survival curves of 93 patients treated with adoptive cell transfer using autologous TIL. The results of three consecutive trials using different preparative regimens have been combined in this analysis. Of 20 patients who achieved a complete cancer regression, only one has recurred with a median follow-up of over 8 years.[5]

The 5-year survival of these 93 patients was 29% and was similar regardless of the prior treatments that these patients had received.

Extensive genomic studies have shown that TILs that mediate complete cancer regressions recognize mutated epitopes presented by the cancer.[52] The use of exomic sequencing combined with in vitro tests of antitumor activity can be used to select for T-cell populations reactive against the cancer. This approach has now been utilized to identify T cells used to successfully treat a patient with chemotherapy-refractory cholangiocarcinoma and provides a blueprint for the application of cell transfer therapy for a variety of common epithelial cancers.[54]

The difficulty in obtaining TILs with antitumor activity from cancers other than melanoma has also led to the development of approaches using lymphocytes genetically modified using retroviral transduction to insert antitumor T-cell receptors into the normal lymphocytes of patients.[131]

Genetic Modification of Lymphocytes for Use in Adoptive Cell Therapy: Basic Principles and Applications to Solid Tumors

Efforts are in progress to genetically engineer autologous PBMCs through the introduction of exogenous high avidity receptors that specifically recognize tumor antigens (Fig. 14.8). These cells can then be expanded to large numbers in vitro and be readministered back to the patient similar to TILs in order to mediate tumor regression. The use of gene-modified cells for ACT has resulted in objective clinical responses for a variety of cancer histologies including melanoma, synovial sarcoma, and CD19-positive B-cell malignancies.[6,131–133]

There are two key requirements necessary for the use of gene-modified cells for the treatment of solid cancer. The first is the selection of an appropriate gene transfer method in order to achieve high receptor expression levels in the transferred T cells. For this discussion, we will consider both nonviral and viral-based gene delivery platforms. Generally speaking, there are two categories of nonviral gene transfer, chemical and physical. Chemical gene transfer involves the use of positively charged delivery vehicle such as calcium phosphate, cationic lipids, or polymers to form DNA complexes capable of entering a cell through endocytosis.[134] These reagents benefit from their ease of manufacture and ability to form complexes with large DNA sequences; however, low transfection efficiency of human T cells continues to be an issue.

Physical methods for gene delivery may involve direct delivery of DNA into a cell via microinjection or indirect DNA uptake via electroporation.[135] Electroporation of messenger RNA (mRNA) can achieve high levels of protein expression in cells, comparable to many of the viral-mediated gene delivery systems (gammaretroviral or lentiviral).[135,136] High-throughput electroporators should allow one to gene modify large numbers of T cells ex vivo.[137] mRNA electroporation appears to be most suited for this application, because there is significant loss of cell viability following electroporation of large amounts of DNA.[136] The electroporation of mRNA, although gaining traction as a means of redirecting T cell specificity,[137] provides for transient receptor expression because the mRNA will degrade over time. Currently, it is not clear if stable long-term receptor expression is required to mediate tumor regression. However, the main criticism of the non-viral methods described is the lack of stable gene transfer. To overcome this problem, many investigators are now using transposons such as *sleeping beauty* or *piggybac*.[138] Transposons are mobile DNA gene delivery elements encoding a gene of interest (i.e., TCR or chimeric antigen receptors [CAR]) that can randomly integrate into the genome in the presence of the transposase enzyme, thereby allowing for stable gene expression. This technology is currently being used for the ACT of CAR-modified cells targeting B-cell malignancies (see Fig. 14.8B).[139]

Viral-mediated gene delivery is currently the most common method for the genetic modification of immune cells for cancer ACT. Retroviridae is a family of RNA viruses that, upon entry into cells, undergo a process called reverse transcription whereby the viral RNA is converted into DNA as it stably integrates into the host genome. The two most common retroviral vector systems are based on the gammaretrovirus, Moloney murine leukemia virus (MLV), and the lentivirus, HIV type 1 (see Fig. 14.8B). Gammaretroviral vectors have been used in human clinical applications for over 20 years. The only reported toxicity associated with gammaretroviral engineering of human cells involved the retroviral transduction of hematopoietic stem cells for the treatment of children with severe combined immunodeficiency syndrome (X-SCID).[140] There have been no reports of clonal outgrowth following the retroviral transduction of mature T lymphocytes in adults. Highly active vectors have been generated from a variety of murine retroviruses including spleen focus forming virus (SFFV), myeloproliferative sarcoma virus (MPSV), and the murine stem cell virus (MSCV).[141–147] In most cases, these vectors are replication incompetent, but non–self-inactivating in

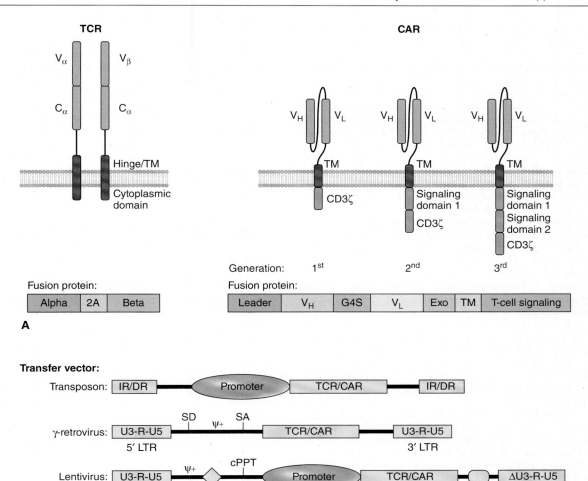

Figure 14.8 Genetic modification of T cells for the treatment of solid cancers. **(A)** In order to gene-modify T cells to confer stable tumor-specific reactivity, one can transduce T cells with an exogenous TCR derived from a naturally occurring or murine T-cell clone or a CAR derived from a tumor-specific monoclonal antibody. The TCR or CAR is synthesized as fusion proteins and inserted into the appropriate gene transfer vector. **(B)** Depending on the transfer vector selected, the T cells are then electroporated (transposon) or transduced (viral vector) to confer tumor specificity. V_α, V_β, and C_α, C_β, TCR alpha and beta chain variable and constant regions, respectively; TM, transmembrane domain; V_H and V_L, immunoglobulin variable regions; 2A and G4S, linker sequences; Exo, extracellular spacer domain; SD, splice donor; SA, splice acceptor; Ψ, packaging signal; LTR, long terminal repeat; U3, unique 3' region; R, repeat region; U5, unique 5' region; RRE, rev response element; cPPT, central polypurine tract; wPRE, woodchuck hepatitis virus posttranscriptional regulatory element; ΔU3, truncated unique 3' region; SIN, self-inactivating.

that the promoter for transgene expression is derived from the viral long terminal repeat (LTR). Self-inactivating (SIN) gammaretroviral vectors have been developed that require an internal promoter to drive transgene expression. The advantage of non-SIN vectors is the ability to use a variety of retroviral packaging cell lines (PG13, Phoenix) engineered to constitutively express gag (capsid protein), pol (reverse transcriptase, integrase, and RNase H enzymes) and env (envelope protein). Transduction of these packaging lines with a non-SIN retroviral vector encoding a transgene allows for the generation of a stable packaging cell line that constitutively releases vector into the medium. This platform is easily scaled up to support large-scale vector production efforts. An alternative to the gammaretroviral vector platform is the lentiviral vector platform. There are some advantages to selecting a lentiviral vector for T-cell engineering in that one can transduce large numbers of minimally stimulated T cells,[148] transfer more complex and larger gene expression cassettes, and yield a potentially safer chromosomal integration profile as compared to gammaretroviruses. However, there has been at least one instance of clonal outgrowth

following lentiviral vector transduction of CD34+ stem cells.[149] Therefore, more data will be needed to better understand the risk of insertional mutagenesis associated with the use of lentiviral vectors. The major disadvantage with using lentiviral vectors for ACT is the lack of a robust packaging cell line, which requires transient vector production and is difficult to scale up.

The first successful application ACT involved the use of autologous T cells genetically modified with a conventional $\alpha\beta$ TCR targeting MART-1 for the treatment of patients with melanoma.[131] The success of this approach relies on the ability to identify naturally occurring TCRs with sufficiently high avidity for the tumor antigen. For this clinical trial, a tumor-specific TCR was cloned directly from melanoma TIL. Exogenous TCR can also be generated from human PBMC following a variety of in vitro sensitization techniques or immunization of transgenic mice expressing HLA molecules. A T-cell clone expressing a low avidity TCR recognizing MART-1 was isolated and the α and β chains cloned into a gammaretroviral vector. The objective response rate from this trial was 13% (2/15).[131] In a follow-up trial with a higher avidity TCR that was cloned from the same melanoma TIL, the objective response rate increased to 30% (6/20).[150] However, patients in this trial experienced significant on-target, off-tumor toxicity with the destruction of normal melanocytes in the skin, eye, and ear. These trials showed the potential to use ACT for the treatment of solid cancers, but also highlight the importance of selecting appropriate tumor antigens to target in order to minimize normal tissue toxicities. Perhaps a better class of antigen to target for ACT would be the cancer testes antigens (CTA) that are expressed only on germ cells during fetal development and then reexpressed on cancers but not other normal tissues with the exception of the testes (see Table 14.1). Because the testes do not express class I MHC molecules, they are protected from any adverse immune response.[151] NY-ESO-1 is a CTA overexpressed on melanoma, as well as a variety of solid epithelial cancers.[152–154] A high-avidity TCR was developed targeting NY-ESO-1 and patients with metastatic melanoma or synovial cell sarcoma were treated following adoptive cell transfer using autologous lymphocytes transduced with a gammaretrovirus encoding this receptor.[6] In updated results from this trial, 8 of 17 patients (47%) with melanoma showed objective tumor responses, two of which were complete responses and ongoing at 51 and 48 months after treatment. Nine of 19 patients (47%) with synovial cell sarcoma showed objective tumor response, only one of which is complete and ongoing at 12 months. Of note, no toxicities were observed in any of these trials. Thus, targeting NY-ESO-1 and other CTAs is an attractive strategy for the application of ACT for the treatment of solid cancers (see Table 14.4 for other trials conducted at the National Cancer Institute, Surgery Branch).

Redirection of T-cell specificity using conventional TCR is constrained by HLA restriction, which limits treatment only to patients expressing a particular MHC haplotype. An alternate approach is to use CAR comprised of an monoclonal antibody single chain variable fragment (scFv) fused in frame to T-cell intracellular signaling domains capable of T-cell activation following antigen-specific binding (see Fig. 14.8A).[155] CARs, unlike conventional TCRs, are not MHC restricted but are limited by the requirement for the tumor antigen to be expressed on the cell surface. CARs can also recognize carbohydrate and lipid moieties further expanding their application. To date, there has been limited success using CAR-based ACT for the treatment of solid cancers. In 2008, the first successful CAR trial targeting the disialoganglioside, GD2, for the treatment of neuroblastoma was reported.[156] In this trial, 4 out of 8 patients (50%) with evaluable tumor experienced tumor regression or necrosis with one complete responder. In that same year, a second CAR trial targeting CD20 on non-Hodgkin and mantle cell lymphomas was reported.[157] Of the 7 patients treated, one achieved a partial response. Much greater success has now been achieved using a CAR targeting CD19, a molecule expressed on normal B cells and virtually all B-cell lymphomas. In a trial conducted at the National Cancer Institute, Surgery Branch, Kochenderfer et al.[132] first reported that autologous T cells expressing a CAR targeting CD19 was able to mediate tumor regression in a patient with B-cell lymphoma (hematologic malignancies will be discussed in more detail elsewhere). Successfully expanding CAR-based ACT to other cancer histologies has been limited by the inability to identify suitable tumor antigens to target. At the National Cancer Institute, Surgery Branch, there are active clinical programs with CAR targeting the mutated epidermal growth factor receptor, EGFRvIII, expressed on approximately 40% of glioblastomas as well as head and neck cancers[158]; the vascular endothelial growth factor-2 receptor, VEGFR-2, expressed on tumor vasculature[159]; and mesothelin, expressed on the mesothelial lining of the pleura, peritoneum, and pericardium, but overexpressed on mesothelioma, pancreatic, and ovarian cancers.[160] These trials are currently accruing patients; however, no objective clinical responses have been observed to date. A summary of clinical trials at the National Cancer Institute, Surgery Branch using gene-modified autologous T cells for ACT are shown in Table 14.4. ACT can mediate the regression of large, established tumors in humans. Efforts to identify and specifically target novel tumor antigens are currently underway with the hope that ACT using gene-modified T cells will develop into an effective treatment for patients with a variety of solid cancers.

Genetic Modification of Lymphocytes to Treat Hematologic Malignancies

Immunologic therapies can be useful treatments for some hematologic malignancies as demonstrated by the effectiveness of mono-

TABLE 14.4

Surgery Branch, National Cancer Institute Program for the Application of Cell Transfer Therapy to a Wide Variety of Human Cancers

Receptor	Type	Cancers	Status
MART-1	TCR	Melanoma	Closed
gp100	TCR	Melanoma	Closed
NY-ESO-1	TCR	Epithelial & sarcomas	Accruing
CEA	TCR	Colorectal	Closed
CD19	CAR	Lymphomas	Accruing
VEGFR2	CAR	All cancers	Accruing
2G-1	TCR	Kidney	Accruing
IL-12	Cytokine	Adjuvant for all receptors	Accruing
MAGE-A3[a]	TCR	Epithelial	In development
EGFRvIII	CAR	Glioblastoma	Accruing
SSX-2	TCR	Epithelial	In development
Mesothelin	CAR	Pancreas & mesothelioma	Accruing
HPV16 (E6&7)	TCR	Cervical, oropharyngeal	In development

[a] MAGE-A3 TCRs; restricted by HLA-A2, A1, Cw7, DP4—covers 80% of patients.
EGFR, epidermal growth factor receptor; VEGFR2, vascular endothelial growth factor 2.

clonal antibodies in treating B-cell malignancies and the fact that allogeneic hematopoietic stem cell transplantation (alloHSCT) can cure a variety of hematologic malignancies.[161–167] The results with monoclonal antibodies and alloHSCT clearly prove that immunologic therapies have significant activity against hematologic malignancies, but monoclonal antibodies are not curative as single agents,[162,166] and alloHSCT has a substantial transplant-related mortality rate due to infections and an immunologic attack against normal tissues known as graft versus host disease (GVHD).[163,165] The proven curative potential of alloHSCT and the effectiveness of autologous T-cell transfer therapies for melanoma have encouraged the development of autologous T-cell therapies for hematologic malignancies.[125,129,163,165] Genetically engineering T cells to specifically recognize antigens expressed by malignant cells has emerged as a very promising strategy for cancer immunotherapy.[125,129,168]

T cells can be genetically engineered to express either of two types of receptors, CARs[168–171] or natural TCRs.[6,131,172] T cells expressing either a CAR or TCR gain the ability to specifically recognize an antigen.[171,172] CARs are artificial fusion proteins that incorporate antigen recognition domains and T-cell activation domains.[168,170,172] The antigen recognition domains are most often derived from monoclonal antibodies.[168,170,172] Antigen recognition by TCRs is major histocompatibility complex restricted.[125,128] In contrast to TCRs, recognition of antigens by CARs is not dependent on MHC molecules. An advantage of TCRs over CARs is that TCRs can recognize intracellular antigens, whereas CARs can only recognize cell-surface antigens.

Chimeric Antigen Receptors

CARs targeting hematopoietic antigens have been extensively studied in preclinical experiments and early-stage clinical trials.[168,170,172,173] For a protein to be a promising target for CAR-expressing T cells, it should be uniformly expressed on the malignant cells being targeted but not expressed on essential normal cells. Many cell-surface proteins with restricted normal tissue expression patterns have been identified on malignant hematologic cells, and CARs targeting many of these proteins are under development (Table 14.5).

Many factors can affect CAR T-cell therapies. The types of gene-therapy vectors encoding the DNA of the CAR could be an important factor. The types of vectors currently being used in clinical trials of CAR T cells are gammaretroviruses, lentiviruses, and transposon-based systems.[132,133,174–181] The design of the CAR fusion protein is another important factor. CAR fusion proteins include an antigen-recognition domain that is most often derived from an antibody, costimulatory domains such as CD28 and 4-1BB, and T-cell activation domains that are usually derived from the CD3z molecule.[168,170,171,182] Other factors that could impact the effectiveness of CAR T-cell therapies include the cell culture method used to prepare the cells and administration of chemotherapy or radiation therapy prior to the CAR T-cell infusions.[170,178,179] In mouse models, a profound enhancement of the antimalignancy activity of infused T cells occurs when the T-cell infusions are preceded by lymphocyte-depleting chemotherapy or radiation therapy.[183–185] Because chemotherapy can have a direct antimalignancy effect against hematologic malignancies, the administration of chemotherapy prior to infusions of T cells is a confounding factor that must always be kept in mind when interpreting the results of clinical trials of T-cell therapies.

Anti-CD19 Chimeric Antigen Receptors

CD19 is an appealing target antigen for CARs because CD19 is expressed on almost all malignant B cells, but CD19 is not expressed on normal cells except B cells.[186] The first preclinical studies of anti-CD19 CARs utilized either gammaretrovirus vectors[174] or plasmid electroporation[176] to insert genes encoding anti-CD19 CARs into human T cells. These studies and subsequent preclinical work by other groups showed that T cells expressing anti-CD19

TABLE 14.5

Hematologic Antigens Targeted by Genetically-Modified T-Cells

Antigen	Malignancy Expressing Antigen	Targeted by CAR or TCR	References
CD19	B-cell malignancies	CAR	17, 19, 21, 22, 23, 24, 25, 26, 34, 35, 55, 56
CD20	B-cell malignancies	CAR	36, 37, 38
CD22	B-cell malignancies	CAR	39, 40
CD23	B-cell malignancies	CAR	41
ROR1	B-cell malignancies	CAR	42
Kappa light chain	B-cell malignancies	CAR	43
B-cell maturation antigen (BCMA)	Multiple myeloma	CAR	44
Lewis Y antigen	Multiple myeloma and acute myeloid leukemia (AML)	CAR	45, 46
CD123	AML	CAR	47
CD30	Hodgkin lymphoma	CAR	48, 49
CD70	Hodgkin lymphoma	CAR	50
Wilms tumor-1 (WT1)	AML and acute lymphoid leukemia (ALL)	TCR	51
Aurora kinase-A	AML and chronic myeloid leukemia (CML)	TCR	52
Hyaluronan-mediated motility receptor (HMMR)	AML and ALL	TCR	53

CARs could specifically recognize and kill CD19-expressing malignant B cells in vitro and in vivo.[174–176,187] These preclinical studies compared many different CAR signaling moieties, which led most groups to utilize CARs with T-cell activation domains from the CD3z molecule and costimulatory molecules from either CD28 or 4-1BB (CD137).[165,180,182,187,188] Preclinical studies showed that lymphocyte-depleting radiation therapy administered before anti-CD19 CAR T-cell infusions was critical to the antimalignancy activity of CAR T cells.[183] The addition of lymphocyte-depleting radiation therapy prior to infusions of anti-CD19 CAR T cells increased the percentage of mice cured of lymphoma by the CAR T cells from 0% to 100%.[183] Preclinical experiments with anti-CD19 CARs have led to several early-phase clinical trials.

The first clinical trial to demonstrate in vivo activity of anti-CD19 CAR T cells in humans was conducted in the Surgery Branch of the National Cancer Institute.[132] The gammaretroviral vector used in this trial encoded a CAR with a CD28 costimulatory domain. Patients treated on this clinical trial received cyclophosphamide and fludarabine chemotherapy followed by an infusion of anti-CD19 CAR T cells and a short course of intravenous IL-2.[132,181] Clear antigen-specific activity of the anti-CD19 CAR T cells was demonstrated because blood B cells were selectively eliminated from four of the seven evaluable patients for several months.[181] The duration of B-cell depletion in these patients was much longer than the duration of B-cell depletion caused by the chemotherapy that the patients received.[132,181] This study also generated evidence of an antimalignancy effect by the anti-CD19 CAR T cells because six of seven evaluable patients with advanced B-cell malignancies obtained either complete remissions or partial remissions (Fig. 14.9).[181] One of these remissions is ongoing 45 months after treatment, and another remission is ongoing 31 months after treatment. Significant toxicity, including hypotension and neurologic toxicity, occurred during this clinical trial.[181] The severity of these toxicities correlated with the levels of serum inflammatory cytokines.[181] Except for one patient who died with influenza pneumonia, the toxicities were transient, with all toxicities resolving within 3 weeks of the anti-CD19 CAR T-cell infusions.[181]

Investigators at the Memorial Sloan Kettering Cancer Center treated nine patients with chronic lymphocytic leukemia (CLL) or acute lymphocytic leukemia (ALL) by infusing T cells that expressed a CAR with a CD28 costimulatory domain.[179] The gene therapy vector used in this work was a gammaretrovirus.[179] None of three patients treated with CAR T cells alone experienced a regression of leukemia, and CLL regressed in one of four evaluable patients treated with cyclophosphamide followed by an infusion of CAR T cells. Using the same CAR, the same group went on to treat five patients with ALL.[173] Patients received chemotherapy followed by an infusion of anti-CD19 CAR T cells. Four patients had detectable leukemia prior to their CAR T-cell infusions, and all of these patients became minimal residual disease negative after infusion of CAR T cells. Four of five patients on this trial rapidly underwent allogeneic stem cell transplantation after their CAR T-cell infusions.[173]

Investigators at the Baylor College of Medicine conducted clinical trials of anti-CD19 CAR T cells in which each patient simultaneously received infusions of two types of anti-CD19 CAR T cells.[189] One type of T cell expressed a CAR expressing a CD28 costimulatory domain. The other type of T cell was identical except that the CAR it expressed lacked a CD28 domain. Compared to the T cells lacking a CD28 moiety, the T cells expressing a CAR with a CD28 moiety had higher peak blood levels and longer in vivo persistence.[189] Patients on this trial did not receive chemotherapy, and there were no remissions of malignancy or long-term B-cell depletion.[189]

Investigators at the University of Pennsylvania reported results from three patients with CLL who were treated with chemotherapy followed by infusions of anti-CD19 CAR-expressing T cells.[133,180] The CAR used in this study was encoded by a lentiviral vector and contained a costimulatory domain from the 4-1BB molecule. Two

Before treatment

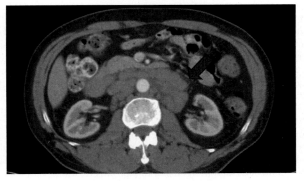

32 days after infusion

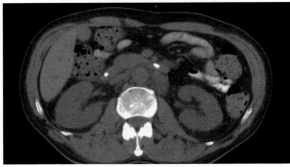

132 days after infusion

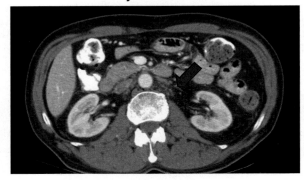

645 days after infusion

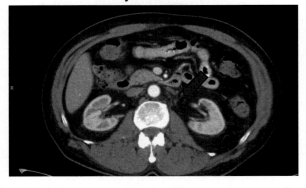

Figure 14.9 Computed tomography (CT) scans show regression of adenopathy in a patient with chronic lymphocytic leukemia (CLL) after treatment with chemotherapy followed by an infusion of autologous anti-CD19 CAR T cells. The time after the cell infusion of each CT scan is indicated. The *arrow* points to a large lymph node mass that resolved completely over time. (Reproduced from Kochenderfer JN, Rosenberg SA. Treating B-Cell cancer with T cells expressing anti-CD19 chimeric antigen receptors. *Nature Rev Clin Oncology* 2013;10:267-276, with permission.)

of the three reported patients obtained prolonged complete remissions.[180] This same CAR design was subsequently evaluated in a clinical trial enrolling patients with ALL.[190] One ALL patient obtained a prolonged complete remission but also experienced significant toxicity that was associated with elevated levels of serum cytokines.[190]

Overall, the early results with anti-CD19 CAR T cells show that this strategy holds great promise to improve the treatment of B-cell malignancies, but anti-CD19 CAR T-cell infusions are also associated with significant toxicity that is usually of short duration. Future progress will require decreasing the toxicity of anti-CD19 CAR T cells while maintaining or enhancing their antimalignancy activity. Parameters that are being studied in an effort to improve anti-CD19 CAR therapy include vector selection, CAR design, cell culture methods, and clinical application.

Chimeric Antigen Receptors and T-Cell Receptors Targeting Hematologic Antigens Other than CD19

CARs and TCRs targeting several hematologic antigens other than CD19 have been evaluated in preclinical or clinical studies. Except for CD19, the B-cell antigen CD20 has been the hematologic antigen most extensively studied as a target of CAR T cells.[191–193] Plasmid electroporation, which is not an optimal method of T-cell genetic modification, was used to transfer the anti-CD20 CAR gene to T cells in these studies. In one trial of anti-CD20 CAR T cells, patients received chemotherapy followed by infusions of T cells expressing a CAR without costimulatory domains.[192] One of seven patients obtained a partial remission that lasted 3 months. In a second trial, patients received chemotherapy followed by anti-CD20 CAR T cells expressing a CAR with both CD28 and 4-1BB costimulatory domains; in this trial, the only evaluable patient obtained a partial remission.[193]

CARs targeting other B-cell antigens including CD22,[157,194] CD23,[195] receptor tyrosine kinase–like orphan receptor-1 (ROR1),[196] and the immunoglobulin kappa light chain[197] have been evaluated in preclinical studies. CARs for treating multiple myeloma are currently being developed. B-cell maturation antigen (BCMA) is expressed on normal and malignant plasma cells, but it is not known to be expressed on other normal cells except for a small subset of mature B cells.[198] CARs targeting BCMA have undergone preclinical testing, and a clinical trial of an anti-BCMA CAR will open soon.[198] Preclinical studies have been performed on CARs targeting the Lewis Y antigen as a treatment for multiple myeloma and acute myeloid leukemia (AML),[199] and activity against AML was recently demonstrated in a phase I clinical trial of a CAR targeting the Lewis Y antigen.[200] CARs targeting the CD123 protein are undergoing preclinical testing for potential use against AML.[201] For Hodgkin lymphoma, CARs have been developed that target the CD30 protein and the CD70 protein, and anti-CD30 CARs are entering early-phase clinical trials.[202–204]

MHC-restricted TCRs targeting some antigens expressed on hematologic malignancies have undergone preclinical testing, but TCRs for treating hematologic malignancies are at a much earlier stage of development than CARs (see Table 14.1). TCRs targeting the Wilms tumor antigen-1 (WT1) are under development to treat ALL and AML.[205] Aurora kinase-A–specific TCRs and hyaluronan-mediated motility receptor (HMMR)-specific TCRs are under preclinical development as leukemia treatments.[206,207]

T-Cell Gene Therapy in the Setting of Allogeneic Hematopoietic Stem Cell Transplantation

A leading cause of death among patients undergoing alloHSCT is relapse of malignancy, and alloHSCT is often complicated by GVHD.[164,165,208] Therefore, a central goal in the field of alloHSCT is to increase the antimalignancy activity of allogeneic T cells without worsening GVHD. One way to accomplish this goal might be to genetically modify T cells to give them the ability to specifically recognize antigens expressed by malignant cells. CARs are well-suited for this task.

Two groups have recently reported promising early results treating B-cell malignancies after alloHSCT with allogeneic donor-derived T cells expressing anti-CD19 CARs.[209,210] Investigators at the National Cancer Institute treated 10 patients with B-cell malignancies that persisted despite alloHSCT and standard donor lymphocyte infusions.[209] Although patients on this trial did not receive chemotherapy before their T-cell infusions, 3 of 10 patients had objective regressions of their malignancies, and 1 patient with CLL remains in CR more than 1 year after treatment.[209] No patient developed GVHD after receiving allogeneic anti-CD19 CAR T cells on this trial.[209] Investigators at the Baylor College of Medicine reported objective antimalignancy responses in two of six patients with relapsed malignancy after infusion of donor-derived allogeneic anti-CD19 CAR T cells that were also specific for viral antigens.[210]

In an effort to improve the safety of infusions of allogeneic lymphocytes by limiting GVHD, investigators have genetically modified T cells to express *suicide genes* that cause death of the T cells containing the suicide gene when certain drugs are administered.[211–214] Suicide gene–expressing T cells are infused to treat malignancy after alloHSCT. This approach has been tested in clinical trials, and rapid abrogation of GVHD has been demonstrated.[211,213,214]

REFERENCES

1. Kenter GG, Welters MJ, Valentijn AR, et al. Vaccination against HPV-16 oncoproteins for vulvar intraepithelial neoplasia. *N Engl J Med* 2009;361: 1838–1847.
2. Gaffen SL, Liu KD. Overview of interleukin-2 function, production and clinical applications. *Cytokine* 2004;28:109–123.
3. Attia P, Phan GQ, Maker AV, et al. Autoimmunity correlates with tumor regression in patients with metastatic melanoma treated with anti-cytotoxic T-lymphocyte antigen-4. *J Clin Oncol* 2005;23:6043–6053.
4. Topalian SL, Hodi FS, Brahmer JR, et al. Safety, activity, and immune correlates of anti-PD-1 antibody in cancer. *N Engl J Med* 2012;366:2443–2454.
5. Rosenberg SA, Yang JC, Sherry RM, et al. Durable complete responses in heavily pretreated patients with metastatic melanoma using T-cell transfer immunotherapy. *Clin Cancer Res* 2011;17:4550–4557.
6. Robbins PF, Morgan RA, Feldman SA, et al. Tumor regression in patients with metastatic synovial sarcoma and melanoma using genetically engineered lymphocytes reactive with NY-ESO-1. *J Clin Oncol* 2011;29:917–924.
7. Chen YT, Scanlan MJ, Sahin U, et al. A testicular antigen aberrantly expressed in human cancers detected by autologous antibody screening. *Proc Natl Acad Sci U S A* 1997;94:1914–1918.
8. Van der Bruggen P, Traversari C, Chomez P, et al. A gene encoding an antigen recognized by cytolytic T lymphocytes on a human melanoma. *Science* 1991;254:1643–1647.
9. van der Bruggen P, Stroobant V, Vigneron N, et al. Peptide database: T cell-defined tumor antigens. *Cancer Immun* 2013. https://www.cancerimmunity.org/peptide/
10. Gnjatic S, Nishikawa H, Jungbluth AA, et al. NY-ESO-1: review of an immunogenic tumor antigen. *Adv Cancer Res* 2006;95:1–30.
11. Chinnasamy N, Wargo JA, Yu Z, et al. A TCR targeting the HLA-A*0201-restricted epitope of MAGE-A3 recognizes multiple epitopes of the MAGE-A antigen superfamily in several types of cancer. *J Immunol* 2011;186:685–696.
12. Morgan RA, Chinnasamy N, Abate-Daga D, et al. Cancer regression and neurological toxicity following anti-MAGE-A3 TCR gene therapy. *J Immunother* 2013;36:133–151.
13. Linette GP, Stadtmauer EA, Maus MV, et al. Cardiovascular toxicity and titin cross-reactivity of affinity-enhanced T cells in myeloma and melanoma. *Blood* 2013;122:863–871.
14. Cox AL, Skipper J, Chen Y, et al. Identification of a peptide recognized by five melanoma-specific human cytotoxic T cell lines. *Science* 1994;264:716–719.

15. Kawakami Y, Eliyahu S, Jennings C, et al. Recognition of multiple epitopes in the human melanoma antigen gp100 by tumor infiltrating T-lymphocytes associated with in vivo tumor regression. *J Immunol* 1995;154:3961–3968.

16. Brichard V, Van Pel A, Wolfel T, et al. The tyrosinase gene codes for an antigen recognized by autologous cytolytic T lymphocytes on HLA-A2 melanomas. *J Exp Med* 1993;178:489–495.

17. Wang RF, Robbins PF, Kawakami Y, et al. Identification of a gene encoding a melanoma tumor antigen recognized by HLA-A31-restricted tumor-infiltrating lymphocytes. *J Exp Med* 1995;181:799–804.

18. Wang R-F, Appella E, Kawakami Y, et al. Identification of TRP-2 as a human tumor antigen recognized by cytotoxic T lymphocytes. *J Exp Med* 1996;184:2207–2216.

19. Kawakami Y, Eliyahu S, Delgado CH, et al. Cloning of the gene coding for a shared human melanoma antigen recognized by autologous T cells infiltrating into tumor. *Proc Natl Acad Sci U S A* 1994;91:3515–3519.

20. Coulie PG, Brichard V, Van Pel A, et al. A new gene coding for a differentiation antigen recognized by autologous cytolytic T lymphocytes on HLA-A2 melanomas. *J Exp Med* 1992;180:35–42.

21. Kawakami Y, Eliyahu S, Sakaguchi K, et al. Identification of the immunodominant peptides of the MART-1 human melanoma antigen recognized by the majority of HLA-A2-restricted tumor infiltrating lymphocytes. *J Exp Med* 1994;180:347–352.

22. Hanada K, Yewdell JW, Yang JC. Immune recognition of a human renal cancer antigen through post-translational protein splicing. *Nature* 2004;427:252–256.

23. Carrington DM, Auffret A, Hanke DE. Polypeptide ligation occurs during post-translational modification of concanavalin A. *Nature* 1985;313:64–67.

24. Paulus H. Protein splicing and related forms of protein autoprocessing. *Annu Rev Biochem* 2000;69:447–496.

25. Vigneron N, Stroobant V, Chapiro J, et al. An antigenic peptide produced by peptide splicing in the proteasome. *Science* 2004;304:587–590.

26. Warren EH, Vigneron NJ, Gavin MA, et al. An antigen produced by splicing of noncontiguous peptides in the reverse order. *Science* 2006;313:1444–1447.

27. Dalet A, Robbins PF, Stroobant V, et al. An antigenic peptide produced by reverse splicing and double asparagine deamidation. *Proc Natl Acad Sci U S A* 2011;108:E323–E331.

28. Michaux A, Larrieu P, Stroobant V, et al. A spliced antigenic peptide comprising a single spliced amino acid is produced in the proteasome by reverse splicing of a longer peptide fragment followed by trimming. *J Immunol* 2014;192:1962–1971.

29. Ikeda H, Lethe B, Lehmann F. Characterization of an antigen that is recognized on a melanoma showing partial HLA loss by CTL expressing an NK inhibitory receptor. *Immunity* 1999;6:199–208.

30. Lundegaard C, Lamberth K, Harndahl M, et al. NetMHC-3.0: accurate web accessible predictions of human, mouse and monkey MHC class I affinities for peptides of length 8-11. *Nucleic Acids Res* 2008;36:W509–W512.

31. Peters B, Sette A. Generating quantitative models describing the sequence specificity of biological processes with the stabilized matrix method. *BMC Bioinformatics* 2005;6:132.

32. Xue BH, Zhang Y, Sosman JA, et al. Induction of human cytotoxic T lymphocytes specific for prostate-specific antigen. *Prostate* 1997;30:73–78.

33. Horiguchi Y, Nukaya I, Okazawa K, et al. Screening of HLA-A24-restricted epitope peptides from prostate-specific membrane antigen that induce specific antitumor cytotoxic T lymphocytes. *Clin Cancer Res* 2002;8:3885–3892.

34. Peoples GE, Goedegeburre PS, Smith R. Breast and ovarian cancer-specific cytotoxic T lymphocytes recognize the same HER2/neu-derived peptide. *Proc Natl Acad U S A* 1995;92:432–436.

35. Zaks TZ, Rosenberg SA. Immunization with a peptide epitope (p369-377) from HER-2/neu leads to peptide-specific cytotoxic T lymphocytes that fail to recognize HER-2/neu+ tumors. *Cancer Res* 1998;58:4902–4908.

36. Vonderheide RH, Hahn WC, Schultze JL, et al. The telomerase catalytic subunit is a widely expressed tumor-associated antigen recognized by cytotoxic T lymphocytes. *Immunity* 1999;10:673–679.

37. Parkhurst MR, Riley JP, Igarashi T, et al. Immunization of patients with the hTERT:540-548 peptide induces peptide-reactive T lymphocytes that do not recognize tumors endogenously expressing telomerase. *Clin Cancer Res* 2004;10:4688–4698.

38. Weinschenk T, Gouttefangeas C, Schirle M, et al. Integrated functional genomics approach for the design of patient-individual antitumor vaccines. *Cancer Res* 2002;62: 5818–5827.

39. Dutoit V, Herold-Mende C, Hilf N, et al. Exploiting the glioblastoma peptidome to discover novel tumour-associated antigens for immunotherapy. *Brain* 2012;135:1042–1054.

40. Walter S, Weinschenk T, Stenzl A, et al. Multipeptide immune response to cancer vaccine IMA901 after single-dose cyclophosphamide associates with longer patient survival. *Nat Med* 2012;18:1254–1261.

41. Theobald M, Biggs J, Dittmer D, et al. Targeting p53 as a general tumor antigen. *Proc Natl Acad Sci U S A* 1995;92:11993–11997.

42. Theoret MR, Cohen CJ, Nahvi AV, et al. Relationship of p53 overexpression on cancers and recognition by anti-p53 T cell receptor-transduced T cells. *Hum Gene Ther* 2008;19:1219–1231.

43. Parkhurst M, Joo J, Riley JP, et al. Characterization of genetically modified T cell receptors that recognize the CEA:691-699 peptide in the context of HLA-A2.1 on human colorectal cancer cells. *Clin Cancer Res* 2009;15:169–180.

44. Parkhurst MR, Yang JC, Langan RC, et al. T cells targeting carcinoembryonic antigen can mediate regression of metastatic colorectal cancer but induce severe transient colitis. *Mol Ther* 2011;19:620–626.

45. Wolfel T, Hauer M, Schneider J, et al. A p16INK4A-insensitive CDK4 mutant targeted by cytolytic T lymphocytes in a human melanoma. *Science* 1995;269:1281–1284.

46. Robbins PF, El-Gamil M, Li YF, et al. A mutated B-catenin gene encodes a melanoma-specific antigen recognized by tumor infiltrating lymphocytes. *J Exp Med* 1996;183:1185–1192.

47. Rubinfeld B, Robbins P, El-Gamil M. Stabilization of beta-catenin by genetic defects in melanoma cell lines. *Science* 1997;275:1790–1792.

48. Mumberg D, Wick M, Schreiber H. Unique tumor antigens redefined as mutant tumor-specific antigens. *Semin Immunol* 1996;8:289–293.

49. Cheever MA, Chen W, Disis ML, et al. T-cell immunity to oncogenic proteins including mutated ras and chimeric bcr-abl. *Ann N Y Acad Sci* 1993;690: 101–112.

50. Castle JC, Kreiter S, Diekmann J, et al. Exploiting the mutanome for tumor vaccination. *Cancer Res* 2012;72:1081–1091.

51. Matsushita H, Vesely MD, Koboldt DC, et al. Cancer exome analysis reveals a T-cell-dependent mechanism of cancer immunoediting. *Nature* 2012;482: 400–404.

52. Robbins PF, Lu YC, El-Gamil M, et al. Mining exomic sequencing data to identify mutated antigens recognized by adoptively transferred tumor-reactive T cells. *Nat Med* 2013;19:747–752.

53. van Rooij N, van Buuren MM, Philips D, et al. Tumor exome analysis reveals neoantigen-specific T-cell reactivity in an ipilimumab-responsive melanoma. *J Clin Oncol* 2013;31:e439–e442.

54. Tran E, Turcotte S, Gros A, et al. Cancer immunotherapy based on mutation-specific CD4+ T cells in a patient with epithelial cancer. *Science* 2014;344:641–645.

55. Koutsky LA, Ault KA, Wheeler CM, et al. A controlled trial of a human papillomavirus type 16 vaccine. *N Engl J Med* 2002;347:1645–1651.

56. Villa LL, Costa RL, Petta CA, et al. Prophylactic quadrivalent human papillomavirus (types 6, 11, 16, and 18) L1 virus-like particle vaccine in young women: a randomised double-blind placebo-controlled multicentre phase II efficacy trial. *Lancet Oncol* 2005;6:271–278.

57. Wolchok JD, Hoos A, O'Day S, et al. Guidelines for the evaluation of immune therapy activity in solid tumors: immune-related response criteria. *Clin Cancer Res* 2009;15:7412–7420.

58. Hoos A, Eggermont AM, Janetzki S, et al. Improved endpoints for cancer immunotherapy trials. *J Natl Cancer Inst* 2010;102:1388–1397.

59. Morgan DA, Ruscetti FW, Gallo R. Selective in vitro growth of T lymphocytes from normal human bone marrows. *Science* 1976;193:1007–1008.

60. Smith KA, Gilbride KJ, Favata MF. Lymphocyte activating factor promotes T-cell growth factor production by cloned murine lymphoma cells. *Nature* 1980;287:853–855.

61. Smith KA, Lachman LB, Oppenheim JJ, et al. The functional relationship of the interleukins. *J Exp Med* 1980;151:1551–1556.

62. Taniguchi T, Matsui H, Fujita T. Structure and expression of a cloned cDNA for human interleukin-2. *Nature* 1983;302:305–307.

63. Rosenberg SA, Grimm EA, McGrogan M, et al. Biological activity of recombinant human interleukin-2 produced in *Escherichia coli*. *Science* 1984;223:1412–1414.

64. Rosenberg SA, Mule JJ, Spiess PJ, et al. Regression of established pulmonary metastases and subcutaneous tumor mediated by the systemic administration of high dose recombinant IL-2. *J Exp Med* 1985;161:1169–1188.

65. Lotze MT, Matory YL, Ettinghausen SE, et al. In vivo administration of purified human interleukin-2. II. Half life, immunologic effects and expansion of peripheral lymphoid cells in vivo with recombinant IL-2. *J Immunol* 1985;135:2865–2875.

66. Rosenberg SA, Lotze MT, Muul LM, et al. Observations on the systemic administration of autologous lymphokine-activated killer cells and recombinant interleukin-2 to patients with metastatic cancer. *N Engl J Med* 1985;313: 1485–1492.

67. Rosenberg SA, Lotze MT, Yang JC, et al. Prospective randomized trial of high-dose interleukin-2 alone or in conjunction with lymphokine-activated killer cells for the treatment of patients with advanced cancer. *J Natl Cancer Inst* 1993;85:622–632.

68. Atkins MB, Sparano J, Fisher RI, et al. Randomized phase II trial of high-dose interleukin-2 either alone or in combination with interferon alfa-2b in advanced renal cell carcinoma. *J Clin Oncol* 1993;11:661–670.

69. Rosenberg SA, Yang JC, White DE, et al. Durability of complete responses in patients with metastatic cancer treated with high-dose interleukin-2: identification of the antigens mediating response. *Ann Surg* 1998;228:307–319.

70. Fyfe G, Fisher R, Sznol M, et al. Results of treatment of 255 patients with metastatic renal cell carcinoma who received high dose proleukin interleukin-2 therapy. *J Clin Oncol* 1995;13:688–696.

71. Fisher RI, Rosenberg SA, Fyfe G. Long-term survival update for high-dose recombinant interleukin-2 in patients with renal cell carcinoma. *Cancer J Sci Am* 2000;6:S55–S57.

72. Yang JC, Sherry RM, Steinberg SM, et al. Randomized study of high-dose and low-dose interleukin-2 in patients with metastatic renal cancer. *J Clin Oncol* 2003;21:3127–3132.

73. Atkins MB, Lotze MT, Dutcher JP, et al. High-dose recombinant interleukin 2 therapy for patients with metastatic melanoma: analysis of 270 patients treated between 1985 and 1993. *J Clin Oncol* 1999;17:2105–2116.

74. Atkins MB, Kunkel L, Sznol M, et al. High-dose recombinant interleukin-2 therapy in patients with metastatic melanoma: long-term survival update. *Cancer J Sci Am* 2000;6:S11–S14.

75. Rosenberg SA, Yang JC, Schwartzentruber DJ, et al. Immunologic and therapeutic evaluation of a synthetic peptide vaccine for the treatment of patients with metastatic melanoma. *Nat Med* 1998;4:321–327.

76. Schwartzentruber DJ, Lawson DH, Richards JM, et al. gp100 peptide vaccine and interleukin-2 in patients with advanced melanoma. *N Engl J Med* 2011;364:2119–2127.

77. Prieto PA, Yang JC, Sherry RM, et al. CTLA-4 blockade with ipilimumab: long-term follow-up of 177 patients with metastatic melanoma. *Clin Cancer Res* 2012;18:2039–2047.

78. Phan GQ, Attia P, Steinberg SM, et al. Factors associated with response to high-dose interleukin-2 in patients with metastatic melanoma. *J Clin Oncol* 2001;19:3477–3482.

79. Rosenberg SA, Yang JC, Topalian SL, et al. Treatment of 283 consecutive patients with metastatic melanoma or renal cell cancer using high-dose bolus interleukin 2. *JAMA* 1994;271:907–913.

80. Rosenberg SA, Lotze MT, Yang JC, et al. Experience with the use of high-dose interleukin-2 in the treatment of 652 cancer patients. *Ann Surg* 1989;210: 474–484.

81. Gemlo BT, Palladino Jr MA, Jaffe HS, et al. Circulating cytokines in patients with metastatic cancer treated with recombinant interleukin 2 and lymphokine-activated killer cells. *Cancer Res* 1988;48:5864–5867.

82. Pockaj BA, Yang JC, Lotze MT, et al. A prospective randomized trial evaluating colloid versus crystalloid resuscitation in the treatment of the vascular leak syndrome associated with interleukin-2 therapy. *J Immunother Emphasis Tumor Immunol* 1994;15:22–28.

83. Klempner MS, Noring R, Mier JW, et al. An acquired chemotactic defect in neutrophils from patients receiving interleukin-2 immunotherapy. *N Engl J Med* 1990;322:959–965.

84. Lee RE, Lotze MT, Skibber JM, et al. Cardiorespiratory effects of immunotherapy with interleukin-2. *J Clin Oncol* 1989;7:7–20.

85. Schwartzentruber DJ. Guidelines for the safe administration of high-dose interleukin-2. *J Immunother* 2001;24:287–293.

86. Kammula US, White DE, Rosenberg SA. Trends in the safety of high dose bolus interleukin-2 administration in patients with metastatic cancer. *Cancer* 1998;83:797–805.

87. Brunet JF, Denizot F, Luciani MF, et al. A new member of the immunoglobulin superfamily—CTLA-4. *Nature* 1987;328:267–270.

88. Linsley PS, Brady W, Urnes M, et al. CTLA-4 is a second receptor for the B cell activation antigen B7. *J Exp Med* 1991;174:561–569.

89. Walunas TL, Lenschow DJ, Bakker CY, et al. CTLA-4 can function as a negative regulator of T cell activation. *Immunity* 1994;1:405–413.

90. Walunas TL, Bakker CY, Bluestone JA. CTLA-4 ligation blocks CD28-dependent T cell activation. *J Exp Med* 1996;183:2541–2550.

91. van Elsas A, Hurwitz AA, Allison JP. Combination immunotherapy of B16 melanoma using anti-cytotoxic T lymphocyte-associated antigen 4 (CTLA-4) and granulocyte/macrophage colony-stimulating factor (GM-CSF)-producing vaccines induces rejection of subcutaneous and metastatic tumors accompanied by autoimmune depigmentation. *J Exp Med* 1999;190:355–366.

92. Hurwitz AA, Yu TF, Leach DR, et al. CTLA-4 blockade synergizes with tumor-derived granulocyte-macrophage colony-stimulating factor for treatment of an experimental mammary carcinoma. *Proc Natl Acad Sci U S A* 1998;95:10067–10071.

93. Phan GQ, Yang JC, Sherry RM, et al. Cancer regression and autoimmunity induced by cytotoxic T lymphocyte-associated antigen 4 blockade in patients with metastatic melanoma. *Proc Natl Acad Sci U S A* 2003;100:8372–8377.

94. Maker AV, Phan GQ, Attia P, et al. Tumor regression and autoimmunity in patients treated with cytotoxic T lymphocyte-associated antigen 4 blockade and interleukin 2: a phase I/II study. *Ann Surg Oncol* 2005;12:1005–1016.

95. Maker AV, Yang JC, Sherry RM, et al. Intrapatient dose escalation of anti-CTLA-4 antibody in patients with metastatic melanoma. *J Immunother* 2006;29:455–463.

96. Beck KE, Blansfield JA, Tran KQ, et al. Enterocolitis in patients with cancer after antibody blockade of cytotoxic T-lymphocyte-associated antigen 4. *J Clin Oncol* 2006;24:2283–2289.

97. Robinson MR, Chan CC, Yang JC, et al. Cytotoxic T lymphocyte-associated antigen 4 blockade in patients with metastatic melanoma: a new cause of uveitis. *J Immunother* 2004;27:478–479.

98. Hodi FS, O'Day SJ, McDermott DF, et al. Improved survival with ipilimumab in patients with metastatic melanoma. *N Engl J Med* 2010;363:711–723.

99. Robert C, Thomas L, Bondarenko I, et al. Ipilimumab plus dacarbazine for previously untreated metastatic melanoma. *N Engl J Med* 2011;364:2517–2526.

100. Wolchok JD, Weber JS, Maio M, et al. Four-year survival rates for patients with metastatic melanoma who received ipilimumab in phase II clinical trials. *Ann Oncol* 2013;24:2174–2180.

101. Yang JC, Hughes M, Kammula U, et al. Ipilimumab (anti-CTLA4 antibody) causes regression of metastatic renal cell cancer associated with enteritis and hypophysitis. *J Immunother* 2007;30:825–830.

102. Kirkwood JM, Lorigan P, Hersey P, et al. Phase II trial of tremelimumab (CP-675,206) in patients with advanced refractory or relapsed melanoma. *Clin Cancer Res* 2010;16:1042–1048.

103. Ribas A, Kefford R, Marshall MA, et al. Phase III randomized clinical trial comparing tremelimumab with standard-of-care chemotherapy in patients with advanced melanoma. *J Clin Oncol* 2013;31:616–622.

104. Ott PA, Hodi FS, Robert C. CTLA-4 and PD-1/PD-L1 blockade: new immunotherapeutic modalities with durable clinical benefit in melanoma patients. *Clin Cancer Res* 2013;19:5300–5309.

105. Keir ME, Butte MJ, Freeman GJ, et al. PD-1 and its ligands in tolerance and immunity. *Annu Rev Immunol* 2008;26:677–704.

106. Dong H, Strome SE, Salomao DR, et al. Tumor-associated B7-H1 promotes T-cell apoptosis: a potential mechanism of immune evasion. *Nat Med* 2002;8:793–800.

107. Brahmer JR, Drake CG, Wollner I, et al. Phase I study of single-agent anti-programmed death-1 (MDX-1106) in refractory solid tumors: safety, clinical activity, pharmacodynamics, and immunologic correlates. *J Clin Oncol* 2010;28:3167–3175.

108. Brahmer JR. Immune checkpoint blockade: the hope for immunotherapy as a treatment of lung cancer? *Semin Oncol* 2014;41:126–132.

109. Topalian SL, Sznol M, McDermott DF, et al. Survival, durable tumor remission, and long-term safety in patients with advanced melanoma receiving nivolumab. *J Clin Oncol* 2014;32:1020–1030.

110. Wolchok JD, Kluger H, Callahan MK, et al. Nivolumab plus ipilimumab in advanced melanoma. *N Engl J Med* 2013;369:122–133.

111. Hamid O, Robert C, Daud A, et al. Safety and tumor responses with lambrolizumab (anti-PD-1) in melanoma. *N Engl J Med* 2013;369:134–144.

112. Brahmer JR, Tykodi SS, Chow LQ, et al. Safety and activity of anti-PD-L1 antibody in patients with advanced cancer. *N Engl J Med* 2012;366:2455–2465.

113. Drake CG, Lipson EJ, Brahmer JR. Breathing new life into immunotherapy: review of melanoma, lung and kidney cancer. *Nat Rev Clin Oncol* 2014;11:24–37.

114. Rosenberg SA, Yang JC, Restifo NP. Cancer immunotherapy: moving beyond current vaccines. *Nat Med* 2004;10:909–915.

115. Klebanoff CA, Acquavella N, Yu Z, et al. Therapeutic cancer vaccines: are we there yet? *Immunol Rev* 2011;239:27–44.

116. Slingluff CL, Yamshchikov G, Neese P, et al. Phase I trial of a melanoma vaccine with gp100 280-288 peptide and tetanus helper peptide in adjuvant: immunologic and clinical outcomes. *Clin Cancer Res* 2001;7:3012–3024.

117. Schaed SG, Klimek VM, Panageas KS, et al. T-cell responses against tyrosinase 368-376(370D) peptide in HLA*A0201+ melanoma patients: randomized trial comparing incomplete Freund's adjuvant, granulocyte macrophage colony-stimulating factor, and QS-21 as immunological adjuvants. *Clin Cancer Res* 2004;8:967–972.

118. Marshall JL, Hoyer RJ, Toomey MA, et al. Phase I study in advanced cancer patients of a diversified prime-and-boost vaccination protocol using recombinant vaccinia virus and recombinant nonreplicating avipox virus to elicit anti-carcinoembryonic antigen immune responses. *J Clin Oncol* 2000;18: 3964–3973.

119. Eder JP, Kantoff PW, Roper K, et al. A phase I trial of a recombinant vaccinia virus expressing prostate-specific antigen in advanced prostate cancer. *Clin Cancer Res* 2003;6:1632–1638.

120. Lurquin C, Lethe B, De Plaen E, et al. Contrasting frequencies of antitumor and anti-vaccine T cells in metastases of a melanoma patient vaccinated with a MAGE tumor antigen. *J Exp Med* 2005;201:249–257.

121. Marincola FM, Rivoltini L, Salgaller ML, et al. Differential anti-MART-1/MelanA CTL activity in peripheral blood of HLA-A2 melanoma patients in comparison to healthy donors: evidence of in vivo priming by tumor cells. *J Immunother Emphasis Tumor Immunol* 1996;19:266–277.

122. Cormier JN, Salgaller ML, Prevette T, et al. Enhancement of cellular immunity in melanoma patients immunized with a peptide from MART-1/Melan A. *Cancer J Sci Am* 1997;3:37–44.

123. Kantoff PW, Higano CS, Shore ND, et al. Sipuleucel-T immunotherapy for castration-resistant prostate cancer. *N Engl J Med* 2010;363:422.

124. Rosenberg SA, Packard BS, Aebersold PM, et al. Use of tumor infiltrating lymphocytes and interleukin-2 in the immunotherapy of patients with metastatic melanoma. Preliminary report. *N Engl J Med* 1988;319:1676–1680.

125. Restifo NP, Dudley ME, Rosenberg SA. Adoptive immunotherapy for cancer: harnessing the T cell response. *Nat Rev Immunol* 2012;12:269–281.

126. Rooney CM, Smith CA, Ng CY, et al. Infusion of cytotoxic T cells for the prevention and treatment of Epstein-Barr virus-induced lymphoma in allogeneic transplant recipients. *Blood* 1998;92:1549–1555.

127. Rosenberg SA, Yannelli JR, Yang JC, et al. Treatment of patients with metastatic melanoma using autologous tumor-infiltrating lymphocytes and interleukin-2. *J Natl Cancer Inst* 1994;86:1159–1166.

128. Dudley ME, Wunderlich JR, Robbins PF, et al. Cancer regression and autoimmunity in patients after clonal repopulation with anti-tumor lymphocytes. *Science* 2002;298:850–854.

129. Dudley ME, Yang JC, Sherry R, et al. Adoptive cell therapy for patients with metastatic melanoma: Evaluation of intensive myeloablative chemoradiation preparative regimens. *J Clin Oncol* 2008;26:5233–5239.

130. Rosenberg SA. Cell transfer immunotherapy for metastatic solid cancer—what clinicians need to know. *Nat Rev Clin Oncol* 2011;8:577–585.

131. Morgan RA, Dudley ME, Wunderlich JR, et al. Cancer regression in patients after transfer of genetically engineered lymphocytes. *Science* 2006;314: 126–129.

132. Kochenderfer JN, Wilson WH, Janik E, et al. Eradication of B-lineage cells and regression of lymphoma in a patient treated with autologous T cells genetically engineered to recognize CD19. *Blood* 2010;116:4099–4102.

133. Porter DL, Levine BL, Kalos M, et al. Chimeric antigen receptor-modified T cells in chronic lymphoid leukemia. *N Engl J Med* 2011;365:725–733.

134. Tiera MJ, Winnik FO, Fernandes JC. Synthetic and natural polycations for gene therapy: state of the art and new perspectives. *Curr Gene Ther* 2006;6:59–71.

135. Birkholz K, Hombach A, Krug C, et al. Transfer of mRNA encoding recombinant immunoreceptors reprograms CD4+ and CD8+ T cells for use in the adoptive immunotherapy of cancer. *Gene Ther* 2009;16:596–604.

CANCER THERAPEUTICS

136. Zhao Y, Zheng Z, Cohen CJ, et al. High-efficiency transfection of primary human and mouse T lymphocytes using RNA electroporation. *Mol Ther* 2006;13:151–159.

137. Li L, Liu LC, Feller S, et al. Expression of chimeric antigen receptors in natural killer cells with a regulatory-compliant non-viral method. *Cancer Gene Ther* 2010;17:147–154.

138. Zhao Y, Moon E, Carpenito C, et al. Multiple injections of electroporated autologous T cells expressing a chimeric antigen receptor mediate regression of human disseminated tumor. *Cancer Res* 2010;70:9053–9061.

139. Ivics Z, Izsvak Z. Transposons for gene therapy! *Curr Gene Ther* 2006;6:593–607.

140. Singh H, Huls H, Kebriaei P, et al. A new approach to gene therapy using Sleeping Beauty to genetically modify clinical-grade T cells to target CD19. *Immunol Rev* 2014;257:181–190.

141. Hacein-Bey-Abina S, von Kalle C, Schmidt M, et al. A serious adverse event after successful gene therapy for X-linked severe combined immunodeficiency. *N Engl J Med* 2003;348:255–256.

142. Riviere I, Brose K, Mulligan RC. Effects of retroviral vector design on expression of human adenosine deaminase in murine bone marrow transplant recipients engrafted with genetically modified cells. *Proc Natl Acad Sci U S A* 1995;92:6733–6737.

143. Maetzig T, Galla M, Baum C, et al. Gammaretroviral vectors: biology, technology and application. *Viruses* 2011;3:677–713.

144. Schambach A, Swaney WP, van der Loo JC. Design and production of retro- and lentiviral vectors for gene expression in hematopoietic cells. *Methods Mol Biol* 2009;506:191–205.

145. Hughes MS, Yu YYL, Dudley ME, et al. Transfer of a TCR gene derived from a patient with a marked antitumor response conveys highly active T-cell effector functions. *Hum Gene Ther* 2005;16:457–472.

146. Zhang X, Godbey WT. Viral vectors for gene delivery in tissue engineering. *Adv Drug Deliv Rev* 2006;58:515–534.

147. Yu SS, Han E, Hong Y, et al. Construction of a retroviral vector production system with the minimum possibility of a homologous recombination. *Gene Ther* 2003;10:706–711.

148. Cavalieri S, Cazzaniga S, Geuna M, et al. Human T lymphocytes transduced by lentiviral vectors in the absence of TCR activation maintain an intact immune competence. *Blood* 2003;102:497–505.

149. Cavazzana-Calvo M, Payen E, Negre O, et al. Transfusion independence and HMGA2 activation after gene therapy of human beta-thalassaemia. *Nature* 2010;467:318–322.

150. Johnson LA, Morgan RA, Dudley ME, et al. Gene therapy with human and mouse T-cell receptors mediates cancer regression and targets normal tissues expressing cognate antigen. *Blood* 2009;114:535–546.

151. Simpson AJ, Caballero OL, Jungbluth A, et al. Cancer/testis antigens, gametogenesis and cancer. *Nat Rev Cancer* 2005;5:625.

152. Hofmann O, Caballero OL, Stevenson BJ, et al. Genome-wide analysis of cancer/testis gene expression. *Proc Natl Acad Sci U S A* 2008;105: 20422–20427.

153. Zhang Y, Wang Z, Liu H, et al. Pattern of gene expression and immune responses to Semenogelin 1 in chronic hematologic malignancies. *J Immunother* 2003;26:461–467.

154. Jungbluth AA, Antonescu CR, Busam KJ, et al. Monophasic and biphasic synovial sarcomas abundantly express cancer/testis antigen NY-ESO-1 but not MAGE-A1 or CT7. *Int J Cancer* 2001;94:252–256.

155. Gross G, Waks T, Eshhar Z. Expression of immunoglobulin-T-cell receptor chimeric molecules as functional receptors with antibody-type specificity. *Proc Natl Acad Sci U S A* 1989;86:10024–10028.

156. Pule MA, Savoldo B, Myers GD, et al. Virus-specific T cells engineered to coexpress tumor-specific receptors: persistence and antitumor activity in individuals with neuroblastoma. *Nat Med* 2008;14:1264–1270.

157. James SE, Greenberg PD, Jensen MC, et al. Antigen sensitivity of CD22-specific chimeric TCR is modulated by target epitope distance from the cell membrane. *J Immunol* 2008;180:7028–7038.

158. Morgan RA, Johnson LA, Davis JL, et al. Recognition of glioma stem cells by genetically modified T cells targeting EGFRvIII and development of adoptive cell therapy for glioma. *Hum Gene Ther* 2012;23:1043–1053.

159. Chinnasamy D, Yu Z, Theoret MR, et al. Gene therapy using genetically modified lymphocytes targeting VEGFR-2 inhibits the growth of vascularized syngenic tumors in mice. *J Clin Invest* 2010;120:3953–3968.

160. Carpenito C, Milone MC, Hassan R, et al. Control of large, established tumor xenografts with genetically retargeted human T cells containing CD28 and CD137 domains. *Proc Natl Acad Sci U S A* 2009;106:3360–3365.

161. Feugier P, Van HA, Sebban C, et al. Long-term results of the R-CHOP study in the treatment of elderly patients with diffuse large B-cell lymphoma: a study by the Groupe d'Etude des Lymphomes de l'Adulte. *J Clin Oncol* 2005;23:4117–4126.

162. Gribben JG, O'Brien S. Update on therapy of chronic lymphocytic leukemia. *J Clin Oncol* 2011;29:544–550.

163. Sorror ML, Sandmaier BM, Storer BE, et al. Long-term outcomes among older patients following nonmyeloablative conditioning and allogeneic hematopoietic cell transplantation for advanced hematologic malignancies. *JAMA* 2011;306:1874–1883.

164. Van BK. Current status of allogeneic transplantation for aggressive non-Hodgkin lymphoma. *Curr Opin Oncol* 2011;23:681–691.

165. Van BK. Stem cell transplantation for indolent lymphoma: a reappraisal. *Blood Rev* 2011;25:223–228.

166. McLaughlin P, Grillo-Lopez AJ, Link BK, et al. Rituximab chimeric anti-CD20 monoclonal antibody therapy for relapsed indolent lymphoma: half of patients respond to a four-dose treatment program. *J Clin Oncol* 1998;16:2825–2833.

167. Bacher U, Klyuchnikov E, Le-Rademacher J, et al. Conditioning regimens for allotransplants for diffuse large B-cell lymphoma: myeloablative or reduced intensity? *Blood* 2012;120:4256–4262.

168. Dotti G, Gottschalk S, Savoldo B, et al. Design and development of therapies using chimeric antigen receptor-expressing T cells. *Immunol Rev* 2014;257:107–126.

169. Eshhar Z, Waks T, Gross G, et al. Specific activation and targeting of cytotoxic lymphocytes through chimeric single chains consisting of antibody-binding domains and the gamma or zeta subunits of the immunoglobulin and T-cell receptors. *Proc Natl Acad Sci U S A* 1993;90:720–724.

170. Kochenderfer JN, Rosenberg SA. Treating B-cell cancer with T cells expressing anti-CD19 chimeric antigen receptors. *Nat Rev Clin Oncol* 2013;10:267–276.

171. Sadelain M, Brentjens R, Riviere I. The basic principles of chimeric antigen receptor design. *Cancer Discov* 2013;3:388–398.

172. Kershaw MH, Westwood JA, Darcy PK. Gene-engineered T cells for cancer therapy. *Nat Rev Cancer* 2013;13:525–541.

173. Brentjens RJ, Davila ML, Riviere I, et al. CD19-targeted T cells rapidly induce molecular remissions in adults with chemotherapy-refractory acute lymphoblastic leukemia. *Sci Transl Med* 2013;5:177ra38.

174. Brentjens RJ, Latouche JB, Santos E, et al. Eradication of systemic B-cell tumors by genetically targeted human T lymphocytes co-stimulated by CD80 and interleukin-15. *Nat Med* 2003;9:279–286.

175. Milone MC, Fish JD, Carpenito C, et al. Chimeric receptors containing CD137 signal transduction domains mediate enhanced survival of T cells and increased antileukemic efficacy in vivo. *Mol Ther* 2009;17:1453–1464.

176. Cooper LJ, Topp MS, Serrano LM, et al. T-cell clones can be rendered specific for CD19: toward the selective augmentation of the graft-versus-B lineage leukemia effect. *Blood* 2003;101:1637–1644.

177. Kebriaei P, Huls H, Jena B, et al. Infusing CD19-directed T cells to augment disease control in patients undergoing autologous hematopoietic stem-cell transplantation for advanced B-lymphoid malignancies. *Hum Gene Ther* 2012;23:444–450.

178. Wang X, Naranjo A, Brown CE, et al. Phenotypic and functional attributes of lentivirus-modified CD19-specific human CD8+ central memory T cells manufactured at clinical scale. *J Immunother* 2012;35:689–701.

179. Brentjens RJ, Rivière I, Park JH, et al. Safety and persistence of adoptively transferred autologous CD19-targeted T cells in patients with relapsed or chemotherapy refractory B-cell leukemias. *Blood* 2011;118:4817–4828.

180. Kalos M, Levine BL, Porter DL, et al. T cells with chimeric antigen receptors have potent antitumor effects and can establish memory in patients with advanced leukemia. *Sci Transl Med* 2011;3:95ra73.

181. Kochenderfer JN, Dudley ME, Feldman SA, et al. B-cell depletion and remissions of malignancy along with cytokine-associated toxicity in a clinical trial of anti-CD19 chimeric-antigen-receptor-transduced T cells. *Blood* 2011;119:2709–2720.

182. Imai C, Mihara K, Andreansky M, et al. Chimeric receptors with 4-1BB signaling capacity provoke potent cytotoxicity against acute lymphoblastic leukemia. *Leukemia* 2004;18:678–684.

183. Kochenderfer JN, Yu Z, Frasheri D, et al. Adoptive transfer of syngeneic T cells transduced with a chimeric antigen receptor that recognizes murine CD19 can eradicate lymphoma and normal B cells. *Blood* 2010;116:3875–3886.

184. North RJ. Cyclophosphamide-facilitated adoptive immunotherapy of an established tumor depends on elimination of tumor-induced suppressor T cells. *J Exp Med* 1982;155:1063–1074.

185. Gattinoni L, Finkelstein SE, Klebanoff CA, et al. Removal of homeostatic cytokine sinks by lymphodepletion enhances the efficacy of adoptively transferred tumor-specific CD8+ T cells. *J Exp Med* 2005;202:907–912.

186. Uckun FM, Jaszcz W, Ambrus JL, et al. Detailed studies on expression and function of CD19 surface determinant by using B43 monoclonal antibody and the clinical potential of anti-CD19 immunotoxins. *Blood* 1988;71:13–29.

187. Kochenderfer JN, Feldman SA, Zhao Y, et al. Construction and preclinical evaluation of an anti-CD19 chimeric antigen receptor. *J Immunother* 2009;32:689–702.

188. Brentjens RJ, Santos E, Nikhamin Y, et al. Genetically targeted T cells eradicate systemic acute lymphoblastic leukemia xeongrafts. *Clin Cancer Res* 2007;13:5426–5435.

189. Savoldo B, Ramos CA, Liu E, et al. CD28 costimulation improves expansion and persistence of chimeric antigen receptor-modified T cells in lymphoma patients. *J Clin Invest* 2011;121:1822–1826.

190. Grupp SA, Kalos M, Barrett D, et al. Chimeric antigen receptor-modified T cells for acute lymphoid leukemia. *N Engl J Med* 2013;368:1509–1518.

191. Jensen MC, Popplewell L, Cooper LJ, et al. Antitransgene rejection responses contribute to attenuated persistence of adoptively transferred CD20/CD19-specific chimeric antigen receptor redirected T cells in humans. *Biol Blood Marrow Transplant* 2010;16:1245–1356.

192. Till BG, Jensen MC, Wang J, et al. Adoptive immunotherapy for indolent non-Hodgkin lymphoma and mantle cell lymphoma using genetically modified autologous CD20-specific T cells. *Blood* 2008;112:2261–2271.

193. Till BG, Jensen MC, Wang J, et al. CD20-specific adoptive immunotherapy for lymphoma using a chimeric antigen receptor with both CD28 and 4-1BB domains: pilot clinical trial results. *Blood* 2012;119:3940–3950.

194. Haso W, Lee DW, Shah NN, et al. Anti-CD22-chimeric antigen receptors targeting B-cell precursor acute lymphoblastic leukemia. *Blood* 2013;121:1165–1174.

195. Giordano Attianese GM, Marin V, Hoyos V, et al. In vitro and in vivo model of a novel immunotherapy approach for chronic lymphocytic leukemia by anti-CD23 chimeric antigen receptor. *Blood* 2011;117:4736–4745.

196. Hudecek M, Schmitt TM, Baskar S, et al. The B-cell tumor-associated antigen ROR1 can be targeted with T cells modified to express a ROR1-specific chimeric antigen receptor. *Blood* 2010;116: 4532–4541.

197. Vera J, Savoldo B, Vigouroux S, et al. T lymphocytes redirected against the kappa light chain of human immunoglobulin efficiently kill mature B lymphocyte-derived malignant cells. *Blood* 2006;108:3890–3897.

198. Carpenter RO, Evbuomwan MO, Pittaluga S, et al. B-cell maturation antigen is a promising target for adoptive T-cell therapy of multiple myeloma. *Clin Cancer Res* 2013;19:2048–2060.

199. Peinert S, Prince HM, Guru PM, et al. Gene-modified T cells as immunotherapy for multiple myeloma and acute myeloid leukemia expressing the Lewis Y antigen. *Gene Ther* 2010;17:678–686.

200. Ritchie DS, Neeson PJ, Khot A, et al. Persistence and efficacy of second generation CAR T cell against the LeY antigen in acute myeloid leukemia. *Mol Ther* 2013;21:2122–2129.

201. Mardiros A, Dos SC, McDonald T, et al. T cells expressing CD123-specific chimeric antigen receptors exhibit specific cytolytic effector functions and antitumor effects against human acute myeloid leukemia. *Blood* 2013;122:3138–3148.

202. Savoldo B, Rooney CM, Di SA, et al. Epstein Barr virus specific cytotoxic T lymphocytes expressing the anti-CD30zeta artificial chimeric T-cell receptor for immunotherapy of Hodgkin disease. *Blood* 2007;110:2620–2630.

203. Hombach A, Heuser C, Sircar R, et al. An anti-CD30 chimeric receptor that mediates CD3-zeta-independent T-cell activation against Hodgkin's lymphoma cells in the presence of soluble CD30. *Cancer Res* 1998;58:1116–1119.

204. Shaffer DR, Savoldo B, Yi Z, et al. T cells redirected against CD70 for the immunotherapy of CD70-positive malignancies. *Blood* 2011;117:4304–4314.

205. Xue SA, Gao L, Hart D, et al. Elimination of human leukemia cells in NOD/SCID mice by WT1-TCR gene-transduced human T cells. *Blood* 2005;106:3062–3067.

206. Nagai K, Ochi T, Fujiwara H, et al. Aurora kinase A-specific T-cell receptor gene transfer redirects T lymphocytes to display effective antileukemia reactivity. *Blood* 2012;119:368–376.

207. Spranger S, Jeremias I, Wilde S, et al. TCR-transgenic lymphocytes specific for HMMR/Rhamm limit tumor outgrowth in vivo. *Blood* 2012;119: 3440–3449.

208. Hale GA, Shrestha S, Le-Rademacher J, et al. Alternate donor hematopoietic cell transplantation (HCT) in non-Hodgkin lymphoma using lower intensity conditioning: a report from the CIBMTR. *Biol Blood Marrow Transplant* 2012;18:1036–1043.

209. Kochenderfer JN, Dudley ME, Carpenter RO, et al. Donor-derived CD19-targeted T cells cause regression of malignancy persisting after allogeneic hematopoietic stem cell transplantation. *Blood* 2013;122:4129–4139.

210. Cruz CR, Micklethwaite KP, Savoldo B, et al. Infusion of donor-derived CD19-redirected virus-specific T cells for B-cell malignancies relapsed after allogeneic stem cell transplant: a phase 1 study. *Blood* 2013;122:2965–2973.

211. Traversari C, Marktel S, Magnani Z, et al. The potential immunogenicity of the TK suicide gene does not prevent full clinical benefit associated with the use of TK-transduced donor lymphocytes in HSCT for hematologic malignancies. *Blood* 2007;109:4708–4715.

212. Tey S, Dotti G, Rooney CM, et al. Inducible caspase 9 suicide gene to improve the safety of allodepleted T cells after haploidentical stem cell transplantation. *Biol Blood Marrow Transplant* 2007;13:924.

213. Ciceri F, Bonini C, Stanghellini MT, et al. Infusion of suicide-gene-engineered donor lymphocytes after family haploidentical haemopoietic stem-cell transplantation for leukaemia (the TK007 trial): a non-randomised phase I-II study. *Lancet Oncol* 2009;10:489–500.

214. Di Stasi A, Tey SK, Dotti G, et al. Inducible apoptosis as a safety switch for adoptive cell therapy. *N Engl J Med* 2011;365:1673–1683.

CANCER THERAPEUTICS

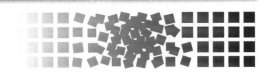

15 Pharmacokinetics and Pharmacodynamics of Anticancer Drugs

Alex Sparreboom and Sharyn D. Baker

INTRODUCTION

Drug selection and therapy considerations in oncology were originally solely based on observations of the effects produced.[1] To overcome some of the limitations of this empirical approach and to answer questions related to considerations of dose, frequency, and duration of drug treatment, it is necessary to understand the events that follow drug administration. Preclinical in vitro and in vivo studies have shown that the magnitude of antitumor response is a function of the concentration of drug,[2] and this has led to the suggestion that the therapeutic objective can be achieved by maintaining an adequate concentration at the site of action for the duration of therapy.[3] However, drugs are rarely directly administered at their sites of action. Indeed, most anticancer drugs are given intravenously or orally, and yet are expected to act in the brain, lungs, or elsewhere. Drugs must, therefore, move from the site of administration to the site of action and, moreover, distribute to all other tissues including organs that eliminate them from the body, such as the kidneys and liver. To administer drugs optimally, knowledge is needed not only of the mechanisms of drug absorption, distribution, and elimination, but also of the kinetics of these processes.[4]

The treatment of human malignancies involving drugs can be divided into two pharmacologic phases, a *pharmacokinetic* phase in which the dose, dosage form, frequency, and route of administration are related to drug level–time relationships in the body, and a *pharmacodynamic* phase in which the concentration of drug at the site(s) of action is related to the magnitude of the effect(s) produced. Once both of these phases have been defined, a dosage regimen can be designed to achieve the therapeutic objective, although additional factors need to be taken into consideration (Fig. 15.1). The clinical application of this approach allows distinctions between pharmacokinetic and pharmacodynamic causes of an unusual drug response. A basic tenet of pharmacokinetics is that the magnitude of both the desired response and toxicity are functions of the drug concentration at the site(s) of action. Accordingly, therapeutic failure results when either the concentration is too low, resulting in ineffective therapy, or is too high, producing unacceptable toxicity. Between these limits of concentrations lies a region associated with therapeutic success, the so-called *therapeutic window*.[5] Because the concentration of a drug at the site of action can rarely be measured directly, with the exception of certain hematologic malignancies, plasma or blood is commonly measured instead as a more accessible alternative.

PHARMACOKINETIC CONCEPTS

A drug's pharmacokinetic properties can be defined by two fundamental processes affecting drug behavior over time, *absorption* and *disposition*.

Absorption

Historically, most anticancer drugs have been administered intravenously; however, the use of orally administered agents is growing with the development of small-molecule targeted cancer therapeutics, such as tyrosine kinase inhibitors.[6] Moreover, drugs may also be administered regionally, for example into the pleural or peritoneal cavities,[7] the cerebrospinal fluid, or intra-arterially into a vessel leading to a cancerous tissue.[8] The process by which the unchanged drug moves from the site of administration to the site of measurement within the body is referred to as *absorption*. Loss at any site prior to the site of measurement contributes to a decrease in the apparent absorption of a drug. For an orally administered agent, this complex series of events involves disintegration of the pharmaceutical dosage form, dissolution, diffusion through gastrointestinal fluids, permeation of the gut membrane, portal circulation uptake, passage through the liver, and, finally, entry into the systemic circulation. The loss of drug as it passes for the first time through organs of elimination, such as the gastrointestinal membranes and the liver, during the absorption process is known as the *first-pass effect*.[9]

The pharmacokinetic parameter most closely associated with absorption is availability or bioavailability (F), defined as the fraction (or percent) of the administered dose that is absorbed intact. Bioavailability can be estimated by dividing the area under the plasma concentration–time curve (AUC) achieved following extravascular administration by the AUC observed after intravenous administration, and can range from 0 to 1.0 (or 0% to 100%).

Disposition

Disposition is defined as all the processes that occur subsequent to absorption of a drug; by definition, the components of disposition are *distribution* and *elimination*. Distribution is the process of reversible transfer of a drug to and from the site of measurement. Any drug that leaves the site of measurement and does not return has undergone elimination, which occurs by two processes, *excretion* and *metabolism*. Excretion is the irreversible loss of the chemically unchanged drug, whereas metabolism is the conversion of drug to another chemical species.

The extent of drug distribution can be determined by relating the concentration obtained with a known amount of drug in the body and is, in essence, a dilution space. The apparent volume into which a drug distributes in the body at equilibrium in called the volume of distribution (V_d), and may or may not correspond to an actual physiologic compartment.

The rate and extent to which a drug distributes into various tissues depend on a number of factors, including hydrophobicity, tissue permeability, tissue-binding constants, binding to serum proteins, and local organ blood flow.[10] Large apparent volumes of distribution are common for agents with high tissue binding or high lipid solubility,

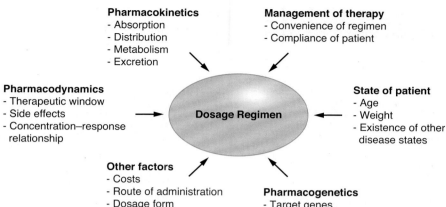

Figure 15.1 Principal determinants of dosage regimen selection for an anticancer drug

although distribution into specific body compartments may be limited by physiologic processes, such as the blood–brain barrier protecting the central nervous system[11,12] or the blood–testes barrier.[13]

Just as V_d is needed as a parameter to relate the concentration to the amount of drug in the body, there is also a need to have a parameter to relate the concentration to the rate of drug elimination, which is known as *clearance* (CL). Of all pharmacokinetic parameters, CL has the most clinical relevance because it defines the key relationship between drug dose and systemic drug exposure (AUC). Derived from V_d and CL is the parameter *elimination rate constant*, which can be regarded as the fractional rate of drug removal. It is, however, more common to refer to the half-life than to the elimination rate constant of a drug. The half-life of a drug is a useful parameter to estimate the time required to reach steady state on a multidose schedule or during a continuous intravenous drug infusion.

Dose Proportionality

When drug concentrations change in strict proportionality to the dose of drug administered, then the condition of dose proportionality (or linear pharmacokinetics) holds. If doubling the dose exactly doubles the plasma concentration or AUC, then pharmacokinetic parameters such V_d, and CL are constant and remain independent of dose and concentration.[14] By strict definition, drugs with linear pharmacokinetics are dose proportional. Dose proportionality is clinically important because it means that dose adjustments will generate predictable changes in systemic drug exposure. For drugs that lack dose proportionality, V_d and CL will demonstrate concentration or time dependence, or both, making it difficult to predict the effect of dose adjustments on drug concentration (Fig. 15.2). Factors that can contribute to a lack of dose proportional pharmacokinetics include saturable oral absorption,[15] capacity-limited distribution or protein binding,[16] and/or saturable metabolism.[17] Dose proportionality of anticancer agents is typically assessed in Phase 1 dose-escalation trials in which small groups of patients are treated at a single dose level using a parallel study design, although the statistical power of such studies to detect deviations from dose proportionality is poor. An alternative, more robust study design is a crossover study in which each patient receives a low dose, an intermediate dose, and a high dose over consecutive cycles of treatment.[18] However, such studies are relatively rare in oncology because of the required use of low, potentially ineffective doses, which may raise ethical concerns for patients.

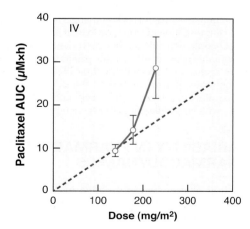

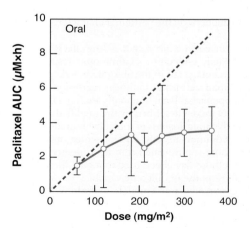

Figure 15.2 Effect of drug dose on systemic exposure to paclitaxel following intravenous (IV) or oral administration in patients with cancer. Data are expressed as mean values (symbols) and standard deviation (error bars). The *dashed line* indicates the hypothetical dose-proportional increase in the area under the plasma concentration time curve (AUC). (Data derived from van Zuylen L, Karlsson MO, Verweij J, et al. Pharmacokinetic modeling of paclitaxel encapsulation in Cremophor EL micelles. *Cancer Chemother Pharmacol* 2001;47:309–318, and Malingre MM, Terwogt JM, Beijnen JH, et al. Phase I and pharmacokinetic study of oral paclitaxel. *J Clin Oncol* 2000;18:2468–2475, respectively.)

TABLE 15.1

Examples of Systemic Exposure as a Pharmacodynamic Marker of Anticancer Drug Effects

Drug	Side Effect	Response/Survival
Carboplatin	Thrombocytopenia	Ovarian cancer
Cisplatin	Nephrotoxicity	Head and neck cancer
Cyclophosphamide	Cardiotoxicity	
Docetaxel	Neutropenia	Non–small-cell lung cancer
Doxorubicin	Neutropenia	
Epirubicin	Neutropenia	
Erlotinib	Skin rash	Non–small-cell lung and head and neck cancer
Etoposide		Non–small-cell lung cancer
5-Fluorouracil	Diarrhea, mucositis	Head and neck cancer
Imatinib		Chronic myeloid leukemia
Irinotecan	Diarrhea, neutropenia	
6-Mercaptopurine		Acute lymphoblastic leukemia
Methotrexate	Mucositis	Acute lymphoblastic leukemia
Nilotinib	Anemia, QT-interval prolongation	
Paclitaxel	Neutropenia	
Sorafenib	Hypertension, hand-foot skin reaction	Renal cell cancer
Sunitinib	Neutropenia	Renal cell cancer
Teniposide		Lymphoma

PHARMACODYNAMIC CONCEPTS

Pharmacodynamic models relate clinical drug effects with drug dose, concentration, or other pharmacokinetic parameters indicative of drug exposures (Table 15.1). In oncology, pharmacodynamic variability may account for substantial differences in clinical outcomes, even when systemic exposures are uniform. Variability in pharmacodynamic response may be heavily influenced by clinical covariates such as age, gender, prior chemotherapy, prior radiotherapy, concomitant medications, or other variables.[19] The pharmacokinetic parameters that are most often correlated with drug effects are markers of drug exposure, such as AUC. In general, the specific parameter used as the independent variable in a pharmacodynamic analysis depends on the particular characteristics of the study drug.

In oncology, pharmacodynamic studies of drug effects have most often focused on toxicity endpoints.[20] Continuous response variables, such as the percentage fall in the absolute blood count from baseline, are easily analyzed using nonlinear regression methods. Dose-limiting neutropenia has been frequently analyzed using a sigmoid maximum effect model described by the modified Hill equation. The pharmacodynamic analysis of subjectively graded clinical endpoints, such as common toxicity criteria scores on a 4-point scale, may require more sophisticated statistical methods.[21,22] Logistical regression methods have been used to model these types of categorical (ordinal) response or outcome variables.

Physiologic pharmacodynamic models describing the severity and time course of drug-related myelosuppression have been derived using population mixed-effect methods for several agents, including paclitaxel[23,24] and pemetrexed.[25] The ability of these models to predict both the severity and duration of drug-induced neutropenia substantially enhances their clinical usefulness.[26] In contrast to small-molecule therapeutics, large-molecule therapeutics such as monoclonal antibodies may not demonstrate toxicities directly related to dose levels. For these agents, a thorough understanding of the pharmacokinetic/pharmacodynamic relationships using modeling approaches may be critical for optimal dose selection.[27]

The antitumor activity of certain chemotherapeutic agents is highly schedule dependent. For such drugs, the dose fractionated over several days can produce a different antitumor response or toxicity profile compared with the same dose given over a shorter period. For example, the efficacy of etoposide in the treatment of small-cell lung cancer is markedly increased when an identical total dose of etoposide is administered by a 5-day divided-dose schedule rather than a 24-hour infusion.[28] Pharmacokinetic analysis in that study showed that both schedules produced very similar overall drug exposure (as measured by AUC), but that the divided-dose schedule produced twice the duration of exposure to an etoposide plasma concentration of >1 μg/mL. This finding has led to the use of prolonged oral administration of etoposide to treat patients with cancer.[29] Similar schedule dependence has been demonstrated for a number of other anticancer agents, notably paclitaxel[30,31] and topotecan.[32] For these agents, the variability in clinically tested treatment schedules is enormous, ranging from short intravenous infusions of less than 30 minutes to 21-day or even 7-week continuous infusion administrations, with large differences in experienced toxicity profiles.

VARIABILITY IN PHARMACOKINETICS/ PHARMACODYNAMICS

There is often a marked variation in drug handling between individual patients, resulting in variability in pharmacokinetic parameters (Fig. 15.3), which will often lead to variability in the pharmacodynamic effects of a given dose of a drug.[33] That is, an identical dose of drug may result in acceptable toxicity in one patient, and unacceptable and possibly life-threatening toxicity in another, or a clinical response in one individual and cancer progression in another. The principal underlying sources of this interindividual pharmacokinetic/pharmacodynamic variability are discussed in the following paragraphs.

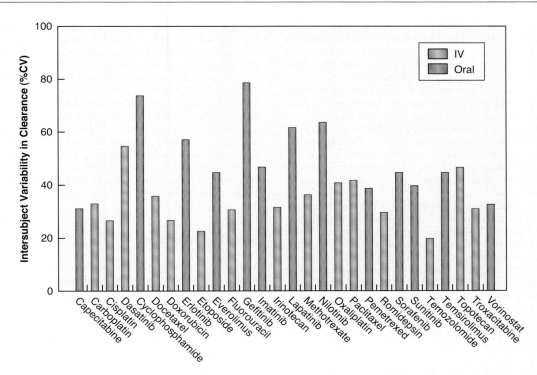

Figure 15.3 Interindividual pharmacokinetic variability of select cytotoxic agents and molecularly targeted agents expressed as a percent coefficient of variation (%CV) in apparent (oral) clearance. IV, intravenous. (Data derived from Mathijssen RH, de Jong FA, Loos WJ, et al. Flat-fixed dosing versus body surface area based dosing of anticancer drugs in adults: does it make a difference? *Oncologist* 2007;12:913–923, and publicly available prescribing information.)

Body Size and Body Composition

The traditional method of individualizing anticancer drug dosage is by using body surface area (BSA).[34] However, the usefulness of normalizing an anticancer drug dose to BSA in adults has been questioned, because, for many drugs, there is no relationship between BSA and CL.[35] Likewise, attempts to replace BSA as a size metric in dose calculation with alternate descriptors such as lean body weight, either in an average population or in individuals at the outer extremes of weight (i.e., frail, severely obese patients) have failed for many anticancer agents.[36,37] It should be pointed out that BSA is a much more important consideration in drug dose calculation for pediatric patients as compared to adults, because of the larger size range in the former population.[38] Based in part on the failure to reduce interindividual pharmacokinetic variability with the use of BSA normalization to obtain a starting dose, many of the more recently developed molecularly targeted agents are currently administered using a flat-fixed dose irrespective of an individual's BSA.[37]

Age

Changes in body composition and organ function at the extremes of age can affect both drug disposition and drug effect.[39] For example, maturational processes in infancy may alter the absorption and distribution of drugs as well as change the capacity for drug metabolism and excretion.[4] The importance of understanding the influence of age on the pharmacokinetics and pharmacodynamics of individual anticancer agents has increased steadily as treatment for the malignancies of infants,[40] adolescents,[41] and the elderly[42] has advanced. Although pediatric cancers remain rare compared with cancers in adults and the elderly population, in particular, optimizing treatment in a patient group with a high cure rate and a long expected survival becomes critical to minimize the incidence of preventable late complications while maintaining efficacy.

Pathophysiologic Changes

Effects of Disease

Pathophysiologic changes associated with particular malignancies may cause dramatic alterations in drug disposition. For example, increases in the clearance of both antipyrine and lorazepam were noted after remission induction compared with the time of diagnosis in children with acute lymphoblastic leukemia (ALL).[43] The clearance of unbound teniposide is lower in children with ALL in relapse than during first remission.[44] Because leukemic infiltration of the liver at the time of diagnosis is common, drugs metabolized by the liver may have a reduced clearance, as has been documented in preclinical models.[45]

Furthermore, in mouse models, certain tumors elicited an acute phase response that coincided with downregulation of human CYP3A4 in the liver as well as the mouse ortholog Cyp3a11.[46] The reduction of murine hepatic Cyp3a gene expression in tumor-bearing mice resulted in decreased Cyp3a protein expression and, consequently, a significant reduction in Cyp3a-mediated metabolism of midazolam. These findings support the possibility that tumor-derived inflammation may alter the pharmacokinetic and pharmacodynamic properties of CYP3A4 substrates, leading to reduced metabolism of drugs in humans.[47] This supports a possible need for disease-specific design of early clinical trials with anticancer drugs,[48] as has been recommended for docetaxel.[49]

Effects of Renal Impairment

The potential impact of pathophysiologic status on interindividual pharmacokinetic variability can be due to either the disease itself or to a dysfunction of specific organs involved in drug elimination. For example, if urinary excretion is an important elimination route for a given drug, any decrement in renal function could lead to decreased drug clearance, which may result in drug accumulation and toxicity.[50] Therefore, it would be logical to decrease the drug dose relative to the degree of impaired renal function in order to maintain plasma concentrations within a target therapeutic window. The best known example of this a priori dose adjustment of an anticancer agent remains carboplatin, which is excreted renally almost entirely by glomerular filtration. Various strategies have been developed to estimate carboplatin doses based on renal function among patients, either using creatinine clearance[51] or glomerular filtration rates as measured by a radioisotope method.[52] The application of these procedures has led to a substantial reduction in pharmacokinetic variability, such that carboplatin is currently one of the few drugs routinely administered to achieve a target exposure rather than on a milligram per square meter or milligram per kilogram basis.

The U.S. Food and Drug Administration (FDA) has developed a guidance on the impact of renal impairment on the pharmacokinetics, dosing, and labeling of drugs.[53] The impact of this guidance has been assessed following a survey of 94 new drug applications for small-molecule new molecular entities approved over the years 2003 to 2007. The survey results indicated that 41% of the applications that included renal impairment study data resulted in a recommendation of dose adjustment in renal impairment.[54] Interestingly, the survey results provided evidence that renal impairment can affect the pharmacokinetics of drugs that are predominantly eliminated by nonrenal processes such as metabolism and/or active transport. The latter finding supports the FDA recommendation to evaluate pharmacokinetic/pharmacodynamic alterations in renal impairment for those drugs that are predominantly eliminated by nonrenal processes, in addition to those that are mainly excreted unchanged by the kidneys. A striking example of a drug in the former category is imatinib, an agent that is predominantly eliminated by hepatic pathways but where predialysis renal impairment is associated with dramatically reduced drug clearance,[55] presumably due to a transporter-mediated process.[56]

Effects of Hepatic Impairment

In contrast to the predictable decline in renal clearance of drugs when glomerular filtration is impaired, it is difficult to make general predictions on the effect of impaired liver function on drug clearance. The major problem is that commonly applied criteria to establish hepatic impairment are typically not good indicators of drug-metabolizing enzyme activity and that several alternative hepatic function tests, such as indocyanine green and antipyrine, have relatively limited value in predicting anticancer drug pharmacokinetics. An alternative dynamic measure of liver function has been proposed, which is based on totaled values (scored to the World Health Organization [WHO] grading system) of serum bilirubin, alkaline phosphatase, and either alanine aminotransferase or aspartate aminotransferase to give a hepatic dysfunction score.[57] Based on pharmacokinetic studies in patients with normal and impaired hepatic function, guidelines have been proposed for dose adjustments of several agents when administered to patients with severe liver dysfunction.[58] It should be emphasized that no uniform criteria have been used in the conduct of these studies and that, ultimately, substantial advances could be made through an a priori determination of the hepatic activity of enzymes of pertinent relevance to the chemotherapeutic drug(s) of interest, as has been done for docetaxel.[59]

Effects of Serum Proteins

The binding of drugs to serum proteins, particularly those that are highly bound, may also have significant clinical implications for a therapeutic outcome.[60] Although protein binding is a major determinant of drug action, it is clearly only one of a myriad of factors that influence the disposition of anticancer drugs.[16] The extent of protein binding is a function of drug and protein concentrations, the affinity constants for the drug–protein interaction, and the number of protein-binding sites per class of binding site. Because only the unbound (or free) drug in plasma water is available for distribution, the therapeutic response will correlate with free drug concentration rather than total drug concentration. Several clinical situations, including liver and renal disease, can significantly decrease the extent of serum binding and may lead to higher free drug concentrations and a possible risk of unexpected toxicity, although the total (free plus bound forms) plasma drug concentrations are unaltered.[61] It is important to realize, however, that after therapeutic doses of most anticancer drugs, binding to serum proteins is independent of drug concentration, suggesting that the total plasma concentration is reflective of the unbound concentration. For some anticancer agents, including etoposide[62] and paclitaxel,[63] however, protein binding is highly dependent on dose and schedule.

Sex Dependence

A number of pharmacokinetic analyses have suggested that male gender is positively correlated with the maximum elimination capacity of various anticancer drugs (e.g., paclitaxel)[8] or with increased clearance (e.g., imatinib)[64] compared with female gender. These observations have added to a growing body of evidence that the pharmacokinetic profile of various anticancer drugs exhibits significant sexual dimorphism, which is rarely considered in the design of clinical trials during oncology drug development.

Drug Interactions

Coadministration of Other Chemotherapeutic Drugs

Favorable and unfavorable interactions between drugs must be considered in developing combination regimens. These interactions may influence the effectiveness of each of the components of the combination, and typically occur when the pharmacokinetic profile of one drug is altered by the other. Such interactions are important in the design of trials evaluating drug combinations because, occasionally, the outcome of concurrent drug administration is diminished therapeutic efficacy or increased toxicity of one or more of the administered agents. Although a recent survey indicated that clinically significant pharmacokinetic interactions are relatively rare in Phase I trials of oncology drug combinations,[65] interactions appear to be more common for combinations of tyrosine kinase inhibitors with cytotoxic chemotherapeutics.[66]

Coadministration of Nonchemotherapeutic Drugs

Many prescription and over-the-counter medications have the potential to cause interactions with anticancer agents by altering their pharmacokinetic characteristics and leading to clinically significant phenotypes. Most clinically relevant drug interactions in this category are due to changes in metabolic routes related to an altered expression or function of cytochrome P450 (CYP) isozymes. This class of enzymes, particularly the CYP3A4 isoform, is responsible for the oxidation of a large proportion of currently approved anticancer drugs. Elevated CYP activity (induction), translated into a more rapid metabolic rate, may result in a decrease in plasma concentrations and to a loss of therapeutic effect. For example, anticonvulsant drugs such as phenytoin, phenobarbital, and carbamazepine can induce drug-metabolizing enzymes and thereby increase the clearance of various anticancer agents.[33]

Conversely, the suppression (inhibition) of CYP activity, for example with ketoconazole,[13,67] may trigger a rise in plasma concentrations and can lead to exaggerated toxicity commensurate with overdose. It should be borne in mind that several pharmacokinetic parameters could be altered simultaneously. Especially in the development of anticancer agents given by the oral route,

TABLE 15.2

Effect of Food on Exposure to Select Oral Anticancer Agents

Drug	Food	Effect on Drug Exposure	Manufacturer's Recommendations
Abiraterone	High-fat meal	↑ AUC 1,000%	Without food
Dasatinib	High-fat meal	↑ AUC 14%	With or without food
Erlotinib	High-fat, high-calorie breakfast	Single dose, ↑ AUC 200% Multiple dose, ↑ AUC 37%–66%	Without food[a]
Gefitinib	High-fat breakfast	↓ AUC 14%, ↓ Cmax 35%	With or without food
	High-fat breakfast	↑ AUC 32%, ↑ Cmax 35%	
Imatinib	High-fat meal	No change	With food and a large glass of water[b]
		Variability (% CV) ↓ 37%	
Lapatinib	Low-fat meal (5% fat, 500 calories)	↑ AUC 167%, ↑ Cmax 142%	Without food[c]
	High-fat meal (50% fat, 1,000 calories)	↑ AUC 325%, ↑ Cmax 203%	
Nilotinib	High-fat meal	↑ AUC 82%	Without food
Sorafenib	Moderate-fat meal (30% fat, 700 calories)	No change in bioavailability	Without food
	High-fat meal (50% fat, 900 calories)	↓ Bioavailability 29%	
Sunitinib	High-fat, high-calorie meal	↑ AUC 18%	With or without food
Everolimus	High-fat meal	↓ AUC 16%, ↓ Cmax 60%	With or without food
Vismodegib	High-fat meal	↑ AUC 74% for single dose; no effect at steady state	With or without food
Vorinostat	High-fat meal	↑ AUC 37%	With food[d]

[a] Recommended without food because the approved dose is the maximum tolerated dose.
[b] Recommended with food to reduce nausea.
[c] Recommended without food to achieve consistent drug exposure; was taken without food in clinical trials.
[d] Was taken with food in clinical trials.
AUC, area under the plasma concentration time curve; Cmax, maximum plasma concentration; CV, coefficient of variation.

oral bioavailability plays a crucial role[9]; this parameter is contingent on adequate absorption and the circumvention of intestinal and, subsequently, hepatic metabolism of the drug. It has been suggested that the prevalence of drug–drug interactions is particularly high in cancer patients receiving oral chemotherapy,[68] especially for agents that are weak bases that exhibit pH-dependent solubility.[69]

An additional consideration is related to a possible influence of food intake on the extent of drug absorption after oral administration, which can increase, decrease, or remain unchanged depending on specific physicochemical properties of the drug in question (Table 15.2). The relatively narrow therapeutic index of most of these agents means that significant inter- and intrapatient variability would predispose some individuals to excessive toxicity or, conversely, inadequate efficacy.[12]

Coadministration of Complementary and Alternative Medicine

Surveys within the past decade estimate the prevalence of complementary and alternative medicine (CAM) use in oncology patients to be as high as 87%, and in many cases the treating physician is not aware of the patients' CAM use.[70] With a larger number of participants to phase I clinical trials[71] using herbal treatments combined with allopathic therapies, the risk for herb–drug interactions is a growing concern, and there is an increasing need to understand possible adverse drug interactions in oncology at the early stages of drug development.

A number of clinically important pharmacokinetic interactions involving CAM and cancer drugs have now been recognized, although causal relationships have not always been established.[72] Most of the observed interactions point to the herbs

affecting several isoforms of the CYP family, either through inhibition or induction. In the context of chemotherapeutic drugs, St. John's wort,[73] garlic,[74] milk thistle,[75] and Echinacea[11] have been formally evaluated for their pharmacokinetic drug–interaction potential in cancer patients. However, various other herbs have the potential to significantly modulate the expression and/or activity of drug-metabolizing enzymes and drug transporters (Table 15.3), including ginkgo, ginseng, and kava.[70] Because of the high prevalence of herbal medicine use, physicians should include herb usage in their routine drug histories in order to have an opportunity to outline to individual patients which potential hazards should be taken into consideration prior to participation in a clinical trial.

Inherited Genetic Factors

The discipline of pharmacogenetics describes differences in the pharmacokinetics and pharmacodynamics of drugs as a result of inherited variation in drug metabolizing enzymes, drug transporters, and drug targets between patients.[76] These inherited variations are occasionally responsible for extensive interpatient variability in drug exposure or effects. Severe toxicity might occur in the absence of a typical metabolism of active compounds, while the therapeutic effect of a drug could be diminished in the case of an absence of activation of a prodrug, such as irinotecan.[77] The importance and detectability of polymorphisms for a given enzyme or transporter depends on the contribution of the variant gene product to pharmacologic response, the availability of alternative pathways of elimination, and the frequency of occurrence of the variant allele. Although many substrates have been identified for the known polymorphic drug metabolizing enzymes

Effects of Common Herbal Products on Exposure to Anticancer Agents

Botanical	Concurrent Chemotherapy/Condition (Suspected Effect)
Ephedra	Avoid with all cardiovascular chemotherapy (synergistic increase in blood pressure)
Ginkgo	Caution with camptothecins, cyclophosphamide, TK inhibitors, epipodophyllotoxins, taxanes, and vinca alkaloids (CYP3A4 and CYP2C19 inhibition); discourage with alkylating agents, antitumor antibiotics, and platinum analogs (free-radical scavenging)
Ginseng	Discourage in patients with estrogen-receptor–positive breast cancer and endometrial cancer (stimulation of tumor growth)
Green tea	Discourage with erlotinib and pazopanib (CYP1A2 induction)
Japanese arrowroot	Avoid with methotrexate (ABC and OAT transporter inhibition)
St. John's wort	Avoid with all concurrent chemotherapy (CYP2B6, CYP2C9, CYP2C19, CYP2E1, CYP3A4, and ABCB1 induction)
Valerian	Caution with tamoxifen (CYP2C9 inhibition), cyclophosphamide, and teniposide (CYP2C19 inhibition)
Kava-kava	Avoid in all patients with preexisting liver disease, with evidence of hepatic injury (herb-induced hepatotoxicity), and/or in combination with hepatotoxic chemotherapy; caution with camptothecins, cyclophosphamide, TK inhibitors, epipodophyllotoxins, taxanes, and Vinca alkaloids (CYP3A4 induction)

TK, tyrosine kinase; CYP, cytochrome P450; ABC, ATP-binding cassette; OAT, organic anion transporter.

and transporters, the contribution of a genetically determined source of interindividual pharmacokinetic variability has been established for only a few cancer chemotherapeutic agents. Most of these cases involve agents for which elimination is critically dependent on a rate-limiting breakdown by a polymorphic enzyme (e.g., 6-mercaptopurine by thiopurine-S-methyltransferase; 5-fluorouracil by dihydropyrimidine dehydrogenase) or when a polymorphic enzyme is involved in the formation of a toxic metabolite (e.g., tamoxifen by CYP2D6).[78]

In addition to drug metabolism, pharmacokinetic processes are highly dependent on the interplay with drug transport in organs such as the intestines, kidneys, and liver. Genetically determined variation in drug transporter function or expression is now increasingly recognized to have a significant role as a determinant of intersubject variability in response to various commonly prescribed drugs.[79] The most extensively studied class of drug transporters are those encoded by the family of ATP-binding cassette (ABC) genes, some of which also play a role in the resistance of malignant cells to anticancer agents. Among the 48 known ABC gene products, ABCB1 (P-glycoprotein), ABCC1 (multidrug-resistance associated protein-1 [MRP1]) and its homologue ABCC2 (MRP2; cMOAT), and ABCG2 (breast cancer resistance protein [BCRP]) are known to influence the oral absorption and disposition of a wide variety of drugs.[80] As a result, the expression levels of these proteins in humans have important consequences for an individual's susceptibility to certain anticancer drug–induced side effects, interactions, and treatment efficacy, for example, in the case of genetic variation in ABCG2 in relation to gefitinib-induced diarrhea.[81]

Similar to the discoveries of functional genetic variations in drug efflux transporters of the ABC family, there have been considerable advances in the identification of inherited variants in transporters that facilitate cellular drug uptake in tissues that play an important role in drug elimination, such as the liver (Fig. 15.4). Among these, members of the organic anion-transporting polypeptides (OATP), organic anion transporters (OAT), and organic cation transporters (OCT) can mediate the cellular uptake of a large number of structurally divergent compounds.[82,83] Accordingly, functionally relevant polymorphisms in these influx transporters may contribute to interindividual and interethnic variability in drug disposition and response,[84] for example, in the case of the impact of polymorphic variants in the OCT1 gene *SLC22A1* on the survival of patients with chronic myeloid leukemia receiving treatment with imatinib.[85]

DOSE-ADAPTATION USING PHARMACOKINETIC/PHARMACODYNAMIC PRINCIPLES

Therapeutic Drug Monitoring

Prolonged infusion schedules of anticancer drugs offer a very convenient setting for dose adaptation in individual patients. At the time required to achieve steady-state concentration, it is possible to modify the infusion rate for the remainder of the treatment course if a relationship is known between this steady-state concentration and a desired pharmacodynamic endpoint. This method has been successfully used to adapt the dose during continuous infusions of 5-fluorouracil and etoposide, and for repeated oral administration of etoposide or repeated intravenous administration of cisplatin.[86] Methotrexate plasma concentrations are routinely monitored to identify patients at high risk of toxicity and to adjust leucovorin rescue in patients with delayed drug excretion. This monitoring has significantly reduced the incidence of serious toxicity, including toxic death, and in fact, has improved outcome by eliminating unacceptably low systemic exposure levels.[87] Therapeutic drug monitoring has also been applied to or is currently under investigation for several more recently developed anticancer drugs, including imatinib[88–90] and sorafenib.[91]

Feedback-Controlled Dosing

It remains to be determined how information on interindividual pharmacokinetic variability can eventually be used to devise an optimal dosage regimen of a drug for the treatment of a given disease in an individual patient. Obviously, the desired objective would be most efficiently achieved if the individual's dosage requirements could be calculated prior to administering the drug. While this ideal cannot be met completely in clinical practice, with the notable exception of carboplatin, some success may be achieved by adopting feedback-controlled dosing. In the adaptive dosage with feedback control, population-based predictive models are used initially, but allow the possibility of dosage alteration based on feedback revision. In this approach, patients are first treated with standard dose and, during treatment, pharmacokinetic information is estimated by a limited-sampling strategy and compared with that predicted from the population model with which treatment was initiated. On the basis of the comparison,

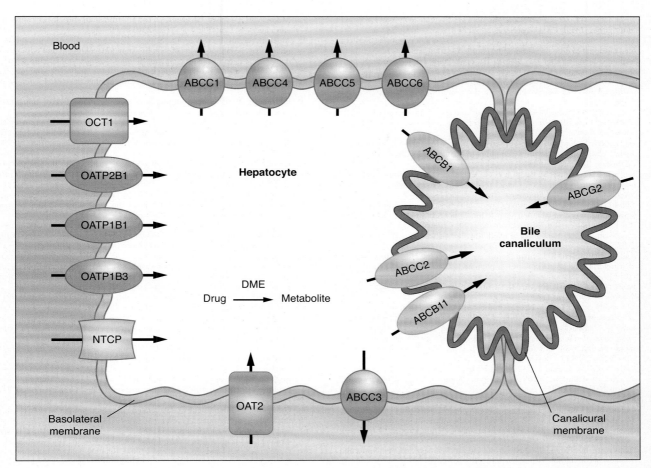

Figure 15.4 Common mechanisms for possible interactions between xenobiotics and anticancer drugs in the liver. DME, drug-metabolizing enzyme(s).

more patient-specific pharmacokinetic parameters are calculated, and dosage is adjusted accordingly to maintain the target exposure measure producing the desired pharmacodynamic effect. Despite its mathematical complexity, this approach may be the only way to deliver the desired and precise exposure of an anticancer agent.

The study of population pharmacokinetics seeks to identify the measurable factors that cause changes in the dose-concentration relationship and the extent of these alterations so that, if these are associated with clinically significant shifts in the therapeutic index, dosage can be appropriately modified in the individual patient. It is obvious that a careful collection of data during the development of drugs and subsequent analyses could be helpful to collect some essential information on the drug. Unfortunately, important information is often lost by failing to analyze this data or due to the fact that the relevant samples or data were never collected. Historically, this has resulted in the notion that tools for the identification of patient population subgroups are inadequate for most of the currently approved anticancer drugs.

However, the use of population pharmacokinetic models is increasingly studied in an attempt to accommodate as much of the pharmacokinetic variability as possible in terms of measurable characteristics. This type of analysis has been conducted for a number of clinically important anticancer drugs, including carboplatin,[92] docetaxel,[93] topotecan,[94] gefitinib,[95] and erlotinib,[96] and provided mathematical equations based on morphometric, demographic, phenotypic enzyme activity, and/or physiologic characteristics of patients, in order to predict drug clearance with an acceptable degree of precision and bias.[97]

REFERENCES

1. DeVita VT, Chu E. A history of cancer chemotherapy. *Cancer Res* 2008; 68:8643–8653.
2. Lieu CH, Tan AC, Leong S, et al. From bench to bedside: lessons learned in translating preclinical studies in cancer drug development. *J Natl Cancer Inst* 2013;105:1441–1456.
3. Sparreboom A, Verweij J. Advances in cancer therapeutics. *Clin Pharmacol Ther* 2009;85:113–117.
4. Fujita KI, Sasaki Y. Optimization of cancer chemotherapy on the basis of pharmacokinetics and pharmacodynamics: from patients enrolled in 'clinical trials' to those in the 'real world'. *Drug Metab Pharmacokin* 2014;29(1):20–28.
5. Liliemark J, Peterson C. Pharmacokinetic optimisation of anticancer therapy. *Clin Pharmacokinet* 1991;21:213–231.
6. Stuurman FE, Nuijen B, Beijnen JH, et al. Oral anticancer drugs: mechanisms of low bioavailability and strategies for improvement. *Clin Pharmacokinet* 2013;52:399–414.

7. Hasovits C, Clarke S. Pharmacokinetics and pharmacodynamics of intraperitoneal cancer chemotherapeutics. *Clin Pharmacokinet* 2012;51:203–224.
8. Cai S, Bagby TR, Forrest ML. Development of regional chemotherapies: feasibility, safety and efficacy in clinical use and preclinical studies. *Ther Deliv* 2011;2:1467–1484.
9. DeMario MD, Ratain MJ. Oral chemotherapy: rationale and future directions. *J Clin Oncol* 1998;16:2557–2567.
10. Zou P, Zheng N, Yang Y, et al. Prediction of volume of distribution at steady state in humans: comparison of different approaches. *Exp Opin Drug Metab Toxicol* 2012;8:855–872.
11. Deeken JF, Loscher W. The blood-brain barrier and cancer: transporters, treatment, and Trojan horses. *Clin Cancer Res* 2007;13:1663–1674.
12. Pitz MW, Desai A, Grossman SA, et al. Tissue concentration of systemically administered antineoplastic agents in human brain tumors. *J Neurooncol* 2011;104:629–638.

13. Mruk DD, Su L, Cheng CY. Emerging role for drug transporters at the blood-testis barrier. *Trends Pharmacol Sci* 2011;32:99–106.

14. Smith BP, Vandenhende FR, DeSante KA, et al. Confidence interval criteria for assessment of dose proportionality. *Pharm Res* 2000;17:1278–1283.

15. Malingre MM, Terwogt JM, Beijnen JH, et al. Phase I and pharmacokinetic study of oral paclitaxel. *J Clin Oncol* 2000;18:2468–2475.

16. Sparreboom A, Chen H, Acharya MR, et al. Effects of alpha1-acid glycoprotein on the clinical pharmacokinetics of 7-hydroxystaurosporine. *Clin Cancer Res* 2004;10:6840–6846.

17. Yamaoka K, Takakura Y. Analysis methods and recent advances in nonlinear pharmacokinetics from in vitro through in loci to in vivo. *Drug Metab Dispos* 2004;19:397–406.

18. van Zuylen L, Karlsson MO, Verweij J, et al. Pharmacokinetic modeling of paclitaxel encapsulation in Cremophor EL micelles. *Cancer Chemother Pharmacol* 2001;47:309–318.

19. Karlsson MO, Molnar V, Bergh J, et al. A general model for time-dissociated pharmacokinetic-pharmacodynamic relationship exemplified by paclitaxel myelosuppression. *Clin Pharmacol Ther* 1998;63:11–25.

20. Zhou Q, Gallo JM. The pharmacokinetic/pharmacodynamic pipeline: translating anticancer drug pharmacology to the clinic. *AAPS J* 2011;13:111–120.

21. Xie R, Mathijssen RH, Sparreboom A, et al. Clinical pharmacokinetics of irinotecan and its metabolites in relation with diarrhea. *Clin Pharmacol Ther* 2002;72:265–275.

22. Xie R, Mathijssen RH, Sparreboom A, et al. Clinical pharmacokinetics of irinotecan and its metabolites: a population analysis. *J Clin Oncol* 2002; 20:3293–3301.

23. Kearns CM, Gianni L, Egorin MJ. Paclitaxel pharmacokinetics and pharmacodynamics. *Sem Oncol* 1995;22:16–23.

24. Minami H, Sasaki Y, Saijo N, et al. Indirect-response model for the time course of leukopenia with anticancer drugs. *Clin Pharmacol Ther* 1998;64:511–521.

25. Latz JE, Schneck KL, Nakagawa K, et al. Population pharmacokinetic/pharmacodynamic analyses of pemetrexed and neutropenia: effect of vitamin supplementation and differences between Japanese and Western patients. *Clin Cancer Res* 2009;15:346–354.

26. Karlsson MO, Anehall T, Friberg LE, et al. Pharmacokinetic/pharmacodynamic modelling in oncological drug development. *Basic Clin Pharmacol Toxicol* 2005;96:206–211.

27. Keizer RJ, Huitema AD, Schellens JH, et al. Clinical pharmacokinetics of therapeutic monoclonal antibodies. *Clin Pharmacokinet* 2010;49:493–507.

28. Slevin ML, Clark PI, Joel SP, et al. A randomized trial to evaluate the effect of schedule on the activity of etoposide in small-cell lung cancer. *J Clin Oncol* 1989;7:1333–1340.

29. Hainsworth JD. Extended-schedule oral etoposide in selected neoplasms and overview of administration and scheduling issues. *Drugs* 1999;58 Suppl 3:51–56.

30. Gelderblom H, Mross K, ten Tije AJ, et al. Comparative pharmacokinetics of unbound paclitaxel during 1- and 3-hour infusions. *J Clin Oncol* 2002;20:574–581.

31. Woodward EJ, Twelves C. Scheduling of taxanes: a review. *Curr Clin Pharmacol* 2010;5:226–231.

32. Soepenberg O, Sparreboom A, Verweij J. Clinical studies of camptothecin and derivatives. *Alkaloid Chem Biol* 2003;60:1–50.

33. Undevia SD, Gomez-Abuin G, Ratain MJ. Pharmacokinetic variability of anticancer agents. *Nat Rev Cancer* 2005;5:447–458.

34. Gurney H. Dose calculation of anticancer drugs: a review of the current practice and introduction of an alternative. *J Clin Oncol* 1996;14:2590–2611.

35. Baker SD, Verweij J, Rowinsky EK, et al. Role of body surface area in dosing of investigational anticancer agents in adults, 1991–2001. *J Natl Cancer Inst* 2002;94:1883–1888.

36. Mathijssen RH, Sparreboom A. Influence of lean body weight on anticancer drug clearance. *Clin Pharmacol Ther* 2009;85:23.

37. Sparreboom A, Wolff AC, Mathijssen RH, et al. Evaluation of alternate size descriptors for dose calculation of anticancer drugs in the obese. *J Clin Oncol* 2007;25:4707–4713.

38. Bartelink IH, Rademaker CM, Schobben AF, et al. Guidelines on paediatric dosing on the basis of developmental physiology and pharmacokinetic considerations. *Clin Pharmacokinet* 2006;45:1077–1097.

39. McLeod HL, Relling MV, Crom WR, et al. Disposition of antineoplastic agents in the very young child. *Br J Cancer* 1992;18:S23–S29.

40. Hutson JR, Weitzman S, Schechter T, et al. Pharmacokinetic and pharmacogenetic determinants and considerations in chemotherapy selection and dosing in infants. *Exp Opin Drug Metab Toxicol* 2012;8:709–722.

41. Veal GJ, Hartford CM, Stewart CF. Clinical pharmacology in the adolescent oncology patient. *J Clin Oncol* 2010;28:4790–4799.

42. Lichtman SM. Pharmacology of aging and cancer: how useful are pharmacokinetic tests? *Interdisc Top Gerontol* 2013;38:104–123.

43. Relling MV, Crom WR, Pieper JA, et al. Hepatic drug clearance in children with leukemia: changes in clearance of model substrates during remission-induction therapy. *Clin Pharmacol Ther* 1987;41:651–660.

44. Evans WE, Rodman JH, Relling MV, et al. Differences in teniposide disposition and pharmacodynamics in patients with newly diagnosed and relapsed acute lymphocytic leukemia. *J Pharmacol Exp Ther* 1992;260:71–77.

45. Powis G, Harris RN, Basseches PJ, et al. Effects of advanced leukemia on hepatic drug-metabolizing activity in the mouse. *Cancer Chemother Pharmacol* 1986;16:43–49.

46. Charles KA, Rivory LP, Brown SL, et al. Transcriptional repression of hepatic cytochrome P450 3A4 gene in the presence of cancer. *Clin Cancer Res* 2006; 12:7492–7497.

47. Moore MM, Chua W, Charles KA, et al. Inflammation and cancer: causes and consequences. *Clin Pharmacol Ther* 2010;87:504–508.

48. Albekairy A, Alkatheri A, Fujita S, et al. Cytochrome P450 3A4FNx011B as pharmacogenomic predictor of tacrolimus pharmacokinetics and clinical outcome in the liver transplant recipients. *Saudi J Gastroenterol* 2013;19:89–95.

49. Franke RM, Carducci MA, Rudek MA, et al. Castration-dependent pharmacokinetics of docetaxel in patients with prostate cancer. *J Clin Oncol* 2010;28:4562–4567.

50. Rahman A, White RM. Cytotoxic anticancer agents and renal impairment study: the challenge remains. *J Clin Oncol* 2006;24:533–536.

51. Egorin MJ, Van Echo DA, Olman EA, et al. Prospective validation of a pharmacologically based dosing scheme for the cis-diamminedichloroplatinum(II) analogue diamminecyclobutanedicarboxylatoplatinum. *Cancer Res* 1985;45: 6502–6506.

52. Calvert AH, Newell DR, Gumbrell LA, et al. Carboplatin dosage: prospective evaluation of a simple formula based on renal function. *J Clin Oncol* 1989;7:1748–1756.

53. Huang SM, Temple R, Xiao S, et al. When to conduct a renal impairment study during drug development: US Food and Drug Administration perspective. *Clin Pharmacol Ther* 2009;86:475–479.

54. Zhang Y, Zhang L, Abraham S, et al. Assessment of the impact of renal impairment on systemic exposure of new molecular entities: evaluation of recent new drug applications. *Clin Pharmacol Ther* 2009;85:305–311.

55. Gibbons J, Egorin MJ, Ramanathan RK, et al. Phase I and pharmacokinetic study of imatinib mesylate in patients with advanced malignancies and varying degrees of renal dysfunction: a study by the National Cancer Institute Organ Dysfunction Working Group. *J Clin Oncol* 2008;26:570–576.

56. Franke RM, Sparreboom A. Inhibition of imatinib transport by uremic toxins during renal failure. *J Clin Oncol* 2008;26:4226–4227.

57. Twelves C, Glynne-Jones R, Cassidy J, et al. Effect of hepatic dysfunction due to liver metastases on the pharmacokinetics of capecitabine and its metabolites. *Clin Cancer Res* 1999;5:1696–1702.

58. Eklund JW, Trifilio S, Mulcahy MF. Chemotherapy dosing in the setting of liver dysfunction. *Oncology (Williston Park)* 2005;19:1057–1063.

59. Hooker AC, Ten Tije AJ, Carducci MA, et al. Population pharmacokinetic model for docetaxel in patients with varying degrees of liver function: incorporating cytochrome P4503A activity measurements. *Clin Pharmacol Ther* 2008;84:111–118.

60. Grandison MK, Boudinot FD. Age-related changes in protein binding of drugs: implications for therapy. *Clin Pharmacokinet* 2000;38:271–290.

61. Sparreboom A, Nooter K, Loos WJ, et al. The (ir)relevance of plasma protein binding of anticancer drugs. *Neth J Med* 2001;59:196–207.

62. Perdaems N, Bachaud JM, Rouzaud P, et al. Relation between unbound plasma concentrations and toxicity in a prolonged oral etoposide schedule. *Eur J Clin Pharmacol* 1998;54:677–683.

63. Sparreboom A, van ZL, Brouwer E, et al. Cremophor EL-mediated alteration of paclitaxel distribution in human blood: clinical pharmacokinetic implications. *Cancer Res* 1999;59:1454–1457.

64. Gardner ER, Burger H, van Schaik RH, et al. Association of enzyme and transporter genotypes with the pharmacokinetics of imatinib. *Clin Pharmacol Ther* 2006;80:192–201.

65. Wu K, House L, Ramirez J, et al. Evaluation of utility of pharmacokinetic studies in phase I trials of two oncology drugs. *Clin Cancer Res* 2013;19:6039–6043.

66. Hu S, Mathijssen RH, de Bruijn P, et al. Inhibition of OATP1B1 by tyrosine kinase inhibitors: in vitro-in vivo correlations. *Br J Cancer* 2014;110(4): 894–898.

67. Kehrer DF, Mathijssen RH, Verweij J, et al. Modulation of irinotecan metabolism by ketoconazole. *J Clin Oncol* 2002;20:3122–3129.

68. van Leeuwen RW, Brundel DH, Neef C, et al. Prevalence of potential drug-drug interactions in cancer patients treated with oral anticancer drugs. *Br J Cancer* 2013;108:1071–1078.

69. Budha NR, Frymoyer A, Smelick GS, et al. Drug absorption interactions between oral targeted anticancer agents and PPIs: is pH-dependent solubility the Achilles heel of targeted therapy? *Clin Pharmacol Ther* 2012;92:203–213.

70. Sparreboom A, Cox MC, Acharya MR, et al. Herbal remedies in the United States: potential adverse interactions with anticancer agents. *J Clin Oncol* 2004;22:2489–2503.

71. Dy GK, Bekele L, Hanson LJ, et al. Complementary and alternative medicine use by patients enrolled onto phase I clinical trials. *J Clin Oncol* 2004;22:4810–4815.

72. Goey AK, Mooiman KD, Beijnen JH, et al. Relevance of in vitro and clinical data for predicting CYP3A4-mediated herb-drug interactions in cancer patients. *Cancer Treat Rev* 2013;39:773–783.

73. Mathijssen RH, Verweij J, De Bruijn P, et al. Effects of St. John's wort on irinotecan metabolism. *J Natl Cancer Inst* 2002;94:1247–1249.

74. Cox MC, Low J, Lee J, et al. Influence of garlic (Allium sativum) on the pharmacokinetics of docetaxel. *Clin Cancer Res* 2006;12:4636–4640.

75. van Erp NP, Baker SD, Zhao M, et al. Effect of milk thistle (Silybum marianum) on the pharmacokinetics of irinotecan. *Clin Cancer Res* 2005;11:7800–7806.

76. Wheeler HE, Maitland ML, Dolan ME, et al. Cancer pharmacogenomics: strategies and challenges. *Nat Rev Genet* 2013;14:23–34.

77. Fujita K, Sparreboom A. Pharmacogenetics of irinotecan disposition and toxicity: a review. *Curr Clin Pharmacol* 2010;5:209–217.

78. Huang RS, Ratain MJ. Pharmacogenetics and pharmacogenomics of anticancer agents. *CA Cancer J Clin* 2009;59:42–55.

79. Evans WE, McLeod HL. Pharmacogenomics—drug disposition, drug targets, and side effects. *N Engl J Med* 2003;348:538–549.

80. Sparreboom A, Danesi R, Ando Y, et al. Pharmacogenomics of ABC transporters and its role in cancer chemotherapy. *Drug Resist Updat* 2003;6:71–84.

81. Cusatis G, Gregorc V, Li J, et al. Pharmacogenetics of ABCG2 and adverse reactions to gefitinib. *J Natl Cancer Inst* 2006;98:1739–1742.

82. Kim RB. Organic anion-transporting polypeptide (OATP) transporter family and drug disposition. *Eur J Clin Invest* 2003;33 Suppl 2:1–5.

83. Smith NF, Figg WD, Sparreboom A. Role of the liver-specific transporters OATP1B1 and OATP1B3 in governing drug elimination. *Exp Opin Drug Metab Toxicol* 2005;1:429–445.

84. Sprowl JA, Mikkelsen TS, Giovinazzo H, et al. Contribution of tumoral and host solute carriers to clinical drug response. *Drug Resist Updat* 2012;15:5–20.

85. Kim DH, Sriharsha L, Xu W, et al. Clinical relevance of a pharmacogenetic approach using multiple candidate genes to predict response and resistance to imatinib therapy in chronic myeloid leukemia. *Clin Cancer Res* 2009;15:4750–4758.

86. Canal P, Chatelut E, Guichard S. Practical treatment guide for dose individualisation in cancer chemotherapy. *Drugs* 1998;56:1019–1038.

87. Evans WE, Relling MV, Rodman JH, et al. Conventional compared with individualized chemotherapy for childhood acute lymphoblastic leukemia. *N Engl J Med* 1998;338:499–505.

88. Blasdel C, Egorin MJ, Lagattuta TF, et al. Therapeutic drug monitoring in CML patients on imatinib. *Blood* 2007;110:1699–1701.

89. Larson RA, Druker BJ, Guilhot F, et al. Imatinib pharmacokinetics and its correlation with response and safety in chronic-phase chronic myeloid leukemia: a subanalysis of the IRIS study. *Blood* 2008;111:4022–4028.

90. Picard S, Titier K, Etienne G, et al. Trough imatinib plasma levels are associated with both cytogenetic and molecular responses to standard-dose imatinib in chronic myeloid leukemia. *Blood* 2007;109:3496–3499.

91. Blanchet B, Billemont B, Cramard J, et al. Validation of an HPLC-UV method for sorafenib determination in human plasma and application to cancer patients in routine clinical practice. *J Pharm Biomed Anal* 2009;49:1109–1114.

92. Chatelut E, Canal P, Brunner V, et al. Prediction of carboplatin clearance from standard morphological and biological patient characteristics. *J Natl Cancer Inst* 1995;87:573–580.

93. Bruno R, Hille D, Riva A, et al. Population pharmacokinetics/pharmacodynamics of docetaxel in phase II studies in patients with cancer. *J Clin Oncol* 1998;16:187–196.

94. Gallo JM, Laub PB, Rowinsky EK, et al. Population pharmacokinetic model for topotecan derived from phase I clinical trials. *J Clin Oncol* 2000;18:2459–2467.

95. Li J, Karlsson MO, Brahmer J, et al. CYP3A phenotyping approach to predict systemic exposure to EGFR tyrosine kinase inhibitors. *J Natl Cancer Inst* 2006;98:1714–1723.

96. Lu JF, Eppler SM, Wolf J, et al. Clinical pharmacokinetics of erlotinib in patients with solid tumors and exposure-safety relationship in patients with non-small cell lung cancer. *Clin Pharmacol Ther* 2006;80:136–145.

97. Mathijssen RH, de Jong FA, Loos WJ, et al. Flat-fixed dosing versus body surface area based dosing of anticancer drugs in adults: does it make a difference? *Oncologist* 2007;12:913–923.

CANCER THERAPEUTICS

Christine M. Walko and Howard L. McLeod

INTRODUCTION

The evolution of understanding cancer biology has yielded many advances that have been translated into cancer treatment. Application of this knowledge has allowed for a shift in chemotherapeutics from traditional cytotoxic agents that worked by killing both healthy and malignant fast growing cells to chemical and biologic therapies aimed at targeting a specific gene or pathway critical to the particular cancer being treated.[1] This age of pathway-directed therapy has been made possible by the increased availability and feasibility of high throughput technology able to provide comprehensive and clinically useful molecular characterization of tumors. Translation of these efforts have resulted in improved degree to disease control for many common cancers including breast, colorectal, lung, and melanoma as well as long-term survival benefits for chronic myelogenous leukemia (CML), gastrointestinal stromal tumors (GIST), and childhood acute lymphoblastic leukemia (ALL).[2]

Pharmacogenomic-guided therapy aims the use information on DNA and RNA integrity to optimize not only the treatment choice for an individual patient, but also the dose and schedule of that treatment. The assessment of both somatic and germ-line mutations contribute to the overall individualization of cancer treatment. Somatic mutations are genetic variations found within the tumor DNA, but not DNA from the normal (germ-line) tissues, which also have functional consequences that influence disease outcomes and/or response to certain therapies. These types of mutations or biomarkers can be classified as either prognostic or predictive. Prognostic biomarkers identify subpopulations of patients with different disease courses or outcomes, independent of treatment. Predictive biomarkers identify subpopulations of patients most likely to have a response to a given therapy.[3] Germ-line mutations are heritable variations found within the individual and, in practical terms, are focused on DNA markers predictive for toxicity or therapeutic outcomes of a particular therapy as well as inheritable risk of certain cancers.[4] Pharmacogenomic mutations in the germ line provide some explanation for the interindividual and interracial variability in drug response and toxicity. For cancer chemotherapy, where cytotoxic agents are administered at doses close to their maximal tolerable dose, and therapeutic windows are relatively narrow, minor differences in individual drug handling may lead to severe toxicities. Therefore, an understanding of the sources of this variability would lead to the possibility of individualizing dosages or influencing clinical decisions that can improve patient care. Pharmacogenomics has putative utility in therapy selection, clinical study design, and as a tool to improve understanding of the pharmacology of a medication.

The term *pharmacogenetics* was initially used to define inherited differences in drug effects and typically focused on individual candidate genes. The field of pharmacogenomics now includes genomewide association studies and is used to describe genetic variations in all aspects of drug absorption, distribution, metabolism, and excretion in addition to drug targets and their downstream pathways.[5] Table 16.1 illustrates some current clinical examples of genotype-guided cancer chemotherapy. Variations in the DNA sequences encoding these proteins may take the form of deletions, insertions, repeats, frameshift mutations, nonsense mutations, and missense mutations, resulting in an inactive, truncated, unstable, or otherwise dysfunctional protein. The most common change involves single nucleotide substitutions, called single-nucleotide polymorphisms (SNP), which occur at approximately 1 per 1,000 base pairs on the human genome. Variability in toxicity or activity can also be mediated by postgenomic events, at the level of RNA, protein, or functional activity.

PHARMACOGENOMICS OF TUMOR RESPONSE

Tumor response to chemotherapy is regulated by a complex, multigenic network of genes that encompasses inherent characteristics of the tumor, differentially activated pathways of cell signaling, proliferation and DNA repair, factors that control drug delivery to the tumor cells (e.g., metabolism, transport), and cell death. These may in turn be modulated by previously administered treatment or drug exposure, which may upregulate target proteins or activate alternative pathways of drug resistance. The polygenic nature of drug response implies that a better understanding of genotype–phenotype associations would require more than the usual single-gene pharmacogenetic strategies employed to date. However, there are instances where the genomic context of a single gene within a cancer will be of high impact for specific therapeutic agents (see Table 16.1).

Pathway Directed Anticancer Therapy

One of the earliest success stories illustrating pathway-driven therapeutics is with CML. The hallmark chromosomal abnormality of this disease is the translocation of chromosomes 9 and 22 that ultimately produces the fusion gene *BCR-ABL*. This discovery in 1960 eventually led to the development of the targeted tyrosine-kinase inhibitor (TKI) imatinib and its subsequent Food and Drug Administration (FDA) approval for treatment of CML in 2001.[6] The International Randomized Study of Interferon and STI571 (IRIS) trial began enrollment in 2000 and compared imatinib with interferon and low-dose cytarabine, which was the previous standard of care for newly diagnosed patients with chronic-phase CML. All efficacy endpoints favored imatinib, including complete cytogenetic response of 76.2% with imatinib compared with 14.5% with interferon (p <0.001).[7] Overall survival (OS) after 60 months of follow-up was 89% with imatinib.[8] This example is just one of many where a once fatal disease can now be considered more akin to a chronic disease, requiring a daily medication and regular physician follow-up, similar to hypertension or diabetes. Drug development has also kept pace with these advances and now several other agents, including dasatinib, nilotinib, bosutinib, and ponatinib, have joined imatinib as treatment options for CML.

The idea of changing treatment focus from a disease-based model to a pathway-driven model is also evolving. Human epidermal

TABLE 16.1

Clinical Examples of Genotype-Guided Cancer Chemotherapy

Somatic Mutation Examples		
Drug Target	**Drug(s)**	**Malignancy**
EML4-ALK	Crizotinib	Non–small-cell lung cancer
BCR-ABL	Dasatinib, imatinib, nilotinib, bosutinib, ponatinib	Chronic myelogenous leukemia
BRAF	Vemurafenib, dabrafenib	Melanoma
Epidermal growth factor receptor (EGFR)	Erlotinib, afatinib	Non–small-cell lung cancer
HER2	Trastuzumab, lapatinib, pertuzumab, Ado-trastuzumab emtansine	Breast cancer, gastric cancer
Janus kinase 2 (JAK2)	Ruxolitinib	Myelofibrosis
Kirsten rat sarcoma viral oncogene (KRAS)	Cetuximab, panitumumab	Colorectal cancer
Rearranged during transfection (RET)	Vandetanib	Medullary thyroid cancer
Germ-Line Mutation Examples		
Gene Mutation	**Drug**	**Effect**
Cytochrome P450 (CYP) 2C19	Voriconazole	Decreased serum levels of active drug and potential decreased efficacy in patients with high enzyme levels (ultrarapid metabolizers)
CYP2D6	Tamoxifen, codeine, ondansetron	Decreased production of active metabolite and potential decreased efficacy in patients with low enzyme levels
Dihydropyrimidine dehydrogenase (DPYD)	5-Fluorouracil	Decreased elimination and increased risk of myelosuppression, diarrhea, and mucositis in patients with low enzyme levels
Glucose-6-phosphate dehydrogenase (G6PD)	Rasburicase	Risk of severe hemolysis in patients with G6PD deficiency
Thiopurine methyltransferase (TPMT)	Mercaptopurine, thioguanine, azathioprine	Decreased methylation of the active metabolite resulting decreased elimination and increased risk of neutropenia in patients with low enzyme levels
UDP-glucuronosyltransferase (UGT) 1A1	Irinotecan	Decreased glucuronidation of the active metabolite resulting decreased elimination and increased risk of neutropenia and diarrhea in patients with low enzyme levels

CANCER THERAPEUTICS

growth factor receptor 2 (HER2) is a transmembrane receptor tyrosine kinase that is overexpressed or amplified in up to 25% of breast cancers. Trastuzumab is a humanized monoclonal antibody directed against HER2 and demonstrated improved response rates (RR) and time to disease progression in patients with metastatic HER2 positive breast cancer and improved disease-free survival (DFS) and OS in HER2-positive breast cancer patients treated with adjuvant trastuzumab.[9] Several additional agents are now available to target the HER2 pathway and vary in their pharmacology and mechanism of action. Lapatinib is an oral TKI directed against HER2 and the epidermal growth factor receptor (EGFR), pertuzumab is a humanized monoclonal antibody that binds at a different location than trastuzumab and inhibits the dimerization and subsequent activation of HER2 signaling, and ado-trastuzumab emtansine is an antibody-drug conjugate that targets HER2-positive cells and then releases the cytotoxic antimitotic agent emtansine through liposomal degradation of the linking compound. All of these agents illustrate the progress and pharmacologic diversity of pathway-directed therapy and remain as standard of care options for HER2-positive breast cancer in either the adjuvant and/or metastatic settings.[10] HER2 expression is not limited to breast cancer, however. Though less common, HER2 expression is seen in numerous solid tumors including bladder, gastric, prostate and non–small-cell lung cancer with varying

degrees of incidence depending on the method of detection. Based on results from a large, open-label phase III randomized, international trial of 594 patients with gastric or gastroesophageal junction cancer expressing HER2 by either immunohistochemistry or gene amplification by fluorescence in situ hybridization, trastuzumab is also approved for treatment of metastatic gastric or gastroesophageal junction adenocarcinoma that expresses HER2. Patients randomized to chemotherapy in combination with trastuzumab had a median OS of 13.8 months compared with 11.1 months in the patients receiving chemotherapy alone (hazard ratio [HR], 0.74; 0.60 to 0.91, p = 0.0046).[11] Numerous examples also support that pathway-directed therapy will cross the boundaries of disease sites and that tumor genetics will become one of the biggest determining factors for treatment.

Simple expression of the drug target does not always translate into desired clinical outcomes though. Cetuximab and panitumumab are monoclonal antibodies directed against EGFR; however, it was found that colorectal cancer (CRC) patients who did not have detectable EGFR still experienced responses to these agents similar in extent to EGFR-positive patients. Kirsten rat sarcoma viral oncogene (KRAS) is a downstream effector of the EGFR pathway. Ligand binding to EGFR on the cell surface activates pathway signaling through the KRAS-RAF-mitogen-activated protein kinase (MAPK) pathway, which is thought to control cell growth, differentiation, and apoptosis.[12] Eventually it was found that CRC patients with a KRAS mutation did not derive benefit from cetuximab or panitumumab. The RR in CRC receiving either cetuximab or panitumumab who were KRAS wild type was 10% to 40% compared with near zero percent in those with KRAS mutations.[13] This finding was the result of a retrospective analysis of small group of patients and was confirmed in large, prospective trials. Additionally, it underscores the importance of tissue collection for biomarker assessment in trials with novel therapeutics. A recent clinical trial genomic analysis suggests that mutations in *NRAS* may also have value in predicting the utility of EGFR antibody therapy in colorectal cancer. Although the predictive value of KRAS mutation status in colorectal cancer has been well established in clinical trials, the role of KRAS in lung cancer and other malignancies is less well elucidated. Lung cancers harboring KRAS mutations have been shown to have less clinical benefit from the EGFR-targeted erlotinib in some trials, although this has not consistently been the case across all trials. Additionally, lung cancer KRAS mutation status does not appear to reproducibly predict clinical benefit from the EGFR-targeted monoclonal antibodies, as is the case in colorectal cancer.[14] Unlike the HER2 example discussed previously, the clinical application of some genetic mutations will differ between tissue of origin.

Deeper investigations and understandings of mutations driving oncogenic pathways can also elucidate mechanisms of resistance and practical therapeutic strategies for treatment and prevention. Approximately half of all cutaneous melanomas carry mutations in *BRAF*, with the most common being the V600E mutation. Vemurafenib is a TKI directed against mutated BRAF that demonstrated improvements in both progression-free survival (PFS) and OS when compared with the cytotoxic agent dacarbazine in previously untreated patients with metastatic melanoma carrying the BRAF V600E mutation. Vemurafenib demonstrated a 63% relative reduction in the risk of death compared with dacarbazine (p <0.001) along with a higher response rate (48% compared with 5% for dacarbazine).[15] Based on these results, vemurafenib was the first BRAF targeted TKI approved by the FDA and was soon joined by dabrafenib. Although dramatic responses to these agents have been observed, relapse almost universally occurs after a median of 6 to 8 months. Activating BRAF mutations, like V600E, result in uncontrolled activity of the MAPK pathway through activation of the downstream kinase MEK, which when phosphorylated, subsequently activates extracellular signal-regulated kinase (ERK), which ultimately translocates to the cell nucleus, resulting in cell proliferation and survival (Fig. 16.1).[16] An assessment of serial biopsies from patients treated with vemurafenib suggested numerous mechanisms for acquired resistance, including the appearance of secondary mutations in MEK.[17] This finding supports the clinical rationale for using combination therapy with a BRAF and a MEK inhibitor. The combination of dabrafenib (BRAF inhibitor) and trametinib (MEK inhibitor) was assessed in 247 metastatic melanoma patients with BRAF V600 mutations compared with dabrafenib alone. Median PFS was 9.4 months in the combination group compared with 5.8 months in the patients who received single agent therapy (HR, 0.39; 0.25 to 0.62, p <0.001). A complete or partial response was also higher in the combination therapy group (76% compared with 54%, p = 0.03). The occurrence of cutaneous squamous cell carcinoma, a known side effect of single-agent BRAF inhibitor therapy due to paradoxical activation of RAF in nonmutated cells, was also decreased in the combination therapy group (7% compared with 19%, p = 0.09), further supporting the evidence of downstream inhibition.[18] Although combination therapy does prolong the time to disease progression, resistance still occurs in patients through a variety of mechanisms. Utilization of sequential biopsies and a genetic assessment will help to inform rationale combination and sequential pathway-driven therapy trials that will ultimately aid in better understanding and mitigation of common mechanism of resistance.

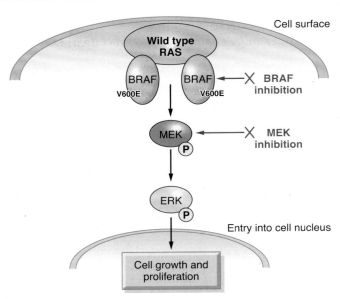

Figure 16.1 MAPK pathway in BRAF mutated melanoma. The BRAF V600E mutation results in activation of the MAPK pathway independent of growth factor binding, initially by phosphorylation (P) of MEK. MEK subsequently phosphorylates ERK. ERK then translocates to the cell nucleus and causes transcription of cellular factors, resulting in cell proliferation and survival. Because one mechanism of resistance to BRAF inhibition is through mutations in MEK, inhibition at both the upstream target of BRAF and the downstream site of MEK can prolong the clinical benefit of the BRAF inhibitor.

Although advances in basic science and drug development have translated many oncogenic driver mutations across tumor types into pathway-directed therapy, this is not the case for the majority. There are numerous examples of functionally relevant recurrent driver mutations that affect protein targets that are not currently druggable. Regardless of malignancy, one of the most commonly mutated tumor suppressors is the protein p53. Mutations can result in p53 acquiring oncogenic functions that enable proliferation, invasion, metastasis, and cell survival as well as coordinating with different proteins, such as EGFR, to enhance or inhibit its effects. However, a clinical application of p53 mutation data or directly targeting p53 has been limited, to date.[19] *PIK3CA* encodes a catalytic subunit of phophoinositol-3 kinase (PI3K), which includes four distinct subfamily kinases involved in regulating cell growth, motility, proliferation, and survival. Direct inhibitors of the kinase, as well as downstream targets, including AKT (protein kinase B [PKB]) and mammalian target of rapamycin (mTOR), are being assessed to target these mutations. Therapeutic challenges include understanding the complex signaling network germane to each cancer and the role of kinases in each subfamily.[20] Both the examples of p53 and PI3K illustrate the challenge of translating the multitude of somatic mutations into applications of available therapeutic agents.

Application of Genomewide Gene Expression Profiling to Guide Therapy

Single gene approaches may not reflect the overall complexity of genetic regulation of chemotherapy responses. Genomic strategies using global gene expression data are able to provide a more complete picture of the tumor through disease classification.[21] These strategies may identify subgroups of patients with early disease that need adjuvant chemotherapy, those who will not benefit from standard therapy, or help with the selection of chemotherapy from a menu of potentially active agents. Oncotype Dx is a 21-gene assay with 16 tumor-associated genes and 5 reference genes used to predict the risk of distant local recurrence in estrogen receptor (ER)-positive, HER2-negative patients with node-negative or select node-positive breast cancer. Additionally, the test also provides predictive information on which patients may benefit from the addition of chemotherapy to hormonal therapy alone. The test ultimately reports a recurrence score (RS) on a continuous scale from zero to 100. Patients with an RS <18 are considered low risk, with a 10-year distant recurrence rate (DRR) of 6.8% (95% confidence interval [CI], 4 to 9.6); RS scores of 18 to 30 are at intermediate risk, with a 10-year DRR of 14.3% (CI, 8.3 to 20.3); and RS scores ≥31 are at high risk, with a 10-year DRR of 30.5% (CI, 23.6 to 37.4).[22] Additionally, high-risk patients have the largest benefit from the addition of chemotherapy to hormonal therapy (HR, 0.26; 0.13 to 0.53), whereas low-risk patients have little benefit from the addition of chemotherapy and could consider hormonal treatment alone (HR, 1.31; 0.46 to 3.78). Intermediate risk patients are harder to classify, and clinical trials are underway to further address treatment recommendations for this group of patients.[23] These type of assays are also in development and in clinical trials for a variety of other solid tumor and hematologic malignancies.

Genetic-Guided Therapy Practical Issues in Somatic Analysis

Currently, targeted DNA capture is the most common type of somatic genetic screening and involves focusing on a few relevant candidate genes followed by deeper sequencing. These types of techniques can reveal common genes associated with a particular malignancy but also may uncover a signaling pathway that would not be obviously associated with a particular histology or tumor site. Application of a next-generation sequencing assay in 40 CRC and 24 non–small-cell lung cancer (NSCLC) tissue samples that assessed 145 cancer-relevant genes demonstrated that somatic mutations were seen in 98% of the CRC tumors and 83% of the NSCLCs (Fig. 16.2).[24] The evolution of sequencing strategies and decreasing costs has made whole genome sequencing more available in the clinical setting, and several companies offer commercially available tumor profiling services. Several limitations exist that currently restrict the broad clinical implementation of these assays, however. Although germ-line genetic assessments can be done on a peripheral blood sample or buccal swab, somatic assessments typically require biopsy tissue, which is often in limited supply and of varying quality or may not be feasible depending on the site of the cancer. Ongoing studies are assessing the

value of liquid biopsies of circulating tumor DNA.[25] Optimizing and creating uniformity in quality control of gene panel or whole-genome assessment is also needed to decrease the reporting of uncertain or erroneous identification of mutations. Once sequencing is completed, a predictive analysis is needed for the 25% to 80% of instances where variants of unknown significance are identified in genes of interest. Translation of genomic sequencing into clinical practice will require a diverse team, including pathologists, medical oncologists, surgical oncologists, information technologists, geneticists, and pharmacologists.

PHARMACOGENOMICS OF CHEMOTHERAPY DRUG TOXICITY

A drug's disposition and pharmacodynamic effects can be influenced by a number of variables, including patient age, diet, concomitant medications, and underlying disease processes. However, an individual's genetic constitution is an important regulator of variability in drug effect. Differences in drug effects are more pronounced between individuals compared to within an individual. Indeed, studies in monozygotic and dizygotic twins identified that 20% to 80% of the variation in drug disposition is mediated by inheritance.[26] Drug-metabolizing enzymes, cellular transporters, and tissue receptors are governed by genetic variation.

Advances in the treatment of most common malignancies have resulted in the availability of multiple distinct combination chemotherapy regimens with similar or equal anticancer efficacy. Therefore, differences in systemic toxicity have become a major determinant in the selection of therapy. The majority of pharmacogenomic examples affecting adverse events or efficacy from cytotoxic drugs involve hepatic metabolizing enzymes that detoxify or biotransform xenobiotics.[27,28]

Thiopurine Methyltransferase

One of the best-studied pharmacogenetic syndrome involves the metabolism of the thiopurine drugs—6-mercaptopurine (6MP), 6-thioguanine, and azathioprine—which have wide applications, including maintenance therapy for childhood ALL and adult leukemias. These prodrugs must be activated to thioguanine nucleotides in order to have antiproliferative effects. However, most of the variability in the formation of active metabolites is mediated by methylation via thiopurine methyltransferase (TPMT).[29] TPMT is a cytosolic enzyme that catalyzes S-methylation of thiopurine agents, resulting in an inactive metabolite. Erythrocyte TPMT activity has a trimodal distribution, with 90% of patients having high activity, 10% intermediate activity, and 0.3% with very low or no detectable activity. TPMT deficiency results in higher intracellular activation of 6MP to form thioguanine nucleotides, resulting in severe or fatal hematologic toxicity from standard doses of therapy.[30] The variable activity results from polymorphism in the TPMT gene, located on chromosome locus 6p22.3. Genetic variants at codon 238 (TPMT*2), codon 719 (TPMT*3C), or both codons 460 and 719 (TPMT*3A) are the most clinically significant, accounting for 95% of the patients with reduced TPMT activity.[31] Heterozygotes (one wild type and one variant allele) are common (10% of patients), and have elevated levels of active metabolites (twofold more than homozygous wild type), and required more cumulative dose reductions of 6MP for maintenance ALL chemotherapy compared to homozygous wild-type patients (Fig. 16.3).[32] Patients with a homozygous variant TPMT genotype are at a fourfold risk of severe toxicity, compared with wild-type patients.[31] TPMT genotype tests are now available commercially in a Clinical Laboratory Improvement Amendments (CLIA)-certified environment. To date, patients homozygous for TPMT variant alleles appear to tolerate 10%, and heterozygotes appear to tolerate 65% of the recommended doses of 6MP, with no apparent

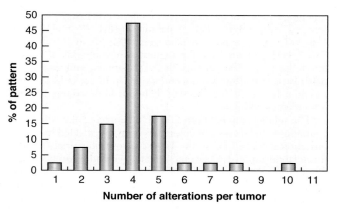

Figure 16.2 Number of alterations per tumor. Deep sequencing of 145 genes in 40 colorectal cancers found a spectrum of incidence of somatic mutations, with more than half occurring in genes that are *druggable* with medication that is either FDA approved or in late stage clinical development.

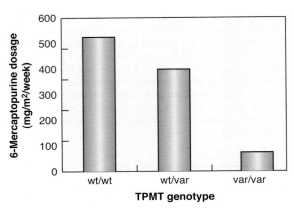

Figure 16.3 Relationship between TPMT genotype and required 6MP dose. Compared with homozygous wild-type patients, those heterozygous for a thiopurine methyltransferase (TPMT) variant allele generally require at least a 30% dose reduction in 6MP, whereas homozygous variant patients require substantial dose reductions of approximately 90% that of wild-type patients.

decrease in clinical efficacy (Fig. 16.3).[32] This has formed the basis for prospective, TPMT genotype-guided dosing of 6MP to avoid severe toxicity. Clinical Pharmacogenomics Implementation Consortium (CPIC) Guidelines recommend that homozygous wild-type patients be started at the full standard dose. Heterozygous patients should start with reduced doses at 30% to 70% of the full dose with adjustments made after 2 to 4 weeks based on myelosuppression and disease-specific guidelines. Homozygous variant patients should start with 10% of the full dose due to the extremely high levels of the active metabolite and potential for fatal toxicity at standard doses. Adjustments should be made after 4 to 6 weeks based on myelosuppression and disease-specific guidelines.[33]

Dihydropyrimidine Dehydrogenase (DPD)

Although 5-fluorouracil (5FU) has been available for over 40 years, it remains the cornerstone of colorectal cancer chemotherapy, both in the adjuvant and metastatic settings. Additionally, the oral prodrug capecitabine ultimately undergoes activation to 5FU and is commonly used in gastrointestinal and breast malignancies. 5FU is a prodrug that is activated intracellularly to 5-fluoro-2'-deoxyuridine monophosphate (5FdUMP), which inhibits thymidylate synthase (TS), among other mechanisms of action. TS inhibition results in impaired de novo pyrimidine synthesis and suppression of DNA synthesis. Approximately 85% of a 5FU dose is catabolized by dihydropyrimidine dehydrogenase (DPD) to inactive metabolites. Therefore, DPD is a primary regulator of 5FU activity. DPD deficiency has been described, resulting in higher 5FU blood levels, greater formation of active metabolites, and severe or fatal clinical toxicity, predominately myelosuppression, mucositis, and cerebellar toxicity.[34] In theory, this toxicity could be reduced or avoided by screening for DPD activity in surrogate tissues, such as peripheral mononuclear cells. However, the technical requirements for preparation of these samples make it impractical for many practice sites. Understanding the molecular basis for DPD deficiency will provide an approach for prospective identification of patients at high risk for severe 5FU toxicity. The gene encoding DPD is composed of 23 exons, and at least 23 SNPs have been found.[35] Studies in DPD-deficient patients have identified several distinct molecular variants associated with low enzyme activity. Many of these are rare, and base substitutions, splicing defects, and frame shift mutations, have been described. The prevalent variation is the splice recognition site in intron 14 (DPYD*2A), where a G to A substitution results in the skipping of exon 14, resulting in an inactive enzyme.[36–38] This polymorphism

has been associated with severe DPD deficiency in heterozygous patients, with a homozygous genotype associated with a mental retardation syndrome. Patients with severe 5FU toxicity may harbor one or more variant alleles of DPD, and a recent study showed that 61% of cancer patients experiencing severe 5FU toxicities had decreased DPD activity in peripheral mononuclear cells, and DPYD*2A was commonly found.[39] In the patients with grade 4 neutropenia, 50% harbored at least one DPYD*2A. It is estimated that in the Caucasian population, homozygotes for the variant alleles have an incidence of 0.1% and heterozygotes occur at an incidence of 0.5% to 2%. There are additional DPD mutations that have been associated with impaired enzyme activity, including DPYD*3 and DPYD*13. CPIC guidelines recommend standard dosing for homozygous wild-type patients. Reducing the dose by at least 50% in heterozygous patients (*1/*2A) is recommended, followed by dose adjustment based on toxicity and/or pharmacokinetic testing. The use of an alternative agent is recommended in homozygous-variant patients (*2A/*2A).[34] There are many patients with severe 5FU toxicity that have normal DPD activity. This highlights that many factors, including multiple genes, are potential causes of 5FU toxicity, and there will not be one simple test to avoid this important clinical problem.

Cytochrome P450 2D6

Tamoxifen is a selective estrogen-receptor modulator used in ER-positive breast cancer in both the localized and metastatic settings. It is the drug of choice for premenopausal women and is a treatment option, along with aromatase inhibitors, for postmenopausal women. The low cost of tamoxifen also makes it a preferred therapy regardless of menopausal status in numerous countries. Tamoxifen metabolism is complex, with extensive metabolism through numerous phase I and II enzymes that produce several primary and secondary metabolites and their corresponding isomers, each possessing different antiestrogen effects.[40] The primary active metabolite is believed to be endoxifen, which is produced by the CYP3A4/5 mediated-conversion of tamoxifen to N-desmethyltamoxifen, which is then further converted to endoxifen (4-hydroxy-N-desmethyltamoxifen) via cytochrome P450 2D6 (CYP2D6). A direct relationship between endoxifen concentration and its antiestrogen effects has been demonstrated, potentially suggesting that a threshold concentration may be needed for optimal clinical effect.[41] CYP2D6 is highly polymorphic, with more than 80 allelic CYP2D6 variants described. These alleles vary in enzyme activity and prevalence with respect to race and ethnicity.[42] Based on genotype, patients can be classified by phenotype into ultrarapid metabolizers (UM; approximately 1% to 2% of patients [common alleles include *1xN, *2xN]) who carry more than two functional allele copies, extensive metabolizers (EM; 77% to 92% [e.g., *1, *2]), intermediate metabolizers (IM; 2% to 11% [e.g., *10, *17, *41]), or poor metabolizers (PM; 5% to 10% [*3, *4, *5]).[43] UM patients have the highest concentrations of endoxifen, followed by EM patients, then IM patients, and finally, PM patients have the lowest concentration. Up to a sixfold variation in endoxifen levels may be seen between homozygous PM and homozygous EM patients.[40]

The relationship between CYP2D6 genotype, endoxifen concentrations, and disease outcomes has been investigated in numerous clinical trials. One of the largest retrospective trials assessed this relationship in 1,325 women treated with adjuvant tamoxifen 20 mg daily. Approximately 46% of the patients were classified as EM, 48% were IM, and 5.9% were PM. A statistically significant increased risk of disease recurrence was seen in the IM and PM patients compared with the EM patients (HR, 1.40; 95% CI, 1.04 to 1.90 for IM; and HR 1.90, 95% CI, 1.10 to 3.28 for PM).[44] A large meta-analysis of 4,973 tamoxifen-treated patients across 12 international studies conducted by the International Tamoxifen Pharmacogenomics Consortium also supported this relationship.

CYP2D6 PM phenotypes were associated with decreased DFS (HR 1.25, 95% CI, 1.06 to 1.47, p = 0.009) when only considering the data from trials with postmenopausal women with ER-positive breast cancer who received tamoxifen 20 mg daily for 5 years.[45]

Not all trial results have been consistent, however, and dosing guidelines for genotype-guided therapy do not yet exist. Clinical trials do support the potential for genotype-guided therapy. IM patients who received an increased dose of 40 mg daily instead of the standard 20 mg were shown to have endoxifen concentrations similar to that of EM patients (p = 0.25).[46] This suggests that genotype-guided therapy with increased dose recommendations may be feasible, but additional prospective trials are needed to determine the clinical efficacy of this intervention.

CONCLUSIONS AND FUTURE DIRECTIONS

Genomic-driven cancer medicine is being translated into clinical practice through increased understanding of somatic mutations in a specific tumor that can be translated to pathway-directed therapeutics as well as germ-line mutations that affect the pharmacokinetics and pharmacodynamics of individual medications. For the practicing oncologist, knowledge of pharmacogenomics is necessary because therapeutic decisions of drug selection and dosage are being based on more molecularly and genetically defined variables than the current phenotypic information of tumor type,

immunohistochemistry, and body surface area. Health-care policy changes preferring the bundling of care and reimbursement based on diagnosis coding may further drive individualized therapy where the goal is to optimize both treatment responses while minimizing toxicity. However, with advances always come challenges. Reimbursement for multiplex genomic testing is not universal, so deciding who and when to initiate testing is a consideration. Optimizing turnaround time, especially for referral patients who have had biopsies performed elsewhere, will require requesting this archived tissue prior to or during the initial patient visit to facilitate minimizing treatment delays. Although some variants have strong evidence supporting treatment recommendations, many currently do not yet. Multidisciplinary committees charged with reviewing the level of evidence for each genetic result and providing clinically actionable recommendations will be essential for translating these multigene tumor assay results into routine clinical practice. Decision tools and development of treatment guidelines will further assist with routine integration of this technology, especially for oncologists at smaller practice sites. Oncology fellowship training programs will also need to be expanded to ensure competence of new practitioners in the area of genomic-guided therapies.

Regardless of these challenges, the treatment paradigm of genomic-driven medicine and individualizing therapy has permitted the field of oncology to move beyond the limitations of nonselective cytotoxic therapy and toward the more optimal selection and dosing of oncology agents.

REFERENCES

1. McLeod HL. Cancer pharmacogenomics: early promise, but concerted effort needed. *Science* 2013;339:1563–1566.
2. Garraway LA. Genomics-driven oncology: framework for an emerging paradigm. *J Clin Oncol* 2013;31:1806–1814.
3. Mandrekar SJ, Sargent DJ. Predictive biomarker validation in practice: lessons from real trials. *Clin Trials* 2010;7:567–573.
4. Evans WE, Relling MV. Pharmacogenomics: translating functional genomics into rational therapeutics. *Science* 1999;286:487–491.
5. Wang L, McLeod HL, Weinshilboum RM. Genomics and drug response. *N Engl J Med* 2011;364:1144–1153.
6. Druker BJ. Translation of the Philadelphia chromosome into therapy for CML. *Blood* 2008;112:4808–4817.
7. O'Brien SG, Guilhot F, Larson RA, et al. Imatinib compared with interferon and low-dose cytarabine for newly diagnosed chronic-phase chronic myeloid leukemia. *N Engl J Med* 2003;348:994–1004.
8. Druker BJ, Guilhot F, O'Brien SG, et al. Five-year follow-up of patients receiving imatinib for chronic myeloid leukemia. *N Engl J Med* 2006;355:2408–2417.
9. Hudis CA. Trastuzumab—mechanism of action and use in clinical practice. *N Engl J Med* 2007;357:39–51.
10. Figueroa-Magalhaes MC, Jelovac D, Connolly RM, et al. Treatment of HER2-positive breast cancer. *Breast* 2014;23:128–136.
11. Bang YJ, Van Cutsem E, Feyereislova A, et al. Trastuzumab in combination with chemotherapy versus chemotherapy alone for treatment of HER2-positive advanced gastric or gastro-oesophageal junction cancer (ToGA): a phase 3, open-label, randomised controlled trial. *Lancet* 2010;76:687–697.
12. Bardelli A, Siena S. Molecular mechanisms of resistance to cetuximab and panitumumab in colorectal cancer. *J Clin Oncol* 2010;28:1254–1261.
13. Jimeno A, Messersmith WA, Hirsch FR, et al. KRAS mutations and sensitivity to epidermal growth factor receptor inhibitors in colorectal cancer: practical application of patient selection. *J Clin Oncol* 2009;27:1130–1136.
14. Roberts PJ, Stinchcombe TE, Der CJ, et al. Personalized medicine in non-small-cell lung cancer: is KRAS a useful marker in selecting patients for epidermal growth factor receptor-targeted therapy? *J Clin Oncol* 2010;28:4769–4777.
15. Chapman PB, Hauschild A, Robert C, et al. Improved survival with vemurafenib in melanoma with BRAF V600E mutation. *N Engl J Med* 2011;364:2507–2516.
16. Dhillon AS, Hagan S, Rath O, et al. MAP kinase signalling pathways in cancer. *Oncogene* 2007;26:3279–3290.
17. Trunzer K, Pavlick AC, Schuchter L, et al. Pharmacodynamic effects and mechanisms of resistance to vemurafenib in patients with metastatic melanoma. *J Clin Oncol* 2013;31:1767–1774.
18. Flaherty KT, Infante JR, Daud A, et al. Combined BRAF and MEK inhibition in melanoma with BRAF V600 mutations. *N Engl J Med* 2012;367:1694–1703.
19. Muller PA, Vousden KH. p53 mutations in cancer. *Nat Cell Biol* 2013;15:2–8.
20. Clarke PA, Workman P. Phosphatidylinositide-3-kinase inhibitors: addressing questions of isoform selectivity and pharmacodynamic/predictive biomarkers in early clinical trials. *J Clin Oncol* 2012;30:331–333.

21. Ramaswamy S, Golub T. DNA microarrays in clinical oncology. *J Clin Oncol* 2002;20:1932–1941.
22. Paik S, Shak S, Tang G, et al. A multigene assay to predict recurrence of tamoxifen-treated, node-negative breast cancer. *N Engl J Med* 2004;351:2817–2826.
23. Paik S, Tang G, Shak S, et al. Gene expression and benefit of chemotherapy in women with node-negative, estrogen receptor-positive breast cancer. *J Clin Oncol* 2006;24:3726–3734.
24. Lipson D, Capelletti M, Yelensky R, et al. Identification of new ALK and RET gene fusions from colorectal and lung cancer biopsies. *Nat Med* 2012;18:382–384.
25. Diaz LA Jr, Bardelli A. Liquid biopsies: genotyping circulating tumor DNA. *J Clin Oncol* 2014;32:579–586.
26. Watters J, McLeod H. Cancer pharmacogenomics: current and future applications. *Biochim Biophys Acta* 2003;1603:99–111.
27. Evans W, Relling M. Pharmacogenomics: translating functional genomics into rational therapeutics. *Science* 1999;286:487–491.
28. Deenen MJ, Cats A, Beijnen H, et al. Part 2: pharmacogenetic variability in drug transport and phase I anticancer drug metabolism. *Oncologist* 2011;16:820–834.
29. Krynetski E, Evans W. Drug methylation in cancer therapy: lessons from the TPMT polymorphism. *Oncogene* 2003;22:7403–7413.
30. McLeod H, Krynetski EY, Relling MV, et al. Genetic polymorphism of thiopurine methyltransferase and its clinical relevance for childhood acute lymphoblastic leukemia. *Leukemia* 2000;14:567–572.
31. Evans W, Hon YY, Bomgaars L, et al. Preponderance of thiopurine S-methyltransferase deficiency and heterozygosity among patients intolerant to mercaptopurine or azathioprine. *J Clin Oncol* 2001;19:2293–2301.
32. Relling M, Hancock ML, Rivera GK, et al. Mercaptopurine therapy intolerance and heterozygosity at the thiopurine S-methyltransferase gene locus. *J Natl Cancer Inst* 1999;91:2001–2008.
33. Relling MV, Gardner EE, Sandborn WJ, et al. Clinical pharmacogenetics implementation consortium guidelines for thiopurine methyltransferase genotype and thiopurine dosing: 2013 update. *Clin Pharmacol Ther* 2013;93:324–325.
34. Caudle KE, Thorn CF, Klein TE, et al. Clinical Pharmacogenetics Implementation Consortium guidelines for dihydropyrimidine dehydrogenase genotype and fluoropyrimidine dosing. *Clin Pharmacol Ther* 2013;94:640–645.
35. McLeod H, Collie-Duguid ES, Vreken P, et al. Nomenclature for human DPYD alleles. *Pharmacogenetics* 1998;8:455–459.
36. Wei X, Elizondo G, Sapone A, et al. Characterization of the human dihydropyrimidine dehydrogenase gene. *Genomics* 1998;51:391–400.
37. Ridge S, Sludden J, Wei X, et al. Dihydropyrimidine dehydrogenase pharmacogenetics in patients with colorectal cancer. *Br J Cancer* 1998;77:497–500.
38. Johnson M, Wang K, Diasio R. Profound dihydropyrimidine dehydrogenase deficiency resulting from a novel compound heterozygote genotype. *Clin Cancer Res* 2002;8:768–774.
39. Van Kuilenburg A, Meinsma R, Zoetekouw L, et al. Increased risk of grade IV neutropenia after administration of 5-fluorouracil due to a dihydropyrimidine dehydrogenase deficiency: high prevalence of the IVS14+1g>a mutation. *Int J Cancer* 2002;101:253–258.

40. Mürdter TE, Schroth W, Bacchus-Gerybadze L, et al. Activity levels of tamoxifen metabolites at the estrogen receptor and the impact of genetic polymorphisms of phase I and II enzymes on their concentration levels in plasma. *Clin Pharmacol Ther* 2011;89:708–717.

41. Desta Z, Ward BA, Soukhova NV, et al. Comprehensive evaluation of tamoxifen sequential biotransformation by the human cytochrome P450 system in vitro: prominent roles for CYP3A and CYP2D6. *J Pharmacol Exp Ther* 2004;310:1062–1075.

42. Bradford LD. CYP2D6 allele frequency in European Caucasians, Asians, Africans and their descendants. *Pharmacogenomics* 2002;3:229–243.

43. Crews KR, Gaedigk A, Dunnenberger HM, et al. Clinical Pharmacogenetics Implementation Consortium (CPIC) guidelines for codeine therapy in the context of cytochrome P450 2D6 (CYP2D6) genotype. *Clin Pharmacol Ther* 2012;91:321–326.

44. Schroth W, Goetz MP, Hamann U, et al. Association between CYP2D6 polymorphisms and outcomes among women with early stage breast cancer treated with tamoxifen. JAMA 2009;302:1429–1436.

45. Province MA, Goetz MP, Brauch H, et al. CYP2D6 genotype and adjuvant tamoxifen: meta-analysis of heterogeneous study populations. *Clin Pharmacol Ther* 2014;95:216–227.

46. Irvin WJ Jr, Walko CM, Weck KE, et al. Genotype-guided tamoxifen dosing increases active metabolite exposure in women with reduced CYP2D6 metabolism: a multicenter study. *J Clin Oncol* 2011;29:3232–3239.

17 Alkylating Agents

Kenneth D. Tew

PERSPECTIVES

Alkylating agents were the first anticancer molecules developed, and they are still used today. After more than 50 years of use, the basic chemistry and pharmacology of this drug family is well understood and has not changed substantially. The family contains six major classes: nitrogen mustards, aziridines, alkyl sulfonates, epoxides, nitrosoureas, and triazene compounds, although a few nonstandard agents have recently been developed. Most epoxides tend to be quite nonspecific with respect to their reactivity and, as such, few have useful clinical characteristics. This chapter provides perspective on how the limited varieties of alkylating agents continue to be useful in the therapeutic management of cancer patients.

The alkylating agents are a diverse group of anticancer agents with the commonality that they react in a manner such that an electrophilic alkyl group or a substituted alkyl group can covalently bind to cellular nucleophilic sites. Electrophilicity is achieved through the formation of carbonium ion intermediates and can result in transition complexes with target molecules. Ultimately, reactions result in the formation of covalent linkages by alkylation with a broad range of nucleophilic groups, including bases in DNA, and these are believed responsible for ultimate cytotoxicity and therapeutic effect. Although the alkylating agents react with cells in all phases of the cell cycle, their efficacy and toxicity result from interference with rapidly proliferating tissues. From a historical perspective, the vesicant properties of mustard gas used during World War I were shown to be accompanied by the suppression of lymphoid and hematologic functions in experimental animals[1] and led to the development of mechlorethamine as the first alkylating agent used in the management of human cancer.[2] Subsequently, a number of related drugs have been developed, and these have roles in the treatment of a range of leukemias, lymphomas, and solid tumors. Most of the alkylating agents cause dose-limiting toxicities to the bone marrow and, to a lesser degree, the intestinal mucosa, with other organ systems also affected contingent on the individual drug, dosage, and duration of therapy. Despite the present trend toward targeted therapies, this class of "nonspecific" drugs maintains an essential role in cancer chemotherapy.

Because of the classic nature of the drug family, there have been relatively few advances in either their use or utility since publication of the previous edition of this book.

CHEMISTRY

Alkylating reactions are generally classified through their kinetic properties as S_N1 (nucleophilic substitution, first order) or S_N2 (nucleophilic substitution, second order) (Fig. 17.1). The first-order kinetics of the S_N1 reactions depend on the concentration of the original alkylating agent. The rate-limiting step is the initial formation of the reactive intermediate, and the rate is essentially independent of the concentration of the substrate. The S_N2 alkylation reaction is a bimolecular nucleophilic displacement with second-order kinetics, where the rate depends on the concentration of both alkylating agent and target nucleophile. Reactivity of electrophiles[3] suggests that the rates of alkylation of cellular nucleophiles (including thiols, phosphates, amino and imidazole groups of amino acids, and various reactive sites in nucleic acid bases) are most dependent on their potential energy states, which can be defined as "hard" or "soft," based on the polarizability of their reactive centers.[4] Although the metabolism and metabolites of nitrogen mustards and nitrosoureas differ, the active alkylating species of each is the alkyl carbonium ion (see Fig. 17.1), a highly polarized hard electrophile as a consequence of its highly positive charge density at the electrophilic center. Alkyl carbonium ions will react most readily with hard nucleophiles (possessing a highly polarized negative charge density), where the high-energy transition state (a potential energy barrier to the reaction) is most favorable. In specific terms, an active alkylating species from a nitrogen mustard will demonstrate selectivity for cellular nucleophiles in the following order: (1) oxygen in phosphate groups of RNA and DNA, (2) oxygens of purines and pyrimidines, (3) amino groups of purine bases, (4) primary and secondary amino groups of proteins, (5) sulfur atoms of methionine, and (6) thiol groups of cysteinyl residues of protein and glutathione.[3] The least favored reactions will still occur, but at much slower rates unless they are catalyzed.

Alkylation through highly reactive intermediates (e.g., mechlorethamine) would be expected to be less selective in their targets than the less reactive S_N2 reagents (e.g., busulfan). However, the therapeutic and toxic effects of alkylating agents do not correlate directly with their chemical reactivity. Clinically useful agents include drugs with S_N1 or S_N2 characteristics, and some with both.[5] These differ in their toxicity profiles and antitumor activity, but more as a consequence of differences in pharmacokinetics, lipid solubility, penetration of the central nervous system (CNS), membrane transport, metabolism and detoxification, and specific enzymatic reactions capable of repairing alkylation sites on DNA.

CLASSIFICATION

The major classes of clinically useful alkylating agents are illustrated in Table 17.1 and summarized in the following sections. Doses and schedules of the various agents are shown in Table 17.2.

Alkyl Sulfonates

Busulfan is used for the treatment of chronic myelogenous leukemia. It exhibits S_N2 alkylation kinetics and shows nucleophilic selectivity for thiol groups, suggesting that it may exert cytotoxicity through protein alkylation rather than through DNA. In contrast to the nitrogen mustards and nitrosoureas, busulfan has a greater effect on myeloid cells than lymphoid cells, thus the reason for its use against chronic myelogenous leukemia.[6]

Aziridines

Aziridines are analogs of ring-closed intermediates of nitrogen mustards and are less chemically reactive, but they have

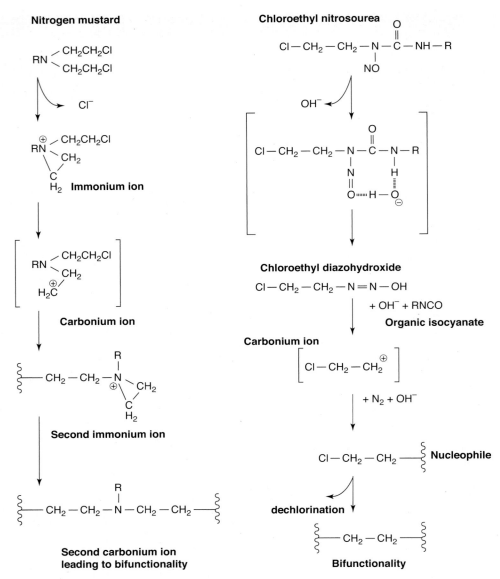

Figure 17.1 Comparative decomposition and metabolism of a typical nitrogen mustard compared to a nitrosourea. Although intermediate metabolites are distinct, the active alkylating species is a carbonium ion in each case. This electrophilic moiety reacts with target cellular nucleophiles.

equivalent therapeutic properties. Thiotepa has been used in the treatment of carcinoma of the breast, ovary, for a variety of CNS diseases, and with increasing frequency as a component of high-dose chemotherapy regimens.[7] Thiotepa and its primary desulfurated metabolite triethylenethiophosphoramide (TEPA) alkylate through aziridine ring openings, a mechanism similar to the nitrogen mustards.

Triazines

Perhaps the newest clinical development in the alkylating agent field is the emergence of temozolomide (TMZ). This agent acts as a prodrug and is an imidazotetrazine analog that undergoes spontaneous activation in solution to produce 5-(3-methyltriazen-1-yl) imidazole-4-carboxamide (MTIC), a triazine derivative. It crosses the blood–brain barrier with concentrations in the CNS approximating 30% of plasma concentrations.[8] Resistance to the methylating agent occurs quite frequently and has adversely affected the rate and durability of the clinical responses of patients. However, because of its favorable toxicity and pharmacokinetics, TMZ is

being combined with numerous other classes of anticancer drugs in an effort to improve response rates in diseases such as malignant melanomas, gliomas, brain metastasis from solid tumors, and refractory leukemias. Many of these trials are currently underway.[9]

Nitrogen Mustards

Bischloroethylamines or nitrogen mustards are extensively administered in the clinic. As an initial step in alkylation, chlorine acts as a leaving group and the β-carbon reacts with the nucleophilic nitrogen atom to form the cyclic, positively charged, reactive aziridinium moiety. Reaction of the aziridinium ring with an electron-rich nucleophile creates an initial alkylation product. The remaining chloroethyl group achieves bifunctionality through the formation of a second aziridinium. Melphalan (L-phenylalanine mustard), chlorambucil, cyclophosphamide, and ifosfamide (see Table 17.1) replaced mechlorethamine as primary therapeutic agents. These derivatives have electron-withdrawing groups substituted on the nitrogen atom, reducing the nucleophilicity of the nitrogen and rendering them less reactive, but enhancing their antitumor efficacy.

TABLE 17.1

Major Classes of Clinically Useful Alkylating Agents

Drug	Main Therapeutic Uses	Clinical Pharmacology	Major Toxicities	Notes
ALKYL SULFONATES				
Busulfan	Bone marrow transplantation, especially in chronic myelogenous leukemia	Bioavailability, 80%; protein bound, 33%; $t_{1/2}$, 2.5 h	Pulmonary fibrosis, hyperpigmentation thrombocytopenia, lowered blood platelet count and activity	Oral or parenteral; high dose causes hepatic veno-occlusive disease
ETHYLENEIMINES/METHYLMELAMINES				
Altretamine		Protein bound, 94%; $t_{1/2}$, 5–10 h	Nausea, vomiting, diarrhea, and neurotoxicity	Not widely used
Thio TEPA	Breast, ovarian, and bladder cancer; also bone marrow transplant	$t_{1/2}$, 2.5 h; urinary excretion at 24 h, 25%; substrate for CYP2B6 and CYP2C11	Myelosuppression	Nadirs of leukopenia, occur 2 wk; thrombocytopenia, 3 wk (correlates with AUC of parent drug)
NITROGEN MUSTARDS				
Mechlorethamine	Hodgkin lymphoma		Nausea, vomiting, myelosuppression	Precursor for other clinical mustards
Melphalan (L-phenylalanine mustard)	Multiple myeloma and ovarian cancer, and occasionally malignant melanoma	Bioavailability 25%–90%; $t_{1/2}$, 1.5 h; urinary excretion at 24 h, 13%; clearance, 9 mL/min/kg	Nausea, vomiting, myelosuppression	Causes less mucosal damage than others in class
Chlorambucil	Chronic lymphocytic leukemia	$t_{1/2}$, 1.5 h; urinary excretion at 24 h, 50%	Myelosuppression, gastrointestinal distress, CNS, skin reactions, hepatotoxicity	Oral
Cyclophosphamide	Variety of lymphomas, leukemias, and solid tumors	Bioavailability, >75%; protein bound, >60%; $t_{1/2}$, 3–12 h; urinary excretion at 24 h, <15%	Nausea and vomiting, bone marrow suppression, diarrhea, darkening of the skin/nails, alopecia (hair loss), lethargy, hemorrhagic cystitis	IV; primary excretion route is urine
Ifosfamide	Testicular, breast cancer; lymphoma (non-Hodgkin); soft tissue sarcoma; osteogenic sarcoma; lung, cervical, ovarian, bone cancer	$t_{1/2}$, 15 h; urinary excretion at 24 h, 15%	As for cyclophosphamide	Ifosfamide is often used in conjunction with mesna to avoid cystinuria
NITROSOUREAS				
Carmustine	Glioma, glioblastoma multiforme, medulloblastoma and astrocytoma, multiple myeloma and lymphoma (Hodgkin and non-Hodgkin)	Bioavailability, 25%; protein bound, 80%; $t_{1/2}$, 30 min	Bone marrow and pulmonary toxicities are a function of lifetime cumulative dose	Clinically, nitrosoureas do not share cross-resistance with nitrogen mustards in lymphoma treatment
Streptozotocin	Cancers of the islets of Langerhans	$t_{1/2}$, 35 min; excreted in the urine (15%), feces (<1%), and in the expired air	Nausea and vomiting; nephrotoxicity can range from transient protein urea and azotemia to permanent tubular damage; can also cause aberrations of glucose metabolism	A natural product from *Streptomyces achromogenes*
TRIAZENES				
Dacarbazine	Malignant melanoma and Hodgkin lymphoma	$t_{1/2}$, 5 h; protein bound, 5% hepatic metabolism	Nausea, vomiting, myelosuppression	IV or IM
Temozolomide	Glioblastoma; astrocytoma; metastatic melanoma	Protein bound, 15%; $t_{1/2}$, 1.8 h; clearance, 5.5 l/h/m^2	Nausea, vomiting, myelosuppression	Oral; derivative of imidazotetrazine, prodrug of dacarbazine; rapidly absorbed

$t_{1/2}$, half-life; TEPA, triethylenethiophosphoramide; AUC, area under curve; CNS, central nervous system; IV, intravenous; IM, intramuscular.

CANCER THERAPEUTICS

TABLE 17.2

Dose and Schedules of Clinically Useful Alkylating Agents

Alkylating Agent	Disease Sites and Dose Ranges Used Clinically	Notes

BCNU (Carmustine)	General antineoplastic
	150–200 mg/m^2 (IV, every 6 wks)
	Cutaneous T-cell lymphoma 200–600 mg
	  (topical solution)
	Adjunct to surgical resection of brain tumor
	  61.6 mg (implant)
		Infusion 1–2 h; in combination, dose usually reduced by
		  25%–50%
		Side effects include irritant dermatitis, telangiectasia,
		  erythema, and bone marrow suppression
		Up to 8 wafers (7.7 mg of carmustine) implanted

Busulfan	Chronic myelogenous leukemia and myeloproliferative disorders 4–8 mg (daily PO) 1.8 mg/m^2 (daily PO) Bone marrow transplant 640 mg/m^2 (daily PO)	Dispensed over 3–4 d, with cyclophosphamide

Carboplatin	Advanced ovarian cancer—monotherapy
	360 mg/m^2 (IV, every 4 wks)
	Ovarian cancer—combination
	300 mg/m^2 (IV, every 4 wks for 6 cycles)
	Ovarian cancer—IP
	200–500 mg/m^2 (IP, 2 L dialysis fluid)
	Ovarian and other sites phase 1/2 setting—
	  high-dose therapy
	800–1,600 mg/m^2 (IV)
		With cyclophosphamide
		Patients usually receive marrow transplantation or
		  peripheral stem cell support

Cisplatin	Metastatic testicular cancer:
	20 mg/m^2/d for 5 d of each cycle (IV)
	Metastatic ovarian cancer:
	75–100 mg/m^2 (IV, once every 4 wks)
	Head and neck cancer:
	100 mg/m^2 (IV)
	Bladder cancer:
	(combination prior to cystectomy)
	50–70; initiate dosing at 50
	mg/m^2 (IV, once every 3–4 wks)
	Metastatic breast cancer:
	20 mg/m^2 (IV, days 1–5 every 3 wks)
	Cervical cancer:
	70 mg/m^2 (IV, dosing cycled every 4 wks)
	Non–small-cell lung cancer:
	75 mg/m^2 (IV, every 3 wks)
	Esophageal cancer:
	75 mg/m^2 on day 1 of wks 1, 5, 8, and 11 (IV)
		With other antineoplastic agents
		With cyclophosphamide (600 mg/m^2 once every 4 wks)
		With vincristine, bleomycin, and fluorouracil
		With methotrexate and fluorouracil
		MVAC regimen (methotrexate, vinblastine, doxorubicin,
		  and cisplatin) used for cervical cancer
		Administration preceded by paclitaxel 135 mg/m^2
		  every 3 wks
		With radiation therapy

Cyclophosphamide	General antineoplastic
	1–5 mg/kg (daily PO)
	40–50 mg/kg (IV, in divided doses over 2–5 d)
	40–50 mg/kg (IV, in divided doses over 2–5 d)
	10–15 mg/kg (IV, every 7–10 d)
	10–15 mg/kg (IV, every 7–10 d)
	3–5 mg/kg (IV twice per wk)
	High-dose regimen in bone marrow transplantation
	  and for other autoimmune disorders
	200 mg/kg (IV)
	1–2.5 mg/kg (daily PO 7–14 d/mo)
		Dose used as monotherapy for patients with no
		  hematologic toxicity

Dacarbazine	General antineoplastic 2–4.5 mg/kg/d (IV) 150 mg/m^2/d (IV)	Administered for 10 d, may be repeated at 4-week intervals With other anticancer agents; treatment lasts 5 d, may be repeated every 4 wks

Etoposide	Testicular cancer
	50–100 mg/m^2/day (IV, slow infusion over
	  30–60+ min for 5 d)
	Small cell lung cancer
	35–50 mg/m^2/day (IV, slow infusion over
	  30–60+ min for 4–5 d)
		Alternatively, 100 mg/m^2/d on days 1, 3, and 5 may
		  be used; doses for combination therapy and are
		  repeated at 3- to 4-wk intervals after recovery from
		  hematologic toxicity
		Doses are for combination therapy and repeated at 3- to
		  4-wk intervals after recovery from hematologic toxicity;
		  oral dose is twice the IV, rounded to the nearest 50 mg

(continued)

TABLE 17.2

Dose and Schedules of Clinically Useful Alkylating Agents *(continued)*

Ifosfamide	General antineoplastic 1.2 g/m^2/d (IV, for 5 consecutive days)	Repeat every 3 wks
Melphalan	Multiple myeloma: 16 mg/m^2 (IV, infusion over 15–20 min) 6 mg (daily PO) Epithelial ovarian cancer: 0.2 mg/kg (daily PO)	2-week intervals for 4 doses, 4-wk intervals thereafter After 2–3 wks treatment, should be discontinued for up to 4 wks, then reinstituted at 2–4 mg/d Daily dose for a 5-d course, repeated every 4–5 wks

Streptozotocin	Pancreatic tumors
	500 mg/m^2/d; 1,000 mg/m^2/d (IV; IV)
		500 mg for 5 consecutive days every 6 wks, 1,000 mg
		  is for 2 wks, followed by an increase in weekly dose
		  not to exceed 1,500 mg/m^2/wk

Temozolomide	Brain tumors 150 mg/m^2 (daily PO)	Dose adjusted on the basis of blood counts
Thiotepa	General antineoplastic: 0.3–0.4 mg/kg (IV) Papillary carcinoma of the bladder: 60 mg/wk for 4 wks (bladder catheter) Control of serous effusions: 0.6–0.8 mg/kg (intracavitary)	Rapid administration given at 1- to 4-wk intervals 30 or 60 mL should be retained for 2 h, so the patient is usually dehydrated prior to administration of the drug

IV, intravenously; PO, by mouth; IP, intraperitoneal.

One distinguishing feature of melphalan is that an amino acid transporter responsible for uptake influences its efficacy across cell membranes.[10] Although a number of glutathione (GSH) conjugates of alkylating agents are effluxed through adenosine triphosphate–dependent membrane transporters,[11] specific uptake mechanisms are generally rare for cancer drugs. Cyclophosphamide and ifosfamide are prodrugs that require cytochrome P-450 metabolism to release active alkylating species. Cyclophosphamide continues to be the most widely used alkylating agent and has activity against a variety of tumors.[12] A cost saving with equivalent therapeutic activity was recently shown in a modified regimen of high-dose cyclophosphamide plus cyclosporine in patients with severe or very severe aplastic anemia.[13]

Nitrosoureas

The nitrosoureas form a diverse class of alkylating agents that have a distinct metabolism and pharmacology that separates them from others.[14] Under physiologic conditions, proton abstraction by a hydroxyl ion initiates spontaneous decomposition of the molecule to yield a diazonium hydroxide and an isocyanate (see Fig. 17.1). The chloroethyl carbonium ion generated is the active alkylating species. Through a subsequent dehalogenation step, a second electrophilic site imparts bifunctionality.[15] Thus, while cross-linking may occur similar to those lesions caused by nitrogen mustards, the chemistry leading to the endpoint is distinct. The isocyanate species generated are also electrophilic, showing nucleophilic selectivity toward sulfhydryl and amino groups that can inhibit a number of enzymes involved in nucleic acid synthesis and thiol balance.[16] Because carbamoylation is considered of minor importance to the therapeutic efficacy of clinically used nitrosoureas, chlorozotocin and streptozotocin were designed to undergo internal carbamoylation at the 1- or 3-OH group of the glucose ring, with the consequence that no carbamoylating species are produced.[17,18] Streptozotocin is also unusual in that most methylnitrosoureas have only modest therapeutic value. However, its lack of bone marrow toxicity and strong diabetogenic effect in animals led to its use in cancer of the pancreas (see Table 17.1).[19] The dose-limiting toxicities in humans are gastrointestinal and renal, but the drug has considerably less hematopoietic toxicity than the other nitrosoureas. Because of their lipophilicity and capacity to cross the blood–brain barrier, the chloroethylnitrosoureas

were found to be effective against intracranially inoculated murine tumors. Indeed, early preclinical studies showed that many mouse tumors were quite responsive to nitrosoureas. The same extent of efficacy was not found in humans. Subsequent analyses demonstrated that an enzyme responsible for repair of O-6-alkyl guanine (O^6-methylguanine-DNA methyltransferase [MGMT], or the Mer/Mex phenotype)[20] was expressed at low levels in mice, but at high levels in humans, a contributory factor in the reduced clinical efficacy of nitrosoureas in humans. In the 1980s, in particular, a number of new nitrosoureas were tested in patients in Europe and Japan, but none established a regular role in standard cancer treatment regimens.

MGMT promoter methylation is crucial in MGMT gene silencing and can predict a favorable outcome in glioblastoma patients receiving alkylating agents.[21] This biomarker is on the verge of entering clinical decision making and is currently used to stratify or even select glioblastoma patients for clinical trials. In other subtypes of glioma, such as anaplastic gliomas, the relevance of MGMT promoter methylation might extend beyond the prediction of chemosensitivity, and could reflect a distinct molecular profile. At this time, the standardization of MGMT assays will be critical in establishing prospective prognostic or predictive effects. In addition, eventual clinical trials will need to determine, for each subtype of glioma, the extent to which methylation patterns are predictive or prognostic and whether such assays could be incorporated into an individualized approach to clinical practice.[21]

CLINICAL PHARMACOKINETICS/ PHARMACODYNAMICS

The pharmacokinetics of the alkylating agents are highly variable depending on the individual agent. Nevertheless, they are generally characterized by high reactivity and short half-lives. Although detailed studies on clinical pharmacology are available,[22] Table 17.1 summarizes some of the primary kinetic characteristics of the major clinically useful drugs. Mechlorethamine is unstable and is administered rapidly in a running intravenous infusion to avoid its rapid breakdown to inactive metabolites. In contrast, chlorambucil and cyclophosphamide are sufficiently stable to be given orally, and are rapidly and completely absorbed from the gastrointestinal tract, whereas others like melphalan have poor and variable

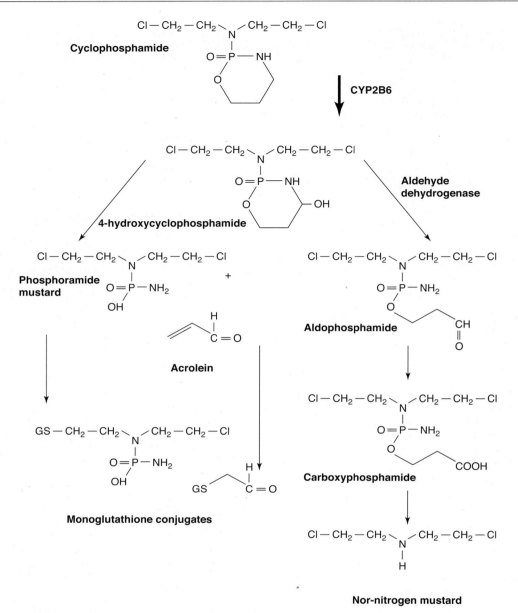

Figure 17.2 Activation and detoxification routes of metabolism for cyclophosphamide.

oral absorption. Cyclophosphamide,[23] ifosfamide, and dacarbazine are unusual in that they require activation by cytochrome P-450 in the liver before they can alkylate cellular constituents. The nitrosoureas also require activation, albeit nonenzymatic. The major route of metabolism of most alkylating agents is spontaneous hydrolysis, although many can also undergo some degree of enzymatic metabolism. This is particularly pertinent for phase II metabolic conversions where reactivity with nucleophilic thiols precedes conversion to mercapturates, with the result that most of the alkylating agents are excreted in the urine. One example of complex multistep metabolism is provided by cyclophosphamide (see Fig. 17.2). Activation by CYP2B6 is followed by the conversion of aldehyde dehydrogenase to reactive alkylating species or possible detoxification through GSH conjugation reactions. The latter is particularly important for acrolein because it is believed to contribute to the bladder toxicities associated with the drug.

The alkylating agents form covalent bonds with a number of nucleophilic groups present in proteins, RNA, and DNA (e.g., amino, carboxyl, sulfhydryl, imidazole, phosphate). Under physiologic conditions, the chloroethyl group of the nitrogen mustards

undergoes cyclization, with the chloride acting as a leaving group forming an intermediate carbonium ion that attacks nucleophilic sites (see Fig. 17.1). Bifunctional alkylating agents (with two chloroethyl side chains) can undergo a subsequent cyclization to form a covalent bond with an adjacent nucleophilic group, resulting in DNA–DNA or DNA–protein cross-links. The N7 or O6 positions of guanine are particularly susceptible and may represent primary targets that determine both the cytotoxic and mutagenic consequences of therapy.[24] The nitrosoureas have a similar, but distinct, mechanism of action, spontaneously forming both alkylating and carbamoylating agents in aqueous media (see Fig. 17.1). The carbamoylating moieties are generally believed to be inconsequential to the therapeutic properties of the nitrosoureas.

THERAPEUTIC USES

The alkylating agents are frequently used in combination therapy to treat a variety of types of cancer. Perhaps the most versatile is cyclophosphamide, whereas the other alkylating agents are of more restricted clinical use. Because of early successes, many disease states are managed with drug combinations that contain several alkylating agents. Cyclophosphamide is employed to treat a variety of immune-related diseases and to purge bone marrow in autologous marrow transplant situations.[25] A general summary of the clinical uses of the primary alkylating agents is shown in Table 17.1.

TOXICITIES

The alkylating agents show significant qualitative and quantitative variability in the sites and severities of their toxicities. The primary dose-limiting toxicity is suppression of bone marrow function, with secondary limiting effects on the proliferating cells of the intestinal mucosa.

Contraindications to the use of alkylating agents would identify patients with severely depressed bone marrow function and patients with hypersensitivity to these drugs. Other listed precautions to these drugs include carcinogenic and mutagenic effects and impairment of fertility. Precaution is also advised in patients with (1) leukopenia or thrombocytopenia, (2) previous exposure to chemotherapy or radiotherapy, (3) tumor cell infiltration of the bone marrow, and (4) impaired renal or hepatic function. These drugs can also increase toxicity in adrenalectomized patients and interfere with wound healing. A brief summary of dose-limiting toxicities is shown in Table 17.1, and a narrative of each follows here.

Nausea and Vomiting

Nausea and vomiting are frequent side effects of alkylating agent therapy and are not well controlled by conventional antiemetics.[24] They are a major source of patient discomfort and a significant cause of lack of drug compliance and even discontinuation of therapy. Frequency and extent are highly variable among patients. The overall frequency of nausea and vomiting is directly proportional to the dose of alkylating agent. The onset of nausea may occur within a few minutes of the administration of the drug or may be delayed for several hours.

Bone Marrow Toxicity

Bone marrow toxicity can involve all of the blood elements, leukocytes, platelets, and red cells.[26] The extent and time course of suppression show marked interindividual fluctuation. Relative platelet sparing is a characteristic of cyclophosphamide treatment. Even at the very high doses (<200 mg/kg) of cyclophosphamide (used in preparation for bone marrow transplantation), some recovery of hematopoietic elements occurs within 21 to 28 days. This stem cell–sparing property is further reflected by the fact that cumulative damage to the bone marrow is rarely seen when cyclophosphamide is given as a single agent, and repeated high doses can be given without progressive lowering of leukocyte and platelet counts. The biochemical basis for the stem cell–sparing effect of cyclophosphamide is related to the presence of high levels of aldehyde dehydrogenase in early bone marrow progenitor cells (see Fig. 17.2). Busulfan is particularly toxic to bone marrow stem cells,[26] and treatment can lead to prolonged hypoplasia. The hematopoietic depression produced by the nitrosoureas is characteristically delayed. The onset of leukocyte and platelet depression occurs 3 to 4 weeks after drug administration and may last an additional 2 to 3 weeks.[22,26] Thrombocytopenia appears earlier and usually is more severe than leukopenia. Even if the nitrosourea is given at 6-week intervals, hematopoietic recovery may not occur between courses, and the drug dose often must be decreased when repeated courses are used.

Renal and Bladder Toxicity

Hemorrhagic cystitis is unique to the oxazaphosphorines (cyclophosphamide and ifosfamide) and may range from a mild cystitis to severe bladder damage with massive hemorrhage.[27] This toxicity is caused by the excretion of toxic metabolites (particularly acrolein) (see Fig. 17.2) in the urine, with subsequent direct irritation of the bladder mucosa. The incidence and severity can be lessened by adequate hydration and continuous irrigation of the bladder with a solution containing 2-mercaptoethane sulfonate (MESNA) and frequent bladder emptying.[26] MESNA is given in divided doses every 4 hours in dosages of 60% of those of the alkylating agent.

At high cumulative doses, all commonly used nitrosoureas can produce a dose-related renal toxicity that can result in renal failure and death.[29] In patients developing clinical evidence of toxicity, increases in serum creatinine usually appear after the completion of therapy and may be first detected up to 2 years after treatment.

Interstitial Pneumonitis and Pulmonary Fibrosis

Long-term busulfan therapy can lead to the gradual onset of fever, a nonproductive cough, and dyspnea, followed by tachypnea and cyanosis, and progressing to severe pulmonary insufficiency and death.[30] If busulfan is stopped before the onset of clinical symptoms, pulmonary function may stabilize, but if clinical symptoms are manifest, the condition may be rapidly fatal. Cyclophosphamide, bischloroethylnitrosourea, and methyl-1-(2-chloroethyl)-3-cyclohexyl-1-nitrosourea in cumulative doses exceeding 1,000 mg/m^2 may also lead to similar side effects.[31] Other alkylating agents, including melphalan, chlorambucil, and mitomycin C, can lead to pulmonary fibrosis after therapy.[32] This effect is probably caused by a direct cytotoxicity of the alkylating agent to pulmonary epithelium, resulting in alveolitis and fibrosis.

Gonadal Toxicity, Teratogenesis, and Carcinogenesis

Alkylating agents can have profound toxic effects on reproductive tissue.[33] A depletion of testicular germ (but not Sertoli) cells is accompanied by aspermia. In patients with a total absence of germ cells, an increase in plasma levels of follicle-stimulating hormone occurs. However, patients in remission and off alkylating agents for 2 to 7 years show complete spermatogenesis, indicating that testicular damage is reversible.

In women, a high incidence of amenorrhea and ovarian atrophy is associated with cyclophosphamide or melphalan therapy.[34] This seems to be age related because it developed after lower doses in older compared with younger patients, and was less likely to be reversible in the older cohort. A pathologic analysis reveals the absence of mature or primordial follicles, and endocrinology studies demonstrate decreased estrogen and progesterone levels and elevated serum follicle-stimulating hormone and luteinizing hormone levels typical of menopause.

The DNA-damaging properties of alkylating agents ensure that they are all teratogenic and carcinogenic to some degree. The administration of alkylating agents during the first trimester of pregnancy presents a definitive risk of a malformed fetus, but the administration of such drugs during the second and third trimesters does not increase the risk of fetal malformation above normal.[35]

Development of second cancer as a consequence of alkylating agent therapy has been documented. For example, a fulminant acute myeloid leukemia characterized by a preceding phase of myelodysplasia is found in some patients treated with melphalan, cyclophosphamide (which is much less leukemogenic than melphalan), chlorambucil, and the nitrosoureas.[33] This circumstance probably reflects the fact that these have been the most widely used of the alkylating agents. Also, the preponderance of patients with multiple myeloma, Hodgkin lymphoma, and carcinoma of the ovary in the reports of leukemogenesis is probably because patients with these diseases may have good responses and are often treated with alkylating agents for a number of years. The rate of occurrence of acute leukemia in patients with ovarian cancer who survive for 10 years after treatment with alkylating agents might be as high as 10%. Acute leukemia has been the most frequently described second malignancy, and it usually develops 1 to 4 years after drug exposure.[36] Other malignancies, including solid tumors, also have been reported to develop in patients treated with alkylating agents.[37]

The last four decades have yielded a significant improvement in the survival of children diagnosed with cancer (5-year survival is approximately 80%). As many as two-thirds of the survivors of childhood malignancies can experience delayed drug toxicities that may be severe or even life threatening. Such complications include impairment in growth and development, neurocognitive dysfunction, cardiopulmonary compromise, endocrine dysfunction, renal impairment, gastrointestinal dysfunction, musculoskeletal sequelae, and second cancers.[38]

Alopecia

The degree of alopecia after cyclophosphamide administration may be quite severe, especially when this drug is used in combination with vincristine sulfate or doxorubicin hydrochloride.[39] Regrowth of hair inevitably occurs after the cessation of therapy, but may be associated with a change in the color and greater curl. Use of a tourniquet or ice pack applied to the scalp during and for a short period after cyclophosphamide administration reduces the impact.

Allergic Reactions

Alkylating agents covalently bind to proteins, and these conjugates can act as haptens and produce allergic reactions.[40] An increasing number of reports of skin eruption, angioneurotic edema, urticaria, and anaphylactic reactions after the systemic administration of alkylating agents have appeared.

Immunosuppression

Alkylating agents suppress both humoral and cellular immunity in a variety of experimental systems.[41] The most immunosuppressive is cyclophosphamide, reported to cause (1) selective suppression of B-lymphocyte function, (2) depletion of B-lymphocytes, and (3) suppression of lymphocyte functions that are mediated by T cells, such as the graft-versus-host response and delayed hypersensitivity. Most intermittent antitumor regimens do not uniformly produce profound immunosuppression, and recovery is usually prompt. Sustained drug treatments can lead to severe lymphocyte depletion and profound immunosuppression and may be accompanied by an increase of viral, fungal, and protozoal infections.[41]

COMPLICATIONS WITH HIGH-DOSE ALKYLATING AGENT THERAPY

At standard doses, alkylating agents produce myelosuppression as their dose-limiting toxicity. Less severe effects on the gastrointestinal epithelium, lungs, bladder, and kidneys may become problems with long-term treatment, but rarely limit initial therapy. For this reason, and because of their steep dose response to tumor-killing curves, the alkylating agents have become a logical tool, either alone or in combination, for high-dose chemotherapy regimens in which bone marrow toxicity is expected, and is accommodated by bone marrow transplantation, stem cell reconstitution from peripheral blood monocytes, and growth factor rescue. In this high-dose setting, toxicities that affect the gut, lungs, liver, and CNS become dose limiting and life threatening.[42] The highly lipid-soluble alkylators, especially ifosfamide, busulfan, the nitrosoureas, and thiotepa, cause CNS dysfunction, including seizures, altered mental status, cerebellar dysfunction, cranial nerve palsies, and coma.[43] High-dose ifosfamide is most frequently the cause of neurotoxicity.[44] Clinical manifestations of grade 4 neurotoxicities were reported in approximately one-fourth of those patients receiving ifosfamide. The side-chain N-linked chloroethyl moiety of ifosfamide (see Table 17.1) is more likely than the bischloroethyl group of cyclophosphamide to undergo oxidation and subsequent N-deethylation and lead to the formation of chloroacetaldehyde. High-dose busulfan is also frequently used in a variety of conditioning regimens for hematopoietic cell transplantation. In this setting, busulfan causes neurotoxicity manifesting in seizures that generally are tonic–clonic in character. Phenytoin has been the preferred drug to treat busulfan-induced seizures, although some emerging clinical data support the use of benzodiazepines, most notably clonazepam and lorazepam, to prevent busulfan-induced seizures. Moreover, the second-generation antiepileptic drug levetiracetam possesses the characteristics of optimal prophylaxis for busulfan-induced seizures.[45] At least one recent study has suggested that a polymorphism in the glutathione S-transferase A2 family may be predictive of transplant-related mortality after allogeneic stem cell transplantation,[46] perhaps indicating that a pharmacogenetic approach might be possible in this disease setting. Moreover, in a preclinical setting, a proteomic analysis identified thioredoxin as a potentially important adjuvant therapy in enhancing donor cell graft enhancement in bone marrow transplantation.[47] The possibility that this approach may benefit patients following alkylating agent–based ablation remains to be tested in a clinical setting.

Cyclophosphamide at doses exceeding 100 mg/kg during a 48-hour period (preparatory to bone marrow transplantation) can cause cardiac toxicity.[48] No evidence exists for cumulative damage to the heart after repeated moderate or low doses of the drug. Cardiac toxicity occurs with greatest frequency in patients older than 50 years or in those previously treated with anthracyclines.[48]

ALKYLATING AGENT–STEROID CONJUGATES

Adapting the rationale that steroid receptors may function to localize and concentrate attached drug species intracellularly in hormone-responsive cancers, a number of synthetic conjugates of nitrogen mustards and steroids have been developed. Of these, two made the transition into clinical use.

Prednimustine is an ester-linked conjugate of chlorambucil and prednisolone designed to function as a prodrug for chlorambucil. Release of the alkylating agent occurs after cleavage by serum esterases,[49] which can release the ester link of prednimustine, producing the hormone and active alkylating drug. The elimination phase of chlorambucil in patient plasma is significantly longer after the administration of prednimustine than after chlorambucil. Estramustine is a carbamate ester–linked conjugate of nor-nitrogen mustard and estradiol. Unlike prednimustine, the pharmacology of estramustine is governed by the presence of the carbamate group in the steroid–mustard linkage. The relative resistance of the carbamate bond to enzymatic cleavage eliminates the alkylating activity of the molecule and conveys an entirely new pharmacology.[50] The crystal structural and mechanism of action studies showed that estramustine has antimitotic activity, an activity shared by some other steroids.[51] Estramustine has found a clinical niche used in combination with other antimitotic drugs in the management of hormone refractory prostate cancer.[52]

DRUG RESISTANCE AND MODULATION

As with all drugs, intrinsic or acquired resistance to alkylating agents occurs and limits the therapeutic utility of this class of anticancer drugs.[53] A plethora of preclinical studies have characterized mechanisms by which cells develop resistance and, to a lesser degree, these have been shown to occur clinically. Because alkylating agents have a narrow therapeutic index, the emergence of resistance can have a significant impact on clinical success. Some of the factors that can contribute to the expression of resistance to alkylating agents include (1) alterations in drug uptake or transport, (2) increased repair of drug-induced nucleic acid damage, (3) failure to activate alkylating agent prodrugs, (4) increased scavenging of drug species by nonessential cellular nucleophiles, (5) increased enzymatic detoxification of drug species, and (6) altered expression of genes coding for cellular commitment to apoptosis.

RECENT DEVELOPMENTS

In the era of directed targeted therapies, the lack of specificity of alkylating agents would seem to limit the likelihood that novel drugs will be forthcoming. High toxicities, narrow therapeutic indices, and chemical instabilities are all properties that consign this drug class to the lower echelons of popularity in drug-discovery platforms. Although covalent bonding to specific target sites is one approach to direct targeting, the random electrophilic attraction toward nucleic acids and proteins is not an optimal property by today's standards. Nevertheless, the relative success of the alkylating agents in gaining therapeutic responses to diseases that are difficult to treat continues to serve as an impetus to use alkylating moieties as a means to kill cells. Some novel agents are presently in development. Cyclophosphamide and ifosfamide were prodrugs synthesized in the hope that high levels of phosphoamidase in epithelial tumors would selectively activate the drugs.[27] Other efforts to improve selectivity have centered on the synthesis of antibody–enzyme conjugates that bind to tumor-specific surface antigens. Enzymes frequently associated with the cell surface include peptidases, nitroreductases, and γ-glutamyl transpeptidase; to some degree, each has been targeted to cleave circulating alkylating prodrugs, thereby in a localized fashion releasing active alkylating species. Antibody-directed enzyme prodrug therapy is exemplified by the use of an antibody linked to the peptidase carboxypeptidase G-2, which releases an active alkylator from an inactive γ-glutamyl conjugate.[54] Linkage of the peptidase to any antibody that localizes selectively to a tumor cell membrane is a viable option. Expression of the peptidase on the cell surface then leads to prodrug activation and cell kill. Such approaches have had limited clinical impact to this time; however, their development does continue.

A further rationale for enhancing tumor-specific delivery takes advantage of the observation that glutathione-S-transferase *pi* (GSTP1-1) is preferentially expressed in a number of solid tumors and some lymphomas. In this case, the prodrug consists of an unusual alkylating agent conjugated to a substituted glutathione peptidomimetic. GSTP initiates the cleavage, thereby creating a cytotoxic alkylating species.[55] The initial canfosfamide design strategy relied on the principle that proton-abstracting sites at the active site of GST could initiate a cleavage reaction that would convert an inactive prodrug into a cytotoxic species. The presence of a histidine residue in proximity to the G binding site was integral to the removal of the sulfhydryl proton from the GSH cosubstrate, resulting in the generation of a nucleophilic sulfide anion. This moiety would be more reactive with electrophiles in the absence of GSH. Unlike other standard nitrogen mustard drugs, canfosfamide contains a tetrakis (chloroethyl) phosphorodiamidate moiety. Other compounds bearing this structure have been shown to be more cytotoxic than a similar structure with a single bis-(chloroethyl) amine group.[56]

As in other nitrogen mustards, the chlorines can act as leaving groups, thus creating aziridinium ions with electrophilic characteristics. Although the exact temporal or sequential formation of the four possible chlorine leaving events is not known, the assumption is that these species possess cytotoxic properties through their capacity to alkylate target nucleophiles, such as DNA bases. Tetrafunctionality could result in the formation of cross-links with bonding distances greater than for bifunctional agents. However, a number of caveats apply to this interpretation. For example, alkylating agents, whether mono-, bi-, or putatively tetrafunctional, generally lead to some form of myelosuppression. A number of clinical trials with canfosfamide have now been completed. These include, phase 1,[57] phase 1/2a,[58] phase 2,[59] and phase 3.[60] The phase 3 study was in platinum refractory ovarian cancer patients and proved negative for enhanced survival. Nevertheless, additional trials are still in progress.

Another targeting approach delivers the gene for a cytochrome P-450 isoenzyme to tumors by viral vector, thereby enhancing specific tumor cell activation of cyclophosphamide.[61] Because this therapy has its base in gene delivery technologies, successful development in humans will await further advances in this arena.

Laromustine is in the sulfonylhydrazine class of alkylating agents. It is presently in clinical development for the treatment of malignancies such as acute myelogenous leukemia (AML).[62] Similar to nitrosoureas, laromustine is a prodrug that yields a chloroethylating and a carbamoylating (methyl isocyanate) species. As with nitrosoureas, the cytotoxicity of laromustine is attributed primarily to the chloroethylating-mediated alkylation of DNA and subsequent interstrand cross-links.[63] The carbamoylating species can inhibit DNA repair and other cellular enzyme systems. Phase 1 trials in patients with solid tumors indicated the expected myelosuppression, although few extramedullary toxicities were observed, indicating potential efficacy in the treatment of hematologic malignancies. Phase 2 trials have been completed in patients with untreated AML, high-risk myelodysplastic syndrome, and relapsed AML. The most encouraging results have been found in patients older than 60 years with poor-risk, de novo AML for which no standard treatment exists. Laromustine is currently in phase 2/3 trials for AML and phase 2 trials for myelodysplastic syndrome and solid tumors.[64] Laromustine appears to be a promising agent in elderly patients who do not respond to or are not fit for intensive chemotherapy.

Although not a new drug, bendamustine is a unique cytotoxic agent with structural similarities to alkylating agents and antimetabolites, but it lacks cross-resistance with other established alkylating agents both in vitro and in the clinic.[65] Its mechanism of action is similar to other mustards in causing DNA intra- and interstrand cross-links. In comparison with other more commonly used alkylating agents, such as cyclophosphamide or phenylalanine mustard, more DNA double-strand breaks are formed at equitoxic dosages. Treatment with bendamustine induces a concentration-dependent apoptosis as evidenced by changes in Bcl-2 and Bax expression profiles in chronic B-cell lymphocytic leukemia.[66] DNA damage produced by bendamustine is repaired via base-excision repair mechanisms, implicating an unusual mode of action, which was recently confirmed through gene expression profiling analyses. This also provided an explanation for the lack of cross-resistance with other alkylating agents, as observed in vitro with anthracycline-resistant breast cancer and cisplatin-resistant ovarian cancer.[66,67]

Clinical studies conducted in Germany more than 30 years ago suggested activity in indolent non-Hodgkin lymphoma. Subsequent American trials showed responses in more than 70% of patients with drug refractory disease, with the implication that bendamustine may be the most effective drug in this patient population. Combinations of bendamustine and rituximab elicited response rates of 90% to 92%, with complete remission in 55% to 60% in follicular and mantle cell lymphoma. Superiority over chlorambucil in previously untreated patients with chronic lymphocytic leukemia (CLL) led to its recent approval for this disease in the United States. Bendamustine is approved in Germany for the treatment of patients with indolent non-Hodgkin lymphoma, CLL, and multiple myeloma. Activity has also been noted in patients with breast cancer and non–small-cell lung cancer.

Bendamustine has been used both as a single agent and in combination with other agents, including etoposide, fludarabine, mitoxantrone, methotrexate, prednisone, rituximab, and vincristine. A multicenter phase 2 trial in lymphomas had an overall response rate of 89%; (35% complete response and 54% partial response). In previously treated patients. the overall response rate was 76% (38% complete response and 38% partial response). The estimated median progression-free survival was 19 months.[67] In CLL patients, the drug is administered at 100 mg/m^2 intravenously over 30 minutes on days 1 and 2 of a 28-day cycle, for up to six cycles. Efficacy relative to first-line therapies other than chlorambucil has not been established. It is also indicated for the treatment of patients with indolent B-cell non-Hodgkin lymphoma that has progressed during, or within, 6 months of treatment with rituximab or rituximab-containing regimens. As with

most alkylating agents, the primary dose-limiting toxicity is myelosuppression; nonhematologic toxicities were mild and included fatigue, nausea, loss of appetite, and vomiting. The optimization of dose and schedule, particularly relative to other drugs, and the management of toxicities has allowed its use in combination with a range of other chemotherapeutic agents, including prednisone, methotrexate, fludarabine, etoposide, mitoxantrone, vinca alkaloids, and rituximab. The availability of bendamustine provides another effective treatment option for patients with lymphoid malignancies, frequently reducing the side effects of the more standard cyclophosphamide, hydroxy doxorubicin, Oncovin, and prednisone (CHOP) regimen.[68] Recent approval by the U.S. Food and Drug Administration has allowed Cephalon, Inc. to market bendamustine under the trade name Treanda and, in combination with mitoxantrone and rituximab, it is now standard of care in indolent lymphomas. Trial results released in 2013 indicated that this combination more than doubled the progression-free survival in this disease[69] and there is early evidence that there may be utility in relapsed or refractory multiple myeloma.[70]

REFERENCES

1. Adair FE, Bagg HJ. Experimental and clinical studies on the treatment of cancer by dichlorethylsulphide (mustard gas). *Ann Surg* 1931;93(1):190–199.
2. Rhoads C. Nitrogen mustards in treatment of neoplastic disease. *JAMA* 1946;131:656–658.
3. Coles B. Effects of modifying structure on electrophilic reactions with biological nucleophiles. *Drug Metab Rev* 1985;15:1307–1334.
4. Pearson R, Songstad J. Application of the principle of hard and soft acids and bases to organic chemistry. *J Am Chem Soc* 1967;89:1827.
5. Ross W. Alkylating agents. In: *Biological Alkylating Agents*. London: Butterworth; 1962.
6. Elson LA. Hematological effects of the alkylating agents. *Ann N Y Acad Sci* 1958;68(3):826–833.
7. Kushner BH, Kramer K, Modak S, et al. Topotecan, thiotepa, and carboplatin for neuroblastoma: failure to prevent relapse in the central nervous system. *Bone Marrow Transplant* 2006;37(3):271–276.
8. Agarwala SS, Kirkwood JM. Temozolomide, a novel alkylating agent with activity in the central nervous system, may improve the treatment of advanced metastatic melanoma. *Oncologist* 2000;5(2):144–151.
9. Tentori L, Graziani G. Recent approaches to improve the antitumor efficacy of temozolomide. *Curr Med Chem* 2009;16(2):245–257.
10. Vistica DT. Cytotoxicity as an indicator for transport mechanism: evidence that murine bone marrow progenitor cells lack a high-affinity leucine carrier that transports melphalan in murine L1210 leukemia cells. *Blood* 1980;56(3):427–429.
11. Dean M, Rzhetsky A, Allikmets R. The human ATP-binding cassette (ABC) transporter superfamily. *Genome Res* 2001;11(7):1156–1166.
12. Sensenbrenner LL, Marini JJ, Colvin M. Comparative effects of cyclophosphamide, isophosphamide, 4-methylcyclophosphamide, and phosphoramide mustard on murine hematopoietic and immunocompetent cells. *J Natl Cancer Inst* 1979;62(4):975–981.
13. Zhang F, Zhang L, Jing L, et al. (2013) High-dose cyclophosphamide compared with antithymocyte globulin for treatment of acquired severe aplastic anemia. *Exp Hematol* 2013;41:328–334.
14. Montgomery JA, James R, McCaleb GS, et al. The modes of decomposition of 1,3-bis(2-chloroethyl)-1-nitrosourea and related compounds. *J Med Chem* 1967;10(4):668–674.
15. Brundrett RB, Cowens JW, Colvin M. Chemistry of nitrosoureas: decomposition of Deuterated 1,3-bis(2-chloroethyl)-1-nitrosourea. *J Med Chem* 1976;19(7):958–961.
16. Tew KD, Kyle G, Johnson A, et al. Carbamoylation of glutathione reductase and changes in cellular and chromosome morphology in a rat cell line resistant to nitrogen mustards but collaterally sensitive to nitrosoureas. *Cancer Res* 1985;45(5):2326–2333.
17. Anderson T, Schein PS, McMenamin MG, et al. Streptozotocin diabetes: correlation with extent of depression of pancreatic islet nicotinamide adenine dinucleotide. *J Clin Invest* 1974;54(3):672–677.
18. Anderson T, McMenamin MG, Schein PS. Chlorozotocin, 2-(3-(2-chloroethyl)-3-nitrosoureido)-D-glucopyranose, an antitumor agent with modified bone marrow toxicity. *Cancer Res* 1975;35(3):761–765.
19. Schein PS, O'Connell MJ, Blom J, et al. Clinical antitumor activity and toxicity of streptozotocin (NSC-85998). *Cancer* 1974;34(4):993–1000.
20. Pieper RO. Understanding and manipulating O6-methylguanine-DNA methyltransferase expression. *Pharmacol Ther* 1997;74(3):285–297.
21. Weller M, Stupp R, Reifenberger G, et al. MGMT promoter methylation in malignant gliomas: ready for personalized medicine? *Nat Rev Neurol* 2010;6(1):39–51.
22. Tew K, Colvin OM, Jones RB. Clinical and high dose alkylating agents. In: Chabner BA, Longo DL, eds. *Cancer: Chemotherapy and Biotherapy: Principles and Practice*. Philadelphia: Lippincott-Raven; 2005: 283.

23. Brookes P, Lawley PD. The reaction of mono- and di-functional alkylating agents with nucleic acids. *Biochem J* 1961;80(3):496–503.
24. Penta JS, Poster DS, Bruno S, et al. Clinical trials with antiemetic agents in cancer patients receiving chemotherapy. *J Clin Pharmacol* 1981;21(8–9 Suppl):11S–22S.
25. Colvin M, Hilton J. Pharmacology of cyclophosphamide and metabolites. *Cancer Treat Rep* 1981;65(Suppl 3):89–95.
26. Elson L. Hematological effects of the alkylating agents. *Ann N Y Acad Sci* 1958;68:826–833.
27. Cox PJ. Cyclophosphamide cystitis—identification of acrolein as the causative agent. *Biochem Pharmacol* 1979;28(13):2045–2049.
28. Andriole GL, Sandlund JT, Miser JS, et al. The efficacy of mesna (2-mercaptoethane sodium sulfonate) as a uroprotectant in patients with hemorrhagic cystitis receiving further oxazaphosphorine chemotherapy. *J Clin Oncol* 1987;5(5):799–803.
29. Schacht RG, Feiner HD, Gallo GR, et al. Nephrotoxicity of nitrosoureas. *Cancer* 1981;48(6):1328–1334.
30. Littler WA, Ogilvie C. Lung function in patients receiving busulphan. *Br Med J* 1970;4(5734):530–532.
31. Mark GJ, Lehimgar-Zadeh A, Ragsdale BD. Cyclophosphamide pneumonitis. *Thorax* 1978;33(1):89–93.
32. Kreisman H, Wolkove N. Pulmonary toxicity of antineoplastic therapy. *Semin Oncol* 1992;19(5):508–520.
33. Kumar R, Biggart JD, McEvoy J, et al. Cyclophosphamide and reproductive function. *Lancet* 1972;1(7762):1212–1214.
34. Miller JJ 3rd, Williams GF, Leissring JC. Multiple late complications of therapy with cyclophosphamide, including ovarian destruction. *Am J Med* 1971;50(4):530–535.
35. Nicholson HO. Cytotoxic drugs in pregnancy: review of reported cases. *J Obstet Gynaecol Br Commonw* 1968;75(3):307–312.
36. Reimer RR, Hoover R, Fraumeni JF Jr, et al. Acute leukemia after alkylating-agent therapy of ovarian cancer. *N Engl J Med* 1977;297(4):177–181.
37. Penn I. Second malignant neoplasms associated with immunosuppressive medications. *Cancer* 1976;37(2 Suppl):1024–1032.
38. Bhatia S, Constine LS. Late morbidity after successful treatment of children with cancer. *Cancer J* 2009;15(3):174–180.
39. Calvert W. Alopecia and cytotoxic drugs. *Br Med J* 1966;2(5517):831.
40. Weiss RB, Bruno S. Hypersensitivity reactions to cancer chemotherapeutic agents. *Ann Intern Med* 1981;94(1):66–72.
41. Santos GW, Sensenbrenner LL, Burke PJ, et al. Marrow transplantation in man following cyclophosphamide. *Transplant Proc* 1971;3(1):400–404.
42. de Jonge ME, Huitema AD, Beijnen JH, et al. High exposures to bioactivated cyclophosphamide are related to the occurrence of veno-occlusive disease of the liver following high-dose chemotherapy. *Br J Cancer* 2006;94(9):1226–1230.
43. Baruchel S, Diezi M, Hargrave D, et al. Safety and pharmacokinetics of temozolomide using a dose-escalation, metronomic schedule in recurrent paediatric brain tumours. *Eur J Cancer* 2006;42(14):2335–2342.
44. Pratt CB, Goren MP, Meyer WH, et al. Ifosfamide neurotoxicity is related to previous cisplatin treatment for pediatric solid tumors. *J Clin Oncol* 1990;8(8):1399–1401.
45. Eberly AL, Anderson GD, Bubalo JS, et al. Optimal prevention of seizures induced by high-dose busulfan. *Pharmacotherapy* 2008;28(12):1502–1510.
46. Bonifazi F, Storci G, Bandini G, et al. Glutathione transferase-A2 S112T polymorphism predicts survival, transplant-related mortality, busulfan and bilirubin blood levels after allogeneic stem cell transplantation. *Haematologica* 2014;99(1):172–179.

47. An N, Janech MG, Bland AM, et al. Proteomic analysis of murine bone marrow niche microenvironment identifies thioredoxin as a novel agent for radioprotection and for enhancing donor cell reconstitution. *Exp Hematol* 2013;41:944–956.

48. Steinherz LJ, Steinherz PG, Mangiacasale D, et al. Cardiac changes with cyclophosphamide. *Med Pediatr Oncol* 1981;9(5):417–422.

49. Bastholt L, Johansson CJ, Pfeiffer P, et al. A pharmacokinetic study of prednimustine as compared with prednisolone plus chlorambucil in cancer patients. *Cancer Chemother Pharmacol* 1991;28(3):205–210.

50. Tew KD, Glusker JP, Hartley-Asp B, et al. Preclinical and clinical perspectives on the use of estramustine as an antimitotic drug. *Pharmacol Ther* 1992;56(3):323–339.

51. Punzi JS, Duax WL, Strong P, et al. Molecular conformation of estramustine and two analogues. *Mol Pharmacol* 1992;41(3):569–576.

52. Hudes GR, Greenberg R, Krigel RL, et al. Phase II study of estramustine and vinblastine, two microtubule inhibitors, in hormone-refractory prostate cancer. *J Clin Oncol* 1992;10(11):1754–1761.

53. Tew K, Houghton JA, Houghton PJ. *Preclinical and Clinical Modulation of Anticancer Drugs.* Boca Raton, FL: CRC Press; 1993.

54. Friedlos F, Davies L, Scanlon I, et al. Three new prodrugs for suicide gene therapy using carboxypeptidase G2 elicit bystander efficacy in two xenograft models. *Cancer Res* 2002;62(6):1724–1729.

55. Tew KD. TLK-286: a novel glutathione S-transferase-activated prodrug. *Expert Opin Investig Drugs* 2005;14(8):1047–1054.

56. Borch RF, Valente RR. Synthesis, activation, and cytotoxicity of aldophosphamide analogues. *J Med Chem* 1991;34(10):3052–3058.

57. Rosen LS, Laxa B, Boulos L, et al. Phase 1 study of TLK286 (Telcyta) administered weekly in advanced malignancies. *Clin Cancer Res* 2004;10(11):3689–3698.

58. Sequist LV, Fidias PM, Temel JS, et al. Phase 1–2a multicenter dose-ranging study of canfosfamide in combination with carboplatin and paclitaxel as first-line therapy for patients with advanced non-small cell lung cancer. *J Thorac Oncol* 2009;4(11):1389–1396.

59. Kavanagh JJ, Gershenson DM, Choi H, et al. Multi-institutional phase 2 study of TLK286 (TELCYTA, a glutathione S-transferase P1-1 activated glutathione analog prodrug) in patients with platinum and paclitaxel refractory or resistant ovarian cancer. *Int J Gynecol Cancer* 2005;15(4):593–600.

60. Vergote I, Finkler N, del Campo J, et al. Phase 3 randomised study of canfosfamide (Telcyta, TLK286) versus pegylated liposomal doxorubicin or topotecan as third-line therapy in patients with platinum-refractory or -resistant ovarian cancer. *Eur J Cancer* 2009;45(13):2324–2332.

61. Chase M, Chung RY, Chiocca EA. An oncolytic viral mutant that delivers the CYP2B1 transgene and augments cyclophosphamide chemotherapy. *Nat Biotechnol* 1998;16(5):444–448.

62. Vey N, Giles F. Laromustine (cloretazine). *Expert Opin Pharmacother* 2010;11(4):657–667.

63. Pigneux A. Laromustine, a sulfonyl hydrolyzing alkylating prodrug for cancer therapy. *IDrugs* 2009;12(1):39–53.

64. Schiller GJ, O'Brien SM, Pigneux A, et al. Single-agent laromustine, a novel alkylating agent, has significant activity in older patients with previously untreated poor-risk acute myeloid leukemia. *J Clin Oncol* 2010;28(5):815–821.

65. Eichbaum M, Bischofs E, Nehls K, et al. Bendamustine hydrochloride—a renaissance of alkylating strategies in anticancer medicine. *Drugs Today (Barc)* 2009;45(6):431–444.

66. Rasschaert M, Schrijvers D, Van den Brande J, et al. A phase I study of bendamustine hydrochloride administered day 1+2 every 3 weeks in patients with solid tumours. *Br J Cancer* 2007;96(11):1692–1698.

67. Weide R, Hess G, Köppler H, et al. High anti-lymphoma activity of bendamustine/mitoxantrone/rituximab in rituximab pretreated relapsed or refractory indolent lymphomas and mantle cell lymphomas: a multicenter phase II study of the German Low Grade Lymphoma Study Group (GLSG). *Leuk Lymphoma* 2007;48(7):1299–1306.

68. Cheson BD, Rummel MJ. Bendamustine: rebirth of an old drug. *J Clin Oncol* 2009;27(9):1492–1501.

69. van der Jagt R. Bendamustine for indolent non-Hodgkin lymphoma in the front-line or relapsed setting: a review of pharmacokinetics and clinical trial outcomes. *Expert Rev Hematol* 2013;6:525–537.

70. Ponisch W, Heyn S, Beck J, et al. Lenalidomide, bendamustine and prednisolone exhibits a favourable safety and efficacy profile in relapsed or refractory multiple myeloma: final results of a phase 1 clinical trial OSHO - #077. *Br J Haematol* 2013;162:202–209.

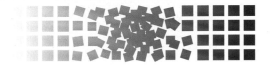

18 Platinum Analogs

Peter J. O'Dwyer and A. Hilary Calvert

INTRODUCTION

The platinum drugs represent a unique and important class of antitumor compounds. Alone or in combination with other chemotherapeutic agents, *cis*-diamminedichloroplatinum (II) (cisplatin) and its analogs have made a significant impact on the treatment of a variety of solid tumors for nearly 40 years. The unique activity and toxicity profile observed with cisplatin in early clinical trials fueled the development of platinum analogs that are less toxic and more active against a variety of tumor types, including those that have developed resistance to cisplatin. In addition to cisplatin, two other platinum complexes are currently approved for use in the United States: *cis*-diamminecyclobutanedicarboxylate platinum (II) (carboplatin) and 1,2-diaminocyclohexaneoxalato platinum (II) (oxaliplatin). Several other analogs with unique activities are in various stages of clinical development, and nedaplatin (Japan) and lobaplatin (China) are locally registered. Progress in the development of superior analogs requires a thorough understanding of the chemical, biologic, pharmacokinetic, and pharmacodynamic properties of this important class of drugs.

HISTORY

The realization that platinum complexes exhibited antitumor activity began serendipitously in a series of experiments to investigate the effect of electromagnetic radiation on the growth of bacteria, carried out by Dr. Barnett Rosenberg and colleagues beginning in 1961.[1,2] Exposure of the bacteria to an electric field resulted in a profound change in their morphology; this effect was found not to be from the electric field, but from electrolysis products produced by the platinum electrodes. An analysis of these products resulted in the identification of the cis-isomer of a platinum coordination complex as the active compound. Tests of *cis*-diamminedichloroplatinum (II) in mice bearing several model tumor types indicated that cisplatin exhibited a broad spectrum of antitumor activity. Although early clinical trials demonstrated responses in several tumor types, particularly testicular cancers, the severe renal and gastrointestinal toxicity caused by the drug nearly led to its abandonment. Work at Memorial Sloan-Kettering[3,4] showed that these effects could be ameliorated, in part, by aggressive prehydration, which rekindled interest in its clinical use. Currently, cisplatin is curative in testicular cancer and significantly prolongs survival in combination regimens for ovarian, lung, head and neck, bladder, and upper gastrointestinal (GI) cancers. Its role is being reexamined in other tumors, too, and especially breast cancer.

PLATINUM CHEMISTRY

Platinum exists primarily in either a 2+ or 4+ oxidation state. These oxidation states dictate the stereochemistry of the ligands surrounding the platinum atom. Platinum (II) compounds exhibit a square planar geometry, in which the ammine ligands (also called carrier groups) are relatively stable, whereas the opposite, more polar ligands (leaving groups) are more easily displaced and

so confer reactivity toward charged macromolecules, including DNA.[5] The stereochemistry of platinum complexes is critical to their antitumor activity as evidenced by the significantly reduced efficacy observed with *trans*-diamminedichloroplatinum (II).

In an aqueous solution, the chloride leaving groups of cisplatin are subject to mono- and diaqua substitution, particularly at chloride concentrations below 100 mmol, which characterize the intracellular environment. The administration of cisplatin in high chloride solutions (normal saline usually), therefore, contributes to stability. Intracellular formation of partially and fully aquated complexes creates the chloroaqua and hydroxoaqua cisplatin species that bind DNA.[6]

PLATINUM COMPLEXES AFTER CISPLATIN

Early in the clinical development of cisplatin, it became clear that its toxicity was a limitation to its therapeutic effectiveness, and that its activity, although striking in certain diseases, did not extend to all cancers. These observations then motivated a search for structural analogs with less toxicity and a different profile of antitumor activity. In addition, the side effects of cisplatin stimulated the development of antiemetics and other supportive care measures for use with chemotherapy. Progress in understanding the chemistry and pharmacokinetics of cisplatin has guided the development of new analogs. In general, modification of the chloride leaving groups of cisplatin results in compounds with different pharmacokinetics and reactivity towards DNA, whereas modification of the carrier ligands alters the activity of the resulting complex. The features of the more important platinum analogs that have been developed are shown in Figure 18.1.

Carboplatin

The carboplatin molecule has the same ammine carrier ligands as cisplatin. Using a murine screen for nephrotoxicity, Harrap and Calvert discovered that substituting a cyclobutanedicarboxylate moiety for the two chloride ligands of cisplatin resulted in a complex with reduced renal toxicity. This observation was translated to the clinic in the form of carboplatin, a more stable and pharmacokinetically predictable analog.[7,8] The results in humans were accurately predicted by the animal models, and marrow toxicity rather than nephrotoxicity was the principal side effect. At effective doses, carboplatin produced less nausea, vomiting, nephrotoxicity, and neurotoxicity than cisplatin. Furthermore, the myelosuppression was closely associated with the pharmacokinetics. The work of Calvert et al.[9] and Egorin and colleagues[10] showed that toxicity can be made more predictable and dose intensity less variable by dosing strategies based on the exposure. Carboplatin was shown to be indistinguishable from cisplatin in its clinical activity in all but a handful of tumor types and is the most frequently used form of platinum in current use. Cisplatin and carboplatin have almost superimposable profiles of activity in the NCI60 cell line screen, which further emphasizes the dependence of spectrum of activity on the carrier ligand.

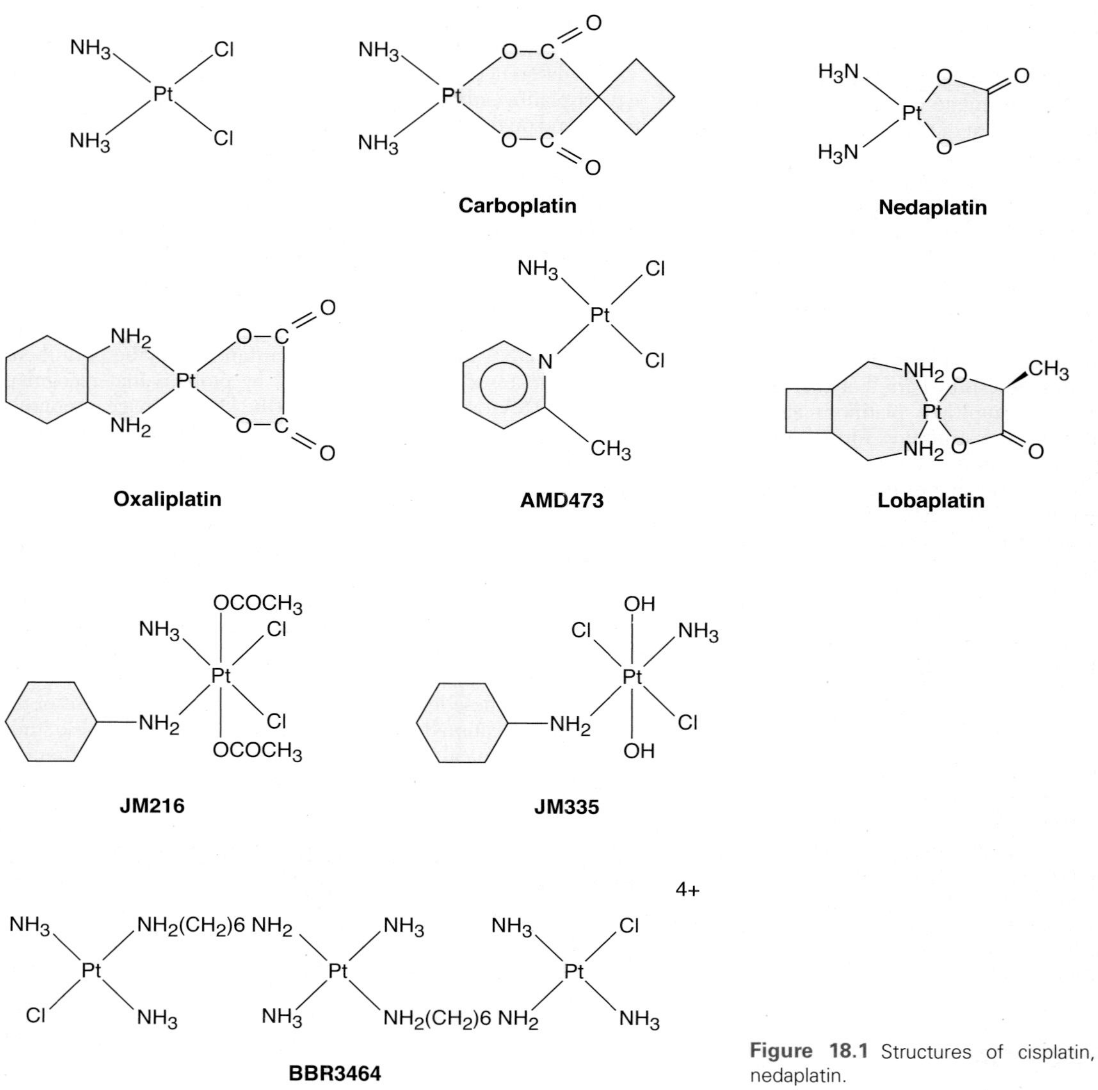

Figure 18.1 Structures of cisplatin, analogs, lobaplatin, and nedaplatin.

Oxaliplatin

Compounds with activity in cisplatin-resistant models emerged from modifications to the carrier group (see left side of the analogs in Fig. 18.1). Connors, in the late 1960s, synthesized platinum co-ordination compounds with varying physicochemical characteristics and found that the series that possessed a diaminocyclohexane (DACH) carrier group was active in models of cancer in vitro[11] and in vivo.[12] Subsequent studies supported the idea that DACH-based platinum complexes were non–cross-resistant with cisplatin, and DACH derivatives exhibited a unique cytotoxicity profile compared to cisplatin and carboplatin in the National Cancer Institute 60 cell line screen.[13–15] After a number of delays, a DACH analog that had been synthesized by Kidani and colleagues in the early 1970s, was developed in the clinic.[13] Oxaliplatin, a coordination compound of a DACH carrier group and an oxalato leaving group, was active in cisplatin-resistant tumor models. Like cisplatin, oxaliplatin preferentially forms adducts at the N7 position of guanine and, to a lesser extent, adenine. However, there is evidence that the three-dimensional structure of the DNA adducts and biologic response(s) they elicit are different from those of cisplatin. Oxaliplatin demonstrated activity in combination with 5-fluorouracil and leucovorin in colon cancer, a disease that is unresponsive to cisplatin. This finding validated the focus on cisplatin-resistant preclinical models to identify new active molecules. Oxaliplatin is approved for the treatment of advanced colorectal cancer, and enhances cure rates in the adjuvant setting. The therapeutic role of oxaliplatin has been found to extend to pancreatic, gastric, and esophageal cancers, in all of which it is the more active platinum derivative.

Nedaplatin and Lobaplatin

Nedaplatin is cis-diammineglycolatoplatinum, developed as a less nephrotoxic second-generation platinum analog, has been shown to be active in a range of tumors similar to that of cisplatin and carboplatin.[16] As a diammine structure, nedaplatin would fall among the cisplatin analogs analyzed in the NCI60 cell line screen,[17] and this activity is therefore anticipated. Lobaplatin is a platinum (II) complex in which the leaving group is lactic acid and the stable ammine ligand is 1,2-bis(aminomethyl)cyclobutane. In a similar way to oxaliplatin the stable ammine ligand may convey some non–cross-resistance compared to cisplatin or carboplatin. It is licensed in China for the breast cancer, small-cell lung cancer, and chronic myelogenous leukemia. It is unique among the platinum drugs for its approval for breast cancer, but there are few published clinical data and no randomized trials. It has not achieved approval in the United States or Europe.

Newer Platinum Structures

The octahedral stereochemistry adopted by platinum (IV) compounds has led investigators to speculate that they may exhibit a different spectrum of activity than that of platinum (II) drugs. Two compounds that were tested clinically without much success are ormaplatin and iproplatin. Two other platinum (IV) compounds that exhibit novel structural features, satraplatin (previously JM216) and JM335 (trans-ammine[cyclohexylamine]dichlorodihydroxo platinum [IV]), underwent more limited development. Satraplatin was the first orally active platinum compound, and showed some activity in lung and ovarian cancers, but despite promising activity in prostate cancer, a phase III trial was not successful.[18,19]

An approach based on the chemistry of the platinum-DNA interaction led to design and synthesis by Farrell et al.[20] of a novel class of compounds containing multiple platinum atoms (see Fig. 18.1). These bi- and trinuclear structures form adducts that span greater distances across the minor groove of DNA and have a profile of cell kill that differs from that of the small molecules. These compounds are unique in that their interaction with DNA is considerably different from that of cisplatin, particularly in the abundance of interstrand cross-links formed. Clinical development of candidate compounds is at a preliminary stage.

Efforts have been made to design novel platinum analogs that can circumvent putative cisplatin resistance mechanisms. An example is cis-amminedichloro(2-methylpyridine) platinum (II) (also known as AMD473 and ZD0473). This compound is a sterically hindered platinum complex that was designed to have minimal reactivity with thiols and thus avoid inactivation by molecules such as glutathione.[21,22] Responses were identified with its use in the clinic, but development was curtailed based on low levels of activity. The recent description of a monofunctional platinum (II) analog, phenanthriplatin, from the lab of Lippard is potentially of great interest, based on both potency in vitro and a mechanistic profile different from existing analogs.[23] A renewed appreciation that chemotherapeutic drugs have a continuing role in managing cancer is likely to prompt additional clinical development of novel platinum structures.

MECHANISM OF ACTION

DNA Adduct Formation

DNA has long been thought to be the major therapeutic target for platinum compounds. The cytotoxic effects are determined, in part, by the structure and relative amount of DNA adducts formed. Cisplatin and its analogs react preferentially at the N7 position of guanine and adenine residues to form a variety of monofunctional and bifunctional adducts.[24] The monoadducts may form intrastrand or interstrand cross-links. The predominant lesions that are formed when platinum compounds bind DNA are d(GpG)Pt intrastrand cross-links. Cisplatin also forms interstrand cross-links between guanine residues located on opposite strands, and these account for less than 5% of the total DNA-bound platinum. The formation of adducts and cross-links has been associated with therapeutic efficacy.[25,26] These adducts may contribute to the drug's cytotoxicity because they impede certain cellular processes that require the separation of both DNA strands, such as replication and transcription. The adducts formed in the reaction between carboplatin and DNA in cultured cells are essentially the same as those of cisplatin; however, higher concentrations of carboplatin are required (20- to 40-fold for cells) to obtain equivalent total platinum-DNA adduct levels due to its slower rate of aquation.[27] Oxaliplatin intrastrand adducts form even more slowly due to a slower rate of conversion from monoadducts; however, they are formed at similar DNA sequences and regions as cisplatin adducts. At equitoxic doses, oxaliplatin forms fewer DNA adducts than does cisplatin. This has been interpreted to mean that oxaliplatin lesions are more cytotoxic than those formed by cisplatin.

The differences observed in cytotoxicity between the diammine (e.g., cisplatin, carboplatin) and DACH platinum compounds may not depend on the type and relative amounts of the adducts formed, but on the overall three-dimensional structure of the adduct and its recognition by various cellular proteins. The major difference between them is the protrusion of the DACH moiety of oxaliplatin into the major groove of DNA, which thus produces a bulkier adduct than that of cisplatin. This bulkier, more hydrophobic adduct seems to be recognized differently by cellular proteins involved in sensing DNA damage.[28] The functional consequences are twofold: Proteins such as polymerases that recognize and participate in reactions on DNA under normal circumstances may be perturbed, whereas processes that are controlled by proteins that recognize damaged DNA may become activated (the DNA damage response). The latter group of proteins function both in the DNA repair process and in cellular signaling toward cell survival/death decisions.

DNA Interstrand Cross-Links

Although the DNA adducts are well-recognized to result in G-G interstrand cross-links, like classical alkylating agents, platinum drugs have the capacity to form intrastrand cross-links, albeit to a lesser degree. By blocking essential aspects of DNA metabolism, such as replication and transcription, intrastrand cross-links are highly cytotoxic. Recent studies have drawn attention both to the cytotoxicity of these lesions, and their differing mechanisms of repair, both replication dependent and independent.[29,30] These studies may have clinical implications in selecting patients for therapy based on the repair competence of tumors.

CELLULAR RESPONSES TO PLATINUM-INDUCED DNA DAMAGE

Multiple cellular outcomes may follow the formation of platinum-DNA adducts, including cell death by apoptosis, necrosis, or mitotic catastrophe, or cell survival by activation of various protective mechanisms including DNA repair, DNA damage signaling pathways, cell cycle arrest, and autophagy (the last may have a dual role, possibly context dependent).

Cell Fate

The cellular effects following DNA binding by platinum drugs have been analyzed. The studies of Sorenson and Eastman,[31] using DNA repair-deficient Chinese hamster ovary (CHO) cells, indicated that passage through the S phase is necessary for G2 arrest and cell death, which suggests that DNA replication on a damaged template may result in the accumulation of further damage. An aberrant mitosis was observed before apoptosis in this model.

DNA Damage Recognition

Among the initiation events that ultimately result in platinum drug–induced cell death are the binding of platinum-DNA damage recognition proteins, which then seed the accumulation of a large protein complex capable both of DNA damage signaling (as to cell cycle proteins to halt replication) and repair of the damaged DNA. Among the DNA-binding proteins are the high-mobility group proteins HMG1 and HMG2.[32–34] These proteins are capable of bending DNA as well as recognizing bent DNA structures, such as that produced by cisplatin, and different specificities for cisplatin and for oxaliplatin adducts are observed in structural studies.[35,36] Other candidate platinum-DNA damage recognition proteins include histone H1, RNA polymerase I transcription upstream binding factor (hUBF), the TATA binding protein (TBP), and proteins involved in mismatch repair (MMR). The MMR complex has been implicated in cisplatin sensitivity.[37] Studies have shown that the MSH2 and MLH1 proteins participate in the recognition of DNA adducts formed by cisplatin, but not oxaliplatin, which could contribute to differences in the cytotoxicity profiles observed between these two platinum complexes.

DNA Damage Signaling

A number of signaling events have been shown to occur after treatment of cells with platinum drugs.[38] For example, the ATM- and Rad3-related (ATR) proteins that are involved in cell-cycle checkpoint activation are activated by cisplatin. These kinases phosphorylate and activate several downstream effectors that regulate cell cycle, DNA repair, cell survival, and apoptosis, including p53, CHK2, and members of the mitogen-activated protein kinase (MAPK) pathway (extracellular signal-related kinase [ERK], c-Jun amino-terminal kinase [JNK], and p38 kinase). Recent data especially implicate signaling through the JNK pathway, and inhibition at the level of JNK seems especially relevant to platinum drug cytotoxicity in vitro and in vivo.[39,40] The pleiotropic nature of this stress response only grows, because each of these molecules subsequently controls the activity and expression of many more proteins. As a result of this complexity, acting in the context of variable genomic tumor aberrations, therapeutic strategies directed to these pathways have been slow to emerge. However, clinical trials to investigate specific inhibitors of DNA damage responses are underway and hold promise. It is also relevant to point out that these signaling pathways affect not just the tumor cell, but also may communicate to cells in the microenvironment, the responses of which may also determine the effectiveness of therapy.

IS DNA THE ONLY TARGET?

Early analyses of the action of cytotoxic drugs included a probe of whether effects on DNA were sufficient to explain drug effects. A pioneer in this field was Tritton,[41] who proposed that effects of DNA-intercalating agents on the plasma membrane could underlie the cytotoxicity of the drug. More recently, enucleated cells were shown to be susceptible to cisplatin, and a seminal paper from Voest and colleagues showed that platinum sensitivity was determined not solely by the accumulation of DNA damage in the tumor cell.[42] In analyzing the contribution of cells in the microenvironment of tumors, he showed that tumor infiltration with mesenchymal stem cells could confer drug resistance. A search for secreted factors defined platinum-induced fatty acids, metabolic products in the thromboxane synthetase, and cyclooxygenase-1 pathways as determining the effectiveness of drug therapy. A proteomic study in cisplatin-sensitive and -resistant cells confirmed the substantial effects of drug exposure on lipid metabolites and their relation to susceptibility. A current focus on therapies

directed to the microenvironment, including immunologic and anti-inflammatory interventions,[43] has the potential to expand our ability to apply platinum drugs in the clinic.

MECHANISMS OF RESISTANCE

The major limitation to the successful treatment of solid tumors with platinum-based chemotherapy is the emergence of drug-resistant tumor cells.[44] Developments in tumor biology have advanced our thinking with regard to how and when these cells emerge; heterogeneity within a tumor even at its earliest diagnosis reflects the emergence of treatment-resistant clones even in advance of selection pressure and the realization that resistance may not be specific to the DNA-damaging drug. Indeed, this may be reflected clinically in the finding that after progression on initial chemotherapy, the use of second-line therapy is usually associated with a shorter duration of response.

Currently described mechanisms of platinum drug resistance (Fig. 18.2) include reduced cellular accumulation, intracellular detoxification, repair of Pt-DNA lesions, increased damage tolerance, and the activation of cellular defense mechanisms such as autophagy. In addition, we have already alluded to exogenous influences on mechanism, as may be mediated by other cells, metabolites, of physicochemical conditions (such as hypoxia) in the tumor microenvironment. It must be acknowledged, however, that our insights are very limited as to why some tumors respond and others do not to platinum chemotherapy. As genome sequencing yields increasing and often surprising revelations about the genes that drive cancers and the complexity inherent in cancers of a single histologic type, it is likely that when associated with outcomes in large patient populations, patterns will emerge to guide selection of therapies.

Reduced Accumulation

Platinum uptake in cells occurs by simple diffusion and by carrier-mediated mechanisms. Inhibition of transport mechanisms has a marked effect on intracellular platinum accumulation, and Howell's group has shown the importance of the copper transporters CTR-1 and CTR-2 in regulating the influx of various platinum analogs in eukaryotic cells.[45,46] The contribution of these mechanisms to clinical platinum drug resistance is being explored.[47] Accumulation may also be influenced by enhanced efflux, and various transport proteins are upregulated in cell lines selected for acquired resistance, and in platinum-resistant ovarian cancers.

Inactivation

Platinum complexes are highly reactive molecules and bind rapidly to multiple cellular macromolecules. Protection from such chemicals in the environment is afforded by cellular thiols, including

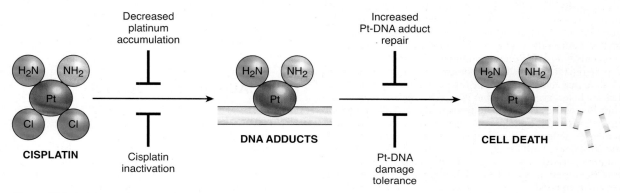

Figure 18.2 Cellular mechanisms of cisplatin resistance.

small peptides such as glutathione (GSH) and larger proteins as exemplified by metallothionein (MT). There are many reports of an association between platinum drug sensitivity and glutathione levels[48–50]; however, reducing intracellular glutathione levels with drugs such as buthionine sulfoximine has resulted in only low to modest potentiation of cisplatin sensitivity.[51] Buthionine sulfoximine was developed for clinical use, and some impact on GSH content of tumors and normal tissues was demonstrated. However, the depletion of GSH was not consistent, and ultimately, the cost of producing the active stereoisomer of the drug was judged prohibitive. Inactivation of the platinum drugs may also occur through binding to the MTs, a family of sulfhydryl-rich, low–molecular-weight proteins that participate in heavy metal binding and detoxification; however, the contribution of MT to clinical platinum drug resistance is unclear, and a therapeutic role has not emerged.

Increased DNA Repair

Once platinum-DNA adducts are formed, cells must either repair or tolerate the damage to survive. In general, the capacity to repair DNA damage seems to play a role in determining a tumor cell's sensitivity to platinum drugs and other DNA-damaging agents. For example, tumors that are unusually sensitive to cisplatin, such as testicular nonseminomatous germ cell tumors, may be deficient in their ability to repair platinum-DNA adducts.[52] The increased repair of platinum-DNA lesions in cisplatin-resistant cell lines as compared to their sensitive counterparts has been shown in several human cancer cell lines, but translation of these observations to the clinic has been difficult. The repair of platinum-DNA adducts appears to occur predominantly by nucleotide excision repair (NER), with a role for MMR under certain circumstances.[53] The molecular basis for the increased repair activity observed in cisplatin-resistant cells is not known precisely, but formation of the ERCC1/XPF protein complex may be a key step. Selvakumaran et al.[54] showed that the downregulation of ERCC-1 using an antisense approach sensitized a platinum-resistant cell line to cisplatin both in vitro and in vivo. There is substantial clinical evidence that implicates *ERCC1* expression in increased NER and cisplatin resistance, and high expression of ERCC1 has been demonstrated to confer a worse outcome after cisplatin treatment in several resistant tumors. The most extensive study of this as a marker has been in non–small-cell lung cancer, results in which were summarized and analyzed by Hubner et al.[55] In gastric cancer also, high levels of ERCC1 are associated with resistance to cisplatin treatment.[56–58] However, a recent reevaluation of discrepant results questioned the reliability of the assays of ERCC1 and their relationship to function.[59] These data suggest that there is a relationship between ERCC1 expression and treatment, but that the lag in marker development precludes implementation of a predictive assay until additional studies have been performed.

Perhaps the most striking evidence that DNA repair is a determinant of platinum drug responses is that breast and ovarian cancers occurring in BRCA1 or BRCA2 mutation carriers are particularly responsive to cisplatin or carboplatin. These cancers are also sensitive to inhibitors of poly(ADP-ribose)polymerase (PARPi), several of which are currently in clinical development. The mechanism of the sensitivity to PARPi has been elucidated. Both the BRCA1 and 2 proteins for part of the homologous recombination repair (HR) system that achieves error-free repair of double strand breaks. Carriers are heterozygous and, therefore, have normal repair function, but loss of the second allele leads to the use of error-prone backup systems and is therefore oncogenic. The cancers that arise are unable to perform HR and, therefore, are sensitive to drugs that induce single strand breaks, such as PARPi.[60,61] A mechanism of resistance to PARPi has been described, which is due to reactivation of the function of the BRCA2 leading to restoration of HR and sensitivity to PARPi.[62] This reactivation is accomplished by an intragenic deletion and the restoration of an open reading frame.

It has further been shown that such revertant cells are resistant to cisplatin as well as PARPi. Finally, recurrent cancers in BRCA2 mutation carriers, which have acquired platinum resistance, have been shown to have undergone reversion of the BRCA2 mutation.[63] This clearly shows that the HR system can be one cause of cisplatin resistance. However, not all cisplatin-resistant patients are also resistant to PARPi,[64] showing that there are multiple other causes of cis/carboplatin resistance.

Combinations of platinum drugs with PARPi are being actively pursued in patients with BRCA-related tumors and also in patients whose tumors are likely to have acquired loss of HR function (poorly differentiated serous ovarian cancer and triple negative breast cancer).

Autophagy

After platinum-DNA adduct formation, the cell detects the DNA damage and initiates signaling through multiple pathways, the effects of which include mobilization of repair proteins; arrest of the cell cycle; altered transcriptional programs; redirection of energy production and consumption; activation of cell death pathways and, simultaneously, of pathways that would counter a cell death decision, and so to permit survival. A process recently characterized to perform the last function is autophagy. Initially described as a mechanism of cell death, autophagy represents a regulated dissolution of cellular elements into a characteristic set of subcellular organelles detectable by electron microscopy and linked by a particular profile of gene expression changes.[65] Multiple stimuli precipitate these changes and have in common scarcity of nutrients that are required for survival, from oxygen and glucose withdrawal to less specific calorie deprivation, and inhibition of metabolic pathways. Autophagy is also a consequence of cytotoxic drug treatment and, more recently, has been appreciated as a means by which cells might survive the stress of cellular insults, and so become resistant to treatment.[66] Amaravadi and colleagues[67] demonstrated that autophagy reversal can sensitize tumors to cytotoxic drugs and several trials of platinum compounds along with the autophagy inhibitor hydroxychloroquine are in progress.

Increased DNA Damage Tolerance

The net result of DNA damage signaling in a sensitive tumor cell is engagement of cell death pathways, including apoptosis, and therapeutic benefit. In a resistant tumor cell, the cell survives as a consequence of one or many of these mechanisms, and this can result in platinum-DNA damage tolerance or multidrug resistance phenotype, or both. Contributors to the tolerance might include deficient DNA MMR (which could excise the adduct if NER failed), enhanced replicative bypass (which essentially ignores the adduct, allowing the cell to survive, but could contribute to the increase in mutation frequency observed in chemotherapy-treated cancers), and altered signaling through stress-related kinases such as JNK, which can both alter transcriptional programs and activate autophagy. Indeed JNK, by phosphorylating Bcl-2 or Bcl-XL, and releasing beclin-1 from inhibition, acts as a key switch to turn on autophagy. The enhanced DNA damage tolerance, in addition to permitting persistence of the cancer cell, may have an additional deleterious effect by fostering further mutagenesis within the tumor, facilitating its evolution to a more malignant phenotype.

CLINICAL PHARMACOLOGY

Pharmacokinetics

The pharmacokinetic differences observed between platinum drugs may be attributed to the structure of their leaving groups. Platinum complexes containing leaving groups that are less easily displaced exhibit reduced plasma protein binding, longer plasma half-lives, and higher rates of renal clearance. These features are

TABLE 18.1

Comparative Parmacokinetics of Platinum Analogs After Bolus or Short Intravenous Infusion

	Cisplatin	Carboplatin	Oxaliplatin
$T_{1/2}\alpha$			
Total platinum	14–49 min	12–98 min	26 min
Ultrafiltrate	9–30 min	8–87 min	21 min
$T_{1/2}\beta$			
Total platinum	0.7–4.6 h	1.3–1.7 h	—
Ultrafiltrate	0.7–0.8 h	1.7–5.9 h	—
$T_{1/2}\gamma$			
Total platinum	24–127 h	8.2–40.0 h	38–47 h
Ultrafiltrate	—	—	24–27 h
Protein binding	>90%	24%–50%	85%
Urinary excretion	23%–50%	54%–82%	>50%

$T_{1/2}\alpha$, half-life of first phase; $T_{1/2}\beta$, half-life of second phase; $T_{1/2}\gamma$, half-life of terminal phase.

evident in the pharmacokinetic properties of cisplatin, carboplatin, and oxaliplatin, which are summarized in Table 18.1. Platinum drug pharmacokinetics have been reviewed.[68]

Cisplatin

After intravenous infusion, cisplatin rapidly diffuses into tissues and is covalently bound to plasma protein. More than 90% of platinum is bound to plasma protein at 4 hours after infusion. The disappearance of ultrafilterable platinum is rapid and occurs in a biphasic fashion. Half-lives of 10 to 30 minutes and 0.7 to 0.8 hours have been reported for the initial and terminal phases, respectively. Cisplatin excretion is dependent on renal function, which accounts for the majority of its elimination. The percentage of platinum excreted in the urine has been reported to be between 23% and 40% at 24 hours after infusion. Only a small percentage of the total platinum is excreted in the bile.

Carboplatin

The differences in pharmacokinetics observed between cisplatin and carboplatin depend primarily on the slower rate of conversion of carboplatin to a reactive species. Thus, the stability of carboplatin results in a low incidence of nephrotoxicity. Carboplatin diffuses rapidly into tissues after infusion; however, it is considerably more stable in plasma. Only 24% of a dose was bound to plasma protein at 4 hours after infusion. The disappearance of platinum from plasma after short intravenous infusions of carboplatin has been reported to occur in a biphasic or triphasic manner. The initial half-lives for total platinum, which vary considerably among several studies, are listed in Table 18.1. The half-lives for total platinum range from 12 to 98 minutes during the first phase ($T_{1/2}\alpha$) and from 1.3 to 1.7 hours during the second phase ($T_{1/2}\beta$). Half-lives reported for the terminal phase range from 8.2 to 40 hours. The disappearance of ultrafilterable platinum is biphasic with $T_{1/2}\alpha$ and $T_{1/2}\beta$ values ranging from 7.6 to 87 minutes and 1.7 to 5.9 hours, respectively. Carboplatin is excreted predominantly by the kidneys, and cumulative urinary excretion of platinum is 54% to 82%, most as unmodified carboplatin. The renal clearance of carboplatin is closely correlated with the glomerular filtration rate (GFR).[69] This observation enabled Calvert et al.[9] to design a carboplatin-dosing formula based on the individual patient's GFR.

Oxaliplatin

After oxaliplatin infusion, platinum accumulates into three compartments: plasma-bound platinum, ultrafilterable platinum, and platinum associated with erythrocytes. When specific and sensitive mass spectrometric techniques are used, oxaliplatin itself is undetectable in plasma, even at end infusion.[70] The active forms of the drug have not been extensively characterized. Approximately 85% of the total platinum is bound to plasma protein at 2 to 5 hours after infusion.[71] Plasma elimination of total platinum and ultrafilterates is biphasic. The half-lives for the initial and terminal phases are 26 minutes and 38.7 hours, respectively, for total platinum and 21 minutes and 24.2 hours, respectively, for ultrafilterable platinum (see Table 18.1).[72] Thus, as with carboplatin, substantial differences between total and free platinum kinetics are not observed. As with cisplatin, a prolonged retention of oxaliplatin is observed in red blood cells. However, unlike cisplatin, oxaliplatin does not accumulate to any significant level after multiple courses of treatment.[71] This may explain why neurotoxicity associated with oxaliplatin is reversible. Oxaliplatin is eliminated predominantly by the kidneys, with more than 50% of the platinum being excreted in the urine at 48 hours.

Pharmacodynamics

Pharmacodynamics relates pharmacokinetic indices of drug exposure to biologic measures of drug effect, usually toxicity to normal tissues or tumor cell kill. Two issues to be addressed in such studies are whether the effectiveness of the drug can be enhanced and whether the toxicity can be attenuated by knowledge of the platinum pharmacokinetics in an individual. These questions are appropriate to the use of cytotoxic agents with relatively narrow therapeutic indices. Toxicity to normal tissues can be quantitated as a continuous variable when the drug causes myelosuppression. Thus, the early studies of carboplatin demonstrated a close relationship of changes in platelet counts to the area under the concentration-time curve (AUC) in the individual. The AUC was itself closely related to renal function, which was determined as creatinine clearance. Based on these observations, Egorin et al.,[10] Calvert et al.,[9] and Chatelut and colleagues[73] derived formulas based on creatinine clearance to predict either the percentage change in platelet count or a target AUC. Application of pharmacodynamically guided dosing algorithms for carboplatin has been widely adopted as a means of avoiding overdosage (by producing acceptable nadir platelet counts) and of maximizing dose intensity in the individual. There is good evidence that this approach can decrease the risk of unacceptable toxicity. Accordingly, a dosing strategy based on renal function is recommended for the use of carboplatin.

A key question is whether maximizing carboplatin exposure in an individual can measurably increase the probability of tumor regression or survival. In an analysis by Jodrell et al.,[74] carboplatin AUC was a predictor of response, thrombocytopenia, and leukopenia. The likelihood of a tumor response increased with increasing AUC up to a level of 5 to 7 mg × hour per milliliter, after which a plateau was reached. Similar results were obtained with carboplatin in combination with cyclophosphamide, and neither response rate nor survival was determined by the carboplatin AUC in a cohort of ovarian cancer patients.[75] As a result, most carboplatin recommended doses are based on an AUC in this range (for every 3 to 4 week schedules), and modifications of these are used for more frequent administration (as in combined chemoradiotherapy regimens).

The relationship of pharmacokinetics to response has been sought by investigating the cellular pharmacology of these agents.[76] The formation and repair of the platinum-DNA adducts in human cells are not easily measured. Schellens and colleagues[77,78] analyzed the pharmacokinetic and pharmacodynamic interactions of cisplatin administered as a single agent. In a series of patients with head and neck cancer, they found that cisplatin exposure (measured as the AUC) closely correlated with both the peak DNA adduct content in leukocytes and the area under the DNA-adduct time curve. These measures were important predictors of response, both individually and in logistic regression analysis. However, as an approach to determine who should or should not be treated with platinum drugs, it seems more likely that genomic analyses will provide guidance in the near future.

Pharmacogenomics

Variability in pharmacokinetics and pharmacodynamics of cytotoxic drugs is an important determinant of therapeutic index. This interindividual variation may be attributed in part to genetic differences among patients. Targeted analyses of germ-line DNA and, increasingly, Genome-wide association studies (GWAS) approaches, have yielded genotypic features associated with results of therapy. Detoxification pathways and DNA repair have emerged as having markers attributable to response of lack of it in response to platinum drugs. Single nucleotide polymorphisms (SNP) in genes related to glutathione metabolism and in several DNA repair genes have been identified in lung cancer, breast cancer, and various GI cancers. A concern is that larger trials have not always confirmed early findings. As yet, informative SNPs that could be used to define therapeutic strategies for individual patients have not yet been defined.

FORMULATION AND ADMINISTRATION

Cisplatin (Platinol)

Cisplatin is administered in a chloride-containing solution intravenously over 0.5 to 2.0 hours. To minimize the risk of nephrotoxicity, patients are prehydrated with at least 500 mL of salt-containing fluid. Immediately before cisplatin administration, mannitol (12.5 to 25.0 g) is given parenterally to maximize urine flow. A diuretic such as furosemide may be used also, along with parenteral antiemetics. These currently include dexamethasone together with a 5-hydroxytryptamine (5-HT$_3$) antagonist. A minimum of 1 L of posthydration fluid is usually given. The intensity of hydration varies somewhat with the dose of cisplatin. High-dose cisplatin (up to 200 mg/m^2 per course) may be administered in a formulation containing 3% sodium chloride, but this method is no longer widely used. Cisplatin may also be administered regionally to increase local drug exposure and diminish side effects. Its intraperitoneal use was defined by Ozols et al.[79] and by Howell and colleagues.[80] Measured drug exposure in the peritoneal cavity is some 50-fold higher compared to levels achieved with intravenous administration. At standard dosages in ovarian cancer patients with low-volume disease, a randomized intergroup trial suggested that intraperitoneal administration is superior to intravenous cisplatin in combination with intravenous cyclophosphamide.[81] The development of combinations of carboplatin and paclitaxel has, however, superseded this technique in the treatment of ovarian cancer, and the intraperitoneal route is now infrequently used. Regional uses also include intra-arterial delivery (as for hepatic tumors, melanoma, and glioblastoma), but none have been adopted as a standard method of treatment. There is growing interest in chemoembolization for the treatment of tumors confined to the liver, and cisplatin is a component of many popular regimens.[82]

Carboplatin (Paraplatin)

Cisplatin treatment over 3 to 6 hours is burdensome for clinical resources and tiring for cancer patients. Previously given as an in-hospital treatment, it is now usually administered in the outpatient setting. The exigencies of the modern health-care environment have contributed to the expanding use of carboplatin as an alternative to cisplatin except in circumstances in which cisplatin is clearly the superior agent. Carboplatin is substantially easier to administer. Extensive hydration is not required because of the lack of nephrotoxicity at standard dosages. Carboplatin is reconstituted

in chloride-free solutions (unlike cisplatin, because chloride can displace the leaving groups) and administered over 30 minutes as a rapid intravenous infusion.

Oxaliplatin (Eloxatin)

Oxaliplatin is also uncomplicated in its clinical administration. For bolus infusion, the required dose is administered in 500 mL of chloride-free diluent over a period of 2 hours. Oxaliplatin is most frequently given as a single dose every 2 weeks (85 mg/m^2) or every 3 weeks (130 mg/m^2), alone or with other active agents. It is common to pretreat patients with active antiemetics, such as a 5-HT$_3$ antagonist, but the nausea is not as severe as with cisplatin. No prehydration is required. Besides a relatively low incidence of myelosuppression, the predominant toxicity of oxaliplatin is cumulative neurotoxicity. The development of an oropharyngeal dysesthesia, often precipitated by exposure to cold, may require prolonging the duration of administration to 6 hours. On occasion, the occurrence of hypersensitivity also requires slowing the infusion.

TOXICITY

A substantial body of literature documents the side effects of platinum compounds. As noted in the section titled History, earlier in this chapter, the toxicity of cisplatin was a driving force both in the search for less toxic analogs and for more effective treatments for its side effects, especially nausea and vomiting. The toxicities associated with cisplatin, carboplatin, and oxaliplatin are described in detail in the following sections and summarized in Table 18.2. Please review the package inserts for these drugs for full prescribing information and delineation of toxic effects.

Cisplatin

The side effects associated with cisplatin (at single doses of more than 50 mg/m^2) include nausea and vomiting, nephrotoxicity, ototoxicity, neuropathy, and myelosuppression. Rare effects include visual impairment, seizures, arrhythmias, acute ischemic vascular events, glucose intolerance, and pancreatitis. The nausea and vomiting stimulated a search for new antiemetics. These effects are currently best managed with 5-HT$_3$ antagonists, usually given with a glucocorticoid, although other combinations of agents are still widely used. In the weeks after treatment, continuous antiemetic therapy may be required. Nephrotoxicity is ameliorated but not completely prevented by hydration. The renal damage to both glomeruli and tubules is cumulative, and after cisplatin treatment, serum creatinine levels are no longer a reliable guide to GFR. An acute elevation of serum creatinine level may follow a cisplatin dose, but this index returns to normal with time. Tubule damage may be reflected in a salt-losing syndrome that also resolves with time.

Ototoxicity is a cumulative and irreversible side effect of cisplatin treatment that results from damage to the inner ear. The initial audiographic manifestation is loss of high-frequency acuity (4,000 to 8,000 Hz). When acuity is affected in the range of speech, cisplatin

TABLE 18.2

Toxicity Profiles of Platinum Analogs in Clinical Use

Toxicity	Cisplatin	Carboplatin	Oxaliplatin
Myelosuppression		X	
Nephrotoxicity	X		
Neurotoxicity	X		X
Ototoxicity	X		
Nausea and vomiting	X	X	X

should be discontinued under most circumstances and carboplatin substituted where appropriate. Peripheral neuropathy is also cumulative, although less common than with agents such as vinca alkaloids. This neuropathy is usually reversible, although recovery is often slow. A number of agents with the potential for protection from neuropathy have been developed, but none is yet used widely.

Carboplatin

Myelosuppression, which is not usually severe with cisplatin, is the dose-limiting toxicity of carboplatin. The drug is most toxic to the platelet precursors, but neutropenia and anemia are frequently observed. The lowest platelet counts after a single dose of carboplatin are observed 17 to 21 days later, and recovery usually occurs by day 28. The effect is dose dependent, but individuals vary widely in their susceptibility. As shown by Egorin et al.[10] and Calvert et al.,[9] the severity of platelet toxicity is best accounted for by a measure of the drug exposure in an individual, the AUC. Both groups derived pharmacologically based formulas to predict toxicity and guide carboplatin dosing. That of Calvert and colleagues targets a particular exposure to carboplatin:

$$\text{Dose (mg)} = \text{target AUC (mg} \cdot \text{min/mL)} \times (\text{GFR mL/min} + 25)$$

This formula has been widely used to individualize carboplatin dosing and permits targeting an acceptable level of toxicity. Patients who are elderly, have a poor performance status, or have a history of extensive pretreatment have a higher risk of toxicity even when dosage is calculated with these methods, but the safety of drug administration has been enhanced. In the combination of carboplatin and paclitaxel, AUC-based dosing has helped to maximize the dose intensity of carboplatin. Dosages some 30% higher than those using a dosing strategy based solely on body surface area may safely be used. A determination of whether this approach to dosing improves outcomes will require a randomized trial.

The other toxicities of carboplatin are generally milder and better tolerated than those of cisplatin. Nausea and vomiting, although frequent, are less severe, shorter in duration, and more easily controlled with standard antiemetics (i.e., prochlorperazine [Compazine]), dexamethasone, lorazepam) than that after cisplatin treatment. Renal impairment is infrequent, although alopecia is common, especially with the paclitaxel-containing combinations. Neurotoxicity is also less common than with cisplatin, although it is observed more frequently with the increasing use of high-dose regimens. Ototoxicity is also less common.

Oxaliplatin

The dose-limiting toxicity of oxaliplatin is sensory neuropathy, a characteristic of all DACH-containing platinum derivatives. This side effect takes two forms. First, a tingling of the extremities, which may also involve the perioral region, that occurs early and usually resolves within a few days. With repeated dosing, symptoms may last longer between cycles, but do not appear to be cumulative or of long duration. Laryngopharyngeal spasms and cold dysesthesias have also been reported but are not associated with significant respiratory symptoms and can be prevented by prolonging the duration of infusion. A second neuropathy, more typical of that seen with cisplatin, affects the extremities and increases with repeated doses. Definitive physiologic characterization of oxaliplatin-induced neuropathy has proven difficult in large studies. Electromyograms performed in six patients treated by Extra et al.[83] revealed an axonal sensory neuropathy, but nerve conduction velocities were unchanged. Specimens from peripheral nerve biopsies performed in this study showed decreased myelination and replacement with collagen pockets. The neurologic effects of oxaliplatin appear to be cumulative in that they become more pronounced and of greater duration with successive cycles; however, unlike those of cisplatin, they are reversible with drug cessation. In a review of 682 patient experiences, Brienza et al.[84] reported that 82% of patients who experienced grade 2 neurotoxicity or higher had their symptoms regress within 4 to 6 months. In a larger adjuvant trial, de Gramont et al.[85] reported that 12% of patients had grade 3 toxicity at the end of a 6-month treatment period and that the majority of these patients had relief, but not always complete resolution of the symptoms, by 1 year later. The persistence of the neurotoxicity has led to approaches to ameliorate it, including the use of protective agents. The use of calcium and magnesium salts intravenously before and after each infusion has been shown to be ineffective. Ototoxicity is not observed with oxaliplatin. Nausea and vomiting do occur and generally respond to 5-HT$_3$ antagonists. Myelosuppression is uncommon and is not severe with oxaliplatin as a single agent, but it is a feature of combinations including this drug. Oxaliplatin therapy is not associated with nephrotoxicity.

REFERENCES

1. Rosenberg B, VanCamp L, Trosko J, et al. Platinum compounds: a new class of potent antitumor agents. *Nature* 1969;222:385–386.
2. Rosenberg B. Fundamental studies with cisplatin. *Cancer* 1985;55:2303–2316.
3. Cvitkovic E, Spaulding J, Bethune V, et al. Improvement of cis-dichlorodiammineplatinum (NSC 119875): therapeutic index in an animal model. *Cancer* 1977;39:1357–1361.
4. Hayes D, Cvitkovic E, Golbey R, et al. High dose cis-platinum diamine dichloride: amelioration of renal toxicity by mannitol diuresis. *Cancer* 1977;39:1372–1381.
5. Roberts J, Thomson A. The mechanism of action of antitumor platinum compounds. *Nucleic Acids Res* 1979;22:71–133.
6. Martin R. Platinum complexes: hydrolysis and binding to N(7) and N(1) of purines. In: Lippert B, ed. *Cisplatin: Chemistry and Biochemistry of a Leading Anticancer Drug.* Zurich: Verlag Helvetica Chimica Acta; 1999:183.
7. Harrap K. Preclinical studies identifying carboplatin as a viable cisplatin alternative. *Cancer Treat Rev* 1985;12:A21–A33.
8. Harrap K. Initiatives with platinum- and quinazoline-based antitumor molecules—Fourteenth Bruce F. Cain Memorial Award Lecture. *Cancer Res* 1995;55:2761–2768.
9. Calvert A, Newell D, Gumbrell L, et al. Carboplatin dosage: prospective evaluation of a simple formula based on renal function. *J Clin Oncol* 1989;7:1748–1756.
10. Egorin M, Echo DV, Olman E, et al. Prospective validation of a pharmacologically based dosing scheme for the cis-diamminedichloroplatinum(II) analogue diamminecyclobutanedicarboxylatoplatinum. *Cancer Res* 1985;45:6502–6506.
11. Connors T, Jones M, Ross W, et al. New platinum complexes with anti-tumour activity. *Chem Biol Interact* 1972;5:415–424.
12. Burchenal J, Kalaker K, Dew K, et al. Rationale for development of platinum analogs. *Cancer Treat Rep* 1979;63:1493–1498.
13. Kidani Y, Inagaki K, Tsukagoshi S. Examination of antitumor activities of platinum complexes of 1,2-diaminocyclohexane isomers and their related complexes. *Gann* 1976;67:921–922.
14. Burchenal J, Irani G, Kern K, et al. 1,2-Diaminocyclohexane platinum derivatives of potential clinical value. *Rec Res Cancer Res* 1980;74:146–155.
15. Rixe O, Ortuzar W, Alvarez M, et al. Oxaliplatin, tetraplatin, cisplatin, and carboplatin: spectrum of activity in drug-resistant cell lines and in the cell lines of the National Cancer Institute's anticancer drug screen panel. *Biochem Pharmacol* 1996;52:1855–1865.
16. Shimada M, Itamochi H, Kigawa J. Nedaplatin: a cisplatin derivative in cancer therapy. *Cancer Manag Res* 2013;5:67–76.
17. Fojo T, Farrell N, Ortuzar W, et al. Identification of non-cross-resistant platinum compounds with novel cytotoxicity profiles using the NCI anticancer drug screen and clustered image map visualizations. *Crit Rev Oncol Hematol* 2005;53:25–34.
18. Bates SE, Amiri-Kordestani L, Giaccone G. Drug development: portals of discovery. *Clin Cancer Res* 2012;18:23–32.
19. Kelland L. The development of orally active platinum drugs. In: Lippert B, ed. *Cisplatin: Chemistry and Biochemistry of a Leading Anticancer Drug.* Zurich: Verlag Helvetica Chimica Acta; 1999:497.
20. Farrell N, Qu Y, Bierbach U, et al. Structure-activity relationships within di- and trinuclear platinum phase-I clinical anticancer agents. In: Lippert B, ed. *Cisplatin: Chemistry and Biochemistry of a Leading Anticancer Drug.* Zurich: Verlag Helvetica Chimica Acta; 1999:477–496.
21. Holford J, Sharp S, Murrer B, et al. In vitro circumvention of cisplatin resistance by the novel sterically hindered platinum complex AMD473. *Br J Cancer* 1998;77:366–373.
22. Flaherty KT, Stevenson JP, Redlinger M, et al. A phase I, dose escalation trial of ZD0473, a novel platinum analogue, in combination with gemcitabine. *Cancer Chemother Pharmacol* 2004;53:404–408.
23. Park GY, Wilson JJ, Song Y, et al. Phenanthriplatin, a monofunctional DNA-binding platinum anticancer drug candidate with unusual potency and cellular activity profile. *Proc Natl Acad Sci U S A* 2012;109:11987–11992.

24. Eastman A. The formation, isolation and characterization of DNA adducts produced by anticancer platinum complexes. *Pharmacol Ther* 1987;34:155–166.

25. Zhu G, Song L, Lippard SJ. Visualizing inhibition of nucleosome mobility and transcription by cisplatin-DNA interstrand crosslinks in live mammalian cells. *Cancer Res* 2013;73:4451–4460.

26. Martens-de Kemp SR, Dalm SU, Wijnolts FM, et al. DNA-bound platinum is the major determinant of cisplatin sensitivity in head and neck squamous carcinoma cells. *PLoS One* 2013;8:e61555.

27. Blommaert F, van Kijk-Knijnenburg H, Dijt F, et al. Formation of DNA adducts by the anticancer drug carboplatin: different nucleotide sequence preferences in vitro and in cells. *Biochemistry* 1995;34:8474–8480.

28. Scheef E, Briggs J, Howell S. Molecular modeling of the intrastrand guanine-guanine DNA adducts produced by cisplatin and oxaliplatin. *Mol Pharmacol* 1999;56:633–643.

29. Enoiu M, Jiricny J, Schärer OD. Repair of cisplatin-induced DNA interstrand crosslinks by a replication-independent pathway involving transcription-coupled repair and translesion synthesis. *Nucleic Acids Res* 2012;40:8953–8964.

30. Zhu G, Song L, Lippard SJ. Visualizing inhibition of nucleosome mobility and transcription by cisplatin-DNA interstrand crosslinks in live mammalian cells. *Cancer Res* 2013;73:4451–4460.

31. Sorenson C, Eastman A. Mechanism of cis-diamminedichloroplatinum (II)-induced cytotoxicity: role of G2 arrest and DNA double-strand breaks. *Cancer Res* 1988;48:4484–4488.

32. Toney J, Donahue B, Kellett P, et al. Isolation of cDNAs encoding a human protein that binds selectively to DNA modified by the anticancer drug cis-diamminedichloroplatinum. *Proc Natl Acad Sci U S A* 1989;86:8328–8332.

33. Bruhn S, Pil P, Essigmann J, et al. Isolation and characterization of human cDNA clones encoding a high mobility group box protein that recognizes structural distortions to DNA caused by binding of the anticancer agent cisplatin. *Proc Natl Acad Sci U S A* 1989;89:2307–2311.

34. Hughes EN, Engelsberg BN, Billings PC. Purification of nuclear proteins that bind to cisplatin-damaged DNA. Identity with high mobility group proteins 1 and 2. *J Biol Chem* 1992;267:13520–13527.

35. Ramachandran S, Temple BR, Chaney SG, et al. Structural basis for the sequence-dependent effects of platinum-DNA adducts. *Nucleic Acids Res* 2009;37:2434–2448.

36. Ramachandran S, Temple B, Alexandrova AN, et al. Recognition of platinum-DNA adducts by HMGB1a. *Biochemistry* 2012;51:7608–7617.

37. Fink D, Zheng H, Nebel S, et al. In vitro and in vivo resistance to cisplatin in cells that have lost DNA mismatch repair. *Cancer Res* 1997;57:1841–1845.

38. Kelland L. The resurgence of platinum-based cancer chemotherapy. *Nat Rev Cancer* 2007;7:573–584.

39. Vasilevskaya IA, Rakitina TV, O'Dwyer PJ. Quantitative effects on c-Jun N-terminal protein kinase signaling determine synergistic interaction of cisplatin and 17-allylamino-17-demethoxygeldanamycin in colon cancer cell lines. *Mol Pharmacol* 2004;65:235–243.

40. Vasilevskaya IA, Selvakumaran M, O'Dwyer PJ. Disruption of signaling through SEK1 and MKK7 yields differential responses in hypoxic colon cancer cells treated with oxaliplatin. *Mol Pharmacol* 2008;74:246–254.

41. Maestre N, Tritton TR, Laurent G, et al. Cell surface-directed interaction of anthracyclines leads to cytotoxicity and nuclear factor kappaB activation but not apoptosis signaling. *Cancer Res* 2001;61:2558–2561.

42. Roodhart JM, Daenen LG, Stigter EC, et al. Mesenchymal stem cells induce resistance to chemotherapy through the release of platinum-induced fatty acids. *Cancer Cell* 2011;20:370–383.

43. Beatty GL, Chiorean EG, Fishman MP, et al. CD40 regulates cancer inflammation and induces regression of pancreatic carcinoma in mice and humans. *Science* 2011;331:1612–1616.

44. Galluzzi L, Senovilla L, Vitale I, et al. Molecular mechanisms of cisplatin resistance. *Oncogene* 2012;31:1869–1883.

45. Lin X, Okuda T, Holzer A, et al. The copper transporter CTR1 regulates cisplatin uptake in Saccharomyces cerevisiae. *Mol Pharmacol* 2002;62:1154–1159.

46. Blair BG, Larson CA, Safaei R, et al. Copper transporter 2 regulates the cellular accumulation and cytotoxicity of cisplatin and carboplatin. *Clin Cancer Res* 2009;15:4312–4321.

47. Samimi G, Varki NM, Wilczynski S, et al. Increase in the expression of the copper transporter ATP7A during platinum drug-based treatment is associated with poor survival in ovarian cancer patients. *Clin Cancer Res* 2003;9:5853–5859.

48. Britten RA, Green JA, Broughton C, et al. The relationship between nuclear glutathione levels and resistance to melphalan in human ovarian tumour cells. *Biochem Pharmacol* 1991;41:647–649.

49. Mistry P, Kelland L, Abel G, et al. The relationships between glutathione, glutathione-S-transferase and cytotoxicity of platinum drugs and melphalan in eight human ovarian carcinoma cell lines. *Br J Cancer* 1991;64:215–220.

50. Godwin A, Meister A, O'Dwyer P, et al. High resistance to cisplatin in human ovarian cancer cell lines is associated with marked increase in glutathione synthesis. *Proc Natl Acad Sci U S A* 1992;89:3070–3074.

51. Hamilton T, Winker M, Louie K, et al. Augmentation of adriamycin, melphalan and cisplatin cytotoxicity in drug-resistant and -sensitive human ovarian cancer cell lines by buthionine sulfoximine mediated glutathione depletion. *Biochem Pharmacol* 1985;34:2583–2586.

52. Koberle B, Grimaldi K, Sunters A, et al. DNA repair capacity and cisplatin sensitivity of human testis tumour cells. *Int J Cancer* 1997;70:551–555.

53. Martin LP, Hamilton TC, Schilder RJ. Platinum resistance: the role of DNA repair pathways. *Clin Cancer Res* 2008;14:1291–1295.

54. Selvakumaran M, Piscarcik DA, Bao R, et al. Enhanced cisplatin cytotoxicity by disturbing the nucleotide excision repair pathway in ovarian cancer cell lines. *Cancer Res* 2003;63:1311–1316.

55. Hubner RA, Riley RD, Billingham LJ, et al. Excision repair cross-complementation group 1 (ERCC1) status and lung cancer outcomes: a meta-analysis of published studies and recommendations. *PLoS One* 2011;6:e25164.

56. De Dosso S, Zanellato E, Nucifora M, et al. ERCC1 predicts outcome in patients with gastric cancer treated with adjuvant cisplatin-based chemotherapy. *Cancer Chemother Pharmacol* 2013;72:159–165.

57. Squires MH 3rd, Fisher SB, Fisher KE, et al. Differential expression and prognostic value of ERCC1 and thymidylate synthase in resected gastric adenocarcinoma. *Cancer* 2013;119:3242–3250.

58. Yamada Y, Boku N, Nishina T, et al. Impact of excision repair cross-complementing gene 1 (ERCC1) on the outcomes of patients with advanced gastric cancer: correlative study in Japan Clinical Oncology Group Trial JCOG9912. *Ann Oncol* 2013;24:2560–2565.

59. Friboulet L, Olaussen KA, Pignon JP, et al. ERCC1 isoform expression and DNA repair in non–small-cell lung cancer. *N Engl J Med* 2013;368:1101–1110.

60. Bryant HE, Schultz N, Thomas HD, et al. Specific killing of BRCA2-deficient tumours with inhibitors of poly(ADP-ribose) polymerase. *Nature* 2005;434:913–917.

61. Farmer H, McCabe1 N, Lord C, et al. Targeting the DNA repair defect in BRCA mutant cells as a therapeutic strategy. *Nature* 2005;434:917–921.

62. Edwards SL, Brough R, Lord CJ, et al. Resistance to therapy caused by intragenic deletion in BRCA2. *Nature* 2008;451:1111–1116.

63. Sakai W, Swisher EM, Karlan BM, et al. Secondary mutations as a mechanism of cisplatin resistance in BRCA2-mutated cancers. *Nature* 2008;451:1116–1121.

64. Gelmon KA, Tischkowitz M, Mackay H, et al. Olaparib in patients with recurrent high-grade serous or poorly differentiated ovarian carcinoma or triple-negative breast cancer: a phase 2, multicentre, open-label, non-randomised study. *Lancet Oncology* 2011;12:852–861.

65. Levine B, Kroemer G. Autophagy in the pathogenesis of disease. *Cell* 2008;132:27–42.

66. Matthew R, Karantza-Wadsworth V, White E. Role of autophagy in cancer. *Nat Rev Cancer* 2007;7:961–967.

67. Amaravadi RK, Yu D, Lum JJ, et al. Autophagy inhibition enhances therapy-induced apoptosis in a Myc-induced model of lymphoma. *J Clin Invest* 2007;117:326–336.

68. Duffull S, Robinson B. Clinical pharmacokinetics and dose optimization of carboplatin. *Clin Pharmacokinet* 1997;33:161–183.

69. Harland S, Newell D, Siddik Z, et al. Pharmacokinetics of cis-diammine-1,1-cyclobutane dicarboxylate platinum(II) in patients with normal and impaired renal function. *Cancer Res* 1984;44:1693–1697.

70. Graham MA, Lockwood GF, Greenslade D, et al. Clinical pharmacokinetics of oxaliplatin: a critical review. *Clin Cancer Res* 2000;6:1205–1218.

71. Gamelin E, Bouil A, Boisdron-Celle M, et al. Cumulative pharmacokinetic study of oxaliplatin, administered every three weeks, combined with 5-fluorouracil in colorectal cancer patients. *Clin Cancer Res* 1997;3:891–899.

72. Extra JM, Marty M, Brienza S, et al. Pharmacokinetics and safety profile of oxaliplatin. *Semin Oncol* 1998;25:13–22.

73. Chatelut E, Canal P, Brunner V, et al. Prediction of carboplatin clearance from standard morphological and biological patient characteristics. *J Natl Cancer Inst* 1995;87:573–580.

74. Jodrell D, Egorin M, Canetta R, et al. Relationships between carboplatin exposure and tumor response and toxicity in patients with ovarian cancer. *J Clin Oncol* 1992;10:520–528.

75. Reyno L, Egorin M, Canetta R, et al. Impact of cyclophosphamide on relationships between carboplatin exposure and response or toxicity when used in the treatment of advanced ovarian cancer. *J Clin Oncol* 1993;11:1156–1164.

76. Shen DW, Pouliot LM, Hall MD, et al. Cisplatin resistance: a cellular self-defense mechanism resulting from multiple epigenetic and genetic changes. *Pharmacol Rev* 2012;64:706–721.

77. Ma J, Verweij J, Planting A, et al. Current sample handling methods for measurement of platinum-DNA adducts in leucocytes in man lead to discrepant results in DNA adduct levels and DNA repair. *Br J Cancer* 1995;71:512–517.

78. Schellens J, Ma J, Planting A, et al. Relationship between the exposure to cisplatin, DNA-adduct formation in leucocytes and tumour response in patients with solid tumours. *Br J Cancer* 1996;73:1569–1575.

79. Ozols R, Corden B, Jacob J, et al. High-dose cisplatin in hypertonic saline. *Ann Intern Med* 1984;100:19–24.

80. Howell S, Pfeifle C, Wung W, et al. Intraperitoneal cis-diamminedichloroplatinum with systemic thiosulfate protection. *Cancer Res* 1983;43:1426–1431.

81. Alberts D, Liu P, Hannigan E, et al. Intraperitoneal cisplatin plus intravenous cyclophosphamide versus intravenous cisplatin plus intravenous cyclophosphamide for stage III ovarian cancer. *N Engl J Med* 1996;335:1950–1955.

82. Solomon B, Soulen M, Baum R, et al. Chemoembolization of hepatocellular carcinoma with cisplatin, doxorubicin, mitomycin-C, Ethiodol, and polyvinyl alcohol: prospective evaluation of response and survival in a US population. *J Vasc Interv Radiol* 1999;10:793–798.

83. Extra J, Marty M, Brienza S, et al. Pharmacokinetics and safety profile of oxaliplatin. *Semin Oncol* 1998;25:13–22.

84. Brienza S, Vignoud J, Itzhaki M, et al. Oxaliplatin (L-OHP): global safety in 682 patients. *Proc Am Soc Clin Oncol* 1995;14:209.

85. André T, Boni C, Mounedji-Boudiaf L, et al. Oxaliplatin, fluorouracil, and leucovorin as adjuvant treatment for colon cancer. *N Engl J Med* 2004;350:2343–2351.

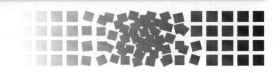

19 Antimetabolites

M. Wasif Saif and Edward Chu

ANTIFOLATES

Reduced folates play a key role in one-carbon metabolism, and they are essential for the biosynthesis of purines, thymidylate, and protein biosynthesis. Aminopterin was the first antimetabolite with documented clinical activity in the treatment of children with acute leukemia in the 1940s. This antifolate analog was subsequently replaced by methotrexate (MTX), the 4-amino, 10-methyl analog of folic acid, which remains the most widely used antifolate analog, with activity against a wide range of cancers (Table 19.1), including hematologic malignancies (acute lymphoblastic leukemia and non-Hodgkin's lymphoma) and many solid tumors (breast cancer, head and neck cancer, osteogenic sarcoma, bladder cancer, and gestational trophoblastic cancer).

Pemetrexed is a pyrrolopyrimidine, multitargeted antifolate analog that targets multiple enzymes involved in folate metabolism, including thymidylate synthase (TS), dihydrofolate reductase (DHFR), glycinamide ribonucleotide (GAR) formyltransferase, and aminoimidazole carboxamide (AICAR) formyltransferase.[1,2] This agent has broad-spectrum activity against solid tumors, including malignant mesothelioma and breast, pancreatic, head and neck, non–small-cell lung, colon, gastric, cervical, and bladder cancers.[3–5]

The third antifolate compound to have entered clinical practice is pralatrexate (10-propargyl-10-deazaaminopterin), a 10-deazaaminopterin antifolate that was rationally designed to bind with higher affinity to the reduced folate carrier (RFC)-1 transport protein, when compared with MTX, leading to enhanced membrane transport into tumor cells. It is also an improved substrate for the enzyme folylpolyglutamyl synthetase (FPGS), resulting in enhanced formation of cytotoxic polyglutamate metabolites.[6,7] When compared with MTX, this analog is a more potent inhibitor of multiple enzymes involved in folate metabolism, including TS, DHFR, and GAR and AICAR formyltransferases. This agent is presently approved for the treatment of relapsed or refractory peripheral T-cell lymphomas.[8]

Mechanism of Action

The antifolate compounds are tight-binding inhibitors of DHFR, a key enzyme in folate metabolism.[1] DHFR plays a pivotal role in maintaining the intracellular folate pools in their fully reduced form as tetrahydrofolates, and these compounds serve as one-carbon carriers required for the synthesis of thymidylate, purine nucleotides, and certain amino acids.

The cytotoxic effects of MTX, pemetrexed, and pralatrexate are mediated by their respective polyglutamate metabolites, with up to 5 to 7 glutamyl groups in a γ-peptide linkage. These polyglutamate metabolites exhibit prolonged intracellular half-lives, thereby allowing for prolonged drug action in tumor cells. Moreover, these polyglutamate metabolites are potent, direct inhibitors of several folate-dependent enzymes, including DHFR, TS, AICAR formyltransferase, and GAR formyltransferase.[1]

Mechanisms of Resistance

The development of cellular resistance to antifolates remains a major obstacle to its clinical efficacy.[9,10] In experimental systems, resistance to antifolates arises from several mechanisms, including an alteration in antifolate transport because of either a defect in the reduced folate carrier or folate receptor systems, decreased capacity to polyglutamate the antifolate parent compound through either decreased expression of FPGS or increased expression of the catabolic enzyme γ-glutamyl hydrolase, and alterations in the target enzymes DHFR and/or TS through increased expression of wild-type protein or overexpression of a mutant protein with reduced binding affinity for the antifolate. Gene amplification is a common resistance mechanism observed in various experimental systems, including tumor samples from patients. In in vitro and in vivo experimental model systems, the levels of DHFR and/or TS protein acutely increase after exposure to MTX and other antifolate compounds. This acute induction of target protein in response to drug exposure is mediated, in part, by a translational regulatory mechanism, which may represent a clinically relevant mechanism for the acute development of cellular drug resistance.

Clinical Pharmacology

The oral bioavailability of MTX is saturable and erratic at doses greater than 25 mg/m². MTX is completely absorbed from parenteral routes of administration, and peak serum levels are achieved within 30 to 60 minutes of administration.

The distribution of MTX into third-space fluid collections, such as pleural effusions and ascitic fluid, can substantially alter MTX pharmacokinetics. The slow release of accumulated MTX from these third spaces over time prolongs the terminal half-life of the drug, leading to potentially increased clinical toxicity. It is advisable to evacuate these fluid collections before treatment and monitor plasma drug concentrations closely.

Renal excretion is the main route of drug elimination, and this process is mediated by glomerular filtration and tubular secretion. About 80% to 90% of an administered dose is eliminated unchanged in the urine. Doses of MTX, therefore, should be reduced in proportion to reductions in creatinine clearance. Renal excretion of MTX is inhibited by probenecid, penicillins, cephalosporins, aspirin, and nonsteroidal anti-inflammatory drugs.

Pemetrexed enters the cell via the RFC system and, to a lesser extent, by the folate receptor protein. As with MTX, it undergoes polyglutamation within the cell to the pentaglutamate form, which is at least 60-fold more potent than the parent compound. This agent is mainly cleared by renal excretion, and in the setting of renal dysfunction, the terminal drug half-life is significantly prolonged to up to 20 hours. Pemetrexed, therefore, should be used with caution in patients with renal dysfunction. In addition, renal excretion is inhibited in the presence of other agents including probenecid, penicillins, cephalosporins, aspirin, and nonsteroidal anti-inflammatory drugs.

TABLE 19.1

Antimetabolites: Indications, Doses and Schedules, and Toxicities

Drug	Main Therapeutic Uses	Main Doses and Schedule	Major Toxicities
Methotrexate	Non-Hodgkin's lymphoma Primary CNS lymphoma Acute lymphoblastic leukemia Breast cancer Bladder cancer Osteogenic sarcoma Gestational trophoblastic cancer	Low dose: 10–50 mg/m^2 IV every 3–4 weeks Low dose weekly: 25 mg/m^2 IV weekly Moderate dose: 100–500 m/m^2 IV every 2–3 weeks High dose: 1–12 gm/m^2 IV over a 3- to 24-hour period every 1–3 weeks Intrathecal (IT): 10–15 mg IT 2 times weekly until CSF is clear, then weekly dose for 2–6 weeks, followed by monthly dose	Mucositis, diarrhea, myelosuppression, acute renal failure, transient elevations in serum transaminases and bilirubin, pneumonitis, neurologic toxicity
Pemetrexed	Mesothelioma Non–small-cell lung cancer	500 mg/m^2 IV, every 3 weeks	Myelosuppression, skin rash, mucositis, diarrhea, fatigue
Pralatrexate	Peripheral T-cell lymphoma	30 mg/m^2 IV, weekly for 6 weeks; cycles repeated every 7 weeks	Myelosuppression, skin rash, mucositis, diarrhea, elevation of serum transaminases and bilirubin, mild nausea/vomiting
5-Fluorouracil	Breast cancer Colorectal cancer Anal cancer Gastroesophageal cancer Hepatocellular cancer Pancreatic cancer Head and neck cancer	Bolus monthly schedule: 425–450 mg/m^2 IV on days 1–5 every 28 days Bolus weekly schedule: 500–600 mg/m^2 IV every week for 6 weeks every 8 weeks Infusion schedule: 2,400–3,000 mg/m^2 IV over 46 hours every 2 weeks 120-hour infusion: 1,000 mg/m^2/d IV on days 1–5 every 21–28 d Protracted continuous infusion: 200–400 mg/m^2/d IV	Nausea/vomiting, diarrhea, mucositis, myelosuppression, neurotoxicity, coronary artery vasospasm, conjunctivitis
Capecitabine	Breast cancer Colorectal cancer Gastroesophageal cancer Hepatocellular cancer Pancreatic cancer	Recommended dose for monotherapy is 1,250 mg/m^2 PO bid for 2 weeks with 1 wk rest May decrease dose of capecitabine to 850–1,000 mg/m^2 bid on days 1–14 to reduce risk of toxicity without compromising efficacy An alternative dosing schedule for monotherapy is 1,250–1,500 mg/m^2 PO bid for 1 week on and 1 week off; this schedule appears to be well tolerated, with no compromise in clinical efficacy Capecitabine should be used at lower doses (850–1,000 mg/m^2 bid on days 1–14) when used in combination with other cytotoxic agents, such as oxaliplatin and lapatinib	Diarrhea, hand-foot syndrome, myelosuppression, mucositis, nausea/vomiting, neurologic toxicity, coronary artery vasospasm
Cytarabine	Hodgkin's lymphoma Non-Hodgkin's lymphoma Acute myelogenous leukemia Acute lymphoblastic leukemia	Standard dose: 100 mg/m^2/day IV on days 1–7 as a continuous IV infusion, in combination with an anthracycline as induction chemotherapy for acute myelogenous leukemia High-dose: 1.5–3.0 gm/m^2 IV q 12 hours for 3 days as a high dose, intensification regimen for acute myelogenous leukemia SC: 20 mg/m^2 SC for 10 days per month for 6 months, associated with IFN-α for treatment of chronic myelogenous leukemia IT: 10–30 mg IT up to 3 times weekly in the treatment of leptomeningeal carcinomatosis secondary to leukemia or lymphoma.	Nausea/vomiting, myelosuppression, cerebellar ataxia, lethargy, confusion, acute pancreatitis, drug infusion reaction, hand-foot syndrome High-dose therapy: noncardiogenic pulmonary edema, acute respiratory distress and *Streptococcus viridans* pneumonia, conjunctivitis, and keratitis
Gemcitabine	Pancreatic cancer Non–small-cell lung cancer Breast cancer Bladder cancer Hodgkin's lymphoma Ovarian cancer Soft tissue sarcoma	Pancreatic cancer: 1,000 mg/m^2 IV every week for 7 weeks with 1 week rest Treatment then continues weekly for 3 weeks followed by 1 week off Bladder cancer: 1,000 mg/m^2 IV on days 1, 8, and 15 every 28 days Non–small-cell lung cancer: 1,000-1,200 mg/m^2 IV on days 1 and 8 every 21 days	Nausea/vomiting, myelosuppression, flulike syndrome, elevation of serum transaminases and bilirubin, pneumonitis, infusion reaction, mild proteinuria, and rarely, hemolytic-uremic syndrome and thrombotic thrombocytopenic purpura

(continued)

TABLE 19.1

Antimetabolites: Indications, Doses and Schedules, and Toxicities *(continued)*

Drug	Main Therapeutic Uses	Main Doses and Schedule	Major Toxicities
6-Mercaptopurine	Acute lymphoblastic leukemia	Induction therapy: 2.5 mg/kg PO daily Maintenance therapy: 1.5–2.5 mg/kg PO daily	Myelosuppression, nausea/vomiting, mucositis and diarrhea, hepatotoxicity, immunosuppression
6-Thioguanine	Acute myelogenous leukemia Acute lymphoblastic leukemia	Induction: 100 mg/m^2 PO every 12 hours on days 1–5, usually in combination with cytarabine Maintenance: 100 mg/m^2 PO every 12 hours on days 1–5, every 4 weeks, usually in combination with other agents Single agent: 1–3 mg/kg PO daily	Myelosuppression, nausea/vomiting, mucositis and diarrhea, hepatotoxicity, immunosuppression
Fludarabine	Chronic lymphocytic leukemia Non-Hodgkin's lymphoma	25 mg/m^2 IV on days 1–5 every 28 days For oral usage, the recommended dose is 40 mg/m^2 PO on days 1–5 every 28 days	Myelosuppression, immunosuppression with increased risk of opportunistic infections, mild nausea/vomiting, hypersensitivity reaction
Cladribine	Hairy cell leukemia Chronic lymphocytic leukemia Non-Hodgkin's lymphoma	Usual dose is 0.09 mg/kg/d IV via continuous infusion for 7 days; one course is usually administered	Myelosuppression, immunosuppression, mild nausea/vomiting, fever
Clofarabine	Acute lymphoblastic leukemia	52 mg/m^2 IV daily for 5 days every 2–6 weeks	Myelosuppression nausea/vomiting, diarrhea, systemic inflammatory response syndrome, increased risk of opportunistic infections, renal toxicity

CNS, central nervous system; IV, intravenously; CSF, cerebrospinal fluid; PO, by mouth; bid, twice daily; SC, subcutaneously; IFN-α, interferon alpha.

As with other antifolate analogs, pralatrexate is transported into the cell by the RFC carrier protein and then metabolized by FPGS to form longer chain polyglutamates, with up to four additional glutamate residues attached to the parent molecule. About 34% of the parent drug is cleared in the urine during the first 24 hours after drug administration. As such, caution is advised when using pralatrexate in patients with renal dysfunction. As with MTX and pemetrexed, the concomitant administration of other agents such as probenecid, penicillins, cephalosporins, aspirin, and nonsteroidal anti-inflammatory drugs, may inhibit renal clearance.

Toxicity

The main side effects of MTX are myelosuppression and gastrointestinal (GI) toxicity, which are usually completely reversed within 14 days, unless drug-elimination mechanisms are impaired. In patients with compromised renal function, even small doses of MTX may result in serious toxicity. MTX-induced nephrotoxicity is thought to result from the intratubular precipitation of MTX and its metabolites in acidic urine. Antifolates may also exert a direct toxic effect on the renal tubules. Vigorous hydration and urinary alkalinization have greatly reduced the incidence of renal failure in patients on high-dose regimens. Acute elevations in hepatic enzyme levels and hyperbilirubinemia are often observed during high-dose therapy, but these levels usually return to normal within 10 days. Methotrexate given concomitantly with radiotherapy may increase the risk of soft tissue necrosis and osteonecrosis.

The original rationale for high-dose MTX therapy was based on the concept of selective rescue of normal tissues by the reduced folate leucovorin (LV). However, recent data suggest that high-dose MTX may also overcome resistance mechanisms caused by impaired active transport, decreased affinity of DHFR for MTX,

increased levels of DHFR resulting from gene amplification, and/or decreased polyglutamation of MTX.

The main toxicities of pemetrexed and pralatrexate include dose-limiting myelosuppression, mucositis, and skin rash, usually in the form of the hand-foot syndrome (HFS). Other toxicities include reversible transaminasemia, anorexia and fatigue syndrome, and GI toxicity. These side effects are reduced by supplementation with folic acid (350 μg orally daily) and vitamin B$_{12}$ (1,000 mg subcutaneously given at least 1 week before starting therapy, and then repeated every three cycles). To date, there is no evidence to suggest that vitamin supplementation adversely affects the clinical efficacy of pemetrexed or pralatrexate.

5-FLUOROPYRIMIDINES

The fluoropyrimidine, 5-fluorouracil (5-FU) was synthesized by Charles Heidelberger in the mid 1950s. Uracil is a normal component of RNA; as such, the rationale leading to the development of the drug was that cancer cells might be more sensitive to *decoy* molecules that mimic the natural compound than normal cells. 5-FU and its derivatives are an integral part of treatment for a broad range of solid tumors (see Table 19.1), including GI malignancies (esophageal, gastric, pancreatic, colorectal, anal, and hepatocellular cancers), breast, head and neck, and skin cancers.[11] It continues to serve as the main backbone for combination regimens used to treat metastatic colorectal cancer (mCRC) and as adjuvant therapy of early-stage colon cancer.

Mechanism of Action

5-FU enters cells via the facilitated uracil base transport mechanism and is then anabolized to various cytotoxic nucleotide forms

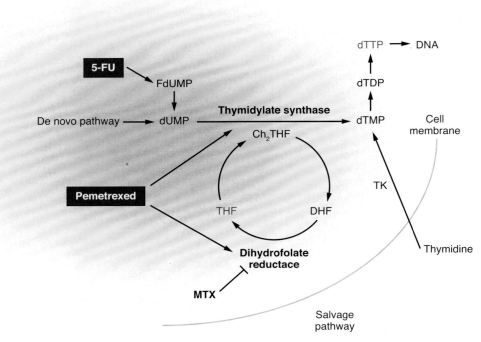

Figure 19.1 Antifolates and 5-fluorouracil (5-FU) sites of action. FdUMP, fluorodeoxyuridine monophosphate; dUMP, deoxyuridine monophosphate; dTTP, deoxythymidine triphosphate; dTDP, deoxyuridine diphosphate; dTMP, deoxythymidine monophosphate; TK, thymidine kinase; CH₂THF, 5,10-methylenetetrahydrofolate; THF, tetrahydrofolate; DHF, dihydrofolate.

by several biochemical pathways. It is thought that 5-FU exerts its cytotoxic effects through various mechanisms, including (1) the inhibition of TS, (2) incorporation into RNA, and (3) incorporation into DNA (Fig. 19.1). In addition to these mechanisms, the genotoxic stress resulting from TS inhibition may also activate programmed cell-death pathways in susceptible cells, which leads to the induction of parental DNA fragmentation.

Mechanisms of Resistance

Several resistance mechanisms to 5-FU have been identified in experimental and clinical settings. Alterations in the target enzyme TS represent the most commonly described mechanism of resistance. In vitro, in vivo, and clinical studies have documented a strong correlation between the levels of TS enzyme activity/TS protein and chemosensitivity to 5-FU. In this regard, cell lines and tumors with higher levels of TS are relatively more resistant to 5-FU. Mutations in the TS protein have been identified that lead to reduced binding affinity of the 5-FU metabolite fluorodeoxyuridine monophosphate (FdUMP) to the TS protein. Reduced expression and/or diminished activity of key activating enzymes may interfere with the formation of cytotoxic 5-FU metabolites. Decreased expression of mismatch repair enzymes, such as human mutL homolog 1 (hMLH1) and human mutS homolog 2 (hMSH2), and increased expression of the catabolic enzyme dihydropyrimidine dehydrogenase (DPD) are associated with fluoropyrimidine resistance. At this time, the relative contribution of each of these mechanisms in the development of cellular resistance to 5-FU in the actual clinical setting remains unclear.

Clinical Pharmacology

5-FU is not orally administered, given its erratic bioavailability resulting from high levels of the catabolic enzyme DPD present

in the gut mucosa. After intravenous bolus doses, metabolic elimination is rapid, with a half-life of 8 to 14 minutes. More than 85% of an administered dose of 5-FU is enzymatically inactivated by DPD, the rate-limiting enzyme in the catabolism of 5-FU.

A pharmacogenetic syndrome has been identified in which partial or compete deficiency in the DPD enzyme is present in 3% to 5% and 0.1% of the general population, respectively. As DPD catalyzes the rate-limiting step in the catabolic pathway of 5-FU, a deficiency of DPD can result in a clinically dangerous increase in the anabolic products of 5-FU. Unfortunately, patients with DPD deficiency do not manifest a phenotype only until they are treated with 5-FU, and in that setting, they can develop severe GI toxicity in the form of mucositis and/or diarrhea, myelosuppression, neurologic toxicity, and in rare cases, death. In patients being treated with 5-FU or any other fluoropyrimidine, it is important to consider DPD deficiency in patients who present with excessive, severe toxicity.[12] It is now increasingly appreciated that DPD mutations are unable to account for all of the observed cases of excessive 5-FU toxicity, because up to 50% of patients who experience 5-FU toxicity will have no documented alterations in the *DPD* gene. Moreover, individuals with normal DPD enzyme activity may be diagnosed with high plasma levels of 5-FU, resulting in increased toxicity. Although DPD enzyme activity can be assayed from peripheral blood mononuclear cells in a specialized laboratory, routine phenotypic and genotypic screenings for DPD deficiency prior to 5-FU therapy are not yet available.

Biomodulation of 5-FU

Significant efforts have focused on enhancing the antitumor activity of 5-FU through biochemical modulation in which 5-FU is combined with various agents, including leucovorin, MTX, N-phosphonacetyl-L-aspartic acid, interferon-α, interferon-γ, and

TABLE 19.2

Toxicities of Different Forms of 5-FU

Route	Schedule	Dose	DLT
IV	Daily × 5, bolus	400–500 (mg/m²/d)	⇓ BM D M
IV	Weekly bolus	450–500 (mg/m²/d)	⇓ BM
IV	Daily × 5, CI	750–1,000 (mg/m²/d)	M D
IV	PCI	200–400 (mg/m²/d)	M HFS
HAI	Daily × 14–21, CI	750–1,000 (mg/m²/d)	M D
IP	32–120 hr	5 nM	M D
Oral (Xeloda)	14–21 d	2,000–2,500 (mg/m²/d)	HFS

DLT, dose limiting toxicity; IV, intravenous; BM, bone marrow; D, diarrhea; M, mucositis; CI, continuous infusion; PCI, protracted continuous infusion; HFS, hand-foot syndrome; HAI, hepatic artery infusion; IP, intraperitoneal.

a whole host of other agents.[13] For the past 20 to 25 years, the reduced folate LV has been the main biochemical modulator of 5-FU. An alternative approach has been to alter the schedule of 5-FU administration. Given the S-phase specificity of this agent, prolonged exposure of tumor cells to 5-FU would increase the fraction of cells being exposed to the drug. Overall response rates are significantly higher in patients treated with infusional schedules of 5-FU than in those treated with bolus 5-FU, and this improvement in response rate has translated into an improved progression-free survival. Moreover, the overall safety profile is improved with infusional regimens. A hybrid schedule of bolus and infusional 5-FU was originally developed in France, and this regimen has shown superior clinical activity compared with bolus 5-FU schedules. This hybrid schedule has now been simplified by using only the 46-hour infusion of 5-FU and completely eliminating the 5-FU bolus doses.

Toxicity

The spectrum of 5-FU toxicity is dose- and schedule-dependent (Table 19.2). The main side effects are diarrhea, mucositis, and myelosuppression. The dermatologic HFS is more commonly observed with infusional 5-FU therapy. Acute neurologic symptoms have also been reported, and they include somnolence, cerebellar ataxia, and upper motor signs. Treatment with 5-FU can, on rare occasions, cause coronary vasospasm, resulting in a syndrome of chest pain, cardiac enzyme elevations, and electrocardiographic changes. Cardiac toxicity seems to be related more to infusional 5-FU than bolus administration.[14]

CAPECITABINE

Capecitabine is an oral fluoropyrimidine carbamate that was rationally designed to allow for selective 5-FU activation in tumor tissue.[15] This oral agent was initially approved in anthracycline- and taxane-resistant breast cancer and subsequently approved for use in combination with docetaxel as second-line therapy in metastatic breast cancer and in combination with lapatinib, a tyrosine-kinase inhibitor of human epidermal growth factor receptor type 2 (HER2) and epidermal growth factor receptor (EGFR) in women with HER2-positive metastatic breast cancer following progression on trastuzumab-based therapy.[16] This agent is also approved by the

U.S. Food and Drug Administration (FDA) for the first-line treatment of mCRC and as adjuvant therapy for stage III colon cancer when fluoropyrimidine therapy alone is preferred.[17] In Europe and throughout much of the world, the combination of capecitabine plus oxaliplatin (XELOX) is approved for the treatment of mCRC as well as for the adjuvant therapy of stage III colon cancer.[18] In addition, recent studies have documented the noninferiority of capecitabine to 5-FU when combined with cisplatin in the treatment of metastatic gastric cancer.

Clinical Pharmacology

Capecitabine is rapidly and extensively absorbed by the gut mucosa, with nearly 80% oral bioavailability. It is inactive in its parent form and undergoes enzymatic conversion via three successive steps. Of note, the third and final step occurs in tumor tissue and involves the conversion of 5′-deoxy-5-fluorouridine to 5-FU by the enzyme thymidine phosphorylase (TP), which is expressed at much higher levels in tumors when compared with corresponding normal tissue. Capecitabine and capecitabine metabolites are primarily excreted by the kidneys, and in contrast to 5-FU, caution must be taken in the presence of renal dysfunction, with appropriate dose modification. The use of capecitabine is absolutely contraindicated in patients whose creatinine clearance is less than 30 mL per minute. The FDA and Roche have added a black box warning and strengthened the precautions section on the capecitabine label about the drug–drug interaction between warfarin and capecitabine-based chemotherapy. It is generally recommended to do weekly monitoring of the coagulation parameters (prothrombin time/international normalized ratio [PT/INR]) for all patients receiving concomitant warfarin and capecitabine, with an appropriate adjustment of warfarin dose.

Toxicity

Similar to what is observed with infusional 5-FU, the main side effects of capecitabine include diarrhea and HFS. Of note, the incidence of myelosuppression, neutropenic fever, mucositis, alopecia, and nausea/vomiting is lower with capecitabine when compared with 5-FU. Elevations in indirect serum bilirubin can be observed, but are usually transient and clinically asymptomatic. Patients in the United States appear to be unable to tolerate as high doses of capecitabine as European patients, either as monotherapy or in combination with other cytotoxic chemotherapy.[19] Although the underlying reasons for this discrepancy are not known, it may in part be related to the increased fortification of the US diet with folate and the increased focus on vitamin and folic acid supplementation.

S-1

S-1 is an oral fluoropyrimidine that consists of tegafur (FT), a prodrug of 5-FU, combined with two 5-FU biochemical modulators: 5-chloro-2,4-dihydroxypyridine (gimeracil or CDHP), a competitive inhibitor of DPD, and oteracil potassium, which inhibits phosphorylation of 5-flurouracil in the GI tract, thereby decreasing serious GI toxicities such as nausea/vomiting, mucositis, and diarrhea.[20] As with other oral agents, S-1 offers several advantages over 5-FU, including ease of administration, no risks associated with use of central venous access such as infection, thrombosis, etc., and reduced toxicities, especially neurotoxicity. Although S-1 has yet to be approved by the FDA, it has been approved for the treatment of gastric cancer, head and neck, colorectal cancer (CRC), non–small-cell lung, breast, pancreatic, and biliary tract cancers in several countries in Asia and for the treatment of advanced gastric cancer in combination with cisplatin in a large number of European countries.

Clinical Pharmacology

S-1 was designed to provide continuous 5-FU plasma exposure comparable to the intravenous (IV) infusion. FT, the 5-FU prodrug, is absorbed in the small intestine and converted to 5-FU through the liver microsomal P-450 metabolizing enzyme system (CYP2A6). Most of the 5-FU is degraded (85%) by DPD, leading to the formation of fluoro-beta-alanine (FBAL).[21] CDHP inhibits DPD, thus allowing higher concentrations of 5-FU to enter the anabolic pathway and enhance its therapeutic effect. Additionally, the inhibition of DPD leads to a decreased amount of FBAL formation, which presumably leads to reduced neurotoxicity. Oteracil is the final component of the S-1 formulation, and it inhibits orotate phosphoribosyltransferase in the GI mucosa, which prevents the formation of fluorouridine monophosphate (FUMP), thereby decreasing GI toxicity.

The maximum tolerated dose was established at 80 mg/m^2 in two divided doses for a Japanese population and 25 mg/m^2 twice a day for a Caucasian population. This interethnic variability of S-1 pharmacokinetics and pharmacodynamics has been attributed to differences in the CYP2A6 genotypes.[22] Studies have demonstrated a high frequency of allelic variants CYP2A6*4, *7, and *9 in East Asians than in Caucasians, which might be associated with reduced enzymatic activity and decreased activation of FT. On the other hand, higher FT metabolism is seen in Caucasian patients due to higher CYP2A6 activity. However, investigators have established similar 5-FU exposure between these two ethnic groups. These findings were explained by higher CDHP exposure in Asians, resulting in increased DPD inhibition and slower catabolism of 5-FU, despite having low CYP2A6 activity, whereas Caucasians had higher CYP2A6 activity but faster 5-FU clearance.

Clinical Toxicity

Clinical studies have shown that the GI toxicities associated with S-1, such as diarrhea, nausea, vomiting, and hyperbilirubinemia, are more prominent in Western patients, whereas hematologic toxicities are more prevalent in Japanese patients. The difference in safety profile cannot be explained by differences in 5-FU exposure, because pharmacokinetic studies have shown that overall drug exposures are similar. A potential explanation might involve interethnic variations in TS promoter enhancer region polymorphisms, which are more frequently seen in Asians or in Caucasians on a higher folate diet.

CYTARABINE

Cytarabine (ara-C) is a deoxycytidine nucleoside analog isolated from the sponge *Cryptotethya crypta*, and it differs from its physiologic counterpart by virtue of a stereotypic inversion of the 2'-hydroxyl group of the sugar moiety.[23] A regimen of ara-C, combined with an anthracycline and given as a 5- or 7-day continuous infusion, is considered the standard induction treatment for acute myeloid leukemia (AML). Ara-C is active against other hematologic malignancies, such as non-Hodgkin's lymphoma, chronic myelogenous leukemia, and acute lymphocytic leukemia (see Table 19.1). However, this agent has absolutely no activity against solid tumors.

Mechanism of Action

Ara-C enters cells via nucleoside transport proteins, the most important one being the equilibrative inhibitor-sensitive (ES) receptor. Once inside the cell, ara-C requires activation for its cytotoxic effects.[23,24] The first metabolic step is the conversion of ara-C to the monophosphate form ara-cytidine monophosphate (ara-CMP) by the enzyme deoxycytidine kinase (dCK) with subsequent phosphorylation to the di- and triphosphate metabolites, respectively. Ara-cytidine triphosphate (ara-CTP) is a potent inhibitor of DNA polymerases α, β, and γ, which in turn interferes with DNA chain elongation, DNA synthesis, and DNA repair. Ara-CTP is also incorporated directly into DNA and functions as a DNA chain terminator, interfering with chain elongation. Catabolism of ara-C involves two key enzymes, cytidine deaminase and deoxycytidylate deaminase. These breakdown enzymes convert ara-C and ara-CMP into the inactive metabolites, ara-uridine (ara-U) and ara-uridine monophosphate (ara-UMP), respectively. The balance between intracellular activation and degradation is critical in determining the amount of drug that is ultimately converted to ara-CTP and, thus, its subsequent cytotoxic and antitumor activity.

Mechanisms of Resistance

Several resistance mechanisms to ara-C have been described. An impaired transmembrane transport, a decreased rate of anabolism, and an increased rate of catabolism may result in the development of ara-C resistance.[23,25,26] The level of cytidine deaminase enzyme activity has been shown to correlate with clinical response in patients with AML undergoing induction chemotherapy with ara-C–containing regimens.

Clinical Pharmacology

Ara-C has poor oral bioavailability given its extensive deamination within the GI tract. Thus, ara-C is administered intravenously via continuous infusion. After administration, ara-C undergoes extensive metabolism in the liver, plasma, and peripheral tissues. Within 24 hours, up to 80% of drug is recovered in the urine as the ara-U metabolite. Ara-C crosses the blood–brain barrier when used at high doses, with cerebrospinal fluid levels between 7% and 14% of plasma levels and reaching peak levels of up to 10 μM.

Toxicity

The toxicity profile of ara-C is highly dependent on the dose and schedule of administration. Myelosuppression is dose-limiting with a standard 7-day regimen. Leukopenia and thrombocytopenia are observed most frequently, with nadirs occurring between days 7 and 14 after drug administration. GI toxicity commonly manifests as a mild-to-moderate degree of anorexia, nausea, and vomiting along with mucositis, diarrhea, and abdominal pain. In rare cases, acute pancreatitis has been observed. The ara-C syndrome has been described in pediatric patients with hematologic malignancies, usually begins within 12 hours after the start of drug infusion, and is characterized by fever, myalgia, bone pain, maculopapular rash, conjunctivitis, malaise, and occasional chest pain.

The administration of ara-C at high doses (2 to 3 g/m^2 with each dose) is associated with profound myelosuppression.[27] Severe GI toxicity in the form of mucositis and/or diarrhea is also observed. Neurologic toxicity is significantly more common with high-dose ara-C than with standard doses, and presents with seizures, cerebral and cerebellar dysfunction, and peripheral neuropathy. Clinical signs of cerebellar dysfunction occur in up to 15% of patients and include dysarthria, dysmetria, and ataxia. Change in alertness and cognitive ability, memory loss, and frontal lobe release signs reflect cerebral toxicity. Despite discontinuation of therapy, clinical recovery is incomplete in up to 30% of affected patients. Pulmonary complications may include noncardiogenic pulmonary edema, acute respiratory distress, and pneumonia, resulting from *Streptococcus viridans* infection. Other side effects associated with high-dose ara-C include conjunctivitis (often responsive to topical corticosteroids), a painful HFS, and rarely, anaphylactic reactions.

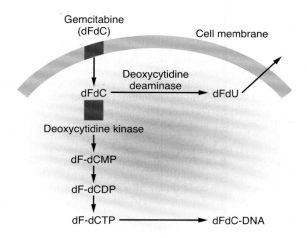

Figure 19.2 Transport and metabolism of gemcitabine. dFdC, gemcitabine; dFdU, 2',2'-difluorodeoxyuridine; dF-dCMP, gemcitabine monophosphate; dF-dCDP, gemcitabine diphosphate; dF-dCTP, gemcitabine triphosphate.

GEMCITABINE

Gemcitabine (2',2'-difluorodeoxycytidine) is a difluorinated deoxycytidine analog. Despite its similarity in structure, metabolism, and mechanism of action to ara-C, the spectrum of antitumor activity of gemcitabine is much broader.[23,28] This compound has significant clinical activity against several human solid tumors, including pancreatic, bile duct, gall bladder, small cell and non–small-cell lung, bladder, ovary, and breast cancers as well as hematologic malignancies, namely Hodgkin's and non-Hodgkin's lymphoma (see Table 19.1).

Mechanism of Action

The transport of gemcitabine into cells requires the nucleoside transporter system. Gemcitabine is inactive in its parent form and requires intracellular activation for its cytotoxic effects. The steps involved in the metabolic activation of gemcitabine are similar to those observed with ara-C, with both drugs being activated by the same enzymatic machinery to the active triphosphate metabolite (see Fig. 19.2). Gemcitabine triphosphate is then incorporated into DNA, resulting in chain termination and the inhibition of DNA synthesis and function, or the triphosphate form can directly inhibit DNA polymerases α, β, and γ, which in turn, interferes with DNA chain elongation, DNA synthesis, and DNA repair. The triphosphate metabolite is also a potent inhibitor of ribonucleotide reductase, which further mediates inhibition of DNA biosynthesis by reducing the levels of key deoxynucleotide pools.[29]

Mechanisms of Resistance

Several mechanisms of resistance to gemcitabine have been described in various preclinical experimental models.[30] Gemcitabine is a polar nucleoside analog that requires the activity of human equilibrative nucleoside transporter 1 (hENT1) to enter cells and exert its cytotoxic effects. Preclinical data in human pancreatic cancer cell lines showed that gemcitabine resistance is negatively correlated with hENT1 expression and can be induced by specific inhibitors of hENT1.[31] Clinical data also support the concept that a lack of hENT1 may be predictive of resistance to gemcitabine. CO-101, a lipid-drug conjugate of gemcitabine, was rationally designed to enter cells independently of hENT1. Unfortunately, two studies in pancreatic cancer failed to show any benefit of CO-101.

Additionally, several enzymes involved in the intracellular metabolism of gemcitabine have been implicated in the development of cellular drug resistance, including reduced expression and/or deficiency in dCK enzyme activity as well as increased expression and/or activity of the catabolic enzymes cytidine deaminase and dCMP deaminase. Recent studies have also identified a subset of CD44-positive cancer stem cells within pancreatic tumors that sustain tumor formation and growth, and are resistant to gemcitabine therapy.[33]

Clinical Pharmacology

Gemcitabine is administered via the intravenous route, typically over a 30-minute intravenous infusion, and it undergoes extensive metabolism by deamination to the catabolic metabolite, difluorodeoxyuridine (dFdU), with more than 90% of the metabolized drug being recovered in urine. Plasma clearance is about 30% lower in women and in elderly patients, and this pharmacokinetic difference may result in an increased risk of toxicity in these respective patient populations. The initial findings from pilot pharmacokinetic studies suggested that gemcitabine, when given at a fixed dose rate (FDR) intravenous infusion of 10 mg/m² per minute, produced the highest accumulation of active dFdCTP metabolites in peripheral blood mononuclear cells, which led to a randomized phase II trial that compared gemcitabine 1,500 mg/m² by FDR or 2,200 mg/m² of gemcitabine over 30 minutes. Although this phase II study suggested an improved overall survival with FDR, a subsequent phase III trial failed to confirm the survival advantage of gemcitabine by FDR over its conventional administration schedule.[34]

Toxicity

Gemcitabine is a relatively well-tolerated drug when used as a single agent. The main dose-limiting toxicity is myelosuppression, with neutropenia more commonly experienced than thrombocytopenia. Toxicity is schedule dependent, with longer infusions producing greater hematologic toxicity. Transient flulike symptoms, including fever, headache, arthralgias, and myalgias, occur in 45% of patients. Asthenia and transient transaminasemia may occur. Renal microangiopathy syndromes, including hemolytic-uremic syndrome and thrombotic thrombocytopenic purpura, have been reported rarely.

6-THIOPURINES

The development of the purine analogs in cancer chemotherapy began in the early 1950s with the synthesis of the thiopurines, 6-mercaptopurine (6-MP) and 6-thioguanine (6-TG). 6-MP has an important role in maintenance therapy for acute lymphoblastic leukemia, whereas 6-TG is active in remission induction and in maintenance therapy for AML (see Table 19.1).

Mechanism of Action

The thiopurines, 6-MP and 6-TG, act similarly with respect to their cellular biochemistry.[34] In their respective monophosphate nucleotide forms, they inhibit enzymes involved in de novo purine synthesis and purine interconversion reactions. The triphosphate nucleotide forms can get directly incorporated into either cellular RNA or DNA, leading to the inhibition of RNA and DNA synthesis and function, respectively.

Mechanisms of Resistance

The development of cellular resistance to 6-thiopurines results from a decreased level of key cytotoxic nucleotide metabolites, either through decreased formation or increased breakdown. Resistant cells have been identified that express either complete or partial deficiency of the activating enzyme hypoxanthine-guanine phosphoribosyltransferase (HGPRT). In clinical samples derived from patients with AML, drug resistance has been associated with increased concentrations of a membrane-bound alkaline phosphatase or a conjugating enzyme, 6-thiopurine methyltransferase (TPMT), the end-result being reduced formation of cytotoxic thiopurine nucleotides. Finally, the decreased expression of mismatch repair enzymes, including hMLH1 and hMSH2, has been associated with cellular drug resistance.

Clinical Pharmacology

Oral absorption of 6-MP is highly erratic, and the relatively poor oral bioavailability is mainly related to rapid first-pass metabolism in the liver. The major route of drug elimination is via metabolism by several enzymatic pathways. 6-MP is oxidized to the inactive metabolite 6-thiouric acid by xanthine oxidase. Enhanced 6-MP toxicity may result from the concomitant administration of 6-MP and the xanthine oxidase inhibitor allopurinol. In patients receiving both 6-MP and allopurinol, the 6-MP dose must be reduced by at least 50% to 75%. 6-MP also undergoes S-methylation by the enzyme TPMT to yield 6-methylmercaptopurine.[35]

6-TG is administered orally in the treatment of AML. Its oral bioavailability is erratic, with peak plasma levels occurring 2 to 4 hours after ingestion. The catabolism of 6-TG differs from 6-MP in that it is not a direct substrate for xanthine oxidase.

TPMT enzyme activity may vary considerably among patients as a result of point mutations or loss of alleles of TPMT.[36] Approximately 0.3% of the Caucasian population expresses either a homozygous deletion or a mutation of both alleles of the *TPMT* gene. In these patients, grossly elevated thiopurine nucleotides concentrations, profound myelosuppression with pancytopenia, and extensive GI symptoms are observed after only a brief course of thiopurine treatment. An estimated 10% of patients may be at increased risk for toxicity because of heterozygous loss of the gene or a mutant allele coding for a less enzymatically active TPMT.

Toxicity

The major dose-related toxicities of the thiopurines are myelosuppression and GI toxicity in the form of nausea/vomiting, anorexia, diarrhea, and stomatitis.[37] In TPMT-deficient patients, dosage reduction to 5% to 25% of the standard dosage is necessary to prevent severe excessive toxicity. Thiopurine hepatotoxicity occurs in up to 30% of adult patients and presents mainly as cholestatic jaundice, although elevations of hepatic transaminases may also be seen. Combinations of thiopurines with other known hepatotoxic agents should be avoided, and liver function should be closely monitored. The thiopurines are also potent suppressors of cell-mediated immunity, and prolonged therapy results in an increased predisposition to bacterial and parasitic infections.

FLUDARABINE

Fludarabine (9-β-D-arabinosyl-2-fluoroadenine monophosphate, F-ara-AMP) is an active agent in the treatment of chronic lymphocytic leukemia (CLL) (see Table 19.1).[38,39] It is also active against indolent non-Hodgkin's lymphoma, prolymphocytic leukemia, cutaneous T-cell lymphoma, and Waldenström macroglobulinemia. This agent has also shown promising activity in mantle cell lymphoma. In contrast to its activity in hematologic malignancies, this compound has virtually no activity against solid tumors.

Mechanism of Action

The active cytotoxic metabolite is the triphosphate metabolite F-ara-ATP, which competes with deoxyadenosine triphosphate (dATP) for incorporation into DNA and serves as a highly effective chain terminator. In addition, F-ara-ATP directly inhibits enzymes involved in DNA replication, including DNA polymerases, DNA primase, DNA ligase I, and ribonucleotide reductase.[37] F-ara-ATP is also incorporated into RNA, causing the inhibition of RNA function, processing, and mRNA translation. In contrast to other antimetabolites, fludarabine is active against nondividing cells. In fact, the primary effect of fludarabine may result from activation of apoptosis, through an as yet ill-defined mechanisms.[39] This finding may explain the activity of fludarabine in indolent lymphoproliferative diseases with relatively low growth fractions.

Mechanisms of Resistance

The decreased expression of the activating enzyme dCK resulting in diminished intracellular formation of F-ara-AMP is one of the main resistance mechanisms identified in preclinical models.[38] A high degree of cross-resistance develops to multiple nucleoside analogs, requiring activation by dCK, including cytarabine, gemcitabine, cladribine, and clofarabine. Reduced cellular transport of drug has also been identified as a resistance mechanism.

Clinical Pharmacology

Peak concentrations of F-ara-A are reached 3 to 4 hours after intravenous administration.[40] The main route of elimination is via the kidneys, with about 25% of a given dose of drug being excreted unchanged in the urine.

Toxicity

Myelosuppression and immunosuppression are the major side effects of fludarabine as highlighted by dose-limiting and possibly cumulative lymphopenia and thrombocytopenia. Suppression of the immune system affects T-cell function more than B-cell function. Fevers, often in the setting of neutropenia, occur in 20% to 30% of patients. Lymphocyte counts, specifically CD4-positive cells, decrease rapidly after the initiation of therapy, and recovery of CD4-positive cells to normal levels may take longer than 1 year. Common opportunistic pathogens include the varicella-zoster virus, *Candida*, and *Pneumocystis carinii*. In general, patients are empirically placed on sulfamethoxazole trimethoprim prophylaxis to prevent the development of *P. carinii* infection.

CLADRIBINE

Cladribine (2-CdA) is a purine deoxyadenosine analog, and it is the drug of choice for hairy cell leukemia with activity in low-grade lymphoproliferative disorders (see Table 19.1).[41,42] Salvage treatment of patients previously treated with interferon-α or splenectomy is as effective as first-line treatment. Retreatment with cladribine results in a complete response in up to 60% of relapsing patients. In addition, this agent has promising activity in patients with CLL and non-Hodgkin's lymphoma.

Mechanism of Action

Upon entry into the cell, 2-CdA undergoes an initial conversion to cladribine-monophosphate (Cd-AMP) via the reaction catalyzed by dCK, and Cd-AMP is subsequently metabolized to the active metabolite, cladribine-triphosphate. The triphosphate metabolite competitively inhibits incorporation of the normal dATP nucleotide into DNA, a process that results in the termination of chain elongation.[43] Progressive accumulation of the triphosphate metabolite leads to an imbalance in deoxyribonucleotide pools, thereby inhibiting further DNA synthesis and repair. Finally, the triphosphate metabolite is a potent inhibitor of ribonucleotide reductase, which further facilitates the inhibition of DNA biosynthesis.

Mechanisms of Resistance

Resistance to 2-CdA has been attributed to altered intracellular drug metabolism. A reduction in the activity of dCK, the enzyme responsible for generating cytotoxic nucleotide metabolites, is a major determinant of acquired resistance. The monophosphate and triphosphate metabolites are dephosphorylated by the cytoplasmic enzyme 5'-nucleotidase. Interestingly, resistant cells derived from a patient with CLL exhibited both low levels of dCK expression and high levels of 5'-nucleotidase.

Clinical Pharmacology

2-CdA is orally bioavailable, with 50% of an administered dose orally absorbed. Approximately 50% of an administered dose of drug is cleared by the kidneys, and 20% to 35% of the drug is excreted unchanged in the urine. Of note, this nucleoside can cross the blood–brain barrier with penetration into the cerebrospinal fluid.

Toxicity

At conventional doses, myelosuppression is dose limiting. After a single course of drug, recovery from thrombocytopenia usually occurs within 2 to 4 weeks, whereas recovery from neutropenia takes place in 3 to 5 weeks. GI toxicities are generally mild, with nausea/vomiting and diarrhea. Mild-to-moderate neurotoxicity occurs in 15% of patients and is at least partly reversible with discontinuation of the drug. Immunosuppression accounts for the late morbidity observed in 2-CdA–treated patients. Lymphocyte counts, particularly CD4-positive cells, decrease within 1 to 4 weeks of drug administration and may remain depressed for several years.[44] After discontinuation of 2-CdA, a median time of up to 40 months may be required for complete recovery of normal CD4-positive counts. Although opportunistic infections occur, they do so less frequently than with fludarabine therapy. Infectious complications correlate with decreases in the CD4-positive count, and they include herpes zoster, *Candida*, *Pneumocystis*, *Pseudomonas aeruginosa*, *Listeria monocytogenes*, *Cryptococcus neoformans*, *Aspergillus*, *P. carinii*, and cytomegalovirus.

CLOFARABINE

Clofarabine is a purine deoxyadenosine nucleoside analog, and it is approved for the treatment of pediatric patients with relapsed or refractory acute lymphoblastic leukemia (see Table 19.1).[45]

Ongoing studies are exploring the benefit of clofarabine alone and in combination with other agents in less heavily pretreated patients and in the use of different dose schedules for other hematologic malignancies.[46]

Mechanism of Action

Clofarabine is inactive in its parent form and, like other purine analogs, it requires intracellular activation by dCK to form the monophosphate nucleotide, which undergoes further metabolism to the cytotoxic triphosphate metabolite. Clofarabine triphosphate is then incorporated into DNA, resulting in chain termination, and inhibition of DNA synthesis and function or the triphosphate form can directly inhibit DNA polymerases α, β, and γ, which in turn, interferes with DNA chain elongation, DNA synthesis, and DNA repair. The triphosphate metabolite is also a potent inhibitor of ribonucleotide reductase, further mediating the inhibition of DNA biosynthesis by reducing the levels of key deoxyribonucleotide pools.

Mechanisms of Resistance

Several resistance mechanisms have been identified in various preclinical systems, and they include decreased activation of the drug through the reduced expression of the anabolic enzyme deoxycytidine kinase, the decreased transport of drug into cells via the nucleoside transporter protein, and the increased expression of CTP synthetase activity resulting in increased concentrations of competing physiologic nucleotide substrate dCTP. To date, the precise resistance mechanism(s) that are relevant in the clinical setting remain to be determined.

Clinical Pharmacology

Approximately 50% to 60% of an administered dose of drug is excreted unchanged in the urine, and the terminal half-life is on the order of 5 hours. To date, the pathways for nonrenal elimination have not been well defined. Caution should be exercised in patients with abnormal renal function, and concomitant use of medications known to cause renal toxicity should be avoided during drug treatment.

Toxicity

Myelosuppression is dose limiting with neutropenia, anemia, and thrombocytopenia. The capillary leak syndrome (systemic inflammatory response syndrome) presents with tachypnea, tachycardia, pulmonary edema, and hypotension.[47] In essence, this adverse event is part of the tumor lysis syndrome and results from rapid cytoreduction of peripheral leukemic cells following treatment.[47] Other side effects may include nausea/vomiting, reversible liver dysfunction (hyperbilirubinemia and elevated serum transaminases), renal dysfunction (approximately 10%), and cardiac toxicity in the form of tachycardia and acute pump dysfunction.

REFERENCES

1. Wright DL, Anderson AC. Antifolate agents: a patent review (2006–2010). *Expert Opin Ther Pat* 2011;21:1293–1308.
2. Chattopadhyay S, Moran RG, Goldman ID. Pemetrexed: biochemical and cellular pharmacology, mechanisms, and clinical applications. *Mol Cancer Ther* 2007;6:404–417.
3. Vogelzang NJ, Rusthoven JJ, Symanowski J, et al. Phase III study of pemetrexed in combination with cisplatin versus cisplatin alone in patients with malignant pleural mesothelioma. *J Clin Oncol* 2003;21:2636–2644.
4. Kindler HL. Systemic treatments for mesothelioma: standard and novel. *Curr Treat Options Oncol* 2008;9:171–179.
5. Joerger M, Omlin A, Cerny T, et al. The role of pemetrexed in advanced non small-cell lung cancer: special focus on pharmacology and mechanism of action. *Curr Drug Targets* 2010;11:37–47.
6. Zain J, O'Connor O. Pralatrexate: basic understanding and clinical development. *Expert Opin Pharmacother* 2010;11:1705–1714.
7. Sirotnak FM, DeGraw JI, Moccio DM, et al. New folate analogs of the 10-deaza-aminopterin series. Basis for structural design and biochemical and pharmacologic properties. *Cancer Chemother Pharmacol* 1984;12:18–25.
8. O'Connor OA. Pralatrexate: an emerging new agent with activity in T-cell lymphomas. *Curr Opin Oncol* 2006;18:591–597.

9. Bertino JR, Göker E, Gorlick R, et al. Resistance mechanisms to methotrexate in tumors. *Oncologist* 1996;1:223–226.

10. Zhao R, Goldman ID. Resistance to antifolates. *Oncogene* 2003;22:7431–7457.

11. Grem JL. 5-Fluorouracil: forty-plus and still ticking. A review of its preclinical and clinical development. *Invest New Drugs* 2000;18:299–313.

12. Saif MW, Ezzeldin H, Vance K, et al. DPYD*2A mutation: the most common mutation associated with DPD deficiency. *Cancer Chemother Pharmacol* 2007;60:503–507.

13. Grem JL. Biochemical modulation of 5-FU in systemic treatment of advanced colorectal cancer. *Oncology (Williston Park)* 2001;15:13–19.

14. Saif MW, Shah MM, Shah AR. Fluoropyrimidine-associated cardiotoxicity: revisited. *Expert Opin Drug Saf* 2009;8:191–202.

15. Saif MW, Eloubeidi MA, Russo S, et al. Phase I study of capecitabine with concomitant radiotherapy for patients with locally advanced pancreatic cancer: expression analysis of genes related to outcome. *J Clin Oncol* 2005;23:8679–8687.

16. Geyer CE, Forster J, Lindquist D, et al. Lapatinib plus capecitabine for HER2-positive advanced breast cancer. *N Engl J Med* 2006;355:2733–2743.

17. Saif MW, Katirtzoglou NA, Syrigos KN. Capecitabine: an overview of the side effects and their management. *Anticancer Drugs* 2008;19:447–464.

18. Van Custem E, Verslype C, Tejpar S. Oral capecitabine: bridging the Atlantic divide in colon cancer treatment. *Semin Oncol* 2005;32:43–51.

19. Haller DG, Cassidy J, Clarke SJ, et al. Potential regional differences for the tolerability profiles of fluoropyrimidines. *J Clin Oncol* 2008;26:2118–2123.

20. Saif MW, Syrigos KN, Katirtzoglou NA. S-1: a promising new oral fluoropyrimidine derivative. *Expert Opin Investig Drugs* 2009;18:335–348.

21. Saif MW, Rosen LS, Saito K, et al. A phase I study evaluating the effect of CDHP as a component of S-1 on the pharmacokinetics of 5-fluorouracil. *Anticancer Res* 2011;31:625–632.

22. Daigo S, Takahashi Y, Fujieda M, et al. A novel mutant allele of the CYP2A6 gene (CYP2A6*11) found in a cancer patient who showed poor metabolic phenotype towards tegafur. *Pharmacogenetics* 2002;12:299–306.

23. Reiter A, Hochhaus A, Berger U, et al. AraC-based pharmacotherapy of chronic myeloid leukaemia. *Expert Opin Pharmacother* 2001;2:1129–1135.

24. Braess J, Wegendt C, Feuring-Buske M, et al. Leukemic blasts differ from normal bone marrow mononuclear cells and CD34+ hematopoietic stem cells in their metabolism of cytosine arabinoside. *Br J Haematol* 1999;105:388–393.

25. Momparler RL, Laliberte J, Eliopoulos N, et al. Transfection of murine fibroblast cells with human cytidine deaminase cDNA confers resistance to cytosine arabinoside. *Anticancer Drugs* 1996;7:266–274.

26. Cai J, Damaraju VL, Groulx N, et al. Two distinct molecular mechanisms underlying cytarabine resistance in human leukemic cells. *Cancer Res* 2008;68:2349–2357.

27. Kern W, Estey EH. High-dose cytosine arabinoside in the treatment of acute myeloid leukemia: review of three randomized trials. *Cancer* 2006;107:116–124.

28. Mini E, Nobili S, Caciagli B, et al. Cellular pharmacology of gemcitabine. *Ann Oncol* 2006;17:v7–v12.

29. Saif MW, Sellers S, Li M, et al. A phase I study of bi-weekly administration of 24-h gemcitabine followed by 24-h irinotecan in patients with solid tumors. *Cancer Chemother Pharmacol* 2007;60:871–882.

30. Bergman AM, Pinedo HM, Peters GJ. Determinants of resistance to 2′, 2′-difluorodeoxycytidine (gemcitabine). *Drug Resist Update* 2002;5:19–33.

31. Saif MW, Lee Y, Kim R. Harnessing gemcitabine metabolism: a step towards personalized medicine for pancreatic cancer. *Ther Adv Med Oncol* 2012;4:341–346.

32. Hong SP, Wen J, Bang S, et al. CD44-positive cells are responsible for gemcitabine resistance in pancreatic cancer cells. *Int J Cancer* 2009;125:2323–2331.

33. Poplin E, Feng Y, Berlin J, et al. Phase III, randomized study of gemcitabine and oxaliplatin versus gemcitabine (fixed-dose rate infusion) compared with gemcitabine (30-minute infusion) in patients with pancreatic carcinoma E6201: a trial of the Eastern Cooperative Oncology Group. *J Clin Oncol* 2009;27:3778–3785.

34. Hande KR. Purine antimetabolites. In: Chabner BA, Longo DL, eds. *Cancer Chemotherapy and Biotherapy: Principles and Practice*, 4th ed. Philadelphia: Lippincott–Raven; 2006: 212.

35. Evans WE. Pharmacogenetics of thiopurine S-methyltransferase and thiopurine therapy. *Ther Drug Monitor* 2004;26:186–191.

36. Wang L, Weinshilboum R. Thiopurine S-methyltransferase pharmacogenetics: insights, challenges, and future directions. *Oncogene* 2006;25:1629–1638.

37. Vora A, Mitchell CD, Lennard L, et al. Toxicity and efficacy of 6-thioguanine versus 6-mercaptopurine in childhood lymphoblastic leukaemia: a randomised trial. *Lancet* 2006;368:1339–1348.

38. Montillo M, Ricci F, Tedeschi A. Role of fludarabine in hematological malignancies. *Expert Rev Anticancer Ther* 2006;6:1141–1161.

39. Gandhi V, Plunkett W. Cellular and clinical pharmacology of fludarabine. *Clin Pharmacokinet* 2002;41:93–103.

40. van den Neste E, Cardoen S, Offner F, et al. Old and new insights into the mechanism of action of two nucleoside analogs active in lymphoid malignancies: flludarabine and cladribine. *Int J Oncol* 2005;27:1113–1124.

41. Gidron A, Tallman MS. 2-CdA in the treatment of hairy cell leukemia: a review of long-term follow-up. *Leuk Lymphoma* 2006;47:2301–2307.

42. Huang P, Robertson LE, Wright S, et al. High molecular weight DNA fragmentation: a critical event in nucleoside analog-induced apoptosis in leukemia cells. *Clin Cancer Res* 1995;1:1005–1013.

43. Grevz N, Saven A. Cladribine: from the bench to the bedside: focus on hairy cell leukemia. *Expert Rev Anticancer Ther* 2004;4:745–757.

44. Seto S, Carrera CJ, Kubota M, et al. Mechanism of deoxyadenosine and 2-chlorodeoxyadenosine toxicity to nondividing human lymphocytes. *J Clin Invest* 1985;75:377–383.

45. Bonate PL, Arthaud L, Cantrell WR Jr, et al. Discovery and development of clofarabine: a nucleoside analogue for treating cancer. *Nat Rev Drug Discov* 2006;5:855–863.

46. Faderi S, Gandhi V, Keating MJ, et al. The role of clofarabine in hematologic and solid malignancies: development of a next generation nucleoside analog. *Cancer* 2005;102:1985–1995.

47. Baytan B, Ozdemir O, Gunes AM, et al. Clofarabine-induced capillary leak syndrome in a child with refractory acute lymphoblastic leukemia. *J Pediatr Hematol Oncol* 2010;32:144–146.

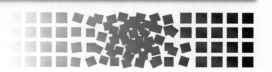

20 Topoisomerase Interactive Agents

Khanh T. Do, Shivaani Kummar, James H. Doroshow, and Yves Pommier

CLASSIFICATION, BIOCHEMICAL, AND BIOLOGIC FUNCTIONS OF TOPOISOMERASES

Nucleic acids (DNA and RNA) being long polymers, topoisomerases fulfill the need for cellular DNA to be densely packaged in the cell nucleus, transcribed, replicated, and evenly distributed between daughter cells following replication without tangles. Topoisomerases are ubiquitous and essential for all organisms as they prevent and resolve DNA and RNA entanglements and resolve DNA supercoiling during transcription and replication. This chapter first summarizes the basic elements necessary to understand the mechanism of action of topoisomerases and their inhibitors. More detailed information can be found in recent reviews[1-7] and two recent books.[8,9] The second part of the chapter summarizes the use of topoisomerase inhibitors as anticancer drugs.

Classification of Topoisomerases

Human cells contain six topoisomerase genes (Table 20.1), which have been numbered historically. The commonly used abbreviations are Top1 for topoisomerases I (Top1mt being the mitochondrial topoisomerase whose gene is encoded in the cell nucleus),[10] Top2 for topoisomerases II, and Top3 for topoisomerases III. Top1 was the first eukaryotic topoisomerase discovered by Champoux and Dulbecco.[11] Topoisomerases solve DNA topologic problems by cutting the DNA backbone and religating without the assistance of any additional ligase. Top1 and Top3 act by cleaving/religating a single strand of the DNA duplex, whereas Top2 enzymes cleave and religate both strands, making a four–base pair reversible staggered cut (Fig. 20.1). It is convenient to remember that odd-numbered topoisomerases (Top1 and Top3) cleave and religate one strand, whereas the even numbered topoisomerases (Top2s) cleave and religate both strands.

Biochemical Characteristics and Cleavage Complexes of the Different Topoisomerases

The DNA cutting/relegation mechanism is common to all topoisomerases and utilizes an enzyme catalytic tyrosine residue acting as a nucleophile and becoming covalently attached to the end of the broken DNA. These catalytic intermediates are referred to as cleavage complexes (see Fig. 20.1B, E). The reverse religation reaction is carried out by the attack of the ribose hydroxyl ends toward the tyrosyl-DNA bond.

Top1 (and Top1mt) attaches to the 3'-end of the break, whereas the other topoisomerases (Top2 and Top3) have opposite polarity and covalently attach to the 5'-end of the breaks (see Table 20.1 [second column] and Fig. 20.1B, E). Topoisomerases have distinct biochemical requirements. Top1 and Top1mt are the simplest, nicking/closing, and relaxing DNA as monomers in the absence of cofactor, and even at ice temperature. Top2 enzymes, on the other hand, are the most complex topoisomerases working as dimers, requiring

ATP binding and hydrolysis, and a divalent metal (Mg^{2+}) for catalysis. Top3 enzymes also require Mg^{2+} for catalysis but function as monomers without ATP requirement. Notably, the DNA substrates differ for Top3 enzymes. Whereas both Top1 and Top2 process double-stranded DNA, the Top3 substrates need to be single-stranded nucleic acids (DNA for Top3α and DNA or RNA for Top3β).[10,12,13]

Differential Topoisomerization Mechanisms: Swiveling Versus Strand Passage, DNA Versus RNA Topoisomerases

Topoisomerases use two main mechanisms to change nucleic topology. The first is by "untwisting" the DNA duplex. This mechanism is unique to Top1, which, by an enzyme-associated single-strand break, allows the broken strand to rotate around the intact strand (see Fig. 20.1B) until DNA supercoiling is dissipated. At this point, the stacking energy of adjacent DNA bases realigns the broken ends, and the 5'-hydroxyl end attacks the 3'-phosphotyrosyl end, thereby relegating the DNA. A remarkable feature of this Top1 untwisting mechanism is its extreme efficiency with a rotation speed around 6,000 rpm and relative independence from torque, thereby allowing full relaxation of DNA supercoiling.[14]

The second topologic mechanism is by "strand passage." This mechanism allows the passage of a double- or a single-stranded DNA (or RNA) through the cleavage complexes. Top2α and Top2β both act by allowing the passage of an intact DNA duplex through the DNA double-strand break generated by the enzymes. After which, Top2 religates the broken duplex. Such reactions permit DNA decatenation, unknotting, and relaxation of supercoils.[3] Top3 enzymes also act by strand passage but only pass one nucleic acid strand through the single-strand break generated by the enzymes. In the case of Top3α, the substrate is a single-stranded DNA segment (such as a double-Holliday junction), whereas in the case of Top3β, the substrate can be a single-stranded RNA segment, with Top3β acting as a RNA topoisomerase.[13,15]

TOPOISOMERASE INHIBITORS AS INTERFACIAL POISONS

Topoisomerase Inhibitors Act as Interfacial Inhibitors by Binding at the Topoisomerase–DNA Interface and Trapping Topoisomerase Cleavage Complexes

Relegation of the cleavage complexes is dependent on the structure of the ends of the broken DNA (i.e., the realignment of the broken ends). Binding the drugs at the enzyme–DNA interface misaligns the ends of the DNA and precludes relegation, resulting in the stabilization of the topoisomerase cleavage complexes (Top1cc and Top2cc). Crystal structures of drug-bound cleavage complexes have firmly established this mechanism for both Top1- and Top2-targeted drugs.[16]

TABLE 20.1

Classification of Human Topoisomerases and Topoisomerase Inhibitors

Type	Polarity	Mechanism	Genes	Proteins	Main Functions	Drugs
IB	3′-PY	Rotation/swiveling	*TOP1*	Top1	DNA supercoiling relaxation, replication, and transcription	Camptothecins, noncamptothecins
			TOP1MT	Top1mt		
IIA	5′-PY	Strand passage ATPase	*TOP2A*	Top2α	Decatenation/replication	Anthracyclines, anthracenediones, epipodophyllotoxins
			TOP2B	Top2β	Transcription	
IA	5′-PY	Strand passage	*TOP3A*	Top3α	DNA replication with BLM	None
			TOP3B	Top3β	RNA topoisomerase	

Top1mt, mitochondrial DNA topoisomerase; BLM, Bloom's syndrome helicare.

It is critical to understand that the cytotoxic mechanism of topoisomerase inhibitors requires the drugs to trap the topoisomerase cleavage complexes rather than block catalytic activity. This sets apart topoisomerase inhibitors from classical enzyme inhibitors such as antifolates. Indeed, knocking out Top1 renders yeast cells totally immune to camptothecin,[17,18] and reducing enzyme levels in cancer cells confers drug resistance. Conversely, in breast cancers, amplification of TOP2A, which is on the same locus as HER2, contributes to the efficacy of doxorubicin.[19] Also, cellular mutations of Top1 and Top2 that renders cells insensitive to the trapping of topoisomerase cleavage complexes produce high resistance to Top1 or Top2 inhibitors. Based on this trapping of cleavage complexes mechanism, we refer to topoisomerase inhibitors as topoisomerase cleavage complex-targeted drugs.

Top1cc-Targeted Drugs (Camptothecin and Noncamptothecin Derivatives) Kill Cancer Cells by Replication Collisions

Top1cc are cytotoxic by their conversion into DNA damage by replication and transcription fork collisions. This explains why cytotoxicity is directly related to drug exposure and why arresting DNA replication protects cells from camptothecin.[20,21] The collisions arise from the fact that the drugs, by slowing down the nicking/closing activity of Top1, uncouple the kinetics of Top1 with the polymerases and helicases, which lead polymerases to collide into Top1cc (Fig. 20.2A). Such collisions have two consequences. They generate double-strand breaks (replication and transcription runoff) and irreversible Top1–DNA adducts (see Fig. 20.2B). The replication double-strand breaks are repaired by homologous recombination, which explains the hypersensitivity of BRCA-deficient cancer cells to Top1cc-targeted drugs.[22] The Top1-covalent complexes can be removed by two pathways, the excision pathway centered around tyrosyl-DNA-phosphodiesterase 1 (TDP1)[23] and the endonuclease pathway involving 3′-flap endonucleases such as XPF-ERCC1.[24] It is also possible that drug-trapped Top1cc directly generate DNA double-strand breaks when they are within 10 base pairs on opposite strands of the DNA duplex or when they occur next to a preexisting single-strand break on the opposite strand. Finally, it is not excluded that topologic defects contribute to the cytotoxicity of Top1cc-targeted drugs (the accumulation of supercoils[25] and the formation of alternative structures such as R-loops) (see Fig. 20.2D).[26]

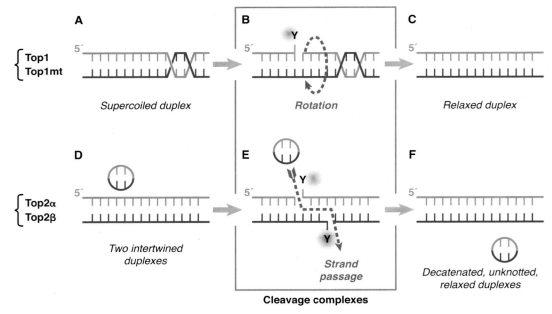

Figure 20.1 Mechanisms of action of topoisomerases. **(A–C)** Topoisomerases I (Top1 for nuclear DNA and Top1mt for mitochondrial DNA) relax supercoiled DNA **(A)** by reversibly cleaving one DNA strand, forming a covalent bond between the enzyme catalytic tyrosine and the 3′ end of the nicked DNA (the Top1 cleavage complex [Top1cc]) **(B)**. This reaction allows the swiveling of the broken strand around the intact strand. Rapid religation allows the dissociation of Top1. **(D–F)** Topoisomerases II (Top2α and Top2β) act on two DNA duplexes **(A)**. They act as homodimers, cleaving both strands and forming a covalent bond between their catalytic tyrosine and the 5′ end of the DNA break (Top2cc) **(E)**. This reaction allows the passage of the intact duplex through the Top2 homodimer *(red dotted arrow)* **(E)**. Top2 inhibitors trap the Top2cc and prevent the normal religation **(F)**.

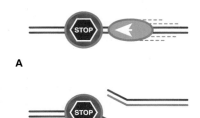

A

Collisions of polymerases and helicases *(green ellipse)*
with trapped Top cleavage complexes *(Stop sign)*
=> Protein-DNA complexes blocking DNA metabolism

B

Conversion of Top1cc into DSB by replication "runoff"
=> Top1 needs to be removed by TDP1
     and /or 3'-flap endonucleases (XPF-ERCC1)
=> DSB repaired by homologous recombination
Top1cc also form DSB when on opposite strands or
opposite to a preexisting single-strand break

Top2cc proteolysis or mechanical disjoining

C

Top2cc readily form DSB when concerted cleavage
on both strands and disjunction of the homodimer

D

Topologic defects resulting from Top sequestration
in the cleavage complexes: accumulation of
=> Supercoils (Top1 and Top2) *(1)*
=> Knots (Top2) *(2)*
=> Catenanes (Top2) *(3)*

Figure 20.2 Mechanisms of action of topoisomerase inhibitors beyond the trapping of topoisomerase cleavage complexes. **(A)** Stalled or slow cleavage complexes lead to collisions with replication and transcription complexes. **(B)** Collisions of replication complexes with Top1cc on the leading strand for DNA synthesis generate DNA double-strand breaks by replication runoff. Top1cc can also form DNA double-strand breaks (DSBs) when they occur opposite to another Top1cc or preexisting nick. **(C)** Top2cc, which are normally held together by Top2 homodimers, can be converted to free DSBs upon Top2cc proteolysis or dimer disjunction. **(D)** Topologic defects resulting from functional topoisomerase deficiencies play a minor role in the anticancer activity of topoisomerase cleavage complex targeted drugs.

CANCER THERAPEUTICS

Cytotoxic Mechanisms of Top2cc-Targeted Drugs (Intercalators and Demethyl Epipodophyllotoxins)

Contrary to camptothecins, Top2 inhibitors kill cancer cells without requiring DNA replication fork collisions. Indeed, even after a 30-minute exposure, doxorubicin and other Top2cc-targeted drugs can kill over 99% of the cells, which is in vast excess of the fraction of S-phase cells in tissue culture (generally less than 50%).[27,28] The collision mechanism in the case of Top2cc-targeted drugs (see Fig. 20.2A) appears to involve transcription and proteolysis of both Top2 and RNA polymerase II.[29] Such situation would then lead to DNA double-strand breaks by disruption of the Top2 dimer interface (see Fig. 20.2C). Alternatively, the Top2 homodimer interface could be disjoined by mechanical tension (see Fig. 20.2C). Yet, it is important to bear in mind that 90% of Top2cc trapped by etoposide are not concerted and, therefore, consist in single-strand breaks,[3,30,31] which is different from doxorubicin, which traps both Top2 monomers and produces a majority of DNA double-strand breaks.[32] Finally, it is not excluded that topologic defects resulting from Top2 sequestration by the drug-induced cleavage complexes could contribute to the cytotoxicity of Top2cc-targeted drugs (see Fig. 20.2D). Such topologic defects would include persistent DNA knots and catenanes, potentially leading to chromosome breaks during mitosis.

TOPOISOMERASE I INHIBITORS: CAMPTOTHECINS AND BEYOND

Camptothecin is an alkaloid identified in the 1960s by Wall and Wani[33] in a screen of plant extracts for antineoplastic drugs. The two water-soluble derivatives of camptothecin containing the active lactone form are topotecan and irinotecan, which are approved by the U.S. Food and Drug Administration (FDA) for the treatment of several cancers. In addition, several Top1cc-targeting drugs are in clinical development, including camptothecin derivatives and formulations (including high–molecular-weight conjugates or liposomal formulations), as well as noncamptothecin compounds that exhibit greater potency or noncross resistance to irinotecan and topotecan in preclinical cancer models.[31,34–36]

Irinotecan

Irinotecan, a prodrug containing a bulky dipiperidine side chain at C-10 (Fig. 20.3), is cleaved by a carboxylesterase-converting enzyme in the liver and other tissues to generate the active metabolite, SN-38. Irinotecan is FDA approved for the treatment of colorectal cancer in the metastatic setting as first-line treatment in combination with 5-fluorouracil/leucovorin (5-FU/LV) and as a single agent in the second-line treatment of progressive colorectal cancer after 5-FU–based therapy (see Table 20.1).[37,38] Newer therapeutic uses of irinotecan include a combination with oxaliplatin and 5-FU as first-line treatment in pancreatic cancer.[39] Irinotecan is additionally used in combination with cisplatin or carboplatin in extensive-stage small-cell lung cancer[40,41] as well as refractory esophageal and gastroesophageal junction (GEJ) cancers, gastric cancer, cervical cancer, anaplastic gliomas and glioblastomas, and non–small-cell lung cancer (Table 20.2). Irinotecan is usually administered intravenously at a dose of 125 mg/m^2 for 4 weeks with a 2-week rest period in combination with bolus 5-FU/LV, 180 mg/m^2 every 2 weeks in combination with an infusion of 5-FU/LV, or 350 mg/m^2 every 3 weeks as a single agent.

Diarrhea and myelosuppression are the most common toxicities associated with irinotecan administration. Two mechanisms explain irinotecan-induced diarrhea. Acute cholinergic effects resulting in abdominal cramping and diarrhea occur within 24 hours of drug administration are the result of acetylcholinesterase inhibition by the prodrug, and can be treated with the administration of atropine. Direct mucosal cytotoxicity with diarrhea is typically observed after 24 hours and can result in significant morbidity. Symptoms are managed with loperamide. Hepatic metabolism and biliary excretion accounts for >70% of the elimination of the administered dose, with renal excretion accounting for the remainder of the dose. SN-38 is glucuronidated in the liver by UGT1A1, and deficiencies in this pathway increase the risk of diarrhea and myelosuppression. Dose reductions are recommended for patients who are homozygous for the UGT1A1*28 allele, for which an FDA-approved test for detection of the UGT1A1*28 allele in patients is available.[42,43] Additionally, dose reductions of irinotecan are recommended for patients with hepatic dysfunction, with bilirubin greater than 1.5 mg/mL.[44]

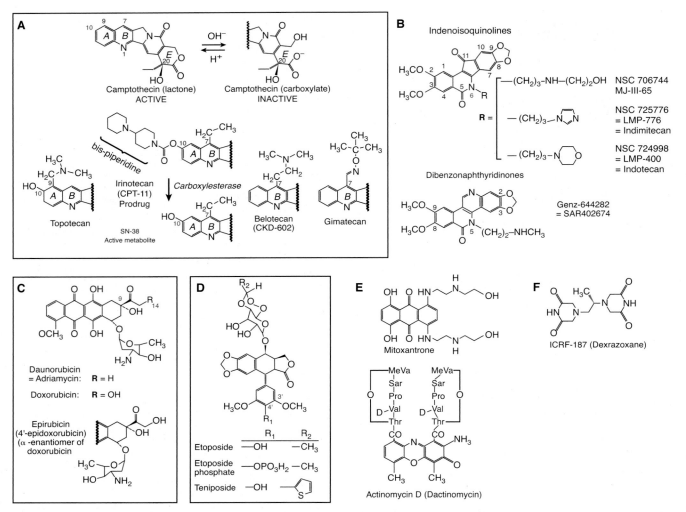

Figure 20.3 Structure of topoisomerase inhibitors. **(A)** Camptothecin derivatives are instable at physiologic pH with the formation of a carboxylate derivative within minutes. Irinotecan is a prodrug and needs to be converted to SN-38 to trap Top1cc. **(B)** Non-camptothecin derivatives in clinical trials. **(C)** Anthracycline derivatives. **(D)** Demethyl epipodophyllotoxin derivatives. **(E)** Other intercalating Top2 inhibitors acting by trapping Top2cc. **(F)** Structure of dexrazoxane, which acts as a catalytic inhibitor of Top2.

Topotecan

Topotecan contains a basic side chain at position C-9 that enhances its water solubility (see Fig. 20.3). Topotecan is approved for the treatment of ovarian cancer,[45] small-cell lung cancer,[46] and as a single agent and in combination with cisplatin for cervical cancer.[47] Additionally, it is active in acute myeloid leukemia (AML) and myelodysplastic syndrome (see Table 20.2). Topotecan is administered intravenously as a single agent at a dose of 1.5 mg/m² as a 30-minute infusion daily for 5 days, followed by a 2-week period of rest for the treatment of solid tumors or at a dose of 0.75 mg/m² as a 30-minute infusion daily for 3 days in combination with cisplatin on day 1, every 3 weeks, for the treatment of cervical cancer.

Myelosuppression is the most common dose-limiting toxicity. Extensive prior radiation or previous bone marrow–suppressive chemotherapy increases the risk of topotecan-induced myelosuppression. Other toxicities include nausea, vomiting, diarrhea, fatigue, alopecia, and transient hepatic transaminitis.

Topotecan and its metabolites are primarily cleared by the kidneys, requiring dose reduction in patients with renal dysfunction. A 50% dose reduction is recommended for patients with moderate renal impairment (creatinine clearance 20 to 39 mL per minute).

There are no formal guidelines for dose reductions in patients with hepatic dysfunction (defined as serum bilirubin >1.5 mg/dL to <10 mg/dL). Topotecan additionally penetrates the blood-brain barrier, achieving concentrations in cerebrospinal fluid that are approximately 30% that of plasma levels.[48]

Camptothecin Conjugates and Analogs

New formulations of camptothecin conjugates and analogs are currently in clinical development in an effort to improve the therapeutic index (Table 20.3). The development of camptothecin conjugates is based on the notion that the addition of a bulky conjugate would allow for a more consistent delivery system and extend the half-life of the molecule.

CRLX101, formerly IT-101, a covalent cyclodextrin-polyethylene glycol copolymer camptothecin conjugate, has plasma concentrations and area under the curve (AUC) that are approximately 100-fold higher than camptothecin, with a half-life in the range of 17 to 20 hours compared to 1.3 hours for camptothecin.[49] It has demonstrated antitumor activity in preclinical studies in irinotecan-resistant tumors with complete tumor regression in human non–small-cell lung cancer, Ewing sarcoma, and

TABLE 20.2

U.S. Food and Drug Administration–Approved Camptothecin Analogs

Irinotecan (Camptosar)	FDA approved for: Metastatic colorectal cancer	First-line therapy in combination with 5-FU/LV	Diarrhea (dose reductions are recommended for patients who are homozygous for the UGT1A1*28 allele)
		Second-line therapy as a single agent	Myelosuppression
	Category 2A[a] recommendations: Pancreatic cancer	First-line therapy in combination with oxaliplatin, 5-FU/LV	
	Extensive-stage small-cell lung cancer	First-line therapy in combination with cisplatin or carboplatin	
	Category 2B[b] recommendations: Esophageal and GEJ cancers, gastric cancer, cervical cancer, anaplastic gliomas and glioblastomas, non–small-cell lung cancer, ovarian cancer		
Topotecan (Hycamtin)	FDA approved for: Cervical cancer	Stage IVB, recurrent, or persistent carcinoma of the cervix not amenable to curative treatment with surgery and/or radiation therapy	Myelosuppression
	Ovarian cancer	After failure of initial therapy	
	Small-cell lung cancer	After failure of initial therapy	
	Class 2B recommendations: AML, MDS		

[a] Category 2A: Recommendations are based upon lower-level evidence, there is uniform National Comprehensive Cancer Network consensus that the intervention is appropriate.

[b] Category 2B: Recommendations are based upon lower-level evidence, there is National Comprehensive Cancer Network consensus that the intervention is appropriate.

MDS, myelodysplastic syndrome.

CANCER THERAPEUTICS

lymphoma xenograft models.[50] Preliminary data from Phase 1 studies indicate that CRLX101 is well tolerated at a dose of 15 mg/m^2 administered in a biweekly administration schedule.[51] It is currently being studied in Phase 2 studies as a single agent and in combination with chemotherapeutic agents in lung, renal cell cancer, and gynecologic malignancies.[52–54]

Etirinotecan pegol (NKTR-102), an irinotecan polymer conjugate, has a longer plasma circulation time with a lower maximum concentration of SN-38 compared with irinotecan. It was evaluated in a Phase 2 study in platinum-resistant refractory epithelial ovarian cancer at a dose of 145 mg/m^2 administered on a schedule of every 21 days; a median progression-free survival of 5.3 months and median overall survival of 11.7 months was observed.[55] Two schedules of administration, 145 mg/m^2 administered every 14 days versus every 21 days, have been tested in a Phase 2 study of NKTR-102 in patients with previously treated metastatic breast cancer.[56] Of the 70 patients evaluated in this study, 20 patients achieved an objective response (29%; 95% confidence interval [CI] 18.4 to 40.6). For both these studies, the most common adverse events

TABLE 20.3

Topoisomerase I Inhibitors in Development

Camptothecin Conjugates	Camptothecin Analogs	Noncamptothecin Agents
CRLX101	Belotecan	Indenoisoquinoline
NKTR-102	Gimatecan	Indotecan (LMP-400)
MM-398	Homocamptothecin	Indimitecan (LMP-776)
	Elomotecan	Dibenzo naphthyridine
	Diflomotecan	Genz-644282

on the 21-day administration schedule were dehydration and diarrhea. Etirinotecan pegol is currently being evaluated in several phase 2 studies in lung cancer, colorectal cancer, and high-grade gliomas,[57–60] with evidence of clinical activity in refractory solid tumors. A Phase 3 trial (The BEACON Study) is underway evaluating NKTR-102 against the physicians' choice in refractory breast cancer.[61]

As an alternative to macromolecular conjugates, attempts have also been made to alter the camptothecin pentacyclic ring structure with modifications of the A and B ring (see Fig. 20.3A) in an effort to improve solubility and enhance antitumor activity. Structure–activity relationship studies have shown that substitutions at the 7, 9, and 10 positions serve to enhance the antitumor activity of camptothecin.[62] Belotecan, a novel camptothecin analog, has a water-solubilizing group at the 7 position of the B ring of camptothecin (see Fig. 20.3A). Several Phase 2 studies have evaluated belotecan in combination with carboplatin in recurrent ovarian cancer[63] and in combination with cisplatin in extensive-stage small-cell lung cancer,[64] demonstrating activity in these cancers; however, these combinations were associated with prominent hematologic toxicities. Phase 2 studies evaluating belotecan as a single agent in patients with recurrent or progressive carcinoma of the uterine cervix failed to show activity.[65] Gimatecan is a lipophilic oral camptothecin analog (see Fig. 20.3A). Pharmacokinetic studies demonstrate that gimatecan is primarily present in plasma as the lactone form (>85%), and has a long half-life of 77.1 +/− 29.6 hours, with an increase in maximum concentration (Cmax) and AUC of three- to six-fold after multiple dosing.[66] Phase 2 studies show that gimatecan has demonstrated activity in previously treated ovarian cancer, with myelosuppression as the main toxicity.[67]

Newer development of analogs have attempted to modify the E-ring through introduction of an electron-withdrawing group at the α position in an effort to overcome the instability of the E-ring while maintaining the binding capability of the camptothecin analog to the Top1-DNA cleavage complex. Collectively called homocamptothecin analogs, two have been tested in clinical trials and include diflomotecan[68] and elomotecan.[69] The dose-limiting toxicity in the Phase I study of elomotecan was neutropenia. A five-member E-ring derivative has also been developed and has reached a Phase 1 clinical trial.[70,71]

Noncamptothecin Topoisomerase I Inhibitors

Noncamptothecin Top1 inhibitors are in clinical development, and include indenoisoquinolines and dibenzonaphthyridines (see Fig. 20.3B). Two indenoisoquinoline derivatives are currently in clinical development, indotecan (LMP400) and indimitecan (LMP776).[72,73] Early in vitro studies show enhanced potency compared with camptothecins, and persistence of Top1 cleavage complexes.[74] Genz-644282, a dibenzonaphthyridine derivative, demonstrated enhanced antitumor activity in preclinical studies[75] and is currently being evaluated in Phase 1 clinical trials.[76]

TOPOISOMERASE II INHIBITORS: INTERCALATORS AND NONINTERCALATORS

Topoisomerase II inhibitors can be classified in two main classes: DNA intercalators, which encompass different chemical classes (Fig. 20.3C, E), and nonintercalators represented by the epipodophyllotoxin derivatives (see Fig. 20.3D). Although both act by trapping Top2 cleavage complexes (Top2cc), DNA intercalators exhibit a second effect as drug concentrations increase above low micromolar values: they block the formation of Top2cc by intercalating into DNA and destabilizing the binding of Top2 to DNA. This explains why Top2α and Top2β are trapped over a relatively narrow concentration range by anthracyclines, and why intercalators have additional effects besides trapping Top2cc, namely inhibition of a broad range of DNA processing enzymes including helicases, polymerase, and even nucleosome destabilization.

Doxorubicin

Doxorubicin and daunorubicin were the first anthracyclines discovered in the 1960s and remain among the most widely used anticancer agents over a broad spectrum of malignancies. Although doxorubicin only differs by one hydroxyl substitution on position 14 (see Fig. 20.3C), doxorubicin has a much broader anticancer activity than daunorubicin. Anthracyclines are natural products derived from *Streptomyces peucetius* variation *caesius*. They were found to target Top2 well after their clinical approval.[77] Subsequent searches for less toxic drugs and formulations led to the approval of liposomal doxorubicin, idarubicin, and epirubicin.

Anthracyclines are flat, planar molecules that are relatively hydrophobic. The quinone structure of anthracyclines (see Fig. 20.3C) enhances the catalysis of oxidation-reduction reactions, thereby promoting the generation of oxygen free radicals, which may be involved in antitumor effects as well as the cardiotoxicity associated with these drugs.[78,79] Anthracyclines are also substrates for P-glycoprotein and Mrp-1, and drug efflux is thought to be a major drug resistance determinant.[80,81]

Doxorubicin is available in a standard salt form and as a liposomal formulation. FDA-labeled indications for standard doxorubicin include acute lymphocytic leukemia (ALL), AML, chronic lymphoid leukemia, Hodgkin lymphoma, non-Hodgkin lymphoma, mantle cell lymphoma, multiple myeloma, mycosis fungoides, Kaposi sarcoma, breast cancer (adjuvant therapy and advanced), advanced prostate cancer, advanced gastric cancer, Ewing sarcoma, thyroid cancer, advanced nephroblastoma,

advanced neuroblastoma, advanced non–small-cell lung cancer, advanced ovarian cancer, advanced transitional cell bladder cancer, cervical cancer, and Langerhans cell tumors. Doxorubicin has activity in other malignancies as well, including soft tissue sarcoma, osteosarcoma, carcinoid, and liver cancer (Table 20.4). Doxorubicin is typically administered at a recommended dose of 30 to 75 mg/m^2 every 3 weeks intravenously.

Major acute toxicities of doxorubicin include myelosuppression, mucositis, alopecia, nausea, and vomiting. Myelosuppression is the acute dose-limiting toxicity. Other toxicities, including diarrhea, nausea, vomiting, mucositis, and alopecia, are dose and schedule related. Prophylactic antiemetics are routinely given with bolus doses of doxorubicin, and longer infusions are associated with less nausea and less cardiotoxicity. Patients should also be warned to expect their urine to redden after drug administration. Doxorubicin is a potent vesicant, and extravasation can lead to severe necrosis of skin and local tissues, requiring surgical debridement and skin grafts. Infusions via a central venous catheter are recommended. Other toxicities of doxorubicin include *radiation recall* and the risk of developing secondary leukemia. *Radiation recall* is an inflammatory reaction at sites of previous radiation and can lead to pericarditis, pleural effusion, and skin rash. Secondary leukemias are thought to be a result of balanced translocations that result from Top2 poisoning by the anthracyclines, albeit to lesser degree than other Top2 poisons, such as the epipodophyllotoxins (see the following).[82]

Anthracyclines are cleared mainly by metabolism to less active forms and by biliary excretion. Less than 10% of the administered dose is cleared by the kidneys. Dose reductions should be made in patients with elevated plasma bilirubin. Doxorubicin should be dose reduced by 50% for plasma bilirubin concentrations ranging from 1.2 to 3.0 mg/dL, by 75% for values of 3.1 to 5.0 mg/dL, and withheld for values greater than 5 mg/dL.

Liposomal Doxorubicin

Doxorubicin is also available in a polyethylene glycol (PEG)ylated liposomal form, which allows for enhancement of drug delivery. Use of liposomal doxorubicin has been associated with less cardiotoxicity even at doses exceeding 500 mg/m^2.[83] Additionally, liposomal doxorubicin produces less nausea and vomiting and relatively mild myelosuppression compared to doxorubicin. Unique to the liposomal formulation is the risk of hand–foot syndrome and an acute infusion reaction manifested by flushing, dyspnea, edema, fever, chills, rash, bronchospasm, and hypertension. These infusion reactions are related to the rate of infusion; therefore, the recommended administration schedule is set at an initial rate of 1 mg per minute for the first 10 to 15 minutes. The rate may be slowly increased to complete infusion over 60 minutes if no reaction occurs. Typical dosing schedules include 50 mg/m^2 intravenous infusion every 4 weeks for four courses in ovarian cancer, 20 mg/m^2 intravenous infusion every 3 weeks in AIDS-related Kaposi sarcoma, and 30 mg/m^2 intravenous infusion in combination with bortezomib to be given on days 1, 4, 8, and 11 every 3 weeks in multiple myeloma.

Daunorubicin

Despite its chemical similarity (see Fig. 20.3C), daunorubicin is considerably less active in solid tumors compared to doxorubicin. It is FDA approved for the treatment of ALL and AML. Daunorubicin is typically administered via intravenous push over 3 to 5 minutes at a dose of 30 to 45 mg/m^2 per day on 3 consecutive days in combination chemotherapy. For induction therapy for pediatric acute lymphoblastic leukemia, daunorubicin is dosed at 25 mg/m^2 intravenously in combination with vincristine and prednisone. In children less than 2 years of age or in those who have a body surface area less than 0.5 m^2, current recommendations are based on

TABLE 20.4

U.S. Food And Drug Administration–Approved Topoisomerase II Inhibitors in Clinical Use

Compound	Tumor Type	Clinical Indication	Major Toxicities
I. Anthracyclines			
Doxorubicin (Adriamycin)	Breast carcinoma	Adjuvant setting with axillary LN involvement following resection of primary breast cancer	Dose-dependent cardiotoxicity Myelosuppression
	ALL AML Wilms' tumor Neuroblastoma Sarcomas Ovarian cancer Transitional cell bladder cancer Thyroid cancer Gastric cancer Hodgkin lymphoma Non-Hodgkin lymphoma	In combination with other cytotoxic agents	
Pegylated liposomal doxorubicin (Doxil)	Ovarian cancer	After failure of platinum-based chemotherapy	Myelosuppression Stomatitis Hand-foot syndrome Dosage reduction recommended with hepatic dysfunction
	AIDS-related Kaposi sarcoma	After failure of prior systemic chemotherapy	
	Multiple myeloma	In combination with bortezomib	
Daunorubicin (Cerubidine)	ALL AML	Induction therapy	Dose-dependent cardiotoxicity Myelosuppression
Epirubicin (Ellence)	Breast cancer	Adjuvant therapy in patients with evidence of axillary node tumor involvement following primary resection	Dose-dependent cardiotoxicity Myelosuppression
Idarubicin (Idamycin)	AML	Induction therapy	Dose-dependent cardiotoxicity Myelosuppression
II. Anthracenediones			
Mitoxantrone (Novantrone)	Prostate cancer AML	Hormone-refractory prostate cancer	Myelosuppression
Dactinomycin (Cosmegen)	Wilms' tumor Rhabdomyosarcoma Ewing sarcoma Nonseminomatous testicular cancer Gestational trophoblastic neoplasia		Myelosuppression
III. Epipodophyllotoxins			
Etoposide (VePesid)	Small-cell lung cancer Testicular cancer	First-line in combination First-line in combination	Myelosuppression
Teniposide (Vumon)	Pediatric lymphoblastic leukemia	Refractory setting	Myelosuppression

LN, lymph node.

body mass index (1 mg/kg) rather than body surface area. A higher dose of daunorubicin at 60 mg/m^2 per day to 90 mg/m^2 per day intravenously for 3 consecutive days is currently recommended as part of the induction combination regimen for the treatment of acute myeloblastic leukemia. Daunorubicin has similar toxicities to doxorubicin, including myelosuppression, cardiac toxicity, nausea, vomiting, alopecia, and is also a vesicant. Daunorubicin is metabolized by the liver and undergoes substantial elimination by the kidneys, requiring dose reductions for both renal and hepatic dysfunction. A 50% dose reduction is recommended for either serum creatinine or bilirubin greater than 3 mg/dL, and a 25% reduction in dose for bilirubin concentrations ranging from 1.2 to 3.0 mg/dL.

Epirubicin

Epirubicin is an epimer of doxorubicin (see Fig. 20.3C) with increased lipophilicity. It is FDA approved for adjuvant therapy of breast cancer but is also used in combination for the treatment of a variety of malignancies. Epirubicin is administered intravenously at doses ranging from 60 to 120 mg/m^2 every 3 to 4 weeks. Epirubicin has a similar toxicity profile to doxorubicin but is overall better tolerated.

In addition to being converted to an enol by an aldose reductase, epirubicin has a unique steric orientation of the C-4 hydroxyl group that allows it to serve as a substrate for conjugation reactions mediated by liver glucuronosyltransferases and sulfatases. As such, dose adjustments are recommended in the setting of hepatic dysfunction. For patients with serum bilirubin of 1.2 to 3 mg/dL or aspartate aminotransferase of 2 to 4 times the upper limit of normal, a 50% dose reduction is recommended. For patients with bilirubin greater than 3 mg/dL or aspartate aminotransferase greater than 4 times the upper limit of normal, a dose reduction of 75% is recommended. Due to limited data, no specific dose recommendations are currently available for patients with renal impairment, although current recommendations are for consideration of dose adjustments in patients with serum creatinine greater than 5 mg/dL.

Idarubicin

Idarubicin is a synthetic derivative of daunorubicin, but lacks the 4-methoxy group (see Fig. 20.3C). It is FDA approved as part of combination chemotherapy regimen for AML and is also active in ALL. It is given intravenously at a dose of 12 mg/m^2 for 3 consecutive days, typically in combination with cytarabine. Idarubicin has similar toxicities as daunorubicin. Its primary active metabolite is idarubicinol, and elimination is mainly through the biliary system and, to a lesser extent, through renal excretion. A 50% dose reduction is recommended for serum bilirubin of 2.6 to 5 mg/dL and idarubicin should not be given if the bilirubin is greater than 5 mg/dL. Additionally, dose reductions in renal impairment are advised, but specific guidelines are not available.

Cardiac Toxicity of Anthracyclines

Anthracyclines are responsible for cardiac toxicities, and special considerations are necessary to minimize this severe side effect. Acute doxorubicin cardiotoxicity is reversible, and clinical signs include tachycardia, hypotension, electrocardiogram changes, and arrhythmias. It develops during or within days of anthracycline infusion, and its incidence can be significantly reduced by slowing doxorubicin infusion rates.

Chronic and delayed cardiotoxicity is more common and more severe because it is irreversible. Chronic cardiotoxicity with congestive heart failure peaks at 1 to 3 months but can occur even years after therapy. Myocardial damage has been shown to occur by several mechanisms. The classical mechanism is by the direct generation of reactive oxygen species (ROS) during the electron transfer from the semiquinone to quinone moieties of the anthracycline,[84] which leads to myocardial damage. ROS can also be generated by mitochondrial damage resulting from drug-mediated inactivation of the oxidative phosphorylation chain because doxorubicin accumulates not only in chromatin, but also in mitochondria.[78,79] A recent study has also related doxorubicin cardiotoxicity to the poisoning of Top2β cleavage complexes in myocardiocytes.[85] Endomyocardial biopsy is characterized by a predominant finding of multifocal areas of patchy and interstitial fibrosis (stellate scars) and occasional vacuolated myocardial cells (Adria cells). Myocyte hypertrophy and degeneration, loss of cross-striations, and the absence of myocarditis are also characteristic of this diagnosis.[86] The incidence of cardiomyopathy is related to both the cumulative dose and the schedule of administration, and predisposition to cardiac damage includes a previous history of heart disease, hypertension, radiation to the mediastinum, age greater than 65 years or younger than 4 years, prior use of anthracyclines or other cardiac toxins, and coadministration of other chemotherapy agents (e.g., paclitaxel, cyclophosphamide, or trastuzumab).[87,88] Sequential administration of paclitaxel followed by doxorubicin in breast cancer patients is associated with cardiomyopathy at total doxorubicin doses above 340 to 380 mg/m^2, whereas the reverse sequence of drug administration did not yield the same systemic toxicities at these doses.[89] When doxorubicin is given in a low-dose weekly regimen (10 to 20 mg/m^2 per week) or by slow continuous infusion over 96 hours, cumulative doses of more than 500 mg/m^2 can be given. Doses of epirubicin less than 1,000 mg/m^2 and daunorubicin

less than 550 mg/m^2 are considered safe. Additionally, liposomal doxorubicin is associated with less cardiac toxicity.

Cardiac function can be monitored during treatment with anthracyclines by electrocardiography, echocardiography, or radionuclide scans. Numerous studies have established the danger of embarking on anthracycline therapy in patients with underlying cardiac disease (e.g., a baseline left ventricular ejection fraction of less than 50%) and of continuing therapy after a documented decrease in the ejection fraction by more than 10% (if this decrease falls below the lower limit of normal). Because anthracycline-induced cardiotoxicity has been related to the generation of free radicals, efforts have been aimed at attenuating this effect through the targeting of redox response and reduction in oxidative stress. Dexrazoxane is a metal chelator that decreases the myocardial toxicity of doxorubicin in breast cancer patients. In two multicenter, double-blind studies, advanced breast cancer patients were randomized to chemotherapy with dexrazoxane or a placebo; dexrazoxane was shown to have a cardioprotective effect based on serial, noninvasive cardiac testing during the course of the trial and is approved for that use by the FDA.[90] Dexrazoxane chelates iron and copper, thereby interfering with the redox reactions that generate free radicals and damage myocardial lipids. Notably, dexrazoxane is also a Top2 catalytic inhibitor (see Fig. 20.3F), which potentially might minimize the therapeutic activity of anthracyclines by interfering with the trapping of Top2 cleavage complexes by anthracyclines.[2,3,91] Other agents currently in use include β-blockers and statins. A recent meta-analysis of 12 randomized controlled trials and 2 observational studies involving the use of agents to prevent the cardiotoxicity associated with anthracyclines demonstrated relatively similar efficacy regardless of which prophylactic treatment was used.[92]

Anthracenediones

Mitoxantrone (see Fig. 20.3E) is currently the only clinically approved anthracenedione. Compared to anthracyclines, mitoxantrone is less cardiotoxic owing to a decreased ability to undergo oxidation-reduction reactions and form free radicals.

Mitoxantrone is FDA approved for the treatment of advanced hormone-refractory prostate cancer[93] and AML.[94] It is typically administered intravenously at a dose of 12 to 14 mg/m^2 every 3 weeks in the treatment of prostate cancer, and at a dose of 12 mg/m^2 in combination with cytosine arabinoside for 3 days in the treatment of AML.

Toxicities are generally less severe compared to doxorubicin and include myelosuppression, nausea, vomiting, alopecia, and mucositis. Cardiac toxicity can be seen at cumulative doses greater than 160 mg/m^2.[95] Mitoxantrone is rapidly cleared from the plasma and is highly concentrated in tissues. The majority of the drug is eliminated in the feces, with a small amount undergoing renal excretion. Dose adjustments for hepatic dysfunction are recommended, but formal guidelines are currently not available.

Dactinomycin

Dactinomycin was the first antibiotic shown to have antitumor activity[96] and consists of a planar phenoxazone ring attached to two peptide side chains. This unique structure allows for tight intercalation into DNA between adjacent guanine–cytosine bases, leading to Top2 and Top1 poisoning and transcription inhibition.[97] Dactinomycin was one of the first drugs shown to be transported by P-glycoprotein, and represents the major mechanism of resistance.[98]

Dactinomycin is FDA approved for Ewing sarcoma,[99] gestational trophoblastic neoplasm,[100] metastatic nonseminomatous testicular cancer,[101] nephroblastoma,[102] and rhabdomyosarcoma.[103] Typically, it is administered intravenously at doses of 15 μg/kg for 5 days in combination with other chemotherapeutic agents for the treatment of nephroblastoma, rhabdomyosarcoma, and Ewing sarcoma; at does of 12 μg/kg intravenously as a single agent in the treatment of gestational trophoblastic neoplasias; and at doses of 1,000 μg/m² intravenously on day 1 as part of a combination regimen with cyclophosphamide, bleomycin, vinblastine, and cisplatin in the treatment of metastatic nonseminomatous testicular cancer. Toxicities include myelosuppression, veno-occlusive disease of the liver, nausea, vomiting, alopecia, erythema, and acne. Additionally, similar to doxorubicin, dactinomycin can cause radiation recall and severe tissue necrosis in cases of extravasation. Dactinomycin is largely excreted unchanged in the feces and urine. Guidelines for dosing in patients with impaired renal or liver function are currently not available.

Epipodophyllotoxins

Epipodophyllotoxins are glycoside derivatives of podophyllotoxin, an antimicrotubule agent extracted from the mandrake plant. Two derivatives, demethylated on the pendant ring (see R1 in Fig. 20.3D), etoposide and teniposide were shown to primarily function as Top2 poisons rather than through antimicrotubule mechanisms.[104,105] Epipodophyllotoxins poison Top2 through a mechanism distinct from that of anthracyclines and other DNA intercalators[106] without intercalating into normal DNA in the absence of Top2. Therefore, they are "cleaner" Top2 inhibitors than the anthracyclines, anthracenediones, and dactinomycin. However, etoposide and teniposide trap Top2 cleavage complexes by base stacking in a ternary complex at the interface of the DNA and the Top2 homodimer. Mechanisms that have been implicated in resistance to etoposide include drug efflux, because epipodophyllotoxins are substrates for P-glycoprotein[107]; altered localization of Top2α; decreased cellular expression of Top2α[108]; and impaired phosphorylation of Top2.[109]

Etoposide

Etoposide (see Fig. 20.3D) is available in intravenous and oral forms. It is FDA approved for the treatment of small-cell lung cancer[110] and refractory testicular cancer.[111] It also has activity in hematologic malignancies and various solid tumors. The intravenous form is generally administered at doses of 35 to 50 mg/m² for 4 to 5 days every 3 to 4 weeks in combination therapy for small-cell lung cancer, and 50 to 100 mg/m² for 5 days every 3 to 4 weeks in combination therapy for refractory testicular cancer. The dose of oral etoposide is usually twice the intravenous dose. Oral bioavailability is highly variable due to dependence on intestinal P-glycoprotein.[112]

The dose-limiting toxicity for etoposide is myelosuppression, with white blood cell count nadirs typically occurring on days 10 to 14. Thrombocytopenia is less common than leukopenia. Additionally, mild to moderate nausea, vomiting, diarrhea, mucositis, and alopecia are associated with etoposide. Among topoisomerase inhibitors, epipodophyllotoxins have the greatest association with secondary malignancies, with etoposide having the highest risk, with an estimated 4% 6-year cumulative risk.[113] The majority of etoposide is cleared unchanged by the kidneys, and a 25% dose reduction is recommended in patients with a creatinine clearance of 15 to 50 mL per minute. A 50% dose reduction is recommended in patients with a creatinine clearance less than 15 mL per minute. Because the unbound fraction of etoposide is dependent on albumin and bilirubin concentrations, dose adjustments for hepatic dysfunction are advised, but consensus guidelines are currently not available.

Teniposide

Teniposide contains a thiophene group in place of the methyl group on the glucose moiety of etoposide (Fig. 20.3D). Teniposide

is FDA approved for refractory pediatric ALL.[114,115] In pediatric ALL studies, doses ranged from 165 mg/m² intravenously in combination with cytarabine to 250 mg/m² intravenously weekly in combination with vincristine and prednisone. Similar to etoposide, the dose-limiting toxicity of teniposide is myelosuppression. Additional toxicities include mild-to-moderate nausea, vomiting, diarrhea, alopecia, and secondary leukemia. Teniposide is associated with greater frequency of hypersensitivity reactions compared to etoposide.

Teniposide is 99% bound to albumin and, as compared to etoposide, undergoes hepatic metabolism more extensively and renal clearance less extensively. No specific guidelines are currently available on dose adjustments for renal or hepatic dysfunction.

THERAPY-RELATED SECONDARY ACUTE LEUKEMIA

One of the major complications of Top2 inhibitor therapies, especially for etoposide and mitoxantrone, is acute secondary leukemia, which occurs in approximately 5% of patients. Therapy-related AMLs (t-AML) are characterized by their relatively rapid onset (they can occur only a few months after therapy) and the presence of recurrent balanced translocations involving the mixed lineage leukemia (MLL) locus on 11q23 and over 50 partner genes.[116] The molecular mechanism is likely from the disjoining of two drug-trapped Top2 cleavage complexes on different chromosomes (see Fig. 20.2C) in relationship with transcription collisions and illegitimate relegation.[117] Top2β, rather than Top2α, has been implicated in the generation of these disjoined cleavage complexes.[117,118]

FUTURE DIRECTIONS

Current challenges in the development of topoisomerase inhibitors lie in the inherent chemical instability of current and established agents. In addition to recent developments designed to enhance the stability with semisynthetic analogs and the development of novel delivery systems in an effort to achieve higher intratumoral concentrations, attention is also being focused on targeting other topoisomerase isoenzymes. Driving this trend has been the recent elucidation of the role of Top2β inhibition in the development of treatment-related cardiotoxicity and secondary AML.[86,117,118] In addition to combination chemotherapy regimens already in use, attempts have also been made for the sequential inhibition of Top1 and Top2. Based on early preclinical models suggesting synergy with sequential inhibition of Top1 and Top2,[120] phase 1 studies have evaluated the sequential administration of topotecan and etoposide in extensive-stage small-cell lung cancer and ovarian cancer, with significant myelosuppression as the dose-limiting toxicity.[121,122] Future rational drug combinations include targeting DNA repair pathways in combination with Top1 inhibition, although further characterization is needed of the specific DNA repair and stress response pathways invoked in response to DNA damage as a result of Top1 inhibition. However, one such attempt of combining topotecan with veliparib, a small molecule inhibitor of poly (ADP-ribose) polymerase, was poorly tolerated due to significant myelosuppression, thus limiting the doses of topotecan that could be safely administered.[123]

Molecular characterization of tumors to better define patient selection and the development of pharmacodynamic biomarkers to monitor the response to treatment and to optimize the combination dose and schedules is needed for the further clinical development of topoisomerase inhibitors. Validated assays have been developed to evaluate topoisomerase 1 levels and levels of plosphorylated histone H2AX (gamma-H2AX) as a marker of DNA damage response to topoisomerase inhibition,[124,125] and are being incorporated in current phase I studies of indenoisoquinolines.[72,73]

REFERENCES

1. Nitiss JL. DNA topoisomerase II and its growing repertoire of biological functions. *Nat Rev Cancer* 2009;9(5):327–337.
2. Nitiss JL. Targeting DNA topoisomerase II in cancer chemotherapy. *Nat Rev Cancer* 2009;9(5):338–350.
3. Pommier Y, Leo E, Zhang H, et al. DNA topoisomerases and their poisoning by anticancer and antibacterial drugs. *Chem Biol* 2010;17(5):421–433.
4. Fortune JM, Osheroff N. Topoisomerase II as a target for anticancer drugs: when enzymes stop being nice. *Prog Nucleic Acid Res Mol Biol* 2000;64:221–253.
5. Wang JC. A journey in the world of DNA rings and beyond. *Annu Rev Biochem* 2009;78:31–54.
6. Wang JC. Cellular roles of DNA topoisomerases: a molecular perspective. *Nat Rev Mol Cell Biol* 2002;3(6):430–440.
7. Champoux JJ. DNA topoisomerases: structure, function, and mechanism. *Annu Rev Biochem* 2001;70:369–413.
8. Wang JC. *Untangling the Double Helix: DNA Entanglements and the Action of DNA Topoisomerases*. Cold Spring Harbor, NY: Cold Spring Harbor Laboratory Press; 2009.
9. Pommier Y. DNA Topoisomerases and cancer. In: Teicher BA, ed. *Cancer Discovery and Development*. New York: Springer & Humana Press; 2012.
10. Zhang H, Barceló JM, Lee B, et al. Human mitochondrial topoisomerase I. *Proc Natl Acad Sci U S A* 2001;98(10):10608–10613.
11. Champoux JJ, Dulbecco R. An activity from mammalian cells that untwists superhelical DNA—a possible swivel for DNA replication (polyoma-ethidium bromide-mouse-embryo cells-dye binding assay). *Proc Natl Acad Sci U S A* 1972;69(1):143–146.
12. Chen SH, Wu CH, Plank JL, et al. Essential functions of C terminus of Drosophila Topoisomerase IIIα in double Holliday junction dissolution. *J Biol Chem* 2012;287(23):19346–19353.
13. Xu D, Shen W, Guo R, et al. Top3β is an RNA topoisomerase that works with fragile X syndrome protein to promote synapse formation. *Nat Neurosci* 2013;16(9):1238–1247.
14. Seol Y, Gentry AC, Osheroff N, et al. Chiral discrimination and writhe-dependent relaxation mechanism of human topoisomerase IIα. *J Biol Chem* 2013;288(19):13695–13703.
15. Stoll G, Pietiläinen OP, Linder B, et al. Deletion of TOP3b, a component of FMRP-containing mRNPs, contributes to neurodevelopmental disorders. *Nat Neurosci* 2013;16(9):1228–1237.
16. Pommier Y, Marchand C. Interfacial inhibitors: targeting macromolecular complexes. *Nat Rev Drug Discov* 2011;11(1):25–36.
17. Nitiss J, Wang JC. DNA topoisomerase-targeting antitumor drugs can be studied in yeast. *Proc Natl Acad Sci U S A* 1988;85(20):7501–7505.
18. Bjornsti MA, Benedetti P, Viglianti GA, et al. Expression of human DNA topoisomerase I in yeast cells lacking yeast DNA topoisomerase I: restoration of sensitivity of the cells to the antitumor drug camptothecin. *Cancer Res* 1989;49(22):6318–6323.
19. Dressler LG, Berry DA, Broadwater G, et al. Comparison of HER2 status by fluorescence in situ hybridization and immunohistochemistry to predict benefit from dose escalation of adjuvant doxorubicin-based therapy in node-positive breast cancer patients. *J Clin Oncol* 2005;23(19):4287–4297.
20. Holm C, Covey JM, Kerrigan D, et al. Differential requirement of DNA replication for the cytotoxicity of DNA topoisomerase I and II inhibitors in Chinese hamster DC3F cell. *Cancer Res* 1989;49(22):6365–6368.
21. Hsiang YH, Lihou MG, Liu LF. Arrest of DNA replication by drug-stabilized topoisomerase I-DNA cleavable complexes as a mechanism of cell killing by camptothecin. *Cancer Res* 1989;49(18):5077–5082.
22. Maede Y, Shimizu H, Fukushima T, et al. Differential and common DNA repair pathways for topoisomerase I- and II-targeted drug in a genetic DT40 repair screen panel. *Mol Cancer Ther* 2014;13(1):214–220.
23. Huang SN, Pommier Y, Marchand C. Tyrosyl-DNA Phosphodiesterase 1(Tdp1) inhibitors. *Expert Opinion Ther Pat* 2011;21(9):1285–1292.
24. Zhang YW, Regairaz M, Seiler JA, et al. Poly(ADP-ribose) polymerase and XPF-ERCC1 participate in distinct pathways for the repair of topoisomerase I-induced DNA damage in mammalian cells. *Nucleic Acids Res* 2011;39(9):3607–3620.
25. Koster DA, Palle K, Bot ES, et al. Antitumor drugs impede DNA uncoiling by topoisomerase I. *Nature* 2007;448(7150):213–217.
26. Sordet O, Redon CE, Guirouilh-Barbat J, et al. Ataxia telangiectasia mutated activation by transcription- and topoisomerase I-induced DNA double-strand breaks. *EMBO Rep* 2009;10(8):887–893.
27. Pommier Y, Zwelling LA, Mattern MR, et al. Effects of dimethyl sulfoxide and thiourea upon intercalator-induced DNA single-strand breaks in mouse leukemia (L1210) cells. *Cancer Res* 1983;43(12 Pt 1):5718–5724.
28. Long BH, Musial ST, Brattain MG. Comparison of cytotoxicity and DNA breakage activity of congeners of podophyllotoxin including VP16-213 and VM26: a quantitative structure-activity relationship. *Biochemistry* 1984;23(6):1183–1188.
29. Ban Y, Ho CW, Lin RK, et al. Activation of a novel ubiquitin-independent proteasome pathway when RNA polymerase II encounters a protein roadblock. *Mol Cell Biol* 2013;33(20):4008–4016.
30. Long BH, Musial ST, Brattain MG. Single- and double-strand DNA breakage and repair in human lung adenocarcinoma cells exposed to etoposide and teniposide. *Cancer Res* 1985;45(7):3106–3112.
31. Pommier Y. Drugging topoisomerases: lessons and challenges. *ACS Chem Biol* 2013;8(1):82–95.
32. Zwelling LA, Michaels S, Erickson LC, et al. Protein-associated deoxyribonucleic acid strand breaks in L1210 cells treated with the deoxyribonucleic acid intercalating agents 4'-(9-acridinylamino) methanesulfon-m-anisidide and adriamycin. *Biochemistry* 1981;20(23):6553–6563.
33. Wall ME, Wani MC. Camptothecin and taxol: discovery to clinic—thirteenth Bruce F. Cain Memorial Award Lecture. *Cancer Res* 1995;55:753–760.
34. Pommier Y. Topoisomerase I inhibitors: camptothecins and beyond. *Nat Rev Cancer* 2006;6(10):789–802.
35. Teicher BA. Next generation topoisomerase I inhibitors: rationale and biomarker strategies. *Biochem Pharmacol* 2008;75(6):1262–1271.
36. Pommier Y, Cushman M. The indenoisoquinoline noncamptothecin topoisomerase I inhibitors: update and perspectives. *Mol Cancer Ther* 2009;8(5):1008–1014.
37. Douillard JY, Cunningham D, Roth AD, et al. Irinotecan combined with fluorouracil compared with fluorouracil alone as first-line treatment for metastatic colorectal cancer: a multicentre randomised trial. *Lancet* 2000;355:1041–1047.
38. Saltz LB, Cox JV, Blanke C, et al. Irinotecan plus fluorouracil and leucovorin for metastatic colorectal cancer. Irinotecan Study Group. *N Engl J Med* 2000;343:905–914.
39. Conroy T, Desseigne F, Tchou M, et al. FOLFIRINOX versus gemcitabine for metastatic pancreatic cancer. *N Engl J Med* 2011;364:1817–1825.
40. Hanna N, Bunn PA Jr, Langer C, et al. Randomized phase III trial comparing irinotecan/cisplatin with etoposide/cisplatin in patients with previously untreated extensive-stage disease small-cell lung cancer. *J Clin Oncol* 2006;24:2038–2043.
41. Schmittel A, Fischer von Weikersthal L, Sebastian M, et al. A randomized phase II trial of irinotecan plus carboplatin versus carboplatin treatment in patients with extended disease small-cell lung cancer. *Ann Oncol* 2006;17:663–667.
42. Iyer L, King CD, Whitington PF, et al. Genetic predisposition to the metabolism of irinotecan (CPT-11). Role of uridine diphosphate glucuronosyltransferase isoform 1A1 in the glucuronidation of its active metabolite (SN-38) in human liver microsomes. *J Clin Invest* 1998;101:847–854.
43. Innocenti F, Undevia SD, Iyer L, et al. Genetic variants in the UDP-glucuronosyltransferase 1A1 gene predict the risk of severe neutropenia of irinotecan. *J Clin Oncol* 2004;22:1382–1388.
44. Schaaf LJ, Hammond LA, Tipping SJ, et al. Phase 1 and pharmacokinetic study of intravenous irinotecan in refractory solid tumor patients with hepatic dysfunction. *Clin Cancer Res* 2006;12:3782–3791.
45. ten Bokkel Huinink W, Gore M, Carmichael J, et al. Topotecan versus paclitaxel for the treatment of recurrent epithelial ovarian cancer. *J Clin Oncol* 1997;15:2183–2193.
46. Ardizzoni A, Hansen H, Dombernowsky P, et al. Topotecan, a new active drug in the second-line treatment of small-cell lung cancer: a phase II study in patients with refractory and sensitive disease. The European Organization for Research and Treatment of Cancer Early Clinical Studies Group and New Drug Development Office, and the Lung Cancer Cooperative Group. *J Clin Oncol* 1997;15:2090–2096.
47. Long HJ 3rd, Bundy BN, Grendys EC Jr, et al. Randomized phase III trial of cisplatin with or without topotecan in carcinoma of the uterine cervix: a Gynecologic Oncology Group Study. *J Clin Oncol* 2005;23:4626–4633.
48. Baker SD, Heideman RL, Crom WR, et al. Cerebrospinal fluid pharmacokinetics and penetration of continuous infusion topotecan in children with central nervous system tumors. *Cancer Chemother Pharmacol* 1996;37:195–202.
49. Schluep T, Cheng J, Khin KT, et al. Pharmacokinetics and biodistribution of the camptothecin-polymer conjugate IT-101 in rats and tumor-bearing mice. *Cancer Chemother Pharmacol* 2006;57:654–662.
50. Young S, Schluep T, Hwang J, et al. CRLX101 (formerly IT-101)-A novel nanopharmaceutical of camptothecin in clinical development. *Curr Bioact Compd* 2011;7:8–14.
51. Weiss GJ, Chao J, Neidhart JD, et al. First-in-human phase 1/2a trial of CRLX101, a cyclodextrin-containing polymer-camptothecin nanopharmaceutical in patients with advanced solid tumor malignancies. *Invest New Drugs* 2013;31:986–1000.
52. University of Chicago. A randomized phase II study of IV Topotecan versus CRLX101 in the second line treatment of recurrent small cell lung cancer. ClinicalTrials.gov Identifier: NCT01803269.
53. Cerulean Pharma Inc. A randomized, phase 2, study to assess the safety and activity of CRLX101, a nanoparticle formulation of camptothecin, in patients with advanced non-small cell lung cancer who have failed one or two previous regimens of chemotherapy. ClinicalTrials Identifier: NCT01380769.
54. Massachusetts General Hospital. A Phase II, 2-stage Trial of CRLX101-202 in recurrent ovarian, tubal and peritoneal cancer. ClinicalTrials.gov Identifier: NCT01652079.
55. Vergote IB, Garcia A, Micha J et al. Randomized multicentre phase II trial comparing two schedules of etirinotecan pegol (NKTR-102) in women with recurrent platinum-resistant/refractory epithelial ovarian cancer. *J Clin Oncol* 2013;31(32):4060–4066.
56. Awada A, Garcia AA, Chan S et al. Two schedules of etirinotecan pegol (NKTR-102) in patients with previously treated metastatic breast cancer: a randomized phase 2 study. *Lancet Oncol* 2013;14(12):1216–1225.
57. Roswell Park Cancer Institute. A phase II study of single agent topoisomerase-I inhibitor polymer conjugate, Etirinotecan Pegol (NKTR-102), in patients with relapsed small cell lung cancer. ClinicalTrials Identifier: NCT01876446.
58. Abramson Cancer Center of the University of Pennsylvania. Phase 2 study of Etirinotecan Pegol (NKTR-102) in the treatment of patients with metastatic and recurrent non-small cell lung cancer (NSCLC) after failure of 2nd line treatment. ClinicalTrials Identifier: NCT01773109.

59. Nektar Therapeutics. A multicentre, open-label, randomized, phase 2 study to evaluate the efficacy and safety of NKTR-102 versus irinotecan in patients with second-line, irinotecan-naive, KRAS-mutant, metastatic colorectal cancer (mCRC). ClinicalTrials Identifier: NCT00856375.

60. Lawrence Recht. A phase II, single arm, open label study of NKTR-102 in bevacizumab-resistant high-grade glioma. ClinicalTrials Identifier: NCT01663012.

61. Nektar Therapeutics. The BEACON study (breast cancer outcomes with NKTR-102): a phase 3 open-label, randomized, multicenter study of NKTR-102 versus treatment of physician's choice (TPC) in patients with locally recurrent or metastatic breast cancer previously treated with an anthracycline, a taxane and capecitabine. ClinicalTrials Identifier: NCT01492101.

62. Basili S, Moro S. Novel camptothecin derivatives as topoisomerase I inhibitors. *Expert Opin Ther Pat* 2009;19:555–574.

63. Choi CH, Lee YY, Song TJ, et al. Phase II study of belotecan, a camptothecin analogue, in combination with carboplatin for the treatment of recurrent ovarian cancer. *Cancer* 2011;117:2104–2111.

64. Rhee CK, Lee SH, Kim JS, et al. A multicentre phase II study of belotecan, a new camptothecin analogue, as a second-line therapy in patients with small cell lung cancer. *Lung Cancer* 2011;72(1):64–67.

65. Hwang JH, Lim MC, Seo SS, et al. Phase II study of belotecan (CKD 602) as a single agent in patients with recurrent or progressive carcinoma of the uterine cervix. *Jpn J Clin Oncol* 2011;41:624–629.

66. Frapolli R, Zucchetti M, Sessa C, et al. Clinical pharmacokinetics of the new oral camptothecin gimatecan: the inter-patient variability is related to alpha1-acid glycoprotein plasma levels. *Eur J Cancer* 2010;46:505–516.

67. Pecorelli S, Ray-Coquard I, Tredan O, et al. Phase II of oral gimatecan in patients with recurrent epithelial ovarian, fallopian tube or peritoneal cancer, previously treated with platinum and taxanes. *Ann Oncol* 2010;21:759–765.

68. Graham JS, Falk S, Samuel LM et al. A multi-centre dose escalation and pharmacokinetic study of diflomotecan in patients with advanced malignancy. *Cancer Chemother Pharmacol* 2009;63:945–952.

69. Trocóniz IF, Cendrós JM, Soto E, et al. Population pharmacokinetic/pharmacodynamics modeling of drug-induced adverse effects of a novel homocamptothecin analog, elomotecan (BN80927), in a Phase I dose finding study in patients with advanced solid tumors. *Cancer Chemother Pharmacol* 2012;70:239–250.

70. Takagi K, Dexheimer TS, Redon C, et al. Novel E-ring camptothecin keto analogues (S38809 and S39625) are stable, potent, and selective topoisomerase I inhibitors without being substrates of drug efflux transporters. *Mol Cancer Ther* 2007;6(12 Pt 1):3229–3238.

71. Lansiaux A, Léonce S, Kraus-Berthier L, et al. Novel stable camptothecin derivatives replacing the E-ring lactone by a ketone function are potent inhibitors of topoisomerase I and promising antitumor drugs. *Mol Pharmacol* 2007;72(2):311–319.

72. National Cancer Institute. A Phase I Study of Indenoisoquinolines LMP400 and LMP776 in Adults With Relapsed Solid Tumors and Lymphomas. ClinicalTrials Identifier: NCT01051635.

73. National Cancer Institute. A phase I trial of weekly Indenoisoquinolines LMP400 in adults with relapsed solid tumors and lymphomas. ClinicalTrials Identifier: NCT01794104.

74. Antony S, Agama KK, Miao ZH, et al. Novel indenoisoquinolines NSC 725776 and NSC 724998 produce persistent topoisomerase I cleavage complexes and overcome multidrug resistance. *Cancer Res* 2007;67:10397–10405.

75. Kurtzberg LS, Roth S, Krumbholz R, et al. Genz-644282, a novel non-camptothecin topoisomerase I inhibitor for cancer treatment. *Clin Cancer Res* 2011;17:2777–2787.

76. Genzyme, a Sanofi Company. Dose Escalation Study to Assess the Safety and Tolerability of Genz-644282 in Patients With Solid Tumors. ClinicalTrials Identifier: NCT00942799.

77. Capranico G, Zunino F, Kohn KW, et al. Sequence-selective topoisomerase II inhibition by anthracycline derivatives in SV40 DNA: relationship with DNA binding affinity and cytotoxicity. *Biochemistry* 1990;29(2):562–569.

78. Davies KJ, Doroshow JH. Redox cycling of anthracyclines by cardiac mitochondria. I. Anthracycline radical formation by NADH dehydrogenase. *J Biol Chem* 1986;261(7):3060–3067.

79. Doroshow JH, Davies KJ. Redox cycling of anthracyclines by cardiac mitochondria. II. Formation of superoxide anion, hydrogen peroxide, and hydroxyl radical. *J Biol Chem* 1986;261:3068–3074.

80. Schneider E, Cowan KH. Multiple drug resistance in cancer therapy. *Med J Aust* 1994;160(6):371–373.

81. Alvarez M, Paull K, Monks A, et al. Generation of a drug resistance profile by quantitation of mdr-1/P-glycoprotein in the cell lines of the National Cancer Institute Anticancer Drug Screen. *J Clin Invest* 1995;95(5):2205–2214.

82. Felix CA, Kolaris CP, Osheroff N. Topoisomerase II and the etiology of chromosomal translocations. *DNA Repair* 2006;5:1093–1108.

83. O'Brien ME, Wigler N, Inbar M, et al. Reduced cardiotoxicity and comparable efficacy in a phase III trial of pegylated liposomal doxorubicin HCl (CAELYX/Doxil) versus conventional doxorubicin for first-line treatment of metastatic breast cancer. *Ann Oncol* 2004;15(3):440–449.

84. Doroshow JH. Effect of anthracycline antibiotics on oxygen radical formation in rat heart. *Cancer Res* 1983;43(2):460–472.

85. Zhang S, Liu X, Bawa-Khalfe T, et al. Identification of the molecular basis of doxorubicin-induced cardiotoxicity. *Nat Med* 2012;18:1639–1642.

86. Speyer J, Wasserheit C. Strategies for reduction of anthracycline cardiac toxicity. *Sem Oncol* 1998;25:525–537.

87. Chanan-Khan A, Srinivasan S, Czuczman MS. Prevention and management of cardiotoxicity from antineoplastic therapy. *J Support Oncol* 2004;2:251–256.

88. Von Hoff DD, Layard MW, Basa P, et al. Risk factors for doxorubicin-induced congestive heart failure. *Ann Intern Med* 1979;91:710–717.

89. Shan K, Lincoff AM, Young JB. Anthracycline-induced cardiotoxicity. *Ann Intern Med* 1996;125:47–58.

90. Swain SM, Whaley FS, Gerber MC, et al. Cardioprotection with dexrazoxane for doxorubicin-containing therapy in advanced breast cancer. *J Clin Oncol* 15(4):1318–1332.

91. Andoh T, Ishida R. Catalytic inhibitors of DNA topoisomerase II. *Biochim Biophys Acta* 1998;1400(1–3):155–171.

92. Kalam K, Marwick TH. Role of cardioprotective therapy for prevention of cardiotoxicity with chemotherapy: a systematic review and meta-analysis. *Eur J Cancer* 2013;49:2900–2909.

93. Tannock IF, Osoba D, Stockler MR, et al. Chemotherapy with mitoxantrone plus prednisone or prednisone alone for symptomatic hormone-resistant prostate cancer: a Canadian randomized trial with palliative end points. *J Clin Oncol* 1996;14:1756–1764.

94. Reece DE, Elmongy MB, Barnett MJ, et al. Chemotherapy with high-dose cytosine arabinoside and mitoxantrone for poor-prognosis myeloid leukemias. *Cancer Invest* 1993;11:509–516.

95. Shenkenberg TD, Von Hoff DD. Mitoxantrone: a new anticancer drug with significant clinical activity. *Ann Intern Med* 1986;105:67–81.

96. Hollstein U. Actinomycin. Chemistry and mechanism of action. *Chem Rev* 1974;74(6):625–652.

97. Wassermann K, Markovits J, Jaxel C, et al. Effects of morpholinyl doxorubicins, doxorubicin, and actinomycin D on mammalian DNA topoisomerases I and II. *Mol Pharmacol* 1990;38(1):38–45.

98. Biedler JL, Riehm H. Cellular resistance to actinomycin D in Chinese hamster cells in vitro: cross-resistance, radioautographic, and cytogenetic studies. *Cancer Res* 1970;30:1174–1184.

99. Jaffe N, Paed D, Traggis D, et al. Improved outlook for Ewing's sarcoma with combination chemotherapy (vincristine, actinomycin D and cyclophosphamide) and radiation therapy. *Cancer* 1976;38(5):1925–1930.

100. Turan T, Karacay O, Tulunay G, et al. Results of EMA/CO (etoposide, methotrexate, actinomycin D, cyclophosphamide, vincristine) chemotherapy in gestational trophoblastic neoplasia. *Int J Gynecol Cancer* 2006;16(3):1432–1438.

101. Early KS, Albert DJ. Single agent chemotherapy (actinomycin D) in the treatment of metastatic testicular carcinoma. *South Med J* 1976;69(8):1017–1021.

102. Fernbach DJ, Martyn DT. Role of dactinomycin in the improved survival of children with Wilm's tumor. *JAMA* 1966;195(1222):1005–1009.

103. Maurer HM, Moon T, Donaldson M, et al. The intergroup rhabdomyosarcoma study: a preliminary report. *Cancer* 1977;40(5):2015–2026.

104. Chen GL, Yang L, Rowe TC, et al. Nonintercalative antitumor drugs interfere with the breakage-reunion reaction of mammalian DNA topoisomerase. *J Biol Chem* 1984;259(21):13560–13566.

105. Long BH, Musial ST, Brattain MG. Comparison of cytotoxicity and DNA breakage activity of cogeners of podophyllotoxin including VP16-213 and VM26: a quantitative structure-activity relationship. *Biochemistry* 1984;23(6):1183–1188.

106. Ross W, Rowe T, Glisson B, et al. Role of topoisomerase II in mediating epipodophyllotoxin-induced DNA cleavage. *Cancer Res* 1984;44:5857–5860.

107. Meresse P, Dechaux E, Monneret C, et al. Etoposide: discovery and medicinal chemistry. *Curr Med Chem* 2004;11:2443–2466.

108. Valkov NI, Gump JL, Engel R, et al. Cell density-dependent VP-16 sensitivity of leukaemic cells is accompanied by the translocation of topoisomerase IIalpha from the nucleus to the cytoplasm. *Br J Haematol* 2000;109:331–345.

109. Takano H, Kohno K, Ono M, et al. Increased phosphorylation of DNA topoisomerase II in etoposide-resistant mutants of human cancer KB cells. *Cancer Res* 1991;51:3951–3957.

110. Sundstrøm S, Bremnes RM, Kaasa S, et al. Cisplatin and etoposide regimen is superior to cyclophosphamide, epirubicin, and vincristine regimen in small-cell lung cancer: results from a randomized phase III trial with 5 years' follow-up. *J Clin Oncol* 2002;20:4665–4672.

111. Nichols CR, Catalano PJ, Crawford ED, et al. Randomized comparison of cisplatin and etoposide and either bleomycin or ifosfamide in treatment of advanced disseminated germ cell tumors: an Eastern Cooperative Oncology Group, Southwest Oncology Group, and Cancer and Leukemia Group B Study. *J Clin Oncol* 1998;16:1287–1293.

112. Leu BL, Huang JD. Inhibition of intestinal P-glycoprotein and effects on etoposide absorption. *Cancer Chemother Pharmacol* 1995;35:432–436.

113. Smith MA, Rubinstein L, Anderson JR, et al. Secondary leukemia or myelodysplastic syndrome after treatment with epipodophyllotoxins. *J Clin Oncol* 1999;17:569–577.

114. Maluf PT, Odone Filho V, Cristofani LM, et al. Teniposide plus cytarabine as intensification therapy and in continuation therapy for advanced nonlymphoblastic lymphomas of childhood. *J Clin Oncol* 1994;12:1963–1968.

115. Rivera G, Bowman WP, Murphy SB, et al. VM-26 with prednisone and vincristine for treatment of refractory acute lymphocytic leukemia. *Med Pediatr Oncol* 1982;10:439–446.

116. Lovett BD, Lo Nigro L, Rappaport EF, et al. Near-precise interchromosomal recombination and functional DNA topoisomerase II cleavage sites at MLL and AF-4 genomic breakpoints in treatment-related acute lymphoblastic leukemia with t(4;11) translocation. *Proc Natl Acad Sci U S A* 2001;98(17):9802–9807.

117. Cowell IG, Sondka Z, Smith K, et al. Model for MLL translocations in therapy-related leukemia involving topoisomerase IIb-mediated DNA strand breaks and gene proximity. *Proc Natl Acad Sci U S A* 2012;109(23):8989–8994.

118. Azarova AM, Lyu YL, Lin CP, et al. Roles of DNA topoisomerases II isozymes in chemotherapy and secondary malignancies. *Proc Natl Acad Sci U S A* 2007;104:11014–11019.

119. Changela A, DiGate RJ, Mondragón A. Structural studies of E. Coli topoisomerase III-DNA complexes reveal a novel type IA topoisomerase-DNA conformational intermediate. *J Mol Biol* 2007;368:105–118.

120. Bertrand R, O'Connor PM, Kerrigan D, et al. Sequential administration of camptothecin and etoposide circumvents the antagonistic cytotoxicity of simultaneous drug administration in slowly growing human colon carcinoma HT-29 cells. *Eur J Cancer* 1992;28A(4–5):743–748.

121. Miller AA, Al Omari A, Murry DJ, et al. Phase I and pharmacologic study of sequential topotecan-carboplatin-etoposide in patients with extensive stage small cell lung cancer. *Lung Cancer* 2006;54:379–385.

122. Rose PG, Markham M, Bell JG, et al. Sequential prolonged oral topotecan and prolonged oral etoposide as second-line therapy in ovarian or peritoneal carcinoma: a phase I Gynecologic Oncology Study Group study. *Gynecol Oncol* 2006;102:236–239.

123. Kummar S, Chen A, Ji J, et al. Phase I study of PARP inhibitor ABT-888 in combination with topotecan in adults with refractory solid tumors and lymphomas. *Cancer Res* 2011;71(17):5626–5634.

124. Pfister TD, Hollingshead M, Kinders RJ, et al. Development and validation of an immunoassay for quantification of topoisomerase I in solid tumor tissues. *PLoS One* 2012;7:e50494.

125. Kinders RJ, Hollingshead M, Lawrence S, et al. Development of a validated immunofluorescence assay for gH2AX as a pharmacodynamics marker of topoisomerase I inhibitor activity. *Clin Cancer Res* 2010;16:5447–5457.

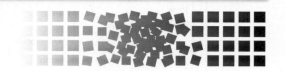

21 Antimicrotubule Agents

Christopher J. Hoimes and Lyndsay N. Harris

MICROTUBULES

Microtubules are vital and dynamic cytoskeletal polymers that play a critical role in cell division, signaling, vesicle transport, shape, and polarity, which make them attractive targets in anticancer regimens and drug design.[1] Microtubules are composed of 13 linear protofilaments of polymerized α/β-tubulin heterodimers arranged in parallel around a cylindrical axis and associated with regulatory proteins such as microtubule-associated proteins, tau, and motor proteins kinesin and dynein.[2] The specific biologic functions of microtubules are due to their unique polymerization dynamics. Tubulin polymerization is mediated by a nucleation-elongation mechanism. One end of the microtubules, termed the *plus end*, is kinetically more dynamic than the other end, termed the *minus end* (Fig. 21.1). Microtubule dynamics are governed by two principal processes driven by guanosine 5′-triphosphate (GTP) hydrolysis: *treadmilling* or *poleward flux* is the net growth at one end of the microtubule and the net shortening at the opposite end, and *dynamic instability*, which is a process in which the microtubule ends switch spontaneously between states of slow sustained growth and rapid depolymerization.[2] Antimicrotubule agents are tubulin-binding drugs that directly bind tubules, inhibitors of tubulin-associated scaffold kinases, or inhibitors of their associated mitotic motor proteins to, ultimately, disrupt microtubule dynamics. They are broadly classified as microtubule stabilizing or microtubule destabilizing agents according to their effects on tubulin polymerization.

TAXANES

Taxanes were the first-in-class microtubule stabilizing drugs. Ancient medicinal attempts at cardiac pharmacotherapy using material from the toxic coniferous yew tree, *Taxus* spp., were likely related to the plant's alkaloid *taxine* effect on sodium and calcium channels. Taxane compounds are the result of a drug screening of 35,000 plant extracts in 1963 that led to the identification of activity from the bark extract of the Pacific yew tree, *Taxus brevifolia*. Paclitaxel was identified as the active constituent with a report of its activity in carcinoma cell lines in 1971.[3] Motivation to identify taxanes derived from the more abundant and available needles of *Taxus baccata* led to the development of docetaxel, which is synthesized by the addition of a side chain to 10-deacetylbaccatin III, an inactive taxane precursor.[4] The taxane rings of paclitaxel and docetaxel are linked to an ester side chain attached to the C13 position of the ring, which is essential for antimicrotubule and antitumor activity. Nanoparticle albumin-bound paclitaxel (nab-paclitaxel) is a formulation that avoids the solvent related side effects of non–water-soluble paclitaxel and docetaxel. Overcoming docetaxel and paclitaxel's susceptibility to the P-glycoprotein efflux pump led to the development of cabazitaxel.[5] Cabazitaxel is synthesized by adding two methoxy groups to the 10-deacetylbaccatin III, which results in

the inhibition of the 5′-triphosphate–dependent efflux pump of P-glycoprotein.

Paclitaxel initially received regulatory approval in the United States in 1992 for the treatment of patients with ovarian cancer after failure of first-line or subsequent chemotherapy (Table 21.1).[1,4] Subsequently, it has been approved for several other indications, including advanced breast cancer after anthracycline-based regimens[6]; combination chemotherapy of lymph node–positive breast cancer in the adjuvant setting[7]; advanced ovarian cancer in combination with a platinum compound; second-line treatment of AIDS-related Kaposi sarcoma; and first-line treatment of non–small-cell lung cancer (NSCLC) in combination with cisplatin[8] (see Table 21.1). In addition to the U.S. Food and Drug Administration (FDA) on-label indications, paclitaxel is widely used for several other tumor types, such as cancers of unknown origin, bladder, esophagus, gastric, head and neck, and cervical cancers. The U.S. patent for paclitaxel expired in 2002, and a generic form of paclitaxel is now available.

Docetaxel was first approved for use in the United States in 1996 for patients with metastatic breast cancer that progressed or relapsed after anthracycline-based chemotherapy, which was later broadened to a general second-line indication (see Table 21.1).[4,6] Subsequently, it received regulatory approval in adjuvant chemotherapy of stage II breast cancer in combination with Adriamycin and cyclophosphamide (TAC)[9], and first-line treatment for locally advanced or metastatic breast cancer.[10] In addition, docetaxel has indications in nonresectable, locally advanced, or metastatic NSCLC after failure of or in combination with cisplatin therapy; metastatic castration-resistant prostate cancer in combination with prednisone[11]; first-line treatment of gastric adenocarcinoma, including gastroesophageal junction adenocarcinoma in combination with cisplatin and 5-fluorouracil (5-FU)[12]; and inoperable locally advanced squamous cell cancer of the head and neck in combination with cisplatin and 5-FU (see Table 21.1). Docetaxel came off patent in 2010 and a generic form is available.

Mechanism of Action

The unique mechanism of action for paclitaxel was initially defined by Schiff et al.[13] in 1979, who showed that it bound to the interior surface of the microtubule lumen at binding sites completely distinct from those of exchangeable GTP, colchicine, podophyllotoxin, and the vinca alkaloids.[14] The taxanes profoundly alter the tubulin dissociation rate constants at both ends of the microtubule, suppressing treadmilling and dynamic instability. Dose-dependent taxane β-tubular binding induces mitotic arrest at the G2/M transition and induces cell death. By stabilizing microtubules, they also can stall ligand-dependent intracellular trafficking, as shown in sequestration of the androgen receptor to the cytosol in metastatic prostate cancer patients treated with docetaxel, and is associated with decreased androgen-regulated gene expression, such as prostate-specific antigen (PSA).[15,16] Peripheral neuropathy is a common dose-limiting toxicity across the antimicrotubule agents and likely is a result of their direct effect on microtubules. Studies

245

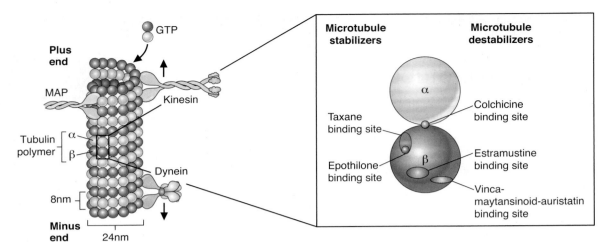

Figure 21.1 Antimicrotubule agents bind tubulin directly or inhibit its associated proteins. Taxanes and epothilones have distinct binding pockets within the same site on the interior surface of the tubule. Estramustine has a distinct site on β-tubulin, although it also directly binds microtubule-associated proteins (MAP). (Adapted from Lieberman M, Marks A. *Mark's Basic Medical Biochemistry: A Clinical Approach.* 3rd ed. Philadelphia: Lippincott Williams & Wilkins; 2009.)

have shown that they inhibit anterograde and/or retrograde fast axonal transport and can explain the demyelinating "dying back" pattern seen and the vulnerability of sensory neurons with the longest axonal projections.[17]

Recent evidence suggests that microtubule inhibitors have collateral effects during interphase that lead to cell death. For instance, paclitaxel-stabilized microtubules serve as a scaffold for the binding of the death-effector domain of pro-caspase-8, and thereby enabling a caspase-8 downstream proteolytic cascade.[18,19] This caspase-8–dependent mechanism also serves as an important basis for the understanding of the loss of function and/or low expression of the breast cancer 1, early onset gene (*BRCA1*) association with resistance to taxane therapy.[20]

Another mechanism of the anticancer effect of taxanes is currently being elaborated and is tied to the B-cell lymphoma-2 (Bcl-2) antiapoptosis family of proteins. Paclitaxel has been shown to cause the phosphorylation of Bcl-2 and the sequestration of Bak and Bim; however, this seemingly cancer-protective phosphorylation needs to be reconciled and likely correlates with Bcl-2–expression levels.[21–23] Interestingly, neutralizing Bcl-2 homology 3 (BH3) domains with compounds such as ABT-737 is synergistic with docetaxel.[24]

Clinical Pharmacology

Paclitaxel

With prolonged infusion schedules (6 and 24 hours), drug disposition is a biphasic process with values for alpha and beta half-lives averaging approximately 20 minutes and 6 hours, respectively.[4] When administered as a 3-hour infusion, the pharmacokinetics are nonlinear and may lead to unexpected toxicity with a small dose escalation, or a disproportionate decrease in drug exposure and loss of tumor response with a dose reduction. Approximately 71% of an administered dose of paclitaxel is excreted in the stool via the enterohepatic circulation over 5 days as either the parent compound or metabolites in humans. Renal clearance of paclitaxel and metabolites is minimal, accounting for 14% of the administered dose. In humans, the bulk of drug disposition is metabolized by cytochrome P-450 mixed-function oxidases—specifically, the isoenzymes CYP2C8 and CYP3A4, which metabolize paclitaxel to hydroxylated 3'p-hydroxypaclitaxel (minor) and 6α-hydroxypaclitaxel (major), as well as dihydroxylated metabolites.

Nanoparticle Albumin-Bound Paclitaxel

Nab-paclitaxel is a solvent-free colloidal suspension made by homogenizing paclitaxel with 3% to 4% albumin under high pressure to form nanoparticles of ~130 nm that disperse in plasma to ~10 nm (see Table 21.1).[25] It received regulatory approval in the United States in 2005 based on results in patients with metastatic breast cancer, and is now also approved in combination with carboplatin for first-line treatment of locally advanced or metastatic NSCLC, and in combination with gemcitabine for first-line treatment of metastatic pancreatic adenocarcinoma.[26–28] The improved responses seen with nab-paclitaxel, when compared to solvent-based paclitaxel, are not fully understood. Nab-paclitaxel likely capitalizes on several mechanisms, which include an improved pharmacokinetic profile with a larger volume of distribution and a higher maximal concentration of circulating, unbound, free drug; improved tumor accumulation by the enhanced permeability and retention (EPR) effect; and receptor-mediated transcytosis via an albumin-specific receptor (gp60) for endothelial transcytosis and binding of secreted protein acidic and rich in cysteine (SPARC) in the tumor interstitium.[29,30] In contrast to cremophor/ethanol (CrEL) solvent-based paclitaxel, nab-paclitaxel exhibits an extensive extravascular volume of distribution exceeding that of water, indicating extensive tissue and extravascular protein distribution. Some studies show that nab-paclitaxel achieves 33% higher drug concentration over CrEL-paclitaxel.[31] Additionally, the maximum concentration (Cmax), the mean plasma half-life of 15 to 18 hours, the area under curve (AUC), and the dose-independent plasma clearance correspond to linear pharmacokinetics over 80 to 300 mg/m[2].[29,32] The improved deposition of a nanoparticle, such as nab-paclitaxel in a tumor tissue, can occur passively through an EPR effect in areas of leaky vasculature, sufficient vascular pore size, and decreased lymphatic flow.[25,33] Once in the tissue, the nab-paclitaxel nanovehicle can deliver the drug locally or benefit from further receptor-mediated targeting to SPARC, which has been shown to be overexpressed, and correlates with disease progression in many tumor types.[34–38] Although preclinical models, as well as one clinical trial, have shown how nanoparticle therapy can benefit from this targeted approach,[39,40] correlative data for nab-paclitaxel is limited. The high stromal SPARC level was associated with longer survival in patients treated with nab-paclitaxel in the phase I/II study of patients with pancreatic cancer; however, this correlative analysis was not included in the phase III trial report and requires validation.[28,41]

TABLE 21.1

Antimicrotubule Agents: Dosages and Toxicities

Chemotherapeutic Agent	Dosage	Indications	Common Toxicities
Paclitaxel	135–200 mg/m^2 IV over 3 h or 135 mg/m^2 IV over 24 h every 3 wk; or 80 mg/m^2 IV over 1 h weekly	Adjuvant therapy of node-positive breast cancer; metastatic breast, ovarian, non–small-cell lung, bladder, esophagus, cervical, gastric, and head and neck cancer; AIDS-related Kaposi sarcoma; cancer of unknown origin	Myelosuppression, hypersensitivity, nausea and vomiting, alopecia, arthralgia, myalgia, peripheral neuropathy
Docetaxel	60–100 mg/m^2 IV over 1 h every 3 wk	Adjuvant therapy of node-positive breast cancer; metastatic breast, gastric, head and neck, prostate, non–small-cell lung, and ovarian cancer	Myelosuppression, hypersensitivity, edema, alopecia, nail damage, rash, diarrhea, nausea, vomiting, asthenia, neuropathy
Cabazitaxel	25 mg/m^2 IV every 3 wk over 1 h	Docetaxel-refractory metastatic castration resistant prostate cancer	Neutropenia, infections, myelosuppression, diarrhea, nausea, vomiting, constipation, abdominal pain, asthenia
Nab-paclitaxel	260 mg/m^2 IV over 30 min every 3 wk; or 125 mg/m^2 IV weekly on days 1, 8, and 15 every 28 d	Metastatic breast cancer, non–small-cell lung cancer, pancreatic cancer	Myelosuppression, nausea, vomiting, alopecia, myalgia, peripheral neuropathy
Ixabepilone	40 mg/m^2 IV over 3 h every 3 wk	Metastatic and locally advanced breast cancer	Myelosuppression, fatigue/asthenia, myalgia/arthralgia, alopecia, nausea, vomiting, stomatitis/mucositis, diarrhea, musculoskeletal pain
Vincristine	0.5–1.4 mg/m^2/wk IV (maximum 2 mg per dose); or 0.4 mg/d continuous infusion for 4 d	Lymphoma, acute leukemia, neuroblastoma, rhabdomyosarcoma, AIDS-related Kaposi sarcoma, multiple myeloma, testicular cancer	Constipation, nausea, vomiting, alopecia, diplopia, myelosuppression
Vinblastine	6 mg/m^2 IV on days 1 and 15 as part of the ABVD regimen; 0.15 mg/kg IV on days 1 and 2 as part of the PVB regimen; 3 mg/m^2 IV as part of days 2, 15, 22 MVAC regimen	Hodgkin and non-Hodgkin lymphoma; Kaposi sarcoma; breast, testicular, bladder, prostate, and renal cell cancer	Myelosuppression, constipation, alopecia, malaise, bone pain
Vinorelbine	25–30 mg/m^2 IV weekly	Non–small-cell lung, breast, cervical, and ovarian cancer	Alopecia, diarrhea, nausea, vomiting, asthenia, neuromyopathy
Estramustine	14 mg/kg PO daily in 3 or 4 divided doses	Metastatic prostate cancer	Nausea, vomiting, gynecomastia, fluid retention
Ado-trastuzumab emtansine	3.6 mg/kg IV every 3 wk	Metastatic breast cancer	Thrombocytopenia, nausea, constipation or diarrhea, peripheral neuropathy, fatigue, increased AST/ALT
Brentuximab vedotin	1.8 mg/kg every 3 wk, maximum dose 180 mg	Refractory Hodgkin lymphoma, refractory systemic anaplastic large cell lymphoma	Neutropenia, anemia, thrombocytopenia, fatigue, fever, peripheral neuropathy

ABVD, doxorubicin (Adriamycin), bleomycin, vinblastine, dacarbazine; PVB, cisplatin, vinblastine, bleomycin; MVAC, methotrexate, vinblastine, doxorubicin (Adriamycin), cisplatin; IV, intravenous; PO, by mouth; AST/ALT, aspartate amniotransferase–alanine amniotransferase.

Docetaxel

The pharmacokinetics of docetaxel on a 1-hour schedule is triexponential and linear at doses of 115 mg/m^2 or less.[4] Terminal half-lives ranging from 11.1 to 18.5 hours has been reported. The most important determinants of docetaxel clearance were the body surface area (BSA), hepatic function, and plasma α_1-acid glycoprotein concentration. Plasma protein binding is high (greater than 80%), and binding is primarily to α_1-acid glycoprotein, albumin, and lipoproteins. The hepatic cytochrome P-450 mixed-function oxidases, particularly isoforms CYP3A4 and CYP3A5, are principally involved in biotransformation. The principal pharmacokinetic determinants of toxicity, particularly neutropenia, are drug exposure and the time that plasma concentrations exceed biologically relevant concentrations. The baseline level of α_1-acid glycoprotein may be elevated as an acute phase reactant in advanced disease and is an independent predictor of response and a major objective prognostic factor of survival in patients with non–small-cell lung cancer treated with docetaxel chemotherapy.

Cabazitaxel

Cabazitaxel is a semisynthetic derivative of the natural taxoid 10-deacetylbaccatin III. It binds to and stabilizes the β-tubulin subunit, resulting in the inhibition of microtubule depolymerization and cell division, cell cycle arrest in the G_2/M phase, and the inhibition of tumor cell proliferation.[5] It is active against diverse cancer cell lines and tumor models that are sensitive and resistant to docetaxel, including prostate, mammary, melanoma, kidney, colon, pancreas, lung, gastric, and head and neck.[5] Cabazitaxel is a poor substrate for the membrane-associated, multidrug resistance P-glycoprotein efflux pump; therefore, is useful for treating docetaxel-refractory prostate cancer for which it gained FDA approval in 2010.[5] In addition, it penetrates the blood–brain barrier.[42] Pharmacokinetics of cabazitaxel is similar to docetaxel; however, cabazitaxel has a larger volume of distribution and a longer terminal half-life (mean 77.3 hours versus 11.2 hours for docetaxel).[43,44]

Tesetaxel

Tesetaxel (DJ-927, XRP6258) is a semisynthetic, orally bioavailable taxane currently in clinical trials in breast, gastric, and prostate cancer. Administration in phase I and II trials has been once per week or every 3 weeks and not associated with hypersensitivity and possibly less neurotoxicity compared to other taxanes. Dose-limiting toxicity has been neutropenia. Overall responses in phase II studies have been 50% and 38% in patients treated for first- and second-line breast cancer, respectively. A phase I/II study in advanced NSCLC showed an overall response rate of 5.6%. Tesetaxel activity is independent of P-glycoprotein expression.[45] Pharmacokinetics on a schedule of every 3 weeks have an AUC of ~1,750 ng/mL per hour, a half life of ~170 hours, and no drug interactions that have been noted.[46]

Drug Interactions

Sequence-dependent pharmacokinetic and toxicologic interactions between paclitaxel and several other chemotherapy agents have been noted. The sequence of cisplatin followed by paclitaxel (on a 24-hour schedule) induces more profound neutropenia than the reverse sequence, which is explained by a 33% reduction in the clearance of paclitaxel after cisplatin.[47] Treatment with paclitaxel on either a 3- or 24-hour schedule followed by carboplatin has been demonstrated to produce equivalent neutropenia and less thrombocytopenia as compared to carboplatin as a single agent, which is not explained by pharmacokinetic interactions. Neutropenia and mucositis are more severe when paclitaxel is administered on a 24-hour schedule before doxorubicin, compared to the reverse sequence, which is most likely due to an approximately 32% reduction in the clearance rates of doxorubicin and doxorubicinol when doxorubicin is administered after paclitaxel. Several agents that inhibit cytochrome P-450 mixed-function oxidases interfere with the metabolism of paclitaxel and docetaxel in human microsomes in vitro; however, the clinical relevance of these findings is not known.[47]

Toxicity

Paclitaxel

The micelle-forming CrEL vehicle, which is required for suspension and intravenous delivery of paclitaxel, causes its nonlinear pharmacokinetics and thereby impacts its therapeutic index. CrEL causes hypersensitivity reactions, with major reactions usually occurring within the first 10 minutes after the first treatment and resolving completely after stopping the treatment. All patients should be premedicated with steroids, diphenhydramine, and an H2 antagonist, although up to 3% will still have reactions. Those who have major reactions have been rechallenged successfully after receiving high doses of corticosteroids.

Neuropathy is the principal toxicity of paclitaxel. Paclitaxel induces a peripheral neuropathy that presents in a symmetric stocking glove distribution, at first transient and then persistent.[48] A neurologic examination reveals sensory loss, and neurophysiologic studies reveal axonal degeneration and demyelination.[48] Compared with cisplatin, a loss of deep tendon reflexes occurs less commonly; however, autonomic and motor changes can occur. Severe neurotoxicity is uncommon when paclitaxel is given alone at doses below 200 mg/m^2 on a 3- or 24-hour schedule every 3 weeks, or below 100 mg/m^2 on a continuous weekly schedule. There is no convincing evidence that any specific measure is effective at ameliorating existing manifestations or preventing the development or worsening of neurotoxicity.[48]

Neutropenia is also frequent with paclitaxel. The onset is usually on days 8 to 11, and recovery is generally complete by days 15 to 21 with an every 3 weeks dosing regimen. Neutropenia is noncumulative, and the duration of severe neutropenia—even in heavily pretreated patients—is usually brief. Severity of neutropenia is related to the duration of exposure above the biologically relevant levels of 0.05 to 0.10 μM/L, and paclitaxel's nonlinear pharmacokinetics should be considered whenever adjusting dose.[49]

The most common cardiac rhythm disturbance, a transient sinus bradycardia, can be observed in up to 30% of patients. Routine cardiac monitoring during paclitaxel therapy is not necessary but is advisable for patients who may not be able to tolerate bradyarrhythmias. Drug-related gastrointestinal effects, such as vomiting and diarrhea, are uncommon. Severe hepatotoxicity and pancreatitis have also been noted rarely. Pulmonary toxicities, including acute bilateral pneumonitis, have been reported. Extravasation of large volumes can cause moderate soft tissue injury. Paclitaxel also induces reversible alopecia of the scalp in a dose-related fashion. Nail disorders have also been reported with paclitaxel use and include ridging, nail bed pigmentation, onychorrhexis, and onycholysis. These side effects have been reported more commonly with dose-intensified paclitaxel regimens.

Recent studies have suggested a role for the adenosine triphosphatase (ATP)-binding cassette (ABC) transporter polymorphisms in the development of neuropathy and neutropenia. Sissung et al.[50] reported that patients carrying two reference alleles for the *ABCB1* (P-glycoprotein, MDR1) 3435C greater than T polymorphism had a reduced risk to develop neuropathy as compared to patients carrying at least one variant allele ($P = .09$). Data from a large controlled trial to evaluate these and other candidate polymorphisms failed to detect a significant association between genotype and outcome or toxicity for any of the genes analyzed, although the correlative studies were retrospective and the sample size was inadequate to rule out smaller differences.[51] A large randomized trial of the CALGB 40101 using an integrated genomewide associate study found two polymorphisms associated with paclitaxel-induced polyneuropathy.[52] Both are involved in nerve development and maintenance, including the hereditary peripheral neuropathy Charcot-Marie-Tooth disease gene, *FGD4*. Further studies are required to adequately assess the role of these variants in predicting toxicity from taxane therapy.

Nab-paclitaxel

Hypersensitivity reactions have not been observed during the infusion period and, therefore, steroid premedications are not necessary. The main dose-limiting toxicities are neutropenia and sensory neuropathy. In a trial comparing weekly paclitaxel 90 mg/m^2 to nab-paclitaxel 150 mg/m^2 to ixabepilone in patients with metastatic breast cancer, there was more hematologic toxicity and peripheral neuropathy in the nab-paclitaxel arm compared to the paclitaxel arm, although median progression-free survival was not significantly different at the 12-month follow-up.[53] This led to dose reductions in 45% of patients in the nab-paclitaxel arm compared with 15% for the paclitaxel arm.[53] Other toxicities include alopecia, diarrhea, nausea and vomiting, elevations in liver enzymes, arthralgia, myalgia, and asthenia.

Docetaxel

Neutropenia is the main toxicity of docetaxel.[4] When docetaxel is administered on an every 3 weeks schedule, the onset of neutropenia is usually noted on day 8, with complete resolution by days 15 to 21. Neutropenia is significantly less when low doses are administered weekly. FDA black box warnings include increased toxicity in patients with abnormal liver function and, in select NSCLC patients that received prior platinum, severe hypersensitivity reactions and severe fluid retention despite dexamethasone at-home premedication.

Hypersensitivity reactions were noted in approximately 31% of patients who received the drug without premedications in early studies.[4] Symptoms include flushing, rash, chest tightness, back pain, dyspnea, and fever or chills. Severe hypotension, bronchospasm, generalized rash, and erythema may also occur.[54] Major reactions usually occur during the first two courses and within minutes after the start of treatment. Signs and symptoms generally resolve within 15 minutes after cessation of treatment, and docetaxel can usually be reinstituted without sequelae after treatment with diphenhydramine and an H2-receptor antagonist. Docetaxel induces a unique fluid retention syndrome characterized by edema, weight gain, and third-space fluid collection. Fluid retention is cumulative and is due to increased capillary permeability. Prophylactic treatment with corticosteroids has been demonstrated to reduce the incidence of fluid retention. Aggressive and early treatment with diuretics has been successfully used to manage fluid retention. Skin toxicity may occur in as many as 50% to 75% of patients; however, premedication may reduce the overall incidence of this effect.[4] Other cutaneous effects include palmar–plantar erythrodysesthesia and onychodystrophy. Docetaxel produces neurotoxicity, which is qualitatively similar to that of paclitaxel; however, neurosensory and neuromuscular effects are generally less frequent and less severe than with paclitaxel. Mild-to-moderate peripheral neurotoxicity occurs in approximately 40% of untreated patients.[55] Asthenia has been a prominent complaint in patients who have been treated with large cumulative doses. Stomatitis appears to occur more frequently with docetaxel than with paclitaxel. Other reported toxicities of note include necrotizing enterocolitis, interstitial pneumonitis, and organizing pneumonia.[56,57]

Cabazitaxel

A phase III multi-institutional study of men with metastatic castration-resistant prostate cancer who had failed docetaxel improved overall median survival on cabazitaxel compared to mitoxantrone.[58] Cabazitaxel was approved by the FDA in June 2010 to treat metastatic castration-resistant prostate cancer in those who had received prior chemotherapy. This was despite a higher rate of adverse deaths (4.9%), a third of which were due to neutropenic sepsis. Cabazitaxel was associated with more grade 3 or 4 neutropenia (82%) than mitoxantrone (58%). Side effects reported in more than 20% of patients treated with cabazitaxel included myelosuppression, diarrhea, nausea, vomiting, constipation, abdominal pain, or asthenia. FDA black box warnings are similar to those for docetaxel.

VINCA ALKALOIDS

The vinca alkaloids have been some of the most active agents in cancer chemotherapy since their introduction 40 years ago. The naturally occurring members of the family, vinblastine (VBL) and vincristine (VCR), were isolated from the leaves of the periwinkle plant *Catharanthus roseus G. Don*. In the late 1950s, their antimitotic and, therefore, cancer chemotherapeutic potential was discovered by groups both at Eli Lilly Research Laboratories and at the University of Western Ontario, and they came into widespread use for the single-agent treatment of childhood hematologic and solid malignancies and, shortly after, for adult hematologic

malignancies (see Table 21.1).[1] Their clinical efficacy in several combination therapies has led to the development of various novel semisynthetic analogs, including vinorelbine (VRL), vindesine (VDS), and vinflunine (VFL).

Mechanism of Action

In contrast to the taxanes, the vinca alkaloids depolymerize microtubules and destroy mitotic spindles.[1] At low but clinically relevant concentrations, VBL does not depolymerize spindle microtubules, yet it powerfully blocks mitosis. This has been suggested to occur as a result of the suppression of microtubule dynamics rather than microtubule depolymerization. This group of compounds binds to the β subunit of tubulin dimers at a distinct region called the vinca-binding domain. Importantly, VBL binding induces a conformational change in tubulin in connection with tubulin self-association. In mitotic spindles, the slowing of the growth and shortening or treadmilling dynamics of the microtubules block mitotic progression. Disruption of the normal mitotic spindle assembly leads to delayed cell cycle progress with chromosomes stuck at the spindle poles and unable to pass from metaphase into anaphase, which eventually induces to apoptosis. The naturally occurring vinca alkaloids VCR and VBL, the semisynthetic analog VRL, and a novel bifluorinated analog VFL have similar mechanisms of action.

Tissue and tumor sensitivities to the vinca alkaloids, which, in part, relate to differences in drug transport and accumulation, also vary. Intracellular or extracellular concentration ratios range from five- to 500-fold depending on the individual cell type, lipophilicity, tissue-specific factors such as tubulin isotype composition, and tissue-specific microtubule-associated proteins (MAP).[59–61] Although the vinca alkaloids are retained in cells for long periods of time and thus may have prolonged cellular effects, intracellular retention is markedly different among the various vinca alkaloids. For instance, VBL appears to be retained in lipophilic tissue much more than either VCR or VDS.[59] Newer theories of antimicrobule agents' mechanism of action have emerged, suggesting that the more important target of these drugs may be the tumor vasculature, as reviewed in the next section.

Clinical Pharmacology

The vinca alkaloids are usually administered intravenously as a brief infusion, and their pharmacokinetic behavior in plasma has generally been explained by a three-compartment model. The vinca alkaloids share many pharmacokinetic properties, including large volumes of distribution, high clearance rates, and long terminal half-lives that reflect the high magnitude and avidity of drug binding in peripheral tissues. VCR has the longest terminal half-life and the lowest clearance rate; VBL has the shortest terminal half-life and the highest clearance rate; and VDS has intermediate characteristics. Although prolonged infusion schedules may avoid excessively toxic peak concentrations and increase the duration of drug exposure in plasma above biologically relevant threshold concentrations, there is little evidence to support the notion that prolonged infusions are more effective than bolus schedules. The longest half-life and lowest clearance rate of VCR may account for its greater propensity to induce neurotoxicity, but there are many other nonpharmacokinetic determinants of tissue sensitivity, as discussed in the previous section.

Vincristine

After conventional doses of VCR (1.4 mg/m^2) given as brief infusions, peak plasma levels approach 0.4 μmol. Plasma clearance is slow, and terminal half-lives that range from 23 to 85 hours have been reported. VCR is metabolized and excreted primarily by the hepatobiliary system. The nature of the VCR metabolites identified to date, as well as the results of metabolic studies in vitro, indicate that VCR metabolism is mediated principally by hepatic cytochrome P-450 CYP3A5.

Vinblastine

The clinical pharmacology of VBL is similar to that of VCR. VBL binding to plasma proteins and formed elements of blood is extensive.[62,63] Peak plasma drug concentrations are approximately 0.4 μm after rapid intravenous injections of VBL at standard doses. Distribution is rapid, and terminal half-lives range from 20 to 24 hours. Like VCR, VBL disposition is principally through the hepatobiliary system with excretion in feces (approximately 95%); however, fecal excretion of the parent compound is low, indicating that hepatic metabolism is extensive.[59]

Vinorelbine

The pharmacologic behavior of VRL is similar to that of the other vinca alkaloids, and plasma concentrations after rapid intravenous administration have been reported to decline in either a biexponential or triexponential manner.[64] After intravenous administration, there is a rapid decay of VRL concentrations followed by a much slower elimination phase (terminal half-life, 18 to 49 hours). Plasma protein binding, principally to α_1-acid glycoprotein, albumin, and lipoproteins, has been reported to range from 80% to 91%, and drug binding to platelets is extensive.[64] VRL is widely distributed, and high concentrations are found in virtually all tissues, except the central nervous system.[64] The wide distribution of VRL reflects its lipophilicity, which is among the highest of the vinca alkaloids. As with other vinca alkaloids, the liver is the principal excretory organ, and up to 80% of VRL is excreted in the feces, whereas urinary excretion represents only 16% to 30% of total drug disposition, the bulk of which is unmetabolized VRL. Studies in humans indicate that 4-O-deacetyl-VRL and 3,6-epoxy-VRL are the principal metabolites, and several minor hydroxy-VRL isomer metabolites have been identified. Although most metabolites are inactive, the deacetyl-VRL metabolite may be as active as VRL. The cytochrome P-450 CYP3A isoenzyme appears to be principally involved in biotransformation.

Vinflunine

VFL is a novel semisynthetic microtubule inhibitor with a fluorinated catharanthine moiety, which translates into lower affinity for the vinca binding site on tubulin and, therefore, different quantitative effects on microtubule dynamics.[65] The low affinity for tubulin may be responsible for its reduced clinical neurotoxicity. Despite this lower affinity, it is more active in vivo than other vinca alkaloids, and resistance develops more slowly. VFL is a new vinca and still under clinical development. Its volume of distribution is large, and has a terminal half-life of nearly 40 hours.[65] The only active metabolite is 4-O-deacetylvinflunine, which has a terminal half-life approximately 5 days longer than that of the parent compound.[65]

Drug Interactions

Methotrexate accumulation in tumor cells is enhanced in vitro by the presence of VCR or VBL, an effect mediated by a vinca alkaloid–induced blockade of drug efflux; however, the minimal concentrations of VCR required to achieve this effect occur only transiently in vivo.[66] The vinca alkaloids also inhibit the cellular influx of the epipodophyllotoxins in vitro, resulting in less cytotoxicity. However, the clinical implications of this potential interaction are unknown. L-asparaginase may reduce the hepatic clearance of the vinca alkaloids, which may result in increased vinca-related toxicity. To minimize the possibility of this interaction, the vinca alkaloids should be given 12 to 24 hours before L-asparaginase. The combined use of mitomycin C and the vinca alkaloids has been associated with acute dyspnea and bronchospasm. The onset of these pulmonary toxicities has ranged from within minutes to hours after treatment with the vinca alkaloids, or up to 2 weeks after mitomycin C.

Treatment with the vinca alkaloids has precipitated seizures associated with subtherapeutic plasma phenytoin concentrations.[66] Reduced plasma phenytoin levels have been noted from 24 hours to 10 days after treatment with VCR and VBL. Because of the importance of the cytochrome P-450 CYP3A isoenzyme in vinca alkaloid metabolism, administration of the vinca alkaloids with erythromycin and other inhibitors of CYP3A may lead to severe toxicity.[67] Concomitantly administered drugs, such as pentobarbital and H$_2$-receptor antagonists, may also influence VCR clearance by modulating hepatic cytochrome P-450 metabolic processes.[66]

Toxicity

Despite close similarities in structure, the vinca alkaloids differ in their safety profiles. Neutropenia is the principal dose-limiting toxicity of VBL and VRL. Thrombocytopenia and anemia occur less commonly. The onset of neutropenia is usually day 7 to 11, with recovery by day 14 to 21, and can be potentiated by hepatic dysfunction. Gastrointestinal autonomic dysfunction, as manifested by bloating, constipation, ileus, and abdominal pain, occur most commonly with VCR or high doses of the other vinca alkaloids. Mucositis occurs more frequently with VBL than with VRL and is least common with VCR. Nausea, vomiting, diarrhea,[31,43,45] and pancreatitis[53,54] also occur to a lesser extent.

VCR principally induces neurotoxicity characterized by a peripheral, symmetric mixed sensory motor and autonomic polyneuropathy.[68,69] Toxic manifestations include constipation, abdominal cramps, paralytic ileus, urinary retention, orthostatic hypotension, and hypertension. Its primary neuropathologic effects are due to interference with axonal microtubule function. Early symmetric sensory impairment and paresthesias can progress to neuritic pain and loss of deep tendon reflexes with continued treatment, which may be followed by foot drop, wrist drop, motor dysfunction, ataxia, and paralysis. Cranial nerves are rarely affected because the uptake of VCR into the central nervous system is low. Severe neurotoxicity occurs infrequently with VBL and VDS. VRL has been shown to have a lower affinity for axonal microtubules than either VCR or VBL, which seems to be confirmed by clinical observations.[70] Mild-to-moderate peripheral neuropathy, principally characterized by sensory effects, occurs in 7% to 31% of patients, and constipation and other autonomic effects are noted in 30% of patients, whereas severe toxicity occurs in 2% to 3%.

In adults, neurotoxicity may occur after treatment with cumulative doses as little as 5 to 6 mg, and manifestations may be profound after cumulative doses of 15 to 20 mg. Patients with delayed biliary excretion or hepatic dysfunction, and those with antecedent neurologic disorders, such as Charcot-Marie-Tooth disease, hereditary and sensory neuropathy type 1, and Guillain-Barré syndrome, are predisposed to neurotoxicity.

The vinca alkaloids are potent vesicants. To decrease the risk of phlebitis, the vein should be adequately flushed after treatment. If extravasation is suspected, treatment should be discontinued, aspiration of any residual drug remaining in the tissues should be attempted, and prompt application of heat (*not* ice) for 1 hour four times daily for 3 to 5 days can limit tissue damage.[71] Hyaluronidase, 150 to 1,500 U (15 U/mL in 6 mL 0.9% sodium chloride solution) subcutaneously, through six clockwise injections in a circumferential manner using a 25-gauge needle (changing the needle with each new injection) into the surrounding tissues may minimize discomfort and latent cellulitis. A surgical consultation to consider early debridement is also recommended. Mild and reversible alopecia occurs in approximately 10% and 20% of patients treated with VLR and VCR, respectively. Acute cardiac ischemia, chest pains without evidence of ischemia, fever, Raynaud syndrome, hand–foot syndrome, and pulmonary and liver toxicity (transaminitis and hyperbilirubinemia) have also been reported with use of the vinca alkaloids. All of the vinca alkaloids can cause a syndrome of inappropriate secretion of antidiuretic hormone (SIADH), and patients who are receiving intensive hydration are particularly prone to severe hyponatremia secondary to SIADH.

MICROTUBULE ANTAGONISTS

Estramustine Phosphate

Estramustine is a conjugate of nor-nitrogen mustard linked to 17β-estradiol by a carbamate ester bridge. Estramustine phosphate received regulatory approval in the United States in 1981 for treating patients with castration-resistant prostate cancer (CRPC). Although the recommended daily dose of estramustine phosphate is 14 mg/kg per day, patients are usually treated in the daily dosing range of 10 to 16 mg/kg in three to four divided daily doses (see Table 21.1). Estramustine has significant activity in CRPC and had been used in combination with VBL or docetaxel. However, phase III trials in patients with CRPC showed that when combined with docetaxel, there is no added benefit to overall survival compared to docetaxel alone.[72,73]

Estramustine binds to β-tubulin at a site distinct from the colchicine and vinca alkaloid binding sites. This agent depolymerizes microtubules and microfilaments, binds to and disrupts MAPs, and inhibits cell growth at high concentrations, resulting in mitotic arrest and apoptosis in tumor cells. The selective accumulation and actions of estramustine phosphate and its metabolite, *estromustine*, in specific tissues appear to be dependent on the expression of the estramustine-binding protein (EMBP). The disposition of estramustine is principally by rapid oxidative metabolism of the parent compound to estromustine. Estromustine concentrations in plasma are maximal within 2 to 4 hours after oral administration, and the mean elimination half-life of estromustine is 14 hours. Estromustine and estramustine are principally excreted in the feces, with only small amounts of conjugated estrone and estradiol detected in the urine (less than 1%).

In general, this agent has a manageable safety profile. Nausea and vomiting are the principal toxicities encountered. In contrast to the taxanes and the vinca alkaloids, myelosuppression is rarely clinically relevant. Common estrogenic side effects include gynecomastia, nipple tenderness, and fluid retention. Thromboembolic complications may occur in up to 10% of patients.

Epothilones

The epothilones are macrolide compounds that were initially isolated from the mycobacterium *Sorangium cellulosum*. They exert their cytotoxic effects by promoting tubulin polymerization and inducing mitotic arrest.[74] In general, the epothilones are more potent than the taxanes. In contrast to the taxanes and vinca alkaloids, overexpression of the efflux protein P-glycoprotein minimally affects the cytotoxicity of epothilones. Epothilones include the natural epothilone B (patupilone; EPO906) and several semisynthetic epothilone compounds such as aza-epothilone B (ixabepilone; BMS-247550), epothilone D (deoxyepothilone B, KOS-862), and a fully synthetic analog, sagopilone (ZK-EPO).[75]

Ixabepilone has been evaluated in several schedules using a cremophor-based formulation and is FDA approved for the treatment of patients with breast cancer.[75] It is active in breast cancer previously treated with paclitaxel or docetaxel. The principal toxicities observed include neutropenia and peripheral neuropathy,

in addition to fatigue, nausea, emesis, and diarrhea.[55,74] It also has been evaluated in other solid tumors such as ovarian, prostate, and renal cell carcinomas.[75] Epothilones are still undergoing evaluations in several clinical trials. Pharmacokinetic studies based on patupilone have shown large volume of distribution (41-fold the total body water) and low body clearance (13% of hepatic blood flow).[76] There do not appear to be active metabolites once the parent drug is hydrolyzed, which is the main elimination pathway.[76]

Maytansinoids and Auristatins: DM1, MMAE

Antibody drug conjugates (ADC) were first attempted with delivery of doxorubicin. Although tissue localization seemed promising, it became clear that the delivery of more potent chemotherapeutics was necessary.[77,78] One of the major advances for the promise of ADC came with the discovery and development of highly potent anticancer compounds such as calicheamicins, maytansinoids, and auristatins.[78] The next necessary advance was a linker that released the drug only when intended, and avoiding, or in some cases capitalizing on, in vivo proteases, oxidizing, or reducing environments. Gemtuzumab ozogamicin was the first ADC using calicheamicin, a potent DNA minor groove binder (and not a microtubule agent), approved in 2000 although withdrawn from the market in 2013 due to failed confirmatory studies. Maytansinoids and auristatins are unrelated, although are both tubulin-binding agents of the vinca binding site and inhibit tubulin polymerization.[78] They are 100- to 1,000-fold more cytotoxic that most cancer chemotherapeutics.[79]

Drug maytansinoid-1 (DM1) is the chemotherapeutic delivered using a thioether linker in the ADC ado-trastuzumab emtansine (T-DM1) that was FDA approved for patients with HER2- positive metastatic breast cancer previously treated with trastuzumab and taxane chemotherapy.[80,81] In the international phase III study, there was a 3.2-month improved progression-free survival among patients that received T-DM1 compared to those receiving standard treatment with capecitabine and lapatinib.[81] Despite a potent chemotherapeutic, the tolerability was much better in the experimental arm, which was dosed at 3.6 mg/kg intravenously every 21 days. The most common side effects in the trial were thrombocytopenia (12.8%), transient transaminitis (4.3%), as well as nausea, fatigue, myalgias, and arthralgias.[81]

Monomethyl auristatin E (MMAE) is linked to a monoclonal antibody against CD30 as an ADC (brentuximab vedotin, SGN35) and approved for refractory Hodgkin lymphoma or anaplastic large cell lymphoma. The linker is a peptide-based substrate for cathepsin-B and thereby designed to detect the lysosome/endosome compartment for drug release.[82,83] Dose-limiting toxicities include thrombocytopenia, hyperglycemia, diarrhea, and vomiting, and the most common side effects in this heavily pretreated population (including autologous stem cell transplant) includes peripheral neuropathy (42%), nausea (35%), and fatigue (34%).[84] The FDA black box warning includes contraindicated use with bleomycin due to increased pulmonary toxicity and the risk of John Cunningham (JC) virus–induced progressive multifocal leukoencephalopathy. Reports of severe pancreatitis are also emerging.[85]

MITOTIC MOTOR PROTEIN INHIBITORS

Aurora Kinase and Pololike Kinase Inhibitors

Aurora kinases are serine/threonine kinases crucial for mitosis in their recruitment of mitotic motor proteins for spindle formation. They are particularly overexpressed in high growth rate tumors. Aurora A and B kinases are expressed globally throughout all tissues, and Aurora C kinase is expressed in testes and participates in meiosis. Aurora A kinase is expressed and frequently amplified in many epithelial tumors and implicated in the microtubule-targeted agent-resistant phenotype.[86] Aurora A kinase interacts with p53, and there is evidence that p53 wild-type tumors are more sensitive to aurora A kinase inhibitors than p53 mutant tumors.[87] MLN-8237 has an IC_{50} of 1 nm for aurora A kinase and >200 nm for aurora B kinase and is in clinical development for treatment-related neuroendocrine prostate cancer.[86,88] The main dose-limiting toxicity of these agents is neutropenia. Pololike kinases (PLKs) are serine or threonine kinases crucial for cell cycle process. Overexpression of PLKs has been shown to be related to histologic grading and poor prognosis in several types of cancer. BI-2536 and ON01910 are PLK inhibitors in early clinical development.[89]

Kinesin Spindle Protein Inhibitor

Ispinesib

Kinesin spindle protein (KSP; also known as EG5) is a kinesin motor protein required to establish mitotic-spindle bipolarity.[90] Several KSP inhibitors have been evaluated in early phase clinical trials. SB-715992 (ispinesib) is a small-molecule inhibitor of KSP ATPase and has been evaluated in two different schedules.[89] The dose-limiting toxicity is neutropenia. Ispinesib was found to be inactive in phase 2 studies evaluating efficacy in patients with castration-resistant and largely docetaxel-resistant prostate cancer, advanced renal cancer, and head and neck cancer.[90–92]

MECHANISMS OF RESISTANCE TO MICROTUBULE INHIBITORS

Drug resistance is often complex and multifaceted and can involve diverse mechanisms such as (1) factors that reduce the ability of drugs to reach their cellular target (e.g., activation of detoxification pathways and decreased drug accumulation); (2) modifications in the drug target; and (3) events downstream of the target (e.g., decreased sensitivity to, or defective, apoptotic signals). Many tubulin binding agents are substrates for multidrug transporters such as P-glycoprotein and the multidrug resistance gene (MDR1).[93,94]

The MDR1-encoded gene product MDR1 (ABC subfamily B1; ABCB1) and MDR2 (ABC subfamily ABCB4) are the best-characterized ABC transporters thought to confer drug resistance to taxanes.[94,95] MDR-related taxane resistance can be reversed by many classes of drugs, including the calcium channel blockers, cyclosporin A, and antiarrhythmic agents.[94,95] However, the clinical utility of this approach has never been proven, despite several clinical trials. The role of ABC transporters in resistance to microtubule inhibitors remains to be determined.[96]

An increasing number of studies suggest that the expression of individual tubulin isotypes are altered in cells resistant to antimicrotubule drugs and may confer drug resistance.[93,97] Inherent differences in microtubule dynamics and drug interactions have been observed with some isotypes in vitro and in vivo.[98] Several taxane-resistant mutant cell lines that have structurally altered α- and β-tubulin proteins and an impaired ability to polymerize into microtubules have also been identified.[99] Mutations of tubulin isotype genes, gene amplifications, and isotype switching have also been reported in taxane-resistant cell lines.[99] In patients, levels of class III β-tubulin have been shown to correlate with response—those with high RNA levels have poor response—and immunohistochemical stains can correlate and may be predictive.[96,100,101] As opposed to taxanes, resistance to vinca alkaloids has been associated with decreased class II β-tubulin expression.[97,98]

MAPs are important structural and regulatory components of microtubules that act in concert to remodel the microtubule network by stabilizing or destabilizing microtubules during mitosis or cytokinesis. Alterations in the activity and/or balance of stabilizing or destabilizing MAPs can profoundly affect microtubule function.[99,102] The overexpression of stathmin, a destabilizing protein, has been reported to decrease sensitivity to paclitaxel and vinblastine.[1] An analysis of predictive or prognostic factors in a large phase 3 study (National Surgical Adjuvant Breast and Bowel Project NSABP-B 28) in patients with node-positive breast cancer showed that MAP-tau, a stabilizing protein, was a prognostic factor; however, it was not predictive for benefit from paclitaxel-based chemotherapy.[1,93] In a separate randomized controlled trial in breast cancer (TAX 307), where the only variable was docetaxel, MAP-tau was also shown to be prognostic, but not predictive of taxane benefit.[103]

Additional studies have shown a correlation with BRCA1 loss measured by gene or protein expression, or gene signatures, with resistance to taxane and sensitivity to DNA-damaging agents (such as cisplatin and anthracyclines).[104–107] BRCA1 is a tumor-suppressor gene with DNA damage response and repair, as well as cell cycle checkpoint activation, which explains why its loss leads to enhanced cisplatin sensitivity.[20] BRCA1 also indirectly regulates microtubule dynamics and stability and can favorably control how microtubules respond to paclitaxel treatment via their association with pro-caspase-8. The loss of BRCA1 can lead to impaired taxane-induced activation of apoptosis due to microtubules that are more dynamic and less susceptible to taxane-induced stabilization and proximity-induced activation of caspase-8 signaling.[20]

In addition to resistance, certain tumor subtypes may be sensitive to the taxane dosing schedule. In two randomized trials of low-dose, weekly paclitaxel, the luminal breast cancer subtype was found to have a better outcome compared with the control arm. This suggests that not only the drug, but also the schedule may influence the response to therapy and that genomic approaches may reveal these insights.[108]

REFERENCES

1. Kavallaris M. Microtubules and resistance to tubulin-binding agents. *Nat Rev Cancer* 2010;10:194–204.
2. Nogales E. Structural insights into microtubule function. *Ann Rev Biophys Biomol Struct* 2001;30:397–420.
3. Wani MC, Taylor HL, Wall ME, et al. Plant antitumor agents. VI. Isolation and structure of taxol, a novel antileukemic and antitumor agent from Taxus brevifolia. *J Am Chem Soc* 1971;93:2325–2327.
4. Rowinsky E, Donehower R. Antimicrotubule agents. In: DeVita VT, Hellmann S, Rosenberg SA, eds. *Cancer: Principles and Practice of Oncology.* 5th ed. Philadelphia: Lippincott-Raven;1997.
5. Vrignaud P, Sémiond D, Lejeune P, et al. Preclinical antitumor activity of cabazitaxel, a semisynthetic taxane active in taxane-resistant tumors. *Clin Cancer Res* 2013;19:2973–2983.
6. Sparano JA. Taxanes for breast cancer: an evidence-based review of randomized phase II and phase III trials. *Clin Breast Cancer* 2000;1:32–40.
7. Mamounas E, Leinbersky B, Bryant J, et al. Paclitaxel after doxorubicin plus cyclophosphamide as adjuvant chemotherapy for node-positive breast cancer: results from NSABP B-28. *J Clin Oncol* 2005;23:3686–3696.
8. Bonomi P, Kim KM, Fairclough D, et al. Comparison of survival and quality of life in advanced non-small-cell lung cancer patients treated with two dose levels of paclitaxel combined with cisplatin versus etoposide with cisplatin: results of an Eastern Cooperative Oncology Group trial. *J Clin Oncol* 2000;18:623–631.
9. Martin M, Pienkowski T, Mackey J, et al. Adjuvant docetaxel for node-positive breast cancer. *N Engl J Med* 2005;352:2302–2313.
10. Jones SE, Erban J, Overmoyer B, et al. Randomized phase III study of docetaxel compared with paclitaxel in metastatic breast cancer. *J Clin Oncol* 2005;23:5542–5551.
11. Tannock IF, de Wit R, Berry WR, et al. Docetaxel plus prednisone or mitoxantrone plus prednisone for advanced prostate cancer. *N Engl J Med* 2004;351:1502–1512.
12. Van Cutsem E, Moiseyenko V, Tjulandin S, et al. Phase III study of docetaxel and cisplatin plus fluorouracil compared with cisplatin and fluorouracil as first-line therapy for advanced gastric cancer: a report of the V325 Study Group. *J Clin Oncol* 2006;24:4991–4997.
13. Schiff PB, Fant J, Horwitz SB. Promotion of microtubule assembly in vitro by taxol. *Nature* 1979;277:665–667.

14. Nogales E. Structural insight into microtubule function. *Annu Rev Biophys Biomol Struct* 2001;30:397–420.

15. Darshan MS, Loftus MS, Thadani-Mulero M, et al. Taxane-induced blockade to nuclear accumulation of the androgen receptor predicts clinical responses in metastatic prostate cancer. *Cancer Res* 2011;71:6019–6029.

16. Hoimes CJ, Kelly WK. Redefining hormone resistance in prostate cancer. *Ther Adv Med Oncol* 2010;2:107–123.

17. LaPointe NE, Morfini G, Brady ST, et al. Effects of eribulin, vincristine, paclitaxel and ixabepilone on fast axonal transport and kinesin-1 driven microtubule gliding: Implications for chemotherapy-induced peripheral neuropathy. *Neurotoxicology* 2013;37:231–239.

18. Mielgo A, Torres VA, Clair K, et al. Paclitaxel promotes a caspase 8-mediated apoptosis through death effector domain association with microtubules. *Oncogene* 2009;28:3551–3562.

19. Komlodi-Pasztor E, Sackett D, Wilkerson J, et al. Mitosis is not a key target of microtubule agents in patient tumors. *Nat Rev Clin Oncol* 2011;8:244–250.

20. Sung M, Giannakakou P. BRCA1 regulates microtubule dynamics and taxane-induced apoptotic cell signaling. *Oncogene* 2014;33(11):1418–1428.

21. Strobel T, Kraeft SK, Chen LB, et al. BAX expression is associated with enhanced intracellular accumulation of paclitaxel: a novel role for BAX during chemotherapy-induced cell death. *Cancer Res* 1998;58:4776–4781.

22. Srivastava RK, Mi QS, Hardwick JM, et al. Deletion of the loop region of Bcl-2 completely blocks paclitaxel-induced apoptosis. *Proc Natl Acad Sci U S A* 1999;96:3775–3780.

23. Dai H, Ding H, Meng XW, et al. Contribution of Bcl-2 phosphorylation to Bak binding and drug resistance. *Cancer Res* 2013;73(23):6998–7008.

24. Oakes SR, Vaillant F, Lim E, et al. Sensitization of BCL-2–expressing breast tumors to chemotherapy by the BH3 mimetic ABT-737. *Proc Natl Acad Sci* 2012;109:2766–2771.

25. Chauhan VP, Stylianopoulos T, Martin JD, et al. Normalization of tumour blood vessels improves the delivery of nanomedicines in a size-dependent manner. *Nat Nanotechnol* 2012;7:383–388.

26. Gradishar W, Tjulandin S, Davidson N, et al. Phase III trial of nanoparticle albumin-bound paclitaxel compared with polyethylated castor oil-based paclitaxel in women with breast cancer. *J Clin Oncol* 2005;23:7794–7803.

27. Socinski MA, Bondarenko I, Karaseva NA, et al. Weekly nab-paclitaxel in combination with carboplatin versus solvent-based paclitaxel plus carboplatin as first-line therapy in patients with advanced non–small-cell lung cancer: final results of a Phase III trial. *J Clin Oncol* 2012;30:2055–2062.

28. Von Hoff DD, Ervin T, Arena FP, et al. Increased survival in pancreatic cancer with nab-paclitaxel plus gemcitabine. *N Engl J Med* 2013;369:1691–1703.

29. Sparreboom A, Scripture CD, Trieu V, et al. Comparative preclinical and clinical pharmacokinetics of a cremophor-free, nanoparticle albumin-bound paclitaxel (ABI-007) and paclitaxel formulated in cremophor (Taxol). *Clin Cancer Res* 2005;11:4136–4143.

30. Yardley DA. nab-Paclitaxel mechanisms of action and delivery. *J Control Release* 2013;170:365–372.

31. Desai N, Trieu V, Yao Z, et al. Increased antitumor activity, intratumor paclitaxel concentrations, and endothelial cell transport of cremophor-free, albumin-bound paclitaxel, ABI-007, compared with cremophor-based paclitaxel. *Clin Cancer Res* 2006;12:1317–1324.

32. Nyman DW, Campbell KJ, Hersh E, et al. Phase I and pharmacokinetics trial of ABI-007, a novel nanoparticle formulation of paclitaxel in patients with advanced nonhematologic malignancies. *J Clin Oncol* 2005;23:7785–7793.

33. Cheng CJ, Saltzman WM. Nanomedicine: downsizing tumour therapeutics. *Nat Nanotechnol* 2012;7:346–347.

34. Infante JR, Matsubayashi H, Sato N, et al. Peritumoral fibroblast SPARC expression and patient outcome with resectable pancreatic adenocarcinoma. *J Clin Oncol* 2007;25:319–325.

35. Kato Y, Nagashima Y, Baba Y, et al. Expression of SPARC in tongue carcinoma of stage II is associated with poor prognosis: an immunohistochemical study of 86 cases. *Int J Mol Med* 2005;16:263–268.

36. Lau CPY, Poon RTP, Cheung ST, et al. SPARC and Hevin expression correlate with tumour angiogenesis in hepatocellular carcinoma. *J Pathol* 2006;210:459–468.

37. Thomas R, True LD, Bassuk JA, et al. Differential expression of osteonectin/SPARC during human prostate cancer progression. *Clin Cancer Res* 2000;6:1140–1149.

38. Watkins G, Douglas-Jones A, Bryce R, et al. Increased levels of SPARC (osteonectin) in human breast cancer tissues and its association with clinical outcomes. *Prostaglandins Leukot Essent Fatty Acids* 2005;72:267–272.

39. Cheng CJ, Saltzman WM. Enhanced siRNA delivery into cells by exploiting the synergy between targeting ligands and cell-penetrating peptides. *Biomaterials* 2011;32:6194–6203.

40. Davis ME, Zuckerman JE, Choi CH, et al. Evidence of RNAi in humans from systemically administered siRNA via targeted nanoparticles. *Nature* 2010;464:1067–1070.

41. Von Hoff DD, Ramanathan RK, Borad MJ, et al. Gemcitabine Plus nab-paclitaxel is an active regimen in patients with advanced pancreatic cancer: a Phase I/II trial. *J Clin Oncol* 2011;29:4548–4554.

42. Mita A, Denis L, Rowinsky E, et al. Phase I and pharmacokinetic study of XRP6258 (RPR 116258A), a novel taxane, administered as a 1-hour infusion every 3 weeks in patients with advanced solid tumors. *Clin Cancer Res* 2009;15:723–730.

43. Diéras V, Lortholary A, Laurence V, et al. Cabazitaxel in patients with advanced solid tumours: results of a Phase I and pharmacokinetic study. *Eur J Cancer* 2013;49:25–34.

44. Mita AC, Denis LJ, Rowinsky EK, et al. Phase I and pharmacokinetic study of XRP6258 (RPR 116258A), a novel taxane, administered as a 1-hour infusion every 3 weeks in patients with advanced solid tumors. *Clin Cancer Res* 2009;15:723–730.

45. Yared JA, Tkaczuk KH. Update on taxane development: new analogs and new formulations. *Drug Des Devel Ther* 2012;6:371–384.

46. Baas P, Szczesna A, Albert I, et al. Phase I/II study of a 3 weekly oral taxane (DJ-927) in patients with recurrent, advanced non-small cell lung cancer. *J Thorac Oncol* 2008;3:745–750.

47. Vigano L, Locatelli A, Grasselli G, et al. Drug interactions of paclitaxel and docetaxel and their relevance for the design of combination therapy. *Invest New Drugs* 2001;19:179–196.

48. Kudlowitz D, Muggia F. Defining risks of taxane neuropathy: insights from randomized clinical trials. *Clin Cancer Res* 2013;19:4570–4577.

49. Henningsson A, Karlsson MO, Viganò L, et al. Mechanism-based pharmacokinetic model for paclitaxel. *J Clin Oncol* 2001;19:4065–4073.

50. Sissung T, Mross K, Steinberg S, et al. Association of ABCB1 genotypes with paclitaxel-mediated peripheral neuropathy and neutropenia. *Eur J Cancer* 2006;42:2893–2896.

51. Marsh S, Paul J, King C, et al. Pharmacogenetic assessment of toxicity and outcome after platinum plus taxane chemotherapy in ovarian cancer: the Scottish Randomised Trial in Ovarian Cancer. *J Clin Oncol* 2007;25:4528–4535.

52. Baldwin RM, Owzar K, Zembutsu H, et al. A genome-wide association study identifies novel loci for paclitaxel-induced sensory peripheral neuropathy in CALGB 40101. *Clin Cancer Res* 2012;18:5099–5109.

53. Rugo H, Barry W, Moreno Aspitia A, et al. CALGB 40502/NCCTG N063H: Randomized phase III trial of weekly paclitaxel (P) compared to weekly nanoparticle albumin bound nab-paclitaxel (NP) or ixabepilone (Ix) with or without bevacizumab (B) as first-line therapy for locally recurrent or metastatic breast cancer (MBC). *J Clin Oncol* 2012;30.

54. Baker J, Ajani J, Scotté F, et al. Docetaxel-related side effects and their management. *Eur J Oncol Nurs* 2009;13:49–59.

55. Lee J, Swain S. Peripheral neuropathy induced by microtubule-stabilizing agents. *J Clin Oncol* 2006;24:1633–1642.

56. Alsamarai S, Charpidou AG, Matthay RA, et al. Pneumonitis related to docetaxel: case report and review of the literature. *In Vivo* 2009;23:635–637.

57. Dumitra S, Sideris L, Leclerc Y, et al. Neutropenic enterocolitis and docetaxel neoadjuvant chemotherapy. *Ann Oncol* 2009;20:795–796.

58. de Bono JS, Oudard S, Ozguroglu M, et al. Prednisone plus cabazitaxel or mitoxantrone for metastatic castration-resistant prostate cancer progressing after docetaxel treatment: a randomised open-label trial. *Lancet* 2010;376:1147–1154.

59. Zhou XJ, Placidi M, Rahmani R. Uptake and metabolism of vinca alkaloids by freshly isolated human hepatocytes in suspension. *Anticancer Res* 1994;14:1017–1022.

60. Zhou J, Giannakakou P. Targeting microtubules for cancer chemotherapy. *Curr Med Chem Anticancer Agents* 2005;5:65–71.

61. Jordan MA, Wilson L. Microtubules as a target for anticancer drugs. *Nat Rev Cancer* 2004;4:253–265.

62. Bender RA, Castle MC, Margileth DA, et al. The pharmacokinetics of [3H]-vincristine in man. *Clin Pharmacol Ther* 1977;22:430–435.

63. Zhou XJ, Martin M, Placidi M, et al. In-vivo and in-vitro pharmacokinetics and metabolism of vinca alkaloids in rat. II. Vinblastine and vincristine. *Eur J Drug Metab Pharmacokinet* 1990;15:323–332.

64. Rowinsky EK, Noe DA, Trump DL, et al. Pharmacokinetic, bioavailability, and feasibility study of oral vinorelbine in patients with solid tumors. *J Clin Oncol* 1994;12:1754–1763.

65. Fumoleau P, Guiu S. New vinca alkaloids in clinical development. *Curr Breast Cancer Rep* 2013;5:69–72.

66. Chan JD. Pharmacokinetic drug interactions of vinca alkaloids: summary of case reports. *Pharmacotherapy* 1998;18:1304–1307.

67. Tobe SW, Siu LL, Jamal SA, et al. Vinblastine and erythromycin: an unrecognized serious drug interaction. *Cancer Chemother Pharmacol* 1995;35:188–190.

68. Peltier A, Russell J. Recent advances in drug-induced neuropathies. *Curr Opin Neurol* 2002;15:633–638.

69. Quasthoff S, Hartung H. Chemotherapy-induced peripheral neuropathy. *J Neurol* 2002;249:9–17.

70. Lobert S, Vulevic B, Correia JJ. Interaction of vinca alkaloids with tubulin: a comparison of vinblastine, vincristine, and vinorelbine. *Biochemistry* 1996;35:6806–6814.

71. Schrijvers DL. Extravasation: a dreaded complication of chemotherapy. *Ann Oncol* 2003;14:iii26–iii30.

72. Petrylak D, Hussain MHA, Tangen C, et al. Docetaxel and estramustine compared with mitoxantrone and prednisone for advanced refractory prostate cancer. *N Engl J Med* 2004;351:1513–1520.

73. Tannock IF, de Wit R, Berry WR, et al. Docetaxel plus prednisone or mitoxantrone plus prednisone for advanced prostate cancer. *N Engl J Med* 2004;351:1502–1512.

74. Lee JJ, Kelly WK. Epothilones: tubulin polymerization as a novel target for prostate cancer therapy. *Nat Clin Pract Oncol* 2009;6:85–92.

75. Kelly WK. Epothilones in prostate cancer. *Urol Oncol* 2011;29:358–365.

76. Kelly K, Zollinger M, Lozac'h F, et al. Metabolism of patupilone in patients with advanced solid tumor malignancies. *Invest New Drugs* 2013;31:605–615.

77. Trail PA, Willner D, Lasch SJ, et al. Cure of xenografted human carcinomas by BR96-doxorubicin immunoconjugates. *Science* 1993;261:212–215.

78. Carter PJ, Senter PD. Antibody-drug conjugates for cancer therapy. *Cancer J* 2008;14:154–169.

79. Doronina SO, Toki BE, Torgov MY, et al. Development of potent monoclonal antibody auristatin conjugates for cancer therapy. *Nat Biotechnol* 2003;21:778–784.

80. Lewis Phillips GD, Li G, Dugger DL, et al. Targeting HER2-positive breast cancer with trastuzumab-DM1, an antibody–cytotoxic drug conjugate. *Cancer Res* 2008;68:9280–9290.

81. Verma S, Miles D, Gianni L, et al. Trastuzumab emtansine for HER2-positive advanced breast cancer. *N Engl J Med* 2012;367:1783–1791.

82. Okeley NM, Miyamoto JB, Zhang X, et al. Intracellular activation of SGN-35, a potent anti-CD30 antibody-drug conjugate. *Clin Cancer Res* 2010;16:888–897.

83. Younes A, Bartlett NL, Leonard JP, et al. Brentuximab vedotin (SGN-35) for relapsed CD30-positive lymphomas. *N Engl J Med* 2010;363:1812–1821.

84. Younes A. Brentuximab vedotin for the treatment of patients with Hodgkin lymphoma. *Hematol Oncol Clin North Am* 2014;28:27–32.

85. Gandhi M, Evens AM, Fenske TS, et al. Pancreatitis in patients treated with brentuximab vedotin: a previously unrecognized serious adverse event. *Blood* 2013;122:4380.

86. Mosquera JM, Beltran H, Park K, et al. Concurrent AURKA and MYCN gene amplifications are harbingers of lethal treatment-related neuroendocrine prostate cancer. *Neoplasia* 2013;15:1–10.

87. Ujhazy P, Stewart D. DNA Repair. *J Thorac Oncol* 2009;4:S1068–S1070.

88. Green MR, Woolery JE, Mahadevan D. Update on aurora kinase targeted therapeutics in oncology. *Expert Opin Drug Discov* 2011;6:291–307.

89. Jackson JR, Patrick DR, Dar MM, et al. Targeted anti-mitotic therapies: can we improve on tubulin agents? *Nat Rev Cancer* 2007;7:107–117.

90. Tang PA, Siu LL, Chen EX, et al. Phase II study of ispinesib in recurrent or metastatic squamous cell carcinoma of the head and neck. *Invest New Drugs* 2008;26:257–264.

91. Beer TM, Goldman B, Synold TW, et al. Southwest oncology group phase II study of ispinesib in androgen-independent prostate cancer previously treated with taxanes. *Clin Genitourin Cancer* 2008;6:103–109.

92. Lee RT, Beekman KE, Hussain M, et al. A university of chicago consortium phase II trial of SB-715992 in advanced renal cell cancer. *Clin Genitourin Cancer* 2008;6:21–24.

93. Perez EA. Microtubule inhibitors: differentiating tubulin-inhibiting agents based on mechanisms of action, clinical activity, and resistance. *Mol Cancer Ther* 2009;8:2086–2095.

94. Gottesman MM, Fojo T, Bates SE. Multidrug resistance in cancer: role of ATP-dependent transporters. *Nat Rev Cancer* 2002;2:48–58.

95. Fojo AT, Menefee M. Microtubule targeting agents: basic mechanisms of multidrug resistance (MDR). *Semin Oncol* 2005;32:S3–S8.

96. Mozzetti S, Ferlini C, Concolino P, et al. Class III beta-tubulin overexpression is a prominent mechanism of paclitaxel resistance in ovarian cancer patients. *Clin Cancer Res* 2005;11:298–305.

97. Drukman S, Kavallaris M. Microtubule alterations and resistance to tubulin-binding agents (review). *Int J Oncol* 2002;21:621–628.

98. Verrills NM, Kavallaris M. Improving the targeting of tubulin-binding agents: lessons from drug resistance studies. *Curr Pharm Des* 2005;11:1719–1733.

99. Orr GA, Verdier-Pinard P, McDaid H, et al. Mechanisms of Taxol resistance related to microtubules. *Oncogene* 2003;22:7280–7295.

100. Monzó M, Rosell R, Sánchez JJ, et al. Paclitaxel resistance in non-small-cell lung cancer associated with beta-tubulin gene mutations. *J Clin Oncol* 1999;17:1786–1793.

101. Seve P, Mackey J, Isaac S, et al. Class III beta-tubulin expression in tumor cells predicts response and outcome in patients with non-small cell lung cancer receiving paclitaxel. *Mol Cancer Ther* 2005;4:2001–2007.

102. Baquero MT, Hanna JA, Neumeister V, et al. Stathmin expression and its relationship to microtubule-associated protein tau and outcome in breast cancer. *Cancer* 2012;118:4660–4669.

103. Baquero MT, Lostritto K, Gustavson MD, et al. Evaluation of prognostic and predictive value of microtubule associated protein tau in two independent cohorts. *Breast Cancer Res* 2011;13(5):R85.

104. Quinn JE, James CR, Stewart GE, et al. BRCA1 mRNA expression levels predict for overall survival in ovarian cancer after chemotherapy. *Clin Cancer Res* 2007;13:7413–7420.

105. Byrski T, Gronwald J, Huzarski T, et al. Response to neo-adjuvant chemotherapy in women with BRCA1-positive breast cancers. *Breast Cancer Res Treat* 2008;108:289–296.

106. Font A, Taron M, Gago JL, et al. BRCA1 mRNA expression and outcome to neoadjuvant cisplatin-based chemotherapy in bladder cancer. *Ann Oncol* 2011;22:139–144.

107. Reguart N, Cardona AF, Carrasco E, et al. BRCA1: a new genomic marker for non-small-cell lung cancer. *Clin Lung Cancer* 2008;9:331–339.

108. Martin M, Prat A, Rodriguez-Lescure A, et al. PAM50 proliferation score as a predictor of weekly paclitaxel benefit in breast cancer. *Breast Cancer Res Treat* 2013;138:457–466.

22 Kinase Inhibitors as Anticancer Drugs

Charles L. Sawyers

INTRODUCTION

In 2001, the first tyrosine-kinase inhibitor imatinib was approved for clinical use in chronic myeloid leukemia. The spectacular success of this first-in-class agent ushered in a transformation in cancer drug discovery from efforts that were largely based on novel cytotoxic chemotherapy agents to an almost exclusive focus on molecularly targeted agents across the pharmaceutical and biotechnology industry and academia. This chapter summarizes this remarkable progress in this field over ~15 years, with the focus on the concepts underlying this paradigm shift as well as the considerable challenges that remain (Table 22.1). Readers in search of more specific details on individual drugs and their indications should consult the relevant disease-specific chapters elsewhere in this volume as well as references cited within this chapter. Readers should also note that the epidermal growth factor receptor (EGFR) and human epidermal growth factor receptor 2 (HER2) receptor tyrosine kinases covered here have also been successfully targeted by monoclonal antibodies that engage these proteins at the cell surface. These drugs, referred to as biologics rather than small molecule inhibitors, are covered in other chapters. The chapter is organized around kinase targets rather than diseases and, intentionally, has a historical flow to make certain thematic points and to illustrate the broad lessons that have been and continue to be learned through the clinical development of these exciting agents.

Perhaps the most stunning discovery from the clinical trials of the Abelson murine leukemia (ABL) kinase inhibitor imatinib was the recognition that tumor cells acquire exquisite dependence on the breakpoint cluster region protein BCR-ABL fusion oncogene, created by the Philadelphia chromosome translocation.[1] Although this may seem intuitive at first glance, consider the fact that the translocation arises in an otherwise normal hematopoietic stem cell, the survival of which is regulated by a complex array of growth factors and interactions with the bone marrow microenvironment. Although BCR-ABL clearly gives this cell a growth advantage that, over years, results in the clinical phenotype of chronic myeloid leukemia, there was no reason to expect that these cells would depend on BCR-ABL for their survival when confronted with an inhibitor. In the absence of BCR-ABL, these tumor cells could presumably rely on the marrow microenvironment, just like their normal, nontransformed neighbors. Thus, it seemed more likely that, by shutting down the driver oncogene, BCR-ABL inhibitors might halt the progression of chronic myeloid leukemia but not eliminate the preexisting tumor cells. In fact, chronic myeloid leukemia (CML) progenitors are eliminated after just a few months of anti–BCR-ABL therapy, indicating they are dependent on the driver oncogene for their survival and have "forgotten" how to return to normal. This phenomenon, subsequently documented in a variety of human malignancies, is colloquially termed *oncogene addiction*.[2] Although the molecular basis for this addiction still remains to be defined, the notion of finding an Achilles' heel for each cancer continues to captivate the cancer research community and has spawned a broad array of efforts to elucidate the molecular identity of these targets and discover relevant inhibitors.

EARLY SUCCESSES: TARGETING CANCERS WITH WELL-KNOWN KINASE MUTATIONS (BCR-ABL, KIT, HER2)

From the beginning, clinical trials of imatinib were restricted to patients with Philadelphia chromosome–positive chronic myeloid leukemia. For what seem like obvious reasons, there was never any serious discussion about treating patients with Philadelphia chromosome–negative leukemia because the assumption was that only patients with the BCR-ABL fusion gene would have a chance of responding. This was clearly a wise decision because hematologic response rates approached 90% and cytogenetic remissions were seen in nearly half of the patients in the early phase studies.[3] It was obvious that the drug worked, and imatinib was approved in record time. Unwittingly, the power of genome-based patient selection was demonstrated in the clinical development of the very first kinase inhibitor. As we will see, it took nearly a decade for this lesson to be fully learned. Today, the much larger clinical experience, with an array of different kinase inhibitors across many tumor types, has led to a much better understanding of the principles that dictate oncogene addiction that, in retrospect, were staring us in the face. Foremost among them is the notion that tumors with a somatic mutation or amplification of a kinase drug target are much more likely to be dependent on that target for survival. Hence, a patient whose tumor has such a mutation is much more likely to respond to treatment with the appropriate inhibitor. This has also led to a new paradigm at the regulatory level of drug approval requiring codevelopment of a *companion diagnostic* (a molecularly based diagnostic test that reliably identifies patients with the mutation) with the new drug.

After chronic myeloid leukemia, the next example to illustrate this principle was gastrointestinal stromal tumor (GIST), which is associated with mutations in the KIT tyrosine-kinase receptor or, more rarely, in the platelet-derived growth factor (PDGF) receptor.[4,5] Serendipitously, imatinib inhibits both KIT and the PDGF receptor; therefore, the clinical test of KIT inhibition in GIST followed quickly on the heels of the success in CML.[6] In retrospect, the rapid progress made in these two diseases was based, in part, on the fact that the driver molecular lesion (BCR-ABL or KIT mutation, respectively) is present in nearly all patients who are diagnosed with these two diseases. The molecular analysis merely confirmed the diagnosis that was made using standard clinical and histologic criteria. Consequently, clinicians could identify the patients most likely to respond based on clinical criteria rather than rely on an elaborate molecular profiling infrastructure to prescreen patients. Consequently, clinical trials evaluating kinase inhibitors in CML and GIST accrued quickly, and the therapeutic benefit became clear almost immediately.

The notion that molecular alteration of a driver kinase determines sensitivity to a cognate kinase inhibitor was further validated during the development of the dual EGFR/HER2 kinase inhibitor lapatinib. Clinical trials of this kinase inhibitor were conducted in women with advanced HER2-positive breast cancer based on earlier success in these same patients with the monoclonal antibody trastuzumab, which targets the extracellular domain of the HER2

TABLE 22.1

Kinase Inhibitors: Approved or Anticipated Approval In 2014

Target	Drug	Approved Indications	Anticipated Future Indications
ALK	Crizotinib Ceritinib	ALK mutant lung cancer	ALK mutant neuroblastoma, anaplastic lymphoma
BCR-ABL	Imatinib Dasatinib Nilotinib Bosutinib Ponatinib	Chronic myeloid leukemia Philadelphia chromosome–positive acute lymphoid leukemia T315 mutation only (ponatinib)	
BRAF	Vemurafenib Dabrafenib	BRAF mutant melanoma	Other BRAF mutant tumors
BTK	Ibrutinib	Chronic lymphocytic leukemia Mantle cell lymphoma	
EGFR	Gefitinib Erlotinib Afatinib	Lung adenocarcinoma with EGFR mutation	
HER2	Lapatinib	Her2$^+$ breast cancer	
JAK2	Ruxolitinib	JAK2 mutant myelofibrosis	
KIT	Imatinib Sunitinib	Gastrointestinal stromal tumor	
MEK	Trametinib	BRAF mutant melanoma	
PI3K delta[a]	Idelalisib	Chronic lymphocytic leukemia Indolent non-Hodgkin lymphoma	
PDGFR- α/β	Imatinib	Chronic myelomonocytic leukemia (with TEL-PDGFR-β fusion) hypereosinophilic syndrome (with PDGFR-β fusion) Dermatofibrosarcoma protuberans	
RET	Vandetanib Sorafenib Cabozantinib	Medullary thyroid cancer	
TORC1	Sirolimus (rapamycin)	Kidney cancer	
(mTOR)	Everolimus Temsirolimus	Breast cancer Tuberous sclerosis	
VEGF Receptor	Sorafenib Sunitinib Axitinib Pazopanib	Kidney cancer Hepatocellular carcinoma (sorafenib only) Pancreatic neuroendocrine tumors (sunitinib)	

[a] Approval is anticipated based on positive phase 3 data and announcement of accepted Food and Drug Administration submission by the sponsor.

kinase. Lapatinib was initially approved in combination with the cytotoxic agent capecitabine for women with resistance to trastuzumab,[7] and then was subsequently approved for frontline use in metastatic breast cancer in combination with chemotherapy or hormonal therapy, depending on estrogen receptor status. A key ingredient that enabled the clinical development of lapatinib was the routine use of HER2 gene amplification testing in the diagnosis of breast cancer, pioneered during the development of trastuzumab several years earlier. This widespread clinical practice allowed for the rapid identification of those patients most likely to benefit. If lapatinib trials had been conducted in unselected patients, the clinical signal in breast cancer would likely have been missed.

The Serendipity of Unexpected Clinical Responses: EGFR in Lung Cancer

In contrast to the logical development of imatinib and lapatinib in molecularly defined patient populations, the EGFR kinase inhibitors gefitinib and erlotinib entered the clinic without the benefit of such a focused clinical development plan. Although considerable preclinical data implicated EGFR as a cancer drug target, there was little insight into which patients were most likely to benefit. The first clue that EGFR inhibitors would have a role in lung cancer came from the recognition by several astute clinicians of remarkable responses in a small fraction of patients with lung adenocarcinoma.[8] Further studies revealed the curious clinical circumstance that those patients most likely to benefit tended to be those who never smoked, women, and those of Asian ethnicity.[9] Clearly, there was a strong clinical signal in a subgroup of patients, who could perhaps be enriched based on these clinical features, but it seemed that a unifying molecular lesion must be present. Three academic groups simultaneously converged on the answer. Mutations in the EGFR gene were detected in the 10% to 15% of patients with lung adenocarcinoma who had radiographic responses.[10–12] It may seem surprising that mutations in a gene as highly visible as EGFR and in such a prevalent cancer had not been detected earlier. But the motivation to search aggressively for EGFR mutations was not there until the clinical responses were seen. Perhaps even more surprising was the failure of the pharmaceutical company sponsors of the two most advanced compounds, gefitinib and erlotinib, to embrace this important discovery and refocus future clinical development plans on patients with EGFR mutant lung adenocarcinoma.

But that was 2004, when the prevailing approach to cancer drug development was an empiric one originally developed (with great success) for cytotoxic agents. Typically, small numbers of patients with different cancers were treated in *all comer* phase I studies (no enrichment for subgroups) with the goal of eliciting a clinical signal in at least one tumor type. A single-agent response rate of 20% to 30% in a disease-specific phase II trial would justify a randomized phase III registration trial, where the typical endpoint for drug approval is time to progression or survival. Cytotoxics were also typically evaluated in combination with existing standard of care treatment (typically approved chemotherapy agents) with the goal of increasing the response rate or enhancing the duration of response. (Note: The use of the past tense here is intentional. As we will see later in this chapter, nearly all cancer drug development today is based on selecting patients with a certain molecular profile.)

The clinical development of gefitinib and erlotinib followed the cytotoxic model. Both drugs had similarly low but convincing single-agent response rates (10% to 15%) in chemotherapy-refractory, advanced lung cancer. Indeed, gefitinib was originally granted accelerated approval by the U.S. Food and Drug Administration (FDA) in 2003 based on the impressive nature of these responses, contingent on the completion of formal phase III studies with survival endpoints.[13] The sponsors of both drugs, therefore, conducted phase III registration studies in patients with chemotherapy-refractory, advanced stage lung cancer but without prescreening patients for EGFR mutation status. (In fairness, these trials were initiated prior to the discovery of EGFR mutations in lung cancer but study amendments could have been considered.) Erlotinib was approved in 2004 on the basis of a modest survival advantage over placebo (the BR.21 trial); however, gefitinib failed to demonstrate a survival advantage in essentially the same patient population.[14,15] This difference in outcome was surprising because the two drugs have highly similar chemical structures and biologic properties. Perhaps the most important difference was drug dose. Erlotinib was given at the maximum tolerated dose, which produces a high frequency of rash and diarrhea. Both side effects are presumed *on target* consequences of EGFR inhibition because EGFR is highly expressed in skin and gastrointestinal epithelial cells. In contrast, gefitinib was dosed slightly lower to mitigate these toxicities, with the rationale that responses were clearly documented at lower doses.

In parallel with the single-agent phase III trials in chemotherapy-refractory patients, both gefitinib and erlotinib were studied as an upfront therapy for advanced lung cancer to determine if either would improve the efficacy of standard *doublet* (carboplatin/paclitaxel or gemcitabine/cisplatin) chemotherapy when all three drugs were given in combination. These trials, termed INTACT-1 and INTACT-2 (gefitinib with either gemcitabine/cisplatin or with carboplatin/paclitaxel) and TRIBUTE (erlotinib with carboplatin/paclitaxel), collectively enrolled over 3,000 patients.[16–18] Excitement in the oncology community was high based on the clear single-agent activity of both EGFR inhibitors. But, both trials were spectacular failures; neither drug showed any benefit over chemotherapy alone. The fact that EGFR mutations are present in only 10% to 15% of patients (i.e., those likely to benefit) provided a logical explanation. The clinical signal from those whose tumors had EGFR mutations was likely diluted out by all the patients whose tumors had no EGFR alterations, many of whom benefited from chemotherapy.

The convergence of the EGFR mutation discovery with these clinical trial results will be remembered as a remarkable time in the history of targeted cancer therapies, not just for the important role of these agents as lung cancer therapies, but also for missteps in deciding that the EGFR genotype should drive treatment selection. Perhaps the most egregious error came from a retrospective

analysis of tumors from patients treated on the BR.21 trial, which concluded that EGFR mutations did *not* predict for a survival advantage.[19] (EGFR gene amplification *was* associated with survival, but only in a univariate analysis.) This conclusion was concerning because less than 30% of patients on the trial had tissue available for EGFR mutation analysis, raising questions about the adequacy of the sample size. Furthermore, the EGFR mutation assay used by the authors was subsequently criticized because a significant number of the EGFR mutations reported in these patients were in residues not previously found by others, who had sequenced thousands of tumors. Many of these mutations were suspected to be an artifact of working from formalin-fixed biopsies. Fortunately, recent advances in DNA mutation detection, using massively parallel next-generation sequencing technology, have largely eliminated this concern. These new platforms are now being used in the clinical setting.

Clinical investigators in Asia, where a greater fraction of lung cancers (roughly 30%) are positive for EGFR mutations, addressed the question of whether mutations predict for clinical benefit in a prospective trial. In this study known as IPASS, gefitinib was clearly superior to standard doublet chemotherapy as frontline therapy for patients with advanced EGFR mutation–positive lung adenocarcinoma.[20] Conversely, EGFR mutation–negative patients fared much worse with gefitinib and benefited from chemotherapy. In addition, EGFR mutation–positive patients had a more favorable overall prognosis regardless of treatment, indicating that EGFR mutation is also a prognostic biomarker. The IPASS trial serves as a compelling example of a properly designed (and executed) biomarker-driven clinical trial. Although the rationale for this clinical development strategy had been demonstrated years earlier with BCR-ABL in leukemia, KIT in GIST, and HER2 in breast cancer, it was difficult to derail the empiric approach that had been used for decades in developing cytotoxic agents.

A Mix of Science and Serendipity: PDGF Receptor–Driven Leukemias and Sarcoma

The discovery of EGFR mutations in lung cancer (motivated by dramatic clinical responses in a subset of patients treated with EGFR kinase inhibitors) is the most visible example of the power of bedside-to-bench science, but it is not the only (or the first) such example from the kinase inhibitor era. Shortly after the approval of imatinib for CML in 2001, two case reports documented dramatic remissions in patients with hypereosinophilic syndrome (HES), a blood disorder characterized by prolonged elevation of eosinophil counts and subsequent organ dysfunction from eosinophil infiltration, when treated with imatinib.[21,22] Although HES resembles myeloproliferative diseases such as CML, the molecular pathogenesis of HES was completely unknown at the time. Reasoning that these clinical responses must be explained by inhibition of a driver kinase, a team of laboratory-based physician/scientists quickly searched for mutations in the three kinases known to be inhibited by imatinib (ABL, KIT, and PDGF receptor). ABL and KIT were quickly excluded, but the PDGF receptor α (PDGFR-α) gene was targeted by an interstitial deletion that fused the upstream FIP1L1 gene to PDGFR-α[23] FIP1L1-PDGFR-α is a constitutively active tyrosine kinase, analogous to BCR-ABL, and is also inhibited by imatinib. As with EGFR-mutant lung cancer, the molecular pathophysiology of HES was discovered by dissecting the mechanism of response to the drug used to treat it.

The HES/FIP1L1-PDGFR-α story serves as a nice bookend to an earlier discovery that the t(5,12) chromosome translocation, found rarely in patients with chronic myelomonocytic leukemia, creates the TEL-PDGFR-β fusion tyrosine kinase.[24] Similar to HES, treatment of patients with t(5,12) translocation-positive leukemias with imatinib has also proven successful.[25] A third example comes from dermatofibrosarcoma protuberans, a sarcoma characterized by a t(17,22) translocation that fuses the COL1A gene to the PDGFB *ligand* (not the receptor). COL1A-PDGFB is oncogenic through autocrine stimulation of the normal PDGF receptor in these tumor cells. Patients with dermatofibrosarcoma protuberans respond to imatinib therapy because it targets the PDGF receptor, just one step downstream from the oncogenic lesion.[26]

Exploiting the New Paradigm: Searching for Other Kinase-Driven Cancers

The benefits of serendipity notwithstanding, the growing number of examples of successful kinase inhibitor therapy in tumors with a mutation or amplification of the drug target begged for a more rational approach to drug discovery and development. In 2002, the list of human tumors known to have mutations in kinases was quite small. Due to advances in automated gene sequencing, it became possible to ask whether a much larger fraction of human cancers might also have such mutations through a brute force approach. To address this question comprehensively, one would have to sequence all of the kinases in the genome in hundreds of samples of each tumor type. Several early pilot studies demonstrated the potential of this approach by revealing important new targets for drug development. Perhaps the most spectacular was the discovery of mutations in the BRAF kinase in over half of patients with melanoma, as well as in a smaller fraction of colon and thyroid cancers.[27] Another was the discovery of mutations in the JAK2 kinase in nearly all patients with polycythemia vera, as well as a significant fraction of patients with myelofibrosis and essential thrombocytosis.[28–30] A third example was the identification of PIK3CA mutations in a variety of tumors, with the greatest frequencies in breast, endometrial, and colorectal cancers.[31] PIK3CA encodes a lipid kinase that generates the second messenger phosphatidyl inositol 3-phosphate (PIP3). PIP3 activates growth and survival signaling through the AKT family of kinases as well as other downstream effectors. Coupled with the well-established role of the phosphatase and tensin homolog (PTEN) lipid phosphatase in dephosphorylating PIP3, the discovery of PIK3CA mutations focused tremendous attention on developing inhibitors at multiple levels of this pathway, as discussed further in the follow paragraphs.

Each of these important discoveries—BRAF, JAK2, and PIK3CA—came from relatively small efforts (less than 100 tumors) and generally focused on resequencing only those exons that coded for regions of kinases where mutations had been found in other kinases (typically, the juxtamembrane and kinase domains). These restricted searches were largely driven by the high cost of DNA sequencing using the Sanger method. In 2006, a comprehensive effort to sequence all of the exons in all kinases in 100 tumors could easily exceed several million dollars. Financial support for such projects could not be obtained easily through traditional funding agencies because the risk/reward was considered too high. Furthermore, substantial infrastructure for sample acquisition, microdissection of the tumors from normal tissue, nucleic acid preparation, high throughput automated sequencing, and computational analysis of the resulting data was essential. Few institutions were equipped to address these challenges. In response, the National Cancer Institute in the United States (in partnership with the National Human Genome Research Institute) and an international group known as the International Cancer Genome Consortium (ICGC) launched large-scale efforts to sequence the complete genomes of thousands of cancers. In parallel, next-generation sequencing technologies resulted in massive reductions in cost, allowing a more comprehensive analysis of much larger numbers of tumors. At the time of this writing, the US effort (called The Cancer Genome Atlas [TCGA]) had reported data on 29 different tumor types (https://tcga-data.nci.nih.gov/tcga/). The international consortium has committed to sequencing 25,000 tumors representing 50 different cancer subtypes.[32] Both groups have enforced immediate release of all sequence information to the research community free of charge so that the entire scientific community can learn from the data. This policy enabled *pan cancer* mutational analyses that give an overall view of the genomic landscape of cancer, serving as a blueprint for the community of cancer researchers and drug developers.[33,34]

Rounding Out the Treatment of Myeloproliferative Disorders: JAK2 and Myelofibrosis

Taken together with the BCR-ABL translocation in CML and FIP1L1-PDGFR-α in HES, the discovery of JAK2 mutations in polycythemia, essential thrombocytosis, and myelofibrosis provided a unifying understanding of myeloproliferative disorders as diseases of abnormal kinase activation. The JAK family kinases are the primary effectors of signaling through inflammatory cytokine receptors and, therefore, had been considered compelling targets for anti-inflammatory drugs. But the JAK2 mutation discovery immediately shifted these efforts toward developing JAK2 inhibitors for myeloproliferative disorders. Because most patients have a common JAK2 V617F mutation, these efforts could rapidly focus on screening for activity against a single genotype. Progress has been rapid. Myelofibrosis was selected as the initial indication (instead of essential thrombocytosis or polycythemia vera) because the time to registration is expected to be the shortest. Currently, ruxolitinib is approved for myelofibrosis based on shrinkage in spleen size as the primary endpoint. Clinical trials in essential thrombocytosis and polycythemia vera (versus hydroxyurea) are ongoing. Other JAK2 inhibitors are also in clinical development.

BRAF Mutant Melanoma: Several Missteps Before Finding the Right Inhibitor

As with JAK2 mutations in myeloproliferative disorders, the discovery of BRAF mutations in patients with melanoma launched widespread efforts to find potent BRAF inhibitors. One early candidate was the drug sorafenib, which had been optimized during drug discovery to inhibit RAF kinases. (Sorafenib also inhibits vascular endothelial growth factor (VEGF) receptors, which led to its approval in kidney cancer, as discussed later in this chapter.) Despite the compelling molecular rationale for targeting BRAF, clinical results of sorafenib in melanoma were extremely disappointing and reduced enthusiasm for pursuing BRAF as a drug target.[35] In hindsight, this concern was completely misguided. Sorafenib dosing is limited by toxicities that preclude achieving serum levels in patients that potently inhibit RAF, but are sufficient to inhibit VEGF receptors. In addition, patients were enrolled without screening for BRAF mutations in their tumors. Although the frequency of BRAF mutations in melanoma is high, the inclusion of patients without the BRAF mutation diluted the chance of seeing any clinical signal. In short, the clinical evaluation of sorafenib in melanoma was poorly designed to test the hypothesis that BRAF is a therapeutic target. The danger is that negative data from such clinical experiments can slow subsequent progress. It is critical to know the pharmacodynamic properties of the drug and the molecular phenotype of the patients being studied when interpreting the results of a negative study.

The fact that RAF kinases are intermediate components of the well-characterized RAS/ mitogen-activated protein (MAP) kinase pathway (transducing signals from RAS to RAF to MEK to ERK) raised the possibility that tumors with BRAF mutations might respond to inhibitors of one of these downstream kinases (Fig. 22.1). Preclinical studies revealed that tumor cell lines with BRAF mutation were exquisitely sensitive to inhibitors of the downstream kinase MEK.[36] (Sorafenib, in contrast, does not show this profile of activity.[37] Thus, proper preclinical screening would have revealed the shortcomings of sorafenib as a BRAF inhibitor.) Curiously, cell lines with a mutation or amplification of EGFR or HER2, which

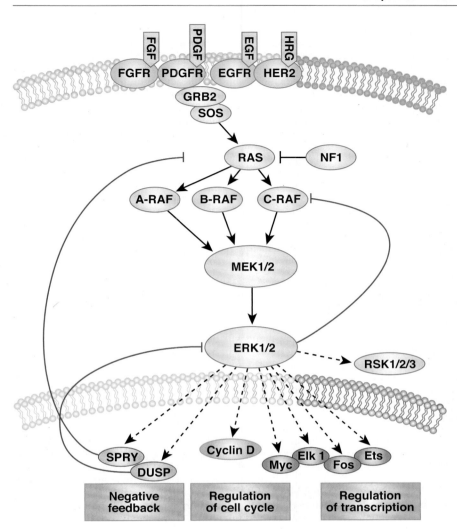

Figure 22.1 The RAS–RAF–MEK–ERK signaling pathway. The classical mitogen-activated protein kinase (MAPK) pathway is activated in human tumors by several mechanisms, including the binding of ligand to receptor tyrosine kinases (RTK), the mutational activation of an RTK, by loss of the tumor suppressor NF1, or by mutations in RAS, BRAF, and MEK1. Phosphorylation and, thus, activation of ERK regulates the transcription of target genes that promote cell cycle progression and tumor survival. The ERK pathway contains a classical feedback loop in which the expression of feedback elements such as SPRY and DUSP family proteins are regulated by the level of ERK activity. Loss of expression of SPRY and DUSP family members due to promoter methylation or deletion is thus permissive for persistently elevated pathway output. In the case of tumors with mutant BRAF, pathway output is enhanced by impaired upstream feedback regulation. FGF, fibroblast growth factor; HRG, heregulin; NF1, neurofibromatosis 1. (From Bernt KM, Zhu N, Sinha AU, et al. MLL-rearranged leukemia is dependent on aberrant H3K79 methylation by DOT1L. *Cancer Cell* 2011;20(1):66–78, with permission.)

CANCER THERAPEUTICS

function upstream in the pathway, were insensitive to MEK inhibition. Even tumor lines with RAS mutations were variably sensitive. In short, the preclinical data made a strong case that MEK inhibitors should be effective in BRAF mutant melanoma, but not in other subtypes. The reason that HER2, EGFR, and RAS mutant tumors were not sensitive to MEK inhibitors is explained, at least in part, by the existence of negative feedback loops that modulate the flux of signal transduction through MEK.[38]

In parallel with the generation of these preclinical findings, clinical trials of several MEK inhibitors were initiated. Patients with various cancers were enrolled in the early studies, but there was a strong bias to include melanoma patients. Significant efforts were made to demonstrate MEK inhibition in tumor cells by measuring the phosphorylation status of the direct downstream substrate ERK using an immunohistochemical analysis of biopsies from patients with metastatic disease. Phase I studies of the two earliest compounds in clinical development (PD325901 and AZD6244) documented reduced phospho-ERK staining at multiple dose levels in several patients for whom baseline and treatment biopsies were obtained.[39,40] (In the following, we will learn that these pharmacodynamic studies, while well intentioned, were not quantitative enough to document the magnitude of MEK inhibition in these patients.) Furthermore, clinical responses were observed in a few patients with BRAF mutant melanoma. Armed with this confidence, a randomized phase II clinical trial of AZD6244 was conducted in advanced melanoma, with the chemotherapeutic agent temozolomide (which is approved for glioblastoma) as the comparator arm. (The clinical development

of PD325901 was discontinued because of safety concerns about ocular and neurologic toxicity.) Disappointingly, patients receiving AZD6244 had no benefit in progression-free survival when compared to temozolomide-treated patients, raising further concerns about the viability of BRAF as a drug target.[41] A closer examination of the data revealed that clinical responses were, indeed, seen in patients receiving AZD6244. The fact that BRAF mutation status was not required for study entry likely diminished the clinical signal in the AZD6244 arm, a lesson learned from the EGFR inhibitor trials in lung cancer. Indeed, a different MEK inhibitor, trametinib, received FDA approval in 2013 based on activity in melanoma patients with the BRAF mutation.[42]

All doubts about BRAF as a target vanished in 2009 to 2010 when dramatic clinical responses were observed with a novel BRAF inhibitor vemurafenib (PLX4032). Like sorafenib, this compound was optimized to inhibit RAF, but with an additional focus on mutant BRAF. Vemurafenib differs dramatically from sorafenib because it potently inhibits BRAF without the additional broad range of activities that sorafenib has against other kinases like the VEGF receptor.[43] The greater selectivity of vemurafenib relative to sorafenib resulted in a much greater tolerability, such that it could be given at high doses while avoiding significant toxicity. The early days of vemurafenib clinical development were plagued by challenges in maximizing the oral bioavailability of the drug.[44] Consequently, the initial phase I clinical trial was temporarily halted to develop a novel formulation (i.e., the coingredients in the drug capsule or tablet that improve solubility and absorption through the gastrointestinal tract). Much higher serum levels were obtained in patients who received the new vemurafenib formation and, shortly thereafter, complete and partial responses were observed in about 80% of the melanoma patients with B-RAF mutant tumors. Strikingly, no activity was observed in patients whose tumors were wild type for BRAF.[45,46] The data were so compelling that vemurafenib was immediately advanced to a phase III registration trial. Similarly impressive responses in BRAF mutant melanoma patients were observed with a second potent RAF inhibitor dabrafenib,[47] providing further proof that BRAF is a important cancer target.

The vemurafenib and dabrafenib data also provide insight into why sorafenib and the early MEK inhibitor trials failed to demonstrate activity. One lesson is the critical importance of achieving adequate target inhibition. Clinical responses with vemurafenib were observed only after the drug was reformulated to achieve substantially higher serum levels. Reductions in phospho-ERK staining (as documented by immunohistochemistry) were documented in the earlier trials but, in retrospect, the assays were not sensitive enough to distinguish between modest (~50%) kinase inhibition versus more complete BRAF or MEK inhibition. Efficacy in preclinical models is significantly improved using doses that give >80% inhibition, and the human trial data suggest that this degree of pathway blockade is also required for a high clinical response rate.[46] Collectively, these experiences illustrate the critical need for quantitative pharmacodynamic assays to measure target inhibition early in clinical development. A second lesson is the importance of genotyping all patients for mutation or amplification of the relevant drug target. Not only does this ensure that a sufficient number of patients with the biomarker of interest are included in the study, but also that the results provide compelling evidence early in clinical development in support (or not) of the preclinical hypothesis.

Getting It Right: ALK and Lung Cancer

The development of the ALK inhibitor crizotinib (PF-02341066) illustrates how an unexpected signal obtained in a small number of patients can quickly shift a program in an entirely new direction with a high probability of success. The key ingredient is this story is a familiar one—a strong molecular hypothesis backed up by clinical response data in a small number of carefully selected patients. Crizotinib emerged from a drug discovery program at Pfizer that was focused on finding inhibitors of the MET receptor tyrosine kinase and entered the clinic with this target as its lead indication.[48] As we previously learned with imatinib, essentially all kinase inhibitors have activity against other targets (so called *off-target* activities), which can sometimes prove to be advantageous. Off-target activities are typically discovered by screening compounds against a large panel of kinases to establish profiles of relative selectivity against the intended target. Off-target activity, potency, and pharmaceutical properties (bioavailability, half-life) are all factors that influence the decision of which compound to advance to clinical development. The primary off-target activity of crizotinib is against the ALK tyrosine kinase.

ALK was first identified as a candidate driver oncogene in 1994 through the cloning of the t(2,5) chromosomal translocation associated with anaplastic large cell lymphoma, which creates the nucleophosmin/anaplastic lymphoma kinase (NPM-ALK) fusion gene.[49] This discovery, together with the demonstration that NPM-ALK causes lymphoma in mice, made a compelling case for ALK as a drug target in this disease. But there was limited interest in developing ALK inhibitors because this particular lymphoma subtype is rare and most commonly found in children. (Companies are generally reluctant to develop drugs solely for pediatric indications because of complexities related to dose selection and additional regulatory guidelines. Efforts to streamline this development process are underway, such as the Creating Hope Act, which provides new incentives for companies to pursue pediatric indications.) In

2007, a different ALK fusion gene called EML4-ALK was discovered in a small fraction of patients with lung adenocarcinoma, with an estimated frequency of 1% to 5%.[50] This discovery did not immediately capture the attention of drug developers, but several academic groups who had already begun testing lung cancer patients seen at their institutions for EGFR mutations simply added an EML4-ALK fusion test to the screening panel. Astute clinical investigators participating in the phase I trial of crizotinib, which was designed to include patients with a broad array of advanced cancers, were aware of the off-target ALK activity and enrolled several lung cancer patients with EML4-ALK fusions in the study. These patients had remarkably dramatic responses.[51] This serendipitous finding in a few ALK-positive patients was confirmed in a larger cohort, resulting in a strongly positive pivotal phase III study in ALK-positive lung cancer, just 2 years after the discovery of the EML4-ALK fusion.[52] Crizotinib is also being evaluated in other diseases associated with genomic alterations in ALK, including large-cell anaplastic lymphoma, neuroblastoma,[53] and inflammatory myofibroblastic sarcoma.[54]

Extending the Model to RET Mutations in Thyroid Cancer: Clinical Responses, But Why?

Subsets of patients with papillary or medullary thyroid cancer have activating mutations or translocations targeting the RET tyrosine-kinase receptor, raising the question of whether RET inhibitors might have a role in this disease.[55] Although no drugs specifically designed to inhibit RET have entered the clinic, four compounds with off-target activity against RET (vandetanib, sorafenib, motesanib, and cabozantinib) have all shown single-agent activity in thyroid cancer studies.[56–60] Vandetanib and cabozantinib are currently approved in medullary thyroid cancer based on improved progression-free survival in phase III registration trials.[61,62] Because all four compounds also inhibit VEGF receptor, it is unclear whether the clinical benefit observed in these studies is explained by inhibition of RET, VEGF receptor, or both. Unlike the crizotinib trials in ALK-positive lung cancer, enrollment in these registration studies was not restricted to patients with RET mutations. In addition to the fact that thyroid cancer patients are not routinely screened for these mutations, the primary reason for including all comers in these studies is that clinical responses are observed in a larger fraction of patients than can be accounted for based on the suspected frequency of an RET mutation. Responses in patients without RET mutation (if they occur) might be explained by mutations in other genes in the RAS-MAP kinase pathway such as BRAF or HRAS, which are found in a substantial fraction of patients and typically do not overlap with RET alterations.[55] Clearly, detailed genotype/response correlations, as demonstrated in lung cancer and melanoma, will clarify the role of these mutations in predicting the response to these drugs. Thyroid cancer is also a compelling indication for the BRAF and MEK inhibitors discussed previously in melanoma.

FLT3 Inhibitors in Acute Myeloid Leukemia: Did the Genomics Mislead Us?

Shortly after the success of imatinib, the receptor tyrosine–kinase FLT3 emerged as a compelling drug candidate based on the presence of activating mutations in about one-third of patients with acute myeloid leukemia.[63] Laboratory studies documented that FLT3 alleles bearing these mutations, which occur as internal tandem duplications (ITD) of the juxtamembrane domain or a point mutation in the kinase domain, function as driver oncogenes in mouse models, giving phenotypes analogous to BCR-ABL.[64] As with RET in thyroid cancer, no compounds had been specifically optimized to target FLT3, but several drugs with off-target FLT3 activity were redirected to acute myeloid leukemia (AML).

Disappointingly, the first three of the compounds tested (midostaurin, lestaurtinib, and sunitinib) showed only marginal single-agent activity in relapsed AML patients, even in those with FLT3 mutations.[65–67] Despite the strong molecular rationale for FLT3 as a driver lesion, questions were raised about the viability of FLT3 as a drug target. Pharmacodynamic studies showed evidence of FLT3 kinase inhibition in tumor cells, but the magnitude and duration of these effects were difficult to quantify, raising the possibility of inadequate target inhibition.[65] Indeed, the dose of all three compounds was limited by toxicities believed to be independent of FLT3. A more pessimistic interpretation was that FLT3, although presumably important for the initiation of AML, was no longer required for tumor maintenance due to the accumulation of additional driver genomic alterations. If true, even a complete FLT3 blockade with a highly selective inhibitor would be expected to fail. But this view was not supported by the fact that clinical responses were observed in the somewhat analogous situation of single-agent ABL kinase inhibitor treatment of CML in blast crisis, where BCR-ABL is just one of many additional genomic alterations that contribute to disease progression, yet complete remissions are observed in many patients.

Despite this pessimism about FLT3 as a viable drug target, several drugs are now advancing toward drug registration trials. Midostaurin, one of the early compounds that showed disappointing single-agent activity in relapsed AML, is being evaluated in a randomized phase III trial in newly diagnosed AML combined with standard induction chemotherapy. A single-arm phase II study showed higher and more durable remission rates in FLT3 mutant patients when compared to historical controls.[68] The second compound, quizartinib (AC220), is a next-generation FLT3 inhibitor with greater potency and specificity and with single-agent activity in FLT3 mutant relapsed AML—precisely the population where midostaurin and others failed.[69,70] The fact that some responder patients have relapsed with drug-resistant gatekeeper mutations in the FLT3 kinase domain provides formal proof that FLT3 is the relevant target.[71] Assuming these compounds prove successful in AML, it will be important to examine their activity in the rare cases of pediatric acute lymphoid leukemia associated with FLT3 mutation. Although the jury is still out on FLT3 inhibitors, the failure of early compounds in AML is reminiscent of the failures of early RAF and MEK inhibitors in melanoma. Collectively, these examples emphasize the importance of using optimized compounds to test a molecularly based hypothesis in patients and to focus enrollment on those patients with the relevant molecular lesion.

Kidney Cancer: Targeting the Tumor and the Host With Mammalian Target of Rapamycin and VEGF Receptor Inhibitors

A recurring theme in this chapter is the critical role of driver kinase mutations in guiding the development of kinase inhibitors. Ironically, several kinase inhibitors have been approved for kidney cancer over the past 5 years in a tumor type with no known kinase mutations. The most common molecular alteration in kidney cancer is a loss of function in the Von Hippel-Lindau (VHL) tumor suppressor gene, resulting in the activation of the hypoxia inducible factor[68] pathway.[72] As a consequence of VHL loss, which normally targets hypoxia-inducible factor (HIF) proteins for proteasomal degradation, HIF-1α and HIF-2α are constitutively active transcription factors that function as oncogenes through activation of an array of downstream target genes. Among these is the angiogenesis factor VEGF, which is secreted by HIF-expressing cells and promotes the development and maintenance of tumor neovasculature. HIF-mediated secretion of VEGF by tumor cells likely explains the highly vascular histopathology of clear cell renal carcinoma. All three currently approved angiogenesis inhibitors (the monoclonal antibody bevacizumab targeting VEGF and the kinase inhibitors sorafenib and sunitinib targeting or its receptor

VEGF receptor) have single-agent clinical activity in clear cell carcinoma.[73–75] The high specificity of bevacizumab for VEGF leaves little doubt that the activity of this drug is explained by antiangiogenic effects. In contrast, the off-target activities of sorafenib and sunitinib include several kinases expressed in kidney tumor cells, stroma, and inflammatory cells (PDGFR, RAF, RET, FLT3, and others). Interestingly, the primary effect of bevacizumab in kidney cancer is disease stabilization, whereas sorafenib and sunitinib have substantial partial response rates. This raises the question of whether the superior antitumor activity of the VEGF receptor kinase inhibitors is due to the concurrent inhibition of other kinases. However, partial responses rates with next-generation VEGF receptor inhibitors (axitinib, pazopanib, and tivozanib), all of which have greater potency and selectivity for the VEGF receptor, are similarly high, and reinforce the importance of the VEGF receptor as the critical target in kidney cancer.[76–78] Pazopanib is approved for advanced kidney cancer, whereas axitinib is approved as second-line therapy.

Two inhibitors of the mammalian target of rapamycin (mTOR) kinase (temsirolimus and everolimus) are also approved for advanced renal cell carcinoma.[79,80] Both temsirolimus and everolimus are known as rapalogs because both are chemical derivatives of the natural product sirolimus (rapamycin). Sirolimus was approved more than 10 years ago to prevent graft rejection in transplant recipients based on its immunosuppressive properties against T cells. Sirolimus also has potent antiproliferative effects against vascular endothelial cells and, on that basis, is incorporated into drug-eluting cardiac stents to prevent coronary artery restenosis following angioplasty.[81] Rapalogs differ from all the other kinase inhibitors discussed in this chapter in that they inhibit the kinase through an allosteric mechanism rather than by targeting the mTOR kinase domain. Because rapalogs also inhibit the growth of cancer cell lines from different tissues of origin, clinical trials were initiated to study their potential role as anticancer agents in a broad range of tumor types. Based on responses in a few phase I patients with different tumor types (including kidney cancer), exploratory phase II studies were conducted in several diseases. Single-agent activity of temsirolimus was observed in a phase II kidney cancer study,[82] then confirmed in a phase III registration trial.[79] The phase III everolimus trial, which was initiated after temsirolimus, was noteworthy because clinical benefit was demonstrated in patients who had progressed on the VEGF receptor inhibitors sorafenib or sunitinib.[80]

In parallel with the empirical clinical development of rapalogs, various laboratories explored the molecular basis for mTOR dependence in cancer cells. mTOR functions at the center of a complex network that integrates signals from growth factor receptors and nutrient sensors to regulate cell growth and size (Fig. 22.2). It does so, in part, by controlling the translation of various mRNAs with complex 5′ untranslated regions into protein. mTOR exists in two distinct complexes known as TOR complex 1 (TORC1) and TORC2. Rapalogs only inhibit the TORC1 complex, which is largely responsible for downstream phosphorylation of targets such as S6K1/2 and 4EBP1/2 that regulate protein translation.[83] The TORC2 complex contributes to the activation of AKT by phosphorylating the important regulatory serine residue S473 and is unaffected by rapalogs.

Two hypotheses have emerged to explain the clinical activity of rapalogs in kidney cancer. The antiproliferative activity of these compounds against endothelial cells suggests an antiangiogenic mechanism, which is consistent with the clinical activity of the VEGF receptor inhibitors. But rapalogs also inhibit the growth of kidney cancer cell lines in laboratory models where the effects on tumor angiogenesis have been eliminated. Interestingly, mRNAs for HIF1/2 are among those whose translation is impaired by rapalogs, and this effect has been implicated as the primary mechanism of rapalog activity in kidney cancer xenograft models.[84] As with the VEGF receptor inhibitors, a detailed molecular annotation of tumors from responders and nonresponders will shed light on these issues.

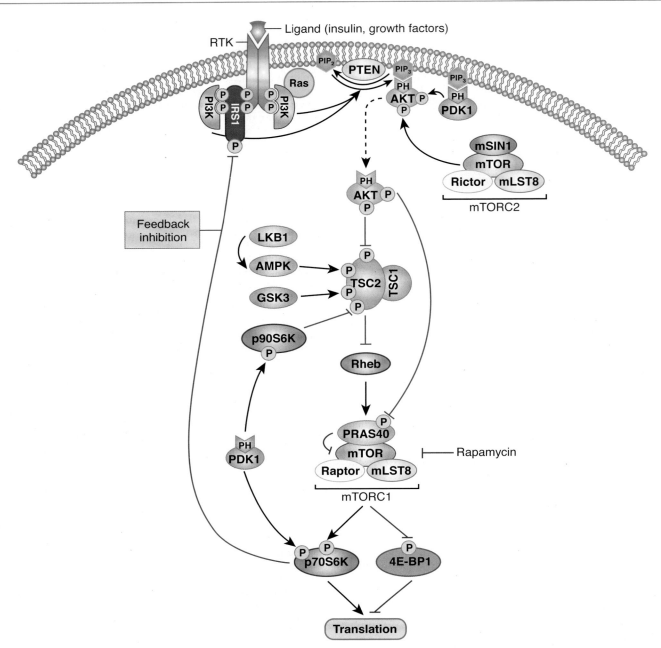

Figure 22.2 Feedback inhibition of the phosphatidylinositol 3-kinase (PI3K) pathway. Activated AKT regulates cellular growth through mammalian target of rapamycin (mTOR), a key player in protein synthesis and translation. mTOR forms part of two distinct complexes known as mTORC1, which contains mTOR, Raptor, mLST8, and PRAS40, and mTORC2, which contains mTOR, Rictor, mLST8, and mSIN1. mTORC1 is sensitive to rapamycin and controls protein synthesis and translation, at least in part, through p70S6K and eukaryotic translation initiation factor 4E–binding protein 1 (4E-BP1). AKT phosphorylates and inhibits tuberous sclerosis complex 2 (TSC2), resulting in increased mTORC1 activity. AKT also phosphorylates PRAS40, thus relieving the PRAS40 inhibitory effect on mTOR and the mTORC1 complex. mTORC2 and 3-phosphoinositide–dependent kinase (PDK1) phosphorylate AKT on Ser473 and Thr308, respectively, rendering it fully active. mTORC1-activated p70S6K can phosphorylate insulin receptor substrate 1 (IRS1), resulting in inhibition of PI3K activity. In addition, PDK1 phosphorylates and activates p70S6K and p90S6K. The latter has been shown to inhibit TSC2 activity through direct phosphorylation. Conversely, LKB1-activated AMP-activated protein kinase (AMPK) and glycogen synthase kinase 3 (GSK3) activate the TSC1/TSC2 complex through direct phosphorylation of TSC2. Thus, signals through PI3K as well as through LKB1 and AMPK converge on mTORC1. Inhibition of mTORC1 can lead to increased insulin receptor–mediated signaling, and inhibition of PDK1 may lead to activation of mTORC1 and may, paradoxically, promote tumor growth. (From Daigle SR, Olhava EJ, Therkelsen CA, et al. Selective killing of mixed lineage leukemia cells by a potent small-molecule DOT1L inhibitor. *Cancer Cell* 2011;20(1):53–65, with permission.)

Other Indications for mTOR Inhibitors: Breast Cancer and Tuberous Sclerosis Complex Mutant Cancers

Two other indications for mTOR have emerged, both based on fundamental insights from laboratory studies but from quite different angles. Preclinical studies of estrogen receptor (ER) therapy in breast cancer suggested that phosphatidylinositol 3-kinase (PI3K) pathway activation may be a mechanism of resistance and that this resistance could be prevented or overcome by combined treatment with ER-based drugs and rapalogs such as everolimus. Based on evidence that some women with progressive disease while receiving the aromatase inhibitor letrozole have clinical benefit from the addition of everolimus, randomized trials were initiated comparing everolimus + exemestane to exemestane alone (called BOLERO-2), or everolimus + tamoxifen to tamoxifen alone (called TAMRAD). Both studies demonstrated substantial improvements in time to progression in women with metastatic breast cancer who had already failed one aromatase inhibitor,[85,86] resulting in FDA approval of the everolimus/exemestane combination. Evidence of cross-talk between the PI3K pathway and hormone receptor signaling (ER in breast cancer, androgen receptor in prostate cancer) provides a molecular rationale for the clinical benefit of combination therapy and is currently under investigation in metastatic prostate cancer.[87]

Yet another indication for rapalog therapy emerged from the genetics of children with tuberous sclerosis caused by a loss of function mutations in tuberous sclerosis complex 1 (TSC1) or TSC2, which encode the proteins hamartin and tuberin that function in the PI3K signaling pathway just upstream of mTOR. Based on laboratory studies showing that TSC1- or TSC2-deficient cells are exquisitely sensitive to rapalogs, a clinical trial was conducted in tuberous sclerosis patients with benign subependymal giant-cell astrocytomas (SEGA) that showed tumor shrinkage in 21 of 28 patients.[88] This genetic dependence on mTOR in tumors with tuberous sclerosis complex (TSC) loss has also been observed in bladder cancer. In a remarkable example of the power of comprehensive DNA sequencing to provide insight into rare clinical phenotypes, investigators examined the tumor genome of the single complete responder patient on a phase II trial of everolimus in bladder cancer and discovered somatic mutations in TSC2 as well as a second gene, NF2, that also controls mTOR activity.[89] This plus other examples of how a retrospective genomic analysis of *extraordinary responders* has led to a national effort to capture these cases, as well as prospective clinical trials of patients with the relevant tumor genotype regardless of histology (called *basket* trials).

It is unclear why rapalogs have failed in other tumor types. One explanation is the concurrence of PI3K pathway mutations with alterations in other pathways that mitigate sensitivity to rapalogs. Another possibility is the disruption of negative feedback loops regulated by mTOR that inhibit signaling from upstream receptor tyrosine kinases. Rapalogs paradoxically *increase* signaling through PI3K due to loss of this negative feedback. A primary consequence is *increased* AKT activation, which signals to an array of downstream substrates that can enhance cell proliferation and survival (other than TORC1, which remains inhibited by rapalog) (see Fig. 22.2). This problem might be overcome by combining rapalogs with an inhibitor of an upstream kinase in the feedback loop, such as HER kinases or the insulinlike growth factor receptor (IGFR), to block this undesired effect of rapalogs on PI3K activation.[90]

DIRECTLY TARGETING THE PI3K PATHWAY

Mutations or copy number alterations (e.g., amplification or deletion of oncogenes or tumor suppressor genes) in PI3K pathway genes (PIK3CA, PIK3R1, PTEN, AKT1, and others) are among the most common abnormalities in cancer. Consequently, intensive efforts at many pharmaceutical companies have been devoted to the discovery of small-molecule inhibitors targeting kinases in the PI3K pathway. Inhibitors of PI3K, AKT, and ATP-competitive (rather than allosteric) inhibitors of mTOR that target both the TORC1 and TORC2 complex are all in clinical development. Phase I clinical trials have, in general, established that the pathway can be efficiently targeted without serious toxicity other than easily manageable effects on glucose metabolism (which is anticipated based on the importance of PI3K signaling in insulin signaling). Unfortunately, there has been no evidence to date of dramatic single-agent clinical activity with any of these agents, although early results with PI3K alpha selective inhibitor BYL719 in PIK3CA mutant breast cancer appear promising.[91]

However, the first approval of a direct PI3K inhibitor in cancer is likely to come in chronic lymphocytic leukemia and in lymphoma, but not on the basis of tumor genomics. Normal and malignant B cells are dependent on PI3K delta as well as Bruton tyrosine kinase (BTK) for proliferation and survival, raising the possibility that inhibitors of these kinases might be broadly active in B-cell malignancies. Concerns about toxicity on normal B cells were alleviated, in part, by the earlier clinical success of the CD20 antibody rituximab in lymphoma, which also eliminates normal circulating B cells, but without significant clinical sequelae. The first such PI3K delta inhibitor, idelalisib, has shown impressive activity in indolent non-Hodgkin lymphoma as a single agent and in relapsed chronic lymphocytic leukemia when given in combination with rituximab. The BTK inhibitor ibrutinib, following a similar clinical development path, was recently approved as second-line therapy for chronic lymphocytic leukemia and for mantle cell lymphoma.[92,93]

COMBINATIONS OF KINASE INHIBITORS TO INDUCT RESPONSE AND PREVENT RESISTANCE

Preclinical studies indicate that combinations of kinase inhibitors are required to realize their full potential as anticancer agents. The most common rationale is to address the problem of concurrent mutations in different pathways that alleviate dependence on a single-driver oncogene. The best examples are cancers with mutations in both the RAS/MAP kinase pathway (RAS or BRAF) and the PI3K pathway (PIK3CA or PTEN). In mouse models, such doubly mutant tumors fail to respond to single-agent treatment with either an AKT inhibitor or a MEK inhibitor. However, combination treatment can give dramatic regressions.[94] Similarly, genetically engineered mice that develop KRAS-driven lung cancer respond only to combination therapy with a PI3K inhibitor and a MEK inhibitor.[95] To date, clinical trials combining different PI3K pathway and RAS/MAP kinase pathway inhibitors have been challenging due to toxicities associated with continuous, concurrent PI3K and RAS/MAP kinase pathway inhibition.

Many of the tumor types discussed in this chapter *do* respond to treatment with a single-agent kinase, but relapse despite continued inhibitor therapy. Research into the causes of "acquired" kinase inhibitor resistance has revealed two primary mechanisms: (1) novel mutations in the kinase domain of the drug target that preclude inhibition, or (2) *bypass* of the driver kinase signal by activation of a parallel kinase pathway. In both cases, the solution is combination therapy to prevent the emergence of resistance. An elegant demonstration of this approach comes from CML where resistance to imatinib is primarily caused by mutations in the BCR-ABL kinase domain.[96,97] The second-generation ABL inhibitors dasatinib and nilotinib are effective against most imatinib-resistant BCR-ABL mutants and were initially approved as single-agent therapy for imatinib-resistant CML.[98,99] Very recently, both drugs have proven superior to imatinib in the upfront treatment of CML due to increased potency and fewer mechanisms of acquired resistance.[100–102] However, one BCR-ABL mutation called T315I is resistant to all three drugs. The third-generation ABL kinase inhibitor ponatinib blocks T315I and showed activity in a phase II clinical trial that included CML patients with the T315I mutation,[103] resulting in FDA approval. However, subsequent reports of severe vascular occlusive events, such as stroke and heart failure, led to withdrawal from the market, followed by approval for restricted use in T315I-mutant patients. Analogous approaches are ongoing in other diseases such as EGFR-mutant lung cancer, where acquired resistance to the frontline kinase inhibitor is also associated with mutations in the target kinase.[104,105] Promising clinical results have been reported with irreversible EGFR inhibitors such as CO-1686 and AZD9291.

The clinical development of kinase inhibitor combinations to prevent acquired resistance is relatively straightforward. Because the frontline drug is already approved, success would be determined by an improvement in response duration using the combination. The situation is more complex when two experimental compounds (e.g., a PI3K pathway inhibitor and a MEK inhibitor) are combined, neither of which shows significant single-agent activity. Older regulatory guidelines required a four-arm study that compared each single agent to the combination and to a control group in order to obtain approval of the combination. Recognizing that this design could discourage drug developers as well as patients from moving forward because it requires a large sample size, the FDA has issued new guidelines for the development of novel combinations that require a two-arm registration study comparing the combination to standard of care http:// www.fda.gov/downloads/Drugs/GuidanceComplianceRegulatory Information/Guidances/UCM236669.pdf. A more challenging issue may be dose optimization and dose schedule that is needed to safely combine two investigational drugs. Much like the development of combination chemotherapy several decades ago, it may be important to select compounds with nonoverlapping toxicities to allow for sufficient doses of each drug to be achieved.

SPECULATIONS ON THE FUTURE ROLE OF KINASE INHIBITORS IN CANCER MEDICINE

The role of genomics in predicting a response to kinase inhibitor therapy is now irrefutable. As the number of kinase driver mutations continues to grow, the field is likely to move away from the current strategy of a *companion diagnostic* for each drug. Rather, comprehensive mutational profiling platforms that query each tumor for hundreds of potential cancer mutations are more likely to emerge as the diagnostic platform. The number of directly *actionable* mutations (meaning the presence of a mutation defines a treatment decision supported by clinical trial data) remains low, but this number will undoubtedly grow. In addition, it is becoming apparent that many patients have rare mutations (defined as rare in that histologic tumor type) but are, in theory, actionable. Because these examples are unlikely to be formally evaluated in clinical trials, many centers have opened *basket* studies (with eligibility based solely on mutation profile) to capture these cases with some reports of remarkable success.

More effort must be devoted to manipulating the dose and schedule of kinase inhibitor therapy to maximize efficacy and minimize toxicity. To date, all kinase inhibitors have been developed based on the assumption that a 24/7 coverage of the target is required for efficacy. Consequently, most compounds are optimized to have a long serum half-life (12 to 24 hours). Phase II doses are then selected based on the maximum tolerated dose determined with daily administration. But a recent clinical of the ABL inhibitor dasatinib in CML indicates that equivalent antitumor activity can be achieved with intermittent therapy.[106] By giving larger doses intermittently, higher peak drug concentrations were achieved that resulted in equivalent and possibly superior efficacy.[107] Similar results were observed in laboratory studies of EGFR inhibitors in EGFR-mutant lung cancer. Clinically robust, quantitative assays of target inhibition are needed to hasten progress in this area.

Although the focus of this chapter is kinase inhibitors, the themes developed here should apply broadly to inhibitors of other cancer targets. Inhibitors of the G-protein coupled receptor smoothened (SMO) in patients with metastatic basal cell carcinoma or medulloblastoma establish that the driver mutation hypothesis extends beyond kinase inhibitors. SMO is a component in the Hedgehog pathway, which is constitutively activated in subsets of patients with basal cell carcinoma and medulloblastoma due to mutations in the Hedgehog ligand-binding receptor Patched-1. Treatment with the SMO inhibitor vismodegib led to impressive responses in basal cell carcinoma and medulloblastoma patients whose tumors had Patched-1 mutations,[108,109] resulting in FDA approval. Other novel cancer targets are emerging from cancer genome sequencing projects. Somatic mutations in the Krebs cycle enzyme isocitrate dehydrogenase (IDH1/2) were found in subsets of patients with glioblastoma, AML, chondrosarcoma, and cholangiocarcinoma,[110–112] and the first IDH2 inhibitor has entered clinical trials in leukemia. Mutations in enzymes involved in chromatin remodeling, such as the histone methyltransferase EZH2, have been reported in lymphoma and have spurred the ongoing development of EZH2 inhibitors.[113,114] Inhibitors of another histone methyltransferase DOT1L, which is required for the maintenance of mixed lineage leukemia (MLL) fusion leukemias, are also in clinical development.[115,116] Kinase inhibitors are just the first wave of molecularly targeted drugs ushered in by our understanding of the molecular underpinnings of cancer cells. There is much more to follow.

REFERENCES

1. Sawyers CL. Shifting paradigms: the seeds of oncogene addiction. *Nat Med* 2009;15(10):1158–1161.
2. Weinstein IB. Cancer. Addiction to oncogenes—the Achilles heal of cancer. *Science* 2002;297(5578):63–64.
3. Druker BJ, Talpaz M, Resta DJ, et al., Efficacy and safety of a specific inhibitor of the BCR-ABL tyrosine kinase in chronic myeloid leukemia. *N Engl J Med* 2001;344(14):1031–1037.
4. Hirota S, Isozaki K, Moriyama Y, et al. Gain-of-function mutations of c-kit in human gastrointestinal stromal tumors. *Science* 1998;279(5350):577–580.
5. Heinrich MC, Corless CL, Duensing A, et al. PDGFRA activating mutations in gastrointestinal stromal tumors. *Science* 2003;299(5607):708–710.
6. Demetri GD, von Mehren M, Blanke CD, et al. Efficacy and safety of imatinib mesylate in advanced gastrointestinal stromal tumors. *N Engl J Med* 2002;347(7):472–480.
7. Geyer CE, Forster J, Lindquist D, et al. Lapatinib plus capecitabine for HER2-positive advanced breast cancer. *N Engl J Med* 2006;355(26):2733–2743.
8. Kris MG, Natale RB, Herbst RS, et al. Efficacy of gefitinib, an inhibitor of the epidermal growth factor receptor tyrosine kinase, in symptomatic patients with non-small cell lung cancer: a randomized trial. *JAMA* 2003;290(16): 2149–2158.
9. Miller VA, Kris MG, Shah N, et al. Bronchioloalveolar pathologic subtype and smoking history predict sensitivity to gefitinib in advanced non-small-cell lung cancer. *J Clin Oncol* 2004;22(6):1103–1109.
10. Paez JG, Jänne PA, Lee JC, et al. EGFR mutations in lung cancer: correlation with clinical response to gefitinib therapy. *Science* 2004;304(5676):1497–1500.
11. Lynch TJ, Bell DW, Sordella R, et al. Activating mutations in the epidermal growth factor receptor underlying responsiveness of non-small-cell lung cancer to gefitinib. *N Engl J Med* 2004;350(21):2129–2139.
12. Pao W, Miller V, Zakowski M, et al. EGF receptor gene mutations are common in lung cancers from "never smokers" and are associated with sensitivity of tumors to gefitinib and erlotinib. *Proc Natl Acad Sci U S A* 2004;101(36): 13306–13311.
13. Cohen MH, Willliams GA, Sridhara R, et al. FDA drug approval summary: gefitinib (ZD1839) (Iressa) tablets. *Oncologist* 2003;8(4):303–306.
14. Shepherd FA, Rodrigues Pereira J, Ciuleanu T, et al. Erlotinib in previously treated non-small-cell lung cancer. *N Engl J Med* 2005;353(2):123–132.

15. Thatcher N, Chang A, Parikh P, et al. Gefitinib plus best supportive care in previously treated patients with refractory advanced non-small-cell lung cancer: results from a randomised, placebo-controlled, multicentre study (Iressa Survival Evaluation in Lung Cancer). *Lancet* 2005;366(9496):1527–1537.

16. Herbst RS, Giaccone G, Schiller JH, et al. Gefitinib in combination with paclitaxel and carboplatin in advanced non-small-cell lung cancer: a phase III trial—INTACT 2. *J Clin Oncol* 2004;22(5):785–794.

17. Giaccone G, Herbst RS, Manegold C, et al. Gefitinib in combination with gemcitabine and cisplatin in advanced non-small-cell lung cancer: a phase III trial—INTACT 1. *J Clin Oncol* 2004;22(5):777–784.

18. Herbst RS, Prager D, Hermann R, et al. TRIBUTE: a phase III trial of erlotinib hydrochloride (OSI-774) combined with carboplatin and paclitaxel chemotherapy in advanced non-small-cell lung cancer. *J Clin Oncol* 2005;23(25):5892–5899.

19. Tsao MS, Sakurada A, Cutz JC, et al. Erlotinib in lung cancer - molecular and clinical predictors of outcome. *N Engl J Med* 2005;353(2):133–144.

20. Mok TS, Wu YL, Thongprasert S, et al. Gefitinib or carboplatin-paclitaxel in pulmonary adenocarcinoma. *N Engl J Med* 2009;361(10):947–957.

21. Schaller JL, Burkland GA. Case report: rapid and complete control of idiopathic hypereosinophilia with imatinib mesylate. *MedGenMed* 2001;3(5):9.

22. Ault P, Cortes J, Koller C, et al. Response of idiopathic hypereosinophilic syndrome to treatment with imatinib mesylate. *Leuk Res* 2002;26(9):881–884.

23. Cools J, DeAngelo DJ, Gotlib J, et al. A tyrosine kinase created by fusion of the PDGFRA and FIP1L1 genes as a therapeutic target of imatinib in idiopathic hypereosinophilic syndrome. *N Engl J Med* 2003;348(13):1201–1214.

24. Golub TR, Barker GF, Lovett M, et al. Fusion of PDGF receptor beta to a novel ets-like gene, tel, in chronic myelomonocytic leukemia with t(5;12) chromosomal translocation. *Cell* 1994;77(2):307–316.

25. Apperley JF, Gardembas M, Melo JV, et al. Response to imatinib mesylate in patients with chronic myeloproliferative diseases with rearrangements of the platelet-derived growth factor receptor beta. *N Engl J Med* 2002;347(7):481–487.

26. Rutkowski P, Van Glabbeke M, Rankin CJ, et al. Imatinib mesylate in advanced dermatofibrosarcoma protuberans: pooled analysis of two phase II clinical trials. *J Clin Oncol* 2010;28(10):1772–1779.

27. Davies H, Bignell GR, Cox C, et al. Mutations of the BRAF gene in human cancer. *Nature* 2002;417(6892):949–954.

28. Baxter EJ, Scott LM, Campbell PJ, et al., Acquired mutation of the tyrosine kinase JAK2 in human myeloproliferative disorders. *Lancet* 2005;365(9464):1054–1061.

29. James C, Ugo V, Le Couédic JP, et al. A unique clonal JAK2 mutation leading to constitutive signalling causes polycythaemia vera. *Nature* 2005;434(7037):1144–1148.

30. Levine RL, Wadleigh M, Cools J, et al. Activating mutation in the tyrosine kinase JAK2 in polycythemia vera, essential thrombocythemia, and myeloid metaplasia with myelofibrosis. *Cancer Cell* 2005;7(4):387–397.

31. Samuels Y, Wang Z, Bardelli A, et al. High frequency of mutations of the PIK3CA gene in human cancers. *Science* 2004;304(5670):554.

32. International Cancer Genome Consortium, Hudson TJ, Anderson W, et al. International network of cancer genome projects. *Nature* 2010;464(7291):993–998.

33. Vogelstein B, Papadopoulos N, Velculescu VE, et al. Cancer genome landscapes. *Science* 2013;339(6127):1546–1558.

34. Lawrence MS, Stojanov P, Mermel CH, et al. Discovery and saturation analysis of cancer genes across 21 tumour types. *Nature* 2014;505(7484):495–501.

35. Eisen T, Ahmad T, Flaherty KT, et al. Sorafenib in advanced melanoma: a Phase II randomised discontinuation trial analysis. *Br J Cancer* 2006;95(5):581–586.

36. Solit DB, Garraway LA, Pratilas CA, et al. BRAF mutation predicts sensitivity to MEK inhibition. *Nature* 2006;439(7074):358–362.

37. McDermott U, Sharma SV, Dowell L, et al. Identification of genotype-correlated sensitivity to selective kinase inhibitors by using high-throughput tumor cell line profiling. *Proc Natl Acad Sci U S A* 2007;104(50):19936–19941.

38. Pratilas CA, Taylor BS, Ye Q, et al. (V600E)BRAF is associated with disabled feedback inhibition of RAF-MEK signaling and elevated transcriptional output of the pathway. *Proc Natl Acad Sci U S A* 2009;106(11):4519–4524.

39. LoRusso PM, Krishnamurthi SS, Rinehart JJ, et al. Phase I pharmacokinetic and pharmacodynamic study of the oral MAPK/ERK kinase inhibitor PD-0325901 in patients with advanced cancers. *Clin Cancer Res* 2010;16(6):1924–1937.

40. Adjei AA, Cohen RB, Franklin W, et al. Phase I pharmacokinetic and pharmacodynamic study of the oral, small-molecule mitogen-activated protein kinase kinase 1/2 inhibitor AZD6244 (ARRY-142886) in patients with advanced cancers. *J Clin Oncol* 2008;26(13):2139–2146.

41. Dummer R, Chapman PB, Sosman JA, et al. AZD6244 (ARRY-142886) vs temozolomide (TMZ) in patients (pts) with advanced melanoma: An open-label, randomized, multicenter, phase II study. *J Clin Oncol* 2008;26(May 20 suppl):9033.

42. Flaherty KT, Robert C, Hersey P, et al. Improved survival with MEK inhibition in BRAF-mutated melanoma. *N Engl J Med* 2012;367(2):107–114.

43. Joseph EW, Pratilas CA, Poulikakos PI, et al. The RAF inhibitor PLX4032 inhibits ERK signaling and tumor cell proliferation in a V600E BRAF-selective manner. *Proc Natl Acad Sci U S A* 2010;107(33):14903–14908.

44. Flaherty K, Puzanov I, Sosman J, et al. Phase I study of PLX4032: proof of concept for V600E BRAF mutation as a therapeutic target in human cancer. *J Clin Oncol* 2009;27(15s):abstract 9000.

45. Flaherty KT, Puzanov I, Kim KB, et al. Inhibition of mutated, activated BRAF in metastatic melanoma. *N Engl J Med* 2010;363(9):809–819.

46. Bollag G, Hirth P, Tsai J, et al. Clinical efficacy of a RAF inhibitor needs broad target blockade in BRAF-mutant melanoma. *Nature* 2010;467(7315):596–599.

47. Hauschild A, Grob JJ, Demidov LV, et al. Dabrafenib in BRAF-mutated metastatic melanoma: a multicentre, open-label, phase 3 randomised controlled trial. *Lancet* 2012;380(9839):358–365.

48. Kwak EL, Camidge DR, Clark J, et al. Clinical activity observed in a phase I dose escalation trial of an oral c-MET and ALK inhibitor, PF-02341066. *J Clin Oncol* 2009;27(Suppl):148s.

49. Morris SW, Kirstein MN, Valentine MB, et al. Fusion of a kinase gene, ALK, to a nucleolar protein gene, NPM, in non-Hodgkin's lymphoma. *Science* 1994;263(5151):1281–1284.

50. Soda M, Choi YL, Enomoto M, et al. Identification of the transforming EML4-ALK fusion gene in non-small-cell lung cancer. *Nature* 2007;448(7153):561–566.

51. Bang Y, Kwak EL, Shaw AT, et al. Clinical activity of the oral ALK inhibitor PF-02341066 in ALK-positive patients with non-small cell lung cancer (NSCLC). *J Clin Oncol* 2010;28:18s.

52. Shaw AT, Kim DW, Nakagawa K, et al. Crizotinib versus chemotherapy in advanced ALK-positive lung cancer. *N Engl J Med* 2013;368(25):2385–2394.

53. Chen Y, Takita J, Choi YL, et al. Oncogenic mutations of ALK kinase in neuroblastoma. *Nature* 2008;455(7215):971–974.

54. Sirvent N,Hawkins AL, Moeglin D, et al. ALK probe rearrangement in a t(2;11;2)(p23;p15;q31) translocation found in a prenatal myofibroblastic fibrous lesion: toward a molecular definition of an inflammatory myofibroblastic tumor family? *Genes Chromosomes Cancer* 2001;31(1):85–90.

55. Fagin JA, Mitsiades N. Molecular pathology of thyroid cancer: diagnostic and clinical implications. *Best Pract Res Clin Endocrinol Metab* 2008;22(6):955–969.

56. Wells SA Jr, Gosnell JE, Gagel RF, et al. Vandetanib for the treatment of patients with locally advanced or metastatic hereditary medullary thyroid cancer. *J Clin Oncol* 28(5):767–772.

57. Lam ET, Ringel MD, Kloos RT, et al. Phase II clinical trial of sorafenib in metastatic medullary thyroid cancer. *J Clin Oncol* 28(14):2323–2330.

58. Kloos RT, Ringel MD, Knopp MV, et al. Phase II trial of sorafenib in metastatic thyroid cancer. *J Clin Oncol* 2009;27(10):1675–1684.

59. Schlumberger MJ, Elisei R, Bastholt L, et al. Phase II study of safety and efficacy of motesanib in patients with progressive or symptomatic, advanced or metastatic medullary thyroid cancer. *J Clin Oncol* 2009;27(23):3794–3801.

60. Kurzrock R, Cohen EE, Sherman SI, et al. Long-term results in a cohort of medullary thyroid cancer (MTC) patients (pts) in a phase I study of XL184 (BMS 907351), an oral inhibitor of MET, VEGFR2, and RET. *J Clin Oncol* 2010;28(Suppl):15s.

61. Wells SA Jr, Robinson BG, Gagel RF, et al. Vandetanib in patients with locally advanced or metastatic medullary thyroid cancer: a randomized, double-blind phase III trial. *J Clin Oncol* 2012;30(2):134–141.

62. Elisei R, Schlumberger MJ, Müller SP, et al. Cabozantinib in progressive medullary thyroid cancer. *J Clin Oncol* 2013;31(29):3639–3646.

63. Sawyers CL. Finding the next Gleevec: FLT3 targeted kinase inhibitor therapy for acute myeloid leukemia. *Cancer Cell* 2002;1(5):413–415.

64. Kelly LM, Qing L, Jeffery L, et al. FLT3 internal tandem duplication mutations associated with human acute myeloid leukemias induce myeloproliferative disease in a murine bone marrow transplant model. *Blood* 2002;99(1):310–318.

65. Stone RM, DeAngelo DJ, Klimek V, et al. Patients with acute myeloid leukemia and an activating mutation in FLT3 respond to a small-molecule FLT3 tyrosine kinase inhibitor, PKC412. *Blood* 2005;105(1):54–60.

66. Knapper S, Burnett AK, Littlewood T, et al. A phase 2 trial of the FLT3 inhibitor lestaurtinib (CEP701) as first-line treatment for older patients with acute myeloid leukemia not considered fit for intensive chemotherapy. *Blood* 2006;108(10):3262–3270.

67. Fiedler W, Serve H, Döhner H, et al. A phase 1 study of SU11248 in the treatment of patients with refractory or resistant acute myeloid leukemia (AML) or not amenable to conventional therapy for the disease. *Blood* 2005;105(3):986–993.

68. Stone RM, Fischer T, Paquette R, et al. A Phase 1b study of midostaurin (PKC412) in combination with daunorubicin and cytarabine induction and high-dose cytarabine consolidation in patients under age 61 with newly diagnosed de novo acute myeloid leukemia: overall survival of patients whose blasts have FLT3 mutations is similar to those with wild-type FLT3. Paper presented at: 2009 American Society of Hematology Annual Meeting; 2009; New Orleans, LA.

69. Zarrinkar PP, Gunawardane RN, Cramer MD, et al. AC220 is a uniquely potent and selective inhibitor of FLT3 for the treatment of acute myeloid leukemia (AML). *Blood* 2009;114(14):2984–2992.

70. Cortes J, et al. AC220, a potent, selective, second generation FLT3 receptor tyrosine kinase inhibitor (RTK), in a first-in-human (FIH) phase 1 AML study. Paper presented at: 2009 American Society of Hematology Annual Meeting; 2009; New Orleans, LA.

71. Smith CC, Wang Q, Chin CS, et al. Validation of ITD mutations in FLT3 as a therapeutic target in human acute myeloid leukaemia. *Nature* 2012;485(7397):260–263.

72. Kaelin WG Jr. The von Hippel-Lindau tumour suppressor protein: O2 sensing and cancer. *Nat Rev Cancer* 2008;8(11):865–873.

73. Yang JC, Haworth L, Sherry RM, et al. A randomized trial of bevacizumab, an anti-vascular endothelial growth factor antibody, for metastatic renal cancer. *N Engl J Med* 2003;349(5):427–434.

74. Escudier B, Eisen T, Stadler WM, et al. Sorafenib in advanced clear-cell renal-cell carcinoma. *N Engl J Med* 2007;356(2):125–134.

75. Motzer RJ, Hutson TE, Tomczak P, et al. Sunitinib versus interferon alfa in metastatic renal-cell carcinoma. *N Engl J Med* 2007;356(2):115–124.

76. Rini BI, Wilding G, Hudes G, et al. Phase II study of axitinib in sorafenib-refractory metastatic renal cell carcinoma. *J Clin Oncol* 2009;27(27):4462–4468.

77. Sonpavde G, Hutson TE, Sternberg CN. Pazopanib, a potent orally administered small-molecule multitargeted tyrosine kinase inhibitor for renal cell carcinoma. *Expert Opin Investig Drugs* 2008;17(2):253–261.

78. Bhargava P, Esteves B, Al-Adhami M, et al. Activity of tivozanib (AV-951) in patients with renal cell carcinoma (RCC): Subgroup analysis from a phase II randomized discontinuation trial (RDT). *J Clin Oncol* 2010;28(suppl):15s.

79. Hudes G, Carducci M, Tomczak P, et al. Temsirolimus, interferon alfa, or both for advanced renal-cell carcinoma. *N Engl J Med* 2007;356(22):2271–2281.

80. Motzer RJ, Escudier B, Oudard S, et al. Efficacy of everolimus in advanced renal cell carcinoma: a double-blind, randomised, placebo-controlled phase III trial. *Lancet* 2008;372(9637):449–456.

81. McKeage K, Murdoch D, Goa FL. The sirolimus-eluting stent: a review of its use in the treatment of coronary artery disease. *Am J Cardiovasc Drugs* 2003;3(3):211–230.

82. Atkins MB, Hidalgo M, Stadler WM, et al. Randomized phase II study of multiple dose levels of CCI-779, a novel mammalian target of rapamycin kinase inhibitor, in patients with advanced refractory renal cell carcinoma. *J Clin Oncol* 2004;22(5):909–918.

83. Guertin DA, Sabatini DM. Defining the role of mTOR in cancer. *Cancer Cell* 2007;12(1):9–22.

84. Thomas GV, Tran C, Mellinghoff IK, et al. Hypoxia-inducible factor determines sensitivity to inhibitors of mTOR in kidney cancer. *Nat Med* 2006;12(1):122–127.

85. Bachelot T, Bourgier C, Cropet C, et al. Randomized phase II trial of everolimus in combination with tamoxifen in patients with hormone receptor-positive, human epidermal growth factor receptor 2-negative metastatic breast cancer with prior exposure to aromatase inhibitors: a GINECO study. *J Clin Oncol* 2012;30(22):2718–2724.

86. Baselga J, Campone M, Piccart M, et al. Everolimus in postmenopausal hormone-receptor-positive advanced breast cancer. *N Engl J Med* 2012;366(6):520–529.

87. Carver BS, Chapinski C, Wongvipat J, et al. Reciprocal feedback regulation of PI3K and androgen receptor signaling in PTEN-deficient prostate cancer. *Cancer Cell* 2011;19(5):575–586.

88. Krueger DA, Care MM, Holland K, et al. Everolimus for subependymal giant-cell astrocytomas in tuberous sclerosis. *N Engl J Med* 2010;363(19):1801–1811.

89. Iyer G, Hanrahan AL, Milowsky MI, et al. Genome sequencing identifies a basis for everolimus sensitivity. *Science* 2012;338(6104):221.

90. O'Reilly KE, Rojo F, She QB, et al. mTOR inhibition induces upstream receptor tyrosine kinase signaling and activates Akt. *Cancer Res* 2006;66(3):1500–1508.

91. Gonzalez-Angulo AM, Juric D, Argilis G, et al. Safety, pharmacokinetics, and preliminary activity of the alpha-specific PI3K inhibitor BYL719: results from the first-in-human study. *J Clin Oncol* 2013;31(15 Suppl):2531.

92. Byrd JC, Furman RR, Coutre SE, et al. Targeting BTK with ibrutinib in relapsed chronic lymphocytic leukemia. *N Engl J Med* 2013;369(1):32–42.

93. Wang ML, Rule S, Martin P, et al. Targeting BTK with ibrutinib in relapsed or refractory mantle-cell lymphoma. *N Engl J Med* 2013;369(6):507–516.

94. She QB, Halilovic E, Ye Q, et al. 4E-BP1 is a key effector of the oncogenic activation of the AKT and ERK signaling pathways that integrates their function in tumors. *Cancer Cell* 18(1):39–51.

95. Engelman JA, Chen L, Tan X, et al. Effective use of PI3K and MEK inhibitors to treat mutant Kras G12D and PIK3CA H1047R murine lung cancers. *Nat Med* 2008;14(12):1351–1356.

96. Gorre ME, Mohammed M, Ellwood K, et al. Clinical resistance to STI-571 cancer therapy caused by BCR-ABL gene mutation or amplification. *Science* 2001;293(5531):876–880.

97. Shah NP, Nicoll JM, Nagar B, et al. Multiple BCR-ABL kinase domain mutations confer polyclonal resistance to the tyrosine kinase inhibitor imatinib (STI571) in chronic phase and blast crisis chronic myeloid leukemia. *Cancer Cell* 2002;2(2):117–125.

98. Shah NP, Tran C, Lee FY, et al. Overriding imatinib resistance with a novel ABL kinase inhibitor. *Science* 2004;305(5682):399–401.

99. Talpaz M, Shah NP, Kantarjian H, et al. Dasatinib in imatinib-resistant Philadelphia chromosome-positive leukemias. *N Engl J Med* 2006;354(24):2531–2541.

100. Kantarjian H, Shah NP, Hochhaus A, et al. Dasatinib versus imatinib in newly diagnosed chronic-phase chronic myeloid leukemia. *N Engl J Med* 2010;362(24):2260–2270.

101. Sawyers CL. Even better kinase inhibitors for chronic myeloid leukemia. *N Engl J Med* 2010;362(24):2314–2315.

102. Saglio G, Kim DW, Issaragrisil S, et al. Nilotinib versus imatinib for newly diagnosed chronic myeloid leukemia. *N Engl J Med* 362(24):2251–2259.

103. Cortes JE, Kim DW, Pinilla-Ibarz J, et al. A phase 2 trial of ponatinib in Philadelphia chromosome-positive leukemias. *N Engl J Med* 2013;369(19):1783–1796.

104. Pao W, Miller VA, Politi KA, et al. Acquired resistance of lung adenocarcinomas to gefitinib or erlotinib is associated with a second mutation in the EGFR kinase domain. *PLoS Med* 2005;2(3):e73.

105. Antonescu CR, Besmer P, Guo T, et al. Acquired resistance to imatinib in gastrointestinal stromal tumor occurs through secondary gene mutation. *Clin Cancer Res* 2005;11(11):4182–4190.

106. Shah NP, Kantarjian HM, Kim DW, et al. Intermittent target inhibition with dasatinib 100 mg once daily preserves efficacy and improves tolerability in imatinib-resistant and -intolerant chronic-phase chronic myeloid leukemia. *J Clin Oncol* 2008;26(19):3204–3212.

107. Shah NP, Kasap C, Weier C, et al. Transient potent BCR-ABL inhibition is sufficient to commit chronic myeloid leukemia cells irreversibly to apoptosis. *Cancer Cell* 2008;14(6):485–493.

108. Von Hoff DD, LoRusso PM, Rudin CM, et al. Inhibition of the hedgehog pathway in advanced basal-cell carcinoma. *N Engl J Med* 2009;361(12):1164–1172.

109. Rudin CM, Hann CL, Laterra J, et al. Treatment of medulloblastoma with hedgehog pathway inhibitor GDC-0449. *N Engl J Med* 2009;361(12):1173–1178.

110. Parsons DW, Jones S, Zhang X, et al. An integrated genomic analysis of human glioblastoma multiforme. *Science* 2008;321(5897):1807–1812.

111. Mardis ER, Ding L, Dooling DJ, et al. Recurring mutations found by sequencing an acute myeloid leukemia genome. *N Engl J Med* 2009;361(11):1058–1066.

112. Ward PS, Patel J, Wise DR, et al. The common feature of leukemia-associated IDH1 and IDH2 mutations is a neomorphic enzyme activity converting alpha-ketoglutarate to 2-hydroxyglutarate. *Cancer Cell* 2010;17(3):225–234.

113. McCabe MT, Ott HM, Ganji G, et al. EZH2 inhibition as a therapeutic strategy for lymphoma with EZH2-activating mutations. *Nature* 2012;492(7427):108–112.

114. Morin RD, Johnson NA, Severson TM, et al. Somatic mutations altering EZH2 (Tyr641) in follicular and diffuse large B-cell lymphomas of germinal-center origin. *Nat Genet* 2010;42(2):181–185.

115. Bernt KM, Zhu N, Sinha AU, et al. MLL-rearranged leukemia is dependent on aberrant H3K79 methylation by DOT1L. *Cancer Cell* 2011;20(1):66–78.

116. Daigle SR, Olhava EJ, Therkelsen CA, et al. Selective killing of mixed lineage leukemia cells by a potent small-molecule DOT1L inhibitor. *Cancer Cell* 2011;20(1):53–65.

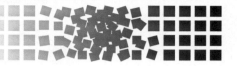

23 Histone Deacetylase Inhibitors and Demethylating Agents

Steven D. Gore, Stephen B. Baylin, and James G. Herman

INTRODUCTION

The past decade has seen an explosive growth, especially at a genome-wide level, in our understanding of the role of chromatin in the normal regulation of gene expression and in the concept of the *epigenome*.[1–3] Concomitant with these advances has been the increasing appreciation of the role of epigenetic abnormalities in the progression of cancer[4–7] and the concept of the *cancer epigenome*. The translational consequences of this research include the possibilities for developing therapies in cancer that target epigenetic abnormalities. These are being explored in clinical trials and several have entered clinical practice.[4,5,7,8] Of these epigenetic abnormalities, the most thoroughly examined is the occurrence of abnormal cytosine guanine (CpG) promoter region DNA methylation and associated altered chromatin involving histone modifications, in the transcriptional silencing of genes, including a group of well-defined tumor suppressor genes.[4,5,7,8] However, targeting epigenetic processes to downregulate the action of overexpressed genes is also an emerging area of research.[9,10] This chapter describes the basis of epigenetic changes in cancer and discusses some of the latest approaches that target epigenetic abnormalities in cancer,[11] including those designed to induce the reexpression of silenced genes, for cancer therapy. The two approaches most mature in development are the inhibition of DNA methyltransferases, which mediate the abnormal promoter DNA methylation, and the inhibition of histone deacetylases, which remove histone modifications associated with active chromatin that alone, or in association with DNA methylation, are associated with transcriptional repression.[4,5,7,8] However, several exciting newer approaches are now in clinical trials and these will be mentioned.

Aberrant gene function and altered patterns of gene expression are key features of cancer.[4] Although genetic alterations remain the best characterized in the development and progression of cancer, increasingly it is appreciated that epigenetic abnormalities cooperate with genetic alterations in multiple ways to cause dysfunction of key regulatory pathways. Through genomic approaches to mutation discovery, there is growing recognition of the frequency of mutations in genes encoding for proteins that regulate the epigenome.[12] This chapter will outline the understanding of how each of these epigenetic alterations contribute to cancer and how derivation of therapeutic approaches may depend on understanding the biology of these changes.

EPIGENETIC ABNORMALITIES AND GENE EXPRESSION CHANGES IN CANCER

Epigenetic changes are defined as heritable alterations of gene expression patterns and cell phenotypes, which are not accompanied by changes in DNA sequence.[13] This definition clearly delineates the two key features of epigenetic regulation important for an understanding of therapies described in this chapter. Specifically, in contrast to genetic alterations (point mutations, deletions, or translocations), epigenetic changes do not alter the coding sequence of targeted genes. Thus, reversal of epigenetic changes can potentially restore the normal function of affected genes and their encoded proteins. Second, the heritable nature of epigenetic changes—that is, the ability of a cell to pass on regulation of gene expression through DNA replication—suggests that such changes, while relatively stable, can be reversed. Thus, therapeutic reprogramming of patterns of gene expression could theoretically result in a long-term change in the cancer cell phenotype, even after the inducing drugs are removed, although to date, this has not been accomplished.

The fundamental unit that determines epigenetic states is the nucleosome that contains an octamer of histone proteins around which approximately 160 base pairs of DNA are wrapped.[13] It is the positioning of these structures, and the three-dimensional aspects of their spacing, and the regulation of this process by posttranslational modifications of the constituent histones that underpins the functions of the epigenome.[13,14]

Abnormal Gene Silencing

One key alteration in cancer, which can be associated with altered epigenetic control, is abnormal gene silencing. Normally, such silencing is fundamental and required at the level of chromatin and DNA methylation regulation for the life of multicellular eukaryotic organisms. The silencing is critical for regulating important biologic processes, including all aspects of development, differentiation, imprinting, and silencing of large chromosomal domains, including the X chromosome of female mammals.[13] For example, the diversity of structure and function of cells derived from epithelial or mesenchymal origin, ultimately differentiating into cells lining the intestine or lung or forming mature granulocytes and myocytes, result from heritable changes in gene expression that are not the result of a change in DNA sequence. Although in many species, silencing can be initiated and maintained solely by processes involving the covalent modifications of histones and other chromatin components, vertebrates utilize an additional layer of gene regulation. This process involves the only natural covalent modification of DNA in humans and is characterized by DNA cytosine methylation that occurs nearly exclusively at the fifth position of the cytosine ring in cytosines preceding guanine, the so-called CpG dinucleotide (Fig. 23.1).[13,15]

Like most biologic processes, the normal patterns of silencing can be altered, resulting in the development of disease states. Thus, activation of genes normally not expressed, or silencing of a gene that should be expressed, can contribute to the dysregulation of gene function that characterizes cancer and, when stably present, represent epigenetic alterations.[4–7] Most studies have focused on the silencing of normally expressed genes. For the purposes of understanding the rationale behind epigenetic therapy, it is important to understand the mechanisms through which such silencing occurs. Alterations in gene expression associated with epigenetic changes that give rise to a growth advantage would be expected to be selected for in the host tissue, leading to progressive dysregulated

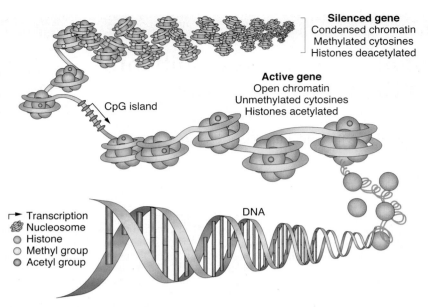

Figure 23.1 Epigenetic regulation of gene expression. In the promoter region, gene expression is controlled by a combination of DNA methylation and chromatin configuration. In normal cells, gene expression is silenced by condensing chromatin, methylating DNA, and deacetylating histones. By contrast, active genes are those with open nucleosome spacing around the transcription start site, are unmethylated, and are associated with acetylated histones. In cancer cells, CpG islands that are rich in cytosine and guanine—and are typically unmethylated to promote gene expression—can be epigenetically silenced by hypermethylation. (Redrawn with permission from Azad N, Zahnow CA, Rudin CM, et al. The future of epigenetic therapy in solid tumours—lessons from the past. *Nat Rev Clin Oncol* 2013;10:256–266.)

growth of the tumor. Such dysregulation is commonly associated with increases in promoter region DNA methylation and is associated with repressive chromatin changes.

Changes in DNA Methylation

The importance of abnormal cytosine methylation and gene silencing has been clearly established in the past 2 decades and been shown convincingly to be involved in cancer development.[4–7] The CpG dinucleotide, usually underrepresented in the genome, is clustered in the promoter regions of approximately 50% of human genes in regions termed *CpG islands*. These regions are largely protected from DNA methylation in normal cells, with the exception of genes on the inactive X chromosome and imprinted genes.[16] This protection is critical, because the methylation of promoter region CpG islands is associated with a loss of gene expression.[4–7] Abnormal de novo DNA methylation of gene promoter CpG islands is a very frequent abnormality in virtually all cancer types and is associated with a process that can serve as an alternative mechanism for loss of tumor suppressor gene function.[4–7] Although a limited number of classic tumor suppressor genes can be affected by this process, a patient's individual cancer may harbor hundreds of such genes.[4–7] Which of these latter genes are drivers of cancer, individually or in groups, versus those which are passengers reflecting only the widespread effects of a global epigenetic abnormality is a leading question in the field and the target of much research.[5,6] A clue to the importance of at least groups of the previous DNA hypermethylated genes may come from the fact that an inordinate number of them are involved in holding normal embryonic and adult stem cells in the self-renewal state and/or rendering such cells refractory to differentiation cues.[17,18] Normally, these genes are then in a poised expression state and can be induced to be activated or repressed as needed for changes in

cell state.[18] Abnormal promoter DNA methylation of such genes renders them more repressed and could be a factor in the fact that cancers inevitably exhibit cell populations with enhanced self-renewal or refractoriness to full differentiation.[18]

Recent studies have also suggested that DNA regions other than promoter CpG islands may undergo changes of DNA methylation in cancer. For example, non–CpG-rich sequences surrounding promoter CpG islands, termed CpG island shores, are abnormally methylated in cancers[19] and may be altered in stem cell populations.[20] Thus, the relative cancer specificity of changes of DNA methylation in multiple CpG regions makes reversal of these changes by targeting DNA methyltransferases, the enzymes that catalyze DNA methylation, logical for cancer therapeutics.

As a key example of the previous points, perhaps the most studied tumor suppressor gene for promoter hypermethylation is the *p16* gene, currently designated *CDKN2A*, a cyclin-dependent kinase inhibitor that functions in the regulation of the phosphorylation of the Rb protein. Hypermethylation associated with loss of expression of the *CDKN2A* gene has been found to be one of the most frequent alterations in neoplasia being common in the lung, head and neck, gliomas, colorectal, and breast carcinomas[21,22] and other cancer types. A member of the same gene family, *p15* or *CDKN2B*, also regulates Rb and is silenced in association with promoter methylation in many forms of leukemia and in the chronic myeloid neoplasm myelodysplastic syndrome (MDS).[23] These two previous changes are of much relevance for the clinical uses of epigenetic therapies discussed later.

As mentioned, many hundreds of genes may be inactivated in a single cancer by promoter methylation,[5,6,18,24] providing potential targets for gene reactivation using epigenetic therapies.[25–27] The latter represents one of the potential ways in which epigenetic therapy may be effective: Multiple genes and gene pathways, all

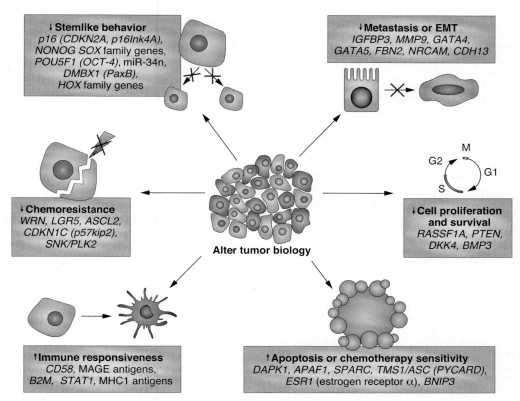

Figure 23.2 Concurrent widespread changes in gene expression with epigenetic therapy. Anticancer efficacy of treatment with epigenetic-modulating agents is associated with extensive changes in gene expression that influence several biologic processes. Gene expression is increased through the direct reversal of epigenetic modifications of genomic DNA, whereas for cancer-promoting genes, gene expression is reduced by the regression of their regulatory genes. EMT, epithelial-membrane transition. (Redrawn with permission from Azad N, Zahnow CA, Rudin CM, et al. The future of epigenetic therapy in solid tumours—lessons from the past. *Nat Rev Clin Oncol* 2013;10:256–266.)

repressed by changes in DNA methylation and chromatin modification, can be reactivated by DNA methyltransferase inhibitors and histone deacetylase (HDAC) inhibitors (HDACi), thereby restoring normal cell cycle control, differentiation, and apoptotic signaling (Fig. 23.2).[8,26,28] In general, methylated CpG islands are not capable of the initiation of transcription unless the methylation signal can be overridden by alterations in factors that modulate chromatin, such as the removal of methylated cytosine-binding proteins. However, reversal of DNA methylation with secondary changes in histone modification or directed reversal of repressive histone modifications represent a target for epigenetic therapies.[8,26,28]

Most studies of DNA methylation, particularly in the study of cancer, have focused on CpG island promoter methylation. However, about 40% of human genes do not contain bona fide CpG islands in their promoters.[29] The primary focus on CpG islands has resulted from the clear demonstration that CpG-island promoter methylation permanently silences genes both physiologically and pathologically in mammalian cells. However, recent work has shown correlations between tissue-specific expression and methylation of non-CpG islands, including, for example, the maspin gene,[30] and as mentioned previously, regions near CpG islands,[19,20] suggesting that many additional genes could be regulated, either normally or abnormally, by changes in DNA methylation.

An exciting new area of DNA methylation research involves the role of this change in regulating gene enhancers: small DNA regions that regulate the expression of multiple target genes.[31–33] The presence of DNA methylation in these areas, which can reside considerable distances from the genes that are being regulated, generally works together with histone modifications to mediate a repressive state for that enhancer.[31–33] The status of enhancers is also emerging as important for cancer risk states.[34]

Chromatin in Gene Regulation

Heritable gene silencing involves the interplay between DNA methylation and histone covalent modifications. Complexes of proteins that can regulate how nucleosomes are positioned perform nucleosomal remodeling.[35–37] What was initially termed the *histone code*, with reference to how histones are modified, has emerged to be much more complex than originally envisioned. An explosion of research findings during the last several years now allows for an appreciation of how the epigenome is controlled by a complex interplay between a myriad of posttranslational histone modifications that occur on key amino acid residues of these proteins.[37] Acetylation, deacetylation, methylation, phosphorylation, and other modifications all modify chromatin structure and thereby alter gene expression.[38] Some of the enzymes that catalyze these modifications include HDACs, histone methyltransferases (HMT), and most recently, histone demethylases.[13,14,39,40] These modifications help establish heritable states at the start site of genes, but also at enhancers and other transcribed DNA regions not encoding for canonical genes. The latter areas contain noncoding RNAs (ncRNAs) and micro-RNAs (miRNAs), which play key modulatory roles for overall gene expression and protein patterns that can be altered in cancer.[41–43] Again, much research is being focused on epigenetic changes in these DNA regions, which may be important to cancer development and, potentially, to cancer management.

A link between covalent histone modifications and DNA methylation has been clearly established.[44–46] In this interaction, cytosine methylation attracts methylated DNA-binding proteins and HDACs to methylated CpG sites during chromatin compaction and gene silencing.[46,47] In addition, the DNA methylation binding protein (MBD2) interacts with the nucleosomal remodeling complex (NuRD) and directs the complex to methylated DNA.[48] This complex also binds HDACs and has recently been identified as a central player for the abnormal silencing of genes associated with promoter DNA hypermethylation in cancer.[47] Thus, the three processes of DNA cytosine methylation, histone modification, and nucleosomal remodeling are intimately linked, and alterations in these processes can result in abnormalities of gene expression in cancer-relevant genes.

Enzymes Regulating DNA Methylation and Histone Acetylation

DNA methylation involves the covalent addition of a methyl group to the 5′ position of cytosine. In mammals, three enzymes have been shown to catalyze this transfer of a methyl group from the methyl donor S-adenosylmethionine. Most of the methyltransferase activity present in differentiated cells is derived from the expression of DNMT1.[49] This enzyme is thought to be most important in maintaining DNA methylation patterns following DNA replication and thus is referred to as a maintenance methyltransferase. However, the enzyme does possess the ability to methylate previously unmethylated DNA sequences (de novo activity).[50] In contrast, the other enzymes, DNMT3a and DNMT3b, are efficient at methylating previously unmethylated DNA and thus are considered de novo methyltransferases. Each of these enzymes possesses a similar catalytic site,[51] a fact important for the inhibition of DNMT enzymes by nucleoside analogs, discussed later in this chapter.

DNA methylation is closely associated with changes in the histone modifications. As previously discussed, histone proteins are the central components of the nucleosome, and modifications of the histone tails of core histones are associated with active or repressed chromatin.[52] Although it is beyond the scope of this chapter to fully discuss the complex series of modifications to the histone tails of histone H3 and H4, a few well-characterized modifications should be mentioned that are relevant to therapies designed to target epigenetic abnormalities in cancer. In reference to currently investigated epigenetic therapies, changes in histone acetylation are of importance. Acetylation of histones H3 and H4 at key amino acids is associated with the active chromatin present at the promoters of transcribed genes, whereas the absence of histone acetylation is associated with repressed, silenced genes.[13,14,53] Histone acetyltransferases (HAT) HDACs have opposing functions to maintain the proper level of histone acetylation for gene expression.[13,14,53] HDACs specifically deacetylate the lysine residues of the histone tails, and this deacetylation is associated with condensation of nucleosome positions in what is termed a closed chromatin formation. This scenario is key to transcriptional repression. There are four classes of HDACs.[53] Class I HDACs are characterized by their similarity to the yeast Rpd3 HDAC. In humans, this class of enzymes includes HDAC1, -2, -3, and -8. These HDACs are thought to be ubiquitously expressed in tissue throughout the body. In contrast, class II HDACs are similar to yeast Hda1 and include HDAC4, -5, -6, -7, -9, and -10, and they have a greater degree of tissue specificity. Class III HDACs are similar to yeast Sir2 and are set apart from the other classes by their dependence on nicotinamide adenine dinucleotide (NAD+) as a cofactor. Finally, class IV includes HDAC11.[53]

Of the previously listed HDACs, class I and 2 HDACs have been most closely tied to gene silencing associated with abnormal promoter DNA hypermethylation.[48] These are bound to the nucleosome remodeling complex, NuRD.[48,49] Experimental decreases in NURD, after use of a DNA demethylating agent, can augment reactivation of many abnormally silenced and DNA hypermethylated genes in colon cancer cells.[48] Manipulation of these HDACs is under study in clinical trials, with and without the use of DNA methyltransferase inhibitors, and is discussed later. Another HDAC, SIRT1 in the class III of these proteins, is also involved with gene silencing.[54,55] This deacetylase has been linked to silencing of DNA hypermethylated genes, and blocking its activity can be associated with reactivation of such genes.[55]

Reversal of Layers of Gene Silencing

The interaction between DNA methylation and HDAC activity and repressive chromatin marks in maintaining aberrant silencing of hypermethylated genes in cancer has therapeutic implications for epigenetic therapies. Experimental evidence suggests that DNA methylation functions as a dominant event that stably establishes transcriptional repression. Inhibition of HDAC activity alone, by potent and specific HDACis, does not generally result in the reactivation of aberrantly silenced and densely hypermethylated genes in tumor cells.[56] In contrast, treatment with HDACis can reactivate densely silenced genes if the cells are first treated with demethylating drugs, such as 5-azacitidine.[56] The clinical implications of this observation are discussed in more detail in the following section (Table 23.1).

DNA Methyltransferase Inhibitors

Originally synthesized as cytotoxic antimetabolite drugs in the 1960s,[57] azacytosine nucleosides were recognized as inhibitors of DNA methylation in the early 1980s. The inhibitors 5-azacitidine (5AC) and 2′-deoxy-5-azacytidine induced muscle, fat, and chondrocyte differentiation in mouse embryo cells, in association with a reversal of DNA methylation.[58,59] The incorporation of azacytosine nucleosides into DNA in lieu of cytosine residues was shown to be associated with inhibition of DNMT activity.[59,60] DNMT inhibition requires the incorporation of decitabine triphosphate into DNA. The incorporated azacytosine nucleoside forms an irreversible inactive adduct with DNMT. The sequential reversal of DNA methylation then results when DNA replication proceeds in the absence of active DNMT.[61] The inhibitor 5AC must be phosphorylated and converted to decitabine diphosphate by ribonucleotide reductase before it can be activated through triphosphorylation, whereas decitabine does not require ribonucleotide reductase. The inhibitor 5AC can also be incorporated into RNA. DNMT2, a misnamed protein that is actually an RNA-specific methyltransferase,[62] becomes inhibited, leading to the depletion of methylated tRNA.[60] This may contribute to the inhibition of protein synthesis and is a potential difference between azacitidine and decitabine.[63] The previous DNA methyltransferase inhibitors not only block the catalytic activities of DNMTs, but also trigger degradation of these proteins, especially DNMTs 1 and 3B.[64–68] This latter activity is potentially important for their activities for gene reexpression because each of these two proteins, experimentally, possess transcriptional repression properties independent of their DNA methylation catalytic sites.[69,70]

The azacytosine nucleosides exhibit complex dose–response characteristics. At low concentrations (0.2 to 1 μM), the epigenetic activities of these drugs predominate, with dose-dependent reversal of DNA methylation[71,72] and induction of terminal differentiation in some systems.[28,71] As concentrations are increased, DNA damage and apoptosis become more prominent.[28,72] Cell lines with 30-fold resistance to the cytotoxic effects of doxifluridine,

TABLE 23.1

Small Molecules Targeting Epigenetic Abnormalities in Clinical Development

Drug	Class	Target	Dose Range	Schedule	Route of Administration
5-Azacitidine	Nucleoside	DNA methyl-transferase	30–75 mg/m^2/d	Daily × 7–14 d/28 d	Subcutaneous or intravenous
2'-Deoxy-5-azacytidine	Nucleoside	DNA methyl-transferase	10–45 mg/m^2/d	Daily × 3–5 d/4–6 wk	Intravenous
SG110	Nucleoside	DNA methyl-transferase	Being determined	Being determined	Subcutaneous
Valproic acid	Small chain fatty acid	Histone deacetylase (class I and II)	25–50 mg/kg/d	Daily	Oral or intravenous
Vorinostat	Hydroxamic acid	Histone deacetylase (class I and II)	400–600 mg/d	Divided doses	Oral
Entinostat	Benzamide	Histone deacetylase (class I)	2–8 mg/m^2	Weekly	Oral
Belinostat	Hydroxamic acid	Histone deacetylase (class I and II)	600–1,000 mg/m^2	Daily × 5/28 d	Intravenous
Romidepsin	Cyclic tetrapeptide	Histone deacetylase (class I and II)	13–18 mg/m^2	Weekly	Intravenous
LBH-589	Hydroxamic acid	Histone deacetylase (class I and II)	5–11 mg/m^2	Daily × 3	Intravenous
MGCD-0103	Benzamide	Histone deacetylase (class I)	40–125 mg/m^2	Twice weekly	Oral
CI-994	Benzamide	Histone deacetylase (class I)	5–8 mg/m^2	Daily	Oral

CANCER THERAPEUTICS

adriamycin, cyclophosphamide (DAC) continue to reverse methylation in response to this nucleoside, suggesting that the methylation reversing and cytotoxic activities of this compound can be separated.[73] The ability of these drugs to inhibit the cell cycle, at least in part through induction of p21$^{WAF1/CIP1}$ expression, complicates the goal of reversing DNA methylation, because the latter requires DNA replication with the azacytosine nucleoside incorporated into the DNA.

The importance of low doses of the two azacytosine nucleosides to achieve a targeted therapeutic effect has been recently explored in a series of laboratory observations. Transient exposure of both leukemia and solid tumor cells to submicromolar doses induce such cells to undergo cellular reprogramming, accompanied by decreases in ability to clone in long-term self-renewal assays and to grow as explants in immune-incompetent mice.[28] These effects occur with partial genome-wide DNA demethylation and changes in gene expression in multiple pathways potentially key for driving tumorigenesis.

The pharmacokinetic properties of the two azacytosine nucleosides are also very important to consider for their clinical use. In this regard, a major potential challenge for their usage is the fact that these drugs are highly unstable in an aqueous solution, resulting in their rapid hydrolysis and resultant inactivation.[74] In clinical practice, the drugs must be administered shortly after reconstitution. The drugs are also metabolized by cytidine deaminase,[74] leading to a short half-life in plasma. When injected subcutaneously, 5AC reaches a maximal plasma concentration at 30 minutes, with a terminal half-life of 1.5 to 2.3 hours.[75,76] At the U.S. Food and Drug Administration (FDA) approved dose of 5AC (75 mg/m^2 administered subcutaneously daily for 7 days), peak plasma concentrations were 3 to 5 μM, which is well within the range of DNMT inhibitory concentrations.[75,76] Intravenous (IV) administration of the same dose has led to higher peak plasma concentrations (11 μM) with a shorter half-life

(approximately 22 minutes).[75] DAC given over 1 hour IV at 15 to 20 mg/m^2 produced plasma concentrations of 1.1 to 1.6 μM during the infusion,[77] whereas in a phase 1 study in patients with thoracic malignancies, patients were treated with escalating doses of decitabine for 72-hour IV infusions for two 35-day cycles. The maximum tolerated total dose was 60 to 75 mg/m^2 with neutropenia as the dose-limiting toxicity. Steady-state plasma concentrations ranged from 25 to 40 nM, which is less than those usually used to induce expression of methylated genes in tissue culture models.[78] An oral formulation of 5AC has also been studied. The oral bioavailability of oral azacitidine ranged from 6% to 20%. Nonetheless, MDS and acute myelogenous leukemia (AML) patients receiving oral azacitidine developed clinical responses similar to patients receiving parenteral azacitidine. Oral azacitidine has also been safely administered on 14-daily and 21-daily schedules repeated monthly. The extended administration of lower daily doses may provide favorable pharmacodynamics of DNA methylation reversal given the need for ongoing cell cycling to effect methylation reversal.[79]

SGI-110 is a dinucleoside that acts as a prodrug for decitabine. This drug is being studied in myelodysplasia and AML.[80]

HISTONE DEACETYLASE INHIBITORS

The increasing recognition of the critical importance of histone modifications in regulating the transcriptional permissively of chromatin has led to intense interest in compounds that can inhibit the activity of HDAC proteins, facilitating the acetylation of lysines associated with transcriptional activation of genes. As with the DNMT inhibitors discussed previously, there are multiple, sometimes dose-dependent, effects of HDACis in preclinical studies. Some of these may truly be epigenetic, others strictly cytotoxic, and others a combination of both.[9,81–84] Some actions of HDACis may relate to altering how chromatin is central to the repair of DNA. Thus, at especially high doses, these compounds can blunt efficient repair and even induce DNA breaks.[84,85] These effects may underlie cell cycle arrest and induction of cell death as is often observed in preclinical studies of HDACis.[81–84]

Perhaps novel uses of these drugs may be inferred by results from recent studies suggesting they could be extremely powerful epigenetic therapy agents when used in proper doses, for targeted purposes, and at key time intervals. Recent studies by Settleman and colleagues[86] suggest that histone acetylation changes, and thus epigenetic mechanisms, could be a key factor for cancer therapy resistance to both targeted therapy agents and conventional chemotherapy. The mechanisms involved may involve the emergence of drug-tolerant stem-like cells.[86] In such cells, gene expression studies suggest that a protein upregulated in resistance is a histone demethylase, which diminishes a key histone modification for active transcription, H3K4methyl.[86] A very similar enzyme has been shown in other studies to be central to self-renewal of stem-like melanoma cells.[87] Key to the therapies under discussion is that, in the previous drug-resistance studies, low doses of HDACis, could reversibly reduce drug-resistant cells induced by the various anticancer drugs.[86] It is essential going forward to sort out which of these effects are dose-related off-target effects and which are desired on-target effects that can be optimized for efficacious therapy strategies.

Types of Histone Deacetylase Inhibitors

Small Chain Fatty Acids

The earliest report of the use of an HDACi to treat leukemia described the treatment of a child with refractory AML with intravenous sodium butyrate, with a concomitant clearance of peripheral blood blast cells and a decrement in bone marrow blasts.[88] No responses developed in a subsequent study of nine AML patients who were treated with intravenous butyrate.[89] Phase 1 studies of sodium phenylbutyrate (NaPB) in MDS and AML explored 7-day continuous infusions administered monthly or biweekly, and 21-day continuous infusions administered monthly.[90,91] At the maximum tolerated dose (375 mg per kilogram per day), the mean steady-state plasma concentration was 0.3 mM, within the range of HDAC inhibition.[90–92] Isolated patients developed hematologic improvement in response to NaPB.

Similar to NaPB, valproic acid (VPA) requires near millimolar concentrations to effectively inhibit HDACs. Of 18 patients with MDS or AML with trilineage dysplasia treated with VPA to target plasma concentrations of 0.3 to 0.7 mM, 6 patients developed hematologic improvement.[93] Of 20 elderly patients with AML treated with VPA, only 11 could remain in control long enough to be considered evaluable for response. Five had improvement in platelet counts.[94] VPA induced hematologic improvement in combination with all-transretinoic acid in two of eight patients treated with AML; a fluorescence in situ hybridization analysis showed definitive evidence of terminal differentiation of the malignant cells.[95] A larger study of this combination induced hematologic response in only 2 of 26 elderly patients with AML.[96] It appears unlikely that the small chain fatty acids will develop an important role in the treatment of malignancy given the availability of HDACis with vastly greater potency.

Hydroxamic Acids

The FDA approved vorinostat as the first commercially available HDACi. The approval was based on activity of this agent in cutaneous T-cell lymphoma (CTCL). Thirty-three patients with a median number of five prior systemic therapy regimens received one of three dose schedules of vorinostat in a single institution study.[97] Eight patients achieved a partial response, with a median time to response of 12 weeks and a median duration of response of 15 weeks. Overall, 45% of patients had relief of pruritus. Fatigue, diarrhea, nausea, and thrombocytopenia were common toxicities. In a multicenter phase 2 trial, 74 patients with relapsed or refractory CTCL were treated with 400 mg daily.[98] Similar to the prior study, 29% of patients responded, consisting almost entirely of partial responses. Median time to response was 56 days, and median duration of response was greater than 6 months. In phase 1 trials, responses to vorinostat have developed in other non-Hodgkin's and Hodgkin's lymphoma cases.[99] More recently, in a trial combining vorinostat with carboplatin and paclitaxel in patients with untreated, advanced, non–small-cell lung cancer (NSCLC), response rates increased significantly from 12.5% to 34%, and a trend to improved progression-free survival and overall survival was observed.[100]

Panobinostat (LBH589), a cinnamic hydroxamic acid HDACi, reduced peripheral blood blast percentage but did not induce remissions in a phase 1 trial of daily times 7 oral dosing in patients with a variety of relapsed hematologic malignancies.[101] Asymptomatic changes in electrocardiographic T waves developed in 80% of treated patients. Gastrointestinal symptoms and thrombocytopenia were common. Panobinostat has recently been approved by the FDA for the treatment of multiple myeloma.[102]

Cyclic Tetrapeptides

Romidepsin is FDA approved for the treatment of CTCL[103] and peripheral T-cell lymphoma.[104,105] Antitumor activity, including tumor lysis syndrome, was demonstrated in a phase 1 study that enrolled patients with chronic lymphocytic leukemia and AML, but no complete or partial remissions were seen.[75] The administration of romidepsin induces electrocardiographic changes, including T-wave flattening and ST-T wave depression in greater than half of the posttreatment tracings; however, no changes in serum cardiac troponin levels or left ventricular ejection fraction have been reported.[106]

Benzamides

Entinostat, formerly known as MS-275, was administered weekly times four to patients with relapsed and refractory AML in a phase 1 study. Infections, unsteady gate, and somnolence were dose-limiting toxicities. No clinical responses developed, although improvements in neutrophil counts were observed.[107] Entinostat did not increase the response rate in patients with higher risk MDS and AML with MDS-related changes when combined with azacitidine compared to azacitidine alone.[108] Most recently, however, studies NSCLC suggest that entinostat could be a valuable therapeutic agent in solid tumors when used with established therapies. When combined with the epidermal growth factor inhibitor erlotinib, in a randomized phase 2 trial for patients with recurrent advanced NSCLC, entinostat was not efficacious alone but appeared to combine with erlotinib to benefit a group of patients whose tumors contained baseline high E-cadherin levels. Overall survival in these latter patients yielded an increased survival benefit of 9.4 versus 5.4 months.[109] Finally, entinostat significantly increased survival when combined with an aromatase inhibitor in a phase 2 trial for patients with breast cancer.[110]

Pharmacodynamic Properties

The administration of oral vorinostat was associated with a transient increase in acetylation of histone H3 in peripheral blood lymphocytes, which peaked at 2 hours post dosing and reverted to baseline by 8 hours; similar changes were observed in the lymph node of a treated patient with lymphoma.[99] Treatment with vorinostat was associated with translocation of phosphorylated signal transducer and activator of transcription 3 (STAT-3) from nucleus to cytoplasm in responding patients and with reduced microvessel density.[97]

Similar changes in the acetylation of histones 2B and 3 were observed in peripheral blood cells from patients treated with LBH589.[101] Romidepsin induced acetylation of H3 and H4 in peripheral blood tumor cells within 4 hours of dosing[111]; of interest, p21[WAF1/CIP1] protein levels also increased, associated with an increase in acetylation of H4 at the p21 promoter (using chromatin immunoprecipitation). Treatment with entinostat led to increased acetylation of H3 and H4 in both peripheral blood and bone marrow. This increase was detectable within 8 hours and remained above baseline throughout the treatment cycle. Thus, this compound may provide the most prolonged inhibition of protein deacetylation of HDACis and is under current investigation.[107] Increases in p21[WAF1/CIP1] and activation of caspase 3 were also demonstrated in these samples.

EPIGENETIC THERAPY FOR HEMATOLOGIC MALIGNANCIES

DNA Methyltransferase Inhibitors

Epigenetic therapy has seen the most widespread use to date and achieved the greatest efficacy in hematologic malignancies. The therapeutic efficacy of 5AC and DAC for patients with the chronic myeloid neoplasm myelodysplasia (MDS) and AML has been well reviewed.[26,27] Their FDA approval for MDS/AML emerged only after doses were reduced, with resultant diminishing toxicities for patients. The successful development of 5AC for the treatment of MDS can be credited largely to Silverman et al.[25,112,114] in the Cancer and Leukemia Group B (CALGB). The inhibitor 5AC had successfully induced the expression of hemoglobin F in patients with sickle cell anemia.[25,112] Viewing this compound as a potential inducer of terminal differentiation, Silverman et al. conducted a series of phase 2 trials of 5AC administered as a continuous intravenous infusion or as subcutaneous injections for the treatment of MDS.[113,114] Based on significant hematologic responses, the group performed a phase 2 trial (CALGB 9221) in which patients with low- and high-risk MDS with significant hematopoietic compromise were randomly assigned to receive subcutaneous 5AC (75 mg/m^2 per day daily for 7 days, repeated on a 28-day cycle) or observation. Patients on the observation arm with progressive disease could cross over to receive 5AC. This study firmly established the ability of 5AC to induce hematologic improvement, and, less frequently, complete and partial responses.[113,115] The median time to development of AML (defined by 30% bone marrow blast cells) or death was greater in the 5AC arm by 9 months (21 versus 12 months); of note, the observation arm included patients who subsequently crossed over to 5AC treatment.

In a subsequent phase 3 trial (AZA001),[116] patients with higher risk myelodysplastic syndromes were randomly assigned one-to-one to receive 5AC (75 mg/m^2 per day for 7 days every 28 days) or conventional care (best supportive care, low-dose cytarabine, or intensive chemotherapy as selected by investigators before randomization). Three hundred fifty-eight patients were randomly assigned to receive 5AC (n = 179) or conventional care regimens (n = 179). After a median follow-up of 21.1 months (interquartile range [IQR] 15.1 to 26.9), median overall survival was 24.5 months (9.9 not reached) for the azacitidine group versus 15.0 months (5.6 to 24.1) for the conventional care group (hazard ratio [HR] 0.58; 95% confidence interval [CI], 0.43 to 0.77; p = 0.0001). At 2 years, on the basis of Kaplan-Meier estimates, 50.8% (95% CI, 42.1 to 58.8) of patients in the 5AC group were

alive compared with 26.2% (95% CI, 18.7 to 34.3) in the conventional care group (p < 0.0001). Median time to AML transformation was 17.8 months (IQR 8.6 to 36.8; 95% CI, 13.6 to 23.6) in the 5AC group compared with 11.5 months (4.9 not reached; 8.3 to 14.5) in the conventional care group (HR 0.50; 95% CI, 0.35 to 0.70; p < 0.0001). Subsequent unplanned analyses of AZA001 included an examination of elderly patients with what would now be classified as AML (blast count 20% to 30%). In these 113 patients, there remains a statistically significant improvement in survival of 24.5 months versus 16.0 months (HR 0.47; 95% CI; p = 0.0001).[117]

The early development of decitabine in MDS took place primarily in Europe under the leadership of Wijermans et al.[118,119] These investigators pursued intravenous scheduling of decitabine administered three times daily for 3 days (45 mg/m^2 per day total dose). This cycle was repeated every 6 weeks. Phase 2 studies suggested a response rate of approximately 50% in MDS patients. In a randomized trial of DAC versus observation, patients with International Prognostic Score risk categories intermediate 1 to high received the previously listed schedule of decitabine or observation. No crossover was allowed in this trial. Response rates reported were: complete response: 9%, partial response: 8%, and hematologic improvement: 13%.[120] A 10% induction death rate occurred, suggesting that this schedule of DAC may be more toxic than the CALGB schedule of 5AC (1% induction mortality). DAC has also been investigated in low-dose daily intravenous dosing[121] and in daily-times-five schedules. The latter appears convenient and well tolerated. A daily-times-five schedule (20 mg/m^2 per day) has been FDA approved[121]; 99 patients with MDS (de novo or secondary) of any French-American-British (FAB) subtype and an International Prognostic Scoring System (IPSS) score equal to or greater than 0.5 were treated, with an overall response rate of 32% (17 complete responses [CR] plus 15 marrow CRs [mCR]).[122] Among patients who improved, 82% demonstrated responses by the end of cycle two. This well-tolerated regimen allows outpatient administration and, as noted previously, provides plasma levels of decitabine that inhibit DNMTs.

The 3-day intravenous schedule of DAC has been studied in two randomized trials compared to supportive care in patients with higher risk MDS. The first trial confirmed the hematologic activity of decitabine in this patient population but failed to show an improvement in survival in the DAC-treated patients.[123] Survival was also not increased in the subsequent trial, performed by the European Organization for Research and Treatment of Cancer (EORTC).[124] The failure of the randomized decitabine trials to show a survival benefit may be partially due to study design. Both randomized trials of 5AC continued treatment until disease progression for patients who did not achieve complete remission; in fact, this meant that most patients received maintenance therapy. In contrast, both randomized trials of decitabine allowed a maximum of eight cycles of treatment. The need for maintenance therapy in patients treated with DNMT inhibitors has not been tested in prospective randomized trials. An additional difference in the conduct of the two sets of DNMT inhibitor trials involves the duration of therapy administered. The median number of cycles of treatment administered in the two randomized trials of decitabine was three, compared to nine in the azacytidine trials. This may reflect greater toxicity of the originally 3-day schedule of decitabine compared to that of the approved schedule of 5AC. Although the differences in survival may reflect differences in trial design and trial conduct, emerging data suggests that despite similarities in methylation reversal, the two drugs differ in other potentially important biologic parameters, which may contribute to clinical outcomes.[62,63,125]

Two randomized phase 3 trials have been published treating elderly AML patients (greater than 20% blasts) with decitabine, both demonstrating improvement in survival that was not statistically significant. In the European study, 233 patients received either

DAC at 15 mg/m^2 × 9 doses over 3 days on 42-day cycles or best supportive care. The patients received a median of 4 cycles (0 to 9), and the overall survival was improved in the decitabine-treated patients, but did not reach statistical significance (median overall survival [OS], 10.1 versus 8.5 months, respectively; HR, 0.88; 95% CI, 0.66 to 1.17; two-sided, log-rank p = 0.38).[126] In the M.D. Anderson Cancer Center–led multicenter trial,[127] 485 patients 65 years or older were randomly assigned to receive decitabine 20 mg/m^2 per day as a 1-hour intravenous infusion for 5 consecutive days every 4 weeks or best supportive care or low-dose cytarabine (20 mg/m^2 per day for 10 days every 4 weeks). There was a similar improvement in OS with decitabine (7.7 months; 95% CI, 6.2 to 9.2) versus the control group (5.0 months; 95% CI, 4.3 to 6.3; p = 0.108; HR, 0.85; 95% CI, 0.69 to 1.04).[127]

The azacytosine nucleosides require prolonged administration to demonstrate hematologic improvement in MDS. Median time to development of first clinical response in the CALGB studies of 5AC was three cycles; 90% of responses developed by cycle six.[114] In the phase 3 trial of decitabine, the median time to response was two cycles,[123] as also seen in the alternative regimen of decitabine.[122] It is, therefore, extremely important when treating patients with azacytosine nucleosides to commit to administering between four and six cycles of therapy before determining whether a patient is responding to treatment. Furthermore, survival benefit is seen even in patients not showing bone marrow improvement for 5AC, perhaps related to decreased transfusion requirements or delayed progression to AML.[116]

Because AML in the context of MDS is arbitrarily defined based on marrow blast count, activity of the azanucleoside analogs in AML should not be surprising. In CALGB 9221, 20 patients were reclassified upon central pathology review as meeting criteria for AML (greater than 30% blasts). Their outcomes were comparable to the overall population in the study.[115] In all three CALGB studies among patients meeting current World Health Organization (WHO) criteria for AML (greater than 20% blasts), a complete response was achieved in 9% and hematologic improvement in 26%.[114] A retrospective review of 20 patients with AML, including 8 patients with bone marrow blasts greater than 29% treated with 5AC, reported a complete remission in 4 patients, a partial response in 5, and a hematologic improvement in 3. The median duration of response was 8 months (range: 3 to 33 months).[128] DAC induced a complete hematologic response in 2 of 20 patients treated who had the blastic phase of chronic myeloid leukemia.[129] These studies suggest activity of the azacytosine nucleosides in the treatment of a subset of AML patients. Current studies do not allow for the determination of whether this subset is limited to MDS-associated AML (AML with MDS-related changes), which tends to have low white blood cell counts and have a low proliferative rate, or whether these compounds are also active for those with AML without a history of antecedent hematologic disorder. Several reports describe the sensitivity MDS and AML, characterized by abnormalities of chromosome 7 and associated with poor outcomes in response to cytarabine-based therapy to azanucleosides. In one nonrandomized retrospective study, survival of such patients following the administration of DNMT inhibitors surpassed survival in response to conventional cytotoxic chemotherapy, similar to the outcomes of AZA001.[130–132]

Although the mechanisms underlying the clinical activity of azacytosine analogs may involve reversal of gene methylation, other actions need to be considered. The administration of DAC has been shown to induce transient decrements of methylation in noncoding regions, including long interspersed nuclear element (LINE) and ALU elements.[133] Early studies that examined methylation reversal of the target gene p15^{INK4B} in response to DAC showed no correlation between methylation reversal and clinical response.[134,135] Clinical responders to DAC developed significantly higher expression of this gene following treatment, and certainly

key biologic roles for this gene and its low basal expression are probable. Moreover, in one study, the clinical response was closely associated with the reversal of methylation of p15 or CDH-1 during the first cycle of treatment with 5AC followed by the HDACi NaPB.[25] In that study, it was noteworthy that the administration of 5AC prior to the addition of an HDACi was associated with the induction of histone acetylation. Although the mechanism underlying this activity is unknown, histone acetylation has been observed following DNA damage due to gamma irradiation.[136] Subsequent studies have found demethylation following treatment with either DAC or 5AC[137–140] but not consistently associated with response.[137,138,140] More work will be required to answer the important mechanistic question underpinning the clinical activity of azacytosine analogs.

Combining Inhibitors in the Treatment of Hematologic Malignancies

It is almost certain that the biggest promise of epigenetic therapy lies in strategies to combine existing and newer drugs with each other and with current chemotherapies and targeted therapies. To date, the example for existing agents is the combination of DNMT inhibitors and HDAC inhibitors based on the hypothesis from the laboratory that this paradigm leads to optimal reexpression of transcriptionally silenced genes with promoter methylation.[56,141] This in vitro treatment paradigm has led to a variety of clinical studies that have attempted to apply this concept to the treatment of hematologic malignancies. Much remains to be determined with regard to its efficacy and precisely what determines this. The first study of sequential DNMT/HDAC inhibitors administered a variety of doses of 5AC for 5 to 14 days followed by 7 days of NaPB by continuous infusion at its maximum tolerated dose to patients with MDS and AML.[25] The combination was well tolerated, and clinical responses were frequent in patients receiving 5AC at 50 mg/m^2 per day daily for 10 days and 25 mg/m^2 per day daily for 14 days, with 5 of 14 patients at those dose schedules achieving complete or partial response.

In a pilot study, 10 patients with MDS or AML were treated with 5AC at 75 mg/m^2 per day daily times seven followed by 5 days of NaPB given at 200 mg per kilogram per day as a 1- to 2-hour infusion. Three patients developed a partial response.[142]

In a similar study, investigators at the M.D. Anderson Cancer Center treated leukemic patients with decitabine (15 mg/m^2 per day IV daily times 10) and concomitant VPA at a variety of doses. Of 54 patients, 12 achieved complete remission or complete remission with incomplete platelet recovery.[143] The inhibitors 5AC, VPA, and all-transretinoic acid have been administered to patients with AML and MDS. Of 33 previously untreated patients, 14 over the age of 60 years developed a complete remission or a complete remission with inadequate platelet recovery.[144] A subsequent study of 5AC and VPA suggests increased efficacy of this combination in high-risk MDS.[145]

Entinostat has been successfully combined with azacytidine in patients with myeloid malignancies.[140] The US Leukemia Intergroup recently completed a randomized phase 2 trial of this combination compared with 5AC alone. In this study, of 149 patients, the primary endpoint of hematologic normalization was statistically similar, with 32% (95% CI, 22% to 44%) of the 5AC group reaching hematologic normalization (HN) versus 27% (95% CI, 17% to 39%) in the AZA + entinostat group. Median overall survivals were 18 months for the AZA group and 13 months for the AZA + entinostat group, but were also not statistically significant.[108] In the latter study, the administration of the combination was associated with less DNA methylation reversal compared to azacitidine monotherapy, likely due to cell cycle inhibitory effects of the HDACi. This highlights the complexity of effectively targeting epigenetic gene regulation.

It remains to be established whether combination therapies are more effective than single-agent demethylating therapies.

Epigenetically Targeted Therapy in Nonhematologic Malignancies

The efficacies that have emerged in the application of epigenetically targeted drugs to hematologic malignancies has spurred interest in using epigenetic therapy for other types of cancer. As outlined as follows, laboratory studies and clinical trials support this approach. Studies in the lab have been directed by lessons learned from therapy in hematologic malignancies, suggesting that low doses of drugs like DAC and 5AC, in the nanomolar range, may avoid excess toxicities due to off-target effects of the drugs and may maximize epigenetic effects of the agents.[28] The desired effects may require minimizing initial cellular cytotoxicity, giving tumor cells time to accrue maximal cellular reprogramming responses to the inhibition of DNMTs.[28] DAC and 5AC are effective only when they have been incorporated into DNA, after which they irreversibly inhibit DNMT catalytic activity and target these proteins for degradation.[64–68] In cell culture and mouse explants, low nanomolar doses appear to induce both human leukemic and solid tumor cells to exhibit blunting of self-renewal and tumorigenic activity of tumor stem-like cells.[28] These preclinical results suggest a key possibility that use of epigenetic therapies might inhibit these latter cell populations, which often are difficult to eradicate and are a factor in resistance to many standard cancer therapies.[146] Exhaustion of such cells over time during therapy with DAC or 5AC might explain the observation that most patients with MDS/AML take several months to reach best response.[147] Leukemic stem cells were not eliminated in one study in MDS and AML patients treated with 5AC in combination with VPA, although their frequency decreased in clinical responders.[148]

Clinical trials for common solid tumors, informed through the previous laboratory studies, have been initiated including phase 2 designs using low-dose strategies with 5AC often combined with use of histone deacetylase inhibitors. Sixty-five patients with advanced, multiply treated NSCLCs were treated with 5AC plus entinostat.[149] Only 3% of patients developed Response Evaluation Criteria (RECIST)-measureable responses; however, these two patients had durable responses, with survival of 3 to 4 years.[149] Upregulation of immunogenic pathways in NSCLC and other solid tumor cells, observed in laboratory studies, suggest a potential for sequencing DNMT inhibitors with immune checkpoint inhibitors.[150] This drug is also reported to induce antitumor responses and immune recognition in a model of pancreatic cancer.[151] Other laboratory results and emerging clinical trials also suggest the promise of combining epigenetic therapy approaches to sensitize cancers other than NSCLC to subsequent therapies. Low-dose DAC appears able to upregulate a key mediator of 5-fluorouracil (5FU) action,

uridine monophosphate (UMP) kinase, in colorectal cancer cell lines.[152] These increases correlated with a reversal of 5FU resistance. Similar to studies discussed previously, DAC plus the HDACi, trichostatin A, decreased marker identified self-renewal populations in ovarian cancer while simultaneously inducing increased sensitivity to cisplatin.[153] In advanced ovarian cancer, 5AC or DAC plus carboplatin have yielded durable responses and induced stable disease in ovarian cancer patients.[154,155] These early results are being extrapolated for verification in larger, ongoing clinical trials.

NEW APROACHES TO EPIGENETIC THERAPY

As we have outlined previously, the emerging promise for epigenetic therapy and the future of the approaches may lie in combinatorial drug strategies. Although this is already being explored with older agents, new drugs for new targets are now entering the picture.[9,11,156–158] In these efforts, several themes we have introduced in this chapter will likely dominate.

Most epigenetic therapies will not induce, when used at truly targeting doses, immediate cytotoxic effects. Therapeutic efficacy based on cellular reprogramming may require significant time to manifest. Clinical trial designs may need adaptation so that effective therapies are not discarded due to premature response evaluations. Finally, the ultimate promise for epigenetic therapy may lie with newer drugs now entering clinical trials. Outcomes with DNMT inhibitors may be improved with alternative scheduling of oral azacitidine or through prolonged pharmacokinetics of the decitabine prodrug SGI110.[79] Also, drugs targeting other proteins including BET family bromodomain proteins are generating much excitement.[9,82,156–159] BET inhibitors may interfere with localization of the oncogene C-MYC to acetylated lysines in regulatory regions of target genes.[9,82,156–159] These inhibitors are now entering clinical trials. Other promising approaches include the use of inhibitors of EZH2, the enzyme in the PcG system, which catalyzes the repressive histone mark H3K27me3.[9,82,156–159] Another clinical trial underway employs targeting of the translocation in which the protein mixed lineage leukemia (MLL) is fused with several targets, such as in infant leukemias. These translocations result in abnormal recruitment of the histone methyltransferase, DOT1L, to target genes like HOXA9.[158] This fusion induces hypermethylation of H3K79 and abnormal activation of MLL target genes.[158,160] Very selective inhibitors of DOT1L are now in clinical trials.

Epigenetically targeted therapies continue to hold great promise that reprogramming of malignant cells could alter approaches to cancer management. Strategies to merge older drugs, which we have focused on in this chapter, with the newer agents briefly discussed in this section, will underpin future trials to test this approach.

REFERENCES

1. Bernstein BE, Meissner A, Lander ES. The mammalian epigenome. *Cell* 2007;128:669–681.
2. Young RA. Control of the embryonic stem cell state. *Cell* 2011;144:940–954.
3. Suva ML, Riggi N, Bernstein BE. Epigenetic reprogramming in cancer. *Science* 2013;339:1567–1570.
4. Herman JG, Baylin SB. Gene silencing in cancer in association with promoter hypermethylation. *N Engl J Med* 2003;349:2042–2054.
5. Jones PA, Baylin SB. The epigenomics of cancer. *Cell* 2007;128:683–692.
6. Baylin SB, Jones PA. A decade of exploring the cancer epigenome — biological and translational implications. *Nat Rev Cancer* 2011;11:726–734.
7. Esteller M. Cancer epigenomics: DNA methylomes and histone-modification maps. *Nat Rev Genet* 2007;8:286–298.
8. Yoo CB, Jones PA. Epigenetic therapy of cancer: past, present and future. *Nat Rev Drug Discov* 2006;5:37–50.
9. Dawson MA, Kouzarides T. Cancer epigenetics: from mechanism to therapy. *Cell* 2012;150:12–27.
10. Dawson MA, Kouzarides T, Huntly BJ. Targeting epigenetic readers in cancer. *N Engl J Med* 2012;367:647–657.
11. Bradner J. New targets for hematologic malignancies. *Clin Adv Hematol Oncol* 2013;11:375–376.
12. You JS, Jones PA. Cancer genetics and epigenetics: two sides of the same coin? *Cancer Cell* 2012;22:9–20.
13. Allis C, Jenuwein T, Reinberg D. *Epigenetics*, Vol. 1. Cold Spring Harbor, NY: Cold Spring Harbor Laboratory Press; 2007.

CANCER THERAPEUTICS

14. Kouzarides T. Chromatin modifications and their function. *Cell* 2007;128: 693–705.

15. Baylin SB, Jones PA. Epigenetic determinants of cancer. In: Allis CD, Jenuwein T, Reinberg D, eds. *Epigenetics.* Cold Spring Harbor, NY: Cold Spring Harbor Laboratory Press; 2006: 457–476.

16. Bird AP. CpG-rich islands and the function of DNA methylation. *Nature* 1986;321:209–213.

17. Morey L, Pascual G, Cozzuto L, et al. Nonoverlapping functions of the Polycomb group Cbx family of proteins in embryonic stem cells. *Cell Stem Cell* 2012;10:47–62.

18. Easwaran H, Johnstone SE, Van Neste L, et al. A DNA hypermethylation module for the stem/progenitor cell signature of cancer. *Genome Res* 2012;22: 837–849.

19. Irizarry RA, Ladd-Acosta C, Wen B, et al. The human colon cancer methylome shows similar hypo- and hypermethylation at conserved tissue-specific CpG island shores. *Nat Genet* 2009;41:178–186.

20. Doi A, Park IH, Wen B, et al. Differential methylation of tissue- and cancer-specific CpG island shores distinguishes human induced pluripotent stem cells, embryonic stem cells and fibroblasts. *Nat Genet* 2009;41:1350–1353.

21. Herman JG, Merlo A, Mao L, et al. Inactivation of the CDKN2/p16/MTS1 gene is frequently associated with aberrant DNA methylation in all common human cancers. *Cancer Res* 1995;55:4525–4530.

22. Merlo A, Herman JG, Mao L, et al. 5′ CpG island methylation is associated with transcriptional silencing of the tumour suppressor p16/CDKN2/MTS1 in human cancers. *Nat Med* 1995;1:686–692.

23. Herman JG, Civin CI, Issa JP, et al. Distinct patterns of inactivation of p15INK4B and p16INK4A characterize the major types of hematological malignancies. *Cancer Res* 1997;57:837–841.

24. Costello JF, Fruhwald MC, Smiraglia DJ, et al. Aberrant CpG-island methylation has non-random and tumour-type-specific patterns. *Nat Genet* 2000;24:132–138.

25. Gore SD, Baylin S, Sugar E, et al. Combined DNA methyltransferase and histone deacetylase inhibition in the treatment of myeloid neoplasms. *Cancer Res* 2006;66:6361–6369.

26. Azad N, Zahnow CA, Rudin CM, et al. The future of epigenetic therapy in solid tumours—lessons from the past. *Nat Rev Clin Oncol* 2013;10:256–266.

27. Issa JP, Kantarjian HM. Targeting DNA methylation. *Clin Cancer Res* 2009;15:3938–3946.

28. Tsai HC, Li H, Van Neste L, et al. Transient low doses of DNA-demethylating agents exert durable antitumor effects on hematological and epithelial tumor cells. *Cancer Cell* 2012;21:430–446.

29. Takai D, Jones PA. Comprehensive analysis of CpG islands in human chromosomes 21 and 22. *Proc Natl Acad Sci U S A* 2002;99:3740–3745.

30. Futscher BW, Oshiro MM, Wozniak RJ, et al. Role for DNA methylation in the control of cell type specific maspin expression. *Nat Genet* 2002;31:175–179.

31. Feldmann A, Ivanek R, Murr R, et al. Transcription factor occupancy can mediate active turnover of DNA methylation at regulatory regions. *PLoS Genet* 2013;9:e1003994.

32. Aran D, Hellman A. Unmasking risk loci: DNA methylation illuminates the biology of cancer predisposition: analyzing DNA methylation of transcriptional enhancers reveals missed regulatory links between cancer risk loci and genes. *Bioessays* 2014;36:184–190.

33. Ziller MJ, Gu H, Muller F, et al. Charting a dynamic DNA methylation landscape of the human genome. *Nature* 2013;500:477–481.

34. Akhtar-Zaidi B, Cowper-Sal-lari R, Corradin O, et al. Epigenomic enhancer profiling defines a signature of colon cancer. *Science* 2012;336:736–739.

35. Kingston R, Tamkun JW. Transcriptional regulation by trithorax group. In: Allis CD, Jenuwein T, Reinberd D, eds. *Epigenetics.* Cold Spring Harbor, NY: Cold Spring Harbor Laboratory Press; 2006: 231–248.

36. Becker PB, Workman JL. Nucleosome remodeling and epigenetics. *Cold Spring Harb Perspect Biol* 2013;5.

37. Petty E, Pillus L. Balancing chromatin remodeling and histone modifications in transcription. *Trends Genet* 2013;29:621–629.

38. Jones PA. Functions of DNA methylation: islands, start sites, gene bodies and beyond. *Nat Rev Genet* 2012;13:484–492.

39. Bannister AJ, Kouzarides T. Reversing histone methylation. *Nature* 2005; 436:1103–1106.

40. Bannister AJ, Kouzarides T. Regulation of chromatin by histone modifications. *Cell Res* 2011;21:381–395.

41. Di Leva G, Garofalo M, Croce CM. MicroRNAs in cancer. *Annu Rev Pathol* 2014;9:287–314.

42. Han BW, Chen YQ. Potential pathological and functional links between long noncoding RNAs and hematopoiesis. *Sci Signal* 2013;6:re5.

43. Xi JJ. MicroRNAs in Cancer. *Cancer Treat Res* 2013;158:119–137.

44. Nan X, Ng HH, Johnson CA, et al. Transcriptional repression by the methyl-CpG-binding protein MeCP2 involves a histone deacetylase complex. *Nature* 1998;393:386–389.

45. Jones PL, Veenstra GJ, Wade PA, et al. Methylated DNA and MeCP2 recruit histone deacetylase to repress transcription. *Nat Genet* 1998;19:187–191.

46. Parry L, Clarke AR. The Roles of the Methyl-CpG Binding Proteins in Cancer. *Genes Cancer* 2011;2:618–630.

47. Lopez-Serra L, Esteller M. Proteins that bind methylated DNA and human cancer: reading the wrong words. *Br J Cancer* 2008;98:1881–1885.

48. Cai Y, Geutjes EJ, de Lint K, et al. The NuRD complex cooperates with DNMTs to maintain silencing of key colorectal tumor suppressor genes. *Oncogene* 2014;33:2157–2168.

49. Bestor TH. Cloning of a mammalian DNA methyltransferase. *Gene* 1998; 74:9–12.

50. Jair KW, Bachman KE, Suzuki H, et al. De novo CpG island methylation in human cancer cells. *Cancer Res* 2006;66:682–692.

51. Rius M, Lyko F. Epigenetic cancer therapy: rationales, targets and drugs. *Oncogene* 2012;31:4257–4265.

52. Jenuwein T, Allis CD. Translating the histone code. *Science* 2001;293: 1074–1080.

53. Bolden JE, Peart MJ, Johnstone RW. Anticancer activities of histone deacetylase inhibitors. *Nat Rev Drug Discov* 2006;5:769–784.

54. Vaquero A, Scher M, Erdjument-Bromage H, et al. SIRT1 regulates the histone methyl-transferase SUV39H1 during heterochromatin formation. *Nature* 2007;450:440–444.

55. Pruitt K, Zinn RL, Ohm JE, et al. Inhibition of SIRT1 reactivates silenced cancer genes without loss of promoter DNA hypermethylation. *PLoS Genet* 2006;2:344–352.

56. Cameron EE, Bachman KE, Myohanen S, et al. Synergy of demethylation and histone deacetylase inhibition in the re-expression of genes silenced in cancer. *Nat Genet* 1999;21:103–107.

57. Sorm F, Piskala A, Cihak A, et al. 5-Azacytidine, a new, highly effective cancer-ostatic. *Experientia* 1964;20:202–203.

58. Taylor SM, Jones PA. Multiple new phenotypes induced in 10T1/2 and 3T3 cells treated with 5-azacytidine. *Cell* 1979;17:771–779.

59. Jones PA, Taylor SM. Hemimethylated duplex DNAs prepared from 5-azacytidine-treated cells. *Nucleic Acids Res* 1981;9:2933–2947.

60. Lu SH, Ohshima H, Bartsch H. Recent studies on N-nitroso compounds as possible etiological factors in oesophageal cancer. *IARC Sci Publ* 1984;947–953.

61. Taylor SM, Jones PA. Mechanism of action of eukaryotic DNA methyltransferase. Use of 5-azacytosine-containing DNA. *J Mol Biol* 1982;162:679–692.

62. Schaefer M, Hagemann S, Hanna K, et al. Azacytidine inhibits RNA methylation at DNMT2 target sites in human cancer cell lines. *Cancer Res* 2009; 69:8127–8132.

63. Hollenbach PW, Nguyen AN, Brady H, et al. A comparison of azacitidine and decitabine activities in acute myeloid leukemia cell lines. *PLoS One* 2010; 5:e9001.

64. Kelly TK, De Carvalho DD, Jones PA. Epigenetic modifications as therapeutic targets. *Nat Biotechnol* 2010;28:1069–1078.

65. Ferguson AT, Vertino PM, Spitzner JR, et al. Role of estrogen receptor gene demethylation and DNA methyltransferase. DNA adduct formation in 5-aza-2′deoxycytidine-induced cytotoxicity in human breast cancer cells. *J Biol Chem* 1997;272:32260–32266.

66. Gabbara S, Bhagwat AS. The mechanism of inhibition of DNA (cytosine-5-)-methyltransferases by 5-azacytosine is likely to involve methyl transfer to the inhibitor. *Biochem J* 1995;307:87–92.

67. Santi DV, Norment A, Garrett CE. Covalent bond formation between a DNA-cytosine methyltransferase and DNA containing 5-azacytosine. *Proc Natl Acad Sci U S A* 1984;81:6993–6997.

68. Ghoshal K, Datta J, Majumder S, et al. 5-Aza-deoxycytidine induces selective degradation of DNA methyltransferase 1 by a proteasomal pathway that requires the KEN box, bromo-adjacent homology domain, and nuclear localization signal. *Mol Cell Biol* 2005;25:4727–4741.

69. Rountree MR, Bachman KE, Baylin SB. DNMT1 binds HDAC2 and a new co-repressor, DMAP1, to form a complex at replication foci. *Nat Genet* 2000;25:269–277.

70. Bachman KE, Rountree MR, Baylin SB. Dnmt3a and Dnmt3b are transcriptional repressors that exhibit unique localization properties to heterochromatin. *J Biol Chem* 2001;276:32282–32287.

71. Jones PA, Taylor SM. Cellular differentiation, cytidine analogs and DNA methylation. *Cell* 1980;20:85–93.

72. Berg T, Guo Y, Abdelkarim M, et al. Reversal of p15/INK4b hypermethylation in AML1/ETO-positive and -negative myeloid leukemia cell lines. *Leuk Res* 2007;31:497–506.

73. Flatau E, Gonzales FA, Michalowsky LA, et al. DNA methylation in 5-aza-2′-deoxycytidine-resistant variants of C3H 10T1/2 C18 cells. *Mol Cell Biol* 1984;4:2098–2102.

74. Chan KK, Giannini DD, Staroscik JA, et al. 5-Azacytidine hydrolysis kinetics measured by high-pressure liquid chromatography and 13C-NMR spectroscopy. *J Pharm Sci* 1979;68:807–812.

75. Gore SD, Weng LJ, Figg WD, et al. Impact of prolonged infusions of the putative differentiating agent sodium phenylbutyrate on myelodysplastic syndromes and acute myeloid leukemia. *Clin Cancer Res* 2002;8:963–970.

76. Yu L, Liu C, Vandeusen J, et al. Global assessment of promoter methylation in a mouse model of cancer identifies ID4 as a putative tumor-suppressor gene in human leukemia. *Nat Genet* 2005;37:265–274.

77. Blum W, Klisovic RB, Hackanson B, et al. Phase I study of decitabine alone or in combination with valproic acid in acute myeloid leukemia. *J Clin Oncol* 2007;25:3884–3891.

78. Schrump DS, Fischette MR, Nguyen DM, et al. Phase I study of decitabine-mediated gene expression in patients with cancers involving the lungs, esophagus, or pleura. *Clin Cancer Res* 2006;12:5777–5785.

79. Garcia-Manero G, Gore SD, Cogle C, et al. Phase I study of oral azacitidine in myelodysplastic syndromes, chronic myelomonocytic leukemia, and acute myeloid leukemia. *J Clin Oncol* 2011;29:2521–2527.

80. Issa JP, Roboz G, Rizzieri D, et al. Abstract LB-214: Interim results from a randomized Phase 1-2 first-in-human (FIH) study of PK/PD guided escalating doses of SGI-110, a novel subcutaneous (SQ) second generation hypomethylating

agent (HMA) in relapsed/refractory MDS and AML. *Cancer Res* 2012;72: LB–214.

81. Mund C, Lyko F. Epigenetic cancer therapy: Proof of concept and remaining challenges. *Bioessays* 2010;32:949–957.

82. Popovic R, Licht JD. Emerging epigenetic targets and therapies in cancer medicine. *Cancer Discov* 2012;2:405–413.

83. Verbrugge I, Johnstone RW, Bots M. Promises and challenges of anticancer drugs that target the epigenome. *Epigenomics* 2011;3:547–565.

84. Robert C, Rassool FV. HDAC inhibitors: roles of DNA damage and repair. *Adv Cancer Res* 2012;116:87–129.

85. Kachhap SK, Rosmus N, Collis SJ, et al. Downregulation of homologous recombination DNA repair genes by HDAC inhibition in prostate cancer is mediated through the E2F1 transcription factor. *PLoS One* 2010;5:e11208.

86. Sharma SV, Lee DY, Li B, et al. A chromatin-mediated reversible drug-tolerant state in cancer cell subpopulations. *Cell* 2010;141:69–80.

87. Villanueva J, Vultur A, Lee JT, et al. Acquired resistance to BRAF inhibitors mediated by a RAF kinase switch in melanoma can be overcome by cotargeting MEK and IGF-1R/PI3K. *Cancer Cell* 2010;18:683–695.

88. Novogrodsky A, Dvir A, Ravid A, et al. Effect of polar organic compounds on leukemic cells. Butyrate-induced partial remission of acute myelogenous leukemia in a child. *Cancer* 1983;51:9–14.

89. Miller AA, Kurschel E, Osieka R, et al. Clinical pharmacology of sodium butyrate in patients with acute leukemia. *Eur J Cancer Clin Oncol* 1987; 23:1283–1287.

90. Gore SD, Weng LJ, Zhai S, et al. Impact of the putative differentiating agent sodium phenylbutyrate on myelodysplastic syndromes and acute myeloid leukemia. *Clin Cancer Res* 2001;7:2330–2339.

91. Gore SD, Weng LJ, Figg WD, et al. Impact of prolonged infusions of the putative differentiating agent sodium phenylbutyrate on myelodysplastic syndromes and acute myeloid leukemia. *Clin Cancer Res* 2002;8:963–970.

92. DiGiuseppe JA, Weng LJ, Yu KH, et al. Phenylbutyrate-induced G1 arrest and apoptosis in myeloid leukemia cells: structure-function analysis. *Leukemia* 1999;13:1243–1253.

93. Kuendgen A, Strupp C, Aivado M, et al. Treatment of myelodysplastic syndromes with valproic acid alone or in combination with all-trans retinoic acid. *Blood* 2004;104:1266–1269.

94. Pilatrino C, Cilloni D, Messa E, et al. Increase in platelet count in older, poor-risk patients with acute myeloid leukemia or myelodysplastic syndrome treated with valproic acid and all-trans retinoic acid. *Cancer* 2005;104:101–109.

95. Fizzotti M, Cimino G, Pisegna S, et al. Detection of homozygous deletions of the cyclin-dependent kinase 4 inhibitor (p16) gene in acute lymphoblastic leukemia and association with adverse prognostic features. *Blood* 1995; 85:2685–2690.

96. Xu GL, Bestor TH, Bourc'his D, et al. Chromosome instability and immunodeficiency syndrome caused by mutations in a DNA methyltransferase gene. *Nature* 1999;402:187–191.

97. Duvic M, Talpur R, Ni X, et al. Phase 2 trial of oral vorinostat (suberoylanilide hydroxamic acid, SAHA) for refractory cutaneous T-cell lymphoma (CTCL). *Blood* 2007;109:31–39.

98. Olsen EA, Kim YH, Kuzel TM, et al. Phase IIb multicenter trial of vorinostat in patients with persistent, progressive, or treatment refractory cutaneous T-cell lymphoma. *J Clin Oncol* 2007;25:3109–3115.

99. O'Connor OA, Heaney ML, Schwartz L, et al. Clinical experience with intravenous and oral formulations of the novel histone deacetylase inhibitor suberoylanilide hydroxamic acid in patients with advanced hematologic malignancies. *J Clin Oncol* 2006;24:166–173.

100. Ramalingam SS, Maitland ML, Frankel P, et al. Carboplatin and Paclitaxel in combination with either vorinostat or placebo for first-line therapy of advanced non-small-cell lung cancer. *J Clin Oncol* 2010;28:56–62.

101. Giles F, Fischer T, Cortes J, et al. A phase I study of intravenous LBH589, a novel cinnamic hydroxamic acid analogue histone deacetylase inhibitor, in patients with refractory hematologic malignancies. *Clin Cancer Res* 2006; 12:4628–4635.

102. Richardson PG, Hungria VTM, Yoon S-S, et al. Panorama 1: A randomized, double-blind, phase 3 study of panobinostat or placebo plus bortezomib and dexamethasone in relapsed or relapsed and refractory multiple myeloma. *ASCO Meeting Abstracts* 2014;32:8510.

103. Piekarz RL, Robey R, Sandor V, et al. Inhibitor of histone deacetylation, depsipeptide (FR901228), in the treatment of peripheral and cutaneous T-cell lymphoma: a case report. *Blood* 2001;98:2865–2868.

104. Coiffier B, Pro B, Prince HM, et al. Romidepsin for the treatment of relapsed/refractory peripheral T-cell lymphoma: pivotal study update demonstrates durable responses. *J Hematol Oncol* 2014;7:11.

105. Coiffier B, Pro B, Prince HM, et al. Results from a pivotal, open-label, phase II study of romidepsin in relapsed or refractory peripheral T-cell lymphoma after prior systemic therapy. *J Clin Oncol* 2012;30:631–636.

106. Piekarz RL, Frye AR, Wright JJ, et al. Cardiac studies in patients treated with depsipeptide, FK228, in a phase II trial for T-cell lymphoma. *Clin Cancer Res* 2006;12:3762–3773.

107. Gojo I, Jiemjit A, Trepel JB, et al. Phase 1 and pharmacologic study of MS-275, a histone deacetylase inhibitor, in adults with refractory and relapsed acute leukemias. *Blood* 2007;109:2781–2790.

108. Prebet T, Sun Z, Figueroa ME, et al. Prolonged administration of azacitidine with or without entinostat for myelodysplastic syndrome and acute myeloid leukemia with myelodysplasia-related changes: results of the US Leukemia Intergroup Trial E1905. *J Clin Oncol* 2014;32:1242–1248.

109. Witta SE, Jotte RM, Konduri K, et al. Randomized phase II trial of erlotinib with and without entinostat in patients with advanced non-small-cell lung cancer who progressed on prior chemotherapy. *J Clin Oncol* 2012;30:2248–2255.

110. Yardley DA, Ismail-Khan RR, Melichar B, et al. Randomized phase II, double-blind, placebo-controlled study of exemestane with or without entinostat in postmenopausal women with locally recurrent or metastatic estrogen receptor-positive breast cancer progressing on treatment with a nonsteroidal aromatase inhibitor. *J Clin Oncol* 2013;31:2128–2135.

111. Byrd JC, Marcucci G, Parthun MR, et al. A phase 1 and pharmacodynamic study of depsipeptide (FK228) in chronic lymphocytic leukemia and acute myeloid leukemia. *Blood* 2005;105:959–967.

112. Charache S, Dover G, Smith K, et al. Treatment of sickle cell anemia with 5-azacytidine results in increased fetal hemoglobin production and is associated with nonrandom hypomethylation of DNA around the gamma-delta-beta-globin gene complex. *Proc Natl Acad Sci U S A* 1983;80:4842–4846.

113. Silverman LR, Holland JF, Weinberg RS, et al. Effects of treatment with 5-azacytidine on the in vivo and in vitro hematopoiesis in patients with myelodysplastic syndromes. *Leukemia* 1993;7:21–29.

114. Silverman LR, McKenzie DR, Peterson BL, et al. Further analysis of trials with azacitidine in patients with myelodysplastic syndrome: studies 8421, 8921, and 9221 by the Cancer and Leukemia Group B. *J Clin Oncol* 2006;24:3895–3903.

115. Silverman LR, Demakos EP, Peterson BL, et al. Randomized controlled trial of azacitidine in patients with the myelodysplastic syndrome: a study of the Cancer and Leukemia Group B. *J Clin Oncol* 2002;20:2429–2440.

116. Fenaux P, Mufti GJ, Hellstrom-Lindberg E, et al. Efficacy of azacitidine compared with that of conventional care regimens in the treatment of higher-risk myelodysplastic syndromes: a randomised, open-label, phase III study. *Lancet Oncol* 2009;10:223–232.

117. Fenaux P, Mufti GJ, Hellstrom-Lindberg E, et al. Azacitidine prolongs overall survival compared with conventional care regimens in elderly patients with low bone marrow blast count acute myeloid leukemia. *J Clin Oncol* 2010;28: 562–569.

118. Wijermans P, Lubbert M, Verhoef G, et al. Low-dose 5-aza-2'-deoxycytidine, a DNA hypomethylating agent, for the treatment of high-risk myelodysplastic syndrome: a multicenter phase II study in elderly patients. *J Clin Oncol* 2000;18:956–962.

119. Wijermans PW, Krulder JW, Huijgens PC, et al. Continuous infusion of low-dose 5-Aza-2'-deoxycytidine in elderly patients with high-risk myelodysplastic syndrome. *Leukemia* 1997;11:1–5.

120. Kantarjian HM, O'Brien S, Cortes J, et al. Results of decitabine (5-aza-2'deoxycytidine) therapy in 130 patients with chronic myelogenous leukemia. *Cancer* 2003;98:522–528.

121. Kantarjian H, Oki Y, Garcia-Manero G, et al. Results of a randomized study of 3 schedules of low-dose decitabine in higher-risk myelodysplastic syndrome and chronic myelomonocytic leukemia. *Blood* 2007;109:52–57.

122. Steensma DP, Baer MR, Slack JL, et al. Multicenter study of decitabine administered daily for 5 days every 4 weeks to adults with myelodysplastic syndromes: the alternative dosing for outpatient treatment (ADOPT) trial. *J Clin Oncol* 2009;27:3842–3848.

123. Kantarjian H, Issa JP, Rosenfeld CS, et al. Decitabine improves patient outcomes in myelodysplastic syndromes: results of a phase III randomized study. *Cancer* 2006;106:1794–1803.

124. WijerMans P, Suciu S, Baila L, et al. Low-dose decitabine versus best supportive care in elderly patients with intermediate or high risk MDS not eligible for intensive chemotherapy: final results of the randomized phase III study (06011) of the EORTC Leukemia and German MDS Study Groups. *ASH Annual Meeting Abstracts* 2008;112:226.

125. Flotho C, Claus R, Batz C, et al. The DNA methyltransferase inhibitors azacitidine, decitabine and zebularine exert differential effects on cancer gene expression in acute myeloid leukemia cells. *Leukemia* 2009;23:1019–1028.

126. Lübbert M, Suciu S, Baila L, et al. Low-dose decitabine versus best supportive care in elderly patients with intermediate- or high-risk myelodysplastic syndrome (MDS) ineligible for intensive chemotherapy: final results of the randomized phase III study (06011) of the European Organisation for Research and Treatment of Cancer Leukemia Group and the German MDS Study Group. *J Clin Oncol* 2011;29:1987–1996.

127. Kantarjian HM, Thomas XG, Dmoszynska A, et al. Multicenter, randomized, open-label, phase III trial of decitabine versus patient choice, with physician advice, of either supportive care or low-dose cytarabine for the treatment of older patients with newly diagnosed acute myeloid leukemia. *J Clin Oncol* 2012;30:2670–2677.

128. Sudan N, Rossetti JM, Shadduck RK, et al. Treatment of acute myelogenous leukemia with outpatient azacitidine. *Cancer* 2006;107:1839–1843.

129. Kantarjian HM, O'Brien SM, Keating M, et al. Results of decitabine therapy in the accelerated and blastic phases of chronic myelogenous leukemia. *Leukemia* 1997;11:1617–1620.

130. Ruter B, Wijermans P, Claus R, et al. Preferential cytogenetic response to continuous intravenous low-dose decitabine (DAC) administration in myelodysplastic syndrome with monosomy 7. *Blood* 2007;110:1080–1082.

131. Raj K, John A, Ho A, et al. CDKN2B methylation status and isolated chromosome 7 abnormalities predict responses to treatment with 5-azacytidine. *Leukemia* 2007;21:1937–1944.

132. Ravandi F, Issa JP, Garcia-Manero G, et al. Superior outcome with hypomethylating therapy in patients with acute myeloid leukemia and high-risk myelodysplastic syndrome and chromosome 5 and 7 abnormalities. *Cancer* 2009;115:5746–5751.

133. Yang AS, Doshi KD, Choi SW, et al. DNA methylation changes after 5-aza-2′-deoxycytidine therapy in patients with leukemia. *Cancer Res* 2006;66:5495–5503.

134. Yang AS, Estecio MR, Doshi K, et al. A simple method for estimating global DNA methylation using bisulfite PCR of repetitive DNA elements. *Nucleic Acids Res* 2004;32:e38.

135. Daskalakis M, Nguyen TT, Nguyen C, et al. Demethylation of a hypermethylated P15/INK4B gene in patients with myelodysplastic syndrome by 5-Aza-2′-deoxycytidine (decitabine) treatment. *Blood* 2002;100:2957–2964.

136. Bakkenist CJ, Kastan MB. DNA damage activates ATM through intermolecular autophosphorylation and dimer dissociation. *Nature* 2003;421:499–506.

137. Borthakur G, Ahdab SE, Ravandi F, et al. Activity of decitabine in patients with myelodysplastic syndrome previously treated with azacitidine. *Leuk Lymphoma* 2008;49:690–695.

138. Shen L, Kantarjian H, Guo Y, et al. DNA methylation predicts survival and response to therapy in patients with myelodysplastic syndromes. *J Clin Oncol* 2010;28:605–613.

139. Figueroa ME, Skrabanek L, Li Y, et al. MDS and secondary AML display unique patterns and abundance of aberrant DNA methylation. *Blood* 2009;114:3448–3458.

140. Fandy TE, Herman JG, Kerns P, et al. Early epigenetic changes and DNA damage do not predict clinical response in an overlapping schedule of 5-azacytidine and entinostat in patients with myeloid malignancies. *Blood* 2009;114:2764–2773.

141. Schuebel KE, Chen W, Cope L, et al. Comparing the DNA hypermethylome with gene mutations in human colorectal cancer. *PLoS Genet* 2007;3:1709–1723.

142. Maslak P, Chanel S, Camacho LH, et al. Pilot study of combination transcriptional modulation therapy with sodium phenylbutyrate and 5-azacytidine in patients with acute myeloid leukemia or myelodysplastic syndrome. *Leukemia* 2006;20:212–217.

143. Garcia-Manero G, Kantarjian HM, Sanchez-Gonzalez B, et al. Phase I/II study of the combination of 5-aza-2′-deoxycytidine with valproic acid in patients with leukemia. *Blood* 2006;108:3271–3279.

144. Soriano AO, Yang H, Faderl S, et al. Safety and clinical activity of the combination of 5-azacytidine, valproic acid, and all-trans retinoic acid in acute myeloid leukemia and myelodysplastic syndrome. *Blood* 2007;110:2302–2308.

145. Voso MT, Santini V, Finelli C, et al. Valproic acid at therapeutic plasma levels may increase 5-azacytidine efficacy in higher risk myelodysplastic syndromes. *Clin Cancer Res* 2009;15:5002–5007.

146. Sharma S, Kelly TK, Jones PA. Epigenetics in cancer. *Carcinogenesis* 2010;31:27–36.

147. Silverman LR, Fenaux P, Mufti GJ, et al. Continued azacitidine therapy beyond time of first response improves quality of response in patients with higher-risk myelodysplastic syndromes. *Cancer* 2011;117:2697–2702.

148. Craddock C, Quek L, Goardon N, et al. Azacitidine fails to eradicate leukemic stem/progenitor cell populations in patients with acute myeloid leukemia and myelodysplasia. *Leukemia* 2013;27:1028–1036.

149. Juergens RA, Wrangle J, Vendetti FP, et al. Combination epigenetic therapy has efficacy in patients with refractory advanced non-small cell lung cancer. *Cancer Discov* 2011;1: 598–607.

150. Wrangle J, Wang W, Koch A, et al. Alterations of immune response of Non-Small Cell Lung Cancer with Azacytidine. *Oncotarget* 2013;4:2067–2079.

151. Shakya R, Gonda TA, Quante M, et al. Hypomethylating therapy in an aggressive stroma-rich model of pancreatic carcinoma. *Cancer Res* 2013;73: 885–896.

152. Humeniuk R, Menon LG, Mishra PJ, et al. Decreased levels of UMP kinase as a mechanism of fluoropyrimidine resistance. *Mol Cancer Ther* 2009;8: 1037–1044.

153. Meng F, Sun G, Zhong M, et al. Anticancer efficacy of the combination of low-dose cisplatin and trichostatin A or 5-aza-2′-deoxycytidine in ovarian cancer cells. Paper presented at: 2012 ASCO Annual Meeting; 2012; Chicago, IL.

154. Matei D, Fang F, Shen C, et al. Epigenetic resensitization to platinum in ovarian cancer. *Cancer Res* 2012;72:2197–2205.

155. Fu S, Hu W, Iyer R, et al. Phase 1b-2a study to reverse platinum resistance through use of a hypomethylating agent, azacitidine, in patients with platinum-resistant or platinum-refractory epithelial ovarian cancer. *Cancer* 2011;117:1661–1669.

156. Chung CW, Coste H, White JH, et al. Discovery and characterization of small molecule inhibitors of the BET family bromodomains. *J Med Chem* 2011;54:3827–3838.

157. Bernt KM, Zhu N, Sinha AU, et al. MLL-rearranged leukemia is dependent on aberrant H3K79 methylation by DOT1L. *Cancer Cell* 2011;20:66–78.

158. Daigle SR, Olhava EJ, Therkelsen CA, et al. Selective killing of mixed lineage leukemia cells by a potent small-molecule DOT1L inhibitor. *Cancer Cell* 2011;20:53–65.

159. Spannhoff A, Hauser AT, Heinke R, et al. The emerging therapeutic potential of histone methyltransferase and demethylase inhibitors. *ChemMedChem* 2009;4:1568–1582.

160. Okada Y, Feng Q, Lin Y, et al. hDOT1L links histone methylation to leukemogenesis. *Cell* 2005;121:167–178.

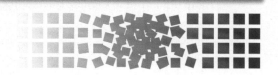

24 Proteasome Inhibitors

Christopher J. Kirk, Brian B. Tuch, Shirin Arastu-Kapur, and Lawrence H. Boise

BIOCHEMISTRY OF THE UBIQUITIN-PROTEASOME PATHWAY

The ubiquitin proteasome system is involved in the degradation of more than 80% of cellular proteins, including those that control cell-cycle progression, apoptosis, DNA repair, and the stress response.[1] A key step in this process is the *tagging* of proteins targeted for degradation with multiple copies of ubiquitin, a 76–amino acid protein whose primary sequence and structure is highly conserved in organisms ranging from yeasts to mammals.[2,3] Once polyubiquitinated, proteins targeted for degradation bind to the 26S proteasome, a holoenzyme composed of two 19S regulatory complexes capping a central 20S proteolytic core. The 20S core is a hollow "barrel" consisting of four stacked heptameric rings. The subunits of the rings are classified as either β subunits (outer two rings) or β subunits (inner two rings). The 19S regulatory complex consists of a lid that recognizes ubiquitinated protein substrates with high fidelity, and a base that contains six adenosine triphosphatases, unfolds protein substrates, removes the polyubiquitin tag, and threads them into the catalytic chamber of the 20S particle in an adenosine triphosphate–dependent manner.[4,5] Unlike typical proteases, the 20S proteasome in eukaryotic cells contains multiple proteolytic activities resulting in the cleavage of protein targets after many different amino acids. In most cells, the 20S core particle contains the catalytic subunits β5 (PSMB5), β1 (PSMB1), and β2 (PSMB2), accounting for chymotrypsin-like (CT-L), caspaselike (C-L), and trypsinlike (T-L) activities, respectively, each differing in their substrate preference.[6] However, in cells of hematopoietic origin, such as lymphocytes and monocytes, the proteasome catalytic subunits are encoded by homologous gene products: LMP7 (PSMB8), LMP2 (PSMB9), and MECL-1 (PSMB10).[7] These immunoproteasome subunits are also induced in nonhematopoietic cells following exposure to inflammatory cytokines such as interferon-γ (IFN-γ) and tumor necrosis factor alpha (TNF-α).[8] In the immunoproteasome, the 19S regulatory complex can be replaced with proteasome activators such as PA28, whose expression is also induced in cells following exposure to IFN-γ. Hybrid proteasomes, both for the catalytic subunits and regulatory particles, have been described.[9]

Given its key role in maintaining cellular homeostasis, the ubiquitin proteasome system appeared to be an unlikely target for pharmaceutical intervention. However, a variety of groundbreaking studies in the 1990s suggested that inhibitors of proteasome function might prove to be viable therapeutic agents.[10] Initial studies used substrate-related peptide aldehydes to investigate the proteolytic functions and specificity of the proteasome.[11] In vitro and in vivo studies with these inhibitors demonstrated their ability to induce apoptosis as well as inhibit tumor growth.[12–15] It was subsequently discovered that several natural products with antitumor activity exert their action via proteasome inhibition, providing additional rationale for the development of selective proteasome inhibitors (PIs).[16,17]

PROTEASOME INHIBITORS

Chemical Classes of Proteasome Inhibitors in Clinical Development

As of the writing of this overview, six different proteasome inhibitors comprising three distinct chemical classes have been tested in clinical trials (Table 24.1) and include: (1) dipeptide boronic acids, (2) peptide epoxy ketones, and (3) β-lactones.[18,19] Bortezomib (PS-341, Velcade), a dipeptide boronic acid, was developed by Millennium Pharmaceuticals (Cambridge, MA) and was the first PI approved for clinical use.[20] Two additional dipeptide boronic acids have entered clinical development, ixazomib/MLN 9708 (Millennium), currently in phase III studies, and delanzomib/CEP-18770 (Teva Pharmaceuticals; Frazer, PA), the clinical development of which has been halted. Carfilzomib (Onyx Pharmaceuticals; San Francisco, CA), a tetrapeptide epoxy ketone, received U.S. Food and Drug Administration (FDA) approval in 2012.[21] A second peptide epoxy ketone proteasome inhibitor, oprozomib (Onyx), entered clinical study in 2010. The third class of proteasome inhibitors, β-lactones, is represented by NPI-0052 (salinosporamide A [Marizomib]) and is currently being developed by Nereus Pharmaceuticals, Inc. (San Diego, CA). The initial approvals for both bortezomib and carfilzomib were in multiple myeloma (MM), a plasma cell neoplasm and the second most common hematologic cancer. However, the activity of PIs in other B-cell neoplasms has resulted in an expansion of the clinical utilization of this drug class.

Preclinical Activity of Proteasome Inhibitors

Each of the three classes of inhibitors has a distinct chemical mechanism of proteasome inhibition.[22] Peptide boronates form stable but reversible tetrahedral intermediates with the γ-hydroxyl (γ-OH) group of the catalytic N-terminal threonine of the proteasome active sites.[23,24] β-lactones also interact with this γ-OH, but form a completely irreversible interaction.[25] Similarly, peptide epoxy ketones form irreversible covalent adducts with the active site threonine but do so via a dual covalent adduction of γ-OH group and the free amine.[26] This interaction is highly specific for N-terminal threonine-containing hydrolases and renders peptide epoxy ketones the most selective proteasome inhibitors yet described.[27,28]

The primary targets of these PIs within the constitutive and immunoproteasomes are the CT-L subunits, β5 and LMP7, respectively. Despite accounting for less than 50% of total protein turnover by the proteasome, these subunits are essential for cell survival.[29] In MM cell lines, inhibiting both subunits (β5 and LMP7) is necessary and sufficient for tumor cell death.[30] Cytotoxicity of other tumor cell types requires the inhibition of multiple active sites beyond the CT-L activity. The combination of inhibitors specific for either the T-L or C-L activities, which have no cytotoxic activity on their own, augments the cytotoxic potential of the CT-L–specific inhibitors.[31,32]

TABLE 24.1

Proteasome Inhibitors in Clinical Development

Agent	Other Names	Drug Class	Stage of Development	Tumor Types	Route of Administration	Dose Levels	Schedule of Administration
Bortezomib	Velcade PS-341	Peptide boronate	FDA/EMEA approved	Multiple myeloma, mantle cell lymphoma	Intravenous, subcutaneous	1.3 mg/m^2	Days 1, 4, 8, & 11 (21-day cycle)
Ixazomib	MLN 9708 MLN 2238	Peptide boronate	Phase III	Multiple myeloma, AL, amyloidosis	Oral	4 mg	Once weekly (21-day cycle)
Delanzomib	CEP-18770	Peptide boronate	Phase I (discontinued)	Multiple myeloma	Intravenous	0.1–1.8 mg/m^2	Days 1, 4, 8, & 11 (21-day cycle)
Carfilzomib	Kyprolis PR-171	Peptide epoxy ketone	FDA approved, phase III	Multiple myeloma	Intravenous	20/27 mg/m^2	Days 1, 2, 8, 9, 15, & 16 (28-day cycle)
Oprozomib	ONX 0912 PR-047	Peptide epoxy ketone	Phase I/II	Multiple myeloma	Oral	150–240 mg (dose escalation ongoing)	Days 1, 2, 8, & 9 (14-day cycle) Days 1–5 (14-day cycle)
Marizomib	NPI-0052 Salinosporamide A	β-lactone	Phase II	Multiple myeloma	Intravenous	0.075–0.6 mg/m^2	Days 1, 4, 8, & 11 (21-day cycle)

EMEA, European Medicines Agency; AL, amyloid light chain.

Given its status as the first proteasome inhibitor approved for marketed use, the antitumor potential and preclinical activity of other proteasome inhibitors have generally been compared to bortezomib.[19] Carfilzomib showed equivalent antitumor activity to bortezomib in vitro against a panel of tumor cell lines under standard culture conditions but was >10-fold more potent at inducing tumor cell death when cells were exposed to drug for a 1-hour pulse, which mimics the pharmacokinetics of both compounds.[33] MLN2238 (the active agent of ixazomib) was active in the same mouse models of human tumors as bortezomib, but demonstrated greater levels of proteasome inhibition in the tumors.[34] In biochemical assays of proteasome activity, delanzomib had an identical potency and subunit activity profile to bortezomib, but in tumor cytotoxicity assays, potency relative to bortezomib was 2- to 10-fold less.[35] In addition, delanzomib appeared to be less cytotoxic than bortezomib to normal cells and had a differential effect on cytokine release in bone marrow stromal cells, suggesting a different pharmacologic activity. Oprozomib is 10-fold less potent than carfilzomib in proteasome activity assays, but showed similar antitumor activity in mouse tumor models.[36,37] Marizomib displayed greater potency against the non–CT-L active sites of the proteasome than bortezomib.[38] Interestingly, this agent synergized with bortezomib in killing tumor cells in vitro.[39] All of the second-generation inhibitors have shown activity in tumor cells made resistant to bortezomib and/or MM cells isolated from patients relapsed from bortezomib-based therapies.[35,36,40–42]

The inhibition of tumor cells with proteasome inhibitors induces cell death via the induction of apoptosis through death effector caspase activation.[10] Although the mechanism underlying the induction of cell death remains to be fully elucidated, extensive research suggests a complex interplay of multiple pathways. PIs have been shown to affect the half-life of the *BH3-only* members of the Bcl-2 family, specifically BH3–interacting-domain death agonist (Bid) and Bcl-2 interacting killer (Bik).[43] Moreover the BH3-only protein NOXA is upregulated at the transcription level by PIs.[44–48] Proteasome inhibition also upregulates the expression of several key cell-cycle checkpoint proteins that include p53 (an inducer of G0/G1 cell-cycle arrest through accumulation of the cyclin-dependent kinase [CDK] inhibitor p27); the CDK inhibitor p21;

mammalian cyclins A, B, D, and E; and transcription factors E2F and Rb.[49,50] The transcription factor nuclear factor kappa B (NF-κB), an important regulator of cell survival and cytokine/growth factor production,[51] is also affected by proteasome inhibition in multiple ways. The net effect on NF-κB signaling is not consistent across various assays and cell lines, and its relative importance in the antitumor effects of PIs remains unclear. Although it is interesting to note that patients whose myeloma harbor NF-κB–activating mutations (~20%) respond better to bortezomib than those without NF-κB–activating mutations.[52–54] In MM cell lines, there is growing evidence that the major determinant of sensitivity to proteasome inhibition is the relative load of protein flux to the proteasome.[55–57] These data suggest that induction of the terminal unfolded protein response may drive cell death. Whether proteotoxic stress induced cell death reflects sensitivity to proteasome inhibitors in other tumor types remains to be determined.

Pharmacokinetics and Pharmacodynamics of Proteasome Inhibitors in Animals

Following intravenous (IV) administration to animals and humans, proteasome activity is inhibited in a dose-dependent fashion within minutes; however, PIs such as bortezomib and carfilzomib are also rapidly cleared from circulation.[55,56,58–61] Recovery of proteasome activity in animals occurs in tissues with a half-life of approximately 24 hours, mirroring the recovery time of cells exposed to sublethal concentrations of PIs in vitro and likely reflecting new protein synthesis.[33,62]

PROTEASOME INHIBITORS IN CANCER

Clinical Activity of Bortezomib

Bortezomib is typically administered on days 1, 4, 8, and 11 of a 3-week cycle either as an IV bolus or subcutaneous administration. Increasing doses of bortezomib inhibit proteasome activity in blood in a dose-dependent fashion, reaching a maximum of 74% inhibition at a dose of 1.38 mg/m^2. Daily dosing schedules in animal studies have been associated with severe toxicity and have not been attempted in humans. In clinical trials, thrombocytopenia and peripheral neuropathy (PN) were common adverse events.[20,63,64] Bortezomib has shown remarkable single-agent antitumor activity in a wide range of B-cell neoplasms, including MM, non Hodgkin lymphoma (NHL), and Waldenström macroglobulinemia (WM). In 2003, bortezomib was approved by the FDA for use as a single agent for the treatment of patients with MM following two prior therapies and who demonstrated disease progression with their most recent therapy. The primary efficacy data for this approval was derived from the SUMMIT trial in which 202 patients with heavily pretreated disease were treated with bortezomib at 1.3 mg/m^2.[65] In this trial, the overall response rate (ORR), defined as patients achieving at least a 50% reduction in serum or urine levels of the myeloma M protein, was 35%. This clinical trial was supported by the CREST trial, in which the activity of 1.3 mg/m^2 dose was determined to be superior to a dose of 1.0 mg/m^2.[66] Bortezomib is also active as a single agent in earlier stage MM patient populations. A single-agent ORR of 38%, with a 6% complete response (CR) rate, was seen in the phase III APEX study in early relapsed MM, with a time to progression (TTP) of 6.2 months and a median duration of response of 8 months.[67] In this study, the major grade 3 and 4 toxicities were PN, 12%; dysesthesia and related symptoms, 8% to 10%; anemia, 8%; diarrhea, 8%; neutropenia, 14%; and fatigue, 12%. In the frontline setting, bortezomib demonstrated a single-agent response rate of 41% (5% CR rate).[68]

Bortezomib is also approved for newly diagnosed MM in combination with velcade, melphalan and prednisone (VMP). The phase III VISTA trial evaluated VMP in patients with untreated MM who were ineligible for high-dose therapy.[69] The addition of bortezomib to the melphalan prednisone (MP) backbone significantly improved response rates in this setting with an ORR of 71% for VMP (including 30% CR) versus 35% (with only 4% CR) for MP.[52] VMP was associated with a TTP of ~24 months, compared with ~16.6 months with MP. After a 5-year follow-up, there was a 31% reduced risk of death for the VMP group versus MP-treated patients.[70]

Bortezomib has also shown promise when combined with other agents in relapsed and refractory MM patients. The combination of bortezomib with pegylated doxorubicin (Doxil, Centocor Ortho Biotech Products, L.P.; Horsham, PA) resulted in an ORR of 79% in relapsed patients, and toxicities were similar to those observed with each agent administered separately.[71] A phase III study in 646 patients with relapsed and refractory MM compared this treatment with bortezomib alone; the combination produced a 44% ORR and extended the TTP from 6 to 9.3 months.[72,73] The combination of bortezomib with revlimid, lenalidomide and dexamethasone (Rd), a standard of care in the treatment of MM, resulted in an ORR of 64% and a median duration of response of 8.7 months.[74] This activity is striking given that 53% of patients had received prior bortezomib and 75% of patients had received prior thalidomide, a closely related analog of lenalidomide. Other agents tested in combination with bortezomib include vorinostat, the anti-CS1 mAb, elotuzumab, the Hsp90 inhibitor tanespimycin, and the Akt inhibitor perifosine.[75]

Frontline combinations with bortezomib in MM patients have shown high ORRs with a notable improvement in CR rates. In longer term studies, CR rates with bortezomib-based combinations have been shown to be associated with improved clinical outcomes.[63,64] A community-based phase IIIb study evaluating bortezomib + dexamethasone (VD) versus bortezomib + thalidomide + dexamethasone (VTD) versus VMP found similar ORR (60%, 70%, and 52%, respectively) and CR rates (13%, 18%, and 15%, respectively).[63] Bortezomib + melphalan + prednisone + thalidomide (VMPT) followed by bortezomib + thalidomide (VT) maintenance resulted in a superior CR rate compared with VMP with no maintenance (34% versus 21%) and improved 2-year progression-free survival (70% versus 58.2%).[64] A protocol modification in this trial involved changing from twice weekly

to weekly bortezomib administration, which yielded similar TTP but reduced the incidence (21% versus 43%) and severity of PN (2% grade 3/4 versus 14%).[64] The bortezomib, lenalidomide, and dexamethasone combination in newly diagnosed MM resulted in a ORR of 100% in 66 patients, 29% of whom achieved a CR.[76]

Bortezomib has also shown activity in other hematologic cancers, most notably mantle cell lymphoma (MCL).[77,78] As a single agent in 155 relapsed and refractory MCL patients, bortezomib yielded an ORR of 33% (8% CR), a median duration of response of 9.2 months, and a TTP of 6.2 months.[78] Toxicities observed were similar to those seen in patients with MM and included thrombocytopenia, PN, and fatigue. When bortezomib was used to treat both newly diagnosed and refractory MCL, a response rate of 46% was observed in both populations,[77] leading to FDA approval late in 2006.

Bortezomib has been tested in a variety of solid tumors in phase I and II studies.[79] Partial responses (PR) were reported in 8% of patients with refractory non–small-cell lung cancer (NSCLC), although the TTP was 1.5 months.[80] Exacerbation of PN was common. Bortezomib was subsequently tested in combination with paclitaxel, irinotecan, and gemcitabine/carboplatin; however, results have not been encouraging. Bortezomib continues to be tested in combination with other agents in a variety of tumor types.[81,82]

Recent clinical activity and preclinical data suggest that proteasome inhibition may extend to nononcology applications. Single-agent bortezomib therapy in kidney transplant patients undergoing antibody-mediated rejection resulted in a reduction of donor-specific antibodies and improved renal function.[83] In mouse models of lupus nephritis, bortezomib resulted in a reduction of pathogenic plasma cells and the prevention of disease progression.[84] These data suggest that PIs may be useful in a wide range of B-cell–mediated diseases. However, toxicities with bortezomib, particularly PN, may prevent wider application of this particular agent.

Carfilzomib

Parallel phase I studies of carfilzomib have been conducted in patients with multiple tumor types, and two phase I dose-finding studies targeting B-cell malignancies have been completed. The first study used daily IV bolus dosing with doses up to 20 mg/m^2 for 5 consecutive days followed by 9 days of rest and resulted in substantial inhibition of proteasome activity.[85] In the second study, carfilzomib was administered daily for 2 days for 3 consecutive weeks (days 1, 2, 8, 9, 15, and 16), followed by 12 days of recovery.[86] Hematologic toxicities were the most frequent adverse events, observed along with transient, noncumulative elevations in serum creatinine, usually with increases in serum urea nitrogen and consistent with a *prerenal* etiology. New onset PN was infrequent. Among 20 evaluable patients (including bortezomib-refractory patients), 4 PRs and 1 minor response were seen. Responses were also durable, lasting more than 1 year in some cases. Although the maximum tolerated dose of carfilzomib was not established in this study, a dose of 20 mg/m^2 was initially selected for the phase II studies.

Based on the phase I studies, an open-label, single-arm, phase II study of single-agent carfilzomib in relapsed and refractory MM was initiated in 2007.[87,88] Carfilzomib was administered as an IV bolus on the twice-weekly dose schedule. Patients enrolled in the initial phase of the study (003-A0) had received a median of five prior therapies, and 78% of patients had grade 1/2 PN at entry.[87] Among 39 evaluable patients in 003-A0, 10 (26%) achieved a minor response or better, including 5 PRs, and 16 additional patients with stable disease. Based on new safety information from phase I studies, the protocol was amended and the carfilzomib dose was escalated to 27 mg/m^2 after the first cycle (003-A1).[89] In this trial, 266 patients were enrolled and all patients had previously been treated with an immunomodulatory agent (IMiD) and bortezomib and were refractory to their last therapy. An ORR of 24% with a median duration of response of 8 months was reported. Adverse events were predominantly hematopoietic (thrombocytopenia, lymphopenia, and anemia) and there was a <1% rate of grade 3 PN, despite 77% having a history of PN. Based on these findings, carfilzomib was granted conditional approval by the FDA in 2012 for the treatment of patients with relapsed and refractory myeloma who had received prior bortezomib and IMiD therapy.

The parallel PX-171-004 trial enrolled patients with relapsed MM following one to three prior treatments and who may have been refractory to one or more of these therapies.[90,91] Of the 155 patients enrolled in this trial, 120 had not received prior bortezomib-based therapy. In patients with relapsed disease, non-hematologic and hematologic toxicity profiles were similar. Despite high rates of baseline PN, reports of worsening neuropathic symptoms were infrequent (2% incidence of grade 3 and no grade 4 events). Carfilzomib demonstrated considerable activity in bortezomib-naïve patients, inducing PR or better in 46% of 54 evaluable patients at 20 mg/m^2 and 53% of patients at 27 mg/m^2.[91] The response rate in patients previously exposed to bortezomib was lower (18%).[90] Responses across groups are durable, typically 8 to 9 months.[90,91]

Based on findings in animal studies in which a 30-minute infusion of carfilzomib resulted in reduced toxicities,[61] the effect of infusional administration was tested in patients with relapsed and refractory myeloma. In a dose escalation study, PX-171-007, the MTD dose of carfilzomib was determined to be 56 mg/m^2, more than twice the dose used in the studies described previously. In a cohort of 24 patients receiving this dose and who had received a median of five prior lines of therapy (including two prior bortezomib-containing regimens), the ORR was 60%.[92] This enhanced efficacy also correlated with a greater level of inhibition of all three subunits of the immunoproteasome measured in isolated peripheral blood mononuclear cells (Lee S, et al., unpublished).[93] This same dose and infusion time is currently being explored in a phase III trial of nearly 900 patients comparing carfilzomib plus low-dose dexamethasone (Cd) to bortezomib plus low-dose dexamethasone (Vd) in MM patients with relapsed disease.

Trials of carfilzomib in combination with other agents in MM have been initiated, including a phase Ib/II safety and efficacy study of carfilzomib in combination with lenalidomide and low-dose dexamethasone (CRd) in relapsed and/or refractory MM. At the maximum planned dose, the ORR was 77% with a median duration of response of 22 months.[94] The CRd combination is now being tested in an international, multicenter, randomized, open-label phase III study in comparison with lenalidomide and low-dose dexamethasone (Rd) in approximately 780 patients with relapsed MM following one to three prior therapies. The CRd regimen has also been explored in newly diagnosed MM patients.[95] When carfilzomib is combined with Rd at a dose of 36 mg/m^2, 62% of the 53 patients treated achieved a CR. In addition, 20 of 21 patients analyzed for signs of minimal residual disease (MRD), utilizing multiparameter flow cytometry were determined to be free of MRD.

Ixazomib

Initial clinical studies of ixazomib involved dose escalation studies in patients with hematologic malignancies and explored both weekly and twice weekly dosing schedules.[96,97] Oral administration resulted in potent proteasome inhibition of ~65%. Clinical activity in patients with relapsed MM was 16%.[98] In patients with newly diagnosed MM, ixazomib plus lenalidomide and low-dose dexamethasone resulted in an ORR of 93% with 24% achieving a CR.[99] This combination is also being investigated in a phase III trial comparing this to Rd in patients with relapsed MM.

Oprozomib

Initial clinical testing of oprozomib in patients with solid tumors investigated a dosing schedule consisting of a 14-day cycle with once daily administration for 5 consecutive days.[100] In patients with relapsed and/or refractory B-cell neoplasms, two dosing schedules are being utilized: the schedule described previously and one involving 2 consecutive days of dosing repeated weekly.[101] Proteasome inhibition following the administration of oprozomib reached >80% and clinical activity was noted in patients with MM and WM. In patients receiving the 5 consecutive day schedule, 5 of 19 MM patients (26%) and 8 of 10 WM patients (80%) achieved a partial response or better. Exploration of the dose and schedule continues as a single agent and in combination with other anti-MM therapies.

Biomarkers for Proteasome Inhibitors

As described previously, PI-based therapies have proven highly effective in the treatment of MM and other B-cell neoplasms. Given that response rates in single-agent trials are generally <50%, there would be a distinct clinical benefit to identify those patients most likely to respond to proteasome inhibition prior to treatment initiation. Gene expression analysis from bone marrow–derived MM tumor cells from 169 bortezomib-treated patients and 70 dexamethasone-treated patients revealed a 100-gene signature that provided a stratification for patients likely to respond that performed better than standard staging systems.[102] However, this signature provided only a modest increase in predictive power for treatment with bortezomib versus dexamethasone. More recently, Keats et al.[54] reanalyzed this dataset based on a pathway analysis of NF-κB and the realization that TRAF3, a key regulatory of the noncanonical NF-κB pathway, is a tumor suppressor in MM cell lines. They found a dramatic enrichment for response to bortezomib in patients with low levels of TRAF3 expression. However, these data remain to be validated in a separate sample set. A transcriptomic analysis of samples derived from single-agent carfilzomib trials suggest that patients with the highest level of immunoglobulin heavy chain expression were the most sensitive to carfilzomib therapy.[103] Similar findings were noted in the expression data from bortezomib-treated patients described previously.[103] These data are supported by phenotypic data from patients progressing on bortezomib-based therapy, in which resistance to bortezomib was associated with a dedifferentiated (and lower immunoglobulin expressing) B-cell phenotype.[104] Taken together, these findings suggest that biomarkers, potentially those involving an analysis of protein load of immunoglobulin expression, may be developed to predict those patients most likely to respond to PIs.

REFERENCES

1. Ciechanover A. Intracellular protein degradation: from a vague idea thru the lysosome and the ubiquitin-proteasome system and onto human diseases and drug targeting. *Biochim Biophys Acta* 2012;1824:3–13.
2. Kopp F, Hendil KB, Dahlmann B, et al. Subunit arrangement in the human 20S proteasome. *Proc Natl Acad Sci U S A* 1997;94:2939–2944.
3. Wilkinson KD. Ubiquitination and deubiquitination: targeting of proteins for degradation by the proteasome. *Semin Cell Dev Biol* 2000;11:141–148.
4. Braun BC, Glickman M, Kraft R, et al. The base of the proteasome regulatory particle exhibits chaperone-like activity. *Nat Cell Biol* 1999;1:221–226.
5. Groll M, Ditzel L, Lowe J, et al. Structure of 20S proteasome from yeast at 2.4 A resolution. *Nature* 1997;386:463–471.
6. Borissenko L, Groll M. 20S proteasome and its inhibitors: crystallographic knowledge for drug development. *Chem Rev* 2007;107:687–717.
7. Kloetzel PM, Ossendorp F. Proteasome and peptidase function in MHC-class-I-mediated antigen presentation. *Curr Opin Immunol* 2004;16:76–81.
8. Griffin TA, Nandi D, Cruz M, et al. Immunoproteasome assembly: cooperative incorporation of interferon gamma (IFN-gamma)-inducible subunits. *J Exp Med* 1998;187:97–104.

9. Tanahashi N, Murakami Y, Minami Y, et al. Hybrid proteasomes. Induction by interferon-gamma and contribution to ATP-dependent proteolysis. *J Biol Chem* 2000;275:14336–14345.

10. Adams J. The proteasome: a suitable antineoplastic target. *Nat Rev Cancer* 2004;4:349–360.

11. Vinitsky A, Michaud C, Powers JC, et al. Inhibition of the chymotrypsin-like activity of the pituitary multicatalytic proteinase complex. *Biochemistry* 1992;31:9421–9428.

12. Orlowski RZ, Eswara JR, Lafond-Walker A, et al. Tumor growth inhibition induced in a murine model of human Burkitt's lymphoma by a proteasome inhibitor. *Cancer Res* 1998;58:4342–4348.

13. Imajoh-Ohmi S, Kawaguchi T, Sugiyama S, et al. Lactacystin, a specific inhibitor of the proteasome, induces apoptosis in human monoblast U937 cells. *Biochem Biophys Res Commun* 1995;217:1070–1077.

14. Shinohara K, Tomioka M, Nakano H, et al. Apoptosis induction resulting from proteasome inhibition. *Biochem J* 1996;317:385–388.

15. Delic J, Masdehors P, Omura S, et al. The proteasome inhibitor lactacystin induces apoptosis and sensitizes chemo- and radioresistant human chronic lymphocytic leukaemia lymphocytes to TNF-alpha-initiated apoptosis. *Br J Cancer* 1998;77:1103–1107.

16. Meng L, Mohan R, Kwok BH, et al. Epoxomicin, a potent and selective proteasome inhibitor, exhibits in vivo antiinflammatory activity. *Proc Natl Acad Sci U S A* 1999;96:10403–10408.

17. Meng L, Kwok BH, Sin N, et al. Eponemycin exerts its antitumor effect through the inhibition of proteasome function. *Cancer Res* 1999;59:2798–2801.

18. Dick LR, Fleming PE. Building on bortezomib: second-generation proteasome inhibitors as anti-cancer therapy. *Drug Discov Today* 2010;15:243–249.

19. Kirk CJ. Discovery and development of second-generation proteasome inhibitors. *Semin Hematol* 2012;49:207–214.

20. Bross PF, Kane R, Farrell AT, et al. Approval summary for bortezomib for injection in the treatment of multiple myeloma. *Clin Cancer Res* 2004;10:3954–3964.

21. Herndon TM, Deisseroth A, Kaminskas E, et al. U.S. Food and Drug Administration approval: carfilzomib for the treatment of multiple myeloma. *Clin Cancer Res* 2013;19:4559–4563.

22. Bennett MK, Kirk CJ. Development of proteasome inhibitors in oncology and autoimmune diseases. *Curr Opin Drug Discov Devel* 2008;11:616–625.

23. Adams J, Behnke M, Chen S, et al. Potent and selective inhibitors of the proteasome: dipeptidyl boronic acids. *Bioorg Med Chem Lett* 1998;8:333–338.

24. Groll M, Berkers CR, Ploegh HL, et al. Crystal structure of the boronic acid-based proteasome inhibitor bortezomib in complex with the yeast 20S proteasome. *Structure* 2006;14:451–456.

25. Groll M, Huber R, Potts BC. Crystal structures of Salinosporamide A (NPI-0052) and B (NPI-0047) in complex with the 20S proteasome reveal important consequences of beta-lactone ring opening and a mechanism for irreversible binding. *J Am Chem Soc* 2006;19:5136–5141.

26. Groll M, Kim KB, Kairies N, et al. Crystal structure of epoxomicin: 20S proteasome reveals a molecular basis for selectivity of a' b'-epoxyketone proteasome inhibitors. *J Am Chem Soc* 2000;122:1237–1238.

27. Kisselev AF, van der Linden WA, Overkleeft HS. Proteasome inhibitors: an expanding army attacking a unique target. *Chem Biol* 2012;19:99–115.

28. Arastu-Kapur S, Anderl JL, Kraus M, et al. Nonproteasomal targets of the proteasome inhibitors bortezomib and carfilzomib: a link to clinical adverse events. *Clin Cancer Res* 2011;17:2734–2743.

29. Kisselev AF, Callard A, Goldberg AL. Importance of the different proteolytic sites of the proteasome and the efficacy of inhibitors varies with the protein substrate. *J Biol Chem* 2006;281:8582–8590.

30. Parlati F, Lee SJ, Aujay M, et al. Carfilzomib can induce tumor cell death through selective inhibition of the chymotrypsin-like activity of the proteasome. *Blood* 2009;114:3439–3447.

31. Britton M, Lucas MM, Downey SL, et al. Selective inhibitor of proteasome's caspase-like sites sensitizes cells to specific inhibition of chymotrypsin-like sites. *Chem Biol* 2009;16:1278–1289.

32. Mirabella AC, Pletnev AA, Downey SL, et al. Specific cell-permeable inhibitor of proteasome trypsin-like sites selectively sensitizes myeloma cells to bortezomib and carfilzomib. *Chem Biol* 2011;18:608–618.

33. Demo SD, Kirk CJ, Aujay MA, et al. Antitumor activity of PR-171, a novel irreversible inhibitor of the proteasome. *Cancer Res* 2007;67:6383–6391.

34. Kupperman E, Lee EC, Cao Y, et al. Evaluation of the proteasome inhibitor MLN9708 in preclinical models of human cancer. *Cancer Res* 2010;70:1970–1980.

35. Piva R, Ruggeri B, Williams M, et al. CEP-18770: A novel, orally active proteasome inhibitor with a tumor-selective pharmacologic profile competitive with bortezomib. *Blood* 2008;111:2765–2775.

36. Chauhan D, Singh AV, Aujay M, et al. A novel orally active proteasome inhibitor ONX 0912 triggers in vitro and in vivo cytotoxicity in multiple myeloma. *Blood* 2010;116:4906–4915.

37. Zhou HJ, Aujay MA, Bennett MK, et al. Design and synthesis of an orally bioavailable and selective peptide epoxyketone proteasome inhibitor (PR-047). *J Med Chem* 2009;52:3028–3038.

38. Chauhan D, Catley L, Li G, et al. A novel orally active proteasome inhibitor induces apoptosis in multiple myeloma cells with mechanisms distinct from Bortezomib. *Cancer Cell* 2005;8:407–419.

39. Chauhan D, Singh A, Brahmandam M, et al. Combination of proteasome inhibitors bortezomib and NPI-0052 trigger in vivo synergistic cytotoxicity in multiple myeloma. *Blood* 2008;111:1654–1664.

40. Chauhan D, Tian Z, Zhou B, et al. In vitro and in vivo selective antitumor activity of a novel orally bioavailable proteasome inhibitor MLN9708 against multiple myeloma cells. *Clin Cancer Res* 2011;17:5311–5321.

41. Kuhn DJ, Chen Q, Voorhees PM, et al. Potent activity of carfilzomib, a novel, irreversible inhibitor of the ubiquitin-proteasome pathway, against preclinical models of multiple myeloma. *Blood* 2007;110:3281–3290.

42. Suzuki E, Demo S, Deu E, et al. Molecular mechanisms of bortezomib resistant adenocarcinoma cells. *PLoS One* 2011;6:e27996.

43. Zhang HG, Wang J, Yang X, et al. Regulation of apoptosis proteins in cancer cells by ubiquitin. *Oncogene* 2004;23:2009–2015.

44. Fernandez Y, Verhaegen M, Miller TP, et al. Differential regulation of noxa in normal melanocytes and melanoma cells by proteasome inhibition: therapeutic implications. *Cancer Res* 2005;65:6294–6304.

45. Nikiforov MA, Riblett M, Tang WH, et al. Tumor cell-selective regulation of NOXA by c-MYC in response to proteasome inhibition. *Proc Natl Acad Sci U S A* 2007;104:19488–19493.

46. Qin JZ, Ziffra J, Stennett L, et al. Proteasome inhibitors trigger NOXA-mediated apoptosis in melanoma and myeloma cells. *Cancer Res* 2005;65:6282–6293.

47. Wang Q, Mora-Jensen H, Weniger MA, et al. ERAD inhibitors integrate ER stress with an epigenetic mechanism to activate BH3-only protein NOXA in cancer cells. *Proc Natl Acad Sci U S A* 2009;106:2200–2205.

48. Mannava S, Zhuang D, Nair JR, et al. KLF9 is a novel transcriptional regulator of bortezomib- and LBH589-induced apoptosis in multiple myeloma cells. *Blood* 2012;119:1450–1458.

49. Koepp DM, Harper JW, Elledge SJ. How the cyclin became a cyclin: regulated proteolysis in the cell cycle. *Cell* 1999;97:431–434.

50. Pagano M, Tam SW, Theodoras AM, et al. Role of the ubiquitin-proteasome pathway in regulating abundance of the cyclin-dependent kinase inhibitor p27. *Science* 1995;269:682–685.

51. Wan F, Lenardo MJ. The nuclear signaling of NF-kappaB: current knowledge, new insights, and future perspectives. *Cell Res* 2010;20:24–33.

52. Annunziata CM, Davis RE, Demchenko Y, et al. Frequent engagement of the classical and alternative NF-kappaB pathways by diverse genetic abnormalities in multiple myeloma. *Cancer Cell* 2007;12:115–130.

53. Chapman MA, Lawrence MS, Keats JJ, et al. Initial genome sequencing and analysis of multiple myeloma. *Nature* 2011;471:467–472.

54. Keats JJ, Fonseca R, Chesi M, et al. Promiscuous mutations activate the noncanonical NF-kappaB pathway in multiple myeloma. *Cancer Cell* 2007;12:131–144.

55. Meister S, Schubert U, Neubert K, et al. Extensive immunoglobulin production sensitizes myeloma cells for proteasome inhibition. *Cancer Res* 2007;67:1783–1792.

56. Obeng EA, Carlson LM, Gutman DM, et al. Proteasome inhibitors induce a terminal unfolded protein response in multiple myeloma cells. *Blood* 2006;107:4907–4916.

57. Shabaneh TB, Downey SL, Goddard AL, et al. Molecular basis of differential sensitivity of myeloma cells to clinically relevant bolus treatment with bortezomib. *PLoS One* 2013;8:e56132.

58. Papadopoulos KP, Burris HA III, Gordon M, et al. A phase I/II study of carfilzomib 2-10-min infusion in patients with advanced solid tumors. *Cancer Chemother Pharmacol* 2013;72:861–868.

59. Papandreou CN, Daliani DD, Nix D, et al. Phase I trial of the proteasome inhibitor bortezomib in patients with advanced solid tumors with observations in androgen-independent prostate cancer. *J Clin Oncol* 2004;22:2108–2121.

60. Wang Z, Yang J, Kirk C, et al. Clinical pharmacokinetics, metabolism, and drug-drug interaction of carfilzomib. *Drug Metab Dispos* 2013;41:230–237.

61. Yang J, Wang Z, Fang Y, et al. Pharmacokinetics, pharmacodynamics, metabolism, distribution, and excretion of carfilzomib in rats. *Drug Metab Dispos* 2011;39:1873–1882.

62. Meiners S, Heyken D, Weller A, et al. Inhibition of proteasome activity induces concerted expression of proteasome genes and de novo formation of mammalian proteasomes. *J Biol Chem* 2003;278:21517–21525.

63. Lonial S, Waller EK, Richardson PG, et al. Risk factors and kinetics of thrombocytopenia associated with bortezomib for relapsed, refractory multiple myeloma. *Blood* 2005;106:3777–3784.

64. Richardson PG, Briemberg H, Jagannath S, et al. Frequency, characteristics, and reversibility of peripheral neuropathy during treatment of advanced multiple myeloma with bortezomib. *J Clin Oncol* 2006;24:3113–3120.

65. Richardson PG, Barlogie B, Berenson J, et al. A phase 2 study of bortezomib in relapsed, refractory myeloma. *N Engl J Med* 2003;348:2609–2617.

66. Jagannath S, Barlogie B, Berenson J, et al. A phase 2 study of two doses of bortezomib in relapsed or refractory myeloma. *Br J Haematol* 2004;127:165–172.

67. Richardson PG, Sonneveld P, Schuster MW, et al. Bortezomib or high-dose dexamethasone for relapsed multiple myeloma. *N Engl J Med* 2005;352:2487–2498.

68. Jagannath S, Brian D, Wolf JL, et al. A phase 2 study of bortezomib as first-line therapy in patients with multiple myeloma. *Blood* 2004;104:333.

69. San Miguel JF, Schlag R, Khuageva NK, et al. Bortezomib plus melphalan and prednisone for initial treatment of multiple myeloma. *N Engl J Med* 2008;359:906–917.

70. San Miguel JF, Schlag R, Khuageva NK, et al. Persistent overall survival benefit and no increased risk of second malignancies with bortezomib-melphalan-prednisone versus melphalan-prednisone in patients with previously untreated multiple myeloma. *J Clin Oncol* 2013;31:448–455.

71. Orlowski RZ, Voorhees PM, Garcia RA, et al. Phase 1 trial of the proteasome inhibitor bortezomib and pegylated liposomal doxorubicin in patients with advanced hematologic malignancies. *Blood* 2005;105:3058–3065.

72. Orlowski RZ, Nagler A, Sonneveld P, et al. Randomized phase III study of pegylated liposomal doxorubicin plus bortezomib compared with bortezomib alone in relapsed or refractory multiple myeloma: combination therapy improves time to progression. *J Clin Oncol* 2007;25:3892–3901.

73. Sonneveld P, Hajek R, Nagler A, et al. Combined pegylated liposomal doxorubicin and bortezomib is highly effective in patients with recurrent or refractory multiple myeloma who received prior thalidomide/lenalidomide therapy. *Cancer* 2008;112:1529–1537.

74. Richardson PG, Xie W, Jagannath S, et al. A phase II trial of lenalidomide, bortezomib and dexamethasone in patients with relapsed and relapsed/refractory myeloma. *Blood* 2014;123:1461–1469.

75. Kapoor P, Ramakrishnan V, Rajkumar SV. Bortezomib combination therapy in multiple myeloma. *Semin Hematol* 2012;49:228–242.

76. Richardson PG, Weller E, Lonial S, et al. Lenalidomide, bortezomib, and dexamethasone combination therapy in patients with newly diagnosed multiple myeloma. *Blood* 2010;116:679–686.

77. Belch A, Kouroukis CT, Crump M, et al. A phase II study of bortezomib in mantle cell lymphoma: the National Cancer Institute of Canada Clinical Trials Group trial IND.150. *Ann Oncol* 2007;18:116–121.

78. Fisher RI, Bernstein SH, Kahl BS, et al. Multicenter phase II study of bortezomib in patients with relapsed or refractory mantle cell lymphoma. *J Clin Oncol* 2006;24:4867–4874.

79. Milano A, Iaffaioli RV, Caponigro F. The proteasome: a worthwhile target for the treatment of solid tumours? *Eur J Cancer* 2007;43:1125–1133.

80. Fanucchi MP, Fossella FV, Belt R, et al. Randomized phase II study of bortezomib alone and bortezomib in combination with docetaxel in previously treated advanced non-small-cell lung cancer. *J Clin Oncol* 2006;24:5025–5033.

81. Ramaswamy B, Phelps MA, Baiocchi R, et al. A dose-finding, pharmacokinetic and pharmacodynamic study of a novel schedule of flavopiridol in patients with advanced solid tumors. *Invest New Drugs* 2012;30:629–638.

82. Luu T, Chow W, Lim D, et al. Phase I trial of fixed-dose rate gemcitabine in combination with bortezomib in advanced solid tumors. *Anticancer Res* 2010;30:167–174.

83. Everly MJ, Everly JJ, Susskind B, et al. Bortezomib provides effective therapy for antibody- and cell-mediated acute rejection. *Transplantation* 2008;86:1754–1761.

84. Neubert K, Meister S, Moser K, et al. The proteasome inhibitor bortezomib depletes plasma cells and protects mice with lupus-like disease from nephritis. *Nat Med* 2008;14:748–755.

85. O'Connor OA, Stewart AK, Vallone M, et al. A phase 1 dose escalation study of the safety and pharmacokinetics of the novel proteasome inhibitor carfilzomib (PR-171) in patients with hematologic malignancies. *Clin Cancer Res* 2009;15:7085–7091.

86. Alsina M, Trudel S, Furman RR, et al. A phase I single-agent study of twice-weekly consecutive-day dosing of the proteasome inhibitor carfilzomib in patients with relapsed or refractory multiple myeloma or lymphoma. *Clin Cancer Res* 2012;18:4830–4840.

87. Jagannath S, Vij R, Stewart AK, et al. An open-label single-arm pilot phase II study (PX-171-003-A0) of low-dose, single-agent carfilzomib in patients with relapsed and refractory multiple myeloma. *Clin Lymphoma Myeloma Leuk* 2012;12:310–318.

88. Siegel DS, Martin T, Wang M, et al. A phase 2 study of single-agent carfilzomib (PX-171-003-A1) in patients with relapsed and refractory multiple myeloma. *Blood* 2012;120:2817–2825.

89. Siegel DS, Martin T, Wang M, et al. Results of PX-171-003-A1, an open-label, single-arm, phase 2 (Ph 2) study of carfilzomib (CFZ) in patients (pts) with relapsed and refractory multiple myeloma (MM). *Blood* 2012;120:2817–2825.

90. Vij R, Siegel DS, Jagannath S, et al. An open-label, single-arm, phase 2 study of single-agent carfilzomib in patients with relapsed and/or refractory multiple myeloma who have been previously treated with bortezomib. *Br J Haematol* 2012;158:739–748.

91. Vij R, Wang M, Kaufman JL, et al. An open-label, single-arm, phase 2 (PX-171-004) study of single-agent carfilzomib in bortezomib-naive patients with relapsed and/or refractory multiple myeloma. *Blood* 2012;119:5661–5670.

92. Papadopoulos K, Capua Siegel DS, Singhal SB, et al. Phase 1b evaluation of the safety and efficacy of a 30-minute IV infusion of carfilzomib in patients with relapsed and/or refractory multiple myeloma. *Blood* 2010;116:3024.

93. Lee SJ, Levitsky K, Parlati F, et al. Clinical activity of carfilzomib correlates with inhibition of multiple proteasome subunits: application of a novel pharmacodynamics assay. (In press).

94. Wang M, Martin T, Bensinger W, et al. Phase 2 dose-expansion study (PX-171-006) of carfilzomib, lenalidomide, and low-dose dexamethasone in relapsed or progressive multiple myeloma. *Blood* 2013;122:3122–3128.

95. Jakubowiak AJ, Dytfeld D, Griffith KA, et al. A phase 1/2 study of carfilzomib in combination with lenalidomide and low-dose dexamethasone as a frontline treatment for multiple myeloma. *Blood* 2012;120:1801–1809.

96. Richardson PG, Baz R, Wang L, et al. Investigational agent MLN9708, an oral proteasome inhibitor, in patients (Pts) with relapsed and/or refractory multiple myeloma (MM): results from the expansion cohorts of a phase 1 dose-escalation study. *Blood* 2011;118:301.

97. Richardson PG, Spencer A, Cannell P, et al. Phase 1 clinical evaluation of twice-weekly marizomib (NPI-0052), a novel proteasome inhibitor, in patients with relapsed/refractory multiple myeloma (MM). *Blood* 2011;118:302.

98. Roy V, Reeder C, LaPlant BR, et al. Phase 2 trial Of single agent MLN9708 in patients with relapsed multiple myeloma not refractory to bortezomib. *Blood* 2013;122:1944.

99. Hofmeister CC, Rosenbaum CA, Htut M, et al. Twice-weekly oral MLN9708 (ixazomib citrate), an investigational proteasome inhibitor, in combination with lenalidomide (len) and dexamethasone (dex) in patients (pts) with newly diagnosed multiple myeloma (MM): final phase 1 results and phase 2 data. *Blood* 2013;122:535.

100. Papadopoulos KP, Mendelson DS, Tolcher AW, et al. A phase I, open-label, dose-escalation study of the novel oral proteasome inhibitor (PI) ONX 0912 in patients with advanced refractory or recurrent solid tumors. *Blood* 2011;29:3075.

101. Kaufman JL, Siegel DS, Vij R, et al. Clinical profile of single-agent modified-release oprozomib tablets in patients (pts) with hematologic malignancies: updated results from a multicenter, open-label, dose escalation phase 1b/2 study. *Blood* 2013;122:3184.

102. Mulligan G, Mitsiades C, Bryant B, et al. Gene expression profiling and correlation with outcome in clinical trials of the proteasome inhibitor bortezomib. *Blood* 2007;109:3177–3188.

103. Loehr A, Degenhardt JD, Kwei KA, et al. Immunoglobulin expression is a major determinant of patient sensitivity to proteasome inhibitors. *Blood* 2013;122:1903.

104. Leung-Hagesteijn C, Erdmann N, Cheung G, et al. Xbp1s-negative tumor B cells and pre-plasmablasts mediate therapeutic proteasome inhibitor resistance in multiple myeloma. *Cancer Cell* 2013;24:289–304.

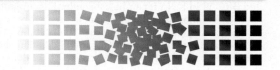

25 Poly (ADP-ribose) Polymerase Inhibitors

Alan Ashworth

INTRODUCTION

Cancer cells may harbor defects in DNA repair pathways leading to genomic instability. This can foster tumorigenesis but also provides a weakness that can be exploited therapeutically. Tumors with compromised ability to repair double-strand DNA breaks by homologous recombination, including those with defects in the *BRCA1* and *BRCA2* genes, are highly sensitive to blockade of the repair of DNA single-strand breaks, via the inhibition of the enzyme poly(ADP-ribose) (PARP). This provides the basis for a *synthetic lethal* approach to cancer therapy, which is showing considerable promise in the clinic.

CELLULAR DNA REPAIR PATHWAYS

DNA is continually damaged by environmental exposures and endogenous activities, such as DNA replication and cellular free-radical generation, which cause diverse lesions including base modifications, double-strand breaks (DSB), single-strand breaks (SSB), and intrastrand and interstrand cross-links.[1] These aberrations are repaired by distinct repair pathways, which are coordinated to maintain the stability and integrity of the genome. This faithful repair of DNA damage is an essential prerequisite for the maintenance of genomic integrity and cellular and organismal viability. Where one DNA strand is affected and the intact complementary strand is available as a template, the base-excision repair (BER), nucleotide-excision repair, or mismatch repair pathways are used and these pathways are highly efficient at repairing damage. DSBs, more problematic than SSBs because the complementary strand is not available as a template, are repaired by the homologous recombination (HR) or nonhomologous end-joining (NHEJ) pathways.[1]

Endogenous base damage, including SSBs, is the most common DNA aberration and it has been estimated that the average cell may repair 10,000 such lesions every day. BER is an important pathway for the repair of SSBs and involves the sensing of the lesion followed by the recruitment of a number of other proteins. PARP-1 (poly[ADP]ribose polymerase) is a critical component of the major "short-patch" BER pathway. PARP is an enzyme, discovered over 40 years ago,[2] that produces large branched chains of poly(ADP) ribose (PAR) from NAD^+. In humans, there are 17 members of the PARP gene family but most of these are poorly characterized.[3,4] The abundant nuclear protein PARP-1 senses and binds to DNA nicks and breaks, resulting in activation of catalytic activity causing poly(ADP)ribosylation of PARP-1 itself as well as other acceptor proteins including histones. This modification may signal the recruitment of other components of DNA repair pathways as well as modify their activity. The highly negatively charged PAR that is produced around the site of damage may also serve as an antirecombinogenic factor. In addition to the BER pathway PARP enzymes have been implicated in numerous cellular pathways.[3,4]

Two main DSB repair pathways are available within eukaryotic cells: NHEJ and HR.[5,6] HR can be further subdivided into the gene conversion (GC) and single-strand annealing (SSA) subpathways.[1]

Both GC and SSA rely on sequence homology for repair whereas NHEJ uses no, or little, homology.[2,3] NHEJ is the most important pathway for the repair of DSBs during G_0, G_1, and early S phases of the cell cycle, although it is likely active throughout the cell cycle.[7,8] This form of DSB repair usually results in changes in DNA sequence at the break site and, occasionally, in the joining of previously unlinked DNA molecules, potentially resulting in gross chromosomal rearrangements such as translocations.[9] GC uses a homologous sequence, preferably the sister chromatid, as a template to resynthesize the DNA surrounding the DSB, and therefore generally results in accurate repair of the break. Repair by GC is critically dependent on the recombinase function of RAD51 and is facilitated by a number of other proteins. SSA also involves the use of homologous sequences for the repair of DSBs, but unlike GC, SSA is RAD51-independent and involves the annealing of DNA strands formed after resection at the DSB. The detailed mechanism of SSA is still obscure but it frequently results in the loss of one of the homologous sequences and deletion of the intervening sequence.[9] SSA is a potentially important pathway of mutagenesis because a significant fraction of mammalian genomes consist of repetitive elements. GC and SSA are cell-cycle regulated and are most active in S-G_2 phases of the cell cycle.[10]

THE DEVELOPMENT OF PARP INHIBITORS

PARP inhibitors were originally developed as chemopotentiators, which are agents that enhance the effects of DNA damage—a common mechanism of action of drugs used to treat cancer. The rationale was that inhibition of the repair of chemotherapy-induced DNA damage might give greater efficacy. Early studies using relatively nonspecific PARP inhibitors such as 3-aminobenzamide, demonstrated potential synergy with alkylating agents.[11] Subsequent studies with more potent PARP inhibitors demonstrated synergy with temozolomide, an observation that was taken into a clinical trial with AG014699,[12] a PARP inhibitor developed by Pfizer. This agent is now being developed by Clovis. Although the major focus of this chapter is the use of PARP inhibitors in synthetic lethal therapeutic strategies, their use in chemopotentiation in combination with chemotherapy remains under active investigation, as described later.

BRCA1 AND *BRCA2* MUTATIONS AND DNA REPAIR

Heterozygous germline mutations in the *BRCA1* and *BRCA2* genes confer a high risk of breast (up to 85% lifetime risk) and ovarian (10% to 40%) cancer in addition to a significantly increased risk of pancreatic, prostate, and male breast cancer.[13] The genes have been classified as tumor suppressors, because the wild-type *BRCA* allele is frequently lost in tumors, a phenomenon that occurs by a variety of mechanisms. The *BRCA1* and *BRCA2* genes encode large proteins that likely function in multiple cellular pathways, including transcription, cell-cycle regulation, and the maintenance of genome integrity. However, the roles of BRCA1 and BRCA2 in DNA repair have been best documented.[14]

BRCA1- and BRCA2-deficient cells are highly sensitive to ionizing radiation and display chromosomal instability, which is likely to be a direct consequence of unrepaired DNA damage.[14] The similar genomic instability in BRCA1- and BRCA2-deficient cells and the interaction of both BRCA1 and BRCA2 with RAD51 suggested a functional link between the three proteins in the RAD51-mediated DNA damage repair process. However, although BRCA2 is directly involved in RAD51-mediated repair, affecting the choice between GC and SSA, BRCA1 acts upstream of these pathways[15]; both GC and SSA are reduced in BRCA1-deficient cells, placing BRCA1 before the branch point of GC and SSA.[15]

BRCA1 has a role in signaling DNA damage and cell-cycle checkpoint regulation,[14,15] whereas BRCA2 has a more direct role in DNA repair itself. BRCA2 is thought to promote genomic stability through a role in the error-free repair of DSBs by GC via association with RAD51. Aberrations in BRCA2-deficient cells arise at least in part by the use of the SSA pathway. NHEJ, however, is apparently unaffected in BRCA2-deficient cells.[14,15] Loss of BRCA2, therefore, results in the repair of DSBs by preferential utilization of an error-prone mechanism, which potentially explains the apparent chromosome instability associated with BRCA2 deficiency.[15]

The physical interaction between BRCA2 and RAD51 is essential for error-free DSB repair. BRCA2 is required for the localization of RAD51 to sites of DNA damage, where RAD51 forms the nucleoprotein filament required for recombination. The foci of the RAD51 protein are apparent in the nucleus after certain forms of DNA damage and these likely represent sites of repair by HR; BRCA2-deficient cells do not form RAD51 foci in response to DNA damage.[15] Two different domains within BRCA2 interact with RAD51, the eight BRC repeats in the central part of the protein and a distinct domain, TR2, at the C-terminus.[16]

PARP-1 INHIBITION AS A SYNTHETIC LETHAL THERAPEUTIC STRATEGY FOR THE TREATMENT OF BRCA-DEFICIENT CANCERS

Synthetic lethality is defined as the situation when a mutation in either of two genes individually has no effect, but combining the mutations leads to death.[17] This effect was first described and studied in genetically tractable organisms such as *Drosophila* and yeast.[17,18] This effect can arise because of a number of different gene–gene interactions. Examples include two genes in separate semiredundant or cooperating pathways, and two genes acting in the same pathway where loss of both critically affects flux through the pathway. The implication is that targeting one of these genes in a cancer where the other is defective should be selectively lethal to the tumor cells but not toxic to the normal cells. In principle, this should lead to a large therapeutic window.[19] The original suggestion that the concept of synthetic lethality could be used in the selection or development of cancer therapeutics came from Hartwell et al.,[18] and from experiments performed in yeast. Synthetic lethal screens have now been performed in a number of model organisms[20] and in human cells,[21] and these have revealed multiple potential gene–gene interactions, some of which could be exploited clinically. However, synthetic lethal therapies have not been clinically used until recently, when evidence has been provided for PARP-1 inhibition as a potential synthetic lethal approach for the treatment of BRCA-mutation–associated cancers.

PARP-1 inhibition causes failure of the repair of SSB lesions but does not affect DSB repair.[22] However, a persistent DNA SSB encountered by a DNA replication fork will cause stalling of the fork and may result in either fork collapse or the formation of a DSB.[23] Therefore, the loss of PARP-1 increases the formation of

DNA lesions that might be repaired by GC. As a loss of function of either BRCA1 or BRCA2 impairs GC,[14,15] a loss of PARP-1 function in a BRCA1- or BRCA2-defective background could result in the generation of replication-associated DNA lesions normally repaired by sister chromatid exchange. If so, this might lead to cell-cycle arrest and/or cell death. Therefore, PARP inhibitors could be selectively lethal to cells lacking functional BRCA1 or BRCA2 but might be minimally toxic to normal cells. This would indicate a synthetic lethal interaction between PARP and BRCA1 or BRCA2. Exemplifying this principle, potent inhibitors of PARP were applied to cells deficient in either BRCA1 or BRCA2. Cell survival assays showed that cell lines lacking wild-type BRCA1 or BRCA2 were extremely sensitive to these agents compared with heterozygous mutant or wild-type cells.[24,25]

To explain these observations, a model was proposed whereby persistent single-strand gaps in DNA caused by PARP inhibition when encountered by a replication fork might trigger fork arrest, collapse, and/or a DSB.[26] Alternatively, PARP-1 trapped on DNA by the inhibition of enzyme activity might also cause a fork collapse. Normally, these DSBs would be repaired by RAD51-dependent GC.[14,15] However, in the absence of BRCA1 or BRCA2, the replication fork cannot be restarted and collapses, causing persistent chromatid breaks. When repaired by the alternative error-prone DSB repair mechanisms of SSA or NHEJ, large numbers of chromatid aberrations would be induced, leading to cell lethality.[26] The idea that the defect in GC is being targeted in BRCA-deficient cells is supported by the demonstration that deficiency in other genes implicated in HR also confers sensitivity to PARP inhibitors.[27] This further suggests that this approach may be more widely applicable in the treatment of sporadic cancers with impairments of the HR pathway or BRCAness[28] (see the following).

INITIAL CLINICAL RESULTS TESTING SYNTHETIC LETHALITY OF PARP INHIBITORS AND BRCA MUTATION

Phase I studies[29] established that olaparib (AstraZeneca, London, UK; formerly KU-0059436, KuDOS Pharmaceuticals, Cambridge, UK) could be administered safely as a single agent at a dose of 400 mg twice per day. Side effects were classified as mild and were unlike those typically experienced with cytotoxic chemotherapy. Significant and durable responses were observed in patients with germ-line BRCA1 or BRCA2 mutations and breast ovary or prostate cancer. Of the 19 mutation carriers enrolled, 9 had an objective response defined by Response Evaluation Criteria in Sold Tumors (RECIST) criteria and 12 had stable disease for more than 4 months in duration. A similar magnitude of clinical responses was observed in an expanded cohort.[30] These observations are impressive because the cohort had been heavily pretreated and most were resistant to a wide range of chemotherapies.[29,30]

Phase II studies were subsequently performed in advanced breast and ovarian cancers arising in BRCA1 and BRCA2 mutation carriers.[31,32] The reported response rate was 41% in the breast study and 52% in the ovarian group; both groups had been heavily pretreated. Again, the drug was well tolerated. Another study of BRCA1/2 carriers with ovarian cancer compared olaparib with pegylated liposomal doxorubicin (PLD).[33] There was no significant difference in the response rates, but there were some differences in the patient characteristics and an unexpectedly high rate of response to PLD.

There are also reports of responses to PARP inhibitors in BRCA2 mutation carriers with prostate[34] and pancreatic[35] cancer. A number of other PARP inhibitors are in clinical development (Table 25.1), and some of these have shown efficacy in the treatment of cancers arising in BRCA1 or BRCA2 mutation carriers.[36,37]

CANCER THERAPEUTICS

TABLE 25.1

PARP Inhibitors in Late Stage Clinical Development

Agent	Company	Phase III Trials
Olaparib	AstraZeneca (formerly KuDOS)	*BRCA*-mutant ovarian cancer
Niraparib	Tesaro (formerly Merck)	Platinum sensitive ovarian cancer *BRCA*-mutant breast cancer
Rucaparib	Clovis (formerly Pfizer)	Platinum sensitive ovarian cancer
Veliparib	AbbVie (formerly Abbot)	Undisclosed
BMN673	BioMarin (formerly Lead)	*BRCA*-mutant breast cancer

Adapted from Garber, K. PARP inhibitors bounce back. *Nat Rev Drug Discov* 2013;12:725–727.

THE USE OF PARP INHIBITORS IN SPORADIC CANCERS

Germline mutations in *BRCA1* or *BRCA2* are relatively common in hereditary breast and ovarian cancer. However, inactivation of *BRCA* genes by mutation in sporadic cancers is rare, at least in breast cancer, which may seem to limit the application of PARP inhibitors to a wider range of patients. However, many tumors display features in common with BRCA-deficient tumors, including similar defects in DNA repair due to either epigenetic mutation of *BRCA1*, such as promoter methylation, or mutation of other components of BRCA-associated pathways.[28] This *BRCA-ness* may make these tumors also susceptible to PARP inhibition.[28] For example, phosphatase and tensin homolog (*PTEN*) mutations, which occur with a frequency estimated at 50% to 80% in sporadic tumors,[38] may cause PARP inhibitor sensitivity in preclinical models, possibly because PTEN-null cells display BRCAness phenotypes, such as the inability to efficiently repair certain forms of DNA damage.[39]

Traditional histopathologic methods and, more recently, gene expression profiling approaches have shown the phenotypic overlap between triple-negative breast cancers, basal-like breast cancers, and *BRCA1* familial breast cancers.[40,41] In gene expression profiling studies, it has been observed that *BRCA1* familial cancers strongly segregate with basal-like tumors and share features such as high-grade and pushing margins.[28,40,41] Although the overlap is not absolute, it leads to the hypothesis that there may be a subset of sporadic breast cancers that exhibits features of BRCAness, including deficiencies in HR and that may be susceptible to treatment with drugs such as PARP inhibitors.[26]

There have been several studies of PARP inhibitors in sporadic ovarian cancer. A study by Lederman[42] showed in a maintenance study following the response to platinum therapy a significant benefit in terms of progression-free survival (PFS) of olaparib compared to placebo. This was even more pronounced when the subgroup of BRCA mutation carriers were examined.[43] In both cases, the overall survival (OS) advantage was less than the PFS, but in the case of the BRCA mutation group, this reached statistical significance. Gelmon[44] also showed activity in sporadic ovarian cancer. In contrast, a study in sporadic triple-negative breast cancer failed to observe any benefit, although the study was small and the patients were heavily pretreated.[44]

Iniparib (initially reported as a PARP inhibitor) showed an overall survival benefit in a Phase II trial of triple-negative breast cancer in combination with gemcitabine and carboplatin compared with chemotherapy alone.[45] However, a subsequent Phase III study showed no improvement in PFS.[45] The reasons for this are uncertain, but significant questions have been raised about whether iniparib is indeed a bona fide PARP inhibitor. Therefore, it is now generally conceded that studies of iniparib have no implications for PARP inhibitors as a drug class.[46]

Which population of patients lacking a *BRCA1* or *BRCA2* mutation might benefit from PARP inhibitors remains unclear. This is likely to require the development of a clinical test to identify prospectively tumors with intrinsic sensitivity. Presently, most efforts are directed at developing assays of DNA repair deficiency.[47]

MECHANISMS OF RESISTANCE TO PARP INHIBITORS

Resistance to targeted therapy frequently occurs, but it was unclear how resistance might arise to a synthetic lethal therapy.[48] Potential mechanisms of resistance to PARP inhibitors have, however, been elucidated both directly in vitro, in mouse models, and in the clinic.[48] An in vitro model for resistance was developed by producing cells from the highly PARP inhibitor–sensitive BRCA2-deficient cell line CAPAN1, which carries a c.6174delT *BRCA2* frameshift mutation. CAPAN1 cells cannot form damage-induced RAD51 foci, are defective for HR, and are extremely sensitive to treatment with PARP inhibitors.[49] PARP inhibitor–resistant clones were highly resistant (over 1,000-fold) to the drug and were also cross-resistant to the DNA cross-linking agent cisplatin, but not to the microtubule-stabilizing drug docetaxel. PARP inhibitors and cisplatin both exert their effects on BRCA-deficient cells by increasing the frequency of misrepaired DSBs in the absence of effective HR. Therefore, this observation indicates that the resistance of PARP inhibitor–resistant clones to PARP inhibitors might be because of restored HR. This contention was supported by the acquisition in PARP inhibitor–resistant clone cells of the ability to form RAD51 foci after PARP inhibitor treatment or exposure to irradiation.

DNA sequencing of PARP inhibitor–resistant clones revealed the unexpected presence of novel *BRCA2* alleles that resulted in the elimination of the c.6174delT mutation and restoration of an open reading frame.[49] Therefore, in this case, resistance arises because of gain of function mutations in the synthetic lethal partner (BRCA2) rather than the direct drug target (PARP). Alternative mechanisms of PARP inhibitor resistance have also been described.[48] A mouse model of *BRCA1*-associated mammary gland cancer demonstrated the efficacy of olaparib in vivo and was used to study mechanisms of resistance.[50] Resistance seemed to be caused by the upregulation of *ABCB1a/b*, which encode P-glycoprotein pumps; this effect could be reversed with the P-glycoprotein inhibitor tariquidar. In addition, other alterations in DNA repair pathways have been proposed to compensate for BRCA1 deficiency resulting in PARP inhibitor deficiency.[48]

Studies of the mechanisms of resistance to PARP inhibitors in patient material are still at an early stage. Initial studies addressed the mechanism of resistance to platinum salts in *BRCA* mutation carriers. Cisplatin and carboplatin are part of the standard of care for the treatment of ovarian cancer, including individuals with *BRCA1* or *BRCA2* mutations. Platinum salts are thought to exert their BRCA-selective effects by a similar mechanism to PARP inhibitors.[15] Clinical observations suggest that *BRCA* mutation carriers with ovarian cancer usually respond better to these agents than patients without *BRCA* mutations[51,52]; however, resistance does eventually occur. To investigate this effect, *BRCA1* and *BRCA2* have been sequenced in tumor material from mutation carriers.[49,53] These studies revealed mutations in *BRCA1* or *BRCA2* that restored the open reading frame and likely contributed to platinum resistance. These observations suggest that specific mutations in *BRCA1* or *BRCA2* and sensitivity to therapeutics in cell lines and patients can be suppressed by intragenic deletion. Presumably, these mutations occur randomly and are then selected for by differential drug sensitivity. Therefore, the best use of these agents is likely to be earlier in the disease process when the disease burden is smaller, which will reduce the probability of resistance based on stochastic genetic reversion. Recently, similar observations of revertant *BRCA* alleles were made in two patients who became resistant after an initial response to olaparib.[54] Although preliminary, these results suggest that this mechanism is responsible for at least some of the clinical resistance observed. Doubtless, as with other targeted therapies, multiple resistance mechanisms will be implicated as further patients are studied.[48]

PROSPECTS

Currently, the treatments for cancers arising in carriers of *BRCA1* or *BRCA2* mutations are the same as those that occur sporadically matched for tumor pathology and age of onset. However, tumors in *BRCA1* or *BRCA2* mutation carriers lack wild-type *BRCA1* or *BRCA2*, but normal tissues retain a single wild-type copy of the relevant gene. This is a potentially targetable alteration that provides the basis for new mechanism-based approaches to the treatment of cancer. The biochemical difference in capacity to carry out HR between the tumor and normal tissues, in a *BRCA1* or

BRCA2 carrier, provides the rationale for this approach. Inhibiting the DNA repair protein PARP results in the generation of specific DNA lesions that require BRCA1 and BRCA2 specialized repair function(s) for their removal. Preclinical data indicate that tumors defective in wild-type BRCA1 or BRCA2 could be much more sensitive to PARP inhibition than unaffected heterozygous tissues, providing a potentially large therapeutic window. The safety and efficacy of this approach is currently being tested in clinical trials, which, if successful, may lead to registration for routine clinical use of one or more PARP inhibitors.[37]

Synthetic lethality by combinatorial targeting of DNA repair pathways may have usefulness as a therapeutic approach beyond familial cancers. The majority of solid tumors also exhibit genomic instability and aneuploidy. This suggests that pathways involved in the maintenance of genomic stability are dysfunctional in a significant proportion of neoplastic disorders.[47] Understanding which specialized DNA damage response and repair pathways are abrogated in sporadic tumor subtypes may allow for the development of therapies that target the residual repair pathways on which the cancer, but not normal tissue, is now completely dependent. These potential therapies may significantly improve response rates while causing fewer treatment-related toxicities. However, these approaches may be associated with mechanism-associated resistance, and careful consideration of their optimal use will be required.

REFERENCES

1. Hoeijmakers JH. Genome maintenance mechanisms for preventing cancer. *Nature* 2001;411:366–374.
2. Chambon P, Weill JD, Mandel P. Nicotinamide mononucleotide activation of new DNA-dependent polyadenylic acid synthesizing nuclear enzyme. *Biochem Biophys Res Commun* 1963;11:39–43.
3. Amé JC, Spenlehauer C, de Murcia G. The PARP superfamily. *Bioessays* 2004;26:882–893.
4. Otto H, Reche PA, Bazan F, et al. In silico characterization of the family of PARP-like poly(ADP-ribosyl)transferases (pARTs). *BMC Genomics* 2005;6:139.
5. van Gent DC, Hoeijmakers JH, Kanaar R. Chromosomal stability and the DNA double-stranded break connection. *Nat Rev Genet* 2001;2:196–206.
6. Shin DS, Chahwan C, Huffman JL, et al. Structure and function of the double-strand break repair machinery. *DNA Repair (Amst)* 2004;3: 863–873.
7. Takata M, Sasaki MS, Sonoda E, et al. Homologous recombination and non-homologous end-joining pathways of DNA double-strand break repair have overlapping roles in the maintenance of chromosomal integrity in vertebrate cells. *EMBO J* 1998;17:5497–5508.
8. Rothkamm K, Krüger I, Thompson LH, et al. Pathways of DNA double-strand break repair during the mammalian cell cycle. *Mol Cell Biol* 2003;23: 5706–5715.
9. Stark JM, Pierce AJ, Oh J, et al. Genetic steps of mammalian homologous repair with distinct mutagenic consequences. *Mol Cell Biol* 2004;24: 9305–9316.
10. Elliott B, Richardson C, Jasin M. Chromosomal translocation mechanisms at intronic alu elements in mammalian cells. *Mol Cell* 2005;17:885–894.
11. Durkacz BW, Omidiji O, Gray DA, et al. (ADP-ribose)n participates in DNA excision repair. *Nature* 1980;283(5747):593–596.
12. Tertoli L, Graziani G. Chemosensitisation by PARP inhibitors in cancer therapy. *Pharmacol Res* 2005;52:25–33.
13. Wooster R, Weber BL. Breast and ovarian cancer. *N Engl J Med* 2003;348: 2339–2347.
14. Gudmundsdottir K, Ashworth A. The roles of BRCA1 and BRCA2 and associated proteins in the maintenance of genomic stability. *Oncogene* 2006;25: 5864–5874.
15. Tutt AN, Lord CJ, McCabe N, et al. Exploiting the DNA repair defect in BRCA mutant cells in the design of new therapeutic strategies for cancer. *Cold Spring Harb Symp Quant Biol* 2005;70:139–148.
16. Lord CJ, Ashworth A. RAD51, BRCA2 and DNA repair: a partial resolution. *Nat Struct Mol Biol* 2007;14:461–462.
17. Dobzhansky T. Genetics of natural populations: Xiii. Recombination and variability in populations of *Drosophila pseudoobscura*. *Genetics* 1946;31:269–290.
18. Hartwell LH, Szankasi P, Roberts CJ, et al. Integrating genetic approaches into the discovery of anticancer drugs. *Science* 1997;278:1064–1068.
19. Kaelin WG Jr. The concept of synthetic lethality in the context of anticancer therapy. *Nat Rev Cancer* 2005;5:689–698.
20. Ooi SL, Pan X, Peyser BD, et al. Global synthetic-lethality analysis and yeast functional profiling. *Trends Genet* 2006;22:56–63.
21. Iorns E, Lord CJ, Turner N, et al. Utilizing RNA interference to enhance cancer drug discovery. *Nat Rev Drug Discov* 2007;6:556–568.

22. Noël G, Giocanti N, Fernet M, et al. Poly(ADP-ribose) polymerase (PARP-1) is not involved in DNA double-strand break recovery. *BMC Cell Biol* 2003;4:7.
23. Haber JE. DNA recombination: the replication connection. *Trends Biochem Sci* 1999;24:271–275.
24. Farmer H, McCabe N, Lord CJ, et al. Targeting the DNA repair defect in BRCA mutant cells as a therapeutic strategy. *Nature* 2005;434:917–921.
25. Bryant HE, Schultz N, Thomas HD, et al. Specific killing of BRCA2-deficient tumours with inhibitors of poly(ADP-ribose) polymerase. *Nature* 2005;434: 913–917.
26. Ashworth A. A synthetic lethal therapeutic approach: PARP inhibitors for the treatment of cancers deficient in double-strand break repair. *J Clin Oncol* 2008;26:3785–3790.
27. McCabe N, Turner NC, Lord CJ, et al. Deficiency in the repair of DNA damage by homologous recombination and sensitivity to poly(ADP-ribose) polymerase inhibition. *Cancer Res* 2006;66:8109–8115.
28. Turner N, Tutt A, Ashworth A. Hallmarks of 'BRCAness' in sporadic cancers. *Nat Rev Cancer* 2004;4:814–819.
29. Fong PC, Boss DS, Yap TA, et al. Inhibition of poly(ADP-ribose) polymerase in tumors from BRCA mutation carriers. *N Engl J Med* 2009;361:123–134.
30. Fong PC, Yap TA, Boss DS, et al. Poly(ADP)-ribose polymerase (PARP) inhibition: frequent durable responses in BRCA carrier ovarian cancer correlating with platinum-free interval. *J Clin Oncol* 2010;28:2512–2519.
31. Audeh MW, Carmichael J, Penson RT, et al. Oral poly(ADP-ribose) polymerase inhibitor olaparib in patients with BRCA1 or BRCA2 mutations and recurrent ovarian cancer: a proof-of-concept trial. *Lancet* 2010;376:245–251.
32. Tutt A, Robson M, Garber JE, et al. Oral poly(ADP-ribose) polymerase inhibitor olaparib in patients with BRCA1 or BRCA2 mutations and advanced breast cancer: a proof-of-concept trial. *Lancet* 2010;376:235–244.
33. Kaye SB, Lubinski J, Matulonis U, et al. Phase II, open-label, randomized, multicenter study comparing the efficacy and safety of olaparib, a poly (ADP-ribose) polymerase inhibitor, and pegylated liposomal doxorubicin in patients with BRCA1 or BRCA2 mutations and recurrent ovarian cancer. *J Clin Oncol* 2012;30:372–379.
34. Sandhu SK, Omlin A, Hylands L et al. Poly (ADP-ribose) polymerase (PARP) inhibitors for the treatment of advanced germline BRCA2 mutant prostate cancer. *Ann Oncol* 2013;24:1416–1418.
35. Fogelman DR, Wolff RA, Kopetz S, et al. Evidence for the efficacy of Iniparib, a PARP–1 inhibitor, in BRCA2-associated pancreatic cancer. *Anticancer Res* 2011;31:1417–1420.
36. Maxwell KN, Domchek SM. Cancer treatment according to BRCA1 and BRCA2 mutations *Nat Rev Clin Oncol* 2012;9:520–528.
37. Garber K. PARP inhibitors bounce back. *Nat Rev Drug Discov* 2013;12: 725–727.
38. Salmena L, Carracedo A, Pandolfi PP. Tenets of PTEN tumor suppression. *Cell* 2008;133:403–414.
39. Mendes-Pereira AM, Martin SA, Brough R, et al. Synthetic lethal targeting of PTEN mutant cells with PARP inhibitors. *EMBO Mol Med* 2009;1:315–322.
40. Foulkes WD, Stefansson IM, Chappuis PO, et al. Germline BRCA1 mutations and a basal epithelial phenotype in breast cancer. *J Natl Cancer Inst* 2003;95:1482–1485.

41. Turner NC, Reis-Filho JS. Basal-like breast cancer and the BRCA1 phenotype. *Oncogene* 2006;25:5846–5853.

42. Ledermann J, Harter P, Gourley C, et al. Olaparib maintenance therapy in platinum-sensitive relapsed ovarian cancer. *N Engl J Med* 2012;366:1382–1392.

43. Ledermann JA, Harter P, Gourley C. Olaparib maintenance therapy in patients with platinum-sensitive relapsed serous ovarian cancer (SOC) and a BRCA mutation (BRCAm). *J Clin Oncol* 2013;31 (suppl; abstr 5505).

44. Gelmon KA, Tischkowitz M, Mackay H, et al. Olaparib in patients with recurrent high-grade serous or poorly differentiated ovarian carcinoma or triple-negative breast cancer: a phase 2, multicentre, open-label, non-randomised study. *Lancet Oncol* 2011;12:852–861.

45. O'Shaughnessy J, Osborne C, Pippen J, et al. Iniparib plus chemotherapy in metastatic triple-negative breast cancer. *N Engl J Med* 2011;3:205–214.

46. Mateo J, Ong M, Tan DS, et al. Appraising iniparib, the PARP inhibitor that never was—what must we learn? *Nat Rev Clin Oncol* 2013;10:688–696.

47. Lord CJ, Ashworth A. The DNA damage response and cancer therapy. *Nature* 2012;481:287–294.

48. Lord CJ, Ashworth A. Mechanisms of resistance to therapies targeting BRCA-mutant cancers. *Nat Med* 2013;19:1381–1388.

49. Edwards S, Brough R, Lord CJ, et al. Resistance to therapy caused by intragenic deletion in BRCA2. *Nature* 2008;451(7182):1111–1115.

50. Rottenberg S, Jaspers JE, Kersbergen A, et al. High sensitivity of *BRCA1*-deficient mammary tumors to the PARP inhibitor AZD2281 alone and in combination with platinum drugs. *Proc Natl Acad Sci U S A* 2008;105:17079–17084.

51. Cass I, Baldwin RL, Varkey T, et al. Improved survival in women with BRCA-associated ovarian carcinoma. *Cancer* 2003;97:2187–2195.

52. Pal T, Permuth-Wey J, Kapoor R, et al. Improved survival in BRCA2 carriers with ovarian cancer. *Fam Cancer* 2007;6:113–119.

53. Sakai W, Swisher EM, Karlan BY, et al. Secondary mutations as a mechanism of cisplatin resistance in BRCA2-mutated cancers. *Nature* 2008;451:1116–1120.

54. Barber LJ, Sandhu S, Chen L, et al. Secondary mutations in BRCA2 associated with clinical resistance to a PARP inhibitor. *J Pathol* 2013;229:422–429.

CANCER THERAPEUTICS

26 Miscellaneous Chemotherapeutic Agents

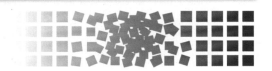

M. Sitki Copur, Scott Nicholas Gettinger, Sarah B. Goldberg, and Hari A. Deshpande

HOMOHARRINGTONINE AND OMACETAXINE

Homoharringtonine and its congener, harringtonine, are cephalotaxine esters isolated from the evergreen tree *Cephalotaxus hainanensis*, which are distributed throughout southern and northeastern China. The two differ only by a single methylene group, but both have a similar activity against murine leukemia.[1] The primary action of homoharringtonine appears to be the inhibition of protein synthesis and chain elongation through binding to 80S ribosome in eukaryotic cells.[2] DNA effects may also be important, involving a block in progression of cells from G1 phase into S phase and from G2 phase into M phase.[3] Homoharringtonine exhibits a triphasic plasma decay with a terminal half-life of 65.3 hours and apparent volume of distribution of 2.4 L/kg.[4] In early phase I studies, homoharringtonine was administered as a 10 to 360 minute infusion daily for 10 days.[5] Dose-limiting cardiovascular toxicity with hypotension began 4 or more hours after drug administration, which was alleviated by interrupting the infusion or by fluid administration and prolonging the duration of administration. Initial clinical studies with homoharringtonine in China showed activity against acute myeloid leukemia (AML) and chronic phase chronic myeloid leukemia (CML).[6] Variable activity was observed in the initial series of phase II trials in pediatric and adult patients with acute leukemia. In early studies of homoharringtonine, a continuous intravenous (IV) infusion at 2.5 mg/m² per day for 10 to 14 days per month induced complete hematologic and cytogenetic responses in 72% and 31% of patients, respectively, with chronic phase CML.[7]

The greater availability of homoharringtonine led to its further testing and the development of a semisynthetic cephalotaxine ester, omacetaxine mepesuccinate.[2] The mechanism of action of omacetaxine includes inhibition of protein synthesis and is independent of direct Bcr-Abl binding. In vitro, it reduces protein levels of the Bcr-Abl oncoprotein and Mcl-1, an antiapoptotic B-cell lymphoma 2 (Bcl-2) family member. The antileukemic effect of omacetaxine is not affected by the presence of mutations in Bcr-Abl.[8] Omacetaxine is absorbed following subcutaneous administration of 1.25 mg/m² twice daily for 11 days with a mean half-life of 6 hours, and a volume of distribution of 141 +/−93.4 L. A phase 2 trial assessed the efficacy of omacetaxine in CML patients with T315I and tyrosine–kinase inhibitor failure. Patients received subcutaneous omacetaxine 1.25 mg/m² twice daily on days 1 through 14, every 28 days until hematologic response or a maximum of 6 cycles, and then days 1 through 7 every 28 days as maintenance. Complete hematologic response was achieved in 77%, with a median response duration of 9.1 months. Of patients, 23% achieved a major cytogenetic response, including a complete cytogenetic response in 16%. Hematologic toxicity included thrombocytopenia (76%), neutropenia (44%), and anemia (39%) and was typically manageable by dose reduction. Nonhematologic adverse events were mostly grade 1/2 and included infection, diarrhea, and nausea.[9]

L-ASPARAGINASE

L-Asparaginase (L-asparagine aminohydrolase, EC 3.5.1.1), which catalyzes the hydrolysis of the essential amino acid L-asparagine to L-aspartic acid and ammonia, is a naturally occurring enzyme in some microorganisms.[10,11] Although cancer cells depend on an exogenous source of L-asparagine for survival, normal cells can synthesize asparagine. In addition to the depletion of L-asparagine, it may exert its antitumor activity through a glutaminase effect, depleting essential glutamine stores and leading to the inhibition of DNA biosynthesis. It comes in three preparations, two of which are native forms purified from bacterial sources, *Escherichia coli* and *Erwinia carotovora*. A third preparation, pegylated (PEG)-L-asparaginase, is a chemically modified form of the enzyme in which native *E. coli* L-asparaginase has been covalently conjugated to polyethylene glycol.[12]

After an intramuscular (IM) injection, peak plasma levels, approximately one-half of those achieved with IV administration, are reached within 14 to 24 hours. Plasma protein binding is 30%. The pharmacokinetics vary depending on the source of the enzyme.[13] Pharmacokinetic studies in newly diagnosed children with acute lymphocytic leukemia (ALL) have shown peak serum concentrations in the range of 1 to 10 IU/mL in 24 to 48 hours of a single dose of 2,500 to 25,000 IU/m² of the enzyme derived from *E. coli*. After a single dose of 25,000 IU/m², peak serum levels are reached within 24 hours. PEG-L-asparaginase, when administered at a dose of 2,500 IU/m², achieves peak drug levels at 72 to 96 hours and has a significantly longer half-life (5.7 days) than the *E. coli* L-asparaginase preparation.[13] Clinical trials have demonstrated the efficacy, safety, and tolerability of PEG-L-asparaginase administered intramuscularly, subcutaneously, or intravenously as part of multiagent chemotherapy regimens in the management of newly diagnosed and relapsed pediatric and adult ALL. L-Asparaginase can antagonize antineoplastic effects of methotrexate if given concurrently or immediately before. These two drugs should be administered sequentially at least 24 hours apart. L-Asparaginase has also been shown to inhibit the metabolic clearance of vincristine and can result in increased neurotoxicity. Toxicity is less pronounced if L-asparaginase is administered after vincristine. Hypersensitivity reactions occur in up to 25% of patients as a skin rash and urticaria or serious anaphylactic reactions. The risk increases with repeat exposure, and as a single-agent use without steroids. PEG-L-asparaginase is less immunogenic than the native nonpegylated forms of the enzyme. A number of other side effects are observed that are secondary to the inhibitory effects of L-asparaginase on cellular protein synthesis. Decreased serum levels of insulin, key lipoproteins, and albumin have been reported. L-Asparaginase can cause alterations in thyroid function tests as early as 2 days after an administered dose, possibly secondary to a reduction in the serum levels of thyroxine-binding globulin. Alterations in coagulation parameters with prolonged thrombin time, prothrombin time, and partial thromboplastin time have been observed. Patients treated with L-asparaginase are at an increased risk for bleeding or thromboembolic

290

events.[14] L-Asparaginase is contraindicated in patients with a prior history of pancreatitis, because there is a 10% incidence of acute pancreatitis. Neurologic toxicity includes lethargy, confusion, agitation, hallucinations, and/or coma. In contrast to the other anticancer agents used to treat ALL, myelosuppression is rare.

BLEOMYCIN

Bleomycin is a glycopeptide antibiotic produced by the bacterium *Streptomyces verticillus*. The most active chemotherapeutical forms are bleomycin A_2 and B_2.[15] The effect of bleomycin is cell cycle specific, because its main effects are mediated in the G_2 and M phases of the cell cycle.[16] The exact mechanism for DNA strand scission has been suggested to be due to bleomycin's chelating of metal ions (primarily iron) and producing a pseudoenzyme that reacts with oxygen to produce superoxide- and hydroxide-free radicals, thus cleaving DNA. Alternatively, bleomycin may bind at specific sites in the DNA strand and induce scission by abstracting the hydrogen atom from the base, resulting in strand cleavage as the base undergoes a Criegee-type rearrangement, or bleomycin may form an alkali-labile lesion.[17] Bleomycin is used in the treatment of Hodgkin lymphoma (as a component of the ABVD and BEACOPP regimen), squamous cell carcinomas, and testicular cancer; in the treatment of plantar warts,[18] as a means of effecting pleurodesis,[19] as well as an intralesional agent with electrochemotherapy in the management of cutaneous malignancies.[20]

The oral bioavailability is poor. It must be administered via IV or IM routes. The initial distribution half-life is 10 to 20 minutes with a terminal half-life of 3 hours. Bleomycin can be administered via the intracavitary route to control malignant pleural effusions or ascites, or both. Approximately 45% to 55% of an administered intracavitary dose of bleomycin is absorbed into the systemic circulation. Elimination is primarily via the kidneys, and approximately 60% to 70% of an administered dose is excreted unchanged in the urine. Dose reductions are required if creatinine clearance is less than 25 mL per minute.

Bleomycin-induced pneumonitis, the dose-limiting toxicity of the drug, occurs in 10% of patients, and is dependent on the cumulative dose.[21] The risk increases in patients older than 70 years and in those who receive a total cumulative dose greater than 400 U. In addition, patients with an underlying lung disease, prior irradiation to the chest or mediastinum, and exposure to high concentrations of inspired oxygen are at increased risk. Increased use of granulocyte colony-stimulating factor (G-CSF) has been paralleled by an increased incidence of bleomycin-induced pulmonary toxicity. The exacerbating effects of G-CSFs seem to be associated with a marked infiltration of activated neutrophils along with the lung injury caused by the direct effects of bleomycin.[22,23] In a retrospective review, 18% of a total of 141 patients with Hodgkin lymphoma treated with a bleomycin-containing regimen developed pulmonary toxicity. G-CSF use was one of the key factors associated with the development of this complication, and omission of bleomycin had no impact on clinical outcomes.[24] Similarly the combination of brentuximab vedotin and ABVD was associated with excessive pulmonary toxicity, indicating that brentuximab vedotin and bleomycin should not be used together.[25]

Patients with bleomycin-induced pulmonary toxicity may present with cough, dyspnea, dry inspiratory crackles, and infiltrates on chest radiograph. Pulmonary function testing is the most sensitive approach to monitor patients, and pulmonary function tests should be obtained at baseline and before each cycle of therapy, with a specific focus on the carbon monoxide diffusion capacity and vital capacity. A decrease greater than 15% in either diffusion capacity of carbon monoxide or vital capacity should mandate immediate discontinuation of bleomycin. Early clinical trials and isolated case reports suggest that bleomycin-induced acute hypersensitivity reactions occur in 1% of patients with lymphoma and less than 0.5% of those with solid tumors. The reactions are mainly characterized by high-grade fever, chills, hypotension, and, in a few cases, cardiovascular collapse, which can lead to death. The exact mechanism of these reactions is unclear, but is thought to be related to the release of endogenous pyrogens from the host cells. Supportive care, including hydration, steroids, antipyretics, and antihistamines, may resolve the symptoms.

Clinicians should monitor their patients for any signs and symptoms of acute hyperpyrexic reactions during bleomycin administration. Because the onset of the reactions can occur with any dose of bleomycin and at any time, routine test dosing does not seem to predict when drug reactions may occur.[26] Mucocutaneous toxicity presents as mucositis, erythema, hyperpigmentation, induration, hyperkeratosis, and skin peeling, which may progress to ulceration, and usually develops in the 2nd and 3rd week of treatment and after a cumulative dose of 150 to 200 U of the drug. Levels of bleomycin hydrolase are relatively low in lung and skin tissue, perhaps offering an explanation as to why these normal tissues are more adversely affected by bleomycin. Myelosuppression and immunosuppression are relatively mild. In rare cases, vascular events, including myocardial infarction, stroke, and Raynaud phenomenon, have been reported.

PROCARBAZINE

Originally prepared as a monoamine oxidase inhibitor, procarbazine is a prodrug, which after oxidation of the hydrazine in the liver, undergoes a complex enzymatic and chemical breakdown to its alkylating and methylating species.[27,28] The precise mechanism of action is uncertain, but may involve damaging the DNA, RNA or transfer RNA, and the inhibition of protein synthesis. Procarbazine is a cell-cycle phase-nonspecific antineoplastic agent. This agent was initially approved by the U.S. Food and Drug Administration (FDA) in 1969 as part of the MOPP (mechlorethamine, vincristine, procarbazine, and prednisone) regimen for the treatment of Hodgkin lymphoma. Since then, it has also demonstrated clinical activity in non-Hodgkin lymphoma, cutaneous T-cell lymphoma, and brain tumors.

Procarbazine is rapidly and completely absorbed from the gastrointestinal tract. Following oral administration, peak drug levels are reached within 10 to 15 minutes. Procarbazine crosses the blood–brain barrier and rapidly equilibrates between plasma and cerebrospinal fluid after oral administration. Peak cerebrospinal fluid drug concentrations are reached within 30 to 90 minutes after drug administration. The biologic half-life of procarbazine hydrochloride in both plasma and cerebrospinal fluid is approximately 1 hour. Procarbazine is metabolized to active and inactive metabolites by chemical breakdown in an aqueous solution and the liver microsomal P-450 system. Approximately 70% of procarbazine is excreted in urine within 24 hours, and less than 5% to 10% of the drug is eliminated in an unchanged form.[29,30]

A careful food and drug history is required before starting a patient on procarbazine therapy, because there are several potential drug–drug and drug–food interactions. Patients should avoid tyramine-containing foods, such as dark beer, wine, cheese, yogurt, bananas, and smoked foods. Procarbazine produces a disulfiramlike reaction with concurrent use of alcohol. Acute hypertensive reactions may occur with coadministration of tricyclic antidepressants and sympathomimetic drugs. Concurrent use of procarbazine with antihistamines and other central nervous system (CNS) depressants can result in CNS and/or respiratory depression.

Dose-limiting toxicity is myelosuppression, more commonly thrombocytopenia, and the nadir in platelet count is generally observed at 4 weeks. Patients with glucose-6-phosphate dehydrogenase deficiency can develop hemolytic anemia while receiving procarbazine therapy. Stepwise dose increments over the first few days of drug administration may minimize gastrointestinal intolerance. On rare occasions, procarbazine may induce interstitial pneumonitis, which mandates the discontinuation of therapy. Azoospermia and infertility after treatment with MOPP can be attributed, in part, to procarbazine. Procarbazine is associated with an increased risk of secondary malignancies, especially acute leukemia.

VISMODEGIB

Vismodegib (Erivedge, GDC-0449, Genentech) is a first-in-class, small-molecule inhibitor of the Hedgehog pathway. It binds to and inhibits smoothened, a transmembrane protein that is involved in Hedgehog signaling.[31] Pharmacodynamic downmodulation in the Hedgehog pathway was shown by a 90% decrease in transcription factor Gli1 mRNA in basal-cell carcinoma biopsy specimens of patients treated for a month. One-month vismodegib treatment also significantly reduced tumor proliferation, as assessed by Ki-67 expression, but did not change apoptosis, as assessed by cleaved caspase 3. The extent of Gli1 downmodulation does not seem to correlate with pharmacokinetic levels of vismodegib in individual patients. Vismodegib is absorbed from the gastrointestinal tract, with an oral bioavailability of 32%. Food does not affect drug exposure. Elimination is mainly hepatic, with excretion in feces. The median steady-state concentration is not changed by increasing the dose from 150 mg to 270 mg, and the median time to steady state is 14 days. The half-life is estimated at 8 days after a single dose. Intermittent doses (e.g., three times per week or once per week) were associated with a decrease of 50% and 80% in effective plasma levels of unbound drug, respectively, thus reinforcing the recommended dose and schedule of 150 mg orally daily.[32] Vismodegib is approved for the treatment of adults with metastatic basal-cell carcinoma that has recurred following surgery or in those who are not candidates for surgery and who are not candidates for radiation.[33]

No dose-limiting toxic effects or grade 5 events have been observed. However, 54% of patients receiving vismodegib discontinued the medication owing to side effects, and only one out of give eligible patients was able to continue vismodegib for 18 months. Abdominal pain, fatigue, weight loss, dysgeusia, and anorexia were reasons for discontinuation of the drug. When vismodegib was withdrawn, dysgeusia and muscle cramps ceased within 1 month, and scalp and body hair started to regrow within 3 months. Other side effects reported include hyponatremia, dyspnea, muscle spasm, atrial fibrillation, aspiration, back pain, corneal abrasion, dehydration, keratitis, lymphopenia, pneumonia, urinary tract infection, and a prolonged QT interval.[34]

ADO-TRASTUZUMAB EMTANSINE

Ado-trastuzumab emtansine (T-DM1), is a HER2-targeted antibody-drug conjugate (ADC). It is a novel compound composed of trastuzumab, a stable thioether linker, and DM1. DM1, a derivative of maytansine, is a microtubule polymerization inhibitor with activity similar to that of vinca alkaloids. T-DM1 is taken up into cells after binding to HER2, allowing for cytotoxic drug delivery specifically to cells overexpressing HER2. It has a drug-to-antibody ratio of approximately 3.5:1. T-DM1 is administered intravenously every 3 weeks and has been tested in a phase I trial at doses ranging from 0.3 to 4.8 mg/kg. The maximally tolerated dose is 3.6 mg/kg, which was the dose used in further phase II–III trials. T-DM1 is metabolized by the liver, via CYP3A4/5, and has a half-life of 3.5 days.[35]

T-DM1 is approved for use in patients with metastatic HER2-positive breast cancer who have received prior trastuzumab and a taxane. This approval was based on the results of the EMILIA trial, which randomized 991 patients with HER2-positive unresectable, locally advanced or metastatic breast cancer to T-DM1 3.6 mg/kg IV every 21 days or lapatinib 1,250 mg daily plus capecitabine 1,000 mg/m^2 on days 1 through 14 every 21 days. All patients were previously treated with trastuzumab and a taxane. T-DM1 resulted in a progression-free survival of 9.6 months compared to 6.4 months for lapatinib plus capecitabine (hazard ratio [HR] 0.65; 95% confidence interval [CI] 0.55 to 0.77; p <0.001). The response rate and overall survival was also higher with T-DM1 compared to lapatinib plus capecitabine.[36]

Although maytansine itself is associated with significant toxicity, T-DM1 is very well tolerated overall, which is likely due to the targeted nature of the compound. Side effects from T-DM1 include thrombocytopenia, hepatotoxicity, hypersensitivity/infusion

reactions, and cardiotoxicity. Nausea, fatigue, headaches, and anemia are also common. The left ventricular ejection fraction should be monitored prior to and at least every 3 months during therapy because of the potential for cardiac dysfunction.

SIROLIMUS AND TEMSIROLIMUS

Sirolimus (rapamycin) was isolated from the soil bacteria *Streptomyces hygroscopicus*, in the mid 1970s.[37] This bacterial macrolide later became the preferred immunosuppressant for kidney transplantation, because it was mildly immunosuppressive; however, in contrast to cyclosporine A, it did not enhance tumor incidence.[38] Sirolimus is the prototypic inhibitor of the mammalian target of rapamycin (mTOR), a serine/threonine protein kinase that is a highly conserved regulatory protein involved in cell-cycle progression, proliferation, and angiogenesis.[39] Signaling pathways both upstream and downstream of mTOR have been shown to be commonly dysregulated in cancer. mTOR functions through two main mechanisms, depending on the presence and activity of the mTOR-associated protein complexes, mTORC1 and mTORC2. Sirolimus and its analog compounds, temsirolimus and everolimus, form a complex with the FK-binding protein (FKBP) and inhibit activation of a subset of mTOR proteins residing within mTORC1. In contrast, mTORC2 holds mTOR in a form that is not as readily inhibited by these rapamycin analogs, and upregulation of mTORC2 may represent a mechanism by which resistance can develop to this class of compounds.

Temsirolimus (CCI-779), a novel functional ester of sirolimus, is a water-soluble dihydroxymethyl propionic acid compound that rapidly undergoes hydrolysis to sirolimus after IV administration, reaching peak concentrations within 0.5 to 2.0 hours.[40] This drug is widely distributed in tissues, and steady-state drug levels are reached in 7 to 8 days. Temsirolimus is metabolized primarily in the liver by CYP3A4 microsomal enzymes to yield sirolimus as the main metabolite. The terminal half-life of temsirolimus is 17 hours, whereas that of sirolimus is approximately 55 hours. When bound to temsirolimus, mTOR is unable to phosphorylate the key protein translation factors, such as 4E-BP1 and S6K1, leading to translational inhibition of several critical regulatory proteins involved in cell-cycle control. Several other cellular proteins involved in the regulation of angiogenesis, such as hypoxia-inducible factor-1α (HIF-1α) and vascular endothelial growth factor (VEGF), are suppressed through mTOR inhibition by temsirolimus.

Phase I studies of temsirolimus have investigated various schedules and doses, ranging from 7.5 mg to 220 mg given as weekly 30-minute infusions.[40] A phase II study in patients with cytokine-refractory renal cell cancer (RCC) investigated the efficacy and safety of three different dose levels (25 mg, 75 mg, and 250 mg, respectively) administered on a weekly schedule. This study showed promising antitumor activity for all three dose levels with no significant difference in efficacy or toxicity.[41] As a result, the 25-mg dose was eventually selected as the monotherapy dose for further study. A phase III randomized trial compared interferon, temsirolimus, and the combination of the two agents in previously untreated patients with advanced RCC who had at least three of six poor prognostic features.[42] Once-weekly IV temsirolimus, 25 mg, prolonged the median overall survival of patients with poor prognostic features by 49% from 7.3 months (95% CI, 6.1 to 8.8 months) in the interferon arm to 10.9 months (95% CI, 8.6 to 12.7 months) in the temsirolimus arm (P = .008). The temsirolimus arm also had a prolonged median progression-free survival of 5.5 months compared to 3.1 months in the interferon arm (P <.001). Moreover, temsirolimus was effective for both clear cell and non–clear cell histologies.[43,44]

Mantle cell lymphoma was the first hematologic malignancy in which mTOR inhibition was explored as a treatment strategy. The rationale for this approach was that mantle cell lymphoma is characterized by overexpression of cyclin D1, which is a cyclin whose expression appears to be tightly regulated by mTOR signaling. The early-phase clinical trials of temsirolimus showed promising activity against non-Hodgkin lymphomas, multiple myeloma, and myeloid leukemias, with some evidence of success thus far.[45]

In terms of the safety profile, the most common adverse events associated with temsirolimus were asthenia and fatigue, dry skin with acneiform skin rash, nausea/vomiting, mucositis, and anorexia. Hyperlipidemia with increased serum triglycerides and/or cholesterol as well as hyperglycemia occur in up to 90% of patients. Allergic, hypersensitivity reactions have been observed in about 10% of patients, and pulmonary toxicity, presenting as increased cough, dyspnea, fever, and pulmonary infiltrates, is a relatively rare event, occurring in less than 1% of patients. However, the risk of pulmonary toxicity increases in patients with an underlying pulmonary disease.[46]

EVEROLIMUS

Everolimus (RAD001) is an orally active hydroxyethyl ether analog of rapamycin that contains a 2-hydroxyethyl chain substitution. This molecule is significantly more water soluble than sirolimus. As with sirolimus and temsirolimus, everolimus targets mTOR by forming a complex with mTOR and FKBP, resulting in inhibition of mTOR activity. Few data are available regarding the actual differences in the ability of temsirolimus and everolimus to inhibit mTOR. One preclinical in vitro study showed that the binding of everolimus to FKBP was approximately threefold weaker than that of sirolimus.[47] In vivo studies, however, have documented similar efficacy of the two agents in terms of immunosuppressive activity as well as antitumor activity. In preclinical models, the administration of everolimus results in the inhibition of mTOR, similar to what has been observed with the other rapamycin analogs.[48] In terms of clinical pharmacology, peak drug levels are achieved within 1 to 2 hours after oral administration, and food with a high fat content reduces oral bioavailability by up to 20%. This compound is metabolized in the liver, mainly by the CYP3A4 system, and six main metabolites have been identified. In general, these metabolites are less active than the parent compound. Elimination is mainly hepatic with excretion in feces, and caution should be used in patients with moderate liver impairment (Child-Pugh class B).[49] In this setting, the daily dose of drug should be reduced to 5 mg. In patients with severe liver dysfunction (Child-Pugh class C), the use of this drug is contraindicated.

Encouraging clinical activity was initially observed in phase 1/2 trials in patients with non–small-cell lung, gastric, and esophageal cancers, sarcomas, pancreatic neuroendocrine tumors, as well as hematologic malignancies.[50–53] Presently, everolimus is indicated and approved for the treatment of adults with advanced RCC after failure with sunitinib or sorafenib; advanced hormone receptor-positive, HER2-negative breast cancer in combination with exemestane; and progressive unresectable, locally advanced, or metastatic neuroendocrine tumors of pancreatic origin (PNET).[54,55] The recommended dose of everolimus for these indications is 10 mg taken orally once daily.

The safety profile of everolimus is similar to what has been observed with temsirolimus. The most common adverse events include asthenia and fatigue, dry skin with acneiform skin rash, nausea/vomiting, mucositis, and anorexia. Hyperlipidemia with increased serum triglycerides and/or cholesterol as well as hyperglycemia occur in up to 90% of patients. Allergic, hypersensitivity reactions have been observed in about 10% of patients, and pulmonary toxicity, presenting as increased cough, dyspnea, fever, and pulmonary infiltrates, are a relatively rare event, occurring in less than 1% of patients. However, the risk of pulmonary toxicity increases in patients with an underlying pulmonary disease.

THALIDOMIDE, LENALIDOMIDE, AND POMALIDOMIDE

Thalidomide and its amino-substituted analogs, lenalidomide and pomalidomide, are small-molecule glutamic acid derivatives that possess a wide range of biologic properties, including immunomodulating, antiangiogenic, and epigenetic effects. They are classified as class I (non–phosphophodiesterase-4 inhibitory) immunomodulatory drugs (IMiDs). Although their primary mechanism of activity against malignancy is uncertain, it is believed that IMiDs exert their anticancer effects both directly on cancer cells and indirectly via effects on the tumor microenvironment and host antitumor immunity. Specific mechanisms include the inhibition of nuclear factor kappa B (NF-κB) transcriptional activity in malignant cells with a resultant decrease in the production of anti-apoptotic molecules; the inhibition of surface adhesion molecule expression on both multiple myeloma cells and bone marrow stromal cells; the inhibition of the production and release of various growth factors (including vascular endothelial growth factor, basic fibroblast growth factor, tumor necrosis factor alpha, and interleukin [IL] 6) that regulate angiogenesis and tumor cell proliferation; and costimulation of IL-2 and interferon gamma (IFN-γ) release with T-helper 1 subset skewing and augmentation of cytotoxic T-cell and natural killer cell effector function.[56,57] Unlike thalidomide, both lenalidomide and pomalidomide result in cell cycle arrest and apoptosis of myeloma cells in vitro, believed in part to be related to epigenetic effects.[58] They are also more potent stimulators of IL-2 and INF-γ production and T-cell proliferation than thalidomide, and appear to additionally inhibit T-regulatory cells.[57] Clinically, lenalidomide has activity in patients with thalidomide-resistant multiple myeloma, and pomalidomide has additional activity in patients with lenalidomide-resistant disease.[59,60] Recently, the protein cereblon (cerebral protein with lon protease), a highly conserved E3 ligase, was recognized as a primary target of IMiDs teratogenic effect, and appears to be an important target of IMiD anticancer activity.[61–63] Efforts are currently under way to evaluate the expression of Cereblon as a predictive biomarker of response to IMiDs.[63] Due to the potential risk of significant teratogenicity, thalidomide, lenalidomide, and pomalidomide can only be prescribed by licensed prescribers who are registered in restricted distribution programs.

Thalidomide

Thalidomide (2-[2,6-dioxopiperidin-3-yl]-2,3-dihydro-1H-isoindole-1,3-dione; Thalomid) is a synthetic glutamic acid derivative that was initially synthesized in 1953. It was used widely in Europe between 1956 and 1962 as a sleeping aid and antiemetic for pregnant women before it was discovered to cause severe congenital malformations. Initial reports of its efficacy in multiple myeloma were published in 1999, and the 200-mg daily dose combined with pulse dexamethasone (40-mg daily dose on days 1 through 4, 9 through 12, and 17 through 20 on a 28-day schedule) was approved by the FDA in 2006 for newly diagnosed multiple myeloma. The use of thalidomide has dropped precipitously in the United States with the FDA approval of more efficacious and less toxic therapies for myeloma. Thalidomide is poorly soluble, and it is absorbed slowly from the gastrointestinal tract, reaching peak plasma concentration in 3 to 6 hours, with 55% to 66% bound to plasma proteins. The exact metabolic route and fate of thalidomide is not known. Thalidomide does not appear to be hepatically metabolized, but rather undergoes spontaneous nonenzymatic hydrolysis in plasma to multiple metabolites, with a half-life of elimination ranging from 5 to 7 hours. These metabolites are believed to be responsible for the antitumor effects of thalidomide. Less than 1% is excreted into the urine as unchanged drug.[64]

Thalidomide frequently causes drowsiness, constipation, and fatigue. Peripheral neuropathy is a common and potentially severe and irreversible side effect occurring in up to 30% of patients. Increased incidences of venous thromboembolic events, such as deep venous thrombosis and pulmonary embolus, have also been observed with thalidomide, particularly when used in combination with dexamethasone or anthracycline-based chemotherapy. Patients who are appropriate candidates may benefit from concurrent prophylactic anticoagulation or aspirin treatment.[65] Other side effects of thalidomide include rash, nausea, dizziness, orthostatic hypotension, bradycardia, and mood changes. In 2013, additional alerts were released linking thalidomide to an increased risk of developing second primary malignancies (both acute myelogenous leukemia and myelodysplastic syndrome) and arterial thromboembolic events.

Lenalidomide

Lenalidomide (3-[4-amino-1-oxo-2,3-dihydro-1H-isoindol-2-yl]piperidine-2,6-dione; Revlimid) is a thalidomide derivative that shares the immunomodulatory and antineoplastic properties of its parent compound. However, lenalidomide appears to be more potent in vitro with less nonhematologic toxicities in clinical studies. It initially received FDA approval (10-mg daily dose) in 2005 for the treatment of patients with transfusion-dependent anemia secondary to low or intermediate risk myelodysplastic syndromes associated with a deletion 5q cytogenetic abnormality, with or without additional cytogenetic abnormalities. In 2006, lenalidomide (25-mg daily dose on days 1 through 21 of a 28-day cycle) in combination with dexamethasone (40-mg daily dose on days 1 through 4, 9 through 12, and 17 through 20 on each 28-day cycle for the first four cycles, then 40 mg daily on days 1 through 4 every 28 days) was approved by the FDA for the treatment of patients with multiple myeloma who had received at least one prior therapy for multiple myeloma. In 2013, lenalidomide 25 mg daily (days 1 through 21 on repeated 28-day cycles) was additionally approved for use in refractory mantle cell lymphoma (after relapse/ progression on two lines of therapy, one of which contained bortezomid). Lenalidomide is administered orally and is rapidly absorbed from the gastrointestinal tract. Maximum plasma concentration is reached 0.625 to 1.5 hours after dosing, with approximately 30% bound to plasma proteins. The half-life of elimination is approximately 3 hours, with little information currently available concerning metabolism. Approximately 70% of an administered dose is excreted unchanged by the kidneys.[66]

Compared with thalidomide, lenalidomide is associated with less sedation, constipation, and peripheral neuropathy. However, myelosuppression in the form of neutropenia and thrombocytopenia can be dose limiting. As with thalidomide, the incidence of thromboembolic events is significant with the combination of dexamethasone and lenalidomide. A pooled analysis of 691 patients enrolled in two randomized studies reported a 12% incidence of thrombotic or thromboembolic events with the combination, compared with 4% with dexamethasone alone.[67]

Pomalidomide

Pomalidomide (4-amino-2-[2,6-dioxopiperidin-3-yl]-2,3-dihydro-1H-isoindole-1,3-dione; Pomalyst) is another thalidomide derivative designed to be more portent and less toxic than both thalidomide and lenalidomide. It is currently FDA approved (4-mg once daily dose orally on days 1 through 21 of a 28-day cycle, with or without dexamethasone) for use in patients with progressive multiple myeloma who have received at least two prior therapies, including lenalidomide and bortezomid. Pomalidomide is administered orally and is rapidly absorbed. Maximum plasma concentration is reached 2 to 3 hours after ingestion, with approximately 12% to 44% protein binding.[68] The half-life of elimination is between 7.5 and 9.5 hours. Pomalidomide is metabolized in the liver, via CYP1A2/CYP3A4 (major) and CYP2C19/CYP2D6 (minor), and excretion occurs primarily through the kidneys (73%; 2% as unchanged drug).

Like lenalidomide, pomalidomide is better tolerated than thalidomide at approved doses with less constipation, fatigue, and neuropathy.[69] The primary toxicity appreciated in myeloma trials has been myelosuppression, particularly neutropenia, which can be dose limiting. The risk of thromboembolic events is similar to that seen with thalidomide and lenalidomide. Unlike thalidomide or lenalidomide, dermatologic toxicity is rare with pomalidomide. A summary of the characteristics of the miscellaneous drugs mentioned in this chapter is provided in Table 26.1. A summary of all hematology oncology drug approvals since the last edition of the textbook can be viewed in Table 26.2.

TABLE 26.1

Miscellaneous Chemotherapeutic Agents

	Main Therapeutic Uses	Clinical Pharmacology	Major Toxicities	Notes
Omacetaxine	CML	Mean half-life of 6 h after subcutaneous injection	Thrombocytopenia, anemia, nausea, diarrhea	Efficacy shown in Bcr-Abl–mutated CML
L-Asparaginase	Pediatric and adult ALL	Peak concentration 7–12 h after IV administration; 30% plasma protein binding; PEG form has longer half-life of 5.7 days; antagonize effects of methotrexate if given before or concurrently	Hypersensitivity reactions, alterations in thyroid function, prolonged PT/PTT, decreased levels of vitamin K–dependent factors, acute pancreatitis	Myelosuppression is rare; hypersensitivity reaction risk increases with repeated exposure and when used as single agent; PEG form is less immunogenic
Bleomycin	Hodgkin disease, neoplastic pleural effusion, non-Hodgkin lymphoma, squamous cell carcinoma of cervix, squamous cell carcinoma of nasopharynx, squamous cell carcinoma of penis, squamous cell carcinoma of the head and neck, squamous cell carcinoma of vulva, testicular cancer	Terminal half-life of 3h; can be given intracavitary; 45%–55% of intracavitary dose absorbed systemically; elimination via kidneys if CrCl <25–35 mL/min dose reduction required	Pulmonary toxicity dose-limiting; more if age >70 y; cumulative dose >400 U; acute hypersensitivity reactions rare (1%); mucositis, erythema, hyperpigmentation	Not myelosuppressive; immunosuppressive; metabolizing enzyme; bleomycin hydrolase enzyme low in lung and skin tissue; G-CSF use seems to exacerbate pulmonary toxicity

(continued)

TABLE 26.1

Miscellaneous Chemotherapeutic Agents *(continued)*

	Main Therapeutic Uses	Clinical Pharmacology	Major Toxicities	Notes
Procarbazine	Hodgkin lymphoma	Rapid complete oral absorption; peak concentration, 10–15 min; crosses blood–brain barrier; half-life 1 h; several drug–drug and food–drug interactions; metabolized by hepatic microsomal P-450 system; 70% excreted in urine	Dose-limiting toxicity is myelosuppression, more commonly thrombocytopenia nadir at 4 wk; G-6PD–deficient patients can develop hemolytic anemia, nausea, vomiting, diarrhea, flulike symptoms, peripheral neuropathy, hypersensitivity reactions	Avoid tyramine-containing foods; disulfiramlike reaction with concurrent alcohol use; hypertensive reaction with concurrent tricyclic antidepressant use; increased risk for azoospermia/infertility and secondary malignancy
Vismodegib	Basal cell carcinoma of the skin	Oral bioavailability 32%; not affected by food	No dose limiting toxicity; abdominal pain, fatigue, weight loss, dysgeusia	Hedgehog-signaling pathway inhibitor
Ado-trastuzumabemtansine	Advanced HER2-positive breast cancer	Peak concentration near the end of infusion metabolized by CYP3A4/5; half-life, 3.5 days	Thrombocytopenia, hepatotoxicity, cardiac toxicity fatigue, nausea	Monitor cardiac function
Temsirolimus	Advanced renal cancer	Peak concentration, 0.5–2 h; widely distributed in tissues; steady-state levels reached in 7–8 d; half-life, 17 h	Asthenia, fatigue, dry skin, acneiform skin rash, mucositis, anorexia, hyperlipidemia, hyperglycemia	Efficacy shown for both clear cell and non–clear-cell histologies; efficacy in hematologic malignancies (mantle cell lymphoma, non-Hodgkin lymphoma, multiple myeloma)
Everolimus	Advanced renal cell carcinoma, breast cancer, pancreatic neuroendocrine tumor	Peak concentration, 1–2 hr; reduced bioavailability with high fat content food; metabolized by CYP3A4 system; mainly hepatic excretion	Asthenia, dry skin, nausea, vomiting, mucositis, hyperlipidemia, hyperglycemia, allergic hypersensitivity reaction, pulmonary toxicity	Contraindicated in Child-Pugh class C patients; encouraging activity in gastric, non–small-cell, lung, esophageal cancers, sarcomas; approved for organ rejection prophylaxis
Thalidomide	Multiple myeloma, erythema nodosum leprosum	Oral absorption slow; peak concentration, 3–6 h; 55%–66% bound to plasma proteins; half-life, 5–7 h; spontaneous nonenzymatic hydrolysis in plasma	Drowsiness, constipation, fatigue, skin rash, increased risk for thromboembolic complications	Pregnancy category X; may be present in semen; serious skin reactions including Stevens-Johnson syndrome
Lenalidomide	Low-to-intermediate risk myelodysplastic syndrome associated with 5q deletion, multiple myeloma	Rapid oral absorption; peak concentration, 0.6–1.5 h; half-life, 3 h; 70% excreted unchanged by kidneys	Less sedation, drowsiness, constipation than thalidomide; myelosuppression; thromboembolic events; peripheral neuropathy	Pregnancy category X; caution in patients with renal function impairment; neutropenia; thrombocytopenia may be dose limiting
Pomalidomide	Multiple myeloma who have received at least two prior therapies	Rapid oral absorption; peak concentration, 2–3 h; half-life, 7.5 h	Myelosuppression; thromboembolic events; skin toxicity rare	Better tolerated than thalidomide; effective in prior bortezomib- and lenalidomide-receiving patients

PT, prothrombin time; PTT, partial thromboplastin time; CrCl, creatinine clearance.

TABLE 26.2

U.S. Food And Drug Administration Hematology Oncology Drug Approvals 2010–2013

Drug/Manufacturer	Indication	Approval Date
Sorafenib (NEXAVAR tablets, Bayer Healthcare Pharmaceuticals Inc.)	For the treatment of locally recurrent or metastatic, progressive, differentiated thyroid carcinoma (DTC) refractory to radioactive iodine treatment.	November 22, 2013
Crizotinib (Xalkori, Pfizer, Inc.) capsules	For the treatment of patients with metastatic non–small-cell lung cancer (NSCLC) whose tumors are anaplastic lymphoma kinase (ALK) positive as detected by an FDA-approved test.	November 20, 2013
Ibrutinib (IMBRUVICA, Pharmacyclics, Inc.)	For the treatment of patients with mantle cell lymphoma (MCL) who have received at least one prior therapy.	November 13, 2013
Obinutuzumab (GAZYVA injection, for intravenous use, Genentech, Inc.; previously known as GA101)	For use in combination with chlorambucil for the treatment of patients with previously untreated chronic lymphocytic leukemia (CLL).	November 1, 2013
Pertuzumab injection (PERJETA, Genentech, Inc.)	For use in combination with trastuzumab and docetaxel for the neoadjuvant treatment of patients with HER2-positive, locally advanced, inflammatory, or early stage breast cancer (either greater than 2 cm in diameter or node positive) as part of a complete treatment regimen for early breast cancer.	September 30, 2013
Paclitaxel protein-bound particles (albumin-bound) (Abraxane for injectable suspension, Abraxis BioScience, LLC, a wholly owned subsidiary of Celgene Corporation)	In combination with gemcitabine for the first-line treatment of patients with metastatic adenocarcinoma of the pancreas.	September 6, 2013
Afatinib (Gilotrif tablets, Boehringer Ingelheim Pharmaceuticals, Inc.)	For the first-line treatment of patients with metastatic NSCLC whose tumors have epidermal growth factor receptor (EGFR) exon 19 deletions or exon 21 (L858R) substitution mutations as detected by an FDA-approved test. The safety and efficacy of afatinib have not been established in patients whose tumors have other EGFR mutations.	July 12, 2013
Denosumab (Xgeva injection, for subcutaneous use, Amgen Inc.)	For the treatment of adults and skeletally mature adolescents with a giant cell tumor of bone that is unresectable or where surgical resection is likely to result in severe morbidity.	June 13, 2013
Lenalidomide capsules (REVLIMID, Celgene Corporation)	For the treatment of patients with MCL whose disease has relapsed or progressed after two prior therapies, one of which included bortezomib.	June 5, 2013
Trametinib (MEKINIST tablet, GlaxoSmithKline, LLC)	For the treatment of patients with unresectable or metastatic melanoma with BRAF V600E or V600K mutation as detected by an FDA-approved test.	May 29, 2013
Dabrafenib (TAFINLAR capsule, GlaxoSmithKline, LLC)	For the treatment of patients with unresectable or metastatic melanoma with BRAF V600E mutation as detected by an FDA-approved test.	May 29, 2013
Radium Ra 223 dichloride (Xofigo Injection, Bayer HealthCare Pharmaceuticals Inc.)	For the treatment of patients with castration-resistant prostate cancer, symptomatic bone metastases, and no known visceral metastatic disease.	May 15, 2013
Erlotinib (Tarceva, Astellas Pharma Inc.)	For the first-line treatment of metastatic NSCLC patients whose tumors have EGFR exon 19 deletions or exon 21 (L858R) substitution mutations.	May 14, 2013
Ado-trastuzumab emtansine (KADCYLA for injection, Genentech, Inc.)	For use as a single agent for the treatment of patients with HER2-positive, metastatic breast cancer who previously received trastuzumab and a taxane, separately or in combination.	February 22, 2013
Pomalidomide (POMALYST capsules, Celgene Corporation)	For the treatment of patients with multiple myeloma who have received at least two prior therapies, including lenalidomide and bortezomib, and have demonstrated disease progression on or within 60 days of completion of the last therapy.	February 8, 2013

(continued)

TABLE 26.2

U.S. Food And Drug Administration Hematology Oncology Drug Approvals 2010–2013 *(continued)*

Drug/Manufacturer	Indication	Approval Date
Doxorubicin hydrochloride liposome injection (Sun Pharma Global FZE), a generic version of DOXIL Injection (doxorubicin hydrochloride liposome; Janssen Products, L.P.)	For the treatment of ovarian cancer in patients whose disease has progressed or recurred after platinum-based chemotherapy and for AIDS-related Kaposi sarcoma after failure of prior systemic chemotherapy or intolerance to such therapy.	February 4, 2013
Bevacizumab (Avastin, Genentech U.S., Inc.)	For use in combination with fluoropyrimidine–irinotecan- or fluoropyrimidine–oxaliplatin-based chemotherapy for the treatment of patients with metastatic colorectal cancer (mCRC) whose disease has progressed on a first-line bevacizumab-containing regimen.	January 23, 2013
Ponatinib (Iclusig tablets, ARIAD Pharmaceuticals, Inc.)	For the treatment of adult patients with chronic phase, accelerated phase, or blast phase chronic myeloid leukemia (CML) that is resistant or intolerant to prior tyrosine–kinase inhibitor (TKI) therapy or Philadelphia chromosome–positive acute lymphoblastic leukemia (Ph+ ALL) that is resistant or intolerant to prior TKI therapy.	December 17, 2012
Abiraterone acetate (Zytiga Tablets, Janssen Biotech, Inc.)	In combination with prednisone for the treatment of patients with metastatic castration-resistant prostate cancer.	December 10, 2012
Cabozantinib (COMETRIQ capsules, Exelixis, Inc.)	For the treatment of patients with progressive metastatic medullary thyroid cancer (MTC). Cabozantinib is a small molecule that inhibits the activity of multiple tyrosine kinases, including RET, MET, and VEGF receptor 2.	November 29, 2012
Omacetaxine mepesuccinate (SYNRIBO for injection, for subcutaneous use, Teva Pharmaceutical Industries Ltd.)	For the treatment of adult patients with chronic or accelerated phase CML with resistance and/or intolerance to two or more TKIs.	October 26, 2012
Paclitaxel protein-bound particles for injectable suspension, albumin-bound (ABRAXANE for injectable suspension; Abraxis Bioscience a wholly owned subsidiary of Celgene Corporation)	For use in combination with carboplatin for the initial treatment of patients with locally advanced or metastatic NSCLC who are not candidates for curative surgery or radiation therapy.	October 11, 2012
Regorafenib (Stivarga tablets, Bayer HealthCare Pharmaceuticals, Inc.)	For the treatment of patients with mCRC who have been previously treated with fluoropyrimidine-, oxaliplatin-, and irinotecan-based chemotherapy, an anti-VEGF therapy, and, if KRAS wild-type, an anti-EGFR therapy.	September 27, 2012
Bosutinib tablets (Bosulif, Pfizer, Inc.)	for the treatment of chronic, accelerated, or blast phase Ph+ CML in adult patients with resistance or intolerance to prior therapy.	September 4, 2012
Enzalutamide (XTANDI Capsules, Medivation, Inc., and Astellas Pharma US, Inc.)	For the treatment of patients with metastatic castration-resistant prostate cancer who have previously received docetaxel.	August 31, 2012
Everolimus tablets for oral suspension (Afinitor Disperz, Novartis Pharmaceuticals Corp.)	For the treatment of pediatric and adult patients with tuberous sclerosis complex (TSC) who have subependymal giant cell astrocytoma (SEGA) that requires therapeutic intervention, but that cannot be curatively resected.	August 30, 2012
Vincristine sulfate LIPOSOME injection (Marqibo, Talon Therapeutics, Inc.)	For the treatment of adult patients with Ph- ALL in second or greater relapse or whose disease has progressed following two or more antileukemia therapies.	August 9, 2012
Ziv-aflibercept injection (ZALTRAP, Sanofi U.S., Inc.)	For use in combination with 5-fluorouracil, leucovorin, irinotecan (FOLFIRI) for the treatment of patients with mCRC that is resistant to or has progressed following an oxaliplatin-containing regimen.	August 3, 2012
Everolimus tablets (Afinitor, Novartis Pharmaceuticals Corporation)	For the treatment of postmenopausal women with advanced hormone receptor–positive, HER2-negative breast cancer in combination with exemestane, after failure of treatment with letrozole or anastrozole.	July 20, 2012

(continued)

CANCER THERAPEUTICS

TABLE 26.2

U.S. Food And Drug Administration Hematology Oncology Drug Approvals 2010–2013 (continued)

Drug/Manufacturer	Indication	Approval Date
Carfilzomib injection (Kyprolis, Onyx Pharmaceuticals)	For the treatment of patients with multiple myeloma who have received at least two prior therapies, including bortezomib and an immunomodulatory agent, and have demonstrated disease progression on or within 60 days of the completion of the last therapy.	July 20, 2012
Cetuximab (Erbitux, ImClone LLC, a wholly owned subsidiary of Eli Lilly and Co.)	For use in combination with FOLFIRI for first-line treatment of patients with K-ras mutation-negative (wild-type), EGFR-expressing mCRC as determined by FDA-approved tests for this use.	July 9, 2012
Pertuzumab injection (PERJETA, Genentech, Inc.)	For use in combination with trastuzumab and docetaxel for the treatment of patients with HER2-positive metastatic breast cancer who have not received prior anti-HER2 therapy or chemotherapy for metastatic disease.	June 8, 2012
Pazopanib tablets (VOTRIENT, a registered Trademark of GlaxoSmithKline)	For the treatment of patients with advanced soft tissue sarcoma (STS) who have received prior chemotherapy.	April 26, 2012
Everolimus (Afinitor tablets, Novartis)	For the treatment of adults with renal angiomyolipoma, associated with TSC who do not require immediate surgery.	April 26, 2012
Imatinib mesylate tablets (Gleevec, Novartis Pharmaceuticals)	For the adjuvant treatment of adult patients following complete gross resection of Kit (CD117)-positive gastrointestinal stromal tumors (GIST).	January 31, 2012
Vismodegib (ERIVEDGE Capsule, Genentech, Inc.)	For the treatment of adults with metastatic basal cell carcinoma or with locally advanced basal cell carcinoma that has recurred following surgery or who are not candidates for surgery and who are not candidates for radiation.	January 30, 2012
Axitinib tablets (Inlyta, Pfizer, Inc.)	For the treatment of advanced renal cell carcinoma after failure of one prior systemic therapy.	January 27, 2012
Glucarpidase injection (Voraxaze, BTG International Inc.)	For the treatment of toxic plasma methotrexate concentrations (> 1 μmol/L) in patients with delayed methotrexate clearance due to impaired renal function.	January 17, 2012
Asparaginase Erwinia chrysanthemi (Erwinaze, injection, EUSA Pharma [USA], Inc.)	As a component of a multiagent chemotherapeutic regimen for the treatment of patients with ALL who have developed hypersensitivity to E. coli–derived asparaginase.	November 18, 2011
Ruxolitinib (Jakafi oral tablets, Incyte Corporation)	For the treatment of intermediate and high risk myelofibrosis, including primary myelofibrosis, postpolycythemia vera myelofibrosis, and postessential thrombocythemia myelofibrosis.	November 16, 2011
Cetuximab (Erbitux, ImClone LLC, a wholly-owned subsidiary of Eli Lilly and Company)	In combination with platinum-based therapy plus 5-fluorouracil (5-FU) for the first-line treatment of patients with recurrent locoregional disease and/or metastatic squamous cell carcinoma of the head and neck (SCCHN).	November 7, 2011
Eculizumab (Soliris, Alexion, Inc.)	For the treatment of pediatric and adult patients with atypical hemolytic uremic syndrome (aHUS).	September 23, 2011
Denosumab (Prolia, Amgen Inc.)	As a treatment to increase bone mass in patients at high risk for fracture receiving androgen-deprivation therapy (ADT) for nonmetastatic prostate cancer or adjuvant aromatase inhibitor (AI) therapy for breast cancer.	September 16, 2011
Crizotinib (XALKORI Capsules, Pfizer Inc.)	For the treatment of patients with locally advanced or metastatic NSCLC that is ALK-positive as detected by an FDA-approved test.	August 26, 2011

(continued)

TABLE 26.2

U.S. Food And Drug Administration Hematology Oncology Drug Approvals 2010–2013 (continued)

Drug/Manufacturer	Indication	Approval Date
Brentuximab vedotin (Adcetris for injection, Seattle Genetics, Inc.)	For treatment of patients with Hodgkin lymphoma after failure of autologous stem cell transplant (ASCT) or after failure of at least two prior multiagent chemotherapy regimens in patients who are not ASCT candidates and treatment of patients with systemic anaplastic large cell lymphoma (ALCL) after failure of at least one prior multiagent chemotherapy regimen.	August 19, 2011
Vemurafenib tablets (ZELBORAF, Hoffmann-La Roche Inc.)	For the treatment of patients with unresectable or metastatic melanoma with the BRAFV600E mutation as detected by an FDA-approved test.	August 17, 2011
Sunitinib (Sutent capsules, Pfizer, Inc.)	For the treatment of progressive, well-differentiated pancreatic neuroendocrine tumors (pNET) in patients with unresectable, locally advanced, or metastatic disease.	May 20, 2011
Everolimus (Afinitor tablets, Novartis Pharmaceuticals Corporation)	For the treatment of progressive PNET in patients with unresectable, locally advanced, or metastatic disease.	May 5, 2011
Abiraterone acetate (Zytiga tablets, Centocor Ortho Biotech, Inc.)	For use in combination with prednisone for the treatment of patients with metastatic castration-resistant prostate cancer (mCRPC) who have received prior chemotherapy containing docetaxel.	April 28, 2011
Vandetanib tablets (Vandetanib tablets, AstraZeneca Pharmaceuticals LP)	For the treatment of symptomatic or progressive medullary thyroid cancer in patients with unresectable, locally advanced, or metastatic disease.	April 6, 2011
Peginterferon alfa-2b (Sylatron, Schering Corporation, Kenilworth, NJ 07033)	For the treatment of patients with melanoma with microscopic or gross nodal involvement within 84 days of definitive surgical resection including complete lymphadenectomy.	March 29, 2011
Ipilimumab injection (YERVOY, Bristol-Myers Squibb Company)	For the treatment of unresectable or metastatic melanoma.	March 25, 2011
Rituximab (Rituxan, Genentech, Inc.)	For maintenance therapy in patients with previously untreated follicular, CD-20 positive, B-cell non-Hodgkin lymphoma who achieve a response to rituximab in combination with chemotherapy.	January 28, 2011
Eribulin mesylate (Halaven injection, Eisai Inc.)	For the treatment of patients with metastatic breast cancer who have previously received an anthracycline and a taxane in either the adjuvant or metastatic setting, and at least two chemotherapeutic regimens for the treatment of metastatic disease.	November 15, 2010
Everolimus (Afinitor, Novartis), an mTOR inhibitor	For patients with SEGA associated with tuberous sclerosis (TS) who require therapy but who are not candidates for surgical resection.	October 29, 2010
Dasatinib (Sprycel, Bristol-Myers Squibb)	For the treatment of newly diagnosed adult patients with Ph+ CML in chronic phase (CP-CML).	October 28, 2010
Trastuzumab (Herceptin, Genentech, Inc.)	In combination with cisplatin and a fluoropyrimidine (capecitabine or 5-FU), for the treatment of patients with HER2-overexpressing metastatic gastric or gastroesophageal (GE) junction adenocarcinoma, who have not received prior treatment for metastatic disease.	October 20, 2010
Nilotinib (Tasigna capsules, Novartis Pharmaceuticals Corporation)	For the treatment of adult patients with newly diagnosed Ph+ CP-CML.	June 17, 2010
Cabazitaxel (Jevtana injection, Sanofi-Aventis)	For use in combination with prednisone for treatment of patients with metastatic hormone-refractory prostate cancer (mHRPC) previously treated with a docetaxel-containing regimen.	June 17, 2010

CANCER THERAPEUTICS

REFERENCES

1. Powell RG, Weisleder D, Smith CR, et al. Antitumor alkaloids from *Cephalotaxus harringtonia* structure and activity. *J Pharm Sci* 1972;61:1227–1230.
2. Huang MT. Harringtonine, an inhibitor of initiation of protein biosynthesis. *Mol Pharmacol* 1975;11:511–519.
3. Baaske DM, Heinstein P. Cytotoxicity and cell cycle specificity of homoharrintonine. *Antimicrob Agents Chemother* 1977;12:298–300.
4. Savaraj N, Lu K, Dimery I, et al. Clinical pharmacology of homoharringtonine. *Cancer Treat Rep* 1986;70:1403–1407.
5. Neidhart JA, Young DC, Derocher D, et al. Phase I trial of homoharringtonine. *Cancer Treat Rep* 1983;67:801–804.
6. Grem JL, Cheson BD, King SA, et al. Cephalotaxine esters: antileukemic advance of therapeutic failure. *J Natl Cancer Inst* 1988;80:1095–1103.
7. O'Brien S, Kantarjian H, Keating M, et al. Homoharringtonine therapy indices responses in patients with chronic myelogenous leukemia in late chronic phase. *Blood* 1995;86:3322–3326.
8. Legros L, Hayette S, Nicolini FE, et al. BCR-ABL(T315I) transcript disappearance in an imatinib-resistant CML patient treated with homoharringtonine: a new therapeutic challenge? *Leukemia* 2007;21(10):2204–2206.
9. Jorge Cortes J, Lipton JF, Rea D, et al. Phase 2 study of subcutaneous omacetaxine mepesuccinate after TKI failure in patients with chronic-phase CML with T315I mutation. *Blood* 2012;120:2573–2580.
10. Labrou NE, Papageorgiou AC, Avramis VI. Structure-function relationships and clinical applications of L-Asparaginases. *Curr Med Chem* 2010;17:2183–2195.
11. Verma N, Kumar K, Kaur G, et al. L-Asparaginase: a promising chemotherapeutic agent. *Crit Rev Biotechnol* 2007;27:45–62.
12. Zeidan A, Wang ES, Wetzler M. Pegasparaginase: where do we stand? *Expert Opin Biol Ther* 2009;9:111–119.
13. Avramis VI, Panosyan EH. Pharmacokinetic/pharmacodynamic relationships of asparaginase formulations: the past, the present and recommendations for the future. *Clin Pharmacokinet* 2005;44:367–393.
14. Appel WE, Hop WC, Pieters R. Changes in hypercoagulability by asparaginase: a randomized study between two asparaginases. *Blood Coagul Fibrinolysis* 2006;17:139–146.
15. Evans WE, Yee GC, Crom WR, et al. Clinical pharmacology of bleomycin and cisplatin. *Head Neck Surg* 1981;4:98–110.
16. Chen J, Stubbe J. Bleomycins: towards better therapeutics. *Nat Rev Cancer* 2005;2:102–112.
17. Hecht SM. Bleomycin: new perspectives on the mechanism of action. *J Nat Prod* 2000;63:158–168.
18. Lewis TG, Nydorf ED. Intralesional bleomycin for warts: a review. *J Drugs Dermatol* 2006;5:499–504.
19. Shaw P, Agarwal R. Pleurodesis for malignant pleural effusions. *Cochrane Database Syst Rev* 2004;(1):CD002916.
20. Good LM, Miller MD, High WA. Intralesional agents in the management of cutaneous malignancy. *J Am Acad Dermatol* 2011;64:413–422
21. Kawai K, Akaza H. Bleomycin-induced pulmonary toxicity in chemotherapy for testicular cancer. *Expert Opin Drug Saf* 2003;2:587–596.
22. Azulay E, Herigault S, Levame M, et al. Effect of granulocyte colony-stimulating factor on bleomycin-induced acute lung injury and pulmonary fibrosis. *Crit Care Med* 2003;31:1442–1448.
23. Adachi K, Suzuki M, Sugimoto T, et al. Effects of granulocyte colony-stimulating factor on the kinetics of inflammatory cells in the peripheral blood and pulmonary lesions during the development of bleomycin-induced lung injury in rats. *Exp Toxicol Pathol* 2003;55:21–32.
24. Martin WG, Ristow KM, Habermann TM, et al. Bleomycin pulmonary toxicity has a negative impact on the outcome of patients with Hodgkin's lymphoma. *J Clin Oncol* 2005;23:7614–7620.
25. Younes A, Connors JM, Park SI et al. Brentuximab vedotin combined with ABVD or AVD for patients with newly diagnosed Hodgkin's lymphoma: a phase 1, open-label, dose-escalation study. *Lancet Oncol* 2013;14:1348–1356.
26. Lam MS. The need for routine bleomycin test dosing in the 21st century. *Ann Pharmacother* 2005;39:1897–1902.
27. Swaffar DS, Horstman MG, Jaw JY, et al. Methylazoxyprocarbazine, the active metabolite responsible for the anticancer activity of procarbazine against L1210 leukemia. *Cancer Res* 1989;49:2442–2447.
28. Patterson LH, Murray GI. Tumour cytochrome P450 and drug activation. *Curr Pharm Des* 2002;8:1335–1347.
29. Swaffar DS, Pomerantz SC, Harker WG, et al. Non-enzymatic activation of procarbazine to active cytotoxic species. *Oncol Res* 1992;4:49–58.
30. Preiss R, Baumann F, Regenthal R, et al. Plasma kinetics of procarbazine and azo-procarbazine in humans. *Anticancer Drugs* 2006;17:75–80.
31. Von Hoff DD, LoRusso PM, Rudin CM, et al. Inhibition of the hedgehog pathway in advanced basal-cell carcinoma. *N Engl J Med* 2009;361:1164–1172.
32. Rudin CM. Vismodegib. *Clin Cancer Res* 2012;18:1–5.
33. U.S. Food and Drug Administration. News & Events: FDA News Release: FDA approves new treatment for most common types of skin cancer. http://www.fda.gov/NewsEvents/Newsroom/PressAnnouncements/ucm289545.htm. Published January 30, 2012. Updated January 31, 2012.
34. Tang JY, Mackay-Wiggan JM, Aszterbaum M, et al. Inhibiting the Hedgehog Pathway in patients with the basal-cell nevus syndrome. *N Engl J Med* 2012;366:2180–2188.

35. Krop IE, Beeram M, Modi S, et al. Phase I study of trastuzumab-DM1, an HER2 antibody-drug conjugate, given every 3 weeks to patients with HER2-positive metastatic breast cancer. *J Clin Oncol* 2010;28:2698–2704.
36. Verma S, Miles D, Gianni L, et al. Trastuzumab emtansine for HER2-positive advanced breast cancer. *N Engl J Med* 2012;367:1783–1791.
37. Sehgal SN, Baker H, Vézina C. Rapamycin (AY-22,989), a new antifungal antibiotic. II. Fermentation, isolation and characterization. *J Antibiot (Tokyo)* 1975;28:727–732.
38. Sehgal SN, Molnar-Kimber K, Ocain TD, et al. Rapamycin: a novel immunosuppressive macrolide. *Med Res Rev* 1994;14:1–22.
39. Wullschleger S, Loewith R, Hall MN. TOR signaling in growth and metabolism. *Cell* 2006;124:471–484.
40. Raymond E, Alexandre J, Faivre S, et al. Safety and pharmacokinetics of escalated doses of weekly intravenous infusion of CCI-779, a novel mTOR inhibitor in patients with cancer. *J Clin Oncol* 2004;22:2336–2347.
41. Zeng Z, Sarbassov dos D, Samudio IJ, et al. Rapamycin derivatives reduce mTORC2 signaling and inhibit AKT activation in AML. *Blood* 2007;109:3509–3512.
42. Kapoor A, Figlin RA. Targeted inhibition of mammalian target of rapamycin for the treatment of advanced renal cell carcinoma. *Cancer* 2009;115:3618–3630.
43. Atkins MB, Hidalgo M, Stadler WM, et al. Randomized phase II study of multiple dose levels of CCI-779, a novel mammalian target of rapamycin kinase inhibitor, in patients with advanced refractory renal cell carcinoma. *J Clin Oncol* 2004;22:909–918.
44. Hudes G, Carducci M, Tomczak P, et al. Temsirolimus, interferon alfa, or both for advanced renal-cell carcinoma. *N Engl J Med* 2007;356:2271–2281.
45. Smith SM, van Besien K, Karrison T, et al. Temsirolimus has activity in non-mantle cell non-Hodgkin's lymphoma subtypes: The University of Chicago phase II consortium. *J Clin Oncol* 2010;28:4740–4746.
46. Duran I, Siu LL, Oza AM, et al. Characterization of the lung toxicity of the cell cycle inhibitor temsirolimus. *Eur J Cancer* 2006;42:1875–1880.
47. Schuler W, Sedrani R, Cottens S, et al. SDZ RAD, a new rapamycine derivative: pharmacological properties in vitro and in vivo. *Transplantation* 1997;64:36–42.
48. Dudkin L, Dilling MB, Cheshire PJ, et al. Biochemical correlates of mTOR inhibition by the rapamycin ester CCI-779 and tumor growth inhibition. *Clin Cancer Res* 2001;7:1758–1764.
49. Kirchner GI, Meier-Wiedenbach I, Manns MP. Clinical pharmacokinetics of everolimus. *Clin Pharmacokinet* 2004;43:83–95.
50. Doi T, Muro K, Boku N, et al. Multicenter phase II study of everolimus in patients with previously treated metastatic gastric cancer. *J Clin Oncol* 2010;28:1904–1910.
51. Yao JC, Lombard-Bohas C, Baudin E, et al. Daily oral everolimus activity in patients with metastatic neuroendocrine tumors after failure of cytotoxic chemotherapy: a phase II trial. *J Clin Oncol* 2010;28:69–76.
52. Yee KW, Zeng Z, Konopleva M, et al. Phase I/II study of the mammalian target of rapamycin inhibitor everolimus(RAD001) in patients with relapsed or refractory hematological malignancies. *Clin Cancer Res* 2008;12:5165–5173.
53. Okuno S. Mammalian target of rapamycin inhibitors in sarcomas. *Curr Opin Oncol* 2006;18:360–362.
54. Yao JC, Shah MH, Ito T, et al. Everolimus for advanced pancreatic neuroendocrine tumors. *N Engl J Med* 2011;364:514–523.
55. Baselga J, Campone M, Piccart M, et al. Everolimus in postmenopausal hormone-receptor-positive advanced breast cancer. *N Engl J Med* 2012;366:520–529.
56. Shortt J, Hsu AK, Johnstone RW. Thalidomide-analogue biology: immunological, molecular and epigenetic targets in cancer therapy. *Oncogene* 2013;32:4191–4202.
57. Zhu YX, Kortuem KM, Stewart AK. Molecular mechanism of action of immune-modulatory drugs thalidomide, lenalidomide and pomalidomide in multiple myeloma. *Leuk Lymphoma* 2013;54:683–687.
58. Escoubet-Lozach L, Lin IL, Jensen-Pergakes K, et al. Pomalidomide and lenalidomide induce p21 WAF-1 expression in both lymphoma and multiple myeloma through a LSD1-mediated epigenetic mechanism. *Cancer Res* 2009;69:7347–7356.
59. Madan S, Lacy MQ, Dispenzieri A, et al. Efficacy of retreatment with immunomodulatory drugs (IMiDs) in patients receiving IMiDs for initial therapy of newly diagnosed multiple myeloma. *Blood* 2011;118:1763–1765.
60. Lacy MQ, Tefferi A. Pomalidomide therapy for multiple myeloma and myelofibrosis: an update. *Leuk Lymphoma* 2011;52:560–566.
61. Ito T, Ando H, Suzuki T, et al. Identification of a primary target of thalidomide teratogenicity. *Science* 2010;327:1345–1350.
62. Zhu YX, Braggio E, Shi CX, et al. Cereblon expression is required for the antimyeloma activity of lenalidomide and pomalidomide. *Blood* 2011;118:4771–4779.
63. Lopez-Girona A, Mendy D, Ito T, et al. Cereblon is a direct protein target for immunomodulatory and antiproliferative activities of lenalidomide and pomalidomide. *Leukemia* 2012;26:2326–2335.
64. Schuster SR, Kortuem KM, Zhu YX, et al. Cereblon expression predicts response, progression free and overall survival after pomalidomide and

dexamethasone therapy in multiple myeloma. *ASH Ann Meeting Abstracts* 2012;120:194.

65. Bennett CL, Angelotta C, Yarnold PR, et al. Thalidomide- and lenalidomide-associated thromboembolism among patients with cancer. *JAMA #2006;296:* 2558–2560.

66. Rao KV. Lenalidomide in the treatment of multiple myeloma. *Am J Health Syst Pharm* 2007;64:1799–1807.

67. Lenalidomide. Drugs@FDA. Food and Drug Administration Web site. http://www.accessdata.fda.gov/drugsatfda_docs/label/2009/021880s006s016s017lbl.pdf. Published December 2008.

68. Pomalidomide. Drugs@FDA. Food and Drug Administration Web site. http://www.accessdata.fda.gov/drugsatfda_docs/label/2013/204026lbl.pdf. Revised February 2013.

69. Lacy MQ, McCurdy AR. Pomalidomide. *Blood* 2013;122:2305–2309.

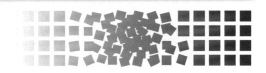

27 Hormonal Agents

Matthew P. Goetz, Charles Erlichman, Charles L. Loprinzi, and Manish Kohli

INTRODUCTION

Hormonal agents are commonly used as a treatment of hormonally responsive cancers, such as breast, prostate, or endometrial carcinomas. Other uses for some hormonal therapies include the treatment of paraneoplastic syndromes, such as carcinoid syndrome, and symptoms caused by cancer, including anorexia. This chapter discusses the major hormonal agents for such therapy, first with an overview of their use in practice, then with more detailed pharmacologic information regarding them (Table 27.1).

SELECTIVE ESTROGEN RECEPTOR MODULATORS

Tamoxifen

Tamoxifen continues to be an important hormonal therapy for the prevention and treatment of breast cancer worldwide. The continued importance of tamoxifen is reflected in the fact that it is the only hormonal agent approved by the U.S. Food and Drug Administration (FDA) for the prevention of premenopausal breast cancer,[1] the treatment of ductal carcinoma in situ (DCIS),[2] and the treatment of surgically resected premenopausal estrogen receptor (ER)–positive breast cancer.[3]

The standard daily dose of tamoxifen is 20 mg, and the optimal duration depends on the underlying clinical setting. Although the recommended duration in the prevention and DCIS settings is 5 years, recently published prospective studies have demonstrated that for the adjuvant treatment of invasive breast cancer, a duration of 10 years (compared to 5 years) further reduced the risk of breast cancer mortality and improved overall survival.[4]

The most common toxicity from tamoxifen is hot flashes, affecting approximately 50% of treated women. These hot flashes are of varying intensity and duration. Tamoxifen-induced hot flashes appear to increase over the first 3 months of therapy and then plateau. They appear to be more prominent in women with a history of hot flashes or estrogen replacement use. Tamoxifen-induced hot flashes can be ameliorated by a number of different pharmacotherapies, including low doses of megestrol[5]; antidepressants such as venlafaxine,[6] desvenlafaxine,[7] citalopram,[8] escitalopram,[9] and paroxetine[10]; and the anticonvulsant drugs gabapentin[11] and pregabalin.[12] There is evidence that drugs that inhibit CYP2D6 (e.g., paroxetine) alter the metabolic activation of tamoxifen to endoxifen, a critical metabolite associated with in vivo tamoxifen efficacy.[13]

The estrogenic properties of tamoxifen are responsible for both beneficial and deleterious side effects. Tamoxifen increases the incidence of endometrial cancer in postmenopausal (but not premenopausal) women, with the increase in the annual incidence of endometrial cancer being approximately 2.58 (ratio of incidence rates).[14] The absolute risk depends on the duration of tamoxifen administration. For women who receive 10 years of adjuvant tamoxifen, the cumulative risk is 3.1% (mortality, 0.4%) versus 1.6% (mortality, 0.2%) for 5 years of tamoxifen.[4] The incidence of a rarer form of uterine cancer, uterine sarcoma, is also increased after tamoxifen use.[15] This form of endometrial cancer comprises approximately 15% of all uterine malignancies that develop after tamoxifen use.[15] Beneficial estrogenic effects from tamoxifen include a decrease in total cholesterol[16] and the preservation of bone density in postmenopausal women.[17] In premenopausal women, however, tamoxifen has a negative effect on bone density.[18] Although most patients do not complain of vaginal symptoms, a few complain of vaginal dryness, whereas others have increased vaginal secretions and discharge, the latter of which is an indication of the estrogenic activity of tamoxifen on the vagina. In the Arimidex, Tamoxifen, Alone or in Combination (ATAC) trial, a commonly observed tamoxifen side effect was vaginal bleeding, leading to a higher hysterectomy rate for patients randomized to tamoxifen (5%) compared to anastrozole (1%).[19] An uncommon effect from tamoxifen is retinal toxicity. This drug can also increase the risk of cataracts. However, no difference in the rate of vision-threatening ocular toxicity has been seen among prospectively treated tamoxifen patients.[20] Tamoxifen predisposes patients to thromboembolic phenomena, especially if used with concomitant chemotherapy. Depression has also been described, but the association with tamoxifen is not clear. Although liver cancers have been noted in laboratory animals, there is no established association between tamoxifen and liver cancers in humans.

Pharmacology

Tamoxifen acts by blocking estrogen stimulation of breast cancer cells, inhibiting both translocation and nuclear binding of the ER. This alters transcriptional and posttranscriptional events mediated by this receptor.[21] Tamoxifen has agonistic, partial agonistic, or antagonistic effects depending on the species, tissue, or endpoints that have been assessed. Additionally, there are marked differences between the antiproliferative properties of tamoxifen and its metabolites.[22]

Resistance to tamoxifen can be intrinsic or acquired, and the potential mechanisms for this resistance are reviewed in the following paragraphs. At each step of the signal transduction pathway with which tamoxifen or its metabolites interferes, there is the potential for an alteration in response. The most important factor appears to be the level of ER, which is highly predictive for a response to tamoxifen. Tamoxifen is ineffective in ER-negative breast cancer. Although decreased or absent expression of the progesterone receptor (PR) is associated with a worse prognosis, the relative risk reduction in tamoxifen-treated patients is the same regardless of the presence or absence of the PR.

Following binding to the ER, subsequent translocation of the tamoxifen/ER complex to the nucleus and binding to an estrogen-response element may occur. This binding prevents transcriptional activation of estrogen-responsive genes. Laboratory and clinical data have demonstrated that ER-positive breast cancers that overexpress HER2 may be less responsive to tamoxifen and

TABLE 27.1

Overview of Major Hormonal Agents Used in Cancer

Class of Drug	Individual Drug	Dose	Route of Delivery	Frequency of Delivery
Selective estrogen receptor modulator	Tamoxifen	20 mg	Oral	Once daily
	Toremifene	60 mg	Oral	Once daily
	Raloxifene	60 mg	Oral	Once daily
Aromatase inhibitor	Anastrozole	1 mg	Oral	Once daily
	Letrozole	2.5 mg	Oral	Once daily
	Exemestane	25 mg	Oral	Once daily
Estrogen receptor downregulator	Fulvestrant	500 mg	IM	Once monthly
Luteinizing hormone releasing hormone agonist	Goserelin	7.5	IM	Once monthly[a]
	Leuprolide	3.6	IM	Once monthly[a]
GnRH antagonist	Degarelix	240 mg loading dose	SC	80 mg SC monthly maintenance dose
Antiandrogen	Flutamide	250 mg	Oral	Three times daily
	Bicalutamide	50 mg	Oral	Once daily
	Nilutamide	300 mg for 30 d then 150 mg	Oral	Once daily
Cytochrome P45017 alpha inhibitors	Abiraterone Acetate	1,000 mg (four 250 mg capsules)	Oral	Once Daily
AR "super antagonists"	Enzalutamide	160–240 mg	Oral	Daily
Androgen	Fluoxymesterone	10 mg	Oral	Twice daily
Estrogen	Estradiol	10 mg	Oral	Up to three times daily
Somatostatin analog	Octreotide	Varies	SC or IV	Up to three times daily[b]
Progestational agents	Megestrol	Varies	Oral	Once daily
	Medroxyprogesterone acetate	Varies	Oral or IM	Varies

[a] Longer acting depot preparations (every 3 months) are available.
[b] Depot formulations are available.
IM, intramuscular; SC, subcutaneous; GnRH, gonadotropin-releasing hormone; CYP, cytochrome P-450; AR, androgen receptor.

to hormonal therapy in general.[23–26] In these tumors, ligand-independent activation of the ER by mitogen-activated protein kinase (MAPK) pathways may contribute to resistance.[27–29] In addition, the expression of AIB1, an estrogen-receptor coactivator, has been associated with tamoxifen resistance in patients whose breast cancers overexpress HER2.[30] In some cases, resistance may result from a decrease or loss of ER expression.[31,32] Although mutations in the ER ligand binding domain (LBD) are rare in newly diagnosed breast cancer, ER mutations are present in up to 20% of recurrent breast cancers.[33–36] These mutations lead to a conformational change in the LBD, which mimics the conformation of activated ligand-bound receptor and constitutive, ligand-independent transcriptional activity, resulting in resistance to hormonal therapy. Preclinical studies suggest that some of these mutations, although insensitive to aromatase inhibitors, retain sensitivity to higher dose selective estrogen-receptor modulators (SERM), such as endoxifen, as well as fulvestrant.[35]

The carcinogenic potential of tamoxifen has been recognized in rat studies[37–39] and in humans (endometrial cancer).[40] It has been proposed that the generation of reactive intermediates that bind covalently to macromolecules underlies the process. Such reactive intermediates have been demonstrated in vitro.[40–43] In addition, the induction of covalent DNA adducts in rat livers treated with tamoxifen has been reported.[44] Both constitutive and inducible cytochrome P-450 (CYP) enzymes have been implicated in the formation of metabolites with tamoxifen,[45,46] and the flavone-containing monooxygenase has been implicated in the formation of the N-oxide of tamoxifen. Reactive intermediates from

such metabolic steps are being evaluated for their carcinogenic potential in vitro and in vivo.

Multiple studies to evaluate tumor gene expression profiling have identified gene expression patterns or specific genes associated with resistance to tamoxifen therapy. A commonly utilized gene expression assay, Oncotype DX 21 gene assay (Genomic Health, Redwood City, California), measures the expression of genes known to be involved in estrogen signaling (e.g., ER, PR), HER2, proliferation (e.g., Ki-67), and others. In multiple different data sets, the recurrence score has been associated with a higher risk of breast cancer recurrence in patients treated with hormonal therapy (e.g., tamoxifen or aromatase inhibitors) without concomitant chemotherapy.[47–49]

The pharmacokinetics of tamoxifen is complex. The chemical structure and metabolic pathway of tamoxifen are shown in Figure 27.1. Metabolic activation of tamoxifen is associated with greater pharmacologic activity. The two most active tamoxifen metabolites are 4-hydroxytamoxifen (4-OH tamoxifen) and 4-OH-N-desmethyltamoxifen (endoxifen). A series of studies carried out to characterize endoxifen pharmacology have demonstrated that it has equivalent potency in vitro to 4-hydroxytamoxifen in ER-α and -beta (ER-β) binding,[50] for the suppression of ER-dependent human breast cancer cell line proliferation,[22,50] and in global ER-responsive gene expression.[51] A recent study suggests that endoxifen's effect on the ER may differ from 4-hydroxytamoxifen based on the observation of ER-α degradation.[52]

In women who receive tamoxifen at a dose of 20 mg per day, plasma endoxifen steady-state concentrations are generally 6 to

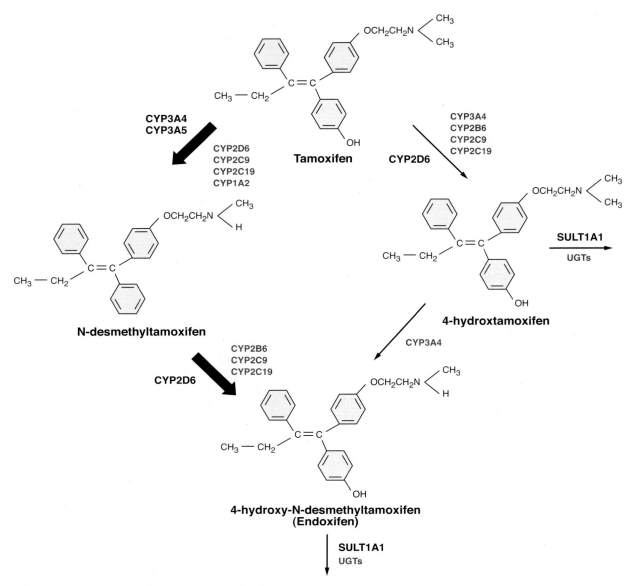

Figure 27.1 Metabolic pathway of tamoxifen biotransformation. (From Sideras K, Ingle JN, Ames MM, et al. Coprescription of tamoxifen and medications that inhibit CYP2D6. *J Clin Oncol* 2010;28:2768–2776.)

10 times higher than 4-hydroxytamoxifen.[53] Although the metabolism of tamoxifen to 4-OH-tamoxifen is catalyzed by multiple enzymes, endoxifen is formed predominantly by the CYP2D6-mediated oxidation of N-desmethyltamoxifen, the most abundant tamoxifen metabolite (see Fig. 27.1).[54] Multiple clinical studies have demonstrated that common *CYP2D6* genetic variation (leading to low or absent CYP2D6 activity) or the drug-induced inhibition of CYP2D6 significantly lowers endoxifen concentrations.[53,55] The *CYP2D6* gene is highly polymorphic, with more than 70 major alleles with four well-defined phenotypes: poor metabolizers (PM), intermediate metabolizers (IM), extensive metabolizers (EM), and ultrarapid metabolizers (UM).

The clinical studies to evaluate the association between *CYP2D6* polymorphisms and tamoxifen outcomes have yielded conflicting results. Initial[56] and follow-up data[57,58] demonstrated that CYP2D6 PM had an approximately two- to threefold higher risk of breast cancer recurrence (compared to CYP2D6 EM) and these data led an FDA special emphasis panel to recommend a tamoxifen label change to incorporate data that the *CYP2D6* genotype was an important biomarker associated with tamoxifen

efficacy.[5] However, this label change has been delayed, in part because of conflicting data from secondary analyses of 5-year tamoxifen prospective trials (ATAC,[59] BIG 1-98,[60] and ABCSG8[61]) as well as meta-analyses,[62] which demonstrate that the *CYP2D6* genotype is associated with tamoxifen efficacy when tamoxifen is administered as monotherapy for the adjuvant treatment of postmenopausal, ER-positive breast cancer. Additional support for the importance of endoxifen concentrations came from a secondary analysis of a prospective study, which demonstrated a higher risk of recurrence for women with low endoxifen concentrations.[13]

Many drugs are known to inhibit CYP2D6 activity. In tamoxifen-treated women, the coadministration of potent CYP2D6 inhibitors, such as paroxetine, converts a patient with normal CYP2D6 metabolism to a phenotypic PM.[63] Many other clinically important drugs have been reported to inhibit the CYP2D6 enzyme system, but their effects on tamoxifen metabolism have not been prospectively studied. As with the data regarding *CYP2D6* genotype, the data regarding CYP2D6 inhibitors has additionally been controversial, including two studies that reported opposite findings with regard to CYP2D6 inhibitor use and breast cancer recurrence or death.[64,65] Although the *CYP2D6* data remain controversial, we conclude that until results from prospective adjuvant studies are available, women should be counseled regarding the potential impact of the *CYP2D6* genotype on the effectiveness of adjuvant tamoxifen, and potent CYP2D6 inhibitors should be avoided. Additional caution should be used with drugs that induce CYP3A, such as rifampicin, as a these drugs have been demonstrated to substantially reduce (up to 86%) the concentrations of tamoxifen and its metabolites.[66]

Strategies to overcome low endoxifen concentrations include dose escalation of tamoxifen to 40 mg per day, which has been demonstrated to significantly increase endoxifen concentrations,[67,68] as well as the direct administration of endoxifen itself. The latter strategy is ongoing in multiple different clinical trials, and early reports suggest clinical activity in aromatase inhibitors (AI)-resistant breast cancer.[69]

Following the metabolic activation of tamoxifen, the hydroxylated metabolites undergo both glucuronidation and sulfation. Peak plasma levels of tamoxifen (maximum concentration [Cmax]) are seen 3 to 7 hours after oral administration. Assuming an oral bioavailability of 30%, the volume of distribution has been calculated to be 20 L/kg, and plasma clearance ranges from 1.2 to 5.1 L per hour.[70] The terminal half-life of tamoxifen has been reported to range between 4 and 11 days.[71,72] The elimination half-life of tamoxifen increases with successive doses, which is consistent with saturable kinetics.[71,73] The drug's distribution in tissues is extensive. Levels of the parent drug and metabolites have been reported to be higher in tissue than in plasma in animal studies.[74,75] Reports of tamoxifen concentrations 10- to 60-fold higher than plasma concentrations in the liver, lungs, brain, pancreas, skin, and bones are reported.[76,77] Elevated levels of tamoxifen with biliary obstruction have been reported.[78]

Tamoxifen has been reported to interact with warfarin,[73,79–81] digitoxin, phenytoin,[82] and medroxyprogesterone.[73] Tamoxifen-induced activation of human transcription factor pregnane X receptor (hPXR), resulting in the induction of CYP3A4, may increase the elimination of concomitantly administered CYP3A substrates,[83] such as anastrozole.[84]

Toremifene

Toremifene is an agent similar to tamoxifen. It is available in the United States for the treatment of patients with metastatic breast cancer, and is approved in other countries for the adjuvant treatment of ER-positive breast cancer. Clinical trials have demonstrated no difference in either disease-free or overall survival when toremifene was compared with tamoxifen for the treatment of ER-positive breast cancer,[85,86] and evidence exists for major cross-resistance between tamoxifen and toremifene.[87,88]

Pharmacology

Toremifene is an antiestrogen with a chemical structure that differs from that of tamoxifen by the substitution of a chlorine for a hydrogen atom that is retained when toremifene undergoes metabolism.[89] Like tamoxifen, toremifene is metabolized by CYP3A,[90] with a secondary metabolism to form hydroxylated metabolites that appear to have similar binding affinities to 4-OH tamoxifen.[89,91] The importance of these metabolites or the role of metabolism to the hydroxylated metabolites is unknown, but may play a role given the structural similarity of toremifene to tamoxifen. Although the oral bioavailability has not been defined, toremifene's oral absorption appears to be good. The time to peak plasma concentrations after oral administration ranges from 1.5 to 6.0 hours,[92] with the terminal half-lives for toremifene and one metabolite, 4-hydroxytoremifene, being 5 to 6 days.[93,94] The apparent clearance is 5.1 L per hour. The terminal half-life for the major metabolite, N-desmethyltoremifene, is 21 days.[95] The time to reach plasma steady-state concentrations is 1 to 5 weeks. Plasma protein binding is more than 99%. As with tamoxifen, toremifene is present at higher concentrations in tissues compared to plasma with a high apparent volume of distribution (958 L). Seventy percent of the drug is excreted in feces as metabolites. Studies in patients with impaired liver function or those on anticonvulsants known to induce CYP3A have demonstrated that hepatic dysfunction decreases the clearance of toremifene and N-desmethyltoremifene,[95] whereas those patients on anticonvulsants had an increased clearance. Although toremifene appeared to be less carcinogenic than tamoxifen in preclinical models,[43,96,97] of the rates of endometrial cancer in the adjuvant studies have been similar to tamoxifen.[85]

Raloxifene

Raloxifene is an estrogen agonist and antagonist originally developed to treat osteoporosis. Large placebo-controlled randomized trials demonstrated reduced rates of osteoporosis and a reduction in new breast cancers in treated women, leading to the development of a second-generation breast cancer chemoprevention trial (National Surgical Adjuvant Breast and Bowel Project, NSAPB P2) in which raloxifene was compared with tamoxifen in high-risk postmenopausal women. In this study, tamoxifen was superior to raloxifene in terms of both invasive and noninvasive cancer events, but was associated with a higher risk of thromboembolic events and endometrial cancer.[98]

Pharmacology

Raloxifene is partially estrogenic in bone[99] and lowers cholesterol.[100] It is antiestrogenic in mammary tissue[101,102] and uterine tissue.[103]

The pharmacokinetics of raloxifene have been studied principally in postmenopausal women.[104–106] Pharmacokinetic parameters of raloxifene show considerable interindividual variation. Limited information is available on the pharmacokinetics of raloxifene in individuals with hepatic impairment, renal impairment, or both.

Raloxifene is rapidly absorbed from the gastrointestinal tract. Because raloxifene undergoes extensive first-pass glucuronidation, oral bioavailability of unchanged drug is low. Although approximately 60% of an oral dose is absorbed, the absolute bioavailability as unchanged raloxifene is only 2%. However, systemic availability of raloxifene may be greater than that indicated in bioavailability studies, because circulating glucuronide conjugates are converted back to the parent drug in various tissues.

After the oral administration of a single 120- or 150-mg dose of raloxifene hydrochloride, peak plasma concentrations of raloxifene and its glucuronide conjugates are achieved at 6 hours and 1 hour, respectively. After the oral administration of radiolabeled raloxifene, less than 1% of total circulating radiolabeled material in plasma represents the parent drug.

Results of a single-dose study in patients with liver dysfunction indicate that plasma raloxifene concentrations correlate with serum bilirubin concentrations and are 2.5 times higher than individuals with normal hepatic function. In postmenopausal women who received raloxifene in clinical trials, plasma concentrations of raloxifene and the glucuronide conjugates in those with renal impairment (i.e., estimated creatinine clearance values as low as 23 mL per minute) were similar to values in women with normal renal function.

Raloxifene and its monoglucuronide conjugates are more than 95% bound to plasma proteins. Raloxifene binds to albumin and α_1-acid glycoprotein. Raloxifene undergoes extensive first-pass metabolism to the glucuronide conjugates raloxifene 4′-glucuronide, 6-glucuronide, and 6,4′-diglucuronide. UGT1A1 and -1A8 have been found to catalyze the formation of both the 6-β-and 4′-β-glucuronides, whereas UGT1A10 formed only the 4′-β-glucuronide.[107] The metabolism of raloxifene does not appear to be mediated by CYP enzymes (such as CYP2D6), because metabolites other than glucuronide conjugates have not been identified.

The plasma elimination half-life of raloxifene at steady state averages 32.5 hours (range, 15.8 to 86.6 hours). Raloxifene is excreted principally in feces as an unabsorbed drug and via biliary elimination as glucuronide conjugates, which, subsequently, are metabolized by bacteria in the gastrointestinal tract to the parent drug. After oral administration, less than 0.2% of a raloxifene dose is excreted as the parent compound and less than 6% as glucuronide conjugates in urine.

Fulvestrant

Fulvestrant is an ER antagonist that has no known agonist activity and results in ER downregulation.[108–111] Like tamoxifen, fulvestrant competitively binds to the ER but with a higher affinity—approximately 100 times greater than that of tamoxifen,[108,112–114]—thus preventing endogenous estrogen from exerting its effect in target cells.

Results from two phase III clinical trials using the 250 mg per month dose demonstrated fulvestrant to be as effective as anastrozole in the treatment of postmenopausal women with advanced hormone receptor–positive breast cancer previously treated with antiestrogen therapy (mainly tamoxifen).[112–116] In the setting of first-line hormone-responsive metastatic breast cancer, a randomized phase III clinical trial to compare tamoxifen to fulvestrant (250 mg per month) demonstrated no differences in response or time to progression.[117] Because of pharmacology data (discussed in the following paragraphs), the 500 mg per day dose was developed. A randomized trial comparing the 250 mg per month with 500 mg per month dose demonstrated a 4-month improvement in median overall survival advantage for the higher dose.[118] For this reason, the higher dose is now the standard recommended dose.

Fulvestrant is well tolerated. The most common drug-related events (greater than 10% incidence) from the randomized phase III studies were injection-site reactions and hot flashes. Common events (1% to 10% incidence) included asthenia, headache, and gastrointestinal disturbances such as nausea, vomiting, and diarrhea, with minor gastrointestinal disturbances being the most commonly described adverse event.

Pharmacology

Fulvestrant is a steroidal molecule derived from E_2 with an alkylsulphonyl side chain in the 7-α position (Fig. 27.2). Because fulvestrant is poorly soluble and has low and unpredictable oral bioavailability, a parenteral formulation of fulvestrant was developed in an attempt to maximize delivery of the drug.[111] The intramuscular formulation provides prolonged release of the drug over several weeks. The pharmacokinetics of three different single doses of fulvestrant (50, 125, and 250 mg) have been published.[111] In this phase I/II multicenter study, postmenopausal women with primary breast cancer who were awaiting curative surgery received either fulvestrant, tamoxifen, or placebo. After single intramuscular injections of fulvestrant, the time of maximal concentration (t_{max}) ranged from 2 to 19 days, with the median being 7 days for each dose group. At the interval of 28 days, Cmin values were two- to fivefold lower than the Cmax values. For most patients in the 125- and 250-mg dose groups, significant levels of fulvestrant were still measurable 84 days after administration. Pharmacokinetic modeling of the pooled data from the 250-mg cohort was best described by a two-compartment model in which a longer terminal phase began approximately 3 weeks after administration. Because of the long time needed to reach a steady state, the 500-mg loading dose regimen was prospectively studied and determined to be superior to the 250 mg per month dose, both in terms of steady state concentrations achieved within 1 month[119]as well as progression-free and overall survival.[118]

AROMATASE INHIBITORS

At menopause, the synthesis of ovarian hormones ceases. However, estrogen continues to be converted from androgens (produced by the adrenal glands) by aromatase, an enzyme of the CYP superfamily. Aromatase is the enzyme complex responsible for the final step in estrogen synthesis via the conversion of androgens, androstenedione and testosterone, to estrogens, estrone (E_1) and E_2. This biologic pathway served as the basis for the development of the antiaromatase class of compounds. Alterations in aromatase expression have been implicated in the pathogenesis of estrogen-dependent disease, including breast cancer, endometrial cancer, and endometriosis. The importance of this enzyme is also highlighted by the fact that selective aromatase inhibitors are commonly used as first-line therapy for the treatment of postmenopausal women with estrogen-responsive breast cancer. Aminoglutethimide was the first clinically used aromatase inhibitor. When it became available, it was used to cause a *medical adrenalectomy*. Because of the lack of selectivity for aromatase and the resultant suppression of aldosterone and cortisol, aminoglutethimide is no longer recommended for treating metastatic breast cancer. Aminoglutethimide is also occasionally used to try to reverse excess hormone production by adrenocortical cancers.[120]

Aromatase (cytochrome P-450 19 [CYP19]) is encoded by the *CYP19* gene, which is highly polymorphic. Some of these variants are functionally important[121] and may have clinical significance.[122,123]

Aromatase inhibitors have been classified in a number of different ways, including first, second, and third generation; steroidal and nonsteroidal; and reversible (ionic binding) and irreversible (suicide inhibitor, covalent binding).[124] The nonsteroidal aromatase inhibitors include aminoglutethimide (first generation), rogletimide and fadrozole (second generation), and anastrozole, letrozole, and vorozole (third generation). The steroidal aromatase inhibitors include formestane (second generation) and exemestane (third generation).

Steroidal and nonsteroidal aromatase inhibitors differ in their modes of interaction with, and their inactivation of, the aromatase enzyme. Steroidal inhibitors compete with the endogenous

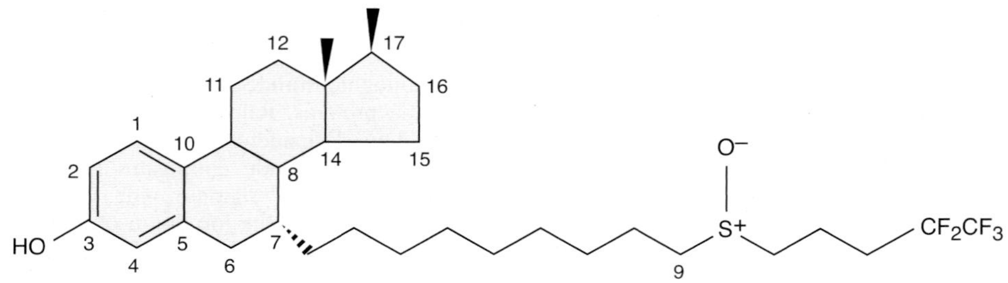

Figure 27.2 Structure of fulvestrant.

substrates, androstenedione and testosterone, for the active site of the enzyme and are processed into intermediates that bind irreversibly to the active site, causing irreversible enzyme inhibition.[19] Nonsteroidal inhibitors also compete with the endogenous substrates for access to the active site, where they then form a reversible bond to the heme iron atom so that enzyme activity can recover if the inhibitor is removed; however, inhibition is sustained whenever the inhibitor is present.[19]

Letrozole and Anastrozole

Both letrozole and anastrozole have been extensively studied in the metastatic and adjuvant settings. When compared to tamoxifen, both letrozole and anastrozole have demonstrated superior response rates and progression-free survival in the metastatic setting.[124,125] In the adjuvant setting, two trials have been performed and demonstrated superiority in terms of relapse-free survivals of both anastrozole (ATAC)[126] and letrozole (BIG 1-98).[127] Additionally, anastrozole has been studied in a sequential approach, and the sequence of tamoxifen followed by anastrozole is superior to 5 years of tamoxifen alone.[128] Anastrozole has recently been compared to placebo in women at an increased risk of developing breast cancer and was demonstrated to significantly reduce the incidence of invasive breast cancer.[129]

The side effects of both anastrozole and letrozole are similar and include arthralgias and myalgias in up to 50% of patients. Both letrozole and anastrozole are associated with a higher rate of bone fracture, compared with the tamoxifen.[130] At the present time, minimal long-term (longer than 5 years) clinical data regarding the effect of aromatase inhibitors on bones are available. When offering anastrozole for extended periods of time to patients with early breast cancer, attention to bone health is paramount, and bone density should be monitored in all patients. Prospective studies have demonstrated that bisphosphonates prevent aromatase-inhibitor–induced bone loss and a meta-analysis presented at the 2013 San Antonio Breast Cancer Symposium demonstrated that bisphosphonates reduce bone recurrences and prolong overall survival. Therefore, bisphosphonates should be considered in AI-treated patients, both in those with and without an increased risk of bone fractures.

A meta-analysis of toxicities comparing aromatase inhibitors with tamoxifen has demonstrated a 30% increase in grade 3 and 4 cardiac events with aromatase inhibitors.[131] However, prospective data demonstrate no differences in myocardial events comparing anastrozole with placebo, although an increase in hypertension was observed.[129]

No impact has been seen with anastrozole on adrenal steroidogenesis at up to 10 times the clinically recommended dose.[132] Although letrozole may decrease basal and adrenocorticotropic hormone–stimulated cortisol synthesis,[133,134] the clinical effect appears to be minimal. Aromatase inhibitors appear to have differential effects on lipids. In a study of over 900 patients with metastatic disease, anastrozole showed no marked effect on lipid profiles compared with baseline.[135] Conversely, the administration of letrozole in women with advanced breast cancer resulted in significant increases in total cholesterol and low-density lipoprotein, from baseline, after 8 and 16 weeks of therapy.[136] In the Breast International Group 1-98 trial, more women who received letrozole experienced grade 1 hypercholesterolemia compared to women who received tamoxifen.[127]

Letrozole is a nonsteroidal aromatase inhibitor with a high specificity for the inhibition of estrogen production (Fig. 27.3). Letrozole is 180 times more potent than aminoglutethimide as an inhibitor of aromatase in vitro. Aldosterone production in vitro is inhibited by concentrations 10,000 times higher than those required for inhibition of estrogen synthesis.[137,138] In a normal male volunteer study, letrozole was shown to decrease E_2 and serum E_1 levels to 10% of baseline with a single 3-mg dose. In phase I

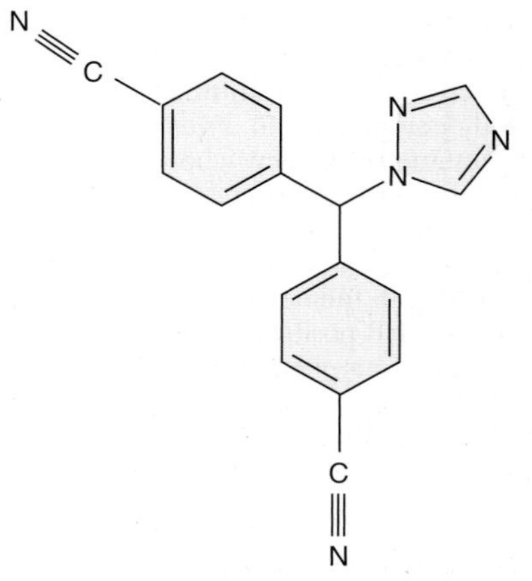

Figure 27.3 Structure of letrozole.

studies, letrozole caused a significant decline in plasma E_1 and E_2 within 24 hours of a single oral dose of 0.1 mg.[139,140] After 2 weeks of treatment, the blood levels of E_2, E_1, and estrone sulfate were suppressed 95% or more from baseline. This continued over the 12 weeks of therapy. There was no apparent alteration in plasma levels of cortisol and aldosterone with letrozole or after corticotropin stimulation.[139] In postmenopausal women with advanced breast cancer, the drug did not have any effect on follicle-stimulating hormone (FSH), luteinizing hormone (LH), thyrotropin (previously thyroid-stimulating hormone), cortisol, 17-α-hydroxyprogesterone, androstenedione, or aldosterone blood concentrations.[141,142]

Anastrozole is a nonsteroidal aromatase inhibitor that is 200-fold more potent than aminoglutethimide.[143] No effect on the adrenal glands has been detected. In human studies, the t_{max} is 2 to 3 hours after oral ingestion.[144] Elimination is primarily via hepatic metabolism, with 85% excreted by that route and only 10% excreted unchanged in urine. The main circulating metabolite is triazole after cleavage of the two rings in anastrozole by N-dealkylation. Linear pharmacokinetics have been observed in the dose range of 1 to 20 mg and do not change with repeat dosing. The terminal half-life is approximately 50 hours, and steady-state concentrations are achieved in approximately 10 days with once-a-day dosing and are three to four times higher than peak concentrations after a single dose. Plasma protein binding is approximately 40%.[145] In one study, anastrozole 1 mg and 10 mg daily, inhibited in vivo aromatization by 96.7% and 98.1%, respectively, and plasma E_1 and E_2 levels were suppressed 86.5% and 83.5%, respectively, regardless of dose.[146] Thus, 1 mg of anastrozole achieves near maximal aromatase inhibition and plasma estrogen suppression in breast cancer patients.

A recent prospective study to evaluate the pharmacokinetics of anastrozole (1 mg per day) demonstrated large interindividual variations in plasma anastrozole and anastrozole metabolite concentrations, as well as pretreatment and postdrug plasma E_1, E_2, and E_1 conjugate and estrogen precursor (androstenedione and testosterone) concentrations.[147] Further research is needed to determine the basis for the wide variability in the pharmacokinetics of anastrozole and whether these findings are clinically relevant.

Exemestane

Exemestane has a steroidal structure and is classified as a type 1 aromatase inhibitor, also known as an *aromatase inactivator*, because it irreversibly binds with and permanently inactivates the enzyme.[134] Exemestane has been compared to tamoxifen in both the metastatic and adjuvant settings. In the setting of tamoxifen-refractory metastatic breast cancer, exemestane is superior to megestrol acetate, as demonstrated in a phase III trial in which improvements in both median time to tumor progression and median survival were observed.[148] In the adjuvant setting, the international exemestane study compared 2 to 3 years of tamoxifen with 2 to 3 years of exemestane in women who had previously competed 2 to 3 years of adjuvant tamoxifen. In this trial, a switch to exemestane resulted in superior disease-free and overall survival in the hormone receptor–positive subtype. Furthermore, exemestane has been compared with the nonsteroidal agent anastrozole in the adjuvant treatment of ER-positive breast cancer, and there were no differences in disease-free or overall survival.[149] Finally, exemestane has been compared to placebo in patients at increased risk of breast cancer, and a significant reduction in the risk of developing invasive breast cancer was observed.[150]

Side Effects of Exemestane

Although preclinical studies have suggested that exemestane prevented bone loss in ovariectomized rats,[151] the Intergroup Exemestane adjuvant trial still demonstrated a higher rate of bone fracture for patients randomized to the exemestane arm and there were no differences in fracture rates comparing anastrozole with exemestane.[149] Side effects, including arthralgias and myalgias, appear to be similar to the other AIs. With regard to steroidogenesis, no impact on either cortisol or aldosterone levels was seen in a small study after the administration of exemestane for 7 days.[152] Finally, exemestane has weak androgenic properties, and its use at higher doses has been associated with steroidal-like side effects, such as weight gain and acne.[153,154] However, these side effects have not been observed with the FDA-approved dose (25 mg per day).[155]

Pharmacology

Exemestane is administered once daily by mouth, with the recommended daily dose being 25 mg. The time needed to reach maximal E_2 suppression is 7 days,[156] and its half-life is 27 hours.[157] At daily doses of 10 to 25 mg, exemestane suppresses estrogen concentrations to 6% to 15% of pretreatment levels. This activity is more pronounced than that produced by formestane and comparable to that produced by the nonsteroidal AIs, anastrozole and letrozole.[158–160] Exemestane does not appear to affect cortisol or aldosterone levels when evaluated after 7 days of treatment based on dose-ranging studies, including doses from 0.5 to 800 mg.[152] Exemestane is metabolized by CYP3A4.[134] Although drug–drug interactions have not been formally reported for exemestane, there is the potential for interactions with drugs that affect CYP3A4.[134]

GONADOTROPIN-RELEASING HORMONE ANALOGS

Gonadotropin-releasing hormone (GnRH) analogs result in a *medical orchiectomy* in men and are used as a means of providing androgen ablation for hormone-sensitive and castration refractory metastatic prostate cancer.[161] Because the initial agonist activity of GnRH analogs can cause a *tumor flare* from temporarily increased androgen levels, concomitant use of the antiandrogen flutamide or bicalutamide has been used to prevent this effect. GnRH analogs can also cause tumor regressions in hormonally responsive breast cancers[162] and have received FDA approval for the treatment of metastatic breast cancer in premenopausal women. Data suggest that these drugs may be useful as adjuvant therapy of premenopausal women with resected breast cancer.[163] The use of these drugs in combination with tamoxifen or exemestane in premenopausal women with primary breast cancer is the subject of large, ongoing, international clinical trials. The primary toxicities of GnRH analogs are secondary to the ablation of sex steroid

concentrations and include hot flashes, sweating, and nausea.[164] These symptoms can be reversed with low doses of progesterone analogs.[5] In males treated with GnRH analogs for prostate cancer, an alternate strategy of intermittent schedule of GnRH administration may result in improved tolerability and quality of life, with comparable efficacy compared with continuous GnRH analog administration in well-selected advanced prostate cancer patient cohorts.[165] However, in a recent trial comparing intermittent with continuous androgen ablation in newly diagnosed metastatic hormone sensitive prostate cancer patients, a greater risk for death from an intermittent strategy could not be conclusively ruled out although intermittent therapy resulted in small improvements in quality of life.[166]

GnRH analogs available for clinical use include goserelin[167,168] and leuprolide.[169] Both are available in depot intramuscular preparations to be given at monthly intervals. The recommended monthly dose of leuprolide is 7.5 mg and of goserelin is 3.6 mg. There are also longer acting depot preparations to be administered every 3, 4, 6, and 12 months.

Pharmacology

Analogs of the decapeptide GnRH[167,169,170] have been synthesized by modifications of position 6 in which the l-glycine has been exchanged for a d-amino acid and the C-terminal amino acid has been either replaced by an ethylamide or substituted for a modified amino acid. These changes increase the affinity of the analog for the GnRH receptor and decrease the susceptibility to enzymatic degradation. There is an amino acid structure of GnRH with the substitutions for leuprolide and goserelin. Initial administration of these compounds results in stimulation of gonadotropin release. However, prolonged administration has led to profound inhibition of the pituitary–gonadal axis.[170] Plasma E_2 and progesterone are consistently suppressed to postmenopausal or castrate levels after 2 to 4 weeks of treatment with goserelin or leuprolide.[164,171] These drugs are administered intramuscularly or subcutaneously in a parenteral sustained-release microcapsule preparation, because parenteral administration of the parent drug is otherwise associated with rapid clearance. The GnRH analogs are metabolized in the liver, kidney, hypothalamus, and pituitary gland by neutral peptidase cleavage of the peptide bond between the tyrosine in the 5 position and the amino acid in position 6 and by a postproline-cleaving enzyme that cleaves the peptide bond between proline in the 9 position and the glycine-NH_2 in the 10 position. Substitutions at the glycine 6 position and modification of the C-terminal make these analogs more resistant to this enzymatic cleavage.

Leuprolide is approximately 80 to 100 times more potent than endogenous GnRH. It induces castrate levels of testosterone in men with prostate cancer within 3 to 4 weeks of drug administration after an initial sharp increase in LH and FSH. The mechanisms of action include pituitary desensitization after a reduction in pituitary GnRH receptor binding sites and possibly a direct antitumor effect in ER-positive human breast cancer cells.[169] The depot form results in a dose rate of 210 µg per day of leuprolide. Peak concentrations of the depot form, achieved approximately 3 hours after drug administration, have been reported to range between 13.1 and 54.5 µg/L. There appears to be a linear increase in the area under the curve (AUC) for doses of 3.75, 7.5, and 15.0 mg in the depot form. The parenteral bioavailability of subcutaneously injected leuprolide is 94%. The volume of distribution ranges from 27.4 to 37.1 L. In human studies, leuprolide urinary excretion as a metabolite was the primary route of clearance.

Goserelin is approximately 100 times more potent than the naturally occurring GnRH. Like leuprolide, it causes the stimulation of LH and FSH acutely, and with subsequent administration, GnRH receptor numbers decrease, and the pituitary becomes desensitized with decreasing LH and FSH levels. Castrate levels of testosterone are achieved within 1 month. In women, goserelin inhibits ovarian androgen production, but serum levels of dehydroepiandrosterone sulfate and, to a lesser extent, androstenedione, are preserved. In vitro, goserelin has demonstrated antitumor activity in estrogen-dependent MCF7 human breast cancer cells and LNCaP2 prostate cancer cells. The drug is released at a continuous mean rate of 120 μg per day in the depot form, with peak concentrations in the range of 2 to 3 μg/L achieved. The mean volume of distribution in six patients has been reported to be 13.7 L,[172] which is consistent with extracellular fluid volume. Goserelin is principally excreted in the urine, with a mean total body clearance of 8 L per hour in patients with normal renal function. The total body clearance is reduced by approximately 75%, with renal dysfunction and the elimination half-life increased two- or threefold. However, dose adjustment for renal insufficiency does not appear to be necessary. The 5 to 10 hexapeptide and the 4 to 10 hexapeptide were detected in urine in animal studies.[173] The terminal half-life of goserelin is approximately 5 hours after subcutaneous injection. Protein binding is low, and no known drug interactions have been documented.

GONADOTROPIN-RELEASING HORMONE ANTAGONISTS

Modification to the structure of GnRH has resulted in the development of GnRH antagonist compounds that are currently being used in the treatment of prostate cancer. Abarelix was initially approved by the FDA in 2003 as the first depot-injectable GnRH antagonist, but was subsequently withdrawn in 2005. Degarelix is a synthetically modified compound with GnRH antagonist activity that was approved for use by the FDA in 2008 for the management of prostate cancer.[174] Its effect in prostate cancer treatment is to block the GnRH receptor, and thereby prevent the trigger for the production of LH, which mediates androgen synthesis. In contrast to GnRH analogs, degarelix does not cause *tumor flare* symptoms secondary to temporary increased androgen production. A large randomized clinical trial demonstrated that degarelix was associated with a rapid and sustained reduction in serum testosterone, prostate-specific antigen (PSA), FSH, and LH levels, with a loading dose of 240 mg subcutaneously, followed by a monthly maintenance dose of 80 mg[175] with comparable efficacy to leuprolide.[176] The most common side effects (greater than 10%) were hot flashes and pain at the injection site[176] when patients were provided degarelix for a 12-month period. It is unknown if degarelix will have a similar chronic side effect profile known to be associated with long-term GnRH analog use.

Pharmacology

The recommended loading dose of degarelix is 240 mg, administered as two injections of 120 mg each subcutaneously. Monthly maintenance doses of 80 mg as a 20 mg/mL solution is started 28 days after the loading dose. In an analysis of pharmacokinetic/pharmacodynamic (PK/PD) properties of degarelix in 60 healthy males, after a single subcutaneous dose, a terminal half life of 47 days was observed.[177] PK properties of degarelix have been evaluated when administered as a subcutaneous depot of drug as a gel in six different doses to 48 healthy males and when administered intravenously. Using data from several clinical trials, the rate of drug diffusion from subcutaneous administration results in detectable drug up to 60 days after a single dose compared to less than 4 days when the drug is injected intravenously.

ANTIANDROGENS

Flutamide

The antiandrogen flutamide is used in men with metastatic prostate cancer either as initial therapy, combined with GnRH analog

administration, or when the metastatic prostate cancer is unresponsive, despite androgen ablation therapy. The recommended dose is 250 mg by mouth three times a day. In patients whose prostate cancer is growing despite flutamide use, stopping flutamide can sometimes cause a flutamide-withdrawal response.

The most common toxicity seen with flutamide is diarrhea, with or without abdominal discomfort. Gynecomastia, which can be tender, frequently occurs in men who are not receiving concomitant androgen ablation therapy.[178] Flutamide can rarely cause hepatotoxicity, a condition that is reversible if detected early, but this toxicity can also be fatal.[179] There is no accepted, clinically recommended testing schedule to screen for flutamide-induced hepatotoxicity other than being aware of this phenomenon and testing for liver function if hepatic symptoms develop.

Pharmacology

Flutamide is a pure antiandrogen with no intrinsic steroidal activity.[180] Flutamide's mechanism of action is as an androgen-receptor antagonist. This binding prevents dihydrotestosterone binding and subsequent translocation of the androgen-receptor complex into the nuclei of cells. Because it is a pure antiandrogen, it acts only at the cellular level. The administration of flutamide alone leads to increased LH and FSH production and a concomitant increase in plasma testosterone and E_2 levels. Plasma protein binding ranges between 94% and 96% for flutamide and between 92% and 94% for 2-hydroxyflutamide, its major metabolite. When the drug is administered three times a day, steady state levels are achieved by day 6. The elimination half-life at steady state is 7.8 hours, and 2-hydroxyflutamide achieves concentrations 50 times higher than the parent drug at steady state and has equal or greater potency than that of flutamide.[180] The elimination half-life for the metabolite is 9.6 hours. The high plasma concentrations of 2-hydroxyflutamide, as compared with flutamide, suggest that the therapeutic benefits of flutamide are mediated primarily through its active metabolite.[181]

Bicalutamide

Bicalutamide is another nonsteroidal antiandrogen that has been approved by the FDA for use in the United States. The recommended dose is one 50-mg tablet per day. One randomized trial reported that bicalutamide compared favorably with flutamide in patients with advanced prostate cancer.[182] Bicalutamide appears to be relatively well tolerated and is associated with a lower incidence of diarrhea than is flutamide.

Pharmacology

Bicalutamide has a binding affinity to the androgen receptor in the rat prostate that is four times greater than that of 2-hydroxyflutamide.[183,184] In vivo, bicalutamide caused a marked inhibition of growth of accessory sex organs in rats, with a potency 5 to 10 times greater than that of flutamide. Unlike flutamide, bicalutamide did not cause a significant increase in LH or testosterone in rats. In humans, the drug has a long plasma half-life of 5 to 7 days, so it may be administered on a weekly schedule. Pharmacokinetics of the drug showed a dose-dependent increase in mean peak plasma concentrations, and the AUC increased linearly with the dose. The half-life of bicalutamide in humans was approximately 6 days, and the drug clearance was not saturable at plasma concentrations up to 1,000 ng/mL. Daily dosing of the drug led to an approximately tenfold accumulation after 12 weeks of administration. In contrast to results in rats, serum concentrations of testosterone and LH increased significantly from baseline at all dose levels tested in humans. Whereas serum FSH concentrations remained essentially unchanged, the median serum E_2 concentrations increased significantly.[185]

Nilutamide

Nilutamide represents the third variation of an antiandrogen available for use in patients with prostate cancer. The observation of unique toxicities, night blindness, and pulmonary toxicity has limited its use.

NOVEL ANTIANDROGENS

Although testosterone depletion remains an unchallenged standard for advanced stage hormone-sensitive disease, evidence has emerged that *castration-recurrent* prostate cancer remains androgen receptor (AR) dependent and is neither *hormone refractory* nor *androgen independent*, which were commonly used terms to define the progression of advanced stage disease following androgen deprivation therapy. Recognition of AR functioning despite the paucity of circulating androgens is evidenced by the elevation of AR messenger RNA in castration-recurrent tumor tissue relative to androgen-dependent tumors and reexpression of some androgen-regulated genes during clinical castration resistance. Recently, the AR axis has been the focus of therapeutic targeting.

Abiraterone Acetate

After the failure of initial androgen manipulation with GnRH analogs and peripheral antiandrogens, prostate cancer continues to respond to a variety of second- and third-line hormonal interventions. Based on this observation, CYP17, a key enzyme in androgen and estrogen synthesis, was targeted using ketoconazole, which is a weak, reversible, and nonspecific inhibitor of CYP17 resulting in modest antitumor activity of short durability. More recently, abiraterone, a more potent (i.e., 20 times more than ketoconazole), selective, and irreversible inhibitor of CYP17, has been investigated in castration-recurrent prostate cancer, and significant objective responses have been observed.[186] Chemically, it is a 3-pyridyl steroid pregnenolone–derived compound available in an oral prodrug form of abiraterone acetate. Its main toxicity is from symptoms of mineralocorticoid excess (including hypokalemia, hypertension, and fluid overload), because continuous CYP17 blockade results in raising adrenocorticotrophic hormone (ACTH) levels that increase steroid levels upstream of CYP17, including corticosterone and deoxycorticosterone. These adverse effects are best avoided by the coadministration of steroids.

The established dose of abiraterone is 1,000 mg a day (four 250 mg tablets). Following oral administration of abiraterone acetate, the median time to maximum plasma abiraterone concentrations is 2 hours. At the dose of 1,000 mg daily, steady state values (mean $\pm$ standard deviation [SD]) of Cmax were 226 ± 178 ng/mL and of AUC were 1173 ± 690 ng.hr/mL. Abiraterone is highly bound (>99%) to the human plasma proteins, albumin and alpha-1 acid glycoprotein. The apparent steady state volume of distribution (mean $\pm$ SD) is $19,669 \pm 13,358$ L. No major deviation from dose proportionality was observed in the dose range of 250 mg to 1,000 mg. However, the exposure was not significantly increased when the dose was doubled from 1,000 to 2,000 mg (8% increase in mean AUC). The two main circulating metabolites of abiraterone in human plasma are abiraterone sulfate (inactive) and N-oxide abiraterone sulfate (inactive), which each account for about 43% of exposure. CYP3A4 and SULT2A1 are enzymes involved in the formation and conjugation of N-oxide abiraterone.

Enzalutamide

Enzalutamide is a new diarylthiohydantoin compound that binds AR with an affinity that is several-fold greater than the antiandrogens bicalutamide and flutamide. This class of novel AR inhibitor also disrupts the nuclear translocation of AR and impairs DNA binding to androgen response elements and the recruitment of coactivators.[187] In early clinical trials, promising results have been observed in castrate refractory and chemotherapy-resistant settings. The major metabolite of enzalutamide is N-desmethyl enzalutamide, and CYP2C8 is responsible for the formation of the active metabolite, N-desmethyl enzalutamide. Enzalutamide pharmacokinetics, in the studied dose range between 30 mg to 480 mg, exhibited a linear, two-compartmental model with first-order kinetics. In patients with mCRPC, the mean (% coefficient of variation [CV]) predose Cmin values for enzalutamide and N-desmethyl enzalutamide were 11.4 (25.9%) μg/mL and 13.0 (29.9%) μg/mL, respectively. Enzalutamide is mainly metabolized by CYP2C8 and CYP3A4. Doses ranging from 30 to 600 mg daily have been evaluated, with dose-limiting toxicities including fatigue, seizure, asthenia, anemia, and arthralgia occurring at higher dose levels. At present, enzalutamide has been approved for treating advanced castrate-recurrent prostate cancer[188] after a failure of docetaxel chemotherapy at a dose of 160 mg (four, 40 mg oral capsules). Clinical trials are ongoing to evaluate the efficacy of enzalutamide in castrate-recurrent patients who are chemotherapy naïve.

Galeterone and Orteronel

Novel CYP17 inhibitors that are more selective for 17,20-lyase over 17 α-hydroxylase are currently being developed. Orteronel (TAK-700) is an example of a highly selective 17,20 lyase, which is currently undergoing phase III clinical trials in a pre- and post-chemotherapy castrate-recurrent setting after the failure of androgen-deprivation therapy.[189] Other novel agents being developed include galeterone, which is an inhibitor of CYP 17 α-hydroxylase and C17,20 lyase. Survival mechanisms of prostate cancer cells targeted by galeterone include its binding to AR, competitive inhibition of testosterone binding, and a reduction in the quantity of AR protein within the prostate cancer cells. It can also enhance the degradation of constitutively active splice variants. Therefore, taken together, it diminishes the ability of the cells to respond to the low levels of androgenic growth signals. This agent is currently in early clinical safety and efficacy testing for advanced stage prostate cancer.

OTHER SEX STEROID THERAPIES

Fluoxymesterone

Fluoxymesterone is an androgen that has been used in women with metastatic breast cancer who have hormonally responsive cancers and who have progressed on other hormonal therapies such as tamoxifen, an aromatase inhibitor, or megestrol acetate. The usual dose is 10 mg given twice daily. Although the overall response rate is low for fluoxymesterone used in this clinical situation,[190] there are some patients who have substantial antitumor responses lasting for months or even years.

Toxicities associated with fluoxymesterone are those that would be expected with an androgen: hirsutism, male-pattern baldness, voice lowering (hoarseness), acne, enhanced libido, and erythrocytosis. Fluoxymesterone can also cause elevated liver function test results in some patients and, rarely, has been associated with hepatic neoplasms.

Pharmacology

Fluoxymesterone is a chlorinated synthetic analog of testosterone with potent androgenic and anabolic activity in humans. Limited pharmacologic information is available on this agent. Colburn,[191] using a radioimmunoassay, studied two patients after a single oral administration of a 50-mg dose. Peak serum concentrations were achieved between 1 and 3 hours after administration, with the average peak concentrations being 335 ng/mL. By 5 hours after drug administration, serum levels had declined to approximately 50% of the peak concentration. Urinary excretion of a 10-mg dose can be detected for 24 hours, and at least 6-hydroxy, 4-ene, 3-β, and 11-hydroxy metabolites of fluoxymesterone have been detected.[192]

Estrogens: Diethylstilbestrol and Estradiol

Diethylstilbestrol (DES) had been the primary hormonal therapy for postmenopausal metastatic breast cancer. Randomized comparative trials demonstrated it had a similar response rate to that of tamoxifen.[193,194] However, based on these trials, DES use was supplanted by tamoxifen, primarily because DES has more toxicity. DES is occasionally used in metastatic breast cancer patients who have hormonally sensitive cancers that have failed to respond to multiple other hormonal therapies. The usual dose in this situation is 15 mg per day, either as a single dose or as divided doses. DES was also used as androgen ablation therapy in men with metastatic prostate cancer.[195] Doses of approximately 3 mg per day result in testosterone levels that are seen in an anorchid state.

DES toxicities include nausea and vomiting, breast tenderness, and a darkening of the nipple–areolar complex. DES increases the risk of thromboembolic phenomenon, which may result in life-threatening complications. Although DES is not clinically available in the United States, similar antitumor effects and toxicities are seen with estradiol, with a target dose of 10 mg by mouth three times a day. The pharmacology of E_2 has been extensively described elsewhere.[196]

Medroxyprogesterone and Megestrol

Medroxyprogesterone and megestrol are 17-OH-progesterone derivatives differing in a double bond between C6 and C7 positions in megestrol. Historically, megestrol was used as a hormonal agent for patients with advanced breast cancer, usually at a total daily dose of 160 mg. Additionally, it is still used for the treatment of hormonally responsive metastatic endometrial cancer, at a dose of 320 mg per day. In addition, doses of 160 mg per day are occasionally used as a hormonal therapy for prostate cancer.[197] Megestrol has also been extensively evaluated for the treatment of anorexia/cachexia related to cancer or AIDS.[198–201] Various dosages ranging from 160 to 1,600 mg per day have been used. A prospective study has demonstrated a dose–response relationship with doses up to 800 mg per day.[202] Low dosages of megestrol (20 to 40 mg per day) have been shown to be an effective means of reducing hot flashes in women with breast cancer and in men who have undergone androgen ablation therapy.[5] Although megestrol had historically been commonly administered four times per day, the long terminal half-life supports once-per-day dosing.

Megestrol is a relatively well-tolerated medication, with its most prominent side effects being appetite stimulation and resultant weight gain. Although these may be beneficial effects in patients with anorexia/cachexia, they can be important problems in patients with breast or endometrial cancers. Another side effect of megestrol acetate is the marked suppression of adrenal steroid production by suppression of the pituitary–adrenal axis.[203] Although this appears to be asymptomatic in the majority of patients, reports suggest that this adrenal suppression can cause clinical problems in some patients.[204] This drug has been abruptly stopped for decades without the recognition of untoward sequelae in patients, and it seems reasonable to continue this practice. Nonetheless, if Addisonian signs or symptoms develop after drug discontinuation, corticosteroids should be administered.

Furthermore, if patients who receive megestrol have a significant infection, experience trauma, or undergo surgery, then corticosteroid coverage should be administered. There appears to be a slightly increased incidence of thromboembolic phenomena in patients receiving megestrol alone.[202] This risk appears to be higher if megestrol is administered with concomitant cytotoxic therapy.[205] There are conflicting reports regarding megestrol-causing edema.[206] If it does, the edema is generally minimal and easily handled with a mild diuretic. Megestrol may cause impotence in some men.[207] The incidence of this is controversial, although it is generally agreed that this is a reversible situation. Megestrol can cause menstrual irregularities, the most prominent of which is withdrawal menstrual bleeding within a few weeks of drug discontinuation.[5] Although nausea and vomiting have sometimes been attributed as a toxicity of this drug, there are data to demonstrate that this drug has antiemetic properties.[200,201,205] In terms of magnitude, megestrol appears to decrease both nausea and vomiting in advanced-stage cancer patients by approximately two thirds.

Medroxyprogesterone has many of the same properties, clinical uses, and toxicities as megestrol acetate. It has never been commonly used in the United States for the treatment of breast cancer but has been used more in Europe. Medroxyprogesterone is available in 2.5- and 10-mg tablets and in injectable formulations of 100 and 400 mg/L. Dosing for the treatment of metastatic breast or prostate cancer has commonly been 400 mg per week or more and 1,000 mg per week or more for metastatic endometrial cancer. Injectable or daily oral doses have been used for controlling hot flashes.

Pharmacology

The exact mechanism of antitumor effect of medroxyprogesterone and megestrol is unclear. These drugs have been reported to suppress adrenal steroid synthesis,[208] suppress ER levels,[209] alter tumor hormone metabolism,[210] enhance steroid metabolism,[211] and directly kill tumor cells.[212] In addition, progestins may influence some growth factors,[213] suppress plasma estrone sulfate formation, and, at high concentrations, inhibit P-glycoprotein.

The oral bioavailability of these progestational agents is unknown, although absorption appears to be poor for medroxyprogesterone relative to megestrol.

The terminal half-life for megestrol is approximately 14 hours,[214,215] with a t_{max} of 2 to 5 hours after oral ingestion.[216] The AUC for a single megestrol dose of 160 mg is between 2.5- and 8-fold higher than that for single-dose medroxyprogesterone at 1,000 mg with a radioactive dose of megestrol; 50% to 78% is found in the urine after oral administration, and 8% to 30% is found in the feces.

Metabolism and excretion of medroxyprogesterone have been incompletely characterized. In humans, 20% to 50% of a [^{3}H]medroxyprogesterone dose is excreted in the urine and 5% to 10% in the stool after intravenous administration.[217–219] Metabolism of medroxyprogesterone occurs via hydroxylation, reduction, demethylation, and combinations of these reactions.[220] The major urinary metabolite is a glucuronide. Less than 3% of the dose is excreted as unconjugated medroxyprogesterone in humans. Clearance of medroxyprogesterone has been reported to range between 27 and 70 L per hour.[219] The initial volume of distribution is between 4 and 8 L in humans. The mean terminal half-life is 60 hours. The t_{max} for medroxyprogesterone occurs 2 to 5 hours after oral administration. Medroxyprogesterone appears to be concentrated in the small intestine, the colon, and in adipose tissue in human autopsy studies.[221] Drug interactions of medroxyprogesterone have been reported with aminoglutethimide, which decreases plasma medroxyprogesterone levels.[222] Medroxyprogesterone may reduce the concentration of the N-desmethyltamoxifen metabolite concentration. Progestational agents also may increase plasma warfarin levels.[223] These reports are consistent with CYP3A being the site of interaction.

OTHER HORMONAL THERAPIES

Octreotide

Octreotide is a somatostatin analog that is administered for the treatment of carcinoid syndrome and other hormonal excess syndromes associated with some pancreatic islet cell cancers and acromegaly. Response rates (measured in terms of a reduction in diarrhea and flushing) are high and can last for several months to years. Occasionally, antitumor responses temporarily related to octreotide are seen with these tumors. Octreotide may be useful to alleviate 5-fluorouracil–associated diarrhea.[224–226]

Octreotide can be administered intravenously or subcutaneously. Initial doses of 50 μg are given two to three times on the first day. The dose is titrated upward, with a usual daily dose of 300 to 450 μg per day for most patients. A depot preparation is available, allowing doses to be administered at monthly intervals. Octreotide is generally well tolerated overall. It appears to cause more toxicity in acromegalic patients, with such problems as bradycardia, diarrhea, hypoglycemia, hyperglycemia, hypothyroidism, and cholelithiasis.

Pharmacology

Octreotide is an 8-amino acid synthetic analog of the 14-amino acid peptide somatostatin.[227] Octreotide has a similar high affinity for somatostatin receptors, as does its parent compound, with a concentration that inhibits the receptor by 50% in the subnanomolar range. Octreotide inhibits insulin, glucagon, pancreatic polypeptide, gastric inhibitory polypeptide, and gastrin secretion. It has a much longer duration of action than the parent compound because of its greater resistance to enzymatic degradation. Its absorption after subcutaneous administration is rapid, and bioavailability is 100% after subcutaneous injection. Peak concentrations of 4 μg/L after a 100-μg dose occur within 20 to 30 minutes of subcutaneous injection and are 20% to 40% of the corresponding intravenous injection. Both peak concentration and AUC for octreotide increase linearly with dose. The total body clearance in healthy volunteers is 9.6 L per hour. Hepatic metabolism of octreotide accounts for 30% to 40% of the drug's disposition, and 11% to 20% is excreted unchanged in the urine. The volume of distribution ranges between 18 and 30 L, and the terminal half-life is reported to be between 72 and 98 minutes. Sixty-five percent of the drug is protein bound primarily to the lipoprotein fraction.[227,228] Because of the short half-life, classic octreotide is administered subcutaneously two or three times per day.[229] A slow-release form of octreotide, designed for once-per-month administration, controls the symptoms of carcinoid syndrome at least as well as three-times-per-day octreotide.[230]

REFERENCES

1. Fisher B, Costantino JP, Wickerham DL, et al. Tamoxifen for the prevention of breast cancer: current status of the National Surgical Adjuvant Breast and Bowel Project P-1 study. *J Natl Cancer Inst* 2005;97:1652–1662.
2. Fisher B, Dignam J, Wolmark N, et al. Tamoxifen in treatment of intraductal breast cancer: National Surgical Adjuvant Breast and Bowel Project B-24 randomised controlled trial. *Lancet* 1999;353:1993–2000.
3. Colleoni M, Gelber S, Goldhirsch A, et al. Tamoxifen after adjuvant chemotherapy for premenopausal women with lymph node-positive breast cancer: International Breast Cancer Study Group Trial 13-93. *J Clin Oncol* 2006;24:1332–1341.
4. Davies C, Pan H, Godwin J, et al. Long-term effects of continuing adjuvant tamoxifen to 10 years versus stopping at 5 years after diagnosis of oestrogen receptor-positive breast cancer: ATLAS, a randomised trial. *Lancet* 2013;381:805–816.
5. Loprinzi CL, Michalak JC, Quella SK, et al. Megestrol acetate for the prevention of hot flashes. *N Engl J Med* 1994;331:347–352.
6. Loprinzi CL, Kugler JW, Sloan JA, et al. Venlafaxine in management of hot flashes in survivors of breast cancer: a randomised controlled trial. *Lancet* 2000;356:2059–2063.
7. Archer DF, Dupont CM, Constantine GD, et al. Desvenlafaxine for the treatment of vasomotor symptoms associated with menopause: a double-blind, randomized, placebo-controlled trial of efficacy and safety. *Am J Obstet Gynecol* 2009;200:238.e1–238e10.
8. Barton DL, LaVasseur BI, Sloan JA, et al. Phase III, placebo-controlled trial of three doses of citalopram for the treatment of hot flashes: NCCTG trial N05C9. *J Clin Oncol* 2010;28:3278–3283.
9. Freeman EW, Guthrie KA, Caan B, et al. Efficacy of escitalopram for hot flashes in healthy menopausal women: a randomized controlled trial. *JAMA* 2011;305:267–274.
10. Stearns V, Beebe KL, Iyengar M, et al. Paroxetine controlled release in the treatment of menopausal hot flashes: a randomized controlled trial. *JAMA* 2003;289:2827–2834.
11. Pandya KJ, Morrow GR, Roscoe JA, et al. Gabapentin for hot flashes in 420 women with breast cancer: a randomised double-blind placebo-controlled trial. *Lancet* 2005;366:818–824.
12. Loprinzi CL, Qin R, Balcueva EP, et al. Phase III, randomized, double-blind, placebo-controlled evaluation of pregabalin for alleviating hot flashes, N07C1. *J Clin Oncol* 2010;28:641–647.
13. Madlensky L, Natarajan L, Tchu S, et al. Tamoxifen metabolite concentrations, CYP2D6 genotype, and breast cancer outcomes. *Clin Pharmacol Ther* 2011;89:718–725.
14. Tamoxifen for early breast cancer: an overview of the randomised trials. Early Breast Cancer Trialists' Collaborative Group. *Lancet* 1998;351:1451–1467.
15. Wickerham DL, Fisher B, Wolmark N, et al. Association of tamoxifen and uterine sarcoma. *J Clin Oncol* 2002;20:2758–2760.
16. Dewar JA, Horobin JM, Preece PE, et al. Long term effects of tamoxifen on blood lipid values in breast cancer. *BMJ* 1992;305:225–226.
17. Love RR, Mazess RB, Barden HS, et al. Effects of tamoxifen on bone mineral density in postmenopausal women with breast cancer. *N Engl J Med* 1992;326:852–856.
18. Powles TJ, Hickish T, Kanis JA, et al. Effect of tamoxifen on bone mineral density measured by dual-energy x-ray absorptiometry in healthy premenopausal and postmenopausal women. *J Clin Oncol* 1996;14:78–84.
19. Buzdar A, Howell A, Cuzick J, et al. Comprehensive side-effect profile of anastrozole and tamoxifen as adjuvant treatment for early-stage breast cancer: long-term safety analysis of the ATAC trial. *Lancet Oncol* 2006;7:633–643.
20. Gorin MB, Day R, Costantino JP, et al. Long-term tamoxifen citrate use and potential ocular toxicity. *Am J Ophthalmol* 1998;125:493–501.
21. Tonetti DA, Jordan VC. Possible mechanisms in the emergence of tamoxifen-resistant breast cancer. *Anticancer Drugs* 1995;6:498–507.
22. Lim YC, Desta Z, Flockhart DA, et al. Endoxifen (4-hydroxy-N-desmethyl-tamoxifen) has anti-estrogenic effects in breast cancer cells with potency similar to 4-hydroxy-tamoxifen. *Cancer Chemother Pharmacol* 2005;55:471–478.
23. Benz CC, Scott GK, Sarup JC, et al. Estrogen-dependent, tamoxifen-resistant tumorigenic growth of MCF-7 cells transfected with HER2/neu. *Breast Cancer Res Treat* 1993;24:85–95.
24. Borg A, Baldetorp B, Ferno M, et al. ERBB2 amplification is associated with tamoxifen resistance in steroid-receptor positive breast cancer. *Cancer Lett* 1994;81:137–144.
25. Houston SJ, Plunkett TA, Barnes DM, et al. Overexpression of c-erbB2 is an independent marker of resistance to endocrine therapy in advanced breast cancer. *Br J Cancer* 1999;79:1220–1226.
26. Lipton A, Ali SM, Leitzel K, et al. Serum HER-2/neu and response to the aromatase inhibitor letrozole versus tamoxifen. *J Clin Oncol* 2003;21:1967–1972.
27. Bunone G, Briand PA, Miksicek RJ, et al. Activation of the unliganded estrogen receptor by EGF involves the MAP kinase pathway and direct phosphorylation. *Embo J* 1996;15:2174–2183.
28. Kato S, Endoh H, Masuhiro Y, et al. Activation of the estrogen receptor through phosphorylation by mitogen-activated protein kinase. *Science* 1995;270:1491–1494.
29. Pietras RJ, Arboleda J, Reese DM, et al. HER-2 tyrosine kinase pathway targets estrogen receptor and promotes hormone-independent growth in human breast cancer cells. *Oncogene* 1995;10:2435–2446.
30. Osborne CK, Bardou V, Hopp TA, et al. Role of the estrogen receptor coactivator AIB1 (SRC-3) and HER-2/neu in tamoxifen resistance in breast cancer. *J Natl Cancer Inst* 2003;95:353–361.
31. Encarnacion CA, Ciocca DR, McGuire WL, et al. Measurement of steroid hormone receptors in breast cancer patients on tamoxifen. *Breast Cancer Res Treat* 1993;26:237–246.
32. Watts CK, Handel ML, King RJ, et al. Oestrogen receptor gene structure and function in breast cancer. *J Steroid Biochem Mol Biol* 1992;41:529–536.
33. Zhang QX, Borg A, Wolf DM, et al. An estrogen receptor mutant with strong hormone-independent activity from a metastatic breast cancer. *Cancer Res* 1997;57:1244–1249.
34. Toy W, Shen Y, Won H, et al. ESR1 ligand-binding domain mutations in hormone-resistant breast cancer. *Nat Genet* 2013;45:1439–1445.
35. Robinson DR, Wu YM, Vats P, et al. Activating ESR1 mutations in hormone-resistant metastatic breast cancer. *Nat Genet* 2013;45:1446–1451.

36. Merenbakh-Lamin K, Ben-Baruch N, Yeheskel A, et al. D538G mutation in estrogen receptor-alpha: a novel mechanism for acquired endocrine resistance in breast cancer. *Cancer Res* 2013;73:6856–6864.

37. Fendl KC, Zimniski SJ. Role of tamoxifen in the induction of hormone-independent rat mammary tumors. *Cancer Res* 1992;52:235–237.

38. Williams GM. Tamoxifen experimental carcinogenicity studies: implications for human effects. *Proc Soc Exp Biol Med* 1995;208:141–143.

39. Williams GM, Iatropoulos MJ, Djordjevic MV, et al. The triphenylethylene drug tamoxifen is a strong liver carcinogen in the rat. *Carcinogenesis* 1993;14:315–317.

40. Rutqvist LE, Johansson H, Signomklao T, et al. Adjuvant tamoxifen therapy for early stage breast cancer and second primary malignancies. Stockholm Breast Cancer Study Group. *J Natl Cancer Inst* 1995;87:645–651.

41. Mani C, Kupfer D. Cytochrome P-450-mediated activation and irreversible binding of the antiestrogen tamoxifen to proteins in rat and human liver: possible involvement of flavin-containing monooxygenases in tamoxifen activation. *Cancer Res* 1991;51:6052–6058.

42. Mani C, Pearce R, Parkinson A, et al. Involvement of cytochrome P4503A in catalysis of tamoxifen activation and covalent binding to rat and human liver microsomes. *Carcinogenesis* 1994;15:2715–2720.

43. Styles JA, Davies A, Lim CK, et al. Genotoxicity of tamoxifen, tamoxifen epoxide and toremifene in human lymphoblastoid cells containing human cytochrome P450s. *Carcinogenesis* 1994;15:5–9.

44. Han XL, Liehr JG. Induction of covalent DNA adducts in rodents by tamoxifen. *Cancer Res* 1992;52:1360–1363.

45. Mani C, Hodgson E, Kupfer D. Metabolism of the antimammary cancer antiestrogenic agent tamoxifen. II. Flavin-containing monooxygenase-mediated N-oxidation. *Drug Metab Dispos* 1993;21:657–661.

46. Mani C, Gelboin HV, Park SS, et al. Metabolism of the antimammary cancer antiestrogenic agent tamoxifen. I. Cytochrome P-450-catalyzed N-demethylation and 4-hydroxylation. *Drug Metab Dispos* 1993;21:645–656.

47. Albain KS, Barlow WE, Shak S, et al. Prognostic and predictive value of the 21-gene recurrence score assay in postmenopausal women with node-positive, oestrogen-receptor-positive breast cancer on chemotherapy: a retrospective analysis of a randomised trial. *Lancet Oncol* 2010;11:55–65.

48. Dowsett M, Cuzick J, Wale C, et al. Prediction of risk of distant recurrence using the 21-gene recurrence score in node-negative and node-positive postmenopausal patients with breast cancer treated with anastrozole or tamoxifen: a TransATAC study. *J Clin Oncol* 2010;28:1829–1834.

49. Paik S, Shak S, Tang G, et al. A multigene assay to predict recurrence of tamoxifen-treated, node-negative breast cancer. *N Engl J Med* 2004;351:2817–2826.

50. Johnson MD, Zuo H, Lee KH, et al. Pharmacological characterization of 4-hydroxy-N-desmethyl tamoxifen, a novel active metabolite of tamoxifen. *Breast Cancer Res Treat* 2004;85:151–159.

51. Lim YC, Li L, Desta Z, et al. Endoxifen, a secondary metabolite of tamoxifen, and 4-OH-tamoxifen induce similar changes in global gene expression patterns in MCF-7 breast cancer cells. *J Pharmacol Exp Ther* 2006;318:503–512.

52. Wu X, Hawse JR, Subramaniam M, et al. The tamoxifen metabolite, endoxifen, is a potent antiestrogen that targets estrogen receptor alpha for degradation in breast cancer cells. *Cancer Res* 2009;69:1722–1727.

53. Jin Y, Desta Z, Stearns V, et al. CYP2D6 genotype, antidepressant use, and tamoxifen metabolism during adjuvant breast cancer treatment. *J Natl Cancer Inst* 2005;97:30–39.

54. Desta Z, Ward BA, Soukhova NV, et al. Comprehensive evaluation of tamoxifen sequential biotransformation by the human cytochrome P450 system in vitro: prominent roles for CYP3A and CYP2D6. *J Pharmacol Exp Ther* 2004;310:1062–1075.

55. Stearns V, Johnson MD, Rae JM, et al. Active tamoxifen metabolite plasma concentrations after coadministration of tamoxifen and the selective serotonin reuptake inhibitor paroxetine. *J Natl Cancer Inst* 2003;95:1758–1764.

56. Goetz MP, Rae JM, Suman VJ. Pharmacogenetics of tamoxifen biotransformation is associated with clinical outcomes of efficacy and hot flashes. *J Clin Oncol* 2005;23:9312–9318.

57. Schroth W, Antoniadou L, Fritz P, et al. Breast cancer treatment outcome with adjuvant tamoxifen relative to patient CYP2D6 and CYP2C19 genotypes. *J Clin Oncol* 2007;25:5187–5193.

58. Schroth W, Goetz MP, Hamann U, et al. Association between CYP2D6 polymorphisms and outcomes among women with early stage breast cancer treated with tamoxifen. *JAMA* 2009;302:1429–1436.

59. Rae JM, Drury S, Hayes DF, et al. CYP2D6 and UGT2B7 genotype and risk of recurrence in tamoxifen-treated breast cancer patients. *J Natl Cancer Inst* 2012;104:452–460.

60. Regan MM, Leyland-Jones B, Bouzyk M, et al. CYP2D6 genotype and tamoxifen response in postmenopausal women with endocrine-responsive breast cancer: the breast international group 1-98 trial. *J Natl Cancer Inst* 2012;104:441–451.

61. Goetz MP, Suman VJ, Hoskin TL, et al. CYP2D6 metabolism and patient outcome in the Austrian Breast and Colorectal Cancer Study Group trial (ABCSG) 8. *Clin Cancer Res* 2013;19:500–507.

62. Province MA, Goetz MP, Brauch H, et al. CYP2D6 Genotype and adjuvant tamoxifen: meta-analysis of heterogeneous study populations. *Clin Pharmacol Ther* 2014;95:216–227.

63. Borges S, Desta Z, Li L, et al. Quantitative effect of CYP2D6 genotype and inhibitors on tamoxifen metabolism: implication for optimization of breast cancer treatment. *Clin Pharmacol Ther* 2006;80:61–74.

64. Dezentje VO, van Blijderveen NJ, Gelderblom H, et al. Effect of concomitant CYP2D6 inhibitor use and tamoxifen adherence on breast cancer recurrence in early-stage breast cancer. *J Clin Oncol* 2010;28:2423–2429.

65. Kelly CM, Juurlink DN, Gomes T, et al. Selective serotonin reuptake inhibitors and breast cancer mortality in women receiving tamoxifen: a population based cohort study. *BMJ* 2010;340:c693.

66. Binkhorst L, van Gelder T, Loos WJ, et al. Effects of CYP induction by rifampicin on tamoxifen exposure. *Clin Pharmacol Ther* 2012;92:62–67.

67. Irvin WJ Jr., Walko CM, Weck KE, et al. Genotype-guided tamoxifen dosing increases active metabolite exposure in women with reduced CYP2D6 metabolism: a multicenter study. *J Clin Oncol* 2011;29:3232–3239.

68. Kiyotani K, Mushiroda T, Imamura CK, et al. Dose-adjustment study of tamoxifen based on CYP2D6 genotypes in Japanese breast cancer patients. *Breast Cancer Res Treat* 2012;131:137–145.

69. Goetz MP, Suman VA, Reid JR, et al. A first-in-human phase I study of the tamoxifen (TAM) metabolite, Z-endoxifen hydrochloride (Z-Endx) in women with aromatase inhibitor (AI) refractory metastatic breast cancer (MBC) (NCT01327781). *Cancer Res* 2013;73(24 Suppl): Abstract nr PD3-4.

70. Lien EA, Anker G, Lonning PE, et al. Decreased serum concentrations of tamoxifen and its metabolites induced by aminoglutethimide. *Cancer Res* 1990;50:5851–5857.

71. Adam HK, Patterson JS, Kemp JV. Studies on the metabolism and pharmacokinetics of tamoxifen in normal volunteers. *Cancer Treat Rep* 1980;64:761–764.

72. Patterson JS, Settatree RS, Adam HK, et al. Serum concentrations of tamoxifen and major metabolite during long-term nolvadex therapy, correlated with clinical response. *Eur J Cancer Suppl* 1980;1:89–92.

73. Camaggi CM, Strocchi E, Canova N, et al. Medroxyprogesterone acetate (MAP) and tamoxifen (TMX) plasma levels after simultaneous treatment with 'low' TMX and 'high' MAP doses. *Cancer Chemother Pharmacol* 1985;14:229–231.

74. Lien EA, Solheim E, Lea OA, et al. Distribution of 4-hydroxy-N-desmethyltamoxifen and other tamoxifen metabolites in human biological fluids during tamoxifen treatment. *Cancer Res* 1989;49:2175–2183.

75. Lien EA, Solheim E, Ueland PM. Distribution of tamoxifen and its metabolites in rat and human tissues during steady-state treatment. *Cancer Res* 1991;51:4837–4844.

76. Daniel P, Gaskell SJ, Bishop H, et al. Determination of tamoxifen and biologically active metabolites in human breast tumours and plasma. *Eur J Cancer Clin Oncol* 1981;17:1183–1189.

77. Robinson SP, Langan-Fahey SM, Johnson DA, et al. Metabolites, pharmacodynamics, and pharmacokinetics of tamoxifen in rats and mice compared to the breast cancer patient. *Drug Metab Dispos* 1991;19:36–43.

78. DeGregorio MW, Wiebe VJ, Venook AP, et al. Elevated plasma tamoxifen levels in a patient with liver obstruction. *Cancer Chemother Pharmacol* 1989;23:194–195.

79. Lodwick R, McConkey B, Brown AM. Life threatening interaction between tamoxifen and warfarin. *Br Med J (Clin Res Ed)* 1987;295:1141.

80. Ritchie LD, Grant SM. Tamoxifen-warfarin interaction: the Aberdeen hospitals drug file. *BMJ* 1989;298:1253.

81. Tenni P, Lalich DL, Byrne MJ. Life threatening interaction between tamoxifen and warfarin. *BMJ* 1989;298:93.

82. Rabinowicz AL, Hinton DR, Dyck P, et al. High-dose tamoxifen in treatment of brain tumors: interaction with antiepileptic drugs. *Epilepsia* 1995;36:513–515.

83. Desai PB, Nallani SC, Sane RS, et al. Induction of cytochrome P450 3A4 in primary human hepatocytes and activation of the human pregnane X receptor by tamoxifen and 4-hydroxytamoxifen. *Drug Metab Dispos* 2002;30:608–612.

84. Dowsett M, Cuzick J, Howell A, et al. Pharmacokinetics of anastrozole and tamoxifen alone, and in combination, during adjuvant endocrine therapy for early breast cancer in postmenopausal women: a sub-protocol of the 'Arimidex and tamoxifen alone or in combination' (ATAC) trial. *Br J Cancer* 2001;85:317–324.

85. Pagani O, Gelber S, Price K, et al. Toremifene and tamoxifen are equally effective for early-stage breast cancer: first results of International Breast Cancer Study Group Trials 12-93 and 14-93. *Ann Oncol* 2004;15:1749–1759.

86. Hayes DF, Van Zyl JA, Hacking A, et al. Randomized comparison of tamoxifen and two separate doses of toremifene in postmenopausal patients with metastatic breast cancer. *J Clin Oncol* 1995;13:2556–2566.

87. Stenbygaard LE, Herrstedt J, Thomsen JF, et al. Toremifene and tamoxifen in advanced breast cancer—a double-blind cross-over trial. *Breast Cancer Res Treat* 1993;25:57–63.

88. Vogel CL, Shemano I, Schoenfelder J, et al. Multicenter phase II efficacy trial of toremifene in tamoxifen-refractory patients with advanced breast cancer. *J Clin Oncol* 1993;11:345–350.

89. Kangas L. Review of the pharmacological properties of toremifene. *J Steroid Biochem* 1990;36:191–195.

90. Berthou F, Dreano Y, Belloc C, et al. Involvement of cytochrome P450 3A enzyme family in the major metabolic pathways of toremifene in human liver microsomes. *Biochem Pharmacol* 1994;47:1883–1895.

91. Simberg NH, Murai JT, Siiteri PK. In vitro and in vivo binding of toremifene and its metabolites in rat uterus. *J Steroid Biochem* 1990;36:197–202.

92. Kohler PC, Hamm JT, Wiebe VJ, et al. Phase I study of the tolerance and pharmacokinetics of toremifene in patients with cancer. *Breast Cancer Res Treat* 1990;16 Suppl:S19–S26.

93. Tominaga T, Abe O, Izuo M. A phase I study of toremifene. *Breast Cancer Res Treat* 1990;16 (Suppl):27.

94. Wiebe VJ, Benz CC, Shemano I, et al. Pharmacokinetics of toremifene and its metabolites in patients with advanced breast cancer. *Cancer Chemother Pharmacol* 1990;25:247–251.

CANCER THERAPEUTICS

95. Anttila M, Laakso S, Nylanden P, et al. Pharmacokinetics of the novel antiestrogenic agent toremifene in subjects with altered liver and kidney function. *Clin Pharmacol Ther* 1995;57:628–635.

96. Hard GC, Iatropoulos MJ, Jordan K, et al. Major difference in the hepatocarcinogenicity and DNA adduct forming ability between toremifene and tamoxifen in female Crl:CD(BR) rats. *Cancer Res* 1993;53:4534–4541.

97. Montandon F, Williams GM. Comparison of DNA reactivity of the polyphenylethylene hormonal agents diethylstilbestrol, tamoxifen and toremifene in rat and hamster liver. *Arch Toxicol* 1994;68:272–275.

98. Vogel VG, Costantino JP, Wickerham DL, et al. Update of the National Surgical Adjuvant Breast and Bowel Project Study of Tamoxifen and Raloxifene (STAR) P-2 Trial: Preventing Breast Cancer. *Cancer Prev Res (Phila)* 2010;3:696–706.

99. Delmas PD, Balena R, Confravreux E, et al. Bisphosphonate risedronate prevents bone loss in women with artificial menopause due to chemotherapy of breast cancer: a double-blind, placebo-controlled study. *J Clin Oncol* 1997;15:955–962.

100. Draper MW, Flowers DE, Huster WJ, et al. A controlled trial of raloxifene (LY139481) HCl: impact on bone turnover and serum lipid profile in healthy postmenopausal women. *J Bone Miner Res* 1996;11:835–842.

101. Anzano MA, Peer CW, Smith JM, et al. Chemoprevention of mammary carcinogenesis in the rat: combined use of raloxifene and 9-cis-retinoic acid. *J Natl Cancer Inst* 1996;88:123–125.

102. Gottardis MM, Jordan VC. Antitumor actions of keoxifene and tamoxifen in the N-nitrosomethylurea-induced rat mammary carcinoma model. *Cancer Res* 1987;47:4020–4024.

103. Black LJ, Jones CD, Falcone JF. Antagonism of estrogen action with a new benzothiophene derived antiestrogen. *Life Sci* 1983;32:1031–1036.

104. Allerheiligen S, Geiser J, Knadler M. Raloxifen (RAL) pharmacokinetics and the associated endocrine effects in premenopausal women treated during the follicular, ovulatory, and luteal phases of the menstrual cycle. *Pharmaceut Res* 1996;13:S430.

105. Forgue ST, Rudy AC, Knadler MP. Raloxifene pharmacokinetics in healthy postmenopausal women. *Pharmaceut Res* 1996;13:S430.

106. Ni L, Allerheiligen S, Basson R. Pharacokinetics of raloxifene in men and postmenopausal women volunteers. *Pharmaceut Res* 1996;13:S430.

107. Kemp DC, Fan PW, Stevens JC. Characterization of raloxifene glucuronidation in vitro: contribution of intestinal metabolism to presystemic clearance. *Drug Metab Dispos* 2002;30:694–700.

108. Coopman P, Garcia M, Brunner N, et al. Anti-proliferative and anti-estrogenic effects of ICI 164,384 and ICI 182,780 in 4-OH-tamoxifen-resistant human breast-cancer cells. *Int J Cancer* 1994;56:295–300.

109. Howell A, DeFriend DJ, Robertson JF, et al. Pharmacokinetics, pharmacological and anti-tumour effects of the specific anti-oestrogen ICI 182780 in women with advanced breast cancer. *Br J Cancer* 1996;74:300–308.

110. Howell A, Osborne CK, Morris C, et al. ICI 182,780 (Faslodex): development of a novel, "pure" antiestrogen. *Cancer* 2000;89:817–825.

111. Robertson JF, Odling-Smee W, Holcombe C, et al. Pharmacokinetics of a single dose of fulvestrant prolonged-release intramuscular injection in postmenopausal women awaiting surgery for primary breast cancer. *Clin Ther* 2003;25:1440–1452.

112. Piccart M, Parker LM, Pritchard KI. Oestrogen receptor downregulation: an opportunity for extending the window of endocrine therapy in advanced breast cancer. *Ann Oncol* 2003;14:1017–1025.

113. Wakeling AE, Bowler J. Steroidal pure antioestrogens. *J Endocrinol* 1987;112: R7–R10.

114. Wakeling AE, Dukes M, Bowler J. A potent specific pure antiestrogen with clinical potential. *Cancer Res* 1991;51:3867–3873.

115. Howell A, Robertson JF, Quaresma Albano J, et al. Fulvestrant, formerly ICI 182,780, is as effective as anastrozole in postmenopausal women with advanced breast cancer progressing after prior endocrine treatment. *J Clin Oncol* 2002;20:3396–3403.

116. Osborne CK, Pippen J, Jones SE, et al. Double-blind, randomized trial comparing the efficacy and tolerability of fulvestrant versus anastrozole in postmenopausal women with advanced breast cancer progressing on prior endocrine therapy: results of a North American trial. *J Clin Oncol* 2002;20:3386–3395.

117. Howell A, Robertson JF, Abram P, et al. Comparison of fulvestrant versus tamoxifen for the treatment of advanced breast cancer in postmenopausal women previously untreated with endocrine therapy: a multinational, double-blind, randomized trial. *J Clin Oncol* 2004;22:1605–1613.

118. Leo AD, Jerusalem G, Petruzelka L, et al. Final overall survival: fulvestrant 500 mg vs 250 mg in the randomized CONFIRM trial. *J Natl Cancer Inst* 2014;106:djt337.

119. McCormack P, Sapunar F. Pharmacokinetic profile of the fulvestrant loading dose regimen in postmenopausal women with hormone receptor-positive advanced breast cancer. *Clin Breast Cancer* 2008;8:347–351.

120. Schteingart DE, Cash R, Conn JW. Amino-glutethimide and metastatic adrenal cancer. Maintained reversal (six months) of Cushing's syndrome. *JAMA* 1996;198:1007–1010.

121. Ma CX, Adjei AA, Salavaggione OE, et al. Human aromatase: gene resequencing and functional genomics. *Cancer Res* 2005;65:11071–11082.

122. Colomer R, Monzo M, Tusquets I, et al. A single-nucleotide polymorphism in the aromatase gene is associated with the efficacy of the aromatase inhibitor letrozole in advanced breast carcinoma. *Clin Cancer Res* 2008;14:811–816.

123. Wang L, Ellsworth KA, Moon I, et al. Functional genetic polymorphisms in the aromatase gene CYP19 vary the response of breast cancer patients to neoadjuvant therapy with aromatase inhibitors. *Cancer Res* 2010;70:319–328.

124. Goss PE, Ingle JN, Martino S, et al. A randomized trial of letrozole in postmenopausal women after five years of tamoxifen therapy for early-stage breast cancer. *N Engl J Med* 2003;349:1793–1802.

125. Mouridsen H, Gershanovich M, Sun Y, et al. Phase III study of letrozole versus tamoxifen as first-line therapy of advanced breast cancer in postmenopausal women: analysis of survival and update of efficacy from the International Letrozole Breast Cancer Group. *J Clin Oncol* 2003;21:2101–2109.

126. Howell A, Cuzick J, Baum M, et al. Results of the ATAC (Arimidex, Tamoxifen, Alone or in Combination) trial after completion of 5 years' adjuvant treatment for breast cancer. *Lancet* 2005;365:60–62.

127. Thurlimann B, Keshaviah A, Coates AS, et al. A comparison of letrozole and tamoxifen in postmenopausal women with early breast cancer. *N Engl J Med* 2005;353:2747–2757.

128. Jakesz R, Jonat W, Gnant M, et al. Switching of postmenopausal women with endocrine-responsive early breast cancer to anastrozole after 2 years' adjuvant tamoxifen: combined results of ABCSG trial 8 and ARNO 95 trial. *Lancet* 2005;366:455–462.

129. Cuzick J, Sestak I, Forbes JF, et al. Anastrozole for prevention of breast cancer in high-risk postmenopausal women (IBIS-II): an international, double-blind, randomised placebo-controlled trial. *Lancet* 2014;383:1041–1048.

130. Baum M, Budzar AU, Cuzick J, et al. Anastrozole alone or in combination with tamoxifen versus tamoxifen alone for adjuvant treatment of postmenopausal women with early breast cancer: first results of the ATAC randomised trial. *Lancet* 2002;359:2131–2139.

131. Amir E, Seruga B, Nira S, et al. Toxicity of adjuvant endocrine therapy in postmenopausal breast cancer patients: a systematic review and meta-analysis. *J Natl Cancer Inst* 2011;103:1299–1309.

132. Plourde PV, Dyroff M, Dukes M. Arimidex: a potent and selective fourth-generation aromatase inhibitor. *Breast Cancer Res Treat* 1994;30:103–111.

133. Bisagni G, Cocconi G, Scaglione F, et al. Letrozole, a new oral non-steroidal aromatase inhibitor in treating postmenopausal patients with advanced breast cancer. A pilot study. *Ann Oncol* 1996;7:99–102.

134. Buzdar AU. Pharmacology and pharmacokinetics of the newer generation aromatase inhibitors. *Clin Cancer Res* 2003;9:468S–472S.

135. Dewar JA, Nabholtz JM, Bonneterre J, et al. The effect of anastrozole (Arimidex) on serum lipids: data from a randomized comparison of anastrozole (AN) versus tamoxifen (TAM) in postmenopausal (PM) women with advanced breast cancer (ABC). *Breast Cancer Res Treat* 2000;64:51.

136. Elisaf MS, Bairaktari ET, Nicolaides C, et al. Effect of letrozole on the lipid profile in postmenopausal women with breast cancer. *Eur J Cancer* 2001;37:1510–1513.

137. Bhatnagar AS, Hausler A, Schieweck K. Inhibition of aromatase in vitro and in vivo by aromatase inhibitors. *J Enzyme Inhib* 1990;4:179–186.

138. Bhatnagar AS, Hausler A, Schieweck K, et al. Highly selective inhibition of estrogen biosynthesis by CGS 20267, a new non-steroidal aromatase inhibitor. *J Steroid Biochem Mol Biol* 1990;37:1021–1027.

139. Demers LM. Effects of Fadrozole (CGS 16949A) and Letrozole (CGS 20267) on the inhibition of aromatase activity in breast cancer patients. *Breast Cancer Res Treat* 1994;30:95–102.

140. Lipton A, Demers LM, Harvey HA, et al. Letrozole (CGS 20267). A phase I study of a new potent oral aromatase inhibitor of breast cancer. *Cancer* 1995;75:2132–2138.

141. Iveson TJ, Smith IE, Ahern J, et al. Phase I study of the oral nonsteroidal aromatase inhibitor CGS 20267 in postmenopausal patients with advanced breast cancer. *Cancer Res* 1993;53:266–270.

142. Trunet PF, Muller PH, Bhatnagar A. Phase I study in healthy male volunteers with the non-steroidal aromatase inhibitor GCS 20267. *Eur J Cancer* 1990;26:173.

143. Dukes M, Edwards PN, Large M, et al. The preclinical pharmacology of "Arimidex" (anastrozole; ZD1033)—a potent, selective aromatase inhibitor. *J Steroid Biochem Mol Biol* 1996;58:439–445.

144. Yates RA, Dowsett M, Fisher GV, et al. Arimidex (ZD1033): a selective, potent inhibitor of aromatase in postmenopausal female volunteers. *Br J Cancer* 1996;73:543–548.

145. Lonning PE, Geisler J, Dowsett M. Pharmacological and clinical profile of anastrozole. *Breast Cancer Res Treat* 1998;49:S53–S57.

146. Geisler J, King N, Dowsett M, et al. Influence of anastrozole (Arimidex), a selective, non-steroidal aromatase inhibitor, on in vivo aromatisation and plasma oestrogen levels in postmenopausal women with breast cancer. *Br J Cancer* 1996;74:1286–1291.

147. Ingle JN, Buzdar AU, Schaid DJ, et al. Variation in anastrozole metabolism and pharmacodynamics in women with early breast cancer. *Cancer Res* 2010;70:3278–3286.

148. Kaufmann M, Bajetta E, Dirix LY, et al. Exemestane is superior to megestrol acetate after tamoxifen failure in postmenopausal women with advanced breast cancer: results of a phase III randomized double-blind trial. The Exemestane Study Group. *J Clin Oncol* 2000;18:1399–1411.

149. Goss PE, Ingle JN, Pritchard KI, et al. Exemestane versus anastrozole in postmenopausal women with early breast cancer: NCIC CTG MA.27—a randomized controlled phase III trial. *J Clin Oncol* 2013;31:1398–1404.

150. Goss PE, Ingle JN, Ales-Martinez JE, et al. Exemestane for breast-cancer prevention in postmenopausal women. *N Engl J Med* 2011;364:2381–2391.

151. Goss PE, Grynpas M, Qi S, et al. The effects of exemestane on bone and lipids in the ovariectomized rat. *Breast Cancer Res Treat* 2001;69:224.

152. Evans TR, Di Salle E, Ornati G, et al. Phase I and endocrine study of exemestane (FCE 24304), a new aromatase inhibitor, in postmenopausal women. *Cancer Res* 1992;52:5933–5939.

153. Bajetta E, Zilembo N, Noberasco C, et al. The minimal effective exemestane dose for endocrine activity in advanced breast cancer. *Eur J Cancer* 1997;33:587–591.

154. Michaud LB, Buzdar AU. Risks and benefits of aromatase inhibitors in postmenopausal breast cancer. *Drug Saf* 1999;21:297–309.

155. Coombes RC, Hall E, Gibson LJ, et al. A randomized trial of exemestane after two to three years of tamoxifen therapy in postmenopausal women with primary breast cancer. *N Engl J Med* 2004;350:1081–1092.

156. Demers LM, Lipton A, Harvey HA, et al. The efficacy of CGS 20267 in suppressing estrogen biosynthesis in patients with advanced stage breast cancer. *J Steroid Biochem Mol Biol* 1993;44:687–691.

157. Spinelli R, Jannuzzo MG, Poggesi I, et al. Pharmacokinetics (PK) of Aromasin (Exemestane, EXE) after single and repeated doses in healthy postmenopausal volunteers (HPV). *Eur J Cancer* 1999;35:S295.

158. Buzdar A, Howell A. Advances in aromatase inhibition: clinical efficacy and tolerability in the treatment of breast cancer. *Clin Cancer Res* 2001;7:2620–2635.

159. Johannessen DC, Engan T, Di Salle E, et al. Endocrine and clinical effects of exemestane (PNU 155971), a novel steroidal aromatase inhibitor, in postmenopausal breast cancer patients: a phase I study. *Clin Cancer Res* 1997;3:1101–1108.

160. Jones S, Vogel C, Arkhipov A, et al. Multicenter, phase II trial of exemestane as third-line hormonal therapy of postmenopausal women with metastatic breast cancer. Aromasin Study Group. *J Clin Oncol* 1999;17:3418–3425.

161. Ahmann FR, Citrin DL, deHaan HA, et al. Zoladex: a sustained-release, monthly luteinizing hormone-releasing hormone analogue for the treatment of advanced prostate cancer. *J Clin Oncol* 1987;5:912–917.

162. Corbin A. From contraception to cancer: a review of the therapeutic applications of LHRH analogues as antitumor agents. *Yale J Biol Med* 1982;55:27–47.

163. Kaufmann M, Jonat W, Blamey R, et al. Survival analyses from the ZEBRA study. Goserelin (Zoladex) versus CMF in premenopausal women with node-positive breast cancer. *Eur J Cancer* 2003;39:1711–1717.

164. Harvey HA, Lipton A, Max DT, et al. Medical castration produced by the GnRH analogue leuprolide to treat metastatic breast cancer. *J Clin Oncol* 1985;3:1068–1072.

165. Abrahamsson PA. Potential benefits of intermittent androgen suppression therapy in the treatment of prostate cancer: a systematic review of the literature. *Eur Urol* 2010;57:49–59.

166. Hussain M, Tangen CM, Berry DL, et al. Intermittent versus continuous androgen deprivation in prostate cancer. *N Engl J Med* 2013;368:1314–1325.

167. Brogden RN, Faulds D. Goserelin. A review of its pharmacodynamic and pharmacokinetic properties and therapeutic efficacy in prostate cancer. *Drugs Aging* 1995;6:324–343.

168. Vogelzang NJ, Chodak GW, Soloway MS, et al. Goserelin versus orchiectomy in the treatment of advanced prostate cancer: final results of a randomized trial. Zoladex Prostate Study Group. *Urology* 1995;46:220–226.

169. Plosker GL, Brogden RN. Leuprorelin. A review of its pharmacology and therapeutic use in prostatic cancer, endometriosis and other sex hormone-related disorders. *Drugs* 1994;48:930–967.

170. Nillius SJ. *The Therapeutic Uses of Gonadotropin-Releasing Hormone and Its Analogues.* London: Butterworth; 1981.

171. Klijn JG, DeJong FH, Blankenstein MA. Anti-tumor and endocrine effects of chronic LHRH agonist treatment (buserelin) with or without tamoxifen in premenopausal metastatic breast cancer. *Breast Cancer Res Treat* 1984;4:209.

172. Clayton RN, Bailey LC, Cottam J, et al. A radioimmunoassay for GnRH agonist analogue in serum of patients with prostate cancer treated with D-Ser (tBu)6 AZA Gly10 GnRH. *Clin Endocrinol (Oxf)* 1985;22:453–462.

173. Chrisp P, Goa KL. Goserelin. A review of its pharmacodynamic and pharmacokinetic properties, and clinical use in sex hormone-related conditions. *Drugs* 1991;41:254–288.

174. Samant MP, Hong DJ, Croston G, et al. Novel gonadotropin-releasing hormone antagonists with substitutions at position 5. *Biopolymers* 2005;80:386–391.

175. Van Poppel H, Tombal B, de la Rosette JJ, et al. Degarelix: a novel gonadotropin-releasing hormone (GnRH) receptor blocker—results from a 1-yr, multicentre, randomised, phase 2 dosage-finding study in the treatment of prostate cancer. *Eur Urol* 2008;54:805–813.

176. Klotz L, Boccon-Gibod L, Shore ND, et al. The efficacy and safety of degarelix: a 12-month, comparative, randomized, open-label, parallel-group phase III study in patients with prostate cancer. *BJU Int* 2008;102:1531–1538.

177. Steinberg M. Degarelix: a gonadotropin-releasing hormone antagonist for the management of prostate cancer. *Clin Ther* 2009;31:2312–2331.

178. Brogden RN, Clissold SP. Flutamide. A preliminary review of its pharmacodynamic and pharmacokinetic properties, and therapeutic efficacy in advanced prostatic cancer. *Drugs* 1989;38:185–203.

179. Wysowski DK, Freiman JP, Tourtelot JB, et al. Fatal and nonfatal hepatotoxicity associated with flutamide. *Ann Intern Med* 1993;118:860–864.

180. Brogden RN, Chrisp P. Flutamide. A review of its pharmacodynamic and pharmacokinetic properties, and therapeutic use in advanced prostatic cancer. *Drugs Aging* 1991;1:104–115.

181. Radwanski E, Perentesis G, Symchowicz S, et al. Single and multiple dose pharmacokinetic evaluation of flutamide in normal geriatric volunteers. *J Clin Pharmacol* 1989;29:554–558.

182. Schellhammer PF, Sharifi R, Block NL, et al. A controlled trial of bicalutamide versus flutamide, each in combination with luteinizing hormone-releasing hormone analogue therapy, in patients with advanced prostate carcinoma. Analysis of time to progression. CASODEX Combination Study Group. *Cancer* 1996;78:2164–2169.

183. Furr BJ. Casodex (ICI 176,334)—a new, pure, peripherally-selective anti-androgen: preclinical studies. *Horm Res* 1989;32:69.

184. Furr BJ. Casodex: preclinical studies. *Eur Urol* 1990;18:2.

185. Kennealey GT, Furr BJ. Use of the nonsteroidal anti-androgen Casodex in advanced prostatic carcinoma. *Urol Clin North Am* 1991;18:99–110.

186. Attard G, Reid AH, A'Hern R, et al. Selective inhibition of CYP17 with abiraterone acetate is highly active in the treatment of castration-resistant prostate cancer. *J Clin Oncol* 2009;27:3742–3748.

187. Tran C, Ouk S, Clegg NJ, et al. Development of a second-generation antiandrogen for treatment of advanced prostate cancer. *Science* 2009;324:787–790.

188. Scher HI, Fizazi K, Saad F, et al. Increased survival with enzalutamide in prostate cancer after chemotherapy. *N Engl J Med* 2012;367:1187–1197.

189. Zhu H, Garcia JA. Targeting the adrenal gland in castration-resistant prostate cancer: a case for orteronel, a selective CYP-17 17,20-lyase inhibitor. *Curr Oncol Rep* 2013;15:105–112.

190. Kennedy BJ. Hormonal therapies in breast cancer. *Semin Oncol* 1974;1:119–130.

191. Colburn WA. Radioimmunoassay for fluoxymesterone (Halotestin). *Steroids* 1975;25:43–52.

192. Kammerer RC, Merdink JL, Jagels M, et al. Testing for fluoxymesterone (Halotestin) administration to man: identification of urinary metabolites by gas chromatography-mass spectrometry. *J Steroid Biochem* 1990;36:659–666.

193. Ingle JN, Ahmann DL, Green SJ, et al. Randomized clinical trial of diethylstilbestrol versus tamoxifen in postmenopausal women with advanced breast cancer. *N Engl J Med* 1981;304:16–21.

194. Stewart HJ, Forrest AP, Gunn JM, et al. The tamoxifen trial - a double-blind comparison with stilboestrol in postmenopausal women with advanced breast cancer. *Eur J Cancer* 1980;Suppl 1:83–88.

195. Byar DP. Proceedings: The Veterans Administration Cooperative Urological Research Group's studies of cancer of the prostate. *Cancer* 1973;32:1126–1130.

196. Loose-Mitchell DS, Stancel GM. *Estrogens and Progestins.* 10 ed. New York: McGraw-Hill; 2001.

197. Bonomi P, Pessis D, Bunting N, et al. Megestrol acetate used as primary hormonal therapy in stage D prostatic cancer. *Semin Oncol* 1985;12:36–39.

198. Bruera E, Macmillan K, Kuehn N, et al. A controlled trial of megestrol acetate on appetite, caloric intake, nutritional status, and other symptoms in patients with advanced cancer. *Cancer* 1990;66:1279–1282.

199. Feliu J, Gonzalez-Baron M, Berrocal A, et al. Usefulness of megestrol acetate in cancer cachexia and anorexia. A placebo-controlled study. *Am J Clin Oncol* 1992;15:436–440.

200. Loprinzi CL, Ellison NM, Schaid DJ, et al. Controlled trial of megestrol acetate for the treatment of cancer anorexia and cachexia. *J Natl Cancer Inst* 1990;82:1127–1132.

201. Tchekmedyian NS, Hickman M, Siau J, et al. Megestrol acetate in cancer anorexia and weight loss. *Cancer* 1992;69:1268–1274.

202. Loprinzi CL, Michalak JC, Schaid DJ, et al. Phase III evaluation of four doses of megestrol acetate as therapy for patients with cancer anorexia and/or cachexia. *J Clin Oncol* 1993;11:762–767.

203. Loprinzi CL, Jensen MD, Jiang NS, et al. Effect of megestrol acetate on the human pituitary-adrenal axis. *Mayo Clin Proc* 1992;67:1160–1162.

204. Leinung MC, Liporace R, Miller CH. Induction of adrenal suppression by megestrol acetate in patients with AIDS. *Ann Intern Med* 1995;122:843–845.

205. Rowland KM Jr., Loprinzi CL, Shaw EG, et al. Randomized double-blind placebo-controlled trial of cisplatin and etoposide plus megestrol acetate/placebo in extensive-stage small-cell lung cancer: a North Central Cancer Treatment Group study. *J Clin Oncol* 1996;14:135–141.

206. Loprinzi CL, Johnson PA, Jensen M. Megestrol acetate for anorexia and cachexia. *Oncology* 1992;49:46–49.

207. Von Roenn JH, Armstrong D, Kotler DP, et al. Megestrol acetate in patients with AIDS-related cachexia. *Ann Intern Med* 1994;121:393–399.

208. Alexieva-Figusch J, Blankenstein MA, Hop WC, et al. Treatment of metastatic breast cancer patients with different dosages of megestrol acetate; dose relations, metabolic and endocrine effects. *Eur J Cancer Clin Oncol* 1984;20:33–40.

209. Tseng L, Gurpide E. Effects of progestins on estradiol receptor levels in human endometrium. *J Clin Endocrinol Metab* 1975;41:402–404.

210. Gurpide E, Tseng L, Gusberg SB. Estrogen metabolism in normal and neoplastic endometrium. *Am J Obstet Gynecol* 1977;129:809–816.

211. Gordon GG, Altman K, Southren AL, et al. Human hepatic testosterone A-ring reductase activity: effect of medroxyprogesterone acetate. *J Clin Endocrinol Metab* 1971;32:457–461.

212. Allegra JC, Kiefer SM. Mechanisms of action of progestational agents. *Semin Oncol* 1985;12:3–5.

213. Ewing TM, Murphy LJ, Ng ML, et al. Regulation of epidermal growth factor receptor by progestins and glucocorticoids in human breast cancer cell lines. *Int J Cancer* 1989;44:744–752.

214. Adlercreutz H, Eriksen PB, Christensen MS. Plasma concentration of megestrol acetate and medroxyprogesterone acetate after single oral administration to healthy subjects. *J Pharm Biomed Anal* 1983;1:153.

215. Martin F, Adlercreutz H, eds. *Aspects of Megestrol Acetate and Medroxyprogesterone Acetate Metabolism.* New York: Raven Press; 1977.

216. Gaver RC, Pittman KA, Reilly CM, et al. Bioequivalence evaluation of new megestrol acetate formulations in humans. *Semin Oncol* 1985;12:17–19.

217. Fotherby K, Kamyab S, Littleton P. Metabolism of synthetic progestational compounds in humans. *J Reprod Fertil* 1968;5:51–61.

218. Fukushima DK, Ievin J, Liang JS, et al. Isolation and partial synthesis of a new metabolite of medroxyrogesterone acetate. *Steroids* 1979;34:57–72.

219. Utaaker E, Lundgren S, Kvinnsland S, et al. Pharmacokinetics and metabolism of medroxyprogesterone acetate in patients with advanced breast cancer. *J Steroid Biochem* 1988;31:437–441.

220. Sturm G, Haberlein H, Bauer T, et al. Mass spectrometric and high-performance liquid chromatographic studies of medroxyprogesterone acetate metabolites in human plasma. *J Chromatogr* 1991;562:351–362.

221. Pannuti F, Camaggi CM, Strocchi E, eds. *Medroxyprogesterone Acetate Pharmacokinetics*. New York: Raven Press; 1984.

222. Lundgren S, Lonning PE, Aakvaag A, et al. Influence of aminoglutethimide on the metabolism of medroxyprogesterone acetate and megestrol acetate in postmenopausal patients with advanced breast cancer. *Cancer Chemother Pharmacol* 1990;27:101–105.

223. Lundgren S, Kvinnsland S, Utaaker E, et al. Effect of oral high-dose progestins on the disposition of antipyrine, digitoxin, and warfarin in patients with advanced breast cancer. *Cancer Chemother Pharmacol* 1986;18:270–275.

224. Cascinu S, Fedeli A, Fedeli SL, et al. Control of chemotherapy-induced diarrhoea with octreotide in patients receiving 5-fluorouracil. *Eur J Cancer* 1992;28:482–483.

225. Cascinu S, Fedeli A, Fedeli SL, et al. Octreotide versus loperamide in the treatment of fluorouracil-induced diarrhea: a randomized trial. *J Clin Oncol* 1993;11:148–151.

226. Gebbia V, Carreca I, Testa A, et al. Subcutaneous octreotide versus oral loperamide in the treatment of diarrhea following chemotherapy. *Anticancer Drugs* 1993;4:443–445.

227. Harris AG. Somatostatin and somatostatin analogues: pharmacokinetics and pharmacodynamic effects. *Gut* 1994;35:S1–S4.

228. Chanson P, Timsit J, Harris AG. Clinical pharmacokinetics of octreotide. Therapeutic applications in patients with pituitary tumours. *Clin Pharmacokinet* 1993;25:375–391.

229. Marbach P, Briner U, Lemaire M. From somatostatin to Sandostatin: pharmacodynamics and pharmacokinetics. *Digestion* 1993;54:9–13.

230. Rubin J, Ajani J, Schirmer W, et al. Octreotide acetate long-acting formulation versus open-label subcutaneous octreotide acetate in malignant carcinoid syndrome. *J Clin Oncol* 1999;17:600–606.

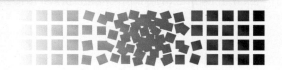

28 Antiangiogenesis Agents

Cindy H. Chau and William Douglas Figg, Sr.

INTRODUCTION

Blood vessels are indispensable for tumor growth and metastasis, and the formation of a new network of blood vessels from the existing vasculature, termed *angiogenesis*, is one of the essential hallmarks of cancer development.[1] Indeed, it was over 70 years ago that the existence of tumor-derived factors responsible for promoting new vessel growth was postulated,[2] and that tumor growth is essentially dependent on vascular induction and the development of a neovascular supply.[3] By the late 1960s, Dr. Judah Folkman and colleagues[4] had begun the search for a tumor angiogenesis factor. In the 1971 landmark report, Folkman[5] proposed that inhibition of angiogenesis by means of holding tumors in a nonvascularized dormant state would be an effective strategy to treat human cancer, and hence laid the groundwork for the concept behind the development of *antiangiogenesis* agents. This fostered the search for angiogenic factors, regulators of angiogenesis, and antiangiogenic molecules over the next few decades and shed light on angiogenesis as an important therapeutic target for the treatment of cancer and other diseases.

A decade has passed since the regulatory approval of the first antiangiogenic drug bevacizumab, and while initial results were regarded as highly promising, clinical evidence indicated that antiangiogenic therapy also had limitations. Successful development and clinical translation of this novel class of agents depends on the complete understanding of the biology of angiogenesis and the regulatory proteins that govern this angiogenic process, topics that have been covered in greater detail in another section of this textbook. This chapter will briefly review the mechanisms underlying tumor angiogenesis followed by an in-depth discussion of antiangiogenic therapy, the modes of action of angiogenesis inhibitors, and the successes and challenges of this treatment modality.

UNDERSTANDING THE ANGIOGENIC PROCESS

Angiogenic Switch and Regulatory Proteins

Tumor development and progression depend on angiogenesis. Recruitment of new blood vessels to the tumor site is required for the delivery of nutrients and oxygen to the cancerous growths and for the removal of waste products.[6] Cancer cells promote angiogenesis at an early stage of tumorigenesis, beginning with the release of molecules that send signals to the surrounding normal host tissue and stimulate the migration of microvascular endothelial cells (EC) in the direction of the angiogenic stimulus. These angiogenic factors not only mediate EC migration, but also EC proliferation and microvessel formation in tumors undergoing the switch to the angiogenic phenotype.[7] Experimental evidence for this *angiogenic switch* was observed when hyperplastic islets in transgenic mice (RIP-Tag model) switch from small (<1 mm), white microscopic dormant tumors to red, rapidly growing tumors.[7] Dormant tumors have been discovered during autopsies of individuals who died of causes other than cancer.[8] These autopsy studies suggest that the vast majority of microscopic in situ cancers never switch to the angiogenic phenotype during a normal lifetime. Such incipient tumors are usually not neovascularized and can remain harmless to the host for long periods of time as microscopic lesions that are in a state of dormancy.[9,10] These nonangiogenic tumors cannot expand beyond the initial microscopic size and cannot become clinically detectable, lethal tumors until they have switched to the angiogenic phenotype[11–13] through neovascularization and/or blood vessel cooption.[14] Depending on the tumor type and the environment, this switch can occur at different stages of the tumor progression pathway and ultimately depends on a net balance of positive and negative regulators. Thus, the angiogenic phenotype may result from the production of growth factors by tumor cells and/or the downregulation of negative modulators.

Changes in this angiogenic balance affecting the levels of activator and inhibitor molecules dictate whether an EC will be in a quiescent or an angiogenic state. Normally, the inhibitors predominate, thereby blocking growth. Once the balance shifts in favor of the angiogenic state, proangiogenic factors prompts the activation, growth, and division of vascular ECs, resulting in the formation of new blood vessels. Activated ECs produce and release matrix metalloproteinases (MMP) into the surrounding tissue to break down the extracellular matrix to allow the ECs to migrate and organize themselves into hollow tubes that eventually evolve into a mature network of blood vessels. Proangiogenic factors or positive regulators of angiogenesis include vascular endothelial growth factor (VEGF), basic fibroblast growth factor (PlGF), platelet-derived growth factor (PDGF), placental growth factor, transforming growth factor-β, pleiotrophins, and others.[15] Activation of the hypoxia-inducible factor 1 (HIF-1) via tumor-associated hypoxic conditions is also involved in the upregulation of several angiogenic factors.[16] The angiogenic switch also involves the downregulation of angiogenesis suppressor proteins, which include endostatin, angiostatin, thrombospondin, and others.[17,18] Most notably, however, is the link between many oncogenes and angiogenesis and the significant role oncogenes play in driving the angiogenic switch.[19,20] These proangiogenic oncogenes not only induce the expression of stimulators, but may also downregulate inhibitors of angiogenesis.[21]

Endogenous Inhibitors of Angiogenesis

The infrequency of microscopic in situ tumors that actually undergo the angiogenic switch (<1%) suggests that naturally occurring endogenous inhibitors exist in the body to defend against the angiogenic switch in pathologic conditions and to limit physiologic angiogenesis.[9] These circulating endogenous inhibitors could also prevent microscopic metastases from growing into visible tumors. Early studies by Langer et al.[22,23] demonstrated the possible existence of such inhibitors through the extraction of a functional inhibitor from cartilage, a tissue that is poorly vascularized. Since then, dozens of endogenous angiogenesis inhibitors have been identified, some of which are listed in Table 28.1.[17,18,24] Many of the endogenous inhibitors of angiogenesis that have been discovered to date are proteolytically cleaved fragments of larger proteins that are members of either the clotting/coagulation system

TABLE 28.1

Examples of Endogenous Inhibitors of Angiogenesis

Alphastatin

Angiostatin

Antithrombin III (cleaved)

Arrestin

Canstatin

Endostatin

Interferon alpha/beta (IFN-α/β)

2-Methoxyestradiol (2-ME)

Pigment epithelial-derived factor (PEDF)

Platelet factor 4 (PF-4)

Tetrahydrocortisol-S

Thrombospondin 1

Tissue inhibitor of metalloproteinase 2 (TIMP-2)

Tumstatin

Vasohibin

or members of the extracellular matrix family of glycoproteins. Endostatin is the most well-studied endogenous angiogenesis inhibitor.[25,26] Other potent endogenous angiogenesis inhibitors include thrombospondin-1[27] and tumstatin.[28] The discovery of vasohibin, an endogenous inhibitor that is selectively induced in ECs by proangiogenic stimulatory growth factors such as VEGF, demonstrated the existence of an intrinsic and EC-specific feedback inhibitor control mechanism,[29,30] whereas most endogenous inhibitors of angiogenesis are extrinsic to ECs. More recently, a second endothelium-produced negative regulator of angiogenesis has been discovered, the Dll4-Notch signaling system.[31,32] Both intrinsic factors have since been shown to control tumor angiogenesis by an autoregulatory or negative-feedback mechanism. The Dll4-Notch axis has emerged as a critical regulator of tumor angiogenesis, and inhibitors of this pathway (e.g., demcizumab, the anti-Dll4 monoclonal antibody) are currently being investigated in early phase trials of solid tumors.[33]

Perhaps the most compelling genetic evidence that endogenous inhibitors suppress pathologic angiogenesis was observed in studies using mice deficient in tumstatin, endostatin, or thrombospondin 1 (TSP-1).[34] These experiments demonstrate that normal physiologic levels of the inhibitors can retard the tumor growth and that their absence leads to enhanced angiogenesis and increased tumor growth by two- to threefold, strongly suggesting that endogenous inhibitors of angiogenesis can act as endothelium-specific tumor suppressors. The connection between a tumor suppressor protein and angiogenesis is best illustrated by the classic tumor suppressor p53. p53 inhibits angiogenesis by increasing the expression of TSP-1[35] by repressing VEGF[36] and basic fibroblast growth factor–binding protein,[37] and by degrading HIF-1,[38] which blocks the downstream induction of VEGF expression. New evidence suggests that p53 also indirectly downregulates VEGF expression via the retinoblastoma pathway in a p21-dependent manner during sustained hypoxia.[39] Furthermore, p53-mediated inhibition of angiogenesis may also occur in part via the antiangiogenic activity of endostatin and tumstatin.[40] This landmark finding clearly demonstrates that p53 not only controls cell proliferation, but can also repress tumor angiogenesis through enzymatic mobilization of these endogenous angiogenesis inhibitor proteins to prevent ECs from being recruited into the dormant, microscopic tumors, thereby preventing the switch to the angiogenic phenotype.[41] The discovery that these endogenous angiogenesis inhibitors can suppress the growth of primary tumors

raises the possibility that such inhibitors might also be able to slow tumor metastasis. Indeed, the inhibition of angiogenesis by angiostatin significantly reduced the rate of metastatic spread.

DRUG DEVELOPMENT OF ANGIOGENESIS INHIBITORS

The first angiogenesis inhibitor was reported in 1980 and involved the low-dose administration of interferon α (IFN-α).[42–44] Over the next decade, several compounds were discovered to have potent antiangiogenic activity, including protamine and platelet factor 4,[45] trahydrocortisol,[46] and the fumagillin analog TNP-470.[47] The proof of concept that targeting angiogenesis is an effective strategy for treating cancer came with the approval of the first angiogenesis inhibitor, bevacizumab, by the U.S. Food and Drug Administration (FDA). Since then, several antiangiogenic agents have received FDA approval for cancer treatment (Table 28.2), and three additional agents (pegaptanib, ranibizumab, and aflibercept) are approved for the treatment of wet age-related macular degeneration.

Rationale for Antiangiogenic Therapy

Antiangiogenic therapy stems from the fundamental concept that tumor growth, invasion, and metastasis are angiogenesis dependent; thus, blocking blood vessel recruitment to starve primary and metastatic tumors is a rational approach. The microvascular EC recruited by a tumor has become an important second target in cancer therapy. Unlike the cancer cell (the primary target of cytotoxic chemotherapy), which is genetically unstable with unpredictable mutations, the genetic stability of ECs may make them less susceptible to acquired drug resistance.[48] Moreover, ECs in the microvascular bed of a tumor may support 50 to 100 tumor cells. Coupling this amplification potential together with the lower toxicity of most angiogenesis inhibitors results in the use of antiangiogenic therapy, which should be significantly less toxic than conventional chemotherapy. However, the variable responses of antiangiogenic therapy observed in different tumor types and the fact that angiogenesis inhibitors have not delivered the benefits initially envisaged suggest that the precise mechanism of action of angiogenesis inhibitors is complex and remains incompletely understood.

Modes of Action of Antiangiogenic Agents

Various strategies for the development of antiangiogenic drugs have been investigated over the years, with these agents being classified into several different categories depending on their modes of action. Some inhibit ECs directly, whereas others inhibit the angiogenesis signaling cascade or block the ability of ECs to break down the extracellular matrix. Inhibitors may block one main angiogenic protein, two or three angiogenic proteins, or have a broad-spectrum effect by blocking a range of angiogenic regulators that can be located in both the tumor and ECs.[49] In some cases, the antiangiogenic activity is discovered as a secondary function after the drug has received regulatory approval for a different primary function. For example, bortezomib is a proteasome inhibitor that is approved for multiple myeloma and was later found to possess antiangiogenic activity via inhibiting VEGF. Some smallmolecule drugs may display their antiangiogenic activity through inducing the expression of endogenous angiogenesis inhibitors such as celecoxib, a cyclooxygenase-2 (COX-2) inhibitor, which inhibits angiogenesis by increasing levels of endostatin.[25]

Some drugs possess antiangiogenic properties but with mechanisms that are not completely understood, such as thalidomide and its analogs, lenalidomide and pomalidomide, referred to as immunomodulatory drugs. Thalidomide was originally shown to inhibit angiogenesis by D'Amato et al.[50] in 1994 and this was subsequently confirmed in several different in vitro and ex vivo

TABLE 28.2

Antiangiogenic Agents that Have Received U.S. Food and Drug Administration Approval for Cancer Treatment

Drug	Class	Mechanism (Cellular Targets)	Year of Approval	Indications	Dosages
Bevacizumab (Avastin)	Anti-VEGF mAB	VEGF	2004	First- and second-line metastatic CRC	5 mg/kg IV q2wk + bolus IFL; 10 mg/kg IV q2wk + FOLFOX4
			2006	First-line NSCLC	15 mg/kg IV q3wk + carboplatin/paclitaxel
			2009	Second-line GBM	10 mg/kg IV q2wk
			2009	Metastatic RCC	10 mg/kg IV q2wk + IFN
			2013	Second-line metastatic CRC (after prior bevacizumab-containing regimen)	5 mg/kg IV q2wk or 7.5 mg/kg IV q3wk + fluoropyrimidine–irinotecan or fluoropyrimidine-oxaliplatin–based regimen
Ziv-aflibercept (Zaltrap, VEGF Trap)	Anti-VEGF mAB	VEGFA, VEGFB, PIGF1, PIGF2	2012	Metastatic CRC (after prior oxaliplatin-containing regimen)	4 mg/kg IV q2wk (1-hr infusion)
Sorafenib (Nexavar, BAY439006)	Small-molecule TKI	VEGFR2, VEGFR3, PDGFR, FLT3, c-Kit	2005	Advanced RCC	400 mg PO bid (w/o food)
			2007	Unresectable HCC	400 mg PO bid (w/o food)
			2013	RAI-refractory DTC	400 mg PO bid (w/o food)
Sunitinib (Sutent, SU11248)	Small-molecule TKI	VEGFR1, VEGFR2, VEGFR3, PDGFR, FLT3, c-Kit, RET	2006	Imatinib-resistant or -intolerant GIST	50 mg PO qd, 4 wk on/2 wk off
			2006	Advanced RCC	50 mg PO qd, 4 wk on/2 wk off
			2011	Advanced pNET	37.5 mg PO qd
Pazopanib (Votrient)	Small-molecule TKI	VEGFR1, VEGFR2, VEGFR3, PDGFR, Itk, Lck, c-Fms	2009	Advanced RCC	800 mg PO qd (w/o food)
			2012	Advanced soft tissue sarcoma	800 mg PO qd (w/o food)
Vandetanib (Caprelsa)	Small molecule TKI	RET, VEGFR, EGFR, BRK, TIE2	2011	Advanced MTC	300 mg PO qd
Axitinib (Inlyta)	Small molecule TKI	VEGFR1, VEGFR2, VEGFR3	2012	Advanced RCC (after failure of prior therapy)	5 mg PO bid
Cabozantinib (XL184, Cometriq)	Small molecule TKI	MET, VEGFR2, RET, KIT, AXL, FLT3	2012	Progressive, metastatic MTC	140 mg PO qd (w/o food)
Regorafenib (Stivarga)	Small molecule TKI	RET, VEGFR1, VEGFR2, VEGFR3, TIE2, KIT, PDGFR	2012	Previously treated metastatic CRC	160 mg PO qd × 21days (q28-day cycle)
			2013	GIST	160 mg PO qd × days 1–21 (q28-day cycle)
Temsirolimus (Torisel)	mTOR inhibitor	mTOR	2007	Advanced RCC	25 mg IV qwk (infused over 30–60 min)
Everolimus (Afinitor, RAD-001)[a]	mTOR inhibitor	mTOR	2009	Second-line advanced RCC (after VEGFR TKI failure)	10 mg PO qd
			2010	SEGA associated w/TSC	4.5 mg/m^2 PO qd
			2011	pNET	10 mg PO qd
			2012	Advanced HR+, HER2- breast cancer	10 mg PO qd
			2012	AML associated w/TSC	10 mg PO qd

[a] Afinitor Disperz (everolimus tablets for oral suspension) was approved in 2012 for children aged 1 and older who have SEGA + TSC.
mAB, monoclonal antibody; CRC, colorectal cancer; IV, intravenous; IFL, irinotecan, 5-fluorouracil, and leucovorin; FOLFOX4, 5-flourouracil, leucovorin, and oxaliplatin; NSCLC, non–small-cell lung cancer; GBM, glioblastoma multiforme; RCC, renal cell carcinoma; VEGFA, vascular endothelial growth factor A; PIGF, placental growth factor; TKI, tyrosine–kinase inhibitor; VEGFR, VEGF receptor; PDGFR, platelet-derived growth factor receptor; FLT, Fms-like tyrosine kinase; c-Kit, stem cell factor receptor; HCC, hepatocellular carcinoma; RAI, radioactive iodine; DTC, differentiated thyroid carcinoma; PO, orally; RET, glial cell line-derived neurotrophic factor receptor; pNET, pancreatic neuroendocrine tumor; GIST, gastrointestinal stromal tumor; qd, every day; Itk, interleukin-2 receptor inducible T-cell kinase; Lck, leukocyte-specific protein tyrosine kinase; c-Fms, transmembrane glycoprotein receptor tyrosine kinase; bid, twice daily; EGFR, epidermal growth factor receptor; BRK, protein tyrosine kinase 6; MTC, medullary thyroid cancer; mTOR, mammalian target of rapamycin; SEGA, subependymal giant cell astrocytoma; TSC, tuberous sclerosis complex; HR, hormone receptor; HER2, human epidermal growth factor receptor 2; AML, angiomyolipoma.

assays.[51–54] Interestingly, unlike other mechanisms of action, the antiangiogenic activity of thalidomide is believed to require enzymatic activation. The extent to which the antiangiogenic properties of thalidomide and its analogs play a role in its antimyeloma activity is not clearly understood. Several mechanisms have been proposed that involve the downregulation of cytokines in EC, the inhibition of EC proliferation, the decrease in the level of circulating ECs, or the modulation of adhesion molecules between the multiple myeloma cells and the endogenous bone marrow stromal cells, thereby decreasing the production of VEGF and interleukin 6 (IL-6).[55–59] The immunomodulatory agents are discussed in greater detail in another section of this textbook. Examples of the various types of angiogenesis inhibitors are highlighted in Table 28.3.

Drugs with antiangiogenic activity may be classified as either direct or indirect angiogenesis inhibitors. A direct angiogenesis inhibitor blocks vascular ECs from proliferating, migrating, or increasing their survival in response to proangiogenic proteins. They target the activated endothelium directly and inhibit multiple angiogenic proteins. Examples of direct angiogenesis inhibitors include many of the endogenous inhibitors of angiogenesis, such as endostatin, angiostatin, and TSP-1. Indirect angiogenesis inhibitors decrease or block expression of a tumor cell product, neutralize the tumor product itself, or block its receptor on ECs. The limitation to indirect inhibitors is that, over time, tumor cells may acquire mutations that lead to increased expression of other proangiogenic proteins that are not blocked by the indirect inhibitor. This may give the appearance of drug resistance and warrants the addition of a second antiangiogenic agent, one that would target the expression of these upregulated proangiogenic proteins. Examples of drugs that interfere with the angiogenesis-signaling pathway include the anti-VEGF monoclonal antibodies and small-molecule tyrosine–kinase inhibitors. These drugs target the major signaling pathways in tumor angiogenesis: VEGF, PDGF, and their respective receptors, as well as other growth factors and/or signaling pathways.

VEGF (also known as vascular permeability factor) is a potent proangiogenic growth factor and its expression is upregulated by most cancer cell types. It stimulates EC proliferation, migration, and survival as well as induces increased vascular permeability. The different forms of VEGF bind to transmembrane receptor tyrosine kinases (RTK) on ECs: VEGFR1 (Flt-1), VEGFR2 (KDR/Flk-1 or kinase insert domain receptor/fetal liver kinase 1), or VEGFR3 (Flt-4).[60] This results in receptor dimerization, activation, and autophosphorylation of the tyrosine–kinase domain, thereby triggering downstream signaling pathways. Other signaling molecules that may represent attractive therapeutic targets include PDGF and the angiopoietins (Ang1, Ang2). PDGF-B/PDGF receptor (R)-β plays an important role in the recruitment of pericytes and maturation of the microvasculature.[61] Ang2, which binds the Tie-2 receptor, is mostly expressed in tumor-induced neovasculature, whereby its selective inhibition results in reduced EC proliferation.[62] The angiopoietins are also involved in lymphangiogenesis, the formation of new lymphatic vessels, which plays a key role in tumor metastasis. An increased Ang2/Ang1 ratio correlates with tumor angiogenesis and poor prognosis in many cancers, thus making the angiopoietins an attractive therapeutic target. Angiopoietin inhibitors are currently under investigation in the preclinical and clinical setting.

Other strategies for targeting angiogenesis involve the tumor microenvironment. Breakdown of the extracellular matrix is required to allow ECs to migrate into surrounding tissues and proliferate into new blood vessels; thus, drugs that target MMPs, enzymes that catalyze the breakdown of the matrix, can also inhibit angiogenesis. However, clinical development of MMP inhibitors (MMPI) has yielded disappointing results.[63–66]

Integrins are cell surface adhesion molecules that play an essential role in cell–cell and cell–matrix adhesion as well as in transmitting signals important for cell migration, invasion, proliferation, and survival. The involvement of integrin in tumor angiogenesis was demonstrated in studies that show the β-4 subunit of integrin promoting endothelial migration and invasion.[67] Agents that target integrins (inhibitors of $\alpha_v\beta_3$ and $\alpha_v\beta_5$) have been evaluated as potential therapeutic options and include etaracizumab, cilengitide, and intetumumab. However, all three integrin inhibitors have proven to be largely ineffective in various early and late stage cancer trials.[68–73] In summary, the downstream effects of antiangiogenic agents, in addition to blocking angiogenesis, may involve inducing vessel regression, promoting sensitization to radiotherapy and chemotherapy by depriving ECs of VEGF's prosurvival signals, and inhibiting the recruitment of proangiogenic bone marrow–derived cells as well as reducing the self-renewal capability of cancer stem cells.[74]

CLINICAL UTILITY OF APPROVED ANTIANGIOGENIC AGENTS IN CANCER THERAPY

The following section reviews the current FDA-approved angiogenesis inhibitors (Table 28.2). These agents include: (1) the monoclonal anti-VEGF antibodies (bevacizumab and ziv-aflibercept); (2) small-molecule tyrosine–kinase inhibitors (TKI) (sorafenib, sunitinib, pazopanib, vandetanib, axitinib, cabozantinib, and regorafenib); and (3) the mammalian target of rapamycin (mTOR) inhibitors (temsirolimus and everolimus), as examples of drugs that possess antiangiogenic activity. Other approved drugs that also inhibit angiogenesis as a secondary function, such as thalidomide, are discussed in greater detail in another section of this textbook and are presented in Table 28.3.

Anti-VEGF Therapy

Bevacizumab

Bevacizumab is a recombinant humanized anti–VEGF-A monoclonal antibody that received FDA approval in February 2004 for use in combination therapy with fluorouracil-based regimens for

---

TABLE 28.3

Examples of Drugs that Possess Antiangiogenic Activity or Inhibit Angiogenesis as a Secondary Function

Drug	Class
Cetuximab Panitumumab Trastuzumab	EGFR/HER monoclonal antibodies
Gefitinib Erlotinib	EGFR small-molecule tyrosine–kinase receptor inhibitors
Everolimus Temsirolimus	mTOR inhibitors
Thalidomide Lenalidomide Pomalidomide	Immunomodulatory agents
Belinostat (PXD101) LBH589 Vorinostat (SAHA)	HDAC inhibitors
Celecoxib	COX-2 inhibitors
Bortezomib	Proteasome inhibitors
Zoledronic acid	Bisphosphonates
Rosiglitazone	PPAR-γ agonists
Doxycycline	Antibiotic

EGFR, epidermal growth factor receptor; mTOR, mammalian target of rapamycin HDAC, histone deacetylase; COX-2, cyclooxygenase-2; PPAR, peroxisome proliferator–activated receptor.

metastatic colorectal cancer. Bevacizumab binds VEGF and prevents the interaction of VEGF to its receptors (Flt-1 and KDR) on the surface of ECs. It is the first antiangiogenic agent clinically proven to extend survival following a large, randomized, double-blind, phase III study in which bevacizumab was administered in combination with bolus irinotecan, 5-fluorouracil, and leucovorin (IFL) as first-line therapy for metastatic colorectal cancer (CRC).[75] In 2006, its approval extended to first- or second-line treatment of patients with metastatic carcinoma of the colon or rectum. This recommendation is based on the demonstration of a statistically significant improvement in overall survival (OS) in patients receiving bevacizumab plus FOLFOX4 (5-flourouracil, leucovorin, and oxaliplatin) when compared to those receiving FOLFOX4 alone. In January 2013, it was further approved to treat mCRC for second-line treatment when used with fluoropyrimidine-based (combined with irinotecan or oxaliplatin) chemotherapy after disease progression following a first-line treatment with a bevacizumab-containing regimen based on clinical benefits observed in the randomized phase III study (ML18147).[76] Despite the benefit in the metastatic setting, the addition of bevacizumab did not improve clinical outcomes in the adjuvant setting in CRC.[77,78] In 2006, bevacizumab received an additional approval for use in combination with carboplatin and paclitaxel, and is indicated for first-line treatment of patients with unresectable, locally advanced, recurrent, or metastatic nonsquamous, non–small-cell lung cancer (NSCLC) based on the demonstration of a statistically significant improvement in OS in patients in the bevacizumab arm compared to those receiving chemotherapy alone.[79] In February 2008, the FDA granted a conditional, accelerated approval for bevacizumab to be used in combination with paclitaxel for the treatment of patients who have not received chemotherapy for metastatic human epidermal growth factor receptor 2 (*HER2*)-negative breast cancer. However, additional clinical trials were conducted and the new data showed only a small effect on progression free survival (PFS) without evidence of an improvement in OS or a clinical benefit to patients sufficient to outweigh the risks; thus, the FDA rescinded its approval and removed the breast cancer indication from the drug's label in November 2011.[80–82] This controversial decision continues to be debated with ongoing subgroup analyses to identify patients who would likely benefit from bevacizumab.

Bevacizumab received another accelerated approval as a single agent for patients with glioblastoma multiforme (GBM) with progressive disease following therapy in May 2009. The approval was based on the demonstration of durable objective response rates observed in two single-arm trials, AVF3708g and NCI 06-C-0064E.[83] Currently, no data have shown whether bevacizumab improves disease-related symptoms or survival in people previously treated for GBM. Moreover, phase III trials of bevacizumab in newly diagnosed GBM (RTOG 8025 and AVAglio) have shown a 3- to 4-month improvement of PFS, but no OS advantage over the standard of care.[84] The AVAglio trial improved patients' quality of life, whereas the RTOG 0825 did not and instead increased the burden of symptoms with a negative impact on cognition. Although these two studies showed that bevacizumab had a modest benefit as the initial therapy for GBM, it remained effective to treat recurrences where treatment options are limited. In July 2009, bevacizumab was approved for use in combination with IFN-α for the treatment of patients with metastatic renal cell carcinoma (RCC). Results from the AVOREN trial demonstrated a 5-month improvement in median PFS in patients treated with bevacizumab plus IFN-α-2a versus IFN-α-2a plus placebo.[85] Another phase III trial (CALGB 90206) of bevacizumab plus IFN-α versus IFN-α monotherapy was conducted in patients with previously untreated, metastatic clear cell RCC. Median PFS was 8.4 months versus 4.9 months in favor of the bevacizumab arm.[86] Both studies did not demonstrate a statistically significant advantage in OS.[87,88]

Clinical studies of bevacizumab in combination with oxaliplatin-containing and 5-fluorouracil–based regimens have shown that combination therapy is well tolerated with toxicity not being substantially greater than that of the chemotherapy alone.[89] Side effects included grade 3 hypertension, grade 1 or 2 proteinuria, a slight increase (less than two percentage points) in grade 3 or 4 bleeding, and impaired surgical wound healing in patients who underwent surgery during treatment with bevacizumab. However, potentially life-threatening events (e.g., arterial and venous thromboembolic events, gastrointestinal perforation, hemoptysis, risk of ovarian failure) have occurred in some patients, thus requiring close patient monitoring in individuals who are at greater risk of adverse events.[90] In a recent meta-analysis of RCTs, bevacizumab in combination with chemotherapy or biologic therapy, compared with chemotherapy alone, was associated with increased treatment-related mortality.[91]

Although four phase III randomized studies have demonstrated improvements in PFS for ovarian cancer (OC)—two first-line trials (GOG 218 and ICON7) and two in recurrent OC [*platinum-resistant* (AURELIA Trial) or *platinum-sensitive* (OCEANS Trial)]—the role of bevacizumab in OC remains controversial. Bevacizumab is approved for use in combination with chemotherapy in the first- and second-line treatment of advanced OC in Europe, but it is not currently licensed in the United States for this indication. Mature OS data and predictive biomarkers are key to defining the subsets of patients who will most like benefit from this therapy. More recently, a randomized, phase III trial (GOG240) has demonstrated for the first time that bevacizumab can prolong OS and PFS for women with advanced, recurrent, or persistent cervical cancer that was not curable with standard chemotherapy. At the time of writing, there are currently over 400 actively recruiting, ongoing trials investigating the clinical benefits of bevacizumab in combination with chemotherapeutic regimens or as adjuvant therapy in various stages and types of cancer (http://clinicaltrial.gov).

Ziv-aflibercept

Ziv-aflibercept (previously known as aflibercept or VEGFTrap) is a recombinant humanized fusion protein of the extracellular domains of VEGF receptor 1 (VEGFR1) and VEGFR2 with the constant region (Fc) of human immunoglobulin (Ig)G1 that binds to VEGF-A, VEGF-B, PlGF1, and PlGF2, thereby preventing these ligands from binding to and activating their cognate receptors.[92] Ziv-aflibercept has a higher VEGF-A binding affinity and more potent blockade of VEGFR1 or VEGFR2 activation than bevacizumab.[93] In tumor models, ziv-aflibercept exerts its antiangiogenic effects through regressing tumor vasculature and size, remodeling or normalizing surviving vasculature, and inhibiting ascites formation.[94] In August 2012, ziv-aflibercept received regulatory approval for use in combination with 5-fluorouracil, leucovorin, and irinotecan (FOLFIRI) for the treatment of patients with metastatic CRC that is resistant to or that has progressed following treatment with an oxaliplatin-containing regimen. Results from the pivotal phase III VELOUR trial showed that ziv-aflibercept plus FOLFIRI statistically and significantly improved PFS (median PFS, 6.90 versus 4.67 months, respectively), OS (median OS, 13.50 versus 12.06 months, respectively), and overall response rates (19% versus 11.1%, respectively) relative to placebo plus FOLFIRI.[95] Toxicities related to ziv-aflibercept were consistent with those expected from the anti-VEGF drug class. The frequency of vascular-related adverse events appeared to be higher with ziv-aflibercept than bevacizumab treatment when compared across trials. Current clinical data are insufficient to directly compare ziv-aflibercept and bevacizumab in the first- or second-line setting for metastatic CRC.

Tyrosine–Kinase Inhibitor Therapy

Sorafenib

Sorafenib is a small-molecule Raf kinase and VEGF receptor kinase (VEGFR2 and VEGFR3) inhibitor. It has been shown to exhibit broad-spectrum effects on multiple targets (PDGF receptor (PDGFR), stem cell factor (c-KIT) receptor, p38) that affect the maintenance of the tumor vasculature and angiogenesis.[96] In December 2005, the FDA granted approval for sorafenib, which is considered the first multikinase inhibitor, for the treatment of patients with advanced RCC. Safety and efficacy of sorafenib was proven in the largest randomized phase III study conducted in advanced RCC that showed prolong PFS in favor of sorafenib.[97,98] In November 2007, sorafenib was approved for the treatment of patients with unresectable hepatocellular carcinoma (HCC) based on the study results in patients with advanced HCC who had not received previous systemic treatment. Median survival and the time to radiologic progression were nearly 3 months longer for patients treated with sorafenib than for those given placebo.[99] In November 2013, sorafenib received a new indication under the FDA's priority review program for the treatment of locally recurrent or metastatic, progressive differentiated thyroid carcinoma (DTC) refractory to radioactive iodine (RAI) treatment based on positive results from the phase III DECISION trial. Treatment with sorafenib improved PFS (the primary endpoint of the trial) by 41% compared with placebo (10.8 versus 5.8 months, respectively; hazard ratio [HR], 0.587, 95% confidence interval [CI] [0.454 to 0.758]; p <0.0001).[100] The overall response rates were 12% for patients who received sorafenib versus 1% for the placebo arm. Although only about 5% to 15% of thyroid cancer patients become refractory to RAI, no standard treatments are available and, thus, sorafenib is the first agent specifically approved for RAI-resistant DTC. Sorafenib was generally well tolerated with a predictable safety profile. Common adverse events include diarrhea, rash/desquamation, fatigue, hand–foot skin reaction, alopecia, and nausea/vomiting. Grade 3/4 adverse events were 38% for sorafenib versus 28% for placebo. Sorafenib-induced hypertension occurred in patients with metastatic RCC. The treatment-related hypertension was noted to be a class effect observed not only with VEGFR inhibitors, but also with the VEGF monoclonal antibody as well.[90] No significant relationship between previously described mediators of blood pressure and the magnitude of increase was found in a study evaluating the mechanism of sorafenib-induced hypertension in patients.[101]

Sunitinib

Sunitinib (SU11248) is a small-molecule, multitargeted TKI that exhibits potent antitumor and antiangiogenic activity and inhibits VEGFR-1, -2, -3, c-KIT, PDGFR; FLT-3; colony-stimulating factor receptor type 1 receptor; and the glial cell line–derived neurotrophic factor receptor. It was rationally designed and chosen for its high bioavailability and its nanomolar-range potency against the antiangiogenic RTKs. Sunitinib received its first U.S. regulatory approval in 2006 for the treatment of gastrointestinal stromal tumor (GIST) after disease progression on, or intolerance to, imatinib and accelerated approval for the treatment of advanced RCC.[102] Sunitinib demonstrated significant efficacy (prolonged median time to progression) in imatinib-resistant or -intolerant GIST in a randomized phase III trial.[103] The accelerated approval for RCC was based on durable partial responses, with a response rate of 26% to 37%, and a median duration of response of 54 weeks from two phase II, single-arm trials of patients with cytokine-refractory RCC.[104] The accelerated approval was converted to regular approval in 2007 following confirmation of an improvement in PFS and OS in a phase III trial of sunitinib for first-line treatment of patients with treatment-naïve, metastatic RCC.[105,106] In May 2011, the drug received a new indication for the treatment of progressive, well-differentiated pancreatic neuroendocrine tumors (pNET) in patients with unresectable, locally advanced, or metastatic disease. The randomized phase III trial was discontinued early after the independent data monitoring committee observed more serious adverse events and deaths in the placebo group as well as a difference in PFS favoring sunitinib. The median PFS for patients treated with sunitinib was 10.2 months,

compared with 5.4 months for patients treated with placebo (HR, 0.427, 95% CI, 0.271 to 0.673], p <0.001).[107] Common adverse effects, including diarrhea, mucositis, asthenia, skin abnormalities, and altered taste, were more common in patients receiving sunitinib. In addition, a decrease in left ventricular ejection fraction and severe hypertension were also more commonly reported in the sunitinib arm. Grade 3 or 4 treatment-emergent adverse events were reported in 56% versus 51% of patients on sunitinib versus placebo, respectively.

Pazopanib

Pazopanib is a second-generation, multitargeted TKI that binds to VEGFR-1, -2, -3, PDGFR-α and -β, c-KIT, and several other key proteins responsible for angiogenesis, tumor growth, and cell survival. Pazopanib exhibited in vivo and in vitro activity against tumor growth, and early clinical trials demonstrated potent antitumor and antiangiogenic activity.[108] A phase III clinical trial in treatment-naïve and cytokine-pretreated patients with advanced and/or metastatic RCC showed a significant improvement in PFS and tumor response compared with placebo,[109] leading to the approval of pazopanib in the United States in October 2009. A recent, randomized phase III trial (COMPARZ) compared the efficacy and safety of pazopanib and sunitinib as first-line therapy involving patients with metastatic RCC and demonstrated that both pazopanib and sunitinib have similar efficacy, but the safety and quality-of-life profiles favor pazopanib.[110] In April 2012, pazopanib was approved for the treatment of patients with metastatic nonadipocytic soft tissue sarcoma who have received prior chemotherapy following a phase III trial that demonstrated a statistically significant improvement in PFS. The median PFS was 4.6 months for patients receiving pazopanib versus 1.6 months for the placebo arm.[111] The drug is generally well tolerated, with the most common adverse events being diarrhea, fatigue, anorexia, hypertension, and hair depigmentation, as well as laboratory abnormalities in elevated aspartate aminotransferase and alanine aminotransferase. Pazopanib has shown clinical activity in a variety of tumors, including breast cancer, thyroid cancer, HCC, and cervical cancer.[112] Ongoing phase II and III trials are further evaluating pazopanib in these malignancies.

Vandetanib

Vandetanib is an oral, small-molecule TKI that inhibits the activity of RET kinase, VEGFR, epidermal growth factor receptor (EGFR), protein tyrosine kinase 6 (BRK), TIE2, members of the ephrin (EPH) receptors kinase family, and members of the Src family of tyrosine kinases.[113] Vandetanib reduced endothelial cell migration, proliferation, survival, and angiogenesis in vitro, and it decreased tumor vessel permeability and inhibited tumor growth and metastasis in vivo. In April 2011, vandetanib received U.S. regulatory approval for the treatment of symptomatic or progressive medullary thyroid cancer (MTC) in patients with unresectable, locally advanced, or metastatic disease. Until the approval of vandetanib, no systemic therapy was approved for the treatment of unresectable MTC, making it the first molecularly targeted agent approved for this disease. Results of a randomized phase III trial of patients with unresectable, locally advanced, or metastatic MTC demonstrated statistically significant and clinically meaningful improvements in PFS for vandetanib compared with placebo (HR, 0.46; 95% CI, 0.31 to 0.69; p <0.001).[114] Common grade 3 and 4 toxicities (>5%) were diarrhea and/or colitis, hypertension and hypertensive crisis, fatigue, hypocalcemia, rash, and corrected QT interval (QTc) prolongation. Given the toxicity profile, which includes QTc prolongation and sudden death, vandetanib is only available through a restricted distribution program. Vandetanib is also the first targeted drug to show evidence of efficacy in a randomized phase II trial in patients with locally advanced or metastatic differentiated thyroid carcinoma,[115] and a phase III trial is currently underway. Early phase studies are also being conducted in solid tumors, including GIST and kidney and pancreatic cancers.

Axitinib

Axitinib is a potent and selective second-generation inhibitor of VEGFR-1, -2, and -3. The in vitro half-maximal inhibitory concentration (IC50) of axitinib is 10-fold lower for the VEGF family of receptors than for other TKIs such as pazopanib, sunitinib, or sorafenib.[116] In January 2012, axitinib received approval for the treatment of advanced RCC after the failure of one prior systemic therapy based on a phase III trial (AXIS) comparing the efficacy and safety of axitinib versus sorafenib as a second-line treatment for metastatic RCC.[117,118] The median PFS was 6.7 months with axitinib compared to 4.7 months with sorafenib (HR, 0.67; 95% CI, 0.54, 0.81; one-sided p <0.0001). This improvement in PFS was greater in the cytokine-pretreated subgroup in comparison with the sunitinib-pretreated subgroup. The most frequent adverse events with axitinib were diarrhea (all grade), hypertension (all grade), fatigue, decreased appetite, nausea, and dysphonia. Moreover, hypertension, nausea, dysphonia, and hypothyroidism were more common with axitinib, whereas palmar–plantar erythrodysesthesia, alopecia, and rash were more frequent with sorafenib. A phase III trial (AGILE) comparing axitinib with sorafenib as first-line therapy in patients with treatment-naïve metastatic RCC demonstrated no significant difference in median PFS between patients treated with axitinib or sorafenib.[119] Additionally, axitinib is being studied as a single agent as well as in combination with chemotherapy across several tumor types including HCC, NSCLC, and pancreatic and thyroid cancers.

Cabozantinib

Cabozantinib (XL184) is a small-molecule TKI with potent activity toward the MET receptor and VEGFR2, as well as a number of other receptor tyrosine kinases, including RET, KIT, AXL, and FLT-3. MET is the only known receptor for hepatocyte growth factor (HGF), and its signaling activity plays a key role in tumorigenic growth, metastasis, and therapeutic resistance. The dysregulated expression and/or activation of MET and HGF have been implicated in the development of numerous human cancers including glioma; melanoma; and hepatocellular, renal, gastric, pancreatic, prostate, ovarian, breast, and lung cancers, and is often correlated with poor prognosis.[120] Recent studies have determined that the MET pathway plays an important role in the development of resistance to VEGF pathway inhibition and that the use of VEGFR inhibitors, such as sunitinib, sorafenib, or a VEGFR2-targeting antibody, can result in the development of an aggressive tumor phenotype characterized by increased invasiveness and metastasis.[121–123] Thus, there is an advantage to targeting both the MET and VEGF pathways to disrupt angiogenesis, tumorigenesis, and cancer progression. In November 2012, cabozantinib received U.S. regulatory approval for progressive metastatic MTC based on the phase III trial that demonstrated a statistically significant PFS prolongation for the cabozantinib-treatment arm.[124] The estimated median PFS was 11.2 months for cabozantinib versus 4.0 months for placebo (HR, 0.28; 95% CI, 0.19 to 0.40; p <0.001). Manageable toxicities included diarrhea, palmar–plantar erythrodysesthesia, decreased weight and appetite, nausea, and fatigue. Cabozantinib has been effective against several solid cancers, including MTC, breast, NSCLC, melanoma, and liver cancer, and is currently being studied in clinical trials in a number of tumor types, with the most significant results observed in the reduction of bone metastatic lesions in castration-resistant prostate cancer.[125]

Regorafenib

Regorafenib is a small-molecule TKI of multiple membrane-bound and intracellular kinases including RET, VEGFR1, VEGFR2, VEGFR3, KIT, PDGFR-α, PDGFR-β, FGFR1, FGFR2, TIE2, DDR2, TrkA, Eph2A, RAF-1, BRAF, BRAFV600E, SAPK2, PTK5, and Abl pathways.[126] Regorafenib is structurally related to sorafenib and differs from the latter by the presence of a fluorine atom in the center phenyl ring, resulting in higher inhibitory potency against various proangiogenic receptors than sorafenib, including VEGFR2 and FGFR1. In September 2012, regorafenib was approved for the treatment of patients with mCRC who have been previously treated with fluoropyrimidine-, oxaliplatin-, and irinotecan-based chemotherapy, with an anti-VEGF therapy, and if KRAS wild type, with an anti-EGFR therapy. The phase III CORRECT trial that resulted in approval of the drug demonstrated a median OS of 6.4 months in the regorafenib group versus 5.0 months in the placebo group (HR, 0.77; 95% CI, 0.64 to 0.94; one-sided p = 0.0052).[127] Regorafenib is the first TKI with survival benefits in mCRC that has progressed after all standard therapies. In February 2013, it received another indication for the treatment of patients with locally advanced, unresectable, or metastatic GIST who have been previously treated with imatinib and sunitinib. This was based on positive findings of the phase III GRID trial that demonstrated a median PFS of 4.8 months for regorafenib and 0.9 months for placebo (HR, 0.27, 95% CI, 0.19 to 0.39; p <0.0001).[128] In both studies, regorafenib provided significant improvements in PFS to highly refractory patient populations who have progressed on standard treatments. The most common adverse events that were grade 3 or higher and related to regorafenib were hand–foot skin reaction, fatigue, diarrhea, hypertension, and rash or desquamation. Its clinical development as a single agent or in combination with standard chemotherapeutic agents in various malignant tumors is ongoing and includes a phase III trial in patients with HCC whose disease has progressed after treatment with sorafenib.

mTOR Inhibitors

The mTOR pathway is a central component of the PI3K/Akt signaling pathway and a regulator of many biologic processes that are essential for angiogenesis, cell proliferation, and metabolism.[129] Inhibition of the mTOR kinase prevents downstream signaling via the Akt pathway, resulting in inhibition of protein translation and cell growth. mTOR plays a key role in angiogenesis and specifically regulates the expression of HIF-1, which is upregulated by the loss of the von Hippel–Lindau gene in RCC. In May 2007, temsirolimus was approved for the treatment of advanced RCC. Efficacy and safety were demonstrated in a phase III study in previously untreated patients (n = 626) with poor risk features of metastatic RCC assigned to one of three treatment arms: IFN-α alone, temsirolimus 25 mg alone, or the combination of temsirolimus (15 mg) and IFN-α.[130] Single-agent temsirolimus was associated with a statistically significant improvement in OS when compared with IFN; the addition of temsirolimus to IFN did not improve OS. The results of the phase III INTORSECT trial compared the efficacy of temsirolimus and sorafenib in the second-line treatment of metastatic RCC after disease progression on sunitinib demonstrated that temsirolimus did not improve survival over sorafenib in the second-line setting.[131] The significant OS difference in favor of sorafenib (stratified HR, 1.31; 95% CI, 1.05 to 1.63; two-sided p = 0.01) suggested that VEGFR inhibition may be a better option than mTOR inhibitors for patients progressing on sunitinib. The most common adverse reactions that occurred were rash, asthenia, mucositis, nausea, edema, and anorexia. Rare, but serious adverse reactions associated with temsirolimus included interstitial lung disease, bowel perforation, and acute renal failure.

Everolimus (RAD001) was approved in March 2009 for patients with advanced RCC whose disease had progressed on VEGFR-targeted therapy (sunitinib or sorafenib). Efficacy was demonstrated in a phase 3 trial that study met its primary endpoint with a median PFS of 4.9 and 1.9 months in the everolimus and placebo arms, respectively (HR, 0.33; p <0.0001).[132] Everolimus is also indicated for subependymal giant cell astrocytoma (SEGA) associated with tuberous sclerosis complex (TSC), renal angiomyolipoma with TSC, progressive neuroendocrine tumors of pancreatic origin, and advanced hormone receptor-positive, HER2-negative breast cancer in combination with exemestane.[133] The most common adverse reactions were stomatitis, infections, asthenia, fatigue, cough, and diarrhea. The most common grade 3/4 adverse reactions were infections, dyspnea, fatigue, stomatitis, dehydration, pneumonitis, abdominal pain, and asthenia. Both temsirolimus and everolimus are currently being evaluated in phase I through III studies of various cancer types. By downregulating HIF-1 in the tumor cell, mTOR inhibitors may complement the effects of TKIs at the level of the EC; thus, the combination of mTOR inhibitors with other targeted agents such as bevacizumab or sorafenib/sunitinib are also being investigated.

On the Horizon: Anti-VEGFR2 Monoclonal Antibody

Ramucirumab (IMC-1121B) is a fully human IgG1 monoclonal antibody that binds with high affinity to the extracellular VEGF-binding domain of VEGFR-2. In a phase III trial (REGARD), ramucirumab monotherapy conferred a statistically significant benefit in OS and PFS compared to placebo in patients with advanced gastric or gastroesophageal junction adenocarcinoma in the second-line setting with an acceptable safety profile.[134] The survival advantage is the first to be elicited by a single-agent biologic treatment in this setting and, based on these findings, the FDA has assigned a priority review designation for ramucirumab. An ongoing phase III trial (RAINBOW) of ramucirumab in combination with chemotherapy as second-line treatment for patients with advanced gastric cancer is currently underway, and preliminary results demonstrated the trial met both its primary (OS) and secondary (PFS) endpoints. In April 2014, the U.S. FDA approved ramucirumab for use as a single agent for the treatment of patients with advanced or metastatic, gastric or gastroesophageal junction adenocarcinoma with disease progression on or after prior treatment with fluoropyrimidine- or platinum-containing chemotherapy. The recommended ramucirumab dose and schedule is 8 mg/kg administered as a 60-minute intravenous infusion every 2 weeks. The drug also marginally improved survival in the second-line treatment of NSCLC in an ongoing phase III (REVEL) trial.

COMBINATION THERAPIES

Tumor angiogenesis is a highly complex process involving multiple growth factors and their receptor signaling pathways. Based on current evidence, with a few exceptions, effective therapy will probably rely on a combinatorial approach that involves targeting multiple pathways simultaneously. However, a recent study has demonstrated that simultaneous inhibition of the VEGF and EGF pathways in combination with chemotherapy shortens rather than prolongs PFS as compared to inhibition of the VEGF pathway alone in combination with chemotherapy.[135] Whether other targeted agents exhibit beneficial effects when combined with VEGF inhibitors remains to be investigated. Moreover, a number of studies have shown that antiangiogenic agents in combination with chemotherapy or radiotherapy result in additive or synergistic effects. Several models have been proposed to explain the mechanism responsible for this potentiation, keying in on the chemosensitizing effects of antiangiogenic therapy.[136] One hypothesis is that antiangiogenic therapy may normalize the tumor vasculature, thus resulting in improved oxygenation, better blood perfusion, and consequently, improved delivery of chemotherapeutic drugs.[137] A second model suggests that chemotherapy delivered at low doses and at close, regular intervals with no extended drug-free break periods preferentially damages ECs in the tumor neovasculature,[138,139] and suppresses circulating endothelial progenitor cells.[140,141] This regimen, also called metronomic

chemotherapy, sustains antiangiogenic activity and reduces acute toxicity.[142] Thus, the efficacy of metronomic chemotherapy may increase when administered in combination with specific antiangiogenic drugs. Another model addresses the use of antiangiogenic drugs to slow down tumor cell repopulation between successive cycles of cytotoxic chemotherapy.[143] This model underscores the importance of timing and sequence in achieving the maximal therapeutic benefit from combination therapies. In fact, a preclinical study in murine tumor models demonstrated that the administration of sunitinib markedly reduced chemotherapy-induced bone marrow toxicity, suggesting that the sequential treatment regimen (delivery of antiangiogenics followed by chemotherapy) showed superior survival benefits compared with the simultaneous administration of two drugs.[144] Finally, other mechanisms that might also contribute to the synergism include angiogenesis inhibitor–induced tumor blood vessel regression, the prevention of tumor coopting of vessels from surrounding healthy tissues, and the formation of abnormal vessels in the tumor microenvironment.[145] Nevertheless, it remains a challenge to determine why bevacizumab has proved largely ineffective as a single agent, whereas VEGF RTK inhibitors have repeatedly failed in randomized phase III trials when used in combination with chemotherapy. Furthermore, an additional challenge is to determine the optimal dose and duration of antiangiogenic drugs as well as the impact of drug sequencing in combination regimens. Studies are warranted to delineate the discrepancy of bevacizumab's efficacy in the macrometastatic versus micrometastatic disease settings.[146,147]

BIOMARKERS OF ANTIANGIOGENIC THERAPY

Antiangiogenic therapy has created a need to develop effective biomarkers to assess the activity of these inhibitors. Biomarkers of tumor angiogenesis activity are important to guide clinical development of these agents and to select patients most likely to benefit from this approach. Although there are currently no validated biomarkers for clinically assessing the efficacy of or selecting patients who will respond to antiangiogenic therapies, a number of candidate markers, including tissue, imaging, and circulating biomarkers, are emerging that need to be prospectively validated.[148,149] Several avenues are currently being investigated and include tumor biopsy analysis, microvessel density, noninvasive vascular imaging modalities (positron-emission tomography, dynamic contrast-enhanced magnetic resonance imaging), and measuring circulating biomarkers (levels of angiogenic factors in serum, plasma, urine, or circulating ECs and their precursors).[150–152] Recent research efforts have focused on identifying genetic and toxicity biomarkers to predict which patients will benefit from anti-VEGF/VEGFR therapy and identify patients at risk of adverse events. The existence of VEGF single-nucleotide polymorphisms (SNP) and their association with clinical outcomes may be predictive of patient response to bevacizumab. A recent study identified a locus in VEGFR1 that correlated with increased VEGFR1 expression and poor bevacizumab treatment outcomes.[153] Moreover, a breast cancer study (E2100) reported the VEGF-2578 AA and VEGF-1154 AA genotypes predicted an improved median OS, whereas the VEGF-634 CC and VEGF-1498 TT genotypes predicted protection from grade 3/4 hypertension in the combination-treatment arm.[154] The degree of hypertension can serve as a predictive biomarker of survival in patients after bevacizumab or TKI treatment. Although an association between hypertension and anti-VEGF therapy has been described, the clinical implications of this association and the predictive value of hypertension remains to be validated prospectively. A retrospective analysis of hypertension and efficacy outcomes was conducted in seven large phase III trials (n = 6,486 patients) and, in six of seven studies, early treatment-related blood pressure increase was neither predictive of clinical benefit from bevacizumab nor prognostic for the course of the disease.[155] However, one study (AVF2107g) showed early increased blood pressure was associated with longer PFS and OS. Because genetics play a significant role in modifying the risk of hypertension,[156] it remains to be determined whether polymorphisms in the VEGF/VEGFR pathway may function as potential biomarkers to predict the association between treatment-related hypertension and response to anti-VEGF therapy, as previously implicated in the E2100 trial.[154] Other biomarkers of response include elevated VEGF and placental growth factor levels,[148,152] whereas biomarkers of resistance, including circulating basic fibroblast growth factor, stromal cell-derived factor 1α, and viable circulating endothelial cells, increased when tumors escaped treatment.[157] A first prospective biomarker study (MERiDiAN) in metastatic breast cancer is currently underway to evaluate the impact of bevacizumab in patients stratified for plasma short VEGF-A isoforms. If validated, these findings could help identify which subgroup of patients should receive antiangiogenic therapy and could lead the way to possible future tailoring of individualized antiangiogenic therapy.

RESISTANCE TO ANTIANGIOGENIC THERAPY

Despite a decade of trials with angiogenesis inhibitors, clinical experience reveals that VEGF-targeted therapy often prolongs the survival of cancer patients by only months because tumors elicit evasive resistance.[145,158] Resistance to VEGF inhibitors may be observed in late-stage tumors when tumors regrow during treatment after an initial period of growth suppression from these antiangiogenic agents. This resistance involves the reactivation of tumor angiogenesis and increased expression of other proangiogenic factors. As the disease progresses, it is possible that redundant pathways might be implicated, with VEGF being replaced by other angiogenic pathways, warranting the addition of a second angiogenesis inhibitor that would target these secondary growth factors and/or their activated receptor pathways, or the use of a multitargeted TKI antiangiogenic drug (e.g., sunitinib, sorafenib).

However, resistance to these drugs eventually occurs, implicating the existence of additional pathways mediating resistance to antiangiogenic therapies. Moreover, tumor cells bearing genetic alterations of the *p53* gene may display a lower apoptosis rate under hypoxic conditions, which might reduce their reliance on vascular supply and, therefore, their responsiveness to antiangiogenic therapy.[159] The selection and overgrowth of tumor-variant cells that are hypoxia resistant and, thus, less dependent[159] on angiogenesis and vasculature remodeling, resulting in vessel stabilization,[160] could also explain the resistance to antiangiogenic drugs. Other possible mechanisms for acquired resistance include tumor vessels becoming less sensitive to antiangiogenic agents, tumor regrowth via rebound revascularization, and vessel cooption.[161–166] Perhaps one of the most intriguing findings is that, although ECs are assumed to be genetically stable, they may under some circumstances harbor genetic abnormalities and thus acquire resistance as well.[167,168]

Recent studies report that VEGF-targeted therapies not only induce primary tumor shrinkage and inhibit tumor progression, but can also initiate mechanisms that increase malignancy to promote tumor invasiveness and metastasis.[122,123,169] These mechanisms of resistance to antiangiogenic therapy involve tumor- and host-mediated pathways and may allow for differential efficacy in different stages of disease progression.[163] Specifically, antiangiogenic drug–resistance mechanisms involve pathways mediated by the tumor, whether intrinsic or acquired in response to therapy or by the host, which is either responding directly to therapy or indirectly to tumoral cues. Taken together, antiangiogenic therapy can enhance tumor invasiveness and metastasis to facilitate and/or accelerate disease in microscopic tumors and, hence, reduce OS benefit. Understanding the mechanisms of resistance, whether intrinsic or acquired, after exposure to antiangiogenic drug treatment is essential for developing strategies that will allow for optimal exploitation of VEGF inhibitors. It is equally important to identify biomarkers of drug resistance and factors mediating this resistance because the development of reliable biomarkers can be invaluable to monitor the development of evasive resistance to angiogenesis inhibitors.

CANCER THERAPEUTICS

REFERENCES

1. Hanahan D, Weinberg RA. Hallmarks of cancer: the next generation. *Cell* 2011;144:646–674.
2. Ide AG, Baker NH, Warren SL. Vascularization of the Brown Pearce rabbit epithelioma transplant as seen in the transparent ear chamger. *Am J Roentgenol* 1939;42:891–899.
3. Algire GH, Chalkley HW, Legallais FY, et al. Vascular reactions of normal and malignant tissues in vivo. I. Vascular reactions of mice to wounds and to normal and neoplastic transplants. *J Natl Cancer Inst* 1945;6:73–85.
4. Folkman J, Merler E, Abernathy C, et al. Isolation of a tumor factor responsible for angiogenesis. *J Exp Med* 1971;133:275–288.
5. Folkman J. Tumor angiogenesis: therapeutic implications. *N Engl J Med* 1971;285:1182–1186.
6. Papetti M, Herman IM. Mechanisms of normal and tumor-derived angiogenesis. *Am J Physiol Cell Physiol* 2002;282:C947–C970.
7. Hanahan D, Folkman J. Patterns and emerging mechanisms of the angiogenic switch during tumorigenesis. *Cell* 1996;86:353–364.
8. Black WC, Welch HG. Advances in diagnostic imaging and overestimations of disease prevalence and the benefits of therapy. *N Engl J Med* 1993;328:1237–1243.
9. Folkman J, Kalluri R. Cancer without disease. *Nature* 2004;427:787.
10. Weidner N, Semple JP, Welch WR, et al. Tumor angiogenesis and metastasis—correlation in invasive breast carcinoma. *N Engl J Med* 1991;324:1–8.
11. Holmgren L, O'Reilly MS, Folkman J. Dormancy of micrometastases: balanced proliferation and apoptosis in the presence of angiogenesis suppression. *Nat Med* 1995;1:149–153.
12. Naumov GN, Bender E, Zurakowski D, et al. A model of human tumor dormancy: an angiogenic switch from the nonangiogenic phenotype. *J Natl Cancer Inst* 2006;98:316–325.
13. Udagawa T, Fernandez A, Achilles EG, et al. Persistence of microscopic human cancers in mice: alterations in the angiogenic balance accompanies loss of tumor dormancy. *Faseb J* 2002;16:1361–1370.
14. Holash J, Maisonpierre PC, Compton D, et al. Vessel cooption, regression, and growth in tumors mediated by angiopoietins and VEGF. *Science* 1999;284:1994–1998.
15. Relf M, LeJeune S, Scott PA, et al. Expression of the angiogenic factors vascular endothelial cell growth factor, acidic and basic fibroblast growth factor, tumor growth factor beta-1, platelet-derived endothelial cell growth factor, placenta growth factor, and pleiotrophin in human primary breast cancer and its relation to angiogenesis. *Cancer Res* 1997;57:963–969.
16. Carmeliet P, Dor Y, Herbert JM, et al. Role of HIF-1alpha in hypoxia-mediated apoptosis, cell proliferation and tumour angiogenesis. *Nature* 1998;394:485–490.
17. Folkman J. Endogenous angiogenesis inhibitors. *Apmis* 2004;112:496–507.
18. Nyberg P, Xie L, Kalluri R. Endogenous inhibitors of angiogenesis. *Cancer Res* 2005;65:3967–3979.
19. Rak J, Yu JL. Oncogenes and tumor angiogenesis: the question of vascular "supply" and vascular "demand". *Semin Cancer Biol* 2004;14:93–104.
20. Bottos A, Bardelli A. Oncogenes and angiogenesis: a way to personalize antiangiogenic therapy? *Cell Mol Life Sci* 2013;70:4131–4140.
21. Rak J, Yu JL, Klement G, et al. Oncogenes and angiogenesis: signaling three-dimensional tumor growth. *J Investig Dermatol Symp Proc* 2000;5:24–33.
22. Langer R, Brem H, Falterman K, et al. Isolations of a cartilage factor that inhibits tumor neovascularization. *Science* 1976;193:70–72.
23. Langer R, Conn H, Vacanti J, et al. Control of tumor growth in animals by infusion of an angiogenesis inhibitor. *Proc Natl Acad Sci U S A* 1980;77:4331–4335.
24. Ribatti D. Endogenous inhibitors of angiogenesis: a historical review. *Leuk Res* 2009;33:638–644.
25. Folkman J. Antiangiogenesis in cancer therapy—endostatin and its mechanisms of action. *Exp Cell Res* 2006;312:594–607.
26. Karamouzis MV, Moschos SJ. The use of endostatin in the treatment of solid tumors. *Expert Opin Biol Ther* 2009;9:641–648.
27. Lawler J. Thrombospondin-1 as an endogenous inhibitor of angiogenesis and tumor growth. *J Cell Mol Med* 2002;6:1–12.
28. Maeshima Y, Manfredi M, Reimer C, et al. Identification of the anti-angiogenic site within vascular basement membrane-derived tumstatin. *J Biol Chem* 2001;276:15240–15248.
29. Kerbel RS. Vasohibin: the feedback on a new inhibitor of angiogenesis. *J Clin Invest* 2004;114:884–886.
30. Sato Y. The vasohibin family: a novel family for angiogenesis regulation. *J Biochem* 2013;153:5–11.

31. Noguera-Troise I, Daly C, Papadopoulos NJ, et al. Blockade of Dll4 inhibits tumour growth by promoting non-productive angiogenesis. *Nature* 2006;444:1032–1037.

32. Ridgway J, Zhang G, Wu Y, et al. Inhibition of Dll4 signalling inhibits tumour growth by deregulating angiogenesis. *Nature* 2006;444:1083–1087.

33. Kuhnert F, Kirshner JR, Thurston G. Dll4-Notch signaling as a therapeutic target in tumor angiogenesis. *Vasc Cell* 2011;3:20.

34. Sund M, Hamano Y, Sugimoto H, et al. Function of endogenous inhibitors of angiogenesis as endothelium-specific tumor suppressors. *Proc Natl Acad Sci U S A* 2005;102:2934–2939.

35. Dameron KM, Volpert OV, Tainsky MA, et al. Control of angiogenesis in fibroblasts by p53 regulation of thrombospondin-1. *Science* 1994;265:1582–1584.

36. Zhang L, Yu D, Hu M, et al. Wild-type p53 suppresses angiogenesis in human leiomyosarcoma and synovial sarcoma by transcriptional suppression of vascular endothelial growth factor expression. *Cancer Res* 2000;60:3655–3661.

37. Sherif ZA, Nakai S, Pirollo KF, et al. Downmodulation of bFGF-binding protein expression following restoration of p53 function. *Cancer Gene Ther* 2001;8:771–782.

38. Ravi R, Mookerjee B, Bhujwalla ZM, et al. Regulation of tumor angiogenesis by p53-induced degradation of hypoxia-inducible factor 1alpha. *Genes Dev* 2000;14:34–44.

39. Farhang Ghahremani M, Goossens S, Nittner D, et al. p53 promotes VEGF expression and angiogenesis in the absence of an intact p21-Rb pathway. *Cell Death Differ* 2013;20:888–897.

40. Teodoro JG, Parker AE, Zhu X, et al. p53-mediated inhibition of angiogenesis through up-regulation of a collagen prolyl hydroxylase. *Science* 2006;313:968–971.

41. Folkman J. Tumor suppression by p53 is mediated in part by the antiangiogenic activity of endostatin and tumstatin. *Sci STKE* 2006;2006:pe35.

42. Brouty-Boye D, Zetter BR. Inhibition of cell motility by interferon. *Science* 1980;208:516–518.

43. Dvorak HF, Gresser I. Microvascular injury in pathogenesis of interferon-induced necrosis of subcutaneous tumors in mice. *J Natl Cancer Inst* 1989;81:497–502.

44. Sidky YA, Borden EC. Inhibition of angiogenesis by interferons: effects on tumor- and lymphocyte-induced vascular responses. *Cancer Res* 1987;47:5155–5161.

45. Taylor S, Folkman J. Protamine is an inhibitor of angiogenesis. *Nature* 1982;297:307–312.

46. Crum R, Szabo S, Folkman J. A new class of steroids inhibits angiogenesis in the presence of heparin or a heparin fragment. *Science* 1985;230:1375–1378.

47. Ingber D, Fujita T, Kishimoto S, et al. Synthetic analogues of fumagillin that inhibit angiogenesis and suppress tumour growth. *Nature* 1990;348:555–557.

48. Kerbel RS. Inhibition of tumor angiogenesis as a strategy to circumvent acquired resistance to anti-cancer therapeutic agents. *Bioessays* 1991;13:31–36.

49. Folkman J. Angiogenesis: an organizing principle for drug discovery? *Nat Rev Drug Discov* 2007;6:273–286.

50. D'Amato RJ, Loughnan MS, Flynn E, et al. Thalidomide is an inhibitor of angiogenesis. *Proc Natl Acad Sci U S A* 1994;91:4082–4085.

51. Bauer KS, Dixon SC, Figg WD. Inhibition of angiogenesis by thalidomide requires metabolic activation, which is species-dependent. *Biochem Pharmacol* 1998;51:1827–1834.

52. Figg WD. The 2005 Leon I. Goldberg Young Investigator Award Lecture: development of thalidomide as an angiogenesis inhibitor for the treatment of androgen-independent prostate cancer. *Clin Pharmacol Ther* 2006;79:1–8.

53. Kenyon BM, Browne F, D'Amato RJ. Effects of thalidomide and related metabolites in a mouse corneal model of neovascularization. *Exp Eye Res* 1997;64:971–978.

54. Price DK, Ando Y, Kruger EA, et al. 5'-OH-thalidomide, a metabolite of thalidomide, inhibits angiogenesis. *Ther Drug Monit* 2002;24:104–110.

55. Dredge K, Marriott JB, Macdonald CD, et al. Novel thalidomide analogues display anti-angiogenic activity independently of immunomodulatory effects. *Br J Cancer* 2002;87:1166–1172.

56. Gupta D, Treon SP, Shima Y, et al. Adherence of multiple myeloma cells to bone marrow stromal cells upregulates vascular endothelial growth factor secretion: therapeutic applications. *Leukemia* 2001;15:1950–1961.

57. Ng SS, Gutschow M, Weiss M, et al. Antiangiogenic activity of N-substituted and tetrafluorinated thalidomide analogues. *Cancer Res* 2003;63:3189–3194.

58. Zhang H, Vakil V, Braunstein M, et al. Circulating endothelial progenitor cells in multiple myeloma: implications and significance. *Blood* 2005;105:3286–3294.

59. De Sanctis JB, Mijares M, Suarez A, et al. Pharmacological properties of thalidomide and its analogues. *Recent Pat Inflamm Allergy Drug Discov* 2010;4:144–148.

60. Ferrara N, Gerber HP, LeCouter J. The biology of VEGF and its receptors. *Nat Med* 2003;9:669–676.

61. Lindahl P, Johansson BR, Leveen P, et al. Pericyte loss and microaneurysm formation in PDGF-B-deficient mice. *Science* 1997;277:242–245.

62. Oliner J, Min H, Leal J, et al. Suppression of angiogenesis and tumor growth by selective inhibition of angiopoietin-2. *Cancer Cell* 2004;6:507–516.

63. Fingleton B. MMPs as therapeutic targets—still a viable option? *Semin Cell Dev Biol* 2008;19:61–68.

64. Roy R, Yang J, Moses MA. Matrix metalloproteinases as novel biomarkers and potential therapeutic targets in human cancer. *J Clin Oncol* 2009;27:5287–5297.

65. Shi ZG, Li JP, Shi LL, et al. An updated patent therapeutic agents targeting MMPs. *Recent Pat Anticancer Drug Discov* 2012;7:74–101.

66. Gialeli C, Theocharis AD, Karamanos NK. Roles of matrix metalloproteinases in cancer progression and their pharmacological targeting. *FEBS J* 2011;278:16–27.

67. Nikolopoulos SN, Blaikie P, Yoshioka T, et al. Integrin beta4 signaling promotes tumor angiogenesis. *Cancer Cell* 2004;6:471–483.

68. Bradley DA, Daignault S, Ryan CJ, et al. Cilengitide (EMD 121974, NSC 707544) in asymptomatic metastatic castration resistant prostate cancer patients: a randomized phase II trial by the prostate cancer clinical trials consortium. *Invest New Drugs* 2011;29:1432–1440.

69. Desgrosellier JS, Cheresh DA. Integrins in cancer: biological implications and therapeutic opportunities. *Nat Rev Cancer* 2010;10:9–22.

70. Hersey P, Sosman J, O'Day S. A randomized phase 2 study of etaracizumab, a monoclonal antibody against integrin alpha(v)beta(3), + or − dacarbazine in patients with stage IV metastatic melanoma. *Cancer* 2010;116:1526–1534.

71. Heidenreich A, Rawal SK, Szkarlat K, et al. A randomized, double-blind, multicenter, phase 2 study of a human monoclonal antibody to human alphanu integrins (intetumumab) in combination with docetaxel and prednisone for the first-line treatment of patients with metastatic castration-resistant prostate cancer. *Ann Oncol* 2013;24:329–336.

72. O'Day S, Pavlick A, Loquai C, et al. A randomised, phase II study of intetumumab, an anti-alphav-integrin mAb, alone and with dacarbazine in stage IV melanoma. *Br J Cancer* 2011;105:346–352.

73. Stupp R, Hegi M, Gorlia T, et al. Standard chemoradiotherapy ± cilengitide in newly diagnosed glioblastoma (GBM): updated results and subgroup analyses of the international randomized phase III CENTRIC trial (EORTC trial #26071-22072/Canadian Brain Tumor Consortium). Program and abstracts presented at: 2013 European Cancer Congress; 2013; Amsterdam.

74. Ellis LM, Hicklin DJ. VEGF-targeted therapy: mechanisms of anti-tumour activity. *Nat Rev Cancer* 2008;8:579–591.

75. Hurwitz H, Fehrenbacher L, Novotny W, et al. Bevacizumab plus irinotecan, fluorouracil, and leucovorin for metastatic colorectal cancer. *N Engl J Med* 2004;350:2335–2342.

76. Bennouna J, Sastre J, Arnold D, et al. Continuation of bevacizumab after first progression in metastatic colorectal cancer (ML18147): a randomised phase 3 trial. *Lancet Oncol* 2013;14:29–37.

77. Allegra CJ, Yothers G, O'Connell MJ, et al. Phase III trial assessing bevacizumab in stages II and III carcinoma of the colon: results of NSABP protocol C-08. *J Clin Oncol* 2011;29:11–16.

78. de Gramont A, Van Cutsem E, Schmoll HJ, et al. Bevacizumab plus oxaliplatin-based chemotherapy as adjuvant treatment for colon cancer (AVANT): a phase 3 randomised controlled trial. *Lancet Oncol* 2012;13:1225–1233.

79. Sandler A, Gray R, Perry MC, et al. Paclitaxel-carboplatin alone or with bevacizumab for non-small-cell lung cancer. *N Engl J Med* 2006;355:2542–2550.

80. Miles DW, Chan A, Dirix LY, et al. Phase III study of bevacizumab plus docetaxel compared with placebo plus docetaxel for the first-line treatment of human epidermal growth factor receptor 2-negative metastatic breast cancer. *J Clin Oncol* 2010;28:3239–3247.

81. Robert NJ, Dieras V, Glaspy J, et al. RIBBON-1: randomized, double-blind, placebo-controlled, phase III trial of chemotherapy with or without bevacizumab for first-line treatment of human epidermal growth factor receptor 2-negative, locally recurrent or metastatic breast cancer. *J Clin Oncol* 2011;29:1252–1260.

82. Brufsky AM, Hurvitz S, Perez E, et al. RIBBON-2: a randomized, double-blind, placebo-controlled, phase III trial evaluating the efficacy and safety of bevacizumab in combination with chemotherapy for second-line treatment of human epidermal growth factor receptor 2-negative metastatic breast cancer. *J Clin Oncol* 2011;29:4286–4293.

83. Cohen MH, Shen YL, Keegan P, et al. FDA drug approval summary: bevacizumab (Avastin) as treatment of recurrent glioblastoma multiforme. *Oncologist* 2009;14:1131–1138.

84. Soffietti R, Trevisan E, Ruda R. What have we learned from trials on antiangiogenic agents in glioblastoma? *Expert Rev Neurother* 2014;14:1–3.

85. Escudier B, Pluzanska A, Koralewski P, et al. Bevacizumab plus interferon alfa-2a for treatment of metastatic renal cell carcinoma: a randomised, double-blind phase III trial. *Lancet* 2007;370:2103–2111.

86. Rini BI, Halabi S, Rosenberg JE, et al. Bevacizumab plus interferon alfa compared with interferon alfa monotherapy in patients with metastatic renal cell carcinoma: CALGB 90206. *J Clin Oncol* 2008;26:5422–5428.

87. Escudier B, Bellmunt J, Negrier S, et al. Phase III trial of bevacizumab plus interferon alfa-2a in patients with metastatic renal cell carcinoma (AVOREN): final analysis of overall survival. *J Clin Oncol* 2010;28:2144–2150.

88. Rini BI, Halabi S, Rosenberg JE, et al. Phase III trial of bevacizumab plus interferon alfa versus interferon alfa monotherapy in patients with metastatic renal cell carcinoma: final results of CALGB 90206. *J Clin Oncol* 2010;28:2137–2143.

89. Hurwitz H, Saini S. Bevacizumab in the treatment of metastatic colorectal cancer: safety profile and management of adverse events. *Semin Oncol* 2006;33:S26–S34.

90. Chen HX, Cleck JN. Adverse effects of anticancer agents that target the VEGF pathway. *Nat Rev Clin Oncol* 2009;6:465–477.

91. Ranpura V, Hapani S, Wu S. Treatment-related mortality with bevacizumab in cancer patients: a meta-analysis. *JAMA* 2011;305:487–494.

92. Holash J, Davis S, Papadopoulos N, et al. VEGF-Trap: a VEGF blocker with potent antitumor effects. *Proc Natl Acad Sci U S A* 2002;99:11393–11398.

93. Papadopoulos N, Martin J, Ruan Q, et al. Binding and neutralization of vascular endothelial growth factor (VEGF) and related ligands by VEGF Trap, ranibizumab and bevacizumab. *Angiogenesis* 2012;15:171–185.

94. Gaya A, Tse V. A preclinical and clinical review of aflibercept for the management of cancer. *Cancer Treat Rev* 2012;38:484–493.

95. Van Cutsem E, Tabernero J, Lakomy R, et al. Addition of aflibercept to fluorouracil, leucovorin, and irinotecan improves survival in a phase III randomized trial in patients with metastatic colorectal cancer previously treated with an oxaliplatin-based regimen. *J Clin Oncol* 2012;30:3499–3506.

96. Wilhelm SM, Carter C, Tang L, et al. BAY 43-9006 exhibits broad spectrum oral antitumor activity and targets the RAF/MEK/ERK pathway and receptor tyrosine kinases involved in tumor progression and angiogenesis. *Cancer Res* 2004;64:7099–7109.

97. Escudier B, Eisen T, Stadler WM, et al. Sorafenib in advanced clear-cell renal-cell carcinoma. *N Engl J Med* 2007;356:125–134.

98. Escudier B, Eisen T, Stadler WM, et al. Sorafenib for treatment of renal cell carcinoma: Final efficacy and safety results of the phase III treatment approaches in renal cancer global evaluation trial. *J Clin Oncol* 2009;27:3312–3318.

99. Llovet JM, Ricci S, Mazzaferro V, et al. Sorafenib in advanced hepatocellular carcinoma. *N Engl J Med* 2008;359:378–390.

100. Brose MS, Nutting C, Jarzab B, et al. Sorafenib in locally advanced or metastatic patients with radioactive iodine refractory differentiated thyroid cancer: the phase III DECISION trial. *J Clin Oncol* 2013;31.

101. Veronese ML, Mosenkis A, Flaherty KT, et al. Mechanisms of hypertension associated with BAY 43-9006. *J Clin Oncol* 2006;24:1363–1369.

102. Goodman VL, Rock EP, Dagher R, et al. Approval summary: sunitinib for the treatment of imatinib refractory or intolerant gastrointestinal stromal tumors and advanced renal cell carcinoma. *Clin Cancer Res* 2007;13:1367–1373.

103. Demetri GD, van Oosterom AT, Garrett CR, et al. Efficacy and safety of sunitinib in patients with advanced gastrointestinal stromal tumour after failure of imatinib: a randomised controlled trial. *Lancet* 2006;368:1329–1338.

104. Motzer RJ, Michaelson MD, Redman BG, et al. Activity of SU11248, a multitargeted inhibitor of vascular endothelial growth factor receptor and platelet-derived growth factor receptor, in patients with metastatic renal cell carcinoma. *J Clin Oncol* 2006;24:16–24.

105. Motzer RJ, Hutson TE, Tomczak P, et al. Sunitinib versus interferon alfa in metastatic renal-cell carcinoma. *N Engl J Med* 2007;356:115–124.

106. Motzer RJ, Hutson TE, Tomczak P, et al. Overall survival and updated results for sunitinib compared with interferon alfa in patients with metastatic renal cell carcinoma. *J Clin Oncol* 2009;27:3584–3590.

107. Raymond E, Dahan L, Raoul JL, et al. Sunitinib malate for the treatment of pancreatic neuroendocrine tumors. *N Engl J Med* 2011;364:501–513.

108. Kumar R, Knick VB, Rudolph SK, et al. Pharmacokinetic-pharmacodynamic correlation from mouse to human with pazopanib, a multikinase angiogenesis inhibitor with potent antitumor and antiangiogenic activity. *Mol Cancer Ther* 2007;6:2012–2021.

109. Sternberg CN, Davis ID, Mardiak J, et al. Pazopanib in locally advanced or metastatic renal cell carcinoma: results of a randomized phase III trial. *J Clin Oncol* 2010;28:1061–1068.

110. Motzer RJ, Hutson TE, Cella D, et al. Pazopanib versus sunitinib in metastatic renal-cell carcinoma. *N Engl J Med* 2013;369:722–731.

111. van der Graaf WT, Blay JY, Chawla SP, et al. Pazopanib for metastatic soft-tissue sarcoma (PALETTE): a randomised, double-blind, placebo-controlled phase 3 trial. *Lancet* 2012;379:1879–1886.

112. Schutz FA, Choueiri TK, Sternberg CN. Pazopanib: Clinical development of a potent anti-angiogenic drug. *Crit Rev Oncol Hematol* 2011;77:163–171.

113. Thornton K, Kim G, Maher VE, et al. Vandetanib for the treatment of symptomatic or progressive medullary thyroid cancer in patients with unresectable locally advanced or metastatic disease: U.S. Food and Drug Administration drug approval summary. *Clin Cancer Res* 2012;18:3722–3730.

114. Wells SA, Jr., Robinson BG, Gagel RF, et al. Vandetanib in patients with locally advanced or metastatic medullary thyroid cancer: a randomized, double-blind phase III trial. *J Clin Oncol* 2012;30:134–141.

115. Leboulleux S, Bastholt L, Krause T, et al. Vandetanib in locally advanced or metastatic differentiated thyroid cancer: a randomised, double-blind, phase 2 trial. *Lancet Oncol* 2012;13:897–905.

116. Gross-Goupil M, Francois L, Quivy A, et al. Axitinib: a review of its safety and efficacy in the treatment of adults with advanced renal cell carcinoma. *Clin Med Insights Oncol* 2013;7:269–277.

117. Rini BI, Escudier B, Tomczak P, et al. Comparative effectiveness of axitinib versus sorafenib in advanced renal cell carcinoma (AXIS): a randomised phase 3 trial. *Lancet* 2011;378:1931–1939.

118. Motzer RJ, Escudier B, Tomczak P, et al. Axitinib versus sorafenib as second-line treatment for advanced renal cell carcinoma: overall survival analysis and updated results from a randomised phase 3 trial. *Lancet Oncol* 2013;14:552–562.

119. Hutson TE, Lesovoy V, Al-Shukri S, et al. Axitinib versus sorafenib as first-line therapy in patients with metastatic renal-cell carcinoma: a randomised open-label phase 3 trial. *Lancet Oncol* 2013;14:1287–1294.

120. Graveel CR, Tolbert D, Vande Woude GF. MET: a critical player in tumorigenesis and therapeutic target. *Cold Spring Harb Perspect Biol* 2013;5.

121. Shojaei F, Lee JH, Simmons BH, et al. HGF/c-Met acts as an alternative angiogenic pathway in sunitinib-resistant tumors. *Cancer Res* 2010;70:10090–10100.

122. Ebos JM, Lee CR, Cruz-Munoz W, et al. Accelerated metastasis after short-term treatment with a potent inhibitor of tumor angiogenesis. *Cancer Cell* 2009;15:232–239.

123. Paez-Ribes M, Allen E, Hudock J, et al. Antiangiogenic therapy elicits malignant progression of tumors to increased local invasion and distant metastasis. *Cancer Cell* 2009;15:220–231.

124. Elisei R, Schlumberger MJ, Muller SP, et al. Cabozantinib in progressive medullary thyroid cancer. *J Clin Oncol* 2013;31:3639–3646.

125. Smith DC, Smith MR, Sweeney C, et al. Cabozantinib in patients with advanced prostate cancer: results of a phase II randomized discontinuation trial. *J Clin Oncol* 2013;31:412–429.

126. Strumberg D, Schultheis B. Regorafenib for cancer. *Expert Opin Investig Drugs* 2012;21:879–889.

127. Grothey A, Van Cutsem E, Sobrero A, et al. Regorafenib monotherapy for previously treated metastatic colorectal cancer (CORRECT): an international, multicentre, randomised, placebo-controlled, phase 3 trial. *Lancet* 2013;381:303–312.

128. Demetri GD, Reichardt P, Kang YK, et al. Efficacy and safety of regorafenib for advanced gastrointestinal stromal tumours after failure of imatinib and sunitinib (GRID): an international, multicentre, randomised, placebo-controlled, phase 3 trial. *Lancet* 2013;381:295–302.

129. Gibbons JJ, Abraham RT, Yu K. Mammalian target of rapamycin: discovery of rapamycin reveals a signaling pathway important for normal and cancer cell growth. *Semin Oncol* 2009;36 Suppl 3:S3–S17.

130. Hudes G, Carducci M, Tomczak P, et al. Temsirolimus, interferon alfa, or both for advanced renal-cell carcinoma. *N Engl J Med* 2007;356:2271–2281.

131. Hutson TE, Escudier B, Esteban E, et al. Randomized phase III trial of temsirolimus versus sorafenib as second-line therapy after sunitinib in patients with metastatic renal cell carcinoma. *J Clin Oncol* 2014;32:760–767.

132. Motzer RJ, Escudier B, Oudard S, et al. Efficacy of everolimus in advanced renal cell carcinoma: a double-blind, randomised, placebo-controlled phase III trial. *Lancet* 2008;372:449–456.

133. Lebwohl D, Anak O, Sahmoud T, et al. Development of everolimus, a novel oral mTOR inhibitor, across a spectrum of diseases. *Ann N Y Acad Sci* 2013;1291:14–32.

134. Fuchs CS, Tomasek J, Yong CJ, et al. Ramucirumab monotherapy for previously treated advanced gastric or gastro-oesophageal junction adenocarcinoma (REGARD): an international, randomised, multicentre, placebo-controlled, phase 3 trial. *Lancet* 2014;383:31–39.

135. Tol J, Koopman M, Cats A, et al. Chemotherapy, bevacizumab, and cetuximab in metastatic colorectal cancer. *N Engl J Med* 2009;360:563–572.

136. Kerbel RS. Antiangiogenic therapy: a universal chemosensitization strategy for cancer? *Science* 2006;312:1171–1175.

137. Jain RK. Normalization of tumor vasculature: an emerging concept in antiangiogenic therapy. *Science* 2005;307:58–62.

138. Browder T, Butterfield CE, Kraling BM, et al. Antiangiogenic scheduling of chemotherapy improves efficacy against experimental drug-resistant cancer. *Cancer Res* 2000;60:1878–1886.

139. Klement G, Baruchel S, Rak J, et al. Continuous low-dose therapy with vinblastine and VEGF receptor-2 antibody induces sustained tumor regression without overt toxicity. *J Clin Invest* 2000;105:R15–R24.

140. Bertolini F, Paul S, Mancuso P, et al. Maximum tolerable dose and low-dose metronomic chemotherapy have opposite effects on the mobilization and viability of circulating endothelial progenitor cells. *Cancer Res* 2003;63:4342–4346.

141. Mancuso P, Colleoni M, Calleri A, et al. Circulating endothelial-cell kinetics and viability predict survival in breast cancer patients receiving metronomic chemotherapy. *Blood* 2006;108:452–459.

142. Kerbel RS, Kamen BA. The anti-angiogenic basis of metronomic chemotherapy. *Nat Rev Cancer* 2004;4:423–436.

143. Hudis CA. Clinical implications of antiangiogenic therapies. *Oncology (Williston Park)* 2005;19:26–31.

144. Zhang D, Hedlund EM, Lim S, et al. Antiangiogenic agents significantly improve survival in tumor-bearing mice by increasing tolerance to chemotherapy-induced toxicity. *Proc Natl Acad Sci U S A* 2011;108:4117–4122.

145. Kerbel RS. Tumor angiogenesis. *N Engl J Med* 2008;358:2039–2049.

146. Mountzios G, Pentheroudakis G, Carmeliet P. Bevacizumab and micrometastases: Revisiting the preclinical and clinical rollercoaster. *Pharmacol Ther* 2014;141:117–124.

147. Ebos JM, Kerbel RS. Antiangiogenic therapy: impact on invasion, disease progression, and metastasis. *Nat Rev Clin Oncol* 2011;8:210–221.

148. Jain RK, Duda DG, Willett CG, et al. Biomarkers of response and resistance to antiangiogenic therapy. *Nat Rev Clin Oncol* 2009;6:327–338.

149. Murukesh N, Dive C, Jayson GC. Biomarkers of angiogenesis and their role in the development of VEGF inhibitors. *Br J Cancer* 2010;102:8–18.

150. Davis DW, McConkey DJ, Abbruzzese JL, et al. Surrogate markers in antiangiogenesis clinical trials. *Br J Cancer* 2003;89:8–14.

151. Wehland M, Bauer J, Magnusson NE, et al. Biomarkers for anti-angiogenic therapy in cancer. *Int J Mol Sci* 2013;14:9338–9364.

152. Lambrechts D, Lenz HJ, de Haas S, et al. Markers of response for the antiangiogenic agent bevacizumab. *J Clin Oncol* 2013;31:1219–1230.

153. Lambrechts D, Claes B, Delmar P, et al. VEGF pathway genetic variants as biomarkers of treatment outcome with bevacizumab: an analysis of data from the AViTA and AVOREN randomised trials. *Lancet Oncol* 2012;13:724–733.

154. Schneider BP, Wang M, Radovich M, et al. Association of vascular endothelial growth factor and vascular endothelial growth factor receptor-2 genetic polymorphisms with outcome in a trial of paclitaxel compared with paclitaxel plus bevacizumab in advanced breast cancer: ECOG 2100. *J Clin Oncol* 2008;26:4672–4678.

155. Hurwitz HI, Douglas PS, Middleton JP, et al. Analysis of early hypertension and clinical outcome with bevacizumab: results from seven phase III studies. *Oncologist* 2013;18:273–280.

156. Levy D, Ehret GB, Rice K, et al. Genome-wide association study of blood pressure and hypertension. *Nat Genet* 2009;41:677–687.

157. Batchelor TT, Sorensen AG, di Tomaso E, et al. AZD2171, a pan-VEGF receptor tyrosine kinase inhibitor, normalizes tumor vasculature and alleviates edema in glioblastoma patients. *Cancer Cell* 2007;11:83–95.

158. Sennino B, McDonald DM. Controlling escape from angiogenesis inhibitors. *Nat Rev Cancer* 2012;12:699–709.

159. Yu JL, Rak JW, Coomber BL, et al. Effect of p53 status on tumor response to antiangiogenic therapy. *Science* 2002;295:1526–1528.

160. Glade Bender J, Cooney EM, Kandel JJ, et al. Vascular remodeling and clinical resistance to antiangiogenic cancer therapy. *Drug Resist Updat* 2004;7:289–300.

161. Bergers G, Hanahan D. Modes of resistance to anti-angiogenic therapy. *Nat Rev Cancer* 2008;8:592–603.

162. Crawford Y, Ferrara N. Tumor and stromal pathways mediating refractoriness/resistance to anti-angiogenic therapies. *Trends Pharmacol Sci* 2009;30:624–630.

163. Ebos JM, Lee CR, Kerbel RS. Tumor and host-mediated pathways of resistance and disease progression in response to antiangiogenic therapy. *Clin Cancer Res* 2009;15:5020–5025.

164. Kerbel RS, Yu J, Tran J, et al. Possible mechanisms of acquired resistance to anti-angiogenic drugs: implications for the use of combination therapy approaches. *Cancer Metastasis Rev* 2001;20:79–86.

165. Shojaei F, Ferrara N. Role of the microenvironment in tumor growth and in refractoriness/resistance to anti-angiogenic therapies. *Drug Resist Updat* 2008;11:219–230.

166. Sweeney CJ, Miller KD, Sledge GW Jr. Resistance in the anti-angiogenic era: nay-saying or a word of caution? *Trends Mol Med* 2003;9:24–29.

167. Hida K, Hida Y, Amin DN, et al. Tumor-associated endothelial cells with cytogenetic abnormalities. *Cancer Res* 2004;64:8249–8255.

168. Streubel B, Chott A, Huber D, et al. Lymphoma-specific genetic aberrations in microvascular endothelial cells in B-cell lymphomas. *N Engl J Med* 2004;351:250–259.

169. Loges S, Mazzone M, Hohensinner P, et al. Silencing or fueling metastasis with VEGF inhibitors: antiangiogenesis revisited. *Cancer Cell* 2009;15:167–170.

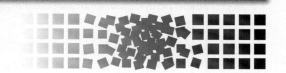

29 Monoclonal Antibodies

Hossein Borghaei, Matthew K. Robinson, Gregory P. Adams, and Louis M. Weiner

INTRODUCTION

Antibody-based therapeutics are important components of the cancer therapeutic armamentarium. Early antibody therapy studies attempted to explicitly target cancers based on the structural and biologic properties that distinguish neoplastic cells from their normal counterparts. The immunogenicity and inefficient effector functions of the first-generation murine monoclonal antibodies (MAb) that were evaluated in clinical trials limited their effectiveness.[1–3] Patients developed human antimouse antibody (HAMA) responses against the therapeutic agents that rapidly cleared it from the body and limited the number of times the therapy could be administered. The development of engineered chimeric, humanized, and fully human MAbs has identified a number of important and useful applications for antibody-based cancer therapy. Currently, the U.S. Food and Drug Administration (FDA) has approved 14 MAbs and MAb-conjugates for the treatment of cancer (Table 29.1) and many more are under evaluation in late-stage clinical trials.[4] Antibodies provide an important means by which to exploit the immune system by specifically recognizing and directing antitumor responses.

Antibodies are produced by B cells and arise in response to exposures to a variety of structures, termed antigens, as a result of a series of recombinations of V, D, and J germline genes. Immunoglobulin-G (IgG) molecules are most commonly employed as the working backbones of current therapeutic monoclonal antibodies, although various other isotypes of antibodies have specialized functions (e.g., IgA molecules play important roles in mucosal immunity, IgE molecules are involved in anaphylaxis). The advent of hybridoma technology by Kohler and Milstein[5] made it possible to produce large quantities of antibodies with high purity and monospecificity for a single binding region (epitope) on an antigen.

The mechanisms that antibody-based therapeutics employ to elicit antitumor effects include focusing components of the patient's immune system to attack tumor cells[6,7] and methods to alter signal transduction pathways that drive tumor progression.[8,9] Antibody-based conjugates employ the targeting specificity of antibodies to deliver toxic compounds, such as chemotherapeutics, specifically to the tumor sites.

IMMUNOGLOBULIN STRUCTURE

Structural and Functional Domains

An IgG molecule is typically divided into three domains consisting of two identical antigen-binding (Fab) domains connected to an effector or Fc domain by a flexible hinge sequence. Figure 29.1 shows the structure of an IgG molecule. IgG antibodies are comprised of two identical light chains and two identical heavy chains, with the chains joined by disulfide bonds, resulting in a bilaterally symmetrical complex. The Fab domains mediate the binding of

IgG molecules to their cognate antigens and are composed of an intact light chain and half of a heavy chain. Each chain in the Fab domain is further divided into variable and constant regions, with the variable region containing hypervariable, or complementarity determining regions (CDR) in which the antigen-contact residues reside. The light and heavy chain variable regions each contain three CDRs (CDR1, CDR2, and CDR3). All six CDRs form the antigen-binding pocket and are collectively defined in immunologic terms as the idiotype of the antibody. In the majority of cases, the variable heavy chain CDR3 plays a dominant role in binding.[10]

The different isotypes of immunoglobulins are defined by the structure and function of their Fc domains. The Fc domain, composed of the CH2 and CH3 regions of the antibody's heavy chains, is the critical determinant of how an antibody mediates effector functions, transports across cellular barriers, and persists in circulation.[7,11]

MODIFIED ANTIBODY-BASED MOLECULES

Advances in antibody engineering and molecular biology have facilitated the development of many novel antibody-based structures with unique physical and pharmacokinetic properties (see Fig. 29.1). These include chimeric human-murine antibodies with human-constant regions and murine-variable regions,[12] humanized antibodies in which murine CDR sequences have been grafted into human IgG molecules, and entirely human antibodies derived from human hybridomas and, more recently, from transgenic mice expressing human immunoglobulin genes.[13] An accepted naming scheme based on "stems" was developed by the World Health Organization's International Nonproprietary Names (INN) for pharmaceuticals and is employed in the United States (Table 29.2). Engineering has also facilitated the development of antibody-based fragments. In addition to the classic, enzymatically derived Fab and F(ab')$_2$ molecules, a plethora of promising IgG-derivatives have been developed that retain antigen-binding properties of intact antibodies (see Fig. 29.1; for review see Robinson et al.[14]). The basic building block for these molecules is the 25 kDa, monovalent single-chain Fv (scFv) that is comprised of the variable domains (V_H and V_L) of an antibody fused together with a short peptide linker. Novel, bispecific antibody-based structures can facilitate binding to two tumor antigens or bridge tumor cells with immune effector cells to focus antibody-dependent cell-mediated cytotoxicity (ADCC) or killing by T cells. An example of the former is MM-111, a bispecific gene-fused molecule composed of an anti-HER2 scFv connected to an anti-HER3 scFv via a modified form of human serum albumin.[15] Examples of the latter mechanism include small scFv-based bispecific T-cell engagers (BiTE) such as the anti-CD3/anti-CD19 molecule blinatumomab[16] and larger MAb-based antibodies such as catumaxomab, a rat/mouse anti-CD3/EpCAM bispecific MAb produced via quadroma technology.[17] Both classes of bispecifics endow selectivity and targeting properties that are not obtainable with natural antibody formats.

TABLE 29.1

FDA Approved Antibodies for the Treatment of Cancer

Generic Name (Trade Name)	Origin	Isotype (Conjugate)	Indication	Target	Initial Approval
Unconjugated MAbs					
Rituximab (Rituxan)	Chimeric	IgG1	NHL	CD20	1997
Trastuzumab (Herceptin)	Humanized	IgG1	BrCa	HER2	1998
Alemtuzumab (Campath-1H)	Humanized	IgG1	CLL	CD52	2001
Cetuximab (Erbitux)	Chimeric	IgG1	CRC, SCCHN	EGFR	2004
Bevacizumab (Avastin)	Humanized	IgG1	CRC, NSCLC, RCC, GBM	VEGF	2004
Panitumumab (Vectibix)	Human (XenoMouse)	IgG2	CRC	EGFR	2006
Ofatumumab (Arzerra)	Human (XenoMouse)	IgG1	CLL	CD20	2009
Denosumab (Prolia/Xgeva)	Human	IgG2	Metastasis-related SREs, ADT/AI-associated osteoporosis, GCT	RANKL	2010
Pertuzumab (Perjeta)	Humanized	IgG1	BrCa	HER2	2012
Immunoconjugates					
Gemtuzumab ozogamicin (Mylotarg)	Humanized	IgG4 (calicheamicin)	AML	CD33	2000[a]
Ibritumomab tiuxetan (Zevalin)	Murine	IgG1 (^{90}Y)	NHL	CD20	2002
Tositumomab (Bexxar)	Murine	IgG2A (^{131}I)	NHL	CD20	2003
Brentuximab vedotin (Adcetris)	Chimeric	IgG1 (MMAE)	HL, sALCL	CD30	2011
Ado-trastuzumab emtansine (Kadcyla)	Humanized	IgG1 (DM1)	BrCa	HER2	2013

[a] Withdrawn from the US market in June 2010.
NHL, non-Hodgkin lymphoma; BrCa, breast cancer; CLL, chronic lymphocytic leukemia; CRC, colorectal cancer; SCCHN, squamous cell carcinoma of head and neck; EGFR, epidermal growth factor receptor; NSCLC, non–small-cell lung cancer; RCC, renal cell carcinoma; GBM, glioblastoma multiforme; VEGF, vascular endothelial growth factor; SREs, skeletal-related events; ADT, androgen deprivation therapy; AI, aromatase inhibitor; GCT, giant cell tumor; RANKL, RANK ligand; AML, acute myelogenous leukemia; ^{90}Y, yttrium-90; ^{131}I, iodine-131; MMAE, Monomethyl auristatin E; HL, Hodgkin lymphoma; sALCL, systemic anaplastic large-cell lymphoma.

IgG

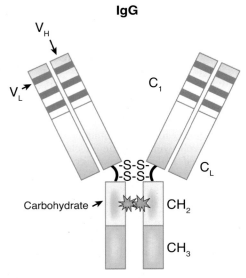

Figure 29.1 Structure of an IgG. C, constant; V, variable; H, heavy chain; L, light chain.

TABLE 29.2

Rules for Naming MAb for the Treatment of Cancer

The International Nonproprietary Names (INN) for monoclonal antibodies (MAbs) are composed of "stems" that indicate their origin, specificity, and modifications. The names include a random prefix to provide distinction from other names, a substem indicating the target specificity (-t[u]- for tumor), a substem indicating the species of origin (see the following) and a suffix (-mab), which indicates the presence of an immunoglobulin variable domain.

Substem Indication of the Species on Which the Immunoglobulin Sequence Is Based	
-o-	mouse
-xi-	chimeric
-zu-	humanized
-xizu-	chimeric/humanized
-u-	human

FACTORS REGULATING ANTIBODY-BASED TUMOR TARGETING

Antibody Size

Nonuniform distribution of systemically administered antibody is generally observed in biopsied specimens of solid tumors. Heterogeneous tumor blood supply limits uniform antibody delivery to tumors, and elevated interstitial pressures in the center of tumors oppose inward diffusion.[18] This high interstitial pressure slows the diffusion of molecules from their vascular extravasation site in a size-dependent manner.[19,20] The relatively large transport distances in the tumor interstitium also substantially increase the time required for large IgG macromolecules to reach target cells.[21]

Tumor Antigens

Access to the target antigen is undoubtedly a critical determinant of therapeutic effect of antibody-based applications. Such access is regulated by the heterogeneity of antigen expression by tumor cells. Shed antigen in the serum, tumor microenvironment, or both may saturate the antibody's binding sites and prevent binding to the cell surface. Alternatively, a rapid internalization of an antibody/antigen complex, although critical for antibody–drug conjugates (ADC), may deplete the quantity of cell surface MAb capable of initiating ADCC or cytotoxic signal transduction events. Finally, target antigens are normally *tumor associated* rather than *tumor specific*. Tumor-specific antigens are both highly desirable and rare. Typically, such antigens arise as a result of unique tumor-based genetic recombinations, such as clonal immunoglobulin idiotypes expressed on the surface of B-cell lymphomas.[22]

Antibody affinity for its target antigen has complex effects on tumor targeting. The *binding-site barrier* hypothesis postulates that antibodies with extremely high affinity for target antigen would bind irreversibly to the first antigen encountered upon entering the tumor, which would limit the diffusion of the antibody into the tumor and accumulate instead in regions surrounding the tumor vasculature.[23,24] Similarly, in tumor spheroids, the in vitro penetration of engineered antibodies is primarily limited by internalization and degradation.[25] The valence of an antibody molecule can increase the functional affinity of the antibody through an avidity effect.[26–28]

Half-Life/Clearance Rate

The concentration of intact IgG in mammalian serum is maintained at constant levels with half-lives of IgGs measured in days. This homeostasis is regulated in part by the major histocompatibility complex (MHC)-class I–related Fc receptor, FcRn (n = neonatal), a saturable, pH-dependent salvage mechanism that regulates quality and quantity of IgG in serum. This mechanism can be exploited via mutations in the Fc portion of an IgG to modulate IgGs pharmacokinetics.[29,30] Indeed, multiple strategies have been developed to increase the serum persistence of antibody-based fragments and other classes of protein therapeutics.[14,31]

Glycosylation

IgGs undergo N-linked glycosylation at the conserved Asn residue at position 297 within the C_H2 domain of the constant region. Glycosylation status of the residue has long been known to impact the ability of IgGs to bind effector ligands such as FcγR and C1q, which, in turn, affects their ability to participate in Fc-mediated functions such as ADCC and complement-dependent cytotoxicity (CDC).[32–34] The glycosylation of MAbs can be altered to increase ADCC by producing them in a cell line engineered to express β(1,4)-N-acetylglucosaminyltransferase III (GnTIII), the enzyme required to add the bisecting GlcNAc residues.[33] Defucosylation of antibody Fc domains is also associated with enhanced ADCC, and in a recently completed multicenter phase II trial of a defucosylated anti-CC chemokine receptor 4 (CCR4), MAb was associated with meaningful antitumor activity, including complete responses and enhanced progression-free survival (PFS).[35]

UNCONJUGATED ANTIBODIES

The majority of monoclonal antibodies approved for clinical use display intrinsic antitumor effects that are mediated by one or more of the following mechanisms.

Cell-Mediated Cytotoxicity

As components of the immune system, effector cells such as natural killer (NK) cells and monocytes/macrophages represent natural lines of defense against oncologically transformed cells. These effector cells express Fcγ receptors (FcγR) on their cell surfaces, which interact with the Fc domain of IgG molecules. This family is comprised of three classes (type I, II, and III) that are further divided into subclasses (IIa/IIb and IIIa/IIIb).[36] Recognition of transformed cells by immune effector cells leads to cell-mediated killing through processes such as ADCC and phagocytosis, as shown in Figure 29.2, and can be mediated by FcγRI (CD64), a high affinity receptor capable of binding to monomeric IgG, or FcγRII (CD32) and FcγRIII (CD16), which are low affinity receptors that preferentially bind multimeric complexes of IgG. Signaling through type I, IIa, and IIIa receptors results in the activation of effector cells due to associated immunoreceptor tyrosine-based activation motifs (ITAM), whereas the engagement of type IIb receptors inhibits cell activation through associated immunoreceptor tyrosine-based inhibitory motifs (ITIM).[36] Clinical results support the idea that ADCC can play a role in the efficacy of antibody-based therapies. Naturally occurring polymorphisms in FcγRs alter their affinity for human IgG1 and have been linked to clinical response.[37,38] A polymorphism in the FCGR3A gene results in either a valine or phenylalanine at position 158 of FcγRIIIa. Human IgG1 binds more strongly to FcγRIIIa-158V than FcγRIIIa-158F, and likewise to NK cells from individuals that are either homozygous for 158F or heterozygous for this polymorphism.[39] The FcγRIIIa-158v was a predictor of early response and was associated with improved PFS.

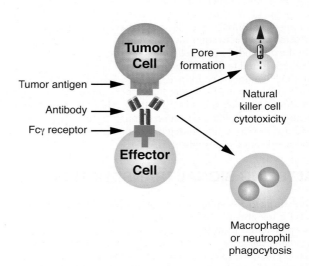

Figure 29.2 Antibody-dependent cellular cytotoxicity. The antibody engages the tumor antigen and the Fc domain binds to cellular Fc receptors to bridge effector and target cells. This bridging induces effector cell activation, resulting in natural killer cell cytotoxicity or phagocytosis by neutrophils, monocytes, or macrophages.

A second polymorphism, FcγRIIa-131H/R, did not predict early response but was an independent predictor of time to progression (TTP).[38] Taken together, these data suggest that modulating the affinity of MAbs for FcγRIIIa, FcγRIIa, or both may increase the efficacy of therapeutic MAbs.

Each class of FcγR exhibits a characteristic specificity for IgG subclasses.[40] Many groups have focused on modifying the Fc domain of IgGs to optimize the engagement of subclasses of FcγR and the induction of ADCC, based on the findings of Shields et al.,[29] who performed a series of mutagenesis experiments to map the residues required for IgG1-FcγR interaction. Antibodies such as ocrelizumab, a humanized version of rituximab, have increased binding to low affinity FcγRIIIa variants and are now in clinical trials.

An alternative to modifying the Fc region of MAbs is to create bispecific antibodies (bsAbs) that recognize both a tumor-associated antigen and a *trigger antigen* present on the surface of an immune effector cell.[43] Simultaneous engagement of both antigens can redirect the cytotoxic potential of the effector cell against the tumor.[41–43] Such antibodies are capable of eliciting effector function against tumor cell lines in vitro and in animal models. Two HER-2 directed bispecific antibodies, 2B1 and MDX-H210, have been tested in phase I clinical trials.[44,45]

Bispecific antibodies have a number of distinctive properties, including flexible choices of cytotoxic trigger molecules,[46] recruitment of effector function in the presence of excess IgG,[42] and custom tailoring of the affinity of the bsAb to match effector cell characteristics. These advantages have been facilitated by improved methods of bsAb production.[47] BiTE antibodies represent a novel class of bispecific, single-chain Fv antibodies.[48] Promising results have been seen in early phase clinical trials with at least two BiTE antibodies, one of which, blinatumomab, targets CD19/CD3.[49] Promising phase I results have also been reported in an interim analysis of an anti-EpCAM/anti-CD3 MT110 BiTE in the setting of advanced lung and gastrointestinal tumors.[50]

Complement-Dependent Cytotoxicity

In addition to cell-mediated killing (see previous), MAbs can recruit the complement cascade to kill cells via CDC. Although IgM is the most effective isotype for complement activation, it is not widely used in clinical oncology. Similar to ADCC, the human IgG subclass used to construct a therapeutic MAb dictates its ability to elicit CDC; IgG1 is extremely efficient at fixing complement, in contrast to IgG2 and IgG4.[51] Antibodies activate complement through the classical pathway, by engaging multiple C1q to trigger activation of a cascade of serum proteases, which kill the antibody-bound cells.[52,53] The anti-CD20 MAb rituximab has been found to depend in part on CDC for its *in vivo* efficacy.[54] Antibody engineering approaches have identified residues in the $C_{H}2$ domain of the Fc region that either suppress or enhance the ability of rituximab to bind C1q and activate CDC.[55] The ability to manipulate complement fixation through engineering approaches warrants *in vivo* testing to determine the impact of these changes on the efficacy and toxicity of MAbs.

ALTERING SIGNAL TRANSDUCTION

Growth factor receptors represent a well-established class of targets for therapeutic intervention. Normal signaling through these receptors often leads to mitogenic and prosurvival responses. Unregulated signaling, as seen in a number of common cancers due to receptor overexpression, promotes tumor cell growth and insensitivity to chemotherapeutic agents. Clinically relevant MAbs can modulate signaling through their target receptors to normalize cell growth rates and sensitize tumor cells to cytotoxic agents. The binding of cetuximab or panitumumab to the epidermal growth factor receptor (EGFR) physically blocks ligand binding[56] and

prevents the receptor from assuming the extended conformation required for dimerization.[57] Pertuzumab binds to the dimerization domain of HER-2, thereby sterically inhibiting subsequent receptor heterodimerization with other ligand-bound family members.[58] Alternatively, signaling through growth factor receptors can be indirectly modified by MAbs that bind to activating ligands, as is seen with the anti–vascular endothelial growth factor (VEGF) MAb, bevacizumab.[59]

IMMUNOCONJUGATES

MAbs that are not capable of directly eliciting antitumor effects, either by altering signal transduction or directing immune system cells, can still be effective against tumors by delivering cytotoxic payloads. MAbs have been employed to deliver a wide variety of agents, including chemotherapy, toxins, radioisotopes, and cytokines (for review see Adams and Weiner[60]). In theory, the appropriate combination of toxic agents and MAbs could lead to a synergistic effect. For example, delivery of a therapeutic radioisotope by a MAb would be significantly enhanced if, by binding to its target antigen, the MAb also activated a signaling event that increased the target cell's sensitivity to ionizing radiation.

Catalytic toxins derived from plants catalytic toxins derived from plants (e.g., ricin) and microorganisms (e.g., Pseudomonas) represent two classes of cytotoxic agent that have been investigated for their utility in immunoconjugate strategies.[61] Although there are promising preclinical studies,[62] few successful clinical trials have been reported using this approach. In a phase I clinical trial in hairy cell leukemia patients who were resistant to cladribine, 11 of 16 patients exhibited complete remissions with minimal side effects with an anti-CD22 immunotoxin with a truncated form of *Pseudomonas exotoxin*.[63] Clinical trials with other immunotoxins have been associated with unacceptable neurotoxicity[64] and life-threatening vascular leak syndrome.[65]

Immunocytokine fusions have also been investigated as an approach to direct the patient's immune response to his or her own tumor.[66] A number of cytokines have been incorporated into antibody-based constructs, including interleukin-2 (IL-2),[67,68] interferon γ (IFN-γ),[69] tumor necrosis factor α (TFN-α),[69] VEGF,[70] and IL-12.[71]

Antibody–Drug Conjugates

The first ADC, gemtuzumab ozogamicin (Mylotarg), was approved by the FDA in 2000 for the treatment of patients with relapsed CD33-positive acute myeloid leukemia, but was voluntarily withdrawn from the US market by its manufacturer in 2010 after a confirmatory phase III trial (SWOG S0106) recommended, based on results of a planned interim analysis, that Mylotarg randomizations be terminated due to a lack of efficacy in the presence of enhanced toxicity.[72] Although two additional randomized trials[73,74] suggested that some patient populations may benefit from Mylotarg therapy, the drug remains off the market in the United States.

The majority of ADCs under development employ potent cytotoxic agents that block the polymerization of tubulin (e.g., auristatins or maytansines) or damage DNA (e.g., calicheamicins or pyrrolobenzodiazepines) by employing a variety of linkers and conjugation strategies.[75] A variety of ADCs specific for a wide range of oncology targets are currently in clinical evaluation, with the majority of the more advanced agents being tested in the setting of diffuse malignancies.[76] The majority of these employ auristatins or maytansines as their payloads. Early observations suggest that cumulative, dose-related peripheral sensory neuropathy can result when auristatins are conjugated to an antibody via a cleavable linker, and dose-limiting thrombocytopenia can result when auristatins and maytansinoids are conjugated to the antibody via an uncleavable linker.[76,77]

Two ADCs are now approved for use in clinical practice. Ado-trastuzumab emtansine (T-DM1, Kadcyla), an ADC composed of the anti-HER2 MAb trastuzumab linked to DM1,[78] is now approved for the treatment of patients with refractory HER2/neu expressing breast cancers. The other, brentuximab vedotin (SGN-35, Adcetris), is an ADC consisting of the anti-CD30 chimeric MAb cAC10 that is linked to three to five molecules of the microtubule-disrupting agent Monomethyl auristatin E. At this point, this drug is approved for use in patients with recurrent systemic anaplastic large cell lymphoma. The clinical data associated with both of these ADCs will be discussed in subsequent sections of this chapter.

Antibodies also can be used to target liposome-encapsulated drugs[79] and other cytotoxic agents, such as antisense RNA[80] or radionuclides to tumors.

Radioimmunoconjugates

Two anti-CD20 radioimmunoconjugates have been FDA approved for radioimmunotherapy (RIT) of non-Hodgkin lymphoma (NHL). Ibritumomab (Zevalin) and tositumomab (Bexxar) are murine MAbs labeled with yttrium-90 (^{90}Y) and iodine-131 (^{131}I), respectively. Both are associated with impressive clinical efficacy.[81,82] Although these radioimmunoconjugates are effective therapeutics, cumbersome logistics surrounding their administration have significantly limited their use. Despite significant preclinical evidence supporting the use of RIT for solid malignancies, clinical results have not demonstrated consistent antitumor activity.[60]

ANTIBODIES APPROVED FOR USE IN SOLID TUMORS

Trastuzumab

Trastuzumab (Herceptin) is a humanized IgG1[83] that targets domain IV of the HER2/ErbB2 member of the EGFR/ErbB family of receptor tyrosine kinases. Gene amplification as judged by fluorescence in situ hybridization (FISH) with concomitant overexpression of HER2 protein measured by immunohistochemistry (IHC) is seen in approximately 25% of breast cancers.[84,85] HER2 amplification and overexpression is now recognized to also be a critical driver in a subset (7% to 34%) of gastric cancers.[86] Trastuzumab inhibits tumor cell growth by binding to HER2 and blocking the unregulated HER2 signaling that is associated with its high level overexpression.

Trastuzumab became the first FDA-approved monoclonal antibody for the treatment of solid tumors based on a series of studies carried out in the setting of HER2-positive metastatic breast cancer.[87,88] A subsequent phase III trial investigating trastuzumab in combination with cytotoxic chemotherapy demonstrated an improved response rate compared to chemotherapy alone, from 25.0% to 57.3% with a taxane regimen.[89]

Trastuzumab is also approved for use in the adjuvant setting based on an approximately 50% reduction in recurrence after 1 year in multiple phase III trials.[90–92] Myocardial dysfunction, seen with anthracycline therapy, was observed with increased frequency in patients receiving antibody alone[93] or with doxorubicin or epirubicin.

Recognition of HER2 as a driver in a subset of gastric cancers led to an open-label, randomized, phase III trial (ToGA) that investigated the addition of trastuzumab to standard of care chemotherapy[94] and showed increased median overall survival with higher levels of HER2 expression. A study by Gomez-Martin et al.[95] in 99 patients with metastatic gastric cancer being treated with first-line trastuzumab plus chemotherapy identified a mean HER2/CEP17 ratio of 4.7 to be an optimal cut-off to discriminate between trastuzumab-sensitive and refractory patients.

Pertuzumab

Pertuzumab (Perjeta) is a humanized IgG1 MAb that binds to domain II of HER2 and blocks ligand-dependent dimerization of HER2 with other members of the EGFR family.[96] Pertuzumab, in combination with trastuzumab and docetaxel, is approved for use as first-line therapy in HER2-positive metastatic breast cancer patients. Use of the combination is also approved for the treatment of HER2-positive, locally advanced, inflammatory, or high-risk early breast cancer (>2 cm node negative or node positive) in the neoadjuvant setting.

FDA-approval of pertuzumab was based on results of a phase III trial (CLEOPATRA) of 808 patients with locally recurrent, unresectable, or metastatic breast cancer randomized to receive trastuzumab plus docetaxel with or without the addition of pertuzumab. Inclusion of pertuzumab increased the independently assessed PFS by 6.1 months from 12.4 to 18.5 (hazard ratio [HR], 0.62 (95% confidence interval [CI], 0.51, 0.75), p <0.0001], with a trend toward improved overall survival[97] that reached statistical significance (p = 0.0008) after an additional year of follow-up.[98] The addition of pertuzumab did increase rates of grade 3 adverse events (AE), but it did not adversely affect cardiac function. Accelerated approval was granted for use of pertuzumab in combination with trastuzumab and docetaxel for the neoadjuvant treatment of high-risk early-stage breast cancer. This approval was based on results from a four-arm, open-label phase II study of 417 patients randomized to receive trastuzumab plus docetaxel, pertuzumab plus docetaxel, pertuzumab plus trastuzumab, or the triple combination. The triple combination improved the pathologic complete response (pCR) rate by 17.8% over the trastuzumab plus docetaxel arm (39.3% versus 21.5%) in the pertuzumab arm.[99] Follow-up studies to confirm a correlation between pCR and long-term clinical benefit are ongoing.

Cetuximab

Cetuximab (Erbitux) targets the EGFR. This chimeric IgG1 binds to domain III of the EGFR, with roughly a tenfold higher affinity than either EGF or transforming growth factor α (TGF-α) ligands and thereby inhibits ligand-induced activation of this tyrosine kinase receptor. Cetuximab may also function to downregulate EGFR-dependent signaling by stimulating EGFR internalization.[100] Cetuximab is approved for the treatment of colorectal cancer (CRC) and, more recently, for the treatment of squamous cell cancer of the head and neck (SCCHN).

The efficacy and safety of cetuximab against CRC was demonstrated alone and in combination with irinotecan in a phase II, multicenter, randomized, and controlled trial of 329 patients.[101] The combination of irinotecan plus cetuximab increased both the overall response and the median duration of response as compared to cetuximab alone. Additionally, patients with irinotecan refractory disease responded to treatment with the combination regimen. Recent studies in patients with colorectal cancers have indicated that patients with KRAS mutations in codon 12 or 13 should not receive anti-EGFR therapy.[101,102]

An international, multicenter, phase III trial comparing definitive radiotherapy to radiotherapy plus cetuximab in SCCHN demonstrated that EGFR blockade with radiotherapy significantly reduced the risk of locoregional failure by 32% and the risk of death by 26%. In advanced stage non–small-cell lung cancer (NSCLC) expressing EGFR, the combination of cetuximab and standard doublet chemotherapy (cisplatin plus vinorelbine) was studied in a prospective randomized phase III trial.[103] The addition of cetuximab was associated with a slight, but statistically significant, benefit in overall survival over chemotherapy alone (median overall survival 10.1 versus 11.3 months). A similar study using the carboplatin plus paclitaxel backbone in combination with cetuximab did not meet its primary endpoint of improved PFS, although cetuximab-treated patients exhibited higher objective response rates.[104] Therefore, the benefit of adding cetuximab to standard chemotherapy for patients with advanced NSCLC is unclear.

Panitumumab

Panitumumab (Vectibix) is a fully human IgG2 monoclonal antibody that binds to EGFR. Similar to cetuximab, panitumumab inhibits EGFR activation by blocking the binding of EGF and TGF-α. However, it does so by binding to EGFR with a higher affinity than cetuximab (5×10^{-11} M versus 1×10^{-10} M). As previously mentioned, the IgG2 class of antibodies does not induce activation of the immune system cell via the Fc-receptor mechanism, so panitumumab's primary action appears to be interference with EGFR–ligand interactions.

A phase III trial of 463 patients with metastatic colorectal cancer compared panitumumab plus best supportive care (BSC) to BSC alone.[105] A partial-response rate of 8% and a stable-disease rate of 28% were reported for the panitumumab arm compared with a 10% stable-disease rate in the best supportive care arm of the study. As with cetuximab, patients with metastatic colorectal cancers who have KRAS mutations in codons 12 or 13 are not routinely offered therapy with panitumumab.[106]

Bevacizumab

Bevacizumab (Avastin or rhuMAb VEGF) is a humanized monoclonal antibody targeting VEGF. VEGF is a critical determinant of tumor angiogenesis, a process that is a necessary component of tumor invasion, growth, and metastasis. VEGF expression by invasive tumors has been shown to correlate with vascularity and cellular proliferation and is prognostic for several human cancers.[107–109] Interestingly, the inhibition of VEGF signaling via bevacizumab treatment may normalize tumor vasculature, promoting a more effective delivery of chemotherapy agents.[110] Bevacizumab is approved for use as a first-line therapy for metastatic colorectal cancer and NSCLC when given in combination with appropriate cytotoxic chemotherapy regimens. Phase III clinical trials leading to the approval of bevacizumab for the treatment of colorectal cancer demonstrated improved response rates from 35% to 45% compared to fluorouracil (5-FU)–based chemotherapy alone. Enhanced response durations and improved patient survival were seen in patients treated with chemotherapy plus bevacizumab as compared to patients receiving chemotherapy alone.[111] A survival benefit was also seen in the setting of NSCLC. A randomized phase III trial (ECOG 4599) of paclitaxel and carboplatin with or without bevacizumab in patients with advanced nonsquamous NSCLC led to a significant improvement in median survival (12.5 months versus 10.2 months; p = 0.0075) for patients in the bevacizumab arm,[112] with significantly higher response rates. A higher incidence of bleeding was associated with bevacizumab (4.5% versus 0.7%). Five of 10 treatment-related deaths occurred as a result of hemoptysis, all in the bevacizumab arm.

A phase III trial randomized 722 patients with metastatic breast cancer with no prior chemotherapy for advanced disease to either paclitaxel or paclitaxel and bevacizumab.[113] PFS was significantly better in the paclitaxel plus bevacizumab arm (median, 11.8 versus 5.9 months; HR for progression, 0.60; p <0.001) with an increased response rate (36.9% versus 21.2%, p <0.001). Overall survival, however, was similar. In contrast,[114] in a randomized phase III trial, capecitabine/bevacizumab increased response rates compared with capecitabine alone in 462 anthracycline and taxane pretreated metastatic breast cancer patients but did not meet its primary endpoint of improved PFS. Overall survival and time to deterioration in quality of life were comparable in both treatment groups.

Bevacizumab has not demonstrated activity in the adjuvant colorectal and breast cancer settings.[115,116] There was no improvement in overall survival between the two groups and the rate of invasive disease-free survival was also not significantly different between the treatment groups.

Bevacizumab is also approved for the management of recurrent glioblastomas based on results of phase II studies.[117]

Ado-Trastuzumab Emtansine

Ado-trastuzumab emtansine (T-DM1, Kadcyla) is an ADC composed of the anti-HER2 MAb trastuzumab linked to DM1, a highly potent derivative of maytansine, through a stable thioether linker.[78]

Based on two single-agent phase II trials of T-DM1[118,119] that demonstrated single-agent activity in the setting of metastatic breast cancer, two separate phase III studies were conducted. The 991 patient EMILIA trial demonstrated that T-DM1 significantly prolongs both PFS and overall survival as compared to a regimen of lapatinib plus capecitabine when used in the setting of metastatic breast cancer that had progressed after treatment with trastuzumab plus a taxane.[120] Grade 3 and worse AEs were lower in the T-DM1 arm (200, 40.8%) as compared to the lapatinib plus capecitabine arm (278, 57%). Results are still awaited from the ongoing MARIANNE trial that is assessing first-line efficacy and safety of T-DM1 alone and T-DM1 plus pertuzumab versus trastuzumab plus taxane (NCT01120184).

Denosumab

Denosumab (Xgeva) is a fully human IgG2 RANK ligand (RANKL) neutralizing antibody. Denosumab is FDA-approved for use in adults and skeletally mature adolescents who have either surgically unsalvageable giant cell tumors of the bone (GCTB) or where resection is anticipated to result in severe morbidity. Approval was based in part on two open-label, phase II trials examining subcutaneous administration of 120 mg q4 week with additional loading doses on days 8 and 15 of the first cycle.[121,122] Serious adverse events were seen in 9% of patients (n = 25). Of 187 patients, 47 (25%) exhibited partial objective responses based on modified Response Evaluation Criteria in Solid Tumors (RECIST) criteria.

Denosumab is also approved in for use in two supportive care settings based on three randomized, double-blind, placebo-controlled phase III trials evaluating its efficacy versus zoledronic acid[123–125] to reduce bone metastasis-related skeletal-related events (SRE). Based on data from two phase III trials, a second formulation and dosing schedule of denosumab is approved to increase bone mass in prostate cancer[126] and breast cancer[127] patients at high risk for bone fracture due to hormone-ablation therapies.

ANTIBODIES USED IN HEMATOLOGIC MALIGNANCIES

Rituximab

Rituximab (Rituxan) is a chimeric anti-CD20 monoclonal antibody that was the first MAb to be approved by the FDA for use in human malignancy.[128,129] Studies have shown that multiple doses can be safely administered, and *in vitro* studies have demonstrated multiple mechanisms by which anti-CD20 antibodies can lead to cell death.[130] Efficacy of rituximab monotherapy is well established.[131]

Rituximab has been tested in conjunction with chemotherapy based on supportive preclinical data.[132,133] The combination of rituximab with cyclophosphamide, doxorubicin, vincristine, and prednisolone (CHOP) resulted in a 95% overall response rate (55% complete response, 40% partial response) among 40 patients with low-grade or follicular B-cell non–Hodgkin lymphoma, with molecular complete remissions observed.[134] A long-term study of elderly patients with previously untreated diffuse large-cell lymphoma randomized to either CHOP chemotherapy plus rituximab (R-CHOP) or CHOP alone demonstrated a significant improvement in event-free survival, PFS, disease-free survival, and overall survival for the combination arm.[135] No significant differences in long-term toxicity were noted.

Low-grade B-cell lymphoma patients possessing the 158V/V polymorphism in FcγRIII experience superior response rates and outcomes when treated with rituximab.[37,38] These findings signify that antibody Fc domain::Fc receptor interactions underlie at least some of the clinical benefit of rituximab, and indicate a possible role for ADCC that depends on such interactions.

A combination of active agents (such as lenalidomide and thalidomide) that are also immune modulating may be additive with rituximab,[136] and perhaps synergize by increasing ADCC.[137] Cytokines such as interleukin-2 (IL-2), IL-12, or IL-15 and myeloid growth factors may also enhance therapeutic antibody activity as suggested by preclinical data demonstrating that IL-2 can promote NK cell proliferation and activation and can enhance rituximab activity[138] and clinical efficacy.[139,140] Myeloid growth factors, in combination with rituximab, may also activate ADCC.[141] Alternative approaches to induce effector cell activity by combining Toll-like receptors (TLR) agonists, such as CpG oligonucleotides, have been investigated.[142] Altering the balance of proapoptotic and antiapoptotic signals could generate more rituximab-induced cytotoxicity. BCL-2 downregulation by antisense oligonucleotides was found to enhance rituximab efficacy in preclinical testing.[143,144] However, small molecules that bind to the BH-3 domain common to many members of the BCL-2 family of proteins may be better therapeutic agents.[145–147]

Ofatumumab

The anti-CD20 ofatumumab[148] is a fully human antibody that binds an epitope on CD20 distinct from that bound by rituximab and is engineered for better complement activation, although it induces less ADCC. Ofatumumab has received regulatory approval for the treatment of patients with fludarabine-refractory chronic lymphocytic leukemia (CLL). In a recently reported, planned interim analysis that included 138 CLL patients with treatment-refractory disease or bulky (>5 cm) lymphadenopathy, treatment with ofatumumab led to an overall response rate (primary endpoint) of 47% in patients with bulky disease and 5% in patients refractory to both alemtuzumab and fludarabine.[149]

Additional humanized anti-CD20 antibodies (veltuzumab[150] and ocrelizumab) are under development.

Alemtuzumab

Alemtuzumab (Campath-1H) targets the CD52 glycopeptide, which is highly expressed on T and B lymphocytes. It has been tested as a therapeutic agent for CLL and promyelocytic leukemias, as well as other non–Hodgkin lymphomas.

Brentuximab Vedotin

Brentuximab vedotin (SGN-35, Adcetris) is an ADC consisting of the anti-CD30 chimeric MAb cAC10 that is linked to three to five molecules of the microtubule-disrupting agent Monomethyl auristatin E (MMAE). MMAE is a highly potent derivative of dolastatin. Linkage of MMAE to cAC10 occurs through a protease-cleavable linter.[151] Brentuximab vedotin is approved for treating systemic, chemotherapy-refractory anaplastic large-cell lymphomas (sALCL). It is also approved to treat patients with Hodgkin lymphoma who have progressed after an autologous stem cell transplant (ASCT). Patients ineligible for ASCT must have failed two prior multidrug chemotherapy regimens.

Brentuximab vedotin received accelerated approval in 2011 based in part on the results of two phase II trials. In a multicenter trial conducted by Pro et al.,[152] 58 patients with relapsed or refractory sALCL received brentuximab vedotin (1.8 mg per kilogram per week), and 86% of patients achieved objective response. Complete responses occurred in 57% of patients, with a median duration of 13.2 months. An additional 17 patients (29%) had partial responses. Median overall response was 12.6 months. Most common grade 3 and 4 adverse events (AE) were neutropenia (21%), thrombocytopenia (14%), and peripheral sensory neuropathy (12%). A similar trial, in Hodgkin lymphoma, was reported by Younes et al.[153] Patients (n = 102) that had failed ASCT received brentuximab vedotin on the same schedule as listed previously and were assessed for the objective response rate. In this setting, 75% of patients had objective responses, with 34% being complete remissions. The median duration of complete responses was 20.5 months, and 31 patients were progression free after a median follow-up of 1.5 years. Phase III trials to assess the known risk of neuropathy (AETHERA) and to confirm overall clinical benefit seen in the phase II trials (ECHELON-2, or ClinicalTrials.gov Identifier NCT01712490) are ongoing.

CONCLUSION

In the 35 years since Kohler and Milstein first developed the hybridoma technology that enabled antibody-based therapeutics, the field has made remarkable progress. Numerous antibody-based molecules are currently in clinical trials and many more are in development. Multiple therapeutic antibodies have a proven clinical benefit and have been licensed by the FDA. The thoughtful application of advances in cancer biology and antibody engineering suggest that this progress will continue.

REFERENCES

1. Badger CC, Anasetti C, Davis J, et al. Treatment of malignancy with unmodified antibody. *Pathol Immunopathol Res* 1987;6:419–434.
2. Khazaeli MB, Conry RM, Lobuglio AF. Human immune-response to monoclonal-antibodies. *J Immunother Emphasis Tumor Immunol* 1994;15:42–52.
3. Lee J, Fenton BM, Koch CJ, et al. Interleukin 2 expression by tumor cells alters both the immune response and the tumor microenvironment. *Cancer Res* 1998;58:1478–1485.
4. Reichert JM, Dhimolea E. The future of antibodies as cancer drugs. *Drug Discov Today* 2012;17:954–963.
5. Kohler G, Milstein C. Continuous cultures of fused cells secreting antibody of predefined specificity. *Nature* 1975;256:495–497.
6. Houghton AN, Mintzer D, Cordon-Cardo C, et al. Mouse monoclonal IgG3 antibody detecting GD3 ganglioside: a phase I trial in patients with malignant melanoma. *Proc Natl Acad Sci U S A* 1985;82:1242–1246.
7. Steplewski Z, Lubeck MD, Koprowski H. Human macrophages armed with murine immunoglobulin G2a antibodies to tumors destroy human cancer cells. *Science* 1983;221:865–867.
8. Trauth BC, Klas C, Peters AM, et al. Monoclonal antibody-mediated tumor regression by induction of apoptosis. *Science* 1989;245:301–305.
9. Yang XD, Jia XC, Corvalan JR, et al. Eradication of established tumors by a fully human monoclonal antibody to the epidermal growth factor receptor without concomitant chemotherapy. *Cancer Res* 1999;59:1236–1243.
10. Komissarov AA, Calcutt MJ, Marchbank MT, et al. Equilibrium binding studies of recombinant anti-single-stranded DNA Fab. Role of heavy chain complementarity-determining regions. *J Biol Chem* 1996;271:12241–12246.
11. Ghetie V, Popov S, Borvak J, et al. Increasing the serum persistence of an IgG fragment by random mutagenesis. *Nat Biotechnol* 1997;15:637–640.
12. LoBuglio AF, Wheeler RH, Trang J, et al. Mouse/human chimeric monoclonal antibody in man: kinetics and immune response. *Proc Natl Acad Sci U S A* 1989;86:4220–4224.
13. Kudo T, Saeki H, Tachibana T. A simple and improved method to generate human hybridomas. *J Immunol Methods* 1991;145:119–125.
14. Robinson MK, Weiner LM, Adams GP. Improving monoclonal antibodies for cancer therapy. *Drug Dev Res* 2004;61:172–187.
15. Denlinger CS, Beeram M, Tolcher AW, et al. A phase I/II and pharmacologic study of MM-111 in patients with advanced, refractory HER2-positive (HER2+) cancers. *J Clin Oncol* 2010;28:15s.
16. Nagorsen D, Bargou R, Ruttinger D, et al. Immunotherapy of lymphoma and leukemia with T-cell engaging BiTE antibody blinatumomab. *Leuk Lymphoma* 2009;50:886–891.
17. Goere D, Flament C, Rusakiewicz S, et al. Potent immunomodulatory effects of the trifunctional antibody catumaxomab. *Cancer Res* 2013;73:4663–4673.
18. Jain RK. Transport of molecules in the tumor interstitium: a review. *Cancer Res* 1987;47:3039–3051.

19. Jain RK. Physiological barriers to delivery of monoclonal antibodies and other macromolecules in tumors. *Cancer Res* 1990;50:814s–819s.

20. Jain RK, Baxter LT. Mechanisms of heterogeneous distribution of monoclonal antibodies and other macromolecules in tumors: significance of elevated interstitial pressure. *Cancer Res* 1988;48:7022–7032.

21. Jain RK. Transport of molecules across tumor vasculature. *Cancer Metastasis Rev* 1987;6:559–593.

22. Miller RA, Maloney DG, Warnke R, et al. Treatment of B-cell lymphoma with monoclonal anti-idiotype antibody. *N Engl J Med* 1982;306:517–522.

23. Fujimori K, Covell DG, Fletcher JE, et al. A modeling analysis of monoclonal antibody percolation through tumors: a binding site barrier. *J Nucl Med* 1990;31:1191–1198.

24. Rudnick SI, Lou J, Shaller CC, et al. Influence of affinity and antigen internalization on the uptake and penetration of Anti-HER2 antibodies in solid tumors. *Cancer Res* 2011;71:2250–2259.

25. Thurber GM, Wittrup KD. Quantitative spatiotemporal analysis of antibody fragment diffusion and endocytic consumption in tumor spheroids. *Cancer Res* 2008;68:3334–3341.

26. Adams GP, Tai MS, McCartney JE, et al. Avidity-mediated enhancement of in vivo tumor targeting by single-chain Fv dimers. *Clin Cancer Res* 2006;12:1599–1605.

27. Wolff EA, Schreiber GJ, Cosand WL, et al. Monoclonal antibody homodimers: enhanced antitumor activity in nude mice. *Cancer Res* 1993;53:2560–2565.

28. Werlen RC, Lankinen M, Offord RE, et al. Preparation of a trivalent antigen-binding construct using polyoxime chemistry: improved biodistribution and potential for therapeutic application. *Cancer Res* 1996;56:809–815.

29. Shields RL, Namenuk AK, Hong K, et al. High resolution mapping of the binding site on human IgG1 for Fc gamma RI, Fc gamma RII, Fc gamma RIII, and FcRn and design of IgG1 variants with improved binding to the Fc gamma R. *J Biol Chem* 2001;276:6591–6604.

30. Kenanova V, Olafsen T, Crow DM, et al. Tailoring the pharmacokinetics and positron emission tomography imaging properties of anti-carcinoembryonic antigen single-chain Fv-Fc antibody fragments. *Cancer Res* 2005;65:622–631.

31. McDonagh CF, Huhalov A, Harms BD, et al. Antitumor activity of a novel bispecific antibody that targets the ErbB2/ErbB3 oncogenic unit and inhibits heregulin-induced activation of ErbB3. *Mol Cancer Ther* 2012;11:582–593.

32. Lund J, Takahashi N, Pound JD, et al. Multiple interactions of IgG with its core oligosaccharide can modulate recognition by complement and human Fc gamma receptor I and influence the synthesis of its oligosaccharide chains. *J Immunol* 1996;157:4963–4969.

33. Umana P, Jean-Mairet J, Moudry R, et al. Engineered glycoforms of an antineuroblastoma IgG1 with optimized antibody-dependent cellular cytotoxic activity. *Nat Biotechnol* 1999;17:176–180.

34. Wright A, Morrison SL. Effect of glycosylation on antibody function: implications for genetic engineering. *Trends Biotechnol* 1997;15:26–32.

35. Ishida T, Joh T, Uike N, et al. Defucosylated anti-CCR4 monoclonal antibody (KW-0761) for relapsed adult T-cell leukemia-lymphoma: a multicenter phase II study. *J Clin Oncol* 2012;30:837–842.

36. Raghavan M, Bjorkman PJ. Fc receptors and their interactions with immunoglobulins. *Annu Rev Cell Dev Biol* 1996;12:181–220.

37. Cartron G, Dacheux L, Salles G, et al. Therapeutic activity of humanized anti-CD20 monoclonal antibody and polymorphism in IgG Fc receptor FcgammaRIIIa gene. *Blood* 2002;99:754–758.

38. Weng WK, Levy R. Two immunoglobulin G fragment C receptor polymorphisms independently predict response to rituximab in patients with follicular lymphoma. *J Clin Oncol* 2003;21:3940–3947.

39. Koene HR, Kleijer M, Algra J, et al. Fc gammaRIIIa-158V/F polymorphism influences the binding of IgG by natural killer cell Fc gammaRIIIa, independently of the Fc gammaRIIIa-48L/R/H phenotype. *Blood* 1997;90:1109–1114.

40. Gessner JE, Heiken H, Tamm A, et al. The IgG Fc receptor family. *Ann Hematol* 1998;76:231–248.

41. Keler T, Graziano RF, Mandal A, et al. Bispecific antibody-dependent cellular cytotoxicity of HER2/neu-overexpressing tumor cells by Fcgamma receptor type I-expressing effector cells. *Cancer Res* 1997;57:4008–4014.

42. Weiner LM, Holmes M, Richeson A, et al. Binding and cytotoxicity characteristics of the bispecific murine monoclonal antibody 2B1. *J Immunol* 1993;151:2877–2886.

43. Shalaby MR, Shepard HM, Presta L, et al. Development of humanized bispecific antibodies reactive with cytotoxic lymphocytes and tumor cells overexpressing the HER2 protooncogene. *J Exp Med* 1992;175:217–225.

44. Valone FH, Kaufman PA, Guyre PM, et al. Phase Ia/Ib trial of bispecific antibody MDX-210 in patients with advanced breast or ovarian cancer that overexpresses the proto-oncogene HER-2/neu. *J Clin Oncol* 1995;13:2281–2292.

45. Weiner LM, Clark JI, Davey M, et al. Phase I trial of 2B1, a bispecific monoclonal antibody targeting c-erbB-2 and FcgammaRIII. *Cancer Res* 1995;55:4586–4593.

46. Liu MA, Kranz DM, Kurnick JT, et al. Heteroantibody duplexes target cells for lysis by cytotoxic T lymphocytes. *Proc Natl Acad Sci U S A* 1985;82:8648–8652.

47. Carter P. Bispecific human IgG by design. *J Immunol Methods* 2001;248:7–15.

48. Mack M, Riethmuller G, Kufer P. A small bispecific antibody construct expressed as a functional single-chain molecule with high tumor cell cytotoxicity. *Proc Natl Acad Sci U S A* 1995;92:7021–7025.

49. Bargou R, Leo E, Zugmaier G, et al. Tumor regression in cancer patients by very low doses of a T cell-engaging antibody. *Science* 2008;321:974–977.

50. Fiedler W, Hönemann D, Ritter B, et al. Safety and pharmacology of the EpCAM/CD3-bispecific BiTE antibody MT110 in patients with metastatic colorectal, gastric, and lung cancer. *Eur J Cancer* 2009;7:136–137.

51. Presta LG. Engineering antibodies for therapy. *Curr Pharm Biotechnol* 2002;3:237–256.

52. Makrides SC. Therapeutic inhibition of the complement system. *Pharmacol Rev* 1998;50:59–87.

53. Walport MJ. Complement, First of two parts. *N Engl J Med* 2001;344:1058–1066.

54. Di Gaetano N, Cittera E, Nota R, et al. Complement activation determines the therapeutic activity of rituximab in vivo. *J Immunol* 2003;171:1581–1587.

55. Idusogie EE, Presta LG, Gazzano-Santoro H, et al. Mapping of the C1q binding site on Rituxan, a chimeric antibody with a human IgG1 Fc. *J Immunol* 2000;164:4178–4184.

56. Sunada H, Magun BE, Mendelsohn J, et al. Monoclonal antibody against epidermal growth factor receptor is internalized without stimulating receptor phosphorylation. *Proc Natl Acad Sci U S A* 1986;83:3825–3829.

57. Li S, Schmitz KR, Jeffrey PD, et al. Structural basis for inhibition of the epidermal growth factor receptor by cetuximab. *Cancer Cell* 2005;7:301–311.

58. Franklin MC, Carey KD, Vajdos FF, et al. Insights into ErbB signaling from the structure of the ErbB2-pertuzumab complex. *Cancer Cell* 2004;5:317–328.

59. Presta LG, Chen H, O'Connor SJ, et al. Humanization of an anti-vascular endothelial growth factor monoclonal antibody for the therapy of solid tumors and other disorders. *Cancer Res* 1997;57:4593–4599.

60. Adams GP, Weiner LM. Monoclonal antibody therapy of cancer. *Nat Biotechnol* 2005;23:1147–1157.

61. Reiter Y, Pastan I. Recombinant Fv immunotoxins and Fv fragments as novel agents for cancer therapy and diagnosis. *Trends Biotechnol* 1998;16:513–520.

62. Kreitman RJ, Wang QC, FitzGerald DJ, et al. Complete regression of human B-cell lymphoma xenografts in mice treated with recombinant anti-CD22 immunotoxin RFB4(dsFv)-PE38 at doses tolerated by cynomolgus monkeys. *Int J Cancer* 1999;81:148–155.

63. Kreitman RJ, Wilson WH, Bergeron K, et al. Efficacy of the anti-CD22 recombinant immunotoxin BL22 in chemotherapy-resistant hairy-cell leukemia. *N Engl J Med* 2001;345:241–247.

64. Pai LH, Bookman MA, Ozols RF, et al. Clinical evaluation of intraperitoneal Pseudomonas exotoxin immunoconjugate OVB3-PE in patients with ovarian cancer. *J Clin Oncol* 1991;9:2095–2103.

65. Baluna R, Vitetta ES. Vascular leak syndrome: a side effect of immunotherapy. *Immunopharmacology* 1997;37:117–132.

66. Lode HN, Xiang R, Becker JC, et al. Immunocytokines: a promising approach to cancer immunotherapy. *Pharmacol Ther* 1998;80:277–292.

67. Hornick JL, Khawli LA, Hu P, et al. Pretreatment with a monoclonal antibody/interleukin-2 fusion protein directed against DNA enhances the delivery of therapeutic molecules to solid tumors. *Clin Cancer Res* 1999;5:51–60.

68. Lode HN, Xiang R, Duncan SR, et al. Tumor-targeted IL-2 amplifies T cell-mediated immune response induced by gene therapy with single-chain IL-12. *Proc Natl Acad Sci U S A* 1999;96:8591–8596.

69. Sharifi J, Khawli LA, Hu P, et al. Generation of human interferon gamma and tumor necrosis factor alpha chimeric TNT-3 fusion proteins. *Hybrid Hybridomics* 2002;21:421–432.

70. Halin C, Niesner U, Villani ME, et al. Tumor-targeting properties of antibody-vascular endothelial growth factor fusion proteins. *Int J Cancer* 2002;102:109–116.

71. Halin C, Rondini S, Nilsson F, et al. Enhancement of the antitumor activity of interleukin-12 by targeted delivery to neovasculature. *Nature Biotechnol* 2002;20:264–269.

72. Petersdorf SH, Kopecky KJ, Slovak M, et al. A phase 3 study of gemtuzumab ozogamicin during induction and postconsolidation therapy in younger patients with acute myeloid leukemia. *Blood* 2013;121:4854–4860.

73. Burnett AK, Hills RK, Milligan D, et al. Identification of patients with acute myeloblastic leukemia who benefit from the addition of gemtuzumab ozogamicin: results of the MRC AML15 trial. *J Clin Oncol* 2011;29:369–377.

74. Castaigne S, Pautas C, Terre C, et al. Effect of gemtuzumab ozogamicin on survival of adult patients with de-novo acute myeloid leukaemia (ALFA-0701): a randomised, open-label, phase 3 study. *Lancet* 2012;379:1508–1516.

75. Ducry L, Stump B. Antibody-drug conjugates: linking cytotoxic payloads to monoclonal antibodies. *Bioconjug Chem* 2010;21:5–13.

76. Lambert JM. Drug-conjugated antibodies for the treatment of cancer. *Br J Clin Pharmacol* 2013;76:248–262.

77. van de Donk NW, Dhimolea E. Brentuximab vedotin. *MAbs* 2012;4:458–465.

78. LoRusso PM, Weiss D, Guardino E, et al. Trastuzumab emtansine: a unique antibody-drug conjugate in development for human epidermal growth factor receptor 2-positive cancer. *Clin Cancer Res* 2011;17:6437–6447.

79. Park JW, Hong K, Kirpotin DB, et al. Anti-HER2 immunoliposomes: enhanced efficacy attributable to targeted delivery. *Clin Cancer Res* 2002;8:1172–1181.

80. Rodriguez M, Coma S, Noe V, et al. Development and effects of immunoliposomes carrying an antisense oligonucleotide against DHFR RNA and directed toward human breast cancer cells overexpressing HER2. *Antisense Nucleic Acid Drug Dev* 2002;12:311–325.

81. Juweid ME. Radioimmunotherapy of B-cell non-Hodgkin's lymphoma: from clinical trials to clinical practice. *J Nucl Med* 2002;43:1507–1529.

82. Witzig TE, White CA, Wiseman GA, et al. Phase I/II trial of IDEC-Y2B8 radioimmunotherapy for treatment of relapsed or refractory CD20(+) B-cell non-Hodgkin's lymphoma. *J Clin Oncol* 1999;17:3793–3803.

83. Carter P, Presta L, Gorman CM, et al. Humanization of an anti-p185HER2 antibody for human cancer therapy. *Proc Natl Acad Sci U S A* 1992;89:4285–4289.

84. Slamon DJ, Clark GM, Wong SG, et al. Human breast cancer: correlation of relapse and survival with amplification of the HER-2/neu oncogene. *Science* 1987;235:177–182.

85. Dawood S, Broglio K, Buzdar AU, et al. Prognosis of women with metastatic breast cancer by HER2 status and trastuzumab treatment: an institutional-based review. *J Clin Oncol* 2010;28:92–98.

86. Tanner M, Hollmen M, Junttila TT, et al. Amplification of HER-2 in gastric carcinoma: association with Topoisomerase IIalpha gene amplification, intestinal type, poor prognosis and sensitivity to trastuzumab. *Ann Oncol* 2005;16:273–278.

87. Baselga J, Tripathy D, Mendelsohn J, et al. Phase II study of weekly intravenous recombinant humanized anti-p185HER2 monoclonal antibody in patients with HER2/neu-overexpressing metastatic breast cancer. *J Clin Oncol* 1996;14:737–744.

88. Cobleigh MA, Vogel CL, Tripathy D, et al. Multinational study of the efficacy and safety of humanized anti-HER2 monoclonal antibody in women who have HER2-overexpressing metastatic breast cancer that has progressed after chemotherapy for metastatic disease. *J Clin Oncol* 1999;17:2639–2648.

89. Slamon D, Leyland-Jones B, Shak S, et al. Addition of Herceptin™ (humanized anti-HER2 antibody) to first line chemotherapy for HER2 overexpressing metastatic breast cancer (HER21/MBC) markedly increases anticancer activity: a randomized multinational controlled phase III trial. *Proc Am Soc Clin Oncol* 1998;17:A377.

90. Piccart-Gebhart MJ, Procter M, Leyland-Jones B, et al. Trastuzumab after adjuvant chemotherapy in HER2-positive breast cancer. *N Engl J Med* 2005;353:1659–1672.

91. Romond EH, Perez EA, Bryant J, et al. Trastuzumab plus adjuvant chemotherapy for operable HER2-positive breast cancer. *N Engl J Med* 2005;353:1673–1684.

92. Smith I, Procter M, Gelber RD, et al. 2-year follow-up of trastuzumab after adjuvant chemotherapy in HER2-positive breast cancer: a randomised controlled trial. *Lancet* 2007;369:29–36.

93. Ewer MS, Gibbs HR, Swafford J, et al. Cardiotoxicity in patients receiving transtuzumab (Herceptin): primary toxicity, synergistic or sequential stress, or surveillance artifact? *Semin Oncol* 1999;26:96–101.

94. Bang YJ, Van Cutsem E, Feyereislova A, et al. Trastuzumab in combination with chemotherapy versus chemotherapy alone for treatment of HER2-positive advanced gastric or gastro-oesophageal junction cancer (ToGA): a phase 3, open-label, randomised controlled trial. *Lancet* 2010;376:687–697.

95. Gomez-Martin C, Plaza JC, Pazo-Cid R, et al. Level of HER2 gene amplification predicts response and overall survival in HER2-positive advanced gastric cancer treated with trastuzumab. *J Clin Oncol* 2013;10:4445–4452.

96. Agus DB, Akita RW, Fox WD, et al. Targeting ligand-activated ErbB2 signaling inhibits breast and prostate tumor growth. *Cancer Cell* 2002;2:127–137.

97. Baselga J, Cortes J, Kim SB, et al. Pertuzumab plus trastuzumab plus docetaxel for metastatic breast cancer. *N Engl J Med* 2012;366:109–119.

98. Swain SM, Kim SB, Cortes J, et al. Pertuzumab, trastuzumab, and docetaxel for HER2-positive metastatic breast cancer (CLEOPATRA study): overall survival results from a randomised, double-blind, placebo-controlled, phase 3 study. *Lancet Oncol* 2013;14:461–471.

99. Gianni L, Pienkowski T, Im YH, et al. Efficacy and safety of neoadjuvant pertuzumab and trastuzumab in women with locally advanced, inflammatory, or early HER2-positive breast cancer (NeoSphere): a randomised multicentre, open-label, phase 2 trial. *Lancet Oncol* 2012;13:25–32.

100. Waksal HW. Role of an anti-epidermal growth factor receptor in treating cancer. *Cancer Metastasis Rev* 1999;18:427–436.

101. Van Cutsem ELI, D'haens G. KRAS status and efficacy in the first-line treatment of patients with metastatic colorectal cancer (metastatic CRC) treated with FOLFIRI with or without cetuximab: The CRYSTAL experience. Abstract 2. *J Clin Oncol* 2008;26:5s.

102. Bokemeyer CBI, Hartmann JT. KRAS status and efficacy of first-line treatment of patients with metastatic colorectal (metastatic CRC) with FOLFOX with or without cetuximab: The OPUS experience. Abstract 4000. *J Clin Oncol* 2008;26:178s.

103. Pirker R, Pereira JR, Szczesna A, et al. Cetuximab plus chemotherapy in patients with advanced non-small-cell lung cancer (FLEX): an open-label randomised phase III trial. *Lancet* 2009;373:1525–1531.

104. Lynch TJ, Patel T, Dreisbach L, et al. Cetuximab and first-line taxane/carboplatin chemotherapy in advanced non-small-cell lung cancer: results of the randomized multicenter phase III trial BMS099. *J Clin Oncol* 2010;28:911–917.

105. Gibson TB, Ranganathan A, Grothey A. Randomized phase III trial of panitumumab, a fully human anti-epidermal growth factor receptor monoclonal antibody, in metastatic colorectal cancer. *Clin Colorectal Cancer* 2006;6:29–31.

106. Amado RG, Wolf M, Peeters M, et al. Wild-type KRAS is required for panitumumab efficacy in patients with metastatic colorectal cancer. *J Clin Oncol* 2008;26:1626–1634.

107. Brown LF, Berse B, Jackman RW, et al. Expression of vascular permeability factor (vascular endothelial growth factor) and its receptors in breast cancer. *Hum Pathol* 1995;26:86–91.

108. Obermair A, Kohlberger P, Bancher-Todesca D, et al. Influence of microvessel density and vascular permeability factor/vascular endothelial growth factor expression on prognosis in vulvar cancer. *Gynecol Oncol* 1996;63:204–209.

109. Takahashi Y, Tucker SL, Kitadai Y, et al. Vessel counts and expression of vascular endothelial growth factor as prognostic factors in node-negative colon cancer. *Arch Surg* 1997;132:541–546.

110. Jain RK. Normalization of tumor vasculature: an emerging concept in antiangiogenic therapy. *Science* 2005;307:58–62.

111. Hurwitz H, Fehrenbacher L, Novotny W, et al. Bevacizumab plus irinotecan, fluorouracil, and leucovorin for metastatic colorectal cancer. *N Engl J Med* 2004;350:2335–2342.

112. Sandler A, Gray R, Perry MC, et al. Paclitaxel-carboplatin alone or with bevacizumab for non-small-cell lung cancer. *N Engl J Med* 2006;355:2542–2550.

113. Miller K, Wang M, Gralow J, et al. Paclitaxel plus bevacizumab versus paclitaxel alone for metastatic breast cancer. *N Engl J Med* 2007;357:2666.

114. Miller KD, Chap LI, Holmes FA, et al. Randomized phase III trial of capecitabine compared with bevacizumab plus capecitabine in patients with previously treated metastatic breast cancer. *J Clin Oncol* 2005;23:792–799.

115. Allegra CJ, Yothers G, O'Connell MJ, et al. Initial safety report of NSABP C-08: A randomized phase III study of modified FOLFOX6 with or without bevacizumab for the adjuvant treatment of patients with stage II or III colon cancer. *J Clin Oncol* 2009;27:3385–3390.

116. Cameron D, Brown J, Dent R, et al. Adjuvant bevacizumab-containing therapy in triple-negative breast cancer (BEATRICE): primary results of a randomised, phase 3 trial. *Lancet Oncol* 2013;14:933–942.

117. Kreisl TN, Kim L, Moore K, et al. Phase II trial of single-agent bevacizumab followed by bevacizumab plus irinotecan at tumor progression in recurrent glioblastoma. *J Clin Oncol* 2009;27:740–745.

118. Burris HA 3rd, Rugo HS, Vukelja SJ, et al. Phase II study of the antibody drug conjugate trastuzumab-DM1 for the treatment of human epidermal growth factor receptor 2 (HER2)-positive breast cancer after prior HER2-directed therapy. *J Clin Oncol* 2011;29:398–405.

119. Krop IE, LoRusso P, Miller KD, et al. A phase II study of trastuzumab emtansine in patients with human epidermal growth factor receptor 2-positive metastatic breast cancer who were previously treated with trastuzumab, lapatinib, an anthracycline, a taxane, and capecitabine. *J Clin Oncol* 2012;30:3234–3241.

120. Verma S, Miles D, Gianni L, et al. Trastuzumab emtansine for HER2-positive advanced breast cancer. *N Engl J Med* 2012;367:1783–1791.

121. Thomas D, Carriere P, Jacobs I. Safety of denosumab in giant-cell tumour of bone. *Lancet Oncol* 2010;11:815.

122. Chawla S, Henshaw R, Seeger L, et al. Safety and efficacy of denosumab for adults and skeletally mature adolescents with giant cell tumour of bone: interim analysis of an open-label, parallel-group, phase 2 study. *Lancet Oncol* 2013;14:901–908.

123. Fizazi K, Carducci M, Smith M, et al. Denosumab versus zoledronic acid for treatment of bone metastases in men with castration-resistant prostate cancer: a randomised, double-blind study. *Lancet* 2011;377:813–822.

124. Henry DH, Costa L, Goldwasser F, et al. Randomized, double-blind study of denosumab versus zoledronic acid in the treatment of bone metastases in patients with advanced cancer (excluding breast and prostate cancer) or multiple myeloma. *J Clin Oncol* 2011;29:1125–1132.

125. Stopeck AT, Lipton A, Body JJ, et al. Denosumab compared with zoledronic acid for the treatment of bone metastases in patients with advanced breast cancer: a randomized, double-blind study. *J Clin Oncol* 2010;28:5132–5139.

126. Smith MR, Egerdie B, Hernandez Toriz N, et al. Denosumab in men receiving androgen-deprivation therapy for prostate cancer. *N Engl J Med* 2009;361:745–755.

127. Ellis GK, Bone HG, Chlebowski R, et al. Randomized trial of denosumab in patients receiving adjuvant aromatase inhibitors for nonmetastatic breast cancer. *J Clin Oncol* 2008;26:4875–4882.

128. Maloney D, Grillo-López A, Bodkin D, et al. IDEC-C2B8: results of a phase I multiple-dose trial in patients with relapsed non-Hodgkin's lymphoma. *J Clin Oncol* 1997;15:3266–3274.

129. Maloney D, Grillo-López A, White C, et al. IDEC-C2B8 (Rituximab) anti-CD20 monoclonal antibody therapy in patients with relapsed low-grade non-Hodgkin's lymphoma. *Blood* 1997;90:2188–2195.

130. Shan D, Ledbetter J, Press O. Signaling events involved in anti-CD20-induced apoptosis of malignant human B cells. *Cancer Immunol Immunother* 2000;48:673–683.

131. Coiffier B, Haioun C, Ketterer N, et al. Rituximab (anti-CD20 monoclonal antibody) for the treatment of patients with relapsing or refractory aggressive lymphoma: a multicenter phase II study. *Blood* 1998;92:1927–1932.

132. Czuczman MS, Grillo-López AJ, White CA, et al. Treatment of patients with low-grade B-cell lymphoma with the combination of chimeric anti-CD20 monoclonal antibody and CHOP chemotherapy. *J Clin Oncol* 1999;17:268–276.

133. Demidem A, Lam T, Alas S, et al. Chimeric anti-CD20 (IDEC-C2B8) monoclonal antibody sensitizes a B cell lymphoma cell line to cell killing by cytotoxic drugs. *Cancer Biother Radiopharm* 1997;12:177–186.

134. Gribben JG, Freedman A, Woo SD, et al. All advanced stage non-Hodgkin's lymphomas with a polymerase chain reaction amplifiable breakpoint of bcl-2 have residual cells containing the rearrangement at evaluation and after treatment. *Blood* 1991;78:3275–3280.

135. Feugier P, Van Hoof A, Sebban C, et al. Long-term results of the R-CHOP study in the treatment of elderly patients with diffuse large B-cell lymphoma: a study by the Groupe d'Etude des Lymphomes de l'Adulte. *J Clin Oncol* 2005;23:4117–4126.

136. Kaufmann H, Raderer M, Wohrer S, et al. Antitumor activity of rituximab plus thalidomide in patients with relapsed/refractory mantle cell lymphoma. *Blood* 2004;104:2269–2271.

137. Reddy N, Hernandez-Ilizaliturri FJ, Deeb G, et al. Immunomodulatory drugs stimulate natural killer-cell function, alter cytokine production by dendritic cells, and inhibit angiogenesis enhancing the anti-tumour activity of rituximab in vivo. *Br J Haematol* 2008;140:36–45.

138. Hooijberg E, Sein JJ, van den Berk PC, et al. Eradication of large human B cell tumors in nude mice with unconjugated CD20 monoclonal antibodies and interleukin 2. *Cancer Res* 1995;55:2627–2634.

139. Friedberg JW, Neuberg D, Gribben JG, et al. Combination immunotherapy with rituximab and interleukin 2 in patients with relapsed or refractory follicular non-Hodgkin's lymphoma. *Br J Haematol* 2002;117:828–834.

140. Khan KD, Emmanouilides C, Benson DM Jr., et al. A phase 2 study of rituximab in combination with recombinant interleukin-2 for rituximab-refractory indolent non-Hodgkin's lymphoma. *Clin Cancer Res* 2006;12:7046–7053.

141. van der Kolk LE, Grillo-López AJ, Baars JW, et al. Treatment of relapsed B-cell non-Hodgkin's lymphoma with a combination of chimeric anti-CD20 monoclonal antibodies (rituximab) and G-CSF: final report on safety and efficacy. *Leukemia* 2003;17:1658–1664.

142. Warren TL, Dahle CE, Weiner GJ. CpG oligodeoxynucleotides enhance monoclonal antibody therapy of a murine lymphoma. *Clin Lymphoma* 2000;1:57–61.

143. Smith MR, Jin F, Joshi I. Enhanced efficacy of therapy with antisense BCL-2 oligonucleotides plus anti-CD20 monoclonal antibody in scid mouse/human lymphoma xenografts. *Mol Cancer Ther* 2004;3:1693–1699.

144. Ramanarayanan J, Hernandez-Ilizaliturri FJ, Chanan-Khan A, et al. Pro-apoptotic therapy with the oligonucleotide Genasense (oblimersen sodium) targeting Bcl-2 protein expression enhances the biological anti-tumour activity of rituximab. *Br J Haematol* 2004;127:519–530.

145. van Delft MF, Wei AH, Mason KD, et al. The BH3 mimetic ABT-737 targets selective Bcl-2 proteins and efficiently induces apoptosis via Bak/Bax if Mcl-1 is neutralized. *Cancer Cell* 2006;10:389–399.

146. Paoluzzi L, Gonen M, Gardner JR, et al. Targeting Bcl-2 family members with the BH3 mimetic AT-101 markedly enhances the therapeutic effects of chemotherapeutic agents in in vitro and in vivo models of B-cell lymphoma. *Blood* 2008;111:5350–5358.

147. Nguyen M, Marcellus RC, Roulston A, et al. Small molecule obatoclax (GX15-070) antagonizes MCL-1 and overcomes MCL-1-mediated resistance to apoptosis. *Proc Natl Acad Sci U S A* 2007;104:19512–19517.

148. Coiffier B, Lepretre S, Pedersen LM, et al. Safety and efficacy of ofatumumab, a fully human monoclonal anti-CD20 antibody, in patients with relapsed or refractory B-cell chronic lymphocytic leukemia: a phase 1-2 study. *Blood* 2008;111:1094–1100.

149. Wierda WG, Kipps TJ, Mayer J, et al. Ofatumumab as single-agent CD20 immunotherapy in fludarabine-refractory chronic lymphocytic leukemia. *J Clin Oncol* 2010;28:1749–1755.

150. Stein R, Qu Z, Chen S, et al. Characterization of a new humanized anti-CD20 monoclonal antibody, IMMU-106, and its use in combination with the humanized anti-CD22 antibody, epratuzumab, for the therapy of non-Hodgkin's lymphoma. *Clin Cancer Res* 2004;10:2868–2878.

151. Senter PD, Sievers EL. The discovery and development of brentuximab vedotin for use in relapsed Hodgkin lymphoma and systemic anaplastic large cell lymphoma. *Nat Biotechnol* 2012;30:631–637.

152. Pro B, Advani R, Brice P, et al. Brentuximab vedotin (SGN-35) in patients with relapsed or refractory systemic anaplastic large-cell lymphoma: results of a phase II study. *J Clin Oncol* 2012;30:2190–2196.

153. Younes A, Gopal AK, Smith SE, et al. Results of a pivotal phase II study of brentuximab vedotin for patients with relapsed or refractory Hodgkin's lymphoma. *J Clin Oncol* 2012;30:2183–2189.

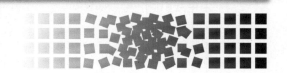

30 Assessment of Clinical Response

Antonio Tito Fojo and Susan E. Bates

INTRODUCTION

Approaches to response assessments have become increasingly important over the past decade as the drug development pipeline has steadily increased in volume. In 2012, an estimated 981 medicines were in development for cancer, and the number is certainly higher today.[1] The challenge is, first, how to measure the activity of an agent in the research setting, and, second, how to measure activity in the standard of care setting.

The "modern era" of drug development began in 1976 when 16 experienced oncologists treating lymphoma gathered to decide what would be considered a reliable measure of response to a therapy.[2] Each oncologist measured 12 *simulated tumor masses* employing *usual clinical methods* (i.e., calipers or rulers). A principal goal was to identify the amount of shrinkage that *could not* be ascribed to operator error and that *would not* be found if a *placebo* was administered. Moertel and Hanley recommended that *to avoid error, a 50% reduction in the product of perpendicular diameters be employed as the criterion for efficacy.*[2] It was from this beginning that our current methodologies of response assessment evolved. The important point to note is that the decision to use a 50% reduction in the product of perpendicular diameters as a measure of efficacy was made so as to reduce error and *not because it represented a value that conferred clinical benefit.*

From Calipers and Rulers in Lymphoma to the Bidimensional World Health Organization Criteria

In 1981, five years after the Moertel and Hanley report,[2] a World Health Organization (WHO) initiative developed standardized approaches for the "reporting of response, recurrence and disease-free interval."[3] The WHO criteria, like Moertel and Hanley, recommended that malignant disease be measured in two dimensions. Complete response (CR) was defined as the disappearance of all known disease, and a partial response (PR) was scored if there occurred a "50% decrease in the sum of the products of the perpendicular diameters of the multiple lesions." Thus, the 50% reduction initially chosen as an operationally optimal value became institutionalized as the threshold for declaring efficacy in the majority of cancers. This measure of efficacy was perpetuated in 2000 with the now widely used Response Evaluation Criteria in Solid Tumors (RECIST), but shifting to one dimension.[4] The authors noted "the definition of a partial response, in particular, is an arbitrary convention—there is no inherent meaning for an individual patient of a 50% decrease in overall tumor load." Nevertheless, the threshold chosen—a 30% reduction in one dimension—was comparable in volume to the 50% decrease in the sum of the products of the perpendicular diameters and thus perpetuated the 1976 standard. In spite of its arbitrary origins, the 50% reduction has held up over time. But the major impact of the WHO criteria was that it marked the beginning of a common language of response. These criteria have been revisited and refined over time, as technology

and medicine advanced. Table 30.1 compares the WHO criteria with those of RECIST 1.0 and RECIST 1.1 and three modifications of RECIST, whereas Figure 30.1 provides a visual presentation of the RECIST threshold required to qualify as response or progression.[3–9]

ASSESSING RESPONSE

RECIST 1.1

The RECIST 1.0 guidelines were updated as RECIST 1.1 in 2009, with a number of differences between the two response criteria highlighted. RECIST 1.1 preserves the same categories of response found in RECIST 1.0:

- Complete response: Complete disappearance of all disease
- Partial response: ≥30% reduction in the sum of the longest diameter of target lesions
- Stable disease: Change not meeting criteria for response or progression
- Progression: ≥20% increase in the sum of the longest diameter of target lesions

However, a decade of experience with RECIST identified several problems with the criteria, some of which could be corrected. In RECIST 1.0, minimum size varied between 1 and 2 cm depending on technique; in RECIST 1.1, a 1-cm lesion is the minimum measurable. In RECIST 1.0, 10 lesions were to be measured, 5 per organ; RECIST 1.1 reduced that to 5 lesions, 2 per organ. Response criteria in RECIST 1.0 did not address lymph nodes; in RECIST 1.1, lymph nodes decreasing to <1 cm in their short axis could constitute a complete response. Disease progression in nontarget disease was further defined to indicate that in addition to a 20% increase in target lesions over the smallest sum on study, there must be an absolute increase of 5 mm, and that an increase of a single nontarget lesion should not trump an overall disease status assessment based on target lesions.

Variations of the RECIST Criteria

The RECIST criteria have been widely used for standardizing the reporting of clinical trial results and have improved reproducibility. However, the increasing precision and codification of RECIST has led to recognition of its limitations. For example, there are unique challenges in central nervous system (CNS) disease, relating response to tumor size measurements based on contrast enhancement. Pseudoprogression refers to an increase in contrast enhancement due to a transient increase in vascular permeability after irradiation, whereas pseudoresponse is a decrease in contrast enhancement that may occur due to a reduction in vascular permeability following corticosteroids or an antiangiogenic agent such as bevacizumab.[10–12] The McDonald criteria, traditionally used in determining glioma response based

TABLE 30.1

Key Features of Response Criteria

	WHO[3]	RECIST 1.0[4]	RECIST 1.1[5]	CNS RANO Criteria[7]	RECIST Mesothelioma[8]	RECIST Immunotherapy[9]
Dimension	Uni- and bidimensional	Unidimensional	Unidimensional	Bidimensional	Unidimensional	Bidimensional
Measurable Lesion	Not defined	Longest diameter, ≥20 mm with most modalities; ≥10 mm with spiral CT	Longest diameter ≥10 mm on CT or on skin if using calipers; ≥20 mm if using CXR	Two perpendicular diameters of contrast enhancing lesions ≥10 mm	Tumor thickness perpendicular to chest wall or mediastinum, measured in two positions at three levels on transverse cuts of CT scan	Longest perpendicular diameters
Measurable Lymph Nodes	Not defined	Not defined	≥15 mm short axis	—	—	—
Disease Burden to be Assessed at Baseline	All (not specified)	Measurable target lesions up to 10 total (5 per organ); other lesions nontarget	Measurable target lesions up to 5 total (2 per organ); other lesions nontarget	Two to five lesions in patients with several lesions	Pleural disease in perpendicular diameter; nodal, subcutaneous, and other bidimensional lesions measured unidimensionally as per the RECIST criteria	5 lesions per organ, up to 10 visceral lesions and five cutaneous lesions
Sum	*Sum of the products* of bidimensional diameters or sum of linear unidimensional diameters	Sum of longest diameters of all measurable lesions	Sum of the longest diameters of target lesions with only exception use of short axis for lymph nodes	Sum of the products of perpendicular diameters of all measurable enhancing target lesions	Sum of the six measurements defines a pleural unidimensional measure	SPD with new lesions incorporated into baseline; tumor burden = $SPD_{index\ lesions}$ + $SPD_{new\ lesions}$
Complete Response	Disappearance all known disease	Disappearance all known disease	Disappearance all known disease; lymph nodes <10 mm	—	Disappearance all target lesions with no evidence of tumor elsewhere	Disappearance all lesions in two consecutive observations
Partial Response	≥50% decrease	≥30% decrease; all other no evidence of progression	≥30% decrease; all other disease, no evidence of progression	≥50% reduction; stable or decreased steroid use compared to baseline	≥30% reduction in total tumor measurement	≥50% decrease compared with baseline in two observations
Response Confirmation?	≥4 weeks apart	≥4 weeks apart	≥4 weeks apart (if response primary end point); no, if secondary endpoint	≥4 weeks apart	Repeat on two occasions ≥4 weeks apart	≥4 weeks apart

(continued)

TABLE 30.1

Key Features of Response Criteria *(continued)*

	WHO[3]	RECIST 1.0[4]	RECIST 1.1[5]	CNS RANO Criteria[7]	RECIST Mesothelioma[8]	RECIST Immunotherapy[9]
Progressive Disease	≥25% increase in size of one or more measurable lesions or appearance of new lesions	≥20% increase, taking as reference smallest sum in study; or appearance of new lesions	≥20% increase, with absolute increase ≥5 mm, taking as reference smallest sum in study; or appearance of new lesions	≥25%, or any new lesions	≥20% increase in the total tumor measurement over the nadir measurement, or the appearance of one or more new lesions	≥25% increase compared with nadir confirmed ≥4 weeks apart; up to five new lesions (≥5 × 5 mm) per organ incorporated into tumor burden
	Nonmeasurable disease: Estimated increase of ≥25%	Nonmeasurable disease: unequivocal progression	Nonmeasurable disease: unequivocal progression	Nonmeasurable disease: >5 mm increase in maximal diameter; ≥25% increase in SPD; or significant increase in nonenhancing lesions on same or lower dose of corticosteroids	—	New, nonmeasurable lesions (i.e., <5 × 5 mm) do not define progression
Stable Disease	Stable disease or non-PR and non-PD ≥4 weeks	Non-PR, non-PD; minimum time defined by protocol	Non-PR, non-PD; minimum time defined by protocol	—	Non-PR, non-PD	Non-irPR, non-irPD

CXR, Chest X-ray; SPD, sum of products of two largest perpendicular diameters; PD, progressive disease; irPR, immune-related partial response; irPD, immune-related progressive disease.

CANCER THERAPEUTICS

on two-dimensional measurements, have been recently updated as part of the Response Assessment in Neuro-Oncology (RANO) response criteria and extended to include a response assessment for metastatic CNS disease.[7,13]

Other examples where RECIST is limited include mesothelioma, gastrointestinal stromal tumors (GIST), hepatocellular cancers, among others. The pleural disease of mesothelioma increases in depth while following the pleural surface. GIST tumors may remain unchanged in size after treatment, whereas the center of the tumor mass undergoes necrosis, and progression may occur in the remaining rim.[14] Hepatocellular cancers are often treated with local–regional therapy in which the goal is tumor necrosis and treatment failure occurs in surviving viable tumor.[15] Different

strategies have emerged to quantify these diseases, including modifications of RECIST, quantifying positron-emission tomography (PET) imaging, and biomarker criteria, as will be discussed. The RECIST adaptation for mesothelioma, growing along the pleural surface, is to measure the diameter perpendicular to the chest wall or mediastinum, and to measure at three levels.[8] The adaptation for hepatocellular cancer following local therapy is measurement of the longest diameter of the tumor that shows enhancement on the arterial phase of the scan, bypassing the dense, homogeneous Lipiodol-containing necrotic area.[15]

Investigators have also observed that following immunotherapy, tumor lesions may increase in size due to the increased infiltration of T cells, even meeting criteria for RECIST-defined progressive

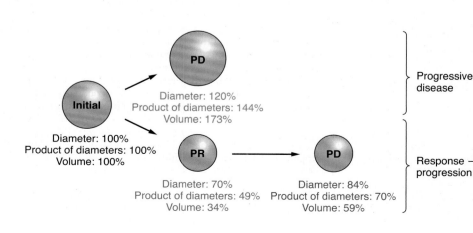

Figure 30.1 RECIST thresholds in three parameters: diameter, product of diameters, and volume. In the figure, spheres meeting RECIST criteria for progressive disease (PD) and for PR are shown with the percentage relative to the baseline calculated for each parameter. To meet the threshold for PD, the longest diameter must increase to 120%, which is equivalent to a 144% increase in the product of the perpendicular diameters and a 173% increase in the volume of a sphere. Although PR definitions are almost identical to those employed with WHO, RECIST has a higher threshold to meet PD.[6]

disease (PD). Previously radiographically undetectable lesions may appear. Departing from conventional RECIST, which defines any new lesion as PD, the immune response criteria allow the appearance of new lesions, adding them to the total tumor burden.[9] An increase in total tumor burden of >25% relative to baseline or nadir is required to define PD.

International Working Group Criteria for Lymphoma

Revised guidelines for lymphoma assessment were promulgated by the International Working Group (IWG) in 2007.[16] These guidelines incorporated 18F-fluorodeoxyglucose (FDG)-PET assessments in metabolically active lymphomas.[16] Although a CR requires the complete disappearance of detectable disease, a posttreatment residual mass is permitted if it is negative on FDG-PET and was positive at baseline. For lymphomas that are not consistently FDG avid, or if FDG avidity is unknown, a CR requires that nodes >1.5 cm before therapy regress to <1.5 cm, and nodes that were 1.1 to 1.5 cm in long axis and >1.0 cm in the short axis shrink to ≤1.0 cm in short axis. The definition of PR resembles the WHO criteria, in that a ≥50% decrease in the sum of the product of the diameters in up to six nodal masses or in hepatic or splenic nodules must be documented. Although RECIST 1.1 now includes lymph node assessment, the IWG criteria remain the assessment method typically used in lymphoma clinical trials.

ALTERNATE RESPONSE CRITERIA

The previous examples represent attempts to more accurately measure tumor burden. Evolving imaging technology enabling volumetric measurements of tumor masses may eventually resolve some of these problems, but effective therapeutic agents are required to enable validation and utilization of response assessment tools. The lack of an agent that can mediate substantial tumor shrinkage underlies the concept of *clinical benefit response* (CBR) as an endpoint in pancreatic cancer. Clinical benefit was defined as a combination of improvement in pain, performance status, and weight; the assessment of CBR supported the U.S. Food and Drug Administration (FDA) approval of gemcitabine in pancreatic cancer.[17,18] Better therapies for pancreatic cancer that result in tumor shrinkage or eradication should include and then eclipse clinical benefit.

Response criteria may be specific to a particular disease or clinical setting. Some diseases by their nature require specific strategies for response assessment.

Severity-Weighted Assessment Tool Score in Cutaneous T-Cell Lymphoma

Cutaneous T-cell lymphoma (CTCL) is a disease that can involve the entire epidermis, or comprise individual skin lesions varying widely in severity rather than size. The severity-weighted assessment tool (SWAT) assigns a factor for skin lesion severity—patch, plaque, or tumor—multiplies this factor by the percent of skin involved with each lesion type and then adds these together. This complex system formed the basis of the FDA approval of vorinostat for CTCL.[19]

Pathologic Complete Response in Breast Cancer

One unique response endpoint is the assessment of breast cancer treated in the neoadjuvant setting. The purpose of neoadjuvant therapy is to improve survival, render locally advanced cancer amenable to surgery, or to aid in breast conservation. In that setting, the absence of cancer cells in resected breast tissue has been used to define a pathologic complete response (pCR). The rate of pCR has been proposed as a surrogate endpoint for event-free survival (EFS) or overall survival (OS) to support approval of new agents or combinations of agents tested in clinical trials.[20] In a pooled analysis of 11,955 patients enrolled on 12 neoadjuvant trials, individual patients with pCR had improved EFS and OS.[21] However, at the trial level, pCR rates did not correlate with EFS or OS, a problem likely due to heterogeneity of breast cancer subtypes among the trials. Despite this, pCR rates were recently used to support the approval of pertuzumab and trastuzumab in the neoadjuvant setting.[21,22]

Computed Tomography-Based Tumor Density

One approach, often called the Choi criteria, advocates assessing tumor response in GIST, renal cell cancer, or hepatocellular cancer based on density on computed tomography (CT) scans (Table 30.2). This variation was prompted by the evident response to treatment with imatinib but with minimal tumor shrinkage.[23] The Choi criteria are still considered exploratory in GIST,[24,25] and it is too soon to know of benefits in other histologies.[26,27] Further study should determine its utility, although it will likely be confined to specific tumor types with specific drugs.

FDG-PET

Although widely used in clinical practice, FDG-PET has become part of standardized response criteria for clinical trials only in lymphoma (see Table 30.2). In solid tumors, FDG-PET can aid in the detection of new or recurrent sites of disease, and can be used as an adjunct during assessments for disease progression when using RECIST criteria.[5] Although FDG uptake is a powerful diagnostic tool and its uptake reflects a tumor's metabolic activity, it has some limitations: Some tumors have variable FDG avidity; differences can occur due to variations in patient activity, carbohydrate intake, blood glucose, and timing; and there are several benign sources of uptake, including inflammatory and postsurgical sites. Multiple methods of quantitating FDG-PET and assessing response have been proposed, but to date there is no consensus, particularly regarding the definition of a metabolic response.[28–33]

The two most widely used response criteria—the European Organisation for the Research and Treatment of Cancer (EORTC) criteria and PET Response Criteria in Solid Tumors (PERCIST) (see Table 30.2)—have been evaluated in specific disease types, but unifying FDG-PET response criteria remains a challenge in anticancer drug development.[28,30] We would note that, as shown in Figure 30.1, a 30% reduction in the diameter of a sphere—the magnitude of change required to score a response according to RECIST—represents a 65% decrease in volume. If an standardized uptake value (SUV) decrease is directly equated to a volume decrease, a reduction of 25% translates to a 10% reduction in diameter, a value that likely constitutes an insufficient response.

Serum Biomarkers of Response

The ideal response assessment method is an assay that could measure tumor quantity by a simple blood test (see Table 30.2). Circulating protein biomarkers have been identified and studied for several decades for screening, early detection of recurrent disease, determining prognosis, selecting therapy, and monitoring response to therapy. These serum tumor markers are to be distinguished from the assays determining the presence of an overexpressed or mutated molecular target. With the successful launch of therapies against such molecular targets, there has been increased interest in the assays needed to select therapy for individual patients (predictive biomarkers). The analytical and clinical validation of such assays, along with determination of their clinical utility, has created a new regulatory paradigm known as *companion diagnostics*.[34,35] This investment in the development of predictive markers for companion diagnostics has reduced the focus on protein biomarkers of treatment response relative to older literature.

As a result, there are few clinically validated biomarkers of response.[36] In addition to issues regarding sensitivity and specificity, their use and development has also been hindered by the often

TABLE 30.2

Alternate Response Criteria: Biomarkers

Criterion	Baseline	Response	Progression
CA-125 in ovarian cancer (GCIG criteria)[43]	CA 125 >2× ULN	CA 125 decline ≥50% confirmed at 28 days	2× nadir OR 2× ULN if normalized on therapy on two occasions 1 wk apart
PSA in prostate cancer (PSA WG1)[45,a]	PSA ≥5 ng/mL and documentation of two consecutive increases in PSA 1 wk apart	PSA decline of 50% from baseline (measured twice 3–4 wks apart)	After decrease from baseline, a 50% increase AND an increase ≥5 ng/mL, or back to baseline, whichever is lower
PSA in prostate cancer (PCWG2)[46,a]	PSA ≥2.0 ng/mL; estimate pretreatment PSA-DT: Need ≥3 values ≥4 wks apart	Report percent change from baseline (rise or fall) at 12 weeks, and separately, the maximal change (rise or fall) at any time using a waterfall plot	PSA increase ≥25% and absolute increase by ≥2 ng/mL above the nadir, confirmed by a second value ≥3 wks later (i.e., confirmed rising trend) OR PSA increase ≥25% and ≥2 ng/mL above baseline >12 wks
hCG and AFP in testicular cancer[50–51]		Decrease consistent with marker half-life: 2–3 d for hCG, 5–7 d for AFP	Rising levels usually indicate need to change therapy
Choi Criteria for CT Imaging			
Choi criteria[24–27]		≥10% decrease in tumor size OR ≥15% reduction in tumor density	An increase in tumor size ≥10% and does not meet criteria of PR by tumor attenuation on CT
FDG-PET Criteria			
EORTC criteria[29–31]	ROI should be drawn, SUV calculated	**CMR:** Complete resolution of uptake **PMR:** SUV reduction ≥25% **SMD:** SUV increase <25% and decrease <15%	**PMD:** SUV increase >25% in regions defined on baseline, or appearance of new FDG-avid lesions
PERCIST criteria[29]	SUL peak >1.5× normal liver	**CMR:** Complete resolution of uptake **PMR:** SUL reduction ≥30%	**PMD:** SUL increase >30% in regions defined on baseline, or appearance of new FDG avid lesions

[a] Guidelines for PSA assessment have evolved from those of the PSAWG1, where responses were dichotomized based on the percent decline, to those in the PCWG2 where PSA response is considered a continuous variable. Recently, emphasis has shifted to assessing PSA doubling time.
CA-125, cancer antigen 125; GCIG, Gynecologic Cancer InterGroup; ULN, upper limit of normal; PSA, prostate-specific antigen; PSAWG1, PSA Working Group 1; PCWG2, Prostate Cancer Working Group 2; PSA-DT, PSA-doubling time; hCG, human chorionic gonatropin; AFP, alpha-fetoprotein; EORTC, European Organisation for the Research and Treatment of Cancer; ROI, regions of interest; SUV, standardized uptake value; CMR, complete metabolic response; PMR, partial metabolic response; SMD, stable metabolic disease; PMD, progressive metabolic disease; PERCIST, PET response criteria in solid tumors; SUL, SUV normalized to lean body mass.

limited efficacy of therapies; response biomarkers are of little value without highly effective primary and salvage therapies. For example, a recent clinical trial indicates that in *asymptomatic patients* with ovarian cancer whose only evidence of disease progression is an isolated rising CA-125, nothing is gained by instituting treatment before there is other evidence of progression.[37,38]

■ **Cancer Antigen 125 (CA-125):** Despite recognized limitations, CA-125 is widely used. For example, the Gynecologic Cancer InterGroup (GCIG) criteria have evolved to help determine whether a patient's tumor has responded to therapy.[39–41] Response is defined as a 50% decline from an elevated baseline value, whereas progression is defined as a doubling over the nadir or the upper limit of normal.[42] In clinical practice, CA-125 levels are followed as part of standard management, but making clinical decisions on marker changes alone is not recommended.[43]

■ **Prostate-Specific Antigen (PSA):** Similar issues have confronted investigators caring for patients with prostate cancer. The PSA Working Group 1 (PCWG1) guidelines, first published in

1999, established PSA criteria, particularly for use in patients with disease that was difficult to quantify.[44] There followed a second working group (PCWG2) that recommended plotting the percent PSA change for each patient in a waterfall plot so as to avoid creating a dichotomous variable from the changes in PSA.[45] PCWG2 also recommended keeping patients on trial until evidence of a change in clinical status—either symptomatic or radiographic progression. The latter addressed concerns with patients in whom PSA changes did not reflect clinical status, particularly those with transient increases in the first 12 weeks of a new therapy.

■ **Human Chorionic Gonadotropin (hCG) and alpha fetoprotein (AFP):** Because testicular cancer is a highly curable disease with validated biomarkers, outcome assessment has focused on the rapid detection of patients whose tumors have a poor response to therapy. Because both markers have relatively short half-lives—2 to 3 days for hCG and 5 to 7 days for serum AFP—the rate of decline can be determined. Various methods have demonstrated that a rapid decline or early normalization of marker levels is indicative of a good outcome, without any one method achieving widespread acceptance.[46–48] Nonetheless, the 2010 American Society of Clinical Oncology (ASCO) guidelines on serum tumor markers concluded there was still insufficient evidence to recommend changing therapy solely on the basis of a slow marker decline.[49] Rising levels after two cycles of therapy (outside the first week of treatment when rises can be due to tumor lysis) can be considered an indication to change the treatment plan.[49,50]

Circulating Tumor Cells and Circulating Tumor DNA

Two response endpoints under recent investigation show a potential to detect the impact of therapy. One is the measurement of circulating tumor cells (CTC) in the bloodstream, enriched by one or more capture strategies, including one that has received FDA approval.[51] The number of CTCs in the blood has been shown to be prognostic, with higher levels conferring a poor prognosis, and to correlate with a response to therapy. A second approach is the determination of levels of circulating tumor DNA (ctDNA) in the blood. This is detected by quantitating the number of DNA molecules carrying a given mutation or gene rearrangement in the blood, typically detected through targeted sequencing of common mutations, or of a previously identified *mutation signature* or gene rearrangement. The amount of ctDNA appears to correlate with tumor burden, increases with stage, and in one study, was deemed more sensitive than CTC detection.[52–54] Whether these tests will ultimately prove to be more sensitive and accurate than the serum biomarkers discussed previously remains to be determined. Because targeted sequencing can be very sensitive, one concern is that false-positive ctDNA detection may occur after treatment, or intermittently in the setting of enlarging tumor masses. At the least, detection of CTCs and ctDNA is advancing our understanding of cancer biology, as studies reveal evidence of metastatic heterogeneity, clonal heterogeneity, and emergence of resistance mutations in clinical samples.

DETERMINING OUTCOME

The response measures described previously represent different approaches to quantitate tumor burden. What happens after those data are obtained varies depending on the clinical setting. In the community, less emphasis is placed on strict criteria. In the setting of a clinical trial, tumor size is measured and the response categorized. For FDA submission, these are but factors in the risk-benefit equation needed for drug approvals. The FDA conveys full approval to new agents based on true *clinical benefit* (i.e., an improvement in a *survival* endpoint or symptom relief).[55] Surrogates for clinical benefit, such as response rate, may support either regular approval or accelerated approval, depending on the setting.

Overall Response Rate, Duration of Response, and Stable Disease

Overall response rate (ORR) is the proportion of patients with a tumor size reduction of a predefined amount for a minimum time period. The FDA has generally defined ORR as the sum of PRs and CRs. Although OS remains the gold standard, ORR is often used both in drug development and in clinical practice to indicate antitumor efficacy of a given therapy. Table 30.3 summarizes the attributes and drawbacks of using ORR as a method of assessment. Using standardized definitions of response, it has been shown that ORR often correlates with OS, although ORR usually explains only a fraction of the variability of the survival

benefits.[56–58] Equally important, however, is the duration of response, a value that is measured from the time of initial response until documented tumor progression, and which assumes added importance when ORR is the endpoint for regulatory approval.

Unlike PR and CR, the FDA has generally not been willing to include *stable disease (SD)*, defined as shrinkage that qualifies as neither response nor progression, as part of the ORR, feeling it is often indicative of the underlying disease biology rather than a drug's therapeutic effect.[55,59] Nevertheless, in reporting data, investigators are increasingly using the term *CBR*, which includes CR + PR + SD and which is a misuse of the term *clinical benefit* because neither CR, PR, or SD are *objective tumor findings* that address the true *clinical benefit* of a therapy.[58,60] In the absence of standardized definitions for SD that are shown to effect meaningful changes in a clinical outcome, SD should not be used as a response endpoint. A better approach is to use nondichotomized response assessments, such as the waterfall plot or one of the kinetic analyses, discussed later.

Progression-Free Survival, Time to Progression, and Time to Treatment Failure

In cancer drug development, one usually finds ORR assessed as an indicator of activity in phase II trials, whereas randomized phase III trials rely on other endpoints such as progression-free survival (PFS) and time to progression (TTP) (see Table 30.3). Although PFS and TTP attempt to assess efficacy in close proximity to a therapy, they score outcomes differently and are not interchangeable. TTP is defined as the time from randomization to *the time of disease progression.*[55] In TTP analyses, *deaths are censored either at the time of death or at an earlier visit.* In contrast, PFS is defined from the time of randomization to the time of *disease progression or death.* Although patients who discontinue trial participation for adverse events might be censored in both analyses, patients who die while on study are censored only in the TTP analysis. Those who favor TTP argue that if a patient dies without their tumor meeting criteria for progression, one cannot accurately estimate when progression might have occurred, so the data should be censored. However, those who favor PFS argue that, in some cases, death might be an adverse effect of the therapy. High-dose therapies represent an example of why PFS might be a preferable (regulatory) endpoint. If in a given tumor there is evidence of a dose-response relationship for an active drug, then high doses may have a greater response. However, such high doses may also be responsible for a greater number of deaths. Assessing only those who survive the high dose therapy and ignoring those who die (i.e., TTP) may lead to the conclusion that the high-dose therapy is more effective. The balance sheet that includes death (i.e., PFS) would clearly demonstrate this efficacy came at too great a price.

Although many have argued that PFS and TTP should be acceptable endpoints for cancer clinical trials, in the majority of tumors there is no convincing evidence PFS is a surrogate for OS, and in those where there is some evidence, its value is arguable.[61] Table 30.3 presents the attributes and drawbacks of PFS and TTP. Note that the definition of progression is often difficult, particularly in some tumor types, and that investigator bias can influence PFS and TTP. Problems with ascertainment bias and censoring, depicted in Figure 30.2, can also impact outcomes.

Alternate endpoints include time to treatment failure (TTF), defined as a composite endpoint measuring time from randomization to discontinuation of treatment for any reason, including disease progression, treatment toxicity, and death. The FDA has not recommended TTF as a regulatory endpoint for drug approval. However, the high rates of censoring due to toxicity seen in phase III clinical trials may lead to a reassessment of this position given that most can agree that not only is efficacy important, but so too is tolerability, and TTF can capture both of these attributes.

TABLE 30.3

A Comparison of Important Cancer Approval Endpoints

Regulatory Evidence	Endpoints	Advantages	Disadvantages
Clinical benefit used for regular approvals	Overall survival (OS)	■ Universally accepted direct measure of clinical benefit ■ Easily measured ■ Includes treatment-related mortality that can obscure benefit in a subset ■ Precisely measured; unambiguous ■ Not dependent on assessment intervals	■ May involve larger studies ■ May require long follow-up ■ May be affected by crossover and/or sequential therapies ■ Includes noncancer deaths
	Symptom endpoints (patient-reported outcomes)	■ Patient perspective of direct clinical benefit	■ Blinding is often difficult ■ Data are frequently missing or incomplete ■ Clinical significance of small changes is unknown ■ Multiple analyses ■ Lack of validated instruments
Surrogates used for accelerated approvals or regular approvals	Disease-free survival (DFS)	■ Smaller sample size and shorter follow-up necessary compared with survival studies	■ Not statistically validated as surrogate for survival in all settings ■ Not precisely measured; subject to assessment bias, particularly in open-label studies ■ Definitions vary among studies
	Objective response rate (ORR)	■ Can be assessed in single-arm studies ■ Assessed earlier and in smaller studies compared with survival studies ■ Effect attributable to drug, not natural history	■ Not a direct measure of benefit ■ Not a comprehensive measure of drug activity ■ Only a subset of patients who benefit
	Complete response (CR)	■ Can be assessed in single-arm studies ■ Durable complete responses can represent clinical benefit ■ Assessed earlier and in smaller studies compared with survival studies ■ Definition of progressive disease (PD) identifies uniform time to end treatment and data capture	■ Not a direct measure of benefit in all cases ■ Not a comprehensive measure of drug activity ■ Small subset of patients with benefit ■ Requires prospective, consistent definition. Meaningful response durations not standardized ■ Definition of PD is arbitrary without evidence it actually represents end of benefit period
	Progression-free survival (PFS) or time to progression (TTP)[a]	■ Smaller sample size and shorter follow-up necessary compared with survival studies ■ Measurement of stable disease included ■ Not confounded by crossover or subsequent therapies ■ Generally based on objective and quantitative assessment	■ Statistically validated as surrogate for survival only in some settings ■ Not precisely measured; subject to assessment bias particularly in open-label studies ■ Definitions vary among studies; little agreement on magnitude of difference that constitutes clinical benefit ■ Requires frequent and consistent radiological or other assessments ■ Involves balanced timing of assessments among treatment arms

[a] Progression-free survival includes all deaths; time to progression censors deaths that occur before progression.
Adapted from U.S. Department of Health and Human Services, Food and Drug Administration, Center for Drug Evaluation and Research (CDER), Center for Biologics Evaluation and Research (CBER). *Guidance from Industry. Clinical Trial Endpoints for the Approval of Cancer Drugs and Biologics.* 2007.
http://www.fda.gov/downloads/Drugs/.../Guidances/ucm071590.pdf.

CANCER THERAPEUTICS

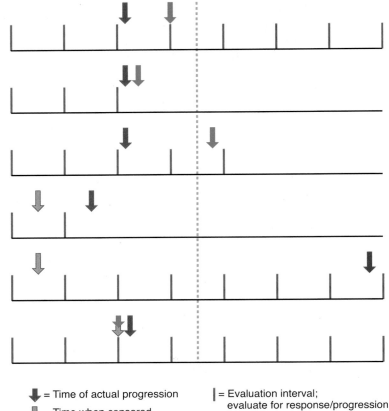

Prespecified evaluation interval
Ideally, disease progression is reported at a prespecified evaluation interval

Ascertainment (evaluation) bias
An earlier evaluation leads to earlier scoring of progression (e.g., concern for symptoms prompt earlier evaluation)

Ascertainment (evaluation) bias
A later evaluation leads to delay in scoring progression (e.g., evaluation delayed by toxicity or treatment delays)

Censoring bias
Patient whose disease would have progressed quickly is censored early. Here censoring is "beneficial."

Censoring bias
Patient whose disease would have progressed late is censored early. Here censoring is "detrimental."

Informative censoring
Central review cannot score progression with available data. Although progression had been scored, the data is instead censored centrally. This is usually "beneficial."

= Time of actual progression
= Time when censored
= Time progression scored

| = Evaluation interval; evaluate for response/progression
⋮ = Median PFS/TTP

Figure 30.2 The potential problems encountered when PFS is used as an endpoint. Ideally, as depicted at the *top*, response assessment will be conducted at a prespecified time. However, the date at which progression is scored may suffer from either ascertainment or censoring bias. Ascertainment bias can occur if either an evaluation occurs before the prespecified date or if it is delayed. For example, a clinician concerned about a patient who is not experiencing side effects and has likely been randomized to placebo may be more inclined to investigate symptoms early and document progression before the prespecified time, while delaying the evaluation of a patient randomized to the experimental arm who experiences some toxicity. Similarly, censoring—an increasing problem in randomized trials—may impact the outcome of a given study arm by either censoring patients who would experience early progression (beneficial impact) or censoring those who would have remained progression free for a long time (detrimental impact). Finally, informative censoring can occur when independent radiologic review cannot concur with an investigator's assessment of progression and censors the patient. This outcome is usually beneficial, because a patient who is very close to experiencing progression is censored. (Adapted from Villaruz LC, Socinski MA. The clinical viewpoint: definitions, limitations of RECIST, practical considerations of measurement. *Clin Cancer Res* 2013;19:2629–2636.)

Overall Survival

Defined as the time from randomization to death, OS has been considered the gold standard of clinical trial endpoints (see Table 30.3). In part, this is so because it is unambiguous and does not suffer from interpretation bias. An additional advantage of the survival endpoint is that it can balance the effect of therapies with high treatment-related mortality even if tumor control is substantially better with the new treatment. However, some worry that because patients may receive multiple lines of therapy following the clinical trial, the results may be confounded by those subsequent therapies. The latter concern is often cited as the reason why an advantage in PFS/TTP *disappears* when one looks to OS. But as a review of clinical trials confirms,[62] the magnitude of the difference does not disappear, only the statistical validity (Fig. 30.3).[63,64]

When evaluating a randomized controlled trial, it is important that the OS as well as the PFS analyses are always by intention to treat (ITT). In an ITT analysis, often described as *once randomized, always analyzed*, all patients assigned to a group at the time of randomization are analyzed regardless of what occurred subsequently.[65] An ITT analysis avoids the bias introduced by omitting dropouts and noncompliant patients that can negate randomization and overestimate clinical effectiveness.

Kaplan–Meier Plots

In a typical clinical trial, data are often presented as a Kaplan–Meier plots. In discrete time intervals, the number of patients in each group who are progression free and alive (PFS analysis) or alive (OS analysis) at the end of the interval are counted and divided by the total number of patients in that group at the beginning of the time interval. One excludes from this calculation patients censored for a reason other than progressive disease or death during the same interval. This has the advantage that it allows one to include censored patients in estimates of the probability of PFS or OS up to the point when they were censored (i.e., they are excluded only beyond the point of censoring). In most clinical trials, a fraction of patients are typically censored.

In constructing the Kaplan–Meier plot, probabilities are calculated for each interval of time. The probability of surviving

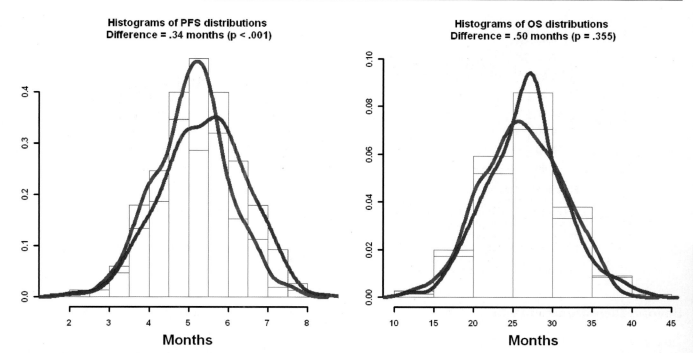

Figure 30.3 Hypothetical distribution of PFS and OS data demonstrating the *disappearance of PFS benefit*. Because chemotherapy does not exert a lasting effect on the underlying tumor biology and because PFS is a shorter interval (measured in increments, not daily as is OS) PFS differences often disappear. The *hypothetical example* shown illustrates this phenomenon. The *left panel* shows a histogram of PFS distributions with a difference of 0.34 months that nevertheless achieves statistical significance over the short interval when PFS is measured. The *right panel* depicts similar histograms for OS captured over a longer time period. Despite a larger absolute difference of 0.5 months, the OS difference does not reach statistical significance. For these hypothetical curves, random number generated data sets (with normal distribution), histograms, and density plots were generated using R version 2.11.1 (2010-05-31).[75] The differences were deliberately chosen to be small, but a similar disappearance can also occur with larger differences. As can be seen, what disappears is not the absolute benefit, but the statistical validity.

progression free or being counted as a survivor to the end of any interval of assessment is the product of the probabilities of surviving in all the preceding assessment intervals multiplied by the probability for the interval of interest. One might ask to what extent the two curves in each study differ. One measure that is of value is the median PFS or OS—a value calculated in most studies from a Kaplan–Meier plot.

Hazard Ratios

Increasingly, however, hazard ratios are cited in preference to the more traditional measures of efficacy such as the median PFS and median OS. *However, because a hazard ratio is a value that has no dimensions, it has very limited value, informing the reader only with regard to the reliability and uniformity of the data.* It does not quantify the magnitude of the benefit. A physician and, especially, a patient want to know the magnitude of the benefit (i.e., the extent to which a life will be prolonged), not what a dimensionless hazard ratio is. By definition, the *hazard ratio* is a ratio of the *hazard rates*. The hazard rate quantifies the likelihood that a patient will experience a *hazardous event* or a hazard during a defined interval of observation, and this is expressed as a rate or percent. For example, if during a given period of observation 20 of 100 patients receiving a reference or control therapy experience progression or death, their hazard rate during this interval is 0.2 (20/100). If during this same interval, only 10 of the 100 patients receiving the experimental therapy experience progression or death, their hazard rate is 0.1 (10/100). In this simple example, the hazard ratio for the interval, calculated as *the ratio of the hazard rates* is 0.5 (0.1/0.2) and indicates the likelihood of experiencing a hazardous event is reduced by 50% in the experimental arm. As commonly presented, and as this simple example illustrates, the lower the

hazard ratio, the better the experimental therapy. To determine whether the hazard ratio has statistical significance, one can (1) use a log-rank test to show that the null hypothesis that the two treatments lead to the same survival probabilities is wrong, or (2) use a parametric approach writing a regression model and fitting the data to the model so that one can establish the hazard ratio for the whole trial and its statistical significance. In many cases, the Cox proportional hazard model is used. Although the ideal hazard ratio would capture the differential benefit throughout the period of study, in practice, the extremes depicted in a Kaplan–Meier plot may not be analyzed.

Forest Plots

Interest in determining whether there is heterogeneity in a treatment effect, such that better outcomes occur in some subgroups, has led to the use of Forest plots to display treatment effects across subgroups. Although simple in concept, these plots are subject to error because subgroups are composed of smaller numbers and the confidence intervals are therefore wider than those for the entire group. The most common presentation includes a vertical line at the *no effect point* (e.g., a hazard ratio of 1.0), with symbols of varying size representing the subgroups, each with its confidence interval depicted by a line that stretches from the symbol to both sides (the symbol size is usually proportional to the size of the subgroup). If the confidence interval for a subgroup crosses the no effect point, this is commonly interpreted (not necessarily correctly) as a lack of effect in the subgroup. *The information one seeks from a Forest plot is whether the effect size for different subgroups varies significantly from the main effect, which is determined by a test for heterogeneity.*[66]

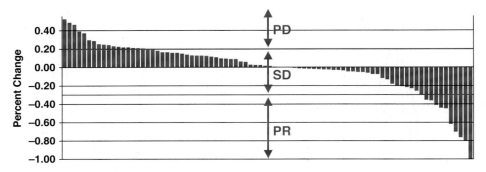

Figure 30.4 Example of a waterfall plot demonstrating for each patient the maximum benefit obtained with the study therapy. Those to the *left* represent patients whose tumors increased, and those on the *right* represent patients whose tumors regressed. The *vertical red lines* at +20% and -30% define the boundaries of stable disease according to RECIST. Ideally, all responses should be confirmed after a period of at least 4 weeks. The example shown is of patients with renal cell carcinoma treated with the microtubule targeting agent ixabepilone. (From Huang H, Menefee M, Edgerly M, et al. A phase II clinical trial of ixabepilone [Ixempra; BMS-247550; NSC 710428], an epothilone B analog, in patients with metastatic renal cell carcinoma. *Clin Cancer Res* 2010;16:1634–1641.)

Beyond Dichotomized Data

Quality of Life

The assessment of cancer patients enrolled on a clinical trial can be said to consist of two sets of endpoints: cancer outcomes and patient outcomes. Cancer outcomes measure the response of the tumor to treatment, the duration of the response, the symptom-free period, and the early recognition of relapse. In contrast, patient outcomes assess the benefit achieved with a given therapy by measuring the increase in survival and the quality of life (QOL) before and after therapy. Unfortunately, physicians tend to concentrate on cancer-related outcomes, often neglecting assessments of QOL. Although a QOL assessment in clinical settings is possible with currently available instruments, there must be continued development and refinement of these instruments. Such development must focus not only on extracting valuable information in an unbiased manner, but also and equally important, developing an instrument that is user friendly and will be completed in a high percentage of encounters.

Waterfall Plots

The arbitrary nature of the 50% cutoff set by Moertel and Hanley and its evolution to the current RECIST threshold of 30%

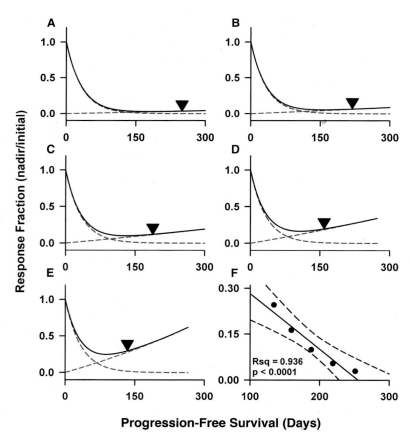

Progression-Free Survival (Days)

Figure 30.5 The effect of the growth rate constant, *g*, on two commonly reported clinical values: maximum tumor shrinkage and PFS. Tumor measurements obtained in patients can be analyzed mathematically. **(A–E)** The *black line* depicts idealized clinical data using tumor quantities measured as patients received chemotherapy. Actually, clinical measurements comprise concurrent tumor regression *(dashed red line)* and growth *(dashed blue line)* that can be described by a rate constant and a first order kinetic equation, $f(t) = \exp^{(-d \cdot t)} + \exp^{(g \cdot t)} - 1$, where *exp* is the base of the natural logarithm, $e = 2.7182...$, and *f* is the percent change in tumor measurement at time *t*, normalized to the value when treatment began. The rate constant *d* accounts for exponential decrease, whereas the rate constant *g* accounts for exponential growth occurring during treatment.[68,69] To demonstrate the correlation between the growth rate, tumor shrinkage and PFS, the *same* regression rate **(*d*)** has been modeled in panels *A* through *E*, whereas the growth rate constant, **g**, *increases* in each successive panel. The *black triangles* depict the point at which tumor size is 20% above the nadir (RECIST definition of PD). As the growth rate increases (i.e., faster tumor growth) from **A** to **E**, the nadir is reached sooner, and the depth of the nadir is less. **(F)** The correlation between PFS and maximum tumor shrinkage (nadir) is shown, plotting the correlation between PFS and response fraction, which is defined as the ratio of nadir to initial value.[68,69] Although idealized plots are given, the curves are based firmly on data obtained from patients enrolled on clinical trials.

reduction in the size of the maximum diameter raises valid queries as to why 30% is valuable and not 29% or 25%. On this background, waterfall plots such as the one shown in Figure 30.4 have become increasingly popular because they depict the benefit or lack thereof in all patients as a continuum of response, rather than a dichotomized response rate.[67] Waterfall plots can be generated from any quantitative assessment. If ctDNA or tumor cells prove to be as quantitative as hoped, the maximum decline could be plotted as a waterfall plot.

Growth Kinetics

Efforts to quantify tumor kinetic parameters from clinical data have been investigated in recent years. Different equations have been applied to describe the two-phase curve based on tumor size as observed in most solid tumor trials, where there is first shrinkage followed by regrowth (Fig. 30.5). These models show exponential tumor shrinkage after treatment, followed by tumor regrowth that is either exponential or linear and have been shown to correlate with OS and to discriminate effective therapies as well as individual patients within trials.[68–73] A major advantage is that more of the data are used, relative to dichotomized response assessment, and regression or growth rates can be determined even in patients who are censored in a Kaplan–Meier analysis. Equations that model both regression and growth rates confirm the clinical intuition that resistant disease is emerging even as overall tumor volume is reduced. Further, "the strategy of studying tumor growth kinetics circumvents one weakness of 'progression criteria,' which is that they inherently dichotomize a complex biological process that may be better characterized using a continuous function."[74] As shown in Figure 30.5, the response of a tumor to a therapy is exemplified by the nadir, the time to the nadir, and the time to progression or PFS, and these are all are all dependent on the growth rate.

REFERENCES

1. America's Biopharmaceutical Research Companies. *Medicines in Development for Cancer.* PhRMA Web site. http://www.phrma.org/sites/default/files/pdf/phrmamedicinesindevelopmentcancer2012.pdf.
2. Moertel CG, Hanley JA. The effect of measuring error on the results of therapeutic trials in advanced cancer. *Cancer* 1976;38:388–394.
3. Miller AB, Hoogstraten B, Staquet M, et al. Reporting results of cancer treatment. *Cancer* 1981;47:207–214.
4. Therasse P, Arbuck SG, Eisenhauer EA, et al. New guidelines to evaluate the response to treatment in solid tumors. European Organization for Research and Treatment of Cancer, National Cancer Institute of the United States, National Cancer Institute of Canada. *J Natl Cancer Inst* 2000;92:205–216.
5. Eisenhauer EA, Therasse P, Bogaerts J, et al. New response evaluation criteria in solid tumours: revised RECIST guideline (version 1.1). *Eur J Cancer* 2009;45:228–247.
6. Mazumdar M, Smith A, Schwartz LH. A statistical simulation study finds discordance between WHO criteria and RECIST guideline. *J Clin Epidemiol* 2004;57:358–365.
7. Wen PY, Macdonald DR, Reardon DA, et al. Updated response assessment criteria for high-grade gliomas: response assessment in neuro-oncology working group. *J Clin Oncol* 2010;28:1963–1972.
8. Byrne MJ, Nowak AK. Modified RECIST criteria for assessment of response in malignant pleural mesothelioma. *Ann Oncol* 2004;15:257–260.
9. Wolchok JD, Hoos A, O'Day S, et al. Guidelines for the evaluation of immune therapy activity in solid tumors: immune-related response criteria. *Clin Cancer Res* 2009;15:7412–7420.
10. Quant EC, Wen PY. Response assessment in neuro-oncology. *Curr Oncol Rep* 2011;13:50–56.
11. Hawkins-Daarud A, Rockne RC, Anderson AR, et al. Modeling tumor-associated edema in gliomas during anti-angiogenic therapy and its impact on imageable tumor. *Front Oncol* 2013;3:66.
12. Fink J, Born D, Chamberlain MC. Pseudoprogression: relevance with respect to treatment of high-grade gliomas. *Curr Treat Options Oncol* 2011;12:240–252.
13. Lin NU, Lee EQ, Aoyama H, et al. Challenges relating to solid tumour brain metastases in clinical trials, part 1: patient population, response, and progression. A report from the RANO group. *Lancet Oncol* 2013;14:e396–e406.
14. Mabille M, Vanel D, Albiter M, et al. Follow-up of hepatic and peritoneal metastases of gastrointestinal tumors (GIST) under Imatinib therapy requires different criteria of radiological evaluation (size is not everything!!!). *Eur J Radiol* 2009;69:204–208.
15. Liu L, Wang W, Chen H, et al. EASL- and mRECIST-evaluated responses to combination therapy of sorafenib with transarterial chemoembolization predict survival in patients with hepatocellular carcinoma. *Clin Cancer Res* 2014;20:1623–1631.
16. Cheson BD, Pfistner B, Juweid ME, et al. Revised response criteria for malignant lymphoma. *J Clin Oncol* 2007;25:579–586.
17. Bernhard J, Dietrich D, Scheithauer W, et al. Clinical benefit and quality of life in patients with advanced pancreatic cancer receiving gemcitabine plus capecitabine versus gemcitabine alone: a randomized multicenter phase III clinical trial—SAKK 44/00-CECOG/PAN.1.3.001. *J Clin Oncol* 2008;26:3695–3701.
18. Burris HA, Moore MJ, Andersen J, et al. Improvements in survival and clinical benefit with gemcitabine as first-line therapy for patients with advanced pancreas cancer: a randomized trial. *J Clin Oncol* 1997;15:2403–2413.
19. Mann BS, Johnson JR, He K, et al. Vorinostat for treatment of cutaneous manifestations of advanced primary cutaneous T-cell lymphoma. *Clin Cancer Res* 2007;13:2318–2322.
20. von Minckwitz G, Untch M, Blohmer JU, et al. Definition and impact of pathologic complete response on prognosis after neoadjuvant chemotherapy in various intrinsic breast cancer subtypes. *J Clin Oncol* 2012;30:1796–1804.
21. Cortazar P, Zhang L, Untch M, et al. Pathological complete response and long-term clinical benefit in breast cancer: the CTNeoBC pooled analysis. *Lancet* 2014 [Epub ahead of print].
22. Bardia A, Baselga J. Neoadjuvant therapy as a platform for drug development and approval in breast cancer. *Clin Cancer Res* 2013;19:6360–6370.
23. Choi H, Charnsangavej C, Faria SC, et al. Correlation of computed tomography and positron emission tomography in patients with metastatic gastrointestinal stromal tumor treated at a single institution with imatinib mesylate: proposal of new computed tomography response criteria. *J Clin Oncol* 2007;25:1753–1759.
24. Schramm N, Englhart E, Schlemmer M, et al. Tumor response and clinical outcome in metastatic gastrointestinal stromal tumors under sunitinib therapy: comparison of RECIST, Choi and volumetric criteria. *Eur J Radiol* 2013;82:951–958.
25. Dudeck O, Zeile M, Reichardt P, et al. Comparison of RECIST and Choi criteria for computed tomographic response evaluation in patients with advanced gastrointestinal stromal tumor treated with sunitinib. *Ann Oncol* 2011;22:1828–1833.
26. Ronot M, Bouattour M, Wassermann J, et al. Alternative response criteria (Choi, European Association for the Study of the Liver, and Modified Response Evaluation Criteria in Solid Tumors [RECIST]) versus RECIST 1.1 in patients with advanced hepatocellular carcinoma treated with sorafenib. *Oncologist* 2014. http://prostatecancer.theoncologist.com/article/alternative-response-criteria-choi-european-association-study-liver-and-modified-response.
27. van der Veldt AA, Meijerink MR, van den Eertwegh AJ, et al. Choi response criteria for early prediction of clinical outcome in patients with metastatic renal cell cancer treated with sunitinib. *Br J Cancer* 2010;102:803–809.
28. Wahl RL, Jacene H, Kasamon Y, et al. From RECIST to PERCIST: evolving considerations for PET response criteria in solid tumors. *J Nucl Med* 2009;50:122S–150S.
29. Shankar LK, Hoffman JM, Bacharach S, et al. Consensus recommendations for the use of 18F-FDG PET as an indicator of therapeutic response in patients in National Cancer Institute Trials. *J Nucl Med* 2006;47:1059–1066.
30. Young H, Baum R, Cremerius U, et al. Measurement of clinical and subclinical tumour response using [18F]-fluorodeoxyglucose and positron emission tomography: review and 1999 EORTC recommendations. European Organization for Research and Treatment of Cancer (EORTC) PET Study Group. *Eur J Cancer* 1999;35:1773–1782.
31. Kramer-Marek G, Capala J. Can PET imaging facilitate optimization of cancer therapies? *Curr Pharm Des* 2012;18:2657–2669.
32. Niederkohr RD, Greenspan BS, Prior JO, et al. Reporting guidance for oncologic 18F-FDG PET/CT imaging. *J Nucl Med* 2013;54:756–761.
33. Liu Y, Litière S, de Vries EG, et al. The role of response evaluation criteria in solid tumour in anticancer treatment evaluation: results of a survey in the oncology community. *Eur J Cancer* 2014;50:260–266.
34. Rubin EH, Allen JD, Nowak JA, et al. Developing precision medicine in a global world. *Clin Cancer Res* 2014;20:1419–1427.
35. Parkinson DR, McCormack RT, Keating SM. Evidence of clinical utility: an unmet need in molecular diagnostics for cancer patients. *Clin Cancer Res* 2014;20:1428–1444.
36. Buyse M, Sargent DJ, Grothey A, et al. Biomarkers and surrogate end points—the challenge of statistical validation. *Nat Rev Clin Oncol* 2010;7:309–317.
37. Karam AK, Karlan BY. Ovarian cancer: the duplicity of CA125 measurement. *Nat Rev Clin Oncol* 2010;7:335–339.

CANCER THERAPEUTICS

38. Rustin GJ, van der Burg ME, Griffin CL, et al. Early versus delayed treatment of relapsed ovarian cancer (MRC OV05/EORTC 55955): a randomised trial. *Lancet* 2010;376:1155–1163.

39. Vergote I, Rustin GJ, Eisenhauer EA, et al. Re: new guidelines to evaluate the response to treatment in solid tumors [ovarian cancer]. Gynecologic Cancer Intergroup. *J Natl Cancer Inst* 2000;92:1534–1535.

40. Guppy AE, Rustin GJ. CA125 response: can it replace the traditional response criteria in ovarian cancer? *Oncologist* 2002;7:437–443.

41. Rustin GJ, Quinn M, Thigpen T, et al. Re: New guidelines to evaluate the response to treatment in solid tumors (ovarian cancer). *J Natl Cancer Inst* 2004; 96:487–488.

42. Rustin GJ, Vergote I, Eisenhauer E, et al. Definitions for response and progression in ovarian cancer clinical trials incorporating RECIST 1.1 and CA 125 agreed by the Gynecological Cancer Intergroup (GCIG). *Int J Gynecol Cancer* 2011;21:419–423.

43. Eisenhauer EA. Optimal assessment of response in ovarian cancer. *Ann Oncol* 2011;22:viii49–viii51.

44. Bubley GJ, Carducci M, Dahut W, et al. Eligibility and response guidelines for phase II clinical trials in androgen-independent prostate cancer: recommendations from the Prostate-Specific Antigen Working Group. *J Clin Oncol* 1999;17:3461–3467.

45. Scher HI, Halabi S, Tannock I, et al. Design and end points of clinical trials for patients with progressive prostate cancer and castrate levels of testosterone: recommendations of the Prostate Cancer Clinical Trials Working Group. *J Clin Oncol* 2008;26:1148–1159.

46. Mazumdar M, Bajorin DF, Bacik J, et al. Predicting outcome to chemotherapy in patients with germ cell tumors: the value of the rate of decline of human chorionic gonadotrophin and alpha-fetoprotein during therapy. *J Clin Oncol* 2001;19:2534–2541.

47. Fizazi K, Culine S, Kramar A, et al. Early predicted time to normalization of tumor markers predicts outcome in poor-prognosis nonseminomatous germ cell tumors. *J Clin Oncol* 2004;22:3868–3876.

48. Toner GC. Early identification of therapeutic failure in nonseminomatous germ cell tumors by assessing serum tumor marker decline during chemotherapy: still not ready for routine clinical use. *J Clin Oncol* 2004;22:3842–3845.

49. Gilligan TD, Seidenfeld J, Basch EM, et al. American Society of Clinical Oncology Clinical Practice Guideline on uses of serum tumor markers in adult males with germ cell tumors. *J Clin Oncol* 2010;28:3388–3404.

50. Albers P, Albrecht W, Algaba F, et al. EAU guidelines on testicular cancer: 2011 update. *Eur Urol* 2011;60:304–319.

51. Yap T, Lorente D, Omlin A, et al. Circulating tumor cells: a multifunctional biomarker. *Clin Cancer Res* 2014;20:2553–2568.

52. Dawson SJ, Tsui DW, Murtaza M, et al. Analysis of circulating tumor DNA to monitor metastatic breast cancer. *N Engl J Med* 2013;368:1199–1209.

53. Punnoose EA, Atwal S, Liu W, et al. Evaluation of circulating tumor cells and circulating tumor DNA in non-small cell lung cancer: association with clinical endpoints in a phase II clinical trial of pertuzumab and erlotinib. *Clin Cancer Res* 2012; 18:2391–2401.

54. Bettegowda C, Sausen M, Leary RJ, et al. Detection of circulating tumor DNA in early- and late-stage human malignancies. *Sci Transl Med* 2014;6:224ra24.

55. Pazdur R. Endpoints for assessing drug activity in clinical trials. *Oncologist* 2008;13:19–21.

56. Buyse M, Thirion P, Carlson RW, et al. Relation between tumour response to first-line chemotherapy and survival in advanced colorectal cancer: a meta-analysis. Meta-Analysis Group in Cancer. *Lancet* 2000;356:373–378.

57. Bruzzi P, Del Mastro L, Sormani MP, et al. Objective response to chemotherapy as a potential surrogate end point of survival in metastatic breast cancer patients. *J Clin Oncol* 2005;23:5117–5125.

58. Vidaurre T, Wilkerson J, Simon R, et al. Stable disease is not preferentially observed with targeted therapies and as currently defined has limited value in drug development. *Cancer J* 2009;15:366–373.

59. McKee AE, Farrell AT, Pazdur R, et al. The role of the U.S. Food and Drug Administration review process: clinical trial endpoints in oncology. *Oncologist* 2010;15:13–18.

60. Ohorodnyk P, Eisenhauer EA, Booth CM. Clinical benefit in oncology trials: is this a patient-centred or tumour-centred end-point? *Eur J Cancer* 2009; 45:2249–2252.

61. Buyse M. Use of meta-analysis for the validation of surrogate endpoints and biomarkers in cancer trials. *Cancer J* 2009;15:421–425.

62. Wilkerson J, Fojo T. Progression-free survival is simply a measure of a drug's effect while administered and is not a surrogate for overall survival. *Cancer J* 2009;15:379–385.

63. Reck M, von Pawel J, Zatloukal P, et al. Overall survival with cisplatin-gemcitabine and bevacizumab or placebo as first-line therapy for nonsquamous non-small-cell lung cancer: results from a randomised phase III trial (AVAiL). *Ann Oncol* 2010;21:1804–1809.

64. Hortobagyi GN, Gomez HL, Li RK, et al. Analysis of overall survival from a phase III study of ixabepilone plus capecitabine versus capecitabine in patients with MBC resistant to anthracyclines and taxanes. *Breast Cancer Res Treat* 2010; 122:409–418.

65. Hennekens C, Buring J. *Epidemiology in Medicine*. 1st ed. Boston: Little, Brown and Co.; 1987.

66. Cuzick J. Forest plots and the interpretation of subgroups. *Lancet* 2005;365:1308.

67. Huang H, Menefee M, Edgerly M, et al. A phase II clinical trial of ixabepilone (Ixempra; BMS-247550; NSC 710428), an epothilone B analog, in patients with metastatic renal cell carcinoma. *Clin Cancer Res* 2010;16:1634–1641.

68. Stein WD, Gulley JL, Schlom J, et al. Tumor regression and growth rates determined in five intramural NCI prostate cancer trials: the growth rate constant as an indicator of therapeutic efficacy. *Clin Cancer Res* 2011;17:907–917.

69. Stein WD, Wilkerson J, Kim ST, et al. Analyzing the pivotal trial that compared sunitinib and IFN-α in renal cell carcinoma, using a method that assesses tumor regression and growth. *Clin Cancer Res* 2012;18:2374–2381.

70. Maitland ML, Wu K, Sharma MR, et al. Estimation of renal cell carcinoma treatment effects from disease progression modeling. *Clin Pharmacol Ther* 2013;93:345–351.

71. Claret L, Girard P, Hoff PM, et al. Model-based prediction of phase III overall survival in colorectal cancer on the basis of phase II tumor dynamics. *J Clin Oncol* 2009;27:4103–4108.

72. Claret L, Gupta M, Han K, et al. Evaluation of tumor-size response metrics to predict overall survival in Western and Chinese patients with first-line metastatic colorectal cancer. *J Clin Oncol* 2013;31:2110–2114.

73. Wang Y, Sung C, Dartois C, et al. Elucidation of relationship between tumor size and survival in non-small-cell lung cancer patients can aid early decision making in clinical drug development. *Clin Pharmacol Ther* 2009;86:167–174.

74. Oxnard GR, Morris MJ, Hodi FS, et al. When progressive disease does not mean treatment failure: reconsidering the criteria for progression. *J Natl Cancer Inst* 2012;104:1534–1541.

75. Team RDC. R: A language and environment for statistical computing. R Foundation for Statistical Computing. Vienna, Austria: R Foundation for Statistical Computing; 2010. http://www.r-project.org.

PART IV

Cancer Prevention and Screening

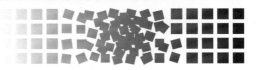

31 Tobacco Use and the Cancer Patient

Graham W. Warren, Benjamin A. Toll, Irene M. Tamí-Maury, and Ellen R. Gritz

INTRODUCTION

Tobacco is commonly described as the largest preventable cause of cancer. Over 50 years ago, tobacco was increasingly recognized as the primary cause of lung cancer, with definitive recognition for tobacco use as a causative factor in the seminal 1964 U.S. Surgeon General's Report (SGR) on Smoking and Health.[1] Recent editions of the SGR have described the widespread adverse health effects of tobacco on a spectrum of diseases, including as a causative agent for a spectrum of cancers.[2,3] Tobacco use is an addiction usually initiated in youth prior to the age of 18 and is driven by the highly addictive drug, nicotine.[4] As related to the cancer patient, considerable work has been conducted to associate tobacco use with the risk of developing cancer and how tobacco cessation can substantially reduce cancer risks. However, there is a relative paucity of effort that has been put forth to identify the effects of smoking on outcomes for cancer patients or to establish methods to help cancer patients quit smoking. Fortunately, in recent years, the importance of tobacco use by the cancer patient has been increasingly recognized as an important health behavior, including a National Cancer Institute (NCI)–sponsored conference on tobacco use in 2010, a joint sponsored NCI–American Association of Cancer Research (AACR)–sponsored workshop at the Institute of Medicine in 2012, and recent recommendations by the AACR and the American Society of Clinical Oncology (ASCO) to address tobacco use in cancer patients.[5,6] The recently released 2014 SGR now provides substantial evidence behind the effects of smoking by cancer patients with the following conclusions[7]:

1. In cancer patients and survivors, the evidence is sufficient to infer a causal relationship between cigarette smoking and adverse health outcomes. Quitting smoking improves the prognosis of cancer patients.
2. In cancer patients and survivors, the evidence is sufficient to infer a causal relationship between cigarette smoking and increased all-cause mortality and cancer-specific mortality.
3. In cancer patients and survivors, the evidence is sufficient to infer a causal relationship between cigarette smoking and increased risk for second primary cancers known to be caused by cigarette smoking, such as lung cancer.
4. In cancer patients and survivors, the evidence is suggestive but not sufficient to infer a causal relationship between cigarette smoking and the risk of recurrence, poorer response to treatment, and increased treatment-related toxicity.

The overall objective of this chapter is to discuss tobacco use by cancer patients, the clinical effects of smoking in cancer patients, methods to address tobacco use by cancer patients, and areas of needed research.

NEUROBIOLOGY OF TOBACCO DEPENDENCE

Nicotine is the primary addictive component of tobacco that increases extracellular concentrations of dopamine in the nucleus accumbens and stimulates the mesolimbic dopaminergic system,[8,9] resulting in nicotine's rewarding effect experienced by tobacco users.[10–12] Dopaminergic neurotransmission may also be involved in the assignment of incentive salience, or stimulus for a pleasure based reward, to tobacco use–related environmental cues[13,14] that may become conditioned reinforcers of tobacco use behaviors. For example, an individual who smokes while drinking their morning coffee may associate coffee, or even holding a coffee cup in their hand, with the reward from smoking. Thus, cigarette smoking is directly linked to external nontobacco-based behavioral stimuli. Activation of the nucleus accumbens has further been implicated in drug reinstatement or relapse.[15,16] Individuals who have quit tobacco use for years have restarted a tobacco habit simply by sitting next to a smoker and being exposed to secondhand smoke. Substantial work has been conducted on the addictive nature of tobacco and nicotine, and readers are referred to several comprehensive reviews on this topic.[9,12,17]

TOBACCO USE PREVALENCE AND THE EVOLUTION OF TOBACCO PRODUCTS

Much of the discussion on tobacco use epidemiology and carcinogenesis is presented in Chapter 4. In brief, the prevalence of cigarette smoking among adults in the United States decreased to 19.0% as compared with 22.8% in 2001, but it did not meet the *Healthy People 2010* objective to reduce smoking prevalence to 12%.[18,19] There have been substantial changes in the landscape of tobacco use over time as a direct consequence of cigarette-centered policies and regulations aiming to reduce the harmful effects and number of deaths caused by smoking.[20–22] Under this new landscape, novel and reemergent noncigarette tobacco products such as cigars, cigarillos, snuff, chewing tobacco, water pipes (hookahs), and other forms of tobacco consumption have been growing in demand as a consequence of aggressive and sophisticated marketing by the tobacco industry.[23] Consumption patterns have also changed due to efforts by the tobacco industry to make cigarettes appear safer, such as low tar or filtered cigarettes, and the inclusion of flavoring (menthol, vanilla, fruits, etc.).[24] Although these efforts may have changed consumption patterns, they have not reduced cancer risk. Large patient cohorts demonstrate that the introduction of low tar and filtered cigarettes actually increased risk by promoting deeper inhalation and higher rates of addiction with no reductions in cancer risk,[24,25] resulting in subsequent changes in lung cancer from centrally located squamous cell cancers to peripherally located nonsquamous cell cancers.

The relatively recent introduction of electronic cigarettes (i.e., e-cigarettes, e-cigs, nicotine vaporizers, or electronic nicotine delivery systems [ENDS]) is noteworthy. These electronic or battery-powered devices activate a heating element that vaporizes a liquid solution contained in a cartridge, and then the user inhales this vapor. Levels of nicotine as well as other chemical additives and flavors in the cartridge are uncertain and vary according to the brand.[26] Although there are no research studies that have evaluated the potential harmful effects of the use of e-cigarettes for cancer patients,[27] organizations such as the World Health Organization have already expressed concerns about the safety of these increasingly popular products.[28,29] To date, e-cigarettes have not been approved by the U.S. Food and Drug Administration (FDA) as therapeutic devices to aid in quitting smoking.[26] Readers are referred to a recent editorial on the use of e-cigarettes by cancer patients[27]; however, it will likely be several years before evidence-based health information is available.

TOBACCO USE BY THE CANCER PATIENT

The prevalence of current smoking among long-term adult cancer survivors appears to have declined in the past decade,[30] but data suggest higher rates of smoking among cancer survivors than in the general population.[30–32] These data are often biased by the fact that assessments in cancer patients may not include cancer patients who were current smokers at the time of death. As a result, estimates of smoking rates in cancer survivors may be misleading and may underestimate true tobacco use patterns for cancer patients. Furthermore, alternative tobacco products are often not assessed in cancer patients. Data from the Childhood Cancer Survivor Study and the 2009 Behavioral Risk Factor Surveillance System indicate that approximately 3% to 8% of cancer survivors use smokeless tobacco products.[33,34] Patients may be attracted to these alternative products due to less social stigma and the nonevidence-based perception that these products are healthier alternatives compared to cigarette smoking.

Continued tobacco use by cancer patients often represents a combined failure by the patient to recognize the need to stop smoking even after a cancer diagnosis and the effort by health-care providers to address tobacco use with evidence-based assessments and tobacco cessation support. Approximately 30% of all cancer patients use tobacco at the time of cancer diagnosis with higher rates in traditionally tobacco-related disease sites, such as head and neck or lung cancers, and lower rates in traditionally nontobacco-related disease sites, such as breast or prostate cancers.[35–44] However, findings from several studies indicate that cancer patients are receptive to smoking cessation interventions even as they continue to smoke.[35,38,45–50]

A cancer diagnosis can be used as a window of opportunity, or *teachable moment*, to intervene and provide assistance in the quitting process.[51] A recent study in 12,000 cancer patients, including 2,700 patients who smoked, capitalized on the teachable moment and demonstrated that less than 3% of patients who were contacted by the cessation program rejected tobacco cessation assistance.[45] However, only 1.2% of patients who received a mailed invitation participated in the program. This highlights the idea that patients may be interested in quitting, but methods such as mailed tobacco cessation information may not yield effective participation by cancer patients. Once enrolled, patients and clinicians must realize that although relapses in the general population usually occur within 1 week of cessation, relapses in cancer patients may be delayed due to cancer treatment–related variables such as surgical or other posttreatment healing.[52] Consequently, it is important to continue offering tobacco assessments and cessation support for cancer survivorship efforts.

Defining Tobacco Use by the Cancer Patient

In dealing with tobacco use by cancer patients, it is important to note that virtually all of the evidence associating tobacco with cancer treatment outcomes deals with smoking. Few studies report associations between other forms of tobacco use (e.g., smokeless, cigars, cigarillos) and outcomes in cancer patients. Furthermore, the definition of smoking across published studies varies substantially.[53] In studies of cancer patients, smoking has been defined as current (e.g., smoking after diagnosis, at diagnosis, in the weeks

before diagnosis, within the 12 months prior to diagnosis, after diagnosis, within the past 10 years), former (e.g., recent, intermediate-, or long-term quit for 1 month, 3 month, 6 month, 12 month, 2 years, 5 years, 10 years), never, quitting after diagnosis, and according to exposure (e.g., multiple pack year cutoffs, Brinkman index, years of smoking, years of smoking within a predefined period of time such as 5 years prior to diagnosis). Though the nonstandard method of addressing tobacco use in cancer patients has been observed in several reports,[54–57] there are no current standard recommendations for the definition of tobacco use by any national organization. There are four primary categories for smoking status:

1. **Never smoking** is typically defined as having smoked less than 100 cigarettes in a person's lifetime and no current cigarette use. These patients are generally considered as a reference group in many studies. Categories 2 through 4 require that a person has smoked at least 100 cigarettes in their lifetime.
2. **Former smoking** is typically defined as no current cigarette use, usually within the past year.
3. **Recent smoking** (or recent quit) is generally defined as having stopped smoking within the recent past, typically for a period of 1 week to 1 year.
4. **Current smoking** is typically defined as smoking one or more cigarettes per day every day or some days.

Ever smoking is a combination of categories 2 through 4 (i.e., former, recent, and current smokers) that has been used to report negative associations between smoking and cancer outcomes in a number of studies.[58–70] Defining smoking according to *ever* smoking status limits the ability to interpret the effects of current smoking on a clinical outcome, and nothing can be done to address a prior tobacco use history. However, defining exposure according to *current* smoking status allows for the analysis of potentially reversible effects as well as for the potential implementation of smoking cessation to prevent the adverse outcomes of smoking on cancer patients. The primary focus for the remainder of this chapter will be on *current* smoking and will include a discussion of methods to address tobacco use with the cancer patient through accurate assessments and structured tobacco cessation support.

THE CLINICAL EFFECTS OF SMOKING ON THE CANCER PATIENT

Cancer treatment is generally defined according to disease site, stage, treatment type (e.g., surgery, chemotherapy [CT], radiotherapy [RT], or biologic therapy), and primary treatment objective, such as cure or palliation. A comprehensive discussion of the effects of smoking on cancer patients is beyond the scope of a single chapter, but the 2014 SGR provides an excellent evidence base, concluding that "the evidence is sufficient to infer a causal relationship between cigarette smoking and adverse health outcomes."[7] Overall, approximately 75% to 80% of studies in the SGR demonstrated a negative association between smoking and outcome, with approximately 65% to 70% of studies demonstrating statistically significant negative associations. This chapter will provide an illustrative review of studies that demonstrate the adverse effects of tobacco across disease sites and treatment modalities (e.g., surgery, CT, RT), and effects will be discussed across the categories of *mortality, recurrence and cancer-related mortality, toxicity*, and *risk of a second primary cancer*. Evidence for the benefits of smoking cessation will also be presented within each section.

The Effect of Smoking on Overall Mortality

Substantial evidence demonstrates that current smoking by cancer patients increases the risk of overall mortality across virtually all cancer disease sites and for all treatment modalities. Currently smoking significantly increased the risk of overall mortality by between 17% to 38% as compared with never, former, and recent quit smokers in a large cohort of patients across 13 disease sites.[71] Similar but larger observations were noted in elderly current smokers from a separate cohort (hazard ratio [HR], 1.72, 95% confidence interval [CI], 1.23 to 2.42).[72] A large analysis of over 20,000 patients treated with surgery demonstrated that current smoking increased mortality by 62% in gastrointestinal cancer patients and by 50% in thoracic cancer patients with a nonsignificant trend in urologic cancer patients.[73] Several larger studies with at least 500 patients demonstrated that current smoking increases mortality in head and neck cancer,[74–77] breast cancer,[78–81] gastrointestinal cancers,[82,83] prostate cancer,[84–87] renal cancer,[88] gynecologic cancers,[89,90] and lung cancer.[91–102] Smaller studies demonstrate similar effects for hematolymphoid cancers such as leukemia and lymphoma.[103,104] Studies suggest that the effects of current smoking on mortality may be dose and time dependent, with higher risks in heavier smokers[105,106] and lesser risks in patients whose time since quitting was longer.[105]

Whereas many reports rely on retrospective chart reviews, several prospective studies demonstrate that current smoking increases mortality.[71] Browman et al.[107] was one of the first prospective studies to demonstrate that current smoking increased mortality by 2.3-fold in patients who continued to smoke during RT as compared with nonsmokers. Results from Radiation Therapy Oncology Group (RTOG) 9003 and 0129 cooperative group trials demonstrated that current smoking increased mortality in advanced head and neck cancer patients treated with RT or concurrent chemoradiotherapy (CRT),[108] with a similar effect noted in 165 cervical cancer patients treated with CRT.[109] In the randomized retinoid chemoprevention trial of 1,190 early stage head and neck cancer patients, current smoking increased mortality by 2.5-fold.[110]

Numerous studies have demonstrated that current smoking increases overall mortality as compared with former and never smokers combined.[72,75,76,101,102,107,108] The adverse effects of smoking compared with former and never smokers not only reflect the negative effects of smoking on mortality as a whole, but also demonstrate that the effects of smoking are reversible. Current smoking increased mortality risk as compared with patients who quit within the year[71] or 1 to 3 months prior to diagnosis.[111,112] Furthermore, in 284 limited-stage small-cell lung cancer patients, patients who quit smoking at or following a cancer diagnosis had a 45% reduction in mortality as compared with current smokers.[113] These studies suggest that the effects of smoking on mortality are reversible.

Collectively, these studies provide significant data associating current smoking with increased overall mortality across most disease sites, tumor stages, treatment modalities, and in both traditionally tobacco-related as well as nontobacco-related cancers. The potential significance of smoking is perhaps best exemplified by Bittner et al.,[114] who analyzed causes of death in prostate cancer patients and demonstrated that more than 90% died of causes other than prostate cancer, but that current smoking increased the risks of non–prostate cancer deaths between 3- and 5.5-fold. As a result, tobacco use and cessation may be of paramount importance to cancers with high cure rates, such as prostate cancer or breast cancer, simply because patients may be at the most risk of death from noncancer-related causes such as heart disease, pulmonary disease, or other diseases related to smoking and tobacco use.

The Effect of Smoking on Cancer Recurrence and Cancer-Related Mortality

The primary objective of cancer therapy is to cure cancer and prevent recurrence. However, smoking has been shown to increase cancer recurrence and cancer-related mortality. Across a broad spectrum of cancer patients, current smoking increased cancer mortality as compared with former and never smokers.[71] Current smoking has been shown to increase cancer mortality in patients with head and neck cancer,[108,115–118] breast cancer,[78,119]

gastrointestinal cancers,[82,120,121] prostate cancer,[41,84,122] gynecologic cancers,[89,90,106,123–125] and lung cancer.[126] Cancer recurrence, whether local or metastatic, is a key driver behind cancer-related mortality. Several studies demonstrate that current smoking increases the risk of recurrence and decreases response across multiple disease sites.[76,84,107,127,128] The effects of smoking on increasing recurrence or cancer-related mortality have also been reported in several relatively rare cancers.[120,129] In a remarkable report of patients with recurrent head and neck cancers treated with salvage surgery, continued smoking after salvage treatment continued to increase the risk of yet another recurrence by 42%.[130] The striking nature of this last study highlights the continued risks even in recurrent cancer patients and the resilience with which some cancer patients will continue to smoke.

The effects of smoking are also noted in premalignant lesions. In patients with high-grade vulvar intraepithelial neoplasia, current smoking increased the risk of persistent disease after therapy by 30-fold.[131] In a prospective trial of progesterone to treat cervical intraepithelial neoplasia (CIN), current smoking increased the risk of progression as compared with former and never smokers combined.[132] A prospective trial of 516 low-grade cervical intraepithelial neoplasia patients demonstrated that current smoking decreased response by 36%, although a similar effect was also noted in former smokers.[133]

As noted with overall mortality, several studies demonstrated that the effects of current smoking are worse than the effects of former smoking[76,86,89,109,127,134–136,137] and that the effects of smoking may be acutely reversible. Several studies also demonstrate that current smoking increases recurrence or cancer mortality, whereas former smoking has no significant effect.[41,78,82,84,85,119,122–124,138] The acutely reversible effects of smoking were shown by Browman et al.[139] who demonstrated that continued smoking increased the risk of cancer-related mortality by 23% as compared with patients who quit within 12 weeks of starting RT. In 284 colorectal cancer patients, smoking at the first postoperative visit increased the risk of cancer mortality by 2.5-fold as compared with all other patients suggesting that smoking after treatment significantly predict for adverse outcome.[121] In a notable study of over 1,400 prostate cancer patients treated with surgery, continued smoking 1 year after treatment increased the risk of recurrence 2.3-fold, but quitting smoking 1 year after treatment did not confer an increased risk of recurrence.[128] Chen et al.[138] demonstrate that patients who continue to smoke before and following a bladder cancer diagnosis have an increased risk of recurrence as compared with patients who quit in the year prior to diagnosis or within the first 3 months after diagnosis. The reversible effects of smoking on recurrence and mortality are consistent with observations on overall mortality and continue to emphasize the benefit of tobacco cessation for cancer patients who smoke at diagnosis.

The Effect of Smoking on Cancer Treatment Toxicity

Discussion of the effects of smoking on cancer treatment toxicity is highly dependent upon disease site, treatment modality (e.g., surgery, CT, RT), and timing of toxicity. Across disease sites and treatments, current smoking has been shown to increase complications from surgery,[140–149] pulmonary complications,[150,151] toxicity from RT,[117,152–156] mucositis,[157] hospitalization,[158] and vasomotor symptoms.[159] One of the largest recent studies in over 20,000 gastrointestinal, pulmonary, and urologic patients demonstrates that former or current smoking increased the risk of surgical site infection, pulmonary complications, or 30-day mortality in a site-specific manner.[73] The effects of current smoking were most significant for pulmonary complications where former smoking had a lesser or nonsignificant effect. In 13,469 lung cancer patients treated with surgery, current smoking increased the risk of postoperative death with no increased risk in former smokers.[160] Current smoking increased the risk of complications, morbidity, or reoperation following esophagectomy, pancreatectomy, or colorectal surgery.[161–163] A study of 836 prostate cancer patients treated with RT demonstrated that current smoking increased abdominal cramps, rectal urgency, diarrhea, incomplete emptying, and sudden emptying between two- and nine-fold,[164] with similar effects noted in 3,489 cervical cancer patients who smoked more than 1 pack per day (PPD).[156]

Several studies have demonstrated that the effects of smoking on cancer treatment toxicity are reversible. Stopping smoking within 3 weeks of surgery reduced wound healing complications in esophageal cancer patients treated with surgery and reconstruction.[165] In 393 T1 laryngeal cancer patients treated with RT, quitting smoking after diagnosis reduced laryngeal complications as compared with continued smoking.[152] In a large study of 7,990 lung cancer patients from the Society of Thoracic Surgeons Database, current smoking increased the risk of pulmonary complications by 80% and hospital mortality 3.5-fold.[151] However, smoking cessation for 2 weeks eliminated the risks for pulmonary complications, and cessation for 1 month eliminated risks for hospital mortality. Vaporciyan et al.[166] also showed that current smoking increased the risk of pulmonary complications 2.7-fold as compared with smoking cessation for at least 1 month prior to surgery. In a striking example of the potentially reversible effects of smoking in 205 head and neck cancer patients treated with RT,[167] 43% of smoking patients treated in the morning experienced Grade 3+ mucositis compared with 72% of smokers treated in the afternoon (p = 0.04). These data suggest that reducing smoking overnight may yield a clinical benefit in reduced toxicity. Whereas all toxicity may not be acutely reversed, these encouraging data show that patients can make clinically meaningful improvements in their health and or cancer treatment within a short time frame by quitting smoking.

The Effect of Smoking on Risk of Second Primary Cancer

Several studies have reported the effects of smoking on the risk of developing a second primary cancer. Park et al.[168] reported on over 14,000 male cancer patients and demonstrated that current smoking increased the risk of developing a second tobacco-related primary cancer twofold, with no increased risk in former smokers. A higher risk was observed in in head and neck cancer patients who smoked more than 10 cigarettes per day, with no increased risk in lighter smokers.[169] Kinoshita et al.[170] showed an 82% increased risk of developing a second primary in gastric cancer patients who are current smokers with no increased risk in former smokers. In the phase III randomized trial of isotretinoin for the prevention of a second primary tumor in 1,190 head and neck cancer patients, current smoking increased the risk of a second primary by 2.2-fold with a nonsignificant trend of 1.6-fold in former smokers.[110] Notably, 39% of patients who reported quitting within the previous year were biochemically confirmed smokers.[171] As a result, these data collectively suggest that some of the increased risk may be biased by continued smoking in patients who deny smoking by self-report.

The effects of smoking on the risk of a second primary cancer are also noted in nontobacco-related cancers and in long-term survivors. In 835 breast cancer patients, smoking increased the risk for the development of lung metastases after breast cancer by more than threefold.[172] Ford et al.[173] demonstrated that breast cancer patients who were former smokers had a threefold increased risk of developing lung cancer, but that current smokers had a 13-fold increased risk. In nearly 1,100 estrogen receptor (ER)-positive breast cancer patients, current smokers had a 1.8-fold increased risk of developing a second contralateral breast cancer, and current smokers at most recent follow-up had a 2.2-fold increased risk, but former smoking at the diagnosis or most recent follow-up had no increased risk.[174] In 2,700 5-year survivors of testicular cancer,

current smokers had a 1.8-fold increased risk of developing a second primary as compared with all other survivors.[175]

There are some studies suggesting that smoking, combined with cytotoxic therapy, may have an additive or synergistic effect on the risk of developing a second primary cancer. In 9,780 prostate cancer patients from the Cancer of the Prostate Strategic Urologic Research Endeavor (CaPSURE) study, RT increased the risk of bladder cancer by 1.6-fold, smoking increased the risk by 2.1-fold, and smoking combined with RT increased risk by 3.7-fold.[176] In ER-positive breast cancer patients, treatment with RT had no significant effect on the risk of developing a contralateral breast cancer, but RT combined with current smoking increased the risk of contralateral cancer by ninefold.[173] In a detailed analysis of Hodgkin lymphoma patients, nonheavy smokers (defined as never, former, and less than one PPD) had a second primary relative risk of between fourfold and sevenfold when treated with CT or RT as compared with patients who received no RT or CT.[177] However, heavy smokers had a sixfold increased risk in the absence of RT and CT and a 17- to 49-fold increased risk when combined with RT and/or CT. These observations suggest that smoking combined with cytotoxic cancer therapy may complement the risk of developing a second primary cancer perhaps through the promotion of mutations induced by CT and/or RT in the presence of tobacco smoke. The potential mechanisms of this effect have not been tested or defined at this time, but the mechanism of tobacco-induced carcinogenesis in prior reports[3] supports these observations.

Human Papilloma Virus, Epidermal Growth Factor Receptor, Anaplastic Lymphoma Kinase, Programmed Cell Death Protein 1, and Smoking

Data over the past decade has shown that head and neck cancers that are human papilloma virus (HPV) positive are known to have an improved prognosis as compared with HPV-negative tumors.[178] Patients who have HPV-positive tumors typically have increased p16 expression and often respond better to conventional cancer therapy, including RT and CT. Many HPV-positive patients are never smokers or have a lighter smoking history. However, smoking was an independent adverse risk factor for both overall and cancer-related mortality with a 1% increase in risk per pack-year smoked.[178] Current smoking increased cancer mortality approximately fivefold even in p16-positive patients treated with surgery.[115] Smoking also increased the risk of developing second primary cancer in both HPV-positive and HPV-negative patients.[179] As a consequence, the presence of HPV does not appear to negate the adverse effects of smoking.

A similar effect is noted in lung cancer patients with epidermal growth factor receptor (EGFR)-mutated or anaplastic lymphoma kinase (ALK)-mutated tumors. As with HPV-positive head and neck cancer patients, lung cancer patients who are light or never smokers have a higher rate of EGFR-positive tumors that may respond to biologic therapy using EGFR tyrosine–kinase inhibitors. At this time, most information regarding EGFR-based therapy for lung cancer reports on the effects of ever smoking demonstrating that ever smokers have a decreased response to EGFR therapy. Early, large, randomized trials demonstrate that Tarceva (erlotinib) and Iressa (gefitinib) provide survival and tumor control benefits specifically in never smokers.[180,181] A very similar pattern is noted for ALK-positive patients with a much higher incidence in never smokers and high response rate to the ALK kinase inhibitor crizotinib.[182] Paik et al.[183] have described the importance of driver mutations in EGFR, ALK, and KRAS demonstrating that smokers have a higher preponderance for K-ras drivers, whereas nonsmokers tend to have EGFR or ALK driver mutations. In general, patients who are smokers may be best served with conventional cancer treatments rather than these biologic therapies, but randomized controlled trials confirming this suggestion are lacking at this time.

Although there are essentially no biologic therapies that have shown to have a better response in smokers, there are exciting data presented at the 2013 European CanCer Organization (ECCO) annual conference, suggesting that anti–programmed cell death protein 1 (PD-1)–based therapies may have a better response rate in smokers.[184] These very preliminary data have yet to be replicated or expanded into randomized trials, but if expanded trials prove effective, they may represent one of the only cancer treatments that may specifically benefit smokers.

Summarizing the Clinical Effects of Smoking on the Cancer Patient

Smoking by cancer patients increases mortality, toxicity, recurrence, and the risk of a second primary cancer. There are four important conclusions, and a fifth implied conclusion, to the evidence previously presented:

1. One or more adverse effects of smoking affect all cancer disease sites.
2. One or more adverse effects of smoking affect all treatment modalities.
3. The effects of current smoking are distinct from an ever or former smoking history.
4. Several lines of evidence demonstrate that many of the effects of smoking are reversible.

Although substantial data demonstrate that smoking by cancer patients increases the risk for one or more outcomes, the largest limitations are the lack of standard tobacco use definitions, the lack of assessing tobacco use in cancer patients at follow-up, and the lack of structured tobacco cessation for cancer patients. Importantly, patients may further misrepresent tobacco use. Several studies suggest that approximately 30% of cancer patients who smoke deny tobacco use.[171,185,186] Marin et al.[187] exemplify the importance of an accurate assessment, demonstrating that patients who self-reported smoking had no significant risk associated with surgical complications; however, biochemical confirmation of smoking significantly increased the risk of surgical wound complications. This highlights the potential discrepancy between the effects of smoking based on subjective versus biochemically confirmed assessments. Due to this discrepancy, the *fifth implied conclusion* is that the adverse effects of smoking and the benefits of cessation may be more pronounced than currently reported in the literature.

ADDRESSING TOBACCO USE BY THE CANCER PATIENT

National Oncology Association Statements and Clinical Practice Guidelines

Professional societies are taking leadership roles in recognizing the need to assess patients' tobacco use and to examine the effects of tobacco use in medical treatment, including the important role of tobacco cessation. The American Medical Association (AMA) passed a resolution supporting documentation of smoking behavior in clinical trials, from trial registration through treatment, follow-up, and to end of the study or death.[188] The Oncology Nursing Society (ONS) has also advocated for assessment and cessation.[189,190] Both the AACR[5,191] and ASCO[6,192] have issued policy statements specifically addressing tobacco use in cancer patients, detailing that clinicians have a responsibility to address tobacco use, that all patients should be screened, that all patients who use tobacco should receive evidence-based tobacco cessation support, and that tobacco use should be included in clinical practice and research. These provide strong counsel to address tobacco use in the general population as well as in cancer patients.

Smoking Cessation Guidelines

Overall, the approach to tobacco cessation for the cancer patient is very similar to the approach for the general population. However, there are a few specific details that are important to consider when approaching the cancer patient who smokes. It is important to recognize that virtually all newly diagnosed cancer patients are faced with a life-changing diagnosis that will require intensive treatment approaches. Treatments, toxicity, and outcomes differ according to disease site and treatment modality. Whereas some cancer patients may have a curable cancer, others may have incurable cancer. Smoking in cancer patients is also often associated with comorbid psychiatric diseases, such as depression, that may affect dependence.[193] The urgency of cessation is also important to consider. If smoking decreases the efficacy of cancer treatment, then every effort should be made to stop tobacco use as soon as possible rather than choosing a quit date several weeks or months after a cancer diagnosis. Patients may also be burdened with a "stigma" associated with certain tobacco-related cancers,[193–197] where they may be viewed by others, or themselves, as causing their cancer due to tobacco use. As a result, the rationale and motivation for quitting tobacco use likely differs among cancer patients, but there is a consistent theme that exists. (1) All patients should be asked about tobacco use with structured assessments; (2) all patients who use tobacco or are at risk for relapse should be offered evidence-based cessation support; and 3) tobacco assessment and cessation support should occur at the time of diagnosis, during treatment, and during follow-up for all cancer patients.

Empiric treatment of tobacco use by cancer patients is fundamentally supported by Public Health Service (PHS) Guidelines that are based on evidence from tobacco cessation efforts in noncancer patients. Originally issued in 1996 and renewed in 2008, *The Clinical Practice Guideline: Treating Tobacco Use and Dependence* is a PHS-sponsored, evidence-based guideline designed to assist health-care providers in delivering and supporting effective smoking cessation treatment.[198,199] The basic recommendation states that clinicians should consistently identify, document, and treat every tobacco user seen in a health-care setting. Details of cessation support range from brief to intensive intervention, but emphasize that consistent repeated cessation support and even brief counseling are effective methods to assist patients with stopping tobacco use. It is important to note that physician-delivered interventions significantly increase long-term abstinence rates.[199] Included are newer effective medication options and strong support for counseling and the use of quit lines as effective intervention strategies. As described in the PHS Guidelines, the principal steps in conducting effective smoking cessation interventions are referred to as The 5 A's:

1. *Ask* about tobacco use for every patient.
2. *Advise* every tobacco user to quit.
3. *Assess* the willingness of patients to quit.
4. *Assist* patients with quitting through counseling and pharmacotherapy.
5. *Arrange* follow-up cessation support, preferably within the first week after the quit date.

There is a strong evidence base for these interventions as documented in the clinical practice guideline.[199]

Implementing Smoking Cessation Into Clinical Practice

An algorithm is provided to guide clinicians in implementing the five A's into clinical cancer care (Fig. 31.1).[5,45,194,199] Included in the algorithm are suggested questions that are useful to accurately assess tobacco use by cancer patients where patients can generally be divided into *current*, *former*, or *never* smokers. The first step (ASK) is to inquire about and document tobacco use behaviors for every

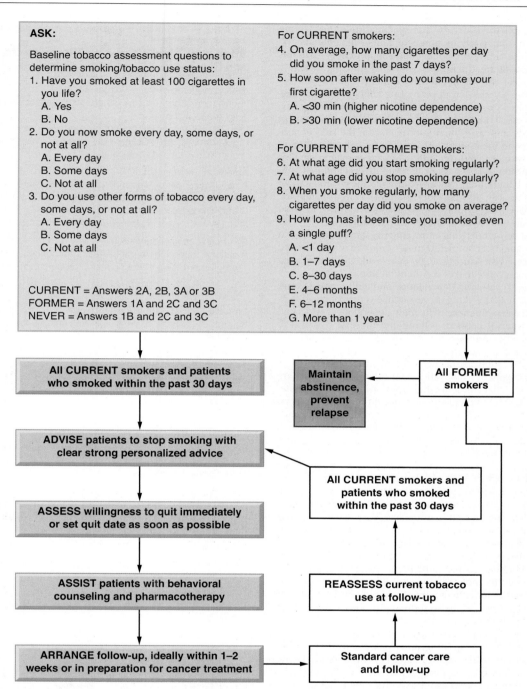

ASK:

Baseline tobacco assessment questions to determine smoking/tobacco use status:
1. Have you smoked at least 100 cigarettes in you life?
   A. Yes
   B. No
2. Do you now smoke every day, some days, or not at all?
   A. Every day
   B. Some days
   C. Not at all
3. Do you use other forms of tobacco every day, some days, or not at all?
   A. Every day
   B. Some days
   C. Not at all

CURRENT = Answers 2A, 2B, 3A or 3B
FORMER = Answers 1A and 2C and 3C
NEVER = Answers 1B and 2C and 3C

For CURRENT smokers:
4. On average, how many cigarettes per day did you smoke in the past 7 days?
5. How soon after waking do you smoke your first cigarette?
   A. <30 min (higher nicotine dependence)
   B. >30 min (lower nicotine dependence)

For CURRENT and FORMER smokers:
6. At what age did you start smoking regularly?
7. At what age did you stop smoking regularly?
8. When you smoke regularly, how many cigarettes per day did you smoke on average?
9. How long has it been since you smoked even a single puff?
   A. <1 day
   B. 1–7 days
   C. 8–30 days
   E. 4–6 months
   F. 6–12 months
   G. More than 1 year

All CURRENT smokers and patients who smoked within the past 30 days

Maintain abstinence, prevent relapse

All FORMER smokers

ADVISE patients to stop smoking with clear strong personalized advice

All CURRENT smokers and patients who smoked within the past 30 days

ASSESS willingness to quit immediately or set quit date as soon as possible

ASSIST patients with behavioral counseling and pharmacotherapy

REASSESS current tobacco use at follow-up

ARRANGE follow-up, ideally within 1–2 weeks or in preparation for cancer treatment

Standard cancer care and follow-up

Figure 31.1 This 5 A's screening and smoking cessation treatment schema for cancer patients may be integrated into clinical oncology practice.

CANCER PREVENTION AND SCREENING

patient at every visit including follow-up visits. Whereas a more comprehensive evaluation is necessary at the first consult, only updates to current tobacco use are needed at follow-up. Including smoking status assessments as a "vital sign" for all patients significantly increases the identification and treatment for patients.[200] Tobacco-use status stickers on paper charts or an automated reminder system for electronic records can increase compliance with tobacco assessments.[45] With the recent Meaningful Use standards that were implemented in 2011, hospitals using an electronic medical record (EMR) are essentially required to document tobacco use.[201] A recent report utilized the EMR to implement mandatory tobacco assessments in cancer patients demonstrating that just a few questions at the initial evaluation and at follow-up could yield high referral.

Less than 1% of referrals were delayed when assessments were repeated on a monthly basis rather than at every clinic visit.[45] These findings reduce the clinical burden and patient fatigue associated with repeated assessments as frequently as every day such as in patients who are treated with daily RT or CT.

At the time of this chapter release, there were no national guidelines for implementation of specific questions to assess tobacco use in cancer patients. However, Figure 31.1 provides effective questions for assessing tobacco use in cancer patients based on advice from published reports.[5,45,194,199] Current, former, and never smokers are identified in a structured manner. Patients who use tobacco within the past 30 days should have structured support to quit tobacco use, maintain abstinence, and prevent relapse.

Although not explicitly stated by any specific guidelines, asking about tobacco use in family members of cancer patients may be important because family members often support cancer patients during and following treatment, but continued smoking by family members can make quitting much more difficult.[202–204]

Advising is the second step in promoting effective tobacco cessation that involves giving clear, strong, and personalized advice to stop tobacco use. This advice should include the importance of quitting smoking, such as explicit information on the risks of continued smoking and the benefits of cessation for cancer treatment outcomes and overall health regardless of cancer diagnosis. This includes a discussion of how it is not "too late" to quit and that quitting will in fact benefit their cancer treatment efficacy and cancer outcome.[5] Patients can also consider the cost savings of stopping a smoking habit. Clinicians must be particularly sensitive to avoid contributing to any perceived blame for the patient's illness.[195–197,205] Clinicians must remember that most patients started smoking in adolescence and did not completely understand the risks associated with tobacco use. At the same time, the severe addiction associated with chronic tobacco use makes it difficult to stop.

The next step is *assessing* dependence and willingness to quit. Asking "How soon after waking do you smoke your first cigarette?" assesses nicotine dependence, with high dependence associated with a shorter interval between waking and the first cigarette.[206] Nicotine dependence is predictive of smoking cessation outcomes and can be used as a good indicator of the intensity of cessation treatment needed, such as the need for pharmacotherapy.[207,208] Determining the patient's motivation and interest in quitting are critical parameters that influence the types of intervention strategies to be employed. Different strategies for quitting are based on the transtheoretical model of change and motivational interviewing stance, which recognizes that unique intervention messages and strategies are needed to optimally promote smoking cessation based on a patient's readiness to quit smoking.[209,210] In the general population, recommendations encourage that clinicians set a target quit date within 30 days. However, for cancer patients, the reader is encouraged to consider an urgent need to stop smoking immediately. If patients are unable to quit immediately, then patients should be encouraged to immediately reduce tobacco use and to set a quit date as soon as possible based on the typical need to start cancer treatment in the immediate future.

Assisting patients with smoking cessation involves clinicians helping the patient design and implement a specific quit plan or broadly enhancing the motivation to quit tobacco. Promoting an effective quit strategy for cancer patients should consist of (1) setting a quit date (immediately or as soon as possible), (2) removing all tobacco-related products from the environment (e.g., cigarettes, ashtrays, lighters), (3) requesting support from family and friends, (4) discussing challenges to quitting, and (5) discussing or prescribing pharmacotherapy where appropriate. Patients should also be provided information on cessation support services (Table 31.1). In the cancer setting, patients can also be informed that smoking cessation is a critical component of cancer care over which they have complete control, thereby conferring some personal control over their cancer care.

Patients who are unwilling to quit should continue to receive repeated assessments and counseling to help motivate patients to quit smoking. These patients should be encouraged to make immediate reductions in tobacco use and work toward abstinence as soon as possible. Clinician education, reassurance, and gentle encouragement can help them to consider changing their smoking behaviors. Specific strategies include discussing the personal relevance of smoking and benefits to cessation, providing support and acknowledging the difficulty of quitting, educating patients about the positive consequences of quitting smoking, and discussing available pharmacologic methods to assist with quitting.[211] The emphasis should be placed on patient autonomy to quit. Motivational strategies for patients unwilling to quit can be employed (e.g., asking open-ended questions, providing affirmations,

TABLE 31.1

Additional Tobacco Cessation Resources for Patients and Clinicians[a]

American Association for Cancer Research
Information about the adverse effects of tobacco and advocacy for tobacco control
(http://www.aacr.org/home/public--media/science-policy--government-affairs/science-policy--government-affairs-committee/tobacco-and-cancer.aspx)

American Cancer Society
A national cancer organization providing brochures and fact sheets on the health effects of tobacco and resources for smoking cessation
(http://www.cancer.org/cancer/cancercauses/tobaccocancer/)

American Legacy Foundation
A national independent public health foundation offering programs to help people quit and resources about the health effects of tobacco use
(http://www.legacyforhealth.org/)

American Society of Clinical Oncology
Resources for tobacco cessation with an emphasis on cancer patients
(http://www.asco.org/practice-research/tobacco-cessation-and-control-resources)

Centers for Disease Control and Prevention
A collection of online resources, information, and materials about quitting tobacco use
(http://www.cdc.gov/TOBACCO/)

North American Quitline Consortium
Information on local and national cessation quitlines, 1-800-QUIT-NOW
(http://www.naquitline.org/)

Smoking Cessation Leadership Center
A collaborative dedicated to disseminating knowledge about the health effects of tobacco and assistance in cessation
(http://smokingcessationleadership.ucsf.edu/)

Smokefree.gov
Tips and resources for people trying to stop smoking
(http://smokefree.gov/)

Tobacco Free Nurses
An organization aimed at engaging nurses in tobacco cessation efforts
(http://www.tobaccofreenurses.org/)

U.S. Department of Health & Human Services, Surgeon General.gov
Tobacco use and cessation information from the Surgeon General
(http://www.surgeongeneral.gov/initiatives/tobacco/index.html)

World Health Organization
An international organization tasked with implementing and monitoring public health with a focus on tobacco control
(http://www.who.int/topics/tobacco/en/)

[a] Current as of December 2013.

reflective listening, summarizing).[198,210,212,213] Table 31.2 provides suggested methods to help clinicians promote tobacco cessation.

The final step in a clinician-delivered smoking cessation intervention involves *arranging* a follow-up contact with the patient. Ideally, cancer patients will follow an immediate quit strategy and follow-up should occur preferably within 1 to 2 weeks. However, a short-term follow-up may also benefit patients who are reluctant to quit smoking. The clinician must remember that a new cancer diagnosis is stressful and patients may rely on continued smoking to

TABLE 31.2

Select Treatment Strategies Used for Tobacco Cessation Treatments

Provide and monitor the use of nicotine replacement or other pharmacotherapy.

Provide education regarding the health effects of tobacco use and its addictive and relapsing nature.

Identify and change environmental and psychological cues for tobacco use.

Generate alternative behaviors for tobacco use.

Assist in optimization of social support for cessation efforts and address tobacco use in family members.

Prevent relapse including the identification of future high-risk situations and plans for specific behaviors in those situations.

Provide motivational interventions as needed throughout treatment.

Identify relaxation techniques such as guided imagery and progressive muscle relaxation.

Provide behavioral strategies to address depressed mood (e.g., increasing pleasurable activities).

Provide crisis intervention including appropriate referrals and emergency intervention if indicated.

Recognize and congratulate patients on success with reducing and/or quitting smoking.

relieve stress, but after absorbing the psychological effects of a new cancer diagnosis, patients may be more receptive to smoking cessation. During follow-up, clinicians should congratulate patients on successful cessation efforts, discuss accomplishments and setbacks, and assess pharmacotherapy use and problems. Patients should not be criticized for returning to smoking; rather, it is critical to create a supportive environment for patients to communicate progress, failure, and personal needs. Framing relapses as a learning experience can be helpful, and patients should be encouraged to set another quit date. Referrals to a psychologist or professionally trained smoking cessation counselor should be considered for patients with numerous unsuccessful quit attempts, comorbid depression, anxiety, additional substance abuse disorders, or inadequate social support.

Clinicians who are not well versed in tobacco cessation should realize that smoking is an extremely difficult addiction to overcome and should recognize the clinical pattern associated with cessation. As patients stop smoking, many will experience symptoms of withdrawal, including dry or sore throat, constipation, cravings to smoke, irritability, anxiety, trouble concentrating, restlessness, increased appetite, depression, and insomnia. In the first few weeks, patients may also report an increase in mucous secretions from the airways, a cough, and other upper respiratory tract symptoms. Patients and clinicians should realize that tobacco cessation requires a concerted effort, may require repeated attempts, and symptoms will not resolve immediately. Clinicians should counsel patients on a repeated basis, recognize success, and provide repeated assistance if patients relapse.

Pharmacologic Treatment for Smoking Cessation

The principles of pharmacotherapy to help patients quit smoking are fundamentally based on reducing the craving associated with nicotine withdrawal. Nicotine replacement therapy (NRT), in the form of patches, lozenges, inhalers, sprays, and gum, varenicline (Chantix), and bupropion (Zyban) are the three principal first-line pharmacotherapies recommended for use either alone or in combination according to PHS Guidelines.[199] Table 31.3 presents information on these first-line agents. Nicotine is the primary addictive substance in tobacco and NRT facilitates smoking cessation by reducing craving and withdrawal that smokers experience during abstinence. NRT also weans smokers off nicotine by providing a lower level and, in some cases, slower infusion of nicotine than smoking.[214] Strong evidence from over 100 randomized clinical trials support the use of NRT to increase the odds of quitting approximately twofold as compared with placebo.[215] Pooled analyses demonstrate that 17% of smokers receiving NRT were able to quit versus 10% with placebo after at least 6 months. Recent evidence further shows that combination therapy, or dual NRT (such as a nicotine patch and lozenge), is a very effective smoking cessation therapy that produces high quit rates.[216,217] Data suggest that activation of the nicotinic acetylcholine receptor (nAChR) may promote tumor development,[218] but evidence suggests that the negative aspects of smoking outweigh these concerns.[219,220] Furthermore, there are no clinical trials reporting negative outcomes for NRT in cancer patients as related to mortality or recurrence. Studies also demonstrate that NRT is not associated with an increased risk of carcinogenesis in the general population.[221,222] As a result, NRT should be used as a clinically proven method to help cancer patients stop smoking.

Antidepressants have been studied as non-nicotine–based pharmacotherapy in part due to depression and psychiatric disease being comorbid conditions in smokers.[223] Bupropion (Zyban) is currently the only FDA-approved antidepressant for the treatment of tobacco dependence.[199] Bupropion inhibits the reuptake of both dopamine and norepinephrine, thereby increasing dopamine and norepinephrine concentrations in the mesolimbic systems.[12,224] Bupropion also antagonizes the nAChR, thereby lowering the rewarding effects of nicotine.[225] Should an abstinent smoker relapse, bupropion may function to reduce the pleasure of cigarette smoking experienced by the smoker[226] and help to prevent further relapse. A meta-analysis found that smokers who received bupropion were twice as likely as those who received placebo to have achieved long-term abstinence at either a 6- or 12-month follow-up.[227]

Varenicline (Chantix) is a α4β2 nAChR partial agonist that produces sustained dopamine release in the mesolimbic system that received FDA approval for treating tobacco dependence in 2006. Sustained dopamine release maintains a normal systemic level of the neurotransmitter, which helps to reduce craving and withdrawal during abstinence.[228] Varenicline also antagonizes the rewarding effects of nicotine. Because varenicline attenuates the pleasure smokers experience from smoking, it may decrease motivation to smoke and protect them from relapse. One of the initially reported randomized clinical trials that compared varenicline (2 mg), bupropion (300 mg), and placebo showed that varenicline was superior to bupropion and placebo, with overall continuous abstinence rates between 10% to 23%.[229] A meta-analysis demonstrated that the 1-mg daily dose approximately doubled, whereas the 2-mg daily dose approximately tripled the likelihood of long-term abstinence at 6 months as compared to placebo.[199] As a result, the 1-mg daily dose can be considered as an alternative should the patient experience significant dose-related side effects. Several meta-analyses have shown that varenicline is superior to bupropion and placebo in the general population.[230–233]

In July 2009, the FDA issued a warning after reports that some patients attempting to quit smoking while using varenicline or bupropion experienced unusual changes in behavior, depressed mood, worsening of depression, or had thoughts of suicide. This has prompted recommendations that health-care providers elicit information about a patient's psychiatric history prior to prescribing varenicline or bupropion to closely monitor changes in mood and behavior during the course of treatment. However,

TABLE 31.3

First-Line Pharmacotherapy Agents for the Treatment of Nicotine Depedence

Agent	Dose	Mechanism	Use
Nicotine Replacement			
Transdermal (patches)	16 h or 24 h 7, 14, or 21 mg 1 patch/d	Steady state NRT to reduce craving and withdrawal	6–10 CPD: 14 mg daily × 8 wks then 7 mg daily × 2 wks >10 CPD: 21 mg daily × 6 wks, then 14 mg × 2 wks, then 7 mg × 2 wks
Gum	2 or 4 mg Max: 24 pieces/d	Short-term NRT to reduce craving and withdrawal	First cigarette >30 min after waking: 2 mg PO q1–2 hr First cigarette <30 min after waking: 4 mg PO q1–2 hr
Lozenge	2 or 4 mg Max: 20 lozenges/d	Short-term NRT to reduce craving and withdrawal	1st cigarette >30 min after waking: 2 mg PO q1–2 hr 1st cigarette <30 min after waking: 4 mg PO q1–2 hr
Nasal spray	0.5 mg/spray Max: 10 sprays/hr or 80 sprays/d	Short-term NRT to reduce craving and withdrawal	1 spray/nostril q1–5 hr
Inhaler	4 mg/cartridge Max: 16 cartridges/d	Short-term NRT to reduce craving and withdrawal	1 cartridge inhaled over 20 min q1.5–6 hr
Bupropion (Zyban)	150 mg	Block nicotinic receptors and reduces reward	1 tablet daily × 3 d, then 1 tablet twice daily for 7–12 wks
Varenicline (Chantix)	0.5 or 1 mg	Dopaminergic reward and partial nicotinic receptor antagonist	0.5 mg daily × 3 d, then 0.5 mg twice daily × 3 d, then 1 mg twice daily

CPD, cigarettes per day; PO, by mouth; NRT, nicotine replacement therapy.

updated recent safety studies examining very large databases (one database of N = 119,546, one database of N = 35,800) regarding safety have shown no difference in neuropsychiatric side effects between varenicline or bupropion as compared to NRT and no increased risk of depression.[234,235] Another prospective study showed no adverse events when treating participants with current or past major depression and also showed higher abstinence rates for the varenicline group as compared to placebo at weeks 9 to 52 (20.3% versus 10.4%, p <0.001).[236] Varenicline should be considered a viable cessation pharmacotherapy for cancer patients.

The clinical practice guideline also identifies two non-nicotine–based medications—clonidine and nortriptyline—as second-line pharmacotherapies for tobacco dependence. A second-line agent is used when a smoker cannot use first-line medications due to either contraindications or lack of effectiveness. Both clonidine, an antihypertensive, and nortriptyline, a tricyclic antidepressant, have been shown to effectively assist smokers achieve abstinence.[227,237] Unfortunately, many patients who quit will eventually relapse, and rates of long-term abstinence remain low. Because smoking poses enormous health risks to individuals and their families, even a modest reduction in smoking may translate into a significant impact on public health. Clinicians should continue to encourage recalcitrant smokers to stop tobacco use and use pharmacotherapy where appropriate with repeated quit attempts.

Empirically Tested Cessation Interventions with Cancer Patients

The overwhelming majority of cessation research has been performed in the general population, but there are several studies that have been performed in cancer patients. Gritz et al.[238] conducted the first physician- or dentist-delivered randomized cessation

intervention comparison in 186 newly diagnosed head and neck cancer patients. Patients were treated with either minimal advice or an enhanced intervention with trained clinicians consisting of strong personalized advice to stop smoking, a contracted quit date, tailored written materials, and booster advice sessions. No significant differences were found between treatments, but a 70.2% continuous abstinence rate was found at 12-month follow-up regardless of treatment condition, suggesting that many cancer patients can benefit from brief physician-delivered advice. A later study by Schnoll et al.,[239] comparing cognitive behavioral treatment with standardized health education advice, also failed to find significant differences in quit rates. All patients received NRT, and quit rates in both groups approached 50% at 1-month follow-up and 40% at 3-month follow-up.

Additional studies, ranging from 15 to 80 patients, examined nurse-delivered cessation interventions for a variety of cancer patients. The lowest cessation rates were found with a single session intervention: a 21% cessation rate in the intervention group versus 14% in the usual care group 6 weeks' postintervention.[240] Higher cessation rates were associated with a more intensive intervention consisting of three inpatient visits, supplementary materials, and five postdischarge follow-up contacts. Additional studies demonstrate higher cessation rates with more intensive intervention (40% to 75%) as compared with usual care (43% to 50%), suggesting more intensive interventions may yield higher cessation rates.[241–243] In general, more intense interventions appear to be more efficacious, but even brief advice is important to achieve tobacco cessation.

In a randomized trial of 432 cancer patients coordinated by the Eastern Cooperative Oncology Group (ECOG) with a physician-delivered intervention (comprised of cessation advice, optional NRT, and written materials) or usual care (unstructured advice from physicians), there were no significant intervention effects and generally low abstinence rates (12% to 15%

at 6 to 12 months).[244] However, patients with head and neck or lung cancer were significantly more likely to have quit smoking compared to patients with tumors that were not smoking related. Analyses of outcomes from the Mayo Clinic Nicotine Dependence Center found that although lung cancer patients were more likely to achieve 6-month tobacco abstinence than controls (22% versus 14%), no significant differences were observed after adjusting for covariates.[245] Garces et al.[246] also found no significant differences in abstinence rates between head and neck cancer patients and controls (33% versus 26%). However, higher abstinence rates were found for both head and neck and lung cancer patients treated within 3 months of diagnosis compared to those treated for more than 3 months after the diagnosis, emphasizing the potential importance of the *teachable moment* at the time of the cancer diagnosis.

The potential importance of addressing smoking combined with considering comorbid disease has been noted in a few studies. In a randomized head and neck cancer patients of usual care versus 9 to 11 sessions of a nurse-administered intervention consisting of cognitive-behavioral therapy and medications, targeting comorbid smoking, drinking, and depression significantly increased quit rates at 6-month follow-up for the intervention group compared to the usual control group (47% versus 31%, p <0.05).[247] In a randomized trial of 246 cancer patients treated with 9 weeks of NRT with or without bupropion, there was no significant difference with the addition of bupropion to NRT, but in patients with depressive symptoms, bupropion increased abstinence rates, lowered withdrawal, and improved quality of life.[248] Patients without depression symptoms did equally well when treated with bupropion versus transdermal nicotine and counseling alone.

Patient recruitment has been a problem noted by some studies, including 5.5 years to accrue 246 patients with telephone screening of over 7,500 potential patients.[249] A pilot trial of varenicline in thoracic oncology patients required screening 1,130 patients to accrue 49 participants randomized to a 12-week course of either varenicline or placebo paired with a behavioral counseling platform of seven sessions.[250] A randomized trial of 185 smoking cancer patients comparing the efficacy of a hospital-based standard care smoking cessation model versus standard care augmented by a behavioral tapering regimen via a handheld device before inpatient hospitalization for cancer surgery demonstrated no difference in quit rates (both 32%,).[251] However, over 29,000 patients were screened to conduct a randomized clinical trial with a smoking cancer patient population. These studies highlight the potential difficulty recruiting participants who smoke, including considerations for the importance of medical comorbidity in guiding smoking cessation treatment, patient mix (multiple tumor sites), treatment status (awaiting treatment to completed treatment), variation in stage of disease, and considering how psychiatric conditions such as depression reflect the difficulty of conducting research in the oncology setting and the importance of these variables in future studies.

Although accruing patients to intervention trials may seem discouraging, several studies demonstrate the benefit of counseling over self-help. Emmons et al.[252] conducted a randomized controlled trial in 796 young adult survivors of pediatric cancer that included six calls, tailored and targeted written materials, and optional NRT as compared with self-help. Significantly higher quit rates were found in the counseling group compared to the self-help group at all reported follow-up time points, including 12 months (15% versus 9%; p <0.01). A randomized trial of a motivational interviewing-based smoking cessation intervention in a south Australian hospital was delivered over a 3-month period, consisted of multiple contacts with a trained counselor, and provided supplementary material tailored to cancer patients with NRT.[253] The control group received brief advice to quit and generic supplementary material. Quit rates did not differ by treatment group (5% to 6% at 3-month follow-up), but the intervention group was significantly more likely to report attempts to quit smoking.

Current Tobacco Assessment and Cessation Support by Oncologists

Access to cessation support is critical to address tobacco use by cancer patients. A recent survey of 58 NCI-designated cancer centers indicated that about 80% reported a tobacco use program available to their patients and about 60% routinely offered educational materials, but less than 50% had a designated individual who provided services.[254] A recent survey of over 1,500 members of the International Association for the Study of Lung Cancer (IASLC)[255] and a parallel study of 1,197 ASCO members[256] observed that approximately 90% of physicians believe that tobacco affects outcomes, tobacco cessation should be a standard part of cancer care, and approximately 80% regularly advise patients to stop using tobacco, but only approximately 40% discuss medications or assist with quitting. Dominant perceived barriers to cessation support were patient resistance to treatment, an inability to get patients to quit, a lack of cessation resources, and a lack of clinician education. These data showed that even motivated clinicians are not regularly providing tobacco cessation support. A recent survey of 155 actively accruing cooperative group clinical trials further demonstrated that only 29% of active trials collected any tobacco use information, 4.5% collected any tobacco use information at follow-up, and none addressed tobacco cessation.[55] Few oncology meetings offer educational workshops or talks, and they are often poorly attended when they are offered.[257] Collectively, these data demonstrate that oncologists are not regularly providing cessation support and that we are not capturing tobacco use information that may be critical to understanding the effects of tobacco on cancer treatment outcomes.

More in-person talks as well as written and Web-based training should be made available, as well as new approaches that move from the traditional 5 A's model delivered by a single professional to referral systems that efficiently connect tobacco users to multiple resources for tobacco cessation.[258–260] The ASCO *Prevention Curriculum* has a chapter devoted to educating oncology healthcare professionals on the evaluation and treatment of tobacco use.[213] Innovative curricula, such as the Texas Tobacco Outreach Education Program (TOEP), are available and can facilitate program development in other states.[261] However, specialty programs in tobacco cessation treatment that are based in cancer centers and other medical centers are valuable resources that need to be further developed.

Addressing tobacco use in cancer patients may be approached in a systematic and efficient manner. A recent report highlighted the potential utility of automated tobacco assessment and smoking cessation using structured assessments in the EMR where all patients were automatically referred to a dedicated cessation program consisting of phone-based cessation support.[45] In 2,700 patients referred for cessation support, half received only a mailing and only 1% contacted the cessation program. However, in the arm with at least five phone call attempts made by the cessation service, 81% of patients were successfully contacted and only 3% refused cessation support. Furthermore, assessments implemented every 4 weeks, rather than more frequent assessments every 2 weeks, resulted in delayed cessation referrals in less than 1% of smokers. This is the first report to try and identify clinically efficient mechanisms of addressing tobacco use that may be useful in clinical practice or research that may be an effective method of increasing patient participation in cessation support, but substantial work is needed to assess who may benefit from low versus high intensity support in such a program.

Examples of Model Tobacco Treatment Programs

Several dedicated tobacco treatment programs at cancer centers have been developed. Table 31.4 contrasts the core elements of

Attributes of Prototypical Tobacco Treatment Programs

Attribute	MDACC	RPCI	Yale	MSKCC
Tobacco assessment of all patients (EMR)	Yes	Yes	Yes	Yes
Automatic referral of all patients	Yes	Yes	No	Yes
In-person counseling	Yes	No	Yes	Yes
Telephone counseling	Yes	Yes	No	Yes
Medications prescribed	Yes	No	Yes	Yes
Biochemical confirmation (CO) testing	Yes	No	Yes	No
Free to patient	Yes	Yes	No	Yes
Third-party payment	No	No	Yes	Yes
Research studies of new treatments	Yes	Yes	Yes	Yes

MDACC, M.D. Anderson Cancer Center, Houston, TX; RPCI, Roswell Park Cancer Institute, Buffalo, NY; Yale, Yale University Hospital, Smilow Cancer Center, New Haven, CT; MSKCC, Memorial Sloan Kettering Cancer Center, New York, NY.

four active model programs at the end of 2013 (University of Texas M.D. Anderson Cancer Center, Roswell Park Cancer Institute, Yale Cancer Center, and Memorial Sloan Kettering Cancer Center), each of which employ different methods to help cancer patients quit smoking. All programs follow the evidence-based 5 A's model described previously from PHS Guidelines.[199] All programs were made available to patients at their respective medical centers and are now designed to evaluate and treat all patients who self-report current tobacco use. Importantly, not all cancer centers can treat smoking cessation in the same manner. Financing of a cessation program is critical and may include institutional funds, state funds, research funds, and third-party billing. Notably, given the broad spectrum of adverse health effects associated with smoking, cancer centers should carefully consider the potential health benefits and cost savings associated with tobacco cessation due to reductions in treatment complications and recurrence associated with smoking by cancer patients. There is no one "correct" way to create and sustain a tobacco treatment program at a cancer center, but at the very least and consistent with evidence, rigorous behavioral counseling should be provided and, if possible, medication management as well.

FUTURE CONSIDERATIONS

Research Considerations

The past several years have shown a surge in activities identifying the effects of tobacco in cancer patients and increasing awareness is being developed for cessation support at cancer centers as well as through several national organizations. There are three fundamental areas of research that need to be expanded:

1. *Evaluating the effects of tobacco use and cessation on clinical cancer outcomes.* The 2014 SGR concluded that smoking caused adverse outcomes in cancer patients,[7] but several limitations remain. Tobacco-use definitions should be standardized and implemented at diagnosis, during treatment, and follow-up. Biochemical confirmation with cotinine or exhaled carbon monoxide may improve the accuracy of tobacco assessment in at-risk groups such as current smokers who are trying to quit or patients who reported quitting in the past year.[171,185,186,262] Although smoking is the predominant form of tobacco consumption, all tobacco products should be considered. A further understanding of the effects of tobacco on the efficacy and toxicity of cancer treatment, tumor response, quality of life, survival, recurrence,

compliance, second primary, and noncancer-related comorbidity is needed. All cancer disease sites and stages are important to consider.

2. *Understanding the effects of tobacco and cessation on cancer biology.* Although not a primary focus of this chapter, tobacco and tobacco-related products increase tumor growth, angiogenesis, migration, invasion and metastasis and decrease response to conventional cancer treatments such as CT and RT. These and other areas are important to consider, including the potential effects on immune-related therapy and vaccine development. *In vivo* models of exposure and cancer response are not well developed, yet are critical to this research area. Work is also needed to assess the effect of emerging tobacco-related products such as e-cigarettes.

3. *Advance understanding of models to increase access to cessation support and increase efficacy of tobacco cessation methods for cancer patients.* This diverse area includes assessing the timing of intervention, intensity, duration, follow-up, and the potential effects of harm-reduction strategies. Cessation pharmacology requires additional consideration in combination with unique approaches to motivational and behavioral counseling in cancer patients. Significant work is needed to disseminate evidence-based cessation support and to assess the cost-effectiveness of different cessation strategies, particularly with regard to improving the cost of cancer care as a whole. Preventing relapse and evaluating the safety of transition to alternative products such as e-cigarettes is equally important and increasingly complex with the addition of new tobacco-related products. Identifying and addressing barriers to effective cessation support is also needed. As related to the cancer patient, clinicians and cessation specialists should consider how their research relates to cancer care. Taking advantage of new integrated medical management systems presents a significant opportunity to improve cessation support access as well as to develop a more effective tracking of patient outcomes.

Policy Implications and Systematic Issues

Several national and international organizations have emphasized the importance of tobacco assessments and cessation for the general population and for cancer patients that include tools to evaluate tobacco use at diagnosis, during treatment, and follow-up appointments, as well as routine support for smoking cessation.[5,6,188–191] In 2012, ASCO, with the contribution of the American Legacy Foundation, published a Tobacco Cessation Toolkit for the oncology setting.[263] This evidence-based guideline intends to help oncology providers integrate tobacco cessation strategies into their patient care. Utilization of the EMR and standardized, automated systems for more efficacious and efficient access to tobacco cessation support has also been suggested,[45] but requires participation by clinicians, institutions, insurers, and health departments. Not only should providers be aware of the need for tobacco cessation and available interventions, but health-care institutions must also build such treatment into their overall system of care. Thus, the identification of patients who smoke or use any alternative tobacco product, referral or direct treatment by providers, billing and reimbursement for treatment provided, and consistent efforts from professional oncology organizations are critically important.[257] The

tremendous public health burden from tobacco-related disability and death has not been countered by a proportional level of funding in tobacco control, cancer treatment research, or public advocacy. Researchers, clinicians, and advocates must come together to persuade policy makers to increase funding in tobacco-related research, treatment, and policy initiatives on behalf of healthy individuals and patients. A united front is critically needed in support of a common agenda that includes both increased tobacco-control efforts and additional funding for disease-related research and treatment. With clinical rationale, guidelines, and advocacy in place, the final steps in effective tobacco control and improving health outcomes are to implement these recommendations into practice.

REFERENCES

1. U.S. Department of Health, Education, and Welfare. *Smoking and Health: Report of the Advisory Committee to the Surgeon General of the Public Health Service*. PHS Publication No. 1103. Washington, D.C.: U.S. Department of Health, Education, and Welfare, Public Health Service, Center for Disease Control; 1964.
2. Office of the Surgeon General, Office on Smoking and Health. *The Health Consequences of Smoking. A Report of the Surgeon General*. Atlanta: Centers for Disease Control and Prevention; 2004.
3. Centers for Disease Control and Prevention, National Center for Chronic Disease Prevention and Health Promotion, Office on Smoking and Health. *How Tobacco Smoke Causes Disease: The Biology and Behavioral Basis for Smoking-Attributable Disease: A Report of the Surgeon General*. Atlanta: Centers for Disease Control and Prevention; 2010.
4. U.S. Department of Health and Human Services. *The Health Consequences of Smoking: Nicotine Addiction. A Report of the Surgeon General*. DHHS Publication No. (CDC) 88-8406. Atlanta: U.S. Department of Health and Human Services, Public Health Service, Centers for Disease Control, National Center for Chronic Disease Prevention and Health Promotion, Office on Smoking and Health; 1988.
5. Toll BA, Brandon TH, Gritz ER, et al. Assessing tobacco use by cancer patients and facilitating cessation: an American Association for Cancer Research policy statement. *Clin Cancer Res* 2013;19:1941–1948.
6. Hanna N, Mulshine J, Wollins DS, et al. Tobacco cessation and control a decade later: American society of clinical oncology policy statement update. *J Clin Oncol* 2013;31:3147–3157.
7. U.S. Department of Health and Human Services. *The Health Consequences of Smoking—50 Years of Progress: A Report of the Surgeon General*. Atlanta: U.S. Department of Health and Human Services, Centers for Disease Control and Prevention, National Center for Chronic Disease Prevention and Health Promotion, Office on Smoking and Health; 2014.
8. Brunzell DH. Preclinical evidence that activation of mesolimbic alpha 6 subunit containing nicotinic acetylcholine receptors supports nicotine addiction phenotype. *Nicotine Tob Res* 2012;14:1258–1269.
9. Benowitz NL. Nicotine addiction. *N Engl J Med* 2010;362:2295–2303.
10. Nestler EJ. Is there a common molecular pathway for addiction? *Nat Neurosci* 2005;8:1445–1449.
11. Dani JA, De Biasi M. Cellular mechanisms of nicotine addiction. *Pharmacol Biochem Behav* 2001;70:439–446.
12. Balfour DJ. The neurobiology of tobacco dependence: a preclinical perspective on the role of the dopamine projections to the nucleus accumbens. *Nicotine Tob Res* 2004;6:899–912.
13. Berridge KC, Robinson TE. What is the role of dopamine in reward: hedonic impact, reward learning, or incentive salience? *Brain Res Brain Res Rev* 1998;28:309–369.
14. Schultz W. Multiple dopamine functions at different time courses. *Annu Rev Neurosci* 2007;30:259–288.
15. Kalivas PW, McFarland K. Brain circuitry and the reinstatement of cocaine-seeking behavior. *Psychopharmacology* 2003;168:44–56.
16. Dani JA, Balfour DJK. Historical and current perspective on tobacco use and nicotine addiction. *Trends Neurosci* 2011;34:383–439.
17. Di Chiara G. Role of dopamine in the behavioural actions of nicotine related to addiction. *Eur J Pharmacol* 2000;393:295–314.
18. Centers for Disease Control and Prevention. Current cigarette smoking among adults—United States, 2011. *MMWR Morb Mortal Wkly Rep* 2012;61:889–894.
19. Centers for Disease Control and Prevention. Cigarette smoking among adults—United States, 2001. *MMWR Morb Mortal Wkly Rep* 2003;52:953–956.
20. Smokefree Laws and Policies. American Lung Association Web site. http://www.lungusa2.org/slati/smokefree_laws.php. Accessed November 25, 2013.
21. Tobacco Policy Project/State Legislated Actions on Tobacco Issues (SLATI). American Lung Association Web site. http://www.lungusa2.org/slati. Accessed November 25, 2013.
22. Tobacco Taxes. American Lung Association Web site. http://www.lungusa2.org/slati/tobacco_taxes.php. Accessed November 25, 2013.
23. Tobacco Situation and Outlook Report, U.S. Department of Agriculture, U.S. Census 1880-2005.
24. Warren GW, Cummings KM. Tobacco and lung cancer: risks, trends, and outcomes in patients with cancer. In: *American Society of Clinical Oncology 2013 Educational Book*. 201; 359–364. ASCO University Web site. http://meetinglibrary.asco.org//content/200-132. Accessed November 25, 2013.
25. Thun MJ, Carter BD, Feskanich D, et al. 50-year trends in smoking-related mortality in the United States. *N Engl J Med* 2013;368:351–364.
26. U.S. Food and Drug Administration. Summary of Results: Laboratory Analysis of Electronic Cigarettes Conducted by FDA. U.S. Food and Drug Administration Web site. http://www.fda.gov/NewsEvents/PublicHealthFocus/ucm173146.htm. Accessed November 25, 2013.
27. Cummings KM, Dresler CM, Field JK, et al. E-cigarettes and cancer patients. *J Thorac Oncol* 2014;9:438–441.
28. Kuschner WG, Reddy S, Mehrotra N, et al. Electronic cigarettes and thirdhand tobacco smoke: two emerging health care challenges for the primary care provider. *Int J Gen Med* 2011;4:115–120.
29. WHO Study Group on Tobacco Product Regulation. WHO Study Group on Tobacco Product Regulation. Report on the scientific basis of tobacco product regulation: third report of a WHO study group. *World Health Organ Tech Rep Ser* 2009;(955):1–41.
30. National Cancer Institute. Cancer Trends Progress Report – 2011/2012 Update. Nation Cancer Institute Web site. http://progressreport.cancer.gov. Published August 2012. Accessed November 25, 2013.
31. Bellizzi KM, Rowland JH, Jeffery DD, et al. Health behaviors of cancer survivors: examining opportunities for cancer control intervention. *J Clin Oncol* 2005;23:8884–8893.
32. Coups EJ, Ostroff JS. A population-based estimate of the prevalence of behavioral risk factors among adult cancer survivors and noncancer controls. *Prev Med* 2005;40:702–711.
33. Klosky JL, Hum AM, Zhang N, et al. Smokeless and dual tobacco use among males surviving childhood cancer: a report from the Childhood Cancer Survivor Study. *Cancer Epidemiol Biomarkers Prev* 2013;22:1025–1029.
34. Underwood JM, Townsend JS, Tai E, et al. Persistent cigarette smoking and other tobacco use after a tobacco-related cancer diagnosis. *J Cancer Surviv* 2012;6:333–344.
35. Walker MS, Vidrine DJ, Gritz ER, et al. Smoking relapse during the first year after treatment for early-stage non-small-cell lung cancer. *Cancer Epidemiol Biomarkers Prev* 2006;15:2370–2377.
36. Gritz ER. Smoking and smoking cessation in cancer patients. *Br J Addict* 1991;86:549–554.
37. Lippman SM, Lee JJ, Karp DD, et al. Randomized phase III intergroup trial of isotretinoin to prevent second primary tumors in stage I non-small-cell lung cancer. *J Natl Cancer Inst* 2001;93:605–618.
38. Ostroff JS, Jacobsen PB, Moadel AB, et al. Prevalence and predictors of continued tobacco use after treatment of patients with head and neck cancer. *Cancer* 1995;75:569–576.
39. Hickey K, Do KA, Green A. Smoking and prostate cancer. *Epidemiol Rev* 2001;23:115–125.
40. Plaskon LA, Penson DF, Vaughan TL, et al. Cigarette smoking and risk of prostate cancer in middle-aged men. *Cancer Epidemiol Biomarkers Prev* 2003;12:604–609.
41. Watters JL, Park Y, Hollenbeck A, et al. Cigarette smoking and prostate cancer in a prospective US cohort study. *Cancer Epidemiol Biomarkers Prev* 2009;18:2427–2435.
42. Alberg AJ, Singh S, May JW, et al. Epidemiology, prevention, and early detection of breast cancer. *Curr Opin Oncol* 2000;12:515–520.
43. Johnson KC, Miller AB, Collishaw NE, et al. Active smoking and secondhand smoke increase breast cancer risk: the report of the Canadian Expert Panel on Tobacco Smoke and Breast Cancer Risk (2009). *Tob Control* 2011;20:e2.
44. Breast Cancer Family Registry; Kathleen Cuningham Consortium for Research into Familial Breast Cancer (Australasia); Ontario Cancer Genetics Network (Canada). Smoking and risk of breast cancer in carriers of mutations in BRCA1 or BRCA2 aged less than 50 years. *Breast Cancer Res Treat* 2008;109:67–75.
45. Warren GW, Marshall JR, Cummings KM, et al. Automated tobacco assessment and cessation support for cancer patients. *Cancer* 2014;120:562–569.
46. Centers for Disease Control and Prevention. Cigarette smoking among adults—United States, 2004. *MMWR Morb Mortal Wkly Rep* 2005;54:1121–1124.

CANCER PREVENTION AND SCREENING

47. Centers for Disease Control and Prevention. Tobacco use among adults—United States, 2005. *MMWR Morb Mortal Wkly Rep* 2006;55:1145–1148.

48. Gritz ER, Nisenbaum R, Elashoff RE, et al. Smoking behavior following diagnosis in patients with stage I non-small cell lung cancer. *Cancer Causes Control* 1991;2:105–112.

49. Chen AM, Vazquez E, Courquin J, et al. Tobacco use among long-term survivors of head and neck cancer treated with radiation therapy. *Psychooncology* 2014;23:190–194.

50. Ostroff J, Garland J, Moadel A, et al. Cigarette smoking patterns in patients after treatment of bladder cancer. *J Cancer Educ* 2000;15:86–90.

51. McBride CM, Emmons KM, Lipkus IM. Understanding the potential of teachable moments: the case of smoking cessation. *Health Educ Res* 2003;18:156–170.

52. Gritz ER, Schacherer C, Koehly L, et al. Smoking withdrawal and relapse in head and neck cancer patients. *Head Neck* 1999;21:420–427.

53. Warren GW, Marshall JR, Cummings KM. Smoking, cancer treatment, and design of clinical trials. *Proc AACR* 2013;54:594.

54. Parsons A, Daley A, Begh R, et al. Influence of smoking cessation after diagnosis of early stage lung cancer on prognosis: systematic review of observational studies with meta-analysis. *BMJ* 2010;340:b5569.

55. Peters EN, Torres E, Toll BA, et al. Tobacco assessment in actively accruing National Cancer Institute Cooperative Group Program Clinical Trials. *J Clin Oncol* 2012;30:2869–2875.

56. Land SR. Methodologic barriers to addressing critical questions about tobacco and cancer prognosis. *J Clin Oncol* 2012;30:2030–2032.

57. Gritz ER, Dresler C, Sarna L. Smoking, the missing drug interaction in clinical trials: ignoring the obvious. *Cancer Epidemiol Biomarkers Prev* 2005;14:2287–2293.

58. Yu GP, Ostroff JS, Zhang ZF, et al. Smoking history and cancer patient survival: a hospital cancer registry study. *Cancer Detect Prev* 1997;21:497–509.

59. Dahlstrom KR, Calzada G, Hanby JD, et al. An evolution in demographics, treatment, and outcomes of oropharyngeal cancer at a major cancer center: a staging system in need of repair. *Cancer* 2012;119:81–89.

60. Molina MA, Cheung MC, Perez EA, et al. African American and poor patients have a dramatically worse prognosis for head and neck cancer: an examination of 20,915 patients. *Cancer* 2008;113:2797–2806.

61. Dragun AE, Huang B, Tucker TC, et al. Disparities in the application of adjuvant radiotherapy after breast-conserving surgery for early stage breast cancer: impact on overall survival. *Cancer* 2011;117:2590–2598.

62. Bostrom PJ, Alkhateeb S, Trottier G, et al. Sex differences in bladder cancer outcomes among smokers with advanced bladder cancer. *BJU Int* 2011;109:70–76.

63. Kroeger N, Klatte T, Birkhäuser FD, et al. Smoking negatively impacts renal cell carcinoma overall and cancer-specific survival. *Cancer* 2011;118:1795–1802.

64. Marks DI, Ballen K, Logan BR, et al. The effect of smoking on allogeneic transplant outcomes. *Biol Blood Marrow Transplant* 2009;15:1277–1287.

65. Gridelli C, Ciardiello F, Gallo C, et al. First-line erlotinib followed by second-line cisplatin-gemcitabine chemotherapy in advanced non-small-cell lung cancer: the TORCH randomized trial. *J Clin Oncol* 2012;30:3002–3011.

66. Maeda R, Yoshida J, Ishii G, et al. Influence of cigarette smoking on survival and tumor invasiveness in clinical stage IA lung adenocarcinoma. *Ann Thorac Surg* 2012;93:1626–1632.

67. Maeda R, Yoshida J, Ishii G, et al. The prognostic impact of cigarette smoking on patients with non-small cell lung cancer. *J Thorac Oncol* 2011;6:735–742.

68. Janjigian YY, McDonnell K, Kris MG, et al. Pack-years of cigarette smoking as a prognostic factor in patients with stage IIIB/IV nonsmall cell lung cancer. *Cancer* 2010;116:670–675.

69. Toyooka S, Takano T, Kosaka T, et al. Epidermal growth factor receptor mutation, but not sex and smoking, is independently associated with favorable prognosis of gefitinib-treated patients with lung adenocarcinoma. *Cancer Sci* 2008;99:303–308.

70. Kawai H, Tada A, Kawahara M, et al. Smoking history before surgery and prognosis in patients with stage IA non-small-cell lung cancer—a multicenter study. *Lung Cancer* 2005;49:63–70.

71. Warren GW, Kasza K, Reid M, et al. Smoking at diagnosis and survival in cancer patients. *Int J Cancer* 2013;132:401–410.

72. Kvale E, Ekundayo OJ, Zhang Y, et al. History of cancer and mortality in community-dwelling older adults. *Cancer Epidemiol* 2011;35:30–36.

73. Gajdos C, Hawn MT, Campagna EJ, et al. Adverse effects of smoking on postoperative outcomes in cancer patients. *Ann Surg Oncol* 2012;19:1430–1438.

74. Duffy SA, Ronis DL, McLean S, et al. Pretreatment health behaviors predict survival among patients with head and neck squamous cell carcinoma. *J Clin Oncol* 2009;27:1969–1975.

75. Farshadpour F, Kranenborg H, Calkoen EV, et al. Survival analysis of head and neck squamous cell carcinoma: influence of smoking and drinking. *Head Neck* 2011;33:817–823.

76. Meyer F, Bairati I, Fortin A, et al. Interaction between antioxidant vitamin supplementation and cigarette smoking during radiation therapy in relation to long-term effects on recurrence and mortality: a randomized trial among head and neck cancer patients. *Int J Cancer* 2008;122:1679–1683.

77. Shen GP, Xu FH, He F, et al. Pretreatment lifestyle behaviors as survival predictors for patients with nasopharyngeal carcinoma. *PLoS One* 2012;7:e36515.

78. Dal Maso L, Zucchetto A, Talamini R, et al. Effect of obesity and other lifestyle factors on mortality in women with breast cancer. *Int J Cancer* 2008;123:2188–2194.

79. Hellmann SS, Thygesen LC, Tolstrup JS, et al. Modifiable risk factors and survival in women diagnosed with primary breast cancer: results from a prospective cohort study. *Eur J Cancer Prev* 2010;19:366–673.

80. Holmes MD, Murin S, Chen WY, et al. Smoking and survival after breast cancer diagnosis. *Int J Cancer* 2007;120:2672–2677.

81. Sagiv SK, Gaudet MM, Eng SM, et al. Active and passive cigarette smoke and breast cancer survival. *Ann Epidemiol* 2007;17:385–393.

82. Phipps AI, Baron J, Newcomb PA. Prediagnostic smoking history, alcohol consumption, and colorectal cancer survival: the Seattle Colon Cancer Family Registry. *Cancer* 2011;117:4948–4957.

83. Huang XE, Tajima K, Hamajima N, et al. Effects of dietary, drinking, and smoking habits on the prognosis of gastric cancer. *Nutr Cancer* 2000;38:30–36.

84. Kenfield SA, Stampfer MJ, Chan JM, et al. Smoking and prostate cancer survival and recurrence. *JAMA* 2011;305:2548–2555.

85. Merrick GS, Butler WM, Wallner KE, et al. Androgen-deprivation therapy does not impact cause-specific or overall survival after permanent prostate brachytherapy. *Int J Radiat Oncol Biol Phys* 2006;65:669–677.

86. Pickles T, Liu M, Berthelet E, et al. The effect of smoking on outcome following external radiation for localized prostate cancer. *J Urol* 2004;171:1543–1546.

87. Taira AV, Merrick GS, Butler WM, et al. Long-term outcome for clinically localized prostate cancer treated with permanent interstitial brachytherapy. *Int J Radiat Oncol Biol Phys* 2011;79:1336–1342.

88. Sweeney C, Farrow DC. Differential survival related to smoking among patients with renal cell carcinoma. *Epidemiology* 2000;11:344–346.

89. Coker AL, DeSimone CP, Eggleston KS, et al. Smoking and survival among Kentucky women diagnosed with invasive cervical cancer: 1995–2005. *Gynecol Oncol* 2009;112:365–369.

90. Modesitt SC, Huang B, Shelton BJ, et al. Endometrial cancer in Kentucky: the impact of age, smoking status, and rural residence. *Gynecol Oncol* 2006;103:300–306.

91. Poullis M, McShane J, Shaw M, et al. Smoking status at diagnosis and histology type as determinants of long-term outcomes of lung cancer patients. *Eur J Cardiothorac Surg* 2012;43:919–924.

92. Kawaguchi T, Tamiya A, Tamura A, et al. Chemotherapy is beneficial for elderly patients with advanced non-small-cell lung cancer: analysis of patients aged 70–74, 75–79, and 80 or older in Japan. *Clin Lung Cancer* 2012;13:442–447.

93. Pirker R, Pereira JR, Szczesna A, et al. Prognostic factors in patients with advanced non-small cell lung cancer: data from the phase III FLEX study. *Lung Cancer* 2012;77:376–382.

94. Ferketich AK, Niland JC, Mamet R, et al. Smoking status and survival in the national comprehensive cancer network non-small cell lung cancer cohort. *Cancer* 2013;119:847–853.

95. Chansky K, Sculier JP, Crowley JJ, et al. The International Association for the Study of Lung Cancer Staging Project: prognostic factors and pathologic TNM stage in surgically managed non-small cell lung cancer. *J Thorac Oncol* 2009;4:792–801.

96. Myrdal G, Lamberg K, Lambe M, et al. Regional differences in treatment and outcome in non-small cell lung cancer: a population-based study (Sweden). *Lung Cancer* 2009;63:16–22.

97. Saito-Nakaya K, Nakaya N, Akechi T, et al. Marital status and non-small cell lung cancer survival: the Lung Cancer Database Project in Japan. *Psychooncology.* 2008;17:869–876.

98. Zhou W, Heist RS, Liu G, et al. Smoking cessation before diagnosis and survival in early stage non-small cell lung cancer patients. *Lung Cancer* 2006;53:375–380.

99. Tsao AS, Liu D, Lee JJ, et al. Smoking affects treatment outcome in patients with advanced nonsmall cell lung cancer. *Cancer* 2006;106:2428–2436.

100. Ebbert JO, Williams BA, Sun Z, et al. Duration of smoking abstinence as a predictor for non-small-cell lung cancer survival in women. *Lung Cancer* 2005;47:165–172.

101. Tammemagi CM, Neslund-Dudas C, Simoff M, et al. Smoking and lung cancer survival: the role of comorbidity and treatment. *Chest* 2004;125:27–37.

102. Nordquist LT, Simon GR, Cantor A, et al. Improved survival in never-smokers vs current smokers with primary adenocarcinoma of the lung. *Chest* 2004;126:347–351.

103. Ehlers SL, Gastineau DA, Patten CA, et al. The impact of smoking on outcomes among patients undergoing hematopoietic SCT for the treatment of acute leukemia. *Bone Marrow Transplant* 2011;46:285–290.

104. Geyer SM, Morton LM, Habermann TM, et al. Smoking, alcohol use, obesity, and overall survival from non-Hodgkin lymphoma: a population-based study. *Cancer* 2010;116:2993–3000.

105. Deleyiannis FW, Thomas DB, Vaughan TL, et al. Alcoholism: independent predictor of survival in patients with head and neck cancer. *J Natl Cancer Inst* 1996;88:542–549.

106. Ngô C, Alran S, Plancher C, et al. Outcome in early cervical cancer following pre-operative low dose rate brachytherapy: a ten-year follow up of 257 patients treated at a single institution. *Gynecol Oncol* 2011;123:248–252.

107. Browman GP, Wong G, Hodson I, et al. Influence of cigarette smoking on the efficacy of radiation therapy in head and neck cancer. *N Engl J Med* 1993;328:159–163.

108. Gillison ML, Zhang Q, Jordan R, et al. Tobacco smoking and increased risk of death and progression for patients with p16-positive and p16-negative oropharyngeal cancer. *J Clin Oncol* 2012;30:2102–2111.

109. Waggoner SE, Darcy KM, Fuhrman B, et al. Association between cigarette smoking and prognosis in locally advanced cervical carcinoma treated with chemoradiation: a Gynecologic Oncology Group study. *Gynecol Oncol* 2006;103:853–858.

110. Khuri FR, Lee JJ, Lippman SM, et al. Randomized phase III trial of low-dose isotretinoin for prevention of second primary tumors in stage I and II head and neck cancer patients. *J Natl Cancer Inst* 2006;98:441–450.

111. Karvonen-Gutierrez CA, Ronis DL, Fowler KE, et al. Quality of life scores predict survival among patients with head and neck cancer. *J Clin Oncol* 2008;26:2754–2760.

112. Sardari Nia P, Weyler J, Colpaert C, et al. Prognostic value of smoking status in operated non-small cell lung cancer. *Lung Cancer* 2005;47:351–359.

113. Chen J, Jiang R, Garces YI, et al. Prognostic factors for limited-stage small cell lung cancer: a study of 284 patients. *Lung Cancer* 2010;67:221–226.

114. Bittner N, Merrick GS, Galbreath RW, et al. Primary causes of death after permanent prostate brachytherapy. *Int J Radiat Oncol Biol Phys* 2008;72:433–440.

115. Haughey BH, Sinha P. Prognostic factors and survival unique to surgically treated p16+ oropharyngeal cancer. *Laryngoscope* 2012;122:S13– S33.

116. Kawakita D, Hosono S, Ito H, et al. Impact of smoking status on clinical outcome in oral cavity cancer patients. *Oral Oncol* 2012;48:186–191.

117. Chen AM, Chen LM, Vaughan A, et al. Tobacco smoking during radiation therapy for head-and-neck cancer is associated with unfavorable outcome. *Int J Radiat Oncol Biol Phys* 2011;79:414–419.

118. Junor E, Kerr G, Oniscu A, et al. Benefit of chemotherapy as part of treatment for HPV DNA-positive but p16-negative squamous cell carcinoma of the oropharynx. *Br J Cancer* 2012;106:358–365.

119. Manjer J, Andersson I, Berglund G, et al. Survival of women with breast cancer in relation to smoking. *Eur J Surg* 2000;166:852–858.

120. Kountourakis P, Correa AM, Hofstetter WL, et al. Combined modality therapy of cT2N0M0 esophageal cancer: the University of Texas M. D. Anderson Cancer Center experience. *Cancer* 2011;117:925–930.

121. Munro AJ, Bentley AH, Ackland C, et al. Smoking compromises cause-specific survival in patients with operable colorectal cancer. *Clin Oncol (R Coll Radiol)* 2006;18:436–440.

122. Gong Z, Agalliu I, Lin DW, et al. Cigarette smoking and prostate cancer-specific mortality following diagnosis in middle-aged men. *Cancer Causes Control* 2008;19:25–31.

123. Kjaerbye-Thygesen A, Frederiksen K, Hogdall EV, et al. Smoking and overweight: negative prognostic factors in stage III epithelial ovarian cancer. *Cancer Epidemiol Biomarkers Prev* 2006;15:798–803.

124. Nagle CM, Bain CJ, Webb PM. Cigarette smoking and survival after ovarian cancer diagnosis. *Cancer Epidemiol Biomarkers Prev* 2006;15:2557–2560.

125. Wright JD, Li J, Gerhard DS, et al. Human papillomavirus type and tobacco use as predictors of survival in early stage cervical carcinoma. *Gynecol Oncol* 2005;98:84–91.

126. Sardari Nia P, Van Marck E, Weyler J, et al. Prognostic value of a biologic classification of non-small-cell lung cancer into the growth patterns along with other clinical, pathological and immunohistochemical factors. *Eur J Cardiothorac Surg* 2010;38:628–636.

127. Hoff CM, Grau C, Overgaard J. Effect of smoking on oxygen delivery and outcome in patients treated with radiotherapy for head and neck squamous cell carcinoma—a prospective study. *Radiother Oncol* 2012;103:38–44.

128. Joshu CE, Mondul AM, Meinhold CL, et al. Cigarette smoking and prostate cancer recurrence after prostatectomy. *J Natl Cancer Inst* 2011;103:835–838.

129. Mai SK, Welzel G, Haegele V, et al. The influence of smoking and other risk factors on the outcome after radiochemotherapy for anal cancer. *Radiat Oncol* 2007;2:30.

130. Kim AJ, Suh JD, Sercarz JA, et al. Salvage surgery with free flap reconstruction: factors affecting outcome after treatment of recurrent head and neck squamous carcinoma. *Laryngoscope* 2007;117:1019–1023.

131. Khan AM, Freeman-Wang T, Pisal N, et al. Smoking and multicentric vulval intraepithelial neoplasia. *J Obstet Gynaecol* 2009;29:123–125.

132. Hefler L, Grimm C, Tempfer C, et al. Treatment with vaginal progesterone in women with low-grade cervical dysplasia: a phase II trial. *Anticancer Res* 2010;30:1257–1261.

133. Matsumoto K, Oki A, Furuta R, et al. Tobacco smoking and regression of low-grade cervical abnormalities. *Cancer Sci* 2010;101:2065–2073.

134. Fleshner N, Garland J, Moadel A, et al. Influence of smoking status on the disease-related outcomes of patients with tobacco-associated superficial transitional cell carcinoma of the bladder. *Cancer* 1999;86:2337–2345.

135. Ioffe YJ, Elmore RG, Karlan BY, et al. Effect of cigarette smoking on epithelial ovarian cancer survival. *J Reprod Med* 2010;55:346–350.

136. Schlumbrecht MP, Sun CC, Wong KN, et al. Clinicodemographic factors influencing outcomes in patients with low-grade serous ovarian carcinoma. *Cancer* 2011;117:3741–3749.

137. Fortin A, Wang CS, Vigneault E. Influence of smoking and alcohol drinking behaviors on treatment outcomes of patients with squamous cell carcinomas of the head and neck. *Int J Radiat Oncol Biol Phys* 2009;74:1062–1069.

138. Chen CH, Shun CT, Huang KH, et al. Stopping smoking might reduce tumour recurrence in nonmuscle-invasive bladder cancer. *BJU Int* 2007;100:281–286.

139. Browman GP, Mohide EA, Willan A, et al. Association between smoking during radiotherapy and prognosis in head and neck cancer: a follow-up study. *Head Neck* 2002;24:1031–1037.

140. Clark JR, McCluskey SA, Hall F, et al. Predictors of morbidity following free flap reconstruction for cancer of the head and neck. *Head Neck* 2007;29:1090–1101.

141. Little SC, Hughley BB, Park SS. Complications with forehead flaps in nasal reconstruction. *Laryngoscope*. 2009;119:1093–1099.

142. Patel RS, McCluskey SA, Goldstein DP, et al. Clinicopathologic and therapeutic risk factors for perioperative complications and prolonged hospital stay in free flap reconstruction of the head and neck. *Head Neck* 2010;32:1345–1353.

143. Baumann DP, Lin HY, Chevray PM. Perforator number predicts fat necrosis in a prospective analysis of breast reconstruction with free TRAM, DIEP, and SIEA flaps. *Plast Reconstr Surg* 2010;125:1335–1341.

144. Goodwin SJ, McCarthy CM, Pusic AL, et al. Complications in smokers after postmastectomy tissue expander/implant breast reconstruction. *Ann Plast Surg* 2005;55:16–19.

145. Bertelsen CA, Andreasen AH, Jorgensen T, et al. Anastomotic leakage after anterior resection for rectal cancer: risk factors. *Colorectal Dis* 2010;12:37–43.

146. Cooke DT, Lin GC, Lau CL, et al. Analysis of cervical esophagogastric anastomotic leaks after transhiatal esophagectomy: risk factors, presentation, and detection. *Ann Thorac Surg* 2009;88:177–184.

147. Richards CH, Platt JJ, Anderson JH, et al. The impact of perioperative risk, tumor pathology and surgical complications on disease recurrence following potentially curative resection of colorectal cancer. *Ann Surg* 2011;254:83–89.

148. Nickelsen TN, Jorgensen T, Kronborg O. Lifestyle and 30-day complications to surgery for colorectal cancer. *Acta Oncol* 2005;44:218–223.

149. Begum FD, Hogdall E, Christensen IJ, et al. Serum tetranectin as a preoperative indicator for postoperative complications in Danish ovarian cancer patients. *Gynecol Oncol* 2010;117:446–450.

150. Joo YH, Sun DI, Cho JH, et al. Factors that predict postoperative pulmonary complications after supracricoid partial laryngectomy. *Arch Otolaryngol Head Neck Surg* 2009;135:1154–1157.

151. Mason DP, Subramanian S, Nowicki ER, et al. Impact of smoking cessation before resection of lung cancer: a Society of Thoracic Surgeons General Thoracic Surgery Database study. *Ann Thorac Surg* 2009;88:362–370.

152. van der Voet JC, Keus RB, Hart AA, et al. The impact of treatment time and smoking on local control and complications in T1 glottic cancer. *Int J Radiat Oncol Biol Phys* 1998;42:247–255.

153. Wedlake LJ, Thomas K, Lalji A, et al. Predicting late effects of pelvic radiotherapy: is there a better approach? *Int J Radiat Oncol Biol Phys* 2010;78:1163–1170.

154. Hocevar-Boltezar I, Zargi M, Strojan P. Risk factors for voice quality after radiotherapy for early glottic cancer. *Radiother Oncol* 2009;93:524–529.

155. Lilla C, Ambrosone CB, Kropp S, et al. Predictive factors for late normal tissue complications following radiotherapy for breast cancer. *Breast Cancer Res Treat* 2007;106:143–150.

156. Eifel PJ, Jhingran A, Bodurka DC, et al. Correlation of smoking history and other patient characteristics with major complications of pelvic radiation therapy for cervical cancer. *J Clin Oncol* 2002;20:3651–3657.

157. Wuketich S, Hienz SA, Marosi C. Prevalence of clinically relevant oral mucositis in outpatients receiving myelosuppressive chemotherapy for solid tumors. *Support Care Cancer* 2012;20:175–183.

158. Zevallos JP, Mallen MJ, Lam CY, et al. Complications of radiotherapy in laryngopharyngeal cancer: effects of a prospective smoking cessation program. *Cancer* 2009;115:4636–4644.

159. Gold EB, Flatt SW, Pierce JP, et al. Dietary factors and vasomotor symptoms in breast cancer survivors: the WHEL Study. *Menopause* 2006;13:423–433.

160. Cheung MC, Hamilton K, Sherman R, et al. Impact of teaching facility status and high-volume centers on outcomes for lung cancer resection: an examination of 13,469 surgical patients. *Ann Surg Oncol* 2009;16:3–13.

161. Zingg U, Smithers BM, Gotley DC, et al. Factors associated with postoperative pulmonary morbidity after esophagectomy for cancer. *Ann Surg Oncol* 2011;18:1460–1468.

162. Kelly KJ, Greenblatt DY, Wan Y, et al. Risk stratification for distal pancreatectomy utilizing ACS-NSQIP: preoperative factors predict morbidity and mortality. *J Gastrointest Surg* 2011;15:250–259.

163. Merkow RP, Bilimoria KY, Cohen ME, et al. Variability in reoperation rates at 182 hospitals: a potential target for quality improvement. *J Am Coll Surg.* 2009;209:557–564.

164. Alsadius D, Hedelin M, Johansson KA, et al. Tobacco smoking and long-lasting symptoms from the bowel and the anal-sphincter region after radiotherapy for prostate cancer. *Radiother Oncol* 2011;101:495–501.

165. Kuri M, Nakagawa M, Tanaka H, et al. Determination of the duration of preoperative smoking cessation to improve wound healing after head and neck surgery. *Anesthesiology* 2005;102:892–896.

166. Vaporciyan AA, Merriman KW, Ece F, et al. Incidence of major pulmonary morbidity after pneumonectomy: association with timing of smoking cessation. *Ann Thorac Surg* 2002;73:420–425.

167. Bjarnason GA, Mackenzie IR, Nabid A, et al. Comparison of toxicity associated with early morning versus late afternoon radiotherapy in patients with head-and-neck cancer: a prospective randomized trial of the National Cancer Institute of Canada Clinical Trials Group (HN3). *Int J Radiat Oncol Biol Phys* 2009;73:166–172.

168. Park SM, Lim MK, Jung KW, et al. Prediagnosis smoking, obesity, insulin resistance, and second primary cancer risk in male cancer survivors: National Health Insurance Corporation Study. *J Clin Oncol* 2007;25:4835–4843.

169. Leon X, del Prado Venegas M, Orus C, et al. Influence of the persistence of tobacco and alcohol use in the appearance of second neoplasm in patients with a head and neck cancer. A case-control study. *Cancer Causes Control* 2009;20:645–652.

170. Kinoshita Y, Tsukuma H, Ajiki W, et al. The risk for second primaries in gastric cancer patients: adjuvant therapy and habitual smoking and drinking. *J Epidemiol* 2000;10:300–304.

171. Khuri FR, Kim ES, Lee JJ, et al. The impact of smoking status, disease stage, and index tumor site on second primary tumor incidence and tumor recurrence in the head and neck retinoid chemoprevention trial. *Cancer Epidemiol Biomarkers Prev* 2001;10:823–829.

CANCER PREVENTION AND SCREENING

172. Scanlon EF, Suh O, Murthy SM, et al. Influence of smoking on the development of lung metastases from breast cancer. *Cancer* 1995;75:2693–2699.

173. Ford MB, Sigurdson AJ, Petrulis ES, et al. Effects of smoking and radiotherapy on lung carcinoma in breast carcinoma survivors. *Cancer* 2003;98:1457–1464.

174. Li CI, Daling JR, Porter PL, et al. Relationship between potentially modifiable lifestyle factors and risk of second primary contralateral breast cancer among women diagnosed with estrogen receptor-positive invasive breast cancer. *J Clin Oncol* 2009;27:5312–5318.

175. van den Belt-Dusebout AW, de Wit R, Gietema JA, et al. Treatment-specific risks of second malignancies and cardiovascular disease in 5-year survivors of testicular cancer. *J Clin Oncol* 2007;25:4370–4378.

176. Boorjian S, Cowan JE, Konety BR, et al. Cancer of the Prostate Strategic Urologic Research Endeavor Investigators. Bladder cancer incidence and risk factors in men with prostate cancer: results from Cancer of the Prostate Strategic Urologic Research Endeavor. *J Urol* 2007;177:883–887.

177. Travis LB, Gospodarowicz M, Curtis RE, et al. Lung cancer following chemotherapy and radiotherapy for Hodgkin's disease. *J Natl Cancer Inst* 2002;94:182–192.

178. Ang KK, Harris J, Wheeler R, et al. Human papillomavirus and survival of patients with oropharyngeal cancer. *N Engl J Med* 2010;363:24–35.

179. Peck BW, Dahlstrom KR, Gan SJ, et al. Low risk of second primary malignancies among never smokers with human papillomavirus-associated index oropharyngeal cancers. *Head Neck* 2012;35:794–799.

180. Herbst RS, Prager D, Hermann R, et al. TRIBUTE: a phase III trial of erlotinib hydrochloride (OSI-774) combined with carboplatin and paclitaxel chemotherapy in advanced non-small-cell lung cancer. *J Clin Oncol* 2005;23:5892–5899.

181. Thatcher N, Chang A, Parikh P, et al. Gefitinib plus best supportive care in previously treated patients with refractory advanced non-small-cell lung cancer: results from a randomised, placebo-controlled, multicentre study (Iressa Survival Evaluation in Lung Cancer). *Lancet* 2005;366:1527–1537.

182. Kwak EL, Bang YJ, Camidge DR, et al. Anaplastic lymphoma kinase inhibition in non-small-cell lung cancer. *N Engl J Med* 2010;363:1693–1703.

183. Paik PK, Johnson ML, D'Angelo SP, et al. Driver mutations determine survival in smokers and never-smokers with stage IIIB/IV lung adenocarcinomas. *Cancer* 2012;118:5840–5847.

184. Soria JC, Cruz C, Bahleda R, et al. Clinical activity, safety and biomarkers of PD-L1 blockade in non-small cell lung cancer (NSCLC): additional analyses from a clinical study of the engineered antibody MPDL3280A (anti-PDL1). Presented at: 2013 European Cancer Congress 2013; 2013; Amsterdam.

185. Morales N, Romano M, Cummings KM, et al. Accuracy of self-reported tobacco use in newly diagnosed cancer patients. *Cancer Causes Control* 2013;24:1223–1230.

186. Warren GW, Arnold SM, Valentino JP, et al. Accuracy of self-reported tobacco assessments in a head and neck cancer treatment population. *Radiother Oncol* 2012;103:45–48.

187. Marin VP, Pytynia KB, Langstein HN, et al. Serum cotinine concentration and wound complications in head and neck reconstruction. *Plast Reconstr Surg* 2008;121:451–457.

188. American Medical Association. Tobacco use or exposure as a variable in clinical research (Resolution 424, A-06).www.ama-assn.org.ama1/pub/upload /mm/475/bot479i406.pdf.

189. Sarna L, Bialous SA. Nursing and tobacco cessation: setting a research agenda. Reports from a national conference. In: *Nursing Research*. Philadelphia: Lippincott Williams & Wilkins; 2006: 4S.

190. Sarna L, Bialous SA, Chan S, et al. International symposia: global perspectives on nursing involvement in tobacco control. Presented in: Oncology Nursing Society, 28th Annual Congress Syllabus, May 1–4, 2003, Denver, Colorado. Denver: Oncology Nursing Society; 2003: 112.

191. Viswanath K, Herbst RS, Land SR, et al. Tobacco and cancer: an American Association for Cancer research policy statement. *Cancer Res* 2010;70(17):3419–3430.

192. American Society of Clinical Oncology. American Society of Clinical Oncology policy statement update: tobacco control—Reducing cancer incidence and saving lives. 2003. *J Clin Oncol* 2003;21:2777–2786.

193. Gritz ER, Fingeret MC, Vidrine DJ, et al. Successes and failures of the teachable moment: smoking cessation in cancer patients. *Cancer* 2006;106:17–27.

194. Gritz ER, Dresler C, Sarna L. Smoking, the missing drug interaction in clinical trials: ignoring the obvious. *Cancer Epidemiol Biomarkers Prev* 2005;14: 2287–2293.

195. Chappel A, Ziebland S, McPherson A, Stigma, shame, and blame experienced by patients with lung cancer: qualitative study. *BMJ* 2004;328:1470.

196. LoConte NK, Else-Quest NM, Eickhoff J, et al. Assessment of guilt and shame in patients with non-small-cell lung cancer compared with patients with breast and prostate cancer. *Clin Lung Cancer* 2008;9:171–178.

197. Wassenaar TR, Eickhoff JC, Jarzemsky DR, et al. Differences in primary care clinicians' approach to non-small cell lung cancer patients compared with breast cancer. *J Thorac Oncol* 2007;2:722–728.

198. Fiore MC, Bailey WC, Cohen SJ, et al. *Quick Reference Guide for Clinicians. Treating Tobacco Use and Dependence*. Rockville, MD: U.S. Department of Health and Human Services, Public Health Services; 2000. http://health.state. tn.us/Downloads/TQL_Quick%20Reference.pdf. Accessed November 25, 2013.

199. Fiore MC, Jaén CR, Baker TB, et al. *Treating Tobacco Use and Dependence: 2008 Update*. Rockville, MD: U.S. Department of Health and Human Services; 2008. http://www.ncbi.nlm.nih.gov/NBK63952/. Accessed November 25, 2013.

200. Fiore MC, Jorenby DE, Schensky AE, et al. Smoking status as the new vital sign: effect on assessment and intervention in patients who smoke. *Mayo Clin Proc* 1995;70:209–213.

201. Blumenthal D, Tavenner M. The "meaningful use" regulation for electronic health records. *N Engl J Med* 2010;363:501–504.

202. Couple approaches to smoking cessation. In: Schmaling KB, Sher TG, eds. *The Psychology of Couples and Illness: Theory, Research, & Practice*. Washington, D.C.: American Psychological Association; 2000: 311–336.

203. Homish GG, Leonard KE. Spousal influence on smoking behaviors in a US community sample of newly married couples. *Soc Sci Med* 2005;61:2557–2567.

204. Hemsing N, Greaves L, O'Leary R, et al. Partner support for smoking cessation during pregnancy: a systematic review. *Nicotine Tob Res* 2012;14:767–776.

205. Tod AM, Joanne R. Overcoming delay in the diagnosis of lung cancer: a qualitative study. *Nurs Stan* 2010;24:35–43.

206. Fagerstrom KO, Schneider NG. Measuring nicotine dependence: a review of the Fagerstrom Tolerance Questionnaire. *J Behav Med* 1989;12:159–182.

207. Baker TB, Piper ME, Bolt DM, et al. Time to first cigarette in the morning as an index of ability to quit smoking: implications for nicotine dependence. *Nicotine Tob Res* 2007;9:S555–S570.

208. Ferguson JA, Patten CA, Schroeder DR, et al. Predictors of 6-month tobacco abstinence among 1224 cigarette smokers treated for nicotine dependence. *Addict Behav* 2003;28:1203–1218.

209. Prochaska JO, DiClemente CC. Stages and processes of self-change of smoking: toward an integrative model of change. *J Consult Clin Psychol* 1983;51: 390–395.

210. Prokhorov AV, Hudmon KS, Gritz ER. Promoting smoking cessation among cancer patients: a behavioral model. *Oncology (Williston Park)* 1997;11: 1807–1813.

211. Toll BA, Rojewski AM, Duncan L, et al. "Quitting smoking will benefit your health": the evolution of clinician messaging to encourage tobacco cessation. *Clin Cancer Res* 2014;20:301–309.

212. Miller WR, Rose GS. Toward a theory of motivational interviewing. *Am Psychol* 2009;64:527–537.

213. Gritz ER, Fingeret MC, Vidrine DJ. Tobacco control in the oncology setting. In: Brawley OW, Khuri FR, Rock CL, eds. ASCO *Cancer Prevention Curriculum*. Alexandria, VA: American Society of Clinical Oncology; 2007.

214. Henningfield JE, Keenan RM. Nicotine delivery kinetics and abuse liability. *J Consult Clin Psychol* 1993;61:743–750.

215. Silagy C, Lancaster T, Stead L, et al. Nicotine replacement therapy for smoking cessation. *Cochrane Database Syst Rev* 2004;(3):CD000146.

216. Piper M, Smith S, Schlam T, et al. A randomized placebo-controlled clinical trial of 5 smoking cessation pharmacotherapies. *Arch Gen Psychiatry* 2009;66:1253–1262.

217. Smith S, McCarthy D, Japuntich S, et al. Comparative effectiveness of 5 smoking cessation pharmacotherapies in primary care clinics. *Arch Intern Med* 2009;169:2148–2155.

218. Warren GW, Singh AK. Nicotine and lung cancer. *J Carcinog* 2013;12:1–8.

219. Myles PS, Iacono GA, Hunt JO, et al. Risk of respiratory complications and wound infection in patients undergoing ambulatory surgery: smokers versus nonsmokers. *Anesthesiology* 2002;97:842–847.

220. Sørensen L, Hørby J, Friis E, et al. Smoking as a risk factor for wound healing and infection in breast cancer surgery. *Eur J Surg Oncol* 2002;28:815–820.

221. Jorgensen ED, Zhao H, Traganos F, et al. DNA damage response induced by exposure of human lung adenocarcinoma cells to smoke from tobacco- and nicotine-free cigarettes. *Cell Cycle* 2010;9:2170–2176.

222. Murray RP, Connett JE, Zapawa LM. Does nicotine replacement therapy cause cancer? Evidence from the Lung Health Study. *Nicotine Tob Res* 2009;11:1076–1082.

223. Hughes JR, Stead LF, Lancaster T. Nortriptyline for smoking cessation: a review. *Nicotine Tob Res* 2005;7:491–499.

224. Ascher JA, Cole JO, Colin JN, et al. Bupropion: a review of its mechanism of antidepressant activity. *J Clin Psychiatry* 1995;56:395–401.

225. Fryer JD, Lukas RJ. Noncompetitive functional inhibition at diverse, human nicotinic acetylcholine receptor subtypes by bupropion, phencyclidine, and ibogaine. *J Pharmacol Exp Ther* 1999;288:88–92.

226. Cryan JF, Bruijnzeel AW, Skjei KL, et al. Bupropion enhances brain reward function and reverses the affective and somatic aspects of nicotine withdrawal in the rat. *Psychopharmacology* 2003;168:347–358.

227. Hughes JR, Stead LF, Lancaster T. Antidepressants for smoking cessation. *Cochrane Database Syst Rev* 2003;(2):CD000031.

228. Coe JW, Brooks PR, Vetelino MG, et al. Varenicline: an alpha4beta2 nicotinic receptor partial agonist for smoking cessation. *J Med Chem* 2005;48:3474–3477.

229. Jorenby DE, Hays JT, Rigotti NA, et al. Efficacy of varenicline, an alpha4beta2 nicotinic acetylcholine receptor partial agonist, vs placebo or sustained-release bupropion for smoking cessation: a randomized controlled trial. *JAMA* 2006;296:56–63.

230. Cahill K, Stead LF, Lancaster T. Nicotine receptor partial agonists for smoking cessation. *Cochrane Database Syst Rev* 2012;4:CD006103.

231. Hoogendoorn M, Welsing P, Rutten-van Mölken MP. Cost-effectiveness of varenicline compared with bupropion, NRT, and nortriptyline for smoking cessation in the Netherlands. *Curr Med Res Opin* 2008;24:51–61.

232. Linden K, Jormanainen V, Linna M, et al. Cost effectiveness of varenicline versus bupropion and unaided cessation for smoking cessation in a cohort of Finnish adult smokers. *Curr Med Res Opin* 2010;26:549–560.

233. Zimovetz EA, Wilson K, Samuel M, et al. A review of cost-effectiveness of varenicline and comparison of cost-effectiveness of treatments for major smoking-related morbidities. *J Eval Clin Pract* 2011;17:288–297.

234. Gibbons RD, Mann JJ. Varenicline, smoking cessation, and neuropsychiatric adverse events. *Am J of Psychiatry* 2013;170:1460–1467.

235. Thomas KH, Martin RM, Davies NM, et al. Smoking cessation treatment and risk of depression, suicide, and self harm in the Clinical Practice Research Datalink: prospective cohort study. *BMJ* 2013;347:f5704.

236. Anthenelli RM, Morris C, Ramey TS, et al. Effects of varenicline on smoking cessation in adults with stably treated current or past major depression: a randomized trial. *Ann Intern Med* 2013;159:390–400.

237. Gourlay SG, Stead LF, Benowitz NL. Clonidine for smoking cessation. *Cochrane Database Syst Rev* 2004;(3):CD000058.

238. Gritz ER, Carr CR, Rapkin D, et al. Predictors of long-term smoking cessation in head and neck cancer patients. *Cancer Epidemiol Biomarkers Prev* 1993;2:261–270.

239. Schnoll RA, Rothman RL, Wielt DB, et al. A randomized pilot study of cognitive-behavioral therapy versus basic health education for smoking cessation among cancer patients. *Ann Behav Med* 2005;30:1–11.

240. Griebel B, Wewers ME, Baker CA. The effectiveness of a nurse-managed minimal smoking-cessation intervention among hospitalized patients with cancer. *Oncol Nurs Forum* 1998;25:897–902.

241. Wewers ME, Bowen JM, Stanislaw AE, et al. A nurse-delivered smoking cessation intervention among hospitalized postoperative patients—influence of a smoking-related diagnosis: a pilot study. *Heart Lung* 1994;23:151–156.

242. Wewers ME, Jenkins L, Mignery T. A nurse-managed smoking cessation intervention during diagnostic testing for lung cancer. *Oncol Nurs Forum* 1997;24:1419–1422.

243. Stanislaw AE, Wewers ME. A smoking cessation intervention with hospitalized surgical cancer patients: a pilot study. *Cancer Nurs* 1994;17:81–86.

244. Schnoll RA, Zhang B, Rue M, et al. Brief physician-initiated quit-smoking strategies for clinical oncology settings: a trial coordinated by the Eastern Cooperative Oncology Group. *J Clin Oncol* 2003;21:355–365.

245. Sanderson Cox L, Patten CA, Ebbert JO, et al. Tobacco use outcomes among patients with lung cancer treated for nicotine dependence. *J Clin Oncol* 2002;20:3461–3469.

246. Garces YI, Schroeder DR, Nirelli LM, et al. Tobacco use outcomes among patients with head and neck carcinoma treated for nicotine dependence: a matched-pair analysis. *Cancer* 2004;101:116–124.

247. Duffy SA, Ronis DL, Valenstein M, et al. A tailored smoking, alcohol, and depression intervention for head and neck cancer patients. *Cancer Epidemiol Biomarkers Prev* 2006;15:2203–2208.

248. Schnoll RA, Martinez E, Tatum KL, et al. A bupropion smoking cessation clinical trial for cancer patients. *Cancer Causes Control* 2010;21:811–820.

249. Martinez E, Tatum KL, Weber DM, et al. Issues related to implementing a smoking cessation clinical trial for cancer patients. *Cancer Causes Control* 2009;20:97–104.

250. Park ER, Japuntich S, Temel J, et al. A smoking cessation intervention for thoracic surgery and oncology clinics: a pilot trial. *J Thorac Oncol* 2011;6:1059–1065.

251. Ostroff JS, Burkhalter JE, Cinciripini PM, et al. Randomized trial of a presurgical scheduled reduced smoking intervention for patients newly diagnosed with cancer. *Health Psychol* 2013 [Epub ahead of print].

252. Emmons KM, Puleo E, Park E, et al. Peer-delivered smoking counseling for childhood cancer survivors increases rate of cessation: the partnership for health study. *J Clin Oncol* 2005;23:6516–6523.

253. Wakefield M, Olver I, Whitford H, et al. Motivational interviewing as a smoking cessation intervention for patients with cancer: randomized controlled trial. *Nurs Res* 2004;53:396–406.

254. Goldstein AO, Ripley-Moffitt CE, Pathman DE, et al. Tobacco use treatment at the U.S. National Cancer Institute's designated Cancer Centers. *Nicotine Tob Res* 2013;15:52–58.

255. Warren GW, Marshall JR, Cummings KM, et al. Practice patterns and perceptions of thoracic oncology providers on tobacco use and cessation in cancer patients. *J Thorac Oncol* 2013;8:543–548.

256. Warren GW, Marshall JR, Cummings KM, et al. Addressing tobacco use in cancer patients: a survey of American Society of Clinical Oncology (ASCO) members. *J Oncol Pract* 2013;9:258–262.

257. Gritz ER, Sarna L, Dresler C, et al. Building a united front: aligning the agendas for tobacco control, lung cancer research, and policy. *Cancer Epidemiol Biomarkers Prev* 2007;16:859–863.

258. Vidrine JI, Shete S, Cao Y, et al. Ask-Advise-Connect: a new approach to smoking treatment delivery in health care settings. *JAMA Intern Med* 2013;173:458–464.

259. Bernstein SL, Jearld S, Prasad D, et al. Rapid implementation of a smokers' quitline fax referral service in an urban area. *J Health Care Poor Underserved* 2009;20:55–63.

260. Sarna L, Bialous SA, Ong MK, et al. Increasing nursing referral to telephone quitlines for smoking cessation using a web-based program. *Nurs Res* 2012;61:433–440.

261. Stancic N, Mullen PD, Prokhorov AV, et al. Continuing medical education: what delivery format do physicians prefer? *J Contin Educ Health Prof* 2003;23:162–167.

262. Society for Research on Nicotine and Tobacco Committee on Biochemical Verification. Biochemical verification of tobacco use and cessation. *Nicotine Tob Res* 2002;4:149–159.

263. American Society of Clinical Oncology. Tobacco Cessation Guide: for Oncology Providers. ASCO Web site. http://www.asco.org/sites/default/files/tobacco_cessation_guide.pdf. Accessed November 25, 2013.

CANCER PREVENTION AND SCREENING

Role of Surgery in Cancer Prevention

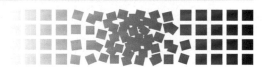

José G. Guillem, Andrew Berchuck, Jeffrey F. Moley, Jeffrey A. Norton,
Sheryl G. A. Gabram-Mendola, and Vanessa W. Hui

INTRODUCTION

Since the heritable component of some cancer predispositions has been linked to mutations in specific genes, clinical interventions have been formulated for mutation carriers within affected families. The primary interventions for mutation carriers for highly penetrant syndromes, such as multiple endocrine neoplasia (MEN), familial adenomatous polyposis (FAP), hereditary nonpolyposis colorectal cancer (CRC), and hereditary breast and ovarian cancer syndromes, are primarily surgical. This chapter is divided into five sections addressing breast (S.G.A.G.), gastric (J.N.), ovarian and endometrial (A.B.), and MENs (J.F.M.) and colorectal (J.G.G., V.W.H.). For each, the clinical and genetic indications and timing of prophylactic surgery and its efficacy, when known, are provided.

Prophylactic surgery in hereditary cancer is a complex process, requiring a clear understanding of the natural history of the disease and variance of penetrance, a realistic appreciation of the potential benefit and consequence of a risk-reducing procedure in an otherwise potentially healthy individual, and the long-term sequelae of such surgical intervention, as well as the individual patient's and family's perception of surgical risk and anticipated benefit.

PATIENTS AT HIGH RISK FOR BREAST CANCER

Identification of Patients at Risk

A detailed family history is the most important tool for identifying individuals at increased risk for hereditary cancers. The US Preventive Services Task Force updated their recommendation for risk assessment, genetic counseling, and genetic testing for asymptomatic women who have not been diagnosed with a BRCA-related cancer. In this update, the use of a risk screening tool is highly recommended to identify appropriate patients for referral for genetic counseling.[1] The American Society of Clinical Oncology has also updated the policy on genetic and genomic testing for cancer susceptibility, and this update includes information on genetic tests of uncertain clinical utility and direct-to-consumer marketing, both of which impact the practice of oncology and preventive medicine.[2] Historically, genetic counseling and testing were offered by health-care providers. However, with the advent of direct-to-consumer marketing, individuals may obtain tests and receive results directly from a company. The American Society of Clinical Oncology still endorses pre- and posttest counseling for thorough disclosure of the impact of testing. Before any woman considers risk-reduction surgery such as bilateral mastectomy or salpingo-oophorectomy, referral to a high-risk or genetic screening program is desirable, as women often overestimate their actual breast cancer risk.[3]

The most common cancer syndromes that place women at risk for breast cancer are BRCA1[4] and BRCA2[5] gene mutations. Other less common syndromes are listed in Table 32.1.[6,7]

Following referral for genetic assessment, three groups of patients emerge.[8] The first consists of those women who have undergone genetic testing and have been found to harbor a mutated gene associated with high penetrance for breast cancer. Given that the possibility of developing breast cancer in this group may be as high as 90%, there is a role for enhanced surveillance or risk-reduction surgery. The American Cancer Society has published guidelines for magnetic resonance imaging (MRI) screening as a method for enhanced surveillance.[9] Women in this first group qualify for such screening, which can be offered annually but scheduled at 6-month intervals with screening mammography to increase the rate of identifying interval cancers. Alternatively, simultaneous screening with MRI and mammography to compare one modality with the other on an annual basis may also be offered. Another choice for this group of women is to pursue bilateral risk-reduction mastectomy with an option for immediate reconstruction. Bilateral salpingo-oophorectomy for BRCA1 and BRCA2 mutation carriers may also be considered, as this procedure has been shown to reduce breast cancer risk by almost 50%.[8,10] This is especially true for BRCA2 mutation carriers, who tend to develop hormone receptor–positive breast cancers.

The second group consists of women with strong family histories suggestive of hereditary breast cancer who test negative for both the BRCA1 and BRCA2 mutations as well as the other described syndromes. In this group, there may not have been a family member with cancer who was tested for the mutation. Therefore, a negative test does not necessarily indicate that a woman's risk is equivalent to that of the general population.[7] There may also be an undetected mutation in such a family, indicating the possibility of higher-than-average risk for that particular woman. These women may or may not qualify for enhanced surveillance with MRI screening,[9] and accurate assessment of their risk may require the use of other risk prediction tools,[3] in addition to evaluating for the presence of lobular carcinoma in situ, atypical lobular hyperplasia, or atypical ductal hyperplasia, and determining if a more intensive surveillance regimen is necessary based on heterogeneously or extremely dense breast tissue on mammography.

The third group consists of women with a strong family history of breast cancer, who for various reasons, have chosen not to pursue genetic testing. These individuals may have other health-related problems, psychological concerns, cost issues, or they may fear perceived medical insurance discrimination. Women in all groups can be educated that with passage of the Genetic Information Nondiscrimination Act in 2008, significant advances have occurred that protect patients from discrimination by employers and health insurers.[11]

Women in the second and third groups may still qualify for bilateral risk-reduction mastectomy and immediate reconstruction. Often, women who elect this path are influenced by their family history or by witnessing breast and/or ovarian cancer deaths in close family members, giving them a significant fear of a breast or ovarian cancer diagnosis. For women in all three groups, the decision of whether to pursue risk-reducing surgery is difficult. Often, the expertise of a cancer clinical psychologist or psychiatrist

TABLE 32.1

Hereditary Carcinoma Syndromes Including Breast Cancer

Syndrome	Chromosome/Gene	Primary Carcinoma	Secondary Carcinoma	Breast Cancer Penetrance
Familial breast cancer/ovarian cancer syndrome	17g21; *BRCA1* Autosomal dominant	Breast cancer, ovarian cancer	Colon, prostate	60%–80%
Familial breast cancer/ovarian cancer syndrome	13q12; *BRCA2* Autosomal dominant	Breast cancer, ovarian cancer	Male breast cancer, endometrial, prostate, oropharyngeal, pancreatic	60%–80%
Li-Fraumeni syndrome	17p13.1 and 22q12.1; *TP53* and *CHEK2* Autosomal dominant	Soft tissue cancers (including breast)	Soft tissue sarcoma, leukemia, osteosarcoma, melanoma, colon, pancreas, adrenal syndrome, cortex, and brain tumors	50%–85% (for all types of cancers in this syndrome)
PTEN hamartoma syndrome (Cowden's)	10q23.31; *PTEN* mutation Autosomal dominant	Breast cancer	Thyroid (follicular) and endometrial carcinoma	25%–50%
Peutz-Jeghers syndrome	19p13.3; *STK11* Autosomal dominant	Gastrointestinal cancers	Esophagus, stomach, small intestine, large bowel, pancreas, lung, ovary, endometrial	29%
Diffuse gastric cancer	16q22.1; *CDH1* Autosomal dominant	Diffuse gastric cancer	Colorectal, lobular breast cancer	39% (lobular breast cancer)
Louis-Bar syndrome	11q22.3; *ATM* Autosomal recessive	Leukemia and lymphoma	Ovarian, breast, gastric, melanoma, leiomyomas, sarcomas	38% (for all types of cancers in the syndrome)

PTEN, phosphatase and tensin homolog.
Data from Lux MP, Fasching PA, Beckmann MW. Hereditary breast and ovarian cancer: review and future perspectives. *J Mol Med* 2006;84:16–28; and Shannon KM, Chittenden A. Genetic testing by cancer site: breast. *Cancer J* 2012;18:310–319.

is enlisted, as risk-reduction mastectomy involves an irreversible procedure with body image and sexual implications.[8]

Updated in 2007, the Society of Surgical Oncology published a position statement on the role of prophylactic mastectomy for patients at high risk for breast cancer, as well as those patients recently diagnosed with breast cancer who are considering contralateral prophylactic breast surgery.[12] For women at high risk, indications fall into three broad categories: presence of a mutation in *BRCA* or other susceptible genes, strong family history with no demonstrable mutation, and histologic risk factors (biopsy-proven atypical ductal hyperplasia, atypical lobular hyperplasia, or lobular carcinoma in situ especially in patients with a strong family history of breast cancer). Recommendations for patients with recently diagnosed breast cancer are similar in that they include the indications for high-risk individuals previously noted, as well as future surveillance challenges for the opposite breast (clinically and mammographically dense breast tissue or diffuse, indeterminate microcalcifications in the contralateral breast). Another important consideration is the need for symmetry in patients with large, ptotic, or disproportionately sized contralateral breasts.

Surgical Issues and Technique

In a single institution's 33-year experience,[13] the risk for breast cancer in both moderate- and high-risk groups of women based on family history was reduced by at least 89% for women who underwent bilateral prophylactic mastectomy. From a technical perspective, in this study, women either had a subcutaneous mastectomy (removal of the majority of breast tissue with sparing of the nipple–areola complex) or total mastectomy (removal of the entire breast through the nipple–areola complex). Most of the recurrences occurred in women undergoing a subcutaneous mastectomy. However, this was the most frequent procedure performed at that time and thus may have contributed to the number of increased recurrences.

Another surgical option for high-risk women is bilateral salpingo-oophorectomy. Among a cohort of women with *BRCA1* and *BRCA2* mutations, this procedure has been associated with a lower risk of mortality from both breast and ovarian cancer.[10] As an additional benefit, this procedure also decreases the risk of breast cancer in this patient population, likely through the mechanism of decreasing hormonal exposure at a younger age.

Contemporary surgical procedures for risk-reducing bilateral mastectomy include total mastectomy, skin-sparing mastectomy (preservation of the skin envelope by removal of the entire breast through a circumareolar incision around the nipple–areola complex), subcutaneous mastectomy, areola-sparing mastectomy (removal of the nipple while sparing the areola), and nipple-sparing mastectomy (removal of entire breast and nipple core tissue but preservation of nipple–areolar skin).[14] Given advances in reconstructive nipple–areolar techniques, it appears that total mastectomy with or without skin-sparing methods reduces the risk of breast cancer to the greatest extent with reasonable cosmesis. More limited and long-term follow-up data are available on areola- and nipple-sparing techniques. The potential limitations of these procedures are distortion of the nipple–areola complex and lack of sensitivity after breast tissue has been completely removed.[8]

Immediate reconstruction is offered to patients and performed in the vast majority undergoing bilateral risk-reduction mastectomy. Choices of reconstruction include a bilateral pedicled or free tissue transverse rectus abdominis muscle flap, a free bilateral deep inferior epigastric perforator flap or superficial inferior epigastric artery flap, bilateral latissimus flaps with or without implant or expanders, or bilateral implant or expander placement alone.[14] Although tissue flap transfer gives a more natural appearance and texture to the reconstructed site, individual body contour drives the ultimate plan for reconstruction. The decision about the type of reconstruction should be made by the plastic surgeon with input from the surgical oncologist, especially for the group of women with breast cancer desiring bilateral mastectomies who may require adjuvant radiation for treatment.

Although the risk reduction is dramatic for bilateral mastectomy, residual breast tissue may be left behind, especially with skin-sparing procedures. Patients should be educated that careful chest wall surveillance is recommended after such a procedure. Local recurrences after bilateral implant reconstruction are reliably detected by clinical examination. Recurrences after reconstruction with autologous tissue present most commonly on the skin 50% to 72% of the time and are detectable by physician examination.[15] Nonpalpable deeper recurrences in this setting are less common, and use of mammography image surveillance may be indicated, especially if significant breast tissue was left behind unintentionally during the bilateral mastectomy procedure. At times, an initial "screening" mammogram may be performed, if significant residual breast tissue is suspected; this should occur well after all healing has taken place to delineate the amount of visible breast tissue on imaging. This drives future decisions of whether to follow a patient with imaging. Finally, all patients should be instructed to return for clinical breast examination with the health provider if any change is noted on the reconstructed breasts, regardless of imaging plan.

Although risk-reduction bilateral mastectomy may be exceedingly beneficial for high-risk women, especially for those testing positive for *BRCA1*, *BRCA2*, or other deleterious mutations, or belonging to a family afflicted with a cancer syndrome, they are never emergent procedures. Along with risk-reduction bilateral salpingo-oophorectomy, risk-reduction bilateral mastectomy resides at the far end of the spectrum of an individual's choices.[16] These procedures should be offered only after appropriate genetic counseling and accurate assessment of a woman's actual risk for breast and ovarian cancer. An in-depth consultation with the patient and her family members is necessary prior to proceeding with an operative plan.

HEREDITARY DIFFUSE GASTRIC CANCER

Gastric cancer is the fourth most common cause of cancer worldwide and is the second leading cause of cancer mortality.[17] Although environmental agents, including *Helicobacter pylori* and diet, are the primary risk factors for this disease, approximately 10% of gastric cancers are a result of familial clustering.[18,19] Histologically, gastric cancers may be classified as either intestinal or diffuse types. The intestinal type histopathology is linked to environmental factors and advanced age. The diffuse type occurs in younger patients and is associated with a familial predisposition. Because of

a decrease in intestinal-type gastric cancers, the overall incidence of gastric cancer has declined significantly in the past 50 years. However, the incidence of diffuse gastric cancer (DGC), which is also called signet ring cell or linitis plastica, has remained stable and, by some reports, may be increasing.

Hereditary DGC (HDGC) is a genetic cancer susceptibility syndrome defined by one of the following: (1) two or more documented cases of DGC in first- or second-degree relatives, with at least one diagnosed before the age of 50; or (2) three or more cases of documented DGC in first- or second-degree relatives, independent of age of onset. The average age of onset of HDGC is 38, and the pattern of inheritance is autosomal dominant.[20] Figure 32.1 shows a pedigree with HDGC.

In 1998, inactivating germline mutations in the E-cadherin gene *CDH1* were identified in three Maori families, each with multiple cases of poorly differentiated DGC.[21] The *CDH1* mutations in these families were inherited in an autosomal dominant pattern, with incomplete but high penetrance. Onset of clinically apparent cancer was early, with the youngest affected individual dying of DGC at the age of 14.[21] Since then, germline mutations of *CDH1* have been identified in 30% to 50% of all patients with HDGC.[19,22] More than 50 mutations have been recognized across diverse ethnic backgrounds, including European, African American, Pakistani, Japanese, Korean, and others.[19] In addition to gastric cancers, germline *CDH1* mutations are associated with increased risk of lobular carcinoma of the breast, and this was the first manifestation of a *CDH1* mutation in one series.[23] *CDH1* is, to date, the only gene implicated in HDGC. Penetrance of DGC in patients carrying a *CDH1* mutation is estimated at 70% to 80%, but may be higher. The need for a systematic study of specimens is supported by recent work by Gaya et al.[24] in which initial total gastrectomy specimens were reported as negative, but detailed sectioning and analysis showed invasive carcinoma.

CDH1 is localized on chromosome 16q22.1 and encodes the calcium-dependent cell adhesion glycoprotein E-cadherin. Functionally, E-cadherin impacts maintenance of normal tissue morphology and cellular differentiation. It is hypothesized that *CDH1* acts as a tumor suppressor gene in HDGC, with loss of function leading to loss of cell adhesion and subsequently to proliferation, invasion, and metastases. Figure 32.2 shows the *CDH1* mutation for the pedigree depicted in Figure 32.1.

The germline *CDH1* mutation is most frequently a truncating mutation. Germline missense mutations are causative in a few HDGC kindreds, but are more often clinically insignificant. In vitro assays for cellular invasion and aggregation may predict the functional impact of missense mutations to aid in this distinction.[22] Within the gastric mucosa, the "second hit" leading to complete loss of E-cadherin function results from *CDH1* promoter methylation, as has been described in sporadic gastric cancer.[25]

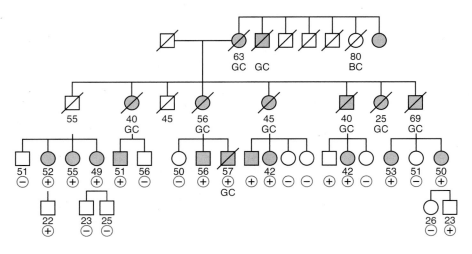

Figure 32.1 A family pedigree showing autosomal dominant inheritance of gastric cancer. Individual mutation testing results for the codon 1003 CDH1 mutation are indicated by + or −. Individuals affected with gastric cancer are *shaded*. (From Norton JA, Ham CM, Van Dam J, et al. CDH1 truncating mutations in the E-cadherin gene: an indication for total gastrectomy to treat hereditary diffuse gastric cancer. *Ann Surg* 2007;245:873.)

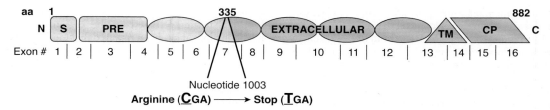

Figure 32.2 The mutation in this kindred is located in the central region of the E-cadherin gene that codes for the extracellular cadherin domains of the protein containing calcium-binding motifs important in the adhesion process. The C → T transition in exon 7 of nucleotide 1003 results in a premature stop codon (R335X), producing truncated peptides that lack the transmembrane and cytoplasmic β-catenin–binding domains essential for tight cell-cell adhesion. *Black* area indicates truncated portion of peptide. N, N-terminus; C, C-terminus; S, signal peptide; PRE, precursor sequence; TM, transmembrane domain; CP, cytoplasmic domain. (From Norton JA, Ham CM, Van Dam J, et al. CDH1 truncating mutations in the E-cadherin gene: an indication for total gastrectomy to treat hereditary diffuse gastric cancer. *Ann Surg* 2007;245:873.)

It remains unclear whether specific *CDH1* mutations are associated with distinctive phenotypic characteristics or rates of penetrance, although this may become apparent as more recurrent mutations are recognized. To date, most mutations identified have been novel and distributed throughout *CDH1*. Recognition of recurrent mutations has usually resulted from independent events; however, there is evidence for the role of founder effects in certain kindreds.[22] At present, it is also unclear whether patients with HDGC without detectable *CDH1* mutations have mutation of a different gene or merely a *CDH1* mutation that has gone unrecognized.

New recommended screening criteria for *CDH1* mutations are as follows:

1. Families with one or more cases of DGC
2. Individuals with DGC before the age of 40 years without a family history
3. Families or individuals with cases of DGC (one case below the age of 50 years) and lobular breast cancer
4. Cases where pathologists detect in situ signet ring cells or pagetoid spread of signet ring cells adjacent to diffuse type gastric cancer[18,26]

As in other familial cancer syndromes, genetic counseling should take place prior to genetic testing so that the family understands the potential impact of the results. After obtaining informed consent, a team comprising a geneticist, gastroenterologist, surgeon, and oncologist should discuss the possible outcomes of testing and the management options associated with each. Genetic testing should first be performed on a family member with HDGC or on a tissue sample if no affected relative is living. In addition to direct sequencing, multiplex ligation-dependent probe amplification is recommended to test for large genomic rearrangements. If a *CDH1* mutation is identified, asymptomatic family members may proceed with genetic testing, preferably by the age of 20.[19] If no mutation is identified in the family member with DGC, the value of testing asymptomatic relatives is low.

Among individuals found to carry a germline *CDH1* mutation, clinical screening is problematic. Histologically, DGC is characterized by multiple infiltrates of malignant signet ring cells, which may underlie normal mucosa.[27] Because these malignant foci are small in size and widely distributed, they are difficult to identify via random endoscopic biopsy. Chromoendoscopy and positron emission tomography have reportedly been used, but the clinical utility of these tools in early detection remains unproven. Lack of a sensitive screening test for HDGC makes early diagnosis extremely challenging. By the time patients are symptomatic and present for treatment, many have diffuse involvement of the stomach or linitis plastica, and rates of mortality are high. Published case reports describe patients who have presented with extensive DGC despite recent normal endoscopy and negative biopsies.[28] The 5-year survival rate for individuals who develop clinically apparent DGC is only 10%, with the majority dying before age 40.

Because of high cancer penetrance, poor outcome, and inadequacy of clinical screening tools for HDGC, prophylactic total gastrectomy is recommended as a management option for asymptomatic carriers of *CDH1* mutations.[18] Although total gastrectomy is performed with prophylactic intent in these cases, most specimens have been found to contain foci of diffuse signet ring cell cancer.[19,28,29] Foci of DGC have been identified even in patients who have undergone extensive negative screening, including high-resolution computed tomography, positron emission tomography scan, chromoendoscopy-guided biopsies, and endoscopic ultrasonography.[19] However, HGDC in asymptomatic *CDH1* carriers is usually completely resected by prophylactic gastrectomy, as pathologic analyses of resected specimens have shown only T1N0 disease.

Because these signet ring cell cancers are multifocal and distributed throughout the entire stomach, especially in the cardia,[30] prophylactic gastrectomy should include the entire stomach, and the surgeon must transect the esophagus and not the proximal stomach. Furthermore, it should be performed by a surgeon experienced in the technical aspects of the procedure and familiar with HDGC. In asymptomatic patients, lymph node metastases have not been observed; therefore, D2 lymph node resection is not necessary. The optimal timing of prophylactic gastrectomy in individuals with *CDH1* mutations is unknown, but recent consensus recommendations indicate that age 20 is reasonable.[18]

Although it is a potentially lifesaving procedure, prophylactic gastrectomy for *CDH1* mutation carries significant risks that must be considered. Overall mortality for total gastrectomy is estimated to be as high as 2% to 4%, although it is estimated to be 1% when performed prophylactically. Patients must also be aware that there is a nearly 100% risk of long-term morbidity associated with this procedure, including diarrhea, dumping, weight loss, and difficulty eating.[19] A recent study of the effects of prophylactic gastrectomy for *CDH1* mutation demonstrated that physical and mental function were normal at 12 months, but specific digestive issues were recognized. Overall, 70% had diarrhea, 63% fatigue, 81% eating discomfort, 63% reflux, 45% eating restrictions, and 44% had altered body image, suggesting that this operation impacted negatively on quality of life.[31] Because of these complications and the fact that lymph node spread has not been observed, some recommend vagus-preserving gastrectomy done either open or laparoscopically. In addition, because the penetrance of *CDH1* mutations is incomplete, some patients who undergo prophylactic gastrectomy would never have gone on to develop clinically significant gastric cancer. Prophylactic gastrectomy has, in fact, been performed on several patients reported to show no evidence of gastric cancer on pathology.[29]

Some individuals with *CDH1* mutations choose not to pursue prophylactic gastrectomy. These individuals should undergo careful surveillance, including biannual chromoendoscopy with biopsies, beginning when they are at least 10 years younger than the youngest family member with DGC was at time of diagnosis. It is recommended that any endoscopically visible lesion is targeted and that six random biopsies are taken from the following regions: antrum, transitional zone, body, fundus, and cardia. Careful white-light examination with targeted and random biopsies combined with detailed histopathology can identify early lesions and help to inform decision making with regard to gastrectomy.[32] Additionally, because women with *CDH1* mutations have a nearly 40% lifetime risk of developing lobular breast carcinoma, they should be carefully screened with annual mammography and breast MRI starting at age 35.[23] They should also do monthly self-examinations and have a breast examination by a physician every 6 months. The same surveillance recommendations are probably appropriate for HDGC families without identifiable *CDH1* mutations, although no current guidelines for this exist.

The emergence of gene-directed gastrectomy as a treatment strategy for patients with HDGC represents the culmination of a successful collaboration between molecular biologists, geneticists, oncologists, gastroenterologists, and surgeons. It is anticipated that the recognition of similar molecular markers in other familial cancer syndromes will transform the approach to the early diagnosis and treatment of a variety of tumors.

SURGICAL PROPHYLAXIS OF HEREDITARY OVARIAN AND ENDOMETRIAL CANCER

Hereditary Ovarian Cancer (*BRCA1, BRCA2*)

Inherited mutations in *BRCA1* and *BRCA2* strongly predispose women to breast cancer and to high-grade serous cancers of the ovary, fallopian tube, and peritoneum.[33,34] About two-thirds are due to *BRCA1* mutations and one-third *BRCA2* mutations, and these account for about 15% to 20% of high-grade serous cases. The lifetime risk of these gynecologic cancers increases from a baseline of 1.5% to about 15% to 25% in *BRCA2* carriers and 30% to 60% in *BRCA1* carriers.[33,34] *BRCA1/2* mutations are rare in most populations (<1 in 500 individuals); one notable exception is the Ashkenazi Jewish population, in which the carrier frequency is 1 in 40.[35] *BRCA1*-associated cases peak in the 50s and *BRCA2*-associated cancers in the 60s.[36] In addition to *BRCA1/2* mutations, germline mutations in a number of other genes in the homologous recombination DNA repair pathway confer high penetrance susceptibility to ovarian cancer (e.g., *RAD51C, RAD51D, BRIP1, PALB2*).[37] This has led to the development of more comprehensive cancer genetic testing panels that are increasingly being used to identify women who are candidates for risk-reducing salpingo-oophorectomy (RRSO).

Genetic testing for inherited high-penetrance mutations in *BRCA1/2* and other genes should be discussed with women who have a significant family history of early onset breast cancer and/or cancers of the ovary, fallopian tube, or peritoneum. Involvement of a genetic counselor prior to testing is helpful, as they have expertise in managing the inherent clinical and social issues. Most *BRCA1/2* mutations involve base deletions or insertions in the coding sequence or splice sites that encode truncated protein products that are clearly dysfunctional. Less frequently, disease-causing mutations may occur that alter a single amino acid, though most of these missense variants represent innocent polymorphisms. The clinical significance of missense mutations can sometimes be elucidated by determining whether they segregate with cancer in other family members. In addition, genomic rearrangements may occur that inactivate *BRCA1* or *BRCA2*, and identification of such alterations requires molecular testing beyond sequencing.

Penetrance of ovarian cancer is not 100% in those with clearly deleterious *BRCA1/2* mutations, but presently it is not possible to provide more precise personalized risk estimates to guide the use of RRSO. However, common variants have been discovered in other genes that appear to affect the risk of ovarian cancer in *BRCA1/2* carriers.[38] Based on the known ovarian cancer risk–modifying loci, it has been reported that the 5% of *BRCA1* carriers at lowest risk have a lifetime risk of ≤28% of developing ovarian cancer, whereas the 5% at highest risk have a ≥63% lifetime risk. In the future, when modifier loci are more completely catalogued, more precise estimates of cancer risk may be provided to individual patients who are considering RRSO.

As about 20% of women with high-grade serous ovarian cancers have *BRCA1/2* mutations, it has been suggested that all of these women undergo genetic testing regardless of family history.[39] Mutational analysis in women with these cancers may increasingly become standard practice as the cost of genetic testing declines. Testing may also be driven by the availability of poly(ADP-ribose) polymerase inhibitor therapy for women whose cancers have germline or sporadic mutations in genes such as *BRCA1/2* and others that are involved in homologous recombination DNA repair.

RRSO is strongly recommended in women who carry *BRCA1/2* mutations because of the high mortality rate of ovarian cancer and the lack of effective screening and prevention approaches. Although screening with pelvic ultrasound and serum CA125 is generally recommended for *BRCA1/2* carriers during their 20s and 30s, it is not proven to reduce ovarian cancer mortality because even early stage high-grade cancers have a very high mortality. Oral contraceptives reduce the risk of ovarian cancer in the general population and appear to have a similar effect in *BRCA1/2* carriers, but this must be balanced against concerns regarding increased breast cancer risks.

The past practice of performing RRSO based solely on family history has been replaced by reliance on genetic testing. Clinical management of women with a strong family history in whom a deleterious germline mutation is not found, or those with variants of uncertain significance, should be resolved on a case-by-case basis. RRSO may be deemed appropriate in some cases, despite the absence of a clearly deleterious mutation. Fortunately, the risk of hereditary ovarian cancer does not rise dramatically until the mid-30s in women with *BRCA1* mutations and the 40s for women with *BRCA2* mutations.[36] As a result, most women are able to complete childbearing prior to undergoing RRSO. It is advisable for *BRCA1* carriers to undergo RRSO around age 35, as there is a 4% risk of ovarian cancer being discovered clinically or at the time of RRSO by age 40.[10] *BRCA2* carriers may choose to delay surgery into their 40s due to their lower risk of ovarian cancer, but this could diminish the protection against breast cancer that is afforded by RRSO. If a mutation carrier, particularly a *BRCA1* carrier, chooses to pursue fertility into her 40s, then she should be counseled that she is at considerable risk of developing a life-threatening cancer that is largely preventable.

Several studies have provided evidence of the efficacy of RRSO. In one early study of *BRCA1/2* carriers, RRSO reduced the rate of breast and ovarian cancer by 75% over several years of follow-up.[40] A separate study in 2002 examined outcome in 551 *BRCA1/2* carriers from various registries.[41] Among 259 women who had undergone RRSO, 6 (2.3%) were found to have stage I ovarian cancer at the time of the procedure and 2 (0.8%) subsequently developed serous peritoneal carcinoma. Among the controls, 58 (20%) women developed ovarian cancer after a mean follow-up of 8.8 years. With the exclusion of the six women whose cancers were diagnosed at surgery, RRSO reduced ovarian cancer risk by 96%. More recently, in 2014, an international registry study of over 5,783 subjects with median follow-up of 5.6 years found that RRSO reduced ovarian, tubal, and peritoneal cancer risk by 80%.[36] There was an estimated lifetime risk of primary peritoneal cancer after RRSO of about 4% for *BRCA1* carriers and 2% for *BRCA2* carriers.[36] The risk of death from all causes was reduced by 77%. A prospective cohort study noted that RRSO was associated with reduction in breast cancer–specific (hazard ratio [HR] = 0.44; 95% confidence interval [CI] = 0.26 to 0.76), ovarian cancer–specific (HR = 0.21; 95% CI = 0.06 to 0.80), and all-cause mortality (HR = 0.40; 95% CI = 0.26 to 0.61).[10]

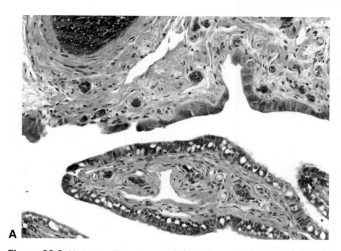 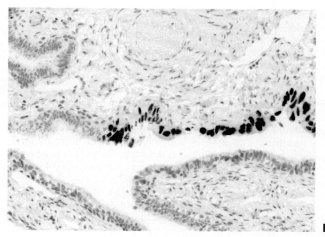

Figure 32.3 Hematoxylin and eosin (**A**) and immunohistochemical staining (**B**) demonstrating overexpression of mutant *TP53* in serous carcinoma in situ of the fallopian tube from a *BRCA1* mutation carrier who underwent risk-reducing bilateral salpingo-oophorectomy.

Removal of the ovaries, as internal organs, usually has little effect on body image and self-esteem, and most *BRCA1/2* mutation carriers elect to undergo RRSO. Insurance payers will almost always pay for RRSO in proven mutation carriers.

RRSO can be performed laparoscopically in most women, with discharge to home the same day. If a laparoscopic approach is problematic due to obesity or adhesions, the surgery can be performed through a small lower abdominal incision. Morbidity including bleeding, infection, and damage to the urinary or gastrointestinal tracts can occur, but the incidence of serious complications is very low. As the fallopian tubes and ovaries are small discrete organs, they are relatively easy to remove completely. Attention should be paid to transecting the ovarian artery and vein proximal to the ovary and tube so that remnants are not left behind. This involves opening the pelvic sidewall peritoneum, visualizing the ureter, and then isolating the ovarian blood supply. If there are adhesions between the adnexa and adjacent structures, careful dissection should be performed to ensure complete removal of the ovaries and fallopian tubes. If the uterus is not removed, care should be taken to remove the entire fallopian tube. A small portion of the tube inevitably will be left in the cornu of the uterus, but the risk of fallopian tube cancer developing in such remnants appears to be negligible.

Though there is not strong evidence that *BRCA1/2* mutations increase uterine cancer risk, many women elect to have the uterus removed as part of the surgical procedure because they have completed their family or have other gynecologic indications. Although the addition of a hysterectomy may increase operative time, blood loss, surgical complications, and hospital stay, it usually can be performed laparoscopically and serious adverse outcomes are infrequent. Furthermore, the likelihood of future exposure to tamoxifen in the context of breast cancer prevention or treatment, which increases endometrial cancer risk two- to three-fold, also argues for concomitant hysterectomy. Women who receive hormone replacement therapy after surgery will require a progestin along with estrogen to protect against the development of endometrial cancer if the uterus is not removed.

In younger women, surgical menopause after RRSO is associated with vasomotor symptoms, vaginal atrophy, decreased libido, and an accelerated onset and incidence of osteoporosis and cardiovascular disease. In premenopausal women who do not have a personal history of breast cancer, estrogen replacement can be administered to ameliorate many of the deleterious effects of premature menopause. Systemic estrogen levels are lower in oophorectomized premenopausal women taking hormone replacement than if the ovaries had been left in place. The therapeutic benefit of oophorectomy in women with breast cancer has long been

appreciated, and more recent studies support the contention that RRSO reduces the risk of breast cancer by about half in *BRCA1/2* carriers.[42] However, a meta-analysis showed that while RRSO was strongly protective against estrogen receptor–positive breast cancer (HR = 0.22), there was no protection against estrogen receptor–negative breast cancer.[42] Many carriers are identified after developing early onset breast cancer, and this group represents the most difficult in which to balance the potential risks and benefits of estrogen replacement therapy.

Early stage high-grade serous cancers and in situ lesions with *TP53* mutations have been identified in the fallopian tubes of some RRSO specimens (Fig. 32.3). This has led to a paradigm shift in which it is now thought that most high-grade serous cancers found in the ovary, fallopian tube, and peritoneum are derived from cells that originate in the tubal fimbria.[43] The frequency of occult malignancies has varied between reports, but appears to be about 3%.[43] In view of this, the pelvis and peritoneal cavity should be examined carefully. Malignant cells also have been found in peritoneal cytologic specimens, and washings of the pelvis should be obtained when performing RRSO. The pathologist should be informed of the indication for surgery and serial sections of the fallopian tubes should be performed to look for the presence of early lesions. Patients found to have occult invasive high-grade serous cancers should be treated with chemotherapy after surgery. Those with in situ lesions appear to have a good outcome without chemotherapy.[44]

Cases of peritoneal serous carcinoma indistinguishable from ovarian cancer have been observed years after RRSO, but the origin of these cancers is unclear. Some may represent recurrences of occult ovarian or tubal cancers. In this regard, retrospective examination of the ovaries and fallopian tubes sometimes has revealed primary cancers that were not originally recognized. In contrast, some of these cancers likely arise directly from fallopian tube cells that have implanted in the peritoneum and subsequently become malignant. Patients who undergo RRSO should be made aware of their residual risk of peritoneal cancer, but there is no evidence that continued surveillance using CA125 and/or ultrasound is beneficial.

HEREDITARY ENDOMETRIAL CANCER (LYNCH SYNDROME)

Although Lynch syndrome (LS, also known as hereditary nonpolyposis CRC syndrome) typically manifests as familial clustering of early onset CRC, there is also an increased incidence of several other types of cancers—most notably endometrial cancer in women.[45] About 3% of endometrial cancers are attributable to inherited mutations in the DNA mismatch repair (MMR) genes that cause LS. Most often, *MSH2* and *MLH1* are implicated, but mutations in *MSH6* and *PMS2* also occur.[45] The risk of ovarian cancer is also significantly increased in LS, but to a lesser degree than in *BRCA1/2* mutation carriers, and accounts for only about 1% of all ovarian cancers.

Cells in which one of the LS genes have been inactivated exhibit a phenomenon called microsatellite instability (MSI).[46] This occurs as DNA mismatches cause shortening or lengthening of repetitive DNA sequences and these mismatches go unrepaired. This results in generation of alleles in the cancer that contain a greater or lesser number of repeats than are present in normal cells from that individual. MSI occurs in most LS-associated colorectal and endometrial cancers.[46] However, MSI is found in about 20% of sporadic cancers that arise in these organs, and in most cases is caused by silencing of the *MLH1* gene due to promoter hypermethylation. Screening strategies for identification of MMR gene alterations in families with LS-associated cancers include analysis of tumor tissue for MSI and/or loss of DNA MMR gene expression using immunohistochemistry (IHC).[46] In cancers with MSI or loss of expression of one of the MMR genes, or in families with pedigrees suggestive of LS, these genes can be sequenced to identify disease-causing mutations, most of which cause truncated protein products.[47] Although it has been suggested that it may be cost-effective to do these tests on all endometrial cancers, this approach has not been widely adopted.[47]

The risk of a woman who carries a LS mutation developing endometrial cancer ranges from 20% to 60% in various reports.[45,48] The risk of ovarian cancer is increased to about 5% to 12%. Whereas the mean age of women with sporadic endometrial cancers is in the early 60s, cancers that arise in association with LS are often diagnosed before menopause, with the average age in the 40s. The clinical features of these endometrial cancers are similar to those of most sporadic cases (well-differentiated, endometrioid histology, early stage), and survival is about 90%. The mean age of onset of ovarian cancer in LS is in the early 40s, and the clinical features of these cancers are generally more favorable than in sporadic cases. They usually are identified at an early stage, are well- or moderately differentiated, have favorable survival, and some occur in the setting of a synchronous endometrial cancer.

Recommendations for screening and risk-reducing surgery in LS are better established for CRC than for extracolonic malignancies.[49] Transvaginal ultrasound has been proposed as a screening test for endometrial cancer (and ovarian cancer), but its efficacy is unproven.[50] Endometrial biopsy is the most sensitive means of diagnosing endometrial cancer, and it has been suggested that this should be employed periodically beginning around age 30 to 35. However, there are no published studies demonstrating that this approach prevents endometrial cancer deaths compared to simply performing a biopsy if abnormal uterine bleeding occurs.

Most experts believe that risk-reducing hysterectomy has a role in the management of some women with LS because of the high incidence of endometrial cancer. The risk of endometrial cancer is low during the prime reproductive years, and the uterus does not serve a vital function once childbearing has been completed. In view of the increased risk of ovarian cancer in LS, concomitant bilateral salpingo-oophorectomy should also be considered. One study demonstrated that there were no cases of endometrial or ovarian cancer in 61 LS carriers who underwent risk-reducing hysterectomy and bilateral salpingo-oophorectomy, while endometrial cancer occurred in 33% and ovarian cancer in 5% who retained their uterus and ovaries.[51] Despite the low risk of death from gynecologic cancers in LS, cost-effectiveness analyses of various approaches suggest that risk-reducing hysterectomy and salpingo-oophorectomy leads to both the lowest cost and the greatest increase in quality-adjusted life-years.[52] Estrogen replacement after removal of the ovaries in premenopausal women with LS is not contraindicated, as there is no evidence that this adversely affects the incidence of other cancers.

Many women with LS elect to undergo risk-reducing colectomy, which provides an opportunity to perform concomitant hysterectomy. Hysterectomy in concert with colectomy, either via laparoscopy or laparotomy, does not greatly increase operative time or surgical complications. If an endometrial biopsy has not been performed preoperatively, an intraoperative inspection of the uterine cavity and possibly frozen section should be performed to exclude the presence of cancer. If cancer is found in the uterus, surgical staging—including sampling of the regional lymph nodes—should be considered in addition to hysterectomy.[53] It is also appropriate to discuss risk-reducing hysterectomy with LS carriers who do not elect to undergo prophylactic colectomy. The operative approach (vaginal versus laparotomy versus laparoscopy) can be determined based on the presence or absence of uterine pathology (e.g., myomas), whether the patient has had prior abdominal surgery, and whether the ovaries are also to be removed.

GYNECOLOGIC CANCER RISK IN VERY RARE HEREDITARY CANCER SYNDROMES

Several very rare hereditary cancer syndromes also increase the risk of gynecologic cancers, and some of these women could potentially benefit from risk-reducing surgery to remove the ovaries and/or uterus. Peutz-Jeghers syndrome is characterized by intestinal polyps and an increased risk of colorectal and breast cancers. This rare syndrome is due to inherited mutations in the *STK11* gene. Affected women also have an increased risk of ovarian sex cord–stromal tumors with annular tubules and adenoma malignum of the cervix. Li-Fraumeni syndrome is caused by inherited mutations in the *TP53* gene, and carriers are predisposed to a number of types of cancers including sarcomas and breast cancer. The risk of ovarian cancer is increased as well, but is not a major cause of cancer in these families. Cowden syndrome is due to germline *PTEN* mutations and increases the risk of several malignancies including breast, thyroid, mucocutaneous, and endometrial cancers. Finally, small cell carcinoma of the ovary, hypercalcemic type, is due to mutations in the *SMARCA4* gene. These highly lethal ovarian cancers occur at a very young age (median 24 years) and present difficult challenges related to timing of RRSO. There are no well-accepted evidence-based guidelines for early detection and prevention of gynecologic cancers in these very rare hereditary cancer syndromes. An awareness of the risk and natural history of gynecologic cancers in these families provides a basis for counseling individual patients.

MULTIPLE ENDOCRINE NEOPLASIA TYPE 2

Gene Carriers

The MEN type 2 syndromes include MEN 2A, MEN 2B, and familial (non-MEN) medullary thyroid carcinoma (FMTC).[54-56] These are autosomal dominant inherited syndromes caused by germline mutations in the *RET* proto-oncogene. Their hallmark is the development of multifocal bilateral medullary thyroid carcinoma (MTC) associated with C-cell hyperplasia. MTCs arise from the thyroid C-cells, also called parafollicular cells. C-cells secrete the hormone calcitonin, a specific tumor marker for MTC. A slow-growing tumor in most cases, MTC causes significant morbidity and death in patients with uncontrolled local or metastatic spread. Large tumor burden is associated with diarrhea and flushing. In the MEN 2 syndromes, there is almost complete penetrance of MTC. Other features are variably expressed, with incomplete penetrance (summarized in Table 32.2).

In MEN 2A, all patients develop MTC. Approximately 42% of affected patients also develop pheochromocytomas, associated with adrenal medullary hyperplasia. Hyperparathyroidism develops in

TABLE 32.2

Clinical Features of Sporadic Medullay Thyroid Carcinoma, Multiple Endocrine Neoplasia 2A, Multiple Endocrine Neoplasia 2B, and Familial Medullay Thyroid Carcinoma

Clinical Setting	Features of MTC	Inheritance Pattern	Associated Abnormalities	Genetic Defect
Sporadic MTC	Unifocal	None	None	Somatic *RET* mutations in >20% of tumors
MEN 2A	Multifocal, bilateral	Autosomal dominant	Pheochromocytomas, hyperparathyroidism, cutaneous lichen amyloidosis, Hirshprung's disease	Germline missense mutations in extracellular cysteine codons of *RET*
MEN 2B	Multifocal, bilateral	Autosomal dominant	Pheochromocytomas, mucosal neuromas, megacolon, skeletal abnormalities	Germline missense mutation in tyrosine kinase domain of *RET*
FMTC	Multifocal, bilateral	Autosomal dominant	None	Germline missense mutations in extracellular or intracellular cysteine codons of *RET*

MTC, medullary thyroid carcinoma; MEN, multiple endocrine neoplasia; FMTC, familial medullary thyroid carcinoma.

10% to 35%. Cutaneous lichen amyloidosis and Hirschsprung's disease are infrequently associated with MEN 2A.[57–60]

MEN 2B appears to be the most aggressive form of hereditary MTC. In MEN 2B, MTC develops in all patients at a very young age (infancy). All affected individuals develop neural gangliomas, particularly in the mucosa of the digestive tract, conjunctiva, lips, and tongue; 40% to 50% develop pheochromocytomas. Patients with MEN 2B may also have megacolon, skeletal abnormalities, and markedly enlarged peripheral nerves. They do not develop hyperparathyroidism.

FMTC is characterized by development of MTC in the absence of any other endocrinopathies. MTC in these patients has a more indolent clinical course. Some individuals with FMTC may never manifest clinical evidence (i.e., symptoms or a lump in the neck), although biochemical testing and histologic evaluation of the thyroid demonstrates MTC.[55,56]

RET Genotype-Phenotype Correlations

Mutations in the *RET* proto-oncogene are responsible for MEN 2A, MEN 2B, and FMTC.[61–64] This gene encodes a transmembrane tyrosine kinase protein.[57,65] The mutations that cause the MEN 2 syndromes are activating gain-of-function mutations affecting constitutive activation of the protein. This is unusual among hereditary cancer syndromes, which are usually caused by loss-of-function mutations in the predisposition gene (e.g., familial polyposis, *BRCA1* and 2, von Hippel-Lindau, and MEN 1). More than 30 missense mutations have been described in patients affected by the MEN 2 syndromes (Fig. 32.4).

There is a relationship between the type of inherited *RET* mutation and presentation of MTC. The most virulent form is seen in patients with MEN 2B. These patients most commonly have a germline mutation in codon 918 of *RET* (ATG->ACG), although other mutations have been described (codon 883 and 922). As noted previously, MTC in MEN 2B has an extremely early age of onset (infancy). Despite its distinctive clinical appearance and associated gastrointestinal difficulties, the disease is often not detected until the patient develops a neck mass. Metastatic spread is usually present at the time of initial treatment, and calcitonin levels often remain elevated postoperatively.

MTC has a variable course in patients with MEN 2A, similar to that of sporadic MTC. Codon 634 and 618 mutations are the most common *RET* mutations associated with MEN 2A, although

mutations at other codons are also observed (see Fig. 32.4). Some patients do extremely well for many years, even with distant metastases, while others develop inanition, symptomatic liver, lung or skeletal metastases, as well as disabling diarrhea. Recurrence in the central neck, with invasion of the airway or great vessels, may cause death.

In patients with FMTC, MTC is usually indolent. These individuals most commonly have mutations of codons 609, 611, 618, 620, 768, 804, or 891, although mutations of other codons have been identified (see Fig. 32.4). Many patients with FMTC are cured by thyroidectomy alone, and even those with persistent elevation of calcitonin levels do well for many years. Occasionally, patients with FMTC survive into the seventh or eighth decade without clinical signs of disease, although pathologic examination of the thyroid will reveal MTC or C-cell hyperplasia.[66]

Risk-Reducing Thyroidectomy in *RET* Mutation Carriers

Genetic counseling and informed consent should be obtained prior to genetic testing. Specific issues that should be covered in genetic counseling sessions include explaining the patterns of heritability, likelihood of expression of different tumors, their prevention and treatment, insurability, nonpaternity, survivor guilt, and others.

It has been shown that *RET* mutation carriers may harbor foci of MTC in the thyroid gland, even when calcitonin levels are normal.[67] While the age of onset and rate of disease progression may differ, the lifetime penetrance of MTC is near 100% in carriers of *RET* mutations associated with MEN 2 syndromes. At-risk individuals who are found to have inherited a *RET* gene mutation are therefore candidates for thyroidectomy, regardless of their plasma calcitonin levels.

The best option for prevention of MTC in *RET* mutation carriers is complete surgical resection prior to malignant transformation. Prophylactic thyroidectomy prior to the development of MTC is the goal in these patients. A number of studies have demonstrated improved biochemical cure rates and/or decreased recurrence rates from early thyroidectomy, performed after positive screening by calcitonin testing or *RET* mutation testing.[68–70]

MEN 2B mutations are the highest risk level, designated level III (see Fig. 32.4).[55,71] Patients with MEN 2B have the most aggressive form of MTC, with invasive disease reported in patients <1 year of age. These patients should have preventative surgery

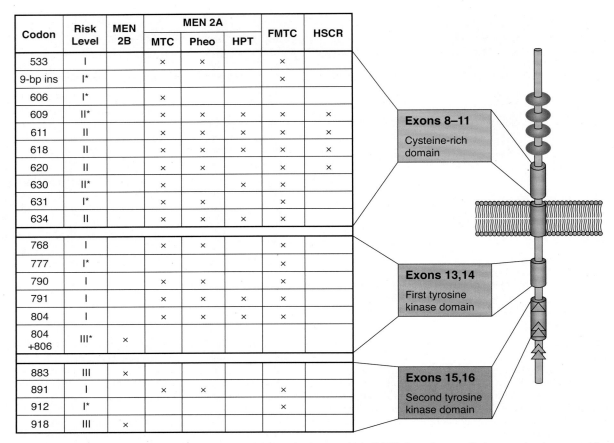

Codon	Risk Level	MEN 2B	MEN 2A			FMTC	HSCR
			MTC	Pheo	HPT		
533	I		×	×		×	
9-bp ins	I*					×	
606	I*		×				
609	II*		×	×	×	×	×
611	II		×	×	×	×	×
618	II		×	×	×	×	×
620	II		×	×		×	×
630	II*		×		×	×	
631	I*		×	×		×	
634	II		×	×	×	×	
768	I		×	×		×	
777	I*					×	
790	I		×	×		×	
791	I		×	×		×	
804	I		×	×	×	×	
804 +806	III*	×					
883	III	×					
891	I		×	×		×	
912	I*					×	
918	III	×					

Exons 8–11
Cysteine-rich domain

Exons 13,14
First tyrosine kinase domain

Exons 15,16
Second tyrosine kinase domain

Figure 32.4 *RET* mutation sites associated with multiple endocrine neoplasia (MEN) 2 syndromes. Codons previously reported in association with MEN-2 syndromes are listed by structural domain within the RET protein. Risk level is based on consensus guidelines or more recent clinical reports. Previously reported phenotypes for each codon are shown. MTC, medullary thyroid carcinoma; Pheo, pheochromocytoma; HPT, hyperparathyroidism; FMTC, familial medullary thyroid carcinoma; HSCR, Hirschsprung's disease. *Asterisk* indicates risk level based on recent clinical reports not available at publication of the consensus guidelines. (From Traugott AL, Moley JF. The RET protooncogene. *Cancer Treat Res* 2010;153:303–319.)

early in the first year of life, if possible. Identification and preservation of parathyroid glands can be extremely difficult in these infants, due to their small size, translucent appearance, and the presence of exuberant thymic and perithyroidal nodal tissue. These procedures should be performed by surgeons experienced in parathyroid and/or pediatric thyroid operations.

Patients with MEN 2A with mutations in codons 634, 620, 618, and 611 are also considered high risk (level II).[55,71] Patients with level II mutations should undergo a total thyroidectomy at 5 to 6 years of age. There is evidence that the risk of lymph node metastasis is very low in patients with MEN 2A under the age of 8, with normal calcitonin levels. Central lymph node dissection is associated with higher risk of hypoparathyroidism, and recurrent laryngeal nerve injury and should be reserved for patients with elevated calcitonin levels.

A larger subset of *RET* mutations, associated with MEN 2A and/or FMTC, is considered the lowest risk (level I).[55,71] These include mutations at codons 768, 790, 791, 804, and 891. For patients with low-risk level I mutations, total thyroidectomy is recommended before age 5 to 10 years. This decision, however, regarding ideal age at preventative thyroidectomy in low-risk mutation carriers, is currently being reviewed, and may be driven by additional clinical data such as the basal or stimulated serum calcitonin level.[72,73] There are no guidelines at present that address the issue of timing of surgery based on calcitonin level, and at present, pentagastrin (the primary calcitonin secretagogue used in testing) is not available in the United States. It is anticipated that within a decade, there will

be enough published data to direct timing of interventions based upon this information. As with the level II mutations, the need for central lymph node dissection should be guided by calcitonin levels and clinical features of the patient and kindred.

Until recently, some groups recommended total thyroidectomy with central neck lymph node dissection and total parathyroidectomy with autotransplantation for all *RET* mutation carriers. Recent studies and personal experience, however, have demonstrated an extremely low likelihood of nodal metastases in patients with MEN 2A or FMTC younger than 8 years of age, and in patients with a normal calcitonin level.[70] Our current strategy is to leave the parathyroid in situ in these patients, if possible.[74] Often, however, the desired complete removal of thyroid tissue results in compromise of parathyroid blood supply. In these situations, autotransplantation of devascularized parathyroid is required. We routinely remove and autotransplant the parathyroid if a central node dissection is done. In parathyroid autotransplantation, parathyroid glands are sliced into 1 mm × 3 mm fragments and autotransplanted into individual muscle pockets in the muscle of the nondominant forearm in patients with MEN 2A, or in the sternocleidomastoid muscle in patients with FMTC or MEN 2B. Patients are maintained on calcium and vitamin D supplementation for 4 to 8 weeks postoperatively.

In a recent series of thyroidectomies performed in 50 individuals with MEN 2A (identified by genetic screening), total thyroidectomy and central node dissection with parathyroidectomy and parathyroid autografting were performed in all patients (Fig. 32.5).[70]

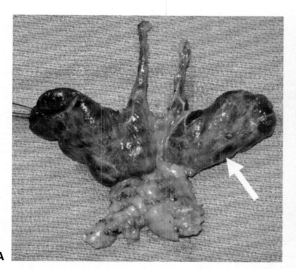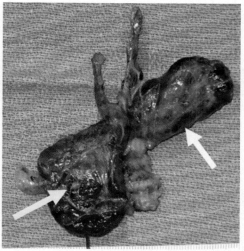

Figure 32.5 Total thyroidectomy specimen with attached central nodes from a patient with germline *RET* mutation and elevated calcitonin levels. Note small visible foci of medullary thyroid carcinoma (*arrows*).

All autografts functioned, but three patients required supplemental calcium. The percentage of individuals requiring calcium supplementation following parathyroidectomy with parathyroid autografting reportedly ranges from 0% to 18%. Parathyroidectomy should be performed in all patients showing gross parathyroid enlargement or biochemical evidence of parathyroid disease at time of surgery. The operating surgeon should have expertise in preservation of parathyroid function. It is important that the surgeon performing an operative procedure for MTC be familiar with the techniques described here. If not, the patient should be referred to a center where these procedures are routinely performed.

Some patients with MEN 2 will be found to have elevated calcitonin levels prior to thyroidectomy. This is usually associated with medullary thyroid carcinoma or C-cell hyperplasia in the gland, and may be associated with lymph node metastases. Much has been written about the correlation between preoperative calcitonin levels and extent of nodal involvement. It has been suggested that preoperative calcitonin level may guide the extent of node dissection. In a study of 300 European patients with MTC, node metastases were not identified when the preoperative basal calcitonin level was <20 pg/ml.[75] Involvement of nodal groups was correlated with basal calcitonin level as follows: ipsilateral central and lateral neck nodes (basal calcitonin >20 pg/ml), contralateral central nodes (basal calcitonin >50 pg/ml), contralateral lateral neck nodes (basal calcitonin >200 pg/ml), and mediastinal nodes (basal calcitonin >500 pg/ml). Based upon these findings, this group (who also wrote the European guidelines) recommends thyroidectomy only if basal calcitonin is <20 pg/ml, ipsilateral central and lateral neck dissection if the calcitonin is 20 to 50 pg/ml, and contralateral central neck dissection if the basal calcitonin is 50 to 200 pg/ml, with the addition of contralateral lateral neck dissection if the calcitonin is 200 to 500 pg/ml. Most experts agree that sternotomy with mediastinal neck dissection should be reserved for patients with image evidence of mediastinal disease. In contrast, most North American surgeons rely heavily upon preoperative ultrasound imaging to map the extent of nodal involvement and determine extent of surgery based upon calcitonin and imaging results.[55,74,76]

Follow-up

Following thyroidectomy, thyroid hormone replacement is required for life. Patients may need several weeks of oral calcium and vitamin D until parathyroid function recovers. Intermittent calcitonin testing may be done to monitor for persistent or recurrent

MTC. The importance of regular monitoring of patients' compliance with thyroid medication following thyroidectomy should not be underestimated. Children and teenagers are frequently noncompliant, and this can be determined by routine measurement of thyroid-stimulating hormone levels. Continued noncompliance can result in growth problems. Occasionally, local human services agencies may need to be involved in particularly difficult cases.

The term "biochemical cure" is used to refer to patients with normal calcitonin levels after surgery for MTC. Complete postoperative normalization of calcitonin has been associated with decreased long-term risk of MTC recurrence, though the evidence is less clear for a survival benefit. A persistent or recurrent elevation in calcitonin indicates residual or recurrent MTC and warrants additional investigation by imaging. However, as most MTC has a fairly indolent course, patients with biochemical evidence of recurrent disease may not have corollary imaging findings for some time.

Conclusions

Identification of *RET* gene mutations in individuals at risk for developing hereditary forms of MTC has simplified management, expanding the scope of indications for surgical intervention. Patients who carry this mutation can be offered operative treatment at a very young age, hopefully before the cancer has developed or spread, and those identified as not having the mutation are spared further genetic and biochemical screening. This achievement marks a new paradigm in surgery: the indication that an operation be performed based on the results of a genetic test. As in the decision to perform any surgical procedure, meticulous preparation and detailed discussion with patient and family must precede the final recommendation. It is also important that the patient and family be involved in preoperative discussions with genetic counselors. Postoperative follow-up for compliance with thyroid medication is important, especially in children and teenagers who are still growing and developing into adults.

FAMILIAL ADENOMATOUS POLYPOSIS, *MYH*-ASSOCIATED POLUPOSIS, AND LYNCH SYNDROME

Inherited CRC syndromes with multiple adenomatous polyps include FAP, *MYH*-associated polyposis (MAP), and LS. In some cases, the diagnosis is suspected because of a striking family history

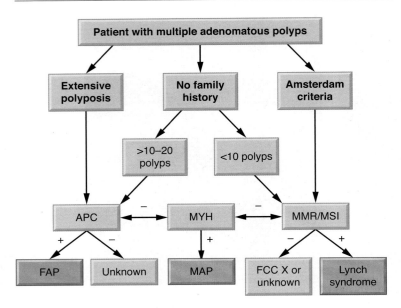

Figure 32.6 Schematic demonstrating the potential genetic workup for a patient with multiple adenomatous colorectal polyps and suspected of having an inherited colorectal cancer syndrome. APC, adenomatous polyposis coli; MMR, mismatch repair; MSI, microsatellite instability; FAP, familial adenomatous polyposis; MAP, *MYH*-associated polyposis; FCC X, familial colorectal cancer syndrome X.

of CRC, while in others, suspicion arises from a very young onset of CRC or florid polyposis.

Although adenomatous polyp burden and family history may suggest one syndrome over another, an initial negative genetic test result should be followed by further evaluation for other syndromes. For example, in clinical practice, a negative adenomatous polyposis coli (*APC*) gene test in a patient with a suspected CRC syndrome is followed by reflex testing for MAP and LS, as shown in Figure 32.6.

FAP is an autosomal dominant syndrome that accounts for <1% of the annual CRC burden, is caused by mutations in the tumor-suppressor *APC* gene. It is characterized by the presence of ≥100 adenomatous polyps in the colorectum, nearly 100% penetrance, and an inevitable risk of CRC if prophylactic colectomy is not performed.[8,77] Patients with a less severe form known as attenuated FAP (AFAP) usually present with <100 colorectal adenomas that tend to be proximally located. MAP is an autosomal recessive syndrome that often presents phenotypically as attenuated polyposis. While an estimated 2% of the general population are mono-allelic carriers of a mutated base-excision-repair *MUTYH* (*MYH*) gene, biallelic germline mutations may account for 9% to 18% of patients with FAP or AFAP phenotypes who have no demonstrable *APC* mutation.[78–80]

LS accounts for 1% to 4% of all newly diagnosed CRC and is attributable to a germline mutation in one of the DNA MMR genes (*MLH1*, *MSH2*, *MSH6*, and *PMS2*).[81–83] Epigenetic silencing of the *MSH2* gene via a 3′-end deletion in *EPCAM* (*TACSTD1*), a neighbor of *MSH2* that plays a role in cell adhesion, also accounts for 20% to 25% of all suspected *MSH2* cases and 1% to 6% of LS cases overall.[84–86] LS is characterized by early age-of-onset CRC, predominance of lesions proximal to the splenic flexure, an increased rate of metachronous CRC, and a unique spectrum of benign and malignant extracolonic tumors. Lifetime risk of CRC in patients with LS may be as high as 80%.[83,87] MSI reflects a deficiency in DNA repair secondary to MMR gene mutation and is a hallmark feature of LS-associated tumors.

Variability in penetrance, phenotypic expression, and certainty of disease development mandate distinctly different surgical approaches in these three syndromes, including the type and timing of risk-reducing colon and rectal surgery.[88]

Familial Adenomatous Polyposis

Surveillance of at-risk family members should begin around age 10 to 15 years with an annual colonoscopy or flexible sigmoidoscopy.[89]

At-risk individuals who belong to families with an AFAP phenotype should undergo colonoscopic screening every 2 to 3 years starting in their late teens. Informative genetic testing is possible in families with a demonstrated *APC* mutation, and mutations are detected in most pedigrees. However, approximately 25% of patients with FAP will have a de novo *APC* mutation.[87] Severity of polyposis should be established during colonoscopy, as the timing of surgery and the risk of developing colorectal is dependent on the extent of polyp burden. Patients with mild polyposis and a correspondingly lower CRC risk can undergo surgery in their late teens. Patients with severe polyposis, a high degree of dysplasia, multiple adenomas >5 mm in size, and symptoms (bleeding, persistent diarrhea, anemia, failure to thrive, psychosocial stress, etc.) should undergo risk-reducing colorectal surgery as soon as is practical after diagnosis.[90,91] However, in carefully selected, fully asymptomatic patients who have small adenomas but a strong family history of aggressive abdominal desmoid disease, consideration can be given to delaying prophylactic colectomy, as the risk of desmoid-related complication may be greater than the risk of CRC development.

The three current surgical options for patients with FAP are total proctocolectomy (TPC) with permanent ileostomy, total colectomy with ileorectal anastomosis (IRA), and proctocolectomy with ileal pouch-anal anastomosis (IPAA). IPAA can be a double-stapled, end-of-pouch-to-anus anastomosis, which may leave behind approximately 1 cm of anal transition zone. An alternative approach, which is preferred when there is carpeting of the anal transition zone with adenomas, is to perform a mucosal stripping of the anal transition zone down to the dentate line followed by a hand-sewn per anal anastomosis of pouch to the dentate line. Selection of the optimal procedure for an individual patient is based on several factors, including characteristics of the FAP syndrome within the patient and family, differences in likely postoperative functional outcome, preoperative anal sphincter status, and patient preference.[8]

TPC with permanent ileostomy, although rarely chosen as a primary procedure, is used in patients with invasive cancer involving the sphincters or levator complex, or patients for whom an IPAA is not technically feasible (secondary to desmoid disease and foreshortening of the small bowel mesentery, making it surgically impossible to bring the ileal pouch to the anus) nor likely to lead to good function such as massive obesity or weak anal sphincters. However, TPC is occasionally chosen as a primary procedure by patients who perceive that their lifestyle would be compromised by the frequent bowel movements (five to six per day) sometimes associated with the IPAA procedure.

In addition to these issues, the key in deciding between an IPAA and an IRA is based primarily on the risk of rectal cancer development if the rectum is left in situ. The risk of rectal cancer following IRA may range from 3% to 10% at 10 years, while the risk for a secondary proctectomy for uncontrolled rectal polyposis ranges from 10% to 61% at 20 years following initial colectomy with IRA.[92–94] The magnitude of risk in an individual patient is, however, related to the overall extent of colorectal polyposis. IRA may be considered for patients with <1,000 colorectal polyps (including those with attenuated FAP) and <20 rectal adenomas, as these individuals have a relatively low risk of developing rectal cancer.[88,93] Patients with severe rectal (>20 adenomas) or colonic (>1,000 adenomas) polyposis, an adenoma >3 cm, or an adenoma with severe dysplasia should ideally undergo a risk-reducing procedure that will include a proctectomy.[90,91,93]

The risk of secondary rectal excision, due to uncontrollable rectal polyposis or rectal cancer, may be estimated by identifying the specific location of the causative *APC* mutation. Patients with mutations located between codons 1250 and 1464 have been shown to have a six-fold increased risk of developing rectal cancer, compared to those with mutations prior to codon 1250 or after codon 1464 (mean number of rectal polyps 42 versus 22, respectively).[8,92] Although the use of the genotype-phenotype relationship to guide patient management may be appealing,[92] it is important to recognize the variability of phenotypic expression that exists even among members of the same family. This suggests that at the current time, the choice between an IRA and an IPAA should be based primarily on clinical (rather than genetic) grounds.[90]

The risk of polyp and cancer development following primary surgery is not limited to patients undergoing IRA. In patients undergoing IPAA, neoplasia may occur at the site of ileal pouch anastomosis; the frequency appears to be greater after stapled anastomosis (28% to 31%) than after mucosectomy and hand-sewn anastomosis (10% to 14%).[95] In the case of neoplasia developing at the anal transition zone after a stapled anastomosis, transanal mucosectomy may be performed, followed by advancement of the pouch to the dentate line. Of additional concern is the development of adenomatous polyps in the ileal pouch, which occurs in approximately 45% of patients by 10-year follow-up.[96] Consequently, depending on polyp burden, lifetime endoscopic surveillance of the rectal remnant (after IRA) every 6 to 12 months or the ileal pouch (after IPAA) every 1 to 3 years is required following either procedure.[89]

Another important consideration in choosing between IPAA and IRA is postoperative bowel function and quality of life. Some studies have associated IPAA with higher frequency of both daytime and nocturnal bowel movements, higher incidence of passive incontinence and incidental soiling, and greater postoperative morbidity.[97] However, long-term follow-up demonstrates a comparable quality of life following IPAA for FAP relative to the patient's preoperative baseline.[98] Therefore, although the choice of procedure must be carefully individualized, because of the risk of rectal cancer associated with IRA, the authors favor IPAA for most patients with FAP whenever feasible. However, an IRA should be considered in specific circumstances, such as when there is mild rectal polyposis (as in AFAP), or a young patient with rectal sparing who is not interested in undergoing the multiple procedures that accompany an IPAA and diverting loop ileostomy, or a young woman interested in having children and trying to avoid the decreased fecundity associated with an IPAA procedure.[99] The use of minimally invasive techniques such as laparoscopy may reduce the risk of infertility associated with IPAA.[100,101] Though a diverting loop ileostomy should be performed in all IPAA procedures, it is not always feasible due to a number of anatomic factors such as body habitus.

Endoscopic surveillance of the rectal segment at 6- to 12-month intervals after the index surgery is recommended, with subsequent surveillance frequencies dependent on the number and size of adenomas observed.[89] Although small (<5 mm) scattered adenomas can be safely observed or removed with biopsy forceps, polyps >5 mm should be removed by snare. However, repeated fulguration and polypectomy over many years can lead to difficulty with subsequent polypectomy, reduced rectal compliance, and difficulty identifying flat cancers in the background of scar tissue. The development of severe dysplasia and/or villous adenomas not amenable to endoscopic removal is indication for proctectomy.

Long-Term Considerations from Extracolonic Manifestations

Despite the reduced risk of CRC-related death following prophylactic colectomy, patients with FAP are still at increased risk of mortality from both rectal cancer and other causes relative to the general population. The three main causes of death following IRA are progression of desmoid disease, stomach and duodenal cancer, and perioperative mortality. Additional FAP-related extraintestinal manifestations include epidermoid cysts, supernumerary teeth, osteomas of the jaw and/or skull, congenital hypertrophy of the retinal pigment epithelium, cancers of the hepatopancreatobiliary tract and genitourinary tract, and thyroid cancer.[102–104]

Desmoids

Desmoids may occur in 10% to 25% of patients with FAP.[105,106] Unlike those found in the general population, FAP-associated desmoids tend to be intra-abdominal and arise following abdominal surgery.[106,107] Although conflicting reports exist, it appears that female patients, those with extracolonic manifestations of FAP, a positive family history of desmoids, and *APC* mutations located at 3' of codon 1440 are at increased risk of developing desmoids.[106,108,109] These tumors often involve the small bowel mesentery as well as the retroperitoneum and are often life-threatening due to invasion or compression of adjacent viscera. Further, recurrence and morbidity rates are high following attempted resection, with recurrent disease often more aggressive than the initial desmoid. Estimated 5-year overall survival for patients with intra-abdominal desmoids causing severe symptoms such as significant pain and septic fistula/abscess, diameter >20 cm or rapidly growing, and/or need for parenteral nutrition is only 53%.[107] Therefore, desmoid resection is evaluated on an individualized case-by-case basis with surgery reserved for highly select cases.

Desmoids that involve the small bowel mesentery may preclude the formation of an IPAA secondary to foreshortening of the small bowel mesentery, especially in patients undergoing proctectomy after an initial IRA.[110] Surgery for intra-abdominal and abdominal wall desmoids should be reserved for limited disease where the likelihood of clear margins is high.

In symptomatic cases where resection of an intra-abdominal desmoid may not be feasible, intestinal bypass or ureteral stenting may be necessary to alleviate bowel or urinary obstruction secondary to mass effect. In addition to surgical intervention, several medical options with variable efficacy are available for the management of desmoid disease and include nonsteroidal anti-inflammatory drugs (e.g., sulindac), selective estrogen receptor modulators (e.g., tamoxifen), immunomodulators (e.g., imatinib, sorafenib, interferon), doxorubin-based cytotoxic chemotherapy, and radiation.

MYH-Associated Polyposis

MAP should be suspected in patients with >10 colorectal adenomas, a weak history of CRC, and no family history of FAP. The diagnosis is confirmed by *MUTYH* (*MYH*) gene testing.[80,88]

Depending on the polyp burden, the management of the colon and rectum of a patient with a biallelic *MYH* mutation can be endoscopic or surgical. If the polyp burden is limited and an endoscopic approach is pursued, colonoscopy should be performed every 1 to 3 years.[87,89] If the polyp burden is not amenable to an endoscopic approach at the time of diagnosis, then a resection is indicated. In most cases in which surgery is deemed necessary, an IRA is sufficient. However, if rectal polyposis is severe, an IPAA may be indicated. Indications for surgery following an endoscopic surveillance program include increasing polyp size or number, or worsening histology.

Extracolonic manifestations of MAP are similar to FAP and include osteomas, desmoids, congenital hypertrophy of the retinal pigment epithelium, as well as cancers of the thyroid, ovary, bladder, sebaceous gland, and breast. In addition, patients with MAP are also at a 4% lifetime risk of developing duodenal cancer and require upper endoscopies every 1 to 3 years beginning as early as ages 18 to 20 years and starting no later than ages 30 to 35 years.[87,89,111]

Lynch Syndrome

Due to the discordance associated with the term hereditary nonpolyposis colorectal cancer, the use of this term has largely been abandoned with reversion back to the eponym LS, which refers to individuals with a predisposition to CRC and other malignancies as a result of a germline MMR mutation.[112] Overall, CRC occurs in up to 80% of patients with LS by their mid-40s.[8,82] Endometrial cancer occurs in 40% to 60%, gastric cancer in 11% to 19%, urinary tract cancer in 5% to 18%, and ovarian cancer in 9% to 15% of affected individuals.[8,82,87]

The Amsterdam criteria and revised Bethesda guidelines[113] (Table 32.3) are used in clinical practice to identify patients at risk for LS who require further genetic evaluation. The Amsterdam criteria, which led to the identification of the LS-causing MMR gene mutations require that there be:

- Three relatives (one a first-degree relative of the other two) with colorectal, endometrial, stomach, ovary, small bowel, ureteral/renal pelvis, brain, hepatobiliary, and/or sebaceous cancer;
- In two or more successive generations;
- With at least one case of cancer diagnosed before the age of 50;
- And that FAP as a diagnosis is excluded.[114]

Though the Amsterdam criteria can be used clinically to identify potential patients with LS, using it alone will result in identification

---

TABLE 32.3

The Revised Bethesda Guidelines for Testing Colorectal Tumors for Microsatellite Instability

Tumors from individuals should be tested for MSI in the following situations:

1. Colorectal cancer diagnosed in a patient who is <50 y of age.
2. Presence of synchronous, metachronous colorectal, or other HNPCC-associated tumors,[a] regardless of age.
3. Colorectal cancer with the MSI-H[b] histology[c] diagnosed in a patient who is <60 y of age.[d]
4. Colorectal cancer diagnosed in one or more first-degree relatives with an HNPCC-related tumor, with one of the cancers being diagnosed under age 50 years.
5. Colorectal cancer diagnosed in two or more first- or second-degree relatives with HNPCC-related tumors, regardless of age.

MSI, microsatellite instability; HNPCC, hereditary nonpolyposis colorectal cancer; MSI-H, microsatellite instability–high.
[a] HNPCC-related tumors include colorectal, endometrial, stomach, ovarian, pancreas, ureter and renal pelvis, biliary tract, and brain (usually glioblastoma as seen in Turcot syndrome) tumors, sebaceous gland adenomas and keratoacanthomas in Muir-Torre syndrome, and carcinoma of the small bowel.
[b] MSI-H in tumors refers to changes in two or more of the five National Cancer Institute–recommended panels of microsatellite markers.
[c] Presence of tumor-infiltrating lymphocytes, Crohn's-like lymphocytic reaction, mucinous/signet ring differentiation, or medullary growth pattern.
[d] There was no consensus among the workshop participants on whether to include the age criteria in guideline 3; participants voted to keep <60 years of age in the guidelines.
From Umar A, Boland CR, Terdiman JP, et al. Revised Bethesda Guidelines for hereditary nonpolyposis colorectal cancer (Lynch syndrome) and microsatellite instability. *J Natl Cancer Inst* 2004;96:261–268.

---

of only 42% of LS mutation carriers.[115] Families meeting Amsterdam criteria but lacking an MMR mutation are referred to as having "familial colorectal cancer type X" and appear to have a lower incidence of colorectal and extracolonic cancers than those with a LS germline MMR mutation (see Fig. 32.6). Of note, they have an increased incidence of left-sided and nonmucinous microsatellite stable tumors.[77,88]

Patients with CRC who belong to pedigrees suspicious for LS should be offered screening by IHC for loss of MMR protein expression or by MSI analysis. As the sensitivity of IHC testing for loss of MMR protein expression is comparable to MSI testing, either approach can be pursued.[112] However, IHC testing is less expensive and can also identify a specific MMR protein loss, which can help target subsequent germline testing. Routine IHC testing for loss of MMR protein in individuals younger than 50 years at the time of CRC diagnosis is feasible and has led to the identification of patients with LS who might otherwise have been missed.[116,117] Patients with MSI-high tumors should undergo testing for germline MMR mutations in *MSH2*, *MLH1*, *MSH6*, and *PMS2*. Reflex IHC and/or MSI testing on all newly diagnosed CRC has been advocated by some expert groups and has been successfully implemented at some institutions.[83,112,118] However, a majority of cancer programs nationwide currently do not have a protocol for reflex testing for LS, citing lack of institutional protocols as well as fear of nonreimbursement.[119] As such, a unified move toward universal testing remains some time away. In families for which tumor tissue is not available, initial germline testing may be considered though the financial burden is not insignificant, with the cost of finding a single LS carrier measuring approximately $58,000 (compared to the $5,000 spent in finding a single LS carrier using IHC screening).[120] As in FAP, a mutation in an affected individual must be established for testing in at-risk individuals to be conclusive.

In lieu of universal testing, several predictive models such as the MMRpredict, MMRpro, and PREMM$_{1,2,6}$ have been devised in order to assess an individual's likelihood of harboring LS.[115,121,122] These models quantify an individual's risk for carrying an *MLH1*, *MSH2*, *or MSH6* germline mutation by using clinical characteristics such as age at onset of CRC and/or other LS-associated cancers, location of CRC, family history, history of synchronous or metachronous CRC, among others. A study of these predictive models demonstrated that they all performed better than the revised Bethesda guidelines in terms of identifying patients with germline mutations for LS.[123] The MMRpredict model appeared to have to be the best predictor, with a sensitivity and specificity for LS of 94% and 91%, respectively. Other validation studies, however, have not demonstrated the superiority of MMRpredict compared to the other aforementioned models.[124,125] It appears that the use of clinical characteristics in combination with MSI or MMR protein expression status in predictive models may potentially improve our ability to establish LS diagnoses in patients with CRC. However, the practicality and applicability of these tools in a clinical setting requires further assessment.

Although development of CRC in LS is not a certainty, the 80% lifetime risk, the 16% to 30% risk of metachronous CRC, and the possibly accelerated adenoma-to-carcinoma sequence mandate consideration of prophylactic surgical options.[82,87,126–129] Patients with LS who have a CRC or more than one advanced adenoma should be offered the options of prophylactic total colectomy with IRA or segmental colectomy with annual postoperative surveillance colonoscopy. Careful surveillance is also necessary after total colectomy and IRA, as the risk of high-risk adenomas and cancer in the retained rectum at a median of 104 months are 11% and 8%, respectively.[126] Although there has been no study demonstrating an improved survival for patients with LS undergoing total colectomy and IRA versus segmental colectomy, mathematical models suggest a slight survival benefit for total colectomy and IRA, especially for individuals under the age of 30.[130,131] In addition, because of increased rates of metachronous CRC development and the risk of multiple abdominal surgeries in those undergoing a segmental resection, a total colectomy and IRA has emerged as the procedure of choice for the index cancer, with consideration for TPC in cases where a high risk of metachronous rectal cancer can be predicted.[126–128] Targeted genetic testing approaches—such as the single amplicon MSH2 A636P mutation test in Ashkenazi Jewish patients with CRC—have demonstrated how a rapid and inexpensive preoperative genetic test can help direct the extent of colon resection.[132]

LS mutation carriers with a normal colon and without a history of CRC may also be offered prophylactic colectomy in highly select situations. One rationale for this approach is the similarity of lifetime cancer risk between patients with APC and MMR gene mutations, and the fact that total abdominal colectomy with IRA produces less functional disturbance than the prophylactic procedure recommended for FAP (TPC with IPAA). However, an alternate strategy for these individuals is surveillance by colonoscopy, which is cost-effective and greatly reduces the rate of CRC development and overall mortality.[133] There is a risk of CRC development in the interval between colonoscopies, though most interval cancers tend to be early stage.[134,135] As such, given that metachronous CRC may develop in as short a duration as a median of 11.3 months,[136] the recommended interval for surveillance colonoscopies is now every 1 to 2 years.[89] While prophylactic colectomy is not routinely recommended, it may be indicated in highly select patients for whom colonoscopic surveillance is not technically possible or in those who refuse to undergo regular surveillance. A decision analysis model suggests that prophylactic subtotal colectomy at age 25 may offer a survival benefit of 1.8 years, compared with surveillance colonoscopy. The benefit of prophylactic colectomy decreases when surgery is delayed until later in life and is negligible when performed at the time of cancer development.[137] Thus, the decision between prophylactic surgery and surveillance for a gene-positive unaffected individual is based on many factors including penetrance of disease in the

TABLE 32.4

Prophylactic Total Abdominal Colectomy and Ileorectal Anastomosis for Lynch Syndrome Patients without Cancer

Pros

- Elimination of colon cancer risk
- Elimination of need for surveillance colonoscopy
- Alleviating patient anxiety over the prospect of colon cancer development

Cons

- Persistence of risk of rectal cancer development
- Rectum still requires flexible endoscopic surveillance
- Patient anxiety of prospect of rectal cancer persists
- Possible altered bowel function
- Risk of surgery and possible associated complications

family, early age-of-onset in affected family members, functional and quality-of-life considerations, and likelihood of compliance with surveillance. Table 32.4 lists some of the pros and cons of a prophylactic colectomy for germline mutation carriers for LS without a history of CRC. Patients with LS and an index rectal cancer should be offered the options of TPC with IPAA or anterior proctosigmoidectomy with primary reconstruction.[128,138] The rationale for TPC is the 10% to 15% associated risk of metachronous colon cancer in the remaining colon following the index rectal cancer. Choosing between the two procedures depends, in part, on the patient's willingness to undergo intensive surveillance of the retained proximal colon, as well as issues regarding quality of life and bowel function.

REFERENCES

1. Moyer VA, US Preventive Services Task Force. Risk Assessment, Genetic Counseling, and Genetic Testing for BRCA-Related Cancer in Women: U.S. Preventive Services Task Force Recommendation Statement. *Ann Intern Med* 2014;160.
2. Robson ME, Storm CD, Weitzel J, et al. American Society of Clinical Oncology policy statement update: genetic and genomic testing for cancer susceptibility. *J Clin Oncol* 2010;28:893–901.
3. Amir E, Freedman OC, Seruga B, et al. Assessing women at high risk of breast cancer: a review of risk assessment models. *J Natl Cancer Inst* 2010;102:680–691.
4. Miki Y, Swensen J, Shattuck-Eidens D, et al. A strong candidate for the breast and ovarian cancer susceptibility gene BRCA1. *Science* 1994;266:66–71.
5. Wooster R, Neuhausen SL, Mangion J, et al. Localization of a breast cancer susceptibility gene, BRCA2, to chromosome 13q12-13. *Science* 1994;265:2088–2090.
6. Lux MP, Fasching PA, Beckmann MW. Hereditary breast and ovarian cancer: review and future perspectives. *J Mol Med* 2006;84:16–28.
7. Shannon KM, Chittenden A. Genetic testing by cancer site: breast. *Cancer J* 2012;18:310–319.
8. Guillem JG, Wood WC, Moley JF, et al. ASCO/SSO review of current role of risk-reducing surgery in common hereditary cancer syndromes. *J Clin Oncol* 2006; 24:4642–4660.
9. Saslow D, Boetes C, Burke W, et al. American Cancer Society guidelines for breast screening with MRI as an adjunct to mammography. *CA Cancer J Clin* 2007;57:75–89.
10. Domchek SM, Friebel TM, Singer CF, et al. Association of risk-reducing surgery in BRCA1 or BRCA2 mutation carriers with cancer risk and mortality. *JAMA* 2010;304:967–975.
11. US Equal Employment Opportunity Commission. Genetic information discrimination. http://www.eeoc.gov/laws/types/genetic.cfm. Accessed January 2, 2014.
12. Society of Surgical Oncology. Position statement on prophylactic mastectomy. http://www.surgonc.org/practice-policy/practice-management/consensus-statements/position-statement-on-prophylactic-mastectomy. Accessed February 1, 2014.
13. Hartmann LC, Schaid DJ, Woods JE, et al. Efficacy of bilateral prophylactic mastectomy in women with a family history of breast cancer. *N Engl J Med* 1999;340:77–84.
14. Eldor L, Spiegel A. Breast reconstruction after bilateral prophylactic mastectomy in women at high risk for breast cancer. *Breast J* 2009;15:S81–S89.
15. Zakhireh J, Fowble B, Esserman LJ. Application of screening principles to the reconstructed breast. *J Clin Oncol* 2010;28:173–180.

16. Gabram SG, Dougherty T, Albain KS, et al. Assessing breast cancer risk and providing treatment recommendations: immediate impact of an educational session. *Breast J* 2009;15:S39–S45.
17. Nadauld LD, Ford JM. Molecular profiling of gastric cancer: toward personalized cancer medicine. *J Clin Oncol* 2013;31:838–839.
18. Bardram L, Hansen TV, Gerdes AM, et al. Prophylactic total gastrectomy in hereditary diffuse gastric cancer: identification of two novel CDH1 gene mutations-a clinical observational study. *Fam Cancer* 2014;13:231–242.
19. Norton JA, Ham CM, Van Dam J, et al. CDH1 truncating mutations in the E-cadherin gene: an indication for total gastrectomy to treat hereditary diffuse gastric cancer. *Ann Surg* 2007;245:873–879.
20. Lynch HT, Grady W, Suriano G, et al. Gastric cancer: new genetic developments. *J Surg Oncol* 2005;90:114–133, discussion 133.
21. Guilford P, Hopkins J, Harraway J, et al. E-cadherin germline mutations in familial gastric cancer. *Nature* 1998;392:402–405.
22. Kaurah P, MacMillan A, Boyd N, et al. Founder and recurrent CDH1 mutations in families with hereditary diffuse gastric cancer. *JAMA* 2007;297:2360–2372.
23. Benusiglio PR, Malka D, Rouleau E, et al. CDH1 germline mutations and the hereditary diffuse gastric and lobular breast cancer syndrome: a multicentre study. *J Med Genet* 2013;50:486–489.
24. Gaya DR, Stuart RC, Going JJ, et al. Hereditary diffuse gastric cancer associated with E-cadherin mutation: penetrance after all. *Eur J Gastroenterol Hepatol* 2008;20:1249–1251.
25. Lee KH, Hwang D, Kang KY, et al. Frequent promoter methylation of CDH1 in non-neoplastic mucosa of sporadic diffuse gastric cancer. *Anticancer Res* 2013;33:3765–3774.
26. Oliveira C, Sousa S, Pinheiro H, et al. Quantification of epigenetic and genetic 2nd hits in CDH1 during hereditary diffuse gastric cancer syndrome progression. *Gastroenterology* 2009;136:2137–2148.
27. Carneiro F, Huntsman DG, Smyrk TC, et al. Model of the early development of diffuse gastric cancer in E-cadherin mutation carriers and its implications for patient screening. *J Pathol* 2004;203:681–687.
28. Huntsman DG, Carneiro F, Lewis FR, et al. Early gastric cancer in young, asymptomatic carriers of germ-line E-cadherin mutations. *N Engl J Med* 2001; 344:1904–1909.
29. Suriano G, Yew S, Ferreira P, et al. Characterization of a recurrent germ line mutation of the E-cadherin gene: implications for genetic testing and clinical management. *Clin Cancer Res* 2005;11:5401–5409.

30. Rogers WM, Dobo E, Norton JA, et al. Risk-reducing total gastrectomy for germline mutations in E-cadherin (CDH1): pathologic findings with clinical implications. *Am J Surg Pathol* 2008;32:799–809.

31. Worster E, Liu X, Richardson S, et al. The impact of prophylactic total gastrectomy on health-related quality of life: a prospective cohort study. *Ann Surg* 2014;260:87–93.

32. Lim YC, di Pietro M, O'Donovan M, et al. Prospective cohort study assessing outcomes of patients from families fulfilling criteria for hereditary diffuse gastric cancer undergoing endoscopic surveillance. *Gastrointest Endosc* 2014;80:78–87.

33. Mavaddat N, Peock S, Frost D, et al. Cancer risks for BRCA1 and BRCA2 mutation carriers: results from prospective analysis of EMBRACE. *J Natl Cancer Inst* 2013;105:812–822.

34. Risch HA, McLaughlin JR, Cole DE, et al. Prevalence and penetrance of germline BRCA1 and BRCA2 mutations in a population series of 649 women with ovarian cancer. *Am J Hum Genet* 2001;68:700–710.

35. Struewing JP, Hartge P, Wacholder S, et al. The risk of cancer associated with specific mutations of BRCA1 and BRCA2 among Ashkenazi Jews. *N Engl J Med* 1997;336:1401–1408.

36. Finch AP, Lubinski J, Moller P, et al. Impact of oophorectomy on cancer incidence and mortality in women with a BRCA1 or BRCA2 mutation. *J Clin Oncol* 2014;32:1547–1553.

37. Walsh T, Casadei S, Lee MK, et al. Mutations in 12 genes for inherited ovarian, fallopian tube, and peritoneal carcinoma identified by massively parallel sequencing. *Proc Natl Acad Sci U S A* 2011;108:18032–18037.

38. Couch FJ, Wang X, McGuffog L, et al. Genome-wide association study in BRCA1 mutation carriers identifies novel loci associated with breast and ovarian cancer risk. *PLoS Genet* 2013;9:e1003212.

39. Schrader KA, Hurlburt J, Kalloger SE, et al. Germline BRCA1 and BRCA2 mutations in ovarian cancer: utility of a histology-based referral strategy. *Obstet Gynecol* 2012;120:235–240.

40. Kauff ND, Satagopan JM, Robson ME, et al. Risk-reducing salpingo-oophorectomy in women with a BRCA1 or BRCA2 mutation. *N Engl J Med* 2002;346:1609–1615.

41. Rebbeck TR, Lynch HT, Neuhausen SL, et al. Prophylactic oophorectomy in carriers of BRCA1 or BRCA2 mutations. *N Engl J Med* 2002;346:1616–1622.

42. Kauff ND, Domchek SM, Friebel TM, et al. Risk-reducing salpingo-oophorectomy for the prevention of BRCA1- and BRCA2-associated breast and gynecologic cancer: a multicenter, prospective study. *J Clin Oncol* 2008; 26:1331–1337.

43. Folkins AK, Jarboe EA, Roh MH, et al. Precursors to pelvic serous carcinoma and their clinical implications. *Gynecol Oncol* 2009;113:391–396.

44. Wethington SL, Park KJ, Soslow RA, et al. Clinical outcome of isolated serous tubal intraepithelial carcinomas (STIC). *Int J Gynecol Cancer* 2013; 23:1603–1611.

45. Bonadona V, Bonaiti B, Olschwang S, et al. Cancer risks associated with germline mutations in MLH1, MSH2, and MSH6 genes in Lynch syndrome. *JAMA* 2011;305:2304–2310.

46. Leenen CH, van Lier MG, van Doorn HC, et al. Prospective evaluation of molecular screening for Lynch syndrome in patients with endometrial cancer ≤70 years. *Gynecol Oncol* 2012;125:414–420.

47. Resnick K, Straughn JM Jr, Backes F, et al. Lynch syndrome screening strategies among newly diagnosed endometrial cancer patients. *Obstet Gynecol* 2009;114:530–536.

48. Watson P, Vasen HF, Mecklin JP, et al. The risk of endometrial cancer in hereditary nonpolyposis colorectal cancer. *Am J Med* 1994;96:516–520.

49. Koornstra JJ, Mourits MJ, Sijmons RH, et al. Management of extracolonic tumours in patients with Lynch syndrome. *Lancet Oncol* 2009;10:400–408.

50. Dove-Edwin I, Boks D, Goff S, et al. The outcome of endometrial carcinoma surveillance by ultrasound scan in women at risk of hereditary nonpolyposis colorectal carcinoma and familial colorectal carcinoma. *Cancer* 2002;94:1708–1712.

51. Schmeler KM, Lynch HT, Chen LM, et al. Prophylactic surgery to reduce the risk of gynecologic cancers in the Lynch syndrome. *N Engl J Med* 2006;354: 261–269.

52. Yang KY, Caughey AB, Little SE, et al. A cost-effectiveness analysis of prophylactic surgery versus gynecologic surveillance for women from hereditary nonpolyposis colorectal cancer (HNPCC) Families. *Fam Cancer* 2011;10:535–543.

53. Pistorius S, Kruger S, Hohl R, et al. Occult endometrial cancer and decision making for prophylactic hysterectomy in hereditary nonpolyposis colorectal cancer patients. *Gynecol Oncol* 2006;102:189–194.

54. Traugott AL, Moley JF. Multiple endocrine neoplasia type 2: clinical manifestations and management. *Cancer Treat Res* 2009;153:321–337.

55. American Thyroid Association Guidelines Task Force, Kloos RT, Eng C, et al. Medullary thyroid cancer: management guidelines of the American Thyroid Association. *Thyroid* 2009;19:565–612.

56. Wells SA Jr, Pacini F, Robinson BG, et al. Multiple endocrine neoplasia type 2 and familial medullary thyroid carcinoma: an update. *J Clin Endocrinol Metab* 2013;98:3149–3164.

57. Eng C, Clayton D, Schuffenecker I, et al. The relationship between specific RET proto-oncogene mutations and disease phenotype in multiple endocrine neoplasia type 2. International RET mutation consortium analysis. *JAMA* 1996;276:1575–1579.

58. Howe JR, Norton JA, Wells SA Jr. Prevalence of pheochromocytoma and hyperparathyroidism in multiple endocrine neoplasia type 2A: results of long-term follow-up. *Surgery* 1993;114:1070–1077.

59. Machens A, Niccoli-Sire P, Hoegel J, et al. Early malignant progression of hereditary medullary thyroid cancer. *N Engl J Med* 2003;349:1517–1525.

60. Gagel RF, Levy ML, Donovan DT, et al. Multiple endocrine neoplasia type 2A associated with cutaneous lichen amyloidosis. *Ann Intern Med* 1989; 111:802–806.

61. Santoro M, Carlomagno F, Romano A, et al. Activation of RET as a dominant transforming gene by germline mutations of MEN2A and MEN2B. *Science* 1995;267:381–383.

62. Mulligan LM, Ponder BA. Genetic basis of endocrine disease: multiple endocrine neoplasia type 2. *J Clin Endocrinol Metab* 1995;80:1989–1995.

63. Mulligan L, Kwok J, Healy C. Germ-line mutations of the RET protoon-cogene in multiple endocrine neoplasia type 2A (MEN 2A). *Nature* 1993; 363:458–460.

64. Donis-Keller H, Dou S, Chi D, et al. Mutations in the RET proto-oncogene are associated with MEN 2A and FMTC. *Hum Mol Genet* 1993;2:851–856.

65. Traugott AL, Moley JF. The RET Protooncogene. *Cancer Treat Res* 2010; 153:303–319.

66. Quayle FJ, Benveniste R, DeBenedetti MK, et al. Hereditary medullary thyroid carcinoma in patients greater than 50 years old. *Surgery* 2004;136:1116–1121.

67. Lips CJ, Landsvater RM, Hoppener JW, et al. Clinical screening as compared with DNA analysis in families with multiple endocrine neoplasia type 2A. *N Engl J Med* 1994;331:828–835.

68. Niccoli-Sire P, Murat A, Baudin E, et al. Early or prophylactic thyroidectomy in MEN 2/FMTC gene carriers: results in 71 thyroidectomized patients. The French Calcitonin Tumours Study Group (GETC). *Eur J Endocrinol* 1999;141:468–474.

69. Rodriguez GJ, Balsalobre MD, Pomares F, et al. Prophylactic thyroidectomy in MEN 2A syndrome: experience in a single center. *J Am Coll Surg* 2002;195: 159–166.

70. Skinner MA, Moley JA, Dilley WG, et al. Prophylactic thyroidectomy in multiple endocrine neoplasia type 2A. *N Engl J Med* 2005;353:1105–1113.

71. Brandi ML, Gagel RF, Angeli A, et al. Guidelines for diagnosis and therapy of MEN type 1 and type 2. *J Clin Endocrinol Metab* 2001;86:5658–5671.

72. Elisei R, Romei C, Renzini G, et al. The timing of total thyroidectomy in RET gene mutation carriers could be personalized and safely planned on the basis of serum calcitonin: 18 years experience at one single center. *J Clin Endocrinol Metab* 2012;97:426–435.

73. Waguespack SG, Rich TA, Perrier ND, et al. Management of medullary thyroid carcinoma and MEN2 syndromes in childhood. *Nat Rev Endocrinol* 2011;7:596–607.

74. Moley JF. Medullary thyroid carcinoma: management of lymph node metastases. *J Natl Compr Canc Netw* 2010;8:549–556.

75. Machens A, Dralle H. Biomarker-based risk stratification for previously untreated medullary thyroid cancer. *J Clin Endocrinol Metab* 2010;95:2655–2663.

76. Solorzano CC, Evans DB. Same-day ultrasound guidance in reoperations for locally recurrent papillary thyroid cancer. *Surgery* 2007;142:973–975.

77. Patel SG, Ahnen DJ. Familial colon cancer syndromes: an update of a rapidly evolving field. *Curr Gastroenterol Rep* 2012;14:428–438.

78. Aretz S, Uhlhaas S, Goergens H, et al. MUTYH-associated polyposis: 70 of 71 patients with biallelic mutations present with an attenuated or atypical phenotype. *Int J Cancer* 2006;119:807–814.

79. Russell AM, Zhang J, Luz J, et al. Prevalence of MYH germline mutations in Swiss APC mutation-negative polyposis patients. *Int J Cancer* 2006; 118:1937–1940.

80. Jasperson KW. Genetic testing by cancer site: colon (polyposis syndromes). *Cancer J* 2012;18:328–333.

81. Hampel H, Frankel WL, Martin E, et al. Screening for the Lynch syndrome (hereditary nonpolyposis colorectal cancer). *N Engl J Med* 2005;352: 1851–1860.

82. Lynch HT, Lynch PM, Lanspa SJ, et al. Review of the Lynch syndrome: history, molecular genetics, screening, differential diagnosis, and medicolegal ramifications. *Clin Genet* 2009;76:1–18.

83. Vasen HF, Blanco I, Aktan-Collan K, et al. Revised guidelines for the clinical management of Lynch syndrome (HNPCC): recommendations by a group of European experts. *Gut* 2013;62:812–823.

84. Niessen RC, Hofstra RM, Westers H, et al. Germline hypermethylation of MLH1 and EPCAM deletions are a frequent cause of Lynch syndrome. *Genes Chromosomes Cancer* 2009;48:737–744.

85. Kuiper RP, Vissers LE, Venkatachalam R, et al. Recurrence and variability of germline EPCAM deletions in Lynch syndrome. *Hum Mutat* 2011;32: 407–414.

86. Rumilla K, Schowalter KV, Lindor NM, et al. Frequency of deletions of EPCAM (TACSTD1) in MSH2-associated Lynch syndrome cases. *J Mol Diagn* 2011;13:93–99.

87. Jasperson KW, Tuohy TM, Neklason DW, et al. Hereditary and familial colon cancer. *Gastroenterology* 2010;138:2044–2058.

88. Steinhagen E, Markowitz AJ, Guillem JG. How to manage a patient with multiple adenomatous polyps. *Surg Oncol Clin N Am* 2010;19:711–723.

89. National Comprehensive Cancer Network. NCCN *Clinical Practice Guidelines in Oncology: Colorectal Cancer Screening*. http://www.nccn.org/professionals /physician_gls/pdf/colorectal_screening.pdf. Accessed February 19, 2014.

90. Vasen HF, Moslein G, Alonso A, et al. Guidelines for the clinical management of familial adenomatous polyposis (FAP). *Gut* 2008;57:704–713.

91. Church J. Familial adenomatous polyposis. *Surg Oncol Clin N Am* 2009; 18:585–598.

92. Nieuwenhuis MH, Bulow S, Bjork J, et al. Genotype predicting phenotype in familial adenomatous polyposis: a practical application to the choice of surgery. *Dis Colon Rectum* 2009;52:1259–1263.

93. Sinha A, Tekkis PP, Rashid S, et al. Risk factors for secondary proctectomy in patients with familial adenomatous polyposis. *Br J Surg* 2010;97:1710–1715.

94. Koskenvuo L, Renkonen-Sinisalo L, Jarvinen HJ, et al. Risk of cancer and secondary proctectomy after colectomy and ileorectal anastomosis in familial adenomatous polyposis. *Int J Colorectal Dis* 2014;29:225–230.

95. Remzi FH, Church JM, Bast J, et al. Mucosectomy vs. stapled ileal pouch-anal anastomosis in patients with familial adenomatous polyposis: functional outcome and neoplasia control. *Dis Colon Rectum* 2001;44:1590–1596.

96. Friederich P, de Jong AE, Mathus-Vliegen LM, et al. Risk of developing adenomas and carcinomas in the ileal pouch in patients with familial adenomatous polyposis. *Clin Gastroenterol Hepatol* 2008;6:1237–1242.

97. Aziz O, Athanasiou T, Fazio VW, et al. Meta-analysis of observational studies of ileorectal versus ileal pouch-anal anastomosis for familial adenomatous polyposis. *Br J Surg* 2006;93:407–417.

98. Fazio VW, Kiran RP, Remzi FH, et al. Ileal pouch anal anastomosis: analysis of outcome and quality of life in 3707 patients. *Ann Surg* 2013;257:679–685.

99. Rajaratnam SG, Eglinton TW, Hider P, et al. Impact of ileal pouch-anal anastomosis on female fertility: meta-analysis and systematic review. *Int J Colorectal Dis* 2011;26:1365–1374.

100. Bartels SA, D'Hoore A, Cuesta MA, et al. Significantly increased pregnancy rates after laparoscopic restorative proctocolectomy: a cross-sectional study. *Ann Surg* 2012;256:1045–1048.

101. Beyer-Berjot L, Maggiori L, Birnbaum D, et al. A total laparoscopic approach reduces the infertility rate after ileal pouch-anal anastomosis: a 2-center study. *Ann Surg* 2013;258:275–282.

102. Steinhagen E, Guillem JG, Chang G, et al. The prevalence of thyroid cancer and benign thyroid disease in patients with familial adenomatous polyposis may be higher than previously recognized. *Clin Colorectal Cancer* 2012;11:304–308.

103. Steinhagen E, Hui VW, Levy RA, et al. Results of a prospective thyroid ultrasound screening program in adenomatous polyposis patients. *Am J Surg* [ePub ahead of print].

104. Jarrar AM, Milas M, Mitchell J, et al. Screening for thyroid cancer in patients with familial adenomatous polyposis. *Ann Surg* 2011;253:515–521.

105. Giardiello FM, Burt RW, Jarvinen H, et al. Familial adenomatous polyposis. In: Bosman FT, Carneiro F, Hruban RH, et al, eds. *Classification of Tumours of the Digestive System*. Lyon: IARC Press; 2010:147–151.

106. Nieuwenhuis MH, Lefevre JH, Bulow S, et al. Family history, surgery, and APC mutation are risk factors for desmoid tumors in familial adenomatous polyposis: an international cohort study. *Dis Colon Rectum* 2011;54:1229–1234.

107. Quintini C, Ward G, Shatnawei A, et al. Mortality of intra-abdominal desmoid tumors in patients with familial adenomatous polyposis: a single center review of 154 patients. *Ann Surg* 2012;255:511–516.

108. Sinha A, Gibbons DC, Phillips RK, et al. Surgical prophylaxis in familial adenomatous polyposis: do pre-existing desmoids outside the abdominal cavity matter? *Fam Cancer* 2010;9:407–411.

109. Schiessling S, Kihm M, Ganschow P, et al. Desmoid tumour biology in patients with familial adenomatous polyposis coli. *Br J Surg* 2013;100:694–703.

110. von Roon AC, Tekkis PP, Lovegrove RE, et al. Comparison of outcomes of ileal pouch-anal anastomosis for familial adenomatous polyposis with and without previous ileorectal anastomosis. *Br J Surg* 2008;95:494–498.

111. Nieuwenhuis MH, Vogt S, Jones N, et al. Evidence for accelerated colorectal adenoma—carcinoma progression in MUTYH-associated polyposis? *Gut* 2012;61:734–738.

112. Palomaki GE, McClain MR, Melillo S, et al. EGAPP supplementary evidence review: DNA testing strategies aimed at reducing morbidity and mortality from Lynch syndrome. *Genet Med* 2009;11:42–65.

113. Umar A, Boland CR, Terdiman JP, et al. Revised Bethesda Guidelines for hereditary nonpolyposis colorectal cancer (Lynch syndrome) and microsatellite instability. *J Natl Cancer Inst* 2004;96:261–268.

114. Vasen HF, Watson P, Mecklin JP, et al. New clinical criteria for hereditary nonpolyposis colorectal cancer (HNPCC, Lynch syndrome) proposed by the International Collaborative group on HNPCC. *Gastroenterology* 1999;116:1453–1456.

115. Barnetson RA, Tenesa A, Farrington SM, et al. Identification and survival of carriers of mutations in DNA mismatch-repair genes in colon cancer. *N Engl J Med* 2006;354:2751–2763.

116. Lee-Kong SA, Markowitz AJ, Glogowski E, et al. Prospective immunohistochemical analysis of primary colorectal cancers for loss of mismatch repair protein expression. *Clin Colorectal Cancer* 2010;9:255–259.

117. Steinhagen E, Shia J, Markowitz AJ, et al. Systematic immunohistochemistry screening for Lynch syndrome in early age-of-onset colorectal cancer patients undergoing surgical resection. *J Am Coll Surg* 2012;214:61–67.

118. Heald B, Plesec T, Liu X, et al. Implementation of universal microsatellite instability and immunohistochemistry screening for diagnosing lynch syndrome in a large academic medical center. *J Clin Oncol* 2013;31:1336–1340.

119. Beamer LC, Grant ML, Espenschied CR, et al. Reflex immunohistochemistry and microsatellite instability testing of colorectal tumors for Lynch syndrome among US cancer programs and follow-up of abnormal results. *J Clin Oncol* 2012;30:1058–1063.

120. Mvundura M, Grosse SD, Hampel H, et al. The cost-effectiveness of genetic testing strategies for Lynch syndrome among newly diagnosed patients with colorectal cancer. *Genet Med* 2010;12:93–104.

121. Chen S, Wang W, Lee S, et al. Prediction of germline mutations and cancer risk in the Lynch syndrome. *JAMA* 2006;296:1479–1487.

122. Kastrinos F, Steyerberg EW, Mercado R, et al. The PREMM(1,2,6) model predicts risk of MLH1, MSH2, and MSH6 germline mutations based on cancer history. *Gastroenterology* 2011;140:73–81.

123. Green RC, Parfrey PS, Woods MO, et al. Prediction of Lynch syndrome in consecutive patients with colorectal cancer. *J Natl Cancer Inst* 2009;101:331–340.

124. Khan O, Blanco A, Conrad P, et al. Performance of Lynch syndrome predictive models in a multi-center US referral population. *Am J Gastroenterol* 2011;106:1822–1827, quiz 1828.

125. Tresallet C, Brouquet A, Julie C, et al. Evaluation of predictive models in daily practice for the identification of patients with Lynch syndrome. *Int J Cancer* 2012;130:1367–1377.

126. Kalady MF, McGannon E, Vogel JD, et al. Risk of colorectal adenoma and carcinoma after colectomy for colorectal cancer in patients meeting Amsterdam criteria. *Ann Surg* 2010;252:507–511, discussion 511–513.

127. Parry S, Win AK, Parry B, et al. Metachronous colorectal cancer risk for mismatch repair gene mutation carriers: the advantage of more extensive colon surgery. *Gut* 2011;60:950–957.

128. Kalady MF, Lipman J, McGannon E, et al. Risk of colonic neoplasia after proctectomy for rectal cancer in hereditary nonpolyposis colorectal cancer. *Ann Surg* 2012;255:1121–1125.

129. Cirillo L, Urso ED, Parrinello G, et al. High risk of rectal cancer and of metachronous colorectal cancer in probands of families fulfilling the Amsterdam criteria. *Ann Surg* 2013;257:900–904.

130. Stupart DA, Goldberg PA, Baigrie RJ, et al. Surgery for colonic cancer in HNPCC: total vs segmental colectomy. *Colorectal Dis* 2011;13:1395–1399.

131. Maeda T, Cannom RR, Beart RW Jr, et al. Decision model of segmental compared with total abdominal colectomy for colon cancer in hereditary nonpolyposis colorectal cancer. *J Clin Oncol* 2010;28:1175–1180.

132. Guillem JG, Glogowski E, Moore HG, et al. Single-amplicon MSH2 A636P mutation testing in Ashkenazi Jewish patients with colorectal cancer: role in presurgical management. *Ann Surg* 2007;245:560–565.

133. Barrow P, Khan M, Lalloo F, et al. Systematic review of the impact of registration and screening on colorectal cancer incidence and mortality in familial adenomatous polyposis and Lynch syndrome. *Br J Surg* 2013;100:1719–1731.

134. Vasen HF, Abdirahman M, Brohet R, et al. One to 2-year surveillance intervals reduce risk of colorectal cancer in families with Lynch syndrome. *Gastroenterology* 2010;138:2300–2306.

135. Stuckless S, Green JS, Morgenstern M, et al. Impact of colonoscopic screening in male and female Lynch syndrome carriers with an MSH2 mutation. *Clin Genet* 2012;82:439–445.

136. Engel C, Rahner N, Schulmann K, et al. Efficacy of annual colonoscopic surveillance in individuals with hereditary nonpolyposis colorectal cancer. *Clin Gastroenterol Hepatol* 2010;8:174–182.

137. Syngal S, Weeks JC, Schrag D, et al. Benefits of colonoscopic surveillance and prophylactic colectomy in patients with hereditary nonpolyposis colorectal cancer mutations. *Ann Intern Med* 1998;129:787–796.

138. Giardiello FM, Allen JI, Axilbund JE, et al. Guidelines on genetic evaluation and management of Lynch syndrome: a consensus statement by the US Multi-Society Task Force on Colorectal Cancer. *Dis Colon Rectum* 2014;57(8):1025–1048.

CANCER PREVENTION AND SCREENING

33 Cancer Risk–Reducing Agents

Dean E. Brenner, Scott M. Lippman, and Susan T. Mayne

WHY CANCER PREVENTION AS A CLINICAL ONCOLOGY DISCIPLINE

Until recently, clinical oncology has been defined as a medical specialty that attempts to intervene in order to slow or reverse the final stage of the cancer process—the clonally derived, genomically damaged, invasive cell mass. Cancer is a long process, a stepwise carcinogenic progression that encompasses critical molecular events that culminate in the loss of key cellular control homeostatic functions (e.g., control of proliferation, apoptosis, invasion, angiogenesis).[1] These events occur prior to and during the morphologic changes that have historically defined neoplasia. Morphologic changes, such as subtle increases in cellular proliferation that progress to early and late precancerous lesions containing dysplastic cells, characterize the carcinogenesis process (Fig. 33.1).[1–3] Opportunities for intervention in this process can include diverse, nonpharmacologic approaches (e.g., obesity management via diet/lifestyle interventions) or pharmacologic interventions (e.g., drugs or nutrients/nonnutrient substances used as drugs) aimed at delaying or reversing the carcinogenesis process prior to or following the appearance of early morphologic changes. Cancer screening and early detection strategies (e.g., surveillance endoscopy, fecal occult blood testing, mammography) identify not only those individuals with early stage, curable malignant transformations, but also those individuals with noninvasive neoplasias who are at risk for progression to transformed invasive malignancies.

Recognizing that cancer is a continuum, oncologists are increasingly expected to be knowledgeable about a diverse array of cancer-related topics including lifestyle behaviors such as diet and exercise, risk assessment, screening, other preventive interventions, in addition to current treatments for advanced malignancy. The understanding, use, and management of interventions designed to delay or reverse the carcinogenesis process have become integral components of the this role.[4]

DEFINING CANCER RISK–REDUCING AGENTS (CHEMOPREVENTION)

Cancer risk reduction, commonly referred to as chemoprevention, is the use of a range of interventions from drugs to isolated dietary components to whole-diet modulation to block, reverse, or prevent the development of invasive cancer.[5,6] Human cancer risk reduction asserts that one can intervene at many steps in the carcinogenic process, which occurs over many years. This prolonged latency provides opportunities to intervene at many time points and at multiple events in the carcinogenic process. Successful deployment of cancer risk–reducing agent interventions requires evidence of reduced cancer-associated incidence and/or mortality.

The concept of field carcinogenesis was first described in the early 1950s as *field cancerization* in squamous cell carcinomas of the head and neck, and subsequently ascribed to many epithelial sites. The field carcinogenesis concept is that patients have a wide surface area of precancerous or cancerous tissue change that can be detected at the gross (oral premalignant lesions, polyps), microscopic (metaplasia, dysplasia), and/or molecular (gene loss or amplification) levels. Recent molecular studies detecting profound genetic alterations in histologically normal tissue from high-risk individuals have provided strong support for the field carcinogenesis concept. The implication of the field effect is that multifocal, genetically distinct, and clonally related premalignant lesions can progress over a broad tissue region.[1] The essence of cancer risk reduction, then, is intervention within the multistep carcinogenic process and throughout a wide field.

IDENTIFYING POTENTIAL CANCER RISK–REDUCING AGENTS

Cancer risk–reducing agent identification results from the synthesis of data from population, basic, translational, and clinical sciences. Findings from all of these disciplines are combined to contribute to the identification of agents with the potential to delay or reverse the carcinogenesis process (see Fig. 33.1).

The Hanahan and Weinberg hallmarks of malignant transformation—self-sufficiency in growth signals, insensitivity to growth-inhibitory signals, evasion of apoptosis, limitless replication potential, sustained angiogenesis, and tissue invasion and metastasis[7]—reflect the loss of cellular signaling control. The molecular damage that results in transformation is triggered by a large array of genetic and environmental stressors such as chronic inflammation, oxidation, inherited genetic mutations, and exogenous environmental exposures. Many such signaling intermediates have common functions in multiple organ sites (see Fig. 33.1). The complexity and overlap of signal transduction pathways suggests that single molecular therapeutic/preventive targets may have limited effectiveness. Interventions aimed at preventing the occurrence of or overcoming the effects of molecular defects in multiple pathways or targets may be required to arrest or reverse carcinogenesis. Using the Hanahan and Weinberg hallmarks, examples of possible targets are shown in Table 33.1.

PRECLINICAL DEVELOPMENT OF CANCER RISK–REDUCING AGENTS

Similar to the development of therapeutic interventions, the assessment of efficacy and toxicity of single chemically synthesized entities, agents designed *in silico*, botanicals, nutrients/nonnutrient substances used as drugs for cancer risk–reducing agent efficacy proceeds through a translational paradigm that identifies efficacy in cell culture models, in live animal models, and in humans. Preclinical models that simulate the carcinogenesis process in target epithelia identify molecular biomarkers for modulation by interventions. These models can be used to identify potential toxicity of interventions and to assess the effect of interventions on the development and progression of preneoplasia/neoplasia.[8]

The U.S. National Cancer Institute's (NCI) PREVENT Cancer Preclinical Drug Development Program is a prime example of a

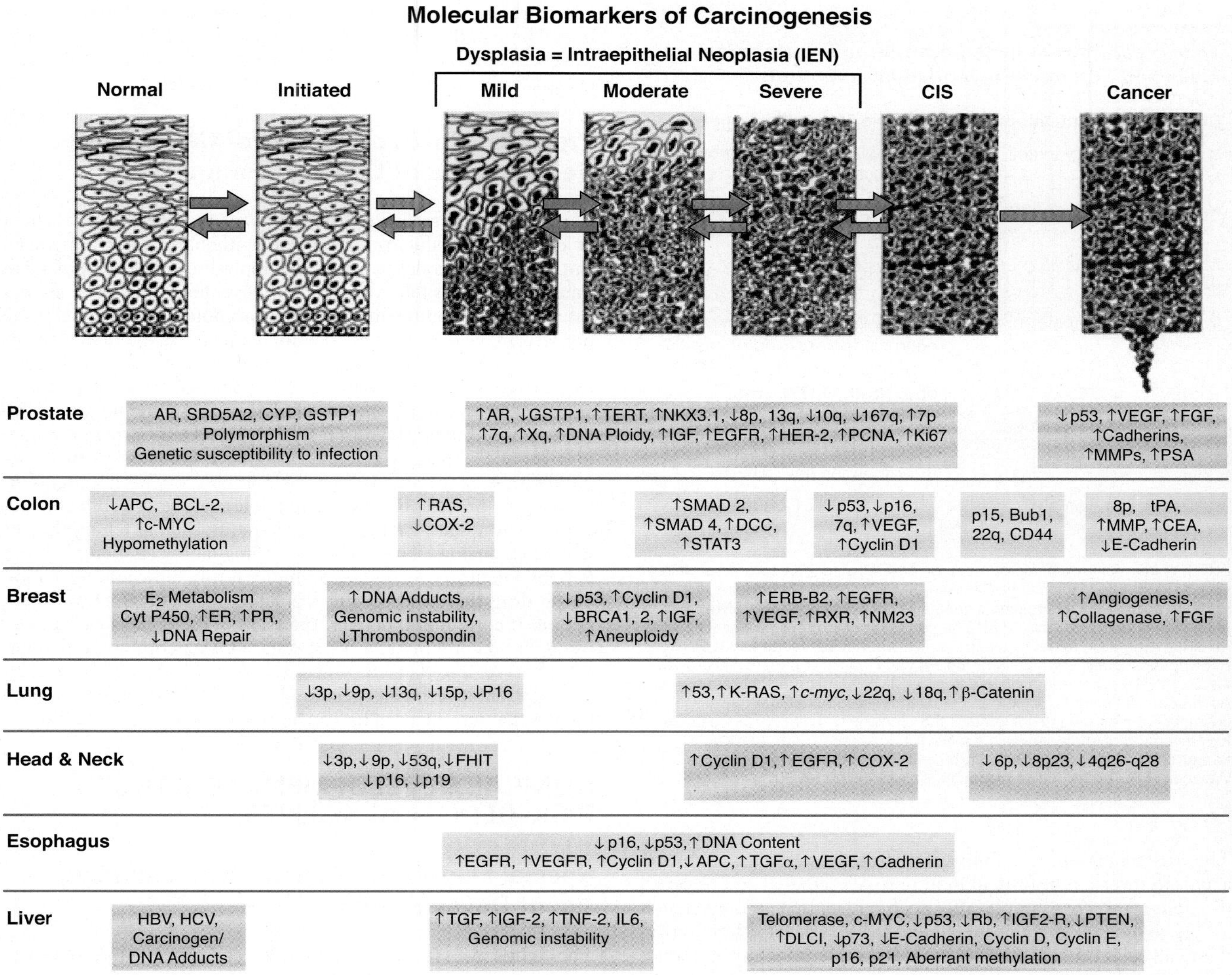

Molecular Biomarkers of Carcinogenesis

Dysplasia = Intraepithelial Neoplasia (IEN)

Organ	Normal	Initiated	Mild	Moderate	Severe	CIS	Cancer
Prostate	AR, SRD5A2, CYP, GSTP1 Polymorphism Genetic susceptibility to infection		↑AR, ↓GSTP1, ↑TERT, ↑NKX3.1, ↓8p, 13q, ↓10q, ↓167q, ↑7p ↑7q, ↑Xq, ↑DNA Ploidy, ↑IGF, ↑EGFR, ↑HER-2, ↑PCNA, ↑Ki67				↓p53, ↑VEGF, ↑FGF, ↑Cadherins, ↑MMPs, ↑PSA
Colon	↓APC, BCL-2, ↑c-MYC Hypomethylation	↑RAS, ↓COX-2		↑SMAD 2, ↑SMAD 4, ↑DCC, ↑STAT3	↓p53, ↓p16, 7q, ↑VEGF, ↑Cyclin D1	p15, Bub1, 22q, CD44	8p, tPA, ↑MMP, ↑CEA, ↓E-Cadherin
Breast	E₂ Metabolism Cyt P450, ↑ER, ↑PR, ↓DNA Repair	↑DNA Adducts, Genomic instability, ↓Thrombospondin	↓p53, ↑Cyclin D1, ↓BRCA1, 2, ↑IGF, ↑Aneuploidy		↑ERB-B2, ↑EGFR, ↑VEGF, ↑RXR, ↑NM23		↑Angiogenesis, ↑Collagenase, ↑FGF
Lung		↓3p, ↓9p, ↓13q, ↓15p, ↓P16		↑53, ↑K-RAS, ↑c-myc, ↓22q, ↓18q, ↑β-Catenin			
Head & Neck		↓3p, ↓9p, ↓53q, ↓FHIT ↓p16, ↓p19		↑Cyclin D1, ↑EGFR, ↑COX-2		↓6p, ↓8p23, ↓4q26-q28	
Esophagus			↓p16, ↓p53, ↑DNA Content ↑EGFR, ↑VEGFR, ↑Cyclin D1, ↓APC, ↑TGFα, ↑VEGF, ↑Cadherin				
Liver	HBV, HCV, Carcinogen/ DNA Adducts		↑TGF, ↑IGF-2, ↑TNF-2, IL6, Genomic instability		Telomerase, c-MYC, ↓p53, ↓Rb, ↑IGF2-R, ↓PTEN, ↑DLCI, ↓p73, ↓E-Cadherin, Cyclin D, Cyclin E, p16, p21, Aberrant methylation		

Figure 33.1 Genetic progression in major cancers. Carcinogenesis is driven by genetic progression. This progression is marked by the appearance of molecular biomarkers in distinctive patterns representing accumulating changes in gene expression and correlating with changes in histologic phenotype as cells move from normal through the early stages of clonal expansion to dysplasia and finally to early invasive, locally advanced, and metastatic cancer. The figure[257] shows candidate molecular biomarkers of genetic progression in seven target organs: the prostate,[300–302] the colon,[2] the breast,[303,304] the lung,[305–307] the head and neck,[308–311] the esophagus,[312,313] and the liver.[314] CIS, carcinoma in situ; AR, androgen receptor; CYP, cytochrome P-450; GSTP1, glutathione S transferase P1; TERT, telomerase reverse transcriptase; NKX3.1, NK 3 transcription factor related, locus 1 (prostate specific, androgren regulated); IGF, insulin-like growth factor; EGFR, epidermal growth factor receptor; HER-2, human epidermal growth factor receptor-2; PCNA, proliferating cell nuclear antigen; VEGF, vascular endothelial growth factor; FGF, fibroblast growth factor; MMP, matrix metalloproteinase; PSA, prostate-specific antigen; APC, adenomatous polyposis coli; BCL-2, B-cell lymphoma 2 gene, apoptosis control; c-MYC, v-myc avian myelocytomatosis viral oncogene homolog; COX-2, cyclooxygenase-2; SMAD, homolog of mothers against decapentaplegic + *C. Elegans* SMA protein; DCC, deleted in colon cancer gene; CEA, carcinoembryonic antigen; ER, estrogen receptor; PR, progesterone receptor; ERB-B2, Receptor tyrosine-protein kinase erbB-2, same as HER-2; RXR, retinoid X receptor; NM23, Nucleoside disphosphate kinase A; K-RAS, Kirsten rat sarcoma viral oncogene homolog; FHIT, fragile histidine triad protein; TGFα, tumor growth factor alpha; HBV, hepatitis B virus; HCV, hepatitis C virus; TNF-2, tumor necrosis factor 2; IL6, interleukin 6; PTEN, phosphatase and tensin homolog. (Figure and revised caption from Kelloff GJ, Lippman SM, Dannenberg AJ, et al. Progress in chemoprevention drug development: the promise of molecular biomarkers for prevention of intraepithelial neoplasia and cancer—a plan to move forward. *Clin Cancer Res* 2006;12:3661–3697, published with permission from the American Association for Cancer Research.)

CANCER PREVENTION AND SCREENING

rational strategy to select promising agents for clinical trials through a stepwise approach of preclinical in vitro testing followed by *in vivo* screening.[8–10] This system involves several phases: biochemical prescreening assays, in vitro efficacy models, in vivo short-term screening, animal efficacy testing, and preclinical toxicology testing.

Biochemical Prescreening Assays

Prescreening assays are a series of short-term, mechanistic assays developed to evaluate the ability of a test compound to modulate biochemical events presumed to be mechanistically linked to carcinogenesis.[8]

These in vitro assays are rapidly completed for potential cancer risk–reducing agents. Examples of such assays include carcinogen-DNA binding, prostaglandin synthesis inhibition, glutathione–S-transferase inhibition, and ornithine decarboxylase inhibition.

In Vitro Efficacy Models

In vitro assays test the cancer risk–reducing activity of a screened compound in four epithelial cell systems (primary rat tracheal epithelial cells, human lung tumor [A427] cells, mouse mammary organ cultures [MMOC], and human foreskin epithelial cells).

TABLE 33.1

Molecular Mechanisms Common to Transforming Cells and Potential Preventive Interventions

Characteristics of Neoplasia	Possible Molecular Targets
Self-sufficiency in cell growth	EGFR, platelet-derived growth factor, MAPK, PI3K
Insensitivity to antigrowth signals	SMADs, pRb, cyclin-dependent kinases, MYC
Limitless replicative potential	hTERT, pRb, p53
Evading apoptosis	Bcl-2, BAX, caspases, Fas, tumor necrosis factor receptor, insulin growth factor/PI3K/Akt, mTOR, p53, NF-κB, PTEN, RAS
Sustained angiogenesis	VEGF, basic fibroblast growth factor, integrins ($\alpha_v\beta_3$), thrombospondin-1, HIF-1α
Tissue invasion and metastases	MMPs, MAPK, E-cadherin

EGFR, epidermal growth factor receptor; MAPK, mitogen-activated protein kinase; PI3K, phosphoinositide 3-kinase; SMAD, drosophila protein, mothers against decapentaplegic gene and the *Elegans* protein SMA; pRb, phosphorylated Rb protein; hTERT, human telomerase reverse transcriptase; mTOR, mammalian target of rapamycin; NF-κB, nuclear factor kappa B; PTEN, phosphatase and tensin homolog; VEGF, vascular endothelial growth factor; HIF-1α, hypoxia-inducible factor-1α; MMP, Matrix metalloproteinases. Adapted from Kelloff GJ, Lippman SM, Dannenberg AJ, et al. Progress in chemoprevention drug development: the promise of molecular biomarkers for prevention of intraepithelial neoplasia and cancer—a plan to move forward. *Clin Cancer Res* 2006;12:3661–3697 and derived from Hanahan D, Weinberg RA. The hallmarks of cancer. *Cell* 2000;100:57–70.

The assays measure the ability of potential cancer risk–reducing agents to reverse transformation in normal epithelial cells exposed to carcinogens. For example, after treatment with a carcinogen such as 7,12-demethylbenz(a)anthracene, MMOCs develop lesions similar to alveolar nodules that are considered precancerous in mouse mammary glands in vivo.[11] Pretreatment of organ cultures before carcinogen exposure measures the effect of cancer risk–reducing agents in the initiation stage of carcinogenesis, whereas treatment

after carcinogen exposure measures activity during tumor promotion. Three of these assays (using rat tracheal epithelial, A427, and MMOC cells) have shown predictive values of 76% to 83% for cancer risk–reducing agent efficacy in in vivo models.[8]

Preclinical In Vivo Models for Cancer Risk–Reducing Agent Efficacy Testing

Animal models remain a crucial link in the efficacy assessment of cancer risk–reducing agents for epithelial cancer. Chemical carcinogenesis models provide the reproducible development of tumors in animals following the administration of a known chemical initiator or combination initiator/promoter and have been the primary in vivo screening tool for cancer risk–reducing agents (Table 33.2A).[12,13] Carcinogenesis models employing genetically engineered mice permit the interrogation of targeted pathways and the corresponding efficacy of cancer risk–reducing agents. Although useful for mechanistic studies, knockout or genetic mutational models create accelerated neoplastic progression that does not accurately recapitulate the more complex, stepwise, human carcinogenesis process. Recombinant alleles can be driven by the addition of drug-sensitive regulatory elements, such as tetracycline or tamoxifen analogs. The drug-sensitive regulatory elements achieve temporal control over a gene promoter through the administration of the drug that binds to the regulatory element. Such a system permits the inhibition or overexpression of the organ-specific gene using Cre recombinase, a site-specific DNA recombinase that targets DNA regions flanked by loxP sequences. Tables 33.2A and 2B list representative organ-specific chemical and transgenic mouse models that may be used for cancer risk–reducing agent testing.

CLINICAL DEVELOPMENT OF CANCER RISK–REDUCING AGENTS

Special Features of Cancer Risk–Reducing Agent Development

The clinical efficacy assessment of cancer risk–reducing agents employs phased testing (phase I to III) models used for development of drugs[14] but with crucial differences in study design and end points. Special features for the clinical development of

TABLE 33.2A

Chemical Carcinogenesis Models Used for Screening of Cancer Risk–Reducing Agents for Common Epithelial Neoplasms in Animals

Organ Site	Species	Carcinogen	End Point
Colon	Rat, mouse	Azoxymethane (AOM)	Aberrant crypts, adenomas, adenocarcinomas
Lung	Mouse	N—butyl-N-(4-hydroxylbutyl)nitrosamine (NNK); benzo[a]pyrene; cigarette smoke	Adenomas, adenocarcinomas
	Hamster	Methylnitrosourea (MNU)	Squamous cell carcinomas
	Mouse	N-nitroso-tris-chloroethylurea	Squamous cell carcinomas
Breast	Rat	Dimethylbenz[a]anthracene (DMBA); MNU	Adenocarcinomas, adenomas
Prostate	Rat	MNU + testosterone	Adenocarcinomas
Bladder	Rat, mouse	N-butyl-N-(4-hydroxybutyl)nitrosamine (OH-BBN)	Transitional cell carcinoma
Pancreas	Hamster	N-nitrobis-(2-oxopropyl)amine (BOP)	Ductal carcinomas
Head and neck	Rat	4-nitroquinoline-1-oxide (4-NQO)	Tongue squamous cell carcinomas
	Mouse	DMBA	Squamous cell carcinomas
Esophagus	Rat	Dimethylbenz[a]anthracene	Squamous cell carcinomas
	Rat	Esophagogastroduodenal anastomosis + iron	Adenocarcinomas

Adapted from Steele VE, Lubet RA. The use of animal models for cancer chemoprevention drug development. *Semin Oncol* 2010;37:327–338.

TABLE 33.2B			
Selected Transgenic Animal Models for Carcinogenesis Evaluation			
Organ Site	**Genes Targeted**	**End Point**	**References**
Colon	*Apc, Lrig1, gp130, Stat3, Smad3, Wnt-β-catenin, villin, TGFBR2, Kras, Ink4a*	Adenomas and adenocarcinomas	(258, 259)
Lung	*KrasG12D, KrasG12Vgeo, PTEN, Braf*V600E, *cRaf, Egfr* L858R±T790M, *PIK3CA*, EMLA4-ALK fusion *Rb. P53*	Adenomas and adenocarcinomas Small cell	(260)
Breast	Mouse mammary tumor virus long terminal repeat promoter (MMTV) driven *BRCA1, p53, ERα,* aromatase, *TGFα, Her2/neu, wnt*, PELP-1, AIB-1	DCIS, adenocarcinomas	(261)
Prostate	Probasin promotor driving SV40 large T antigen (*TRAMP/LADY*), *c-Myc, TMPRSS-ERG, Akt, Wnt-β-catenin*, androgen receptor *Nkx3.1, FGFR1, TGF, PTEN*	Prostate intraepithelial neoplasia, neuroendocrine tumors (TRAMP); adenocarcinomas (*c-Myc, TMPRESS-ERG, Akt, Wnt*, androgen receptor) Adenocarcinomas	(262)
Pancreas	*KrasG12D* alone, *LSL-Kras, PDX-1, R26Notch, Tif1γ* Combined *PDX-1, LSL-Kras, LSL-Trp53*; combined *PDX-1, Brca2, LSL-Kras Trp53*; *KrasG12D* on *Mist1* locus; *PDX-1, KrasG12D+ Ink4a/Arf* or *Smad4*; *Ptf1a, KrasG12D, TGFBR2*	Pancreatic intraepithelial neoplasia Pancreatic adenocarcinoma	(263)

Note: Most models are mouse models. Such models will permit efficacy testing of specific pathway targets using single agent interventions, combinations, or multimechanism-based natural products.

cancer risk–reducing agents create the following challenges to be overcome: (1) the need for large therapeutic index (doses associated with potential toxicity of an intervention need to substantially exceed doses aimed at delaying or reversing transformation) for use in individuals who are asymptomatic yet may benefit from an extended (years) treatment course; (2) the long latency to malignant transformation (an assessment of effectiveness based on the reduction in cancer incidence requires studies lasting for years and involving thousands of participants); (3) adherence (once-daily dosing regimens using interventions that have sufficiently long half-lives may minimize the impact of a missed dose yet maintain the biologic impact on the physiologic target; minimal toxicity and strong psychological commitment to preventive goals also enhance adherence[15]); and (4) complex risk assessment for cancer (individuals with highly penetrant but infrequent, germ-line genetic susceptibility to breast and colon cancers[16,17] are excellent candidates for cancer risk–reducing agents and are likely to accept some toxicity for reduced cancer risk). For individuals at more modestly increased risk (e.g., long-term, current smokers; persons with a family history of cancer; women with mammographically dense breasts), quantitative risk assessment algorithms may be useful in the future to identify optimal cancer risk–reducing agents. The refinement of cancer risk calculators for breast,[18] colon,[19] and prostate cancer[20] promises to appropriately select high-risk individuals for cancer risk–reducing agents such that anticipated benefits exceed potential risks.

Biomarkers as Cancer Risk–Reducing Agent Targets and Efficacy End Points

A biomarker is a characteristic that is measured and evaluated as an indicator of normal biologic processes, pathogenic processes, or pharmacologic responses to therapeutic interventions.[21] A surrogate end point for cancer prevention assumes that a measured biologic feature will predict the presence or future development of a cancer outcome.[22] Biomarkers enable a reduction in the size and duration of an intervention trial by replacing a rare or distal end point with a more frequent, proximate end point.[23] Intraepithelial

neoplasia has served and continues to serve as a biomarker for invasive malignancy (Table 33.3). Although many advocate the use of intraepithelial neoplasia-based biomarkers as regulatory surrogate end points, others caution that intraepithelial neoplasias may not serve as sufficiently robust surrogate biomarkers for cancer incidence or mortality.[24]

In order to be useful as end points for cancer risk–reducing agent efficacy testing as regulatory end points, any biomarker must have statistical accuracy, precision, and effectiveness of results[24] that demonstrate prediction of a *hard* disease end point—cancer incidence or mortality. An independent validation data set must address defined standards of validation that minimize bias in the study design and the populations studied.[25] The biomarker must be generalizable to the specific clinical or screening population (Table 33.4).

Phases of Cancer Risk–Reducing Agent Development

Phase I cancer risk–reducing agent trials define an optimal cancer risk–reducing agent dose. An optimal cancer risk–reducing agent dose is one that is usually nontoxic, scheduled once daily, and modulates a tissue, cellular, or serum biomarker of drug activity (e.g., the dose of aspirin that inhibits prostaglandin production in a target tissue site). The definition of a maximum tolerated dose is not an essential end point of a phase I cancer risk–reducing agent trial. Higher, yet nontoxic doses may lower cancer risk–reducing agent efficacy. For example, β-carotene at high doses has pro-oxidant activity and may enhance the carcinogenesis process, whereas at low doses, it is a potent antioxidant and differentiating agent.[26]

Phase II cancer risk–reducing agent trials begin to define cancer risk–reduction efficacy. These short-term (6 months to 1 year) treatment periods gather evidence of risk reduction by assessing drug effects on tissue, cellular, or blood surrogate markers of carcinogenesis. Phase IIa trials are nonrandomized, biomarker modulation trials. Phase IIb trials are randomized, placebo-controlled trials of several hundred subjects testing, for example, whether a risk-reducing agent reduces recurrence of a previously resected intraepithelial neoplastic lesion as the primary end point. Cellular dynamic

TABLE 33.3

Common Intraepithelial Neoplasias

Epithelium	Intraepithelial Neoplasia	References
Colon and rectum	Adenoma	(264)
Lower esophagus	Barrett esophagus	(265)
Upper esophagus	Squamous dysplasia	(266, 267)
Skin: Squamous/basal cell	Actinic keratosis	(268)
Skin: Pigmented	Dysplastic nevus	(269)
Cervix	Cervical intraepithelial neoplasia	(270)
Head and neck	Leukoplakia/oral epithelial dysplasia	(271)
Prostate	Prostate intraepithelial neoplasia (PIN), intraductal carcinoma of the prostate	(272)
Lung	Bronchial dysplasia	(273)
Pancreas	Pancreatic intraepithelial neoplasia	(274)

(e.g., proliferation, apoptotic index), biochemical, or molecular (e.g., p53, cyclin D) end points may be used as secondary end points. Preoperative or *window of opportunity trials* enroll subjects for brief study periods prior to obtaining tissue by a planned resection of an invasive neoplasm. Such designs permit the exploration of biomarker modulation in the invasive neoplasm and in contiguous epithelial fields proximal and distal to the invasive neoplasm.[27]

Phase III cancer risk–reducing agent trials define reduction in a hard cancer end point such as cancer incidence or mortality. Such trials, using large, higher risk populations in a randomized, double-blinded intervention, are designed to identify a standard of preventive care for a given risk population. For example, trials of tamoxifen for the reduction of breast cancer incidence,[28,29] finasteride for the reduction of prostate cancer incidence,[30] and β-carotene for the reduction of lung cancer incidence[31] serve as examples of well-conducted, definitive phase III cancer risk–reducing agent clinical trials.

Some investigators consider randomized, controlled clinical trials with an end point sufficient for regulatory review as phase III.

TABLE 33.4

Characteristics of Biomarkers for Use as End Points in Cancer Risk–Reducing Agent Efficacy Assessment

- Variability of expression between phases of the carcinogenesis process
- Detected early in the carcinogenesis process
- Genetic progression or protein pathway based
- Target of modulation by preventive interventions
- Changes in biomarker linked to reduction in incident cancer of epithelial target
- Changes in biomarker linked to clinical benefit
- Can be quantified directly or via closely related activity such as a downstream target or upstream kinase
- Measurable in an accessible biosample (preferably urine, serum, saliva, stool, or breath)
- High throughput, technically feasible, analytical procedure with strong quality assurance/quality control procedures
- Cost-effective

Using such a definition, a clinical trial with an end point of reduction in adenoma recurrence is considered a phase III trial. Other investigators define phase III cancer risk–reducing agent trials as randomized, controlled clinical trials with a cancer incidence or mortality end point. This controversy causes confusion in the literature. For the purpose of clarity in this textbook, the latter definition of phase III trial is used—a prospective, randomized, controlled clinical trial with a cancer incidence or mortality end point. Randomized, controlled clinical trials with a surrogate biomarker end point such as an intraepithelial neoplasia (e.g., adenoma) are defined as phase IIb cancer risk–reducing agent trials.

MICRONUTRIENTS

Definition

Micronutrients comprise a large, diverse group of molecules typically ingested as part of the diet that play roles in normal human biology. This group of compounds has been investigated extensively as cancer risk–reducing agents in purified forms (i.e., supplements), as components of multiagent cocktails, and occasionally, as components of food extracts/other mixtures. Although retinoids are not micronutrients per se, they are related to retinol (vitamin A) and share certain properties with carotenoids, which are diet derived and, therefore, included along with micronutrients.

Retinoids, Carotenoids, and Antioxidant Nutrients

Overview and Mechanisms

Retinoids are the natural derivatives and synthetic analogs of vitamin A.[32] Cancer risk–reduction intervention studies have evaluated the parent compound (retinol, typically given as retinyl acetate or palmitate), naturally occurring retinoids such as all-trans–retinoic acid (ATRA) and 13-cis-retinoic acid (13cRA), and also synthetic retinoids such as etretinate and fenretinide (4-hydroxy[phenyl]retinamide [4HPR]). These agents have been of interest for cancer risk reduction for decades. Mechanistically, retinoids have been shown to modulate cellular growth and differentiation, as well as apoptosis.[32] A large body of research indicates that retinoids have activity in the promotion and progression phases of carcinogenesis, including extensive evidence of efficacy in the setting of premalignant lesions, leading to their evaluation in human Phase III trials. Nuclear retinoic acid receptors mediate many of the retinoid-signaling effects; however, retinoids interact with other signaling pathways, such as estrogen signaling in breast cancer.[33]

Carotenoids are a group of naturally occurring plant pigments, only some of which are found in appreciable levels in the human diet and human tissues, including beta-carotene, alpha-carotene, lycopene, lutein, and β-cryptoxanthin.[34] Of these, the most widely studied carotenoids for cancer risk reduction are beta-carotene and lycopene. Beta-carotene has the highest pro–vitamin A activity of the carotenoids, but alpha-carotene and β-cryptoxanthin also possess pro–vitamin A activity. Other carotenoids, such as lycopene, do not possess vitamin A activity but are known to have potent antioxidant activity, particularly with regard to singlet oxygen quenching.[35] Furthermore, eccentric cleavage products of beta-carotene,[36] as well as other non-pro–vitamin A carotenoids such as lycopene (e.g., apocarotenals, apocarotenoic acids) appear to be biologically active and may also act via retinoid-signaling pathways.[37]

Because of the known antioxidant function of carotenoids, they are often studied for risk-reducing efficacy in combination with other antioxidant nutrients, especially vitamins E and C and selenium (sometimes as a cocktail, versus placebo). Thus, we will consider this group of nutrients first, followed by other micronutrients that are thought to act via different mechanisms and/or pathways.

Epidemiology

A large body of literature indicates that people who consume greater amounts of carotenoids from foods (primarily fruits and vegetables) and people with higher serum or plasma levels of various carotenoids have a lower risk for various cancers.[38] In particular, according to the systematic review of the literature conducted by the World Cancer Research Fund/American Institute for Cancer Research,[38] foods containing carotenoids are "probably" associated with lower risks of cancers of the mouth/pharynx/larynx and lung; foods containing beta-carotene are "probably" associated with lower risks of cancers of the esophagus; and foods containing lycopene are "probably" associated with lower risks of prostate cancer. Preformed retinol intake is inconsistently associated with risks of various cancers but that, in part, likely reflects confounding, because dietary sources of preformed retinol primarily include foods of animal origin (e.g., liver, eggs, milk). Vitamin C in the diet comes primarily from the consumption of fruits and vegetables; therefore, vitamin C and carotenoids often trend together in epidemiologic findings. Vitamin E, in contrast, is found in different foods, especially nuts, seeds, and vegetable oils; intake and blood concentrations are somewhat inconsistently associated with cancer risk.[39] Selenium, being a trace mineral, is difficult to measure in the diet, but higher selenium status has been associated with a lower risk of certain cancers, although the results are not entirely consistent.[39]

Preclinical In Vivo Models

In preclinical models, retinoids induce differentiation as well as arrest proliferation[33] of various cancers, making them attractive agents for cancer risk reduction.[40] The International Agency for Research on Cancer reviewed the preclinical research involving beta-carotene, concluding that there was "sufficient" evidence of cancer preventive activity, particularly involving mouse skin tumor models and the hamster buccal pouch model.[41] Notably, there was inconsistent evidence of efficacy in respiratory tract models. Lycopene has been evaluated in numerous cell culture systems and in a variety of models of prostate carcinogenesis, including chemically induced, orthotopic implantation, transgenic, and xenotransplantation, with mixed evidence of efficacy.[42] Evidence, primarily from cell culture studies, suggests that lycopene metabolites may be at least partially responsible for anticarcinogenic activity.[37]

Clinical Trials: Retinoids, Carotenoids, and Antioxidant Nutrients

Retinoids, carotenoids, and antioxidant nutrients have been evaluated in the setting of preneoplasia/neoplasia in many different organ sites, as will be discussed. Of the many clinical trials of retinoids and carotenoids/other antioxidant nutrients, key trials with cancer incidence/recurrence as primary outcomes are tabulated (see Tables 33.5 and 33.6) and reviewed.

Clinical Efficacy in the Upper Airway

Many trials of cancer risk–reducing agents have been done in the setting of squamous cell carcinomas of the head and neck, in large part because of the substantial clinical problem of relatively high rates of recurrences and second primary tumors in curatively treated cancer patients. Early work demonstrated that high-dose 13cRA (50 to 100 mg/m^2 per day) produced no significant differences in disease recurrence (local, regional, or distant) but significantly lowered the rate of second primary invasive neoplasms,[43] with the benefits persisting for at least 5 years.[44] Substantial retinoid toxicity, however, including skin dryness and peeling, cheilitis, conjunctivitis, and hypertriglyceridemia, was evident in a large proportion of patients. Subsequent trials thus used lower doses of retinoids (13cRA or a synthetic retinoid, etretinate), but failed to show efficacy in reducing second primary tumor formation (Table 33.5).[45,46]

Supplemental beta-carotene has also been studied as a single agent and in combination with other agents for the prevention of second primary cancers of the mouth and throat (Table 33.6). One trial of beta-carotene alone observed no harm or benefit[47]; another observed nonsignificantly fewer second head and neck cancers but more lung cancers[48]; and a third gave beta-carotene with α-tocopherol (400 IU per day).[49] In the third trial, beta-carotene was discontinued early due to adverse findings from lung cancer prevention trials (see the following); however, after a median follow-up of 6.5 years, all-cause mortality was increased, which the authors attributed to the supplemental α-tocopherol. As will be discussed later, adverse effects of antioxidant nutrients are not limited to head and neck cancer patients; potential mechanisms for adverse effects are discussed further.

Clinical Efficacy in the Lung (Lower Airway)

Reversal of Metaplasia or Dysplasia. Active smokers and recent quitters have multiple preinvasive metaplastic and dysplastic lesions in the pulmonary tree. Most of these lesions resolve upon smoking cessation, but some remain and progress to invasive neoplasms. Unfortunately, micronutrient or retinoid interventions have not demonstrated preventive efficacy in most rigorous trials in patients with early lesions. For example, a US trial randomized 755 asbestos workers to receive beta-carotene (50 mg per day) and retinol (25,000 IU every other day) versus placebo; sputum atypia was not reduced after 5 years.[50] As another example, eligible smokers with lung metaplasia or dysplasia were randomized to 6 months of 13cRA or placebo. The extent of metaplasia decreased similarly (in approximately 50% of subjects) in both study arms.[51] Only smoking cessation was associated with a significant reduction in the metaplasia index during the 6-month intervention.

Prevention of Invasive Neoplasms. Large, phase III efficacy trials of beta-carotene plus other micronutrients for primary prevention of lung cancer have been completed, as summarized in Table 33.6. The Alpha-Tocopherol, Beta-carotene (ATBC) Trial involved 29,133 men from Finland who were heavy cigarette smokers at entry.[52] In a two-by-two factorial design, participants were randomized to receive either supplemental α-tocopherol, beta-carotene, the combination, or placebo. Unexpectedly, participants receiving beta-carotene (alone or in combination with α-tocopherol) had a statistically significant 18% increase in lung cancer incidence and an 8% increase in total mortality relative to participants receiving placebo. α-Tocopherol had no effect.

The finding of an increased incidence of lung cancer in the beta-carotene–supplemented smokers was replicated in the Carotene and Retinol Efficacy Trial (CARET), a large randomized trial of supplemental beta-carotene plus retinol versus placebo in asbestos workers and smokers.[53] This trial was terminated early, but, at the time of termination, overall lung cancer incidence was increased by 28% in the supplemented subjects and total mortality was also increased by 17%. In contrast, the Physicians' Health Study (PHS) of supplemental beta-carotene versus placebo in 22,071 male US physicians reported no significant effect—positive or negative—of 12 years of supplementation of beta-carotene on total cancer, lung cancer, or cardiovascular disease (see Table 33.6).[54] Two other trials involving supplemental beta-carotene alone (the Women's Health Study[55]) or with other antioxidant nutrients (the Medical Research Council/British Heart Foundation Heart Protection Study[56]) on overall cancer incidence also failed to observe efficacy.

Prevention of Second Primary Invasive Neoplasms. EUROSCAN was a multicenter trial employing a two-by-two factorial design to test retinyl palmitate and N-acetylcysteine (also a compound with known antioxidant activity) in preventing second primary invasive neoplasms in patients with early stage cancers

TABLE 33.5

Larger, Randomized Trials of Retinoids in Human Cancer Risk Reduction with Cancer Outcomes[a,b]

Population	Drug (Dose)	End Point	Outcomes	References
United States, prior HNSCC	13cRA (50–100 mg/m²/d)	Second primary tumor	Significant reduction in second primary tumors at 32 and 55 mos; however, substantial toxicity	(43, 44)
France, prior HNSCC	Etretinate (50/25 mg/d)	Second primary tumor	No difference	(46)
United States, prior HNSCC	13cRA (30 mg/d)	Second primary tumor	No difference	(45)
Europe, prior HNSCC, NSCLC	Vitamin A (300,000/150,000 IU/d) +/− N-acetylcysteine	Second primary tumor	No difference	(57)
United States, Prior NSCLC	13cRA (30 mg/d)	Second primary tumor	No difference, but second primary tumors were lower in nonsmokers on drug but higher in smokers on drug	(58)
Italy, prior breast cancer	4HPR (200 mg/d) No treatment	Contralateral breast cancer	Nonsignificant reduction; premenopausal women did better but opposite in postmenopausal women	(60)
United States, prior BCC	13cRA (10 mg/d)	Second basal cell carcinoma	No difference	(65)
United States, prior actinic keratosis	Retinol (25,000 IU/d)	Skin cancer incidence	Reduction in squamous cell carcinomas but not basal cell carcinomas	(67)
United States, prior BCC/ SCC of the skin	13cRA (5–10 mg/d) Retinol (25,000 IU/d)	Second skin cancer	No significant difference for either agent	(66)
Netherlands, renal transplant patients	Acitretin (30 mg/d)	Skin cancer	Significant reduction	(64)
United States, aggressive SCC of the skin	13cRA (1 mg/kg/d) + interferon alpha	Second primary tumors and tumor recurrences	No effect	(275)
United States, prior bladder TCC	Megadose vitamins (40,000 IU retinol/d) versus RDA vitamins	Recurrence	Significant reduction in recurrence	(73)
United States, prior bladder TCC	4HPR (200 mg/d)	Recurrence	No difference	(72)

[a] Trials of retinoids that also included beta-carotene are listed under Table 33.2 only.
[b] Versus placebo unless otherwise indicated.
HNSCC, head and neck squamous cell carcinoma; NSLC, non–small-cell lung cancer; BCC, basal cell carcinoma; TCC, transitional cell carcinoma; RDA, recommended dietary allowance.

of the head and neck or lung. None of the interventions reduced second airway primary invasive neoplasms.[57] The Lung Intergroup Trial randomized patients with surgically resected lung cancer to 13cRA versus placebo and found no significant differences between the two arms in second primary tumors.[58] Notably, smoking status modified the effect of the 13cRA intervention, which was harmful in current smokers yet beneficial in former smokers.

Thus, phase III trials of both carotenoids/antioxidants and retinoids indicate that these agents overall do not reduce the risk of developing invasive lung cancers, nor do they prevent the development of second primary invasive neoplasms. However, the finding that former smokers seemed to benefit from both 13cRA[58] and beta-carotene[53] is intriguing. Mechanistic work suggests this interaction is real rather than chance (see the following), suggesting that (1) risk-reduction in smokers is especially challenging,[59] and (2) trials in former smokers may merit consideration.

Clinical Efficacy in the Breast

Moon et al.[40] first showed that fenretinide was a promising cancer risk–reducing agent for the breast, having a high therapeutic index and synergistic interaction with tamoxifen in mammary carcinogenesis model studies. This laboratory work led to a large-scale randomized trial of fenretinide (versus no treatment) for 5 years to prevent contralateral breast cancer in women aged 30 to 70 years with a history of resected early breast cancer and no prior adjuvant therapy.[60] The intervention produced no significant overall effect, although fenretinide reduced contralateral and ipsilateral breast cancer rates in premenopausal women, with an opposite (adverse) trend observed in postmenopausal women. The reduced incidence of second breast cancer in premenopausal patients persisted with longer follow-up.[61]

Retinoid X receptor (RXR)–selective retinoids are also being evaluated in preclinical and clinical studies. Ongoing work suggests that combination treatment may represent a promising new strategy to suppress both estrogen receptor–negative and estrogen receptor–positive breast tumors, and the combination of retinoids with antiestrogens may be particularly effective.[62]

Clinical Efficacy in the Skin

Retinoids have been widely studied for cancer risk–reducing efficacy in skin. Early work was done in patients who have substantial skin cancer risk either due to xeroderma pigmentosum or medication-induced immunosuppression for transplants. For example, 13cRA reduced skin cancer by 63% in patients with

TABLE 33.6

Randomized Trials of Antioxidant Nutrients in Human Cancer Risk Reduction with Cancer Outcomes[a]

Population	Drug (Dose)	End Point	Outcomes	References
United States, prior head/neck cancer	Beta-carotene (50 mg/d)	Second primary head and neck cancers	Nonsignificant reduction in second head and neck cancer, increase in lung cancer	(48)
Italy, prior head/neck cancer	Beta-carotene (75 mg/d) for 3 mos with 1 mo off	Second primary head and neck cancers	No effect on second primary tumors, nonsignificant decrease in death	(47)
Canada, prior head/neck cancer	30 mg beta-carotene/d + 400 IU vitamin E/d	Deaths	Beta-carotene discontinued, mortality increased at end of trial	(49)
Finland, male smokers	20 mg beta-carotene/d +/− 50 mg vitamin E/d	Lung cancer	Lung cancer increased with beta-carotene, no effect vitamin E	(52)
United States, smokers and asbestos workers	Beta-carotene (30 mg/d) + retinol (25,000 IU/d)	Lung cancer	Lung cancer increased with beta-carotene + vitamin A	(53)
United States, resected stage I non–small-cell lung cancer	Selenized yeast, 200 µg/d versus placebo	Second primary cancer	No effect	(276)
United States, male physicians	Beta-carotene (50 mg every other day)	Total cancer	No effect	(54)
United States, female health professionals	Beta-carotene (50 mg/ every other day)	All cancers	No effect	(55)
United Kingdom, adults at risk for coronary heart disease	20 mg beta-carotene/d + 600 mg vitamin E/d + 250 mg vitamin C/d	Total cancers	No effect	(56)
United States, prior skin cancer	50 mg beta-carotene/d	Second skin cancer	No effect	(68)
Australia	Beta-carotene (30 mg/d)	Incident squamous cell skin cancer incident basal cell skin cancer	No effect	(69)
United States, prior skin cancer	200 µg selenium/d	Second skin cancer	No effect, with longer follow-up became adverse	(70)
Linxian County, China, general population	15 mg beta-carotene/d + 30 mg vitamin E/d + 50 µg selenium/d	Stomach cancer death Esophageal cancer death	Significant decrease in stomach cancer death; no effect on esophageal cancer death	(75)
Linxian County, China, esophageal dysplasia	Multivitamin/multimineral + 15 mg beta-carotene/d	Stomach cancer death Esophageal cancer death	No effect	(78)
United States, males	200 µg selenium/d +/− 400 IU vitamin E/d	Prostate cancer incidence	No effect; with longer follow-up vitamin E became adverse	(84)
United States, male physicians II	500 mg vitamin C/d + 400 IU vitamin E every other day	Prostate cancer incidence, total cancer incidence	No effect	(86)

[a] All versus placebo.

xeroderma pigmentosum; however, severe, acute mucocutaneous toxicity with the 13cRA occurred.[63] Also, the preventive effect of the retinoid was lost after stopping retinoid therapy. In renal transplant patients, acitretin (30 mg per day) reduced the numbers of premalignant lesions, the number of patients with skin cancer, and the cumulative number of skin cancers.[64]

In lower risk populations, low-dose 13cRA (10 mg per day)[65] and retinol or 13cRA alone did not reduce the recurrence of basal or squamous cell skin cancers,[66] although retinol alone reduced squamous but not basal cell carcinomas in patients with prior actinic keratoses.[67]

Beta-carotene (50 mg per day), in a randomized trial did not reduce the recurrence of nonmelanoma skin cancers.[68] Consistent with findings in the lung, the risk was increased by 44% in current smokers randomized to beta-carotene but not in never smokers randomized to beta-carotene as compared with placebo.

Supplemental beta-carotene (30 mg per day) also did not prevent basal cell carcinoma or squamous cell carcinoma of the skin in an Australian trial.[69]

Clark et al.[70] randomized patients with a history of nonmelanoma skin cancer to 200 µg per day selenium or placebo.[70] Selenium did not reduce the incidence of second skin cancers; a further report of this trial with longer follow-up[71] indicated that there was instead a significant increase in total nonmelanoma skin cancer (hazard ratio [HR] = 1.17; 95% confidence interval [CI], 1.02 to 1.34) and squamous cell skin cancer (HR = 1.25; 95% CI, 1.03 to 1.51).

Clinical Efficacy in the Bladder

A trial of fenretinide (200 mg per day orally for 12 months) versus placebo was conducted for preventing tumor recurrence in patients with nonmuscle-invasive bladder transitional cell carcinoma after transurethral resection with or without adjuvant intravesical bacillus Calmette-Guérin; recurrence rates were similar in both groups.[72] Another trial randomized 65 patients with biopsy-confirmed transitional cell carcinoma of the bladder to a multivitamin (recommended dietary allowance [RDA] levels) alone or supplemented with 40,000 IU retinol, 100 mg pyridoxine, 2,000 mg ascorbic acid, 400 U of α-tocopherol, and 90 mg zinc.[73] The 5-year estimate of tumor recurrence was 91% in the RDA arm versus 41% in the higher-dose nutrient arm ($p = 0.0014$).

Clinical Efficacy in the Cervix

Randomized trials include four with beta-carotene (alone or with other antioxidant nutrients), and five with retinoids. Only one of these trials, involving ATRA,[74] found a significant treatment effect. This trial administered a 0.372% ATRA solution by collagen sponge in a cervical cap delivery system. There was a higher complete response rate in the ATRA group (43%) than the placebo group (27%; $p = 0.041$) among the 141 patients with moderate dysplasia; no significant differences in dysplasia regression rates between the two study arms were detected in patients with severe dysplasia. The investigators experienced substantial losses to follow-up in this patient population.

Clinical Efficacy in the Esophagus and Stomach

Certain regions of China (Huixian and Linxian) have strikingly high incidence rates of esophageal and gastric cancers. Two trials were done in Linxian County; one was a general population trial that tested the efficacy of four different nutrient combinations at inhibiting the development of esophageal and gastric cancers.[75] Those who were given the combination of beta-carotene, vitamin E, and selenium had a 13% reduction in total cancer deaths, a 4% reduction in esophageal cancer deaths, and a 21% reduction in gastric cancer deaths (see Table 33.6). None of the other nutrient combinations reduced gastric or esophageal cancer deaths significantly in this trial. The treatment benefit has been shown to persist for 10 years postintervention, with greater efficacy seen in participants under age 55 years.[76] This finding stands in contrast to most other antioxidant nutrient supplement intervention trials, suggesting that the applicability of these results for populations with adequate nutritional status and for other tumor sites may be limited.[77]

The other Linxian trial evaluated a multivitamin/multimineral preparation plus beta-carotene (15 mg per day) in residents with esophageal dysplasia.[78] There was no clear evidence of efficacy, although confidence intervals were wide.

Clinical Efficacy in the Colon/Rectum

Of the randomized trials aimed at the prevention of recurrent colorectal adenomas with micronutrients that have been completed, some used beta-carotene alone[79] or with other nonmicronutrient interventions.[80] Others evaluated beta-carotene with and without supplemental vitamins C and E.[81] None of the trials observed benefit with supplementation. A subsequent report from one trial noted that alcohol intake and cigarette smoking modified the efficacy of beta-carotene.[82] Among nonsmokers and nondrinkers, beta-carotene was associated with a significant decrease in the risk of one or more recurrent adenomas (relative risk [RR] = 0.56). Among persons who smoked and also drank more than one alcoholic drink per day, beta-carotene significantly increased the risk of recurrent adenoma (RR = 2.07).

Clinical Efficacy in the Prostate

Because oxidative stress may play a role in the etiology of prostate cancer, several antioxidant nutrients, including vitamin E, selenium, and lycopene, have been of interest for preventing prostate cancer. The largest trial to date of these nutrients is the Selenium and Vitamin E Cancer Prevention Trial (SELECT), which tested selenium and vitamin E in a two-by-two factorial design for the primary prevention of prostate cancer. Despite preliminary indications of prostate cancer risk–reducing efficacy for selenium (from a trial of selenium for skin cancer[70]) and vitamin E (from a trial of vitamin E to prevent lung cancer[83]), there was no evidence of efficacy.[84] With extended follow-up, the nonsignificant adverse effect of vitamin E became significantly adverse.[85] Negative/neutral findings also were reported for vitamins E and C and prostate and total cancer in the PHS II randomized controlled trial.[86]

The carotenoid lycopene has generated much interest with regard to prostate cancer risk, and several intervention trials have been conducted based on lycopene supplements. These studies have been small, short term, based on intermediate end points, and often lack adequate control groups. The use of a tomato sauce–based intervention is arguably a better approach to evaluate, based on animal data indicating that tomato powder (which includes lycopene along with other phytochemicals), but not lycopene alone, was effective at inhibiting prostate carcinogenesis.[87]

Mechanisms for Ineffective Retinoid and Carotenoid Cancer Risk–Reducing Activity

There are now a number of trials demonstrating that supplemental beta-carotene/retinoids given to current smokers can produce increases rather than reductions in cancer incidence. In tobacco users, beta-carotene and other carotenoids may produce oxidative carotenoid breakdown products that alter retinoid metabolism and signaling pathways, along with pro-oxidation.[88] For retinoids such as 13cRA, smoking may induce genetic and epigenetic changes in the lung that affect retinoid activity; for example, tobacco smoking can affect RAR-β expression.[58] The adverse effects of supplemental nutrients are not limited to smokers; α-tocopherol increased rather than reduced prostate cancer in SELECT (which had relatively few smokers) and selenium increased prostate cancer among men without a baseline selenium deficiency.[89] This may be a consequence of the relatively high doses used in SELECT,[77] but certainly calls into question the notion that reducing oxidative stress is a pivotal cancer risk–reduction strategy, even in nonsmokers.

It has become clear that reactive oxygen species (ROS), such as hydrogen peroxide, can act as important physiologic regulators of intracellular signaling pathways.[90,91] Data in mouse models have shown that vitamin E accelerates lung tumor growth by disrupting the ROS–p53 axis, potentially by removing oxidative damage to DNA, which can serve as a potent stimulus for p53 activation.[92] Although some of the large cancer risk–reducing trials may have failed in their primary objective, they may indirectly contribute to a clearer understanding of cancer biology, leading to the recognition that the role of oxidative stress and ROS in human disease is much more nuanced than originally hypothesized.[93]

As for the retinoids, these agents are generally too toxic to be used as single agents for risk-reducing efficacy; however, a major area of ongoing research is examining retinoids (low doses) given in combination with other agents, especially those that regulate the epigenome, such histone deacetylase (HDAC) inhibitors.[33]

Folic Acid and Other B Vitamins

Overview and Mechanisms. Folate is a water-soluble B vitamin found in foods, whereas folic acid is the synthetic form found in supplements and fortified foods. Adequate folate is critical for DNA methylation, repair, and synthesis.[94,95] The methylation status of genes can play a key role in gene silencing and gene expression, lending plausibility to the idea that folate could be a key nutrient in regulating cell growth and proliferation.

Epidemiology. Epidemiologic studies have linked low folate intake with higher risk of several cancers, most notably colorectal cancer.[96] Long-term use of multivitamin supplements, which are a major source of folate and other B vitamins, has been associated with a reduction in the risk of colon cancer in some studies, including recent (postfortification) findings.[97–99] Supporting an anticancer role of folate is that genotypes for methylene tetrahydrofolate reductase, an enzyme known to be involved in folate metabolism, predict the risk of colon cancer dependent on folate intake or status.[100] Vitamin B$_6$ has been less studied in relation to cancer than folate, but some epidemiologic studies suggest that vitamin B$_6$ may be important for colorectal cancer.[101,102] A higher risk of cancer related to deficiencies of these vitamins has been suggested for alcohol drinkers.[103]

Clinical Trials: Folic Acid and B Vitamins.

Risk-reducing efficacy for supplemental folic acid has been primarily evaluated in the setting of prevention of recurrent colorectal adenomas (i.e., in patients with prior adenomas). Of six randomized trials of folic acid, two small trials reported suggestions of benefit of folic acid supplementation.[104,105] However, benefits were not observed in two much larger trials, the Aspirin/Folate Polyp Prevention Study (AFPPS) (dose: 1 mg of folic acid daily)[106] and the United Kingdom Colorectal Adenoma Prevention (ukCAP) trial (dose: 500 μg of folic acid daily).[107] AFPPS found indications of an increased risk for advanced lesions and multiple adenomas with prolonged treatment and follow-up. A third large trial, the Nurses Health Study/Health Professionals Follow-up Study (NHS/HPFS) folic acid polyp prevention trial, showed no overall risk reduction.[108] The most recent trial, done in a Chinese population >50 years of age,[109] reported that 1 mg folic acid per day reduced sporadic colorectal adenomas when compared to no intervention (not a placebo-controlled study). One possible explanation for the discrepancy of the Chinese trial versus North American and European trials is the baseline plasma folate status. In the Chinese trial, the mean baseline folate concentration of 5 ng/mL[109] was half of the reported 10 ng/mL in a United States trial,[106] where folate fortification of the food supply occurs.

Calcium and Vitamin D

Overview and Mechanisms.

There are two major forms of vitamin D: ergocalciferol (D$_2$) and cholecalciferol (D$_3$). Vitamin D$_2$ is absorbed through dietary sources such as fortified milk products, and D$_3$ is synthesized via ultraviolet (UV) B light isomerization of 7-dehydrocholestrol in the epidermis.[110] Vitamin D$_3$ is converted to calcitriol (1, 25-[OH]$_2$ D$_3$) in a two-step process requiring both hepatic and renal hydroxylation. Calcitriol binds to the vitamin D receptor, which translocates to the nucleus and binds to multiple gene promoter sites. Through this mechanism, vitamin D regulates cytoplasmic signaling pathways that impact cellular differentiation and growth through proteins such as Ras and mitogen-activated protein kinase (MAPK), protein lipase A, prostaglandins, cyclic adenosine monophosphate (AMP), protein kinase A, and phosphatidyl inositol 3 kinase.[110] 1,25(OH)$_2$D$_3$ regulates cellular proliferation and apoptosis. For example, 1,25(OH)$_2$D$_3$ can induce cleavage of caspase 3, poly (ADP-ribose) polymerase (PARP), and MAPK, leading to apoptosis. 1,25(OH)$_2$D$_3$ inhibits the expression and phosphorylation of Akt, a key regulator of cellular proliferation. The differentiation properties of 1,25(OH)$_2$D$_3$ are mediated through transcriptional activation of the CDK inhibitor p21. The effects of vitamin D on multiple signal transduction pathways operational in cancer cells are reviewed by Deeb et al.[111]

Epidemiology.

Observational epidemiologic studies have shown a relatively consistent inverse association between low calcium intake, including that from supplements, and increased colorectal and colon cancer risk.[112,113] Vitamin D exposure is typically assessed by measuring 25(OH)vitamin D in plasma because exposure is derived not only from diet and supplements, but also from cutaneous synthesis following dermal exposure to UV radiation. A large number of observational studies have evaluated the association between vitamin D status and cancer risk, as systematically reviewed by the Agency for Healthcare Research and Quality (AHRQ).[114] The evidence is inconsistent for most cancer sites, with the exception of studies showing that individuals with lower blood vitamin D levels have a higher risk of colorectal cancer or adenoma. Although some observational studies have reported that higher serum vitamin D is associated with lower breast cancer risk, the association is inconsistent.[114,115] Also, there are some studies suggesting high serum vitamin D is associated with increases in certain cancers, particularly pancreatic cancer.[116]

Clinical Trials: Calcium and Vitamin D

Clinical Efficacy in the Colon. Baron et al.[117] randomized subjects with a recent history of colorectal adenomas to either calcium carbonate (1,200 mg per day of elemental calcium) or placebo. Results showed significant benefit for the calcium arm (adjusted RR = 0.81; 95% CI, 0.67 to 0.99; p = 0.04). In a smaller, similar study of calcium gluconolactate and carbonate (2 g elemental calcium daily), the adjusted odds ratio (OR) for adenoma recurrence was 0.66 (95% CI, 0.38 to 1.17; p = 0.16) for calcium treatment,[118] and while not statistically significant, it was similar to the data of Baron et al.[117]

In the largest trial of calcium and vitamin D with primary cancer end points (e.g., colon, breast), the US Women's Health Initiative (WHI) evaluated the combination of 400 IU of vitamin D per day plus 1,000 mg of calcium per day in 36,282 postmenopausal women. For colon cancer, there was no benefit observed,[119] although the mean baseline intake of calcium was already very high (more than 1,151 mg per day). With regard to vitamin D as a single agent, there was also no suggestion of benefit for colon cancer incidence in a 5-year British trial of vitamin D (100,000 IU every 4 months) that reported colon cancer incidence,[120] although this was not a primary end point.

Clinical Efficacy in the Breast. Vitamin D has received considerable attention for a possible role in the prevention of breast cancer,[121] although no trials have yet investigated vitamin D as a single agent for breast cancer risk reduction. The large WHI trial gave a combination of calcium and vitamin D, as noted previously, and there was no significant effect of this combination on breast cancer risk (HR, 0.96; 95% CI, 0.85 to 1.09).[122] Lappe et al.[123] conducted a trial that examined the relation between calcium plus vitamin D (1,100 IU per day) supplementation (versus calcium alone or placebo) in 1,179 healthy postmenopausal women in Nebraska.[123] Although fracture was the primary outcome of the trial, total cancer incidence was reportedly lower in the calcium plus vitamin D group, although the number of end points was very small (n = 50 total cancers observed during the follow-up). An ongoing randomized trial of vitamin D and omega-3 fatty acids (the **VIT**amin D and OmegA-3 Tria**L** [VITAL]) among 20,000 participants is expected to provide more definitive data on a possible role of vitamin D in the prevention of breast and other cancers.[124]

Summary and Conclusion: Micronutrients

Certain agents, including the retinoids, beta-carotene, folic acid, calcium plus vitamin D, vitamin E, and selenium, have received substantial attention for a possible role in reducing the risk of cancer in humans. As reviewed herein, some of the trials have observed statistically significant reductions in the risk of the primary end point (e.g., retinoids in skin carcinogenesis models, calcium in colorectal adenomas, antioxidant nutrients in Linxian, China, for gastric cancer prevention), whereas others have observed statistically significant increases in the risk of the primary end points (beta-carotene and retinoid lung cancer prevention trials in smokers, vitamin E and prostate cancer, selenium and nonmelanoma skin cancer). Considering the completed trials, there is clear evidence against the general use of nutrient *supplements* for cancer prevention, which is

CANCER PREVENTION AND SCREENING

the conclusion also reached by the World Cancer Research Fund/American Institute for Cancer Research.[38] Note that there is no evidence that food sources of these nutrients increase risk.

Having noted that, there are other key themes emerging from this growing body of research. One such theme is that nutrient supplementation may be of benefit to some but not all. One such population that may benefit includes persons who are low in the nutrient of interest at baseline.[77] This was initially suggested in the Linxian Country trial (done in a micronutrient-deficient population), with growing support from subgroup analyses of several completed trials.[77] However, the hypothesis that nutrient supplementation can reduce cancer risk in subgroups selected based on inadequate nutritional status has, to date, not been formally evaluated in intervention trials.

Another consistent theme is that lifestyle factors (e.g., smoking) and genetics (polymorphisms) may determine who is most likely to benefit from supplementation. Trial data will likely be increasingly mined to identify genetic profiles associated with both better outcomes (risk prediction) and response to intervention.[125,126] Ultimately, a more personalized approach to cancer risk reduction may emerge, consistent with the movement toward a more personalized approach for cancer treatment.

Finally, nearly all of these trials initiate intervention with older adults (who are more likely to develop cancer end points during the follow-up); but, animal models suggest that the timing of exposure may likely be quite relevant. For example, folic acid may protect against initiation, but may also promote the proliferation of existing neoplasms.[127] Thus, the dose, form (food versus supplement), timing, and nutritional and lifestyle characteristics may all be relevant in affecting the efficacy of risk-reducing interventions involving nutrients and related substances. Further research, drawing upon newer tools now available through the field of nutritional genomics, will be needed to gain greater clarity on the heterogeneous biologic effects observed in nutrient-based risk reduction.

ANTI-INFLAMMATORY DRUGS

Mechanism

Nonsteroidal anti-inflammatory drugs (NSAIDs) represent a class of drugs that reduce cellular inflammation through multiple mechanisms, the most prominent of them being the modulation of eicosanoid metabolism.[128] Eicosanoids are metabolites of dietary fatty acids, primarily linoleic acid. Linoleic acid is metabolized to arachidonic acid, which is stored in the lipid membrane and, once mobilized from the membrane, further metabolized by prostaglandin-H synthases (PGHS) 1 and 2 to PGD_2, PGE_2, $PGF_{2\alpha}$, PGI_2, or thromboxane A_2 (TxA_2) by specific synthases. Leukotriene pathways involve the conversion of arachidonic acid to leukotriene A_4 by 5-lipoxygenase and subsequent hydrolysis of leukotriene A_4 to other downstream leukotrienes. Newly formed prostaglandins function primarily through binding to prostaglandin receptors (EP receptors), releasing coupled G-proteins to elicit responses in the same or neighboring cells.[129]

Prostaglandins (PG) play crucial roles in controlling cellular proliferation, apoptosis, cellular invasiveness, and angiogenesis and in modulating immunosuppression.[129] Because PGE_2 is the most abundant PG in tumors, reducing local concentrations of PGE_2 may be a pivotal cancer preventive strategy.[129]

PGHS-independent mechanisms of NSAID action may, at least in part, explain NSAID preventive efficacy.[130] A diverse group of NSAIDs inhibit apoptosis via multiple mechanisms. Among the more prominent of these mechanisms is the inhibition of cyclic guanosine monophosphate (cGMP) phosphodiesterase activity, attenuation of beta-catenin mRNA through suppressing transcription of the *CTNNB1* gene, and activation of c-Jun N-terminal kinase 1.[130] NSAIDs activate peroxisome proliferator–activated receptor (PPAR)γ, leading to increased E-cadherin

expression and reduced colony formation in vitro, while reducing PPARδ, leading to reduced resistance to apoptosis.[130] Selective cyclooxygenase 2 (COX-2) inhibitors inhibit Akt signaling and induce apoptosis of human colorectal and prostate cancer cells in vitro in a COX-2–independent manner via the inhibition of phosphoinositide-dependent kinase-1 (PDK-1). NSAIDs inhibit nuclear factor kappa B (NF-κB) at pharmacologic concentrations and key cellular proliferation signaling intermediates such as activator protein 1 (AP-1) and other intermediates of the MAPK pathway.[130] The impact of NSAIDs on carcinogenic events driven by these upstream pathways in humans as opposed to preliminary in vitro or in vivo models remains unclear.

Epidemiology

Pooled analyses of 34 controlled trials of aspirin 75 mg to 100 mg daily (69,224 participants), conducted primarily for cardiovascular disease reduction, observed reduced cancer deaths (OR, 0.63; 95% CI, 0.49 to 0.82). Most of the benefit occurred after 5 years follow-up.[131] In a pooled analysis of 150 case control and 45 cohort studies, in addition to a reduced risk of death from colorectal cancer (OR, 0.58; 95% CI, 0.44 to 0.78), chronic and frequent (once daily or more) use of aspirin also reduced the risk of death from esophageal (OR, 0.58; 95% CI, 0.44 to 0.76), gastric (OR, 0.61; 95% CI, 0.40 to 0.93), and breast (OR, 0.81; 95% CI, 0.72 to 0.93) cancers.[132] An analysis of 662,624 men and women enrolled in the American Cancer Society's Cancer Prevention Study II found that aspirin taken at least 16 times per month over a 6-year period conferred a 40% reduced risk of colorectal cancer mortality.[133] Both the 46,363 male patients of the Health Professional Study[134] and the 82,911 patients of the Nurse's Health Study[135] suggest that prolonged use (>10 years) of 325 mg of aspirin twice weekly or more reduces colorectal cancer risk (RR, 0.77; 95% CI, 0.67 to 0.88, from the Nurse's Health Study). Daily NSAID intake is associated with a 40% reduction (OR, 0.56; 95% CI, 0.43 to 0.73) in the risk of esophageal adenocarcinoma.[136]

Evidence in Preclinical In Vivo Carcinogenesis Models

NSAIDs, including aspirin, indomethacin, piroxicam, sulindac, ibuprofen, and ketoprofen, suppress colonic tumorigenesis induced chemically (1,2-dimethylhydrazine or its metabolites) or transgenically (Min^+).[137,138] The selective COX-2 inhibitors were the most efficacious colon tumorigenesis inhibitors in both chemical and transgenic rodent models.[139,140] In preclinical models, NSAIDs affect the onset and progression of cancers in the stomach, skin, breast, lung, prostate, and urinary bladder, although the evidence is more limited than for colon cancers.[141]

Clinical Trials

Key clinical trials of NSAIDs for the prevention of colorectal cancer are summarized in Table 33.7. Sulindac reduced the size and number of preexisting adenomas in patients with familial adenomatous polyposis but did not suppress the development of new adenomas,[142] whereas the selective COX-2 inhibitor, celecoxib, suppressed the development of new adenomatous polyps in patients with familial adenomatous polyposis.[143] Although these results are promising, reports of invasive neoplasms developing in familial adenomatous polyposis patients being treated with sulindac[144] raise the question of whether NSAIDs preferentially alter the formation or regression of those adenomas less likely to progress to invasive adenocarcinomas, as compared to those more likely to progress.

Randomized, double-blinded placebo controlled trials of NSAIDs as cancer risk–reducing agents for colorectal adenocarcinoma (see Table 33.7) have confirmed that aspirin suppresses

TABLE 33.7

Summary of Clinical Trials of Nonsteroidal Anti-Inflammatory Drugs as Colorectal Cancer Risk–Reducing Agents

Population	Drug (Dose), Duration	Phase	Endpoint	Outcome	References
Gene Associated					
Familial adenomatous polyposis (FAP)	Sulindac (300–400 mg/d, divided doses)	IIb	Polyp regression	Colorectal and duodenal polyps regressed in ~50%	(277, 278) (279)
Hereditary nonpolyposis colon cancer (Lynch syndrome)	Aspirin 600 mg/d, resistant starch	III	Cancer	≥2 yr, hazard ratio (HR) colon cancer 0.41; 95% CI, 0.19–0.86; all cancers Incidence rate ratio 0.37; 95% CI, 0.18–0.78; no effect of starch	(280, 281)
Sporadic Risk					
Previous adenomatous polyps, healthy subjects	Aspirin (40, 81, 325, 650 mg once per day)	I, IIa	Dose-biomarker	Aspirin dose of 81 mg daily sufficient to suppress colorectal mucosal prostaglandin E_2	(282–284)
Previous adenomatous polyps	Sulindac (300 mg), 4 mos	IIb	Polyp regression	Sulindac did not significantly decrease the number or size of polyps	(146)
Previous adenomatous polyps	Piroxicam (7.5 mg), 2 yr	IIb	Polyp recurrence	Colorectal mucosal PGE_2 reduced in piroxicam treated arm, unacceptable toxicity	(145)
Prior colorectal cancer	Aspirin (325 mg once per day), 3 yr	IIb	Polyp recurrence	Aspirin use associated with delayed development of adenomatous polyps	(285)
Previous adenomatous polyps	Aspirin (81 mg once per day or 325 mg once per day) and/or folate, 3 yr	IIb	Polyp recurrence	Low-dose aspirin reduced the recurrence of adenomatous polyps	(286)
Previous adenomatous polyps	Celecoxib and rofecoxib	IIb	Polyp recurrence	Celecoxib and rofecoxib reduced the recurrence of adenomatous polyps, unacceptable toxicity	(148–150)

adenoma recurrence in patients previously treated for adenomas or for cancer. Neither sulindac nor piroxicam alone suppressed adenoma formation in high-risk, sporadic populations at tolerable doses.[145,146] Sulindac, in combination with difluoromethylornithine, has potent colorectal anticarcinogenesis effects.[147] Selective COX-2 inhibitors (celecoxib, rofecoxib) reduce the recurrence of adenomas by one-third in all patients previously treated for adenomas and by one-half in patients with previously resected large (≥1 cm) adenomas,[148–150] but they are too toxic as cancer risk–reducing agents due to their cardiovascular toxicity.[151,152] Although most NSAIDs (piroxicam, indomethacin) have sufficient gastrointestinal (GI) toxicity to reduce their acceptability as cancer risk–reducing agents,[153,154] the long-term administration of low-dose aspirin in vascular prevention trials demonstrates acceptable GI toxicity.[155]

Up to 40% of individuals screened for colorectal neoplasms will have an adenomatous polyp detected and removed, yet only 10% of these lesions will progress to invasive neoplasms. To date, prospective NSAID trials of only 2 to 3 years cannot substitute for cancer incidence or mortality end points. Given the 10-year latency between adenoma formation and a cancer event, prospective trials sufficiently powered to detect colorectal cancer incidence end points are unlikely in the future.[156] Alternatively, a follow-up of patients randomized on trials of aspirin in the prevention of vascular events in the 1980s and 1990s offers secondary analysis opportunities. In a pooled analysis of three prospective vascular end point cohort studies, 20-year low-dose aspirin treatments reduced cancer deaths from all solid tumors (OR, 0.69; CI, 0.54 to 0.88) and from lung and esophageal adenocarcinomas (OR, 0.66; CI, 0.56 to 0.77).[155] Despite this, the U.S. Preventive Services Task Force (USPSTF) does not recommend the use of aspirin or NSAIDs as cancer risk–reducing agents for normal risk populations, preferring adherence to colorectal cancer screening recommendations (fecal occult blood testing and endoscopy).[153,154,157]

Minimal prospective cancer risk reduction data are available at other epithelial organ sites. Ketorolac, given as a 1% rinse solution, did not reduce the size or histology of leukoplakia lesions.[158] Celecoxib reduces the Ki67 labeling index and increases the expression of nuclear survivin without significantly changing the cytoplasmic survivin in bronchial biopsies of smokers.[159] Cancer prevention trials of aspirin as interventions for delaying progression from intraepithelial neoplasias in other epithelial sites remain ongoing for the lower esophagus.[136] No prospective, randomized trials or data are available for breast, prostate, or gynecologic cancer prevention.

EPIGENETIC TARGETING AGENTS (SELECTIVE ESTROGEN RECEPTOR MODULATORS, 5α-STEROID REDUCTASE INHIBITORS, POLYAMINE INHIBITORS)

Posttranslational pathway targets remain a fertile source of chemopreventive strategies. Phase III data support cancer risk–reduction agent efficacy of selective estrogen receptor modulators (SERM) and 5α-steroid reductase inhibitors for breast and prostate cancer prevention, respectively. Inhibitors of the polyamine pathway may be useful preventives for colorectal cancer.

Selective Estrogen Receptor Modulators

Mechanism

SERMs function as estrogen receptor (ER) agonists and antagonists depending on the SERM structure and target tissue. Predominant ERα receptors occur in the human uterus, cortical bone, and the liver; whereas predominant ERβ receptors occur in blood vessels, cancellous bone, the whole brain, and immune cells.[160,161] During carcinogenesis, the amount of ERα increases while the amount of ERβ decreases in breast tissues.[162] Ideally, a desirable SERM for cancer prevention will function as an antiestrogen in the breast and uterus, but a partial estrogen agonist in skeletal, cardiovascular, central nervous system (CNS), GI tract, and vaginal tissues. In addition, an ideal SERM will not have procoagulant effects and will not cause perimenopausal symptoms such as hot flashes.[162]

Tamoxifen. Tamoxifen is a triphenylethylene compound developed for the treatment of ER-positive breast cancer in the 1960s and 1970s.[163,164] Tamoxifen inhibits the initiation and promotion phases of breast carcinogenesis in the dimethylbenzanthracene chemical carcinogenesis model.[164,165] When tamoxifen binds to ERβ, which then binds to an AP-1 type gene promoter, it functions as an estrogen agonist. When bound to ERα, which binds to an estrogen response element (ERE) target gene promoter, tamoxifen functions as an estrogen antagonist.[162,166] Tamoxifen has estrogen antagonist effects in the human breast; partial estrogen agonist effects in bone, the cardiovascular system, and CNS; and predominant estrogen agonist effects in the uterus, liver, and vagina. The estrogen agonist effects in the liver and uterus result in tamoxifen's toxicities of thromboembolism and endometrial cancer, respectively. The clinical finding that tamoxifen reduces the incidence of contralateral second primary breast cancers during adjuvant treatment regimens catalyzed the push for its development as a cancer risk–reduction agent.[167,168]

Raloxifene. The benzothiophene structure of raloxifene confers a different tissue-specific ER-binding profile than the triphenylethylene tamoxifen. Raloxifene has greater estrogen agonist activity in bone but reduced estrogen agonist activity in the uterus. Raloxifene was studied for the treatment and prevention of osteoporosis in a large, pivotal trial (the Multiple Outcomes of Raloxifene Evaluation [MORE]) and was found to reduce the rate of vertebral fracture as compared to placebo in postmenopausal women.[169]

Lasofoxifene and Arzoxifene. Lasofoxifene and arzoxifene are third-generation SERMs developed as more potent blockers of bone resorption with the goal of reducing the risk of fractures, breast cancer, and heart disease while minimizing the SERM-induced risk of endometrial hyperplasia in postmenopausal women. Both agents proved potent in vitro and in preliminary clinical trials for bone fracture prevention.[170–173]

Selective Estrogen Receptor Modulators as Risk-Reducing Agents for Breast Cancer Prevention

Efficacy. Table 33.8 summarizes the phase III data for SERM-based breast cancer–risk reduction. In a systematic review of MEDLINE and Cochrane databases through December, 2012, the USPSTF identified seven trials of tamoxifen or raloxifene that showed a reduced incidence of invasive breast cancer by 7 to 9 cases in 1,000 women over 5 years compared to placebo.[174] Tamoxifen is more effective than raloxifene; it reduces breast cancer incidence more than raloxifene by 5 cases in 1,000 women. Both drugs reduce the incidence of ER-positive breast cancer, but neither reduces the risk of ER-negative breast cancer. Neither drug reduced breast cancer–specific or all cause mortality rates. Based on benefit–risk models, women with estimated 5-year risks of breast cancer of 3% or greater are likely to benefit from treatment.[175] Using similar

TABLE 33.8

Phase III, Randomized, Controlled Clinical Trials of SERMs for the Prevention of Breast Cancer

Study	Drug and Daily Dose	N =	Treatment Duration (Years)	Entry Criteria	Overall Outcome HR (95% CI)	References
NSABP P-1	Tamoxifen 20 mg Placebo	13,388	5	Gail model: 5 yr predicted risk of ≥1.66%	0.52 (0.42–0.64)	(28,287)
IBIS-I	Tamoxifen 20 mg Placebo	7,139	5	>Twofold relative risk	0.72 (0.58–0.90)	(288)
Marsden	Tamoxifen 20 mg Placebo	2,471	8	Family history	0.87 (0.63–1.21)	(289)
Italian	Tamoxifen 20 mg Placebo	5,408	5	Normal risk, hysterectomy	0.67 (0.59–0.76)	(290)
NSABP P-2 (STAR)	Raloxifene 60 mg Tamoxifen 20 mg	19,747	5	Gail model: 5 yr predicted risk of ≥1.66%	RR Raloxifene versus tamoxifen 1.02 (0.81–1.28)	(29)
MORE/CORE	Raloxifene 60 mg Placebo Raloxifene 120 mg Placebo	7,705 6,511	5	Normal risk, postmenopausal with osteoporosis	0.42 (0.29–0.60)	(291,292)
RUTH	Raloxifene 60 mg Placebo	10,101	5	Normal risk, postmenopausal with risk of coronary heart disease	0.67(0.47–0.96)	(179)
PEARL	Lasofoxifene 0.5 mg Lasofoxifene 0.25 mg Placebo	8,856	5	Normal risk, postmenopausal, with osteoporosis	0.25 mg: 0.82 (0.45–1.49) 0.5 mg: 0.21 (0.05–0.55)	(170)
GENERATIONS	Arzoxifene 20 mg Placebo	9,354	4	Normal risk, postmenopausal, with osteoporosis	0.42 (0.25–0.68)	(172)

Table and data adapted from Cuzick J, Sestak I, Bonanni B, et al. Selective oestrogen receptor modulators in prevention of breast cancer: an updated meta-analysis of individual participant data. *Lancet* 2013;381:1827–1834.

analysis methods as the USPSTF, the American Society of Clinical Oncology recommends the use of tamoxifen (20 mg per day orally for 5 years) or raloxifene (60 mg per day orally for 5 years) "in premenopausal women who are age ≥35 years with a 5-year projected absolute breast cancer risk ≥1.66% according to the NCI Breast Cancer Risk Assessment Tool (or equivalent measures), or with lobular carcinoma in situ."[176] Tamoxifen reduces the risk of in situ (preinvasive) breast neoplasms (lobular carcinoma in situ, ductal carcinoma in situ) by 50%.[177,178] The reduction during treatment persists for at least 5 years after treatment.[177,178] Raloxifene does not reduce the risk of in situ breast neoplasms.

Data from two trials designed to evaluate the safety and efficacy of lasofoxifene (PEARL)[170,171] and arzoxifene (GENERATIONS)[172,173] as bone fracture preventives have been analyzed for breast cancer–risk reduction. Their effect at reducing breast cancer incidence was captured in secondary analyses (see Table 33.8). Neither lasofoxifene nor arzoxifene have been evaluated in phase III randomized controlled breast cancer prevention trials. Arzoxifene development has been discontinued in the United States.

Toxicity Profiles. Tamoxifen causes a twofold increase in the risk of endometrial adenocarcinoma (RR, 2.13; 95% CI, 1.36 to 3.32) and is related to more benign gynecologic conditions, uterine bleeding, and surgical procedures than the placebo controls, whereas raloxifene did not increase the risk for endometrial cancer or uterine bleeding.[174] Tamoxifen causes a twofold increase in thromboembolic events (RR, 1.93; 95% CI, 1.41 to 2.64), whereas raloxifene causes a 60% increase in risk of venous thromboembolism (RR, 1.60; 95% CI, 1.15 to 2.23).[174] Raloxifene does not differ from tamoxifen in risk of fractures, other cancers, or cardiovascular events.[177] Raloxifene's lower risk of endometrial adenocarcinomas compared to tamoxifen needs to be weighed against the increased risk of stroke seen in in the MORE/CORE trials (see Table 33.8).[179] Raloxifene's effectiveness in the community may also be compromised by its poor bioavailability (2%) due to rapid phase II enzyme metabolism in the gut and liver,[180] whereas tamoxifen is more bioavailable and has active metabolites that permit a prolonged drug effect. Missed raloxifene doses may potentially compromise efficacy and prevention outcomes in widespread, community use.

Aromatase Inhibitors. In adjuvant clinical trials for breast cancer, aromatase inhibitors (anastrozole, exemestane, letrozole) given after 5 years of tamoxifen enhance the reduction of breast cancer recurrence in the contralateral breast compared to tamoxifen alone.[181] In a phase I cancer risk–reducing agent trial, letrozole reduced the Ki-67 proliferation index of breast epithelial cells aspirated from high-risk women.[182] Exemestane reduced the overall risk of ER-positive invasive breast cancer (Table 33.9). It did not reduce the risk of noninvasive breast neoplasms or ER-negative breast cancer.[183] Exemestane has no increased risk of venous thromboembolism, endometrial cancer, fracture, or cataract,[183] but losses in bone mineral density and cortical thickness of the distal tibia and radius occurred after 2 years of treatment despite calcium and vitamin D supplementation.[184] The results of the

International Breast Cancer Intervention Study II (IBIS-II), comparing anastrozole with placebo, are similar to those reported for exemestane.[185] Compared to exemestane, anastrozole decreases the incidence of ductal carcinoma in situ (DCIS), whereas exemestane does not. Neither aromatase inhibitor increased survival compared to placebo controls. The American Society of Clinical Oncology recommends exemestane for breast cancer prevention in addition to tamoxifen and raloxifene.

Use Counseling. Despite the widespread evidence of breast cancer preventive efficacy for tamoxifen and raloxifene, only 3% to 20% of eligible high-risk women agree to take tamoxifen for primary prevention.[186] The low willingness of eligible women to take tamoxifen for 5 years demonstrates the issue of risk benefit for cancer risk–reducing agents. Women with high short-term risk (5 year Gail risk of >3%)—for example, those with ER-positive atypical hyperplasia, lobular carcinoma in situ, and the majority of non–high-grade ductal carcinoma in situ lesions—have an acceptable risk to benefit ratio and are the most likely to benefit from a 5-year cancer risk–reducing agent intervention with a SERM.[175,176] The toxicity profile of aromatase inhibitors differs from SERMs. Although aromatase inhibitors may have a more favorable risk to benefit profile than SERMs, long-term outcomes and toxicity experience for aromatase inhibitor risk-reducing agent intervention are not available to date. In the National Surgical Adjuvant Breast and Bowel Project, tamoxifen-treated women with a *BRCA2* mutation but not a *BRCA1* mutation had reduced cancer incidence,[187] but subsequent data from another group have found reduced cancer risk in women with both BRCA mutations.[188] Data remain insufficient to recommend the use of SERMs for risk reduction in women with BRCA mutations.

5α-Steroid Reductase Inhibitors

Mechanism

Prostate cancers require androgens to proliferate and evade apoptosis. The primary nuclear androgen responsible for the maintenance of epithelial function is dihydrotestosterone. The testes and adrenal gland synthesize dihydrotestosterone by the conversion of testosterone by 5α-steroid reductase types 1 and 2 isozymes. Dihydrotestosterone binds to intracellular androgen receptors to form a complex that binds to DNA hormone response elements controlling cellular proliferation and apoptosis. Finasteride, a selective, competitive inhibitor of type 2 5α-steroid reductase,[189] inhibits proliferation in the transformed prostate cell. In the 3,2′-dimethyl-4-aminobiphenyl (DMAB), methylnitrosourea (MNU), and testosterone chemical carcinogenesis models in rats, finasteride reduces prostate tumor incidence by close to six-fold. Finasteride appears to be more effective in the promotion phase of prostate carcinogenesis.[190] Dutasteride inhibits both 5α-steroid reductase inhibitor[190] types 1 and 2 isoforms and has similar anticarcinogenesis activity in preclinical models to finasteride.

TABLE 33.9

Phase III, Randomized, Controlled Clinical Trials of Aromatase Inhibitors for the Prevention of Breast Cancer

Study	Drug and Daily Dose	N =	Treatment Duration (Years)	Entry Criteria	Overall Outcome HR (95% CI)	References
MAP.3	Exemestane 25 mg Placebo	4,560	5	Gail model 5 yr predicted risk of ≥2.3%	0.35 (0.18–0.70)	(183)
IBIS-II	Anastrozole 1 mg Placebo	3,851	5	RR twofold higher than general population or Tyrer-Cuzick 10-yr risk >5%	0.47 (0.32–0.68)	(185)

TABLE 33.10

Phase III, Randomized, Controlled Clinical Trials of 5α-Steroid Reductase Inhibitors for the Prevention of Prostate Cancer

Study	Drug and Daily Dose	N =	Treatment Duration (Years)	Entry Criteria	Overall Outcome HR (95% CI)	References
PCPT	Finasteride 5 mg Placebo	18,880	7	Age ≥55 y, PSA ≤3 ng/mL	0.70 (0.65–0.76)	(30, 193)
REDUCE	Dutaseride 0.5 mg Placebo	6,729	4	Age 50–75 y, PSA 2.5–10.0 ng/mL, core biopsies within 6 mos	RR = 0.77 (0.70–0.85)	(192)

PSA, prostate specific antigen.

Cancer Risk–Reducing Agent Activity

Randomized, placebo-controlled cancer incidence end point risk-reducing agent clinical trials demonstrated that finasteride and dutasteride reduced the incidence of prostate cancer by approximately 22% (Table 33.10).[30,191,192] Patients who are treated with either drug yet progress to transformed neoplasms develop more tumors of a high Gleason grade (7 to 10) compared to the placebo arm (22%). After 18 years of follow-up, no significant differences in overall survival or survival after prostate cancer diagnosis were found in the finasteride-treated group compared to the placebo-treated group.[193] Sexual function side effects (e.g., erectile dysfunction, loss of libido, gynecomastia) were more common in the finasteride- or dutasteride-treated groups.[30,192]

The 5α-steroid reductase inhibitors, finasteride and dutasteride, prevent or delay carcinogenesis progression in the prostate, yet progression of high-grade lesions is unaffected. Use of finasteride for a period of 7 years reduced the incidence of prostate cancer but did not significantly affect mortality.[193] Increasing the diagnosis of low-grade prostate cancer through prostate-specific antigen (PSA) testing or intervention with a drug with a minimal toxicity profile without reducing mortality is of no benefit and "all forms of therapy cause considerable burden to the patient and to society."[193]

SIGNAL TRANSDUCTION MODIFIERS

Both cancer therapy and cancer prevention have investigated drugs that modify specific targets in signal transduction pathways. Although the emphasis in drug development has focused on cancer treatment, interventions aimed at modulating signal transduction pathways promise new approaches to interventions in the carcinogenic process. Because of the complexity of signaling systems, the inhibition of single targets may not be effective or may cause unacceptable toxicity.

Difluoromethylornithine

Mechanism

Polyamines (spermidine, spermine, and the diamine, putrescine) are required to maintain cellular growth and function.[194] In mammalian cells, polyamine inhibition by genetic mutation or pharmaceutical agents is associated with virtual cessation in cellular growth. Difluoromethylornithine (DFMO) is an enzyme-activated irreversible inhibitor of ornithine decarboxylase (which is trans-activated by the c-MYC oncogene and cooperates with the RAS oncogene in malignant transformation).[195]

Evidence in Preclinical In Vivo Carcinogenesis Models

Extensive preclinical data has found that DFMO prevents tumor promotion in a variety of systems, including skin, mammary, colon, cervical, and bladder carcinogenesis models.[194] Synergistic or additive activity with retinoids, butylated hydroxyanisole, tamoxifen, piroxicam, and fish oil has been demonstrated with low concentrations of DFMO.[194]

Clinical Trials

In phase I prevention trials, DFMO at a dose of 0.5 mg/m² per day reduced tissue polyamines in the colon and skin[196,197] and causes regression of cervical intraepithelial neoplasia when used topically,[198] but does not reduce tissue polyamines or other biomarkers of cellular proliferation in the human breast.[199] As a single agent, DFMO has anticarcinogenic activity for nonmelanoma skin cancers, primarily basal cell carcinoma. In combination with an NSAID (sulindac), DFMO reduced adenoma recurrences, suggesting a synergistic reduction of colorectal cancer risk (Table 33.11). Preliminary data suggest some cancer risk–reducing agent activity for the lower esophagus and the prostate (see Table 33.11).[200]

Statins

Mechanism

Statins are hydroxyl-3-methylglutaryl coenzyme A (HMG-CoA) reductase inhibitors that inhibit the conversion of HMG-CoA to mevalonate, a cholesterol precursor. The statins are a class of medications with similar structures but with variable moieties that can result in hydrophilic forms (e.g., pravastatin, rosuvastatin) and lipophilic forms (e.g., lovastatin, simvastatin, fluvastatin, atorvastatin).[201] Statins decrease the risk of cancer in preclinical studies by inhibiting RAS- and RHO-mediated cell proliferation, upregulating cell cycle inhibitors (e.g., p21 and p27), and inducing apoptosis of transformed cells and the inhibition of angiogenesis.[202]

Evidence in Preclinical In Vivo Carcinogenesis Models

Lipophilic statins delay progression of pancreatic intraepithelial neoplasias and the growth of pancreatic carcinoma xenografts. Atorvastatin alone and in combination with NSAIDs reduced colonic adenoma and adenocarcinoma incidence and multiplicity by half in rodent transgenic and chemical carcinogenesis models. Lovastatin reduced lung adenoma multiplicity but not incidence.[201]

Clinical Trials

Although several large trials of pravastatin or simvastatin on cardiovascular disease risk with cancer as secondary end points have shown no benefit for reducing cancer risk with follow-ups between 18 months to 4 years, these trials were not adequately powered to examine cancer end points.[201] Several case control studies evaluating statin effects have shown a significant association with lower risk of colorectal adenocarcinoma with odds ratios ranging from 0.53 to 0.91 for arzoxifene. A secondary analysis of a celecoxib prevention trial demonstrated no statin protection against colorectal

TABLE 33.11

Summary of Clinical Trials of Difluoromethylornithine as a Cancer Risk–Reducing Agent

Population	Dose per Day, Duration	Phase	Endpoint	Outcome	References
Low risk bladder cancer (Ta. T1. Grades 1 or 2)	1 gm versus placebo × 1 year	III	Bladder cancer recurrence	Did not prevent or delay recurrence	(293)
Prostate risk: men with family history prostate cancer, age 35–70 yr	500 mg versus placebo × 1 yr	IIb	Prostate volume, polyamines, PSA	10-fold reduction of prostate size increase over 1 yr compared to placebo, PSA reduction not significant	(294)
Nonmelanoma skin cancer	500 mg/m^2 versus placebo × 4–5 y	III	New nonmelanoma skin cancers	Lower rate of basal cell carcinomas per year (0.28 versus 0.40); persistent reduction in nonmelanoma skin cancers, not statistically significant	(295, 296)
Colon adenomas	DFMO: 500 mg Sulindac: 150 mg versus placebo × 3 y	IIb	Adenoma recurrence	RR for adenoma recurrence for DFMO/sulindac treatment 5 0.30 (0.18–0.49)	(147)

PSA, prostate specific antigen.

neoplasms.[203] The Women's Health Initiative (prospective longitudinal cohort of 159,319 women) found that lovastatin was associated with a lower risk of developing colorectal cancer (HR = 0.62; 95% CI, 0.39 to 0.99).[204] Prospective longitudinal studies have shown mixed results. The PHS reported statin use was inversely associated with prostate cancer (adjusted RR, 0.51),[205] whereas the Nurse's Health Study showed no association with risk of breast cancer.[206] Interventional trials to determine statin preventive efficacy for colon and breast cancer are ongoing.[201] Statins may be effective risk-reducing agents in individuals with the A/A variant of the predominant T/T genotype of rs12654264 of the HMG-CoA reductase gene.[207]

Bisphosphonates

Mechanism

Bisphosphonates are pyrophosphate analogs with a central phosphorus-carbon-phosphorus bond that resists bone degradation preventing bone loss and fractures. Second- and third-generation amino bisphosphonates (pamidronic, alendronic, risedronic, ibandronic, and zoledronic acids) inhibit farnesyl diphosphate synthase downstream of HMG-CoA reductase, leading to decreased posttranslational prenylation of GTP-binding proteins such as RAS and Rho. Amino bisphosphonates inhibit cell proliferation, angiogenesis, and cell cycle arrest while inducing apoptosis.[201]

Evidence in In Vivo Preclinical and Clinical Models

HER2-transgenic mice treated with zoledronic acid had increased tumor-free survival and overall survival. Zoledronic acid suppressed bone, lung, and liver metastases when treated prior to an injection of breast cancer cells.[201] The short-term use of bisphosphonates is associated with reduced breast cancer incidence in case control studies[208,209] and prospective cohort studies (HR = 0.68; 95% CI, 0.52 to 0.88 in a prospective cohort study).[210] Randomized trials of amino-bisphosphonates in postmenopausal women with breast cancer treated for 1 year have found a reduction of breast cancer risk in the contralateral breast (HR = 0.39; 95% CI, 0.18 to 0.88).[211] Case control data suggesting a bisphosphonate-associated reduction in colorectal cancer risk have not been confirmed by prospective cohort studies (i.e., Women's Health Initiative, Nurse's Health Study).[201]

Metformin

Mechanism

Metformin, an oral antidiabetic drug in the biguanide class, is the first-line drug of choice for the treatment of type 2 diabetes.[212] Cancers are more common in diabetics and obese individuals than their normal weight and normoglycemic counterparts, leading to the hypothesis that elevated serum insulin concentrations promote cancer risk.[213,214] Insulin and insulin-like growth factors (IGF1 and 2) stimulate cellular DNA synthesis, proliferation, and tumor growth through phosphoinositide-3 kinase (PI3K), mammalian target of rapamycin (mTOR), and the RAS-MAPK signaling pathways.[213] Metformin activates the adenosine monophosphate-activated protein kinase (AMPK) via LKB1, a protein-threonine kinase that has tumor-suppressor activity.[201] Metformin anticarcinogenesis activity appears to be broad and includes downregulation of erbB-2 and epidermal growth factor receptor (EGFR) expression, inhibiting the phosphorylation of erbB family members, IGF1R, Akt, mTOR, and STAT3 in vivo. Low doses of metformin inhibit the self-renewal/proliferation of cancer stem cells in breast, colon, and pancreatic models.[215,216]

Evidence in Preclinical In Vivo Carcinogenesis Models

Metformin reduces tobacco carcinogen–induced tumors in mice, and pancreatic premalignant and malignant tumors in hamsters.[201] However, metformin's anticarcinogenic activity appears dependent on the dose and the induced carcinogenesis process. Metformin promoted carcinogenesis in MNU-induced rat breast cancers, MMTV-Neu ER-negative breast cancers, OH-BBN induced bladder cancer, and Min$^+$ mouse intestinal tumors using nonobese rodents.[217] Metformin cancer risk–reducing agent effects may be limited to obesity- and diabetes-associated carcinogenesis mechanisms.

Clinical Trials

Two large retrospective cohort studies have shown that metformin therapy is associated with a reduced risk of solid tumors by 25% to 30%.[201] The Women's Health Imitative observed a lower incidence of invasive breast cancer in metformin-treated women with type 2 diabetes mellitus.[218] Phase II window of opportunity randomized trials have shown reduced proliferation and increased apoptosis in resected tissue of breast cancer patients.[201]

Diet-Derived Natural Products

Mechanism

Polyphenolic phytochemicals, such as curcumin, resveratrol, epigallocatechin gallate (EGCG), genistein, and ginger, are attractive as cancer risk–reducing agents for their low toxicity and multimechanism anticarcinogenic properties. They have anti-inflammatory activity, in part through scavenging of ROS, modulation of protein kinase signal transduction pathways (e.g., STAT-3, HER2/neu, MAPK, and Akt), and downstream inhibition of eicosanoid synthesis potentially due to upstream inhibition of NF-κB and PPAR or direct blockade or inhibition of eicosanoid-metabolizing enzymes.[219–221] Curcumin, and presumably other polyphenolics, downregulate stem cell driver signaling systems Wnt, Hedgehog, and Notch with subsequent reductions of breast, pancreatic, and colonic stem cell self-renewal.[222,223]

Omega-3 fatty acids (derived from marine products) compete with omega-6 fatty acid substrates for eicosanoid-metabolizing enzymes with subsequent tissue reduction of these inflammatory mediators.[224,225] These fatty acids have other diverse anticarcinogenic mechanisms (e.g., G-protein inhibition, changes in membrane physical characteristics that alter transmembrane signaling protein dynamics) that make them attractive as cancer risk–reducing agents.[226,227]

Whole berries, black raspberries, and strawberries contain mixtures of multiple anticarcinogenic compounds such as ellagic acid, anthocyanins, and tocopherols.[228] Research-grade berries are grown in a standardized cultivation environment and assayed for key components to ensure year-to-year reproducibility despite yearly climatologic variation. Berries have potent stabilization of methylation properties in addition to the expected anti-inflammatory and antioxidative properties associated with the prominent components.[229,230]

Preclinical and Clinical Anticarcinogenesis Efficacy. Diverse diet-derived natural products have moderate-to-strong anticarcinogenic effects in both chemical and transgenic rodent carcinogenesis models (Table 33.12). Phase I clinical trials of curcumin detected little parent compound in plasma or tissues, raising the possibility of biologically active conjugates or deconjugation at the target site.[231–233] Resveratrol's plasma bioavailability exceeds that of curcumin and ginger, and partitions into human colon tissue at 10-fold concentrations compared to plasma.[219,234,235] No natural products have been studied in large prospective, cancer incidence risk–reduction trials. Using intraepithelial biomarker end points in human phase II trials, berry formulations reduce esophageal dysplasia and oral leukoplakia.[236,237] Curcumin reduces the number of colon aberrant crypt foci in human smokers.[238]

ANTI-INFECTIVES

Many infectious agents are known causes of human cancers, including the human hepatitis viruses, hepatitis B virus (HBV) and hepatitis C virus (HCV) for hepatocellular carcinoma[239]; Helicobacter pylori for gastric adenocarcinoma[240]; human papilloma viruses (HPV) for cervical, anal, vulva, penis, and oral cavity and pharynx carcinomas[241]; herpes virus-8 for Kaposi sarcoma[242]; Epstein-Barr virus for Burkitt and other lymphomas[243]; liver flukes for cholangiocarcinoma[244]; and schistosomes for bladder carcinoma.[245] The success of the HPV vaccine at reducing the incidence of intraepithelial neoplasia of the cervix is one example that demonstrates the potential of immunochemoprevention for epithelial targets for which an etiologic agent can be identified.

Helicobacter pylori

Intestinal-type gastric adenocarcinoma arises through a multistep process that begins with chronic gastritis initiated by H. pylori, progressing through gastric mucosal atrophy, intestinal metaplasia to dysplasia, and ultimately, to adenocarcinoma.[246] H. pylori infects 50% of the world's population.[240] Infection occurs early in life, remains quiescent, and may be associated with chronic gastritis of variable intensity but with minimal symptoms. Although the majority of H. pylori organisms remain in the gastric mucous layer, 10% adhere to the gastric mucosa through adhesion BabA, an outer membrane protein that binds to the Lewis-B histo-blood group antigen.[240] Progression to atrophic gastritis and peptic ulcer disease (occurs in 10% to 15% of infected individuals) requires other bacterial and host cofactors.[245,246] Infection with H. pylori is associated with an OR of 2.7 to 6.0 for gastric cancer; CagA increases this risk by 20- to 40-fold. The risk of developing gastric adenocarcinoma with an H. pylori infection is estimated to be 1% to 3%.[245,246]

The eradication of H. pylori with antibiotics and anti-inflammatory agents—for example, amoxicillin, metronidazole, and bismuth subsalicylate—increases the rate of regression of nonmetaplastic gastric atrophy and intestinal metaplasia in geographically diverse regions.[247,248] A combination of a 2-week course of a proton pump inhibitor (omeprazole) and an antibiotic (amoxicillin) reduced the risk of gastric cancer in a high-risk population in China (OR = 0.61; (95% CI, 0.36 to 0.96) for 14.7 years after the treatment.[249] The sequence of giving proton pump inhibitors and antibiotic therapy does not alter the treatment outcome. In addition to contributing to gastric cancer risk, H. pylori infections may also contribute to pancreatic cancer risk.[250] Because H. pylori infections are so widespread, mass eradication campaigns in high-risk regions are being considered.[251] However, complicating this is that H. pylori infections have also been associated with a reduced risk of both esophageal adenocarcinoma and gastric cardia carcinoma.[252]

MULTIAGENT APPROACHES TO CANCER RISK REDUCTION

In the transition to molecularly targeted interventions, combinations of targets that logically address critical carcinogenic pathways may have greater efficacy than single agents. For example, previously demonstrated interactive signaling of EGFRs and COX-2 experiments in Min+ mice[253] demonstrates cancer preventive synergism. Combining atorvastatin with selective or nonselective COX inhibitors enhanced the inhibition of azoxymethane-induced colon carcinogenesis in F344 rats and reduced the dose of the combined drugs required to achieve a reduction of colon carcinogenesis.[254]

DFMO plus sulindac inhibited adenoma formation in a phase IIb trial of 375 patients with a prior history of adenomas followed for 36 months (see Table 33.11).[147] Cardiovascular-adverse outcomes were higher in DFMO/sulindac-treated patients who had preexisting high baseline cardiovascular risk; however, the cardiovascular-adverse events were similar to placebo in moderate or low cardiovascular risk patients.[255] Using IGF-1 as a biomarker, Guerrieri-Gonzaga et al.[256] showed that the combination of low-dose tamoxifen with low-dose fenretinide is safe but not synergistic. As more data accumulate from in vivo models, combined drugs aimed at specific targets in coordinated signaling pathways will enter clinical biomarker-based trials. Optimal doses, toxicity, and biomarker modulation data will select those combinations useful for risk reduction trials and, ultimately, generalized use in at-risk populations.

TABLE 33.12

Selected Diet-Derived Natural Products with Cancer Risk–Reducing Activity

Nutritional Extract	Source	Mechanisms	In Vivo Anticarcinogenesis Efficacy	Human Trials	References
Curcumin ([1E,6E]-1,7-bis-[4-hydroxy-3-methoxyphenyl]-1,6-heptadiene-3,5-dione/diferuloylmethane)	Turmeric, rhizome of *Curcuma longa*	Inhibits: PGE_2 synthesis via direct binding to COX-2 and through inhibition of NF-κB; angiogenesis. ErbB2 transduction; PI3K-Akt transduction; Inhibits stem cell self renewal Agonist: vitamin D receptor	Colon, breast, skin	Phase I: Poor bioavailability due to biotransformation in gut, enterohepatic cycling of metabolites; Phase IIa: reduced aberrant crypt foci	(219, 238)
Resveratrol (3,5,4'-trihydroxy-trans-stilbene)	Grapes, mulberries, peanuts, and *Cassia quinquangulata* plants	Inhibits: Carcinogen activation via inhibition of phase I isozyme, eicosanoids via direct binding; NF-κB; Nrf2. Acts as a caloric restriction mimetic, activates the histone deacetylase SIRT1 and AMPK	Colorectal, breast, pancreas, skin, and prostate	Phase I: 1 g dose generated peak concentration ~2 µM, conjugates 10-fold higher; resveratrol tissue concentrations 10-fold higher than plasma; Phase IIa: Small reduction in IGF-1 and IGFBP-1	(220, 234)
Ginger (gingerols, paradols, shagaols)	Rhizome of *Zingiber officinale*	Induces apoptosis via caspase-3 mechanisms; Inhibits NF-κB activation and downstream COX-2 expression; reduces iNOS expression and ornithine decarboxylase activity	Colon, breast, skin, oral cavity, liver	Phase I: 2 g dose nontoxic; Phase IIa: Small reductions in PGE_2, increased Bax in upper colon crypt	(235, 297, 298)
Green tea (epigallocatechin gallate, other catechins)	Green tea extract	Inhibits: PI3K-Akt transduction, IGF-1, IGFBP-3; NK-κB; catenin reduces methylation via inhibition of DNA methyltransferase 1	Lung, prostate, skin, colorectal	Phase IIa: 500–1,000 mg/m^2 × 12 wk reduced oral premalignant lesions in 50%; Phase IIb: 2.5 g × 1 yr reduced colorectal adenoma recurrence by 50%	(221)
Omega-3 fatty acids (eicosapentaenoic acid; docosahexaenoic acid)	Fish oil	Reduction of inflammation via eicosanoid reduction; direct binding to G receptor proteins; PPAR activation; induction of anti-inflammatory lipid mediators (resolvins, protectins, maresins)	Colon, breast, prostate	Phase II: 4–7 mg/d reduced colon adenomas in familial adenomatous polyposis; ongoing trials for sporadic; extensive case control studies	(226, 299)
Berries	Black raspberries, strawberries	Reduction of methylation via inhibition of methyltransferases, re-regulated Wnt; inhibits NF-κB; inhibits cyclooxygenases; inhibits proliferation	Esophageal squamous cell, colon, skin	Phase IIb: Freeze dried strawberries reduced esophageal dysplasia; Phase IIa: Blackberry gel reduced leukoplakia	(228, 229, 236, 237)

IGFBP-1, insulin growth factor binding protein-1; iNOS, inducible isoform of nitric oxide synthase.

CANCER PREVENTION AND SCREENING

REFERENCES

1. Vogelstein B, Papadopoulos N, Velculescu VE, et al. Cancer genome landscapes. *Science* 2013;339:1546–1558.
2. Fearon ER, Vogelstein B. A genetic model for colorectal tumorigenesis. *Cell* 1990;61:759–767.
3. Sidransky D. Emerging molecular markers of cancer. *Nat Rev Cancer* 2002; 2:210–219.
4. Lippman SM, Levin B, Brenner DE, et al. Cancer prevention and the American Society of Clinical Oncology. *J Clin Oncol* 2004;22:3848–3851.
5. Wattenberg L. Chemoprevention of cancer. *Cancer Res* 1985;45:1–8.
6. Greenwald P, Kelloff G. The role of chemoprevention in cancer control. *IARC Scientific Publications (Lyon)* 1996;139:13–22.
7. Hanahan D, Weinberg RA. The hallmarks of cancer. *Cell* 2000;100:57–70.
8. Steele VE, Boone CW, Lubet RA, et al. Preclinical drug development paradigms for chemopreventives. *Hematol Oncol Clin North Am* 1998;12:943–961.
9. Perloff M, Steele VE. Early-phase development of cancer prevention agents: challenges and opportunities. *Cancer Prev Res (Phila)* 2013;6:379–383.
10. National Cancer Institute. PREVENT Cancer Preclinical Drug Development Program. National Cancer Institute Web site. http://prevention.cancer.gov/programs-resources/programs/prevent. Accessed December 7, 2013.
11. Mehta RG, Naithani R, Huma L, et al. Efficacy of chemopreventive agents in mouse mammary gland organ culture (MMOC) model: a comprehensive review. *Curr Med Chem* 2008;15:2785–2825.
12. Hoenerhoff MJ, Hong HH, Ton TV, et al. A review of the molecular mechanisms of chemically induced neoplasia in rat and mouse models in National Toxicology Program bioassays and their relevance to human cancer. *Toxicol Pathol* 2009;37:835–848.
13. Steele VE, Lubet RA. The use of animal models for cancer chemoprevention drug development. *Semin Oncol* 2010;37:327–338.
14. Shureiqi I, Reddy P, Brenner DE. Chemoprevention: general perspective. *Crit Rev Oncol Hematol* 2000;33:157–167.
15. Becker M. Adherence to prescribed therapies. *Med Care* 1985;23:539–554.
16. Miki Y, Swensen J, Shattuck-Eidens D, et al. A strong candidate for the breast and ovarian cancer susceptibility gene BRCA1. *Science* 1994;266:66–71.
17. Powell SM, Petersen GM, Krush AJ, et al. Molecular diagnosis of familial adenomatous polyposis. *N Engl J Med* 1993;329:1982–1987.
18. Meads C, Ahmed I, Riley RD. A systematic review of breast cancer incidence risk prediction models with meta-analysis of their performance. *Breast Cancer Res Treat* 2012;132:365–377.
19. Kastrinos F, Steyerberg EW, Balmana J, et al. Comparison of the clinical prediction model PREMM(1,2,6) and molecular testing for the systematic identification of Lynch syndrome in colorectal cancer. *Gut* 2013;62:272–279.
20. Ankerst DP, Boeck A, Freedland SJ, et al. Evaluating the PCPT risk calculator in ten international biopsy cohorts: results from the Prostate Biopsy Collaborative Group. *World J Urol* 2012;30:181–187.
21. National Institutes of Health, U.S. Food and Drug Administration. *Biomarkers and Surrogate Endpoints: Advancing Clinical Research and Applications*. Bethesda, MD: National Insitutes of Health; 1999.
22. Schatzkin A, Freedman LS, Schiffman MH, et al. Validation of intermediate end points in cancer research. *J Natl Cancer Inst* 1990;82:1746–1752.
23. Prentice R. Surrogate endpoints in clinical trials: definition and operational criteria. *Statistics Med* 1989;8:431–440.
24. Ransohoff DF. Rules of evidence for cancer molecular-marker discovery and validation. *Nat Rev Cancer* 2004;4:309–314.
25. Pepe MS, Feng Z, Janes H, et al. Pivotal evaluation of the accuracy of a biomarker used for classification or prediction: standards for study design. *J Natl Cancer Inst* 2008;100:1432–1438.
26. Pryor WA, Stahl W, Rock CL. Beta carotene: from biochemistry to clinical trials. *Nutr Rev* 2000;58:39–53.
27. Brenner DE, Hawk E. Trials and tribulations of interrogating biomarkers to define efficacy of cancer risk reductive interventions. *Cancer Prev Res (Phila)* 2013;6:71–73.
28. Fisher B, Costantino J, Wickerham D, et al. Tamoxifen for prevention of breast cancer: report of the National Surgical Adjuvant Breast and Bowel Project P-1 study. *J Natl Cancer Inst* 1998;90:1371–1388.
29. Vogel VG, Costantino JP, Wickerham DL, et al. Update of the National Surgical Adjuvant Breast and Bowel Project Study of Tamoxifen and Raloxifene (STAR) P-2 Trial: Preventing breast cancer. *Cancer Prev Res (Phila)* 2010;3:696–706.
30. Thompson IM, Goodman PJ, Tangen CM, et al. The influence of finasteride on the development of prostate cancer. *N Engl J Med* 2003;349:215–224.
31. Omenn G, Goodman G, Thornquist M, et al. Effects of a combination of beta carotene and vitamin A on lung cancer and cardiovascular disease. *N Engl J Med* 1996;334:1150–1155.
32. Lotan R. Retinoids in cancer chemoprevention. *Faseb J* 1996;10:1031–1039.
33. Tang X-H, Gudas LJ. Retinoids, retinoic acid receptors, and cancer. *Annu Rev Pathol* 2011;6:345–364.
34. Khachik F, Beecher, G, Smith JC Jr. Lutein, lycopene, and their oxidative metabolites in chemoprevention of cancer. *J Cell Biochem* 1995;22:236–246.
35. Di Mascio P, Kaiser S, Sies H. Lycopene as the most efficient biological carotenoid singlet oxygen quencher. *Arch Biochem Biophys* 1989;274:532–538.
36. Eroglu A, Hruszkewycz DP, dela Sena C, et al. Naturally occurring eccentric cleavage products of provitamin A beta-carotene function as antagonists of retinoic acid receptors. *J Biol Chem* 2012;287:15886–15895.
37. Ford NA, Erdman JW Jr. Are lycopene metabolites metabolically active? *Acta Biochim Pol* 2012;59:1–4.
38. World Cancer Research Fund, American Institute for Cancer Research. *Food, Nutrition, Physical Activity, and the Prevention of Cancer: A Global Perspective*. Washington, DC: AICR; 2007.
39. Panel on Dietary Antioxidants and Related Compounds, Subcommittees on Upper Reference Levels of Nutrients and Interpretation and Uses of DRIs, Standing Committee on the Scientific Evaluation of Dietary Reference Intakes, Food and Nutrition Board, Institute of Medicine. *Dietary Reference Intakes for Vitamin C, Vitamin E, Selenium, and Carotenoids*. Washington, DC: National Academy Press; 2000.
40. Moon RC, Mehta RG, Rao KVN. Retinoids and cancer in experimental animals. In: Sporn MB, Roberts AB, Goodman DS, eds., *The Retinoids*. 2nd ed. New York: Raven Press; 1994: 573–595.
41. International Agency for Research on Cancer World Health Organization. *Carotenoids*. Lyon: International Agency for Research on Cancer; 1998.
42. Holzapfel NP, Holzapfel BM, Champ S, et al. The potential role of lycopene for the prevention and therapy of prostate cancer: from molecular mechanisms to clinical evidence. *Int J Mol Sci* 2013;14:14620–14646.
43. Hong WK, Lippman SM, Itri LM, et al. Prevention of second primary tumors with 13cRA in squamous-cell carcinoma of the head and neck. *N Engl J Med* 1990;323:795–801.
44. Benner SE, Pajak TF, Lippman SM, et al. Prevention of second primary tumors with isotretinoin in patients with squamous cell carcinoma of the head and neck: long term follow-up. *J Natl Cancer Inst* 1994;86:140–141.
45. Khuri FR, Lee JJ, Lippman SM, et al. Randomized phase III trial of low-dose isotretinoin for prevention of second primary tumors in stage I and II head and neck cancer patients. *J Natl Cancer Inst* 2006;98:441–450.
46. Bolla M, Lefur R, Ton Van J, et al. Prevention of second primary tumours with etretinate in squamous cell carcinoma of the oral cavity and oropharynx. Results of a multicentric double-blind randomised study. *Eur J Cancer* 1994;30A: 767–772.
47. Toma S, Bonelli L, Sartoris A, et al. beta-carotene supplementation in patients radically treated for stage I-II head and neck cancer: results of a randomized trial. *Oncol Rep* 2003;10:1895–1901.
48. Mayne ST, Cartmel B, Baum M, et al. Randomized trial of supplemental beta-carotene to prevent second head and neck cancer. *Cancer Res* 2001;61:1457–1463.
49. Bairati I, Meyer F, Jobin E, et al. Antioxidant vitamins supplementation and mortality: a randomized trial in head and neck cancer patients. *Int J Cancer* 2006;119:2221–2224.
50. McLarty JW, Holiday DB, Girard WM, et al. Beta-carotene, vitamin A and lung cancer chemoprevention: results of an intermediate endpoint study. *Am J Clin Nutr* 1995;62:1431S–1438S.
51. Lee JS, Lippman SM, Benner SE, et al. Randomized placebo-controlled trial of isotretinoin in chemoprevention of bronchial squamous metaplasia. *J Clin Oncol* 1994;12:937–945.
52. The Alpha-Tocopherol Beta Carotene Cancer Prevention Study Group. The effect of vitamin E and beta carotene on the incidence of lung cancer and other cancers in male smokers. *N Engl J Med* 1994;330:1029–1035.
53. Omenn GS, Goodman G, Thornquist M, et al. Chemoprevention of lung cancer: the beta-Carotene and Retinol Efficacy Trial (CARET) in high-risk smokers and asbestos-exposed workers. *IARC Sci Publ* 1996;67–85.
54. Hennekens CH, Buring JE, Manson JE, et al. Lack of effect of long-term supplementation with beta carotene on the incidence of malignant neoplasms and cardiovascular disease. *N Engl J Med* 1996;334:1145–1149.
55. Lee IM, Cook NR, Manson JE, et al. Beta-carotene supplementation and incidence of cancer and cardiovascular disease: the Women's Health Study. *J Natl Cancer Inst* 1999;91:2102–2106.
56. Heart Protection Study Collaborative Group. MRC/BHF Heart Protection Study of antioxidant vitamin supplementation in 20,536 high-risk individuals: a randomised placebo-controlled trial. *Lancet* 2002;360:23–33.
57. van Zandwijk N, Dalesio O, Pastorino U, et al. EUROSCAN, a randomized trial of vitamin A and N-acetylcysteine in patients with head and neck cancer or lung cancer. For the European Organization for Research and Treatment of Cancer Head and Neck and Lung Cancer Cooperative Groups. *J Natl Cancer Inst* 2000;92:977–986.
58. Lippman SM, Lee JJ, Karp DD, et al. Randomized phase III intergroup trial of isotretinoin to prevent second primary tumors in stage I non-small-cell lung cancer. *J Natl Cancer Inst* 2001;93:605–618.
59. Mayne ST, Lippman SM. Cigarettes: a smoking gun in cancer chemoprevention. *J Natl Cancer Inst* 2005;97:1319–1321.
60. Veronesi U, De Palo G, Marubini E, et al. Randomized trial of fenretinide to prevent second breast malignancy in women with early breast cancer. *J Natl Cancer Inst* 1999;91:1847–1856.
61. De Palo G, Mariani L, Camerini T, et al. Effect of fenretinide on ovarian carcinoma occurrence. *Gynecol Oncol* 2002;86:24–27.
62. Uray IP, Brown PH. Chemoprevention of hormone receptor-negative breast cancer: new approaches needed. *Recent Results Cancer Res* 2011;188:147–162.
63. Kraemer KH, DiGiovanna JJ, Moshell AN, et al. Prevention of skin cancer in xeroderma pigmentosum with the use of oral isotretinoin. *N Engl J Med* 1988;318:1633–1637.
64. Bouwes Bavinck JN, Tieben LM, Van Der Woude FJ, et al. Prevention of skin cancer and reduction of keratotic skin lesions during acitretin therapy in renal

transplant recipients: a double-blind, placebo-controlled study. *J Clin Oncol* 1995;13:1933–1938.

65. Tangrea JA, Edwards BK, Taylor PR, et al. Long-term therapy with low-dose isotretinoin for prevention of basal cell carcinoma: a multicenter clinical trial Isotretinoin-Basal Cell Carcinoma Study Group. *J Natl Cancer Inst* 1992;84:328–332.

66. Levine N, Moon TE, Cartmel B, et al. Trial of retinol and isotretinoin in skin cancer prevention: a randomized, double-blind, controlled trial. Southwest Skin Cancer Prevention Study Group. *Cancer Epidemiol Biomarkers Prev* 1997;6:957–961.

67. Moon TE, Levine N, Cartmel B, et al. Effect of retinol in preventing squamous cell skin cancer in moderate-risk subjects: a randomized, double-blind, controlled trial. Southwest Skin Cancer Prevention Study Group. *Cancer Epidemiol Biomarkers Prev* 1997;6:949–956.

68. Greenberg ER, Baron JA, Stukel TA, et al. A clinical trial of beta carotene to prevent basal-cell and squamous-cell cancers of the skin. The Skin Cancer Prevention Study Group. *N Engl J Med* 1990;323:789–895.

69. Green A, Williams G, Neale R, et al. Daily sunscreen application and beta-carotene supplementation in prevention of basal-cell and squamous-cell carcinomas of the skin: a randomised controlled trial. *Lancet* 1999;354:723–729.

70. Clark LC, Combs GF Jr, Turnbull BW, et al. Effects of selenium supplementation for cancer prevention in patients with carcinoma of the skin. A randomized controlled trial. Nutritional Prevention of Cancer Study Group. *JAMA* 1996;276:1957–1963.

71. Duffield-Lillico AJ, Slate EH, Reid ME, et al. Nutritional Prevention of Cancer Study Group. Selenium supplementation and secondary prevention of nonmelanoma skin cancer in a randomized trial. *J Natl Cancer Inst* 2003;95:1477–1481.

72. Sabichi AL, Lerner SP, Atkinson EN, et al. Phase III prevention trial of fenretinide in patients with resected non-muscle-invasive bladder cancer. *Clin Cancer Res* 2008;14:224–229.

73. Lamm DL, Riggs DR, Shriver JS, et al. Megadose vitamins in bladder cancer: a double-blind clinical trial. *J Urol* 1994;151:21–26.

74. Meyskens FL Jr, Surwit E, Moon TE, et al. Enhancement of regression of cervical intraepithelial neoplasia II (moderate dysplasia) with topically applied all-trans-retinoic acid: a randomized trial. *J Natl Cancer Inst* 1994;86:539–543.

75. Blot WJ, Li JY, Taylor PR, et al. Nutrition intervention trials in Linxian, China: supplementation with specific vitamin/mineral combinations, cancer incidence, and disease-specific mortality in the general population. *J Natl Cancer Inst* 1993;85:1483–1492.

76. Qiao YL, Dawsey SM, Kamangar F, et al. Total and cancer mortality after supplementation with vitamins and minerals: follow-up of the Linxian General Population Nutrition Intervention Trial. *J Natl Cancer Inst* 2009;101:507–518.

77. Mayne ST, Ferrucci LM, Cartmel B. Lessons learned from randomized clinical trials of micronutrient supplementation for cancer prevention. *Annu Rev Nutr* 2012;32:369–390.

78. Li JY, Taylor PR, Li B, et al. Nutrition intervention trials in Linxian, China: multiple vitamin/mineral supplementation, cancer incidence, and disease-specific mortality among adults with esophageal dysplasia. *J Natl Cancer Inst* 1993;85:1492–1498.

79. Kikendall JW, Mobarhan S, Nelson R, et al. Oral beta carotene does not reduce the recurrence of colorectal adenomas [Abstract]. *Am J Gastroenterol* 1991;36:1356.

80. MacLennan R, Macrae F, Bain C, et al. Randomized trial of intake of fat, fiber, and beta carotene to prevent colorectal adenomas. *J Natl Cancer Inst* 1995;87:1760–1766.

81. Greenberg ER, Baron JA, Tosteson TD, et al. A clinical trial of antioxidant vitamins to prevent colorectal adenoma. Polyp Prevention Study Group. *N Engl J Med* 1994;331:141–147.

82. Baron JA, Cole BF, Mott L, et al. Neoplastic and antineoplastic effects of beta-carotene on colorectal adenoma recurrence: results of a randomized trial. *J Natl Cancer Inst* 2003;95:717–722.

83. Heinonen OP, Albanes D, Virtamo J, et al. Prostate cancer and supplementation with alpha-tocopherol and beta-carotene: incidence and mortality in a controlled trial. *J Natl Cancer Inst* 1998;90:440–446.

84. Lippman SM, Klein EA, Goodman PJ, et al. Effect of selenium and vitamin E on risk of prostate cancer and other cancers: the Selenium and Vitamin E Cancer Prevention Trial (SELECT). *JAMA* 2009;301:39–51.

85. Klein EA, Thompson IM Jr, Tangen CM, et al. Vitamin E and the risk of prostate cancer: the Selenium and Vitamin E Cancer Prevention Trial (SELECT). *JAMA* 2011;306:1549–1556.

86. Gaziano JM, Glynn RJ, Christen WG, et al. Vitamins E and C in the prevention of prostate and total cancer in men: the Physicians' Health Study II randomized controlled trial. *JAMA* 2009;301:52–62.

87. Boileau TW, Liao Z, Kim S, et al. Prostate carcinogenesis in N-methyl-N-nitrosourea (NMU)-testosterone-treated rats fed tomato powder, lycopene, or energy-restricted diets. *J Natl Cancer Inst* 2003;95:1578–1586.

88. Goralczyk R. Beta-carotene and lung cancer in smokers: review of hypotheses and status of research. *Nutr Cancer* 2009;61:767–774.

89. Kristal AR, Darke AK, Morris JS, et al. Baseline Selenium Status and Effects of Selenium and Vitamin E Supplementation on Prostate Cancer Risk. *J Natl Cancer Inst* 2014;106:djt456.

90. Stone JR, Yang S. Hydrogen peroxide: a signaling messenger. *Antioxid Redox Signal* 2006;8:243–270.

91. Finkel T. Signal transduction by reactive oxygen species. *J Cell Biol* 2011;194:7–15.

92. Sayin V, Ibrahim M, Larsson E, et al. Antioxidants accelerate lung cancer progression in mice. *Sci Transl Med* 2014;6:ra15.

93. Mayne ST. Oxidative stress, dietary antioxidant supplements, and health: is the glass half full or half empty? *Cancer Epidemiol Biomarkers Prev* 2013;22:2145–2147.

94. Duthie SJ, Narayanan S, Blum S, et al. Folate deficiency in vitro induces uracil misincorporation and DNA hypomethylation and inhibits DNA excision repair in immortalized normal human colon epithelial cells. *Nutr Cancer* 2000;37:245–251.

95. Blount BC, Mack MM, Wehr CM, et al. Folate deficiency causes uracil misincorporation into human DNA and chromosome breakage: implications for cancer and neuronal damage. *Proc Natl Acad Sci U S A* 1997;94:3290–3295.

96. Giovannucci E. Epidemiologic studies of folate and colorectal neoplasia: a review. *J Nutr* 2002;132:2350S–2355S.

97. White E, Shannon JS, Patterson RE. Relationship between vitamin and calcium supplement use and colon cancer. *Cancer Epidemiol Biomarkers Prev* 1997;6:769–774.

98. Jacobs EJ, Connell CJ, Patel AV, et al. Multivitamin use and colon cancer mortality in the Cancer Prevention Study II cohort (United States). *Cancer Causes Control* 2001;12:927–934.

99. Gibson TM, Weinstein SJ, Pfeiffer RM, et al. Pre- and postfortification intake of folate and risk of colorectal cancer in a large prospective cohort study in the United States. *Am J Clin Nutr* 2011;94:1053–1062.

100. Chen J, Giovannucci E, Kelsey, K, et al. A methylenetetrahydrofolate reductase polymorphism and the risk of colorectal cancer. *Cancer Res* 1996;56:4862–4864.

101. Larsson S, Giovannucci, E, Wolk A. Vitamin B6 intake, alcohol consumption, and colorectal cancer: a longitudinal population-based cohort of women. *Gastroenterology* 2005;128:1830–1837.

102. Wei E, Giovannucci E, Selhub J, et al. Plasma vitamin B6 and the risk of colorectal cancer and adenoma in women. *J Natl Cancer Inst* 2005;97:684–692.

103. Giovannucci E, Rimm EB, Ascherio A, et al. Alcohol, low-methionine-low-folate diets, and risk of colon cancer in men. *J Natl Cancer Inst* 1995;87:265–273.

104. Jaszewski R, Misra S, Tobi M, et al. Folic acid supplementation inhibits recurrence of colorectal adenomas: a randomized chemoprevention trial. *World J Gastroenterol* 2008;14:4492–4498.

105. Paspatis GA, Karamanolis DG. Folate supplementation and adenomatous colonic polyps. *Dis Colon Rectum* 1994;37:1340–1341.

106. Cole BF, Baron JA, Sandler RS, et al. Folic acid for the prevention of colorectal adenomas: a randomized clinical trial. *JAMA* 2007;297:2351–2359.

107. Logan RF, Grainge MJ, Shepherd VC, et al. Aspirin and folic acid for the prevention of recurrent colorectal adenomas. *Gastroenterology* 2008;134:29–38.

108. Wu K, Platz EA, Willett WC, et al. A randomized trial on folic acid supplementation and risk of recurrent colorectal adenoma. *Am J Clin Nutr* 2009;90:1623–1631.

109. Gao Q-Y, Chen H-M, Chen Y-X, et al. Folic acid prevents the initial occurrence of sporadic colorectal adenoma in Chinese older than 50 years of age: a randomized clinical trial. *Cancer prevention research (Phila)* 2013;6:744–752.

110. Ramnath N, Kim S, Christensen PJ. Vitamin D and lung cancer. *Expert Rev Respir Med* 2011;5:305–309.

111. Deeb KK, Trump DL, Johnson CS. Vitamin D signalling pathways in cancer: potential for anticancer therapeutics. *Nat Rev Cancer* 2007;7:684–700.

112. McCullough M, Robertson AS, Rodriguez C, et al. Calcium, vitamin D, dairy products, and risk of colorectal cancer in the cancer prevention study II nutrition cohort (United States). *Cancer Causes Control* 2003;14:1–12.

113. Wu K, Willett WC, Fuchs CS, et al. Calcium intake and risk of colon cancer in women and men. *J Natl Cancer Inst* 2002;94:437–446.

114. Chung M, Balk EM, Brendel M, et al. *Vitamin D and Calcium: A Systematic Review of Health Outcomes.* Evidence Report No. 183 (Prepared by the Tufts Evidence-based Practice Center). Rockville, MD: Agency for Healthcare Research and Quality; 2009.

115. World Health Organization, International Agency for Research on Cancer. Vitamin D and Cancer. Working Group Reports, Volume 5. Lyon, France: IARC; 2008.

116. Stolzenberg-Solomon RZ, Jacobs EJ, Arslan AA, et al. Circulating 25-hydroxyvitamin D and risk of pancreatic cancer: Cohort Consortium Vitamin D Pooling Project of Rarer Cancers. *Am J Epidemiol* 2010;172:81–93.

117. Baron J, Beach M, Mandel JS, et al. Calcium supplements for the prevention of colorectal adenomas. The Calcium Polyp Prevention Study Group. *N Engl J Med* 1999;340:101–107.

118. Bonithon-Kopp C, Kronborg O, Giacosa A, et al. Calcium and fibre supplementation in prevention of colorectal adenoma recurrence: a randomized intervention trial. *Lancet* 2000;356:1300–1306.

119. Wactawski-Wende J, Kotchen JM, Anderson GL, et al. Calcium plus vitamin D supplementation and the risk of colorectal cancer. *N Engl J Med* 2006;354:684–696.

120. Trivedi DP, Doll R, Khaw KT. Effect of four monthly oral vitamin D3 (cholecalciferol) supplementation on fractures and mortality in men and women living in the community: randomised double blind controlled trial. *BMJ* 2003;326:469.

121. Cui Y, Rohan TE. Vitamin D, calcium, and breast cancer risk: a review. *Cancer Epidemiol Biomarkers Prev* 2006;15:1427–1437.

122. Chlebowski RT, Johnson KC, Kooperberg C, et al. Calcium plus vitamin D supplementation and the risk of breast cancer. *J Natl Cancer Inst* 2008;100:1581–1591.

123. Lappe JM, Travers-Gustafson D, Davies KM, et al. Vitamin D and calcium supplementation reduces cancer risk: results of a randomized trial. *Am J Clin Nutr* 2007;85:1586–1591.

124. Manson JE, Bassuk SS, Lee IM, et al. The VITamin D and OmegA-3 TriaL (VITAL): rationale and design of a large randomized controlled trial of vitamin D and marine omega-3 fatty acid supplements for the primary prevention of cancer and cardiovascular disease. *Contemp Clin Trials* 2012;33: 159–171.

125. Wu X, Spitz MR, Lee JJ, et al. Novel susceptibility loci for second primary tumors/recurrence in head and neck cancer patients: large-scale evaluation of genetic variants. *Cancer Prev Res (Phila)* 2009;2:617–624.

126. Platz EA. Is prostate cancer prevention with selenium all in the genes? *Cancer Prev Res (Phila)* 2010;3:576–578.

127. Miller JW, Ulrich CM. Folic acid and cancer—where are we today? *Lancet* 2013;381:974–976.

128. Thun MJ, Henley SJ, Patrono C. Nonsteroidal anti-inflammatory drugs as anti-cancer agents: mechanistic, pharmacologic, and clinical issues. *J Natl Cancer Inst* 2002;94:252–266.

129. Wang D, Mann JR, DuBois RN. The role of prostaglandins and other eico-sanoids in the gastrointestinal tract. *Gastroenterology* 2005;128:1445–1461.

130. Gurpinar E, Grizzle WE, Piazza GA. COX-Independent Mechanisms of Cancer Chemoprevention by Anti-Inflammatory Drugs. *Front Oncol* 2013;3:181.

131. Rothwell PM, Wilson M, Price JF, et al. Effect of daily aspirin on risk of cancer metastasis: a study of incident cancers during randomised controlled trials. *Lancet* 2012;379:1591–1601.

132. Rothwell PM, Price JF, Fowkes FG, et al. Short-term effects of daily aspirin on cancer incidence, mortality, and non-vascular death: analysis of the time course of risks and benefits in 51 randomised controlled trials. *Lancet* 2012;379:1602–1612.

133. Thun MJ, Namboodiri MM, Heath C Jr. Aspirin use and reduced risk of fatal colon cancer. *N Engl J Med* 1991;325:1593–1596.

134. Chan AT, Giovannucci EL, Meyerhardt JA, et al. Aspirin dose and duration of use and risk of colorectal cancer in men. *Gastroenterology* 2008;134:21–28.

135. Chan AT, Giovannucci EL, Meyerhardt JA, et al. Long-term use of aspirin and nonsteroidal anti-inflammatory drugs and risk of colorectal cancer. *JAMA* 2005;294:914–923.

136. Liao LM, Vaughan TL, Corley DA, et al. Nonsteroidal anti-inflammatory drug use reduces risk of adenocarcinomas of the esophagus and esophagogastric junction in a pooled analysis. *Gastroenterology* 2012;142:442–452.

137. Pollard M, Luckert PH. Effect of indomethacin on intestinal tumor induced in rats by the acetate derivative of dimethylnitrosamine. *Science* 1981;214:558–559.

138. Jacoby RF, Marshall DJ, Newton MA, et al. Chemoprevention of spontaneous intestinal adenomas in the Apc Min mouse model by the nonsteroidal anti-inflammatory drug piroxicam. *Cancer Res* 1996;56:710–714.

139. Kawamori T, Rao C, Seibert K, et al. Chemopreventive effect of celecoxib, a specific cyclooxygenase-2 inhibitor on colon carcinogenesis. *Cancer Res* 1998;58:409–412.

140. Oshima M, Dinchuk JE, Kargman SL. Suppression of intestinal polyposis in Apc delta 716 knockout ice by inhibition of cyclooxygenase 2 (COX-2). *Cell* 1996;87:803–809.

141. Anderson WF, Umar A, Viner JL, et al. The role of cyclooxygenase inhibitors in cancer prevention. *Curr Pharm Des* 2002;8:1083–1062.

142. Giardiello FM, Yang VW, Hylind LM, et al. Primary chemoprevention of familial adenomatous polyposis with sulindac. *N Engl J Med* 2002;346:1054–1059.

143. Steinbach G, Lynch PM, Phillips RK. The effect of celecoxib, a cyclooxygenase-2 inhibitor, in familial adenomatous polyposis. *N Engl J Med* 2000;342:1946–1952.

144. Thorson AG, Lynch HT, Smyrk TC. Rectal cancer in FAP patient after sulindac. *Lancet* 1994;343:180.

145. Calaluce R, Earnest DL, Heddens D, et al. Effects of piroxicam on prostaglandin E2 levels in rectal mucosa of adenomatous polyp patients: a randomized phase IIb trial. *Cancer Epidemiol Biomarkers Prev* 2000;9:1287–1292.

146. Ladenheim J, Garcia G, Titzer D, et al. Effects of sulindac on sporadic colonic polyps. *Gastroenterology* 1995;108:1083–1087.

147. Meyskens FL Jr, McLaren CE, Pelot D, et al. Difluoromethylornithine plus sulindac for the prevention of sporadic colorectal adenomas: a randomized placebo-controlled, double-blind trial. *Cancer Prev Res (Phila)* 2008;1:32–38.

148. Arber N, Eagle CJ, Spicak J, et al. Celecoxib for the prevention of colorectal adenomatous polyps. *N Engl J Med* 2006;355:885–895.

149. Bertagnolli MM, Eagle CJ, Zauber AG, et al. Celecoxib for the prevention of sporadic colorectal adenomas. *N Engl J Med* 2006;355:873–884.

150. Baron JA, Sandler RS, Bresalier RS, et al. A randomized trial of rofecoxib for the chemoprevention of colorectal adenomas. *Gastroenterology* 2006;131: 1674–1682.

151. Bresalier RS, Sandler RS, Quan H, et al. Cardiovascular events associated with rofecoxib in a colorectal adenoma chemoprevention trial. *N Engl J Med* 2005; 352:1092–1102.

152. Solomon SD, McMurray JJ, Pfeffer MA, et al. Cardiovascular risk associated with celecoxib in a clinical trial for colorectal adenoma prevention. *N Engl J Med* 2005;352:1071–1080.

153. Rostom A, Dube C, Lewin G, et al. Nonsteroidal anti-inflammatory drugs and cyclooxygenase-2 inhibitors for primary prevention of colorectal cancer: a systematic review prepared for the U.S. Preventive Services Task Force. *Ann Intern Med* 2007;146:376–389.

154. Dube C, Rostom A, Lewin G, et al. The use of aspirin for primary prevention of colorectal cancer: a systematic review prepared for the U.S. Preventive Services Task Force. *Ann Intern Med* 2007;146:365–375.

155. Rothwell PM, Fowkes FG, Belch JF, et al. Effect of daily aspirin on long-term risk of death due to cancer: analysis of individual patient data from randomised trials. *Lancet* 2011;377:31–41.

156. Rothwell PM. Aspirin in prevention of sporadic colorectal cancer: current clinical evidence and overall balance of risks and benefits. *Recent Results Cancer Res* 2013;191:121–142.

157. U.S. Preventive Services Task Force. Routine aspirin or nonsteroidal anti-inflammatory drugs for the primary prevention of colorectal cancer: U.S. Preventive Services Task Force recommendation statement. *Ann Intern Med* 2007; 146:361–364.

158. Mulshine JL, Atkinson JC, Greer RO, et al. Randomized, double-blind, placebo-controlled phase IIb trial of the cyclooxygenase inhibitor ketorolac as an oral rinse in oropharyngeal leukoplakia. *Clin Cancer Res* 2004;10:1565–1573.

159. Mao JT, Fishbein MC, Adams B, et al. Celecoxib decreases Ki-67 proliferative index in active smokers. *Clin Cancer Res* 2006;12:314–320.

160. Bord S, Horner A, Beavan S, et al. Estrogen receptors alpha and beta are differentially expressed in developing human bone. *J Clin Endocrinol Metab* 2001;86:2309–2314.

161. Kuiper GG, Carlsson B, Grandien K, et al. Comparison of the ligand binding specificity and transcript tissue distribution of estrogen receptors alpha and beta. *Endocrinology* 1997;138:863–870.

162. Fabian CJ, Kimler BF. Selective estrogen-receptor modulators for primary prevention of breast cancer. *J Clin Oncol* 2005;23:1644–1655.

163. Jordan VC. SERMs: meeting the promise of multifunctional medicines. *J Natl Cancer Inst* 2007;99:350–356.

164. Jordan VC. Tamoxifen (ICI46,474) as a targeted therapy to treat and prevent breast cancer. *Br J Pharmacol* 2006;147:S269–S276.

165. Jordan VC. Effect of tamoxifen (ICI 46,474) on initiation and growth of DM-BA-induced rat mammary carcinomata. *Eur J Cancer* 1976;12:419–424.

166. Jordan VC. Chemoprevention of breast cancer with selective oestrogen-receptor modulators. *Nat Rev Cancer* 2007;7:46–53.

167. Cuzick J, Baum M. Tamoxifen and contralateral breast cancer. *Lancet* 1985;2:282.

168. Fisher B, Redmond C. New perspective on cancer of the contralateral breast: a marker for assessing tamoxifen as a preventive agent. *J Natl Cancer Inst* 1991;83:1278–1280.

169. Ettinger B, Black DM, Mitlak BH, et al. Reduction of vertebral fracture risk in postmenopausal women with osteoporosis treated with raloxifene: results from a 3-year randomized clinical trial. Multiple Outcomes of Raloxifene Evaluation (MORE) Investigators. *JAMA* 1999;282:637–645.

170. LaCroix AZ, Powles T, Osborne CK, et al. Breast cancer incidence in the randomized PEARL trial of lasofoxifene in postmenopausal osteoporotic women. *J Natl Cancer Inst* 2010;102:1706–1715.

171. Cummings SR, Ensrud K, Delmas PD, et al. Lasofoxifene in postmenopausal women with osteoporosis. *N Engl J Med* 2010;362:686–696.

172. Cummings SR, McClung M, Reginster JY, et al. Arzoxifene for prevention of fractures and invasive breast cancer in postmenopausal women. *J Bone Miner Res* 2011;26:397–404.

173. Powles TJ, Diem SJ, Fabian CJ, et al. Breast cancer incidence in postmenopausal women with osteoporosis or low bone mass using arzoxifene. *Breast Cancer Res Treat* 2012;134:299–306.

174. Nelson HD, Smith ME, Griffin JC, et al. Use of medications to reduce risk for primary breast cancer: a systematic review for the U.S. Preventive Services Task Force. *Ann Intern Med* 2013;158:604–614.

175. Moyer VA. Medications for risk reduction of primary breast cancer in women: U.S. Preventive Services Task Force recommendation statement. *Ann Intern Med* 2013;159:698-708.

176. Visvanathan K, Hurley P, Bantug E, et al. Use of pharmacologic interventions for breast cancer risk reduction: American Society of Clinical Oncology clinical practice guideline. *J Clin Oncol* 2013;31:2942–2962.

177. Vogel VG, Costantino JP, Wickerham DL, et al. Carcinoma in situ outcomes in National Surgical Adjuvant Breast and Bowel Project Breast Cancer Chemoprevention Trials. *J Natl Cancer Inst Monogr* 2010;2010:181–186.

178. Cuzick J, Sestak I, Bonanni B, et al. Selective oestrogen receptor modulators in prevention of breast cancer: an updated meta-analysis of individual participant data. *Lancet* 2013;381:1827–1834.

179. Barrett-Connor E, Mosca L, Collins P, et al. Effects of raloxifene on cardiovascular events and breast cancer in postmenopausal women. *N Engl J Med* 2006;355:125–137.

180. Snyder KR, Sparano N, Malinowski JM. Raloxifene hydrochloride. *Am J Health Syst Pharm* 2000;57:1669–1675.

181. Goss PE, Ingle JN, Martino S, et al. A randomized trial of letrozole in post-menopausal women after five years of tamoxifen therapy for early-stage breast cancer. *N Engl J Med* 2003;349:1793–1802.

182. Fabian CJ, Kimler BF, Zalles CM, et al. Reduction in proliferation with six months of letrozole in women on hormone replacement therapy. *Breast Cancer Res Treat* 2007;106:75–84.

183. Goss PE, Ingle JN, Ales-Martinez JE, et al. Exemestane for breast-cancer prevention in postmenopausal women. *N Engl J Med* 2011;364:2381–2391.

184. Cheung AM, Tile L, Cardew S, et al. Bone density and structure in healthy postmenopausal women treated with exemestane for the primary prevention of breast cancer: a nested substudy of the MAP.3 randomised controlled trial. *Lancet Oncol* 2012;13:275–284.

185. Cuzick J, Sestak I, Forbes JF, et al. Anastrozole for prevention of breast cancer in high-risk postmenopausal women (IBIS-II): an international, double-blind, randomised placebo-controlled trial. *Lancet* 2014;383:1041–1048.

186. Waters EA, McNeel TS, Stevens WM, et al. Use of tamoxifen and raloxifene for breast cancer chemoprevention in 2010. *Breast Cancer Res Treat* 2012;134:875–880.

187. King MC, Wieand S, Hale K, et al. Tamoxifen and breast cancer incidence among women with inherited mutations in BRCA1 and BRCA2: National Surgical Adjuvant Breast and Bowel Project (NSABP-P1) Breast Cancer Prevention Trial. *JAMA* 2001;286:2251–2256.

188. Gronwald J, Tung N, Foulkes WD, et al. Tamoxifen and contralateral breast cancer in BRCA1 and BRCA2 carriers: an update. *Int J Cancer* 2006; 118:2281–2284.

189. Hess-Wilson JK, Knudsen KE. Endocrine disrupting compounds and prostate cancer. *Cancer Lett* 2006;241:1–12.

190. Andriole G, Bostwick D, Civantos F, et al. The effects of 5alpha-reductase inhibitors on the natural history, detection and grading of prostate cancer: current state of knowledge. *J Urol* 2005;174:2098–2104.

191. Thompson IM, Tangen CM, Goodman PJ, et al. Chemoprevention of prostate cancer. *J Urol* 2009;182:499–507.

192. Andriole GL, Bostwick DG, Brawley OW, et al. Effect of dutasteride on the risk of prostate cancer. *N Engl J Med* 2010;362:1192–1202.

193. Thompson IM Jr, Goodman PJ, Tangen CM, et al. Long-term survival of participants in the prostate cancer prevention trial. *N Engl J Med* 2013;369: 603–610.

194. Gerner EW, Meyskens FL Jr. Polyamines and cancer: old molecules, new understanding. *Nat Rev Cancer* 2004;4:781–792.

195. Meyskens FL Jr, Gerner EW. Development of difluoromethylornithine (DFMO) as a chemoprevention agent. *Clin Cancer Res* 1999;5:945–951.

196. Love R, Carbone P, Verma A, et al. Randomized phase I chemoprevention dose seeking study of alpha-difluoromethylornithine. *J Natl Cancer Inst* 1993;85: 732–737.

197. Alberts DS, Dorr RT, Einspahr JG, et al. Chemoprevention of human actinic keratoses by topical 2-(difluoromethyl)-dl-ornithine. *Cancer Epidemiol Biomarkers Prev* 2000;9:1281–1286.

198. Meyskens FL Jr, Surwit E, Moon TE, et al. Enhancement of regression of cervical intraepithelial neoplasia II (moderate dysplasia) with topically applied all-trans-retinoic acid: randomized trial. *J Natl Cancer Inst* 1994;86: 539–543.

199. Fabian CJ, Kimler BF, Brady DA, et al. A phase II breast cancer chemoprevention trial of oral alpha-difluoromethylornithine: breast tissue, imaging, and serum and urine biomarkers. *Clin Cancer Res* 2002;8:3105–3117.

200. Jeter JM, Alberts DS. Difluoromethylornithine: the proof is in the polyamines. *Cancer Prev Res (Phila)* 2012;5:1341–1344.

201. Gronich N, Rennert G. Beyond aspirin-cancer prevention with statins, metformin and bisphosphonates. *Nat Rev Clin Oncol* 2013;10:625–642.

202. Moyad MA. Why a statin and/or another proven heart healthy agent should be utilized in the next major cancer chemoprevention trial: part II. *Urologic Oncol* 2004;22:472–477.

203. Bertagnolli MM, Hsu M, Hawk ET, et al. Statin use and colorectal adenoma risk: results from the adenoma prevention with celecoxib trial. *Cancer Prev Res (Phila)* 2010;3:588–596.

204. Simon MS, Rosenberg CA, Rodabough RJ, et al. Prospective analysis of association between use of statins or other lipid-lowering agents and colorectal cancer risk. *Ann Epidemiol* 2012;22:17–27.

205. Platz EA, Leitzmann MF, Visvanathan K, et al. Statin drugs and risk of advanced prostate cancer. *J Natl Cancer Inst* 2006;98:1819–1825.

206. Eliassen AH, Colditz GA, Rosner B, et al. Serum lipids, lipid-lowering drugs, and the risk of breast cancer. *Arch Intern Med* 2005;165:2264–2271.

207. Lipkin SM, Chao EC, Moreno V, et al. Genetic variation in 3-hydroxy-3-methylglutaryl CoA reductase modifies the chemopreventive activity of statins for colorectal cancer. *Cancer Prev Res (Phila)* 2010;3:597–603.

208. Rennert G. Bisphosphonates: beyond prevention of bone metastases. *J Natl Cancer Inst* 2011;103:1728–1729.

209. Rennert G, Pinchev M, Rennert HS. Use of bisphosphonates and risk of postmenopausal breast cancer. *J Clin Oncol* 2010;28:3577–3581.

210. Chlebowski RT, Chen Z, Cauley JA, et al. Oral bisphosphonate use and breast cancer incidence in postmenopausal women. *J Clin Oncol* 2010;28: 3582–3590.

211. Monsees GM, Malone KE, Tang MT, et al. Bisphosphonate use after estrogen receptor-positive breast cancer and risk of contralateral breast cancer. *J Natl Cancer Inst* 2011;103:1752–1760.

212. Kirpichnikov D, McFarlane SI, Sowers JR. Metformin: an update. *Ann Intern Med* 2002;137:25–33.

213. Pollack MN. Insulin, insulin-like growth factors, insulin resistance, and neoplasia. *Am J Clin Nutr* 2007;86:s820–s822.

214. Evans JM, Donnelly LA, Emslie-Smith AM, et al. Metformin and reduced risk of cancer in diabetic patients. *BMJ* 2005;330:1304–1305.

215. Zhu P, Davis M, Blackwelder A, et al. Metformin selectively targets tumor initiating cells in erbB-2 overexpressing breast cancer models. *Cancer Prev Res (Phila)* 2014;7:199–210.

216. Lonardo E, Cioffi M, Sancho P, et al. Metformin targets the metabolic achilles heel of human pancreatic cancer stem cells. *PLoS One* 2013;8:e76518.

217. Grubbs C, Clapper M, Reid J, et al. *Metformin Promotes Tumorigenesis in Animal Models of Cancer Prevention.* Washington, DC: American Association for Cancer Research; 2013.

218. Chlebowski RT, McTiernan A, Wactawski-Wende J, et al. Diabetes, metformin, and breast cancer in postmenopausal women. *J Clin Oncol* 2012;30: 2844–2852.

219. Heger M, van Golen RF, Broekgaarden M, et al. The molecular basis for the pharmacokinetics and pharmacodynamics of curcumin and its metabolites in relation to cancer. *Pharmacol Rev* 2014;66:222–307.

220. Whitlock NC, Baek SJ. The anticancer effects of resveratrol: modulation of transcription factors. *Nutr Cancer* 2012;64:493–502.

221. Lambert JD. Does tea prevent cancer? Evidence from laboratory and human intervention studies. *Am J Clin Nutr* 2013;98:1667S–1675S.

222. Kakarala M, Brenner DE, Korkaya H, et al. Targeting breast stem cells with the cancer preventive compounds curcumin and piperine. *Breast Cancer Res Treat* 2010;122:777–785.

223. Norris L, Karmokar A, Howells L, et al. The role of cancer stem cells in the anti-carcinogenicity of curcumin. *Mol Nutr Food Res* 2013;57:1630–1637.

224. Zou H, Yuan C, Dong L, et al. Human cyclooxygenase-1 activity and its responses to COX inhibitors are allosterically regulated by nonsubstrate fatty acids. *J Lipid Res* 2012;53:1336–1347.

225. Wada M, Delong CJ, Hong YH, et al. Enzymes and receptors of prostaglandin pathways with arachidonic acid- vs. eicosapentaenoic acid-derived substrates and products. *J Biol Chem* 2007;282:22254–22266.

226. Laviano A, Rianda S, Molfino A, et al. Omega-3 fatty acids in cancer. *Curr Opin Clin Nutr Metab Care* 2013;16:156–161.

227. Cockbain AJ, Toogood GJ, Hull MA. Omega-3 polyunsaturated fatty acids for the treatment and prevention of colorectal cancer. *Gut* 2012;61:135–149.

228. Stoner GD, Wang LS, Casto BC. Laboratory and clinical studies of cancer chemoprevention by antioxidants in berries. *Carcinogenesis* 2008;29:1665–1674.

229. Wang LS, Dombkowski AA, Seguin C, et al. Mechanistic basis for the chemopreventive effects of black raspberries at a late stage of rat esophageal carcinogenesis. *Mol Carcinog* 2011;50:291–300.

230. Wang LS, Kuo CT, Stoner K, et al. Dietary black raspberries modulate DNA methylation in dextran sodium sulfate (DSS)-induced ulcerative colitis. *Carcinogenesis* 2013;34:2842–2850.

231. Ireson C, Orr S, Jones DJ, et al. Characterization of metabolites of the chemopreventive agent curcumin in human and rat hepatocytes and in the rat in vivo, and evaluation of their ability to inhibit phorbol ester-induced prostaglandin E2 production. *Cancer Res* 2001;61:1058–1064.

232. Ireson CR, Jones DJ, Orr S, et al. Metabolism of the cancer chemopreventive agent curcumin in human and rat intestine. *Cancer Epidemiol Biomarkers Prev* 2002;11:105–111.

233. Vareed SK, Kakarala M, Ruffin MT, et al. Pharmacokinetics of curcumin conjugate metabolites in healthy human subjects. *Cancer Epidemiol Biomarkers Prev* 2008;17:1411–1417.

234. Gescher A, Steward WP, Brown K. Resveratrol in the management of human cancer: how strong is the clinical evidence? *Ann N Y Acad Sci* 2013;1290:12–20.

235. Stoner GD. Ginger: is it ready for prime time? *Cancer Prev Res (Phila)* 2013;6:257–262.

236. Stoner GD, Wang LS. Chemoprevention of esophageal squamous cell carcinoma with berries. *Top Curr Chem* 2013;329:1–20.

237. Mallery SR, Zwick JC, Pei P, et al. Topical application of a bioadhesive black raspberry gel modulates gene expression and reduces cyclooxygenase 2 protein in human premalignant oral lesions. *Cancer Res* 2008;68:4945–4957.

238. Carroll RE, Benya RV, Turgeon DK, et al. Phase IIa clinical trial of curcumin for the prevention of colorectal neoplasia. *Cancer Prev Res (Phila)* 2011;4: 354–364.

239. Seeff LB, Hoofnagle JH. Epidemiology of hepatocellular carcinoma in areas of low hepatitis B and hepatitis C endemicity. *Oncogene* 2006;25:3771–3777.

240. Fox JG, Wang TC. Inflammation, atrophy, and gastric cancer. *J Clin Invest* 2007;117:60–69.

241. Saslow D, Castle PE, Cox JT, et al. American Cancer Society Guideline for human papillomavirus (HPV) vaccine use to prevent cervical cancer and its precursors. *CA Cancer J Clin* 2007;57:7–28.

242. Mohanna S, Maco V, Bravo F, et al. Epidemiology and clinical characteristics of classic Kaposi's sarcoma, seroprevalence, and variants of human herpesvirus 8 in South America: a critical review of an old disease. *Int J Infect Dis* 2005;9:239–250.

243. Castillo JJ, Reagan JL, Bishop KD, et al. Viral lymphomagenesis: from pathophysiology to the rationale for novel therapies. *Br J Haematol* 2014;165: 300–315.

244. Al-Bahrani R, Abuetabh Y, Zeitouni N, et al. Cholangiocarcinoma: risk factors, environmental influences and oncogenesis. *Ann Clin Lab Sci* 2013;43: 195–210.

245. Mostafa MH, Sheweita SA, O'Connor PJ. Relationship between schistosomiasis and bladder cancer. *Clin Microbiol Rev* 1999;12:97–111.

246. Zivny J, Wang TC, Yantiss R, et al. Role of therapy or monitoring in preventing progression to gastric cancer. *J Clin Gastroenterol* 2003;36:S50–S60.

247. Correa P, Fontham ET, Bravo JC, et al. Chemoprevention of gastric dysplasia: randomized trial of antioxidant supplements and anti-helicobacter pylori therapy. *J Natl Cancer Inst* 2000;92:1881–1888.

248. Wong BC, Zhang L, Ma JL, et al. Effects of selective COX-2 inhibitor and Helicobacter pylori eradication on precancerous gastric lesions. *Gut* 2012;61:812–818.

249. Ma JL, Zhang L, Brown LM, et al. Fifteen-year effects of Helicobacter pylori, garlic, and vitamin treatments on gastric cancer incidence and mortality. *J Natl Cancer Inst* 2012;104:488–492.

250. Risch HA, Lu L, Kidd MS, et al. Helicobacter pylori seropositivities and risk of pancreatic carcinoma. *Cancer Epidemiol Biomarkers Prev* 2014;23: 172–178.

251. Mazzoleni LE, Francesconi CF, Sander GB. Mass eradication of *Helicobacter pylori*: feasible and advisable? *Lancet* 2011;378:462–464.

252. Whiteman DC, Parmar P, Fahey P, et al. Association of Helicobacter pylori infection with reduced risk for esophageal cancer is independent of environmental and genetic modifiers. *Gastroenterology* 2010;139:73–83.

253. Torrance CJ, Jackson PE, Montgomery E, et al. Combinatorial chemoprevention of intestinal neoplasia. *Nat Med* 2000;6:1024–1028.

254. Reddy BS, Wang CX, Kong AN, et al. Prevention of azoxymethane-induced colon cancer by combination of low doses of atorvastatin, aspirin, and celecoxib in F 344 rats. *Cancer Res* 2006;66:4542–4546.

255. Zell JA, Pelot D, Chen WP, et al. Risk of cardiovascular events in a randomized placebo-controlled, double-blind trial of difluoromethylornithine plus sulindac for the prevention of sporadic colorectal adenomas. *Cancer Prev Res (Phila)* 2009;2:209–212.

256. Guerrieri-Gonzaga A, Robertson C, Bonanni B, et al. Preliminary results on safety and activity of a randomized, double-blind, 2 x 2 trial of low-dose tamoxifen and fenretinide for breast cancer prevention in premenopausal women. *J Clin Oncol* 2006;24:129–135.

257. Kelloff GJ, Lippman SM, Dannenberg AJ, et al. Progress in chemoprevention drug development: the promise of molecular biomarkers for prevention of intraepithelial neoplasia and cancer—a plan to move forward. *Clin Cancer Res* 2006;12:3661–3697.

258. Washington MK, Powell AE, Sullivan R, et al. Pathology of rodent models of intestinal cancer: progress report and recommendations. *Gastroenterology* 2013;144:705–717.

259. Nandan MO, Yang VW. Genetic and chemical models of colorectal cancer in mice. *Curr Colorectal Cancer Rep* 2010;6:51–59.

260. Kwon MC, Berns A. Mouse models for lung cancer. *Mol Oncol* 2013;7:165–177.

261. Kirma NB, Tekmal RR. Transgenic mouse models of hormonal mammary carcinogenesis: advantages and limitations. *J Steroid Biochem Mol Biol* 2012;131:76–82.

262. Irshad S, Abate-Shen C. Modeling prostate cancer in mice: something old, something new, something premalignant, something metastatic. *Cancer Metastasis Rev* 2013;32:109–122.

263. Herreros-Villanueva M, Hijona E, Cosme A, et al. Mouse models of pancreatic cancer. *World J Gastroenterol* 2012;18:1286–1294.

264. Winawer SJ, Zauber AG, Ho MN, et al. Prevention of colorectal cancer by colonoscopic polypectomy. The National Polyp Study Workgroup. *N Engl J Med* 1993;329:1977–1981.

265. Spechler S. Barrett's esophagus. *Semin Oncol* 1994;21:431–437.

266. Shen O, Liu S, Dawsey S, et al. Cytologic screening for esophageal cancer: results from 12,877 subjects from a high risk population in China. *Int J Cancer* 1993;54:185–188.

267. Taylor P, Li B, Dawsey S, et al. Prevention of esophageal cancer: the nutrition intervention trials in Linxian, China. Linxian Nutrition Intervention Trials Study Group. *Cancer Res* 1994;54:2029s–2031s.

268. Sober A, Burstein J. Precursors to skin cancer. *Cancer* 1995;75:645–650.

269. Tucker M, Halpern A, Holly E, et al. Clinically recognized dysplastic nevi. A central risk factor for cutaneous melanoma. *JAMA* 1997;277:1439–1444.

270. Gustafsson L, Adami H-O. Natural history of cervical neoplasia: consistent results obtained by an identification technique. *Br J Cancer* 1989;60:132–137.

271. Cawson R. Premalignant lesions in the mouth. *Br Med Bull* 1975;31:164–180.

272. Zhou M. Intraductal carcinoma of the prostate: the whole story. *Pathology* 2013; 45:533–539.

273. Saccomanno G, Archer VE, Auerbach O, et al. Development of carcinoma of the lung as reflected in exfoliated cells. *Cancer* 1974;33:256–270.

274. Cooper CL, O'Toole SA, Kench JG. Classification, morphology and molecular pathology of premalignant lesions of the pancreas. *Pathology* 2013;45:286–304.

275. Brewster AM, Lee JJ, Clayman GL, et al. Randomized trial of adjuvant 13-cis-retinoic acid and interferon alfa for patients with aggressive skin squamous cell carcinoma. *J Clin Oncol* 2007;25:1974–1978.

276. Karp DD, Lee SJ, Keller SM, et al. Randomized, double-blind, placebo-controlled, phase III chemoprevention trial of selenium supplementation in patients with resected stage I non-small-cell lung cancer: ECOG 5597. *J Clin Oncol* 2013;31:4179–4187.

277. Labayle D, Fischer D, Vielh P. Sulindac causes regression of rectal polyps in familial adenomatous polyposis. *Gastroenterology* 1991;101:635–639.

278. Giardiello FM, Hamilton SR, Krush AJ, et al. Treatment of colonic and rectal adenomas with sulindac in familial adenomatous polyposis. *N Engl J Med* 1993;328:1313–1316.

279. Nugent KP, Farmer KC, Sipgelman AD, et al. Randomized controlled trial of the effect of sulindac on duodenal and rectal polyposis and cell proliferation in patients with familial adenomatous polyposis. *Br J Surg* 1993;80:1618–1619.

280. Mathers JC, Movahedi M, Macrae F, et al. Long-term effect of resistant starch on cancer risk in carriers of hereditary colorectal cancer: an analysis from the CAPP2 randomised controlled trial. *Lancet Oncol* 2012;13:1242–1249.

281. Burn J, Gerdes AM, Macrae F, et al. Long-term effect of aspirin on cancer risk in carriers of hereditary colorectal cancer: an analysis from the CAPP2 randomised controlled trial. *Lancet* 2011;378:2081–2087.

282. Ruffin MT, Krishnan K, Rock CL, et al. Suppression of human colorectal mucosal prostaglandins: determining the lowest effective aspirin dose. *J Natl Cancer Inst* 1997;89:1152–1160.

283. Krishnan K, Ruffin MT, Normolle D, et al. Colonic mucosal prostaglandin E2 and cyclooxygenase expression before and after low aspirin doses in subjects at high risk or at normal risk for colorectal cancer. *Cancer Epidemiol Biomarkers Prev* 2001;10:447–453.

284. Sample D, Wargovich M, Fischer SM, et al. A dose-finding study of aspirin for chemoprevention utilizing rectal mucosal prostaglandin E(2) levels as a biomarker. *Cancer Epidemiol Biomarkers Prev* 2002;11:275–279.

285. Sandler RS, Halabi S, Baron JA, et al. A randomized trial of aspirin to prevent colorectal adenomas in patients with previous colorectal cancer. *N Engl J Med* 2003;348:883–890.

286. Baron JA, Cole BF, Sandler RS, et al. A randomized trial of aspirin to prevent colorectal adenomas. *N Engl J Med* 2003;348:891–899.

287. Fisher B, Costantino JP, Wickerham DL, et al. Tamoxifen for the prevention of breast cancer: current status of the National Surgical Adjuvant Breast and Bowel Project P-1 study. *J Natl Cancer Inst* 2005;97:1652–1662.

288. Cuzick J, Forbes JF, Sestak I, et al. Long-term results of tamoxifen prophylaxis for breast cancer—96-month follow-up of the randomized IBIS-I trial. *J Natl Cancer Inst* 2007;99:272–282.

289. Powles TJ, Ashley S, Tidy A, et al. Twenty-year follow-up of the Royal Marsden randomized, double-blinded tamoxifen breast cancer prevention trial. *J Natl Cancer Inst* 2007;99:283–290.

290. Veronesi U, Maisonneuve P, Rotmensz N, et al. Tamoxifen for the prevention of breast cancer: Late results of the Italian randomzied tamoxifen prevention trial among women with hysterectomy. *J Natl Cancer Inst* 2007;99:727–737.

291. Cauley JA, Norton L, Lippman ME, et al. Continued breast cancer risk reduction in postmenopausal women treated with raloxifene: 4-year results from the MORE trial. Multiple outcomes of raloxifene evaluation. *Breast Cancer Res Treat* 2001;65:125–134.

292. Martino S, Cauley JA, Barrett-Connor E, et al. Continuing outcomes relevant to Evista: breast cancer incidence in postmenopausal osteoporotic women in a randomized trial of raloxifene. *J Natl Cancer Inst* 2004;96:1751–1761.

293. Messing E, Kim KM, Sharkey F, et al. Randomized prospective phase III trial of difluoromethylornithine vs placebo in preventing recurrence of completely resected low risk superficial bladder cancer. *J Urol* 2006;176:500–504.

294. Simoneau AR, Gerner EW, Nagle R, et al. The effect of difluoromethylornithine on decreasing prostate size and polyamines in men: results of a year-long phase IIb randomized placebo-controlled chemoprevention trial. *Cancer Epidemiol Biomarkers Prev* 2008;17:292–299.

295. Bailey HH, Kim K, Verma AK, et al. A randomized, double-blind, placebo-controlled phase 3 skin cancer prevention study of {alpha}-difluoromethyl-ornithine in subjects with previous history of skin cancer. *Cancer Prev Res (Phila)* 2010;3:35–47.

296. Kreul SM, Havighurst T, Kim K, et al. A phase III skin cancer chemoprevention study of DFMO: long-term follow-up of skin cancer events and toxicity. *Cancer Prev Res (Phila)* 2012;5:1368–1374.

297. Zick SM, Ruffin MT, Djuric Z, et al. Quantitation of 6-, 8- and 10-gingerols and 6-shogaol in human plasma by high-performance liquid chromatography with electrochemical detection. *Int J Biomed Sci* 2010;6:233–240.

298. Zick SM, Turgeon DK, Vareed SK, et al. Phase II study of the effects of ginger root extract on eicosanoids in colon mucosa in people at normal risk for colorectal cancer. *Cancer Prev Res (Phila)* 2011;4:1929–1937.

299. Hull MA. Nutritional agents with anti-inflammatory properties in chemoprevention of colorectal neoplasia. *Recent Results Cancer Res* 2013;191:143–156.

300. Nelson WG, De Marzo AM, Isaacs WB. Prostate cancer. *N Engl J Med* 2003;349:366–381.

301. von Knobloch R, Konrad L, Barth PJ, et al. Genetic pathways and new progression markers for prostate cancer suggested by microsatellite allelotyping. *Clin Cancer Res* 2004;10:1064–1073.

302. Palapattu GS, Sutcliffe S, Bastian PJ, et al. Prostate carcinogenesis and inflammation: emerging insights. *Carcinogenesis* 2005;26:1170–1181.

303. Dontu G, Liu S, Wicha MS. Stem cells in mammary development and carcinogenesis: implications for prevention and treatment. *Stem Cell Rev* 2005;1:207–213.

304. Liu S, Dontu G, Mantle ID, et al. Hedgehog signaling and Bmi-1 regulate self-renewal of normal and malignant human mammary stem cells. *Cancer Res* 2006;66:6063–6071.

305. Wistuba II, Lam S, Behrens C, et al. Molecular damage in the bronchial epithelium of current and former smokers. *J Natl Cancer Inst* 1997;89:1366–1373.

306. Massion PP, Carbone DP. The molecular basis of lung cancer: molecular abnormalities and therapeutic implications. *Respir Res* 2003;4:12.

307. Mao C, Koutsky LA, Ault KA, et al. Efficacy of human papillomavirus-16 vaccine to prevent cervical intraepithelial neoplasia: a randomized controlled trial. *Obstet Gynecol* 2006;107:18–27.

308. Califano J, van der Riet P, Westra W, et al. Genetic progression model for head and neck cancer: implications for field cancerization. *Cancer Res* 1996;56:2488–2492.

309. Califano J, Westra WH, Meininger G, et al. Genetic progression and clonal relationship of recurrent premalignant head and neck lesions. *Clin Cancer Res* 2000;6:347–352.

310. Braakhuis BJ, Tabor MP, Kummer JA, et al. A genetic explanation of Slaughter's concept of field cancerization: evidence and clinical implications. *Cancer Res* 2003;63:1727–1730.

311. Ha PK, Benoit NE, Yochem R, et al. A transcriptional progression model for head and neck cancer. *Clin Cancer Res* 2003;9:3058–3064.

312. Barrett MT, Sanchez CA, Prevo LJ, et al. Evolution of neoplastic cell lineages in Barrett oesophagus. *Nat Genet* 1999;22:106–109.

313. Reid BJ, Levine DS, Longton G, et al. Predictors of progression to cancer in Barrett's esophagus: baseline histology and flow cytometry identify low- and high-risk patient subsets. *Am J Gastroenterol* 2000;95:1669–1676.

314. Thorgeirsson SS, Grisham JW. Molecular pathogenesis of human hepatocellular carcinoma. *Nat Genet* 2002;31:339–346.

34 Cancer Screening

Otis W. Brawley and Howard L. Parnes

INTRODUCTION

Cancer screening refers to a test or examination performed on an asymptomatic individual. The goal is not simply to find cancer at an early stage, nor is it to diagnose as many patients with cancer as possible. The goal of cancer screening is to prevent death and suffering from the disease in question through early therapeutic intervention.

The assumption that early detection improves outcomes can be traced back to the concept that cancer inexorably progresses from a small, localized, primary tumor to local–regional spread, to distant metastases and death. This linear model of disease progression predicts that early intervention would reduce cancer mortality.

Cancer screening was an element of the "periodic physical examination," as espoused by the American Medical Association in the 1920s.[1] It consisted of palpation to find a mass or enlarged lymph nodes and auscultation to find a rub or abnormal sound. Today, screening has grown to include radiologic testing, the measurement of serum markers of disease, and even molecular testing. A positive screening test leads to further diagnostic testing, which might lead to a cancer diagnosis.

The intuitive appeal of early detection accounts for the emphasis that has long been placed on screening. However, it is not widely understood that screening tests are always associated with some harm (e.g., anxiety, financial costs) and may actually cause substantial harm (e.g., invasive follow-up diagnostic or therapeutic procedures). Because screening is, by definition, done in healthy people, all early detection tests should be carefully studied and their risk–benefit ratio determined before they are adopted for widespread usage.

Screening is a public health intervention. However, some draw a distinction between screening an individual within the doctor–patient relationship and mass screening, a program aimed at screening a large population. The latter may involve advertising campaigns to encourage people to be screened for a particular cancer at a shopping mall or at a community event, such as state fair.

Screening may be either *opportunistic* (i.e., a patient sees a health-care provider who chooses to screen or not to screen) or *programmatic*. Programmatic refers to a standardized approach with algorithms for screening and follow-up as well as recall of patients for regular routine screening with quality control measures. Programmatic screening is usually more effective.

PERFORMANCE CHARACTERISTICS

The degree to which a screening test can discriminate between individuals with and without a particular disease is described by its performance characteristics. These include the a test's sensitivity, specificity, positive predictive value (PPV), and negative predictive value (NPV) (Table 34.1). It should be noted that these measures relate to the accuracy of a screening test; they do not provide any information regarding a test's efficacy or effectiveness.

- Sensitivity is the proportion of persons designated positive by the screening test among all individuals who have the disease: true positive (TP)/(TP + false negative [FN]).
- Specificity is the proportion of persons designated negative by the screening test among all individuals who do not have the disease: true negative TN/(TN + false positive [FP]).
- Positive predictive value is the proportion of individuals with a positive screening test who have the disease: (TP)/(TP + FP).
- Negative predictive value is the proportion of individuals with a negative screening test who do not have the disease: (TN)/(TN + false negative [FN]).[2]

For a given screening test, sensitivity and specificity are inversely related. For example, as one lowers the threshold for considering a serum prostate-specific antigen (PSA) level to represent a *positive* screen, the sensitivity of the test increases and more cancers will be detected. This increased sensitivity comes at the cost of decreased specificity (i.e., more men without cancer will have *positive* screenings tests and, therefore, will be subjected to unnecessary diagnostic procedures).

Some screening tests, such as mammograms, are more subjective and operator dependent than others. For this reason, the sensitivity and specificity of screening mammography varies among radiologists. For a given radiologist, the lower his or her threshold for considering a mammogram to be suspicious, the higher the sensitivity and lower the specificity will be for them. However, mammography can have both a higher sensitivity and higher specificity in the hands of a more experienced versus a less experienced radiologist.

As opposed to sensitivity and specificity, the PPV and NPV of a screening test are dependent on disease prevalence. PPV is also highly responsive to small increases in specificity. As shown in Table 34.2, given a disease prevalence of 5 cases per 1,000 (0.005), the PPV of a hypothetical screening test increases dramatically as specificity goes from 95% to 99.9%, but only marginally as sensitivity goes from 80% to 95%. Given a disease prevalence of only 1 per 10,000 (0.0001), the PPV of the same test is poor even at high sensitivity and specificity. The positive association between breast cancer prevalence and age is the major reason why screening mammography is a better test (higher PPV) for women aged 50 to 59 than for women 40 to 49 years of age.

ASSESSING SCREENING TESTS AND OUTCOMES

Screening Test Results

Lead time bias occurs whenever screening results in an earlier diagnosis than would have occurred in the absence of screening.

TABLE 34.1

Performance Characteristics of a Screening Test

Sensitivity is the proportion designated positive by the screening test among all individuals who have the disease.

$$\frac{TP}{TP + FN}$$

Specificity is the proportion designated negative by the screening test among all those who do not have the disease.

$$\frac{TN}{TN + FP}$$

Positive predictive value is the proportion of individuals with a positive test who have the disease.

$$\frac{TP}{TP + FP}$$

Negative predictive value is the proportion of individuals with a negative test negative who do not have the disease.

$$\frac{TN}{TN + FN}$$

TP, true positive, the condition present and the test is positive; FN, false negative, the condition is present and the test is negative; FP, false positive, the condition is absent and the test is positive; TN, true negative, the condition is absent and test is negative.

Because survival is measured *from the time of diagnosis*, an earlier diagnosis, by definition, increases survival. Unless an effective intervention is available, lead time bias has no impact on the natural history of a disease and death will occur at the same time it would have in the absence of early detection (Fig. 34.1).

Length bias is a function of the biologic behavior of a cancer. Slower growing, less aggressive cancers are more likely to be detected by a screening test than faster growing cancers, which are more likely to be diagnosed due to the onset of symptoms between scheduled screenings (interval cancers). Length bias has an even greater effect on survival statistics than lead time bias (Fig. 34.2).

Overdiagnosis is an extreme form of length bias and represents pure harm. It refers to the detection of tumors, often through highly sensitive modern imaging modalities and other diagnostic tests, that fulfill the histologic criteria for malignancy

TABLE 34.2

Positive Predictive Value Given Varying Sensitivity and Specificity and Prevalence

Prevalence 0.005		Sensitivity %		
		80	90	95
Specificity %	95	7	8	9
	99	29	31	32
	99.9	80	82	83
Prevalence 0.0001		Sensitivity %		
		80	90	95
Specificity %	95	0.2	0.2	2.0
	99	0.8	0.9	0.9
	99.9	0.7	8.0	9.0

PPV improves dramatically in response to small changes in specificity. Changes in specificity influence PPV much more than changes in sensitivity. Note the influence of prevalence on PPV. Screening tests do not perform as well in populations with a low prevalence of disease.

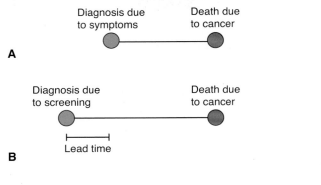

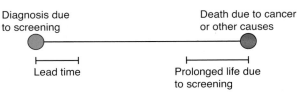

Lead Time Bias

(A) Diagnosis due to symptoms — Death due to cancer

(B) Diagnosis due to screening — Death due to cancer; Lead time

(C) Diagnosis due to screening — Death due to cancer or other causes; Lead time; Prolonged life due to screening

Figure 34.1 Survival is the time from cancer diagnosis to death. **(A)** Lead time bias occurs when screening results in an earlier diagnosis. Without screening, a patient is diagnosed with cancer due to symptoms. **(B)** With screening, the patient is often diagnosed earlier. When screening and treatment do not prolong life, the screened patient can have a longer survival solely due to the earlier diagnosis. The survival increase is pure lead time bias. **(C)** When screening and treatment are beneficial, the patient is diagnosed before the onset of symptoms and the patient lives beyond the point in which death would have occurred without screening.

but are not biologically destined to harm the patient (see Fig. 34.2).

There are two categories of overdiagnosis: the detection of histologically defined *cancers* not destined to metastasize or harm the patient, and the detection of cancers not destined to metastasize or cause harm *in the life span of the specific patient*. The importance of this second category is illustrated by the widespread practice in the United States of screening elderly patients with limited life expectancies, who are thus unlikely to benefit from early cancer diagnosis.

Overdiagnosis occurs with many malignancies, including lung, breast, prostate, renal cell, melanoma, and thyroid cancers.[3] Neuroblastoma provides one of the most striking examples of overdiagnosis.[4] Urine vanillylmandelic acid (VMA) testing is a highly sensitive screening test for the detection of this pediatric disease. After screening programs in Germany, Japan, and Canada showed marked increases in the incidence of this disease without a concomitant decline in mortality, it was noticed that nearby areas that did not screen had similar death rates with lower incidence.[4,5] It is now appreciated that screen-detected neuroblastomas have a very good prognosis with minimal or no treatment. Many actually regress spontaneously.

Stage shift—i.e., a cancer diagnosis at an earlier stage than would have occurred in the absence of screening—is necessary, but not sufficient, for a screening test to be effective in terms of reducing mortality. Both lead time bias and length bias contribute to this phenomenon. Although it is tempting to speculate that diagnosis at an earlier stage must confer benefit, this is not necessarily the case. For example, a substantial proportion of men treated with radical prostatectomy for what appears to be a localized prostate cancer relapse after undergoing surgery. Conversely, some men who are treated with definitive therapy would never have gone on to develop metastatic disease in the absence of treatment.

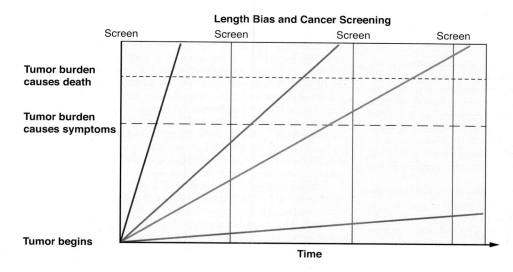

Figure 34.2 Length bias and cancer screening. The *red line* is indicative of a fast-growing tumor that is not amenable to regular screening. The *blue line* is indicative of a fast-growing tumor that can be diagnosed by screening or later by symptoms; death may possibly be prevented by treatment. The *green line* is a slower growing but potentially deadly cancer that can be detected by symptoms or several screenings and treated, possibly preventing death. The *orange line* is indicative of a very slow growing tumor that would never cause death and would never need treatment despite being screen detected. This is classic overdiagnosis.

Selection bias occurs when enrollees in a clinical study differ from the general population. In fact, people who voluntarily participate in clinical trials tend to be healthier than the general population, perhaps due to a greater interest in health and healthcare research. Screening studies tend to enroll individuals healthier than the general population. This so-called *healthy volunteer effect*[6,7] can introduce a powerful bias if not adequately controlled for by randomization procedures.

Assessing Screening Outcomes

The usual primary goal of cancer screening is to reduce mortality from the disease in question (a reduction in disease-specific mortality). Screening studies generally do not have sufficient statistical power to assess the impact of screening for a specific malignancy on overall mortality. (Lung cancer screening provides an exception to this rule; see the following.) As discussed previously, the fact that a screening test increases the percentage of people diagnosed with early stage cancer and decreases that of late stage cancer (stage shift) is not equivalent to proof of mortality reduction. Further, due to the healthy volunteer effect, case control and cohort studies cannot provide definitive evidence of mortality benefit. Prospective, randomized clinical trials are required to address this issue. In such trials, volunteers are randomized to be screened or not and are then followed longitudinally to determine if there is a difference in disease-specific or overall mortality.

A reduction in mortality rates or in the risk of death is often stated in terms of relative risk. However, this method of reporting may be misleading. It is preferable to report both the relative and absolute reduction in mortality. For example, the European Randomized Study of Screening for Prostate Cancer (ERSPC) showed that screening reduced the risk of prostate cancer death by 20%. However, this translates into only 1 prostate cancer death averted per 1,000 men screened (5 prostate cancer deaths per 1,000 men not screened versus 4 prostate cancer deaths per 1,000 men screened) and a relatively modest lifetime reduction in the absolute risk of prostate cancer death of only 0.6%, from 3.0% to 2.4%.[8]

PROBLEMS WITH RANDOMIZED TRIALS

It is important to acknowledge that even prospective, randomized trials can have serious methodologic shortcomings. For example, imbalances caused by flaws in the randomization scheme can prejudice the outcome of a trial. Other flaws include so-called *drop-in* or *contamination*, in which some participants on the control arm get the intervention. Patients on the intervention arm may also *drop out* of the study. Both drop-ins and drop-outs reduce the statistical power of a clinical trial.

In the United States, it is now considered standard to obtain informed consent before randomization takes place. However, there have been several published studies that randomized participants from rosters of eligible subjects such as census lists. In these trials, informed consent was obtained after randomization and only among those randomized to the screening arm of the study. Those randomized to the control arm were not contacted, and indeed, did not know they were in a clinical trial. They were followed through national death registries. Although the study was analyzed on an intent-to-screen basis, this method can still introduce biases. For example, only patients on the intervention arm had access to the screening facility and staff for counseling and treatment if diagnosed; those in the control group were more likely to be treated in the community as opposed to high-volume centers of excellence and were less likely to be treated with surgery and more likely to be treated with hormones alone than those on the screened arm. The study arms would also tend to differ in their knowledge of the disease, which may contribute to an overestimate of the benefits of a screening test.[9]

Virtually every screening test is a balance between known harms and potential benefits. The most important risk of screening is the detection and subsequent treatment of a cancer that would never have come to clinical detection or harmed the patient in the absence of screening (i.e., overdiagnosis and overtreatment). Treatment can cause emotional and physical morbidity and even death.[10] Even when screening has a net mortality benefit, there can be considerable harm. For example, in the recent randomized trial of spiral lung computed tomography (CT) scan, approximately 27,000 current smokers and former smokers were given three annual low-dose CT scans. More than 20% had a *positive* screening CT scan, necessitating further testing. About 1,000 subsequently underwent invasive diagnostic procedures and 16 deaths were reported within 60 days of the procedure.[11] It is not known how many of these deaths were directly related to the screening.

It can be dangerous to extrapolate estimates of benefit from one population to another. In particular, studies showing that a radiographic test is beneficial to average risk individuals may not mean that it is beneficial to a population at high risk, and vice versa. For example, women at high risk for breast cancer due to an inherited mutation of a DNA repair gene may be at higher risk for radiation-induced cancer from mammographies compared to the general population; a screening test (e.g., spiral lung CT scan), shown to be efficacious in a high-risk population of heavy smokers may result in net harm if applied to a low or average risk population.

SCREENING GUIDELINES AND RECOMMENDATIONS

A number of organizations develop cancer screening recommendations or guidelines. These organizations use varying methods. The Institute of Medicine (IOM) has released two reports to establish standards for developing trustworthy clinical practice guidelines and conducting systematic evidence reviews that serve as their basis.[12,13] The U.S. Preventive Services Task Force (USPSTF) and the American Cancer Society (ACS) are two organizations that issue respected and widely used cancer guidelines (Table 34.3). Both have changed their methods to comply with the IOM standards.

The USPSTF is a panel of experts in prevention and evidence-based medicine.[14] They are primary care providers specializing in internal medicine, pediatrics, family practice, gynecology and obstetrics, nursing, and health behavior. The task force process begins by conducting an extensive structured scientific evidence review. The task force then develops recommendations for primary care clinicians and health-care systems. They adhere to some of the highest standards for recommending a screening test. They are very much concerned with the question, "Does the evidence supporting a screening test demonstrate that the benefits outweigh its harms?"

The ACS guidelines date back to the 1970s. The current process for making guidelines involves commissioning academics to do an independent systematic evidence review. A single generalist group digests the evidence review, listens to public input, and writes the guidelines. The ACS panel tries to clearly articulate the benefits, limitations, and harms associated with a screening test.[15]

BREAST CANCER

Mammographies, clinical breast examinations (CBE) by a health-care provider, and breast self-examinations (BSE) have long been advocated[16] for the early detection of breast cancer. In recent years, ultrasound, magnetic resonance imaging (MRI), and other technologies have been added to the list of proposed screening modalities.

Mammographic screening was first advocated in the 1950s. The Health Insurance Plan (HIP) Study was the first prospective, randomized clinical trial to formally assess its value in reducing death from breast cancer. In this study, started in 1963, about 61,000 women were randomized to three annual mammograms with clinical breast examination versus no screening, which was the standard practice at that time. HIP first reported that mammography reduced breast cancer mortality by 30% at about 10 years after study entry. With 18 years of follow-up, those in the screening arm had a 25% lower breast cancer mortality rate.[16]

Nine additional prospective randomized studies have been published. These studies provide the basis for the current consensus that screening women 40 to 75 years of age does reduce the relative risk of breast cancer death by 10% to 25%. The 10 studies demonstrate that the risk–benefit ratio is more favorable for women over 50 years of age. Mammography has also been shown to be operator dependent, with better performance characteristics (higher sensitivity and specificity and lower FP rates) reported by high-volume centers (Table 34.4).

It is important to note that every one of these studies has some flaws and limitations. They vary in the questions asked and their findings. The Canadian screening trial suggests mammographies and clinical breast examinations do not decrease risk of death for woman aged 40 to 49 and that mammographies add nothing to CBEs for women age 50 to 59 years.[17] On the other extreme, the Kopparberg Sweden study suggests that mammographies are associated with a 32% reduction in the risk of death for women aged 40 to 74 years.[18]

To date, no study has shown that BSEs decrease mortality. BSEs have been studied in two large randomized trials. In one, approximately 266,000 Chinese women were randomized to receive intensive BSE instruction with reinforcements and reminders compared to a control group receiving no instruction on BSE. At 10 years of follow-up, there was no difference in mortality, but the intervention arm had a significantly higher incidence of benign breast lesions diagnosed and breast biopsies preformed. In the second study, 124,000 Russian women were randomized to monthly BSEs versus no BSEs. There was no difference in mortality rates, despite the BSE group having a higher proportion of early stage tumors and a significant increase in the proportion of cancer patients surviving 15 years after diagnosis.

Ultrasonography is primarily used in the diagnostic evaluation of a breast mass identified by palpation or mammography. There is little evidence to support the use of ultrasound as an initial screening test. This modality is highly operator dependent and time consuming, with a high rate of FP findings.[19] An MRI is used for screening women at elevated breast cancer risk due to BRCA1 and BRCA2 mutations, Li-Fraumeni syndrome, Cowden disease, or a very strong family history. MRI is more sensitive but less specific than mammography, leading to a high FP rate and more unnecessary biopsies, especially among young women.[20] The impact of MRI breast screening on breast cancer mortality has not yet been determined.

Thermography, an infrared imaging technology, has some advocates as a breast cancer screening modality despite a lack of evidence from several small cohort studies.[21] Nipple aspirate cytology and ductal lavage have also been suggested as possible screening methods. Both should be considered experimental at this time.[22]

Effectiveness of Breast Cancer Screening

Breast cancer screening has been associated with a dramatic rise in breast cancer incidence. At the same time, there has been a dramatic decrease in breast cancer mortality rates. However, in the United States and Europe, incidence-by-stage data show a dramatic increase in the proportion of early stage cancers without a concomitant decrease in the incidence of regional and metastatic cancers.[23] These findings are at odds with the clinical trials data and raise questions regarding the extent to which early diagnosis is responsible for declining breast cancer mortality rates.

From 1976 to 2008, the incidence of early-stage breast cancer for American women aged 40 and older increased from 112 to 234 per 100,000. This is a rise of 122 cases per 100,000, whereas the absolute decrease in late-stage cancers was only 8 cases per 100,000 (from 102 to 94 cases per 100,000). These data raise questions regarding the magnitude of benefit, as well as the potential risks, of breast cancer screening. The discrepancy between the magnitude of the increase of early disease and the decrease of late-stage cancer and cancer mortality suggests that a proportion of invasive breast cancers diagnosed by screening represents overdiagnosis. These data suggest that overdiagnosis accounts for up to 31% of all breast cancers diagnosed by screening.[24] Others have estimated that up to 50% of breast cancers detected by screening mammography are overdiagnosed cancers. In an exhaustive review of the screening literature, a panel of experts concluded that overdiagnosis does exist and estimated it to be 11% to 19% of breast cancers diagnosed by screening.[25]

A confounding factor with regard to the mortality benefits of breast cancer screening is the improvement that has occurred in breast cancer treatment over this period of time. The effects of the advances in therapy are supported by cancer modeling studies. Indeed, the Cancer Intervention and Surveillance Modeling Network (CISNET), supported by the U.S. National Cancer Institute (NCI), has estimated that two-thirds of the observed breast cancer mortality reduction is attributable to modern therapy, rather than to screening.[26]

TABLE 34.3

Screening Recommendations for Normal-Risk Asymptomatic Subjects

Cancer Type	Test or Procedure	American Cancer Society	U.S. Preventive Services Task Force
Breast	Self-examination	Women ≥20 years: Breast self-exam is an option	"D"
	Clinical examination	Women 20–39 years: Perform every 3 years Women ≥40 years: Perform annually	Women ≥40 years: "I" (as a stand alone without mammography)
	Mammography	Women ≥40 years: Screen annually for as long as the woman is in good health	Women 40–49 years: The decision should be an individual one, and take patient context/values into account ("C") Women 50–74 years: Every 2 years ("B") Women ≥75 years: "I"
	MRI	Women >20% lifetime risk of breast cancer: Screen with MRI plus mammography annually Women 15%–20% lifetime risk of breast cancer: Discuss option of MRI plus mammography annually Women <15% lifetime risk of breast cancer: Do not screen annually with MRI	"I"
Cervical	Pap test (cytology)	Women ages 21–29 years: Screen every 3 years Women 30–65 years: Acceptable approach to screen with cytology every 3 years (see HPV test) Women <21 years: No screening Women >65 years: No screening following adequate negative prior screening Women after total hysterectomy for noncancerous causes: Do not screen	Women ages 21–65 years: Screen every 3 years ("A") Women <21 years: "D" Women >65 years, with adequate, normal prior Pap screenings: "D" Women after total hysterectomy for noncancerous causes: "D"
	HPV test	Women <30 years: Do not use HPV testing Women ages 30–65 years: Preferred approach to screen with HPV and cytology cotesting every 5 years (see Pap test) Women >65 years: No screening following adequate negative prior screening Women after total hysterectomy for noncancerous causes: Do not screen	Women ages 30–65 years: Screen in combination with cytology every 5 years if woman desires to lengthen the screening interval (see Pap test) ("A") Women <30 years: "D" Women >65 years, with adequate, normal prior Pap screenings: "D" Women after total hysterectomy for noncancerous causes: "D"
Colorectal	Sigmoidoscopy	Adults ≥50 years: Screen every 5 years Note: For all CRC screening tests, stop screening when benefits are unlikely due to life-limiting comorbidity.	Adults 50–75 years: Every 5 years in combination with high-sensitivity fecal occult blood testing (FOBT) every 3 years ("A")[a] Adults 76–85 years: "C" Adults ≥85 years: "D"
	Fecal occult blood testing (FOBT)	Adults ≥50 years: Screen every year with high sensitivity guaiac based FOBT or fecal immunochemical test (FIT) only	Adults 50–75 years: Annually, for high-sensitivity FOBT ("A") Adults 76–85 years: "C" Adults ≥85 years: "D"
	Colonoscopy	Adults ≥50 years: Screen every 10 years	Adults 50–75 years: every 10 years ("A") Adults 76–85 years: "C" Adults ≥85 years: "D"
	Fecal DNA testing	Adults ≥50 years: Screen, but interval uncertain	"I"
	Fecal immunochemical testing (FIT)	Adults ≥50 years: Screen every year	"I"
	CT colonography	Adults ≥50 years: Screen every 5 years	"I"
Lung	Complete skin examination by clinician or patient	Men and women, 55–74 years, with ≥30 pack-year smoking history, still smoking or have quit within past 15 years: Discuss benefits, limitations, and potential harms of screening. Only perform screening in facilities with the right type of CT scanner and with high expertise/specialists.	"I" ("B" draft recommendation issued for public comment in July 2013)

(continued)

TABLE 34.3

Screening Recommendations for Normal-Risk Asymptomatic Subjects *(continued)*

Cancer Type	Test or Procedure	American Cancer Society	U.S. Preventive Services Task Force
Ovary	CA-125 Transvaginal ultrasound	There is no sufficiently accurate test proven effective in the early detection of ovarian cancer. For women at high risk of ovarian cancer and/or who have unexplained, persistent symptoms, the combination of CA-125 and transvaginal ultrasound with pelvic exam may be offered.	"D" "D"
Prostate	Prostate-specific antigen (PSA)	Starting at age 50, men should talk to a doctor about the pros and cons of testing so they can decide if testing is the right choice for them. If African American or have a father or brother who had prostate cancer before age 65, men should have this talk starting at age 45. How often they are tested will depend on their PSA level.	Men, all ages: "D"
	Digital rectal examination (DRE)	As for PSA; if men decide to be tested, they should have the PSA blood test with or without a rectal exam.	No individual recommendation
Skin	Complete skin examination by clinician or patient	Self-examination monthly; clinical exam as part of routine cancer-related checkup	"I"

Note: Summary of the screening procedures recommended for the general population by the American Cancer Society and the U.S. Preventive Services Task Force. These recommendations refer to asymptomatic persons who have no risk factors for the cancer, other than age or gender.
[a] USPSTF lettered recommendations are defined as follows:
"A": The USPSTF recommends the service, because there is high certainty that the net benefit is substantial.
"B": The USPSTF recommends the service, because there is high certainty that the net benefit is moderate or moderate certainty that the net benefit is moderate to substantial.
"C": The USPSTF recommends selectively offering or providing this service to individual patients based on professional judgment and patient preferences. There is at least moderate certainty that the net benefit is small.
"D": The USPSTF recommends against the service, because there is moderate or high certainty that the service has no net benefit or that the harms outweigh the benefits.
"I": The USPSTF concludes that the current evidence is insufficient to assess the balance of benefits and harms of the service.

Questions have also been raised regarding the quality of the randomized screening trials that demonstrated the mortality benefits of mammography and clinical breast examination because these trials suffered from a variety of design flaws. In some, randomization methods were suboptimal, others reported varying numbers of participants over the years, and still others had substantial contamination (drop-ins). Perhaps more importantly, most trials were started and concluded before the widespread use of more advanced mammographic technology, before the modern era of adjuvant therapy, and before the advent of targeted therapy.

Although randomized control trials (RCT) remain the gold standard for assessing the benefits of a clinical intervention, they cannot take into account improvements in both treatment and patient awareness that occurred over time. For this reason, observational and modeling studies can provide important, complementary information.

One systematic review of 17 published population-based and cohort studies compared breast cancer mortality in groups of women aged 50 to 69 years who started breast cancer screening at different times. Although these studies are subject to methodologic limitations, only four suggested that breast cancer screening reduced the relative risk of breast cancer mortality by 33% or more and five suggested no benefit from screening. The review concluded that breast cancer screening likely reduces the risk of breast cancer death by no more than 10%.[27]

Even with these limitations, a systematic review of the data sponsored by the USPSTF concluded that regular mammography reduces breast cancer mortality in women aged 40 to 74 years.[28] The task force also concluded that the benefits of mammography are most significant in women aged 50 to 74 years.

Screening Women Age 40 to 49

Experts disagree about the utility of screening women in their forties. In the HIP Randomized Control Trial, women who entered at age 40 to 49 years had a mortality benefit at 18 years of follow-up. However, to a large extent, the mortality benefit among those aged 45 to 49 years at entry was driven by breast cancers diagnosed after they reached age 50 years.[16]

Mammography, like all screening tests, is more efficient (higher PPV) for the detection of disease in populations with higher disease prevalence (see Table 34.2). Mammography is, therefore, a better test in women age 50 to 59 years than it is among women age 40 to 49 years because the risk of breast cancer increases with age. Mammography is also less optimal in women age 40 to 49 years compared to women 50 to 59 years of age for the following reasons:

- A larger proportion have increased breast density, which can obscure lesions (lower sensitivity).
- Younger women are more likely to develop aggressive, fast-growing breast cancers that are diagnosed between regular screening visits. By definition, these *interval cancers* are not screen detected.[29]

The USPSTF meta-analysis of eight large randomized trials suggested a 15% relative reduction in mortality (relative risk [RR], 0.85; 95% confidence interval [CI], 0.75 to 0.96) from mammography screening for women aged 40 to 49 years after 11 to 20 years of follow-up. This is equivalent to a needing to invite 1,904 women to screenings over 10 years to prevent one breast cancer death. Studies, however, show that more than half of women aged 40 to 49 years screened annually over a 10-year period will have an FP mammogram necessitating further evaluation, often including biopsy. In addition, estimates of overdiagnosis in this group range from 10% to 40% of diagnosed invasive cancers.[30]

In an effort to decrease FP rates, some have suggested screening every 2 years rather than yearly. Comparing biennial with annual screening, the CISNET Model consistently shows that biennial screening of women ages 40 to 70 only marginally decreases the number of lives saved while halving the false positive rate.[29] Notably, the Swedish two-county trial, which had a planned 24-month screening interval (the actual interval was 33 months) reported one

TABLE 34.4

Randomized Controlled Trials

Study	Randomization	Sample Size	Intervention and Age at Entry	Follow-up	Finding
Health Insurance Plan, United States 1963[a,b]	Individual	60,565–60,857	MMG and CBE for 3 years Age 40–64 years	18 years	RR 0.77 (95% CI: 0.61–0.97)
Malmo, Sweden 1976[c,d]	Individual	42,283	Two-view MMG every 18–24 months × 5 Age 45–69 years	12 years	RR 0.81 (95% CI: 0.62–1.07)
Ostergotland (County E of Two-County Trial) Sweden 1977[e-g]	Geographic cluster	38,405–39,034 study 37,145–37,936 control	Three single-view MMG every 2 years women, Age 40–50 years Every 33 months women, Age 50–74	12 years	RR 0.82 (95% CI: 0.64–1.05)
Kopparberg (County W of Two-County Trial) Sweden 1977[e-g]	Geographic cluster	38,562–39,051 intervention 18,478–18,846 control	Three single-view MMG every 2 years women, Age 40–50 years Every 33 months women, Age 50–74 years	12 years	RR 0.68 (95% CI: 0.52–0.89)
Edinburgh, United Kingdom[h]	Cluster by physician practice	23,266 study 21,904 control	Initially, two-view MMG and CBE Then annual CBE with single-view MMG years 3, 5, and 7, Age 45–64 years	10 years	RR 0.84 (95% CI: 0.63–1.12)
NBSS-1, Canada 1980[i,j]	Individual	25,214 study (100% screened after entry CBE) 25,216 control	Annual two-view MMG and CBE for 4–5 years, Age 40–49 years	13 years	RR 0.97 (95% CI: 0.74–1.27)
NBSS-2, Canada 1980[i,j]	Individual	19,711 study (100% screened after entry CBE) 19,694 control	Annual two-view MMG and CBE versus CBE, Age 50–59 years	11–16 years (mean 13 years)	RR 1.02 (95% CI: 0.78–1.33)
Stockholm, Sweden 1981[k]	Cluster by birth date	40,318–38,525 intervention group 19,943–20,978 control group	Single view MMG every 28 months × 2 Age 40–64 years	8 years	RR 0.80 (95%) CI: 0.53–1.22)
Gothenberg, Sweden 1982[d]	Complex	21,650 invited 29,961 control	Initial two-view MMG, then single-view MMG every 18 months × 4 Single read first three rounds, then double-read, Age 39–59 years	12–14 years	RR 0.79 (95% CI 0.58–1.08) In the evaluation phase RR 0.77 (95% CI 0.60–1.00) In follow-up phase
Age Trial[l]	Individual	160,921 (53,884 invited; 106,956 not invited)	Invited group aged 48 and younger offered annual screening by MMG (double-view first screen, then single mediolateral oblique view thereafter); 68% accepted screening on the first screen an 69% and 70% were reinvited (81% attended at least one screen) Age 39–41 years	10.7 years	RR 0.83 (95% CI: 0.66–1.04)

[a] Shapiro S, Venet W, Strax P, et al. Ten- to fourteen-year effect of screening on breast cancer mortality. *J Natl Cancer Inst* 1982;69:349–355.
[b] Shapiro S. Periodic screening for breast cancer: the HIP Randomized Controlled Trial. Health Insurance Plan. *J Natl Cancer Inst Monogr* 1997:27–30.
[c] Andersson I, Aspegren K, Janzon L, et al. Mammographic screening and mortality from breast cancer: the Malmo mammographic screening trial. *BMJ* 1988;297:943–948.
[d] Nystrom L, Rutqvist LE, Wall S, et al. Breast cancer screening with mammography: overview of Swedish randomised trials. *Lancet* 1993;341:973–978.
[e] Tabar L, Fagerberg CJ, Gad A, et al. Reduction in mortality from breast cancer after mass screening with mammography. Randomised trial from the Breast Cancer Screening Working Group of the Swedish National Board of Health and Welfare. *Lancet* 1985;1:829–832.
[f] Tabar L, Fagerberg G, Duffy SW, Day NE. The Swedish two county trial of mammographic screening for breast cancer: recent results and calculation of benefit. *J Epidemiol Community Health* 1989;43:107–114.
[g] Tabar L, Fagerberg G, Duffy SW, et al. Update of the Swedish two-county program of mammographic screening for breast cancer. *Radiol Clin North Am* 1992;30:187–210.
[h] Roberts MM, Alexander FE, Anderson TJ, et al. Edinburgh trial of screening for breast cancer: mortality at seven years. *Lancet* 1990;335:241–246.
[i] Miller AB, To T, Baines CJ, Wall C. The Canadian National Breast Screening Study-1: breast cancer mortality after 11 to 16 years of follow-up. A randomized screening trial of mammography in women age 40 to 49 years. *Ann Intern Med* 2002;137:305–312.
[j] Miller AB, Wall C, Baines CJ, et al. Twenty five year follow-up for breast cancer incidence and mortality of the Canadian National Breast Screening Study: randomised screening trial. *BMJ* 2014;348–366.
[k] Frisell J, Eklund G, Hellstrom L, et al. Randomized study of mammography screening—preliminary report on mortality in the Stockholm trial. *Breast Cancer Res Treat* 1991;18:49–56.
[l] Moss SM, Cuckle H, Evans A, et al. Effect of mammographic screening from age 40 years on breast cancer mortality at 10 years' follow-up: a randomised controlled trial. *Lancet* 2006;368:2053–2060.

CANCER PREVENTION AND SCREENING

of the greatest reductions in breast cancer mortality among the RCTs conducted to date.

Screening Women at High Risk

There is interest in creating risk profiles as a way of reducing the inconveniences and harms of screening. It might be possible to identify women who are at greater risk of breast cancer and refocus screening efforts on those most likely to benefit.

Risk factors for breast cancer include the following:

- Extremely dense breasts on mammography or a first-degree relative with breast cancer are each associated with at least a twofold increase in breast cancer risk
- Prior benign breast biopsy, second-degree relatives with breast cancer, or heterogeneously dense breasts each increase risk 1.5- to twofold
- Current oral contraceptive use, nulliparity, and age at first birth 30 years and older increase risk 1- to 1.5-fold.[31]

Importantly, these are risk factors for breast cancer diagnosis, not breast cancer mortality. Few studies have assessed the association between these factors and death from breast cancer; however, reproductive factors and breast density have been shown to have limited influence on breast cancer mortality.[32,33]

Genetic testing for *BRCA1* and *BRCA2* mutations and other markers of breast cancer risk has identified a group of women at high risk for breast cancer. Unfortunately, when to begin and the optimal frequency of screening have not been defined. Mammography is less sensitive at detecting breast cancers in women carrying *BRCA1* and *BRCA2* mutations, possibly because such cancers occur in younger women in whom mammography is known to be less sensitive.

MRI screening may be more sensitive than mammography in women at high risk, but specificity is lower. MRIs are associated with both an increase in FP and an increase in the detection of smaller cancers, which are more likely to be biologically indolent. The impact of MRIs on breast cancer mortality with or without concomitant use of mammographies has not been evaluated in a randomized controlled trial.

Breast Density

It is well established that mammogram sensitivity is lower in women with heterogeneously dense or very dense breasts.[29,32] However, at this time, there are no clear guidelines regarding whether or how screening algorithms should take breast density into account.

In the American College of Radiology's Imaging Network (ACRIN)/NCI 666 Trial, breast ultrasound was offered to women with increased mammographic breast density and, if either test was positive, they were referred for a breast biopsy.[34] The radiologists performing the ultrasounds were not aware of the mammographic findings. Mammography detected 7.6 cancers per 1,000 women screened; ultrasound increased the cancer detection rate to 11.8 per 1,000. However, the PPV for mammography alone was 22.6%, whereas the PPV for mammography with ultrasound was only 11.2%.

It has yet to be determined whether supplemental imaging reduces breast cancer mortality in women with increased breast density. Although it continues to be strongly advocated by some, systematic reviews have concluded that the evidence is currently insufficient to recommend for or against this approach.[35] There are also a number of barriers to supplemental imaging, including inconsistent insurance coverage, lack of availability in many communities, concerns about cost-effectiveness (particularly with regard to MRI), and the increased FP rate associated with supplemental imaging leading to unnecessary biopsies.[36]

Newer technologies may improve screening accuracy for women with dense breasts. Compared to conventional mammography, full field digital mammography (FFDM) appears to have less FPs. This could reduce the number of women needing supplemental imaging and biopsies.[37] Digital breast tomosynthesis (DBT) uses x-rays and a digital detector to generate cross-sectional images of the breasts. Data are limited, but compared to mammograms, DBT appears to offer increased sensitivity and a reduction in the recall rates.[38] Another potential supplementary imaging modality currently under investigation is three-dimensional (3-D) automated breast ultrasound, and having screening ultrasounds performed by technologists rather than radiologists.

Ductal Carcinoma In Situ

The incidence of noninvasive ductal carcinoma in situ (DCIS) has increased more than fivefold since 1970 as a direct consequence of widespread screening mammographies.[39] DCIS is a heterogeneous condition with low- and intermediate-grade lesions taking a decade or more to progress. Nevertheless, women with this diagnosis are uniformly subjected to treatment. A better understanding of this entity and an increased ability to predict its biologic behavior may enable more judicious, personalized treatment of DCIS.

There is little evidence that the early detection and aggressive treatment of low- and intermediate-grade DCIS reduces breast cancer mortality. The standard of care for all grades of DCIS is lumpectomy with radiation or mastectomy, followed by tamoxifen for 5 years. Interestingly, patterns of care studies indicate that mastectomy rates are increasing,[40] and that women are more often choosing double mastectomies for the treatment of DCIS.[41] Genomic characterization will hopefully lead to the identification of a subset of noninvasive cancers that can be treated less aggressively or even observed.

Harms

The harms and disadvantages of mammography screening include overdiagnosis, FP tests, FN tests, and the possibility of radiation-induced breast cancer.

The fact that mammography screening has increased the incidence of localized disease without a significant change in metastatic disease at the time of diagnosis suggests that there is some degree of overdiagnosis. The risk of overdiagnosis is greatest at the first screening[3] and varies with patient age, tumor type, and grade of disease.

FP screening tests lead to substantial inconvenience and anxiety in addition to unnecessary invasive biopsies with their attendant complications. In the United States, about 10% of all women screened for breast cancer are called back for additional testing, and less than half of them will be diagnosed with breast cancer.[39] The risk of a FP mammogram is greater for women under the age of 50.[37]

FN tests delay diagnosis and provide false reassurance. They are more common in younger women and in women with dense breasts.[42,43] Certain histologic subtypes are also more difficult to see on mammogram. Mucinous and lobular tumors and rapidly growing tumors tend to blend in with normal breast architecture.[44]

A typical screening mammogram provides approximately 4 mSv of radiation. It has been estimated that annual mammographies will cause up to 1 case of breast cancer per 1,000 women screened from age 40 to age 80 years. Radiation exposure at younger ages causes a greater risk of breast cancer.[45] There is also concern that ionizing radiation from mammographies might disproportionately increase the breast cancer risk for women with certain *BRCA1* or *BRCA2* mutations, because these genes are related to DNA repair.[46]

Recommendations

Women at Average Risk

The ACS and most other medical groups recommend that average risk women undergo a CBE every 3 years starting at age 20 and that women 40 years of age and over should undergo CBEs and screening mammograms annually. Women should be informed of the benefits, limitations, and harms associated with breast cancer screening. A mammography will not detect all breast cancers, and some breast cancers detected with mammographies may still have a poor prognosis. The harms associated with breast cancer screening also include the potential for FP results, causing substantial anxiety. When abnormal findings cannot be resolved with additional imaging, a biopsy is required to rule out the possibility of breast cancer. A majority of biopsies are benign. Finally, some breast cancers detected by a mammography may be biologically indolent, meaning they would not have caused a problem or have been detected in a woman's lifetime had she not undergone a mammography.

The USPSTF, the American College of Physicians, and the Canadian Task Force on the Periodic Health Examination recommend routine screening beginning at age 50 years.[30,47,48] For women aged 40 to 49 years of age, these groups advise physicians to enter into a discussion with the patient. The physician and patient should take into account individual risks and concerns before deciding to screen.[47]

An Advisory Committee on Cancer Prevention in the European Union recommends that women between the ages of 50 and 69 years be offered mammogram screening in an organized screening program with quality assurance.[49] This committee says women aged 40 to 49 years should be advised of the potential harms of screening and, if mammographic screening is offered, it should be performed with strict quality standards and double reading.

Women at High Risk

The ACS has issued guidelines for women who were known or likely carriers of a *BRCA* mutation and other rarer high-risk genetic syndromes, or at high risk for other reasons.[50] Annual screening mammographies and MRIs starting at age 30 is recommended for women:

- With a known *BRCA* mutation
- Who are untested but have a first-degree relative with a *BRCA* mutation
- Who had been treated with radiation to the chest for Hodgkin disease
- Who have an approximately 20% to 25% or greater lifetime risk of breast cancer based on specialized breast cancer risk estimation models.

COLON CANCER SCREENING

Colorectal cancer screening with the rigid sigmoidoscope dates back to the late 1960s. The desire to examine the entire colon led to the use of a barium enema and the development of fecal occult blood tests. With the development of fiber optics, flexible sigmoidoscopies and, later, colonoscopies were employed. Today, fecal occult blood testing (FOBT), stool DNA testing, flexible sigmoidoscopies, colonoscopies, and CT colonographies and, occasionally, barium enemas are all used in colorectal cancer screening. MRI colonoscopy is in development.

Screening examinations of the colon and rectum can find cancer early, but also find precancerous polyps. Randomized trials have demonstrated that endoscopic polypectomies reduce the incidence of colorectal cancer by about 20%.[51–53]

FOBT was the first colorectal screening test studied in a prospective randomized clinical trial. The Minnesota Colon Cancer Control Study randomized 46,551 adults to one of three arms: annual FOBTs, biennial screening, or usual care. A rehydrated guaiac test was used. With 13 years of follow-up, the annual screened arm had a 33% relative reduction in colorectal cancer mortality compared to the usual care group.[54] At 18 years of follow-up, the biennially screened group had a 21% reduction in colorectal cancer

mortality.[55] This study would subsequently show that stool blood testing was associated with a 20% reduction in colon cancer incidence.[51] These results were confirmed by two other randomized trials.[56,57] A reduction in colon cancer–specific mortality persisted in the Minnesota trial through 30 years of follow-up. Overall mortality was not affected.

Rehydration increases the sensitivity of FOBT at the expense of lowering specificity.[58] Indeed, rehydrated specimens have a very high FP rate. Overall, 1% to 5% of FOBTs are positive, but only 2% to 10% of those with a positive FOBT have cancer.

Fecal immunochemical tests (FIT) are stool tests that do not react to hemoglobin in dietary products. They appear to have higher sensitivity and specificity for colorectal cancer when compared to nonrehydrated FOBT tests.[59]

Fecal DNA testing is an emerging modality. These tests look for DNA sequences specific to colorectal polyps and colorectal cancer. They may have increased sensitivity and specificity compared to FOBT. Although fecal DNA tests appear to find cancer, the body of evidence on their ability to reduce colorectal cancer mortality is limited due to a lack of study. This test has been intermittently available.

Flexible sigmoidoscopies are, of course, limited to an examination of the rectum and sigmoid colon. A prospective randomized trial of once-only flexible sigmoidoscopies demonstrated a 23% reduction in colorectal cancer incidence and a 31% reduction in colorectal cancer mortality after a median 11.2 years of follow-up.[60] In the NCI's Prostate, Lung, Colorectal, and Ovarian Cancer Screening Trial (PLCO), there was a 21% reduction in colorectal cancer incidence and a 26% reduction in colorectal cancer mortality with two sigmoidoscopies done 3 to 5 years apart compared with the usual care group after a median follow-up of 11.9 years.[53] In both studies, there was no effect on proximal lesions (i.e., right and transverse colon) due to the limited reach of the scope. It is estimated that flexible sigmoidoscopies can find 60% to 80% of cancers and polyps found by colonoscopies.[61]

In two meta-analyses of five randomized controlled trials of sigmoidoscopies, there was an 18% relative reduction in colorectal cancer incidence and a 28% relative reduction in colorectal cancer mortality.[62,63] Participants ranged in age from 50 to 74 years. Follow-up ranged from 6 to 13 years.

The *colonoscopy* has become the preferred screening method of many, although there have been no prospective, randomized trials of colonoscopy screening. A positive FOBT, FIT, fecal DNA test, or sigmoidoscopy warrants a follow-up diagnostic colonoscopy. Perhaps the best support for colonoscopy screening is indirect evidence from the Minnesota Colon Cancer Control Study, which required that all participants with a positive stool blood test have diagnostic imaging of the entire colon. In the Minnesota study, more than 40% of those screened annually eventually received a colonoscopy. One can also make the argument that the sigmoidoscopy studies indirectly support the efficacy of colonoscopy screening, although it can be argued that embryologic and epidemiologic evidence indicate that the right and left colon are biologically distinct and, therefore, the mortality benefits from sigmoidoscopies do not constitute proof that a colonoscopy would similarly reduce mortality from proximal colon lesions.

In studies involving repeat colonoscopies by a second physician, 21% of all adenomas were missed, including 26% of 1 to 5 mm adenomas and 2% of adenomas 10 mm or more in length.[64] Other limitations of colonoscopies include the inconvenience of the bowel preparation and the risk of bowel perforation (about 3 out of 1,000 procedures, overall, with nearly all of the risk among patients who undergo colonoscopic polypectomies). The cost of the procedure and the limited number of physicians who can do the procedure are also of concern.

A *CT colonography* or *virtual* colonoscopy allows a physician to visually reproduce the endoscopic examination on a computer screen. A CT colonography involves the same prep as a colonoscopy, but is less invasive. It might have a higher compliance rate.

In experienced hands, the sensitivity of a CT colonography for the detection of polyps ≥6 mm appears to be comparable to that of a colonoscopy. In a meta-analysis of 30 studies, 2-D and 3-D CT colonographies performed equally well.[65]

The disadvantages of a CT colonography include the fact that it requires a colonic prep and a finding on CT requires a follow-up diagnostic colonoscopy. The rate of extracolonic findings of uncertain significance is high (~15% to 30%), and each one must be evaluated, thereby contributing to additional expense and potential morbidity. The long-term, cumulative radiation risk of repeated colonography screenings is also a concern.

Current Recommendations

The ACS, the American College of Gastroenterology, the American Gastroenterological Association, the American Society for Gastrointestinal Endoscopy, and the American College of Radiology have issued joint colorectal cancer guidelines. These groups consider FOBT, FIT, rigid and flexible sigmoidoscopies, colonoscopies, and CT colonographies to all be reasonable screening methodologies.

They recommend the following: (1) Screening modalities be chosen based on personal preference and access, and (2) average risk adults should begin colorectal cancer screening at age 50 years with *one* of the following options:

1. Annual high sensitivity FOBT or FIT
2. A flexible sigmoidoscopy every 5 years
3. A colonoscopy every 10 years
4. A double contrast barium enema every 5 years
5. A CT colonography every 5 years

No test is of unequivocal superiority. Patient preferences should be incorporated into screening in order to increase compliance. The guidelines also stress that a single screening examination is far from optimal and that patients should be in a program of regular screening.

Although some colorectal cancers are diagnosed in persons under the age of 50 years, screening persons age 40 to 49 years has low yield.[66] The guidelines also state that patients with less than a 10-year life expectancy should not be screened.

The USPSTF issued colorectal cancer screening guidelines in 2008.[67] The guidelines were based on a systematic literature review and decision models. The task force concluded that three screening strategies appear to be equivalent for adults age 50 to 75 years:

1. An annual FOBT with a sensitive test
2. A flexible sigmoidoscopy every 5 years, with a sensitive FOBT every 3 years
3. A colonoscopy every 10 years

The task force recommends that patients age 76 to 85 years be evaluated individually for screening. They found "insufficient evidence" to recommend CT colonographies or fecal DNA testing.

Patients at Increased Risk of Colorectal Cancer

Patients can have higher than average risk of colorectal cancer due to familial or hereditary factors and clinical conditions such as inflammatory bowel disease. These patients technically undergo surveillance and not screening. Nevertheless, there are few clinical studies to guide recommendations. Guidelines have been created based on professional opinion and an understanding of the biology of colorectal cancer (Table 34.5).[68]

OTHER CANCERS OF THE GASTROINTESTINAL TRACT

There are no widely accepted screening guidelines for cancers of the esophagus, stomach, pancreas, and liver. However, surveillance is advocated for some patients at high risk.

Esophageal Cancer Screening

Esophageal cancer screening has centered on endoscopic examinations for those at high risk due to chronic, severe gastroesophageal reflux disease.[69] Some physicians advocate routine endoscopic surveillance of patients with Barrett esophagus. At this time, there is no evidence that such surveillance is effective at reducing cancer mortality.

TABLE 34.5

Colon Cancer Screening Recommendations for People with Familial or Inherited Risk

Familial Risk Category	Screening Recommendation
First-degree relative[a] affected with *colorectal cancer* or an *adenomatous polyp* at age ≥60 years, or two second-degree relatives[b] affected with colorectal *cancer*	Same as average risk but starting at age 40 years
Two or more first-degree relatives with *colon cancer*, or a single first-degree relative with *colon cancer* or *adenomatous polyps* diagnosed at an age <60 years	Colonoscopy every 5 years, beginning at age 40 years or 10 years younger than the earliest diagnosis in the family, whichever comes first
One second-degree or any third-degree relative[b,c] with *colorectal cancer*	Same as average risk
Gene *carrier* or *at risk* for familial adenomatous polyposis[d]	Sigmoidoscopy annually, beginning at age 10–12 years[e]
Gene carrier or at risk for HNPCC	Colonoscopy, every 1–2 years, beginning at age 20–25 years or 10 years younger than the earliest case in the family, whichever comes first

[a] First-degree relatives include patients, siblings, and children.
[b] Second-degree relatives include grandparents, aunts, and uncles.
[c] Third-degree relatives include great-grandparents and cousins.
[d] Includes the subcategories of familial adenomatous polyposis, Gardner syndrome, some Turcot syndrome families, and attenuated adenomatous polyposis coli (AAPC).
[e] In AAPC, colonoscopy should be used instead of sigmoidoscopy because of the preponderance of proximal colonic adenomas. Colonoscopy screening in AAPC should probably begin in the late teens or early 20s.
HNPCC, hereditary nonpolyposis colon cancer.
From Winawer S, Fletcher R, Rex D, et al. Colorectal cancer screening and surveillance: clinical guidelines and rationale: update based on new evidence. *Gastroenterology* 2003;124:544–560, with permission.

Gastric Cancer Screening

Barium-meal photofluorography, serum pepsinogen, and gastric endoscopy have been proposed as screening methods for the early detection of gastric cancer. There are no randomized trials evaluating the impact of these modalities on gastric cancer mortality. Indeed, screening with barium-meal photofluorography has been studied in high-risk populations for more than 40 years without clear evidence of benefit.

Time-trend analysis and case control studies of gastric endoscopy have suggested a decrease in gastric cancer mortality among those at high risk in screened versus unscreened individuals; however, a large observational study in a high-risk population failed to demonstrate a benefit.[70,71]

Although widespread gastric screenings cannot be advocated, there may be justification for endoscopic screenings of high-risk populations. Candidates for screening might include elderly individuals with atrophic gastritis or pernicious anemia, patients who have had partial gastrectomy,[72] those with a history of sporadic adenomas, and patients with familial adenomatous polyposis or hereditary nonpolyposis colon cancer.

Pancreatic Cancer Screening

At this time, there are no data from prospective clinical trials to support a role for pancreatic cancer screening. Some patients with an extensive family history have undergone periodic CT scanning of the abdomen, but this approach has not been shown to reduce pancreatic cancer mortality. There is an ongoing search for screening biomarkers. There is a need to follow large cohorts prospectively after collecting and storing biologic samples to identify biomarkers of risk.[73]

Liver Cancer Screening

Screening for liver cancer or hepatocellular carcinoma (HCC) has focused on very high-risk individuals, such as those with cirrhosis.[54] To date, trial results are unreliable due to small study sizes and a lack of randomization.

Serum alpha-fetoprotein (AFP), a fetal-specific glycoprotein antigen, is an HCC tumor marker used in screening. It is not specific to HCC because it may be elevated in hepatitis, pregnancy, and some germ cell tumors. AFP has variable sensitivity and has not been tested in any randomized clinical trial with a mortality end point.

In one prospective, 16-year, population-based observational study, screening was done on 1,487 Alaska natives with chronic hepatis B virus (HBV) infection. The survival of those with screen-detected HCC was compared with a historical group of clinically diagnosed HCC patients.[74] With a target of AFP determination every 6 months, there was a 97% sensitivity and 95% specificity for HCC. Such high sensitivity and specificity have not been found in other studies. It is not known if AFP screening decreases HCC mortality.[75]

Hepatic ultrasound has been used as an additional method for detection of HCC. This procedure is operator dependent with variable sensitivity and specificity. Ultrasound screening is commonly used in patients with hepatitis and cirrhosis.[76,77]

Interest in CT scanning has grown due to the limitations of AFP and ultrasound. CT scans may be a more sensitive test for HCC than ultrasound or AFP.[75]

GYNECOLOGIC CANCER

Cervical Cancer Screening

Dr. George Papanicolaou first introduced the Pap smear or Pap test in the early 1940s. The test was widely adopted based on its ability to identify squamous premalignancies and malignancies (from the ectodermal cervix) and glandular dysplasia and adenocarcinomas (from the endocervix). It is, however, more sensitive at detecting squamous lesions.

The Pap test was introduced before the advent of the prospective, randomized clinical trial and, therefore, has never been so tested. However, a number of observational studies over the past 60 years support the effectiveness of this screening test.[78,79] Multiple ecologic studies have shown an inverse correlation between the introduction of Pap testing in a given country and reductions in both cervical cancer incidence and mortality.[80] Importantly, mortality reductions in these studies have been proportional to the intensity of screening. In one series, more than half of women diagnosed with cervical cancer either had never had a Pap test or had not been screened within 5 years of diagnosis.[80]

Cervical cytology has evolved over the years. The original Pap smear used an ectocervical spatula to apply a specimen ("smear") to glass slides. It later included an endocervical brush. The smear was fixed, stained, and manually examined under a microscope. That method is still used today, but a liquid-based/thin-layer system capable of being analyzed by computer is gaining in popularity.[81]

Human papillomavirus (HPV) 16 and 18 are the cause of more than 70% of cervical cancers. Thirteen other HPV subtypes are known to be associated with cervical cancer. With increasing understanding of the role of HPV in cervical disease, interest in developing tests to determine the presence of HPV DNA and RNA has grown. HPV screening can be used along with cytology (*cotesting*), in response to an abnormal cytologic test (*reflexive testing*), or as a stand-alone test. One advantage of the liquid-based/thin-layer tests over the older smears is that it makes reflexive testing easier to perform. An abnormal cytology screen can be objectively verified by testing for the presence of the HPV virus without calling the patient back.

HPV testing is especially useful because of its negative predictive value. Although a positive test for HPV infection is not diagnostic of cervical disease, a negative HPV test strongly suggests that the abnormal Pap does not represent a premalignant condition.

The utility of the HPV test is limited in younger women because one-third or more of women in their 20s have active cervical infections at any given time. The overwhelming majority of these infections and resultant dysplasia will regress and resolve within 8 to 24 months. For women over the age of 30, screening for the presence of HPV DNA or RNA appears to be superior to cytology in identifying women at risk for cervical dysplasia and cancer.[82] An HPV infection in women over the age of 30 is more likely to be persistent and clinically significant.[83] The risk of cervical cancer also increases with age, and most cervical cancer deaths occur in women over 50 years of age.

Cytologic Terminology

The terminology of the Pap smear has changed over time. The traditional cytologic categories were mild, moderate, and severe dysplasia and carcinoma in situ. *Mild* correlated with cervical intraepithelial neoplasia (CIN)1 histology on biopsy; *moderate* usually indicated CIN2; and *severe* dysplasia indicated CIN3 or carcinoma in situ.

There was some subjectivity and some overlap, especially in the area of mild and moderate dysplasia. The NCI sponsored the development of the Bethesda system in 1988. This system provides an assessment of the adequacy of the cervical specimen and a way of categorizing and describing the Pap smear findings. It more effectively and uniformly communicates cytology results from the laboratory to the patient caregiver. The Bethesda system was modified in 1991 and again in 2001.[84] Today, more than 40 international professional societies have endorsed the Bethesda system.

The Bethesda system recognizes both squamous and glandular cytologic abnormalities.

Squamous cell abnormalities include:

- Atypical squamous cells (ASC), which are categorized as either:
  - Of undetermined significance (ASC-US)
  - Cannot exclude high-grade squamous intraepithelial lesions (ASC-H)
- Low-grade squamous intraepithelial lesion (LSIL), which correlates with histologic CIN1
- High-grade squamous intraepithelial lesion (HSIL), which correlates with histologic CIN2, CIN3, and carcinoma in situ

Glandular cell abnormalities (features suggestive of adenocarcinoma) include:

- Atypical glandular cells (AGC): endocervical, endometrial, or not otherwise specified
- AGCs, favor neoplastic
- Endocervical or not otherwise specified
- Endocervical adenocarcinoma in situ (AIS)
- Adenocarcinoma

ASCs differ from normal cells but do not meet criteria for LSIL or HSIL. A small proportion of ASC-US smears are from CIN1 lesions; a smaller proportion are from CIN2 or 3. LSILs are usually due to a transient HPV infection. HSILs are more likely to be due to a persistent HPV infection and are more likely to progress to cervical cancer than LSILs.

The Lower Anogenital Squamous Terminology (LAST) project of the College of American Pathology and the American Society for Colposcopy and Cervical Pathology has proposed that histologic cervical findings be described using the same terminology as cytologic findings.[85]

Women under the age of 30 who have not received the HPV vaccine have a high incidence of HPV infection[86] and the highest prevalence of CIN. However, the overwhelming majority of these HPV infections and associated CIN will spontaneously regress.[87,88] Due to the high regression rates, cervical screening and treatment in women aged 20 to 24 years appear to have little or no impact on the incidence of invasive cervical cancer. It is estimated that about 6% of CIN1 lesions progress to CIN3, and 10% to 20% of CIN3 lesions progress to invasive cancer.[89]

The Atypical Squamous Cells of Undetermined Significance (ASCUS)-LSIL Triage Study (ALTS) evaluated women with abnormal Pap smears.[90] The investigators concluded that women with ASC-US should be tested for HPV. Those who are HPV positive should receive a colposcopy. In addition, because most women with LSIL or HSIL had an HPV infection, an immediate colposcopy and a biopsy of lesions was recommended.[91] HPV DNA testing is very sensitive for identifying CIN2 or worse pathology. Among women 30 to 69 years of age, the sensitivity of the Pap test with HPV testing was 95% compared with 55% for the Pap test alone.[92]

Performance Characteristics of Cervical Cytology

The sensitivity of cytology varies and is a function of the adequacy of the cervical specimen. It is also affected by the age of the woman and the experience of the cytologist. The addition of HPV testing increases the number of women referred for a colposcopy. Not surprisingly, sensitivity is improved by serial examinations over time versus a single screen.

Screening Recommendations

Cervical screening, like other screening tests, is associated with some degree of overdiagnosis as evidenced by the phenomenon of spontaneous regression (see previous) and, therefore, potential harm from overtreatment, such as cervical incompetence, which may reduce fertility and the ability to carry a pregnancy to term. Because dysplasia takes years to progress to cervical cancer,

increasing the screening interval can reduce overdiagnosis and excessive treatment without decreasing screening efficacy.

In 2012, the ACS, the American Society for Colposcopy and Cervical Pathology (ASCCP), and the American Society for Clinical Pathology (ASCP) issued joint screening guidelines.[93] These guidelines recommend different surveillance strategies and options based on a woman's age, screening history, risk factors, and choice of screening tests. The following are the recommendations for a woman at average risk.

- Screening for cervical cancer should begin at 21 years of age. Women aged 21 to 29 years should receive cytology screening (with either conventional cervical cytology smears or liquid-based cytology) every 3 years. HPV testing should not be performed in this age group (although it can be used to follow-up a diagnosis of ASC-US). Women under 21 years of age should not be screened regardless of their age of sexual initiation.
- For women aged 30 to 65 years, the preferred approach is to be screened every 5 years with both HPV testing and cytology (cotesting). It is also acceptable to continue screening every 3 years with cytology alone.
- Women should discontinue screening after age 65 years if they have had three consecutive negative cytology tests or two consecutive negative HPV test results within the 10-year period before ceasing screening, with the most recent test occurring within the last 5 years.
- Women who have undergone a hysterectomy for noncancerous conditions do not need to undergo cervical cancer screening.
- Women, regardless of age, should NOT be screened annually by any screening method.
- Women who have received HPV vaccinations should still be screened according to the previously listed schedule.

Screening in Low Resource Countries

Cytology and HPV testing is not widely available in much of the world. Cervical cancer remains a leading cause of death in many of these areas. Visual inspection of the cervix is a low-tech method of screening that is now recognized as having the potential to save thousands of lives per year. A clustered, randomized trial in India compared one-time cervical visual inspection and immediate colposcopy, biopsy, and/or cryotherapy (where indicated) versus counseling on cervical cancer deaths in women aged 30 to 59 years. After 7 years of follow-up, the age-standardized rate of death due to cervical cancer was 39.6 per 100,000 person-years in the intervention group versus 56.7 per 100,000 person-years in unscreened controls.[94,95] This was the first prospective randomized clinical trial to evaluate cervical cancer screening.

Ovarian Cancer Screening

Modalities proposed for ovarian cancer screening include the bimanual pelvic examination, serum CA-125 antigen measurement, and transvaginal ultrasound (TVU). The bimanual pelvic examination is subjective and not very reproducible, but serum CA-125 can be objectively measured. Unfortunately, CA-125 is neither sensitive nor specific. It is elevated in only about half of women with ovarian cancer and may be elevated in a number of nonmalignant diseases (e.g., diverticulosis, endometriosis, cirrhosis, normal menstruation, pregnancy, uterine fibroids).[96–98] TVU has shown poor performance in the detection of ovarian cancer in average and high-risk women.[99] There is interest in the analysis of serum proteomic patterns, but this should be considered experimental.[100,101]

The combination of CA-125 and TVU has been assessed in two large, prospective randomized trials. The U.S. trial, the Prostate Lung Colorectal and Ovarian trial (PLCO), enrolled

78,216 women of average risk age 55 to 74 years.[102,103] Participants were randomized to receive annual examinations with CA-125 (at entry and then annually for 5 years) and TVU (at entry and then annually for 3 years) (n = 39,105), or usual care (n = 39,111). Participants were followed for a maximum of 13 years, with mortality from ovarian cancer as the main study outcome. At the conclusion of the study, the number of deaths from ovarian cancer was similar in each group. There were 3.1 ovarian cancer deaths per 10,000 women years in the screened group versus 2.6 deaths per 10,000 women years in the control group (RR = 1.18; 95% CI, 0.82 to 1.71).[103]

The U.K. Collaborative Trial of Ovarian Cancer Screening (UKCTOCS) is a randomized trial assessing the efficacy of CA-125 and TVU in more than 200,000 postmenopausal women. In this trial, CA-125 is being used as a first-line test and TVU as a follow-up test using a risk of ovarian cancer algorithm (ROCA).[104] The ROCA measures changes in CA-125 over time rather than using a predefined cut point.[105] ROCA is believed to improve sensitivity for smaller tumors without measurably increasing the FP rate. A mortality assessment is expected in 2015.[106]

No organization currently recommends screening average risk women for ovarian cancer. In 2012, the USPSTF recommended against screening for ovarian cancer, concluding that there was "adequate evidence" that (1) annual screening with TVU and CA-125 does not reduce ovarian cancer mortality and (2) screening for ovarian cancer can lead to important harms, mainly surgical interventions in women without ovarian cancer.[107]

Women at High Risk for Ovarian Cancer

Although no study has shown a mortality benefit for ovarian cancer screening of high-risk individuals, a National Institutes of Health (NIH) consensus panel concluded that it was prudent for women with a known hereditary ovarian cancer syndrome, such as BRCA1/2 mutations or HNPCC, to have annual rectovaginal pelvic examinations, CA-125 determinations, and TVU until childbearing is completed or at least until age 35 years, at which time a prophylactic bilateral oophorectomy is recommended.[108]

Endometrial Cancer Screening

There is insufficient evidence to recommend endometrial cancer screening either for women at average risk or for those at increased risk due to a history of unopposed estrogen therapy, tamoxifen therapy, late menopause, nulliparity, infertility or failure to ovulate, obesity, diabetes, or hypertension.[109] The ACS recommends that women be informed about the symptoms of endometrial cancer—in particular, vaginal bleeding and spotting—after the onset of menopause. Women should be encouraged to immediately report these symptoms to their physician.

Women at High Risk for Endometrial Cancer

Women with a suspected autosomal-dominant predisposition to colon cancer (e.g. Lynch syndrome), should consider undergoing an annual endometrial biopsy to evaluate endometrial histology, beginning at age 35 years.[110,111] This is based only on *expert opinion*, given the paucity of clinical trial data. Women should be informed about the potential benefits, harms, and limitations of testing for early endometrial cancer.

LUNG CANCER SCREENING

Lung cancer screening programs using chest radiographs (CXR) and sputum cytology began in the late 1940s.[112] An evaluation of these programs showed that screening led to the diagnosis of an increased number of cancers, an increased proportion of early stage cancers, and a larger proportion of screen-diagnosed patients surviving more than 5 years.

These findings led many to advocate for mass lung cancer screening, whereas others called for a prospective, randomized trial with a lung cancer mortality endpoint.[113] The Mayo Lung Project (MLP), which began in 1971, was such a trial. More than 9,200 male smokers were enrolled and randomized to either have sputum cytology collected and CXRs done every 4 months for 6 years or to have these same tests performed annually.

At 13 years of follow-up, there were more early stage cancers in the intensively screened arm (n = 99) than in the control arm (n = 51), but the number of advanced tumors was nearly identical (107 versus 109, respectively).[114] Despite an increase in 5-year survival (35% versus 15%) intensive screening was not associated with a reduction in lung cancer mortality (3.2 versus 3.0 deaths per 1,000 person-years, respectively).[115]

The impact of screening on cancer incidence persisted through nearly 20 years of follow-up. There were 585 lung cancers diagnosed on the intensive screening arm versus 500 on the control arm (p = 0.009) and intensive screening continued to be associated with a significant increase in disease-specific survival. However, a concomitant decrease in lung-cancer mortality did not emerge with long-term follow-up (4.4 lung cancer deaths per 1,000 person-years in the intensively screened arm versus 3.9 per 1,000 person-years in the control arm).[116] This suggests that some lung cancers diagnosed by screening would not have resulted in death had they not been detected (i.e., overdiagnosis).[116]

Two other large, randomized studies of CXR and sputum cytology were conducted in the United States during the same time period. All three studies evaluated different screening schedules rather than screening versus no screening. Paradoxically, a meta-analysis of the three studies found that more frequent screening was associated with an increase (albeit not statistically significant), rather than a decrease, in lung cancer mortality when compared with less frequent screening.[117] A study conducted in Czechoslovakia in the 1980s also failed to show a reduction in lung cancer mortality with CXR screening.[118]

More recently, the NCI conducted the PLCO trial at 10 sites across the United States. This was a prospective, randomized trial of nearly 155,000 men and women, aged 55 to 74 years. Participants were randomized to receive annual, single-view, posteroanterior CXRs for 4 years versus routine care. With 13 years of follow-up, no significant difference in lung cancer mortality was observed. A total of 1,213 lung cancer deaths occurred on the intervention arm versus 1,230 in the control group (RR, 0.99; 95% CI, 0.87 to 1.22).[119]

Low-dose computerized tomography (LDCT) is an appealing technology for lung cancer screening. It uses an average of 1.5 mSv of radiation to perform a lung scan in 15 seconds. A conventional CT scan uses 8 mSv of radiation and takes several minutes. The LDCT image is not as sharp as the conventional image, but sensitivity and specificity for the detection of lung lesions are similar.

As in the early chest radiograph trials, a number of single-arm LDCT studies reported a substantial increase in the number of early stage lung cancers diagnosed. These studies also demonstrated that 5-year survival rates were increased in screened compared to unscreened populations.

These findings led to the conduct of several randomized trials of LDCT for the early detection of lung cancer. The largest, longest, and first to report a mortality end point is the National Lung Screening Trial (NLST). In this trial, approximately 53,000 persons were randomized to receive three annual LDCT scans or single-view posteroanterior CXRs. Eligible participants were current and former smokers between 55 and 74 years of age at the time of randomization with at least a 30 pack-year smoking history; former smokers were eligible if they had quit smoking within the previous 15 years.

With a median follow-up of 6.5 years, 13% more lung cancers were diagnosed and a 20% (95% CI, 6.8 to 26.7; p = 0.004) relative reduction in lung cancer mortality was observed in the LDCT arm compared to the CXR arm.[11] This corresponds to rates of death from lung cancer of 247 and 309 per 100,000 person-years, respectively.[11] Another important finding from the NLST was a 6.7% (95% CI, 1.2 to 13.6; p = 0.02) decrease in death from any cause in the LDCT group.

NLST participants were at high risk for developing lung cancer based on their smoking history. Indeed, 25% of all participant deaths were due to lung cancer. A further analysis of the NLST shows that screening prevented the greatest number of lung cancer deaths among participants who were at the highest risk but prevented very few deaths among those at the lowest risk. These findings provide empirical support for risk-based screening.[120]

LDCT screening is clearly promising, but there are some notable caveats. The risk of a FP finding in the first screen was 21%. Overall, after three CT scans, 39.1% of participants had at least one positive screening result. Of those who screened positive, the FP rate was 96.4% in the LDCT group.[11] Positive results require additional workup, which can include conventional CT scans, a needle biopsy, bronchoscopy, mediastinoscopy, or thoracotomy. These diagnostic procedures are associated with anxiety, expense, and complications (e.g., pneumo- or hemothorax after a lung biopsy). In the LDCT study arm, there were 16 deaths within 60 days of an invasive diagnostic procedure. Of the 16 deaths, 6 ultimately did not have cancer. Although it is not known whether these deaths were directly caused by the invasive procedure, such findings do give pause. Although the radiation dose from LDCT is low, the possibility that this screening test could cause radiation-induced cancers is at least a theoretical concern. The possibility of this long-term phenomenon will have to be assessed in future analyses.

The CXR lung screening studies suggested that there is a reservoir of biologically indolent lung cancer and that a percentage of screen-detected lung cancers represent overdiagnosis. The estimated rate of overdiagnosis in the long-term follow-up of the Mayo Lung Study and the other CXR studies was 17 to 18.5%.[121] Similarly, it is estimated that 18.5% of the cancers diagnosed on the LDCT arm of the NLST represented overdiagnosis.[122]

There are estimates that widespread, high-quality screening has the potential to prevent 12,000 lung cancer deaths per year in the United States.[123] However, the NLST was performed at 33 centers specifically chosen for their expertise in the screening, diagnosis, and treatment of lung cancer. It is not known whether the widespread adoption of LDCT lung cancer screening will result in higher complication rates and a less favorable risk–benefit ratio.

Although LDCT lung cancer screening should clearly be considered for those at high risk of the disease, those at lower risk are equally likely to suffer the harms associated with screening but less likely to reap the benefits.

Following the announcement of the NLST results, the ACS, the American College of Chest Physicians (AACP), the American Society of Clinical Oncology (ASCO), and the National Comprehensive Cancer Network (NCCN) recommended that clinicians should initiate a discussion about lung cancer screening with patients who would have qualified for the trial. That is:

- Age 55 to 74 years
- At least a 30 pack-year smoking history
- Currently smoke or have quit within the past 15 years
- Relatively good health

Core elements of this discussion should include the benefits, uncertainties, and harms associated with screening for lung cancer with LDCT. Adults who choose to be screened should enter an organized screening program at an institution with expertise in LDCT screening, with access to a multidisciplinary team skilled in the evaluation, diagnosis, and treatment of abnormal lung lesions. If such a program is not available, the risks of harm due to screening may be greater than the benefits.[124,125] The guidelines recommend an annual LDCT screening with the caveat that participants in NLST had only three annual screens.

The USPSTF guidelines give LDCT a grade B recommendation, concluding that there is moderate certainty that annual screening for lung cancer with LDCT is of moderate net benefit in asymptomatic persons at high risk for lung cancer based on age, total cumulative exposure to tobacco smoke, and years since quitting.

PROSTATE CANCER SCREENING

Hugh Hampton Young first advocated the early detection of prostate cancer with a careful digital rectal examination (DRE) in 1903. Screening for prostate cancer with the DRE and serum PSA was first advocated in the mid 1980s and became commonplace by 1992. PSA screening is directly responsible for prostate cancer becoming the most common nonskin cancer in American men.

PSA is a glycoprotein produced almost exclusively by the epithelial component of the prostate gland. This protein was discovered in the late 1970s, and a serum test to measure circulating levels was developed in the early 1980s. Although PSA is prostate specific, it is not prostate cancer specific and may be elevated in a variety of conditions (e.g., benign prostatic hyperplasia, inflammation and following trauma to the gland, the presence of prostate cancer).

The PSA test has been widely advocated for prostate cancer screening because it is objective, easily measured, reproducible, noninvasive, and inexpensive. Although PSA screening increases the detection of potentially curable disease, there is substantial debate about the overall utility of the test. This is because PSA screening introduces substantial lead time and length bias as well as being associated with a high FN and FP rates and having a low positive predictive value. The prostate cancer conundrum was best summarized by the distinguished urologist, Willet Whitmore when he said, "Is cure necessary for those in whom it is possible? Is cure possible for those in whom it is necessary?"[126]

Observational studies suggest that the problem of prostate cancer overdiagnosis precedes the PSA era. In a landmark analysis with 20-year follow-up, only a small proportion of 767 men, diagnosed with localized prostate cancer in the 1970s and early 1980s and followed expectantly, died from prostate cancer: 4% to 7% of those with Gleason 2 to 4 tumors, 6% to 11% of those with Gleason 5 disease, and 18% to 30% of men with Gleason 6 cancer.[127]

Although obviously present in the pre-PSA era, overdiagnosis increased substantially after the introduction of PSA screening. This is illustrated by an examination of the prostate cancer incidence and mortality rates in Washington state and Connecticut. Due to the earlier uptake of PSA screening, the incidence of prostate cancer in Washington increased to twice that of Connecticut during the 1990s. However, mortality rates remained similar throughout the decade and, in fact, have remained similar to this day. The Surveillance, Epidemiology, and End Results (SEER) cancer registries show that, over the last 2 decades, a larger proportion of men living in western Washington have been diagnosed with prostate cancer and definitively treated, without a concomitant reduction in prostate cancer mortality compared to that of men living in Connecticut.[128]

Additional evidence of the potential for overdiagnosis comes from the unexpectedly large number of men diagnosed with prostate cancer in the Prostate Cancer Prevention Trial (PCPT). The PCPT was a prospective, randomized, placebo-controlled trial of finasteride for prostate cancer prevention. Men were screened annually during this trial, and those who had not been diagnosed with prostate cancer after 7 years on-study were asked to undergo an end-of-study prostate biopsy. Of 4,692 men on the placebo arm whose prostate cancer status had been determined by biopsy or transurethral resection (TURP), 24.4% were diagnosed with prostate cancer. Given that the lifetime risk of prostate cancer mortality in the United States is less than 3%, it is clear that many men harbor indolent prostate cancer and, therefore, are at risk of being overdiagnosed.

The unexpectantly high rate of positive end-of-study biopsies in men with PSA levels less than or equal to 4.0 ng/mL provided a more accurate assessment of disease prevalence and thus a more accurate assessment of PSA sensitivity than was previously possible. Of the 2,950 men on the placebo arm of the PCPT with PSA levels consistently less than or equal to 4 ng/mL who underwent end-of-study biopsies, 449 (15.2%) were diagnosed with prostate cancer. Accordingly, a PSA level <4.0 ng/mL is more likely to be a *false* negative. Because Sensitivity = True Positives / (True Positives + False Negatives), a higher FN rate means a lower sensitivity at any given PSA threshold. This has prompted some to advocate using a lower PSA threshold for recommending biopsies. However, although lowering the PSA threshold from 4.0 to 2.5 ng/mL increases the sensitivity from 24% to 42.8%, it reduces specificity from 92.7% to an unacceptably low 80%.[129]

In the PCPT, cancer was found on end-of-study biopsies at all PSA levels (e.g., including 10% of biopsies in men with PSA levels between 0.6 and 1.0 ng/mL and 6% of biopsies in men with PSA levels between 0 and 0.6 were positive), suggesting a continuum of prostate cancer risk and no cut point with simultaneously high sensitivity and high specificity. High-grade disease was also documented at all PSA levels, albeit at an overall frequency of only 2.3% of men with PSAs <4 ng/mL.[130,131]

Does Prostate Cancer Treatment Prevent Deaths?

In order for screening to work, treatment has to work. The first prospective, randomized studies showing that any prostate cancer treatment saves lives were published in the late 1990s. These studies demonstrated an overall survival benefit for the addition of long-term androgen deprivation to radiation therapy in men with locally advanced, high-risk prostate cancer.[132]

The value of surgery for localized disease was assessed by the Scandinavian Prostate Cancer Group 4 study (SPCG-4). In this trial, 695 men with clinically localized prostate cancer were prospectively randomized to receive radical prostatectomy (RP) or watchful waiting (WW). In the expectant management group, hormonal therapy was given at the time of symptomatic metastases. About 60% of those enrolled had low-grade, 23% had moderate-grade, 5% had high-grade tumors, and 12% had tumors of unknown grade. At a median follow-up of 12.8 years, the RP group had significantly lower overall (RR 0.75; p = 0.007) and prostate cancer–specific mortality (RR 0.62; p = 0.01), with 14.6% of the PR group and 20.7% of the WW group having died of prostate cancer. The number needed to treat or prevent one prostate cancer death was 15. The survival benefit associated with RP was similar before and after 9 years of follow-up and for men with low and high-risk disease. However, a subset analysis suggested that the mortality benefit of surgery was limited to men less than 65 years of age. An important limitation of this trial is that 75% of the study participants had palpable disease, only 12% had nonpalpable disease, and only 5% of the cancers had been screen detected. It is, therefore, difficult to apply these data to the US prostate cancer population, which is dominated by nonpalpable, screen-detected disease.[133]

In contrast to the SPCG-4, the Prostate Intervention versus Observation Trial (PIVOT) was conducted in the United States during the early PSA era. In this study, 731 men with screen-detected prostate cancer were randomized to receive RP or WW. Of the participants, 50% had nonpalpable disease and, using established criteria for PSA levels, grade, and tumor stage, 43% of men had low-risk, 36% had intermediate-risk, and 21% had high-risk prostate cancer. With a median follow-up of 12 years, during which time 48.4% (354 of 731) of the study participants had died, RP was associated with statistically insignificant 2.9% and 2.6% absolute reductions in overall and prostate cancer–specific mortality,

respectively. Subgroup analyses suggested mortality benefits for men with PSA values greater than 10 ng/mL and for those with intermediate- and high-risk disease.[134]

The Prospective Randomized Screening Trials

The PLCO Cancer Screening Trial was a multicenter, phase III trial conducted in the United States by the NCI. In this trial, nearly 77,000 men age 55 to 74 years were randomized to receive annual PSA testing for 6 years or usual care. At 13 years of follow-up, a nonsignificant increase in cumulative prostate cancer mortality was observed among men randomized to annual screening (RR, 1.09; 95% CI, 0.87 to 1.36).[135] The most important limitation of this trial was the high rate of PSA testing among men randomized to the control arm. This *drop-in* or *contamination* served to reduce the statistical power of the study to detect differences in outcome between the two arms. It has also been argued that, due to the high rate of PSA screening on the control arm, PLCO effectively compared regular prostate cancer screening to opportunistic screening rather than comparing screening to no screening.

The ERSPC is a multicenter trial initiated in 1991 in the Netherlands and Belgium; five additional European countries joined between 1994 and 1998.[136,137] The frequency of PSA testing was every 4 years in all countries except Sweden, in which it was every 2 years. The study results were initially reported in 2009 and updated in 2012.[136,137] Although the overall analysis of 182,160 men, aged 50 to 74, did not show a reduction in prostate cancer–specific mortality, screening was associated with a significant decrease in prostate cancer mortality in the prespecified core age group, 55 to 69 years, which included 162,243 men. After a median follow-up of 11 years, a 21% relative reduction of prostate cancer death (RR, 0.79; 95% CI, 0.68 to 0.91) was observed in this group. In absolute terms, prostate cancer mortality was reduced from 5 to 4 men per 1,000 screened and 37 men had to be diagnosed to avert one prostate cancer death. It remains to be seen whether the benefits of screening will increase with continued follow-up.

The recruitment and randomization procedures of the ERSPC differed among countries. Notably, potential participants in Finland, Sweden, and Italy were identified from population registries and underwent randomization *before* written informed consent was obtained. In some trials, men on the control arm were not aware they were in the study. Therefore, men on the intervention arm in these countries were more likely to be cared for at high-volume referral centers. This may have contributed to the higher proportion of men on the screening arm, with clinically localized cancer being treated with RPs.[138]

In a separate report on 20,000 men randomized to screening or a control group in Göteborg, Sweden, there was a 40% (95% CI, 1.50 to 1.80) risk reduction at 14 years of follow-up.[139] They reported 293 (95% CI, 177 to 799) needed to be screened and 12 needed to be diagnosed in order to prevent one prostate cancer death. Three-fourths of the men in this report and 89% of the prostate cancer deaths were included in the published ERSPC analysis. Given this, these data do not constitute independent evidence of the efficacy of prostate cancer screening.

The other site to report separately was in Finland. A total of 80,144 men were randomized to a screening or usual care arm. At 12 years after randomization, there was no statistical difference in risk of prostate cancer death (hazard ratio [HR] = 0.85; 95% CI, 0.69 to 1.04).[140] Possible explanations as to why Sweden and Finland would have such different outcomes include differences in the frequency of screening (every 2 years versus every 4 years, respectively) and the higher background rate of death from prostate cancer in the control group in the Goteborg cohort. Given that the mortality data from these two cohorts have been largely included in the ERSPC analyses, they do not provide independent evidence of the efficacy of prostate cancer screening.

The decline in prostate cancer mortality in the United States since the introduction of PSA screening 2 decades ago is often offered as evidence supporting a mortality benefit for prostate cancer screening. However, prostate cancer mortality rates have also declined in many countries that have not widely adopted screening.[141] Thus, it is likely that improvements in treatment have contributed, at least in part, to the observed decline in prostate cancer mortality. Another possible contributing factor may be the World Health Organization (WHO) algorithm for adjudicating cause of death. A change occurred just as mortality rates began to go up in the late 1970s, and WHO changed back to the older algorithm in 1991 when prostate cancer mortality began declining in many countries.[142] All of these factors, including a beneficial effect from screening, may be contributing to the declining prostate cancer mortality rates in the United States.

Screening Recommendations

The topic of prostate cancer screening tends to evoke strong emotional reactions. Although the intuitive appeal of early detection is undeniable and screening may save some lives, the magnitude of the mortality reduction is relatively small, whereas the harms associated with screening can be substantial. Whether the potential benefits outweigh the known harms is a question that each man must answer for himself based on his individual preferences.

Several professional organizations in the United States, Europe, and Canada have recently reviewed the screening data and issued screening guidelines. All acknowledge that legitimate concerns remain regarding the risk–benefit ratio of prostate cancer screening. There is also general agreement that prostate cancer screening should only be done in the context of fully informed consent and that men should know that experts do not agree as to whether the benefits of screening for this disease outweigh the harms. Most recommend against mass screening in public meeting places, malls, churches, etc.

In 2009, the American Urological Association (AUA) PSA Best Practice Statement was published, which stated, "Given the uncertainty that PSA testing results in more benefit than harm, a thoughtful and broad approach to PSA is critical. Patients need to be informed of the risks and the benefits of testing before it is undertaken. The risks of over-detection and over-treatment should be included in this discussion."[143]

In 2010, the ACS updated their guidelines, stating that the balance of benefits and harms related to prostate cancer early detection are uncertain and the existing evidence is insufficient to support a recommendation for or against the routine use of PSA screening.[144] The ACS called for discussion and shared decision making within the physician–patient relationship.

The most recent 2012 USPSTF guidelines recommend against the use of PSA screening on the basis that there is moderate certainty that the harms of PSA testing outweigh the benefits and, on that basis, recommended against PSA-based screening for all men.[14] The task force did acknowledge that some men will continue to request screening and some physicians will continue to offer it. Like the ACS and AUA, they state that screening under such circumstances should respect patient preferences.

In 2013, the AUA conducted a systematic review of over 300 studies. They recommended against screening men younger than 40 years of age, and against screening average-risk men age 40 to 54 years, most men over 70 years of age, and men with a life expectancy of less than 10 to 15 years. They recommend that screening decisions be individualized for higher risk men ages 40 to 54 years and men over 70 years of age who are in excellent health. They placed primacy on shared decision making versus physician judgments about the balance of benefits and harms at the population level.[145] Even for men aged 55 to 69 years, the AUA concluded that the quality of evidence for benefits associated with screening was moderate, whereas the quality of the evidence for harm was high. They recommended shared decision making for this group, in whom they have concluded the benefits may outweigh the harm.

SKIN CANCER SCREENING

Assessments of skin cancer screening have focused on melanoma end points with very little attention to screening for nonmelanoma skin cancer. A systematic review of skin cancer screening studies examining the available evidence through mid 2005 concluded that direct evidence of improved health outcomes associated with skin cancer screening is lacking.[146]

No randomized, clinical trial of skin cancer screening has been attempted. However, several observational studies have suggested that melanoma screening might reduce mortality. For example, a decrease in melanoma mortality did occur after a Scottish campaign to promote awareness of the signs of suspicious skin lesions and encourage early self-referral. However, uncontrolled, ecologic studies such as this provide a relatively low level of evidence, because it is not possible to determine whether the observed mortality reduction was due to screening or other factors.

More recently, the Skin Cancer Research to Provide Evidence for Effectiveness of Screening project, or SCREEN project, compared a region of Germany in which intensive skin cancer screening was performed to areas of Germany without intensive screening. Approximately 360,000 residents of the Schleswig-Holstein region aged 20 years and older participated. They chose either to be screened by a nondermatologist physician trained in skin examinations or by a dermatologist. Almost 16,000 biopsies were performed and 585 melanomas were diagnosed. Overall, 1 in 23 participants had an excisional skin biopsy and 620 persons needed to be screened to detect one melanoma. This screening effort led to a 16% and 38% increase in melanoma incidence among men and women, respectively, compared to 2 years earlier. The melanoma incidence rate returned to preprogram levels after the program ended. Of the screen-detected melanomas, 90% were less than 1 mm thick. Screening was performed in 2003 to 2004, and melanoma mortality in this region subsequently declined. In 2008, it was nearly 50% lower in both men and women compared to the rest of Germany.[147,148]

Recommendations of Experts

Skin cancer screening recommendations are based on *expert opinion*, given the absence of a randomized clinical trial data and limited observational studies. The ACS recommends monthly skin self-examinations and a yearly clinical skin examination as part of a routine cancer-related checkup.[149] The USPSTF finds insufficient evidence to recommend for or against either routine skin cancer screening of the general population by primary care providers or counseling patients to perform periodic skin self-examinations. The task force does recommend that clinicians "remain alert" for skin lesions with malignant features when performing a physical examination for other purposes, particularly in high-risk individuals. The American Academy of Dermatology recommends that persons at highest risk (i.e., those with a strong family history of melanoma and multiple atypical nevi), perform frequent self-examination and seek a professional evaluation of the skin at least once per year.[150]

High-risk individuals are persons with multiple nevi or atypical moles. There is consensus they should be educated about the need for frequent surveillance by a trained health-care provider beginning at an early age. In the United States, Australia, and Western Europe, Caucasian men age 50 years and over account for nearly half of all melanoma cases. There is some discussion that melanoma early detection efforts should be focused on this population.

REFERENCES

1. Collen MF, Dales LG, Friedman GD, et al. Multiphasic checkup evaluation study. 4. Preliminary cost benefit analysis for middle-aged men. *Prev Med* 1973; 2:236–246.
2. Prorok PC, Kramer BS, Gohagan JK. Screening theory and study design: the basics. In: Kramer B, Prorok P, eds. *Cancer Screening.* New York: Marcel Dekker; 1999: 29–53.
3. Welch HG, Black WC. Overdiagnosis in cancer. *J Natl Cancer Inst* 2010; 102:605–613.
4. Yamamoto K, Hayashi Y, Hanada R, et al. Mass screening and age-specific incidence of neuroblastoma in Saitama Prefecture, Japan. *J Clin Oncol* 1995;13:2033–2038.
5. Woods WG, Gao RN, Shuster JJ, et al. Screening of infants and mortality due to neuroblastoma. *N Engl J Med* 2002;346:1041–1046.
6. Friedman GD, Collen MF, Fireman BH. Multiphasic Health Checkup Evaluation: a 16-year follow-up. *J Chronic Dis* 1986;39:453–463.
7. Pinsky PF, Miller A, Kramer BS, et al. Evidence of a healthy volunteer effect in the prostate, lung, colorectal, and ovarian cancer screening trial. *Am J Epidemiol* 2007;165:874–881.
8. Boyle P, Brawley OW. Prostate cancer: current evidence weighs against population screening. *CA Cancer J Clin* 2009;59:220–224.
9. Autier P, Boyle P, Buyse M, et al. Is FOB screening really the answer for lowering mortality in colorectal cancer? *Recent Results Cancer Res* 2003;163: 254–263.
10. de Boer AG, Taskila T, Ojajarvi A, et al. Cancer survivors and unemployment: a meta-analysis and meta-regression. *JAMA* 2009;301:753–762.
11. Aberle DR, Adams AM, Berg CD, et al. Reduced lung-cancer mortality with low-dose computed tomographic screening. *N Engl J Med* 2011;365: 395–409.
12. Eden J, Levit L, Berg A, et al., eds. *Finding What Works in Health Care: Standards for Systematic Reviews.* Washington DC: The National Academies Press; 2011.
13. Graham R, Mancher M, Wolman DM, et al. Medicine CoSfDTCPGIo. Washington, DC: The National Academies; 2011.
14. Moyer VA. Screening for prostate cancer: U.S. Preventive Services Task Force recommendation statement. *Ann Intern Med* 2012;157:120–134.
15. Brawley O, Byers T, Chen A, et al. New American Cancer Society process for creating trustworthy cancer screening guidelines. *JAMA* 2011;306:2495–2499.
16. Shapiro S. Periodic screening for breast cancer: the HIP Randomized Controlled Trial. Health Insurance Plan. *J Natl Cancer Inst Monogr* 1997:27–30.
17. Miller AB, Wall C, Baines CJ, et al. Twenty five year follow-up for breast cancer incidence and mortality of the Canadian National Breast Screening Study: randomised screening trial. *BMJ* 2014;348:g366.
18. Tabar L, Fagerberg G, Duffy SW, et al. Update of the Swedish two-county program of mammographic screening for breast cancer. *Radiol Clin North Am* 1992;30: 187–210.
19. Moy L, Slanetz PJ, Moore R, et al. Specificity of mammography and US in the evaluation of a palpable abnormality: retrospective review. *Radiology* 2002;225:176–181.
20. Lord SJ, Lei W, Craft P, et al. A systematic review of the effectiveness of magnetic resonance imaging (MRI) as an addition to mammography and ultrasound in screening young women at high risk of breast cancer. *Eur J Cancer* 2007;43:1905–1917.
21. Wishart GC, Campisi M, Boswell M, et al. The accuracy of digital infrared imaging for breast cancer detection in women undergoing breast biopsy. *Eur J Surg Oncol* 2010;36:535–540.
22. Dooley WC, Ljung BM, Veronesi U, et al. Ductal lavage for detection of cellular atypia in women at high risk for breast cancer. *J Natl Cancer Inst* 2001;93:1624–1632.
23. Autier P, Boniol M, Middleton R, et al. Advanced breast cancer incidence following population-based mammographic screening. *Ann Oncol* 2011;22:1726–1735.
24. Bleyer A, Welch HG. Effect of three decades of screening mammography on breast-cancer incidence. *N Engl J Med* 2012;367:1998–2005.
25. Marmot MG, Altman DG, Cameron DA, et al. The benefits and harms of breast cancer screening: an independent review. *Br J Cancer* 2013;108:2205–2240.
26. Berry DA, Cronin KA, Plevritis SK, et al. Effect of screening and adjuvant therapy on mortality from breast cancer. *N Engl J Med* 2005;353:1784–1792.
27. Harris R, Yeatts J, Kinsinger L. Breast cancer screening for women ages 50 to 69 years a systematic review of observational evidence. *Prev Med* 2011;53: 108–114.
28. Nelson HD, Tyne K, Naik A, et al. Screening for breast cancer: an update for the U.S. Preventive Services Task Force. *Ann Intern Med* 2009;151:727–737.
29. Mandelblatt JS, Cronin KA, Bailey S, et al. Effects of mammography screening under different screening schedules: model estimates of potential benefits and harms. *Ann Intern Med* 2009;151:738–747.
30. U.S. Preventive Services Task Force. Screening for breast cancer: U.S. Preventive Services Task Force recommendation statement. *Ann Intern Med* 2009;151:716–726.
31. Nelson HD, Zakher B, Cantor A, et al. Risk factors for breast cancer for women aged 40 to 49 years: a systematic review and meta-analysis. *Ann Intern Med* 2012;156:635–648.
32. Barnett GC, Shah M, Redman K, et al. Risk factors for the incidence of breast cancer: do they affect survival from the disease? *J Clin Oncol* 2008;26: 3310–3316.

33. Gierach GL, Ichikawa L, Kerlikowske K, et al. Relationship between mammographic density and breast cancer death in the Breast Cancer Surveillance Consortium. *J Natl Cancer Inst* 2012;104:1218–1227.
34. Berg WA, Blume JD, Cormack JB, et al. Combined screening with ultrasound and mammography vs mammography alone in women at elevated risk of breast cancer. *JAMA* 2008;299:2151–2163.
35. Gartlehner G, Thaler K, Chapman A, et al. Mammography in combination with breast ultrasonography versus mammography for breast cancer screening in women at average risk. *Cochrane Database Syst Rev* 2013;4:CD009632.
36. Tice JA, O'Meara ES, Weaver DL, et al. Benign breast disease, mammographic breast density, and the risk of breast cancer. *J Natl Cancer Inst* 2013;105: 1043–1049.
37. Kerlikowske K, Hubbard RA, Miglioretti DL, et al. Comparative effectiveness of digital versus film-screen mammography in community practice in the United States: a cohort study. *Ann Intern Med* 2011;155:493–502.
38. Haas BM, Kalra V, Geisel J, et al. Comparison of tomosynthesis plus digital mammography and digital mammography alone for breast cancer screening. *Radiology* 2013;269:694–700.
39. Rosenberg RD, Yankaskas BC, Abraham LA, et al. Performance benchmarks for screening mammography. *Radiology* 2006;241:55–66.
40. Gomez SL, Lichtensztajn D, Kurian AW, et al. Increasing mastectomy rates for early-stage breast cancer? Population-based trends from California. *J Clin Oncol* 2010;28:e155–e157.
41. Tuttle TM, Jarosek S, Habermann EB, et al. Increasing rates of contralateral prophylactic mastectomy among patients with ductal carcinoma in situ. *J Clin Oncol* 2009;27:1362–1367.
42. Rosenberg RD, Hunt WC, Williamson MR, et al. Effects of age, breast density, ethnicity, and estrogen replacement therapy on screening mammographic sensitivity and cancer stage at diagnosis: review of 183,134 screening mammograms in Albuquerque, New Mexico. *Radiology* 1998;209:511–518.
43. Kerlikowske K, Grady D, Barclay J, et al. Effect of age, breast density, and family history on the sensitivity of first screening mammography. *JAMA* 1996;276: 33–38.
44. Porter PL, El-Bastawissi AY, Mandelson MT, et al. Breast tumor characteristics as predictors of mammographic detection: comparison of interval- and screen-detected cancers. *J Natl Cancer Inst* 1999;91:2020–2028.
45. Ronckers CM, Erdmann CA, Land CE. Radiation and breast cancer: a review of current evidence. *Breast Cancer Res* 2005;7:21–32.
46. Pijpe A, Andrieu N, Easton DF, et al. Exposure to diagnostic radiation and risk of breast cancer among carriers of BRCA1/2 mutations: retrospective cohort study (GENE-RAD-RISK). *BMJ* 2012;345:e5660.
47. Qaseem A, Snow V, Sherif K, et al. Screening mammography for women 40 to 49 years of age: a clinical practice guideline from the American College of Physicians. *Ann Intern Med* 2007;146:511–515.
48. Tonelli M, Connor Gorber S, Joffres M, et al. Recommendations on screening for breast cancer in average-risk women aged 40-74 years. *CMAJ* 2011;183: 1991–2001.
49. Recommendations on cancer screening in the European Union. Advisory Committee on Cancer Prevention. *Eur J Cancer* 2000;36:1473–1478.
50. Saslow D, Boetes C, Burke W, et al. American Cancer Society guidelines for breast screening with MRI as an adjunct to mammography. *CA Cancer J Clin* 2007;57:75–89.
51. Mandel JS, Church TR, Bond JH, et al. The effect of fecal occult-blood screening on the incidence of colorectal cancer. *N Engl J Med* 2000;343: 1603–1607.
52. Nishihara R, Wu K, Lochhead P, et al. Long-term colorectal-cancer incidence and mortality after lower endoscopy. *N Engl J Med* 2013;369: 1095–1105.
53. Schoen RE, Pinsky PF, Weissfeld JL, et al. Colorectal-cancer incidence and mortality with screening flexible sigmoidoscopy. *N Engl J Med* 2012;366: 2345–2357.
54. Mandel JS, Bond JH, Church TR, et al. Reducing mortality from colorectal cancer by screening for fecal occult blood. Minnesota Colon Cancer Control Study. *N Engl J Med* 1993;328:1365–1371.
55. Mandel JS, Church TR, Ederer F, et al. Colorectal cancer mortality: effectiveness of biennial screening for fecal occult blood. *J Natl Cancer Inst* 1999;91:434–437.
56. Hardcastle JD, Chamberlain JO, Robinson MH, et al. Randomised controlled trial of faecal-occult-blood screening for colorectal cancer. *Lancet* 1996;348: 1472–1477.
57. Kronborg O, Fenger C, Olsen J, et al. Randomised study of screening for colorectal cancer with faecal-occult-blood test. *Lancet* 1996;348:1467–1471.
58. Ahlquist DA, Wieand HS, Moertel CG, et al. Accuracy of fecal occult blood screening for colorectal neoplasia. A prospective study using Hemoccult and HemoQuant tests. *JAMA* 1993;269:1262–1267.
59. Levin B, Brooks D, Smith RA, et al. Emerging technologies in screening for colorectal cancer: CT colonography, immunochemical fecal occult blood tests, and stool screening using molecular markers. *CA Cancer J Clin* 2003;53:44–55.
60. Atkin WS, Edwards R, Kralj-Hans I, et al. Once-only flexible sigmoidoscopy screening in prevention of colorectal cancer: a multicentre randomised controlled trial. *Lancet* 2010;375:1624–1633.
61. Levin TR. Flexible sigmoidoscopy for colorectal cancer screening: valid approach or short-sighted? *Gastroenterol Clin North Am* 2002;31:1015–1029.

CANCER PREVENTION AND SCREENING

62. Littlejohn C, Hilton S, Macfarlane GJ, et al. Systematic review and meta-analysis of the evidence for flexible sigmoidoscopy as a screening method for the prevention of colorectal cancer. *Br J Surg* 2012;99:1488–1500.

63. Elmunzer BJ, Hayward RA, Schoenfeld PS, et al. Effect of flexible sigmoidoscopy-based screening on incidence and mortality of colorectal cancer: a systematic review and meta-analysis of randomized controlled trials. *PLoS Med* 2012;9:e1001352.

64. van Rijn JC, Reitsma JB, Stoker J, et al. Polyp miss rate determined by tandem colonoscopy: a systematic review. *Am J Gastroenterol* 2006;101:343–350.

65. Rosman AS, Korsten MA. Meta-analysis comparing CT colonography, air contrast barium enema, and colonoscopy. *Am J Med* 2007;120:203–210.

66. Imperiale TF, Wagner DR, Lin CY, et al. Using risk for advanced proximal colonic neoplasia to tailor endoscopic screening for colorectal cancer. *Ann Intern Med* 2003;139:959–965.

67. U.S. Preventive Services Task Force. Screening for colorectal cancer: U.S. Preventive Services Task Force recommendation statement. *Ann Intern Med* 2008;149:627–637.

68. Winawer S, Fletcher R, Rex D, et al. Colorectal cancer screening and surveillance: clinical guidelines and rationale-Update based on new evidence. *Gastroenterology* 2003;124:544–560.

69. Quintero E, Castells A, Bujanda L, et al. Colonoscopy versus fecal immunochemical testing in colorectal-cancer screening. *N Engl J Med* 2012;366:697–706.

70. Murakami R, Tsukuma H, Ubukata T, et al. Estimation of validity of mass screening program for gastric cancer in Osaka, Japan. *Cancer* 1990;65:1255–1260.

71. Kampschoer GH, Fujii A, Masuda Y. Gastric cancer detected by mass survey. Comparison between mass survey and outpatient detection. *Scand J Gastroenterol* 1989;24:813–817.

72. Stael von Holstein C, Eriksson S, Huldt B, et al. Endoscopic screening during 17 years for gastric stump carcinoma. A prospective clinical trial. *Scand J Gastroenterol* 1991;26:1020–1026.

73. Shaukat A, Mongin SJ, Geisser MS, et al. Long-term mortality after screening for colorectal cancer. *N Engl J Med* 2013;369:1106–1114.

74. McMahon BJ, Bulkow L, Harpster A, et al. Screening for hepatocellular carcinoma in Alaska natives infected with chronic hepatitis B: a 16-year population-based study. *Hepatology* 2000;32:842–846.

75. Chalasani N, Horlander JC Sr, Said A, et al. Screening for hepatocellular carcinoma in patients with advanced cirrhosis. *Am J Gastroenterol* 1999;94:2988–2993.

76. Sherman M, Peltekian KM, Lee C. Screening for hepatocellular carcinoma in chronic carriers of hepatitis B virus: incidence and prevalence of hepatocellular carcinoma in a North American urban population. *Hepatology* 1995;22:432–438.

77. Dodd GD 3rd, Miller WJ, Baron RL, et al. Detection of malignant tumors in end-stage cirrhotic livers: efficacy of sonography as a screening technique. *AJR Am J Roentgenol* 1992;159:727–733.

78. Laara E, Day NE, Hakama M. Trends in mortality from cervical cancer in the Nordic countries: association with organised screening programmes. *Lancet* 1987;1:1247–1249.

79. Christopherson WM, Lundin FE Jr, Mendez WM, et al. Cervical cancer control: a study of morbidity and mortality trends over a twenty-one-year period. *Cancer* 1976;38:1357–1366.

80. Janerich DT, Hadjimichael O, Schwartz PE, et al. The screening histories of women with invasive cervical cancer, Connecticut. *Am J Public Health* 1995;85:791–794.

81. Sawaya GF, McConnell KJ, Kulasingam SL, et al. Risk of cervical cancer associated with extending the interval between cervical-cancer screenings. *N Engl J Med* 2003;349:1501–1509.

82. Sankaranarayanan R, Nene BM, Shastri SS, et al. HPV screening for cervical cancer in rural India. *N Engl J Med* 2009;360:1385–1394.

83. Vesco KK, Whitlock EP, Eder M, et al. In: *Screening for Cervical Cancer: A Systematic Evidence Review for the US Preventive Services Task Force*. Rockville, MD: Agency for Healthcare Research and Quality; 2011.

84. Solomon D, Davey D, Kurman R, et al. The 2001 Bethesda System: terminology for reporting results of cervical cytology. *JAMA* 2002;287:2114–2119.

85. Darragh TM, Colgan TJ, Thomas Cox J, et al. The Lower Anogenital Squamous Terminology Standardization project for HPV-associated lesions: background and consensus recommendations from the College of American Pathologists and the American Society for Colposcopy and Cervical Pathology. *Int J Gynecol Pathol* 2013;32:76–115.

86. Ho GY, Bierman R, Beardsley L, et al. Natural history of cervicovaginal papillomavirus infection in young women. *N Engl J Med* 1998;338:423–428.

87. Holowaty P, Miller AB, Rohan T, et al. Natural history of dysplasia of the uterine cervix. *J Natl Cancer Inst* 1999;91:252–258.

88. Richardson H, Kelsall G, Tellier P, et al. The natural history of type-specific human papillomavirus infections in female university students. *Cancer Epidemiol Biomarkers Prev* 2003;12:485–490.

89. Melnikow J, Nuovo J, Willan AR, et al. Natural history of cervical squamous intraepithelial lesions: a meta-analysis. *Obstet Gynecol* 1998;92:727–735.

90. Cox JT, Schiffman M, Solomon D. Prospective follow-up suggests similar risk of subsequent cervical intraepithelial neoplasia grade 2 or 3 among women with cervical intraepithelial neoplasia grade 1 or negative colposcopy and directed biopsy. *Am J Obstet Gynecol* 2003;188:1406–1412.

91. Guido R, Schiffman M, Solomon D, et al. Postcolposcopy management strategies for women referred with low-grade squamous intraepithelial lesions or human papillomavirus DNA-positive atypical squamous cells of undetermined significance: a two-year prospective study. *Am J Obstet Gynecol* 2003;188:1401–1405.

92. Mayrand MH, Duarte-Franco E, Rodrigues I, et al. Human papillomavirus DNA versus Papanicolaou screening tests for cervical cancer. *N Engl J Med* 2007;357:1579–1588.

93. Saslow D, Solomon D, Lawson HW, et al. American Cancer Society, American Society for Colposcopy and Cervical Pathology, and American Society for Clinical Pathology screening guidelines for the prevention and early detection of cervical cancer. *CA Cancer J Clin* 2012;62:147–172.

94. Sankaranarayanan R, Esmy PO, Rajkumar R, et al. Effect of visual screening on cervical cancer incidence and mortality in Tamil Nadu, India: a cluster-randomised trial. *Lancet* 2007;370:398–406.

95. Szarewski A. Cervical screening by visual inspection with acetic acid. *Lancet* 2007;370:365–366.

96. Johnson CC, Kessel B, Riley TL, et al. The epidemiology of CA-125 in women without evidence of ovarian cancer in the Prostate, Lung, Colorectal and Ovarian Cancer (PLCO) Screening Trial. *Gynecol Oncol* 2008;110:383–389.

97. Duffy MJ, Bonfrer JM, Kulpa J, et al. CA125 in ovarian cancer: European Group on Tumor Markers guidelines for clinical use. *Int J Gynecol Cancer* 2005;15:679–691.

98. Moss EL, Hollingworth J, Reynolds TM. The role of CA125 in clinical practice. *J Clin Pathol* 2005;58:308–312.

99. Fishman DA, Cohen L, Blank SV, et al. The role of ultrasound evaluation in the detection of early-stage epithelial ovarian cancer. *Am J Obstet Gynecol* 2005;192:1214–1221.

100. Kobayashi E, Ueda Y, Matsuzaki S, et al. Biomarkers for screening, diagnosis, and monitoring of ovarian cancer. *Cancer Epidemiol Biomarkers Prev* 2012;21:1902–1912.

101. Ren J, Cai H, Li Y, et al. Tumor markers for early detection of ovarian cancer. *Expert Rev Mol Diagn* 2010;10:787–798.

102. Prorok PC, Andriole GL, Bresalier RS, et al. Design of the Prostate, Lung, Colorectal and Ovarian (PLCO) Cancer Screening Trial. *Control Clin Trials* 2000;21:273S–309S.

103. Buys SS, Partridge E, Black A, et al. Effect of screening on ovarian cancer mortality: the Prostate, Lung, Colorectal and Ovarian (PLCO) Cancer Screening Randomized Controlled Trial. *JAMA* 2011;305:2295–2303.

104. Menon U, Gentry-Maharaj A, Hallett R, et al. Sensitivity and specificity of multimodal and ultrasound screening for ovarian cancer, and stage distribution of detected cancers: results of the prevalence screen of the UK Collaborative Trial of Ovarian Cancer Screening (UKCTOCS). *Lancet Oncol* 2009;10:327–340.

105. Drescher CW, Shah C, Thorpe J, et al. Longitudinal screening algorithm that incorporates change over time in CA125 levels identifies ovarian cancer earlier than a single-threshold rule. *J Clin Oncol* 2013;31:387–392.

106. Sharma A, Apostolidou S, Burnell M, et al. Risk of epithelial ovarian cancer in asymptomatic women with ultrasound-detected ovarian masses: a prospective cohort study within the UK collaborative trial of ovarian cancer screening (UKCTOCS). *Ultrasound Obstet Gynecol* 2012;40:338–344.

107. Moyer VA. Screening for ovarian cancer: U.S. Preventive Services Task Force reaffirmation recommendation statement. *Ann Intern Med* 2012;157:900–904.

108. NIH consensus conference. Ovarian cancer. Screening, treatment, and follow-up. NIH Consensus Development Panel on Ovarian Cancer. *JAMA* 1995;273:491–497.

109. Smith RA, von Eschenbach AC, Wender R, et al. American Cancer Society guidelines for the early detection of cancer: update of early detection guidelines for prostate, colorectal, and endometrial cancers. Also: update 2001—testing for early lung cancer detection. *CA Cancer J Clin* 2001;51:38–75.

110. Burke W, Petersen G, Lynch P, et al. Recommendations for follow-up care of individuals with an inherited predisposition to cancer. I. Hereditary nonpolyposis colon cancer. Cancer Genetics Studies Consortium. *JAMA* 1997;277:915–919.

111. Gull B, Karlsson B, Milsom I, et al. Can ultrasound replace dilation and curettage? A longitudinal evaluation of postmenopausal bleeding and transvaginal sonographic measurement of the endometrium as predictors of endometrial cancer. *Am J Obstet Gynecol* 2003;188:401–408.

112. Scamman CL. Follow-up study of lung cancer suspects in a mass chest X-ray survey. *N Engl J Med* 1951;244:541–544.

113. Croswell JM, Ransohoff DF, Kramer BS. Principles of cancer screening: lessons from history and study design issues. *Semin Oncol* 2010;37:202–215.

114. Fontana RS, Sanderson DR, Taylor WF, et al. Early lung cancer detection: results of the initial (prevalence) radiologic and cytologic screening in the Mayo Clinic study. *Am Rev Respir Dis* 1984;130:561–565.

115. Fontana RS, Sanderson DR, Woolner LB, et al. Screening for lung cancer. A critique of the Mayo Lung Project. *Cancer* 1991;67:1155–1164.

116. Marcus PM, Bergstralh EJ, Zweig MH, et al. Extended lung cancer incidence follow-up in the Mayo Lung Project and overdiagnosis. *J Natl Cancer Inst* 2006;98:748–756.

117. Manser R, Wright G, Hart D, et al. Surgery for early stage non-small cell lung cancer. *Cochrane Database Syst Rev* 2005:CD004699.

118. Kubik A, Parkin DM, Khlat M, et al. Lack of benefit from semi-annual screening for cancer of the lung: follow-up report of a randomized controlled trial on a population of high-risk males in Czechoslovakia. *Int J Cancer* 1990;45:26–33.

119. Oken MM, Hocking WG, Kvale PA, et al. Screening by chest radiograph and lung cancer mortality: the Prostate, Lung, Colorectal, and Ovarian (PLCO) randomized trial. *JAMA* 2011;306:1865–1873.

120. Kovalchik SA, Tammemagi M, Berg CD, et al. Targeting of low-dose CT screening according to the risk of lung-cancer death. *N Engl J Med* 2013;369:245–254.

121. Kubik AK, Parkin DM, Zatloukal P. Czech Study on Lung Cancer Screening: post-trial follow-up of lung cancer deaths up to year 15 since enrollment. *Cancer* 2000;89:2363–2368.

122. Patz EF Jr, Pinsky P, Gatsonis C, et al. Overdiagnosis in low-dose computed tomography screening for lung cancer. *JAMA Intern Med* 2014;174:269–274.

123. Ma J, Ward EM, Smith R, et al. Annual number of lung cancer deaths potentially avertable by screening in the United States. *Cancer* 2013;119:1381–1385.

124. Wender R, Fontham ET, Barrera E Jr, et al. American Cancer Society lung cancer screening guidelines. *CA Cancer J Clin* 2013;63:107–117.

125. Bach PB, Mirkin JN, Oliver TK, et al. Benefits and harms of CT screening for lung cancer: a systematic review. *JAMA* 2012;307:2418–2429.

126. Montie JE, Smith JA. Whitmoreisms: memorable quotes from Willet F. Whitmore, Jr, M.D. *Urology* 2004;63:207–209.

127. Albertsen PC, Hanley JA, Fine J. 20-year outcomes following conservative management of clinically localized prostate cancer. *JAMA* 2005;293:2095–2101.

128. Lu-Yao G, Albertsen PC, Stanford JL, et al. Screening, treatment, and prostate cancer mortality in the Seattle area and Connecticut: fifteen-year follow-up. *J Gen Intern Med* 2008;23:1809–1814.

129. Thompson IM, Chi C, Ankerst DP, et al. Effect of finasteride on the sensitivity of PSA for detecting prostate cancer. *J Natl Cancer Inst* 2006;98:1128–1133.

130. Thompson IM, Pauler DK, Goodman PJ, et al. Prevalence of prostate cancer among men with a prostate-specific antigen level < or =4.0 ng per milliliter. *N Engl J Med* 2004;350:2239–2246.

131. Thompson IM, Ankerst DP, Chi C, et al. Operating characteristics of prostate-specific antigen in men with an initial PSA level of 3.0 ng/ml or lower. *JAMA* 2005;294:66–70.

132. Widmark A, Klepp O, Solberg A, et al. Endocrine treatment, with or without radiotherapy, in locally advanced prostate cancer (SPCG-7/SFUO-3): an open randomised phase III trial. *Lancet* 2009;373:301–308.

133. Bill-Axelson A, Holmberg L, Ruutu M, et al. Radical prostatectomy versus watchful waiting in early prostate cancer. *N Engl J Med* 2011;364:1708–1717.

134. Wilt TJ, Brawer MK, Jones KM, et al. Radical prostatectomy versus observation for localized prostate cancer. *N Engl J Med* 2012;367:203–213.

135. Andriole GL, Crawford ED, Grubb RL 3rd, et al. Prostate cancer screening in the randomized Prostate, Lung, Colorectal, and Ovarian Cancer Screening Trial: mortality results after 13 years of follow-up. *J Natl Cancer Inst* 2012;104:125–132.

136. Schroder FH, Hugosson J, Roobol MJ, et al. Screening and prostate-cancer mortality in a randomized European study. *N Engl J Med* 2009;360:1320–1328.

137. Schroder FH, Hugosson J, Roobol MJ, et al. Prostate-cancer mortality at 11 years of follow-up. *N Engl J Med* 2012;366:981–990.

138. Wolters T, Roobol MJ, Steyerberg EW, et al. The effect of study arm on prostate cancer treatment in the large screening trial ERSPC. *Int J Cancer* 2010;126:2387–2393.

139. Hugosson J, Carlsson S, Aus G, et al. Mortality results from the Goteborg randomised population-based prostate-cancer screening trial. *Lancet Oncol* 2010;11:725–732.

140. Kilpelainen TP, Tammela TL, Malila N, et al. Prostate cancer mortality in the Finnish randomized screening trial. *J Natl Cancer Inst* 2013;105:719–725.

141. Center MM, Jemal A, Lortet-Tieulent J, et al. International variation in prostate cancer incidence and mortality rates. *Eur Urol* 2012;61:1079–1092.

142. Boyle P. Screening for prostate cancer: have you had your cholesterol measured? *BJU Int* 2003;92:191–199.

143. Greene KL, Albertsen PC, Babaian RJ, et al. Prostate specific antigen best practice statement: 2009 update. *J Urol* 2009;182:2232–2241.

144. Wolf AM, Wender RC, Etzioni RB, et al. American Cancer Society guideline for the early detection of prostate cancer: update 2010. *CA Cancer J Clin* 2010;60:70–98.

145. Carter HB. American Urological Association (AUA) guideline on prostate cancer detection: process and rationale. *BJU Int* 2013;112:543–547.

146. Wolff T, Tai E, Miller T. Screening for skin cancer: an update of the evidence for the U.S. Preventive Services Task Force. *Ann Intern Med* 2009;150:194–198.

147. Katalinic A, Waldmann A, Weinstock MA, et al. Does skin cancer screening save lives?: an observational study comparing trends in melanoma mortality in regions with and without screening. *Cancer* 2012;118:5395–5402.

148. Breitbart EW, Waldmann A, Nolte S, et al. Systematic skin cancer screening in Northern Germany. *J Am Acad Dermatol* 2012;66:201–211.

149. Smith RA, Brooks D, Cokkinides V, et al. Cancer screening in the United States, 2013: a review of current American Cancer Society guidelines, current issues in cancer screening, and new guidance on cervical cancer screening and lung cancer screening. *CA Cancer J Clin* 2013;63:88–105.

150. U.S. Preventive Services Task Force. Screening for skin cancer: U.S. Preventive Services Task Force recommendation statement. *Ann Intern Med* 2009;150:188–193.

CANCER PREVENTION AND SCREENING

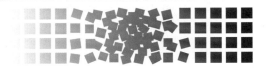

35 Genetic Counseling

Ellen T. Matloff and Danielle C. Bonadies

INTRODUCTION

Clinically based genetic testing has evolved from an uncommon analysis ordered for the rare hereditary cancer family to a widely available tool ordered on a routine basis to assist in surgical and radiation decision making, chemoprevention, and surveillance of the patient with cancer, as well as management of the entire family. The evolution of this field has created a need for accurate cancer genetic counseling and risk assessment. Extensive coverage of this topic by the media, including Angelina Jolie's public disclosure of her *BRCA1+* status in May 2013, and widespread advertising by commercial testing laboratories have further fueled the demand for counseling and testing.

Cancer genetic counseling is a communication process between a health-care professional and an individual concerning cancer occurrence and risk in his or her family.[1] The process, which may include the entire family through a blend of genetic, medical, and psychosocial assessments and interventions, has been described as a bridge between the fields of traditional oncology and genetic counseling.[1]

The goals of this process include providing the client with an assessment of individual cancer risk, while offering the emotional support needed to understand and cope with this information. It also involves deciphering whether the cancers in a family are likely to be caused by a mutation in a cancer gene and, if so, *which one*. There are >30 hereditary cancer syndromes, many of which can be caused by mutations in different genes. Therefore, testing for these syndromes can be complicated. Advertisements by genetic testing companies bill genetic testing as a simple process that can be carried out by health-care professionals with no training in this area; however, there are many genes involved in cancer, the interpretation of the test results is often complicated, the risk of result misinterpretation is great and associated with potential liability, and the emotional and psychological ramifications for the patient and family can be powerful.[2,3] A few hours of training by a company generating a profit from the sale of these tests does not adequately prepare providers to offer their own genetic counseling and testing services.[4] Furthermore, the delegation of genetic testing responsibilities to office staff and, recently, mammography technicians, is alarming and likely presents a huge liability for these ordering physicians, their practices, and their institutions.[5,6] *Providers should proceed with caution before taking on the role of primary genetic counselor for their patients.*

Counseling about hereditary cancers differs from *traditional* genetic counseling in several ways. Clients seeking cancer genetic counseling are rarely concerned with reproductive decisions, which are often the primary focus in traditional genetic counseling, but are instead seeking information about their own and other relatives' chances of developing cancer.[1] Additionally, the risks given are not absolute but change over time as the family and personal history changes and the patient ages. The risk reduction options available are often radical (e.g., chemoprevention or prophylactic surgery), and are not appropriate for every patient at every age. The surveillance and management plan must be tailored to the patient's age, childbearing status, menopausal status, risk category, ease of screening, and personal preferences and will likely change over time with the patient. The ultimate goal of cancer genetic counseling is to help the patient reach the decision best suited to her personal situation, needs, and circumstances.

There are now a significant number of referral centers across the country specializing in cancer genetic counseling, and the numbers are growing. However, some experts insist that the only way to keep up with the overwhelming demand for counseling will be to educate more physicians and nurses in cancer genetics. The feasibility of adding another specialized and time-consuming task to the clinical burden of these professionals is questionable, particularly with average patient encounters of 19.5 and 21.6 minutes for general practitioners and gynecologists, respectively.[7,8] A more practical goal is to better educate clinicians in the area of risk assessment so that they can screen their patient populations for individuals at high risk for hereditary cancer and refer them on to comprehensive counseling and testing programs. Access to genetic counseling is no longer an issue because there are now internet, phone, and satellite-based telemedicine services available (Table 35.1), with most major health insurance companies now covering these services[9–11] and several requiring them.[12]

WHO IS A CANDIDATE FOR CANCER GENETIC COUNSELING?

Only 5% to 10% of most cancer is thought to be caused by single mutations within autosomal-dominant inherited cancer susceptibility genes.[13] The key for clinicians is to determine which patients are at greatest risk to carry a hereditary mutation. There are seven critical risk factors in hereditary cancer (Table 35.2). The first is early age of cancer onset. This risk factor, *even in the absence of a family history*, has been shown to be associated with an increased frequency of germline mutations in many types of cancers.[14] The second risk factor is the presence of the same cancer in multiple affected relatives on the same side of the pedigree. These cancers do not need to be of similar histologic type in order to be caused by a single mutation. The third risk factor is the clustering of cancers known to be caused by a single gene mutation in one family (e.g., breast/ovarian/pancreatic cancer or colon/uterine/ovarian cancers). The fourth risk factor is the occurrence of multiple primary cancers in one individual. This includes multiple primary breast or colon cancers as well as a single individual with separate cancers known to be caused by a single gene mutation (e.g., breast and ovarian cancer in a single individual). Ethnicity also plays a role in determining who is at greatest risk to carry a hereditary cancer mutation. Individuals of Jewish ancestry are at increased risk to carry three specific *BRCA1/2* mutations.[15] The presence of a cancer that presents unusually—in this case, breast cancer in a male—represents a sixth risk factor and is important even when it is the only risk factor present. Finally, the last risk factor is pathology. Certain types of cancer are overrepresented in hereditary cancer families. For example, medullary and triple negative breast

TABLE 35.1

How to Find a Genetic Counselor for Your Patient

American Board of Genetic Counselors

https://abgcmember.goamp.com/Net/ABGCWcm/Find_
Counselor/ABGCWcm/PublicDir.aspx?hkey=0ad511c0-
d9e9-4714-bd4b-0d73a59ee175

http://bit.ly/1kzTbk9
Directory of board-certified genetic counselors

InformedDNA

www.informeddna.com
(800) 975-4819
*A nationwide network of independent genetic counselors
that use telephone and internet technology to bring genetic
counseling to patients and providers. Covered by many
insurance companies.*

National Society of Genetic Counselors

www.nsgc.org (click "Find a Counselor" button)
(312) 321-6834
*For a listing of genetic counselors in your area who specialize
in cancer.*

National Cancer Institute Cancer Genetics Services Directory

www.cancer.gov/cancertopics/genetics/directory
(800) 4-CANCER
*A free service designed to locate providers of cancer risk
counseling and testing services.*

cancers (where the estrogen, progesterone and Her2 receptors are all negative, often abbreviated ER-/PR-/Her2) are overrepresented in *BRCA1* families,[16,17] and the National Comprehensive Cancer Network (NCCN) BRCA testing guidelines now include individuals diagnosed with a triple negative breast cancer <age 60 years.[18] However, breast cancer patients without these pathologic findings are *not* necessarily at lower risk to carry a mutation. In contrast, patients with a borderline or mucinous ovarian carcinoma are at lower risk to carry a *BRCA1* or *BRCA2* mutation[19] and may instead

TABLE 35.2

Risk Factors that Warrant Genetic Counseling for Hereditary Cancer Syndromes

1. Early age of onset (e.g., <50 years for breast, colon, and uterine cancer)
2. Multiple family members on the same side of the pedigree with the same cancer
3. Clustering of cancers in the family known to be caused by a single gene mutation (e.g., breast/ovarian/pancreatic; colon/uterine/ovarian; colon cancer/polyps/desmoid tumors/osteomas)
4. Multiple primary cancers in one individual (e.g., breast/ovarian cancer; colon/uterine; synchronous/metachronous colon cancers; <15 gastrointestinal polyps; <5 hamartomatous or juvenile polyps)
5. Ethnicity (e.g., Jewish ancestry for breast/ovarian cancer syndrome)
6. Unusual presentation of cancer/tumor (e.g., breast cancer in a male; medullary thyroid cancer; retinoblastoma; even one sebaceous carcinoma or adenoma)
7. Pathology (e.g., triple negative [ER/PR/Her-2] breast cancer <60; medullary breast cancers are overrepresented in women with hereditary breast and ovarian cancer; a colon tumor with an abnormal microsatellite instability (MSI) or immunohistochemistry (IHC) result increases the risk for a hereditary colon cancer syndrome)

carry a mutation in a different gene. It is already well-established that medullary thyroid carcinoma, sebaceous adenoma or carcinoma, adrenocortical carcinoma before the age of 25 years, and multiple adenomatous, hamartomatous, or juvenile colon polyps are indicative of other rare hereditary cancer syndromes.[11,20] These risk factors should be viewed in the context of the entire family history, and must be weighed in proportion to the number of individuals who have not developed cancer. The risk assessment is often limited in families that are small or have few female relatives; in such families, a single risk factor may carry more weight.

A less common, but extremely important, finding is the presence of unusual physical findings or birth defects that are known to be associated with rare hereditary cancer syndromes. Examples include benign skin findings, autism, large head circumference[20,21] and thyroid disorders in Cowden syndrome, odontogenic keratocysts in Gorlin syndrome,[22] and desmoid tumors or dental abnormalities in familial adenomatous polyposis (FAP).[23] These and other findings should prompt further investigation of the patient's family history and consideration of a referral to genetic counseling.

In this chapter, the breast/ovarian cancer counseling session with a female patient will serve as a paradigm by which all other sessions may follow broadly.

COMPONENTS OF THE CANCER GENETIC COUNSELING SESSION

Precounseling Information

Before coming in for genetic counseling, the counselee should be informed about what to expect at each visit, and what information he/she should collect ahead of time. The counselee can then begin to collect medical and family history information and pathology reports that will be essential for the genetic counseling session.

Family History

An accurate family history is undoubtedly one of the most essential components of the cancer genetic counseling session. Optimally, a family history should include at least three generations; however, patients do not always have this information. For each individual affected with cancer, it is important to document the exact diagnosis, age at diagnosis, treatment strategies, and environmental exposures (i.e., occupational exposures, cigarettes, other agents).[24] The current age of the individual, laterality, and occurrence of any other cancers must also be documented. Cancer diagnoses should be confirmed with pathology reports whenever possible. A study by Love et al.[25] revealed that individuals accurately reported the primary site of cancer only 83% of the time in their first degree relatives with cancer, and 67% and 60% of the time in second and third degree relatives, respectively. It is common for patients to report a uterine cancer as an ovarian cancer, or a colon polyp as an invasive colorectal cancer. These differences, although seemingly subtle to the patient, can make a tremendous difference in risk assessment. Individuals should be asked if there are any consanguineous (inbred) relationships in the family, if any relatives were born with birth defects or mental retardation, and whether other genetic diseases run in the family (e.g., Fanconi anemia, Cowden syndrome), because these pieces of information could prove to be important in reaching a diagnosis.

The most common misconception in family history taking is that somehow a maternal family history of breast, ovarian, or uterine cancer is more significant than a paternal history. Conversely, many still believe that a paternal history of prostate cancer is more significant than a maternal history. Few cancer genes discovered thus far are located on the sex chromosomes and, therefore, both maternal and paternal history are significant and must be explored thoroughly. It has also become necessary to elicit the spouse's personal and family history of cancer. This has bearing on the cancer status of common children, but may also determine if children are at increased risk for a serious recessive genetic disease such as Fanconi anemia.[26] Children who inherit two copies of a BRCA2 mutation (one from each parent) are now known to have this serious disorder characterized by defective DNA repair and high rates of birth defects, aplastic anemia, leukemia, and solid tumors.[26] Patients should be encouraged to report changes in their family history over time (e.g., new cancer diagnoses, genetic testing results in relatives), because this may change their risk assessment and counseling.

A detailed family history should also include genetic diseases, birth defects, mental retardation, multiple miscarriages, and infant deaths. A history of certain recessive genetic diseases (e.g., ataxia telangiectasia, Fanconi anemia) can indicate that healthy family members who carry just one copy of the genetic mutation may be at increased risk to develop cancer.[26,27] Other genetic disorders, such as hereditary hemorrhagic telangiectasia, can be associated with a hereditary cancer syndrome caused by a mutation in the same gene—in this case, juvenile polyposis.[28]

Dysmorphology Screening

Congenital anomalies, benign tumors, and unusual dermatologic features occur in a large number of hereditary cancer predisposition syndromes. Examples include osteomas of the jaw in FAP, palmar pits in Gorlin syndrome, and papillomas of the lips and mucous membranes in Cowden syndrome. Obtaining an accurate past medical history of benign lesions and birth defects, and screening for such dysmorphology can greatly impact diagnosis, counseling, and testing. For example, BRCA1/2 testing is inappropriate in a patient with breast cancer who has a family history of thyroid cancer and the orocutaneous manifestations of Cowden syndrome.

Risk Assessment

Risk assessment is one of the most complicated components of the genetic counseling session. It is crucial to remember that risk assessment changes over time as the person ages and as the health statuses of their family members change. Risk assessment can be broken down into three separate components.

- What is the chance that the counselee will develop the cancer observed in his/her family (or a genetically related cancer such as ovarian cancer due to a family history of breast cancer)?
- What is the chance that the cancers in this family are caused by a single gene mutation?
- What is the chance that we can identify the gene mutation in this family with our current knowledge and laboratory techniques?

Cancer clustering in a family may be due to genetic and/or environmental factors, or may be coincidental because some cancers are very common in the general population.[29] Although inherited factors may be the primary cause of cancers in some families, in others, cancer may develop because an inherited factor increases the individual's susceptibility to environmental carcinogens. It is also possible that members of the same family may be exposed to similar environmental exposures due to shared geography or patterns in behavior and diet that may increase the risk of cancer.[30] Therefore, it is important to distinguish the difference between a familial pattern of cancer (due to environmental factors or chance) and a hereditary pattern of cancer (due to a shared genetic mutation). Emerging research is also evaluating the role and clinical utility of more common low-penetrance susceptibility genes and single nucleotide polymorphisms (SNP) that may account for a proportion of familial cancers.[31]

Several models are available to calculate the chance that a woman will develop breast cancer, including the Gail and Claus models.[32,33] Computer-based models are also available to help determine the chance that a BRCA mutation will be found in a family.[34] At first glance, many of these models appear simple and easy to use, and it may be tempting to exclusively rely on these models to assess cancer risk. However, each model has its strengths and weaknesses, and the counselor needs to understand the limitations well and know which are validated, which are considered problematic, when a model will not work on a particular patient, or when another genetic syndrome should be considered. For example, none of the existing models are able to factor in other risks that may be essential in hereditary risk calculation (e.g., a sister who was diagnosed with breast cancer after radiation treatment for Hodgkin disease).

The risk of a detectable mutation will also vary based on cancer history and the degree of relationship to an affected family member. For example, family members with early-onset breast cancer have a higher likelihood of testing positive than unaffected family members. Therefore, the risk assessment process should include a discussion of which family member is the best candidate for testing.

DNA Testing

DNA testing is now available for a variety of hereditary cancer syndromes. However, despite misrepresentation by the media, testing is feasible for only a small percentage of individuals with cancer. DNA testing offers the important advantage of presenting clients with *actual risks* instead of the empiric risks derived from risk calculation models. DNA testing can be very expensive; full sequencing and rearrangement testing of the BRCA1/2 genes currently averages $2,500, and full panel testing costs up to $7,000 per patient. Importantly, testing should begin in an affected family member whenever possible to maximize scientific accuracy. Most insurance companies now cover cancer genetic testing in families where the test is medically indicated.

One of the most crucial aspects of DNA testing is accurate result ordering and interpretation. Unfortunately, errors in ordering and interpretation are the greatest risk of genetic testing and are very common.[35] Emerging data reveal that between 30% to 50% of genetic tests are ordered inappropriately, which is problematic for patients, clinicians, and insurers.[36-38] Recent data demonstrate that many medical providers have difficulty interpreting even basic pedigrees and genetic test results.[33-35] Additional studies have demonstrated that an inaccurate interpretation of genetic testing has been shown to result in inappropriate medical management recommendations, unnecessary prophylactic surgeries, a massive waste of health-care dollars, psychosocial distress, and false reassurance for patients.[2,3]

Interpretations are becoming increasingly complicated as more tests and gene panels become available. For example, one study demonstrated that approximately 25% of high-risk families that were BRCA1 and BRCA2 negative by commercially available sequencing were found to carry a deletion or duplication in one of these genes, or a mutation in another gene.[39]

This is particularly concerning in an era in which testing companies are canvassing physicians, and now mammography technicians, and encouraging them to perform their own counseling and testing. The potential impact of test results on the patient and his/her family is great and, therefore, accurate interpretation of the results is paramount. Professional groups have recognized this and have adopted standards encouraging clinicians to refer patients to genetics experts to ensure proper ordering and interpretation of genetic tests. The U.S. Preventive Services Task Force recommends that women whose family history is suggestive of a BRCA mutation be referred for genetic counseling before being offered genetic testing.[40] The American College of Surgeons' Commission on Cancer standards include "cancer risk assessment, genetic counseling and testing services provided to patients either on site or by referral, by a qualified genetics professional."[4] In an effort to reduce errors, some insurance companies are requiring genetic counseling by a certified genetic counselor before testing for hereditary breast or colon cancer syndromes.[12]

Results can fall into a few broad categories. It is important to note that a negative test result can actually be interpreted in three different ways, detailed in #2, #3, and #4, which follows.

1. Deleterious mutation "positive." When a deleterious mutation in a well-known cancer gene is discovered, the cancer risks for the patient and her family are relatively straightforward. However, with the development of multigene panels and the inclusion of many lesser known genes, the risks of detecting a mutation within a gene whose cancer risks are ill defined and medical management options unknown is much greater. Even for well-known genes, the risks are not precise and should be presented to patients as a risk range.[41,42] When a true mutation is found, it is critical to test both parents (whenever possible) to determine from which side of the family the mutation is originating, even when the answer appears obvious.

2. True negative. An individual does not carry the deleterious mutation found in her family, which ideally, has been proven to segregate with the cancer family history. In this case, the patient's cancer risks are usually reduced to the population risks.

3. Negative. A mutation was not detected, and the cancers in the family are not likely to be hereditary based on the personal and family history assessment. For example, a patient is diagnosed with breast cancer at age 38 years and comes from a large family with no other cancer diagnoses and relatives who died at old ages of other causes.

4. Uninformative. A mutation cannot be found in affected family members of a family in which the cancer pattern appears to be hereditary; there is likely an undetectable mutation within the gene, or the family carries a mutation in a different gene. If, for example, the patient developed breast cancer at age 38 years, has a father with breast cancer, and has a paternal aunt who developed breast and ovarian cancers before age 50 years, a negative test result would be almost meaningless. It would simply mean that the family has a mutation that could not be identified with our current testing methods or a mutation in another cancer gene. The entire family would be followed as high risk.

5. Variant of uncertain significance. A genetic change is identified, the significance of which is unknown. It is possible that this change is deleterious or completely benign. It may be helpful to test other *affected* family members to see if the mutation segregates with disease in the family. If it does not segregate, the variant is less likely to be significant. If it does, the variant is more likely to be significant. Other tools, including a splice site predictor, in conjunction with data on species conservation and amino acid difference scores, can also be helpful in determining the likelihood that a variant is significant. It is rarely helpful (and can be detrimental) to test *unaffected* family members for such variants. The rates of variants of uncertain significance vary greatly depending on the reporting protocols of the lab and the genes analyzed. Creation of open databases through a nationwide movement called Free the Data will likely improve variant reporting for all laboratories.

In order to pinpoint the mutation in a family, an affected individual most likely to carry the mutation should be tested first whenever possible. This is most often a person affected with the cancer in question at the earliest age. Test subjects should be selected with care, because it is possible for a person to develop sporadic cancer in a hereditary cancer family. For example, in an early-onset breast cancer family, it would not be ideal to first test a woman diagnosed with breast cancer at age 65 years because she may represent a sporadic case.

If a mutation is detected in an affected relative, other family members can be tested for the same mutation with a great degree of accuracy. Family members who do not carry the mutation found in their family are deemed true negative. Those who are found to carry the mutation in their family will have more definitive information about their risks to develop cancer. This information can be crucial in assisting patients in decision making regarding surveillance and risk reduction.

If a mutation is not identified in the affected relative, it usually means that either the cancers in the family are (1) not hereditary, or (2) caused by an undetectable mutation or a mutation in a different gene. A careful review of the family history and the risk factors will help to decipher whether interpretation 1 or 2 is more likely. Additional genetic testing may need to be ordered at this point. In cases in which the cancers appear hereditary and no mutation is found, DNA banking should be offered to the proband for a time in the future when improved testing may become available. A letter indicating exactly who in the family has access to the DNA should accompany the banked sample.

The genetic counseling result disclosure session should also include a detailed discussion of which other family members would benefit from genetic counseling and testing and referral information. This can apply not only to families who have been found to carry a deleterious mutation, but may also prove useful in other families (e.g., test a higher risk relative or determine segregation of a variant within a family).

The penetrance of mutations in cancer susceptibility genes is also difficult to interpret. Initial estimates derived from high-risk families provided very high cancer risks for *BRCA1* and *BRCA2* mutation carriers.[43] More recent studies done on populations that were not selected for family history have revealed lower penetrances.[44] Because exact penetrance rates cannot be determined for individual families at this time, and because precise genotype/phenotype correlations remain unclear, it is prudent to provide patients with a range of cancer risk and to explain that their risk probably falls somewhere within this spectrum. This can prove challenging for genes that lack published long-term data on cancer associations and risks.

Female carriers of *BRCA1* and *BRCA2* mutations have a 50% to 85% lifetime risk to develop breast cancer and between a 15% to 60% lifetime risk to develop ovarian cancer.[15,42,43] It is important to note that the classification "ovarian cancer" also includes cancer of the fallopian tubes and primary peritoneal carcinoma.[44,45] *BRCA2* carriers also have an increased lifetime risk of male breast cancer, pancreatic cancer, and possibly, melanoma.[46,47]

Options for Surveillance, Risk Reduction, and Tailored Treatment

The cancer risk counseling session is a forum to provide counselees with information, support, options, and hope. Mutation carriers can be offered: earlier and more aggressive surveillance, chemoprevention, and/or prophylactic surgery. Detailed management options for *BRCA* carriers are discussed in this chapter.

Surveillance recommendations are evolving with newer techniques and additional data. At this time, it is recommended that individuals at increased risk for breast cancer, particularly those who carry a *BRCA* mutation, have annual mammograms beginning at age 25 years, with a clinical breast exam by a breast specialist, a yearly breast magnetic resonance imaging (MRI) with a clinical breast exam by a breast specialist, and a yearly clinical breast exam by a gynecologist.[48,49] It is suggested that the mammogram and MRI be spaced out around the calendar year so that some intervention is planned every 6 months. Recent data suggest that MRI may be safer and more effective in *BRCA* carriers <40 years of age and may someday replace mammograms in this population.[50]

BRCA carriers may take a selective estrogen-receptor modulator (SERM) or aromatase inhibitor in hopes of reducing their risks of developing breast cancer. These medications have been proven effective in women at increased risk due to a positive family history of breast cancer.[51-53] There are limited data on the effectiveness of such medications in unaffected BRCA carriers[54-56]; however, there are some data to suggest that BRCA carriers taking tamoxifen as treatment for a breast cancer reduce their risk of a contralateral breast cancer.[57] Additionally, the majority of BRCA2 carriers who develop breast cancer develop an estrogen-positive form of the disease,[58] and it is hoped that this population will respond especially well to chemoprevention. Further studies in this area are necessary before drawing conclusions about the efficacy of chemoprevention in this population. Prophylactic bilateral mastectomy reduces the risk of breast cancer by >90% in women at high-risk for the disease.[59] Before genetic testing was available, it was not uncommon for entire generations of cancer families to have at-risk tissues removed without knowing if they were *personally* at increased risk for their familial cancer. Fifty percent of unaffected individuals in hereditary cancer families will *not* carry the inherited predisposition gene and can be spared prophylactic surgery or invasive high-risk surveillance regimens. Therefore, it is clearly not appropriate to offer prophylactic surgery until a patient is referred for genetic counseling and, if possible, testing.[60]

Women who carry BRCA1/2 mutations are also at increased risk to develop second contralateral and ipsilateral primaries of the breast.[61] These data bring into question the option of breast conserving surgery in women at high risk to develop a second primary within the same breast. For this reason, the BRCA1/2 carrier status can have a profound impact on surgical decision making,[62] and many patients have genetic counseling and testing immediately after diagnosis and before surgery or radiation therapy. Those patients who test positive and opt for prophylactic mastectomy can often be spared radiation and the resulting side effects that can complicate reconstruction. Approximately 30% to 60% of previously irradiated patients who later opt for mastectomy with reconstruction report significant complications or unfavorable cosmetic results.[62,63]

Women who carry BRCA1/2 mutations are also at increased risk to develop ovarian, fallopian tube, and primary peritoneal cancer, even if no one in their family has developed these cancers. Surveillance for ovarian cancer includes transvaginal ultrasounds and CA-125 testing; however, the effectiveness of such surveillance in detecting ovarian cancers at early, more treatable stages has not been proven in any population. Oral contraceptives reduce the risk of ovarian cancer in all women, including BRCA carriers.[64] Recent data indicate that the impact of this intervention on increasing breast cancer risk, if any, is low.[56,65] Given the difficulties in screening and in the treatment of ovarian cancer, the risk/benefit analysis likely favors the use of oral contraceptives in young carriers of BRCA1/2 mutations[30] who are not yet ready to have their ovaries removed. Prophylactic bilateral salpingo-oophorectomy (BSO) is currently the most effective means to reduce the risk of ovarian cancer and is recommended to BRCA1/2 carriers by the age of 35 to 40 or when childbearing is complete.[66] Specific operative and pathologic protocols have been developed for this prophylactic surgery.[67] In BRCA1/2 carriers whose pathologies come back normal, this surgery is highly effective at reducing the subsequent risk of ovarian cancer.[68] A decision analysis, comparing various surveillance and risk-reducing options available to BRCA carriers, has shown an increase in life expectancy if BSO is pursued by age 40.[69] Emerging data indicate that most ovarian cancers begin in the fallopian tube, and that salpingectomy may someday be sufficient in reducing ovarian cancer risk in young women; however, more data are needed before this option is offered to patients outside of clinical trials.[70] A relatively small percentage of women who pursue BSO may develop primary peritoneal carcinoma.[44,71] There has been some debate about whether BRCA1/2 carriers should also opt for total abdominal hysterectomy (TAH) due to the fact that small stumps of the fallopian tubes remain after BSO alone. The question of whether BRCA carriers are at increased risk for uterine serous papillary carcinoma (USPC) has also been raised.[72-74] If a relationship does exist between BRCA mutations and uterine

cancer, the risk appears to be low and not elevated over that of the general population.[75] Removing the uterus may make it possible for a BRCA carrier to take unopposed estrogen or tamoxifen in the future without the risk of uterine cancer, but this surgery is associated with a longer recovery time and has more side effects than does BSO alone. Each patient should be counseled about the pros and cons of each procedure and the risks associated with premature menopause before having surgery.[76]

A secondary, but important, reason for female BRCA carriers to consider prophylactic oophorectomy is that it also significantly reduces the risk of a subsequent breast cancer, particularly if they have this surgery before menopause.[77,78] The reduction in breast cancer risk remains even if a healthy premenopausal carrier elects to take low-dose hormone-replacement therapy (HRT) after this surgery[79]. Early data suggest that tamoxifen, in addition to premenopausal oophorectomy, in BRCA carriers may have little additional benefit in terms of breast cancer risk reduction.[80] Research is needed in balancing quality of life issues secondary to estrogen deprivation with cancer risk reduction in these young female BRCA1/2 carriers.

New developments are also emerging in the treatment and, possibly, the prevention of BRCA-related cancers. Early data revealed that breast and ovarian cancers in BRCA carriers were particularly sensitive to treatment with poly adenosine diphosphate (ADP)-ribose polymerases (PARP) inhibitors in combination with chemotherapy.[81,82] New trials are focusing on which chemotherapeutic regimens are most effective in mutation carriers. More data are needed on larger cohorts of patients and are currently being studies in multiple clinical trials.

Genetic counseling and testing is also available for dozens of cancer syndromes, including Lynch syndrome, von Hippel-Lindau syndrome, multiple endocrine neoplasias, and familial adenomatous polyposis. Surveillance and risk reduction for patients who are known mutation carriers for such conditions may decrease the associated morbidity and mortality of these syndromes.

Follow-up

A follow-up letter to the patient is a concrete means of documenting the information conveyed in the sessions so that the patient and his/her family members can review it over time. This letter should be sent to the patient and health-care professionals to whom the patient has granted access to this information. A follow-up phone call and/or counseling session may also be helpful, particularly in the case of a positive test result. Some programs provide patients with an annual or biannual newsletter updating them on new information in the field of cancer genetics or patient support groups. It is now recommended that patients return for follow-up counseling sessions months, or even years, after their initial consult to discuss advances in genetic testing and changes in surveillance and risk reduction options. This can be beneficial for individuals who have been found to carry a hereditary predisposition, for those in whom a syndrome/mutation is suspected but yet unidentified, and for those who are ready to move forward with genetic testing. Follow-up counseling is also recommended for patients whose life circumstances have changed (e.g., preconception, after childbearing is complete), who are preparing for prophylactic surgery, or who are ready to discuss the family genetics with their children.

ISSUES IN CANCER GENETIC COUNSELING

Psychosocial Issues

The psychosocial impact of cancer genetic counseling cannot be underestimated. Just the process of scheduling a cancer risk counseling session may be quite difficult for some individuals with a family history who are not only frightened about their own cancer risk, but also are reliving painful experiences associated with the cancer of their loved ones.[13] Counselees may be faced with an onslaught of emotions, including anger, fear of developing cancer, fear of disfigurement and dying, grief, lack of control, negative body image, and a sense of isolation.[24] Some counselees wrestle with the fear that insurance companies, employers, family members, and even future partners will react negatively to their cancer risks. For many, it is a double-edged sword as they balance their fears and apprehensions about dredging up these issues with the possibility of obtaining reassuring news and much needed information.

A person's perceived cancer risk is often dependent on many "nonmedical" variables. They may estimate that their risk is higher if they look like an affected individual, or share some of their personality traits.[24] Their perceived risks will vary depending on if their relatives were cancer survivors or died painful deaths from the disease. Many people wonder not *if* they are going to get cancer, but *when*.

The counseling session is an opportunity for individuals to express why they believe they have developed cancer, or why their family members have cancer. Some explanations may revolve around family folklore, and it is important to listen to and address these explanations rather than dismiss them.[24] In doing this, the counselor will allow the clients to alleviate their greatest fears and to give more credibility to the medical theory. Understanding a patient's perceived cancer risk is important, because that fear may *decrease* surveillance and preventive health-care behaviors.[83] For patients and families who are moving forward with DNA testing, a referral to a mental health-care professional is often very helpful. Genetic testing has an impact not only on the patient, but also on his/her children, siblings, parents, and extended relatives. This can be overwhelming for an individual and the family, and should be discussed in detail prior to testing.

To date, studies conducted in the setting of pre- and postgenetic counseling have revealed that, at least in the short term, most patients do not experience adverse psychological outcomes after receiving their test results.[84,85] In fact, preliminary data have revealed that individuals in families with known mutations who seek testing seem to fare better psychologically at 6 months than those who avoid testing.[84] Among individuals who learn they are *BRCA* mutation carriers, anxiety and distress levels appear to increase slightly after receiving their test results but returned to pretest levels in several weeks.[86] Although these data are reassuring, it is important to recognize that genetic testing is an individual decision and will not be right for every patient or every family.

Presymptomatic Testing in Children

Presymptomatic testing in children has been widely discussed, and most concur that it is appropriate only when the onset of the condition regularly occurs in childhood or if there are useful interventions that can be applied.[87] For example, genetic testing for mutations in the *BRCA* genes and other adult-onset diseases is generally limited to individuals who are >18 years of age. The American College of Medical Genetics states that if the "medical or psychosocial benefits of a genetic test will not accrue until adulthood . . . genetic testing generally should be deferred."[88] In contrast, the DNA-based diagnosis of children and young adults at risk for hereditary medullary thyroid carcinoma (MTC) is appropriate and has improved the management of these patients.[89] DNA-based testing for MTC is virtually 100% accurate and allows at-risk family members to make informed decisions about prophylactic thyroidectomy. FAP is a disorder that occurs in childhood and in which mortality can be reduced if detection is presymptomatic.[90] Testing is clearly indicated in these instances.

Questions have been raised about the parents' right to demand testing for adult-onset diseases, and this is now happening regularly

with direct-to-consumer tests and whole exome testing of children.[91] The risks of such testing to the child, and the child's right *not* to be tested must be considered. Whenever childhood testing is not medically indicated, it is preferable that testing decisions are postponed until the children are adults and can decide for themselves whether to be tested.

Confidentiality

The level of confidentiality surrounding cancer genetic testing is paramount due to concerns of genetic discrimination. Careful consideration should be given to the confidentially of family history information, pedigrees, genetic test results, pathology reports, and the carrier status of other family members as most hospitals and clinicians transition to electronic medical records systems. The goal of electronic records is to share information about the patient with his/her entire health-care team. However, genetics is a unique specialty that involves the whole family. Patient's charts often contain Health Insurance Portability and Accountability Act (HIPAA)–protected health information and genetic test results for many other family members. This information may not be appropriate to enter into an electronic record. The unique issues of genetics services need to be considered when designing electronic medical record standards.

Confidentiality of test results *within* a family can also be of issue, because genetic counseling and testing often reveals the risk statuses of family members other than the patient. Under confidentiality codes, the patient needs to grant permission before at-risk family members can be contacted. For this reason, many programs have built in a "share information with family members" clause to their informed consent documents. It has been questioned whether or not a family member could sue a health-care professional for negligence if they were identified at high risk yet not informed.[92] Most recommendations have stated that the burden of confidentiality lies between the provider and the patient. However, more recent recommendations state that confidentiality *should* be violated if the potential harm of not notifying other family members outweighs the harm of breaking a confidence to the patient.[93] There is no patent solution for this difficult dilemma, and situations must be considered on a case-by-case basis with the assistance of the in-house legal department and ethics committee.

Insurance and Discrimination Issues

When genetic testing for cancer predisposition first became widely available, the fear of health insurance discrimination by both patients and providers was one of the most common concerns.[94,95] It appears that the risks of health insurance discrimination were overstated and that almost no discrimination by health insurers has been reported.[96] HIPAA banned the use of genetic information as a preexisting condition.[97,98] In May of 2008, Congress passed the Genetic Information Nondiscrimination Act (GINA, HR 493), which provides broad protection of an individual's genetic information against health insurance and employment discrimination.[99] In addition, the Heath Care and Education Reconciliation Act of 2010 (HR 4872) prohibits group health plans from denying insurance based on preexisting conditions and from increasing premiums based on health status.[100] Health-care providers can now more confidently reassure their patients that genetic counseling and testing will not put them at risk of losing group or individual health insurance.

More and more patients are choosing to submit their genetic counseling and/or testing charges to their health insurance companies. In the past few years, more insurance companies have agreed to pay for counseling and/or testing,[101] perhaps in light of data that show these services reduce errors related to ordering and interpreting genetic testing and that decision analyses have revealed subsequent prophylactic surgeries to be cost effective.[102] The risk of life or disability insurance discrimination, however, is more realistic. Patients should be counseled about such risks before they pursue genetic testing.

Reproductive Issues

Reproductive technology in the form of preimplantation genetic diagnosis, prenatal testing, or sperm sorting are options[103] for men and women with a hereditary cancer syndrome, but are requested by few patients for adult-onset conditions in which there are viable options for surveillance and risk reduction. Importantly, if a BRCA2 carrier is considering having a child, it is important to assess the spouse's risk of also carrying a BRCA2 mutation. If the spouse is of Jewish ancestry or has a personal or family history of breast, ovarian, or pancreatic cancer, BRCA testing should be considered and a discussion of the risk of Fanconi anemia in a child with two BRCA2 mutations should take place.[104]

RECENT ADVANCES AND FUTURE DIRECTIONS

Cancer genetic counseling and testing were thrust into the national spotlight in the spring of 2013 when Hollywood icon Angelina Jolie publically disclosed that she was a BRCA1 carrier. One month later the Supreme Court unanimously ruled against gene patents. Referrals for genetic testing spiked across the country and have not returned to baseline levels at most centers. Within hours of the ruling, other labs began offering less expensive and more comprehensive BRCA testing, dramatically changing the marketplace of genetic testing for hereditary breast cancer.

All laboratories that have entered the BRCA marketplace have done so by including BRCA1 and BRCA2 in gene panels. These panels simultaneously analyze groups of genes that contribute to increased risk for breast, colon, ovarian, uterine, and other cancers. The cost of this technology continues to decrease with some multigene panels costing just a few hundred dollars *less* than traditional BRCA testing (~$4,000). Some panels include only well-known genes (e.g., p53, APC, MLH1), although many include lesser known genes (e.g., BRIP1, NBN, MRE11A) for which cancer risks are ill defined and medical management options are unknown. Because testing for these genes is new to the clinical setting, it is expected to take several years to compile accurate cancer risk estimates and appropriate recommendations for surveillance and risk reduction. Furthermore, the rate of *variants of uncertain significance* will likely be more common in the lesser known genes. These changes have increased the complexity of genetic testing exponentially. In response, several state and one national insurance company have mandated genetic counseling by certified providers before they will cover cancer genetic testing. In a surprising response, the American Society of Clinical Oncology (ASCO) opposed this insurer's decision, despite more than a decade's worth of data demonstrating that the majority of physicians do not have the time or expertise to offer genetic counseling and testing[38,105-108]. The AMA will decide whether to back the ASCO resolution in June 2014.

Some companies are now offering direct-to-consumer (DTC) genetic testing via websites. The accuracy of some of these DTC genetic tests are in question, and the leading company, 23andMe, has recently come under fire by the U.S. Food and Drug Administration.[105]

Maintaining high standards for thorough genetic counseling, informed consent, and accurate result interpretation will be paramount in reducing potential risks and maximizing the benefits of genetic technology in the next century.

REFERENCES

1. Peters J. Breast cancer genetics: relevance to oncology practice. *Cancer Control* 1995;2:195–208.
2. Brierley KL, Campfield D, Ducaine W, et al. Errors in delivery of cancer genetics services: implications for practice. *Conn Med* 2010;74:413–423.
3. Brierley KL, Blouch E, Cogswell W, et al. Adverse events in cancer genetic testing: medical, ethical, legal, and financial implications. *Cancer J* 2012;18:303–309.
4. American College of Surgeons, Commission on Cancer: Cancer Program Standards 2012: Ensuring Patient-Centered Care. http://www.facs.org/cancer/coc/programstandards2012.html Accessed on December 3, 2012.
5. Yale Cancer Genetic Counseling Program. Mammography techs ordering their own genetic testing? It appears our suspicion was correct. yalecancergeneticcounseling.blogspot.com October 2, 2013. http://yalecancergeneticcounseling.blogspot.com/2013/10/mammography-techs-ordering-their-own.html
6. Lubin IM, Caggana M, Constantin C, et al. Ordering molecular genetic tests and reporting results: practices in laboratory and clinical settings. *J Mol Diagn* 2008;10:459–468.
7. Weeks WB, Wallace AE. Time and money: a retrospective evaluation of the inputs, outputs, efficiency, and incomes of physicians. *Arch Intern Med* 2003;163(8):944–948.
8. Doksum T, Bernhardt BA, Holtzman NA. Does knowledge about the genetics of breast cancer differ between nongeneticist physicians who do or do not discuss or order BRCA testing? *Genet Med* 2003;5:99–105.
9. Rosenthal ET. Shortage of genetics counselors may be anecdotal, but need is real. *Oncology Times* 2007;29:34–36.
10. Informed Medical Decisions. Adult Genetics: Genetic counseling for your health concerns. Available at: http://www.informeddna.com/index.php/patients/adult-genetics.html. Accessed August 24, 2009.
11. Informed Medical Decisions. News: Aetna Press Release: Aetna to offer access to confidential telephonic cancer genetic counseling to health plan members. Available at: http://www.informeddna.com/images/stories/news_articles/aetna%20press%20release%20bw.pdf. Accessed August 24, 2009.
12. Schneider, ME. Cigna to require counseling for some genetic tests. Internal Medicine News Digital Network. July 26, 2013. http://www.internalmedicinenews.com/single-view/cigna-to-require-counseling-for-some-genetic-tests/efd4f421df8b46ba2208da423adf198d.html
13. Claus E, Schildkraut J, Thompson W, et al. The genetic attributable risks of breast and ovarian cancer. *Cancer* 1996;77:2318–2324.
14. Loman N, Johannsson O, Kristoffersson U. Family history of breast and ovarian cancers and BRCA1 and BRCA2 mutations in a population-based series of early-onset breast cancer. *J Natl Cancer Inst* 2001;93:1215.
15. Struewing J, Hartge P, Wacholder S. The risk of cancer associated with specific mutations of BRCA1 and BRCA2 among Ashkenazi Jews. *N Engl J Med* 1997;336:1401–1408.
16. Eisinger F, Jacquemier J, Charpin C, et al. Mutations at BRCA1: the medullary breast carcinoma revisited. *Cancer Res* 1998;58:1588–1592.
17. Kandel M, Stadler Z, Masciari S, et al. Prevalence of BRCA1 mutations in triple negative breast cancer. Paper presented at: 2006 42nd Annual ASCO Meeting; 2006; Atlanta, GA.
18. National Comprehensive Cancer Network Clinical Guidelines in Oncology: Genetics/Familial High-Risk Assessment - Breast and Ovarian Cancer. http://www.nccn.org/professionals/physician_gls/f_guidelines.asp#detection Accessed November 2, 2012.
19. Risch H, McLaughlin J, Cole D, et al. Population BRCA1 and BRCA2 mutation frequencies and cancer penetrances: a kin-cohort study in Ontario, Canada. *JNCI* 2006;98:1694–706.
20. Matloff E, Brierley K, Chimera C. A clinician's guide to hereditary colon cancer. *Cancer J* 2004;10(5):280–287.
21. Pilarski R. Cowden syndrome: a critical review of the clinical literature. *J Genet Couns* 2009 Feb;18:13–27.
22. Varga EA, Pastore M, Prior T, et al. The prevalence of PTEN mutations in a clinical pediatric cohort with autism spectrum disorders, developmental delay, and macrocephaly. *Genet Med* 2009;11:111–117.
23. Gorlin R. Nevoid basal-cell carcinoma syndrome. *Medicine* 1987;66(2):98–113.
24. Schneider K. *Counseling About Cancer: Strategies for Genetic Counseling.* 2nd ed. Wiley-Liss; 2001.
25. Love R, Evan A, Josten D. The accuracy of patient reports of a family history. *J Chronic Dis* 1985;38(4):289–293.
26. Alter B, Rosenberg P, Brody L. Clinical and molecular features associated with biallelic mutations in FANCD1/BRCA2. *J Med Genet* 2007;44:1–9.
27. Thompson D, Duedal S, Kirner J, et al. Cancer risks and mortality in heterozygous ATM mutation carriers. *J Natl Cancer Inst* 2005;97:813–822.
28. Korzenik J, Chung D, Digumarthy S, at al. Case 33-2005: a 43 year-old man with lower gastrointestinal bleeding. *N Engl J Med* 2005;353:1836–1844.
29. American Cancer Society. *Cancer Facts and Figures 2009.* Atlanta, GA: American Cancer Society; 2009.

30. Olopade O, Weber B. Breast cancer genetics: toward molecular characterization of individuals at increased risk for breast cancer. Part II. PPO Updates 1998;12:1–8.

31. Stratton MR, Rahman N. The emerging landscape of breast cancer susceptibility. *Nat Genet* 2008;40:17–22.

32. Gail M, Brinton L, Byar D. Projecting individualized probabilities of developing breast cancer for white females who are being examined annually. *J Natl Cancer Inst* 1989;81:1879–1886.

33. Claus E, Risch N, Thompson W. Autosomal dominant inheritance of early-onset breast cancer. *Cancer* 1994;73:643.

34. Parmigiani G, Berry D, Aguilar O. Determining carrier probabilities for breast cancer susceptibility genes BRCA1 and BRCA2. *Am J Hum Genet* 1998;62:145–158.

35. Friedman S. *Thoughts from FORCE: Comments Submitted to the Secretary's Advisory Committee on Genetics Health and Society*. http://facingourrisk.wordpress.com/2008/12/03/comments-submitted-to-the-secretarys-advisory-committee-on-genetics-health-and-society/. Accessed April 6, 2010.

36. UnitedHealth. *Personalized Medicine: Trends and Prospects for the New Science of Genetic Testing and Molecular Diagnostics*. Working Paper 7. Minnetonka, MN: UnitedHealth Center for Health Reform & Modernization; March 2012.

37. ARUP Laboratories. *Value of Genetic Counselors in the Laboratory*. Salt Lake City: ARUP Laboratories; March 2011.

38. Plon SE, Cooper HP, Parks B, et al. Genetic testing and cancer risk management recommendations by physicians for at-risk relatives. *Genet Med* 2011;13:148–154.

39. Walsh T. *More Than 25% of Breast Cancer Families with Wild-Type Results from Commercial Genetic Testing of BRCA1 and BRCA2 Are Resolved by BROCA Sequencing of All Known Breast Cancer Genes*. Paper presented at: 2013 American Society of Human Genetics Meeting Session #19; 2013; Boston, MA.

40. U.S. Preventive Services Task Force. *Genetic Risk Assessment and BRCA Mutation Testing for Breast and Ovarian Cancer Susceptibility*. Rockville, MD: Agency for Healthcare Research and Quality; 2013. http://www.uspreventiveservicestaskforce.org/uspstf12/brcatest/brcatestfinalrs.htm. Accessed June 2, 2014.

41. King MC, Marks JH, Mandell JB, et al. Breast and ovarian cancer risks due to inherited mutations in BRCA1 and BRCA2. *Science* 2003;302:643–646.

42. Antoniou A, Pharoah PD, Narod S, et al. Average risks of breast and ovarian cancer associated with BRCA1 or BRCA2 mutations detected in case Series unselected for family history: a combined analysis of 22 studies. *Am J Hum Genet* 2003;72:1117–1130.

43. Ford D, Easton D, Bishop D, et al. Risks of cancer in BRCA1 mutation carriers. *Lancet* 1994;343:692–695.

44. Piver M, Jishi M, Tsukada Y. Primary peritoneal carcinoma after prophylactic oophorectomy in women with a family history of ovarian cancer. *Cancer* 1993;71:2751–2755.

45. Aziz S, Kuperstein G, Rosen B. A genetic epidemiological study of carcincoma of the fallopian tube. *Gynecol Oncol* 2001;80:341–345.

46. van Asperen C, Brohet R, Meijers-Heijboer, et al. Cancer risks in BRCA2 families: estimates for sites other than breast and ovary. *J Med Genet* 2005;42:711–719.

47. Breast Cancer Linkage Consortium. Cancer risks in BRCA2 mutation carriers. *J Natl Cancer Inst* 1999;91:1310–1316.

48. Warner E, Plewes D, Hill K, et al. Surveillance of BRCA1 and BRCA2 mutation carriers with magnetic resonance imaging, ultrasound, mammography, and clinical breast examination. *JAMA* 2004;202:1317–1325.

49. Kriege M, Brekelmans CT, Boetes C, et al. Efficacy of MRI and mammography for breast-cancer screening in women with a familial or genetic predisposition. *N Engl J Med* 2004;29:351:427–437.

50. Kuhl C, Weigel S, Schrading S, et al. Prospective multicenter cohort study to refine management recommendations for women at elevated familial risk of breast cancer: the EVA Trial. *J Clin Oncol* 2010;1450–1457.

51. Powles T, Ashley S, Tidy A, et al. Twenty-year follow-up of the Royal Marsden randomized, double-blinded tamoxifen breast cancer prevention trial. *J Natl Cancer Inst* 2007;99:283–290.

52. Cuzick J, Forbes J, Sestak I, et al. Long-term results of tamoxifen prophylaxis for breast cancer: 96 month follow-up of the randomized IBIS-I trial. *J Natl Cancer Inst* 2007;99:272–282.

53. Goss PE, Ingle JN, Alés-Martínez JE, et al. Exemestane for breast-cancer prevention in postmenopausal women. *N Engl J Med* 2011;364:2381.

54. Fisher B, Constantino J, Wickerman D. Tamoxifen for the prevention of breast cancer: report of the National Surgical Adjuvant Breast and Bowel Project P-1 Study. *J Natl Cancer Inst* 1998;90:1371–1388.

55. King MC, Wieand S, Hale K. Tamoxifen and breast cancer incidence among women with inherited mutations in BRCA1 and BRCA2. *JAMA* 2001;286:2251–2256.

56. Narod S, Brunet J, Ghadirian P. Tamoxifen and risk of contralateral breast cancer in BRCA1 and BRCA2 mutation carriers: a case-control study. *Lancet* 2000;356:1876–1881.

57. Phillips KA, Milne RL, Rookus MA, et al. Tamoxifen and risk of contralateral breast cancer for BRCA1 and BRCA2 mutation carriers. *J Clin Oncol* 2013;31:3091–3099.

58. Lakhani S, van de Vijver M, Jacquemier J, et al. The pathology of familial breast cancer: predictive value of immunohistochemical markers estrogen receptor, progesterone receptor, HER-2, and p53 in patients with mutations in BRCA1 and BRCA2. *J Clin Oncol* 2002;20:2310–2318.

59. Hartmann L, Schaid D, Woods J. Efficacy of bilateral prophylactic mastectomy in women with a family history of breast cancer. *N Engl J Med* 1999;340:77–84.

60. Matloff E. The breast surgeon's role in BRCA1 and BRCA2 testing. *Am J Surg* 2000; 180:294–298.

61. Turner B, Harold E, Matloff E, et al. BRCA1/BRCA2 germline mutations in locally recurrent breast cancer patients after lumpectomy and radiation therapy: Implications for breast-conserving management in patients with BRCA1/BRCA2 mutations. *J Clin Oncol* 1999;17:3017–3024.

62. Contant CM, et al. Clinical experience of prophylactic mastectomy followed by immediate breast reconstruction in women at hereditary risk of breast cancer (HBOC) or a proven BRCA1 or BRCA2 germ-line mutation. *Eur J Surg Oncol* 2002;28:627–632.

63. Forman DL, Chiu J, Restifo RJ, et al. Breast reconstruction in previously irradiated patients using tissue expanders and implants: a potentially unfavorable result. *Ann Plast Surg* 1998;40:360–363.

64. McLaughlin J, Risch H, Lubinski J, et al. Reproductive risk factors for ovarian cancer in carriers of BRCA1 or BRCA2 mutations: a case-control study. *Lancet* 2007;8:26–34.

65. Milne R, Knight J, John E, et al. Oral contraceptive use and risk of early-onset breast cancer in carriers and noncarriers of BRCA1 and BRCA2 mutations. *Cancer Epidemiol Biomarkers Prev* 2005;14:350–356.

66. Domchek S, Friebel T, Neuhausen S, et al. Mortality reduction after risk-reducing bilateral salpingo-oophorectomy in a prospective cohort of BRCA1 and BRCA2 mutation carriers. *Lancet Oncol* 2006;7:223–229.

67. Powel CB, Kenley E, Chen LM, et al. Risk-reducing salpingo-oophorectomy in BRCA mutation carriers: role of serial sectioning in the detection of occult malignancy. *J Clin Oncol* 2005;23:127–132.

68. Finch A, Beiner M, Lubinski J, et al. Salpingo-oophorectomy and the risk of ovarian, fallopian tube, and peritoneal cancers in women with a BRCA1 or BRCA2 mutation. *JAMA* 2006;296:185–192.

69. Kurian AW, Sigal BM, Plevritis SK. Survival analysis of cancer risk reduction strategies for BRCA1/2 mutation carriers. *J Clin Oncol* 2010;10;28:222–231.

70. Kwon JS, Tinker A, Pansegrau G, et al. Prophylactic salpingectomy and delayed oophorectomy as an alternative for BRCA mutation carriers. *Obstet Gynecol* 2013;121:14–24.

71. American College of Obstetricians and Gynecologists. ACOG committee opinion. Breast–ovarian cancer screening. Number 176, October 1996. Committee on Genetics. The American College of Obstetricians and Gynecologists. *Int J Gynaecol Obstet* 1997;56:82–83.

72. Hornreich G, Beller U, Lavie O. Is uterine serous papillary carcinoma a BRCA1 related disease? Case report and review of the literature. *Gynecol Oncol* 1999;75(2):300–304.

73. Levine D, Lin P, Barakat R. Risk of endometrial carcinoma associated with BRCA mutation. *Gynecol Oncol* 2001;80(3):395–398.

74. Goshen R, Chu W, Elit L. Is uterine papillary serous adenocarcinoma a manifestation of the hereditary breast-ovarian cancer syndrome? *Gynecol Oncol* 2000;79(3):477–481.

75. Boyd J. The breast, ovarian, and other cancer genes. *Gynecol Oncol* 2001; 80(3):337–340.

76. Campfield Bonadies D, Moyer A, Matloff ET. What I wish I'd known before surgery: BRCA carriers' perspectives after bilateral salipingo-oophorectomy. *Fam Cancer* 2011;10:79–85.

77. Rebbeck T, Lynch H, Neuhausen S, et al. Prophylactic oophorectomy in carriers of BRCA1 or BRCA2 mutations. *N Engl J Med* 2002;346:1616–1622.

78. Kauff N, Satagopan J, Robson M, et al. Risk-reducing salpingo-oophorectomy in women with a BRCA1 or BRCA2 mutation. *N Engl J Med* 2002;346:1609–1615.

79. Rebbeck T, Friebel T, Wagner T, et al. Effect of short-term hormone replacement therapy on breast cancer risk reduction after bilateral prophylactic oophorectomy in BRCA1 and BRCA2 mutation carriers: the PROSE study group. *J Clin Oncol* 2005;23:7804–7810.

80. Gronwald J, Tung N, Foulkes W, et al. Tamoxifen and contralateral breast cancer in BRCA1 and BRCA2 carriers: an update. *Int J Cancer* 2006;118:2281–2284.

81. Fong PC, Boss DS, Yap TA, et al. Inhibition of Poly (ADPRibose) Polymerase in Tumors from BRCA Mutation Carriers. *N Engl J Med* 2009;361:1–12.

82. Inglhart JD, Silver DP. Synthetic lethality – a new direction in cancer-drug development. *N Engl J Med* 2009;361:1–3.

83. Kash K, Holland J, Halper M, et al. Psychological distress and surveillance behaviors of women with a family history of breast cancer. *J Natl Cancer Inst* 1992;84:24–30.

84. Lerman C, Hughes C, Lemon S. What you don't know can hurt you: adverse psychologic effects in members of BRCA1-linked and BRCA2-linked families who decline genetic testing. *J Clin Oncol* 1998;16:1650–1654.

85. Croyle R, Smith K, Botkin J. Psychological responses to BRCA1 mutation testing: preliminary findings. *Health Psychol* 1997;16:63–72.

86. Hamilton JG, Lobel M, Moyer A. Emotional distress following genetic testing for hereditary breast and ovarian cancer: a meta-analytic review. *Health Psychol* 2009;28:510–518.

87. Clayton E. Removing the shadow of the law from the debate about genetic testing of children. *Am J Med Genet* 1995;57:630–634.

88. ASHG/ACMG. Points to consider: ethical, legal, and psychosocial implications of genetic testing in children and adolescents. American Society of Human Genetics Board of Directors, American College of Medical Genetics Board of Directors. *Am J Hum Genet* 1995;57:1233–1241.

89. Ledger G, Khosia S, Lindor N, et al. Genetic testing in the diagnosis and management of multiple endocrine neoplasia type II. *Ann Intern Med* 1995; 122:118–124.

CANCER PREVENTION AND SCREENING

90. Rhodes M, Bradburn D. Overview of screening and management of familial adenomatous polyposis. *Br J Surg* 1992;33:125–123.

91. Howard HC, Avard D, Borry P. Are the kids really all right? Direct-to-consumer genetic testing in children: are company policies clashing with professional norms? *Eur J Hum Genet* 2011;19:1122–1126.

92. Tsoucalas C. Legal aspects of cancer genetics - screening, counseling, and registers. In: Lynch H, Kullander S, eds. *Cancer Genetics in Women*. Vol I. Boca Raton, FL: CRC Press, Inc.; 1987:9.

93. American Society of Human Genetics. ASHG Statement: professional disclosure of familial genetic information. *Am J Hum Genet* 1998;62:474–483.

94. Bluman L, Rimer B, Berry D. Attitudes, knowledge, and risk perceptions of women with breast and/or ovarian cancer considering testing for BRCA1 and BRCA2. *J Clin Oncol* 1999; 17:1040–1046.

95. Matloff E, Shappell H, Brierley K, et al. What would you do? Specialists' perspectives on cancer genetic testing, prophylactic surgery and insurance discrimination. *J Clin Oncol* 2000;18:2484–2492.

96. Hall MA, Rich SS. Patients' fear of genetic discrimination by health insurers: the impact of legal protections *Genet Med* 2000:2:214–221.

97. Leib JR, Hoodfar E, Larsen Haidle J, Nagy R. The new genetic privacy law. *Community Oncol* 2008;5:351–354.

98. Hudson KL, Holohan JD, Collins FS. Keeping pace with the times — the Genetic Information Nondiscrimination Act of 2008. *N Engl J Med* 2008;358:2661–2663.

99. The Genetic Information Nondiscrimination Act of 2008 (H.R. 493). Library of Congress Web site. http://beta.congress.gov/bill/110th-congress/house-bill/493. Accessed June 2, 2014.

100. The Health Care and Education Affordability Reconciliation Act of 2010 (H.R. 4872). Library of Congress Web site. http://beta.congress.gov/bill/111th-congress/house-bill/4872: Accessed June 2, 2014.

101. Manley S, Pennell R, Frank T. Insurance coverage of BRCA1 and BRCA2 sequence analysis. *J Genet Couns* 1998;7:A462.

102. Grann V, Whang W, Jabcobson J, et al. Benefits and costs of screening Ashkenazi Jewish women for BRCA1 and BRCA2. *J Clin Oncol* 1999;17: 494–500.

103. Offit K, Kohut K, Clagett B, et al. Cancer genetic testing and assisted reproduction. *J Clin Oncol* 2006;24:4775–4782.

104. Offit K, Levran O, Mullaney B, et al. Shared genetic susceptibility to breast cancer, brain tumors, and Fanconi anemia. *J Natl Cancer Inst* 2003;95(20): 1548–1551.

105. Greendale K, Pyeritz RE. Empowering primary care health professionals in medical genetics: How soon? How fast? How far? *Am J Med Genet* 2001;106:223–232.

106. Wilkins-Haug L, Hill LD, Power ML, et al. Gynecologists' training, knowledge, and experiences in genetics: a survey. *Obstet Gynecol* 2000;95:421–424.

107. Wood ME, Stockdale A, Flynn BS. Interviews with primary care physicians regarding taking and interpreting the cancer family history. *Fam Pract* 2008; 25:334–340.

108. Bellcross CA, Kolor K, Goddard K, et al. Awareness and utilization of BRCA1/2 testing among U.S. primary care physicians. *Am J Prev Med* 2011;40:61–66.

109. Pollack A. F.D.A. Orders genetic testing firm to stop selling DNA analysis service. *New York Times*. November 25, 2013. http://www.nytimes.com/2013/11/26/business/fda-demands-a-halt-to-a-dna-test-kits-marketing.html?_r=0

PART V

Cancers of the Gastrointestinal Tract

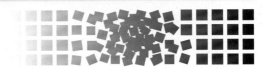

36 Molecular Biology of the Esophagus and Stomach

Anil K. Rustgi

INTRODUCTION

This chapter will deal with the molecular biology of esophageal and gastric cancers. The reader is referred to Chapters 37 and 38 for detailed information about the epidemiology, etiology, pathology, clinical manifestations, diagnosis, and therapy of esophageal and gastric cancers. There are several key aspects in the elucidation of the genetic basis of esophageal and gastric cancers through molecular biology approaches. These include, but are not limited to, new insights into underlying pathogenesis, possibilities for risk stratification and prognosis, correlations with traditional pathology classification schemes, the development of new diagnostics, and potential applications in molecular imaging and therapy. In considering the genetic underpinnings of esophageal and gastric cancers, critical appraisal is required of oncogenes, tumor suppressor genes, and DNA mismatch repair genes as they modulate, either positively or negatively, growth factor receptor–mediating signaling cascades, transcription of target genes, and cell-cycle progression. These molecular networks conspire to influence cellular behaviors, such as proliferation, differentiation, apoptosis, senescence, and response to stress and injury. The exquisite equilibrium that is the signature of normal cellular homeostasis is perturbed in uncontrolled cell growth, resulting in the eventual evolution of premalignant stages and malignant transformation. However, the time required for malignant transformation varies, depending on cellular- and tissue-specific context, and is affected by environmental factors.

The salient features of tumorigenesis and the acquisition of the malignant phenotype that are required, as described by Hanahan and Weinberg,[1] include growth signal autonomy, the ability to surmount antigrowth signals, the evasion of apoptosis, unlimited replicative ability, angiogenesis, and invasion and metastatic potential. More recently, the role of inflammation in carcinogenesis has gained much attention.

MOLECULAR BIOLOGY OF ESOPHAGEAL CANCER

The vast majority of esophageal cancers are of two subtypes: esophageal squamous cell cancer (ESCC) and esophageal adenocarcinoma (EAC). ESCC is preceded by squamous dysplasia, whereas EAC is preceded by a Barrett esophagus (BE) or an incomplete intestinal metaplasia of the normal squamous epithelium of the esophagus (Fig. 36.1). A BE undergoes transition from low-grade and high-grade dysplasia before progressing into EAC. ESCC and EAC have common and divergent genetic features as manifest by alterations in canonical oncogenes and tumor suppressor genes in somatic cells of tumors (Table 36.1). However, inherited predisposition to ESCC is rare, as described in *tylosis palmaris et plantaris*. Although the gene mutation for

tylosis has remained elusive, the region of allelic deletion is on chromosome 17p.[2] Similarly, there is no classic syndrome that distinguishes familial BE or familial EAC. That being said, studies continue to analyze families with BE in an effort to identify relevant genes or single-nucleotide polymorphisms. It is estimated that about 7% of patients with BE may have a family history. In a model-free linkage analysis of concordant-affected and discordant sibling pairs with BE/EAC, and tested independently prospectively in BE/EAC patients (and ancestry-matched controls), three genes—*MSR1, ASCC1,* and *CTHRC1*—were associated with BE/EAC.[3] An initial genome-wide association study (GWAS) revealed that common variants at chromosome 16q24.1 (the closest gene is *FOXF1*, which may be involved in esophageal organogenesis) and major histocompatibility complex (MHC) locus (chromosome 6p21) are associated with BE.[4] Subsequently, another GWAS revealed new susceptibility loci in BE/EAC in the following chromosomes and genes: chromosome 19p13-*CRTC1* (encoding cAMP repsonse element binding protein [CREB]-regulated transcription coactivator) gene; chromosome 9q22-*BARX1* gene, which is a transcription factor important in esophageal and gastric organogenesis; and chromosome 3p14- near the *FOXP1* gene, which regulates esophageal development).[5]

Epidermal Growth Factor Receptor

The epidermal growth factor receptor (EGFR) family of receptor tyrosine kinases stimulates a number of signal transduction cascades (e.g., *Ras/Raf/MEK/ERK, PI3K/AKT*) that regulate diverse cellular processes, such as proliferation, differentiation, survival, migration, and adhesion. These signaling pathways are important in normal cellular homeostasis, but aberrant activation of the EGFR members is crucial in esophageal carcinogenesis. This family of receptors comprises EGFR (also referred to as *erbB1, erbB2, erbB3,* and *erbB4*). The receptors have the ability to homo- or heterodimerize on engagement with one of several ligands: transforming growth factor α (TGF-α), EGF, amphiregulin, heparin-binding EGF-like growth factor, betacellulin, and epiregulin. The tyrosine phosphorylation of homo- or heterodimers of EGFRs creates docking sites for signaling proteins or adapter proteins. EGFR is commonly overexpressed in early-stage esophageal cancer, and overexpression correlates with a poor prognosis.[6–9] EGFR overexpression is typically due to increased engagement with ligands and decreased turnover. However, the mutation of a tyrosine residue in the cytoplasmic domain is rare. Increased expression of TGF-α and EGF has been detected in BE, EAC, and ESCC.[10–14] EGFR overexpression may predict a poor response to chemoradiotherapy[15,16] and is associated with decreased survival in patients with squamous cell carcinoma.[15] Furthermore, EGFR overexpression was associated with recurrent disease and diminished overall survival in patients undergoing an esophagectomy for ESCC.[16,17]

Normal esophagus ⟶ Squamous dysplasia ⟶ Squamous cell cancer

Normal esophagus ⟶ Intestinal metaplasia ⟶ Low-grade dysplasia ⟶ High-grade dysplasia ⟶ Adenocarcinoma

Figure 36.1 Progression of stages in esophageal squamous cell cancer and esophageal adenocarcinoma.

Cyclin D1 and p16INK4a

Cyclins, cyclin-dependent kinases (CDK), and cyclin-dependent kinase inhibitors (CDKi [such as p15, p16, p21, and p27]) regulate the mammalian cell cycle. During the G1 phase, the cyclin D1 oncogene complexes with either CDK4 or CDK6 to phosphorylate the retinoblastoma (pRb) tumor suppressor protein and, in so doing, relieves the negative regulatory effect of pRb, allowing the E2F family of transcription factors to propel the cell cycle toward the G1/S phase transition.[18] Toward the late G1 phase, cyclin E complexes with CDKs to phosphorylate p107, which is related to pRb, and liberates more E2F members to navigate the cell cycle into S phase. As with EGFR, cyclin D1 overexpression is found in premalignant lesions, such as esophageal squamous dysplasia or BE, and the majority of early-stage ESCC or EAC.[19,20] Additionally, cyclin D1 overexpression correlates with poor outcomes and survival as well as poor response to chemotherapy.[21,22]

Although cyclin D1 overexpression accounts for cyclin D1 dysregulation, other mechanisms include mutations in cyclin D1 and mutations in Fbx4, which is the E3 ligase for cyclin D1, thereby preventing degradation of cyclin D1 in the cytoplasm and reimportation into the nucleus, where it exerts its oncogenic effects.[23]

In a similar vein, *p16INK4a* is an early genetic alteration, via promoter hypermethylation, point mutation, or allelic deletion, in BE and EAC, but interestingly, is a late event in ESCC. Loss of heterozygosity of 9p21, the locus for both p16 and p15, has been demonstrated with high frequency in both dysplastic Barrett epithelium and Barrett adenocarcinoma (90% and more than 80% of cases, respectively).[24,25] Promoter hypermethylation, which prevents tumor suppressor function by blocking transcription, has been documented and correlates with the degree of dysplasia in BE. It is present in up to 75% of specimens with high-grade dysplasia and is found in almost 50% of patients with adenocarcinoma of the esophagus.[24,26] Point mutations of p16 in ESCC have been found, and promoter hypermethylation has been noted in up to 50% of these tumors.[27,28] An *Rb* gene mutation is not found in either type of esophageal neoplasm, but allelic loss of 13q, where the locus of the *Rb* gene resides, is found in up to 50% of patients with Barrett adenocarcinoma and squamous cell carcinoma.[29] This can correlate with diminished or loss of pRb protein in BE with dysplasia, EAC, and ESCC.[30]

TP53 Tumor Suppressor Gene

TP53 is the most commonly known mutated gene in human cancer.[31–33] *TP53* is a tumor suppressor that interrupts the G1 phase to evaluate and permit the repair of damaged DNA, which may arise from environmental exposure (e.g., irradiation, ultraviolet light) or cellular stress.[34] In the face of irreparable damage, *p53* induces apoptosis. The *p53* transcription factor binds DNA to activate or suppress a large repertoire of target genes.[35] *TP53* mutations induce the loss of cell-cycle checkpoints and promote genomic instability. The majority of *TP53* mutations occur in the DNA-binding region, and more than 80% of them are missense mutations resulting in loss of wild-type *p53* function.[36] Wild-type TP*p53* has a short half-life and is difficult to detect by immunohistochemistry; a mutation in *p53* results in the stabilization of the protein and allows for easier detection by immunohistochemistry.

The detection of the mutated p53 protein by immunohistochemistry has been demonstrated with increasing frequency during histologic progression from BE (5%) through dysplasia (65% to 75%) to frank adenocarcinoma (up to 90%).[37–39] Thus, the *p53* mutation or loss of heterozygosity appears early in BE and EAC. Both mutant p53 protein detected by immunohistochemistry and specific *p53* gene mutations detected by genomic sequencing have been identified in 40% to 75% of patients with ESCC.[40–42] The presence of a *p53* point mutation correlates with a response to induction chemoradiotherapy and predicted survival after esophagectomy in patients with either ESCC or EAC.[43]

Telomerase Activation

The maintenance of telomere length allows DNA replication to be sustained indefinitely. The aberrant expression of telomerase has been observed in most esophageal cancers examined to date.[43] Morales et al.[44] observed increased telomerase expression in 100% of adenocarcinoma and BE cases with high-grade dysplasia. Telomerase activation is important, but alternative mechanisms to maintain the length of telomeres may operate in these cancers as well.[45]

Tumor Invasion and Metastasis

The loss of cell–cell adhesion can lead to both invasion and metastases. Alterations in expression of E-cadherin, a cell–cell adhesion molecule, or its associated catenins (e.g., p120 catenin or p120ctn) disrupt cell–cell interactions, which results in the potential for tumor progression.[46] Reduced expression of E-cadherin has been correlated with progression from BE, to dysplasia, and finally to adenocarcinoma, and is also observed in ESCC.[47,48]

Models of Esphageal Squamous Cell Cancer and Esophageal Adenocarcinoma

Advances in the diagnosis and therapy of esophageal neoplasms will ultimately be fostered through cell lines, xenotransplantation mouse models, surgically based rodent models, and genetically engineered mouse models. There is a vast array of cell lines established from primary and metastatic human esophageal cancers that allow the perturbation of gene expression to gauge effects on cellular behavior. Recently, organotypic (three-dimensional) cell culture models, which mimic human tissue, have revealed that the combination of EGFR and mutant *p53* results in the transformation of human esophageal epithelial

TABLE 36.1
Common Molecular Genetic Alterations Observed in Esophageal and Gastric Cancers
Oncogenes
Epidermal growth factor receptor (*EGFR*)
Cyclin D1
Tumor Suppressor Genes
P16INK4a
TP53
E-cadherin
p120 catenin
DNA Mismatch Repair Genes (*hMLH1, hMSH2*)
Mismatch repair instability

cells immortalized with human telomerase reverse transcriptase (hTERT).[49]

In transgenic mice in which cyclin D1 is targeted to the esophagus, esophagi reveal evidence of dysplasia that evolves into squamous cell cancer on crossbreeding the mice with *p53* loss.[50] More recently, the conditional knockout of p120ctn in the esophagi of mice results in invasive ESCC.[51] Rodents have also been treated with nitrosamines to yield esophageal papillomas and ESCC.[52]

A classic rodent model involves a total gastrectomy followed by an esophagojejunostomy.[53] This creates a milieu whereby the esophagus is exposed to high concentrations of bile (*nonacid reflux*) with the development of BE and EAC. Recently, two genetically engineered mouse models have changed our views of BE and EAC. The targeted expression of the interleukin-1β, a cytokine, to the mouse esophagi, results in esophageal and gastroesophageal inflammation, the development of BE, and long latency to EAC.[54] However, the time for EAC development is hastened by adding bile acid to drinking water consumed by the mice or by crossbreeding these mice with mice null for the *p16INK4a* allele.[54] Another model involves the global knockout of p63, which is important in squamous stem cells and progenitor cells, revealing Barrett-like cells in the postnatal period when the mice die from other causes.[55] In each of these two models, the cells that give rise to the Barrett cells or Barrettlike cells migrate from the gastric–squamous forestomach junction to the junction–distal esophagus.[54,55]

Functional Genomics

The underlying fate switch between ESCC and EAC may also be influenced by the expression and function of *lineage*-specific transcriptional factors as demonstrated through functional genomics. To that end, SOX2, found to be part of an amplicon on chromosome 3q26.33 in human ESCC, fosters growth of these cancers. This may have implications in the therapy of human ESCC.[56] Similarly, GATA6, a known transcriptional factor, has been reported to be overexpressed in EAC.[57] Exome and whole-genome sequencing of EAC has revealed >20 genes that are mutated significantly, some of which include newly identified chromatin-modifying factors.[58]

MOLECULAR BIOLOGY OF GASTRIC CANCER

The most common type of gastric cancer is adenocarcinoma, of which there are two subtypes: intestinal and diffuse. They are distinguished by different anatomic locations within the stomach, variable clinical outcomes, and different pathogenesis. The intestinal type of sporadic gastric adenocarcinoma has a hallmark progression from normal gastric epithelium, to chronic atrophic gastritis (typically due to *Helicobacter pylori* infection), to intestinal metaplasia (which has some overlapping but also different features than intestinal metaplasia of BE), to dysplasia, to cancer (Fig. 36.2). Diffuse-type gastric adenocarcinoma is even more invasive and aggressive in its behavior, has overlap with lobular-type breast cancer, and may be highlighted by E-cadherin loss.

Inherited Susceptibility

Case-control studies have observed consistent—up to threefold—increases in risk for gastric cancer among relatives of patients with gastric cancer.[59,60] Studies of monozygotic twins have even shown a slight trend toward increased concordance of gastric cancers compared with dizygotic twins.[61,62] Large families with an autosomal dominant, highly penetrant inherited predisposition for the development of gastric cancer are rare. However, early-onset diffuse gastric cancers have been described and linked to the E-cadherin/CDH1 locus on chromosome 16q and associated with mutations in this gene.[63] This seminal finding has been confirmed in other studies with gastric cancers at a relatively high (67% to 83%) penetrant rate.[64–67] Thus, E-cadherin mutation testing should be considered in the appropriate clinical setting. In fact, prophylactic gastrectomy should be strongly considered in families with germ-line E-cadherin mutation even without gross mucosal abnormalities by endoscopic examination of the stomach.[68] Recently, germ-line alpha-catenin mutations have been described as well in these families.[69]

Lynch syndrome, or hereditary nonpolyposis colon cancer, involves germ-line mutations of DNA mismatch repair genes.[70] Gastric adenocarcinoma may be observed in some families with Lynch syndrome. Gastric cancers have also been noted to occur in patients with familial adenomatous polyposis and Peutz-Jeghers syndrome.[70]

Role of *Helicobacter pylori* Infection and Other Host–Environmental Factors

As a commensal organism, H. pylori infection is widely prevalent throughout the world. Despite its classification by the World Health Organization as a class I carcinogen, infection with H. pylori does not typically lead to gastric cancer. This underscores the importance of other factors, such as virulence, environmental factors, and host factors, as well as genetic polymorphisms (e.g., interleukin-1β, a potent inhibitor of acid secretion).[71] The blood group A phenotype has been reported to be associated with gastric cancers.[72,73] H. pylori may adhere to the Lewis blood group antigen, indicating a factor for increased risk for gastric cancer.[74] Small variant alleles of a mucin gene, *Muc1*, were found to be associated with gastric cancer patients when compared with a blood donor control population.[75] Epstein-Barr virus infection has been noted in a certain type of gastric carcinoma (lymphoepithelioid type), although the importance of this is unclear.[76]

Molecular Genetic Alterations

In contrast to ESCC, EAC, pancreatic cancer, and colon cancer, in which certain oncogenes and tumor suppressor genes are altered with high frequency, such degree of alteration is not observed in sporadic gastric cancers. A reasonably prevalent alteration is microsatellite instability, the result of changes in DNA mismatch repair genes (see Table 36.1). Microsatellite instability and associated alterations of the *TGF-β II receptor, IGFRII, BAX, E2F-4, hMSH3,* and *hMSH6* genes are found in a subset of gastric carcinomas.[77–81] Microsatellite instability has been found in 13% to 44% of sporadic gastric carcinomas.[82] A high degree of microsatellite instability occurs in gastric cancers of the intestinal type, reduced involvement of lymph nodes, enhanced lymphoid infiltration, and better prognosis.[83] This is reminiscent of colon cancers associated with Lynch syndrome.

The *p53* tumor suppressor gene is consistently altered in most gastric cancers.[84] In a study of the promoter region of p16 in gastric cancers, a significant number (41%) exhibited CpG island methylation.[85] Many cases with hypermethylation of promoter regions displayed the phenotype with a high degree of microsatellite instability and multiple sites of methylation, including the *hMLH1* promoter region.[86]

E-cadherin may be down-regulated in gastric carcinogenesis by a point mutation, allelic deletion, or promoter methylation.[87,88]

Normal gastric mucosa ⟶ chronic atrophic gastritis ⟶ Intestinal metaplasia ⟶ Low-grade dysplasia ⟶ High-grade dysplasia ⟶ Adenocarcinoma

Figure 36.2 Progression of stages in intestinal-type gastric adenocarcinoma.

In addition, during the epithelial–mesenchymal transition, E-cadherin transcription can be silenced by transcriptional factors such as Snail and Slug. However, it is not clear if the epithelial–mesenchymal transition is an important process in gastric carcinogenesis, as is believed to be the case, for example, in breast cancer.

Alterations in a number of other oncogenes and tumor suppressor genes have been described in a very small subset of gastric cancers by polymerase chain reaction–based or immunohistochemical analysis, but the variability in methods and lack of uniformity in quality control make these observations less compelling. Current efforts in deep sequencing of gastric adenocarcinomas through the Cancer Genome Tumor Atlas (CGTA) consortium should reveal new insights in the near future.

Models of Gastric Cancer

Genetically engineered mouse models of gastric cancer have emerged in rapid fashion in recent years, indicating that activated Wnt signaling and induced downstream effectors, p53 inactivation, APC gene inactivation, Smad4 gene inactivation, and gastrin are critical factors.[89–92] Gastric cancers in these protean mouse models are facilitated by concomitant infection with Helicobacter.[93–96] Furthermore, the recruitment of bone marrow stem cells may augment the effects of Helicobacter infection during gastric carcinogenesis.[96] Recently, it has been demonstrated that overexpression of interleukin-1β in mice results in gastric inflammation and cancer, with concomitant recruitment of immature myeloid cells (also referred to as *myeloid-derived suppressor cells*).[97]

REFERENCES

1. Hanahan D, Weinberg RA. The hallmarks of cancer. *Cell* 2011;144:646–674.
2. Risk JM, Field EA, Field JK, et al. Tylosis oesophageal cancer mapped. *Nat Genet* 1994;8:319–321.
3. Orloff M, Peterson C, He X, et al. Germline mutations in MSR1, ASCC1, and CTHRC1 in patients with Barrett esophagus and esophageal adenocarcinoma. *JAMA* 2011;306:410–419.
4. Su Z, Gay LJ, Strange A, et al. Common variants at the MHC locus and at chromosome 16q24.1 predispose to Barrett's esophagus. *Nat Genet* 2012;44:1131–1136.
5. Levine DM, Ek WE, Zhang R, et al. A genome-wide association study identifies new susceptibility loci for esophageal adenocarcinoma and Barrett's esophagus. *Nat Genet* 2013;45:1487–1493.
6. al-Kasspooles M, Moore JH, Orringer MB, et al. Amplification and overexpression of the EGFR and erbB-2 genes in human esophageal adenocarcinomas. *Int J Cancer* 1993;54:213–219.
7. Torzewski M, Sarbia M, Verreet P, et al. The prognostic significance of epidermal growth factor receptor expression in squamous cell carcinomas of the oesophagus. *Anticancer Res* 1997;17:3915–3919.
8. Inada S, Koto T, Futami K, et al. Evaluation of malignancy and the prognosis of esophageal cancer based on an immunohistochemical study (p53, E-cadherin, epidermal growth factor receptor). *Surg Today* 1999;29:493–503.
9. Rusch V, Mendelsohn J, Dmitrovsky E. The epidermal growth factor receptor and its ligands as therapeutic targets in human tumors. *Cytokine Growth Factor Rev* 1996;7:133–141.
10. Jankowski J, McMenemin R, Hopwood D, et al. Abnormal expression of growth regulatory factors in Barrett's oesophagus. *Clin Sci (Lond)* 1991;81:663–668.
11. Yoshida K, Kuniyasu H, Yasui W, et al. Expression of growth factors and their receptors in human esophageal carcinomas: regulation of expression by epidermal growth factor and transforming growth factor alpha. *J Cancer Res Clin Oncol* 1993;119:401–407.
12. Jankowski J, Hopwood D, Wormsley KG. Flow-cytometric analysis of growth-regulatory peptides and their receptors in Barrett's oesophagus and oesophageal adenocarcinoma. *Scand J Gastroenterol* 1992;27:147–154.
13. Brito MJ, Filipe MI, Linehan J, et al. Association of transforming growth factor alpha (TGFA) and its precursors with malignant change in Barrett's epithelium: biological and clinical variables. *Int J Cancer* 1995;60:27–32.
14. Yacoub L, Goldman H, Odze RD. Transforming growth factor-alpha, epidermal growth factor receptor, and MiB-1 expression in Barrett's-associated neoplasia: correlation with prognosis. *Mod Pathol* 1997;10:105–112.
15. Itakura Y, Sasano H, Shiga C, et al. Epidermal growth factor receptor overexpression in esophageal carcinoma: an immunohistochemical study correlated with clinicopathologic findings and DNA amplification. *Cancer* 1994;74:795–804.
16. Hickey K, Grehan D, Reid IM, et al. Expression of epidermal growth factor receptor and proliferating cell nuclear antigen predicts response of esophageal squamous cell carcinoma to chemoradiotherapy. *Cancer* 1994;74:1693–1698.
17. Kitagawa Y, Ueda M, Ando N, et al. Further evidence for prognostic significance of epidermal growth factor receptor gene amplification in patients with esophageal squamous cell carcinoma. *Clin Cancer Res* 1996;2:909–914.
18. Deshpande A, Sicinski P, Hinds PW. Cyclins and CDKs in development and cancer: a perspective. *Oncogene* 2005;24:2909–2915.
19. Arber N, Lightdale C, Rotterdam H, et al. Increased expression of the cyclin D1 gene in Barrett's esophagus. *Cancer Epidemiol Biomarkers Prev* 1996;5:457–459.
20. Roncalli M, Bosari S, Marchetti A, et al. Cell cycle-related gene abnormalities and product expression in esophageal carcinoma. *Lab Invest* 1998;78:1049–1057.
21. Shamma A, Doki Y, Shiozaki H, et al. Cyclin D1 overexpression in esophageal dysplasia: a possible biomarker for carcinogenesis of esophageal squamous cell carcinoma. *Int J Oncol* 2000;16:261–266.
22. Sarbia M, Bektas N, Muller W, et al. Expression of cyclin E in dysplasia, carcinoma, and nonmalignant lesions of Barrett esophagus. *Cancer* 1999;86:2597–2601.
23. Barbash O, Zamfirova P, Lin DI, et al. Mutations in Fbx4 inhibit dimerization of the SCF(Fbx4) ligase and contribute to cyclin D1 overexpression in human cancer. *Cancer Cell* 2008;14(1):68–78.
24. Wong DJ, Barrett MT, Stoger R, et al. p16INK4a promoter is hypermethylated at a high frequency in esophageal adenocarcinomas. *Cancer Res* 1997;57:2619–2622.
25. Klump B, Hsieh CJ, Holzmann K, et al. Hypermethylation of the CDKN2/p16 promoter during neoplastic progression in Barrett's esophagus. *Gastroenterology* 1998;115:1381–1386.
26. Xing EP, Nie Y, Wang LD, et al. Aberrant methylation of p16INK4a and deletion of p15INK4b are frequent events in human esophageal cancer in Linxian, China. *Carcinogenesis* 1999;20:77–84.
27. Maesawa C, Tamura G, Nishizuka S, et al. Inactivation of the CDKN2 gene by homozygous deletion and de novo methylation is associated with advanced stage esophageal squamous cell carcinoma. *Cancer Res* 1996;56:3875–3878.
28. Boynton RF, Huang Y, Blount PL, et al. Frequent loss of heterozygosity at the retinoblastoma locus in human esophageal cancers. *Cancer Res* 1991;51:5766–5769.
29. Coppola D, Schreiber RH, Mora L, et al. Significance of Fas and retinoblastoma protein expression during the progression of Barrett's metaplasia to adenocarcinoma. *Ann Surg Oncol* 1999;6:298–304.
30. Ikeguchi M, Oka S, Gomyo Y, et al. Clinical significance of retinoblastoma protein (pRB) expression in esophageal squamous cell carcinoma. *J Surg Oncol* 2000;73:104–108.
31. Joerger AC, Ang HC, Veprintsev DB, et al. Structures of p53 cancer mutants and mechanism of rescue by second-site suppressor mutations. *J Biol Chem* 2005;280:16030–16037.
32. Vogelstein B, Kinzler KW. Cancer genes and the pathways they control. *Nat Med* 2004;10:789–799.
33. Sengupta S, Harris CC. p53: traffic cop at the crossroads of DNA repair and recombination. *Nat Rev Mol Cell Biol* 2005;6:44–55.
34. Hamelin R, Flejou JF, Muzeau F, et al. TP53 gene mutations and p53 protein immunoreactivity in malignant and premalignant Barrett's esophagus. *Gastroenterology* 1994;107:1012–1018.
35. Ramel S, Reid BJ, Sanchez CA, et al. Evaluation of p53 protein expression in Barrett's esophagus by two-parameter flow cytometry. *Gastroenterology* 1992;102:1220–1228.
36. Younes M, Lebovitz RM, Lechago LV, et al. p53 protein accumulation in Barrett's metaplasia, dysplasia, and carcinoma: a follow-up study. *Gastroenterology* 1993;105:1637–1642.
37. Casson AG, Mukhopadhyay T, Cleary KR, et al. p53 gene mutations in Barrett's epithelium and esophageal cancer. *Cancer Res* 1991;51:4495–4499.
38. Gaur D, Arora S, Mathur M, et al. High prevalence of p53 gene alterations and protein overexpression in human esophageal cancer: correlation with dietary risk factors in India. *Clin Cancer Res* 1997;3:2129–2136.
39. Kato H, Yoshikawa M, Miyazaki T, et al. Expression of p53 protein related to smoking and alcoholic beverage drinking habits in patients with esophageal cancers. *Cancer Lett* 2001;167:65–72.
40. Lam KY, Tsao SW, Zhang D, et al. Prevalence and predictive value of p53 mutation in patients with oesophageal squamous cell carcinomas: a prospective clinicopathological study and survival analysis of 70 patients. *Int J Cancer* 1997;74:212–219.
41. Taniere P, Martel-Planche G, Saurin JC, et al. TP53 mutations, amplification of P63 and expression of cell cycle proteins in squamous cell carcinoma of the oesophagus from a low incidence area in Western Europe. *Br J Cancer* 2001;85:721–726.
42. Ribeiro U Jr, Finkelstein SD, Safatle-Ribeiro AV, et al. p53 sequence analysis predicts treatment response and outcome of patients with esophageal carcinoma. *Cancer* 1998;83:7–18.
43. Koyanagi K, Ozawa S, Ando N, et al. Clinical significance of telomerase activity in the non-cancerous epithelial region of oesophageal squamous cell carcinoma. *Br J Surg* 1999;86:674–679.
44. Morales CP, Lee EL, Shay JW. In situ hybridization for the detection of telomerase RNA in the progression from Barrett's esophagus to esophageal adenocarcinoma. *Cancer* 1998;83:652–659.

45. Opitz OG, Suliman Y, Hahn WC, et al. Cyclin D1 overexpression and p53 inactivation immortalize primary oral keratinocytes by a telomerase-independent mechanism. *J Clin Invest* 2001;108(5):725–732.

46. Christofori G, Semb H. The role of the cell-adhesion molecule E-cadherin as a tumour-suppressor gene. *Trends Biochem Sci* 1999;24:73–76.

47. Swami S, Kumble S, Triadafilopoulos G. E-cadherin expression in gastroesophageal reflux disease, Barrett's esophagus, and esophageal adenocarcinoma: an immunohistochemical and immunoblot study. *Am J Gastroenterol* 1995; 90:1808–1813.

48. Takeno S, Noguchi T, Fumoto S, et al. E-cadherin expression in patients with esophageal squamous cell carcinoma: promoter hypermethylation, Snail overexpression, and clinicopathologic implications. *Am J Clin Pathol* 2004;122: 78–84.

49. Okawa T, Michaylira CZ, Kalabis J, et al. The functional interplay between EGFR overexpression, hTERT activation, and p53 mutation in esophageal epithelial cells with activation of stromal fibroblasts induces tumor development, invasion, and differentiation. *Genes Dev* 2007;21:2788–2803.

50. Opitz OG, Harada H, Suliman Y, et al. A mouse model of human oral-esophageal cancer. *J Clin Invest* 2002;110:761–769.

51. Stairs DB, Bayne LJ, Rhoades B, et al. Deletion of p120-catenin results in a tumor microenvironment with inflammation and cancer that establishes it as a tumor suppressor gene. *Cancer Cell* 2011;19:470–483.

52. Siglin JC, Khare L, Stoner GD. Evaluation of dose and treatment duration on the esophageal tumorigenicity of N-nitrosomethylbenzylamine in rats. *Carcinogenesis* 1995;16:259–265.

53. Xu X, LoCicero J 3rd, Macri E, et al. Barrett's esophagus and associated adenocarcinoma in a mouse surgical model. *J Surg Res* 2000;88:120–124.

54. Quante M, Bhagat G, Abrams JA, et al. Bile acid and inflammation activate gastric cardia stem cells in a mouse model of Barrett-like metaplasia. *Cancer Cell* 2012;21:36–51.

55. Wang X, Ouyang H, Yamamoto Y, et al. Residual embryonic cells as precursors of a Barrett's-like metaplasia. *Cell* 2011;145:1023–1035.

56. Bass AJ, Watanabe H, Mermel CH, et al. SOX2 is an amplified lineage-survival oncogene in lung and esophageal squamous cell carcinomas. *Nat Genet* 2009;41:1238–1242.

57. Lin L, Bass AJ, Lockwood WW, et al. Activation of GATA binding protein 6 (GATA6) sustains oncogenic lineage-survival in esophageal adenocarcinoma. *Proc Natl Acad Sci USA* 2012;109:4251–4256.

58. Dulak AM, Stojanov P, Peng S, et al. Exome and whole-genome sequencing of esophageal adenocarcinoma identifies recurrent driver events and mutational complexity. *Nat Genet* 2013;45:478–486.

59. Zanghieri G, Di Gregorio C, Sacchetti C, et al. Familial occurrence of gastric cancer in the 2-year experience of a population-based registry. *Cancer* 1990;66:2047–2051.

60. Mecklin JP, Nordling S, Saario I. Carcinoma of the stomach and its heredity in young patients. *Scand J Gastroenterol* 1988;23:307–311.

61. Gorer P. Genetic interpretation of studies on cancer in twins. *Ann Eugen* 1938;8:219.

62. Lee FI. Carcinoma of the gastric antrum in identical twins. *Postgrad Med J* 1971;47:622–624.

63. Guilford P, Hopkins J, Harraway J, et al. E-cadherin germline mutations in familial gastric cancer. *Nature* 1998;392:402–405.

64. Gayther SA, Gorringe KL, Ramus SJ, et al. Identification of germ-line E-cadherin mutations in gastric cancer families of European origin. *Cancer Res* 1998;58:4086–4089.

65. Yoon KA, Ku JL, Yang HK, et al. Germline mutations of E-cadherin gene in Korean familial gastric cancer patients. *J Hum Genet* 1999;44:177–180.

66. Shinmura K, Kohno T, Takahashi M, et al. Familial gastric cancer: clinicopathological characteristics, RER phenotype and germline p53 and E-cadherin mutations. *Carcinogenesis* 1999;20:1127–1131.

67. Pharoah PD, Caldas C. Incidence of gastric cancer and breast cancer in CDH1 (E-cadherin) mutation carriers from hereditary diffuse gastric cancer families. *Gastroenterology* 2001;121:1348–1353.

68. Lewis FR, Mellinger JD, Hayashi A, et al. Prophylactic total gastrectomy for familial gastric cancer. *Surgery* 2001;130:612–617.

69. Majewski IJ, Kluijt I, Cats A, et al. An α-E-catenin (CTNNA1) mutation in hereditary diffuse gastric cancer. *J Pathol* 2013;229:621–629.

70. Rustgi AK. The genetics of hereditary colon cancer. *Genes Dev.* 2007;21: 2525–2538.

71. El Omar EM, Rabkin CS, Gammon MD, et al. Increased risk of noncardiac gastric cancer associated with proinflammatory cytokine gene polymorphisms. *Gastroenterology* 2003;124:1193–1201.

72. Billington BP. Gastric cancer relationships between blood groups, site, and epidemiology. *Lancet* 1956;2:859–862.

73. Buckwalter JA, Wholwend CB, Colter DC. The association of the ABO blood groups to gastric carcinoma. *Surg Gynecol Obstet* 1957;104:176–179.

74. Borén T, Falk P, Roth KA, et al. Attachment of Helicobacter pylori to human gastric epithelium mediated by blood group antigens. *Science* 1993;262: 1892–1895.

75. Silva F, Carvalho F, Peixoto A, et al. MUC1 polymorphism confers increased risk for intestinal metaplasia in a Colombian population with chronic gastritis. *Eur J Hum Genet* 2003;11:380–384.

76. Lee HS, Chang MS, Yang HK, et al. Epstein-Barr virus-positive gastric carcinoma has a distinct protein expression profile in comparison with Epstein-Barr virus-negative carcinoma. *Clin Cancer Res* 2004;10:1698–1705.

77. Kim SJ, Bang YJ, Park JG, et al. Genetic changes in the transforming growth factor beta (TGF-beta) type II receptor gene in human gastric cancer cells: correlation with sensitivity to growth inhibition by TGF-beta. *Poc Natl Acad Sci U S A* 1994;91:8772–8776.

78. Yamamoto H, Sawai H, Perucho M. Frameshift somatic mutations in gastrointestinal cancer of the microsatellite mutator phenotype. *Cancer Res* 1997;57: 4420–4426.

79. Yin J, Kong D, Wang S, et al. Mutation of hMSH3 and hMSH6 mismatch repair genes in genetically unstable human colorectal and gastric carcinomas. *Hum Mutat* 1997;10:474–478.

80. Souza RF, Appel R, Yin J, et al. Microsatellite instability in the insulin-like growth factor II receptor gene in gastrointestinal tumours. *Nat Genet* 1996;14:255–257.

81. Souza RF, Yin J, Smolinski KN, et al. Frequent mutation of the E2F-4 cell cycle gene in primary human gastrointestinal tumors. *Cancer Res* 1997;57:2350–2353.

82. Seruca R, Santos NR, David L, et al. Sporadic gastric carcinomas with microsatellite instability display a particular clinicopathologic profile. *Int J Cancer* 1995;64:32–36.

83. dos Santos NR, Seruca R, Constancia M, et al. Microsatellite instability at multiple loci in gastric carcinoma: clinicopathologic implications and prognosis. *Gastroentevrology* 1996;110:38–44.

84. Hollstein M, Shomer B, Greenblatt M, et al. Somatic point mutations in the p53 gene of human tumors and cell lines: updated compilation. *Nucleic Acids Res* 1996;24:141–146.

85. Suzuki H, Itoh F, Toyota M, et al. Distinct methylation pattern and microsatellite instability in sporadic gastric cancer. *Int J Cancer* 1999;83:309–313.

86. Toyota M, Ahuja N, Suzuki H, et al. Aberrant methylation in gastric cancer associated with the CpG island methylator phenotype. *Cancer Res* 1999;59: 5438–5442.

87. Ascano JJ, Moskaluk CA, Harper JC, et al. Inactivation of the E-cadherin gene in sporadic diffuse-type gastric cancer. *Mod Pathol* 2001;14:942–949.

88. Grady WM, Willis J, Guilford PJ, et al. Methylation of the CDH1 promoter as the second genetic hit in hereditary diffuse gastric cancer. *Nat Genet* 2000;26:16–17.

89. Taketo MM. Wnt signaling and gastrointestinal tumorigenesis in mouse models. *Oncogene* 2006;25:7522–7530.

90. Fox JG, Dangler CA, Whary MT, et al. Mice carrying a truncated Apc gene have diminished gastric epithelial proliferation, gastric inflammation, and humoral immunity in response to *Helicobacter felis* infection. *Cancer Res* 1997;57:3972–3978.

91. Teng Y, Sun AN, Pan XC, et al. Synergistic function of Smad4 and PTEN in suppressing forestomach squamous cell carcinoma in the mouse. *Cancer Res* 2006;66:6972–6981.

92. Watson SA, Grabowska AM, El-Zaatari M, et al. Gastrin—active participant or bystander in gastric carcinogenesis? *Nat Rev Cancer* 2006;6:936–946.

93. Wang TC, Dangler CA, Chen D, et al. Synergistic interaction between hypergastrinemia and *Helicobacter* infection in a mouse model of gastric cancer. *Gastroenterology* 2000;118:36–47.

94. Rogers AB, Taylor NS, Whary MT, et al. *Helicobacter pylori* but not high salt induces gastric intraepithelial neoplasia in B6129 mice. *Cancer Res* 2005;65:10709–10715.

95. Cai X, Carlson J, Stoicov C, et al. *Helicobacter felis* eradication restores normal architecture and inhibits gastric cancer progression in C57BL/6 mice. *Gastroenterology* 2005;128:1937–1952.

96. Houghton J, Stoicov C, Nomura S, et al. Gastric cancer originating from bone marrow-derived cells. *Science* 2004;306:1568–1571.

97. Tu S, Bhagat G, Cui G, et al. Overexpression of interleukin-1beta induces gastric inflammation and cancer and mobilizes myeloid-derived suppressor cells in mice. *Cancer Cell* 2008;14:408–419.

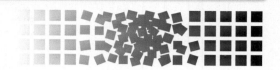

37 Cancer of the Esophagus

Mitchell C. Posner, Bruce D. Minsky, and David H. Ilson

INTRODUCTION

Esophageal cancer is unique among the gastrointestinal tract malignancies because it embodies two distinct histopathologic types: squamous cell carcinoma and adenocarcinoma. Which type of cancer occurs in a given patient or predominates in a given geographic area depends on many variables, including individual lifestyle, socioeconomic pressures, and environmental factors. In recent decades, the United States, along with many other Western countries, has witnessed a profound increase in incidence rates of adenocarcinoma, whereas squamous cell carcinoma continues to predominate worldwide. Although it would seem appropriate to individualize treatment of these tumors, in the past, they have often been managed as a single entity. Although present-day therapeutic interventions have begun to have an impact, with statistically significant improvement in survival over the most recent 3 successive decades, cancer of the esophagus remains a highly lethal disease as evidenced by the case fatality rate of 90%. However, a more thorough understanding of the initiating events, the molecular biologic basis, and treatment successes and failures has begun to spawn a new era of therapy aimed at targeting both adenocarcinoma and squamous cell carcinoma of the esophagus.

EPIDEMIOLOGY

The epidemiology of esophageal cancer is defined by its substantial variability as a function of histologic type, geographic area, gender, race, and ethnic background.[1] Because of the recent increase in incidence rates of adenocarcinoma, especially in the Western hemisphere, epidemiologic studies are now distinguishing between histologic types when reporting results, whereas in the past, incidence rates of esophageal cancer reflected only squamous cell carcinoma. This remains true in high-incidence areas where published rates are not obtained from population-based tumor registries. These high-incidence areas include Turkey, northern Iran, southern republics of the former Soviet Union, and northern China, where incidence rates exceed 100 per 100,000 person-years. Incidence rates of squamous cell carcinoma may vary 200-fold between different populations in the same geographic area because of unique cultural practices. The highest incidence rates for males (more than 15 per 100,000 person-years) reported from population-based tumor registries were in Calvados, France; Hong Kong; and Miyagi, Japan; and the highest rates for females (more than 5 per 100,000 person-years) were in Bombay, India; Shanghai, China; and Scotland.[2]

Esophageal cancer is relatively uncommon in the United States, and the lifetime risk of being diagnosed with the disease remains less than 1%.[3] It was estimated that 17,990 new cases would be identified in 2013, with 15,210 patients expected to die of the disease.[4] Age-adjusted incidence rates are essentially equivalent among African American and Caucasian men (Fig. 37.1), although the predominant histologic type in African American men is squamous cell carcinoma. The incidence rates for African American men peaked in the early 1980s, and since then they have shown a marked decline to the current rate of approximately 7 per 100,000 person-years.[3] Incidence rates among Caucasian men increased up until the year 2000, reflecting the marked increase in the incidence of adenocarcinoma of the esophagus of more than 400% in the past 2 decades, but now have stabilized between 7 and 8 per 100,000 person-years.[3] Although the incidence of esophageal cancer in Caucasian females (1.6 per 100,000) is lower than that in Caucasian males, rates of adenocarcinoma have increased in women by more than 300% during the past 20 years. Similar trends have been noted in Western European countries. This trend of increased incidence of adenocarcinoma of the esophagus has paralleled the upward trend in rates of both gastroesophageal reflux disease and obesity.

A steady decline in esophageal cancer mortality has been noted since the mid-1980s in the non-Caucasian U.S. population, whereas a marked increase in mortality was noted among Caucasian men and women during the same period (Fig. 37.2).[3] The mortality rates among men are markedly higher than women, regardless of race. Although survival rates for all esophageal cancer patients are uniformly dismal, regardless of race or gender, 5-year relative survival rates have significantly improved since the 1970s (5% if diagnosed in 1975 to 1977 versus 19% if diagnosed in 2003 to 2009) based on Surveillance, Epidemiology, and End Results (SEER) population-based tumor registry reporting.[3] There is no survival difference related to cell type (squamous cell carcinoma versus adenocarcinoma).

ETIOLOGIC FACTORS AND PREDISPOSING CONDITIONS

Squamous cell carcinoma and adenocarcinoma of the esophagus share some risk factors, whereas other risk factors are specific to one histologic type or the other.

Tobacco and Alcohol Use

Tobacco and alcohol use are considered the major contributing factors in the development of esophageal cancer worldwide. It is estimated that up to 90% of the risk of squamous cell carcinoma of the esophagus in Western Europe and North America can be attributed to tobacco and alcohol use.[5] Population-based studies demonstrate that tobacco and alcohol use are independent risk factors, and their effects are multiplicative, as evidenced by the association of the highest risk of developing esophageal cancer with heavy use of both agents. Approximately 65% and 57% of squamous cell carcinomas of the esophagus have been attributed to smoking tobacco for longer than 6 months in Caucasian and African American men, respectively, in the United States.[6] There appears to be a dose–response effect related to the duration and intensity of smoking, and, importantly, there is an impressive (up to 50%) reduction in the risk of developing squamous cell carcinoma of the esophagus for those who quit smoking and an inverse relationship between risk and the length of time since cessation of

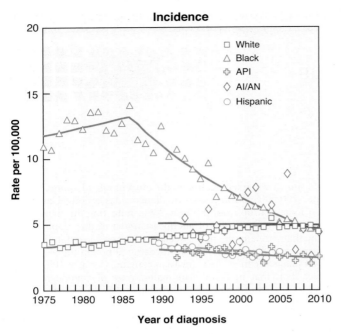

Figure 37.1 Surveillance, Epidemiology and End Results (SEER) age-adjusted esophageal cancer incidence rates in the United States. API, Asian/Pacific Islanders; AI/AN, American Indians/Alaska Natives.

tobacco use.[7] Cigarette smoking in adenocarcinoma of the esophagus leads to a twofold increase in risk for heavy smokers (more than one pack per day).[7,8] Quitting smoking does not appear to decrease the risk of adenocarcinoma, which remains elevated for decades after smoking cessation.[7,8] This suggests that tobacco carcinogens may affect carcinogenesis early on in esophageal adenocarcinoma, and, therefore, the decline in prevalence of smoking in the United States has not had an impact on the risk for the disease. Consistent with this hypothesis, cigarette smoking was recently identified as

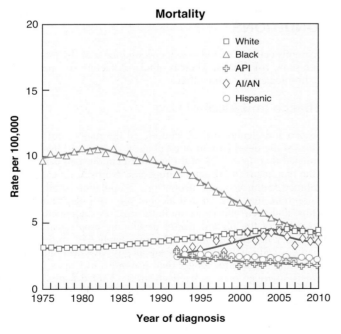

Figure 37.2 Surveillance, Epidemiology and End Results (SEER) age-adjusted esophageal cancer mortality rates in the United States. API, Asian/Pacific Islanders; AI/AN, American Indians/Alaska Natives.

a risk factor for the development of Barrett's esophagus. Specifically, when analyzing data from five case-control studies involving 1,059 patients with Barrett's esophagus, 1,332 patients with gastroesophageal reflux disease (GERD), and 1,143 population-based controls, patients with Barrett's esophagus were significantly more likely to have ever smoked than either control cohort (odds ratio [OR] = 1.67 versus population-based controls; OR = 1.61 versus GERD controls). Furthermore, increasing the pack-years of smoking increased the risk of Barrett's esophagus.[9]

Alcohol is a major contributing factor in the increased risk of esophageal squamous cell carcinoma in Western countries, likely accounting for 80% of squamous cell carcinoma of the esophagus in men in the United States.[6] A dose–response relationship exists between the amount of alcohol ingested and the risk of developing squamous cell carcinoma.[10,11] In most studies, the most commonly consumed beverage in a specific geographic region is the one most frequently associated with increased risk.[1] Although specific carcinogens may be present in a variety of alcoholic beverages, in all likelihood, it is alcohol itself—either as a mechanical irritant, promoter of dietary deficiency, or contributor to susceptibility to other carcinogens—that leads to carcinogenesis. Large population-based case-control studies in both the United States and Australia revealed no relationship between alcohol intake and risk of esophageal adenocarcinoma.[12]

Diet and Nutrition

For both squamous cell carcinoma and adenocarcinoma of the esophagus, case-control studies provide evidence of a protective effect of a diet enriched with fruits and vegetables, especially those eaten raw.[7,13] These food groups contain a number of micronutrients and dietary components such as vitamins A, C, and E; selenium; carotenoids; and fiber, which may prevent carcinogenesis. Deficiencies of the aforementioned nutrients and dietary components (in particular, selenium), have been associated with an increased risk of esophageal squamous cell carcinoma in some parts of the world.[14] Consumption of hot beverages has been suggested as a risk factor for esophageal cancer in South America.[15] More recently, a diet enriched with "animal products and related components" was significantly associated with the development of esophageal carcinoma (OR = 1.64; 95% confidence interval [CI], 1.06 to 2.55), whereas diets high in "vitamins and fiber" and "other polyunsaturated fatty acids and vitamin D" were protective of developing esophageal carcinoma (OR = 0.50 and 0.48, respectively).[16]

Socioeconomic Status

Low socioeconomic status as defined by income, education, or occupation is associated with an increased risk for esophageal squamous cell carcinoma and, to a lesser degree, for adenocarcinoma.[8,17] In the United States, it is estimated that 39% and 69% of squamous cell carcinomas of the esophagus in Caucasian men and African American men, respectively, are related to low annual income.[6] A number of occupational and industrial hazards, including exposure to perchloroethylene (e.g., dry cleaners, metal polishers), combustion products, and fossil fuels (e.g., chimney sweeps, printers, gas station attendants, asphalt and metal workers), silica and metal dust, and asbestos, as well as viral exposure via meat packing and slaughtering, have been suggested as possible risk factors for squamous cell carcinoma but not adenocarcinoma of the esophagus.[2]

Obesity

The prevalence of obesity in the United States markedly increased from 12.8% in the early 1960s to almost 23% between 1988 and 1994.[18] This upward trend parallels that seen for incidence rates of esophageal adenocarcinoma. Increased body mass index (BMI) is a risk factor for adenocarcinoma of the esophagus, and individuals with the highest BMI have up to a sevenfold greater risk of esophageal cancer than those with a low body mass index.[7,19-21] The mechanism by which obesity contributes to an increased risk of esophageal adenocarcinoma is uncertain, although the linkage between obesity and GERD is presumed to be a chief, but not the sole, factor. Recent reports suggest that the presence of abdominal/intra-abdominal or central obesity rather than BMI itself may increase the risk of Barrett's esophagus and, subsequently, esophageal adenocarcinoma.[22-24] Because of the influence of nutritional and socioeconomic factors, the risk of squamous cell carcinoma of the esophagus increases with decreasing BMI.

Gastroesophageal Reflux Disease

GERD has been implicated as one of the strongest risk factors for the development of adenocarcinoma of the esophagus.[25,26] Chronic reflux is associated with Barrett's esophagus, the premalignant precursor of esophageal adenocarcinoma. Population-based case-control studies that examined the relationship between symptomatic reflux and risk of adenocarcinoma of the esophagus have demonstrated that increased frequency, severity, and chronicity of reflux symptoms are associated with a 2- to 16-fold increased risk of adenocarcinoma of the esophagus, regardless of the presence of Barrett's esophagus.[25,26] Trends in incidence rates of GERD during the past 3 decades parallel the time trends of increasing incidence of adenocarcinoma in the United States.

Helicobacter pylori Infection

Infection with *Helicobacter pylori*, and particularly with cagA+ strains, is inversely associated with the risk of adenocarcinoma of the esophagus.[27,28] The mechanism of action is unclear, although an *H. pylori* infection can result in chronic atrophic gastritis, leading to decreased acid production and potentially reducing the development of Barrett's esophagus. Although infection by *H. pylori* cagA+ strains by itself may not increase the risk of squamous cell carcinoma, the concurrent presence of gastric atrophy and *H. pylori* infection has been reported to significantly increase the risk of squamous cell carcinoma.[29] Atrophic gastritis may promote bacterial overgrowth, leading to intragastric nitrosation, with the production of nitrosamines increasing the risk of esophageal squamous cell carcinoma.

Barrett's Esophagus

Barrett's esophagus is defined by the presence of intestinal metaplasia (mucin-producing goblet cells) in columnar cell–lined epithelium that replaces the normal squamous epithelium of the distal esophagus.[30-32] The appearance at endoscopy of salmon-colored columnar epithelium extending about the gastroesophageal junction contrasts with the pale, pink-colored normal squamous epithelium of the esophagus. Although other types of mucosa (gastric, fundic, or junctional type) have been identified in Barrett's esophagus, specialized intestinal metaplasia confirmed by histologic examination of biopsy specimens is required for the diagnosis of Barrett's esophagus. The absolute risk to develop adenocarcinoma in a year, once thought to be 1 in 100, is now estimated to be 0.12% to 0.33%.[33-36] Regardless of this revised absolute risk, Barrett's esophagus remains the single most important risk factor for developing esophageal adenocarcinoma, with a relative risk of 11.3 (95% CI, 8.8 to 14.4), implying that patients with Barrett's esophagus are 11-fold more likely to develop esophageal adenocarcinoma than individuals without Barrett's esophagus. Patients with short- and long-segment Barrett's esophagus are at risk of developing dysplasia and subsequently adenocarcinoma.[37]

The prevalence of Barrett's esophagus in the general population undergoing endoscopy is approximately 1.5%[38]; for those with reflux symptoms, the presence of Barrett's esophagus is 2.3%, and in those without reflux symptoms, it is 1.2%. The utility of screening patients with symptomatic reflux is unproven and unlikely to have a significant impact on reducing death from cancer because 40% of patients with adenocarcinoma of the esophagus have no history of reflux,[25] and fewer than 5% of patients undergoing resection for adenocarcinoma were documented to have Barrett's esophagus before seeking medical attention for their symptomatic cancer.[39] Despite this, the American Gastroenterological Association, the American College of Gastroenterology, and the American Society of Gastrointestinal Endoscopy[40-42] recommend selective screening of patients with GERD and multiple risk factors for esophageal cancer. Both medical and surgical antireflux therapies are effective at reducing or eliminating the symptoms of gastroesophageal reflux, but no clear-cut evidence exists that either therapy reduces the risk of esophageal adenocarcinoma. A randomized Veterans Affairs Cooperative Study of medical and surgical antireflux treatment in patients with severe GERD demonstrated superior control of reflux symptoms in the surgical treatment group but no difference between medical and surgical therapy groups in the incidence of esophageal cancer.[43] Overall survival was significantly decreased in the surgical treatment group as a result of an unexpected excess of deaths from heart disease.

All three U.S. medical societies mentioned previously recommend surveillance endoscopy for patients with the diagnosis of Barrett's esophagus, and the grade of dysplasia determines the endoscopy interval.[40-42] Uncontrolled studies suggest that adenocarcinomas identified by surveillance methods are detected at an earlier stage and are associated with a more favorable outcome after an esophagectomy.[44-46] However, the efficacy of surveillance endoscopy is unclear, and there are no convincing data demonstrating that surveillance prevents cancer or improves life expectancy.[47-49] Macdonald et al.[49] followed 143 patients with Barrett's esophagus for an average of 4.4 years with surveillance endoscopy and identified only one patient with asymptomatic esophageal adenocarcinoma. Similar findings were reported by O'Connor et al.[47] These studies suggest that routine surveillance of patients with Barrett's esophagus is unlikely to alter the natural history of this disease due to the low incidence of adenocarcinoma. Some authors suggest that surgical antireflux therapy causes regression of metaplastic epithelium or interrupts progression from Barrett's esophagus to low-grade and high-grade dysplasia,[50,51] but convincing evidence is lacking. A prospective, randomized trial of medical treatment versus open Nissen fundoplication in patients with Barrett's esophagus with or without low-grade dysplasia showed no statistically significant difference in progression to dysplasia or adenocarcinoma.[52] Observational studies suggest that the use of acid suppressive medial therapy—in particular, proton pump inhibitors—may decrease the risk of progression to either high-grade dysplasia or adenocarcinoma.[53] Progression from intestinal metaplasia to dysplasia in Barrett's esophagus signifies an unequivocal neoplastic change associated with the potential for malignant degeneration. Dysplasia is classified as low grade or high grade. The experience of the pathologist is crucial in correctly diagnosing high-grade dysplasia, which is the most important predictor for esophageal adenocarcinoma.[54] The differentiation of high-grade dysplasia from either low-grade dysplasia, indefinite dysplasia, or absence of dysplasia is straightforward (85% interobserver agreement). However, the diagnosis of low-grade dysplasia as differentiated from either indefinite dysplasia or findings negative for dysplasia is less reproducible (50% to 75% interobserver agreement).[55,56] Any degree of dysplasia warrants endoscopic surveillance. Annual endoscopy is recommended for those patients with low-grade dysplasia, and more frequent screening (i.e., every 3 months) is recommended for those patients with high-grade dysplasia if eradication therapy has not been instituted. The management of high-grade dysplasia is discussed in Treatment of Premalignant and T1 Disease, later in this chapter.

The proposed stepwise carcinogenic sequence in which specialized intestinal metaplasia proceeds to low-grade dysplasia, high-grade dysplasia, and frank carcinoma suggests a potential opportunity for chemoprevention to disrupt the succession to cancer. Buttar et al.,[57] recognizing that carcinogenesis in Barrett's esophagus is associated with the increased expression of cyclooxygenase-2 (COX-2), examined the effect of COX-2 inhibitors on the development of Barrett's esophagus and adenocarcinoma in a preclinical model. Both selective and nonselective COX-2 inhibitors were effective at inhibiting Barrett's esophagus–related adenocarcinoma. A meta-analysis of two cohort and seven case-control studies comprising 1,813 cancer cases demonstrated a protective association between aspirin or nonsteroidal anti-inflammatory drugs (NSAID) and esophageal cancer.[58] These findings suggest that NSAIDs may act as potential chemopreventive agents. A small, phase IIb randomized placebo-controlled trial of celecoxib in 100 patients with Barrett's esophagus and low- or high-grade dysplasia failed to demonstrate a protective effect against progression of Barrett's dysplasia to adenocarcinoma.[59] The ongoing ASPECT trial in the United Kingdom, a phase III randomized study of aspirin and esomeprazole chemoprevention in Barrett's metaplasia, is evaluating the effect of high- and low-dose esomeprazole, with and without low-dose aspirin, on the progression of Barrett's esophagus to high-grade dysplasia or cancer. More than 2,500 patients have been enrolled in this chemoprevention trial with a planned follow-up of at least 8 years.

Tylosis

Tylosis (focal nonepidermolytic palmoplantar keratoderma) is a rare disease inherited in an autosomal-dominant manner that is characterized by hyperkeratosis of the palms and soles and esophageal papillomas. Patients with this condition exhibit abnormal maturation of squamous cells and inflammation within the esophagus and are at extremely high risk of developing esophageal cancer.[60,61] The tylosis esophageal cancer (TOC) gene has been mapped to 17q25 by linkage analysis of pedigrees.[62] The TOC gene is also frequently deleted in sporadic human esophageal cancers.[63,64] Envoplakin, which encodes a protein component of desmosomes that is expressed in esophageal keratinocytes, has been mapped to the TOC region[61]; however, no tylosis-specific mutations involving this gene have been observed.[65]

Plummer–Vinson/Paterson–Kelly Syndrome

Plummer–Vinson syndrome, also known as Paterson–Kelly syndrome, is characterized by iron-deficiency anemia, glossitis, cheilitis, brittle fingernails, splenomegaly, and esophageal webs. Approximately 10% of individuals with Plummer–Vinson/Paterson–Kelly syndrome develop hypopharyngeal or esophageal epidermoid carcinomas.[66] The mechanisms by which these tumors arise have not been fully defined, although nutritional deficiencies as well as chronic mucosal irritation from retained food particles at the level of the webs may contribute to the pathogenesis of these neoplasms.[67]

Caustic Injury

Squamous cell carcinomas may arise in lye strictures, often developing 40 to 50 years after a caustic injury.[68] The majority of these cancers are located in the middle third of the esophagus. The pathogenesis of these neoplasms may be similar to that implicated in esophageal cancers arising in patients with Plummer–Vinson/Paterson–Kelly syndrome. These cancers are often diagnosed late because chronic dysphagia and pain caused by the lye strictures obscure symptoms of esophageal cancer.

Achalasia

Achalasia is an idiopathic esophageal motility disorder characterized by increased basal pressure in the lower esophageal sphincter, incomplete relaxation of this sphincter after deglutition, and aperistalsis of the body of the esophagus. A 16- to 30-fold increase in esophageal squamous cancer risk has been noted in achalasia

patients.[69,70] In a retrospective analysis, Aggestrup et al.[71] observed the development of esophageal carcinomas in 10 of 147 patients undergoing an esophagomyotomy for achalasia. These neoplasms are believed to result from prolonged irritation from retained food in the midesophagus and arise an average of 17 years after the onset of achalasia. The chronic dysphagia and pain attributable to mega-esophagus contributes to their late diagnosis in achalasia patients.[72]

Human Papillomavirus Infection

Human papillomavirus (HPV) infection may contribute to the pathogenesis of esophageal squamous cell cancer in high-incidence areas in Asia and South Africa.[73] This oncogenic virus encodes two proteins (E6 and E7) that sequester the Rb and p53 tumor suppressor gene products. Using polymerase chain reaction techniques, de Villiers et al.[74] detected HPV DNA sequences in 17% of esophageal squamous cell cancers in patients from China. In an additional study using similar techniques, Lavergne and de Villiers[75] identified a broad spectrum of HPV in approximately one-third of esophageal cancer specimens obtained from patients living in high-incidence areas in China and South Africa. Shibagaki et al.[76] detected HPV sequences in 15 of 72 (21%) esophageal cancer specimens obtained from Japanese patients. In contrast, neither evidence of HPV infection nor HPV DNA sequences have been observed in cancers arising in low-incidence areas.[77–80]

Prior Aerodigestive Tract Malignancy

Patients with upper aerodigestive tract cancers develop second primary cancers at a rate of approximately 4% per year.[81] Nearly 10% of secondary neoplasms arising in patients with prior histories of oropharyngeal of lung carcinoma arise in the esophagus.[82–84] Interestingly, p53 mutational analysis of multiple primary cancers of the aerodigestive tract in 17 patients demonstrated complete discordance of the p53 genotype between separate primary tumors from the same patient, which suggests that p53 is not functioning as a tumor susceptibility gene in this setting.[85]

Comparative Genomics

Cancers of the esophagus and stomach are heterogenous and are noted to have genomic instability, as measured by greater somatic copy number alterations when compared with lower gastrointestinal tract tumors.[86] For esophageal and gastroesophageal junction (GEJ) adenocarcinomas, amplification of certain genes rather than gene mutations may be more important drivers of oncogenesis, including targetable kinases such as epidermal growth factor receptor (EGFR), ERBB2, fibroblast growth factor receptor (FGFR)1 and 2, and MET. The most commonly affected genes by mutation include TP53 and CDKN2A.[87] A recent study reported the results of whole-exome sequencing of esophageal adenocarcinoma and esophageal squamous cell carcinoma, and identified notable differences that support the different epidemiology and risk factors for these two distinct diseases.[88] In addition to mutations in TP53, investigators identified NOTCH1 as an important gene in esophageal squamous cell carcinoma development. Also of note, the investigators found conserved mutations in matched samples of Barrett's esophagus and esophageal adenocarcinoma, supporting the progressive molecular pathogenesis of esophageal adenocarcinoma.[88]

APPLIED ANATOMY AND HISTOLOGY

Anatomy

The esophagus bridges three anatomic compartments: the neck, the thorax, and the abdomen (Fig. 37.3). The esophagus extends from the cricopharyngeus muscle at the level of the cricoid

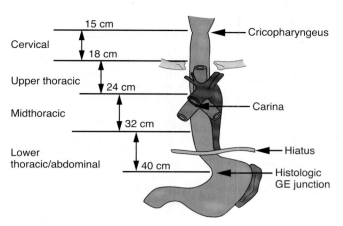

Figure 37.3 Anatomy of the esophagus with landmarks and recorded distance from the incisors used to divide the esophagus into topographic compartments. GE, gastroesophageal.

cartilage to the gastroesophageal junction.[89] The borders of the cervical esophagus span from the cricopharyngeus to the thoracic inlet (approximately 18 cm from the incisors). The remainder of the esophagus is commonly divided into thirds, with the upper third extending from the thoracic inlet to the carina (approximately 24 cm from the incisors), the middle third extending from the carina to the inferior pulmonary veins (32 cm from the incisors), and the distal esophagus traversing the remaining distance into the abdomen to the GEJ (40 cm from the incisors). Squamous cell carcinoma of the esophagus is the predominant histology in the cervical esophagus and upper and middle thirds (above the pulmonary vein) of the thoracic esophagus, whereas adenocarcinoma predominates in the distal esophagus.

Adenocarcinomas of the GEJ present a unique challenge because appropriate management of these tumors as either esophageal or gastric cancers has been uncertain. Siewert et al.[81] have offered a classification system based on demographics, histopathologic variables, and patterns of lymphatic spread that provides clarity, is well established, and has been generally accepted worldwide (Fig. 37.4). In this classification scheme, type I tumors are considered adenocarcinomas of the distal esophagus and type II and III lesions are classified as gastric cancers (cardia and subcardia). This classification system allows for a tailored and consistent surgical approach to these tumors as well as consistency in reporting outcome results associated with therapeutic interventions. However, it should be noted that in the most recent guidelines established by the American Joint Committee on Cancer, GEJ tumors are included under the esophageal cancer staging classification.[90]

The pattern of lymphatic drainage of the esophagus influences the choice of surgical approach, based on tumor location in the esophagus (Fig. 37.5). Tumors of the cervical and upper third of the thoracic esophagus drain to cervical and superior mediastinal lymph nodes. Tumors of the middle third of the esophagus drain both cephalad and caudad with lymph nodes at risk in the paratracheal, hilar, subcarinal, periesophageal, and pericardial nodal basins. Lesions in the distal esophagus primarily drain to lymph nodes in the lower mediastinum and celiac axis region. Because of the extensive lymphatic network within the wall of the esophagus, skip metastases for upper third lesions have been noted in celiac axis nodal basins, and likewise, cervical lymph node metastases have been noted in as many as 30% of patients with distal esophageal lesions. Some surgeons recommend a more radical oncologic procedure, a combined transthoracic and abdominal approach for lesions of the middle and distal esophagus,[91,92] and others recommend a three-field (cervical, mediastinal, and abdominal) lymphadenectomy for all tumors of the middle through distal esophagus.[93,94] However, lymph node metastases are initially limited in an overwhelming majority of patients to regional lymph nodes. Lymph node involvement in lymphatic basins distant from the primary tumor are rarely identified unless metastases to regional lymph nodes have already occurred,[95] which suggests the potential of sentinel lymph node sampling to direct surgical dissection.[96]

Histology

Squamous cell carcinomas account for approximately 40% of esophageal malignancies diagnosed in the United States and the majority of cases arising in high-incidence areas throughout the world.[97] Approximately 60% of these neoplasms are located in the middle third of the esophagus, whereas 30% and 10% arise in the distal third and proximal third of the intrathoracic esophagus, respectively. These tumors are associated with contiguous or noncontiguous carcinoma in situ as well as widespread submucosal lymphatic dissemination.

Adenocarcinomas frequently arise in the context of Barrett's esophagus; because of this, these tumors occur in the distal third of the esophagus. No significant survival differences have been noted in adenocarcinoma patients compared with individuals with squamous cell cancers.

Rarer cancers of the esophagus include squamous cell carcinoma with sarcomatous features, adenoid cystic, and mucoepidermoid carcinomas. These neoplasms are indistinguishable clinically and prognostically from the more common types of esophageal carcinoma.

Small cell carcinomas account for approximately 1% of esophageal malignancies and arise from argyrophilic cells in the basal

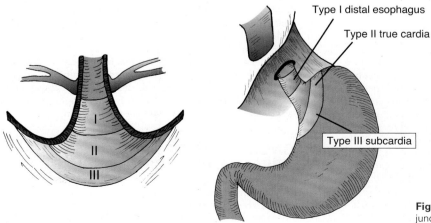

Figure 37.4 Anatomic classification of gastroesophageal junction tumors.

CANCERS OF THE GASTROINTESTINAL TRACT

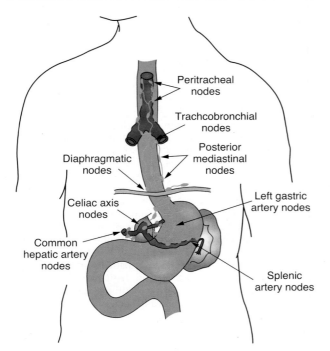

Figure 37.5 Lymphatic drainage of the esophagus with anatomically defined lymph node basins.

layer of the squamous epithelium. These neoplasms are usually located in the middle or lower third of the esophagus and may be associated with an ectopic production of a variety of hormones, including parathormone, secretin, granulocyte colony-stimulation factor, and gastrin-releasing peptide; individuals with these cancers often present with systemic disease.[98–100] Recent series have reported patients with locally advanced disease treated with systemic chemotherapy in combination with either radiation therapy, surgery, or both, with some patients achieving long-term disease-free survival.[101]

Leiomyosarcoma is the most common mesenchymal tumor that affects the esophagus, still accounting for less than 1% of esophageal malignancies. These neoplasms are lower third tumors presenting as bulky masses with hemorrhaging and necrosis. Malignant lymphoma and Hodgkin lymphoma rarely involve the esophagus and is usually secondary to extension from other sites. Patients with AIDS may exhibit Kaposi sarcoma involving the esophagus. Malignant melanoma involving the esophagus is exceedingly rare and presents as a bulky polypoid intraesophageal tumor of varying color depending on melanin production.

NATURAL HISTORY AND PATTERNS OF FAILURE

At presentation, the overwhelming majority of patients have locally or regionally advanced or disseminated cancer, irrespective of histologic type.[4,102] The lack of a serosal envelope and the rich submucosal lymphatic network of the esophagus lead to extensive local infiltration and lymph node involvement. Evidence suggests that occult micrometastases are invariably present, and recurrence patterns confirm that distant failure is a significant and universally fatal component of relapse.[103–107] Bone marrow samples obtained during rib resections performed at an esophagectomy revealed disseminated tumor cells in up to 90% of patients sampled.[108,109] The lung, liver, and bone are the most common sites of distant disease, with depth of tumor invasion and lymph node involvement predictive of tumor dissemination.[89,103,104]

Median survival after esophagectomy for patients with localized disease is 15 to 18 months with a 5-year overall survival rate of 20% to 25%. Patterns of failure after an esophagectomy suggest that both the location of tumor and histologic type may influence the distribution of recurrence. In patients with cancers of the upper and middle thirds of the esophagus, which are predominately squamous cell carcinomas, local–regional recurrence predominates over distant recurrence, whereas in patients with lesions of the lower third, where adenocarcinomas are more frequently located, distant recurrence is more common.[103,104] Only a very small percentage of patients (fewer than 5%) develop a clinically evident recurrence at cervical sites.[95]

The addition of chemotherapy, radiotherapy, or chemoradiation to surgery alters patterns of failure, although reported results are not consistent. Preoperative radiotherapy and preoperative chemoradiation may reduce the rate of local–regional recurrence but have no obvious effect on the rate of distant metastases.[107–111] In two prospective randomized trials recently updated with a long-term follow-up of preoperative chemotherapy plus surgery versus surgery alone that reported patterns of failure, one study showed a slight but not statistically significant decrease in distant relapse with chemotherapy,[105,112] whereas the other demonstrated equivalent distant recurrence rates in both the preoperative chemotherapy and surgery-alone arms.[106,113] Treatment failure patterns after definitive chemoradiation without surgical resection reveal that the concurrent administration of chemotherapy and radiotherapy provides better local control than radiotherapy alone, and that the administration of chemotherapy may reduce systemic recurrence; however, the long-term follow-up of both randomized and nonrandomized patients treated with primary chemoradiation failed to indicate a clear reduction in distant disease recurrence compared with radiation therapy alone.[114] Although the addition of surgery further reduces local failure from 45% to 32%,[115] it does not diminish the systemic recurrence and, in fact, may enhance it by allowing patients to manifest distant disease because they do not succumb to local–regional failure.[116,117] These patterns of relapse suggest that any further improvement in overall outcome for patients with esophageal cancer will be achieved through advances in systemic therapy.

CLINICAL PRESENTATION

The most noticeable symptoms are dysphagia and weight loss. Dysphagia signifies locally advanced disease or distant metastases, or both. Patients describe progressive dysphagia, with initial difficulty in swallowing solids, then liquids. Control of this single symptom impacts most on the patient's quality of life. Patients with squamous cell carcinoma of the esophagus more often have a history of tobacco or alcohol abuse, or both. Weight loss is seen in approximately 90% of patients with squamous cell carcinoma. Patients with adenocarcinoma of the esophagus tend to be Caucasian males from middle to upper socioeconomic classes who are overweight, have a symptomatic gastroesophageal reflux, and have been treated with antireflux therapy.

Approximately 20% of patients experience odynophagia (painful swallowing). Additional presenting symptoms include dull retrosternal pain, bone pain secondary to bone metastases, and cough or hoarseness secondary to paratracheal nodal or recurrent laryngeal nerve involvement. These types of symptoms suggest unresectable locally advanced disease or metastases. Unusual presentations are pneumonia secondary to tracheoesophageal fistula or exsanguinating hemorrhage due to aortic invasion.

DIAGNOSTIC STUDIES AND PRETREATMENT STAGING

Patients with symptoms of dysphagia should undergo an upper endoscopy and a biopsy to establish a tissue diagnosis. Biopsies or cytologic brushings have a diagnostic accuracy approaching 100%.[118,119]

A targeted biopsy can be enhanced by the use of chromoendoscopy techniques using vital dyes, including indigo carmine, Lugol iodine solution, methylene blue, and toluidine blue.[120,121] Autofluorescence imaging and narrow band imaging are emerging endoscopic techniques that allow for a detailed inspection of mucosa.[122–125]

A focused history taking should elicit information on predisposing factors for esophageal cancer, including tobacco use, alcohol use, symptomatic reflux, a diagnosis of Barrett's esophagus, and history of head and neck or thoracic malignancy. Prior surgery on the stomach or colon may influence the choice of reconstructive conduit to restore alimentary continuity at the time of an esophagectomy. Findings on history and physical examination that would prompt further diagnostic testing include hoarseness, cervical or supraclavicular lymphadenopathy, pleural effusion, or new onset of bone pain.

A chest radiography and a liquid oral contrast examination of the esophagus and stomach have been replaced by a computed tomography (CT) scan and a flexible endoscopy. An esophagogastroscopy allows for a precise evaluation of the extent of esophageal and gastric involvement and can precisely measure the distance of the tumor from the incisors to appropriately categorize the tumor's location. An upper endoscopy also allows for the identification of "skip" lesions or second primaries as well as indicates the presence and extent of Barrett's esophagus. A bronchoscopy should be reserved for those patients with tumors of the middle and upper esophagus to rule out invasion of the membranous trachea and possible tracheoesophageal fistula, although an endoscopic ultrasound is now the procedure of choice to identify these unusual manifestations.

Pretreatment staging procedures establish the depth of esophageal wall penetration, regional lymph nodes, and the presence of distant metastases so that patients can be guided to appropriate treatment. A CT scan of the chest and abdomen is mandatory. A recent single institution review of 201 CT scans in 99 patients undergoing staging for esophageal cancer indicated that imaging of the pelvis did not contribute added staging information, and it may not need to be routinely performed.[126] CT scans are highly accurate (approaching 100%) at detecting liver or lung metastases and suggesting peritoneal carcinomatosis (e.g., ascites, omental infiltration, peritoneal tumor studding).[127–129] Accuracy for detecting aortic involvement or tracheobronchial invasion exceeds 90%.[128,130,131] A CT scan is inaccurate in determining T stage and N stage.[127,128,130,132–134] The accuracy of endoscopic ultrasonography (EUS) in determining both T and N stage is a function of its ability to clearly delineate the multiple layers of the esophageal wall[135,136] and its use of multiple criteria, including shape, border pattern, echogenicity, and size, to determine lymph node involvement.[137,138] EUS is superior to CT scans in both T and N staging of esophageal cancer.[139,140] The overall accuracy for T staging is approximately 85%, and for N staging it is approximately 75%.[141] The accuracy of determining lymph node involvement has been increased to 85% to 100% with the use of linear-array EUS with a channel that allows for passage of a needle to perform tissue aspiration for cytology.[134,142,143] EUS is highly operator dependent and is limited in its ability to define relatively superficial lesions as either T1 or T2.[141,144,145] This distinction is critical to allow for the use of minimal resection techniques for T1 lesions and to avoid preoperative chemoradiation for T1 and T2 tumors. Miniprobe high-frequency (20 MHz) sonographic catheters that can be passed through the working channel of the standard endoscope are now being used and provide improved accuracy.[146,148] A new generation of endoscopes that are thin caliber may traverse almost all obstructing lesions, allowing for an EUS assessment.[148] The accuracy of EUS in assessing a response to induction chemoradiation is severely limited, and its use frequently leads to overstaging because the fibrotic changes induced by treatment mimic residual tumor,[149,150] although recent data may indicate some utility for posttherapy EUS.[151]

The fluorine-18 (^{18}F) fluorodeoxyglucose (FDG) positron emission tomography (PET) scan is being widely applied in the management of esophageal cancer. The accuracy of FDG-PET scans in assessing regional lymph nodes falls somewhere between the low and high accuracy of CT scans and EUS, respectively.[152,153] In the detection of distant metastases, an FDG-PET scan is superior to CT, with a sensitivity, specificity, and accuracy all in the range of 80% to 90%.[153,154] PET scans, in combination with CT (PET-CT fusion or hybrid FDG-PET/CT) scans, further improves specificity and accuracy of noninvasive staging.[155] This leads to the detection of unsuspected metastatic disease (upstaging) in 15% of patients, which leads to alteration of the intended treatment plan in at least 20% of patients. Currently, the utility of PET to detect distant disease not identified by other imaging modalities confirms a role for PET that is complementary to other staging procedures, although it should not supplant them.

FDG-PET may also have value in evaluating response to chemotherapy and radiotherapy. Weber et al.[156] demonstrated that decreased FDG uptake significantly correlated with pathologically confirmed response in patients treated with induction chemotherapy before esophagectomy for esophageal adenocarcinoma. A prospective validation study confirmed that a decrease in the standard uptake value of 35% or more during preoperative chemotherapy may predict histologic response and is associated with improved survival and decreased recurrence.[157] Brucher et al.,[158] from the same institution, Technische Universitat Munchen, showed a similar result of decreased FDG uptake in responders compared with nonresponders in patients with squamous cell carcinoma of the esophagus treated with preoperative chemoradiation. The MUNICON trial from the group led by Lordick et al.[159] examined PET scan response during induction chemotherapy in 110 patients with adenocarcinoma of the GEJ. PET scan nonresponders (54 patients) assessed after 2 weeks of induction chemotherapy were referred for immediate surgery rather than continuing with the full 3-month course of preoperative chemotherapy. Survival in these patients (median, 26 months) was comparable to nonresponding patients in a preceding trial (median, 18 months) who continued the full 3 months of chemotherapy prior to surgery, indicating that discontinuation of an ineffective therapy and referral for earlier surgery did not compromise outcome. Survival, however, was inferior in the PET-nonresponding patients compared with the PET responders. Although PET response may identify patients in whom ineffective preoperative therapy should be discontinued, whether or not referral of such patients for alternative chemotherapy, or chemoradiation, is warranted remains to be established. The MUNICON II trial explored whether PET scan nonresponders could have their outcome improved by further treatment with salvage neoadjuvant chemoradiotherapy consisting of single-agent cisplatin combined with 3,000 cGy of radiation therapy followed by surgery. When comparing PET scan nonresponders from MUNICON II treated with additional chemoradiation to nonresponders from the MUNICON trial, the R0 resection rate was not improved and there was no difference in either time to progression or overall survival across trials.[160] The small sample size and the utilization of suboptimal chemotherapy and radiotherapy dosing on the PET scan nonresponder arm make this trial difficult to interpret. One series of patients treated with induction chemotherapy, followed with serial PET scans, identified some patients who progressed on induction chemotherapy. Several of these patients achieved durable disease control, including pathologic complete response, when changed to an alternative chemotherapy during radiation therapy, suggesting that salvage with alternative treatment may be possible.[161] Although pathologic responses on this trial were seen in virtually only early PET scan responding patients, other trials have not shown a clear correlation with early response seen on PET scan during induction chemotherapy with subsequent pathologic response to chemoradiotherapy.[161] Two recent systematic reviews of the current available literature that addressed the evaluation of tumor response by PET scan to neoadjuvant therapy concluded that, although PET scans are the best imaging modality available to assess response, the current data

CALGB 80803 Schema

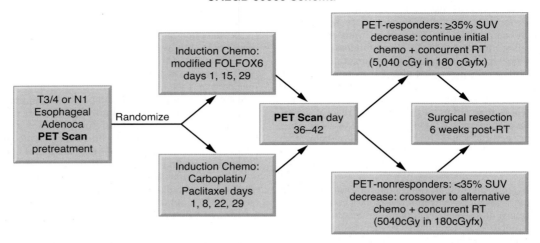

Figure 37.6 Alliance Intergroup randomized phase II trial (CALGB 80803) in resectable adenocarcinoma of the esophagus. SUV, standard update value; RT, radiation therapy.

do not support recommending the routine use of PET scans to guide therapeutic decisions.[162,163] The ALLIANCE Cooperative Group is currently prospectively evaluating the use of PET scans to direct preoperative chemoradiotherapy. Accrual is ongoing to a randomized phase II trial (CALGB 80803) designed to answer the question of whether nonresponders to induction preoperative chemotherapy subsequently treated with a nonoverlapping chemoradiotherapy regimen prior to surgery improves outcome (Fig 37.6).

Minimally invasive surgical techniques (laparoscopy, thoracoscopy, or both) are being used for the staging of both local–regional and distant disease. Performing laparoscopy as the initial procedure at the time of a planned esophagectomy adds little in the way of time and cost to the procedure and allows for the detection of unsuspected distant metastases, which spares the morbidity of laparotomy in 10% to 15% of cases.[164,165] Although studies suggest improved pretreatment staging with minimally invasive surgical approaches,[166–168] such approaches have not been embraced because of the morbidity, length of hospital stay, and cost associated with what is considered an additional procedure.

A study comparing the health-care costs and efficacy of staging procedures, including CT scans, EUS fine-needle aspirations (FNA), PET scans, and thoracoscopies or laparoscopies reported that CT scans plus EUS FNAs were the least expensive and offered the most quality-adjusted life-years on average than all the other strategies. PET scans plus EUS FNAs were somewhat more effective but also more expensive.[169]

PATHOLOGIC STAGING

The most recent guidelines established by the American Joint Committee on Cancer (AJCC) for the staging of esophageal cancer are outlined in Tables 37.1 and 37.2.[90] Changes between the current (seventh edition) and immediate past staging guidelines are highlighted. The tumor location is now defined by the position of the proximal edge of the tumor and is designated as upper, middle, or lower esophagus. Esophagogastric junction tumors are now included in the esophageal cancer staging schema. The primary tumor (T) stage is based on depth of tumor invasion into and through the wall of the esophagus. T stage is now listed as high-grade dysplasia that includes all noninvasive neoplastic epithelium, which was formerly called carcinoma in situ. T1 tumors are now subclassified as T1a (the tumor invades the lamina propria or muscularis mucosae) and T1b (the tumor invades the submucosa). T4 tumors that invade adjacent structures are now subclassified as

TABLE 37.1

Tumor (T), Node (N), Metastasis (M) Staging System for Esophageal Cancer

Primary Tumor (T)

TX	Primary tumor cannot be assessed
T0	No evidence of primary tumor
Tis	High grade dysplasia[a]
T1	Tumor invades lumina propria, muscularis mucosae, or submucosa
T1a	Tumor invades lamina propria or muscularis mucosae
T1b	Tumor invades submucosa
T2	Tumor invades muscularis propria
T3	Tumor invades adventitia
T4	Tumor invades adjacent structures
T4a	Resectable tumor invading pleura, pericardium, or diaphragm
T4b	Unresectable tumor invading other adjacent structures, such as aorta, vertebral body, trachea, etc.

Regional Lymph Nodes (N)

NX	Regional lymph nodes cannot be assessed
N0	No regional lymph node metastasis
N1	Regional lymph node metastasis involving 1 to 2 nodes
N2	Regional lymph node metastases involving 3 to 6 nodes
N3	Regional lymph node metastases involving 7 or more nodes

Distant Metastasis (M)

M0	No distant metastasis (no pathologic M0; use clinic M to complete stage group)
M1	Distant metastasis

[a] High-grade dysplasia includes all noninvasive neoplastic epithelium that was formerly called carcinoma in situ, a diagnosis that is no longer used for columnar mucosae anywhere in the gastrointestinal tract.
Used with permission of the American Joint Committee on Cancer (AJCC), Chicago, Illinois. The original source for this material is the *AJCC Cancer Staging Manual*, Seventh Edition (2010) published by Springer Science and Business Media LLC, www.springer.com, page 109.

TABLE 37.2

Classification of Staging Groupings for Esophageal Cancer

Squamous Cell Carcinoma[a]

Group	T	N	M	Grade	Tumor Location[b]
0	Tis (HGD)	N0	M0	1	Any
IA	T1	N0	M0	1, X	Any
IB	T1	N0	M0	2–3	Any
	T2–3	N0	M0	1, X	Lower, X
IIA	T2–3	N0	M0	1, X	Upper, middle
	T2–3	N0	M0	2–3	Lower, X
IIB	T2–3	N0	M0	2–3	Upper, middle
	T1–2	N1	M0	Any	Any
IIIA	T1–2	N2	M0	Any	Any
	T3	N1	M0	Any	Any
	T4a	N0	M0	Any	Any
IIIB	T3	N2	M0	Any	Any
IIIC	T4a	N1–2	M0	Any	Any
	T4b	Any	M0	Any	Any
	Any	N3	M0	Any	Any
IV	Any	Any	M1	Any	Any

Adenocarcinoma

Group	T	N	M	Grade
0	Tis (HGD)	N0	M0	1, X
IA	T1	N0	M0	1–2, X
IB	T1	N0	M0	3
	T2	N0	M0	1–2, X
IIA	T2	N0	M0	3
IIB	T3	N0	M0	Any
	T1–2	N1	M0	Any
IIIA	T1–2	N2	M0	Any
	T3	N1	M0	Any
	T4a	N0	M0	Any
IIIB	T3	N2	M0	Any
IIIC	T4a	N1–2	M0	Any
	T4b	Any	M0	Any
	Any	N3	M0	Any
IV	Any	Any	M1	Any
Stage unknown				

[a] Or mixed histology including a squamous component, or not otherwise specified.
[b] Location of the primary cancer site is defined by the position of the upper (proximal) edge of the tumor in the esophagus.
Used with permission of the American Joint Committee on Cancer (AJCC), Chicago, Illinois. The original source for this material is the *AJCC Cancer Staging Manual*, Seventh Edition (2010) published by Springer Science and Business Media LLC, www.springer.com, page 109.

T4a (a resectable tumor invading the pleura, pericardium, or diaphragm) and T4b (an unresectable tumor). The nodal (N) stage is determined by the presence of involved regional lymph nodes and is now subclassified according to the number of regional lymph nodes involved. The subclassification of metastasis (M) based on distant lymph node involvement (e.g., celiac node metastases for distal esophageal tumors) is no longer used. An analysis of 336 esophageal cancer patients who underwent resection alone recommended that the AJCC system be revised to take into account the number of involved lymph nodes, and that 18 lymph nodes should be the minimum harvested to provide for an accurate staging.[170] The current AJCC guidelines do not specify the number of lymph nodes to be removed, but instead suggest that the surgeon resect as many lymph nodes as possible while minimizing morbidity. Future refinements in the staging of esophageal cancer may result from incorporation of computational modalities such as nomograms and artificial neural networks that may predict outcome better than the TNM-based staging systems.[171] Successive pathologically determined stage groups are predictive of length of survival.[89,102] Overall survival for adenocarcinoma and squamous cell carcinoma in patients treated with surgery alone, as staged by the new AJCC staging system is outlined in Figure 37.7.[172]

TREATMENT

The paucity of appropriately designed studies to scientifically determine the most effective therapeutic strategy in esophageal cancer fuels an ongoing debate and undermines the potential for achieving consensus. Although there is no disagreement that esophageal resection prevents progression from high-grade dysplasia to invasive carcinoma and is curative for T1 lesions limited to the mucosa, the morbidity and mortality associated with esophagectomy has created appropriate enthusiasm for alternative approaches such as mucosal ablation and endoscopic resection. Surgery has always been considered the most effective way of ensuring both local–regional control and long-term survival for patients with tumors invading into or beyond the submucosa with or without lymph node involvement. Some investigators suggest that extending the limits of resection will further improve an outcome. However, surgery alone or any other single modality fails in most patients, which has led oncologists to embrace chemoradiation and some to question the necessity for surgical intervention. Chemoradiation with or without resection is the most common therapeutic regimen offered to patients with locally advanced (stage II or III) esophageal carcinoma in the United States and its use has increased dramatically in the past decade.[102,173]

Treatment of Premalignant and T1 Disease (Localized to the Mucosa Only)

High-grade dysplasia in Barrett's esophagus is the most powerful predictor of subsequent invasive adenocarcinoma and is associated with a per-year cancer incidence of 6%, thereby warranting therapeutic intervention. The rationale for esophagectomy is that resection completely eradicates the mucosa at risk, which prevents progression to invasive carcinoma. This is supported by older surgical series reporting previously unidentified invasive cancer, which was present in up to 40% of resected specimens.[174–177] The argument against esophagectomies is that most patients with high-grade dysplasia do not develop invasive carcinoma in their lifetimes and, in the era of endoscopic resection, that early cancers can be effectively addressed without an esophagectomy. Those supporting endoscopic methods, ranging from surveillance to mucosal ablative and resection techniques, argue that this allows for the identification of patients with an early invasive lesion that is readily amenable to cure or elimination of the mucosa at risk, thus preventing progression. Indeed, patients with superficial invasive tumors confined to the mucosa, and those with T1a disease in particular, have little or no risk of lymph node metastases[178,179] and are considered candidates for endoscopic therapies.

Surveillance

Endoscopic surveillance is based on the assumptions that the majority of patients will not progress to invasive carcinoma[180] and

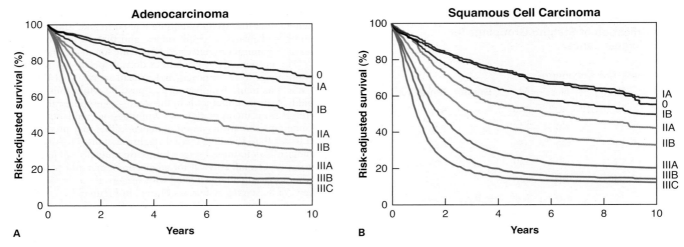

Figure 37.7 Risk-adjusted survival for **(A)** adenocarcinoma and **(B)** squamous cell carcinoma of the esophagus according to stage groups based on the seventh edition of the American Joint Commission on Cancer staging system.

that actual cancers detected by surveillance are at an earlier stage and are therefore curable.[181] Studies demonstrating that patients with Barrett's esophagus–associated adenocarcinomas detected by surveillance have an earlier stage of disease and have better survival than those detected at an initial endoscopy provide supportive evidence for surveillance.[44–46,174] Critics counter this argument with reports identifying invasive adenocarcinoma in up to 45% of esophagectomy specimens from patients with a diagnosis of high-grade dysplasia.[175–177] Proponents of surveillance management argue that these patients were not on an endoscopic surveillance program with strict biopsy criteria, and that strict pathologic criteria of invasive disease (submucosal invasion or beyond) were not utilized.[182]

Proposed guidelines for surveillance include serial endoscopy at 3- to 6-month intervals with multiple four-quadrant biopsies at 1- to 2-cm intervals.[33] The downside of endoscopic vigilance is that in a certain percentage of patients, invasive cancer goes undetected and the patients will not be candidates for potentially curative treatment.[183–185] This must be weighed against the morbidity and mortality of an esophagectomy. It is important to note that the extent of high-grade dysplasia does not predict the presence of occult adenocarcinoma identified at an esophagectomy and, therefore, cannot necessarily be applied to a subjective quantification of disease.[186]

Ablative Methods

The mechanism of action of all mucosal ablative techniques, including photodynamic therapy (PDT), laser ablation, multipolar electrocoagulation, argon plasma coagulation, and radiofrequency ablation, is destruction of the mucosal layer. The premise for managing high-grade dysplasia with endoscopic ablative therapy is that mucosal injury in an acid-controlled environment via proton-pump inhibitors eliminates the premalignant mucosa and resurfaces the esophageal lining with regenerated squamous epithelium.[181]

PDT involves the administration of an inactive photosensitizing agent that, when exposed to light of the proper wavelength, results in oxygen radical production and tissue destruction. Results of a phase III multicenter study that randomized 208 patients on a two to one basis to either PDT plus omeprazole or omeprazole alone demonstrated improved eradication of high-grade dysplasia in the PDT arm (77% versus 39%; p <0.0001) at a 24-month follow-up.[187] A marked reduction in the occurrence of adenocarcinoma was noted in the PDT-treated group (13% versus 28%); however, the results emphasize the risk of development of invasive cancer in a relatively short follow-up interval of 24 months.

These results highlight the limitations of PDT, and due to the complexity of treatment and inconvenience of exposure to photosensitizing agents, PDT has fallen out of favor. Limited experience with thermal ablation for high-grade dysplasia has been reported. Small series of either laser ablation[188–189] or argon plasma coagulation[190,191] of high-grade dysplasia suggest that high-grade dysplasia can be eradicated; however, the follow-up period in these studies was short, and invasive carcinoma has subsequently been documented. Radiofrequency ablation is now considered the preferred ablation technique. A randomized trial in 127 patients with Barrett's esophagus and either low- or high-grade dysplasia assigned patients to either a sham endoscopic procedure or to treatment with radiofrequency ablation.[192] Patients assigned to receive radiofrequency ablation were treated with a circumferential ablation device employing an inflatable cylindrical balloon, bringing electrodes into contact with the esophageal lining, with four applications performed per session, and up to four sessions performed over 9 months. At 12 months, a complete eradication of metaplasia occurred in 77.4% of the radiofrequency ablation patients compared to 2.3% in the control group. Although the development of cancer in either group was uncommon, progression to cancer in the ablation group was significantly less in the control group. More long-term follow-up beyond the 12 months in this trial as well as other confirmatory studies are required.

Endoscopic Mucosal Resection

Endoscopic mucosal resection (EMR) is now considered an essential diagnostic, staging, and therapeutic option available for patients with either high-grade dysplasia or superficial esophageal cancers (T1a). The EMR technique either involves a submucosal injection of fluid to lift and separate the lesion from the underlying muscular layer or the use of suction to trap the lesion into a cylinder, which allows for a full resection and tissue retrieval with a snare or endoscopic knife for appropriate histologic examination. Ell et al.[193] prospectively examined the utility of endoscopic resection in 100 consecutive patients with low-risk adenocarcinoma (no ulceration, mucosal lesion, no vascular or lymphatic invasion, less than 20 mm, and not poorly differentiated). Complete local remission was achieved in 99 of 100 patients; at a median follow-up of 33 months, 11% of patients developed recurrent or metachronous carcinomas, all successfully treated with repeat endoscopic resection. The calculated 5-year survival rate was 98% and no patient died of esophageal cancer. In a previous study from the same group,[194] the complete remission rate in patients with less favorable lesions was 59%, which emphasizes the need to adhere to strict criteria to optimize disease eradication.

A report examining the value of EUS and EUS-guided FNA in patients with high-grade dysplasia or intramucosal cancer considered candidates for endoscopic therapy and demonstrated that 20% of patients had unsuspected lymph node metastases and were therefore deemed unsuitable for endoscopic intervention.[195] These results and similar findings in smaller series examining EMR[196,197] confirm that use of this technique is feasible for the treatment of high-grade dysplasia and carcinoma limited to the mucosa (T1a) and provides an alternative to esophagectomy. Furthermore, one could justifiably conclude that patients carefully screened and confirmed to have mucosa-limited lesions should first be offered EMR prior to considering an esophagectomy.[198,199]

Minimally Invasive Esophagectomy

In an attempt to reduce morbidity and mortality while achieving an equivalent oncologic outcome, minimally invasive techniques for esophageal resection have been designed and continue to be investigated. A variety of minimally invasive approaches have been used for esophagectomies, including laparoscopic, thoracoscopic, combined laparoscopic and thoracoscopic, and hand-assisted techniques and robotic assisted.[200-204] These techniques have been described and are similar in conduct to open procedures of transthoracic and transhiatal esophagectomy (detailed in Surgical Resection) except for the nuances of the minimally invasive approach (Figs. 37.8 and 37.9). These procedures have been applied to the treatment of all stages of potentially resectable esophageal cancer, but until oncologic equivalency to open techniques is confirmed, it would seem to be most applicable in the management of premalignant and early-stage disease.

By far the largest single-institution experience with minimally invasive esophagectomies (MIE) has been reported by Luketich et al.,[205] which included 1,011 consecutive patients, the vast majority (95%) of whom had malignant disease. Approximately equivalent numbers of patients underwent either a three-incision MIE or, more recently, an Ivor Lewis MIE. The median intensive care unit stay was 2 days, the median length of hospital stay was 8 days, 30-day perioperative mortality was 1.7%, and the R0 resection rate was 98%. Median follow-up was only 20 months, and stage-specific

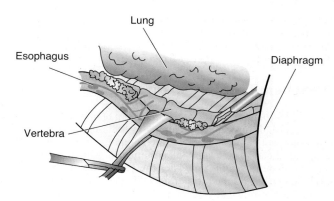

Figure 37.9 Thoracoscopic view and dissection of intrathoracic esophagus.

survival was similar to that reported in a series with open esophagectomies. This group concluded that MIEs are safe and an appropriate surgical approach in experienced hands. The same group reported their experience with 100 consecutive patients with T1 esophageal cancer who underwent esophagectomy, 80% of which were performed via a minimally invasive approach. The 30-day mortality was 0% and a R0 resection was achieved in 99%. N1 disease was present in 21% of patients, the majority of whom (90%) had T1b lesions with submucosal invasion. At a median follow-up of 5.5 years, 5-year overall survival was 62% and 3-year disease-free survival was 80%. The authors concluded that esophagectomies remain the standard of care for patients with T1 esophageal cancer.[206] The results following minimally invasive esophagectomies reported by this group at the University of Pittsburgh are both promising and impressive, but whether they are reproducible in other institutions and therefore more broadly applicable needed to be determined through further study.[207,208] The first, multicenter, randomized controlled trial of MIEs versus open esophagectomies recently reported its short-term results. Patients (n = 115) were randomly assigned to MIEs or open esophagectomies with the primary endpoint of postoperative pulmonary infection within 2 weeks of surgery. MIEs were associated with a statistically significant reduction in pulmonary infections and in length of stay. There was no difference detected in either 30-day or in-hospital mortality, and postoperative complication rates were similar. Patients randomized to the MIE arm had statistically significant longer operative times and decreased operative blood loss. Long-term oncologic outcomes are pending, but R0 resection rates and lymph node retrieval were equivalent between minimally invasive and open approaches.[209]

Nonresection or Ablative Therapy

There is limited experience with the use of radiation or chemoradiation in the curative setting for patients with cT1N0 disease. Sai et al.[210] from Kyoto University treated 34 patients who were either medically inoperable or refused surgery with either external beam alone (64 Gy) or external beam (52 Gy) plus 8 to 12 Gy with brachytherapy. With a median follow-up of 61 months, 5-year results were 59% survival, 68% local relapse-free survival, and 80% cause-specific survival. Treating a similar population of 63 patients with chemoradiation plus brachytherapy, Yamada et al.[211] reported 66% survival, 64% disease-free survival, and 76% cause-specific survival at 5 years. In a recent cohort study of patients with clinical stage T1bN0 esophageal squamous cell carcinoma of the thoracic esophagus, nearly 20% of patients in the surgery cohort of 102 patients had nodal involvement on pathologic inspection. Patients who received definitive chemoradiotherapy (n = 71) had a higher risk of disease recurrence. Local recurrence in the definitive chemoradiotherapy cohort could be controlled by salvage esophagectomy

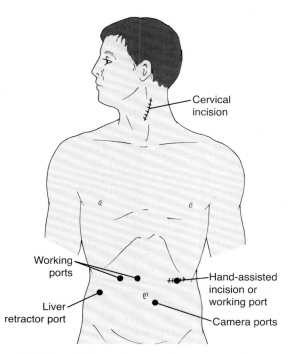

Figure 37.8 Abdominal port sites and incisions used for minimally invasive esophagectomy.

30% of the time, with the remaining ultimately dying of progressive esophageal adenocarcinoma.[212] These data highlight the importance of patient selection in the decision process for local–regional therapy for early stage esophageal carcinoma.

Treatment of Localized Disease

Surgery has traditionally been the treatment of choice for patients with localized, resectable carcinoma of the esophagus and continues to be a component of a more comprehensive approach to esophageal cancer in a substantial number of patients. Failure of surgery alone to significantly alter the natural history of esophageal cancer has resulted in considerable and appropriate enthusiasm for multimodality therapy approaches. The shift toward multimodal treatment is not only theoretically sound, but is also supported by results from phase III randomized trials. Recent trials, unlike their predecessors, which were statistically underpowered and often came to conflicting conclusions about the worth of preoperative therapeutic regimens (radiation, chemotherapy, or chemoradiation), consistently demonstrate benefit to neoadjuvant therapy compared to surgery alone. Results from clinical trials have also brought into question the role of surgery in a multimodal approach to treatment of esophageal cancer, with studies (almost exclusively in squamous cell cancer) suggesting the absence of a survival benefit for the addition of surgery after chemoradiation, despite improved local disease control. Most clinicians and investigators consider some form of combined modality treatment that includes surgery to be the standard of care for localized, resectable esophageal cancer.

Surgical Resection

Decisions regarding surgical technique are routinely based on personal bias, comfort level of the surgeon, and a subjective view of tumor biology because solid evidence from scientifically designed trials is nonexistent. Studies that used health services–linked databases have demonstrated a statistically significant association between performance of surgery in hospitals designated as high-volume esophagectomy institutions with lower complication and mortality rates.[214–217] A study from the Netherlands noted a significant reduction in postoperative morbidity, decrease in length of stay, reduction in in-hospital mortality, and improved 2-year survival following centralization of esophageal resections in high volume units when compared to before the centralization project was introduced.[218] Importantly, the strength of the inverse volume–outcome relationship for esophagectomy has significantly increased over time (2008 to 2009 versus 2000 to 2001) with the adjusted odds ratio of mortality in very low volume hospitals increasing substantially compared to that of very high volume hospitals.[219]

Transhiatal Esophagectomy. The transhiatal route for esophageal resection has gained favor, especially among surgeons in the United States, concurrent with the rising incidence of adenocarcinoma of the distal esophagus, which is readily approachable and effectively dissected through the diaphragmatic hiatus (Table 37.3). The technique is as follows.[220,221] It is prudent to initially perform laparoscopic exploration to rule out disseminated disease and, if it is confirmed, to abort the intended resection before exposing the patient to the risks of laparotomy. Through a midline incision, the stomach is mobilized by dividing all vascular attachments while preserving the right gastroepiploic and right gastric vessels on whose pedicle the reconstructive conduit will be based. The duodenum is fully mobilized via a Kocher maneuver and a pyloric drainage procedure is performed, which has been demonstrated in prospective randomized trials to reduce gastric stasis and minimize pulmonary complications such as aspiration.[222,223] Cautery division of the diaphragmatic crus allows for wide access to the mediastinum and dissection under direct vision of the middle and lower third of the esophagus. A left cervical incision provides

---

TABLE 37.3

Conventional Approaches to Esophageal Resection for Cancer

Transhiatal
- Laparotomy and cervical approach
- Peritumoral or two-field lymph node dissection
- En bloc resection feasible for distal esophageal tumors
- Cervical anastomosis

Transthoracic
- Ivor Lewis
  - Right thoracotomy and laparotomy
  - Peritumoral or two-field lymph node dissection
  - En bloc resection feasible for middle/distal thoracic tumors
- McKeown or "three hole"
  - Right thoracotomy, laparotomy, cervical approach
  - Peritumoral, two-field or three-field lymph node dissection
  - En bloc resection feasible for mid- or distal thoracic tumors
  - Cervical anastomosis
- Left thoracotomy
  - Left thoracotomy with or without cervical approach
  - Peritumoral lymph nodes dissection
  - Intrathoracic or cervical anastomosis
- Left thoracoabdominal
  - Left thoracoabdominal approach
  - Peritumoral or two-field lymph node dissection
  - Intrathoracic anastomosis

---

exposure to the cervical esophagus, and circumferential dissection of the cervical esophagus is carried down to below the thoracic inlet to the upper thoracic esophagus, with care to avoid injury to the recurrent laryngeal nerve. The remainder of the dissection at the level of and superior to the carina is completed by blunt dissection through the esophageal hiatus.

The cervical esophagus is then divided, the stomach and attached intrathoracic esophagus are delivered through the abdominal wound, and a gastric tube, which will serve as the reconstructive conduit, is fashioned using multiple applications of a linear stapling device. The gastric tube is then transposed through the posterior mediastinum to the cervical wound, where a cervical esophagogastric anastomosis is performed. The stomach is considered by most surgeons as the replacement conduit of choice for the resected esophagus. A segment of colon, usually based on the ascending branch of the inferior mesenteric artery, is an effective esophageal substitute if for any reason the stomach is deemed unsuitable for reconstruction or if it is the surgeon's preference. Although the original intent of this approach was not to perform a methodical lymph node dissection, a standard two-field lymphadenectomy (abdominal and lower mediastinal) can readily be achieved, and for that matter, if the surgeon is so inclined, a radical en bloc resection can be performed, as described by Bumm et al.[224]

The stated advantages attributed to the transhiatal approach to esophagectomy include avoidance of a thoracotomy incision, which thereby minimizes pain and subsequent postoperative pulmonary complications; elimination of the lethal complications of mediastinitis associated with an intrathoracic anastomotic leak; and a shorter duration of operation, which results in decreased morbidity and mortality.[221] Limitations and disadvantages of transhiatal esophagectomy include poor visualization of upper and middle thoracic esophageal tumors, increased anastomotic leak rate with subsequent stricture formation, the possibility of chylothorax, and the possibility of recurrent laryngeal nerve injury. The largest experience with transhiatal esophagectomy was reported by Orringer et al.[225] and included 1,525 patients with esophageal

TABLE 37.4

Results of Transhiatal Esophagectomy for Esophageal Cancer

Study (Ref.)	Year	No. of Patients (n)	Histologic Type	Perioperative Mortality (%)	5-Year Survival (%)
Gelfand et al.[227]	1992	160	A	0.9	21
Gertsch et al.[229]	1993	100	A/S	3	23
Vigneswaran et al.[228]	1993	131	A/S	2.3	21
Dudhat and Shinde[231]	1998	80	S	7.5	37
Orringer et al.[226]	1999	800	A/S	4.5	23
Bolton and Teng[230]	2002	124	A/S	1.6	27.3

A, adenocarcinoma; S, squamous cell carcinoma.

cancer, 79% of whom had adenocarcinoma and 21% of whom had squamous cell carcinoma. Tumors were located in the lower third of the esophagus in 82% and in the middle or upper third in 18%. In-hospital mortality was 3%. The most common complications were anastomotic leak (12%) and recurrent laryngeal nerve palsy (4.5%). Leak of a cervical esophageal gastric anastomosis was handled simply, in most patients with opening of the cervical wound, followed by local wound care. Hoarseness from recurrent laryngeal nerve injury resolved spontaneously in 99% of cases. Overall 5-year survival was 29%, and stage-specific 5-year survival was 65% for stage I, 28% for stage II, 29% for stage IIB, and 11% for stage III. These results reflect those reported from other surgical series of transhiatal esophagectomy (Table 37.4).[226–231]

Transthoracic Esophagectomy. The transthoracic esophagectomy has been the most common surgical approach used to resect carcinomas of the esophagus and is the standard procedure against which all other techniques are measured (see Table 37.3). Although a left thoracotomy provides adequate exposure to tumors of the distal esophagus, a right thoracotomy affords access to upper, middle, and distal esophageal lesions and is the preferred route for transthoracic exposure. A right thoracotomy combined with an upper midline laparotomy (Ivor Lewis esophagectomy) is the technique most commonly used for esophageal resection and is briefly described here.[221] The abdominal portion of the procedure duplicates that of the transhiatal approach previously detailed and includes mobilization of the stomach and distal esophagus, upper abdominal lymphadenectomy, pyloromyotomy, and placement of a feeding jejunostomy before abdominal wound closure and repositioning for the thoracic component of the procedure. A muscle-sparing right lateral thoracotomy is performed through the fifth or sixth intercostal space. The azygos vein is divided, the mediastinal pleura incised, the intrathoracic esophagus mobilized, and a mediastinal lymph node dissection performed.

After division of the proximal esophagus in the chest to ensure an adequate margin, the GEJ and stomach are pulled into the thoracic cavity. The stomach is then divided with a linear stapler, the specimen is removed, and an esophagogastric anastomosis is performed. An alternative approach has been described in which the right thoracotomy is the initial stage of the procedure followed by repositioning of the patient supine for an abdominal and left cervical incision to achieve a cervical esophagogastric anastomosis.[232,233] Initial experience with a minimally invasive Ivor Lewis esophagectomy has also been reported.[234]

The transthoracic approach provides direct visualization and exposure of the intrathoracic esophagus, facilitating a wider dissection to achieve a more adequate radial margin around the primary tumor and more thorough lymph node dissection, which theoretically results in a more sound cancer operation. In patients with significant comorbid conditions, the combined effects of an abdominal and thoracic incision may compromise cardiorespiratory function. An intrathoracic anastomotic leak can lead to mediastinitis, sepsis, and death. In addition, esophagitis in the nonresected thoracic esophagus may occur secondary to bile reflux. The three-incision (cervical, thoracic, and abdominal) modification of the procedure effectively eliminates the potential for complications associated with an intrathoracic esophagogastric anastomosis.

Numerous authors have reported results of transthoracic esophagectomy; however, most, if not all, of these reports include patients who were resected via other surgical approaches and underwent a more extended lymphadenectomy (Table 37.5).[235–240] Both overall and stage-specific 5-year survival rates were similar to those seen with a transhiatal esophagectomy. The most reliable data may be derived from prospective randomized trials in which there is a surgery-alone control arm. In only one of those trials[240] was a transthoracic approach the only surgical procedure allowed. In that trial, median survival time on the surgery alone arm was 18.6 months and 5-year survival rate was 26%.

TABLE 37.5

Results of Transthoracic Esophagectomy for Esophageal Cancer

Study (Ref.)	Year	No. of Patients (n)	Histologic Type	Perioperative Mortality (%)	5-Year Survival (%)
Wang et al.[238]	1992	368	S	6.5	7.6
Lieberman et al.[239]	1995	258	A/S	5	27
Adam et al.[237]	1996	597	A/S	6.9	16.3
Sharpe and Moghissi[235]	1996	562	A/S	9	18
Bosset et al.[240]	1997	139	S	3.6	26
Ellis[236]	1999	455	A/S	3.3	24.7

A, adenocarcinoma; S, squamous cell carcinoma.

Transhiatal Versus Transthoracic Esophagectomy. The controversy regarding the optimal surgical approach for esophageal cancer remains unresolved. Two large meta-analyses have compared transhiatal esophagectomy with transthoracic esophagectomy based on collective reviews of numerous individual studies.[241,242] Both reports include studies that compared transhiatal with transthoracic esophagectomies, studies of transhiatal esophagectomies only, and studies of transthoracic esophagectomies only. Rindani et al.[241] reviewed 5,483 patients from 44 series published between 1986 and 1996. Perioperative mortality was significantly higher in the transthoracic esophagectomy group than in the transhiatal group (9.5% versus 6.3%), whereas overall perioperative complications were not significantly different. Transhiatal esophagectomies resulted in a higher incidence of anastomotic leak, anastomotic stricture, and recurrent laryngeal nerve injury. Overall 5-year survival was similar: 24% for transhiatal esophagectomies and 26% for transthoracic esophagectomies. Hulscher et al.[242] performed a collective review of 50 studies performed between 1990 and 1999 yielding 7,527 patients. Postoperative mortality was significantly greater in the transthoracic group than in transhiatal group (9.2% versus 5.7%). Transthoracic esophagectomies were associated with a significantly higher risk of pulmonary complications (18.7% versus 12.7%), whereas patients treated with a transhiatal esophagectomy had a higher anastomotic leak rate (13.6% versus 7.2%). Five-year survival was not significantly different, with a 23% 5-year survival for transthoracic and a 21.7% 5-year survival with transhiatal esophagectomies. A third meta-analysis of over 50 comparative studies with a total of 5,905 patients included studies published up to 2010 and also included the largest randomized controlled trial. In-hospital or 30-day mortality was significantly higher in the transthoracic group (10.6% versus 7.2%) as was pulmonary complications and length of stay (4 days greater). Anastomotic leak (16.9% versus 10.6%), anastomotic stricture and vocal cord paralysis was significantly higher in the transhiatal group. Five-year overall survival was not statistically different between the transthoracic (26.6%) and transhiatal (25.8%) groups.[243] A prospective database based on the Veterans Administration National Surgical Quality Improvement Program analyzed perioperative outcome in 945 patients: 562 who underwent transthoracic esophagectomy and 383 who underwent resection through a transhiatal approach.[244] There was no difference in overall mortality (10% for transthoracic approach versus 9.9% for transhiatal approach) or morbidity (47% for transthoracic versus 49% for transhiatal). A large population-based study evaluated transhiatal and transthoracic esophagectomies through the SEER Medicare-linked database from 1992 to 2002.[245] A lower operative mortality was found after transhiatal esophagectomies (6.7% versus 13.1%). Although observed 5-year survival was higher after a transhiatal esophagectomy, after adjusting for stage, patient, and provider factors, no significant 5-year survival difference was found.

Four phase III trials have prospectively examined the outcomes for patients randomly assigned to undergo either a transhiatal or a transthoracic esophagectomy.[246–249] No definitive conclusions can be drawn from three of these trials because of the extremely small sample size. The trial in the Netherlands, however, deserves special attention. Hulscher et al.[249] randomly assigned 220 patients with middle or distal esophageal carcinoma to undergo either a transhiatal esophagectomy or a transthoracic esophagectomy. The transthoracic group underwent a systematic mediastinal and upper abdominal lymph node dissection. Although the number of lymph nodes retrieved was significantly higher in the transthoracic group (31 versus 16; p <0.001), there was no difference in the radicality of the two procedures with equivalent R0, R1, and R2 resections. Postoperative pulmonary complications, ventilatory time, intensive care unit stay, and hospital stay were significantly higher in those patients assigned to the transthoracic group. Despite the higher perioperative morbidity, there was no statistically significant increase in in-hospital mortality (4% versus 2% for transthoracic versus transhiatal esophagectomy, respectively; p = 0.45).

At a median follow-up of 4.7 years, there were no significant differences between the transhiatal and transthoracic esophagectomy groups with respect to median disease-free interval (1.4 years versus 1.7 years) and median overall survival time (1.8 years versus 2.0 years), respectively. Likewise, no significant differences were noted in local–regional recurrence, distant recurrence, and combined local–regional and distant recurrence for patients randomly allocated to the transthoracic or transhiatal esophagectomy arm. The investigators point out that a trend toward improved disease-free survival (39% versus 27%) and overall survival (39% versus 29%) at 5 years favored the transthoracic approach group. However, a recent update on this study that provided complete 5-year survival data demonstrated that survival was equivalent in patients randomized to either a transhiatal (34%) or transthoracic (36%) resection.[250]

Either the transhiatal or transthoracic procedure can be performed with acceptable morbidity and mortality in experienced hands and, with either technique, the outcome is remarkably similar.

Extended Esophagectomy. In an attempt to improve on the dismal results reflected in high local recurrence rates and poor overall survival with standard transhiatal and transthoracic esophagectomy techniques, some surgeons have examined extending the limits of resection to accomplish a more effective primary tumor excision and lymph node dissection. Two concepts guide the intent of these more extended resections: en bloc resection of the primary tumor with its adjacent surrounding tissue and systematic lymph node dissection, encompassing either two (mediastinal and abdominal) or three (cervical, mediastinal, and abdominal) lymph node basins (Fig. 37.10). Although some investigators have focused and reported separately on en bloc esophagectomies and extended lymphadenectomies, most of the techniques described encompass both components of this "radical" approach. An en bloc esophagectomy involves the resection of middle and lower esophageal tumors with an envelope of adjacent tissue that includes the mediastinal pleura laterally, the pericardium anteriorly, and the azygos vein and thoracic duct posterolaterally with the surrounding periesophageal tissue and lymph nodes. For tumors traversing the esophageal hiatus, a cuff of diaphragm is resected. In addition to a thorough mediastinal lymph node dissection extending from the tracheal bifurcation to the esophageal hiatus, an upper abdominal lymph node dissection incorporating lymph nodes along the portal vein, common hepatic artery, celiac trunk, left gastric artery, and splenic artery is included to achieve a two-field lymph node dissection.[251] A three-field lymph node dissection extends the lymphadenectomy to the superior mediastinum, including nodes along the course of the right and left recurrent laryngeal nerves, and, through a separate collar incision in the neck, completes the dissection with removal of the lower cervical nodes, including the deep external and lateral cervical lymph node basins.[96,97]

Most of the series that examine the utility of extended esophagectomies are retrospective and involve a single institution. Hagen et al.[91] reported on 100 consecutively treated patients who had undergone an en bloc esophagectomy with two-field lymphadenectomies; none of the patients received additional preoperative or postoperative chemotherapy or radiotherapy. The perioperative mortality was 6%, with the most common complications being pneumonia (19%), subphrenic abscess (13%), respiratory failure (9%), anastomotic leak (10%), and empyema (7%). Local recurrence was detected in only one patient and overall actuarial 5-year survival was 52%. Patients with stage III lesions had a 25% actuarial 5-year survival. Altorki et al.[97] reviewed the results of 128 patients who underwent an esophagectomy at a single institution; 61% received an en bloc esophagectomy and the remainder underwent a standard esophageal resection. Approximately 40% of those undergoing the more extended resection had a three-field lymphadenectomy; the others had a systematic two-field lymphadenectomy. The in-hospital mortality for the en bloc resection

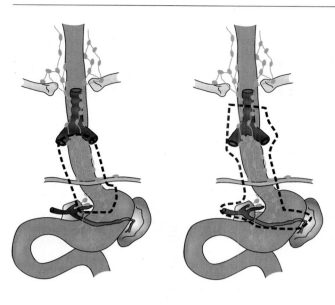
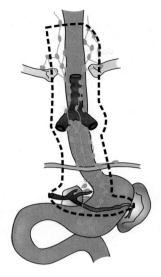

Figure 37.10 *Left to right:* Standard, two-field, and three-field lymphadenectomy.

group was 5.1%, similar to that for those undergoing a standard resection. The most common postoperative complications in the extended resection group were respiratory events (24%) and anastomotic leak (12.8%), but no significant differences were noted in comparison to the standard resection group. Four-year survival for the en bloc group was 41.5% overall and 34.5% for stage III patients, with both of these survival figures markedly better than those for the standard resection group. However, both of the studies described here are single-institution, retrospective analyses for which the results, at least in part, if not completely, can be attributed to selection bias and enhanced staging, leading to stage migration. It is interesting to note that similar results have been achieved without a thoracotomy using a transhiatal approach as described earlier in Transhiatal Esophagectomy.[224]

A group at Cornell University also separately examined 80 patients who underwent an esophagectomy with a three-field lymphadenectomy.[94] Overall 30-day mortality was 5%, with 31% of patients developing major postoperative complications, including the need for reintubation (16%), anastomotic leak (11%), and recurrent laryngeal nerve injury (9%). Overall 5-year survival was 51%. Cervical lymph node metastases were identified in 36% of patients, and the 5-year survival rate for those with positive cervical lymph nodes was 25%. Lerut et al.[252] reported on 174 patients, equally divided between squamous cell and adenocarcinoma histology, who underwent a three-field lymphadenectomy. Hospital mortality was only 1.2%, with an overall mortality of 58%. Five-year survival for stage III patients was 36.8%. Twenty-three percent of patients with adenocarcinoma and 25% of those with squamous cell carcinoma had positive cervical nodes. Five-year survival for patients with positive cervical lymph nodes was 27% and 12%, respectively, for squamous cell and adenocarcinoma histology. The authors suggest that a three-field lymphadenectomy may have a role in patients with squamous cell carcinoma, but this remains investigational for patients with adenocarcinoma. These results, although impressive, may also reflect both selection bias and stage migration. In addition, the expertise required to perform these technically demanding procedures effectively limits their application to specialized centers only and a fraction of the patients who might benefit from these procedures if an actual advantage were proven.

The Hulscher trial, discussed previously, which also employed an en bloc resection of the esophagus, compared to transhiatal esophagectomies, failed to improve outcome.[250] A small study by Nishihira et al.[253] of 62 patients showed an improved, but not statistically significant, survival advantage for extended lymphadenectomies (66.2% versus 48%; $p = 0.19$). Patients in this study were also randomly assigned to receive either chemoradiation or chemotherapy alone after surgery, confounding the interpretation of the results.

The body of evidence confirms that extended resections improve staging and may enhance local–regional control; however, there are no reliable data confirming a survival benefit for these procedures.

Adjuvant Therapy

Preoperative Chemotherapy.
Nearly three-fourths of patients newly diagnosed with esophageal cancer present with locally advanced (stage IIB or III) disease. The poor survival rate achieved with surgery alone, and given the patterns of both local and systemic disease recurrence, has provided the impetus for the evaluation of preoperative (induction) chemotherapy in patients with resectable esophageal cancer.

The benefits of induction chemotherapy include the potential downstaging of the disease to facilitate surgical resection, improvement in local control, relief of dysphagia in patients responding to induction chemotherapy, and the potential eradication of micrometastatic disease. An esophagectomy after induction therapy enables a comprehensive pathologic assessment of treatment response, which may be important in selecting patients for postoperative adjuvant therapy. The disadvantages of preoperative chemotherapy include the potential development of chemotherapy resistance and the delay in definitive treatment with the risk of further spread of the disease. These are important concerns because approximately 50% of patients do not respond to current chemotherapeutic regimens. Further compromise of the patient's already marginal nutritional status due to a delay in local disease control is also of concern when surgery is not the initial treatment.

Trials evaluating the use of induction chemotherapy followed by surgery for the treatment of esophageal cancer have been under way since the late 1970s. This strategy was evaluated in parallel with studies of concurrent chemoradiation followed by surgery or chemoradiation as definitive therapy. Early trials used cisplatin and bleomycin-based chemotherapy.[254–257] Use of cisplatin and 5-fluorouracil (5-FU)[258–262] led to the initiation of randomized trials in the 1980s. For lesions of squamous histology, the response rate to two or three cycles of cisplatin (100 mg/m² on day 1) and 5-FU (1,000 mg/m² per day for 96 or 120 hours) every 3 weeks ranged between 42% and 66%, with a 0% to 10% pathologically confirmed complete-response rate; curative resection rates were between 40% and 80%, and median survival was from 18 to 28 months.[258–262] Lesions were staged with a barium esophagogram and CT scan initially and then again before surgery to assess the response to induction therapy.

TABLE 37.6

Randomized Trials of Preoperative Chemotherapy

Study (Ref.)	Treatment	No. of Patients (n)	Histologic Type	Median Survival (months)	3- or 5-Year Survival (%)
Nygaard et al.[263]	Preop C/B	50	S		3 yr: 3
	Surgery	41			3 yr: 9
Roth et al.[264]	Preop C/VDS/B and adjuvant C/VDS	19	S	9	5 yr: 25
	Surgery	20		9	5 yr: 5
Schlag[265]	Preop C/5-FU	34	S	10	NS
	Surgery	41		10	NS
Boonstra et al.[269]	Preop C/etoposide	86	S	16	5 yr: 26
	Surgery	85		12	5 yr: 17
Kelsen et al. (Intergroup 0013)[105,112]	Preop C/5-FU and adjuvant C/5-FU	213	S/A	15	3 yr: 26
	Surgery	227		16	3 yr: 23
Allum et al.[106,113]	Preop C/5-FU	400	S/A	16.8	5 yr: 23
	Surgery	402	A	13.3	5 yr: 17
Cunningham et al.[266]	Preop/postop ECF	250	A	24	5 yr: 36
	Surgery	253	A	20	5 yr: 23
Ychou et al.[267]	Preop/postop CF	113	A	—	5 yr: 38
	Surgery	111	A	—	5 yr: 24
Schuhmacher et al.[268]	Preop CF	72	A	65	—
	Surgery	72	A	53	—

Preop, preoperative; C, cisplatin; B, bleomycin; VDS, vindesine; S, squamous cell carcinoma; A, adenocarcinoma; ECF, epirubicin/cisplatin; 5-FU, 5-fluorouracil; postop, postoperative.

Nine randomized trials evaluating the use of preoperative chemotherapy in esophageal cancer patients are summarized in Table 37.6.[105,106,263–269] Four of the trials enrolled only patients with squamous cell carcinoma,[263–265,267–269] whereas half to two-thirds of patients enrolled in the two more recent and largest trials (U.S. Intergroup and Medical Research Council) had adenocarcinoma of the esophagus, GEJ, or cardia.[105,106] Another large randomized trial treated mostly gastric cancer, although one-fourth of patients enrolled had adenocarcinoma of the distal esophagus or GEJ.[266] Two recent small European trials treated only adenocarcinoma of the esophagus and stomach with half or more of patients having esophageal or GEJ adenocarcinoma.[267,268]

No improvement in survival was noted in three small trials enrolling fewer than 100 patients each, with the small sample size making study interpretation difficult.[263–266] Boonstra et al.[269] reported a survival advantage for preoperative chemotherapy in the final report of a study initially published in abstract form back in 1997. This study, enrolling 171 patients with squamous cell carcinoma, differed from other trials by requiring a response assessment after two courses of preoperative chemotherapy. Patients showing no response underwent immediate surgery, whereas patients showing a response received two more courses of chemotherapy before surgery. The regimen consisted of cisplatin (80 mg/m^2 on day 1) and etoposide (100 mg/m^2 intravenously on days 1 to 2 and 200 mg/m^2 orally on days 3 to 5). Median overall survival in the surgery arm was 12 months compared to 16 months for surgery plus chemotherapy. Fewer patients went on to surgery after preoperative chemotherapy (89%) compared to patients undergoing immediate surgery (97%). Rates of R0 resection favored the chemotherapy arm, but the difference was nonsignificant ($p = 0.09$). Overall survival was superior with preoperative chemotherapy (hazard ratio [HR], 0.71; $p = 0.03$) with the 5-year survival for chemotherapy plus surgery 26% compared to 17% for surgery alone.

The U.S. Intergroup mounted a large, potentially definitive trial, INT-0113. A total of 467 patients with resectable esophageal cancer were randomly assigned to one of two treatment groups: (1) three cycles of cisplatin and 5-FU followed by surgery and then, for those patients whose resection was curative (R0), two additional cycles of cisplatin and 5-FU as adjuvant treatment; or (2) immediate surgery.[105] In contrast to other trials, a barium esophagogram was the only test required to assess clinical response to preoperative chemotherapy. Thus, it is not surprising that only a 19% response rate was reported. Survival and pattern of failure were the major study end points. No differences were observed between the surgery control group and the preoperative cisplatin and 5-FU group in terms of curative resection rate (59% versus 62%), treatment mortality (6% versus 7%), overall median survival (16.1 months versus 14.9 months), or 3-year survival (26% versus 23%) (Fig. 37.11). Furthermore, the median survival of patients who had a curative resection was the same in both treatment groups (27.4 months versus 25.0 months). The pattern of failure was also similar for the two treatment groups (local recurrence 31% versus 32%, and distant recurrence of 50% versus 41% in the surgery-alone group compared to those receiving induction chemotherapy followed by surgery, respectively). Tumor histologic type did not influence response to treatment. A recent update of the trial reported no late benefit for preoperative chemotherapy.[112] The importance of achieving an R0 resection in the updated analysis was emphasized, with these patients achieving long-term survival, whereas patients with an R1 resection treated only with surgery all died of recurrent disease. The only patients with R1 resection achieving long-term survival were those receiving protocol-permitted postoperative chemoradiotherapy: Among 34 patients treated with surgery alone with R1 resection, 18 received postoperative chemoradiotherapy and 9 (21%) achieved long-term survival. These results indicated that R1 resection patients may be salvaged with postoperative chemoradiotherapy.

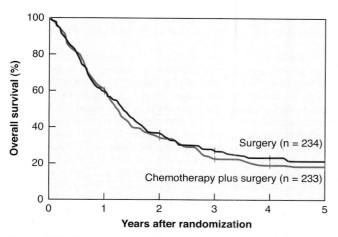

Figure 37.11 Overall survival US Intergroup trial INT-0113 comparing patients randomized to preoperative chemotherapy versus surgery alone.

Although no improvement in survival was demonstrated for preoperative chemotherapy on INT-0113, the trial importantly provides a contemporary surgical experience in the treatment of esophageal squamous carcinoma and adenocarcinoma. Important outcomes in this trial include a postoperative death rate well below 10%, the lack of difference in survival for lesions of different histologic types, and the fact that an R0 curative resection (regardless of treatment) conferred a median survival time of more than 2 years.

In contrast to the results of the 467-patient U.S. Intergroup trial, the Medical Research Council (MRC) Oesophageal Cancer Working Group demonstrated a statistically significant 9% improvement in 2-year survival rate (43% versus 34%) (Fig. 37.12) with preoperative cisplatin and 5-FU.[106] A total of 802 patients, 31% with squamous lesions and 69% with adenocarcinoma or lesions of undifferentiated histologic type, were enrolled. Patients were randomly assigned either to receive two courses of cisplatin (80 mg/m^2) and 5-FU (1,000 mg/m^2 per day, continuous infusion for 4 days) 3 weeks apart followed by surgery or to undergo immediate surgery. The curative resection (R0) rate (60% versus 54%) and the percentage of randomly assigned patients undergoing surgery (92% versus 97%) were similar for the two treatment groups, although the improvement in curative resection rate did reach statistical significance. Patients receiving preoperative chemotherapy had improved median survival (16.8 months versus 13.3 months) and 2-year survival rate (43% versus 34%) (Fig. 37.12). Overall survival was significantly improved with preoperative chemotherapy

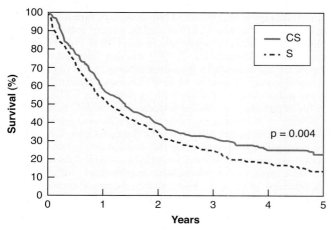

Figure 37.12 Overall survival Medical Research Council (MRC) Oesophageal Cancer Working Group trial comparing patients randomized to preoperative chemotherapy (CS) versus surgery alone (S).

(p = 0.004; HR, 0.79; 95% CI, 0.67 to 0.93). The estimated reduction in risk of death was 21%. The postoperative mortality rate was 10% in both treatment groups. Pathologic complete responses were rare and were reported in 4% of patients undergoing preoperative chemotherapy. These authors recently reported an update of this trial at a median follow-up of 6 years.[113] Although a survival benefit was maintained in the preoperative chemotherapy arm, it had diminished to only 6% at 5 years (23.0% for preoperative therapy versus 17.1% for surgery; HR, 0.84; p = 0.03). There was no difference in pattern of failure—in particular, the development of distant metastatic disease—in the chemotherapy surgery versus surgery alone group, with the authors attributing the survival improvement with preoperative chemotherapy to the enhancement of rate of curative resection. The modest survival improvement with preoperative chemotherapy in this trial update is consistent with a 4.3% survival benefit observed in a recent meta-analysis of preoperative chemotherapy reported in abstract form, in which updated survival data from individual trials were obtained in over 2,000 patients in nine studies.[270]

There is no clear explanation for the discrepancy in survival outcome for the INT and MRC trials, whereas survival of the surgery control groups was essentially the same. The MRC study had the advantage of a larger sample size and greater power to observe a small difference. A greater proportion of patients who received chemotherapy underwent surgery in the MRC study, 92% compared with 80% in the INT trial. Although a microscopically complete resection (R0) was performed in similar proportions in the two trials, the MRC trial indicated a higher rate of R0 resection with preoperative chemotherapy compared to surgery alone. The duration of preoperative chemotherapy in the MRC trial was shorter and may have lessened the risk to patients of disease progression during induction therapy.

Positive results of another recent trial of perioperative chemotherapy in gastric and distal esophagus or GEJ cancer have been reported. In a trial by Cunningham et al.,[266] 503 patients were assigned to three cycles of preoperative and three cycles of postoperative epirubicin/cisplatin/5-FU or surgery alone. Preoperative chemotherapy resulted in significant improvement in patient survival, with a 6-month improvement in progression-free survival, a 4-month improvement in median survival, and a 13% improvement in 5-year overall survival (23% to 36%), all of which are statistically significant. Despite the survival improvement with pre- and postoperative chemotherapy, there was no improvement in the rate of curative resection in patients treated with preoperative chemotherapy compared with surgery alone (66% to 69%), and there were no cases of pathologic complete response to preoperative chemotherapy. Downstaging was also observed with preoperative chemotherapy, with a shift to earlier T and N stage tumors with preoperative chemotherapy compared to surgery alone. Because 26% of patients on this trial had tumors in the GEJ and lower esophagus, the results may apply to locally advanced esophageal cancer. The median follow-up was 47 months in the surgery-alone arm and 49 months in the chemotherapy arm.

Two recent studies from Europe also came to conflicting results for any benefit for preoperative chemotherapy. Ychou and colleagues[267] randomized 234 patients with esophageal, GEJ, or gastric adenocarcinoma to immediate surgery or to perioperative chemotherapy with cisplatin and fluorouracil. Rates of R0 resections were improved with preoperative chemotherapy to 84% compared to 74% for surgery alone (p = 0.04). At a median follow-up of 5.7 years, preoperative chemotherapy improved 5-year survival from 24% to 38%. On the other hand, Schuhmacher and colleagues[268] for the European Organisation for Research and Treatment of Cancer (EORTC) reported a negative trial of 144 patients with GEJ junction or gastric adenocarcinoma randomized to surgery alone or to two 48-day cycles of infusional fluorouracil and cisplatin.[268] In contrast to all earlier studies reported, this trial performed modern presurgical staging including endoscopic ultrasound, CT scan, and laparoscopic staging, and only endoscopic stage T3 to T4 tumors were eligible. The R0 resection was improved from 67% for surgery to 82% for preoperative chemotherapy ($p = 0.036$). At a median follow-up of 4.4 years, median survival was 65 months for the chemotherapy arm versus 63 months for surgery alone (HR, 0.84; $p = 0.466$) and 2-year overall survival was equivalent (70% for surgery alone, and 73% for the chemotherapy arm). Both arms had higher than expected median survival.

Despite the inconsistency of these outcomes, preoperative cisplatin and 5-FU is now the standard of care for resectable esophageal cancers—in particular, adenocarcinoma of the esophagus and GEJ—in the United Kingdom and in much of Europe, whereas this approach has not been generally accepted for esophageal cancer in the United States.

Preoperative Radiation Therapy. The high rate of local failure after esophagectomies engendered interest in the use of radiation therapy in conjunction with surgery. The incidence of local failure in the surgical control arms of randomized trials of preoperative radiation therapy reported by Mei et al.[271] and Gignoux et al.[272] was 12% and 67%, respectively. The local failure rate in the surgical control arm of the randomized trial of postoperative radiation therapy conducted by Teniere et al.[273] was 35% for patients with negative local–regional lymph nodes and 38% for patients with positive local–regional lymph nodes. The surgical control arm of INT-0113 provides a modern, more relevant baseline for the results of surgery alone. As discussed in Preoperative Chemotherapy, there was a 31% local failure rate in patients undergoing an R0 resection and a total local failure rate (including the additional 30% of patients with persistent disease) of 61%. Six randomized trials of preoperative radiation therapy for patients with clinically resectable disease have been reported.[263,271,272,274–276] Overall, preoperative radiation therapy did not increase the resectability rate, and only two series reported local failure rates. Although Mei et al.[271] reported no difference in local failure, Gignoux et al.[272] observed a significantly lower local failure rate in patients who received preoperative radiation therapy than in those treated with surgery alone (46% versus 67%, respectively).

Two trials have reported an improvement in survival. In the series of Nygaard et al.,[263] patients who received preoperative radiation therapy (with or without chemotherapy) had a significant improvement in overall 3-year survival (18% versus 5%; $p = 0.009$). The 48 patients who received preoperative radiation therapy without chemotherapy had a 20% 3-year survival rate; however, this did not reach statistical significance. This was not a pure radiation study, and the benefit may have been partly because of the chemotherapy. A similar improvement in survival was reported by Huang et al.[276] (46% versus 25%). A meta-analysis from the Oesophageal Cancer Collaborative Group also showed no clear evidence of a survival advantage with preoperative radiation therapy.[110]

Design flaws in these trials include the failure to use conventional doses of radiation therapy, the use of split-course radiation therapy, and failure to allow an adequate interval (4 to 8 weeks) between the completion of radiation therapy and surgery. The only study that allows an analysis of the effect of radiation fractionation is a randomized trial performed in France involving patients with squamous cell carcinomas who received chemoradiation using continuous-course versus split-course radiation.[277] The 95 patients who received a continuous-course regimen had a significantly higher local control rate (57% versus 29%) and 2-year event-free survival rate (33% versus 23%), and a borderline, significantly higher 2-year survival rate (37% versus 23%). Because it is less effective than continuous-course therapy, split-course radiation therapy is not recommended.

In summary, because only two of the six series have reported local failure rates, it is difficult to draw firm conclusions regarding the influence of preoperative radiation therapy on local control. Nonrandomized trials[278,279] also reported no survival benefit. Based on the available data from randomized trials, preoperative

radiation therapy does not appear to significantly decrease local failure rate or improve survival in esophageal cancer patients.

Preoperative Chemoradiation. The rationale for trimodal therapy—chemoradiation followed by surgery—is based on the pattern of both local and distant failure associated with surgery alone or chemoradiation without surgery, which are the two treatment options established as standards of care based on data from randomized controlled trials. The results for patients randomly assigned to the surgery control arm of the INT-0113 trial revealed a 61% rate of failure in controlling local disease.[105] Similarly, the two Intergroup trials (RTOG-85-01 and INT-0123) that evaluated nonsurgical treatment (concurrent cisplatin and 5-FU, and radiotherapy), which are discussed in greater detail later in this chapter, showed unacceptably high rates of local failure (44% to 53%).[280,281] Most of the agents active against esophageal cancer (i.e., 5-FU, cisplatin, carboplatin, mitomycin C, paclitaxel, irinotecan, docetaxel, capecitabine, and oxaliplatin) are known to enhance radiosensitivity in cancer cells. Chemotherapy in conjunction with radiotherapy may both sensitize radiation therapy to improve local control as well as impact a reduction on systemic disease recurrence. Treatment with chemoradiation followed by an esophagectomy has the potential to: (1) downstage the disease, (2) increase the rate of complete resection with negative circumferential margins, and (3) eradicate occult micrometastatic disease.

Nonrandomized Trials. Most trials have used 5-FU and cisplatin-based chemotherapy combined with radiation therapy[111,282–301] although more recent trials incorporate paclitaxel, docetaxel, oxaliplatin, or irinotecan in two- or three-drug combination regimens.[101,302–314]

Since the initial trials by Leichman et al.[315] and the Southwest Oncology Group (SWOG-8037),[282] results of many phase II single-institution or multicenter trials of preoperative chemoradiation have been published.[316] Most trials used cisplatin (75 to 100 mg/m^2) and 5-FU (1,000 mg/m^2 per day continuous infusion for 4 or 5 days) with concurrent radiotherapy followed by surgery in 4 to 8 weeks. In most series, the pathologic complete-response rate (based on total number treated) was approximately 25%. The highest pathologic complete-response rates have been reported in trials treating mainly squamous cancers, and as more modern series predominantly treat adenocarcinoma, pathologic complete-response rates are consistently lower. Intensive chemoradiation regimens using hyperfractionated radiotherapy were evaluated by Forastiere et al.,[284,285] Raoul et al.,[295] and Adelstein et al.[292] Some of these regimens achieved higher pathologically determined complete-response rates and survival rates, usually with corresponding increases in acute toxicity. However, no clear advantage to altered fractionation schedules has been shown. The total dose of radiotherapy with concurrent chemotherapy varied from 30 Gy in earlier series up to 60 Gy, followed by surgery. Pathologic complete-response rates are uniformly in the 15% to 20% range with lower doses of radiation,[282,286,297,298] whereas total doses exceeding 50 Gy are associated with increased toxicity and perioperative complications.[296] Doses of 44 to 50 Gy using standard fractionation and concurrent therapy with cisplatin plus 5-FU generally result in pathologic complete-response rates of 25% to 40%[111,284, 286,287,290,292,295,299] and acceptable toxicity with postoperative mortality rates well below 10%. As will be discussed later, the CROSS randomized trial of preoperative chemoradiation used 41.4 Gy and achieved a significant survival benefit with neoadjuvant therapy.[317]

Most trials use conventional fractionation and doses of radiotherapy (45.0 to 50.4 Gy) with concurrent chemotherapy. In addition to overall outcome, some investigators have sought to determine whether preoperative endoscopy with biopsy can accurately assess response to treatment and whether achievement of pathologically confirmed complete response after chemoradiation improves overall survival. Bates et al.[287] reported a 65% 3-year survival rate in patients who achieved a pathologic confirmed complete response, compared with a 25% survival rate in those who did not. In 106 of 262 (41%) patients who achieved a pathologic complete response with preoperative chemoradiation, the 5-year survival was 52% compared with 38% in partial responders ($p <0.001$) and 19% in nonresponders ($p <0.001$).[301]

In other trials with long-term follow-up, investigators observed 5-year survival rates of 60% to 67% and 27% to 32% for those with pathologic complete response and those with residual disease after induction therapy, respectively.[111,284] In addition, the fact that long-term survival was observed in approximately 30% of patients with a residual tumor in the resected specimen suggests that surgery is an important component following chemoradiation.

At present, no methods short of surgical resection can accurately determine which patients will be found to have no residual tumor in the resected esophageal specimen after chemoradiation. Bates et al.[287] noted a 41% false-negative rate with preoperative endoscopy and biopsy. Sarkaria et al.[318] reported the correlation of postchemoradiotherapy endoscopy findings and surgical pathologic findings in 156 patients with esophageal cancer. Although 76% had a biopsy-negative endoscopy after preoperative therapy, only 31% of these patients were found to be pathologic complete responders at subsequent surgery. Chedella et al.[319] reported the results of 284 patients who received preoperative chemoradiation at M.D. Anderson Cancer Center, and at 5 to 6 weeks posttreatment, underwent restaging with endoscopy, biopsy, and PET-CT scan. The 24% of patients who achieved a pathologic complete response (pCR) had a higher median survival compared to those who did not achieve a pCR (95 versus 55 months).[319] Of note, only 31% of patients who achieved a clinical complete response were found to have a pCR.

Yang et al.[320] made similar observations about the accuracy of posttherapy biopsy. Jones et al.[321] reported that CT scans had a sensitivity of 65%, a specificity of 33%, a positive predictive value of 58%, and a negative predictive value of 41% in evaluating pathologic response after preoperative chemoradiation in esophageal cancer patients. Many studies show that EUS performed after chemoradiation is also a poor predictor of complete response because of the inability to distinguish postirradiation fibrosis and inflammation from residual tumor. Reported staging accuracy is below 50%.[323–324]

To further pursue the selective surgical approach as a treatment modality, it will be critical to establish the definition of an adequate response. However, the ability to predict a pCR prior to surgery is variable. A multivariate analysis by Gaca and colleagues[325] reported that posttreatment nodal status ($p = 0.03$), but not the degree of primary tumor response, predicted disease-free survival. Fields et al.[326] reviewed 714 patients treated at Memorial Sloan Kettering Cancer Center (MSKCC) and reported that there was a significant improvement in 5-year survival in the 60 patients who achieved a pCR compared with the 549 who did not (55% versus 35%; $p = 0.036$).[326]

The value of FDG-PET scans for restaging after chemoradiation remains to be established. Several studies of esophageal cancer patients show that an early decrease in FDG uptake after chemotherapy can predict clinical response.[156,327,328] In addition, multiple studies have evaluated the ability of FDG-PET scans to predict a pCR following chemoradiation.[328–332] Flamen et al.[328] evaluated the predictive value of PET scans after chemoradiation in patients receiving preoperative treatment. The sensitivity and positive predictive value of PET scans for identifying a pathologically determined complete response were 67% and 50%, respectively. Both false-positive PET findings (residual FDG activity in an area of intense inflammatory activity on histopathologic analysis) and false-negative findings occurred at the primary tumor site. Vallbohmer et al.[329] treated 119 patients with preoperative chemoradiation (cisplatin, 5-FU, and 36 Gy) and reported a nonsignificant association between major responders and FDG-PET results ($p = 0.056$). However, there was no clear standardized uptake value threshold that predicted a response.

Possible reasons for discrepant findings include the inflammatory effect of chemoradiation as well as a lack of standardization of FDG-PET protocols and techniques and definitions of a pathologic response.

Few studies have reported a long-term follow-up to determine actual survival rates at 5 years. Rates range from 25% reported by Bedenne et al.[297] for a series of 96 patients with squamous cell esophageal cancer to as high as 39% reported by Meredith et al.[301]

Taken together, data from nonrandomized trials accumulated during nearly 3 decades suggest an approximate 5% to 10% improvement in survival compared with historical surgery controls. However, substantially greater improvement in survival is seen in patients who are downstaged to pathologically confirmed complete response or minimal residual disease.

Patterns of failure after chemoradiation and resection are influenced by histologic type, with a greater likelihood of local recurrence for patients with squamous cell carcinoma of the esophagus and predominantly distant recurrence for those with adenocarcinoma of the distal esophagus, GEJ, and cardia. In a literature review of trials of preoperative chemoradiation published between 1980 and 2000, Geh et al.[316] found that the overall risk of relapse was 46%, but that the majority of relapses, 80%, were at distant sites; local–regional recurrence alone constituted only 9% of treatment failures. These cumulative data correspond with individual reports from other major centers[111,287,292,294] and suggest that preoperative chemoradiation followed by surgery leads to better local–regional control than does surgery alone or chemoradiation without surgery.

Newer regimens employing various combinations of 5-FU, cisplatin or oxaliplatin, taxanes, and irinotecan with radiotherapy report pathologic complete-response rates similar to those for previous cisplatin and 5-FU plus radiotherapy preoperative regimens, and rates of survival are also similar.

Meluch et al.[306] reported mature trial results for a combination of carboplatin, 5-FU, and paclitaxel plus concurrent radiotherapy. Among a total of 123 patients, the pathologic complete-response rate was 38%, and after a median follow-up of 45 months, the 3-year survival rate was 41%. Grade 3 or 4 leukopenia (73% of patients), esophagitis (43%), and hospitalization (57%) suggest that this regimen added toxicity without providing incremental improvement in survival. Toxicity on trials of paclitaxel and cisplatin on a once-weekly schedule, with conventional dose fractionation of radiation therapy, have reported lesser degrees of esophagitis.[303,308,333] McCurdy et al.[334] from the M.D. Anderson Cancer Center reported that the addition of taxanes to chemoradiation increased both the FDG-PET scan–determined pulmonary metabolic response and the radiation pneumonitis response compared with non–taxane-containing regimens. Weekly carboplatin combined with weekly paclitaxel and concurrent radiotherapy also appeared to have a favorable toxicity profile in a recent phase II trial treating 54 patients with adenocarcinoma and squamous cell carcinoma of the esophagus, and this regimen formed the basis of the recent Dutch CROSS Trial, which will be discussed.[310,317] The rate of pathologic complete response was 25%. Rates of grade 3 and 4 neutropenia (15%) and esophagitis (8%) were relatively low, but were in agreement with other trials employing a weekly paclitaxel and platinum drug chemotherapy regimen.

Swisher et al.,[308] Ajani et al.,[309] Bains et al.,[307] Ilson et al.,[101] and Rivera et al.[314] have published pilot experiences in the administration of induction chemotherapy before chemoradiotherapy and then surgery as a strategy to increase pathologically determined complete-response rate and to reduce distant failure. Some trials of induction chemotherapy have noted significant relief of patients' dysphagia and the rare need to place feeding tubes for nutritional support in patients.[101,307] The RTOG-0113 performed a phase II randomized trial comparing paclitaxel and 5-FU to paclitaxel and cisplatin plus radiation therapy.[312] Both arms were associated with significant toxicity, and the study did not meet its 1-year survival end point.

In summary, some of these newer regimens appear to be more toxic than cisplatin and 5-FU plus radiotherapy, whereas others suggest a potentially more favorable toxicity profile; the pathologic complete-response rates and survival estimates show no consistent benefit, but longer follow-up is needed. The interpretation of survival rates from these studies must be done cautiously, given the likelihood of stage migration due to the incorporation of EUS and PET scans into routine staging evaluation. Roof et al.[300] reported a single-institution experience of 177 patients treated with either cisplatin, 5-FU, or paclitaxel in combination with cisplatin, 5-FU, and radiation therapy as preoperative treatment in esophageal cancer. The 3-year overall survival was similar for the 5-FU/cisplatin–treated patients (39%) compared with those receiving paclitaxel in combination with 5-FU/cisplatin (42%). Pathologic complete-response rates were also comparable for two-drug (42%) compared with three-drug therapy (37%). In two sequential trials from Urba et al.[335,336] that evaluated two-drug paclitaxel cisplatin therapy plus radiation in one trial, and three-drug 5-FU, cisplatin, and paclitaxel plus radiation in another trial, there was also no difference in pathologic complete-response rates (17% to 19%). These rates of pathologic complete response were significantly lower than other trials reporting pathologic complete-response rates of 37% to 38% for three-drug therapy.[300]

The Eastern Cooperative Oncology Group (ECOG) reported response and survival[337] outcomes in a randomized phase II trial testing two of these combinations (E1201), limited to patients with resectable adenocarcinoma of the distal esophagus, GEJ, and cardia. The two preoperative treatments tested were (1) paclitaxel (50 mg/m^2, 1-hour infusion) followed by cisplatin (30 mg/m^2) on days 1, 8, 15, 22, 29, and concurrent radiotherapy (45 Gy); and (2) cisplatin (30 mg/m^2) followed by irinotecan (65 mg/m^2) on days 1, 8, 22, 29, and concurrent radiotherapy (45 Gy). Patients in each arm proceeded to esophagectomy followed by three cycles of adjuvant paclitaxel and cisplatin (arm 1) or cisplatin and irinotecan (arm 2). Staging with esophageal EUS was an eligibility requirement. A preliminary report indicated comparable rates of pathologic complete response for the two regimens of 15% to 16%, with the lower than expected pathologic complete-response rate likely partly due to the exclusive treatment of adenocarcinoma on this trial.[338] The median survival on the paclitaxel arm was 20.9 months, and 34.9 months on the irinotecan arm (difference nonsignificant). Although the results are comparable to other modern phase II trials in esophageal adenocarcinoma, neither regimen appeared superior to more conventional 5-FU and cisplatin-based therapy.

Randomized Trials. Randomized trials comparing preoperative chemoradiation with surgery alone in patients with clinically resectable disease are listed in Table 37.7.[107,114,240,317,339–344] The series of Le Prise et al.[345] is not included because patients received sequential rather than concurrent chemotherapy and radiotherapy. Most trials combined cisplatin and 5-FU[339–341] or single-agent cisplatin[240] with concurrent radiotherapy.

The Bosset et al.[240] trial was limited to patients with stage I or II squamous cell carcinoma based on a previously defined CT scan staging system, whereas the trials of Urba et al.,[107] Burmeister et al.,[341] Tepper et al.,[342] and van Hagen et al.[317] treated adenocarcinoma and squamous cell carcinoma, and the trial of Walsh et al.[339,340] was designed for locally advanced, resectable adenocarcinoma. A significant difference in the median and 3-year survival rates was observed in the Walsh, Tepper, and Van Hagen et al. trials. It is noteworthy that the pathologically determined complete-response rate was consistent for all studies, 25% to 28%, with the exception of the Burmeister et al. trial, which indicated a statistically significant lower pathologic complete-response rate for adenocarcinoma (9%) compared to squamous cell carcinoma (27%). Van Hagen et al. reported a pathologic complete response rate of 24% for adenocarcinoma and 49% for squamous cell carcinoma. Comparable rates of 3-year survival for patients in each of the investigational treatment groups (30% to 40%) was also observed. Higher 5-year survival rates, however, were reported on the Tepper et al. trial (39%) and the Van Hagen et al. trial (47%).

Urba et al.[107] at the University of Michigan randomly assigned 100 patients (75 with adenocarcinoma, 25 with squamous cell

---

TABLE 37.7

Results of Preoperative Chemoradiation for Esophageal Cancer: Randomized Trials

Study (Ref.)	No. of Patients (n)	Histology	Chemotherapy	RT (Gy)	R0 Resection (%)	Pathologic Complete Response (%)	Median Survival (months)	Overall Survival 3-, and 5-Year Overall Survival (%)
Bosset et al.[240]	282	S	C + RT + surgery	37	78	26	19	5 yr: 26
			Surgery		68		19	5 yr: 26
Walsh et al.[339]	113	A	CF + RT + surgery	40	NS	25	16	3 yr: 32
					NS	—	11	3 yr: 6
Urba et al.[107]	100	S/A	CF + RT + surgery	45	90	28	18	3 yr: 30
			Surgery		90	—	17	3 yr: 16
Burmeister et al.[341]	256	S/A	CF + RT + Surgery	35	80	9 (A) 27 (S)	22	NS
			Surgery	44	59	—	19	NS
Tepper et al.[342]	56	S/A	CF + RT + surgery	50.4	NS	40	54	5 yr: 39
			Surgery		NS	—	22	5 yr: 16
Van Hagen et al.[317]	366	S/A	CaP + RT + surgery	41.4	92	24 (A) 49 (S)	49	3 yr: 58 5 yr: 47
			Surgery		69	—	24	3 yr: 50 5 yr: 34
Lee et al.[343]	102	S	CF + RT + surgery		NS	49	28	3 yr: 46
			Surgery		NS	—	27	3 yr: 46

S, squamous cell carcinoma; C, cisplatin; RT, radiation therapy; A, adenocarcinoma; NS, not stated; Ca, carboplatin; P, paclitaxel.

carcinoma) to receive (1) preoperative cisplatin (20 mg/m² on days 1 to 5 and 17 to 21), vinblastine (1 mg/m² on days 1 to 4 and 17 to 20), 5-FU (300 mg/m² per 24 hours on days 1 to 21), and concurrent radiotherapy (1.5 Gy twice a day to 45 Gy), followed on day 42 by a transhiatal esophagectomy, or (2) immediate surgery. A survival analysis after a median follow-up of 8.2 years for surviving patients revealed a nonsignificant improvement favoring preoperative chemoradiation (3-year survival, 30% versus 16%; $p = 0.15$). A significant decrease in local–regional recurrence as a component of first failure was observed (19% recurrence rate for the combined treatment group versus 42% for the group undergoing immediate surgery; $p = 0.02$). However, there was no difference in the rates of distant metastases, 60% and 65%, respectively. Although overall survival rates were not significantly different, there was a 31% lower risk of death, after adjustment for other prognostic factors, for patients randomly assigned to receive trimodal therapy, which suggests a possible benefit and the need for a trial adequately powered to detect a smaller survival difference. Consistent with phase II trial data, patients who achieved a pathologically confirmed complete response had better survival outcomes, with a median survival time of 50 months and 3-year survival rate of 64%, compared to those with residual disease in the resected specimen, who had a median survival time of 12 months and a 3-year survival rate of 19%. The low statistical power of this trial may have failed to detect a potential modest survival benefit for chemoradiation compared to surgery alone.

In their series, Walsh et al.[339] reported a significant survival advantage for patients receiving preoperative chemoradiation. A total of 113 patients with adenocarcinoma of the esophagus, GEJ, and cardia were randomly assigned to receive (1) two cycles (weeks 1 and 6) of 5-FU (15 mg/kg per 24 hours on days 1 to 5), cisplatin (75 mg/m² on day 7), plus concurrent radiotherapy (2.67 Gy per day to 40 Gy) followed by esophagectomy; or (2) immediate surgery alone. Chemoradiation was well tolerated. The incidence of acute toxicity of grade 3 or higher was 15%. The operative mortality was 9% in the multimodality treatment arm compared with 4% in the surgery control arm. After a median follow-up of surviving patients of 18 months, a significant improvement in both median survival time (16 months versus 11 months; $p = 0.01$) and 3-year survival rate (32% versus 6%; $p = 0.01$) was observed in patients who received preoperative therapy compared with those treated with surgery alone. A major criticism of this trial was the low 3-year survival rate (6%) in the surgical control arm. This probably reflects a patient population with more advanced disease than in those enrolled in the other two trials. CT scan staging was not required. More than 80% of patients had lymph node metastases.[340]

A third randomized trial of preoperative chemoradiation was reported by Bosset et al.[240] of the EORTC. A total of 282 patients with clinically resectable (early stage I and II) squamous cell carcinoma were randomly assigned to undergo either preoperative chemoradiation or surgery alone. The preoperative regimen consisted of five daily fractions of 3.7 Gy each followed by a 2-week rest and another 3.7 Gy for 5 days. Chemotherapy was limited to cisplatin, 80 mg/m², 0 to 2 days before starting each 5 days of radiotherapy. Rates of curative resection were significantly higher in patients undergoing preoperative chemoradiation (81%) compared with immediate surgery (69%). After a median follow-up of 55 months, patients who received preoperative chemoradiation had a significantly better 3-year disease-free survival rate (40% versus 28%) and local disease-free survival (relative risk [RR], 0.6), yet had no improvement in median survival time (19 months) or overall 3-year survival (36%) compared with patients treated with surgery alone. However, this chemoradiation regimen was unconventional in design; not only was the radiation split course and delivered with unusually high doses per fraction, but the doses of chemotherapy would not be considered adequate for systemic therapy. The threefold higher postoperative mortality in the com-

bined modality arm (12%) compared with the surgery-alone arm (4%) may have undercut any potential overall survival benefit for chemoradiation.

The trial reported by Burmeister et al.[341] treated 256 patients with adenocarcinoma and squamous cell carcinoma with either surgery alone, or preoperative cisplatin, 5-FU, and radiation followed by surgery. The combined modality arm received one cycle of 5-FU dosed at 800 mg/m² per day during a 4-day continuous infusion in combination with cisplatin 80 mg/m² on day 1, plus concurrent radiotherapy (2.33 Gy per day to 35 Gy) followed by esophagectomy. Chemoradiation was well tolerated, with the most common toxicities grade 3 or 4 esophagitis (16%) or nausea and vomiting (5%). There was no difference in surgical complications in either treatment group, with an overall operative mortality of 5%. After a median follow-up of 65 months, no significant difference was seen in either median overall survival time (22 months versus 19 months with surgery alone) or 3-year survival rate. The chemoradiation group had a higher rate or curative resection (80%) compared with the surgery-alone arm (59%). Pathologic complete responses were significantly less common in adenocarcinoma (9%) compared with squamous cell carcinoma (27%). A univariate analysis indicated that patients with squamous cell cancer had significantly better progression-free and overall survival when treated with preoperative chemoradiation. The low rate of pathologic complete responses in patients with adenocarcinoma on this trial raises concern about the adequacy of chemotherapy delivered (one cycle) during radiotherapy.

A similar trial was reported by Lee et al.[343] from Korea. A total of 102 patients with squamous cell cancer were randomized to surgery alone versus preoperative therapy with 45.6 Gy (1.2 Gy twice a day) plus 5-FU/cisplatin. There was no difference in median survival (28 months versus 27 months).

The sixth randomized trial by Tepper et al.[342] reported the results of an Intergroup trial led by the Cancer and Leukemia Group B (CALGB-9781), in which patients were randomly assigned to receive either (1) immediate surgery or (2) two cycles of cisplatin, 5-FU, and concurrent radiotherapy (total dose, 50.4 Gy) followed by surgery. This trial, activated in July 1998 and projected to enroll 475 patients, was terminated early because of failure to meet accrual targets. However, follow-up was available in 56 patients ultimately randomized and treated on protocol. With a median follow-up of 6 years, 5-year survival was significantly improved with the addition of preoperative chemoradiation (39% versus 16%; $p = 0.005$). Interpretation of this trial is confounded by the small number of patients treated.

The most contemporary trial recently reported by Van Hagen et al., the CROSS Trial,[317] has for many practitioners established a new standard or care for preoperative chemoradiotherapy. This study randomized 366 patients with squamous cell carcinoma or adenocarcinoma of the esophagus or GEJ to treatment with (1) preoperative carboplatin at an area under the curve of 2 mg/mL per minute and paclitaxel 50 mg/m² once weekly for 5 weeks, and concurrent radiotherapy (1.8 Gy daily to 41.4 Gy in 23 fractions, followed by transthoracic esophagectomy or transhiatal esophagectomy for GEJ cancers, or (2) immediate surgery. Unlike earlier trials, this more modern trial staged all patients by endoscopic ultrasound and CT scan, and patients were required to have either node-positive or T2-3Nany disease. The majority of patients treated had adenocarcinoma (75%), and most tumors involved the distal third of the esophagus (58%). The majority of patients were node positive (65%), and slightly more patients on the chemoradiotherapy arm had T3 tumors (84%) compared to the surgery-alone arm (78%). At a median follow-up of 45 months, the trial showed a significant survival benefit (Fig 37.13) for chemoradiotherapy added to surgery, with a median survival increased from 24 to 49 months (HR, 0.0657; $p = 0.003$), and improvement in 2- and 5-year overall survival (67% and 47% versus 50% and 34%; HR, 0.665). The rate of R0 resection was significantly improved on the chemoradiotherapy arm (95% compared

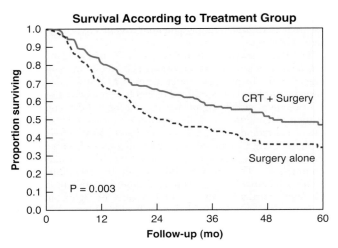

Figure 37.13 Overall survival CROSS trial comparing patients randomized to preoperative chemoradiotherapy (CRT + surgery) versus surgery alone.

to 69%; $p < 0.001$). Pathologic complete responses were seen in 24% of adenocarcinomas and 49% of squamous cancers. Survival benefits were significant for both histologies, but with an even greater benefit for squamous cancers (HR, 0.453) compared to adenocarcinomas (HR, 0.741). Therapy was well tolerated with grade 3 or 4 hematologic toxicity seen in 7% patients, and grade 3 or 4 nonhematologic toxicity seen in less than 13%. There was no difference in either operative morbidity or mortality, and mortality was below 4% in each arm, which is considered consistent and appropriate with modern day surgical outcomes in high-volume centers. Many investigators feel that this well-conducted chemoradiotherapy trial using a well-tolerated, relatively easy to administer therapeutic regimen established a new standard of care for squamous cell carcinomas and adenocarcinomas of the distal esophagus or GEJ.

Some additional insight may be obtained from a small trial reported by Stahl et al.,[344] a multicenter phase III trial directly comparing preoperative chemotherapy to combined chemoradiotherapy followed by surgery in patients with GEJ adenocarcinoma. The trial did not meet accrual goals and randomized only 119 eligible patients with Siewert I to III GEJ adenocarcinoma. The strength of the trial was the rigorous pretherapy staging, including EUS and laparoscopy, and the balance in treatment arms by clinical stage. Patients were assigned to (1) 2.5 cycles of a 6-week schedule of weekly 5-FU 2 g/m², 24-hour infusion and leucovorin 500 mg/m², 2-hour infusion plus biweekly cisplatin 50 mg/m², or (2) two cycles of the same regimen, followed by 3 weeks of radiotherapy given in 15 fractions at a dose of 2 Gy combined with cisplatin 50 mg/m² on day 1 and 8 and etoposide 80 mg/m² on days 3 to 5. The primary end point was 3-year overall survival. Comparable numbers of patients had an R0 resection after chemotherapy (69.5%) compared to chemoradiotherapy (72%). More patients on the chemoradiotherapy arm achieved a pathologic complete response (15.6%) compared to the chemotherapy arm (2.0%), and more patients were node negative (64.4% compared to 36.7%, respectively). Three-year survival trended superior in the chemoradiotherapy group (47.4%) compared to the chemotherapy group (27.7%; $p = 0.07$), and freedom from local tumor progression also favored the chemoradiotherapy group (76.5% versus 59%; $p = 0.06$). More in-hospital deaths occurred in the chemoradiotherapy arm (10.2% versus 3.8%; not statistically significant). The authors concluded that preoperative chemoradiotherapy could be considered a standard of care based on the favorable comparison to preoperative chemotherapy alone.

The accumulated experience from phase II and III trials indicates the following concerning chemoradiation using cisplatin and infusional 5-FU–based therapy followed by an esophagectomy:

- In approximately two-thirds of patients, the disease is downstaged.
- A survival advantage exists for patients experiencing downstaging to pathologically confirmed complete response or minimal residual disease status.
- Surgery appears to be an important component of treatment to eliminate persistent disease after chemoradiation, especially for adenocarcinoma. Of this group, 20% to 30% will be long-term survivors. The higher rates of pathologic complete response for squamous cancers make an argument for primary chemoradiotherapy without surgery, and this issue will be reviewed in the Radiation Therapy section.
- Local–regional control is improved, whereas distant failure is frequent and is the major cause of death.
- Rates of curative resection may be improved with preoperative chemoradiation.

Controversy continues about the optimal management of adenocarcinoma of the distal esophagus or GEJ, in particular the relative merits of preoperative chemotherapy versus combined chemoradiotherapy followed by surgery. Two ongoing randomized trials may shed light on this debate once completed. One trial, the CRITICS trial being run in the Netherlands and Sweden (NCT00407186), assigns patients with adenocarcinoma of the distal esophagus, GEJ, and stomach to all receive pre- and postoperative chemotherapy in addition to surgery; patients are randomized postoperatively to continue to receive either chemotherapy alone, or to chemotherapy combined with postoperative radiotherapy. Another trial, TOPGEAR (NCT01924819), being run by the Australasian Gasto-Intestinal Trials Group (AGITG) will treat patients with esophageal, GEJ, or gastric cancers with perioperative chemotherapy, with patients randomized to receive combined radiation therapy with preoperative chemotherapy or to preoperative chemotherapy alone.

Meta-analyses lend support to the inclusion of chemotherapy and radiation therapy as part of surgical management. Two studies evaluated in a combined analysis randomized trials predominantly of preoperative chemotherapy[346] and preoperative chemotherapy and radiation therapy compared to surgery alone.[347] These studies pooled the results of 11 to 25 randomized trials treating between 2,300 and nearly 4,200 patients. Preoperative chemotherapy improved 2-year survival by 5.1% to 6.3% for preoperative chemotherapy alone, and preoperative combined chemoradiation improved 2-year survival by 8.7%. Because of the toxicity and ongoing controversy about the benefit associated with preoperative combined chemoradiation, the priority should be given to enrolling patients in clinical trials.

Targeted Agents

Limited studies have evaluated the combination of a targeted agent with either definitive, nonoperative chemoradiotherapy, or preoperative chemoradiotherapy. Two pilot trials combining the vascular endothelial growth factor (VEGF) ligand-targeted agent, bevacizumab, added to chemoradiotherapy failed to improve outcome compared to historical controls.[313,348] The EGFR-targeted agent cetuximab was combined with definitive chemoradiotherapy in two recently reported trials. First is the SCOPE-1 trial where 258 patients with stages I through III cancer (25% adenocarcinoma) were randomized to 50 Gy/capecitabine/cisplatin ± cetuximab without planned surgery.[349] The trial was stopped early since it met its futility rules. Patient who received cetuximab had inferior 2-year survival (41% versus 56%) and higher nonheme grade 3+ acute toxicity (79% versus 63%). The second is the recently completed RTOG 0436 trial in which patients with nonoperable esophageal cancer were randomized to 50.4

Gy/paclitaxel ± cetuximab, reported only in abstract form.[350] On this nonoperative trial, of the 328 patients, the majority had adenocarcinoma. There was no difference in outcome with the addition of cetuximab to chemoradiotherapy, with no increase in rates on endoscopic clinical complete response, and no differences in overall survival and no impact on either adenocarcinoma of squamous cell carcinoma histology. These negative results add to the accumulating literature, also discussed in the section on metastatic disease, that currently available EGFR-targeted therapies are ineffective in esophageal cancer. A phase I/II trial combining the HER2-targeted agent trastuzumab with chemoradiotherapy[351] in esophageal cancer led to a randomized phase III trial in esophageal adenocarcinoma being conducted by RTOG (NCT01196390). Patients with esophageal or GEJ adenocarcinoma whose tumors test HER2 positive are randomized to chemoradiotherapy with weekly carboplatin AUCS 2 and paclitaxel 50 mg/m^2 for six doses combined with 50.4 Gy of radiotherapy followed by surgery, with or without the addition of trastuzumab during chemoradiotherapy and as a surgical adjuvant therapy for 1 year after surgery. As will be reviewed in the section covering advanced disease, with the exception of trastuzumab, suitable targets as well as active targeted agents remain to be established in the combined modality treatment of esophageal cancer.

Postoperative Chemotherapy. Administering chemotherapy after surgery to patients who have already received chemotherapy or chemoradiation preoperatively has not been easily achieved in phase II[257,258,299] and phase III trials.[105,264] This is exemplified by the INT-0113 trial, in which only 38% of patients who were candidates for adjuvant cisplatin and 5-FU therapy received the two planned courses.[105]

In Japan, surgery includes the removal of the primary lesion plus extended dissection of lymph nodes in the mediastinum, neck, and abdomen. The Japanese Oncology Group has evaluated postoperative chemotherapy in a series of randomized trials.[352–355] One study of 205 patients who had undergone resection compared observation with two courses of adjuvant cisplatin and vindesine.[354] Median follow-up was 59 months, and the 5-year survival rate was 45% in the control arm and 48% in the adjuvant treatment arm, which indicated no survival benefit from this chemotherapy regimen.

A second trial of adjuvant chemotherapy in 242 patients had the same study design, except that the chemotherapy was cisplatin and 5-FU administered for two courses after curative resection.[353,355] At a median follow-up of 40.4 months, no differences were observed in the 5-year survival estimates (51% versus 61% for adjuvant chemotherapy; $p = 0.3$). The estimated 5-year disease-free survival rate was improved with chemotherapy (58% for the chemotherapy versus 46% for observation; $p = 0.05$). Disease-free survival for node-negative patients was 77% in the surgery-alone group versus 82% in the adjuvant treatment group ($p = 0.3$), and for node-positive patients 35% in the surgery-alone group versus 53% in the adjuvant treatment group ($p = 0.06$). These data suggest that adjuvant chemotherapy may benefit node-positive patients, but this was an unplanned subset analysis on this trial. The ECOG completed a phase II trial (E8296) to evaluate adjuvant therapy consisting of cisplatin (75 mg/m^2) and paclitaxel (175 mg/m^2 during 3 hours) every 3 weeks for four courses in 55 patients with completely resected, T3, or node-positive adenocarcinoma of the esophagus, GEJ, or cardia.[356] The majority (89%) had lymph node involvement. The majority of these (84%) were able to complete all four cycles of chemotherapy. The 2-year survival rate was 60%, which compared favorably with results for contemporary historical controls.[105]

In summary, the available data for postoperative adjuvant chemotherapy suggest a possible prolongation of survival for patients who have had a potentially curative (R0) resection and have lymph node–positive (N1) disease. There are no data to indicate or suggest that the administration of postoperative adjuvant chemotherapy will prolong survival for patients who have undergone a curative resection and have negative nodes (N0). Patients who have positive margins of resection should be considered for postoperative radiation. Those who have had R0 resections but have regional nodal metastases (stages IIB and III) should be enrolled in clinical trials to evaluate adjuvant therapies.

Postoperative Radiation Therapy. Several reports of nonrandomized trials have suggested that postoperative radiation therapy may be effective after esophagectomy. Yamamoto et al.[357] reported a 94% 2-year local control rate in node-positive patients. For patients who underwent a three-field dissection, Hosokawa et al.[358] added intraoperative radiation followed by 45 Gy postoperatively. The 5-year survival rate was 34%.

Two randomized trials were limited to patients treated in the adjuvant setting. Teniere et al.[273] reported the results for 221 patients with squamous cell carcinoma randomly assigned to receive either surgery alone or postoperative radiation therapy (45 to 55 Gy at 1.8 Gy per fraction). Postoperative radiation therapy was found to have no significant impact on survival. In the series of Fok et al.,[359] patients with both squamous cell carcinomas and adenocarcinomas receiving either curative or palliative resections were evaluated; although the total dose of radiation therapy was conventional, the dose per fraction (3.5 Gy) was unconventional. No significant decrease in local failure or distant failure or improvement in the median survival time was achieved with the addition of postoperative radiation therapy.

Postoperative Chemoradiation. The only randomized trial of postoperative chemoradiation is the Intergroup trial INT-0116.[360] Although the goal of this trial was to examine the role of postoperative adjuvant chemoradiation in gastric cancer, 20% of patients had adenocarcinoma of the GEJ. Eligible patients included those with stage IB, II, IIIA, IIIB, or IV nonmetastatic adenocarcinoma of the stomach or GEJ after curative resection. Patients were randomly assigned to receive either observation alone or postoperative chemoradiation consisting of four monthly cycles of bolus 5-FU and leucovorin plus 45 Gy concurrent radiation with cycle two. A total of 603 patients were registered. Pretreatment characteristics were similar in both arms, and most patients had locally advanced disease. Approximately two-thirds of the patients had pT3 or pT4 tumors and approximately 85% had positive local–regional nodes.

Patients randomly assigned to receive postoperative chemoradiation had a significant decrease in local failure as the first site of failure (19% versus 29%) and an increase in median survival (36 months versus 27 months), 3-year relapse-free survival (48% versus 31%), and overall survival (50% versus 41%; $p = 0.005$). Although 17% of patients could not complete all therapy as planned, there was only one treatment-related death. With a median follow-up of 10 years, the improvement in survival with postoperative chemoradiation remains statistically significant.[360] An analysis of the impact of HER2 status in the INT-0116 trial revealed that HER2-negative patients had a survival benefit from chemoradiation whereas patients who underwent surgery only did not.[361]

The other role for postoperative radiation therapy is in cases of positive surgical margins. Based on the RTOG-85-01 trial, patients selected for treatment with postoperative radiation should receive chemoradiation.[280,362,363]

Definitive Chemoradiation

Although definitive chemoradiation is a treatment option for patients with localized resectable esophageal carcinoma, especially those with cervical esophageal squamous cell carcinoma or those not considered ideal resection candidates, this therapeutic approach is discussed in detail in Chemoradiation in the next section.

Treatment of Locally Advanced Disease

Radiation Therapy

The 1996 to 1999 patterns of care study examined 414 patients who received radiation therapy as part of definitive or adjuvant management at 59 institutions.[364] Overall, 51% had adenocarcinoma and 49% had squamous cell carcinoma. With a median follow-up of 8 months, a multivariate analysis revealed that patients who received chemoradiation followed by surgery had a significant decrease in local–regional recurrence (HR, 0.40; p <0.0001) and survival (HR, 0.32; p = 0.001) compared with those who did not undergo surgery. A similar significant decrease in local–regional recurrence (HR, 1.36; p = 0.01) and survival (HR, 1.32; p <0.03) was seen in those patients who received their care at large radiation oncology centers (treating 500 or more new cancer patients per year) compared with small centers (treating fewer than 500 new cancer patients per year). In a similar patterns of care study of 767 patients treated in Japan from 1998 to 2001, 220 (29%) received preoperative or postoperative radiation, or both, with or without chemotherapy.[365]

The effect of histologic type (adenocarcinoma versus squamous cell carcinoma) is unclear. Most series suggest that squamous cell cancers have a higher response rate compared with adenocarcinomas; however, no clear difference in outcome was found. The National Cancer Institute Intergroup has randomized trials that stratify patients by lesion histologic type. Until these data are available, the impact of histologic type cannot be adequately assessed, and it is reasonable to treat both types of lesions in a similar fashion.

Primary Nonsurgical Therapy. Primary therapy for esophageal cancer is either surgical or nonsurgical. The patient population selected for treatment with each modality is usually different. For several reasons, this results in a selection bias against nonsurgical therapy. Patients with unfavorable prognostic features are more commonly selected for treatment with nonsurgical therapy. These features include medical contraindications and primary unresectable or actual metastatic disease. Surgical series report results based on pathologic stage, whereas nonsurgical series report results based on clinical stage. Pathologic staging has the advantage of excluding some patients with metastatic disease not identified during clinical staging. Because some patients treated without surgery are approached in a palliative rather than a curative fashion, the intensity of chemotherapy and the doses and techniques of radiation therapy used may be suboptimal.

The difficulty of accurately staging esophageal cancer preoperatively is discussed in Diagnostic Studies and Pretreatment Staging, earlier in this chapter. The efficacy of FDG-PET scans as a complement to CT scans and EUS must be emphasized. Undetected metastatic disease was identified by PET scans in 15% of patients in the series by Flamen et al.[328] and in 20% of patients in the series by Downey et al.[327]

Radiation Therapy Alone. Many series have reported results of external-beam radiation therapy alone. Most include patients with unfavorable features such as clinical T4 disease and multiple positive lymph nodes. For example, in the series of De-Ren,[366] 184 of the 678 patients had stage IV disease. Overall, the 5-year survival rate for patients treated with conventional doses of radiation therapy alone is 0% to 10%.[362,366,367] The use of radiation therapy as a potentially curative modality requires doses of at least 50 Gy at 1.8 to 2.0 Gy per fraction. Shi et al.[368] reported a 33% 5-year survival rate with the use of late-course accelerated fractionation to a total dose of 68.4 Gy. However, in the radiation-therapy–alone arm of the RTOG-85-01 trial in which patients received 64 Gy at 2 Gy per day with modern techniques, all patients were dead of their disease by 3 years.[280,363]

Collectively, these data indicate that radiation therapy alone should be reserved for palliation or for patients who are medically unable to receive chemotherapy. As is discussed in the following section, the results of chemoradiation are more favorable, and it remains the standard of care.

Definitive Chemoradiation

Conventional Approaches

Comparison of Definitive Chemoradiation and Surgery. There are many single-arm, nonrandomized trials of chemoradiation alone, and they have included patients with disease at a variety of stages.[335–338] Few series examine patients with T1 or T2 disease.[369,370] In the series reported by Coia et al.,[369] patients received 5-FU and mitomycin C concurrently with 60 Gy of radiation therapy. When results for clinical stage I and II disease are combined, the local failure rate was 25%, the 5-year actuarial local relapse-free survival was 70%, and the 5-year actuarial survival was 30%.

Six randomized trials compared radiation therapy alone with chemoradiation.[114,263,280,371–375] Of these six trials, five used suboptimal doses of radiation and three used inadequate doses of systemic chemotherapy, and some studies used sequential chemotherapy and radiotherapy rather than concurrent therapy. For example, in the series of Araujo et al.,[375] patients received only one cycle of 5-FU, mitomycin C, and bleomycin. The EORTC trial used subcutaneous methotrexate.[371] In the Scandinavian trial reported by Nygaard et al.,[263] patients received low doses of chemotherapy (cisplatin, 20 mg/m^2, and bleomycin, 10 mg/m^2, for a maximum of two cycles). An analysis of pooled data from these trials reported a significant local control and survival benefit at 1 year for chemoradiation compared with radiation therapy alone.[376] Chemoradiation was associated with a significant increase in adverse effects, including life-threatening toxicities.

In the ECOG EST-1282 trial,[374] patients who received chemoradiation had a significantly increased median survival compared with those who received radiation alone (15 months versus 9 months; p = 0.04) but experienced no improvement in 5-year survival (9% versus 7%). However, this was not a pure nonsurgical trial because approximately 50% of patients in each arm underwent surgery after receiving 40 Gy of radiation. Furthermore, this decision depended on the individual investigator's preference. The operative mortality was 17%. Finally, the Pretoria trial reported by Slabber et al.,[373] which was limited to a total of 70 patients with T3 squamous cell cancers, used a low-dose (40 Gy) split-course radiation schedule.

The only trial that was designed to deliver adequate doses of systemic chemotherapy with concurrent radiation therapy was the RTOG-85-01 trial reported by Herskovic et al.,[280] and updated by Al-Sarraf et al.[372] This Intergroup trial primarily included patients with squamous cell carcinoma. Patients received four cycles of 5-FU (1,000 mg/m^2 per 24 hour × 4 days) and cisplatin (75 mg/m^2 on day 1). Radiation therapy (50 Gy at 2 Gy per day) was given concurrently with day 1 of chemotherapy. Curiously, cycles three and four of chemotherapy were delivered every 3 weeks (weeks 8 and 11) rather than every 4 weeks (weeks 9 and 13). This intensification may explain, in part, why only 50% of the patients finished all four cycles of the chemotherapy. The control arm was given radiation therapy alone, albeit at a higher dose (64 Gy) than the chemoradiation arm.

Patients who received chemoradiation had a significant improvement in median survival (14 months versus 9 months) and 5-year survival (27% versus 0%; p <0.0001).[344] There was a clear plateau in the survival curve. Minimum follow-up was 5 years, and the 8-year survival was 22%.[114,375] The histologic type did not significantly influence the results: 21% of patients with squamous cell carcinomas (n = 107) were alive at 5 years compared with 13% of patients with adenocarcinoma (n = 23) (p was not significant). Although African Americans had larger primary tumors, all of which were squamous cell cancers, there was no difference in their survival compared with that of Caucasians.[377] The incidence of local failure as the first site of failure (defined as local persistence or recurrence) was also decreased in the chemoradiation arm (47% versus 65%). The protocol was closed early because of the positive results; however, after this early closure, an additional 69 eligible patients were treated with the same chemoradiation regimen. In this nonrandomized combined modality group, the 5-year survival was 14% and local failure was 52%.

Chemoradiation not only improves the results compared with radiation alone but also is associated with a higher incidence of toxicity. In the 1997 report of the RTOG-85-01 trial, patients who received chemoradiation had a higher incidence of acute grade 3 toxicity (44% versus 25%) and acute grade 4 toxicity (20% versus 3%) compared with those who received radiation therapy alone. Including the one treatment-related death (2%), the incidence of total acute grade 3+ toxicity was 66%.[372] The 1999 report examined late toxicity. The incidence of late grade 3+ toxicity was similar in the chemoradiation arm and in the radiation-alone arm (29% versus 23%).[114] However, grade 4+ toxicity remained higher in the combined modality arm (10% versus 2%). Interestingly, the nonrandomized chemoradiation group experienced a similar incidence of late grade 3+ toxicity (28%) but a lower incidence of grade 4 toxicity (4%), and there were no treatment-related deaths.

Based on the positive results from the RTOG-85-01 trial, the conventional nonsurgical treatment for esophageal carcinoma is chemoradiation. Notwithstanding, the local failure rate in the RTOG-85-01 chemoradiation arm was 45%, and there is room for improvement. Therefore, new approaches, such as intensification of chemoradiation and escalation of the radiation dose, have been developed in an attempt to help improve these results.

Randomized Trials. Although there are a number of trials comparing preoperative chemoradiation with surgery alone, there are only two trials that directly compare nonoperative treatment with surgery. One randomized trial compared surgery with radiation alone[378] and one compared surgery with chemoradiation.[379] Both series have small numbers of patients, limited follow-up, and neither report a difference in survival.

Nonrandomized Trials. The positive results of RTOG-85-01, demonstrating a 27% 5-year survival rate for patients treated with definitive chemoradiation compared with no 5-year survival after treatment with radiotherapy alone, is a major advance. This treatment option has influenced the selection of patients for nonsurgical management because it provides an alternative for restoring swallowing function in patients with locally advanced disease for whom resection would likely be palliative.

For patients with earlier-stage disease that appears resectable, definitive chemoradiation may also be appropriate treatment; however, prospective trials comparing this approach with surgery, stratified by stage, have not been performed. Nonetheless, nonrandomized comparisons of contemporary series suggest that the nonsurgical approach offers a survival rate that is the same or better than that achievable with surgery alone. For example, the median survival time and 5-year survival rate were 14 months and 27%, respectively, in the chemoradiation arm of RTOG-85-01, and 20 months and 20%, respectively, in INT-0122.[380] In comparison, the median survival in the surgical control arm of the Dutch trial reported by Kok et al.[269] was 11 months, and the median survival time and 5-year survival rate in the surgical control arm of INT-0113 were 16 months and 20%, respectively. Likewise, the local failure rates were similar. The incidence of local failure (local recurrence plus local persistence of disease) as the first site of failure was 45% in RTOG-85-01 and 39% in INT-0122. If all patients, including patients failing to undergo surgery or patients having an R2 resection are included, the local failure as the first site of failure was 61% on the surgical trial INT-0113, which is actually higher than the 45% reported on RTOG-85-01. The treatment-related mortality rates were also similar (2% in RTOG-85-01, 9% in INT-0122, and 6% in INT-0113).

In summary, the local failure, survival, and treatment-related mortality rates for nonsurgical and surgical therapies are similar. Although the results are comparable, it is clear that both the nonsurgical and surgical approaches have limited success.

Necessity for Surgery After Chemoradiation. Two randomized trials examine whether surgery is necessary after chemoradiation. In the Fédération Francaise de Cancérologie Digestive (FFCD) 9102 trial, 444 patients with clinically resectable T3-4N0-1M0 squamous cell or adenocarcinoma of the esophagus received initial chemoradiation.[116] Patients initially received two cycles of 5-FU, cisplatin, and concurrent radiation (either 46 Gy at 2 Gy per day or split course 15 Gy weeks 1 and 3). The 259 patients who had at least a partial response were then randomized to surgery versus additional chemoradiation, which included three cycles of 5-FU, cisplatin, and concurrent radiation (either 20 Gy at 2 Gy per day or split course 15 Gy). Two-year local control was 66% in the surgery arm versus 57% in the chemoradiation-alone arm. There was no significant difference in 2-year survival (34% versus 40%; $p = 0.44$) or median survival (17.7 months versus 19.3 months) in patients who underwent surgery versus additional chemoradiation. These data suggest that patients who initially respond to chemoradiation should complete chemoradiation rather than stop and undergo surgery. Using the Spitzer index, there was no difference in global quality of life; however, a significantly greater decrease in quality of life was observed in the surgery arm during the postoperative period (7.52 versus 8.45; $p < 0.01$, respectively).[381] A separate analysis revealed that compared with split course radiation, patients who received standard course radiation had improved 2-year local relapse-free survival rates (77% versus 57%; $p = 0.002$) but no significant difference in overall survival (37% versus 31%).[382]

The German Oesophageal Cancer Study Group compared preoperative chemoradiation followed by surgery versus chemoradiation alone.[117] In this trial, 172 eligible patients age 70 years or more with uT3-4N0-1M0 squamous cell cancers of the esophagus were randomized to preoperative therapy (three cycles of 5-FU, leucovorin, etoposide, and cisplatin, followed by concurrent etoposide, cisplatin, plus 40 Gy) followed by surgery versus chemoradiation alone (the same chemotherapy but the radiation dose was increased to 60 to 65 Gy with or without brachytherapy). The pathologic complete response (pCR) rate was 33%. Despite a decrease in 2-year local failure (36% versus 58%; $p = 0.003$), there was no significant difference in 3-year survival (31% versus 24%) for those who were randomized to preoperative chemoradiation followed by surgery versus chemoradiation alone.

The current standard of care is to perform esophagectomy following chemoradiation in patients that can tolerate this approach. However, it is known that a subset of patients will have a complete response to chemoradiation. Further, patients with pCR have improved survival. Data from both Berger et al.[383] and Rohatgi et al.[384] suggest that patients who achieve a pCR had an improvement in survival compared to those who do not (5-year: 48% versus 15%, and median: 133 months versus 34 months, respectively). In these patients, surgical resection may not be necessary and has led to the concept of *selective* surgery after preoperative chemoradiation.

Swisher et al.[385] reported a retrospective analysis of patients who underwent a salvage compared with a planned esophagectomy at the M.D. Anderson Cancer Center from 1987 to 2000. The operative mortality was higher in those who underwent salvage versus planned surgery (15% versus 6%), but there was no difference in survival (25%). Because only 13 patients were identified who had salvage, the results need to be interpreted with caution. This approach formed the basis of a phase II Radiation Therapy Oncology Group (RTOG) trial (RTOG 0246), which prospectively examined the approach of preoperative paclitaxel/CDDP and 50.4 Gy followed by selective surgery in patients with either residual disease or recurrent disease in the absence of distant metastasis. In this trial of 43 patients with locally advanced disease, 21 patients required surgical resection after chemoradiation due to residual

(17 patients) or recurrent (3 patients) disease and one patient by choice.[386] This approach led to a 1-year overall survival of 71% and was closed early because it did not meet the predetermined survival rate of 78%.

Tumor Markers and Predictors of Response to Chemoradiation. It would be helpful to predict which tumors have a higher likelihood of responding to radiation or chemoradiation. Geh et al.[316] performed a systematic review to identify factors associated with a higher rate of pCR in patients receiving preoperative chemoradiation. The analysis was limited to the 26 trials meeting four criteria: (1) at least 20 patients treated, (2) a single chemoradiation regimen was delivered, (3) 5-FU, cisplatin, or mitomycin C–based chemotherapy was used, and (4) there was information on patient numbers, age, resection, and pCR rates. Overall, the pCR rate was 24% and the probability of pCR increased with increasing radiation dose ($p = 0.006$) and the use of a 5-FU-based ($p = 0.003$) or cisplatin-based ($p = 0.018$) regimen. In contrast, increased radiation treatment time ($p = 0.035$) and median age ($p = 0.019$) both decreased the chance of a pCR.

Data from both Berger et al.[383] and Rohatgi et al.[384] suggest that patients who achieve a pCR had an improvement in survival compared with those who do not (5-year, 48% versus 15%, and median, 133 months versus 34 months, respectively). However, the ability to predict a pCR prior to surgery is variable, as discussed earlier. A multivariate analysis by Gaca et al.[387] reported that posttreatment nodal status ($p = 0.03$), but not the degree of primary tumor response, predicted disease-free survival. Studies have linked tumor lymphocytic infiltration as well as the apoptotic index with response to chemoradiation.[388] Additional studies have linked a large number of proteins and genes involved in a wide array of signaling cascades with response to chemoradiation. Examples include alterations in diverse signaling cascades involving PI3 kinase, p53, EGFR, and hypoxia-inducible factor 1 alpha (HIF-1a).[389–394] Unfortunately, the vast majority of these studies lack validation and the specificity required to be used clinically. One recent study generated a micro-RNA signature to predict pCR from tumors in 52 patients treated uniformly with chemoradiation.[395] This signature was then validated in a separate cohort of 72 patients treated similarly. When combined with clinical stage, the area under the curve (AUC) for pathologic complete response (pCR) was 0.77 ($p = 2 \times 10^{-41}$).

Posttreatment imaging does not consistently identify the response. An ultrasound following chemoradiation does not accurately predict a pCR.[396] In contrast, Blackstock et al.[397] reported that the percentage of decrease in standard uptake value measured by 18F-FDG-PET predicted response, and Brucher et al.[398] found that it correlated with survival. McLoughlin et al.[399] treated 81 patients with preoperative chemoradiation and reported that FDG-PET scans were able to predict a pathologic complete response with 62% sensitivity, 44% specificity, and 56% accuracy.

The predictive ability of molecular markers has been examined. In 38 patients with squamous cell carcinoma who received chemoradiation with or without surgery, tumors without *p53* expression and tumors with weak $Bcl-X_L$ expression showed a higher response to chemotherapy (56% and 53%, respectively) than tumors positive for *p53* or with strong $Bcl-X_L$ expression (30% and 32%, respectively; *p* not significant).[400] After preoperative chemoradiation, patients with *p53*-negative tumors had a significantly better mean survival than those with *p53*-positive tumors (31 months versus 11 months; $p = 0.0378$). By multivariate analysis, Pomp et al.[401] found that overexpression of p53 resulted in a decrease in the survival in 69 patients with squamous cell carcinoma or adenocarcinoma treated with radiation alone. In one study, there was a correlation between decreasing levels of four phospholipids and increasing T stage and grade.[402]

Understanding the mechanism of radioresistance through the identification and targeting of molecular pathways by serum protein profiling[403] and the identification of genes involved in apoptosis,[404] activated transcription factor nuclear factor κB (NF-κB),[392]

and microvascular density[405] may offer new opportunities for therapeutic advances.

Intensification of Chemoradiation. The phase II Intergroup trial 0122 (ECOG-PE289/RTOG-90-12) was designed to intensify treatment in the RTOG-85-01 combined modality arm.[381] Both the chemotherapy and radiation therapy in INT-0122 were intensified by 20%.[406] The median survival time was 20 months and the 5-year actuarial survival rate was 20%. Similar toxicities were reported by Ishikura et al.[407] for 139 patients with squamous cell cancers treated with 5-FU, cisplatin, and 60 Gy of radiation. However, the higher radiation dose (64.8 Gy) in INT-0122 was tolerated and compared with the 50.4 Gy of radiation in the Intergroup trial INT-0123, discussed as follows.

A potential advantage of neoadjuvant chemotherapy is the early identification of those patients who may or may not respond to the chemotherapeutic regimen being delivered concurrently with chemoradiation. Ilson et al.[101] have shown that the change in standard update value (SUV) on FDG-PET scan was able to predict which patients showed a response to the full course of chemotherapy followed by chemoradiotherapy. Weider and associates[408] reported similar findings in 38 patients with squamous cell cancers. As discussed previously, the use of an early PET scan during induction chemotherapy to direct subsequent chemotherapy during combined chemoradiotherapy is the subject of an ongoing Alliance Trial.

Amini et al.[409] performed a retrospective review of 141 patients who achieved an initial clinical complete response (cCR) after chemoradiation. By a multivariate analysis, the initial SUV of >10 and poorly differentiated tumors had a significantly higher incidence of in-field failure.[409]

Intensification of the Radiation Dose. Another approach to the dose intensification of chemoradiation is increasing the radiation dose above 50.4 Gy. There are two methods by which to increase the radiation dose to the esophagus: brachytherapy and external-beam radiation therapy.

Brachytherapy. Intraluminal brachytherapy allows for the escalation of the dose to the primary tumor while protecting the surrounding dose-limiting structures such as the lung, heart, and spinal cord.[410] A radioactive source is placed intraluminally via bronchoscopy or a nasogastric tube. Brachytherapy has been used both as primary therapy (usually palliative)[411,412] and as a boost after external-beam radiation therapy or chemoradiation.[413–415] It can be delivered by high-dose rate or low-dose rate.[416] Although there are technical and radiobiologic differences between the two dose rates, there are no clear therapeutic advantages for either.

Series that combine brachytherapy with external-beam radiation therapy or chemoradiation report results similar to those for conventional chemoradiation. Yorozu et al.[415] reported a local failure rate of 57% and a 5-year actuarial survival of 28% in 46 patients with stage T2-3N0-1M0 disease. Even for a more favorable subset of patients with clinical T1 to T2 disease, Yorozu et al.[417] reported a local failure rate of 44% and a 5-year survival of 26%. In the series by Pasquier et al.,[414] local failure was 23% and 5-year survival was 36%. In an updated series by Ishikawa et al.,[418] 59 patients with submucosal esophageal cancer received external-beam therapy followed by brachytherapy in 36 patients with either low-dose rate caesium-137 (^{137}Cs) (17 patients) or high-dose rate iridium-192 (^{192}Ir) (19 patients). Patients selected to receive a brachytherapy boost had a significantly higher 5-year cause specific survival (86% versus 62%; $p = 0.04$).

In the RTOG-92-07 trial, 75 patients with squamous cell cancers (92%) or adenocarcinomas (8%) of the thoracic esophagus received the RTOG-85-01 combined modality regimen (5-FU, cisplatin, and 50 Gy of radiation) followed by a boost during cycle three of chemotherapy with either low-dose rate or high-dose rate intraluminal brachytherapy.[419] Because of low accrual, the low-dose rate option was discontinued and the analysis was limited to patients who received the high-dose rate treatment. High-dose rate brachytherapy was delivered in weekly fractions of 5 Gy during weeks 8, 9, and 10. After the development of several fistulas, the fraction delivered at week 10 was discontinued. Although the complete-response rate was 73%, the rate of local failure was 27%. Rates of acute toxicity were 58% for grade 3, 26% for grade 4, and 8% for grade 5 (treatment-related death). The cumulative incidence of fistula was 18% per year and the crude incidence was 14%. Of the six treatment-related fistulas, three were fatal. Given the significant toxicity, this treatment approach should be used with caution.[420] Based on these and other data, the American Brachytherapy Society has developed guidelines for esophageal brachytherapy.[421–423]

External-Beam Therapy: 2D and 3D Techniques. Because almost all patients in both the INT-0122 trial who started radiation therapy were able to complete the full dose (64.8 Gy), this higher dose of radiation was used in the experimental arm of the Intergroup esophageal trial INT-0123 (RTOG-94-05).[281] In this trial, patients with either squamous cell carcinoma or adenocarcinoma who were selected for nonsurgical treatment were randomly assigned to receive a slightly modified RTOG-85-01 combined modality regimen with 50.4 Gy of radiation versus the same chemotherapy with 64.8 Gy of radiation.

The modifications to the original RTOG-85-01 chemoradiation arm includes (1) using 1.8-Gy fractions to 50.4 Gy rather than 2-Gy fractions to 50 Gy; (2) treating with 5-cm proximal and distal margins for 50.4 Gy rather than treating the whole esophagus for the first 30 Gy followed by a cone down with 5-cm margins to 50 Gy; (3) cycle three of 5-FU and cisplatin did not begin until 4 weeks after the completion of radiation therapy rather than 3 weeks after; and (4) cycles three and four of chemotherapy were delivered every 4 weeks rather than every 3 weeks.

INT-0123 was closed to accrual in 1999 with 218 patients after an interim analysis revealed that it was unlikely that the high-dose arm would achieve superior survival compared with the standard-dose arm: There was no significant difference in median survival time (13.0 months versus 18.1 months) or 2-year survival rate (31% versus 40%) between the high-dose and standard-dose arms.[281] Although 11 treatment-related deaths occurred in the high-dose arm compared with 2 in the standard-dose arm, 7 of the 11 deaths occurred in patients who had received 50.4 Gy or less.

Although the crude incidence of local failure or persistence of local disease (or both) was lower in the high-dose arm than in the standard-dose arm (50% versus 55%), as was the incidence of distant failure (9% versus 16%), these were not significant. Although retrospective data from the M.D. Anderson Cancer Center suggest a positive correlation between radiation dose and local–regional control,[422] the results of the INT-0123 trial maintain the standard dose of 50.4 Gy.

The modifications to the original RTOG-85-01 chemoradiation arm outlined earlier did not adversely affect the local control or survival rate in the control arm of INT-0123. Therefore, the radiation doses and field design used in the control arm of INT-0123 should be used.

Radiation can be intensified not only by increasing the total dose, but also by using accelerated fractionation or hyperfractionation. This approach has revealed modest results. Zaho and colleagues[424] treated 201 patients with squamous cell cancer using 41.4 Gy followed by late-course accelerated hyperfractionation to 68.4 Gy. The results were similar to RTOG 85-01 (38% local failure and 26% 5-year survival). Choi and colleagues[425] treated 46 patients with 5-FU/cisplatin and twice per day radiation using a concurrent boost technique and reported a 37% 5-year survival. Additionally, Lee et al.[343] reported on a trial of 102 patients with locally advanced disease, limited to squamous cell carcinoma, randomized to surgery alone versus preoperative therapy with 45.6 Gy (1.2 Gy twice per day) plus 5-FU/cisplatin. There was no difference in median survival (28 versus 27 months). Thus, although

these approaches appear to be reasonable, there appears to be a significant increase in acute toxicity without any clear therapeutic benefit.

Dose Escalation: Intensity Modulated Radiation Therapy and Protons. A criticism of many dose escalation trials in the definitive management of locally advanced esophageal cancer is the use of conventional two-dimensional (2D) and three-dimensional (3D) radiation techniques. Trials using newer techniques such as intensity-modulated radiation therapy (IMRT) and protons may be able to deliver higher doses of radiation with a more tolerable toxicity profile. Multiple dosimetric studies comparing standard 3D-conformal radiotherapy and IMRT, generally have found improved sparing of the heart, lung, or both using either static field or arc-based IMRT.[426–435] This has led multiple clinical centers to begin the routine use of IMRT in this disease. A retrospective analysis of these data does not suggest an inferior outcome and may provide decreased toxicity versus non-IMRT treatment techniques.[436–438] Investigators at the M.D. Anderson Cancer Center reported the results of 676 patients with locally advanced disease treated with either IMRT (263 patients) or 3D conformal radiation therapy (3DCRT) (413 patients).[436] On a multivariate analysis, IMRT was associated with improved survival ($p = 0.004$), but not cancer-specific survival ($p = 0.86$). The survival difference between 3DCRT and IMRT was thought to be due to a higher level of cardiac deaths ($p = 0.05$) and unexplained deaths ($p = 0.003$) in the 3DCRT patients, suggesting that decreased cardiac dose may have a direct impact on patient outcome. Although this and other comparisons between 3DCRT and IMRT are retrospective, a randomized trial is unlikely, thus the available data may represent the best comparison.

Another theoretical advantage of IMRT is the possibility of dose escalation. With the use of IMRT, a simultaneous integrated boost (SIB) may be performed while maintaining commonly used lung and heart dosimetric constraints. Retrospective data from Zhang and colleagues[422] suggest a positive correlation between radiation dose and local–regional control. This has led to a phase I studying examining this approach in locally advanced disease. However, at this point, based on results of the INT-0123 trial, the standard dose of external beam radiation remains 50.4 Gy.

New Chemoradiation Regimens. Because 75% to 80% of patients die of metastatic disease, advances in systemic therapies are necessary for a further improvement of results. The most widely used chemotherapeutic regimen to be combined with radiation for the treatment of esophageal cancer is 5-FU and cisplatin. A number of new cytotoxic and targeted regimens are being evaluated in both the preoperative and nonoperative setting. These are discussed previously in the section on preoperative chemoradiation regimens.

Palliation of Esophageal Cancer with Radiation Therapy

Palliation of Dysphagia and Bleeding. Many of the series examining dysphagia are retrospective, and most do not use objective criteria to define and assess dysphagia. Some do not report the number of patients presenting with dysphagia or the percentage who receive palliative treatment until the time of death. Furthermore, few series carefully examine other variables that may influence the results, such as histologic type, stage, and location of the primary tumor.

Options for palliation include stents, feeding tubes, chemotherapy, and external-beam radiation therapy or brachytherapy (or both). The selection of the technique is variable and commonly is based on physician preference. In a randomized trial from the Dutch SIREC Study Group of stent versus one 12-Gy fraction of brachytherapy, dysphagia, as measured by a variety of quality-of-life scales, improved more rapidly after stent placement; however, long-term relief was superior after brachytherapy.[412] Median survivals were similar (145 days versus 155 days).

Patients for whom stents fail are commonly treated with palliative radiation. Li et al.[439] reported that the presence of a metal stent increases the radiation dose 5% to 10% at a 0.5-cm depth in the esophageal wall. Therefore, the radiation dose should be decreased by 5% to 10% when a metal stent is in the radiation field. Nishimura et al.[440] reported a high-grade 3+ complication rate in 47 patients who underwent stent placement before or during radiation treatment and recommend that stent placement be delayed until radiation therapy has failed.

As seen in Table 37.8, series have examined the palliative benefits of either radiation alone[371,441–444] or chemoradiation.[406,443,445–450] Overall, external-beam radiation therapy alone provides palliation of dysphagia in 70% to 80% of patients.

The most comprehensive and carefully performed analysis of swallowing function in patients receiving chemoradiation is by Coia et al.[450] Using a swallowing score modified from O'Rourke et al.,[451] they analyzed 102 patients treated with three 5-FU–based combined modality regimens. Before the start of therapy, 95% of patients had some degree of dysphagia. Within 2 weeks after the start of treatment, 45% had improvement in dysphagia, and by the completion of the 6-week therapy, 83% had improvement. Overall, 88% experienced an improvement in dysphagia. The median time to improvement was 4 weeks (range, 1 to 21 weeks), and all but two patients could swallow at least soft or solid foods. Harvey et al.[446] treated 106 patients and reported that 78% had improvement of at least one grade in their dysphagia score; 51% maintained swallowing improvement until the time of last follow-up.

Intraluminal brachytherapy is also an effective, albeit a more limited method, achieving palliation of dysphagia in 35% to 80% of patients and a median survival of 5 months. A major limitation of brachytherapy is the effective treatment distance. The primary isotope is [192]-Ir, which is usually prescribed to treat to a distance of 1 cm from the source. Any portion of the tumor that is more than 1 cm from the source will receive a suboptimal radiation dose, confirmed by pathologic analysis of surgical specimens.[452] Given its limited effective range, brachytherapy is usually not as successful as external-beam radiation therapy in treating the entire tumor volume. However, in a randomized trial, there was no difference in local control or survival with high-dose–rate brachytherapy as opposed to external-beam radiation therapy.[452]

If a patient requires rapid palliation (within a few days), alternative approaches such as laser treatment or stent placement are recommended. Although external-beam radiation with or without chemotherapy takes at least 2 weeks to produce palliation, once palliation is achieved it is more durable than that provided by the other palliative modalities because external-beam radiation treats the problem (the gross tumor mass), not just the symptom. If external-beam radiation is not possible, then intraluminal brachytherapy should be considered because it is an effective modality for decreasing symptoms such as dysphagia and bleeding. Chemotherapy by itself may also substantially relieve dysphagia when used as an initial treatment of metastatic disease.

Treatment in the Setting of Tracheoesophageal Fistula

The presence of a malignant tracheoesophageal fistula usually results in poor survival, although occasionally, patients may survive for a prolonged period. Historically, radiation therapy was believed to be contraindicated for these patients for fear of exacerbating the fistula as the tumor responded. More recently, there have been reports to the contrary. In a Mayo Clinic series, 10 patients with malignant tracheoesophageal fistulas received 30 to 66 Gy external-beam radiation, and the median survival time was 5 months.[453] A series from Japan that treated 24 patients with fistulization to the airway reported ultimate closure of the fistula after chemoradiotherapy in 17 patients, with time to closure ranging from 6 to 280 days.[454]

TABLE 37.8

Palliation of Dysphagia with Radiation Therapy with or without Chemotherapy

Study (Ref.)	No. of Patients	Palliation of Dysphagia[a]	
		At the End of Treatment (%)	Duration
Radiation Therapy Alone			
Wara et al.[441]	103	89	6-mo average
Petrovich et al.[442]	133	87	34% = 6 mo 18% = 3 mo 35% = 3 mo
Roussel et al.[371]	69	70	—
Caspers et al.[444]	127	71	54% until death
Whittington et al.[443]	25	—	5% at 9 mo
Chemoradiation			
Coia et al.[450]	102	88	67%–100% until death
Seitz et al.[445]	35	100[b]	—
Whittington et al.[443]	26	—	87% 3-y actuarial
Algan et al.[447]	8	100	—
Gill et al.[448]	71	60	—
Urba et al.[449]	27	—	59% until death
Izquierdo et al.[406]	25	64	Median, 5 mo
Harvey et al.[446]	106	78	51% until lost follow-up

[a] See text for definition and number of patients presenting with dysphagia.
[b] Patients had dilation or neodymium yttrium-aluminum garnet laser treatment at the start of therapy.

Although the experience is very limited, the data suggest that radiation treatment does not necessarily increase the severity of a malignant tracheoesophageal fistula and it can be administered safely. It is unclear if radiation treatment improves outcome.

Acute and Long-Term Toxicity of Radiation Therapy.

The toxicity of radiation therapy is a function of what the total dose is, what technique is used, and whether the patient has received chemotherapy. Essentially all patients experience lethargy and esophagitis commencing 2 to 3 weeks after the start of radiation therapy; these symptoms usually resolve 1 to 2 weeks after completion of therapy.

The most carefully documented acute toxicity data for patients who receive radiation therapy alone (without chemotherapy) are from the control arm of RTOG-85-01 in which patients received radiation therapy alone to a dose of 64 Gy.[280,372] The incidence of acute grade 3 toxicity was 25% and the incidence of acute grade 4 toxicity was 3%. The incidence of long-term grade 3+ toxicity and long-term grade 4+ toxicity was 23% and 2%, respectively. Radiation therapy can produce esophageal strictures, as can surgery. The total incidence of stricture (benign plus malignant) in patients receiving radiation therapy alone or radiation combined with chemotherapy is 20% to 40% in a modern series and up to 60% in historical series,[455] with up to 50% malignant, associated with recurrence. The incidence of stricture is lower in series in which careful radiation techniques were used. Coia et al.[450] examined a subset of 25 patients who experienced local control and survived at least 1 year. The incidence of benign stricture was 12%. Radiation toxicity is related to dose–volume effects.[456]

One series examined the functional outcomes of benign and malignant strictures.[451] Patients received 45 to 56 Gy and 53% received some form of chemotherapy. Of the 24 patients (30%) who developed a benign stricture, 71% were able to tolerate a full or soft diet and required dilation, with a median interval between dilations of 5 months. Even in the subset of patients who develop a benign stricture, dilation is effective in the majority of patients. In contrast, in the 28% of patients who developed a malignant stricture, dilation was unsuccessful and esophageal intubation was required.

The high incidence of fistula reported in the RTOG-92-07 trial of chemoradiation plus intraluminal brachytherapy (18% actuarial, 14% crude) has not been seen in series using radiation therapy or chemoradiation. The incidence of other long-term grade 3+ toxicities such as pneumonitis or pericarditis is 5%.

The effect of radiation on pulmonary function was examined by Gergel et al.[457] Patients received 39.6 Gy with anterior–posterior fields followed by radiation with oblique fields to a total dose of 50.4 Gy, plus concurrent chemotherapy with oxaliplatin and 5-FU. Results of pulmonary function tests administered before and a median of 16 days after radiation revealed significant declines in diffusing capacity for carbon monoxide and total lung capacity. Investigators at the M.D. Anderson Cancer Center performed retrospective treatment-planning studies on 10 patients and found that IMRT reduced the dose volume of exposed normal lung but had no clinically meaningful differences on the irradiated volumes of spinal cord, heart, liver, or total body integral doses.[426] The impact of respiratory and organ movement on defining target volumes is being investigated.[458,459]

The issue of treatment-related deaths in patients who receive chemoradiation is complex. Although the incidence was only 2% in RTOG-85-01, subsequent trials have reported a higher treatment-related mortality rate (i.e., 9% in INT-0122 and 8% in RTOG-92-07). These mortality rates are lower than the 10% to 15% incidence reported in historical surgical series, although only slightly higher than the 6% reported in the surgical control arm of INT-0113.[105] It is interesting to note that, as the mortality rate with surgery has decreased, there has been a corresponding increase in the treatment-related mortality rate reported in the nonoperative trials. As previously discussed in Primary Nonsurgical Therapy,

this may be partly related to bias in selecting patients to be treated with the nonoperative approach.

Radiation Field Design and Treatment Techniques.

Just as expert surgical skills are required for a successful esophagectomy, radiation field design for esophageal cancer requires careful planning. Historically, the standard radiation dose, based on INT-0123, for patients selected for chemoradiation is 50.4 Gy at 1.8 Gy per fraction. However, recent data from the CROSS trial suggest that 41.4 Gy in the same fractionation may be sufficient to treat in the preoperative setting. As previously described, some investigators have performed dose escalation; however, based on INT-0113, dose escalation above 50.4 Gy should not be performed off protocol. Additionally, radiation should be delivered without treatment breaks, as randomized data from France reveal a higher local control (57% versus 29%) and 2-year survival rate (37% versus 23%) with continuous course compared with split course radiation.[382]

The radiation field should include the primary tumor with 5 cm superior and inferior margins and 2 cm lateral margins. The primary local–regional lymph nodes should receive the same dose. For cervical (proximal) primary tumors (defined as at or proximal to the carina), the treatment volume includes the bilateral supraclavicular nodes, and for GEJ (distal) primaries, the celiac axis nodes should be included.

Treatment Modality.

At many centers, the standard of care in radiotherapy for locally advanced esophageal cancer is 3D conformal radiotherapy using a beam arrangement optimized via CT scan–based planning. However, as mentioned previously, many clinicians have used IMRT with a possible benefit with regard to toxicity and no apparent compromise in oncologic outcome.[436] A comparison of three techniques is shown in Figure 37.14. If IMRT is to be used, careful attention should be given to target delineation. In addition, particularly in the case of distal/GEJ tumors, 4D CT or other forms of motion management should be considered.

Recently, proton radiotherapy has become more available as a treatment modality. By virtue of its physical characteristics, proton radiotherapy is thought to decrease dose to critical structures, in large part by minimizing the low-dose "bath" often seen with IMRT. This is to some degree shown in dosimetric studies, with V5, V10, and V20 to the lung and heart with protons compared to IMRT (see Fig. 37.14). Several studies have examined patient outcome after treating with proton radiotherapy. Sugahara and colleagues[460] examined outcomes in 46 patients with squamous cell carcinoma treated with protons with or without photons to a median total dose of 76 Gy.[460] The 5-year local control rate was for T1: 83%, for T2 through 4: 29%, and for survival T1: 55% and for T2 through 4: 13%. Koyama[461] reported mean actuarial survival rates of 60% for patients with superficial and 39% for those with advanced disease treated with mean total doses of 78 to 81 Gy. The incidence of esophageal ulcer was 67%. In the United States, Lin and colleagues[462] retrospectively reviewed 62 patients treated with proton radiotherapy for locally advanced disease. Overall, 47% were treated with surgical resection following chemoradiation, with a pCR rate in these patients of 28%. In this series, two patients (3.2%) developed symptomatic pneumonitis and an additional two patients died due to treatment-related factors. Proton therapy remains experimental and is currently being evaluated in a randomized trial.

Target Delineation.

Although CT scans can identify adjacent organs and structures, it may be limited in defining the extent of the primary tumor. Leong and colleagues[463] have demonstrated that the addition of PET/CT scan information for treatment planning improved the identification of the gross tumor volume (GTV). The GTV based on CT scan information alone excluded PET-avid disease in 11 of 16 patients (69%), 5 of whom would have resulted in a geographic miss of gross tumor. Thus, in many centers, it is

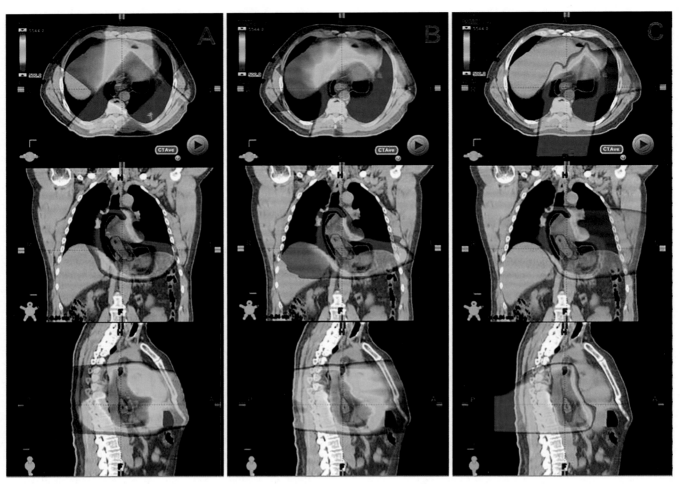

Figure 37.14 Comparative radiation treatment plans. **(A)** 3D-CRT, **(B)** IMRT, and **(C)** proton beam comparison between treatment modalities. In this selected case, both IMRT and protons provide improved lung and cardiac sparing compared to 3D-CRT. Proton beam decreases liver dose compared to other modalities. (Modified from Zhang Z, Liao Z, Jin J, et al. Dose response relationship in locoregional control for patients with stage II–III esophageal cancer treated with concurrent chemotherapy and radiotherapy. *Int J Radiat Oncol Biol Phys* 2005;61:656–664.)

customary to obtain pretreatment FDG-PET scans, not only to identify patients with occult metastatic disease, but also to assist in target delineation. Conversely, MRI has also been suggested to delineate esophageal tumors, although initial studies showed limited benefit in tumor or positive lymph node delineation.[464] Thus, the use of MRI in this context remains experimental. Thus, the current recommendation for target delineation includes using contrasted CT and EGD/EUS findings, as well as FDG-PET.

Limiting Toxicity of Chemoradiation. Depending on the location of the primary tumor, there are a number of sensitive organs that will be in the radiation field. Specifically, the most well-studied organs at risk in the context of treating esophageal cancer include the lungs and heart. Radiation pneumonitis is clearly linked to the dose and volume of lung treated. Various single dosimetric parameters have been proposed to estimate the probability of developing radiation pneumonitis after radiotherapy.[428,465–469] Investigators from the Netherlands compared different normal tissue complication probability (NTCP) models to predict radiation pneumonitis.[468] Using the observed incidence of radiation pneumonitis among breast cancer, malignant lymphoma, and inoperable non–small-cell lung cancer (NSCLC) patients, they found that the underlying local dose-effect relation for radiation pneumonitis was linear. This was better represented by the mean lung dose (MLD) model, rather than a step function model represented by a threshold dose such as V20. In their patient population, the MLD

was the most accurate predictor for the incidence of radiation pneumonitis. Willner and colleagues[466] performed an analysis of pneumonitis risk from dose volume histogram (DVH) parameters among patients treated with 3D conformal radiotherapy.[466] Their data indicated that it is reasonable to disperse the dose outside the target volume over large areas in order to reduce the volumes of lung receiving >40 Gy. They found that reducing the high-dose volume reduces the pneumonitis rate more than a corresponding reduction in the low-dose regions of the DVH. Additionally, Konski and colleagues[470] were able to correlate cardiac toxicity to dosimetric and patient factors. Specifically they recommended a threshold of V20, V30, and V40 below 70%, 65%, and 60%, respectively, to decrease symptomatic cardiac toxicity. In general, practice a MLD <20 Gy is standard. Cardiac dose constraints are not as clearly defined, but a V30 <35% is reasonable.

In the palliative setting, there are a variety of radiation-treatment regimens.[471] The goal is rapid palliation of symptoms and the most common approach is to treat anteroposteriorly and posteroanteriorly, including the primary tumor with 2-cm margins, in 10 3-Gy fractions to a total dose of 30 Gy.

Treatment of Metastatic Disease

A variety of single-agent and combination chemotherapy regimens have been evaluated in patients with recurrent or metastatic carcinoma of the esophagus. Phase II clinical trials in this population have identified drugs with activity that have been integrated into combined modality regimens for the treatment of earlier stage disease. Standard criteria for evaluating treatment response require that serial measurement of disease be possible. For the esophageal cancer patient with metastatic disease to distant organ sites or lymph nodes, treatment response can be reliably assessed using spiral CT scans or MRI. The serial tumor measurement for response assessments in patients with disease limited to the esophagus is less reliable. An endoscopy with brushings and biopsy may be performed to confirm a clinically determined complete response; however, a biopsy is subject to sampling error, and biopsy findings are not a reliable indicator of complete histologic resolution of disease. Whole-body FDG-PET performed before and during or after chemotherapy may be a valuable noninvasive method of predicting tumor response and a favorable treatment outcome. Several studies have shown that a reduction in tumor FDG uptake (median decrease in standardized uptake value) correlates with response and longer survival.[154,158,327] Until the mid-1990s, the accumulated experience with chemotherapy was almost entirely in patients with squamous cell tumors. With the rising incidence of adenocarcinoma of the distal esophagus, GEJ, and cardia in the United States and Western industrialized countries, patients with this histologic type now make up more than half of referrals for chemotherapy. Most trials of new agents and combined modality regimens now include patients with both tumor types. Modern chemotherapy trials in advanced disease also treat gastric adenocarcinoma in concert with adenocarcinoma of the GEJ and distal esophagus, and some trials also include squamous esophageal cancer.

Single-Agent Chemotherapy

Studies of single-agent chemotherapy for esophageal cancer are summarized here. Response data for many of the older drugs have come from broad phase I and II trials conducted in the 1970s and 1980s, which included small numbers of esophageal cancer patients.[472–481] Bleomycin, 5-FU, mitomycin, and cisplatin have been used most frequently because of their single-agent activity and additive or synergistic effects with radiation. Because of the potential for pulmonary toxicity, bleomycin is no longer included in combination regimens, having been replaced by 5-FU. Similarly, mitomycin is used less often because of its toxicity profile, which includes hemolytic–uremic syndrome and cumulative myelosuppression.

Seven trials examined the use of cisplatin for single-agent therapy in esophageal cancer patients,[479,482–487] six of which used dosages ranging from 50 to 120 mg/m^2 every 3 to 4 weeks. The cumulative response rate in patients with metastatic or recurrent disease was 21%. Vinorelbine is a semisynthetic vinca alkaloid that has less neurotoxicity than vincristine and vinblastine. Phase II trials in metastatic squamous cell cancer of the esophagus report response rates of 20% to 25% using weekly or biweekly dosing schedules.[488,489] In a subsequent trial, Conroy et al.[490] evaluated the doublet of vinorelbine and cisplatin. A total of 71 patients with metastatic squamous cell cancer were treated, and a 34% response rate was observed. Vinorelbine was evaluated in a phase II trial in 29 patients with adenocarcinoma of the esophagus who had failed prior chemotherapy, with minor activity (7% response rate) observed.[491]

The taxane paclitaxel has been tested in both adenocarcinoma and squamous cell carcinoma of the esophagus. Paclitaxel promotes the stabilization of microtubules and is a cycle-specific agent affecting cells in the G2/M phase. Paclitaxel also enhances radiation effects and may be both concentration and schedule dependent.[492] Three trials of single-agent paclitaxel have been reported. One used the maximum tolerable dose of 250 mg/m^2, derived from initial phase I trials using a 24-hour infusion schedule.[493] The overall response rate was 32% (34% in 33 patients with adenocarcinoma, and 28% in 18 patients with squamous cell

carcinoma). The second trial tested a regimen of 140 mg/m^2 infused during 96 hours in patients previously treated using a shorter infusion schedule of paclitaxel-containing combination chemotherapy.[494] No responses were observed. The third trial evaluated single-agent paclitaxel administered by a weekly 1-hour infusion at a dose of 80 mg/m^2 in a large multicenter phase 2 setting.[495] A modest response rate of 15% was observed in 65 patients without prior chemotherapy treatment (16% in the 50 patients treated with adenocarcinoma and 13% in the 15 patients treated with squamous cell carcinoma). Limited activity (5%) was seen in patients with prior chemotherapy. Despite the low response rate, the median survival was 274 days, and toxicity, including hematologic toxicity, was minimal.

Docetaxel was evaluated at a dose of 100 mg/m^2, every 3 weeks in a combined esophageal and gastric cancer trial treating 33 patients with gastric cancer and 8 patients with esophageal adenocarcinoma.[496] Two of the eight patients (25%) with esophageal adenocarcinoma had a major response. Overall, grade 4 neutropenia occurred in 88% of patients and neutropenic fever in 46%. A larger trial of docetaxel 75 mg/m^2 in 22 patients with esophageal adenocarcinoma reported a response rate of 18% in chemotherapy-naïve patients and no responses in previously treated patients.[496] Febrile neutropenia occurred in 32% of patients. A recent trial of 70 mg/m^2 every 3 weeks in 49 patients with squamous cell carcinoma reported a 20% response rate.[497] Eighty-eight percent of patients had grade 3 or 4 neutropenia and 18% had febrile neutropenia.

Drugs that have been adequately tested in squamous cell cancer of the esophagus and have response rates less than 5% are the methotrexate analog dichloromethotrexate[498] and trimetrexate,[499,500] and etoposide,[501,502] ifosfamide,[503,504] and carboplatin.[505,506] A more contemporary study of etoposide in untreated patients with squamous cell carcinoma reported a response rate of 19% (5 of 26 patients).[507] Carboplatin has been studied in both adenocarcinoma and squamous cell carcinoma, and, in contrast to the activity of a single agent, responses to carboplatin were observed in only 3 of 59 chemotherapy-naïve patients. Therefore, substitution of single-agent carboplatin for cisplatin is not recommended when treating patients with either adenocarcinomas or squamous cell carcinomas of the esophagus. Nonetheless, carboplatin combination regimens used as part of combination chemotherapy, in chemoradiation (as previously discussed) and in metastatic disease regimens (discussed later), appear to have comparable activity to cisplatin-based therapy.

Topotecan and gemcitabine have been separately evaluated in both histologic tumor types and have been shown to be inactive.[508–510] The topoisomerase II inhibitor irinotecan has been evaluated in two phase II trials in adenocarcinoma of the stomach and GEJ, with a response rate of 15% observed.[511,512]

Combined-Agent Chemotherapy

Older trials (before the mid-1990s) and those in Europe were almost exclusively limited to patients with squamous cell carcinoma. Because esophageal cancer is a relatively uncommon malignancy, many studies include a heterogeneous population of treatment-naïve patients with locally advanced intrathoracic disease as well as patients with recurrent or metastatic disease. Not only is there variation in the patient population, but more recent trials usually limit eligibility to patients with no prior chemotherapy and performance status of 0 or 1. Thus, in the absence of comparative trials, newer regimens may appear more effective.

Most series consist of small numbers of patients; therefore, the 95% CIs are large and nearly all responses are partial. On average, the duration of response ranges from 3 to 6 months.

Trials conducted in the 1980s testing three-drug regimens such as cisplatin, bleomycin, and vindesine[255,513] and cisplatin and mitoguazone combined with vindesine[514] or vinblastine[515] yielded response rates of 30% to 40% in patients with squamous cell carcinoma. Toxicity was primarily moderate myelosuppression. Bleomycin and

TABLE 37.9

Randomized Phase II–III Chemotherapy Trials In Esophageal and GE Junction Cancers

Regimen	Patients (N)	Histologic Type	Response Rate (%)	Overall Survival	Reference
C + 5-FU vs	88	S	35	28 wks	483
C			19	33 wks	
ECF vs	274	A	45	8.9 mos	517
FAMTX			21	5.7 mos	
ECF vs	690	A/S	42	9.4 mos	518
MCF			44	8.7 mos	
ECF vs	1002	A/S	41	9.9 mos	520
ECX vs			46	9.9 mos	
EOF vs			42	9.3 mos	
EOX			48	11.2 mos	
5-FU + O vs	220	A	35	10.7 mos	521
5-FU + C			25	8.8 mos	
5-FU + C vs	316	A	32	9.3 mos	522
Cape + C			46	10.5 mos	
5-FU + C vs	1,053	A	32	7.9 mos	524
S-1 + C			29	8.6 mos	
CF vs	445	A	26	8.6 mos	525
DCF			36	9.2 mos	
5-FU + O +/− D	143	A	49	17.3 mos	526
			28	14.5 mos	
5-FU + C vs	333	A	26	8.7 mos	549
5-FU + Irino			32	9.0 mos	

C, cisplatin; S, squamous cell carcinoma; ECF, epirubicin/cisplatin; FAMTX, 5-FU/doxorubicin/methotrexate; A, adenocarcinoma; EOX, epirubicin/cisplatin or oxaliplatin/5-FU or capecitabine; O, oxaliplatin; Cape, capecitabine; D, docetaxel; Irino, irinotecan.

mitoguazone were subsequently replaced by 5-FU to reduce toxicity and to take advantage of its synergistic activity with cisplatin.

The two-drug combination of cisplatin (100 mg/m^2 on day 1) and 5-FU (1,000 mg/m^2 per day continuous infusion for 96 to 120 hours) has been the standard regimen for 2 decades to treat patients with either squamous cell carcinoma or adenocarcinoma. A 35% response rate was observed in patients with metastatic, recurrent, or locally advanced incurable squamous cell cancer of the esophagus.[483] Higher response rates (in the 40% to 60% range) were reported in trials administering two or three cycles of cisplatin and 5-FU as induction therapy before surgery. The difference in response rates may be related to better performance status, better nutrition, and smaller volume disease in the surgical candidates. Despite the common use in the oncology community of the combination of 5-FU and cisplatin for the treatment of esophageal carcinoma, only one trial conducted by the EORTC has directly addressed the issue of the comparative efficacy of single-agent cisplatin and the combination of 5-FU and cisplatin (Table 37.9).[483] Patients with locally advanced or metastatic squamous cell carcinoma were randomly assigned to receive either cisplatin (100 mg/m^2) plus continuous-infusion 5-FU (1,000 mg/m^2 per day, days 1 to 5) or to cisplatin (100 mg/m^2) alone, with both regimens repeated every 3 weeks. The cisplatin/5-FU arm had a higher response rate (35%) and better median survival (33 weeks) than the cisplatin arm (19% and 28 weeks, respectively), but these findings were not statistically significant. Cisplatin/5-FU was also more toxic, with 16% treatment-related deaths for the combination.

Cisplatin in combination with tegafur uracil (UFT), an oral 5-FU pro-drug combining tegafur with uracil, an inhibitor of the enzyme dihydropyrimidine dehydrogenase that degrades 5-FU,

has also been evaluated in esophageal cancer. A response rate of 46% was reported.[516]

Recent phase III trials have compared the addition of a third agent to cisplatin/5-FU versus cisplatin/5-FU alone. The Royal Marsden group developed the ECF regimen, a combination of epirubicin (50 mg/m^2) and cisplatin (60 mg/m^2) every 3 weeks in combination with daily protracted continuous infusion 5-FU (200 mg/m^2 per day) in gastric cancer. The ECF regimen was compared in a phase III trial in gastric and GEJ adenocarcinoma with a bolus regimen of 5-FU, doxorubicin, and methotrexate (FAMTX) (see Table 37.9).[517] The ECF regimen resulted in a superior response rate (45% versus 21%), failure-free survival (7.4 months versus 3.4 months), and median survival (8.9 months versus 5.7 months) in comparison with FAMTX. The ECF regimen had a tolerable toxicity profile, with less than 10% rates of grade 3 or 4 diarrhea or stomatitis. A more recent trial treating nearly 600 patients with advanced esophageal squamous and adenocarcinoma and gastric adenocarcinoma compared the ECF regimen with a similar regimen substituting mitomycin (7 mg/m^2 every 6 weeks) for epirubicin (see Table 37.9).[518] This trial validated the previously reported response rate and median survival for the ECF regimen (42%, 9.4 months), but the response rate and median survival observed for the mitomycin combination regimen (44%, 8.7 months) were identical to those of ECF. Given that there was no difference in efficacy for the epirubicin- versus mitomycin-containing arms, this study raises the question of whether or not the addition of a third agent makes a difference in outcome when combined with cisplatin and protracted infusion 5-FU. Of the 533 patients enrolled in this trial, 40 had squamous cell carcinoma of the esophagus and the remainder had adenocarcinoma (125, esophagus; 125, gastroesophageal junction; 243, stomach). There was a significantly higher response rate among patients with GEJ cancers than among those with distal gastric cancers (48% versus 37%).

Oxaliplatin, as a potential substitute for cisplatin, and oral capecitabine, as a substitute for 5-FU, have been explored in phase II trials[519] and, more recently, phase III randomized trials in esophageal and gastric adenocarcinoma (see Table 37.9). Cunningham et al.[520] reported results of a 1,000 patient phase III trial in esophageal squamous cell and adenocarcinoma and gastric cancer, evaluating the frontline use of oxaliplatin or capecitabine. This trial compared conventional ECF with the substitution of capecitabine for infusional 5-FU, and oxaliplatin for cisplatin. The trial employed a two-by-two design, with the control arm ECF, and the experimental arms including capecitabine (625 mg/m^2 twice daily) substituted for infusional 5-FU; oxaliplatin (130 mg/m^2) substituted for cisplatin; and a fourth arm with a substitution of both capecitabine and oxaliplatin. Capecitabine was found to be noninferior to 5-FU, and oxaliplatin noninferior to cisplatin, with comparable rates of antitumor response and progression-free survival across the four treatment arms. A toxicity analysis favored oxaliplatin over cisplatin for neutropenia, alopecia, renal toxicity, and thromboembolism. In a planned comparison of ECF to EOX (epirubicin, oxaliplatin, capecitabine), median survival was superior for EOX (11.2 months versus 9.9 months; HR, 0.80; $p = 0.02$). A second phase III trial from the German AIO group compared infusional 5-FU (24-hour infusion) plus leucovorin combined with either oxaliplatin (85 mg/m^2) or cisplatin (50 mg/m^2) once every 2 weeks in 220 patients with metastatic gastroesophageal adenocarcinoma.[521] Like the Cunningham et al. trial, oxaliplatin was found to be noninferior to cisplatin. Oxaliplatin caused significantly less nausea and vomiting, fatigue, renal toxicity, and thromboembolism. Remarkable on both arms of this trial was the relatively low level of grade 3 or 4 toxicities in all categories, running less than 10% to 15%, which was likely due to the 2 weekly schedule of chemotherapy mimicking colorectallike cancer scheduling of chemotherapy. Response rates (24.5% to 34.8%), progression-free (3.9 months versus 5.8 months), and overall survival (8.8 months versus 10.7 months) were comparable between the two treatment arms, although all end points trended higher on the oxaliplatin arm. Lastly, a third phase III trial reported by Kang et al.[522] compared capecitabine (1,000 mg/m^2) twice a day for 14 days to 5-FU (800 mg/m^2 per day continuous infusion) for 5 days, cycled every 3 weeks with cisplatin (80 mg/m^2). Like the Cunningham et al. trial, capecitabine was found to be noninferior to 5-FU. Rates of toxicity on the treatment arms were similar, as were measures of progression-free (5.0 months versus 5.6 months) and overall survival (9.3 months versus 10.5 months). Based on the results of these three phase III trials, the substitution of oxaliplatin for cisplatin, or capecitabine for 5-FU, seems justified. The two-drug regimens in the Al-Batran et al.[521] and Kang et al.[522] trials had favorable toxicity profiles and efficacy compared to the three drug regimens of Cunningham et al., and whether or not epirubicin is required as part of therapy in metastatic disease is unclear.

An alternative oral 5-FU agent, S-1, combines the 5-FU prodrug tegafur with a bowel protectant (oteracil) and an inhibitor of dihydropyrimidine dehydrogenase (gimeracil). A phase III trial conducted in Japan evaluated S-1 40 to 60 mg twice a day for 3 weeks as a single agent, versus S-1 plus cisplatin (60 mg/m^2), cycled once every 5 weeks, in advanced gastric cancer. S-1 plus cisplatin was superior to S-1 alone, with improved rates of response (54% versus 31%), progression-free (6 months versus 4 months), and overall survival (13 months versus 11 months).[523] Based on encouraging data for S-1, a phase III superiority trial comparing S-1 50 mg/m^2 in two daily divided doses for 21 days was compared to infusional 5-FU 1,000 mg/m^2 per day for 5 days, cycled every 28 days (see Table 37.9).[524] Both arms were combined with cisplatin, with a lower dose of cisplatin combined with S-1 (75 mg/m^2) compared to the 5-FU arm (100 mg/m^2). A lower dose of S-1 than that used in the Japanese trials was mandated due to greater toxicity for S-1 reported in Western patients in prior phase I and II trials. The trial failed to demonstrate superiority for the S-1 arm, with

equivalent rates of overall survival (7.9 months versus 8.6 months). The S-1 arm had less toxicity than 5-FU, but the lesser cisplatin dose likely accounted for much of the toxicity differences between the treatment arms. Whether S-1 will be adopted in practice in Western countries has yet to be established.

The addition of docetaxel as a third agent added to 5-FU and cisplatin has also recently been reported in a phase III trial of GEJ and gastric cancer (see Table 37.9). 5-FU dosed at 1,000 mg/m^2 by continuous infusion during 5 days combined with cisplatin (100 mg/m^2) was compared with cisplatin (75 mg/m^2), 5-FU (750 mg/m^2) by continuous infusion during 5 days, and docetaxel (75 mg/m^2) in 445 patients with metastatic gastric and GEJ adenocarcinoma.[525] Docetaxel resulted in a higher response rate and time to progression (36%, 5.6 months) compared with 5-FU and cisplatin (26%, 3.7 months), but only a marginal median survival improvement (0.6 months) was noted for three-drug therapy. Toxicity was substantial in both treatment arms, including hematologic and gastrointestinal toxicity, with 80% of patients receiving the three-drug combination experiencing grade 3 or 4 neutropenia. The recent trials of 5-FU infusion combination chemotherapy indicate improved therapy tolerance and potentially enhanced antitumor activity, employing either a once every 2 week or a more protracted infusion of 5-FU as in the ECF regimen. The addition of a third agent, including epirubicin or docetaxel, to 5-FU and cisplatin may modestly increase response rates and survival, but, in the case of docetaxel combination therapy, may result in substantial therapy-related toxicity. The use of relatively high and relatively toxic doses of cisplatin (75 to 100 mg/m^2) is also called into question, given data from the British phase III ECF trials that indicate potential better therapy tolerance for 60 mg/m^2 without evident compromising of treatment efficacy. The tolerance of a three-drug regimen may also be influenced by patient age. In a phase III trial targeting 143 patients with esophagogastric cancer 65 years or older, Al-Batran and colleagues[526] compared a regimen of biweekly infusional 5-FU and oxaliplatin with or without the addition of docetaxel (see Table 37.9). A higher response rate was reported for triplet therapy with no impact on overall survival, and resulted in much higher rates of toxicity and an actual detriment in quality of life measures compared to two-drug therapy.

Five trials using interferon-α_{2a} (IFN-α_{2a}) as a biomodulator of 5-FU suggested possible benefit.[527–531] These phase 2 trials combined IFN-α_{2a} with 5-FU and with cisplatin combined with continuous-infusion 5-FU, with response rates reported ranging from 27% to 50%, with a suggestion of higher response rates seen in squamous cell carcinoma. Etoposide and cisplatin with or without 5-FU have also undergone a phase II evaluation.[532–534] Combination regimens that include paclitaxel have been evaluated in esophageal cancer patients. In three phase II trials of paclitaxel and cisplatin, response rates ranged from 43% to 50%; activity was comparable in both histologic tumor types, often with severe hematologic toxicity.[535–537] A phase I trial of weekly carboplatin dosed from an area under the curve of 2 to 5 combined with a 1-hour infusion of paclitaxel, 100 mg/m^2, in 40 patients with advanced esophageal and GEJ cancer had an overall response rate of 54%.[538]

The three-drug combination of paclitaxel (175 mg/m^2, 3-hour infusion), combined with cisplatin (20 mg/m^2 daily days 1–5) and 5-FU (1,000 mg/m^2 per day continuous infusion × 120 hours) was evaluated in a multicenter 60 patient trial.[539] A 48% response rate was reported (56% in patients with squamous cell cancer and 46% in patients with adenocarcinoma). Toxicity resulted in unplanned hospitalizations for 48% of patients.

Although the dose and schedule of paclitaxel in combination with other active drugs varies among phase II trials, shorter infusion schedules of paclitaxel, in particular the weekly 1-hour schedule, result in less myelotoxicity.

Other regimens of interest include those containing irinotecan. First reported was the doublet of irinotecan and cisplatin administered in low dose on a weekly schedule.[540] In vitro studies demonstrated sequence-dependent synergy for cisplatin followed by irinotecan, which prevents the removal of cisplatin-induced DNA interstrand cross-links. Two trials yielded encouraging results (51% to

57% response) with a regimen of cisplatin (30 mg/m²) followed by irinotecan (65 mg/m²) administered weekly for 4 weeks, repeated every 6 weeks in adenocarcinoma and squamous cancer.[540,541] Dysphagia and global quality of life were improved in the majority of patients in one of these trials.[540] In both studies, toxicity consisted of myelosuppression, diarrhea, and fatigue. Irinotecan 50 mg/m² combined with weekly cisplatin 25 mg/m² and docetaxel 30 mg/m², days 1 and 8 every 21 days, was studied in a phase II trial in 39 patients with esophagogastric cancer.[542] An encouraging response rate of 54% was observed, with tolerable rates of grade 3 and 4 neutropenia (21%) and diarrhea (26%). However, a recent randomized phase II trial reported only in abstract form compared the chemotherapy regimens FOLFOX, irinotecan and cisplatin, and ECF, all combined with the EGFR-targeted agent cetuximab (Table 37.10).[543] The FOLFOX and ECF arms had similar response rates and overall survival, and the toxicity analysis favored the FOLFOX arm, and has led to further questioning of the contribution of epirubicin to a two-drug combination of oxaliplatin and a fluorinated pyrimidine. Notable, however, was the inferior performance of the irinotecan–cisplatin arm, which had the lowest rates of response and overall survival.

Recent studies exploring non–cisplatin-containing combination regimens have employed the taxanes and irinotecan. Although these trials have indicated encouraging response rates in the phase II setting, substantial hematologic and diarrheal toxicities of these regimens may not offer an advantage over the older cisplatin-containing regimens.[544–548] Docetaxel has been evaluated in combination with irinotecan in four recent phase II trials. Two trials evaluated irinotecan doses of 100 to 160 mg/m² and docetaxel doses of 50 to 60 mg/m² administered once every 3 weeks. Two trials evaluated the day 1 and day 8 schedule of irinotecan (50 to 55 mg/m²) and docetaxel (25 to 35 mg/m²) cycled every 3 weeks. Response rates range from 13 to 30 hematologic toxicity, which exceeded 50% in patients treated on the schedule of once every 3 weeks, seemed to be less using the day 1 and day 8 schedule compared with the once every 3 weeks schedule.

A phase III comparison of cisplatin and infusional 5-FU to the combination of irinotecan and infusional 5-FU was recently reported in advanced esophagogastric cancer (see Table 37.9).[549] Response rates (25.8% to 31.8%) and progression-free (4.2 months versus 5.0 months), and overall survival (8.7 months versus 9.0 months) were comparable for the two regimens. Toxicity favored the irinotecan 5-FU arm. Data from this trial and the oxaliplatin-based studies conducted in Europe have led to greater utilization of both irinotecan and oxaliplatin in combination with infusional 5-FU for the treatment of advanced esophagogastric cancer at European centers.

Docetaxel and either vinorelbine or capecitabine were evaluated in phase II trials in squamous cell carcinoma[550,551] with response rates of 46% to 60%. In summary, recent trials of combination regimens that include paclitaxel or irinotecan appear to have comparable response rates to previous regimens; however, the duration of response remains brief. In addition, the toxicities recorded in some of these phase II single-institution experiences have been excessive.

Targeted Agents

Phase III trials of targeted agents studied alone or in combination with chemotherapy are outlined in Table 37.10. Validation of the activity of a growth factor receptor–targeted agent, trastuzumab, was recently achieved in esophagogastric cancer (see Table 37.10).[552] Over 3,800 patients with gastric or GEJ adenocarcinoma were screened for overexpression of the HER2 receptor by fluorescence in situ hybridization (FISH) and immunohistochemistry; 22.1% tested positive. Five hundred ninety-four patients were ultimately randomized to chemotherapy alone with (1) capecitabine 1,000 mg/m² twice a day for 14 days or (2) infusional 5-FU 800 mg/m² per day for 5 days, combined with cisplatin 80 mg/m² on day 1, cycled every 3 weeks, or to chemotherapy plus trastuzumab 6 mg/kg once every 3 weeks. The majority of patients received capecitabine plus cisplatin as the chemotherapy regimen. All end points were improved with the addition of trastuzumab to chemotherapy, including antitumor response (47.3% versus 34.5%), progression-free survival (6.7 months versus 5.5 months), and overall survival (13.8 months versus 11.1 months) (HR, 0.74; $p = 0.0046$). Toxicity was comparable for the two

---

TABLE 37.10

Phase II–III Randomized Trials of Targeted Agents

Regimen	Patients (N)	Histologic Type	Response Rate (%)	Overall Survival (months)	Reference
Cape-C +/− trastuzumab	584	A	47 35	13.8 11.1	552
FOLFOX vs Irino-C vs ECF + cetuximab	210	A/S	54 46 58	12.4 8.9 11.5	561
EOX +/− panitumumab	553	A	46 42	8.8 11.3	562
Cape-C +/− cetuximab	904	A	29 29	10 10	563
5-FU–C +/− cetuximab	62	S	19 13	9.5 5.5	564
Cape-C +/− bevacizumab	774	A	46 37	12.1 10.1	566
Ramucirumab vs placebo	355	A	3 3	5.2 3.8	567
Everolimus vs placebo	656	A	4 2	5.4 4.3	568

Cape, capecitabine; C, cisplatin; A, adenocarcinoma; FOLFOX, 5-FU + oxaliplatin; Irino-C, irinotecan-cisplatin; ECF, epirubicin/cisplatin; S, squamous cell carcinoma; EOX, epirubicin/cisplatin or oxaliplatin/5-FU or capecitabine.

treatment arms, with no significant cardiotoxicity from trastuzumab other than an asymptomatic, less than 10% drop in left ventricular ejection fraction, which was slightly higher on the trastuzumab arm compared to chemotherapy alone (4.6% versus 1.1%). Based on these results, the inclusion of trastuzumab in the first-line treatment of HER2+ metastatic esophagogastric cancer should now be considered. Based on these data and pilot data combining trastuzumab with chemoradiotherapy in esophageal cancer RTOG has undertaken a phase III trial (RTOG-1010) comparing preoperative chemoradiotherapy with carboplatin and paclitaxel with or without trastuzumab in locally advanced adenocarcinoma of the esophagus and GEJ, as discussed previously.

In patients with localized esophageal adenocarcinoma, HER2+ disease was associated with a significantly lower tumor grade, earlier stage of disease with fewer malignant lymph nodes, and the presence of Barrett's esophagus. These features of HER2+ localized esophageal cancer led to an independent improvement in disease-specific survival (HR, 0.54; 95% CI, 0.35 to 0.84) and overall survival ($p = 0.0022$), suggesting that HER2+ is a favorable prognostic feature in localized esophageal adenocarcinoma.[553]

With evidence for effectiveness of agents targeting the EGFR in NSCLC (including receptor-associated tyrosine-kinase inhibitors) and in colorectal cancer (including monoclonal antibodies blocking the binding of the EGFR ligand), recent phase II trials have evaluated EGFR-targeted agents in esophageal squamous cell and adenocarcinoma. A recent phase II trial of the EGFR tyrosine-kinase inhibitor gefitinib failed to indicate activity for esophageal adenocarcinoma, but limited activity was observed in squamous cell cancer.[554] A second trial indicated some limited activity for adenocarcinoma,[555] but in both trials, most patients experienced early disease progression. A phase II trial of the EGFR tyrosine-kinase inhibitor erlotinib reported a 9% response rate in 44 patients with adenocarcinoma of the GEJ.[556] With these mixed phase II trial results, a recent negative trial for an EGFR tyrosine-kinase inhibitor was reported only in abstract form by Dutton et al.[557] The trial compared best supportive care to treatment with gefitinib in patients with esophageal and GEJ adenocarcinomas progressing on conventional chemotherapy. In this large trial, no difference in overall survival could be demonstrated for gefitinib compared to supportive care alone.

Monoclonal antibodies targeting the EGFR, including cetuximab and panitumumab, have proceeded to phase III trial investigation combined with chemotherapy, based on promising data from phase II trials.[558–560] The randomized phase II trial conducted by the CALGB and ECOG evaluated three modern chemotherapy regimens combined with cetuximab in the first-line treatment of esophageal and GEJ cancer (see Table 37.10),[561] and was discussed previously. The regimens used were weekly irinotecan–cisplatin, ECF, and FOLFOX (5-FU, leucovorin, and oxaliplatin). The trial indicated comparable response rates, progression-free survival, and overall survival for the FOLFOX and ECF plus cetuximab arms, whereas the irinotecan–cisplatin arm was inferior. The final results of this study may not contribute much to the debate about EGFR-targeted agents, because two large phase III trials of these agents combined with chemotherapy failed to improve outcomes. Waddell and colleagues[562] reported results of the REAL-3 trial in esophagogastric cancer, comparing patient treatment with EOX with or without the EGFR antibody panitumumab (see Table 37.10).[562] In the 553 patients treated, although response rates for treatment with or without panitumumab were similar, overall survival was significantly inferior on the panitumumab arm (11.3 versus 8.8 months) and progression-free survival trended inferior for panitumumab (7.4 versus 6.0 months). Toxicity rates were higher on the panitumumab arm, and the chemotherapy starting doses were lower with panitumumab than on the chemotherapy alone arm. Prognostic biomarkers studied on the trial included *KRAS* mutation, *PIK3CA* kinase mutation, and loss of phosphatase and tensin homolog (PTEN). These markers were affected in a tiny minority of patients, and no clear biomarker has emerged from this trial. The potential deleterious effect of adding an EGFR anti-

body to the treatment of esophagogastric cancer was also seen in a recent chemoradiotherapy trial, discussed earlier, in which adding cetuximab to definitive chemoradiotherapy in esophageal cancer also appeared to worsen outcomes.[349] A second negative trial for EGFR-targeted antibodies in advanced disease was reported by Lordick et al. (see Table 37.10).[563] The 904 patients with esophagogastric cancer were randomized to treatment with capecitabine and cisplatin with or without cetuximab. Progression-free survival and overall survival also trended inferior on the cetuximab arm (progression-free survival, 5.6 versus 4.4 months; overall survival, 10.7 versus 9.4 months), and response rates were identical (29%). In contrast to these negative trials, Lorenzen et al.[564] reported results of a small phase II trial in advanced squamous cancer of the esophagus comparing 5-FU–cisplatin with or without cetuximab (see Table 37.10). Outcomes were poor on both arms of the trial; however, response rates and overall survivals were improved on the cetuximab arm (19% versus 13%; 9.5 months versus 5.5 months). A larger phase III trial in squamous cancer of the esophagus is now ongoing (NCT01627379) to evaluate panitumumab combined with 5-FU and cisplatin. RTOG-0436, adding cetuximab to primary chemoradiotherapy in locally advanced esophageal cancer,[350] was discussed earlier, and was also a negative trial for the addition of EGFR-targeted therapy.

Another growth factor receptor pathway under active investigation is the vascular endothelial growth factor (VEGF) receptor pathway, based on trials that demonstrate improved effectiveness for chemotherapy in colorectal cancer when combined with the anti–VEGF-A ligand monoclonal antibody bevacizumab. A recent phase II trial combined bevacizumab at a dose of 15 mg/kg every 3 weeks in combination with a day 1 and day 8 schedule of irinotecan (65 mg/m^2) and cisplatin (30 mg/m^2).[565] The multicenter trial treated 47 patients treated with metastatic adenocarcinoma of the GEJ and more distal gastric cancer. An encouraging response rate of 65% was observed, with a suggestion of improvement in time to tumor progression (8.9 months) compared with historical controls. A phase III trial combining bevacizumab with either 5-FU or capecitabine plus cisplatin in 774 patients with esophagogastric adenocarcinoma was recently reported by Ohtsu and colleagues (see Table 37.10).[566] Despite improvements in progression-free survival (5.3 to 6.7 months) and response rate (37% to 46%), a trend toward improvement in overall survival did not reach statistical significance (10.1 to 12.1 months; HR, 0.87; $p = 0.1002$). Another VEGF-targeted agent, ramucirumab, which blocks ligand binding to the receptor VEGF2, indicated a positive effectiveness in refractory esophagogastric cancer compared to placebo.[567] Fuchs and colleagues[567] randomized 355 patients progressing on 5-FU or platinum-based chemotherapy to best supportive care plus placebo versus best supportive care plus ramucirumab administered once every 2 weeks. Although no significant antitumor responses were seen, overall survival was significantly improved with ramucirumab (3.8 to 5.2 months) and toxicity was limited to a slight increase in hypertension. Results for studies of the combination of ramucirumab with chemotherapy in first- or second-line treatment are pending publication. The positive results for ramucirumab have led to a resurgent interest in the study of VEGF-targeted agents in esophageal cancer.

Finally, a recent large, placebo-controlled trial in chemotherapy refractory esophagogastric cancer compared placebo to the mammalian target of rapamycin (mTOR)–targeted agent everolimus in 656 patients (see Table 37.10).[568] Although progression-free survival was slightly improved with everolimus, there was no improvement in overall survival (5.4 months for everolimus versus 4.3 months for placebo).

STAGE-DIRECTED TREATMENT RECOMMENDATIONS

Although level I evidence is lacking to support ironclad recommendations regarding the most effective treatment of patients grouped by stage in many clinical situations, reasonable trial-generated information exists to suggest appropriate therapeutic interventions for patients grouped under broad staging categories.

Resection remains the standard by which all other treatment options must be measured for patients with high-grade dysplasia in the setting of Barrett's esophagus or T1 disease limited to the mucosa, with the caveat that esophagectomy-associated mortality must be extremely low. EMR may be considered an appropriate first step in addressing patients with mucosa-limited lesions. Intensive long-term endoscopic surveillance for patients with Barrett's esophagus–associated high-grade dysplasia is necessary to limit both cancer- and treatment-related mortality.

An esophagectomy is an appropriate method for treating patients with stage I, II, and III disease. Alternatively, definitive chemoradiation is a therapeutic option for patients with stage II and III disease, especially those who are not considered surgical candidates or who have squamous cell carcinoma at or above the carina. The high rate of persistent or recurrent local–regional disease after definitive chemoradiation suggests that additional local therapy in the form of surgery may be necessary and beneficial. This potential benefit may be realized only if perioperative mortality is minimized. Preoperative chemoradiation has been proven to be more effective than surgery alone, and is now appropriately embraced by US oncologists for patients with resectable stage IIB and III esophageal cancers. Defining more effective regimens must continue to be the focus of well-designed clinical trials. Postoperative chemoradiation should be reserved for patients with resected adenocarcinoma of the GEJ. Preoperative chemotherapy is an accepted standard of care in the United Kingdom but is still considered investigational in the United States. All patients with unresectable or stage IV disease are ideally suited for clinical trials exploring novel therapeutic agents and approaches.

REFERENCES

1. Brown L, Devesa S. Epidemiologic trends in esophageal and gastric cancer in the United States. *Surg Oncol Clin North Am* 2002;11:235–256.
2. Brown LM, Devesa S, Fraumeni JF. Epidemiology of esophageal cancer. In: Posner M, Vokes EE, Weichselbaum RR, eds. *Cancer of the Upper Gastrointestinal Tract*. Hamilton, Ontario: BC Decker; 2002:1.
3. Howlader N, Noone AM, Krapcho M, et al. (eds). SEER Cancer Statistics Review, 1975–2010. Bethesda, MD: National Cancer Institute. SEER Web site. http://seer.cancer.gov/csr/1975_2010/. April 2013.
4. Siegel R, Naishadham D, Jemal A. Cancer Statistics, 2013. *CA Cancer J Clin* 2013;63:11–30.
5. Schottenfeld D. Epidemiology of cancer of the esophagus. *Semin Oncol* 1984;11:92–100.
6. Brown LM, Hoover R, Silverman D, et al. Excess incidence of squamous cell esophageal cancer among US black men: role of social class and other risk factors. *Am J Epidemiol* 2001;153:114–122.
7. Kabat GC, Ng SK, Wynder EL. Tobacco, alcohol intake, and diet in relation to adenocarcinoma of the esophagus and gastric cardia. *Cancer Causes Control* 1993;4:123–132.
8. Gammon MD, Schoenberg JB, Ahsan H, et al. Tobacco, alcohol, and socioeconomic status and adenocarcinomas of the esophagus and gastric cardia. *J Natl Cancer Inst* 1997;89:1277–1284.
9. Cook MB, Shaheen NJ, Anderson LA, et al. Cigarette smoking increases risk of Barrett's esophagus: an analysis of the Barrett's and Esophageal Adenocarcinoma Consortium. *Gastroenterology* 2012;142:744–753.
10. Castellsague X, Munoz N, De Stefani E, et al. Independent and joint effects of tobacco smoking and alcohol drinking on the risk of esophageal cancer in men and women. *Int J Cancer* 1999;82:657–664.
11. Castellsague X, Munoz N, De Stefani E, et al. Smoking and drinking cessation and risk of esophageal cancer (Spain). *Cancer Causes Control* 2000;11:813–818.
12. Pandeya N, Williams G, Green AC, et al. Alcohol consumption and the risks of adenocarcinoma and squamous cell carcinoma of the esophagus. *Gastroenterology* 2009;136:1215–1224.
13. Munoz N, Day NE. Esophageal cancer. In: Schottenfeld D, Fracmeni JF, eds. *Cancer Epidemiology and Prevention*. New York: Oxford University Press; 1996:681.
14. Qiao Y, Dawsey S, Kamangar F, et al. Total and cancer mortality after supplementation with vitamins and minerals: follow-up of the Linxian general population nutrition intervention trial. *J Natl Cancer Inst* 2009;101:507–518.
15. Castellsague X, Munoz N, De Stefani E, et al. Influence of mate drinking, hot beverages and diet on esophageal cancer risk in South America. *Int J Cancer* 2000;88:658–664.
16. Bravi F, Edefonti V, Randi G, et al. Dietary patterns and the risk of esophageal cancer. *Ann Oncol* 2012;23:765–770.
17. Gorey K, Vena JE. Cancer differentials among US blacks and whites: quantitative estimates of socioeconomic-related risks. *J Natl Med Assoc* 1994;86:209–215.
18. National Center for Health Statistics. *Health, United States 2000, with Adolescent Health Chartbook*. Hyattsville, MD: NCHS; 2000.
19. Vaughan TL, Davis S, Kristal A, et al. Obesity, alcohol, and tobacco as risk factors for cancers of the esophagus and gastric cardia: adenocarcinoma versus squamous cell carcinoma. *Cancer Epidemiol Biomarkers Prev* 1995;4:85–92.
20. Brown LM, Swanson CA, Gridley G, et al. Adenocarcinoma of the esophagus: role of obesity and diet. *J Natl Cancer Inst* 1995;87:104–109.
21. Chow WH, Blot WH, Vaughan TL, et al. Body mass index and risk of adenocarcinomas of the esophagus and gastric cardia. *J Natl Cancer Inst* 1998;90:150–155.
22. Edelstein ZR, Farrow DC, Bonner MP, et al. Central adiposity and risk of Barrett's esophagus. *Gastroenterology* 2007;133:403–411.
23. Ryan AM, Duong M, Healy L, et al. Obesity, metabolic syndrome and esophageal adenocarcinoma: epidemiology, etiology and new targets. *Cancer Epidemiol* 2011;35:309–319.
24. Lagergren J. Influence of obesity on the risk of esophageal disorders. *Nat Rev Gastroenterol Hepatol* 2011;8:340–347.
25. Lagergren J, Bergstrom R, Lindgren A, et al. Symptomatic gastroesophageal reflux as a risk factor for esophageal adenocarcinoma. *N Engl J Med* 1999;340:825–831.
26. Chow WH, Finkle WD, McLaughlin JK, et al. The relation of gastroesophageal reflux disease and its treatment to adenocarcinomas of the esophagus and gastric cardia. *JAMA* 1995;274:474–477.
27. Islami F, Kamangar F. *Helicobacter pylori* and esophageal cancer risk: a meta-analysis. *Cancer Prev Res (Phila)* 2008;1:329–338.
28. Kamangar F, Dawsey SM, Blaser MJ, et al. Opposing risks of gastric cardia and noncardiac gastric adenocarciomas associated with *Helicobacter pylori* seropositivity. *J Natl Can Inst* 2006;98:1445–1452.
29. Ye W, Held M, Lagergren J, et al. *Helicobacter pylori* infection and gastric atrophy: risk of adenocarcinoma and squamous cell carcinoma of the esophagus and adenocarcinoma of the gastric cardia. *J Natl Can Inst* 2004;96:388–396.
30. Cameron AJ. Management of Barrett's esophagus. *Mayo Clin Proc* 1998;73:457–461.
31. Spechler SJ. Clinical practice. Barrett's esophagus. *N Engl J Med* 2002;346:836–842.
32. Sampliner RE. Updated guidelines for the diagnosis, surveillance, and therapy of Barrett's esophagus. *Am J Gastroenterol* 2002;97:1888–1895
33. Spechler SJ. Barrett esophagus and risk of esophageal cancer: a clinical review. *JAMA* 2013;310:627–636.
34. Desai TK, Krishnan K, Samala N, et al. The incidence of oesophageal adenocarcinoma in non-dysplastic Barrett's oesophagus: a meta-analysis. *Gut* 2012;61:970–976.
35. Bhat S, Coleman HG, Yousef F, et al. Risk of malignant progression in Barrett's esophagus patients: results from a large population-based study. *J Natl Cancer Inst* 2011;103:1049–1057.
36. Hvid-Jensen F, Pedersen L, Drewes AM, et al. Incidence of adenocarcinoma among patients with Barrett's esophagus. *N Engl J Med* 2011;365:1375–1383.
37. Rudolph RE, Vaughn TL, Storer BE, et al. Effect of segment length on risk for neoplastic progression in patients with Barrett esophagus. *Ann Intern Med* 2000;132:612–620.
38. Ronkainen J, Aro P, Storskrubb T, et al. Prevalence of Barrett's esophagus in the general population: an endoscopic study. *Gastroenterology* 2005;129:1825–1831.
39. Dulai GS, Guha S, Kahn KL, et al. Preoperative prevalence of Barrett's esophagus in esophageal adenocarcinoma: a systematic review. *Gastroenterology* 2002;122:26–33.
40. Spechler SJ, Sharma P, Souza RF, et al. American Gastroenterological Association. American Gastroenterological Association medical position statement on the management of Barrett's esophagus. *Gastroenterology* 2011;140:1084–1091.
41. Katz PO, Gerson LB, Vela MF. Guidelines for the diagnosis and management of gastroesophageal reflux disease. *Am J Gastroenterol* 2013;108:308–328.
42. Evans JA, Early DS, Fukami N, et al. Standards of Practice Committee of the American Society for Gastrointestinal Endoscopy. The role of endoscopy in Barrett's esophagus and other premalignant conditions of the esophagus. *Gastrointest Endosc* 2012;76:1087–1094.
43. Spechler SJ, Lee E, Ahnen D, et al. Long-term outcome of medical and surgical therapies for gastroesophageal reflux disease: follow-up of a randomized controlled trial. *JAMA* 2001;285:2331–2338.
44. Chang LC, Oelschlager BK, Quiroga E, et al. Long-term outcome of esophagectomy for high-grade dysplasia or cancer found during surveillance for Barrett's esophagus. *Gastrointest Surg* 2006;10:341–346.
45. Corley DA, Levin TR, Habel LA, et al. Surveillance and survival in Barrett's adenocarcinomas: a population-based study. *Gastroenterology* 2002;122:633–640.
46. Ferguson MK, Durkin A. Long-term survival after esophagectomy for Barrett's adenocarcinoma in endoscopically surveyed and nonsurveyed patients. *J Gastrointest Surg* 2002;6:29–35.

47. O'Connor JB, Falk GW, Richter JE. The incidence of adenocarcinoma and dysplasia in Barrett's esophagus: report on the Cleveland Clinic Barrett's Esophagus Registry. *Am J Gastroenterol* 1999;94:2037–2042.

48. van der Burgh A, Dees J, Hop WC, et al. Oesophageal cancer is an uncommon cause of death in patients with Barrett's oesophagus. *Gut* 1996;39:5–8.

49. Macdonald CE, Wicks AC, Playford RJ. Final results from 10 year cohort of patients undergoing surveillance for Barrett's oesophagus: observational study. *BMJ* 2000;321:1252–1255.

50. DeMeester SR, DeMeester TR. Columnar mucosa and intestinal metaplasia of the esophagus: fifty years of controversy. *Ann Surg* 2000;231:303–321.

51. Gurski RR, Peters JH, Hagen JA, et al. Barrett's esophagus can and does regress after antireflux surgery: a study of prevalence and predictive features. *J Am Coll Surg* 2003;196:706–712.

52. Faybush EM, Sampliner RE. Randomized trials in the treatment of Barrett's esophagus. *Dis Esophagus* 2005;18:291–297.

53. Singh S, Garg SK, Singh PP, et al. Acid-suppressive medications and risk of oesophageal adenocarcinoma in patients with Barrett's oesophagus: a systematic review and meta-analysis. *Gut* 2013;Nov 12 [Epub ahead of print].

54. Haggitt RC. Barrett's esophagus, dysplasia, and adenocarcinoma. *Hum Pathol* 1994;25:982–993.

55. Skacel M, Petras RE, Gramlich TL, et al. The diagnosis of low-grade dysplasia in Barrett's esophagus and its implications for disease progression. *Am J Gastroenterol* 2000;95:3383–3387.

56. Montgomery E, Bronner MP, Goldblum JR, et al. Reproducibility of the diagnosis of dysplasia in Barrett esophagus: a reaffirmation. *Hum Pathol* 2001;32:368–378.

57. Buttar NS, Wang KK, Leontovich O, et al. Chemoprevention of esophageal adenocarcinoma by COX-2 inhibitors in an animal model of Barrett's esophagus. *Gastroenterology* 2002;122:1101–1112.

58. Maley C. Multistage carciogenesis in Barrett's esophagus. *Cancer Lett* 2007;245:22–32.

59. Heath E, Canto MI, Piantadosi S, et al. Secondary chemoprevention of Barrett's esophagus with celecoxib: results of a randomized trial. *J Natl Cancer Inst* 2007;99:545–557.

60. Ashworth MT, Nash JR, Ellis A, et al. Abnormalities of differentiation and maturation in the oesophageal squamous epithelium of patients with tylosis: morphological features. *Histopathology* 1991;19:303–310.

61. Risk JM, Mills HS, Garde J, et al. The tylosis esophageal cancer (TOC) locus: more than just a familial cancer gene. *Dis Esophagus* 1999;12:173–176.

62. Risk JM, Field EA, Field JK, et al. Tylosis oesophageal cancer mapped. *Nat Genet* 1994;8:319–321.

63. von Brevern M, Hollstein MC, Risk JM, et al. Loss of heterozygosity in sporadic oesophageal tumors in the tylosis oesophageal cancer (TOC) gene region of chromosome 17q. *Oncogene* 1998;17:2101–2105.

64. Iwaya T, Maesawa C, Ogasawara S, et al. Tylosis esophageal cancer locus on chromosome 17q25.1 is commonly deleted in sporadic human esophageal cancer. *Gastroenterology* 1998;114:1206–1210.

65. Risk JM. Envoplakin, a possible candidate gene for focal NEPPK/esophageal cancer (TOC): the integration of genetic and physical maps of the TOC region on 17q25. *Genomics* 1999;59:234–242.

66. Shamma'A MH, Benedict EB. Esophageal webs; a report of 58 cases & an attempt at classification. *N Engl J Med* 1958;259:378–384.

67. Ribeiro U Jr, Posner MC, Safatle-Ribeiro AV, et al. Risk factors for squamous cell carcinoma of the oesophagus. *Br J Surg* 1996;83:1174–1185.

68. Csikos M, Horvath O, Petri A, et al. Late malignant transformation of chronic corrosive oesophageal strictures. *Langenbecks Arch Chir* 1985;365:231–238.

69. Sandler RS, Nyren O, Ekbon A, et al. The risk of esophageal cancer in patients with achalasia. A population-based study. *JAMA* 1995;274:1359–1362.

70. Meijssen MA, Tilanus HW, van Blankenstein M, et al. Achalasia complicated by oesophageal squamous cell carcinoma: a prospective study in 195 patients. *Gut* 1992;33:155–158.

71. Aggestrup S, Holm JC, Sorensen HR. Does achalasia predispose to cancer of the esophagus? *Chest* 1992;102:1013–1016.

72. Loviscek LF, Cenoz MC, Badaloni AE, et al. Early cancer in achalasia. *Dis Esophagus* 1998;11:239–247.

73. Sur M, Cooper K. The role of the human papilloma virus in esophageal cancer. *Pathology* 1998;30:348–354.

74. de Villiers EM, Lavergne D, Chang F, et al. An interlaboratory study to determine the presence of human papillomavirus DNA in esophageal carcinoma from China. *Int J Cancer* 1999;81:225–228.

75. Lavergne D, de Villiers EM. Papillomavirus in esophageal papillomas and carcinomas. *Int J Cancer* 1999;80:681–684.

76. Shibagaki I, Tanaka H, Shimada Y, et al. p53 mutation, murine double minute 2 amplification, and human papillomavirus infection are frequently involved but not associated with each other in esophageal squamous cell carcinoma. *Clin Cancer Res* 1995;1:769–773.

77. Poljak M, Cerar A, Seme K. Human papillomavirus infection in esophageal carcinomas: a study of 121 lesions using multiple broad-spectrum polymerase chain reactions and literature review. *Hum Pathol* 1998;29:266–271.

78. Rugge M, Bovo D, Busatto G, et al. p53 alterations but no human papillomavirus infection in preinvasive and advanced squamous esophageal cancer in Italy. *Cancer Epidemiol Biomark Prev* 1997;6:171–176.

79. Turner JR, Shen LH, Crum CP, et al. Low prevalence of human papillomavirus infection in esophageal squamous cell carcinomas from North America: analysis by a highly sensitive and specific polymerase chain reaction-based approach. *Hum Pathol* 1997;28:174–178.

80. Lagergren J, Wang Z, Bergstrom R, et al. Human papillomavirus infection and esophageal cancer: a nationwide seroepidemiologic case-control study in Sweden. *J Natl Cancer Inst* 1999;91:156–162.

81. Siewert JR, Feith M, Werner M, et al. Adenocarcinoma of the esophagogastric junction. Results of surgical therapy based on anatomic-topographic classification in 1,002 consecutive patients. *Ann Surg* 2000;232:353–361.

82. Leon X, Quer M, Diez S, et al. Second neoplasm in patients with head and neck cancer. *Head Neck* 1999;21:204–210.

83. Levi F, Randimbison L, Te VC, et al. Second primary cancers in patients with lung carcinoma. *Cancer* 1999;86:186–190.

84. Narayana A, Vaughan AT, Fisher SG, et al. Second primary tumors in laryngeal cancer: results of long-term follow-up. *Int J Radiat Oncol Biol Phys* 1998;42:557–562.

85. Ribeiro U, Safatle-Ribeiro AV, Posner MC, et al. Comparative p53 mutational analysis of multiple primary cancers of the upper aerodigestive tract. *Surgery* 1996;120:45–53.

86. Dulak AM, Schumacher SE, van Lieshout J, et al. Gastrointestinal adenocarcinomas of the esophagus, stomach, and colon exhibit distinct patterns of genome instability and oncogenesis. *Cancer Res* 2012;72:4383–4393.

87. Dulak AM, Stojanov P, Peng S, et al. Exome and whole genome sequencing of esophageal adenocarcinoma identifies recurrent driver events and mutational complexity. *Nat Genet* 2013;5:478–486.

88. Agrawal N, Jiao Y, Bettegowda C, et al. Comparative genomic analysis of esophageal adenocarcinoma and squamous cell carcinoma. *Cancer Discov* 2012;2:899–905.

89. American Joint Commission on Cancer. *AJCC Cancer Staging Manual.* 6th ed. New York: Springer Verlag; 2002.

90. Edge SB, Byrd DR, Compton CC, et al. American Joint Commission on Cancer. *AJCC Cancer Staging Manual.* 7th ed. New York: Springer-Verlag; 2009.

91. Hagen JA, DeMeester SR, Peters JH, et al. Curative resection for esophageal adenocarcinoma. Analysis of 100 en bloc esophagectomies. *Ann Surg* 2001;234:520–530.

92. Altorki NK, Girardi L, Skinner DB. En bloc esophagectomy improves survival for stage III esophageal cancer. *J Thorac Cardiovasc Surg* 1997;114:948–955.

93. Akiyama H, Tsurumaru M, Udagawa H, et al. Radical lymph node dissection for cancer of the thoracic esophagus. *Ann Surg* 1994;220:364–372.

94. Altorki N, Kent M, Ferrara C, et al. Three-field lymph node dissection for squamous cell and adenocarcinoma of the esophagus. *Ann Surg* 2002;236:177–183.

95. Feith M, Stein JH, Siewert JR. Pattern of lymphatic spread of Barrett's cancer. *World J Surg* 2003;27:1052–1057.

96. Kitagawa Y, Fujii H, Mukai M, et al. Intraoperative lymphatic mapping and sentinel lymph node sampling in esophageal and gastric cancer. *Surg Oncol Clin North Am* 2002;11:293–304.

97. Blot WJ. Epidemiology and genesis of esophageal cancer. In: Roth J, Ruckdeschel JC, Weisenburger TH, eds. *Thoracic Oncology.* Philadelphia PA: WB Saunders; 1995.

98. Medgyesy CD, Wolff RA, Putnam JB Jr, et al. Small cell carcinoma of the esophagus: the University of Texas M. D. Anderson Cancer Center experience and literature review. *Cancer* 2000;88:262–267.

99. Maier A, Woltsche M, Fell B, et al. Local and systemic treatment in small cell carcinoma of the esophagus. *Oncol Rep* 2000;7:187–192.

100. Kimura H, Konishi K, Maeda K, et al. Highly aggressive behavior and poor prognosis of small-cell carcinoma in the alimentary tract: flow-cytometric analysis and immunohistochemical staining for the p53 protein and proliferating cell nuclear antigen. *Dig Surg* 1999;16:152–157.

101. Ilson DH, Minsky BD, Ku GY, et al. Phase 2 trial of induction and concurrent chemoradiotherapy with weekly irinotecan and cisplatin followed by surgery for esophageal cancer. *Cancer* 2012;118:2820–2827.

102. Daly JM, Karnell LH, Menck HR. National cancer database report on esophageal carcinoma. *Cancer* 1996;78:1820–1828.

103. Mariette C, Balon JM, Piessen G, et al. Pattern of recurrence following complete resection of esophageal carcinoma and factors predictive of recurrent disease. *Cancer* 2003;97:1616–1623.

104. Katayama A, Mafune K, Tanaka Y, et al. Autopsy findings in patients after curative esophagectomy for esophageal carcinoma. *J Am Coll Surg* 2003;196:866–873.

105. Kelsen DP, Ginsberg R, Pajak RF, et al. Chemotherapy followed by surgery compared with surgery alone for localized esophageal cancer. *N Engl J Med* 1998;339:1979–1984.

106. Medical Research Council Oesophageal Cancer Working Group. Surgical resection with or without preoperative chemotherapy in oesophageal cancer: a randomised controlled trial. *Lancet* 2002;359:1727–1733.

107. Urba SG, Orringer MB, Turrisi A, et al. Randomized trial of preoperative chemoradiation versus surgery alone in patients with locoregional esophageal carcinoma. *J Clin Oncol* 2001;19:305–313.

108. O'Sullivan G, Sheehan D, Clarke A, et al. Micrometastases in esophagogastric cancer: high detection rate in resected rib segments. *Gastroenterology* 1999;116:543–548.

109. Bonavina L, Soligo D, Quirici N, et al. Bone marrow-disseminated tumor cells in patients with carcinoma of the esophagus or cardia. *Surgery* 2001;129:15–22.

110. Arnott SJ, Duncan W, Gignoux M, et al. Preoperative radiotherapy in esophageal carcinoma: a meta-analysis using individual patient data (Oesophageal Cancer Collaborative Group). *Int J Radiat Oncol Biol Phys* 1998;41:579–583.

111. Kleinberg L, Knisely J, Heitmiller R, et al. Mature survival results with preoperative cisplatin, protracted infusion 5-fluorouracil, and 44-Gy radiotherapy for esophageal cancer. *Int J Radiat Oncol Biol Phys* 2003;56:328–334.

CANCERS OF THE GASTROINTESTINAL TRACT

112. Kelsen DP, Winter KA, Gunderson LL, et al. Long-term results of RTOG Trial 8911 (USA Intergroup 113): a random assignment trial comparison of chemotherapy followed by surgery compared with surgery alone for esophageal cancer. *J Clin Oncol* 2007;25:3719–3725.

113. Allum WH, Stenning SP, Bancewicz J, et al. Long term results of a randomized trial of surgery with or without preoperative chemotherapy in esophageal cancer. *J Clin Oncol* 2009;27:5062–5067.

114. Cooper JS, Guo MD, Herskovic A, et al. Chemoradiotherapy of locally advanced esophageal cancer: long-term follow-up of a prospective randomized trial (RTOG 85–01). Radiation Therapy Oncology Group. *JAMA* 1999;281:1623–1627.

115. Denham JW, Steigler A, Kilmurray J, et al. Relapse patterns after chemoradiation for carcinoma of the oesophagus. *Clin Oncol (R Coll Radiol)* 2003;15:98–108.

116. Bedenne L, Michel P, Bouche O, et al. Chemoradiation followed by surgery compared to chemoradiation alone in squamous cancer of the esophagus: FFCD 9102. *J Clin Oncol* 2007;25:1160–1168.

117. Stahl M, Stuschke M, Lehmann N, et al. Chemoradiation with and without surgery in patients with locally advanced squamous cell carcinoma of the esophagus. *J Clin Oncol* 2005;23:2310–2317.

118. Cusso X, Mones-Xiol J, Vilardell F. Endoscopic cytology of cancer of the esophagus and cardia: a long-term evaluation. *Gastrointest Endosc* 1989;35:321–323.

119. Zargar SA, Khuroo MS, Jan GM, et al. Prospective comparison of the value of brushings before and after biopsy in the endoscopic diagnosis of gastroesophageal malignancy. *Acta Cytol* 1991;35:549–552.

120. Jung M, Kiesslich R. Chromoendoscopy and intravital staining techniques. *Baillieres Best Pract Res Clin Gastroenterol* 1999;13:11–19.

121. Acosta MM, Boyce HW Jr. Chromoendoscopy—where is it useful? *J Clin Gastroenterol* 1998;27:13–20.

122. Kara M, Peters FP, Fockens P, et al. Endoscopic video-autofluorescence imaging followed by narrow band imaging for detecting early neoplasia in Barrett's esophagus. *Gastrointest Endosc* 2006;64:176–185.

123. Sharma P, Bansal A, Mathur S, et al. The utility of a novel narrow band imaging endoscopy system in patients with Barrett's esophagus. *Gastrointest Endosc* 2006;64:167–175.

124. Ross AS, Noffsinger A, Waxman I. Narrow band imaging directed EMR for Barrett's esophagus with high-grade dysplasia. *Gastrointest Endosc* 2007;65:166–169.

125. Wolfson HC, Crook JE, Krisha M, et al. Prospective, controlled tandem endoscopy study of narrow band imaging for dysplasia detection in Barrett's esophagus. *Gastroenterology* 2008;135:24–31.

126. Gollub MJ, Lefkowitz R, Moskowitz CS, et al. Pelvic CT in patients with esophageal cancer. *AJR Am J Roentgenol* 2005;184:487–490.

127. Lea JW, Prager RL, Bender HW Jr. The questionable role of computed tomography in preoperative staging of esophageal cancer. *Ann Thorac Surg* 1984;38:479–481.

128. Quint LE, Glazer GM, Orringer MB. Esophageal imaging by MR and CT: study of normal anatomy and neoplasms. *Radiology* 1985;156:727–731.

129. Watt I, Stewart I, Anderson D, et al. Laparoscopy, ultrasound and computed tomography in cancer of the oesophagus and gastric cardia: a prospective comparison for detecting intra-abdominal metastases. *Br J Surg* 1989;76:1036–1039.

130. Becker CD, Barbier P, Porcellini B. CT evaluation of patients undergoing tranhiatal esophagectomy for cancer. *J Comput Assist Tomogr* 1986;10:607–611.

131. Vilgrain V, Mompoint D, Palazzo L, et al. Staging of esophageal carcinoma: comparison of results with endoscopic sonography and CT. *Am J Roentgenol* 1990;155:277–281.

132. Picus D, Balfe D, Koehler RE, et al. Computed tomography in the staging of esophageal carcinoma. *Radiology* 1983;146:433–438.

133. Yoon YC, Lee KS, Shim YM, et al. Metastasis to regional lymph nodes in patients with esophageal squamous cell carcinoma: CT versus FDG PET for presurgical detection prospective study. *Radiology* 2003;227:764–770.

134. Romagnuolo J, Scott J, Hawes RH, et al. Helical CT versus EUS with fine needle aspiration for celiac nodal assessment in patients with esophageal cancer. *Gastrointest Endosc* 2002;55:648–654.

135. Aibe T, Fuji T, Okita K, et al. A fundamental study of normal layer structure of the gastrointestinal wall visualized by endoscopic ultrasonography. *Scand J Gastroenterol Suppl* 1986;123:6–15.

136. Tio TL, den Hartog Jager FC, Tytgat GN. The role of endoscopic ultrasonography in assessing local resectability of oesophagogastric malignancies. Accuracy, pitfalls, and predictability. *Scand J Gastroenterol Suppl* 1986;123:78–86.

137. Aibe T, Ito T, Yoshida T, et al. Endoscopic ultrasonography of lymph nodes surrounding the upper GI tract. *Scand J Gastroenterol Suppl* 1986;123:164–169.

138. Catalano MF, Sivak MV Jr, Rice T, et al. Endosonographic features predictive of lymph node metastasis. *Gastrointest Endosc* 1994;40:442–446.

139. Botet JF, Lightdale CJ, Zauber AG, et al. Preoperative staging of gastric cancer: comparison of endoscopic US and dynamic CT. *Radiology* 1991;181:426–432.

140. Tio TL, Cohen P, Coene PP, et al. Endosonography and computed tomography of esophageal carcinoma. Preoperative classification compared to the new (1987) TNM system. *Gastroenterology* 1989;96:1478–1486.

141. Rosch T. Endosonographic staging of esophageal cancer: a review of literature results. *Gastrointest Endosc Clin North Am* 1995;5:537–547.

142. Vazquez-Sequeiros E, Norton ID, Cain JE, et al. Impact of EUS-guided fine-needle aspiration on lymph node staging in patients with esophageal carcinoma. *Gastrointest Endosc* 2001;53:751–757.

143. O'Toole D, Palazzo L, Arotcarena R, et al. Assessment of complications of EUS-guided fine-needle aspiration. *Gastrointest Endosc* 2001;53:470–474.

144. Souquet JC, Napoleon B, Pujol B, et al. Endoscopic ultrasonography in the preoperative staging of esophageal cancer. *Endoscopy* 1994;26:764–766.

145. Yoshikane H, Tsukamoto Y, Niwa Y, et al. Superficial esophageal carcinoma: evaluation by endoscopic ultrasonography. *Am J Gastroenterol* 1994;89:702–707.

146. McLoughlin RF, Cooperberg PL, Mathieson JR, et al. High resolution endoluminal ultrasonography in the staging of esophageal carcinoma. *J Ultrasound Med* 1995;14:725–730.

147. Wu LF, Wang BZ, Feng JL, et al. Preoperative TN staging of esophageal cancer: comparison of miniprobe ultrasonography, spiral CT and MRI. *World J Gastroenterol* 2003;9:219–224.

148. Mallery S, Van Dam J. Increased rate of complete EUS staging of patients with esophageal cancer using the nonoptical, wire-guided echoendoscope. *Gastrointest Endosc* 1999;50:53–57.

149. Willis J, Cooper GS, Isenberg G, et al. Correlation of EUS measurement with pathologic assessment of neoadjuvant therapy response in esophageal carcinoma. *Gastrointest Endosc* 2002;55:655–661.

150. Saltzman JR. Section III: endoscopic and other staging techniques. *Semin Thorac Cardiovasc Surg* 2003;15:180–186.

151. Jost C, Binek J, Schuller JC, et al. Endosonographic radial tumor thickness after neoadjuvant chemoradiation therapy to predict response and survival in patients with locally advanced esophageal cancer: a prospective multicenter phase II study. Swiss Group for Clinical Cancer Research (SAKK 75/02). *Gastrointest Endosc* 2010;7:1114.

152. Flamen P, van Cutsem E, Lerut T, et al. The utility of positron emission tomography with 18F-fluorodeoxyglucose (FDG-PET) to predict the pathologic response and survival of esophageal cancer after preoperative chemoradiation therapy (CRT). *Proc Am Soc Clin Oncol* 2001;20:127a.

153. Luketich JD, Schauer PR, Meltzer CC, et al. Role of positron emission tomography in staging esophageal cancer. *Ann Thorac Surg* 1997;64:765–769.

154. Kole AC, Plukker JT, Nieweg OE, et al. Positron emission tomography for staging of oesophageal and gastroesophageal malignancy. *Br J Cancer* 1998;78:521–527.

155. Plukker JT, van Westreenen JT. Staging in oesophageal cancer. *Best Pract Res Clin Gastroenterol* 2006;20:877–891.

156. Weber WA, Ott K, Becker K, et al. Prediction of response to preoperative chemotherapy in adenocarcinomas of the esophagogastric junction by metabolic imaging. *J Clin Oncol* 2001;19:3058–3065.

157. Ott K, Weber WA, Lordick F, et al. Metabolic imaging predicts response, survival, and recurrence in adenocarcinomas of the esophagogastric junction. *J Clin Oncol* 2006;24:4692–4698.

158. Brucher BL, Weber W, Bauer M, et al. Neoadjuvant therapy of esophageal squamous cell carcinoma: response evaluation by positron emission tomography. *Ann Surg* 2001;233:300–309.

159. Lordick F, Ott K, Krause BJ, et al. PET to assess early metabolic response and to guide treatment of adenocarcinoma of the oesophagogastric junction: the MUNICON phase II trial. *Lancet Oncol* 2007;8:797–805.

160. zum Büschenfelde CM, Herrmann K, Schuster T, et al. 18F-FDG PET-guided salvage neoadjuvant radiochemotherapy of adenocarcinoma of the esophagogastric junction: the MUNICON II trial. *J Nucl Med* 2011;52:1189–1196.

161. Klaeser B, Nitzsche E, Schuller JC, et al. Limited predictive value of FDG-PET for response assessment in the preoperative treatment of esophageal cancer: results of a prospective mutli-center trial (SAKK 75/01). *Onkologie* 2009;32:724–730.

162. Rebollo Aguirre AC, Ramos-Font C, Villegas Portero R, et al. 18F-fluorodeoxiglucose positron emission tomography for the evaluation of neoadjuvant therapy response in esophageal cancer: systematic review of the literature. *Ann Surg* 2009;250:247–254.

163. Kwee R. Prediction of tumor response to neoadjuvant therapy in patients with esophageal cancer with the use of 18F FDG PET: a systematic review. *Radiology* 2010;254:707–717.

164. Dagnini G, Caldironi MW, Marin G, et al. Laparoscopy in abdominal staging of esophageal carcinoma. Report of 369 cases. *Gastrointest Endosc* 1986;32:400–402.

165. Mortensen MB, Scheel-Hincke JD, Madsen MR, et al. Combined endoscopic ultrasonography and laparoscopic ultrasonography in the pretherapeutic assessment of resectability in patients with upper gastrointestinal malignancies. *Scand J Gastroenterol* 1996;31:1115–1119.

166. Luketich JD, Meehan M, Mguyen NT, et al. Minimally invasive surgical staging for esophageal cancer. *Surg Endosc* 2000;14:700–702.

167. Meltzer CC, Luketich JD, Friedman D, et al. Whole-body FDG positron emission tomographic imaging for staging esophageal cancer comparison with computed tomography. *Clin Nucl Med* 2000;25:882–887.

168. Krasna MJ, Jiao X, Mao YS, et al. Thoracoscopy/laparoscopy in the staging of esophageal cancer: Maryland experience. *Surg Laparosc Endosc Percutan Tech* 2002;12:213–218.

169. Wallace MB, Nietert PJ, Earle C, et al. An analysis of multiple staging management strategies for carcinoma of the esophagus: computed tomography, endoscopic ultrasound, positron emission tomography, and thoracoscopy/laparoscopy. *Ann Thorac Surg* 2002;74:1026–1032.

170. Rizk N, Venkatraman E, Park B, et al. The prognostic importance of the number of involved lymph nodes in esophageal cancer: implications for revisions of the American Joint Committee on Cancer staging system. *J Thorac Cardiovasc Surg* 2005;132:1374–1381.

171. Lagarde SM, Ten Kate FJ, Reitsma JB, et al. Prognostic factors in adenocarcinoma of the esophagus or gastroesophageal junction. *J Clin Oncol* 2006;24:4347–4355.

172. Rice TW, Rusch VW, Ishwaran H, et al. Cancer of the esophagus and esophagogastric junction: data-driven staging for the seventh edition of the American Joint Committee on Cancer/International Union Against Cancer Cancer Staging Manuals. Worldwide Esophageal Cancer Collaboration. *Cancer* 2010;116:3763–3773.

173. Merkow RP, Bilimoria KY, McCarter MD. Use of multimodality neoadjuvant therapy for esophageal cancer in the United States: assessment of 987 hospitals. *Ann Surg Oncol.* 2012;19:357–364.

174. Peters JH, Clark GW, Ireland AP, et al. Outcome of adenocarcinoma arising in Barrett's esophagus in endoscopically surveyed and nonsurveyed patients. *J Thorac Cardiovasc Surg* 1994;108:813–821.

175. Heitmiller RF, Redmond M, Hamilton SR. Barrett's esophagus with high-grade dysplasia. An indication for prophylactic esophagectomy. *Ann Surg* 1996;224:66–71.

176. Falk GW, Rice TW, Goldblum JR, et al. Jumbo biopsy forceps protocol still misses unsuspected cancer in Barrett's esophagus with high-grade dysplasia. *Gastrointest Endosc* 1999;49:170–176.

177. Nigro JJ, Hagen JA, DeMeester TR, et al. Occult esophageal adenocarcinoma: extent of disease and implications for effective therapy. *Ann Surg* 1999;230:433–438.

178. Stein HJ, Feith M, Brucher BL, et al. Early esophageal cancer: pattern of lymphatic spread and prognostic factors for long-term survival after surgical resection. *Ann Surg* 2005;242:566–573.

179. Dunbar KB, Spechler SJ. The risk of lymph-node metastases in patients with high-grade dysplasia or intramucosal carcinoma in Barrett's esophagus: a systematic review. *Am J Gastroenterol* 2012;107:850–862.

180. Rastogi A, Puli S, El-Serag HB, et al. Incidence of esophageal adenocarcinoma in patients with Barrett's esophagus and high-grade dysplasia: a meta-analysis. *Gastrointest Endosc* 2008;67:394–398.

181. Pacifico RJ, Want KK. Nonsurgical management of Barrett's esophagus with high-grade dysplasia. *Surg Oncol Clin North Am* 2002;11:321–336.

182. Konda VJ, Ross AS, Ferguson MK. Is the risk of concomitant invasive esophageal cancer in high-grade dysplasia in Barrett's esophagus overestimated? *Clin Gastroenterol Hepatol* 2008;6:159–164.

183. Romagnoli R, Collard JM, Gutschow C, et al. Outcomes of dysplasia arising in Barrett's esophagus: a dynamic view. *J Am Coll Surg* 2003;197:365–371.

184. Levine DS, Haggitt RC, Blout PL, et al. An endoscopic biopsy protocol can differentiate high-grade dysplasia from early adenocarcinoma in Barrett's esophagus. *Gastroenterology* 1993;105:40–50.

185. Cameron AJ. Barrett's esophagus: does the incidence of adenocarcinoma matter? *Am J Gastroenterol* 1997;92:193–194.

186. Dar MS, Goldblum JR, Rice TW, et al. Can extent of high grade dysplasia in Barrett's oesophagus predict the presence of adenocarcinoma at oesophagectomy? *Gut* 2003;52:486–489.

187. Overholt BF, Lightdale CJ, Wang KK, et al. Photodynamic therapy with porfimer sodium for ablation of high-grade dysplasia in Barrett's esophagus: international, partially blinded, randomized phase III trial. *Gastrointest Endosc* 2005;62:488–498.

188. Gossner L, May A, Stolte M, et al. KTP laser destruction of dysplasia and early cancer in columnar-lined Barrett's esophagus. *Gastrointest Endosc* 1999;49:8–12.

189. Sharma P, Jaffe PE, Bhattacharyya A, et al. Laser and multipolar electrocoagulation ablation of early Barrett's adenocarcinoma: long-term follow-up. *Gastrointest Endosc* 1999;49:442–446.

190. Morris CD, Byrne JP, Armstrong GR, et al. Prevention of the neoplastic progression of Barrett's oesophagus by endoscopic argon beam plasma ablation. *Br J Surg* 2001;88:1357–1362.

191. Van Laethem JL, Jagodzinski R, Peny MO, et al. Argon plasma coagulation in the treatment of Barrett's high-grade dysplasia and in situ adenocarcinoma. *Endoscopy* 2001;33:257–261.

192. Shaheen NJ, Sharma P, Overholt BF, et al. Radiofrequency ablation in Barrett's esophagus and dysplasia. *N Engl J Med* 2009;360:2277–2288.

193. Ell C, May A, Pech O, et al. Curative endoscopic resection of early esophageal adenocarciomas (Barrett's cancer). *Gastrointest Endosc* 2007;65:3–10.

194. Ell C, May A, Gossner L, et al. Endoscopic mucosal resection of early cancer and high-grade dysplasia in Barrett's esophagus. *Gastroenterology* 2000;118:670–677.

195. Shami VM, Villaverde A, Stearns L, et al. Clinical impact of conventional endosonography and endoscopic ultrasound-guided fine-needle aspiration in the assessment of patients with Barrett's esophagus and high-grade dysplasia or intramucosal carcinoma who have been referred for endoscopic ablation therapy. *Endoscopy* 2006;38:157–161.

196. Nijhawan K, Wang KK. Endoscopic mucosal resection for lesions with endoscopic features suggestive of malignancy and high-grade dysplasia within Barrett's esophagus. *Gastrointest Endosc* 2000;52:328–332.

197. Yoshida M, Hanashi T, Momma K, et al. Endoscopic mucosal resection for radical treatment of esophageal cancer. *Gan To Kagaku Ryoho* 1995;22:847–854.

198. Chennat J, Konda V, Ross AS, et al. Complete Barrett's eradication endoscopic mucosal resection: an effective treatment modality for high-grade dysplasia and intramucosal carcinoma—an American single-center experience. *Am J Gastroenterol* 2009;104:2684–2692.

199. Bennett C, Vakil N, Bergman J, et al. Consensus statements for management of Barrett's dysplasia and early-stage esophageal adenocarcinoma, based on a Delphi process. *Gastroenterology* 2012;143:336–346.

200. Swanstrom LL, Hansen P. Laparoscopic total esophagectomy. *Arch Surg* 1997;132:943–947.

201. Luketich JD, Schauer PR, Christie NA, et al. Minimally invasive esophagectomy. *Ann Thorac Surg* 2000;70:906–911.

202. Posner MC, Alverdy J. Hand-assisted laparoscopic surgery for cancer. *Cancer J* 2002;8:144–153.

203. Osugi H, Takemura M, Higashino M, et al. Video-assisted thoracoscopic esophagectomy and radical lymph node dissection for esophageal cancer. A series of 75 cases. *Surg Endosc* 2002;16:1588–1593.

204. Dunn DH, Johnson EM, Morphew JA, et al. Robot-assisted transhiatal esophagectomy: a 3-year single-center experience. *Dis Esophagus* 2013;26:159–166.

205. Luketich JD, Pennathur A, Awais O. Outcomes after minimally invasive esophagectomy: review of over 1000 patients. *Ann Surg* 2012;256:95–103.

206. Pennathur A, Farkas A, Krasinskas AM, et al. Esophagectomy for T1 esophageal cancer: outcomes in 100 patients and implications for endoscopic therapy. *Ann Thorac Surg* 2009;87:1048–1054.

207. Law S, Wong J. Use of minimally invasive oesophagectomy for cancer of the oesophagus. *Lancet Oncol* 2002;3:215–222.

208. Wu PC, Posner MC. The role of surgery in the management of oesophageal cancer. *Lancet Oncol* 2003;4:481–488.

209. Biere SS, van Berge Henegouwen MI, Maas KW, et al. Minimally invasive versus open oesophagectomy for patients with oesophageal cancer: a multicentre, open-label, randomised controlled trial. *Lancet* 2012; 379:1887–1892.

210. Sai H, Mitsumor M, Arai K, et al. Long-term results of definitive radiotherapy for stage I esophageal cancer. *Int J Radiat Oncol Biol Phys* 2005;62:1339–1344.

211. Yamada K, Murakami M, Okamoto Y, et al. Treatment results of chemoradiotherapy for clinical stage I (T1N0M0) esophageal carcinoma. *Int J Radiat Oncol Biol Phys* 2006;64:1106–1111.

212. Matoori S, Yanon M, Ishihara R, et al. Comparison between radical esophagectomy and definitive chemoradiotherapy in patients with clinical T1bN0M0 esophageal cancer. *Ann Surg Oncol* 2012;19:2135–2141.

213. Swisher SG, Deford L, Merriman KW, et al. Effect of operative volume on morbidity, mortality, and hospital use after esophagectomy for cancer. *J Thorac Cardiovasc Surg* 2000;119:1126–1132.

214. Begg CB, Cramer LD, Hoskins WJ, et al. Impact of hospital volume on operative mortality for major cancer surgery. *JAMA* 1998;280:1747–1751.

215. Birkmeyer JD, Siewers AE, Finlayson EV, et al. Hospital volume and surgical mortality in the United tates. *N Engl J Med* 2002;346:1128–1137.

216. Verhoef C, van de Weyer R, Schaapveld M, et al. Better survival in patients with esophageal cancer after surgical treatment in university hospitals: a plea for performance by surgical oncologists. *Ann Surg Oncol* 2007;14:1678–1687.

217. Halm EA, Lee C, Chassiin MR. Is volume related to outcome in health care? A systematic review and methodologic critique of the literature. *Ann Intern Med* 2002;137:511–520.

218. Wouters MW, Karin-Kos H, le Cessie S, et al. Centralization of esophageal cancer surgery: does it improve clinical outcomes? *Ann Surg Oncol* 2009;16:1789–1798.

219. Reames BN, Ghaferi AA, Birkmeyer JD, et al. Hospital Volume and Operative Mortality in the Modern Era. *Ann Surg* 2013 Dec 23 [Epub Ahead of Print].

220. Posner MC. Techniques of esophageal resection. In: Posner MC, Vokes EE, Weichselbaum RR, eds. *Cancer of the Upper Gastrointestinal Tract.* Hamilton, Ontario: BC Decker; 2002:1.

221. Park JO, Posner MC. Standard surgical approaches in the management of esophageal cancer. *Surg Oncol Clin North Am* 2002;11:351–363.

222. Fok M, Cheng SW, Wong J. Pyloroplasty versus no drainage in gastric replacement of the esophagus. *Am J Surg* 1991;162:447–452.

223. Urschel JD, Blewett CJ, Young JE, et al. Pyloric drainage (pyloroplasty) or no drainage in gastric reconstruction after esophagectomy: a meta-analysis of randomized controlled trials. *Dig Surg* 2002;19:160–164.

224. Bumm R, Feussner H, Bartels H, et al. Radical transhiatal esophagectomy with two-field lymphadenectomy and endodissection for distal esophageal adenocarcinoma. *World J Surg* 1997;21:822–831.

225. Orringer MB, Marshall B, Chang AC, et al. Two thousand transhiatal esophagectomies: changing trends, lessons learned. *Ann Surg* 2007;246:363–372.

226. Orringer MB, Marshall B, Iannettoni MD. Transhiatal esophagectomy: clinical experience and refinements. *Ann Surg* 1999;230:392–400.

227. Gelfand GA, Finley RJ, Nelems B, et al. Transhiatal esophagectomy for carcinoma of the esophagus and cardia. Experience with 160 cases. *Arch Surg* 1992;127:1164–1167.

228. Vigneswaran WT, Visset J, Paineau J, et al. Transhiatal esophagectomy for carcinoma of the esophagus. *Ann Thorac Surg* 1993;56:838–844.

229. Gertsch P, Vauthey JN, Lustenberger AA, et al. Long-term results of transhiatal esophagectomy for esophageal carcinoma. A multivariate analysis of prognostic factors. *Cancer* 1993;72:2312–2319.

230. Bolton JS, Teng S. Transthoracic or transhiatal esophagectomy for cancer of the esophagus—does it matter? *Surg Oncol Clin North Am* 2002;11:365–375.

231. Dudhat SB, Shinde SR. Transhiatal esophagectomy for squamous cell carcinoma of the esophagus. *Dis Esophagus* 1998;11:226–230.

232. McKeown KC. Total three-stage oesophagectomy for cancer of the oesophagus. *Br J Surg* 1976;63:259–262.

233. Linden A, Sugarbaker DJ. Section V: techniques of esophageal resection. *Semin Thorac Cardiovasc Surg* 2003;15:197–209.

234. Bizekis C, Kent MS, Luketich JD, et al. Initial experience with minimally invasive Ivor Lewis esophagectomy. *Ann Thorac Surg* 2006;82:402–406.

CANCERS OF THE GASTROINTESTINAL TRACT

235. Sharpe DA, Moghissi K. Resectional surgery in carcinoma of the oesophagus and cardia: what influences long-term survival? *Eur J Cardiothorac Surg* 1996;10:359–363.

236. Ellis FH Jr. Standard resection for cancer of the esophagus and cardia. *Surg Oncol Clin North Am* 1999;8:279–294.

237. Adam DJ, Craig SR, Sang CT, et al. Oesophagogastrectomy for carcinoma in patients under 50 years of age. *J R Coll Surg Edinb* 1996;41:371–373.

238. Wang LS, Huang MH, Huang BS, et al. Gastric substitution for resectable carcinoma of the esophagus: an analysis of 368 cases. *Ann Thorac Surg* 1992;53:289–294.

239. Lieberman MD, Shriver CD, Bleckner S, et al. Carcinoma of the esophagus. Prognostic significance of histologic type. *J Thorac Cardiovasc Surg* 1995;109: 130–138.

240. Bosset JF, Gignoux M, Triboulet JP, et al. Chemoradiotherapy followed by surgery compared with surgery alone in squamous cell cancer of the esophagus. *N Engl J Med* 1997;337:161–167.

241. Rindani R, Martin CJ, Cox MR. Transhiatal versus Ivor-Lewis oesophagectomy: is there a difference? *Aust N Z J Surg* 1999;69:187–194.

242. Hulscher JB, Tijssen JG, Obertop H, et al. Transthoracic versus transhiatal resection for carcinoma of the esophagus: a meta-analysis. *Ann Thorac Surg* 2001;72:306–313.

243. Boshier PR, Anderson O, Hanna GB. Transthoracic versus transhiatal esophagectomy for the treatment of esophagogastric cancer: a meta-analysis. *Ann Surg* 2011;254:894–906.

244. Rentz J, Bull D, Harpole D, et al. Transthoracic versus transhiatal esophagectomy: a prospective study of 945 patients. *J Thorac Cardiovasc Surg* 2003;125:1114–1120.

245. Chang AC, Ji J, Birkmeyer NJ, et al. Outcomes after transhiatal and transthoracic esophagectomy for cancer. *Ann Thorac Surg* 2008;85:424–429.

246. Goldminc M, Maddern G, LePrise E, et al. Oesophagectomy by a transhiatal approach or thoracotomy: a prospective randomized trial. *Br J Surg* 1993;80:367–370.

247. Jacobi CA, Zieren HU, Muller JM, et al. Surgical therapy of esophageal carcinoma: the influence of surgical approach and esophageal resection on cardiopulmonary function. *Eur J Cardiothorac Surg* 1997;11:32–37.

248. Chu KM, Law SY, Fok M, et al. A prospective randomized comparison of transhiatal and transthoracic resection for lower-third esophageal carcinoma. *Am J Surg* 1997;174:320–324.

249. Hulscher JB, van Sandick JW, deBoer AG, et al. Extended transthoracic resection compared with limited transhiatal resection for adenocarcinoma of the esophagus. *N Engl J Med* 2002;347:1662–1669.

250. Omloo JM, Lagarde SM, Hulscher JB, et al. Extended transthoracic resection compared with limited transhiatal resection for adenocarcinoma of the mid/distal esophagus: five-year survival of randomized clinical trial. *Ann Surg* 2007;246:992–1000.

251. Skinner DB. En bloc resection for neoplasms of the esophagus and cardia. *J Thorac Cardiovasc Surg* 1983;85:59–71.

252. Lerut T, Nafteux P, Moons J, et al. Three-field lymphadenectomy for carcinoma of the esophagus and gastroesophageal junction in 174 R0 resections: impact on staging, disease-free survival, and outcome: a plea for adaptation of TNM classification in upper-half esophageal carcinoma. *Ann Surg* 2004;240:962–972.

253. Nishihira T, Hirayama K, Mori S. A prospective randomized trial of extended cervical and superior mediastinal lymphadenectomy for carcinoma of the thoracic esophagus. *Am J Surg* 1998;175:47–51.

254. Coonley CJ, Bains M, Hilaris B, et al. Cisplatin and bleomycin in the treatment of esophageal carcinoma. A final report. *Cancer* 1984;54:2351–2355.

255. Kelsen D, Hilaris B, Coonley C, et al. Cisplatin, vindesine, and bleomycin chemotherapy of local-regional and advanced esophageal carcinoma. *Am J Med* 1983;75:645–652.

256. Schlag P, Hermann R, Raeth V, et al. Preoperative chemotherapy in esophageal cancer. A phase II study. *Acta Oncol* 1988;27:811–814.

257. Forastiere AA, Gennis M, Orringer MB, et al. Cisplatin, vinblastine, and mitoguazone chemotherapy for epidermoid and adenocarcinoma of the esophagus. *J Clin Oncol* 1987;5:1143–1149.

258. Carey RW, Hilgenberg AD, Wilkins EW, et al. Long-term follow-up of neoadjuvant chemotherapy with 5-fluorouracil and cisplatin with surgical resection and possible postoperative radiotherapy and/or chemotherapy in squamous cell carcinoma of the esophagus. *Cancer Invest* 1993;11:99–105.

259. Kies MS, Rosen ST, Tsang TK, et al. Cisplatin and 5-fluorouracil in the primary management of squamous esophageal cancer. *Cancer* 1987;60:2156–2160.

260. Ajani JA, Ryan B, Rich TA, et al. Prolonged chemotherapy for localised squamous carcinoma of the oesophagus. *Eur J Cancer* 1992;28A:880–884.

261. Vignoud J, Visset J, Paineau J, et al. Preoperative chemotherapy in squamous cell carcinoma of the esophagus: clinical and pathological analysis, 48 cases. *Ann Oncol* 1990;1:45.

262. Wright CD, Mathiesen DJ, Wain JC, et al. Evolution of treatment strategies for adenocarcinoma of the esophagus and gastroesophageal junction. *Ann Thorac Surg* 1994;58:1574–1578.

263. Nygaard K, Hagen S, Hansen JS, et al. Pre-operative radiotherapy prolongs survival in operable esophageal carcinoma: a randomized, multicenter study of pre-operative radiotherapy and chemotherapy. The second Scandinavian trial in esophageal cancer. *World J Surg* 1992;16:1104–1110.

264. Roth JA, Pass HI, Flanagan MM, et al. Randomized clinical trial of preoperative and postoperative adjuvant chemotherapy with cisplatin, vindesine, and bleomycin for carcinoma of the esophagus. *J Thorac Cardiovasc Surg* 1988;96:242–248.

265. Schlag PM. Randomized trial of preoperative chemotherapy for squamous cell cancer of the esophagus. The Chirurgische Arbeitsgemeinschaft Fuer Onkologie der Deutschen Gesellschaft Fuer Chirurgie Study Group. *Arch Surg* 1992;127:1446–1450.

266. Cunningham D, Allum W, Stenning SP, et al. Perioperative chemotherapy versus surgery alone for resectable gastroesophageal cancer. *N Engl J Med* 2006;355:11–20.

267. Yehou M, Boige V, Pignon JP, et al. Perioperative chemotherapy compared with surgery alone for resectable gastroesophageal adenocarcinoma: an FNLCC and FFCF multicenter phase III trial. *J Clin Oncol* 2011;29:1715–1721.

268. Schuhmacher C, Gretschel S, Lordick F, et al. Neoadjuvant chemotherapy compared with surgery alone for locally advanced cancer of the stomach and cardia: European Organization for Research and Treatment of Cancer randomized Trial 40954. *J Clin Oncol* 2010;28:5210–5218.

269. Boonstra JJ, Kok TC, Wijnhoven BPL, et al. Chemotherapy followed by surgery versus surgery alone in patients with resectable oesophageal squamous cell carcinoma: long-term results of a randomized trial. *BMC Cancer* 2011;11:181.

270. Thirion PG, Michiels S, LeMaitre A, et al. Individual patient data based meta analysis assessing preoperative chemotherapy in resectable oesophageal cancer. *J Clin Oncol* 2007;25:4512.

271. Mei W, Xian-Zhi G, Weibo Y, et al. Randomized clinical trial on the combination of preoperative irradiation and surgery in the treatment of esophageal carcinoma: report on 206 patients. *Int J Radiat Oncol Biol Phys* 1989;16: 325–327.

272. Gignoux M, Roussel A, Paillot B, et al. The value of preoperative radiotherapy in esophageal cancer: results of a study of the EORTC. *World J Surg* 1987;11:426–432.

273. Teniere P, Hay JM, Fingerhut A, et al. Postoperative radiation therapy does not increase survival after curative resection for squamous cell carcinoma of the middle and lower esophagus as shown by a multicenter controlled trial. French University Association for Surgical Research. *Surg Gynecol Obstet* 1991;173:123.

274. Launois B, Delaru D, Campion JP, et al. Preoperative radiotherapy for carcinoma of the esophagus. *Surg Gynecol Obstet* 1981;153:690–692.

275. Arnott SJ, Duncan W, Kerr GR, et al. Low dose preoperative radiotherapy for carcinoma of the oesophagus: results of a randomized clinical trial. *Radiother Oncol* 1993;24:108–113.

276. Huang GJ, Gu XZ, Wang LJ, et al. Combined preoperative irradiation and surgery for esophageal carcinoma. In: Delalrue NC, ed. *International Trends in General Thoracic Surgery*. St. Louis: Mosby; 1988:315.

277. Jacob JH, Seitz JF, Langlois C, et al. Definitive concurrent chemoradiation therapy (CRT) in squamous cell carcinoma of the esophagus (SCCE): preliminary results of a French randomized trial comparing standard vs. split course irradiation (FNLCC-FFCD 9305). *Proc Am Soc Clin Oncol* 1999;18: (abst 270a).

278. Yadava OP, Hodge AJ, Matz LR, et al. Esophageal malignancies: is preoperative radiotherapy the way to go? *Ann Thorac Surg* 1991;51:189–193.

279. Sugimachi K, Matsufuji H, Kai H, et al. Preoperative irradiation for carcinoma of the esophagus. *Surg Gynecol Obstet* 1986;162:174–176.

280. Herskovic A, Martz K, Al-Sarraf M, et al. Combined chemotherapy and radiotherapy compared with radiotherapy alone in patients with cancer of the esophagus. *N Engl J Med* 1992;326:1593–1598.

281. Minsky B, Pajak T, Ginsberg RJ, et al. INT 0123 (Radiation Therapy Oncology Group 94–05) phase III trial of combined-modality therapy for esophageal cancer: high-dose versus standard-dose radiation therapy. *J Clin Oncol* 2002; 20:1167–1174.

282. Poplin E, Fleming T, Leichman L, et al. Combined therapies for squamous-cell carcinoma of the esophagus, a Southwest Oncology Group Study (SWOG-8037). *J Clin Oncol* 1987;5:622–628.

283. Naunheim KS, Petruska P, Roy TS, et al. Preoperative chemotherapy and radiotherapy for esophageal carcinoma. *J Thorac Cardiovasc Surg* 1992;103: 887–893.

284. Forastiere A, Orringer MB, Perez-Tamayo C, et al. Preoperative chemoradiation followed by transhiatal esophagectomy for carcinoma of the esophagus: final report. *J Clin Oncol* 1993;11:1118–1123.

285. Forastiere A, Orringer MB, Perez-Tamayo C, et al. Concurrent chemotherapy and radiation therapy followed by transhiatal esophagectomy for local-regional cancer of the esophagus. *J Clin Oncol* 1990;8:119–127.

286. Hoff SJ, Stewart JL, Murray MK, et al. Preliminary results with neoadjuvant therapy and resection for esophageal carcinoma. *Ann Thorac Surg* 1993;56: 282–286.

287. Bates BA, Detterbeck FC, Bernard SA, et al. Concurrent radiation therapy and chemotherapy followed by esophagectomy for localized esophageal carcinoma. *J Clin Oncol* 1996;14:156–163.

288. Malhaire JP, Labat JP, Lozach P, et al. Preoperative concomitant radiochemotherapy in squamous cell carcinoma of the esophagus: results of a study of 56 patients. *Int J Radiat Oncol Biol Phys* 1996;34:429–437.

289. Stahl M, Wilke H, Fink U, et al. Combined preoperative chemotherapy and radiotherapy in patients with locally advanced esophageal cancer: interim analysis of a phase II trial. *J Clin Oncol* 1996;14:829–837.

290. Forastiere AA, Heitmiler RF, Lee DJ, et al. Intensive chemoradiation followed by esophagectomy for squamous cell and adenocarcinoma of the esophagus. *Cancer J Sci Am* 1997;3:144–152.

291. Jones DR, Detterbeck FC, Egan TM, et al. Induction chemoradiotherapy followed by esophagectomy in patients with carcinoma of the esophagus. *Ann Thorac Surg* 1997;64:185–191.

292. Adelstein DJ, Rice TW, Rybicki LA, et al. Use of concurrent chemotherapy, accelerated fractionation radiation, and surgery for patients with esophageal cancer. *Cancer* 1997;80:1011–1020.

293. Posner MC, Gooding WE, Landreneau RJ, et al. Preoperative chemoradiotherapy for carcinoma of the esophagus and gastroesophageal junction. *Cancer J Sci Am* 1998;4:237–246.

294. Posner MC, Gooding WE, Lew JI, et al. Complete 5-year follow-up of a prospective phase II trial of preoperative chemoradiotherapy for esophageal cancer. *Surgery* 2001;130:620–626.

295. Raoul JL, LePrise E, Meunier B, et al. Neoadjuvant chemotherapy and hyperfractionated radiotherapy with concurrent low-dose chemotherapy for squamous cell esophageal carcinoma. *Int J Radiat Oncol Biol Phys* 1998; 42:29–34.

296. Keller SM, Ryan L, Coia LR, et al. High dose chemoradiotherapy followed by esophagectomy for adenocarcinoma of the esophagus and gastroesophageal junction. Results of a phase II study of the Eastern Cooperative Oncology Group. *Cancer* 1998;83:1908–1916.

297. Bedenne L, Seitz JF, Milan C, et al. Cisplatin, 5-FU and preoperative radiotherapy in esophageal epidermoid cancer. Multicenter phase II FFCD 8804 study. *Gastroenterol Clin Biol* 1998;22:273–281.

298. Laterza E, de'Manzoni G, Tedesco P, et al. Induction chemo-radiotherapy for squamous cell carcinoma of the thoracic esophagus: long-term results of a phase II study. *Ann Surg Oncol* 1999;6:777–784.

299. Heath EI, Burtness BA, Heitmiller RF, et al. Phase II evaluation of preoperative chemoradiation and postoperative adjuvant chemotherapy for squamous cell and adenocarcinoma of the esophagus. *J Clin Oncol* 2000;18:868–876.

300. Roof KS, Coen J, Lynch TJ, et al. Concurrent cisplatin, 5-FU, paclitaxel, and radiation therapy in patients with locally advanced esophageal cancer. *Int J Radiat Oncol Biol Phys* 2006;65:1120–1128.

301. Meredith K, Weber J, Turaga K, et al. Pathologic response after neoadjuvant therapy is the major determinant of survival in patients with esophageal cancer. *Ann Surg Oncol* 2010;17:1159–1167.

302. Leichman LP, Goldman BH, Bohanes PO, et al. S0356: A phase II clinical and a prospective molecular trial with oxaliplatin, fluorouracil, and external-beam radiation therapy before surgery for patients with esophageal adenocarcinoma. *J Clin Oncol* 2011;29:4555–4560.

303. Safran H, Gaissert H, Akerman P, et al. Paclitaxel, cisplatin, and concurrent radiation for esophageal cancer. *Cancer Invest* 2001;19:1–7.

304. Adelstein DJ, Rice TW, Rybicki LA, et al. Does paclitaxel improve the chemoradiotherapy of locoregionally advanced esophageal cancer? A nonrandomized comparison with fluorouracil-based therapy. *J Clin Oncol* 2000;18: 2032–2039.

305. Wright CD, Wain JC, Lynch TJ, et al. Induction therapy for esophageal cancer with paclitaxel and hyperfractionated radiotherapy: a phase I and II study. *J Thorac Cardiovasc Surg* 1997;114:811–815.

306. Meluch AA, Greco FA, Gray JR, et al. Preoperative therapy with concurrent paclitaxel/carboplatin/infusional 5-FU and radiation therapy in locoregional esophageal cancer: final results of a Minnie Pearl Cancer Research Network phase II trial. *Cancer J* 2003;9:251–260.

307. Bains MS, Stojadinovic A, Minsky B, et al. A phase II trial of preoperative combined-modality therapy for localized esophageal carcinoma: initial results. *J Thorac Cardiovasc Surg* 2002;124:270–277.

308. Swisher SG, Ajani JA, Komaki R, et al. Long term outcome of a phase II trial evaluating chemotherapy, chemoradiotherapy, and surgery for locoregionally advanced esophageal cancer. *Int J Radiat Oncol Biol Phys* 2003;57:120–127.

309. Ajani JA, Correa A, Walsh G, et al. Trimodality therapy without a platinum compound for localized carcinoma of the esophagus and gastroesophageal junction. *Cancer* 2010;116:1656–1663.

310. van Meerten E, Muller K, Tilanus HW, et al. Neoadjuvant concurrent chemoradiation with weekly paclitaxel and carboplain for patients with oesophageal cancer: a phase II study. *Br J Cancer* 2006;94:1389–1394.

311. Spigel DR, Greco A, Meluch AA, et al. Phase I/II trial of preoperative oxaliplatin, docetaxel, and capecitabine with concurrent radiation therapy in localized carcinoma of the esophagus or gastroesophageal junction. *J Clin Oncol* 2010;28:2213–2219.

312. Ajani JA, Winter KA, Komaki R, et al. Phase II randomized trial of two nonoperative regimens of induction chemotherapy followed by chemoradiation in patients with localized carcinoma of the esophagus: RTOG 0113. *J Clin Oncol* 2008;26:4551–4556.

313. Ilson D, Goodman KA, Janjigian YY, et al. Phase II trial of bevacizumab, irinotecan, cisplatin and radiation as preoperative therapy in esophageal adenocarcinoma. *J Clin Oncol* 2012;30:(abs 4061).

314. Rivera F, Galan M, Tabernero J, et al. Phase II trial of preoperative irinotecancisplatin followed by concurrent irinotecan-cisplatin and radiotherapy for resectable locally advanced gastric and esophogastric junction adenocarcinoma. *Int J Rad Oncol Biol Phys* 2009;75:1430.

315. Leichman L, Steiger Z, Seydel HG, et al. Preoperative chemotherapy and radiation therapy for patients with cancer of the esophagus: a potentially curative approach. *J Clin Oncol* 1984;2:75–79.

316. Geh JI, Bond SJ, Bentzen SM, et al. Systematic overview of preoperative (neoadjuvant) hemoradiotherapy trials in oesophageal cancer: evidence of a radiation and chemotherapy dose response. *Radiother Oncol* 2006;78: 236–244.

317. Van Hagen P, Hulshof MC, van Lanschot JJ, et al. Preoperative chemoradiotherapy for esophageal or junctional cancer. *N Engl J Med* 2012;366: 2074–2084.

318. Sarkaria IS, Rizk NP, Bains MS, et al. Post-treatment endoscopic biopsy is a poor predictor of pathologic response in patients undergoing chemoradiation therapy for esophageal cancer. *Ann Surg* 2009;249:764–767.

319. Chedella NKS, Suzuki A, Xiao L, et al. Association between clinical complete response and pathological complete response after preoperative chemoradiation in patients with gastroesophageal cancer: analysis in a large cohort. *Ann Oncol* 2013;24:1262.

320. Yang Q, Cleary KR, Yao JC, et al. Significance of post-chemoradiation biopsy in predicting residual esophageal carcinoma in the surgical specimen. *Dis Esophagus* 2004;14:38–43.

321. Jones DR, Parker LA, Detterbeck FC, et al. Inadequacy of computed tomography in assessing patients with esophageal carcinoma after induction chemoradiotherapy. *Cancer* 1999;85:1026–1032.

322. Zuccaro G Jr, Rice TW, Goldblum J, et al. Endoscopic ultrasound cannot determine suitability for esophagectomy after aggressive chemoradiotherapy for esophageal cancer. *Am J Gastroenterol* 1999;94:906–912.

323. Laterza E, deManzoni G, Guglielmi A, et al. Endoscopic ultrasonography in the staging of esophageal carcinoma after preoperative radiotherapy and chemotherapy. *Ann Thorac Surg* 1999;67:1466–1469.

324. Beseth BD, Bedford R, Isacoff WH, et al. Endoscopic ultrasound does not accurately assess pathologic stage of esophageal cancer after neoadjuvant chemoradiotherapy. *Am Surg* 2000;66:827–831.

325. Gaca JG, Petersen RP, Peterson BL, et al. Pathologic nodal status predicts disease-free survival after neoadjuvant chemoradiation for gastroesophageal junction carcinoma. *Ann Surg Oncol* 2006;13:340–346.

326. Fields RC, Strong VE, Gonen M, et al. Recurrence and survival after pathologic complete response to preoperative therapy followed by surgery for gastric or gastroesophageal adenocarcinoma. *Br J Cancer* 2011;104:1840–1847.

327. Downey RJ, Akhurst T, Ilson D, et al. Whole body 18FDG-PET and the response of esophageal cancer to induction therapy: results of a prospective trial. *J Clin Oncol* 2003;21:428–432.

328. Flamen P, Van Cutsem E, Lerut A, et al. Positron emission tomography for assessment of the response to induction radiochemotherapy in locally advanced oesophageal cancer. *Ann Oncol* 2002;13:361–368.

329. Vallböhmer D, Holscher AH, Dietleiin M, et al. [18F] fluorodeoxyglucosepositron emission tomography for the assessment of histologic response and prognosis after completion of neoadjuvant chemoradiation in esophageal cancer. *Ann Surg* 2009;250:888–894.

330. Klayton T, Li T, Yu JQ, et al. The role of qualitative and quantitative analysis of F18-FDG positron emission tomography in predicting pathologic response following chemoradiotherapy in patients with esophageal carcinoma. *J Gastrointest Surg* 2012;43:612–618.

331. Suzuki A, Xiao L, Taketa T, et al. Results of the baseline positron emission tomography can customize therapy of localized esohpageal adenocarcinoma patients who achieve a clinical complete response after chemoradiation. *Ann Oncol* 2013;24:2854–2859.

332. Monjazeb AM, Riedlinger G, Aklilu M, et al. Outcomes of patients with esophageal cancer staged with [18F] fluorodeoxyglucose positron emission tomography (FDG-PET): can postradiochemotherapy FDG-PED predict the utility of resection? *J Clin Oncol* 2010;28:4714–4721.

333. Brenner B, Ilson D, Minsky B, et al. Phase I trial of combined-modality therapy for localized esophageal cancer: escalating doses of continuous-infusion paclitaxel with cisplatin and concurrent radiation therapy. *J Clin Oncol* 2004; 22:45–52.

334. McCurdy M, McAleer MF, Wei W, et al. Induction and concurrent taxanes enhance both the pulmonary metabolic response and the radiation pneumonitis response in patients with esophagus cancer. *Int J Radiat Oncol Biol Phys* 2010;76:816–823.

335. Urba SG, Orringer MB, Ianettonni M, et al. Concurrent cisplatin, paclitaxel, and radiotherapy as preoperative treatment for patients with locoregional esophageal carcinoma. *Cancer* 2003;98:2177–2183.

336. Urba S, Hayman M, Ianettonni M, et al. Preoperative chemoradiation with cisplatin, 5-FU, and paclitaxel followed by surgery and adjuvant chemotherapy for locoregional esophageal cancer. *J Clin Oncol* 2004;22:4029.

337. Kleinberg L, Powell ME, Forastiere AA, et al. Survival outcome of E1201: an Eastern Cooperative Oncology Group randomized phase II trial of neoadjuvant preoperative paclitaxel/cisplatin/radiotherapy or irinotecan/cisplatin/radiotherapy in endoscopy with ultrasound stage esophageal adenocarcinoma. *J Clin Oncol* 2008;26:4532.

338. Kleinberg LR, Eapen S, Hamilton S, et al. E1201: an Eastern Cooperative Oncology Group (ECOG) randomized phase II trial to measure response rate and toxicity of preoperative combined modality paclitaxel/cisplatin/RT or irinotecan/cisplatin/RT in adenocarcinoma of the esophagus. *Int J Rad Oncol Biol Phys* 2006;66:s173.

339. Walsh TN, Noonan N, Hollywood D, et al. A comparison of multimodal therapy and surgery for esophageal adenocarcinoma. *N Engl J Med* 1996; 335:462–467.

340. Walsh TN, Grennell M, Mansoor S, et al. Neoadjuvant treatment of advanced stage esophageal adenocarcinoma increases survival. *Dis Esophagus* 2002;15:121–124.

341. Burmeister BH, Smithers BM, Gebski V, et al. Surgery alone versus chemoradiotherapy followed by surgery for resectable cancer of the oesophagus: a randomised controlled phase III trial. *Lancet Oncol* 2005;6:659–668.

342. Tepper J, Krasna MJ, Niedzwiecki D, et al. Phase III trial of trimodality therapy with cisplatin, fluorouracil, radiotherapy, and surgery compared with surgery alone for esophageal cancer: CALGB 9781. *J Clin Oncol* 2008;26:1086–1092.

343. Lee J, Kim S, Jung H, et al. A single institutional phase III trial of preoperative chemotherapy with hyperfractionation radiotherapy plus surgery versus surgery alone for resectable esophageal squamous cell carcinoma. *Ann Oncol* 2004;15:947–954.

344. Stahl M, Walz MK, Stuschke M, et al. Phase III comparison of preoperative chemotherapy compared with chemoradiotherapy in patients with locally advanced adenocarcinoma of the esophagogastric junction. *J Clin Oncol* 2009;27:851–856.

345. Le Prise E, Etienne PL, Meunier B, et al. A randomized study of chemotherapy, radiation therapy, and surgery versus surgery for localized squamous cell carcinoma of the esophagus. *Cancer* 1994;73:1779–1784.

346. Kaklamanos IG, Walker GR, Ferry K, et al. Neoadjuvant treatment for resectable cancer of the esophagus and gastroesophageal junction: a meta-analysis of randomized clinical trials. *Ann Surg Oncol* 2003;10:754–761.

347. Sjoquist KM, Burmeister BH, Smithers BM, et al. Survival after neoadjuvant chemotherapy or chemoradiotherapy for resectable oesophageal carcinoma: an updated meta-analysis. *Lancet Oncol* 2011;12:681–692.

348. Bendell JC, Meluch A, Peyton J, et al. A phase II trial of preoperative concurrent chemotherapy/radiation therapy plus bevacizumab/erlotinib in the treatment of localized esophageal cancer. *Clin Adv Hematol Oncol* 2012;10:430–437.

349. Crosby T, Hurt CN, Falk S, et al. Chemoradiotherapy with or without cetuximab in patients with oesophageal cancer (SCOPE-1): a multicenter, phase 2/3 randomized trial. *Lancet Oncol* 2013;14:627–637.

350. Suntharalingham M, Winter KW, Ilson D, et al. The initial Report of RTOG 0436: A Phase III Trial evaluating the addition of cetuximab to paclitaxel, cisplatin, and radiation for patients with esophageal cancer treated without surgery. *2014 LBA GI Symposium* 2014.

351. Safran H, Dipretillo T, Akerman P, et al. Phase I/II study of trastuzumab, paclitaxel, cisplatin, and radiation for locally advanced, HER2-over expressing esophageal adenocarcinoma. *Int J Radiat Oncol Biol Phys* 2007;67:405–409.

352. A comparison of chemotherapy and radiotherapy as adjuvant treatment to surgery for esophageal carcinoma. Japanese Esophageal Oncology Group. *Chest* 1993;104:203–207.

353. Iizuka AT, Isono KK, Watanabe H, et al. A randomized trial comparing surgery to surgery plus postoperative chemotherapy for localized squamous carcinoma of the thoracic esophagus: the Japan Clinical Oncology Study Group (JCOG) study. *Proc Am Soc Clin Oncol* 1998;17:282a.

354. Ando N, Iizuka T, Kakegawa T, et al. A randomized trial of surgery with and without chemotherapy for localized squamous carcinoma of the thoracic esophagus: the Japan Clinical Oncology Group Study. *J Thorac Cardiovasc Surg* 1997;114:205–209.

355. Iizuka T. Surgical adjuvant treatment of esophageal carcinoma: a Japanese Esophageal Oncology Group Experience. *Semin Oncol* 1994;21:462–466.

356. Armanios MY, Xu R, Forastiere A, et al. Phase II adjuvant chemotherapy for resected adenocarcinoma of the esophagus, gastro-esophageal (GE) junction and cardia (8296): A trial of the Eastern Cooperative Oncology Group. *Proc Am Soc Clin Oncol* 2003;22:4495–4499.

357. Yamamoto M, Yamashita T, Matsubara T, et al. Reevaluation of postoperative radiotherapy for thoracic esophageal carcinoma. *Int J Radiat Oncol Biol Phys* 1997;37:75–78.

358. Hosokawa M, Shirato H, Ohara K, et al. Intraoperative radiation therapy to the upper mediastinum and nerve-sparing three-field lymphadenectomy followed by external beam radiotherapy for patients with thoracic esophageal carcinoma. *Cancer* 1999;86:6–13.

359. Fok M, Sham JS, Choi D, et al. Postoperative radiotherapy for carcinoma of the esophagus: a prospective, randomized controlled study. *Surgery* 1993;113:138–147.

360. MacDonald J, Benedetti J, Smalley S, et al. Chemoradiation of resected gastric cancer: a 10-year follow-up of the phase III trial INT 0116 (SWOG 9008). *Proc Am Soc Clin Oncol* 2009;27:205s.

361. Gordon MA, Gundacker HM, Benedetti J, et al. Assessment of HER2 gene amplification in adenocarcinomas of the stomach or gastroesophageal junction in the INT-0116/SWOG9008 clinical trial. *Ann Oncol* 2013;24:1754–1761.

362. Okawa T, Kita M, Tanaka M, et al. Results of radiotherapy for inoperable locally advanced esophageal cancer. *Int J Radiat Oncol Biol Phys* 1989;17:49–54.

363. al-Sarraf M, Martz K, Herskovic A, et al. Superiority of chemo-radiotherapy (CT-RT) vs radiotherapy (RT) in patients with esophageal cancer. Final report of an Intergroup randomized and confirmed study. *Proc Am Soc Clin Oncol* 1996;15:abst 206.

364. Suntharalingam M, Moughhan J, Cola LR, et al. Outcome results of the 1996–1999 patterns of care survey of the national practice for patients receiving radiation therapy for carcinoma of the esophagus. *J Clin Oncol* 2005;23:2325–2331.

365. Gomi K, Oguchi M, Hirokawa Y, et al. Process and preliminary outcome of a patterns of care study of esophageal cancer in Japan: patients treated with surgery and radiotherapy. *Int J Radiat Oncol Biol Phys* 2003;56:813–822.

366. De-Ren S. Ten-year follow-up of esophageal cancer treated by radical radiation therapy: analysis of 869 patients. *Int J Radiat Oncol Biol Phys* 1989;16:329–334.

367. Newaishy GA, Read GA, Duncan W, et al. Results of radical radiotherapy of squamous cell carcinoma of the oesophagus. *Clin Radiol* 1982;33:347–352.

368. Shi X, Yao W, Liu T. Late course accelerated fractionation in radiotherapy of esophageal carcinoma. *Radiother Oncol* 1999;51:21–26.

369. Coia LR, Engstrom PF, Paul AR, et al. Long-term results of infusional 5-FU, mitomycin-C and radiation as primary management of esophageal carcinoma. *Int J Radiat Oncol Biol Phys* 1991;20:29–36.

370. Nemoto K, Yamada S, Hareyama M, et al. Radiation therapy for superficial esophageal cancer: a comparison of radiotherapy methods. *Int J Radiat Oncol Biol Phys* 2001;50:639–644.

371. Roussel A, Jacob JH, Jung GM, et al. Controlled clinical trial for the treatment of patients with inoperable esophageal carcinoma: a study of the EORTC Gastrointestinal Tract Cancer Cooperative Group. In: Schlag P, Hohenberger P, Metzger U, eds. *Recent Results in Cancer Research*. Berlin: Springer-Verlag; 1988: 21.

372. al-Sarraf M, Martz K, Herskovic A, et al. Progress report of combined chemoradiotherapy versus radiotherapy alone in patients with esophageal cancer: an Intergroup study. *J Clin Oncol* 1997;15:277–284.

373. Slabber CF, Nel JS, Schoeman L, et al. A randomized study of radiotherapy alone versus radiotherapy plus 5-fluorouracil and platinum in patients with inoperable, locally advanced squamous cancer of the esophagus. *Am J Clin Oncol* 1998;21:462–465.

374. Smith TJ, Ryan LM, Douglass HO, et al. Combined chemoradiotherapy vs. radiotherapy alone for early stage squamous cell carcinoma of the esophagus: a study of the Eastern Cooperative Oncology Group. *Int J Radiat Oncol Biol Phys* 1998;42:269–276.

375. Araujo C, Souhami L, Gil R, et al. A randomized trial comparing radiation therapy versus concomitant radiation therapy and chemotherapy in carcinoma of the thoracic esophagus. *Cancer* 1991;67:2258–2261.

376. Wong RK, Malthaner RA, Zuraw L, et al. Combined modality radiotherapy and chemotherapy in nonsurgical management of localized carcinoma of the esophagus: a practice guideline. *Int J Radiat Oncol Biol Phys* 2003;55:930–942.

377. Streeter OE Jr, Martz KL, Gaspar LE, et al. Does race influence survival for esophageal cancer patients treated on the radiation and chemotherapy arm of RTOG #85-01? *Int J Radiat Oncol Biol Phys* 1999;44:1047–1052.

378. Yu J, Ren R, Sun X, et al. A randomized clinical study of surgery versus radiotherapy in the treatment of resectable esophageal cancer. *Proc Am Soc Clin Oncol* 2006;24:181s.

379. Chiu PWY, Chan ACW, Leung SF, et al. Multicenter prospective randomized trial comparing standard esophagectomy with chemoradiotherapy for treatment of squamous esophageal cancer: early results from the Chinese University Research Group for Esophageal Cancer (CURE). *J Gastrointest Surg* 2005;9:794.

380. Minsky BD, Neuberg D, Kelsen DP, et al. Final report of Intergroup trial 0122 (ECOG PE-289, RTOG 90-12): phase II trial of neoadjuvant chemotherapy plus concurrent chemotherapy and high-dose radiation for squamous cell carcinoma of the esophagus. *Int J Radiat Oncol Biol Phys* 1999;43:517–523.

381. Bonnetain F, Bedenne L, Michel P, et al. Definitive results of a comparative longitudinal quality of life study using the Spitzer index in the randomized multicentric phase III trial FFCD 9102 (surgery vs. radiochemotherapy in patients with locally advanced esophageal cancer). *Proc Am Soc Clin Oncol* 2003;22:250.

382. Crehange G, Maingon P, Peignaux K, et al. Phase III trial of protracted compared with split-course chemoradiation for esophageal cancer: Federation Francophone de Cancerologie Digestive 9102. *J Clin Oncol* 2007;25:4895–4901.

383. Berger AC, Farma J, Scott WJ, et al. Complete response to neoadjuvant chemoradiotherapy in esophageal carcinoma is associated with significantly improved survival. *J Clin Oncol* 2005;23:4330–4337.

384. Rohatgi R, Swisher SG, Correa AM, et al. Histologic subtypes as determinants of outcome in esophageal carcinoma patients with pathologic complete response after preoperative chemoradiotherapy. *Cancer* 2006;106:552–558.

385. Swisher SG, Hofstetter W, Wu TT, et al. Proposed revision of the esophageal cancer staging system to accommodate pathologic response (pP) following preoperative chemoradiation (CRT). *Ann Surg* 2005;241:810–817.

386. Swisher SG, Winter KA, Komaki RU, et al. A phase II study of a paclitaxel-based chemoradiation regimen with selective surgical salvage for resectable locoregionally advanced esophageal cancer: initial reporting of RTOG 0246. *Int J Radiat Oncol Biol Phys* 2012;82:1967–1972.

387. Gaca JG, Petersen RP, Peterson BL, et al. Pathologic nodal status predicts disease-free survival after neoadjuvant chemoradiation for gastroesophageal junction carcinoma. *Ann Surg Oncol* 2006;13:340–346.

388. Morita M, Kuwano H, Araki K, et al. Prognostic significance of lymphocytic infiltration following preoperative chemoradiotherapy and hyperthermia for esophageal cancer. *Int J Radiat Oncol Biol Phys* 2001;49:1259–1266.

389. Alexander BM, Wang XZ, Niemierko A, et al. DNA repair biomarkers predict response to neoadjuvant chemoradiotherapy in esophageal cancer. *Int J Radiat Oncol Biol Phys* 2012;83:164–171.

390. Kuwahara A, Yamamori M, Fujita M, et al. TNFRSF1B A 1466G genotype is predictive of clinical efficacy after treatment with a definitive 5-fluorouracil/cisplatin-based chemoradiotherapy in Japanese patients with esophageal squamous cell carcinoma. *J Exp Clin Cancer Res* 2010;29:100(abstr).

391. Yi Y, Li B, Sun H, et al. Predictors of sensitivity to chemoradiotherapy of esophageal squamous cell carcinoma. *Tumour Biol* 2010;31:333–340.

392. Izzo JG, Malhotra V, Wu TT, et al. Association of activated transcription factor nuclear factor kB with chemoradiation resistance and poor outcome in esophageal carcinoma. *J Clin Oncol* 2006;24:748–754.

393. Izzo JG, Wu TT, Wu X, et al. Cyclin D1 guanine/adenine 870 polymorphism with altered protein expression is associated with genomic instability and aggressive clinical biology of esophageal adenocarcinoma. *J Clin Oncol* 2007;25:698–707.

394. Hildebrandt M, Yang H, Hung M, et al. Genetic variations in the PI3K/PTEN/mTOR pathway are associated with clinical outcomes in esophageal cancer patients treated with chemoradiotherapy. *J Clin Oncol* 2009;27:857–871.

395. Skinner HD, Xu E, Lee JH, et al. A validated miRNA expression profile for response to neoadjuvant therapy in esophageal cancer. *Proc ASCO* 2013;31:4078(abstr).

396. Kalha I, Kaw M, Fukami N, et al. The accuracy of endoscopic ultrasound for restaging esophageal carcinoma after chemoradiation therapy. *Cancer* 2004;101:940–947.

397. Blackstock AW, Farmer MR, Lovato J, et al. A prospective evaluation of the impact of 18-F-fluoro-deoxy-D-glucose positron emission tomography staging on survival for patients with locally advanced esophageal cancer. *Int J Radiat Oncol Biol Phys* 2006;64:455–460.

398. Brucher BL, Becker K, Lordick F, et al. The clinical impact of histopathologic response assessment by residual tumor cell quantification in esophageal squamous cell carcinomas. *Cancer* 2006;106:2119–2127.

399. McLoughlin J, Melis M, Siegel E, et al. Are patients with esophageal cancer who become PET negative after neoadjuvant chemoradiation free of cancer. *J Am Coll Surg* 2008;206:879–886.

400. Sarbia M, Stahl M, Fink U, et al. Expression of apoptosis-regulating proteins and outcome of esophageal cancer patients treated by combined therapy modalities. *Clin Cancer Res* 1998;4:2991–2997.

401. Pomp J, Davelaar J, Blom J, et al. Radiotherapy for oesophagus carcinoma: the impact of p53 on treatment outcome. *Radiother Oncol* 1998;46:179–184.

402. Merchant TE, Minsky BD, Lauwers GY, et al. Esophageal cancer phospholipids correlated with histopathologic findings: a 31P NMR study. *NMR Biomed* 1999;12:184–188.

403. Hayashida Y, Honda K, Osaka Y, et al. Possible prediction of chemoradiosensitivity of esophageal cancer by serum protein profiling. *Clin Cancer Res* 2005;11:8042–8047.

404. Chang JY, Zhang X, Komaki R, et al. Tumor-specific apoptotic gene targeting overcomes radiation resistance in esophageal adenocarcinoma. *Int J Radiat Oncol Biol Phys* 2006;64:1482–1494.

405. Nomiya T, Nemoto K, Miyachi H, et al. Relationships between radiosensitivity and microvascular density in esophageal carcinoma: significance of hypoxic fraction. *Int J Radiat Oncol Biol Phys* 2004;58:589–596.

406. Izquierdo MA, Marcuello E, Gomez de Segura G, et al. Unresectable non-metastatic squamous cell carcinoma of the esophagus managed by sequential chemotherapy (cisplatin and bleomycin) and radiation therapy. *Cancer* 1993;71:287–292.

407. Ishikura S, Nihei K, Ohtsu A, et al. Long-term toxicity after definitive chemoradiotherapy for squamous cell carcinoma of the thoracic esophagus. *J Clin Oncol* 2003;21:2697–2702.

408. Wieder HA, Brucher BL, Zimmermann F, et al. Time course of tumor metabolic activity during chemoradiotherapy of esophageal squamous cell carcinoma and response to treatment. *J Clin Oncol* 2004;22:900–908.

409. Amini A, Ajani J, Komaki R, et al. Factors associated with local-regional failure after definitive chemoradiation for locally advanced esophageal cancer. *Ann Surg Oncol* 2014;21:306–314.

410. Armstrong JG. High dose rate remote afterloading brachytherapy for lung and esophageal cancer. *Sem Radiat Oncol* 1993;4:270–277.

411. Maingon P, d'Hombres A, Truc G, et al. High dose rate brachytherapy for superficial cancer of the esophagus. *Int J Radiat Oncol Biol Phys* 2000;46:71–76.

412. Homs MY, Essink-Bot ML, Borsboom GJ, et al. Quality of life after palliative treatment for oesophageal carcinoma—a prospective comparison between stent placement and single dose chemotherapy. *Eur J Cancer* 2004;40:1862–1871.

413. Okawa T, Dokiya T, Nishio M, et al. Multi-institutional randomized trial of external radiotherapy with and without intraluminal brachytherapy for esophageal cancer in Japan. *Int J Radiat Oncol Biol Phys* 1999;45:623–628.

414. Pasquier D, Mirabel X, Adenis A, et al. External beam radiation therapy followed by high-dose-rate brachytherapy for inoperable superficial esophageal carcinoma. *Int J Radiat Oncol Biol Phys* 2006;65:1456–1461.

415. Yorozu A, Toya K, Dokiya T. Long-term results of concurrent chemoradiotherapy followed by high dose rate brachytherapy for T2-3N0-1M0 esophageal cancer. *Esophagus* 2006;3:1.

416. Caspers RJ, Zwinderman AH, Griffioen G, et al. Combined external beam and low dose rate intraluminal radiotherapy in oesophageal cancer. *Radiother Oncol* 1993;27:7–12.

417. Yorozu A, Dokiya T, Oki Y, et al. Curative radiotherapy with high-dose-rate brachytherapy boost for localized esophageal carcinoma: dose-effect relationship of brachytherapy with the balloon type applicator system. *Radiother Oncol* 1999;51:133–139.

418. Ishikawa H, Nonaka T, Sakurai H, et al. Usefulness of intraluminal brachytherapy combined with external beam radiation therapy for submucosal esophageal cancer: long-term follow-up results. *Int J Rad Oncol Biol Phys* 2010;76:452–459.

419. Gaspar LE, Qian C, Kocha WI, et al. A phase I/II study of external beam radiation, brachytherapy and concurrent chemotherapy in localized cancer of the esophagus (RTOG 92–07): preliminary toxicity report. *Int J Radiat Oncol Biol Phys* 1997;37:593–599.

420. Thomas CR, Berkey BA, Minsky BD, et al. Recursive partitioning analysis of pretreatment variables of 416 patients with locoregional esophageal cancer treated with definitive concomitant chemoradiotherapy on Intergroup and Radiation Therapy Oncology Group trials. *Int J Radiat Oncol Biol Phys* 2004;58:1405–1410.

421. Gaspar LE, Nag S. Herskovic A, et al. American Brachytherapy Society (ABS) consensus guidelines for brachytherapy of esophageal cancer. *Int J Radiat Oncol Biol Phys* 1997;38:127–132.

422. Zhang Z, Liao Z, Jin J, et al. Dose response relationship in locoregional control for patients with stage II–III esophageal cancer treated with concurrent chemotherapy and radiotherapy. *Int J Radiat Oncol Biol Phys* 2005;61:656–664.

423. Wang Y, Shi XH, He SQ, et al. Comparison between continuous accelerated hyperfractionated and late-course accelerated hyperfractionated radiotherapy for esophageal carcinoma. *Int J Radiat Oncol Biol Phys* 2002;54:131–136.

424. Zaho KL, Shi XH, Jiang GL, et al. Late course accelerated hyperfractionated radiotherapy for localized esophageal carcinoma. *Int J Radiat Oncol Biol Phys* 2004;60:123–129.

425. Choi N, Park SD, Lynch T, et al. Twice-daily radiotherapy as concurrent boost technique during chemotherapy cucles in neoadjuvant chemoradiotherapy for resectable esophageal cancer: mature results of a phase II study. *Int J Radiat Oncol Biol* 2004;50:111–122.

426. Chandra A, Guerrero TM, Liu HH, et al. Feasibility of using intensity-modulated radiotherapy to improve lung sparing in treatment planning for distal esophageal cancer. *Radiother Oncol* 2005;77:247–253.

427. Fenkell L, Kaminsky I, Breen S, et al. Dosimetric comparison of IMRT vs. 3D conformal radiotherapy in the treatment of cancer of the cervical esophagus. *Radiother Oncol* 2008;89:287–291.

428. Kole TP, Aghayere O, Kwah J, et al. Comparison of heart and coronary artery doses associated with intensity-modulated radiotherapy versus three-dimensional conformal radiotherapy for distal esophageal cancer. *Int J Radiat Oncol Biol Phys* 2012;83:1580–1586.

429. Yin L, Wu H, Gong J, et al. Volumetric-modulated arc therapy vs. c-IMRT in esophageal cancer: a treatment planning comparison. *World J Gastroenterol* 2012;18:5266–5275.

430. Nicolini G, Ghosh-Laskar S, Shrivastava SK, et al. Volumetric modulation arc radiotherapy with flattening filter-free beams compared with a static gantry IMRT and 3D conformal radiotherapy for advanced esophageal carcinoma: a feasibility study. *Int J Radiat Oncol Biol Phys* 2012;84:553–560.

431. Martin S, Chen JZ, Rashid Dar A, et al. Dosimetric comparison of helical tomotherapy, rapid arc, and a novel IMRT & arc technique for esophagela carcinoma. *Radiother Oncol* 2011;101:431–437.

432. Vivekanandan N, Sriram P, Kumar SA, et al. Volumetric modulated arc therapy for esophageal cancer. *Med Dosim* 2011;37:108–113.

433. Yin Y, Chen J, Xing L, et al. Applications of IMAT in cervical esophageal cancer radiotherapy: a comparison with fixed-field IMRT in dosimetry and implementation. *J Appl Clin Med Phys* 2011;12:3343.

434. Van Benthuysen L, Hales L, Podgorsak MB. Volumetric modulated arc therapy vs. IMRT for the treatment of distal esophageal cancer. *Med Dosim* 2011;36:404–409.

435. Gong Y, Wang S, Zhou L, et al. Dosimetric comparison using different multi-leaf collimators in intensity-modulated radiotherapy for upper thoracic esophageal cancer. *Radiother Oncol* 2010;5:65.

436. Lin SH, Wang L, Myles B, et al. Propensity score-based comparison of long-term outcomes with 3-dimensional conformal radiotherapy vs. intensity-modulated radiotherapy for esophageal cancer. *Int J Radiat Oncol Biol Phys* 2012;84:1078–1085.

437. Wang SL, Liao Z, Liu H, et al. Intensity-modulated radiation therapy with concurrent chemotherapy for locally advanced cervical and upper thoracic esophageal cancer. *World J Gastroenterol* 2006;14:5501–5508.

438. La TH, Minn AY, Su Z, et al. Multimodality treatment with intensity modulated radiation therapy for esophageal cancer. *Dis Esoph* 2010;23:300–308.

439. Li XA, Chibani O, Greenwald B, et al. Radiotherapy dose pertubation of metallic esophageal stents. *Int J Radiat Oncol Biol Phys* 2002;54:1276–1285.

440. Nishimura Y, Nagata K, Katano S, et al. Severe complications in advanced esophageal cancer treated with radiotherapy after intubation of esophageal stents: a questionnaire survey of the Japanese Society for Esophageal Diseases. *Int J Radiat Oncol Biol Phys* 2003;56:1327.

441. Wara WM, Mauch PM, Thomas AN, et al. Palliation for carcinoma of the esophagus. *Radiology* 1976;121:717–720.

442. Petrovich Z, Langholz B, Formenti S, et al. Management of carcinoma of the esophagus: the role of radiotherapy. *Am J Clin Oncol* 1991;14:80–86.

443. Whittington R, Coia LR, Haller DG, et al. Adenocarcinoma of the esophagus and esophagogastric junction: the effects of single and combined modalities on the survival and patterns of failure following treatment. *Int J Radiat Oncol Biol Phys* 1990;19:593–603.

444. Caspers RJ, Welvaart K, Verkes RJ, et al. The effect of radiotherapy on dysphagia and survival in patients with esophageal cancer. *Radiother Oncol* 1988;12:15–23.

445. Seitz JF, Giovannini M, Padaut-Cesana J, et al. Inoperable nonmetastatic squamous cell carcinoma of the esophagus managed by concomitant chemotherapy (5-fluorouracil and cisplatin) and radiation therapy. *Cancer* 1990;66:214–219.

446. Harvey JA, Bessell JR, Beller E, et al. Chemoradiation therapy is effective for the palliative treatment of malignant dysphagia. *Dis Esophagus* 2004;17:260–265.

447. Algan O, Coia LR, Keller SM, et al. Management of adenocarcinoma of the esophagus with chemoradiation alone or chemoradiation followed by esophagectomy: results of sequential nonrandomized phase II studies. *Int J Radiat Oncol Biol Phys* 1995;32:753–761.

448. Gill PG, Denham JW, Jamieson GG, et al. Patterns of treatment failure and prognostic factors associated with the treatment of esophageal carcinoma with chemotherapy and radiotherapy either as sole treatment or followed by surgery. *J Clin Oncol* 1992;10:1037–1043.

449. Urba S, Orringer M, Turrisi A, et al. A randomized trial comparing transhiatal esophagectomy (THE) to preoperative concurrent chemoradiation (CT/XRT) followed by esophagectomy in local regional esophageal carcinoma. *Proc Am Soc Clin Oncol* 1995;14:199.

450. Coia LR, Soffen EM, Schultheiss TE, et al. Swallowing function in patients with esophageal cancer treated with concurrent radiation and chemotherapy. *Cancer* 1993;71:281–286.

451. O'Rourke IC, Tiver K, Bull C, et al. Swallowing performance after radiation therapy for carcinoma of the esophagus. *Cancer* 1988;61:2022–2026.

452. Sur M, Sur R, Cooper K, et al. Morphologic alterations in esophageal squamous cell carcinoma after preoperative high dose rate intraluminal brachytherapy. *Cancer* 1996;77:2200–2205.

453. Gschossmann JM, Bonner JA, Foote RL, et al. Malignant tracheoesophageal fistula in patients with esophageal cancer. *Cancer* 1993;72:1513–1521.

454. Muto M, Ohtsu A, Miyamoto S, et al. Concurrent chemoradiotherapy for esophageal carcinoma with malignant fistulae. *Cancer* 1999;86:1406–1413.

455. Minsky BD. The adjuvant treatment of esophageal cancer. *Sem Radiat Oncol* 1994;4:165–169.

456. Werner-Wasik M, Yorke E, Deasy J, et al. Radiation dose-volume effects in the esophagus. *Int J Radiat Oncol Biol Phys* 2010;76:S86–S93.

457. Gergel TJ, Leichmann LL, Nava HR, et al. Effect of concurrent radiation therapy and chemotherapy on pulmonary function in patients with esophageal cancer: dose-volume histogram analysis. *Cancer J* 2002;8:451–460.

458. Lorchel F, Dumas JL, Noel A, et al. Esophageal cancer: determination of internal target volume for conformal radiotherapy. *Radiother Oncol* 2006;80:327–332.

459. Yaremko B, Guerrero T, McAleer M, et al. Determination of respiratory motion for distal esophagus cancer using four-dimensional computed tomography. *Int J Rad Oncol Biol Phys* 2008;70:145–153.

460. Sugahara S, Tokuuye K, Okumura T, et al. Clinical results of proton beam therapy for cancer of the esophagus. *Int J Radiat Oncol Biol Phys* 2005;61:76–84.

461. Koyama S, Hirohiko T. Proton beam therapy with high dose irradiation for superficial and advanced esophageal carcinomas. *Clin Cancer Res* 2003;9:3571–3577.

462. Lin SH, Komaki R, Liao Z, et al. Proton beam therapy and concurrent chemotherapy for esophageal cancer. *Int J Radiat Oncol Biol Phys* 2012;83:e345–e351.

463. Leong T, Everitt C, Yuen K, et al. A prospective study to evaluate the impact of FDG-PET on CT-based radiotherapy treatment planning for oesophageal cancer. *Radiother Oncol* 2006;78:254–261.

464. Sakurada A, Takahara T, Kwee TC, et al. Diagnostic performance of diffusion-weighted magnetic resonance imaging in esophageal carcinoma. *Eur Radiol* 2009;19:1461–1469.

465. Seppenwoolde Y, Lebesque JV, de Jaeger K, et al. Comparing different NTCP models that predict the incidence of radiation pneumonitis. Normal tissue complication probability. *Int J Radiat Oncol Biol Phys* 2003;55:724–735.

466. Willner J, Jost A, Baier K, et al. A little to a lot or a lot to a little? An analysis of pneumonitis risk from dose-volume histogram parameters of the lung in patients with lung cancer treated with 3-D conformal radiotherapy. *Strahlenther Onkol* 2003;179:548–556.

467. Yorke ED, Jackson A, Rosenzweig KE, et al. Dose-volume factors contributing to the incidence of radiation pneumonitis in non-small-cell lung cancer patients treated with three-dimensional conformal radiation therapy. *Int J Radiat Oncol Biol Phys* 2002;54:329–339.

468. Schallenkamp J, Miller R, Brinkmann D, et al. Incidence of radiation pneumonitis after thoracic irradiation; Dose-Volume correlates. *Int J Radiat Oncol Biol Phys* 2007;67:410–416.

469. Wang S, Liao Z, Wej X, et al. Analysis of clinical and dosimetric factors associated with treatment-related pneumonitis (TRP) in patients with non-small-cell lung cancer (NSCLC) treated with concurrent chemotherapy and three-dimensional conformal radiotherapy (3D-CRT). *Int J Radiat Oncol Biol Phys* 2006;66:1399–1407.

470. Konski A, Li T, Christensen M, et al. Symptomatic cardiac toxicity is predicted by dosimetric and patient factors rather than changes in 18F-FDG PET determination of myocardial activity after chemoradiotherapy for esophageal cancer. *Radiother Oncol* 2012;104:72–77.

471. Rueth NM, Shaw D, D'Cunha J, et al. Esophageal stenting and radiotherapy: a multimodal approach for the palliation of symptomatic malignant dysphagia. *Ann Surg Oncol* 2012;19:4223–4228.

472. Yagoda A, Mukherji B, Young C, et al. Bleomycin, an antitumor antibiotic. Clinical experience in 274 patients. *Ann Intern Med* 1972;77:861–870.

473. Stephens FO. Bleomycin—a new approach in cancer chemotherapy. *Med J Aust* 1973;1:1277–1283.

474. Ravry M, Moertel CG, Schutt AJ, et al. Treatment of advanced squamous cell carcinoma of the gastrointestinal tract with bleomycin (NSC-125066). *Cancer Chemother Rep* 1973;57:493–495.

475. Tancini G, Bajetta E, Bonadonna G. [Bleomycin alone and in combination with methotrexate in the treatment of carcinoma of the esophagus]. *Tumori* 1974;60:65–71.

476. Kolaric K, Maricic Z, Dujmovic I, et al. Therapy of advanced esophageal cancer with bleomycin, irradiation and combination of bleomycin with irradiation. *Tumori* 1976;62:255–262.

477. Lokich JJ, Shea M, Chaffey J. Sequential infusional 5-fluorouracil followed by concomitant radiation for tumors of the esophagus and gastroesophageal junction. *Cancer* 1987;60:275–279.

478. Ezdinli EZ, Gelber R, Desai DV, et al. Chemotherapy of advanced esophageal carcinoma: Eastern Cooperative Oncology Group experience. *Cancer* 1980;46:2149–2153.

479. Engstrom PF, Lavin PT, Klaassen DJ. Phase II evaluation of mitomycin and cisplatin in advanced esophageal carcinoma. *Cancer Treat Rep* 1983;67:713–715.

480. Whitington RM, Close HP. Clinical experience with mitomycin C (NSC-26980). *Cancer Chemother Rep* 1970;54:195–198.

481. Kolaric K, Maricic Z, Roth A, et al. Combination of bleomycin and adriamycin with and without radiation on the treatment of inoperable esophageal cancer. A randomized study. *Cancer* 1980;45:2265–2273.

482. Advani SH, Saikia TK, Swaroop S, et al. Anterior chemotherapy in esophageal cancer. *Cancer* 1985;56:1502–1506.

483. Bleiberg H, Conroy T, Paillot B, et al. Randomised phase II study of cisplatin and 5-fluorouracil (5-FU) versus cisplatin alone in advanced squamous cell oesophageal cancer. *Eur J Cancer* 1997;33:1216–1220.

484. Davis S, Shanmugathasa M, Kessler W. cis-Dichlorodiammineplatinum(II) in the treatment of esophageal carcinoma. *Cancer Treat Rep* 1980;64:709–711.

485. Miller JI, McIntyre B, Hatcher CR Jr. Combined treatment approach in surgical management of carcinoma of the esophagus: a preliminary report. *Ann Thorac Surg* 1985;40:289–293.

486. Panettiere FJ, Leichman LP, Tilchen EJ, et al. Chemotherapy for advanced epidermoid carcinoma of the esophagus with single-agent cisplatin: final report on a Southwest Oncology Group study. *Cancer Treat Rep* 1984;68:1023–1024.

487. Ravry M, Moore M. Phase II pilot study of cisplatinum (II) in advanced squamous cell esophageal cancer. *Proc Am Soc Clin Oncol* 1980;21:353.

488. Conroy T, Etienne PL, Adenis A, et al. Phase II trial of vinorelbine in metastatic squamous cell esophageal carcinoma. European Organization for Research and Treatment of Cancer. Gastrointestinal Treat Cancer Cooperative Group. *J Clin Oncol* 1996;14:164–170.

489. Bidoli P, Stani SC, DeCandis D, et al. Single-agent chemotherapy with vinorelbine for pretreated or metastatic squamous cell carcinoma of the esophagus. *Tumori* 2001;87:299–302.

490. Conroy T, Etienne PL, Adenis A, et al. Vinorelbine and cisplatin in metastatic squamous cell carcinoma of the oesophagus: response, toxicity, quality of life and survival. *Ann Oncol* 2002;13:721–729.

491. Kulke MH, Muzikansky A, Clark J, et al. A Phase II trial of vinorelbine in patients with advanced gastroesophageal adenocarcinoma. *Cancer Invest* 2006;24:346–350.

492. Milas L, Hunter NR, Mason KA, et al. Enhancement of tumor radio response of a murine mammary carcinoma by paclitaxel. *Cancer Res* 1994;54:3506–3510.

493. Ajani JA, Ilson DH, Daugherty K, et al. Activity of taxol in patients with squamous cell carcinoma and adenocarcinoma of the esophagus. *J Natl Cancer Inst* 1994;86:1086–1091.

494. Anderson SE, O'Reilly EM, Kelsen DP, et al. Phase II trial of 96-hour paclitaxel in previously treated patients with advanced esophageal cancer. *Cancer Invest* 2003;21:512–516.

495. Ilson DH, Wadleigh S, Leichman L, et al. Paclitaxel by weekly 1-h infusion in advanced esophageal cancer. *Ann Oncol* 2007;18:898–902.

496. Heath EI, Urba S, Marshall J, et al. Phase II trial of docetaxel chemotherapy in patients with incurable adenocarcinoma of the esophagus. *Invest New Drugs* 2002;20:95–99.

497. Muro K, Hamaguchi T, Ohtsu A, et al. A phase II study of single-agent docetaxel in patients with metastatic esophageal cancer. *Ann Oncol* 2004;15:955–959.

498. Bajorin D, Kelsen D, Heelan R. Phase II trial of dichloromethotrexate in epidermoid carcinoma of the esophagus. *Cancer Treat Rep* 1986;70:1245–1246.

499. Alberts AS, Falkson G, Badata M, et al. Trimetrexate in advanced carcinoma of the esophagus. *Invest New Drugs* 1988;6:319–321.

500. Brown T, Fleming T, Tangen C, et al. A phase II trial of trimetrexate in the treatment of esophageal cancer. A Southwest Oncology Group Trial. *Proc Am Soc Clin Oncol* 1992;11:(abst A479).

501. Coonley C, Bains M, Kelsen DP. VP-16-213 in the treatment of esophageal cancer: a phase II trial. *Cancer Treat Rep* 1983;67:397–398.

502. Radice PA, Bunn PA Jr, Ihde DC. Therapeutic trials with VP-16-213 and VM-26: active agents in small cell lung cancer, non-Hodgkin's lymphomas, and other malignancies. *Cancer Treat Rep* 1979;63:1231–1239.

503. Kok TC, Van Der Gaast A, Splinter TA. Ifosfamide in advanced adenocarcinoma of the oesophagus or oesophageal-gastric junction area. Rotterdam Esophageal Tumor Study Group. *Eur J Cancer* 1991;27:1112–1114.

504. Nanus DM, Kelsen DP, Lipperman R, et al. Phase II trial of ifosfamide in epidermoid carcinoma of the esophagus: unexpectant severe toxicity. *Invest New Drugs* 1988;6:239–241.

505. Mannell A, Winters Z. Carboplatin in the treatment of oesophageal cancer. *S Afr Med J* 1989;76:213–214.

506. Queisser W, Preusser P, Mross KB, et al. Phase II evaluation of carboplatin in advanced esophageal carcinoma. A trial of the phase I/II study group of the Association for Medical Oncology of the German Cancer Society. *Onkologie* 1990;13:190–193.

507. Harstrick A, Bokemeyer C, Preusser P, et al. Phase II study of single-agent etoposide in patients with metastatic squamous-cell carcinoma of the esophagus. *Cancer Chemother Pharmacol* 1992;29:321–322.

508. Sandler AB, Kindler HL, Einhorn LH, et al. Phase II trial of gemcitabine in patients with previously untreated metastatic cancer of the esophagus or gastroesophageal junction. *Ann Oncol* 2000;11:1161–1164.

509. MacDonald JS, Jacobson JL, Ketchel SJ, et al. A phase II trial of topotecan in esophageal carcinoma: a Southwest Oncology Group study (SWOG 9339). *Invest New Drugs* 2000;18:199–202.

510. Asbury RF, Lipsitz S, Graham D, et al. Treatment of squamous cell esophageal cancer with topotecan: an Eastern Cooperative Oncology Group Study (E2293). *Am J Clin Oncol* 2000;23:45–46.

511. Enzinger C, Kulke MH, Clark WH, et al. A phase II trial of irinotecan in patients with previously untreated advanced esophageal and gastric adenocarcinoma. *Dig Dis Sci* 2005;20:2218–2223.

512. Lin L, Hecht JR. A Phase II trial of irinotecan in patients with advanced adenocarcinoma of the gastroesophageal junction. *Proc Am Soc Clin Oncol* 2000;19:1130.

513. Dinwoodie WR, Bartolucci AA, Lyman GH, et al. Phase II evaluation of cisplatin, bleomycin, and vindesine in advanced squamous cell carcinoma of the esophagus: a Southeastern Cancer Study Group Trial. *Cancer Treat Rep* 1986;70:267–270.

514. Kelsen DP, Fein R, Coonley C, et al. Cisplatin, vindesine, and mitoguazone in the treatment of esophageal cancer. *Cancer Treat Rep* 1986;70:255–259.

515. Chapman R, Fleming TR, Van Damme J, et al. Cisplatin, vinblastine, and mitoguazone in squamous cell carcinoma of the esophagus: a Southwest Oncology Group Study. *Cancer Treat Rep* 1987;71:1185–1187.

516. Ogura T, Hiramatsu Y, Araki H, et al. Combined chemotherapy with 5-FU and low dose CDDP for advanced or recurrent cancer of the digestive system and home anti-cancer chemotherapy. *Gan To Kagaku Ryoho* 1995;22:433–438.

517. Webb A, Cunningham D, Scarffe JH, et al. Randomized trial comparing epirubicin, cisplatin, and fluorouracil versus fluorouracil, doxorubicin, and methotrexate in advanced esophagogastric cancer. *J Clin Oncol* 1997;15:261–267.

518. Ross P, Nicholson M, Cunningham D, et al. Prospective randomized trial comparing mitomycin, cisplatin, and protracted venous-infusion fluorouracil (PVI 5-FU) with epirubicin, cisplatin, and PVI 5-FU in advanced esophagogastric cancer. *J Clin Oncol* 2002;20:1996.

519. Mauer AM, Kraut EH, Krauss SA, et al. Phase II trial of oxaliplatin, leucovorin and fluorouracil in patients with advanced carcinoma of the esophagus. *Ann Oncol* 2005;16:1320–1325.

520. Cunningham D, Starling N, Rao S, et al. Capecitabine and oxaliplatin for advanced esophagogastric cancer. *N Engl J Med* 2008;358:36–46.

521. Al-Batran S, Hartmann J, Probst S, et al. Phase III trial in metastatic gastroesophageal adenocarcinoma with fluorouracil, leucovorin plus either oxaliplatin or cisplatin: a study of the Arbeitsgemeinschaft Internistische Onkologie. *J Clin Oncol* 2008;26:1435–1442.

522. Kang YK, Kang KW, Shin DB, et al. Capecitabine/cisplatin versus 5-fluorouracil/cisplatin as first-line therapy in patients with advanced gastric cancer: a randomized phase III noninferiority trial. *Ann Oncol* 2009;20:666–673.

523. Koizumi W, Narahara H, Hara T, et al. S-1 plus cisplatin versus S-1 alone for first line treatment of advanced gastric cancer (SPIRITS Trial): a phase III trial. *Lancet Oncol* 2008;9:215–221.

524. Ajani JR, Correa A, Walsh G, et al. Multicenter phase III comparison of cisplatin/S-1 with cisplatin/infusional fluorouracil in advanced gastric or gastroesophageal adenocarcinoma study: the FLAGS Trial. *J Clin Oncol* 2010;28:1547–1553.

525. Van Cutsem E, Moiseyenko VM, Tjulandin S, et al. Phase III study of docetaxel and cisplatin plus fluorouracil compared with cisplatin and fluorouracil as first-line therapy for advanced gastric cancer: a report of the V325 study group. *J Clin Oncol* 2006;24:4991–4997.

526. Al-Batran SE, Pauligk C, Homann N, et al. The feasibility of triple-drug chemotherapy combination in older adult patients with esophagogastric cancer: a randomized trial of the Abreitsgemeinschaft Internistische Onkologie (FLOT65+). *Eur J Cancer* 2013;49:835–842.

527. Wadler S, Fell S, Haynes H, et al. Treatment of carcinoma of the esophagus with 5-fluorouracil and recombinant alfa-2a-interferon. *Cancer* 1993;71:1726–1730.

528. Ilson DH, Sirott M, Saltz L, et al. A phase II trial of interferon alpha-2A, 5-fluorouracil, and cisplatin in patients with advanced esophageal carcinoma. *Cancer* 1995;75:2197–2202.

529. Wadler S, Haynes H, Beitler J, et al. Phase II clinical trial with 5-FU, interferon-alpha-2b and cisplatin for patients with metastatic or regionally advanced carcinoma of the esophagus. *Cancer* 1996;78:30–34.

530. Kelsen D, Lovett D, Wong J, et al. Interferon alfa-2a and fluorouracil in the treatment of patients with advanced esophageal cancer. *J Clin Oncol* 1992;10:269–274.

531. Bazarbashi S, Rahal M, Raja MA, et al. A pilot trial of combination cisplatin, 5-fluorouracil and interferon-alpha in the treatment of advanced esophageal carcinoma. *Chemotherapy* 2002;48:211–216.

532. Kok TC, Van Der Gaast A, Dees J, et al. Cisplatin and etoposide in oesophageal cancer: a phase II study. Rotterdam Oesophageal Tumour Study Group. *Br J Cancer* 1996;74:980–984.

533. Polee MB, Kok TC, Siersema PD, et al. Phase II study of the combination cisplatin, etoposide, 5-fluorouracil and folinic acid in patients with advanced squamous cell carcinoma of the esophagus. *Anticancer Drugs* 2001;12:513–517.

534. Spiridonidis CH, Laufman LR, Jones JJ, et al. A phase II evaluation of high dose cisplatin and etoposide in patients with advanced esophageal adenocarcinoma. *Cancer* 1996;77:2070–2077.

535. Polee MB, Eskens FA, Van Der Burg ME, et al. Phase II study of bi-weekly administration of paclitaxel and cisplatin in patients with advanced oesophageal cancer. *Br J Cancer* 2002;86:669–673.

536. Polee MB, Verweij J, Siersema PD, et al. Phase I study of a weekly schedule of a fixed dose of cisplatin and escalating doses of paclitaxel in patients with advanced oesophageal cancer. *Eur J Cancer* 2002;38:1495–1500.

537. Ilson DH, Forastiere A, Arquette M, et al. A phase II trial of paclitaxel and cisplatin in patients with advanced carcinoma of the esophagus. *Cancer J* 2000;6:316–323.

538. Polee MB, Sparreboom A, Eskens FA, et al. A Phase I and pharmacokinetic study of weekly paclitaxel and carboplatin in patients with metastatic esophageal cancer. *Clin Cancer Res* 2004;10:1928–1934.

539. Ilson DH, Ajani J, Bhalla K, et al. Phase II trial of paclitaxel, fluorouracil, and cisplatin in patients with advanced carcinoma of the esophagus. *J Clin Oncol* 1998;16:1826–1834.

540. Ilson DH, Saltz L, Enzinger P, et al. Phase II trial of weekly irinotecan plus cisplatin in advanced esophageal cancer. *J Clin Oncol* 1999;17:3270–3275.

541. Ajani JA, Baker J, Pisters PW, et al. CPT-11 plus cisplatin in patients with advanced, untreated gastric or gastroesophageal carcinoma: results of a phase II study. *Cancer* 2002;94:641–646.

542. Enzinger PC, Ryan D, Clark J, et al. Weekly docetaxel, cisplatin, and irinotecan (TPC): results of a multicenter phase II trial in patients with metastatic esophagogastric cancer. *Ann Oncol* 2009;20:475–480.

543. Enzinger PC, Burtness BA, Hollis DR, et al. CALGB 80403 / ECOG 1206: Randomized phase II study of standard chemotherapy plus cetuximab for metastatic esophageal cancer. *J Clin Oncol* 2010;28:15S.

544. Hecht JR, Blanke CD, Benson AB, et al. Irinotecan and paclitaxel in metastatic adenocarcinoma of the esophagus and gastric cardia. *Oncology* 2003;17:13–15.

545. Jatoi A, Tirona MT, Cha SS, et al. A phase II trial of docetaxel and CPT-11 in patients with metastatic adenocarcinoma of the esophagus, gastroesophageal junction, and gastric cardia. *Int J Gastrointest Cancer* 2002;32:115–123.

546. Govindan R, Read W, Faust J, et al. Phase II study of docetaxel and irinotecan in metastatic or recurrent esophageal cancer: a preliminary report. *Oncology (Williston Park)* 2003;17:27–31.

547. Burtness B, Gibson M, Egleston B, et al. Phase II trial of docetaxel-irinotecan combination in advanced esophageal cancer. *Ann Oncol* 2009;20:1242–1248.

548. Lordick F, von Schilling C, Bernhard H, et al. Phase II trial of irinotecan plus docetaxel in cisplatin-pretreated relapsed or refractory oesophageal cancer. *Br J Cancer* 2003;89:630–633.

549. Dank M, Zaluski J, Barone C, et al. Randomized phase III study comparing irinotecan combined with 5-fluorouracil and folinic acid to cisplatin combined with 5-fluorouracil in chemotherapy naive patients with advanced adenocarcinoma of the stomach or esophagogastric junction. *Ann Oncol* 2008;19:1450–1457.

550. Airoldi M, Cortesina G, Giordano C, et al. Docetaxel and vinorelbine: an effective regimen in recurrent squamous cell esophageal carcinoma. *Med Oncol* 2003;20:19–24.

551. Lorenzen S, Duyster RJ, Lersch C, et al. Capecitabine plus docetaxel every 3 weeks in first- and second-line metastatic oesophageal cancer: final results of a phase II trial. *Br J Cancer* 2005;92:2129–2133.

552. Bang YJ, Van Cutsem E, Fevereislova A, et al. Trastuzumab in combination with chemotherapy versus chemotherapy alone for treatment of HER2-positive advanced gastric or gastroesophageal junction cancer (ToGA): a phase 3, open-label, randomized controlled trial. *Lancet* 2010;376:687–697.

553. Yoon HH, Shi Q, Sukov WR, et al. Association of HER2/ErbB2 expression and gene amplification with pathologic features and prognosis in esophageal adenocarcinomas. *Clin Cancer Res* 2012;18:546–554.

554. Janmaat ML, Gallegos-Ruiz MI, Rodriguez JA, et al. Predictive factors for outcome in a phase II study of gefitinib in second line treatment of advanced esophageal cancer patients. *J Clin Oncol* 2006;24:1612–1619.

555. Ferry D, Anderson M, Beddard K, et al. A phase II study of gefitinib monotherapy in advanced esophageal adenocarcinoma: evidence of gene expression, cellular, and clinical response. *Clin Cancer Res* 2007;13:5869–5875.

556. Dragovich T, McCoy S, LaFleur B, et al. Phase II trial of erlotinib in gastroesophageal junction and gastric adenocarcinoma. *J Clin Oncol* 2006;24:4922–4927.

557. Dutton SJ, Blazeby JM, Petty RD, et al. Patient-reported outcomes from a phase III muticenter, randomized double-blind, placebo-controlled trial of gefitinib versus placebo in esophageal cancer progressing after chemotherapy: Cancer Oesophagus Gefitinib (COG). *J Clin Oncol* 2012;30:S34.

558. Pinto C, DiFabio F, Siena S, et al. Phase II study of cetuximab in combination with FOLFIRI in patients with untreated advanced gastric or gastroesophageal junction adenocarcinoma. *Ann Oncol* 2006;18:510–517.

559. Lorenzen S, Schuster T, Porschen R, et al. Cetuximab plus cisplatin 5-fluorouracil versus cisplatin 5-fluorouracil alone in first line metastatic squamous cell carcinoma of the esophagus: a randomized phase II trial. *Ann Oncol* 2009;20:1667–1673.

560. Lordick F, Luber B, Lorenzen S, et al. Cetuximab plus oxaliplatin/leucovorin/5-fluorouracil in first line metastatic gastric cancer: a phase II study. *Br J Cancer* 2010;102:500–505.

561. Enzinger PC, Burtness BA, Hollis DR, et al. CALGB 80403/ECOG 1206: Randomized phase II study of standard chemotherapy plus cetuximab for metastatic esophageal cancer. *J Clin Oncol* 2010;28:15S.

562. Waddell T, Cunningham D, Gonzalez D, et al. Epirubicin, oxaliplatin, and capecitabine with or without panitumumab for patients with previously untreated esophagogastric cancer (REAL-3): a randomized, open-label phase 3 trial. *Lancet Oncol* 2013;14:481.

563. Lordick F, Kang YK, Chung HC, et al. Capecitabine and cisplatin with or without cetuximab for patients with previously untreated gastric cancer (EXPAND): a randomized, open-label phase 3 trial. *Lancet Oncol* 2013;14:490–499.

564. Lorenzen S, Schuster T, Porschen R, et al. Cetuximab plus cisplatin-5-fluorouracil versus cisplatin-5-fluorouracil alone in first-line metastatic squamous cell carcinoma of the esophagus: a randomized phase II study of the Arbeitsgemeinschaft Internistische Onkologie. *Ann Oncol* 2009;20:1667–1673.

565. Shah MA, Ramanathan RA, Ilson DH, et al. Multicenter phase II trial of irinotecan, cisplatin, and Bevacizumab in patients with metastatic gastric or gastroesophageal junction adenocarcinoma. *J Clin Oncol* 2006;24:5201–5206.

566. Ohtsu A, Shah MA, van Cutsem E, et al. Bevacizumab in combination with chemotherapy as first-line therapy in advanced gastric cancer: a randomized, double-blind, placebo-controlled phase III study. *J Clin Oncol* 2011;29:3968–3976.

567. Fuchs CS, Tomasek J, Yang CJ, et al. Ramucirumab monotherapy for previously treated advanced gastric or gastro-esophageal junction adenocarcinoma (REGARD): an international, randomized, multicenter, placebo-controlled, phase 3 trial. *Lancet* 2014;383:31–39.

568. Ohtsu A, Ajani JA, Bai YX, et al. Everolimus in previously treated, advanced gastric cancer: results of the randomized, double-blind, phase III GRANITE-1 Study. *J Clin Oncol* 2013;31:3935–3943.

38 Cancer of the Stomach

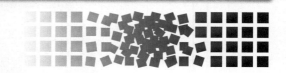

Itzhak Avital, Alexander Stojadinovic, Peter W. T. Pisters, David P. Kelsen, and Christopher G. Willett

INTRODUCTION

Adenocarcinoma of the stomach was the leading cause of cancer-related death worldwide through most of the 20th century. It now ranks second only to lung cancer, and an estimated 870,000 new cases are diagnosed annually, and 650,000 deaths (10% of all cancer deaths) worldwide.[1] In 2011, the epidemiologic data on cancer of the stomach was updated. It now ranks fourth after lung cancer, breast cancer, and colorectal cancer. An estimated 989,600 new cases are diagnosed annually, with 738,000 deaths (10% of all cancer deaths) worldwide.[2] In the West, the incidence of gastric cancer has decreased, potentially because of changes in diet, food preparation, and other environmental factors. The declining incidence has been dramatic in the United States, where this disease ranked sixth as a cause of cancer-related death during the period of 2000 to 2005.[3] It is estimated that in 2009, 21,130 new gastric cancer cases were diagnosed in the United States, with approximately 10,600 deaths.[3] Data was updated for 2014 where an estimated 22,220 new cases will be diagnosed in the United States, with approximately 10,990 deaths.[4] Prognosis remains poor except in a few countries. The explanations for this finding are multifactorial. The lack of defined risk factors, disease-specific symptoms, and the low incidence of gastric cancer has contributed to the late stage at diagnosis seen in most Western countries. In Japan, where gastric cancer is endemic, more patients are diagnosed at an early stage, which is reflected in higher overall survival (OS) rates.

The decline in incidence has been limited to noncardia gastric cancers.[5] The number of newly diagnosed cases of proximal gastric and esophagogastric junction (EGJ) adenocarcinomas has increased six-fold since the mid-1980s.[6] These proximal tumors are thought to be biologically more aggressive and more complex to treat. The only chance of cure is complete surgical resection. However, even after what is believed to be a "curative" gastrectomy, disease recurs in the majority of patients. Efforts to improve these poor results have focused on developing effective pre- and postoperative systemic and regional adjuvant therapies. This chapter details the state-of-the-art regarding the origins, screening, diagnosis, treatment, and palliation of this significant worldwide health problem.

ANATOMIC CONSIDERATIONS

The stomach begins at the gastroesophageal junction and ends at the pylorus (Fig. 38.1). Cancers arising from the proximal greater curvature may directly involve the splenic hilum and tail of pancreas, whereas more distal tumors may invade the transverse colon. Proximal cancers may extend into the diaphragm, spleen, or the left lateral segment of the liver. A recent study reported on the potential benefits and harms of complete resection even when the tumor invades adjacent abdominal visceral structures (pT4b).[7] In this large multicenter cohort series of 2,208 patients who underwent curative intent resection, 206 patients had pT4b tumors and 112 underwent resection of adjacent organs as part of en bloc gastric cancer resection. The overall 5-year survival rate for this group of patients was 27.2%, suggesting that patients do have a chance at long-term survival if their tumor can be removed en bloc with involved adjacent organs, thereby supporting the role of multivisceral resection if required and technically feasible.[7]

The blood supply to the stomach is extensive and is based on vessels arising from the celiac axis (see Fig. 38.1). The right gastric artery arises from the hepatic artery proper (50% to 68%), left hepatic artery (29% to 40%), or from the common hepatic artery (3.2%). The left gastric artery originates from the celiac axis directly (90%) and may arise from the common hepatic artery (2%), splenic artery (4%), or aorta or from the superior mesenteric artery (3%). Both right and left gastric arteries course along the lesser curvature. Along the greater curvature are the right gastroepiploic artery, which originates from the gastroduodenal artery at the inferior border of the proximal duodenum (rarely from the superior mesenteric artery), and the left gastroepiploic artery (highly variable artery), branching from the distal (72%), inferior, middle splenic artery laterally. The short gastric arteries (vasa brevia, five to seven separate vessels) arise directly from the splenic artery or the left gastroepiploic artery. The posterior (dorsal) gastric artery (17% to 68%) may arise from the splenic artery to supply the distal esophagus, cardia, and fundus. The preservation of any of these vessels in the course of a subtotal gastrectomy for carcinoma is not necessary, and the most proximal few centimeters of remaining stomach are well supplied by collateral flow from the lower segmental esophageal arterial arcade. The rich submucosal blood supply of the stomach is an important factor in its ability to heal rapidly and produce a low incidence of anastomotic disruption following radical gastric resection. The venous drainage of the stomach tends to parallel the arterial supply. The venous efflux ultimately passes through the portal venous system, and this is reflected in the fact that the liver is the primary site for distant metastatic spread.

The lymphatic drainage of the stomach is extensive, and distinct anatomic groups of perigastric lymph nodes have been defined according to their relationship to the stomach and its blood supply. There are six perigastric lymph node groups. In the first echelon (stations 1 through 6) are the right and left pericardial nodes (stations 1 and 2). Along the lesser curvature are the lesser curvature nodes (station 3) and the suprapyloric nodes (station 5). Along the greater curvature, the gastroepiploic nodes or greater curvature nodes (station 4), and the subpyloric nodes (station 6). In the second echelon (stations 7 through 12) are the nodes along named arteries, which include the left gastric, common hepatic, celiac, splenic hilum, splenic artery, and hepatoduodenal lymphatics (stations 7 through 12, respectively), which drain into the celiac and periaortic lymphatics. The third echelon (stations 13 through 16) contains the posterior to pancreatic head, superior mesenteric artery, middle colic artery, and para-aortic lymphatics (stations 13 through 16, respectively). Proximally are the lower esophageal lymph nodes; extensive spread of gastric cancer along the intrathoracic lymph channels may be manifested clinically by a metastatic lymph node in the left supraclavicular fossa (Virchow's node) or left axilla (Irish's node). Tumor spread to the lymphatics in the hepatoduodenal ligament can extend along the falciform ligament and result in subcutaneous periumbilical tumor deposits (Sister Mary Joseph's nodes).

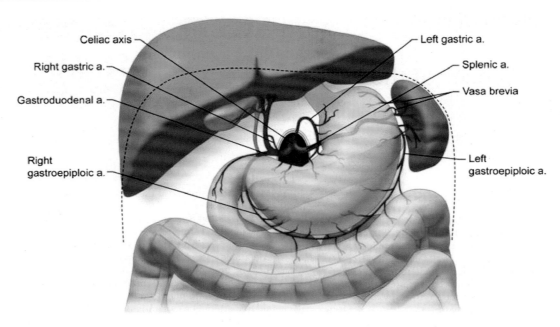

Figure 38.1 Blood supply to the stomach and anatomic relationships of the stomach with other adjacent organs likely to be involved by direct extension of a T4 gastric tumor.

PATHOLOGY AND TUMOR BIOLOGY

Approximately 95% of all gastric cancers are adenocarcinomas. The term *gastric cancer* refers to adenocarcinoma of the stomach. Other malignant tumors are rare and include squamous cell carcinoma, adenoacanthoma, carcinoid tumors, small cell carcinoma, mucinous carcinoma, hepatoid adenocarcinoma, oncocytic (parietal gland) carcinoma, sarcomatoid carcinoma, lymphoepithelioma-like carcinoma, adenocarcinoma with rhabdoid features, gastric carcinoma with osteoclastlike giant cells, neuroendocrine tumor, gastrointestinal stromal tumor, or leiomyosarcoma.[8] Although no normal lymphoid tissue is found in the gastric mucosa, the stomach is the most common site for lymphomas of the gastrointestinal tract. The increased awareness of association between mucosa-associated lymphoid tissue lymphomas and *Helicobacter pylori* may explain, in part, the rise in incidence,[9] although the incidence of mucoas-associated lymphoid tissue gastric lymphomas is decreasing likely because of effective treatment against *H. pylori*.[10]

In terms of pathogenesis, two new concepts are worth mentioning: bone marrow participation in gastric carcinogenesis and gastric cancer stem cells. It has been hypothesized that the gastric epithelial cells acquiring abnormal phenotype (resembling intestinal epithelium) originate from gastric stem cells localized to the only cell replication zone of the gastric glands (i.e., the isthmus). However, Houghton et al.,[11] Stoicov et al.,[12,13] and Li et al.[14] demonstrated in a rodent model of *Helicobacter*-induced gastric cancer that the entire cancer mass was derived from cells originating in the bone marrow. This interesting phenomenon was observed by other authors studying solid cancers in patients receiving bone marrow transplantation.[15] Recent evidence proposes the existence of cancer stem cells or stemlike cancer cells in various cancers. Although controversial, cancer stem cells are defined as cancer cells with the exclusive ability to initiate tumors, metastasize, and self-renew tumors. In gastric cancer, several investigators suggested the existence of gastric cancer stem cells (i.e., CD44+) and side population cells.[16,17] These cells showed relative resistance to chemotherapy and radiation, and exclusive ability to initiate tumors. These important observations might lead to novel approaches to the diagnosis and treatment of gastric cancer in the next decade.

HISTOPATHOLOGY

Several staging schemas have been proposed based on the morphologic features of gastric tumors. The Borrmann classification divides gastric cancer into five types depending on macroscopic appearance. Type I represents polypoid or fungating cancers, type II encompasses ulcerating lesions surrounded by elevated borders, type III represents ulcerated lesions infiltrating the gastric wall, type IV includes diffusely infiltrating tumors, and type V gastric cancers are unclassifiable cancers.[18] The gross morphologic appearance of gastric cancer and the degree of histologic differentiation are not independent prognostic variables. Ming[19] has proposed a histomorphologic staging system that divides gastric cancer into either a prognostically favorable expansive type or a poor prognosis infiltrating type. Based on an analysis of 171 gastric cancers, the expansive-type tumors were uniformly polypoid or superficial on gross appearance, whereas the infiltrative tumors were almost always diffuse. Grossly ulcerated lesions were divided between the expansive or infiltrative forms. Broder's classification of gastric cancer grades tumors histologically from 1 (well-differentiated) to 4 (anaplastic). Bearzi and Ranaldi[20] have correlated the degree of histologic differentiation with the gross appearance of 41 primary gastric cancers seen on endoscopy. Ninety percent of protruding or superficial cancers were well differentiated (Broder's grade 1), whereas almost half of all ulcerated tumors were poorly differentiated or diffusely infiltrating (Broder's grades 3 and 4).

The most widely used classification of gastric cancer is by Laurén.[21] It divides gastric cancers into either intestinal or diffuse forms. This classification scheme, based on tumor histology, characterizes two varieties of gastric adenocarcinomas that manifest distinctively different pathology, epidemiology, genetics, and etiologies. The intestinal variety represents a differentiated cancer with a tendency to form glands similar to other sites in the gastrointestinal tract, but in particular the colon type; hence the intestinal type. In contrast, the diffuse form exhibits very little cell cohesion with a predilection for extensive submucosal spread and early metastases. Although the diffuse-type cancers are associated with a worse outcome than the intestinal type, this finding is not independent of tumor, node, and metastasis (TNM) stage. The molecular pathogenesis of these two distinct forms of gastric cancer is also different. Although the intestinal type represents

H. pylori–initiated multistep progression with less defined progressive genetic alterations, the diffuse type main carcinogenic event is loss of expression of E-cadherin (*CDH1* gene). E-cadherin is a molecule involved in cell-to-cell adhesion; loss of its expression leads to noncohesive growth, hence the diffuse type. In tumors that display both intestinal and diffuse phenotypes, the *CDH1* mutation and loss of E-cadherin function are observed only within the diffuse phenotype.[22]

PATTERNS OF SPREAD

Carcinomas of the stomach can spread by local extension to involve adjacent structures and can develop lymphatic metastases, peritoneal metastases, and distant metastases. These extensions can occur by the local invasive properties of the tumor, lymphatic spread, or hematogenous dissemination. The initial growth of the tumor occurs by penetration into the gastric wall, extension through the wall, within the wall longitudinally,[23] and subsequent involvement of an increasing percentage of the stomach. The two modes of local extension that can have major therapeutic implications are tumor penetration through the gastric serosa, where the risk of tumor invasion of adjacent structures or peritoneal spread is increased, and lymphatic involvement. Zinninger[24] has evaluated spread within the gastric wall and has found a wide variation in its extent. Tumor spread is often through the intramural lymphatics or in the subserosal layers.[23] Local extension can also occur into the esophagus or the duodenum.[25] Duodenal extension is rare (0.5% to 1.8% of all resected cases),[26] portrays poor prognosis, and is principally through the muscular layer by direct infiltration and through the subserosal lymphatics, but is not generally to any great extent.[27] Extension into the esophagus occurs primarily through the submucosal lymphatics.[28]

Local extension does not occur solely by radial intramural spread but also by deep invasion through the wall to adjacent structures[23] (omentum, spleen, adrenal gland, diaphragm, liver, pancreas, or colon). Many studies report that 60% to 90% of patients had primary tumors penetrating the serosa or invading adjacent organs and that at least 50% had lymphatic metastases. In the largest series reporting on 10,783 patients with gastric cancer from Korea, 57% of the patients had lymph node metastasis, and the average number of involved lymph nodes was five.[29,30] Of the 1,577 primary gastric cancer cases admitted to Memorial Sloan Kettering Cancer Center (MSKCC) between July 1, 1985, and June 30, 1998, 60% of the 1,221 resected cases had evidence of serosal penetration and 68% had positive nodes. Lymph node metastases were found in 18% of pT1 lesions, and 60% of pT2 lesions after R0 resection in 941 patients. The highest incidence of lymphatic metastasis was seen in tumors diffusely involving the entire stomach. Tumors located at the gastroesophageal junction also had a high incidence relative to other sites.[31]

The pattern of nodal metastases also varies depending on the location of the primary site. In a study, reporting on 1,137 patients with early gastric cancer (EGC), tumors located in the upper, middle, and lower third of the stomach had 12%, 10%, and 8% nodal involvement, respectively. The most common nodal station metastases for the upper, middle, and lower third of the stomach were stations 3 (lesser curvature), 3/4/7 (lesser/greater curvature/left gastric artery), and 3/4/6 (lesser/greater curvature/infrapyloric), respectively.[32] Earlier studies that included more advanced gastric cancers showed that the left gastric artery nodes were at increased risk for nodal metastases independent of tumor location.[32,33]

Gastric cancer recurs in multiple sites, locoregionally and systemically. Patterns of failure are variable. These differences are likely related to the patient cohorts evaluated, the time at which failure was determined, and the method of determination of failure patterns. Recent series from the MSKCC and Korea do shed light on modern patterns of failure.[31,34] In the report from MSKCC, recurrence patterns of 1,038 patients who underwent R0 gastrectomy with D2 lymphadenectomy (61%) were analyzed; complete data on recurrence were available in 367 (74%) of 496 patients who experienced recurrence. The locoregional area was involved in 199 (54%) patients. Distant sites were involved in 188 (51%) patients, and peritoneal recurrence was detected in 108 (29%) patients. More than one site of recurrence was detected: distal, peritoneal, and locoregional recurrences in 9 (2.5%); locoregional and peritoneal in 34 (9.3%); locoregional and distant in 61 (16.6%); and distant and peritoneal in 15 (4.1%) patients. On multivariate analysis, peritoneal recurrence was associated with female gender, advanced T stage, and distal and diffuse type tumors; locoregional recurrence was associated with proximal location, early T stage, and intestinal type tumors. In the study from Korea, recurrence patterns were analyzed in 2,038 patients who were treated with potentially curative gastrectomy.[34] Of 508 patients who developed recurrence, 33% involved locoregional sites, 44% were peritoneal, and 38% were distant. At time of presentation, 35% of patients presented with distant metastasis, with 4% to 14% having liver metastases.[35,36]

CLINICAL PRESENTATION AND PRETREATMENT EVALUATION

Signs and Symptoms

Because of the vague, nonspecific symptoms that characterize gastric cancer, many patients are diagnosed with advanced-stage disease. Patients may have a combination of signs and symptoms such as weight loss (22% to 61%)[37]; anorexia (5% to 40%); fatigue, epigastric discomfort, or pain (62% to 91%); and postprandial fullness, heart burn, indigestion, nausea, and vomiting (6% to 40%). None of these unequivocally indicates gastric cancer. In addition, patients may be asymptomatic (4% to 17%).[38] Weight loss and abdominal pain are the most common presenting symptoms at initial encounter.[39–41] Weight loss is a common symptom, and its clinical significance should not be underestimated. Dewys et al.[42] found that in 179 patients with advanced gastric cancer, >80% of patients had a >10% decrease in body weight before diagnosis. Furthermore, patients with weight loss had a significantly shorter survival than did those without weight loss.[40]

In some patients, symptoms may suggest the presence of a lesion at a specific location. Up to 25% of the patients have history/symptoms of peptic ulcer disease.[39] A history of dysphagia or pseudoachalasia may indicate the presence of a tumor in the cardia with extension through the gastroesophageal junction.[43] Early satiety is an infrequent symptom of gastric cancer but is indicative of a diffusely infiltrative tumor that has resulted in loss of distensibility of the gastric wall. Delayed satiety and vomiting may indicate pyloric involvement. Significant gastrointestinal bleeding is uncommon with gastric cancer; however, hematemesis does occur in approximately 10% to 15% of patients, and anemia in 1% to 12% of patients. Signs and symptoms at presentation are often related to spread of disease. Ascites, jaundice, or a palpable mass indicate incurable disease.[40] The transverse colon is a potential site of malignant fistulization and obstruction from a gastric primary tumor. Diffuse peritoneal spread of disease frequently produces other sites of intestinal obstruction. A large ovarian mass (Krukenberg's tumor) or a large peritoneal implant in the pelvis (Blumer's shelf), which can produce symptoms of rectal obstruction, may be palpable on pelvic or rectal examination.[37,44] Nodular metastases in the subcutaneous tissue around the umbilicus (Sister Mary Joseph's node) or in peripheral lymph nodes such as in the supraclavicular area (Virchow's node) or axillary region (Irish's node) represent areas in which a tissue diagnosis can be established with minimal morbidity.[45] There is no symptom complex that occurs early in the evolution of gastric cancer that can identify individuals for further diagnostic measures. However, alarming symptoms (dysphagia,

CANCERS OF THE GASTROINTESTINAL TRACT

weight loss, and palpable abdominal mass) are independently associated with survival; increased number and the specific symptom is associated with mortality.[40,41]

Screening

A list of risk factors associated with gastric cancer is outlined in Table 38.1. These factors might be use for risk stratification in screening programs. Mass screening programs for gastric cancer have been most successful in high-risk areas, especially in Japan.[46] A variety of screening tests have been studied in Japanese patients, with a sensitivity and specificity of approximately 90%.[40] Screening typically includes serology for *H. pylori*, the use of double-contrast barium radiographs, or upper endoscopy with risk stratification (OLGA staging system for gastric cancer risk[46,47]).

Ohata et al.[48] reported on 4,655 asymptomatic patients with an average age of 50 years old who were followed for 7.7 years. Atrophic gastritis was identified using pepsinogen and *H. pylori* testing: 2,341 (52%) were *H. pylori*–positive with nonatrophic gastritis, 967 (21%) were *H. pylori*–negative without atrophic gastritis, 1,316 (28%) were *H. pylori*–positive with atrophic gastritis,

and 31 (0.7%) had severe atrophic gastritis. The rates of gastric cancer development per population per year were 107/100,000 for *H. pylori*–positive with nonatrophic gastritis, 0/100,000 for *H. pylori*–negative without atrophic gastritis, 238/100,000 for *H. pylori*–positive with atrophic gastritis, and 871/100,000 for severe atrophic gastritis. Thus the number of endoscopies needed to detect one cancer was 1/1,000, 0/1,000, 1/410, and 1/114, respectively. Similar data were reported on 6,985 patients by Watabe et al.[49] Surveillance in endemic populations is clinically important because EGC has a very high cure rate with surgical treatment. However, the fact that gastric cancer remains one of the top causes of death in Japan indicates the limitations of a mass-screening program when the entire population at risk is not effectively screened. However, more recent studies indicate that for surveillance programs to be effective and feasible from an economical perspective, they should be instituted only in high-risk populations (>20/100,000 incidence of disease) and include the following components: detection and eradication of *H. pylori*, serum pepsinogen (pepsinogen I/II ratio), endoscopy with biopsy, and risk stratification before and after *H. pylori* eradication using a system such as the OLGA staging system for gastric cancer risk. Such programs are expected to avoid long-term repeated screening of approximately 70% of the population who are at low risk of developing gastric cancer.[46,50–52] A US study found that screening and eradication of *H. pylori* in Japanese Americans is cost-effective in preventing gastric cancer.[53] These findings were confirmed by two studies from the United Kingdom.[54,55]

PRETREATMENT STAGING

Tumor Markers

Most gastric cancers have at least one elevated tumor marker, but some benign gastric diseases show elevated serum tumor markers as well. Tumor markers in gastric cancer continue to have limited diagnostic usefulness, with their role more informative in follow-up after primary treatment. The most commonly used markers are serum carcinoembryonic antigen (CEA), cancer antigen (CA) 19-9, CA 50, and CA 72-4. There is wide variation in the reported serum levels of these markers; positive CEA and CA 19-9 levels varied from 8% to 58% and 4% to 65%, respectively. Overall, the sensitivity of each serum tumor marker alone as a diagnostic marker of gastric cancer is low. However, when the levels are elevated, it does usually correlate with stage of disease. Combining CEA with other markers, such as CA 19-9, CA 72-4, or CA 50, can increase sensitivity compared with CEA alone.[56–62]

In a large study evaluating serum CEA, α-fetoprotein, human chronic gonadotropin-β, CA 19-9, CA 125, as well as tissue staining for *HER2* in gastric cancer patients, only human chronic gonadotropin-β level >4 IU/L and a CA 125 level ≥350 U/mL had prognostic significance. Elevated serum tumor marker levels in gastric cancer before chemotherapy may reflect not just tumor burden but also biology of disease.

Endoscopy

Endoscopy is the best method to diagnose gastric cancer as it visualizes the gastric mucosa and allows biopsy for a histologic diagnosis. Chromoendoscopy helps identify mucosal abnormalities through topical mucosal stains. Magnification endoscopy is used to magnify standard endoscopic fields by 1.5- to 150-fold. Narrow band imaging affords enhanced visualization of the mucosal microvasculature. Confocal laser endomicroscopy permits in vivo, three-dimensional microscopy including subsurface structures with diagnostic accuracy, sensitivity, and specificity of 97%, 90%, and 99.5%, respectively.[63–65]

TABLE 38.1
Factors Associated with Increased Risk of Developing Stomach Cancer

Acquired Factors
- Nutritional
  - High salt consumption
  - High nitrate consumption
  - Low dietary vitamin A and C
  - Poor food preparation (smoked, salt cured)
  - Lack of refrigeration
  - Poor drinking water (well water)
- Occupational
  - Rubber workers
  - Coal workers
- Cigarette smoking
- *Helicobacter pylori* infection
- Epstein-Barr virus
- Radiation exposure
- Prior gastric surgery for benign gastric ulcer disease
- Prior treatment for mucosa-associated lymphoid tissue lymphoma

Genetic Factors
- Type A blood
- Pernicious anemia
- Family history without known genetic factors (first-degree relative with gastric cancer)
- Hereditary diffuse gastric cancer (*CDH1* mutation)
- Familial gastric cancer
- Hereditary nonpolyposis colon cancer
- Familial adenomatous polyposis
- Li-Fraumeni syndrome
- *BRCA1* and *BRAC2*
- Precursor lesions
  - Adenomatous gastric polyps
  - Chronic atrophic gastritis
  - Dysplasia
  - Intestinal metaplasia
  - Menetrier disease
- Ethnicity (in the United States, gastric cancer is more common among Asian/Pacific Islanders, Hispanics and African Americans)
- Obesity (the strength of this link is not clear)

Endoscopic ultrasound (EUS) is a tool for preoperative staging and selection for neoadjuvant therapy. It is used to assess the T and N stage of primary tumors. A study of 225 patients from MSKCC found that the concordance between EUS and pathology was lower than expected. The accuracy for individual T and N stage were 57% and 50%, respectively. However, the combined assessment of N stage and serosal invasion identified 77% of the patients at risk of disease-related death after curative resection.[66] Other investigators compared the accuracy of EUS with that of multidetector computed tomography (MDCT) and magnetic resonance imaging (MRI) and found that the overall accuracy was 65% to 92% (EUS), 77% to 89% (MDCT), and 71% to 83% (MRI) for T stage, and 55% to 66% (EUS), 32% to 77% (MDCT) for N stage, respectively. The corresponding sensitivity and specificity for serosal involvement were 78% to 100% (EUS), 83% to 100% (MDCT), and 89% to 93% (MRI) for T stage, and 68% to 100% (EUS), 80% to 97% (MDCT), and 91% to 100% (MRI) for N stage, respectively.[65,67]

Computed Tomography

Once gastric cancer is suspected, a triphasic CT with oral and intravenous contrast of the abdomen, chest, and pelvis is imperative. In a study of 790 patients who underwent MDCT prior to surgery, the overall accuracy in determining T stage was 74% (T1 46%, T2 53%, T3 86%, and T4 86%), and for N staging it was 75% (N0 76%, N1 69%, and N2 80%). The sensitivity, specificity, and accuracy for lymph node metastasis were 86%, 76%, and 82%, respectively.[68] MDCT with thin-sliced multiplanar reconstruction (MPR) and water filling is increasingly used. The accuracy rate for advanced gastric cancer was 96% and for EGC it was 41%. An improvement on axial CT and MPR-MDCT was the addition of staging with three-dimensional MPR-MDCT. The detection rate for MPR with virtual gastroscopy was 98%. MPR-MDCT with combined water and air distention is superior to conventional axial imaging.[69]

Magnetic Resonance Imaging

MRI is not used routinely in preoperative staging of gastric cancer. Several studies have demonstrated that CT and MRI are comparable in terms of accuracy and understaging.[70,71] However, MRI is a useful modality to further characterize liver lesions identified on preoperative CT staging workup.

Positron Emission Tomography

Whole-body 2-[18F]-fluoro-2-deoxyglucose (FDG) positron emission tomography (PET) is being applied increasingly in the evaluation of gastrointestinal malignancies. In gastric cancer, approximately half of the primary tumors are FDG-negative; the diffuse (signet cell) subtype was most likely to be non-FDG avid, likely because of decreased expression of the glucose transporter-1 (Glut-1).[72] In patients with non-FDG–avid primary tumor, FDG-PET/CT is not useful.[72–76] PET/CT was tested as a tool to predict response to neoadjuvant chemotherapy. Ott et al.[77] reported 90% 2-year survival in patients with PET-defined response (<35% decrease standardized uptake value [SUV]) versus 25% for patients not responding to PET. PET response could be detected as early as 14 days. At least 60% of the patients were PET-nonresponding patients and thus could have been spared further chemotherapy. Authors of the MUNICON trial reported on patients who were PET nonresponders by day 14 after cisplatin and fluorouracil (5-FU) (CF) neoadjuvant chemotherapy, and subsequently were sent for surgery, and patients who were PET responders and continued 3 months of neoadjuvant therapy before surgery. The PET-responding patients had a survival benefit (hazard ratio [HR] = 2.13; p <0.15). In PET-nonresponding patients, stopping the chemotherapy did not affect long-term survival.[78] Recent studies, including one large meta-analysis, showed that in terms of diagnostic accuracy and lymph node staging EUS, MDCT, MRI, and PET/CT are comparable modalities. There were no significant differences between mean sensitivities and specificities.[79,80] Even in patients whose tumors were FDG-avid, FDG-PET/CT scans did not identify occult peritoneal disease (0 of 18), but did identify extraperitoneal M1 disease in nine patients with bone (n = 2), liver (n = 4), and retroperitoneal lymph node (n = 3) involvement. In patients with FDG-avid tumors, PET may be useful in detecting metastatic disease and follow-up for recurrence. Interestingly, the presence of Glut-1– and FDG-avid gastric cancers may be associated with decreased OS.[72] The role of PET/CT in the primary staging of gastric cancer remains to be established; its role might be better defined in advanced disease.

In a prospective study of 113 patients who were clinically staged as locally advanced but nonmetastatic gastric cancer (T3-T4, Nx or N+, M0), investigators found that FDG-PET/CT did identify occult metastatic disease in about 10% of patients. In this study, FDG-PET/CT did not identify occult peritoneal disease, suggesting a necessary role for laparoscopy in preoperative staging of locally advanced gastric cancer. A cost evaluation was also performed, and it suggested that if FDG-PET/CT is included as part of the staging algorithm, that would result in an estimated cost savings of approximately $13,000 US dollars per patient.[81]

Staging Laparoscopy and Peritoneal Cytology

Staging laparoscopy with peritoneal lavage should be an integral part of the pretreatment staging evaluation of patients believed to have localized gastric cancer. Current noninvasive modalities used in preoperative staging of gastric cancer have sensitivities significantly lower than 100%, particularly in cases of low-volume peritoneal carcinomatosis.[82–84] Current CT techniques cannot consistently identify low-volume macroscopic metastases that are ≤5 mm in size. Laparoscopy directly inspects the peritoneal and visceral surfaces for detection of CT-occult, small-volume metastases. Staging laparoscopy also allows for assessment of peritoneal cytology and laparoscopic ultrasound. Laparoscopic staging is done to spare nontherapeutic operations and for potential stratification in various trials.[85]

The rate of detection of CT-occult M1 disease by laparoscopy depends on the quality of CT scanning and interpretation.[86] Muntean et al.[87] reported on 98 patients with primary gastric cancer: 45 underwent staging laparoscopy with subsequent surgery and 53 went directly to surgery. An unnecessary laparotomy was avoided in 38% of the patients. The overall sensitivity and specificity were 89% and 100%, respectively. Nonetheless, even high-quality MDCT is insufficiently sensitive for detection of low-volume extragastric disease and thus CT, EUS, and laparoscopy are complementary staging studies.[88,89]

The value of peritoneal cytology as a preoperative staging tool in patients with gastric cancer who are potential candidates for curative resection by EUS and CT has been examined by several investigators. Bentrem et al.[90] reported on 371 patients who underwent R0 resection, 6.5% of whom had positive cytology after staging laparoscopy. Median survival of patients with positive cytology was 14.8 versus 98.5 months for patients with negative cytology findings (p <0.001). Positive cytology predicted death from gastric cancer (relative risk = 2.7; p <0.001) and is tantamount to M1 disease. Several groups confirmed these findings and concluded that staging laparoscopy with peritoneal cytology can change the management of gastric cancer in 6.5% to 52% of patients.[85,91–94]

Laparoscopy can be performed as a separate staging procedure prior to definitive treatment planning or immediately prior to planned laparotomy for gastrectomy. When performed as a separate procedure, laparoscopy has the disadvantage of the additional risks and expense of a second general anesthetic. However, separate procedure laparoscopy allows the additional staging information including cytology acquired at laparoscopy to be reviewed and discussed with the patient and in multidisciplinary treatment group prior to definitive treatment planning. Laparoscopic ultrasound (LUS) and "extended laparoscopy" are techniques that may increase the diagnostic yield of laparoscopy. Preliminary results reveal conflicting data on the added benefit of LUS and extended laparoscopy.[95–97] Further prospective studies will be required to evaluate the cost-benefit relationship of LUS and extended laparoscopy in the routine or selective workup of patients with gastric cancer.

Although laparoscopic staging is thought to detect CT-occult metastatic disease in approximately 40% of patients and spares nontherapeutic operations in approximately one-third of patients with gastric cancer, one needs to remember that tumor biology, not staging, will eventually guide outcomes. Clearly, not all patients benefit from preoperative laparoscopic staging; therefore, future studies should address the issue of selective laparoscopy based on noninvasive staging (i.e., patients with T1 tumors). Staging laparoscopy with or without cytology should be considered only if therapy will be altered consequent to information obtained by laparoscopy.[82]

STAGING, CLASSIFICATION, AND PROGNOSIS

For patients with surgically treated gastric adenocarcinoma, both pathologic staging (American Joint Committee on Cancer [AJCC]/International Union Against Cancer [UICC] or Japanese system) and classification of the completeness of resection (R classification) should be done. Although not formal components of the stage grouping, the AJCC recommends collection of additional prognostic factors: tumor location, serum CEA and CA 19.9, and histopathologic grade and type.[98]

American Joint Committee on Cancer/International Union Against Cancer Tumor, Node, Metastasis Staging

The AJCC/UICC TNM staging system for gastric cancer is outlined in Table 38.2.[98] The AJCC/UICC stage-stratified survival rates of 10,601 patients treated by surgical resection from the Surveillance, Epidemiology, and End Results program 1973 to 2005 public-use file diagnosed in years 1991 to 2000 are shown in Fig. 38.2. Several definitions in the most recent version of the AJCC (2010) differ from the previous version (2002). Tumors arising at the EGJ including Siewert type I or arising in the stomach ≤5 cm from the EGJ and crossing into the EJG including Siewert types II and III are staged using the TNM system for esophageal adenocarcinoma. Gastric tumors lying ≤5 cm from the EGJ but that do not cross the EGJ into the esophagus are staged as gastric cancer.[98]

In the AJCC/UICC staging system, tumor (T) stage is determined by depth of tumor invasion into the gastric wall and extension into adjacent structures (Fig. 38.3). The relationship between T stage, the overall stage, and survival is well defined (see Fig. 38.2). Nodal stage (N) is based on the number of involved lymph nodes, a criterion that may predict outcome more accurately than the location of involved lymph nodes.[99,100] Tumors with 1 to 2 involved nodes are classified as pN1, 3 to 6 involved nodes are classified as pN2, and those with 7 or more involved nodes are classified as pN3 (N3a has 7 to 15 nodes and N3b has ≥16 nodes). The use of numerical thresholds for nodal classification has gained increasing acceptance, although the extent of lymphadenectomy and rigor of pathologic assessment may affect results.[101,102] The nodal numerical threshold approach is based on observations that

TABLE 38.2

American Joint Committee on Cancer Staging of Gastric Cancer 2010: Definition of Tumor, Nodes, Metastasis

Primary Tumor (T)

TX	Primary tumor cannot be assessed
T0	No evidence of primary tumor
Tis	Carcinoma in situ: intraepithelial tumor without invasion of the lamina propria
T1	Tumor invades lamina propria, muscularis mucosae, or submucosa
T1a	Tumor invades lamina propria or muscularis mucosae
T1b	Tumor invades submucosa
T2	Tumor invades muscularis propria
T3	Tumor penetrates subserosal connective tissue without invasion of visceral peritoneum or adjacent structures
T4	Tumor invades serosa (visceral peritoneum) or adjacent structures
T4a	Tumor invades serosa (visceral peritoneum)
T4b	Tumor invades adjacent structures

Regional Lymph Nodes (N)

NX	Regional lymph node(s) cannot be assessed
N0	No regional lymph node metastasis
N1	Metastasis in 1 to 2 regional lymph nodes
N2	Metastasis in 3 to 6 regional lymph nodes
N3	Metastases in more than 7 regional lymph nodes
N3a	Metastasis in 7–15 regional nodes
N3b	Metastasis in 16 or more regional nodes

Distant Metastasis (M)

MX	Presence of distant metastasis cannot be assessed
M0	No distant metastasis
M1	Distant metastasis

Stage Grouping

O	Tis	N0	M0
IA	T1	N0	M0
IB	T2	N0	M0
	T1	N1	M0
IIA	T3	N0	M0
	T2	N1	M0
	T1	N2	M0
IIB	T4a	N0	M0
	T3	N1	M0
	T2	N2	M0
	T1	N3	M0
IIIA	T4a	N1	M0
	T3	N2	M0
	T2	N3	M0
IIIB	T4b	N0	M0
	T4b	N1	M0
	T4a	N2	M0
	T3	N3	M0
IIIC	T4b	N2	M0
	T4b	N3	M0
	T4a	N3	M0
IV	Any T	Any N	M1

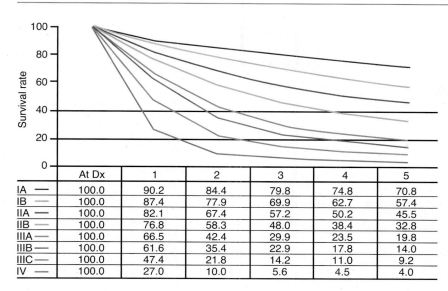

	At Dx	1	2	3	4	5
IA —	100.0	90.2	84.4	79.8	74.8	70.8
IB —	100.0	87.4	77.9	69.9	62.7	57.4
IIA —	100.0	82.1	67.4	57.2	50.2	45.5
IIB —	100.0	76.8	58.3	48.0	38.4	32.8
IIIA —	100.0	66.5	42.4	29.9	23.5	19.8
IIIB —	100.0	61.6	35.4	22.9	17.8	14.0
IIIC —	100.0	47.4	21.8	14.2	11.0	9.2
IV —	100.0	27.0	10.0	5.6	4.5	4.0

Figure 38.2 Disease-specific survival by American Joint Committee on Cancer stage grouping. *Numbers* beneath x-axis indicate patients at risk. (From Crew KD, Neugut AI. Epidemiology of gastric cancer. *World J Gastroenterol* 2006;12:354, with permission.)

survival decreases as the number of metastatic lymph nodes increases,[103,104] and that survival significantly decreases at three or more involved[103] lymph nodes and again at seven or more involved lymph nodes.[30,105]

Given the reliance on numerical thresholds for nodal staging, it is extremely important that adequate number of lymph nodes are retrieved surgically and examined pathologically. However, recent reports document poor compliance with AJCC staging primarily because the number of lymph nodes removed and/or examined (≤15) was insufficient.[104,106] Positive peritoneal cytology is classified as M1. Ratio-based lymph node classification (number of positive nodes over number of total nodes resected and evaluated) is an alternative to the threshold-based system currently utilized by the AJCC/UICC staging systems. It may minimize the confounding effects of regional variations in the extent of lymphadenectomy and pathologic evaluation on lymph node staging and thereby

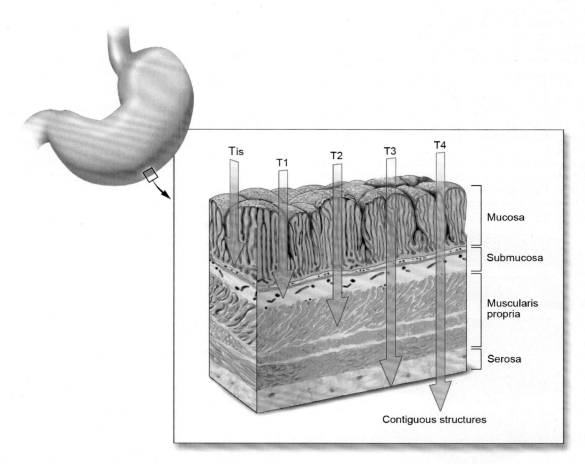

Figure 38.3 Definition of American Joint Committee on Cancer/International Union Against Cancer T stage based on depth of penetration of the gastric wall.

reduce stage migration.[107–109] Sun et al.[108] evaluated the ratio between metastatic and examined lymph nodes (RML) in a group of 2,159 patients who underwent curative gastrectomy. The anatomic location, number of positive lymph nodes (AJCC/UICC), and RML were analyzed for staging accuracy and relationship to survival. RML was an independent prognostic factor for survival and reduced stage migration. These findings were confirmed by several investigators reporting on approximately 2,000 patients treated by R0 gastrectomy.[107,109–112]

Japanese Staging System

The most recent *Japanese Classification for Gastric Carcinoma* was published in 1998.[113–116] The Japanese classification and staging system is more detailed than the AJCC/UICC staging system and places more emphasis on the distinction between clinical, surgical, pathologic, and "final" staging (prefixes "c," "s," "p," and "f," respectively). For example, a surgically treated and staged patient with locally advanced, nonmetastatic gastric cancer might be staged as pT3, pN2, sH0, sM0, stage f-IIIB (where H0 denotes no hepatic metastases and the "f" prefix denotes final clinicopathologic stage). The Japanese classification system also includes a classification system for EGC (Fig. 38.4).

In the combined superficial types, the type occupying the largest area should be described first, followed by the next type (e.g., IIc + III). Type 0I and type 0IIa are distinguished as follows: type 0I, the lesion has a thickness of more than twice that of the normal mucosa; type 0IIa, the lesion has a thickness up to twice that of the normal mucosa.

Similar to the AJCC/UICC staging system, primary tumor (T) stage in the Japanese system is based on the depth of invasion and extension to adjacent structures, as outlined in Table 38.3.[117] However, the assignment of lymph node (N) stage involves much more rigorous pathologic assessment than is required for AJCC/UICC staging. The Japanese system extensively classifies 18 lymph node regions into four N categories (N0 to N3) depending on their relationship to the primary tumor and anatomic location.[118] Most perigastric lymph nodes (nodal stations 1 through 6) are considered group N1. Lymph nodes situated along the proximal left gastric artery (station 7), common hepatic artery (station 8), celiac axis (station 9), splenic artery (station 11), and proper hepatic artery (station 12) are defined as group N2. Para-aortic lymph nodes (station 16) are defined as group N3. However, some lymph nodes, even perigastric nodes for specific tumor locations, can be regarded as M1 disease (i.e., involvement of station 2 in the case of antral tumors). This is because their involvement in antral tumors is rare and portrays a poor prognosis.[117]

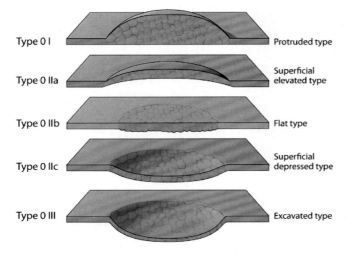

Figure 38.4 Japanese classification system for early gastric cancer.

Type 0 I	Protruded type
Type 0 IIa	Superficial elevated type
Type 0 IIb	Flat type
Type 0 IIc	Superficial depressed type
Type 0 III	Excavated type

TABLE 38.3

Japanese Gastric Cancer Association Staging System

Tumor Stage

T1	Tumor invasion of mucosa and/or muscularis mucosa or submucosa
T2	Tumor invasion of muscularis propria or subserosa
T3	Tumor penetration of serosal
T4	Tumor invasion of adjacent structures
TX	Unknown

Nodal Stage

N0	No evidence of lymph node metastasis
N1	Metastasis to group 1 lymph nodes, but no metastasis to groups 2 to 3 lymph nodes
N2	Metastasis to group 2 lymph nodes, but no metastasis to group 3 lymph nodes
N3	Metastasis to group 3 lymph nodes
NX	Unknown

Hepatic Metastasis Stage (H)

H0	No liver metastasis
H1	Liver metastasis
HX	Unknown

Peritoneal Metastasis Stage (P)

P0	No peritoneal metastasis
P1	Peritoneal metastasis
PX	Unknown

Peritoneal Cytology Stage (CY)

CY0	Benign/indeterminate cells on peritoneal cytology[a]
CY1	Cancer cells on peritoneal cytology
CYX	Peritoneal cytology was not performed

Other Distant Metastasis (M)

M0	No other distant metastases (although peritoneal, liver, or cytologic metastases may be present)
M1	Distant metastases other than the peritoneal, liver, or cytologic metastases
MX	Unknown

Stage Grouping

	N0	N1	N2	N3
T1	IA	IB	II	
T2	IB	II	IIIA	
T3	II	IIIA	IIIB	IV
T4	IIIA	IIIB		
H1, P1, CY1, M1				

[a] Cytology believed to be "suspicious for malignancy" should be classified as CY0.
Adapted from Japanese Gastric Cancer Association. Japanese Classification of Gastric Carcinoma - 2nd English Edition. *Gastric Cancer* 1998;1:10.

The Japanese staging system also includes elements not included in the AJCC/UICC system (see Table 38.3). These are macroscopic descriptions of the tumor (EGC subtype or Borrmann type for more advanced tumors), extent of peritoneal metastases (classified as P0-1), extent of hepatic metastases (H0-1), and peritoneal cytology findings (CY0-1). Recent comparison of the

Japanese and AJCC/UICC staging systems in 731 patients suggests that both are comparable.[119] However, older studies suggest that the AJCC/UICC system more accurately estimates prognosis.[101]

Classification of Esophagogastric Junction Cancers

EGJ cancers (i.e., tumors with a definitive component involving the EGJ) are no longer classified by the AJCC as gastric cancers per se. They are briefly reviewed here for historical reasons. Siewert and Stein[120] classified adenocarcinomas of the EGJ (Siewert classification) into three distinct clinical entities that arise within 5 cm of the EGJ: type I arises in the distal esophagus and may infiltrate the EGJ from above, type II arises in the cardia or the EGJ, and type III arises in the subcardial stomach and may infiltrate the EGJ from below. The assignment of tumors to one of these subtypes is based on morphology and the anatomic location of the epicenter of the tumor. The Siewert classification has important therapeutic implications.[121] The lymphatic drainage routes differ for type I versus types II and III lesions. The lymphatic pathways from the lower esophagus pass both cephalad and caudad. In contrast, the lymphatic drainage from the cardia and subcardial regions is caudad. Thus, the Siewert classification provides a practical means for choosing among surgical options. For type I tumors, esophagectomy is required, whereas types II and III tumors can be treated by transabdominal gastrectomy.[121,122]

Resection Classification

The R classification system indicates the amount of residual disease left after tumor resection.[123] R0 indicates no gross or microscopic residual disease, R1 indicates microscopic residual disease (positive margins), and R2 signifies gross residual disease. The R classification has implications for individual patient care and clinical research. Results of clinical trials that include surgery should include information on R status. Readers should be aware of the dual use of the "R" terminology in the gastric cancer literature. Prior to 1995, the Japanese staging and treatment vernacular included an "R level," which described the extent of lymphadenectomy. The latter is now classified by "D" (for dissection) level.

GASTRIC CANCER NOMOGRAMS: PREDICTING INDIVIDUAL PATIENT PROGNOSIS AFTER POTENTIALLY CURATIVE RESECTION

Kattan et al.[103] have developed a nomogram for predicting individual patient 5-year disease-specific survival using established prognostic factors derived from a population of 1,039 patients with gastric cancer treated by R0 surgical resection without neoadjuvant therapy at a single institution (nomograms@mskcc.org). Clinicopathologic factors incorporated in the nomogram include age and gender, primary tumor site, Laurén classification, numbers of positive and negative lymph nodes resected, and depth of invasion. This nomogram was subsequently validated by several authors. Peeters et al.[124] found that the nomogram prognosticates better then the AJCC staging system. Novotny et al.[125] validated the nomogram in 862 patients from Germany and the Netherlands; Strong et al.[126] compared outcomes using the nomogram in 711 patients from the United States and 1,646 patients from Korea. This tool may be useful for individual patient counseling regarding the use of adjuvant therapy, follow-up scheduling, and clinical trial eligibility assessment, and is available for personal handheld computer devices at www.nomograms.org.

Recently, a large retrospective cohort study of 1,273 patients who underwent resection revealed that having a positive family history of gastric cancer (defined as a self-reported history of cancer in first-degree relatives) was associated with significant reduction in disease-free survival (DFS; $p = 0.012$), relapse-free survival ($p = 0.006$), and OS ($p = 0.005$) when compared with those who did not have a family history of gastric cancer. The improvement in outcomes was more pronounced among patients with stage III or IV gastric cancer, with significant adjusted HRs for DFS (HR = 0.49; 95% confidence interval [CI] = 0.29 to 0.84), relapse-free survival (HR = 0.47; 95% CI = 0.30 to 0.87), and OS (HR = 0.47; 95% CI = 0.26 to 0.84), respectively.[127]

TREATMENT OF LOCALIZED DISEASE

Stage I Disease (Early Gastric Cancer)

Classification of Early Gastric Cancer and Risk for Nodal Metastases

The Japanese Research Society for Gastric Cancer has classified EGCs based on endoscopic criteria first established for the description of T1 tumors. The current classification system is used for both in situ and invasive tumors and categorizes tumors based on endoscopic findings as follows: protruded, type 0I; superficial elevated, type 0IIa; flat, type 0IIb; superficial depressed, type 0IIc; and excavated, type 0III (see Fig. 38.4). The English language version of the Japanese EGC classification contains excellent color photos of these subtypes.[128] This classification system is important in describing patients treated by newer gastric-sparing approaches for EGC, such as endoscopic mucosal resection (EMR).[114–116,129] The risk for lymph node metastasis is important when evaluating treatment options for patients with EGC. The frequency and anatomic distribution of nodal disease are related to the depth of tumor invasion. In a Japanese series of >5,000 patients who underwent gastrectomy with lymph node dissection for EGC, none of the 1,230 patients with well-differentiated intramucosal tumors <3 cm in diameter (regardless of ulceration) had lymph node metastases.[130] None of the 929 patients with EGC without ulceration had nodal metastases, irrespective of tumor size. In contrast, in the subset of >2,000 patients with tumors that invaded the submucosa, the frequencies of lymph node involvement for tumors ≤1.0 cm, 1.1 to 2.0 cm, 2.1 to 3.0 cm, and >3.0 cm were 7.9%, 13.3%, 15.6%, and 23.3%, respectively. Thus, once tumors penetrate into the submucosa, the risk for nodal metastasis increases with tumor size.[131–137] The estimates of the frequency of nodal disease in EGC are based on conventional light-microscopic histologic assessment. However, the use of more sensitive techniques such as serial sectioning of individual lymph nodes, immunohistochemistry, or reverse transcriptase-polymerase chain reaction may increase the frequency of detection of occult micrometastatic disease.[138] The clinical significance of micrometastasis remains unknown.

Endoscopic Mucosal Resection

A subset of patients with EGC can undergo an R0 resection without lymphadenectomy or gastrectomy. The Japanese have popularized EMR for EGC. This approach involves the submucosal injection of fluid to elevate the lesion and facilitate complete mucosal resection under endoscopic guidance. Most centers reporting significant experience with EMR are in Japan. There is less experience with EMR in Western countries. Only patients with tumors that have extremely low metastatic potential should be offered EMR. These are generally well-differentiated, superficial type IIa or IIc lesions, <3 cm in diameter, and located in an easily manipulated area. Tumors invading the submucosa are at increased risk for metastasizing to lymph nodes and are not usually considered candidates for EMR.

Recently, Bennett et al.[139] reviewed the available data reporting on EMR for EGC. No randomized controlled trial (RCT) reported on EMR. The indications for EMR are well-differentiated lesions, size ≤20 mm in elevated type, ≤10 mm in depressed type, no ulceration, and limited to the mucosa.[140] The incidence of lymph node metastases for such lesions is approximately 1%. Complete resection of selected EGCs can be accomplished in a majority of cases (73.4% to 98%).[139,141,142]

Two retrospective reports indicated that EMR can reduce the risk of local residual tumor, and repeat EMR is an effective option.[143,144] Recurrence after EMR varies with type of EGC. Ida et al.[145] reported on 412 patients: 8 of 199 (4.0%) had recurrence of lesions size 20 to 40 mm; 5 patients were retreated by EMR and 3 underwent open surgery; and none had lymph node metastasis. Patients (0/305) with lesions ≤20 mm did not have recurrence. Complication rates associated with EMR are low. Bleeding and perforation are reported in 0% to 20.5% and 0% to 5.2 % of patients, respectively.[141,146–149] The reported morbidity and mortality rates in patients undergoing open surgery (n = 256) versus EMR (n = 56) were 0.8% and 7.8% versus 0% and 16%, repsectively.[139,150]

Fukase et al.[151,152] reported on the long-term outcomes of patients undergoing open surgery (n = 116) versus EMR (n = 59). For patients age 65 year or under, the 5- and 10-year survival rates were 100% and 91.7% versus 92.8% and 92.8%, with open surgery and EMR, respectively. For patients older than 65 years of age, the 5- and 10-year survival rates were 100% and 75% versus 80.8% and 80.8%, respectively. The differences were not statistically significant. Similar results were reported by Park et al.[153] and Kim et al.[154]

There are emerging variations of EMR techniques, including the cap suction and cut versus a ligating device. As outcome studies accumulate demonstrating favorable survival, EMR is emerging as the definitive management of selected EGCs and is not just reserved for patients in whom gastrectomy cannot be considered. However, RCTs are needed to establish an outcome advantage over open surgery.[140,155–165]

Limited Surgical Resection

Given the low rate of nodal involvement for patients with EGC, limited resection may be a reasonable alternative to gastrectomy for some patients. There are no well-accepted pretreatment criteria for selection of patients for limited resection. Based on available pathology studies, patients with small (<3 cm) intramucosal tumors and those with nonulcerated intramucosal tumors of any size may be candidates for EMR or limited resection. Surgical options for these patients may include gastrotomy with local excision. This procedure should be performed with full-thickness mural excision (to allow accurate pathologic assessment of T status) and is often aided by intraoperative gastroscopy for tumor localization. Formal lymph node dissection is not required in these patients.

Gastrectomy

Gastrectomy with lymph node dissection should be considered for patients with EGC who cannot be treated with EMR or limited surgical resection, and/or patients who have intramucosal tumors with poor histologic differentiation, or size >3 cm, or who have tumor penetration into the submucosa or beyond. Gastrectomy with lymph node dissection allows for adequate pathologic staging and local therapy for these patients at increased risk of nodal metastasis. Dissection of level I lymph nodes is a reasonable minimum standard at this time for higher risk EGCs. The roles for nodal "sampling" without formal node dissection (D0 dissection) and sentinel lymph node (SLN) mapping and biopsy in the treatment of EGC remain undefined at this time.

Stage II and Stage III Disease

Surgery

Surgical resection of the primary tumor and regional lymph nodes is the cornerstone of treatment for patients with localized gastric cancer. However, for stage II and III disease, surgery is necessary but often not sufficient for cure. The general therapeutic goal is to achieve a microscopically complete resection (R0). A complete discussion of all the technical details of gastric resection and reconstruction is beyond the scope of this chapter. However, specific surgical issues of oncologic significance are addressed here, including the extent of gastrectomy, extent of regional lymph node dissection, and role of partial pancreatectomy and splenectomy. Additional technical details can be found in surgical atlases and the section "Technical Treatment-Related Issues."

Extent of Resection for Mid- and Distal Gastric Cancers. The extent of gastrectomy required for satisfactory primary tumor treatment depends primarily on the gross and microscopic status of surgical margins. For most clinical situations, a 5-cm grossly negative margin around the tumor and microscopically negative surgical margin (R0) are the treatment goals. When gastrectomy is performed with curative intent, frozen-section assessment of proximal and distal resection margins should be used intraoperatively to improve the likelihood that an R0 resection has been attained. Three relatively small prospective RCTs have compared total gastrectomy with partial (subtotal) gastrectomy for distal gastric cancer.[166–168] Overall morbidity, mortality, and oncologic outcome were comparable in each of these RCTs. When the general oncologic goal of an R0 resection can be achieved by a gastric-preserving approach, partial gastrectomy is preferred over total gastrectomy. This is particularly relevant for distal gastric cancers, for which a gastric-preserving R0 approach may minimize the risks of specific sequelae of total gastrectomy such as early satiety, weight loss, and the need for vitamin B_{12} supplementation.

Extent of Resection for Proximal Gastric Cancer. There are many choices for surgical management of adenocarcinomas arising at the EGJ or in the proximal stomach (Siewert types II and III). Many abdominal surgeons have advocated transabdominal approaches with resection of the lower esophagus and proximal stomach or total gastrectomy. Surgeons trained in thoracic surgery have frequently advocated a combined abdominal and thoracic procedure (often termed *esophagogastrectomy*) with an intrathoracic or cervical anastomosis between the proximal esophagus and the distal stomach, or a procedure termed *transhiatal (or blunt) esophagectomy* (THE), which involves resection of the esophagus and EGJ with mediastinal dissection performed in a blunt fashion through the esophageal hiatus of the diaphragm. When THE is performed for adenocarcinoma of the EGJ, gastrointestinal continuity is restored by low cervical anastomosis of the stomach (usually advanced through the esophageal bed in the posterior mediastinum) to the cervical esophagus. Selection among the options has been dependent primarily on individual surgeon training and experience.

The optimal surgical procedure for patients with localized tumors of the EGJ and proximal stomach is a matter of considerable debate. A recently completed Dutch RCT compared transthoracic esophagogastrectomy (TTEG, with abdominal and thoracic incisions) with THE in 220 patients with adenocarcinoma of the esophagus and EGJ.[169] Although this trial was designed for patients with esophageal cancer, 40 (18%) of the patients had adenocarcinomas of the EGJ (Siewert type II), and the operations evaluated are among those considered for patients with Siewert type II or III cancers. Perioperative morbidity was higher after THE, but there was no significant difference in in-hospital mortality compared with TTEG. Although median overall, disease-free, and quality-adjusted survival did not differ significantly between the groups, there was a trend toward improved OS at 5 years with TTEG. These results are judged equivocal, and there is currently no consensus on the optimal surgical approach for patients with Siewert type II tumors.[170] Until longer follow-up of the Dutch trial is available and/or additional RCTs are performed, the surgical approach to these patients will continue to be individualized and determined by a constellation of factors including surgeon factors (training and experience), patient factors (age, comorbid conditions, and functional status), and tumor factors (pretreatment T and N stage).

Extent of Lymphadenectomy. There has been intense debate surrounding the extent of lymphadenectomy. It involves at least two important issues: (1) adequate staging in terms of the number of lymph nodes resected surgically and examined pathologically, and (2) adequate therapy (i.e., do some forms of lymphadenectomy result in better outcomes?).[171–182]

Single-institution reports suggest that the number of pathologically positive lymph nodes is of prognostic significance,[100,102,180,183–185] and that removal and pathologic analysis of at least 15 lymph nodes is required for adequate pathologic staging.[99,186] Indeed, the current AJCC staging system accounts for these issues and therefore requires analysis of ≥16 lymph nodes to assign a pathologic N stage.[187] The possible therapeutic benefit of extended lymph node dissection D2 versus D1 dissection has been the focus of six RCTs, which are summarized in Table 38.4.[167,188–193] These trials were performed because retrospective and prospective nonrandomized evidence suggested that extended lymph node dissection may be associated with improved long-term survival.[194] The RCTs tested the hypothesis that removal of additional pathologically positive lymph nodes (not generally removed as part of a standard lymph node dissection) improves survival. The larger RCTs attempted to follow what are referred to as the "Japanese rules" for lymph node classification and dissection that govern the extent of nodal dissection required based on anatomic location of the primary tumor.[195] Using these Japanese definitions, the RCTs compared limited lymphadenectomy of the perigastric lymph nodes (D1 dissection) to en bloc removal of second-echelon lymph nodes (D2 dissection). At least two of the completed trials are underpowered for their primary end point, OS.[167,188] The trials from the Medical Research Council (MRC) of the United Kingdom[189] and the Dutch Gastric Cancer Group[190] have received the most attention and discussion.

The MRC trial registered 737 patients with gastric adenocarcinoma; 337 (46%) patients were ineligible by staging laparotomy because of advanced disease, and 400 (54%) patients were randomized at the time of laparotomy to undergo D1 (200) or D2 (200) lymph node dissection. Postoperative morbidity was significantly greater in the D2 group (46% versus 28%; p <0.001), and in-hospital mortality rates were also significantly higher in the D2 group than in the D1 group (13% versus 6%, p <0.04).[189] The most frequent postoperative complications were related to anastomotic leakage (D2 26% versus D1 11%), cardiac complications (8% versus 2%), and respiratory complications (8% versus 5%). The excess morbidity and mortality seen in the D2 group were thought to be related to the routine use of distal (left) pancreatectomy and splenectomy. Partial pancreatectomy and splenectomy were performed to maximize clearance of lymph nodes at the splenic hilum, primarily for patients with proximal tumors; however, many surgeons now believe that adequate lymph node dissection can be performed with pancreas- and spleen-preserving techniques. Long-term follow-up analysis of patients in the MRC trial demonstrated comparable 5-year OS rates of 35% and 33% in the D1 and D2 dissection groups, respectively. Survival based on death from gastric cancer as the event was also similar in the D1 and D2 groups (HR = 1.05; 95% CI = 0.79 to 1.39), as was recurrence-free survival (HR = 1.03; 95% CI = 0.82 to 1.29). The authors concluded that classic Japanese-style D2 lymphadenectomy (with partial pancreatectomy and splenectomy) offered no survival advantage over D1 lymphadenectomy.

The Dutch Gastric Cancer Group conducted a larger RCT with optimal surgical quality control comparing D1 to D2 lymph node dissection for patients with gastric adenocarcinoma that was updated in 2010 after 15-year follow-up.[196] Between 1989 and July 1993, 1,078 patients were entered, of whom 996 patients were eligible; 711 patients were randomized to D1 dissection (n = 380) or

D2 dissection (n = 331). To maximize surgical quality control, all operations were monitored.[197] Initially, this oversight was done by a Japanese surgeon who trained a group of Dutch surgeons, who in turn acted as supervisors during surgery at 80 participating centers. Notwithstanding the extraordinary efforts to ensure quality control of the two types of lymph node dissection, both noncompliance (not removing all lymph node stations) and contamination (removing more than was indicated) occurred, thus blurring the distinction between the two operations and confounding the interpretation of the oncologic end points.[196,198] The postoperative morbidity rate was higher in the D2 group (43% versus 25%; p <0.001), the reoperation rate was also higher at 18% (59/331) versus 8% (30/380), and the mortality rate was also significantly higher in the D2 group (10% versus 4%; p = 0.004). Patients treated with D2 dissection also required a longer hospitalization.[199] As in the MRC trial, partial pancreatectomy and splenectomy were performed en passant in the D2 group. Five-year survival rates were similar in the two groups: 45% for the D1 group and 47% for the D2 group (95% CI for the difference = −9.6% to 5.6%). The subset of patients who had R0 resections, excluding those who died postoperatively, had cumulative risks of relapse at 5 years of 43% with D1 dissection and 37% with D2 dissection (95% CI for the difference = −2.4% to 14.4%).

The Dutch investigators concluded that there was no role for the routine use of D2 lymph node dissection in patients with gastric cancer. At 15-year follow-up, 174/711 (25%) patients were alive, all but one without recurrence. The OS was 21% (82/711) and 29% (92 patients) for the D1 and D2 groups, respectively (p = 0.34). Interestingly, gastric cancer–specific death was higher in the D1 group 48% (182/380) versus 37% (123/331). Local recurrence was higher in the D1 group 22% (82/380) versus 12% (40/331), and regional recurrence 19% (73/380) versus 13% (43/331). The authors concluded that after 15 years of follow-up, D2 lymphadenectomy is associated with lower locoregional recurrence and gastric cancer–specific death rates than D1 lymphadenectomy. D2 resection is also associated with higher postoperative mortality, morbidity, and reoperation rates. Examining the results after 15-year follow-up and given the data regarding gastric cancer–specific mortality, local recurrence, and regional recurrence, the authors revised their original conclusion: "Because spleen-preserving D2 resection is safer in high-volume centers, it is the recommended surgical approach for patients with potentially curable gastric cancer."[196]

Degiuli et al.[191] reported on the Italian Gastric Cancer Study Group experience with a prospective randomized trial comparing pancreas-sparing D1 versus D2. There were 76 patients randomized to undergo D1 and 86 D2 resections. Complication rates were higher in the D2 group: 16.3% versus 10.5%. Postoperative mortality was higher in the D1 group: 1.3% versus 0% in the D2 group. Thus far, no survival data are available. The authors concluded that, in experienced hands, the morbidity and mortality can be as low as shown by Japanese surgeons.

Wu et al.[192] reported on a randomized trial comparing D1 versus D3 dissections.[199] There were no operative deaths, and morbidity was only 12%. At median follow-up of 94.5 months, D3 showed better overall 5-year survival of 59.5% (95% CI = 50.3 to 68.7) versus 53.6% (95% CI = 44.2 to 63.0; p = 0.041), and a trend toward better DFS at 5 years: 40.3% versus 50.6% (p = 0.197). Only 13% had pancreas or splenic resection as compared with 23% in the Dutch trial. The authors concluded that D3 as compared to D1 offers survival benefit. As far as the authors of this chapter understand, this is the first RCT to demonstrate survival advantage for more extensive lymphadenectomy (D3). As such, it requires careful examination. Roggin and Posner[200] have critically reviewed the work by Wu et al.[192] One controversial element of this trial was the use of OS versus gastric cancer–specific survival; 17/111 (15%) of the reported deaths were not related to tumor recurrence, resulting in very small survival benefit.

Interpretation of the existing level 1 evidence is encumbered by a number of issues that have been discussed in detail elsewhere.[171,172] The primary concerns relate to whether (1) the increased operative

TABLE 38.4

Prospective Randomized Trials Comparing D1 Versus D2 and D3 Resection for Potentially Curable Gastric Carcinoma

Study (Ref.)	Extent of Lymphadenectomy		
	D1	**D2**	***P* Value**
Groote Schuur Hospital, Cape Town, 1988[188]			
Number of patients	22	21	—
Length of operation (h)	1.7 ± 0.6	2.33 ± 0.7	<0.005
Transfusions (units/group)	4	25	<0.05
Postoperative stay (d)	9.3 ± 4.7	13.9 ± 9.7	<0.05
5-y overall survival (log rank test)	0.69	0.67	NS
Prince of Wales Hospital, Hong Kong, 1994[167]			
Number of patients	25	29	—
Length of operation (h)	140	260	<0.05
Operative blood loss (ml)	300	600	<0.05
Postoperative stay	8	16	<0.05
Median survival (d)	1,511	922	<0.05
Medical Research Council Trial, United Kingdom, 1999[189,193]			
Number of patients	200	200	—
Operative mortality (%)	6.5	13	<0.04
Postoperative complications (%)	28	46	<0.001
5-y overall survival (%)	35	3	NS
Dutch Gastric Cancer Trial, The Netherlands, 1999 (2009, 15-y F/U update)[190,196]			
Number of patients	380	331	—
Operative mortality rate (%)	4	10	0.004
Postoperative complications (%)	25	43	<0.001
Postoperative stay (d)	18	25	<0.001
5-y overall survival (%)	45	47	NS
11-y F/U overall survival (%)	30	35	0.53
11-y F/U survival (perioperative death excluded)	32	39	0.10
15y F/U overall survival	21	29	0.34
15y F/U gastric cancer–specific death	48	37	0.01
Italian Gastric Cancer Study Group, 2004[191]			
Number of patients	76	86	—
Operative mortality rate (%)	1.3	0	NS
Postoperative complication (%)	10.5	16.3	0.29
Postoperative stay (d)	12	12	NS
5-y overall survival	NS	NS	NS
Yang-Ming University, Taiwan, 2006[192]			
Number of patients	110	111, D3	
Operative mortality rate (%)	0	0	
Postoperative complication (%)	10.1	17.1	0.012
Postoperative stay (d)	15	19.6	0.001
5-y overall survival	53.6	59.5	0.041

NS, not stated; F/U, follow-up.

mortality associated with protocol-mandated partial pancreatectomy and splenectomy for patients with proximal tumors undergoing D2 dissection prevented identification of a potential therapeutic impact of extended lymph node dissection, and (2) the phenomena of noncompliance and contamination led to homogenization of the operative procedures to such an extent that the fundamental hypothesis was not tested. Owing to these interpretation issues, the question of a possible therapeutic benefit of D2 dissection remains unsettled.

Many Japanese gastric surgeons have considered the caveats associated with the MRC and Dutch trials and believe that, notwithstanding inherent patient selection and stage migration biases,[171,196,198,201,202] the existing retrospective data provide sufficient proof of a clinical benefit of D2 dissection. On this basis, D2 dissection has been adopted as the standard of care for patients with localized, higher-risk gastric cancer in many centers in Japan and some specialized centers in the West.[203] The Japanese Clinical Oncology Group (JCOG-9501) has investigated an even more aggressive surgical approach in an RCT evaluating standard D2 versus D2-plus (para-aortic node dissection [PAND]) in the management of completely resected (R0) T2–4 gastric cancer.[204,205] Between July 1995 and April 2001, 523 patients from 25 institutions were registered. Patients were randomized intraoperatively to undergo D2 lymphadenectomy alone (263 patients) or D2 lymphadenectomy plus PAND (260 patients). The primary end point was OS. Postoperative morbidity was higher in the PAND group (28% versus. 21%; $p = 0.07$), and mortality was similar at 0.8% in each group. Five-year OS for patients undergoing PAND was 70.3% versus 69.2% (HR = 1.03; $p = 0.85$). There was no significant difference in recurrence-free survival. The authors concluded that, as compared to D2 lymphadenectomy, PAND when added to D2 lymphadenectomy does not improve survival rates.

Another Japanese study compared D2 with extended PAND (D4).[206] This trial randomized patients to undergo gastrectomy with D2 ($n = 135$) or D4 ($n = 134$) lymphadenectomy. The 5-year survival rates were 52.6% versus 55%, respectively ($p = 0.8$). The authors concluded that prophylactic D4 dissection is not recommended. In an RCT, a Western group from Poland investigated D2 dissection versus extended D2 dissection defined according to the Japanese Gastric Cancer Association classification.[207] They randomized 275 patients with gastric cancer to gastrectomy with D2 ($n = 141$) versus D2 + lymphadenectomy ($n = 134$). The overall postoperative morbidity and mortality were similar and did not differ statistically. Survival data are not available at this time.[207] Thus, the limits of radical surgery have been reached in Japan and the pendulum has swung back toward D2 dissection in clinical settings in which this can be safely performed.[201]

In summary, lymph nodes should be considered as indicators that the gate was opened rather than as the gate keepers for cure.[208] None of the prospective RCT trials executed in the West demonstrated survival advantage for more extensive lymphadenectomy. However, none of these studies were powered enough to detect single-digit difference in 5-year OS. Several non-a priori planned subgroup analyses were done and showed some survival advantage for certain subgroups. These analyses cannot be used to form evidence-based medicine, but should be used to form hypotheses for further RCT studies. In high-volume specialty centers, spleen- and pancreas-preserving D2 dissection is performed safely, and can potentially result in decreased gastric cancer–specific mortality based on 15 years of follow-up from the Dutch study (D2 37% versus 48%; $p = 0.01$).[196]

A recently published RCT from the multicenter Italian Gastric Cancer Study Group compared D1 to D2 lymphadenectomy for gastric adenocarcinoma with primary outcome of OS over median follow-up of 8.8 years.[209] There was no significant difference in OS (5-year OS = 66.5% versus 64.2%), operative morbidity (12% versus 17.9%), and mortality (3% versus 2.2%) in patients undergoing D1 and D2 gastrectomy; however, subgroup analysis suggested a trend toward improved disease-specific survival with D2 gastrectomy in patients with advanced T-stage (pT2-4) and node-positive disease (5-year disease-specific survival: D1 versus D2 = 38% versus 59%; $p = 0.055$).

A systematic review and meta-analysis of eight RCTs encompassing over 2,000 patients (D1, $n = 1,042$; D2, $n = 1,002$) evaluated the safety and efficacy of extended lymphadenectomy in gastric cancer.[210] A significant increase in operative morbidity and mortality was evident in patients undergoing extended D2 lymphadenectomy, with a trend in decreased disease-specific mortality in those having spleen- and pancreas-preserving gastrectomy. Longer-term survival is required to ascertain oncologically relevant outcome benefit with D2 gastrectomy.

Partial Pancreatectomy and Splenectomy Resect or Preserve? Partial (left, distal) pancreatectomy and splenectomy have been performed as part of D2 lymph node dissection to remove the lymph nodes along the splenic artery (station 11) and lymph nodes within the splenic hilum (station 12), primarily for patients with tumors located in the proximal and midstomach. Indeed, partial pancreatectomy and splenectomy were required for patients with proximal tumors in the D2 arm of the Dutch and MRC RCTs but were required only for direct tumor extension in the D1 arm. In the Dutch and MRC D1 versus D2 randomized trials, splenectomy was associated with increased risk of surgical complications and operative mortality. In addition, a multivariate analysis suggested that splenectomy is associated with inferior long-term survival. The frequent performance of splenectomy (e.g., 30% of patients in the D2 arm versus 3% in the D1 arms of the Dutch trial) in the patient undergoing extended D2 lymphadenectomy, with its associated adverse effects on both short- and long-term mortality, confounds the interpretation of the Dutch and MRC RCTs. Thus, the hypothesis that spleen- and pancreas-preserving D2 lymph node dissection improves survival remains unproven. There is an evolving consensus that splenectomy should be performed only in cases with intraoperative evidence of direct tumor extension into the spleen, or its hilar vasculature, or when the primary tumor is located in the proximal stomach along the greater curvature.[211] Partial pancreatectomy should be performed only in cases of direct tumor extension to the pancreas.

Recent reports have described pancreas- and spleen-preserving forms of D2 dissection.[212–218] This organ-preserving modification of classic D2 dissection allows for dissection of some station 11 and 12 lymph nodes without the potential adverse effects of pancreatectomy and/or splenectomy. In a small single-institution RCT recently reported from Chile, Csendes et al.[219] randomized 187 patients with localized proximal gastric adenocarcinoma to treatment by total gastrectomy with D2 lymph node dissection plus splenectomy or total gastrectomy with D2 lymphadenectomy alone. Operative mortality was similar in both groups (splenectomy group, 3%; control group, 4%). However, septic complication rates were higher in the splenectomy arm than in the control arm ($p < 0.04$). There was no difference in 5-year OS between study groups, although it is not clear that the trial was designed with survival as the primary end point. Other investigators confirmed these findings.[218,220,221]

The JCOG is conducting a multi-institutional RCT (JCOG 0110-MF) comparing D2 dissection with and without splenectomy for patients diagnosed with proximal gastric cancer.[222] The hypothesis to be tested is that 5-year OS of patients treated by extended D2 dissection *without* splenectomy is 5% less than that of patients treated by D2 dissection *with* splenectomy. With a planned accrual of 500 patients, this design will provide 70% power to reject the null hypothesis when 5-year OS is 3% greater following splenic preservation compared with splenectomy.[222] The results of this trial will better define the short- and long-term effects of splenectomy for patients with proximal gastric cancers undergoing extended lymphadenectomy.

In an effort to reduce operative morbidity and mortality without compromising oncologic outcome in patients undergoing extended lymphadenectomy for gastric adenocarcinoma, eight clinical trials have compared laparoscopic to open gastrectomy with D2 lymph node dissection. A meta-analysis was conducted of these eight trials, which enrolled nearly 1,500 patients with gastric cancer to assess the feasibility and safety of laparoscopic total gastrectomy with D2 lymphadenectomy compared to the same operation done in the standard open manner.[223] The laparoscopic technique was associated with significantly longer operative time, less operative blood loss, fewer analgesic requirements, earlier return of bowel function, shorter hospital stay, and reduced operative morbidity (relative risk = 0.70; 95% CI = 0.50 to 0.98; p = 0.035). The total number of lymph nodes removed surgically and analyzed pathologically as well as operative mortality was not significantly different between groups. Further well-designed clinical RCTs are warranted to define the role of laparoscopic gastrectomy and extended lymphadenectomy for gastric adenocarcinoma. (A more detailed discussion follows in the section titled "Minimally Invasive Surgery for Gastric Resection.")

Laparoscopy clearly has a role in the complete staging of disease in patients with gastric adenocarcinoma and the detection of radiologically occult macroscopic, or microscopic peritoneal cytology positive-only metastasis. Laparoscopy and peritoneal cytology are important for accurate staging and the detection of occult metastatic disease. This methodology adds value to modern imaging techniques, for positive microscopic peritoneal cytology-only disease is tantamount to macroscopic M1 disease in terms of oncologic outcome.

A recent international multidisciplinary expert panel created statements to define processes of care relevant to the perioperative management of patient with gastric cancer.[224] Ten processes were deemed essential to maintaining quality of care:

1. CT of the abdomen and pelvis is part of preoperative staging.
2. PET scans are not routinely indicated.
3. Adjuvant therapy should be considered.
4. Clinical trials should be conducted and patients considered for participation.
5. Treatment decision making should involve a multidisciplinary team.
6. Hospitals must have sufficient systems in place to support the care of patients with gastric cancer.
7. Sixteen or more lymph nodes should be resected and staged pathologically.
8. Surgery should only be performed to palliate major symptoms in the setting of metastatic disease.
9. Surgeons experienced in the treatment of gastric cancer should be performing the operations.
10. These surgeons should also have advanced laparoscopic surgery experience for laparoscopic gastric resection.

These processes were deemed to be of indeterminate necessity for maintaining quality of care:

1. Diagnostic laparoscopy before treatment
2. Multidisciplinary approach to patients with linitis plastica
3. Genetic testing for diffuse gastric cancer, family history, or age <45 years at time of diagnosis
4. Endoscopic removal of select T1aN0 lesions
5. D2 lymphadenectomy in curative intent cases
6. D1 lymphadenectomy for EGC or patients with comorbidities
7. Frozen section analysis of gastric resection margins
8. Nonemergent cases performed in a hospital with a volume of >15 gastric cancer resections per year
9. By a surgeon who performs more than six gastric resections per year

Individualized Assessments of Lymph Node Involvement.

Recent attention has focused on methods of individual assessment of risk of lymphatic spread. These techniques offer the possibility of tailoring surgical therapy for an individual patient based on clinico-pathologic risk assessment of the primary tumor and/or preoperative or intraoperative identification of SLNs, or primary draining lymph nodes. At present, at least three approaches to individual nodal risk assessment have been evaluated: computer modeling, preoperative endoscopic peritumoral injection, and SLN biopsy.

Preoperative Computer Modeling of Individual Patient Nodal Involvement. Kampschoer et al.[225] have developed a computer program to estimate the probability of spread to specific nodal regions for an individual patient using his or her pretreatment clinicopathologic data. The program incorporated data on tumor size, depth of infiltration, primary tumor location, grade, type, and macroscopic appearance of primary tumors from 2,000 patients with surgically resected gastric cancers treated at the National Cancer Center of Tokyo. The data set used for matching individual patient data is continuously updated and now includes >8,000 patients. This computer model has been validated in non-Japanese patients in Germany[226] and Italy.[227] In the United States, Hundahl et al.[228] retrospectively applied this computer model to evaluate the surgical treatment of patients entered into the intergroup trial of adjuvant 5-FU–based chemoradiation. The Kampschoer et al.[225] program was used to estimate the likelihood of disease in undissected regional node stations, defining the sum of these estimates as the Maruyama index of unresected disease. Fifty-four percent of participating patients underwent D0 lymphadenectomy. The median index was 70 (range = 0 to 429). In contrast to D level, the Maruyama index proved to be an independent prognostic factor of survival, even with adjustment for the potentially linked variables of T stage and number of positive nodes. More recent and smaller studies confirmed these findings.[229–231]

Preoperative Endoscopic Peritumoral Injection. The hypothesis that peritumoral injection of compounds designed to optimize lymph node dissection improves lymph node clearance was addressed in a small RCT evaluating preoperative endoscopic vital dye staining with CH40 prior to D2 dissection. The frequency of positive lymph nodes in patients injected with CH40 before D2 dissection was greater than that observed in patients treated by D2 dissection alone.[232] This approach optimized the yield of lymph node dissection presumably by directing surgeons to include specific lymph nodes in the dissection that might have otherwise been left in situ and/or by directing pathologists to examine specific areas of the lymphadenectomy specimens. Further prospective studies of this approach are required to confirm the feasibility of this technique and to assess its impact on intraoperative decision making regarding the extent of lymphadenectomy and accuracy of specimen dissection and nodal retrieval in anatomic pathology.

Sentinel Lymph Node Biopsy. The goal of SLN biopsy is to identify the node or nodes believed to be the first peritumoral lymph nodes in the orderly spread of gastric adenocarcinoma from the primary site to the regional lymph nodes. Sampling of this lymph node(s) may allow for prediction of the nodal status of the entire lymph node basin, possibly obviating extended nodal dissection and its attendant morbidity in patients found to have a negative SLN. Recent pilot studies have evaluated the feasibility, sensitivity, and specificity of SLN biopsy for patients with gastric cancer.[233–242] These pilot studies demonstrated that SLN identification is feasible in approximately 95% of patients. However, most patients with gastric cancer have multiple "sentinel" nodes, with mean numbers of SLNs per patient ranging from 2.6 to 6.3. The aggregate experience to date suggests that among patients with pathologically involved lymph nodes, SLN results in false-negative assessment of pathologic regional nodal status in 11% to 60% of patients. Thus, the preliminary data available suggest that SLN biopsy cannot reliably replace lymph node dissection as a means of accurately staging regional nodal basins in gastric adenocarcinoma.[243–247]

In a large study of nearly 400 patients, the ability and accuracy of SLNs was examined in a prospective, multicenter phase 2 study.[248] Patients with early T stage gastric cancer (cT1 or cT2, tumor <4 cm) were evaluated with SLN mapping, followed by gastrectomy and D2 dissection. The SLN mapping technique identified 57 patients who had nodal involvement, of which 53 had true positive SLNs, resulting in 99% accuracy. Though further validation is needed, these results are quite encouraging.

The JCOG multicenter trial (JCOG-0302) assessed the feasibility and accuracy of indocyanine green (ICG) SLN mapping at time of surgery prior to gastrectomy and lymphadenectomy for EGC (T1).[249] Single sections of ICG-stained SLNs were examined intraoperatively using frozen section with hematoxylin and eosin stain. The primary study end point was the proportion of false-negative SLNs. Study accrual was halted after 440 of the planned 1,550 patients were enrolled when the proportion of false negatives was found to be unexpectedly and unacceptably high (46%). The authors appropriately concluded that SLN mapping and biopsy using ICG and intraoperative single nodal frozen section evaluation using hematoxylin and eosin staining is inappropriate for clinical use in EGC.

Volume-Outcome Relationships for Gastrectomy. Recent studies have established a clear relationship between institutional gastrectomy volume and perioperative mortality rates—the so-called volume-outcome relationship. The recent analysis of a national database by Birkmeyer et al.[250–252] of 31,854 patients who underwent gastrectomy between 1994 and 1999 demonstrated an inverse relationship between institutional gastrectomy volume and operative mortality rates. The odds ratio for gastrectomy-related death was lowest among patients treated within hospitals in the highest gastrectomy volume quintile (odds ratio = 0.72; 95% CI = 0.63 to 0.83). A separate analysis evaluating surrogate end points for morbidity demonstrated that gastrectomy at high-volume centers was associated with the shortest duration of hospital stay and the lowest readmission rates.[253–256] Similar findings were noted by Hannan et al.[257] in an analysis of the New York State Department of Health's administrative database. Their analysis of 3,711 patients who underwent gastrectomy between 1994 and 1997 included adjustments for covariates such as age, demographic variables, organ metastasis, socioeconomic status, and comorbidities. Patients who had a gastrectomy at hospitals in the highest-volume quartile had an absolute risk-adjusted mortality rate that was 7.1% (p <0.0001) lower than those treated at hospitals in the lowest-volume quartile, although the overall mortality rate for gastrectomy was only 6.2%.

These studies demonstrate that the risk-adjusted mortality rates for gastrectomy are significantly lower when gastrectomy is performed by high-volume providers.[258–261] It is likely that the variations in gastrectomy-related mortality rates relate in part to surgeon training and their patient age-volume[262–264] and experience with the procedure. Data on gastrectomy volume obtained from general surgeons undergoing recertification after a minimum of 7 years in practice demonstrate that the mean number of gastric resections performed by recertifying general surgeons in the United States is only 1.4 per year.[265] Thus, given the data supporting a relationship between hospital and provider volumes and the morbidity and mortality rate of gastric resection, there are reasons to consider regionalization of the surgical treatment of gastric cancers.

Outcome in Japan Versus Western Countries. Stage-stratified survival rates for gastric adenocarcinoma are higher in Japan than in most Western countries. The reasons for this are complex, are incompletely understood, and cannot be fully addressed within the context of a chapter covering all aspects of gastric cancers.

Important differences in the epidemiology of gastric cancer may contribute to observed differences in outcome in Japan versus Western countries. First, the better-prognosis intestinal-type (Laurén classification)[266] tumors are seen more commonly in Japan, whereas the diffuse-type cancers (poorer prognosis) are more frequent in Western series. These regional differences in the frequencies of intestinal and diffuse cancers are believed to be related to the higher incidence of *H. pylori* infection and atrophic gastritis in Japan. Second, poorer-prognosis proximal gastric cancers are less frequent in Japan.[267–269] Indeed, the progressive increase in proximal gastric cancers observed in the West has not been observed in Japanese populations.

Regional differences in the diagnostic criteria for EGC also may contribute to regional differences in observed outcome. In Japan, gastric carcinoma is diagnosed based on its structural and cytologic features without consideration of invasion of the lamina propria. In contrast, Western pathologists consider invasion of the lamina propria to be an essential element of the diagnosis of carcinoma.[270–274] As a consequence, unequivocally neoplastic noninvasive lesions are classified as carcinoma in Japan, but as dysplasia by Western pathologists.[270] To overcome these differences, the Padvova,[275] Vienna,[276] and Revised Vienna[276] classifications have recently been proposed. However, until there is worldwide consensus and implementation of uniform diagnostic criteria for EGC, comparative assessments of the outcome of patients with EGC treated in Japan and Western countries should acknowledge the selection bias associated with different diagnostic criteria.

Stage migration is a well-documented factor contributing to the stage-specific differences in outcome between Japanese and Western patients.[277] Stage migration arises because there is widespread use of extensive D2 or D3 lymphadenectomy combined with rigorous pathologic assessment of the lymphadenectomy specimen in Japan. More accurate stage assignment of Japanese patients leads to secondary stage migration—improvement in stage-specific survival without improvement in OS. The frequency and impact of stage migration were quantified by the Dutch Gastric Cancer Group in their RCT comparing D1 and D2 lymph node dissection.[190,278] Stage migration occurred in 30% of patients in the D2 group, and the stage-specific decreases in survival rates attributable to stage migration were 3% for AJCC/UICC stage I disease, 8% for stage II, 6% for stage III, and 12% for stage IIIB, with the more accurately staged D2 group having higher survival rates.[278]

In addition to regional differences in epidemiology, diagnostic criteria for EGC, and stage migration, other factors may contribute to the observed differences in stage-stratified survival. Such factors may include genetic, environmental, and biologic differences between Japanese and Western patients and tumors. These factors have been less well studied, but were addressed in a comprehensive review by Davis and Sano.[279]

Outcome in Korea Versus Western Countries. A separate evaluation was performed comparing gastric cancer survival following curative intent resection in Korea versus the United States.[126] This study compared two independent, single-institution prospectively maintained databases from 1995 to 2005: one from MSKCC (n = 711 curatively resected patients who did not receive neoadjuvant therapy) and another from St. Mary's Hospital in Seoul, South Korea (n = 1,646 patients, also curatively resected without receiving preoperative therapy). All patients had a D2 dissection and adequate nodal staging. There were notable differences in the two cohorts: patients from the United States were more likely to have proximal tumors and more advanced stage compared with patients resected in Korea. However, when controlling for all known risk factors, stage for stage, patients from Korea still had better OS (HR = 1.3; 95% CI = 1.0 to 1.7; p = 0.05). These data cannot exclude differences in underlying cancer biology as a potential explanation for the observed differences in survival in gastric cancer between patients treated in Korea versus those treated in the United States.

Minimally Invasive Surgery for Gastric Resection

The utilization of laparoscopy in gastric surgery has been increasing over the past decade. There are a plethora of non-RCTs reporting on laparoscopic distal gastrectomy, total gastrectomy, and D2 dissection, and practically every open procedure has been tested using laparoscopy. We will review here the available data from published RCTs. There are no RCTs reporting on total gastrectomies.[280] None of the current RCTs reporting on laparoscopy in gastric cancer are of sufficient quality and magnitude to be considered "practice changing." Huscher et al.[281,282] reported on the largest RCT testing laparoscopic ($n = 29$) versus open ($n = 30$) subtotal gastrectomy for distal gastric cancer. After 5 years of follow-up, overall morbidity and mortality were equivalent. Laparoscopic resection resulted in less blood loss, shorter hospital stay, longer operative time, and earlier resumption of oral intake; these were reported by other authors as well.[283,284] There was no difference in the number of lymph nodes harvested. Overall 5-year and DFS did not differ significantly. The authors concluded that laparoscopic subtotal gastrectomy is feasible and has similar short- and long-term outcomes as open surgery.

Kim et al.[285] reported on laparoscopy-assisted distal gastrectomy (LADG) versus open distal gastrectomy (ODG) for early gastric cancer. This trial was designed to test the 5-year survival utilizing noninferiority design. The interim analysis showed less blood loss ($p < 0.001$), reduced amount of analgesic used ($p < 0.019$), shorter hospital stay ($p < 0.0001$), fewer number of lymph nodes harvested in the LADG arm ($p < 0.05$), and improved short-term quality of life (QOL) parameters on global health ($p < 0.0001$). The authors concluded that comparison of LADG with ODG resulted in improved QOL outcomes in patients followed up to 3 months. The authors have now reported long-term follow-up data.[286] In this study, the authors evaluated 2,976 patients who were treated with either laparoscopic gastrectomy (1,477 patients) or open gastrectomy (1,499 patients) between April 1998 and December 2005. With a median follow-up of 70.8 months, there was no difference in survival between the two resection methodologies, with the exception that for stage IA gastric cancer, laparoscopic gastrectomy had a improved survival (95.3% 5-year survival) versus open gastrectomy (90.3% 5-year survival) ($p < 0.001$).[286] Recently, Ohtani et al.[287] performed meta-analysis of RCT that compared LADG versus ODG for EGC. Their report confirmed the results from Kim et al.[286] and Lee and Han.[288]

A recent update and meta-analysis analyzed data on 784 patients enrolled in eight RCTs[289] comparing laparoscopy-assisted to open gastrectomy for resectable gastric cancer. Despite the fact that operative time was significantly prolonged in the laparoscopy group and that analgesic use, operative blood loss, nodal yield, morbidity (overall and anastomotic), and mortality were *no* different when compared with open gastrectomy, there were a number of clinically important benefits observed in those undergoing minimally invasive surgery. Pulmonary morbidity (odds ratio = 0.43; 95% CI = 0.20 to 0.93; $p = 0.03$), duration of postoperative ileus (missing data = -0.23; 95% CI = -0.41 to -0.05), and hospital stay (missing data = -1.72; 95% CI = -3.40 to 0.04) were significantly reduced in the laparoscopy-assisted gastrectomy group. The survival benefit of minimally invasive surgery in resectable gastric cancer has yet to be definitively demonstrated.[289]

Laparoscopy is another tool in the armamentarium of the surgical oncologist. The question is not whether it can be done laparoscopically, certainly it can; the question is whether it should be done in patients with gastric adenocarcinoma. Recently, a meta-analysis of six clinical trials (658 patients) compared laparoscopic versus open gastrectomy for distal EGC.[290] In this analysis, the authors noted significant reductions in postoperative complications and length of hospital stay in the laparoscopic group, whereas the open gastrectomy group had less operating time and a greater number of lymph nodes harvested. There were no notable differences in the time to return of bowel function, incidence of wound infection, postoperative abscess formation, or anastomotic leak or pulmonary complications, suggesting that there may be some advantages of the laparoscopic approach. The oncologic equivalence, however, has not been adequately tested. Whether the energy, time, and capital invested in developing laparoscopic surgery for gastric

cancer is worth it is the relevant question particularly in an era of skyrocketing medical costs. Certainly, beyond the short term there seems to be no advantage of laparoscopic surgery in gastric cancer. In view of the reported morbidity and mortality in specialty centers, the advantage gained by laparoscopic gastric resection over the first few days underlines the question of whether we should invest more in innovative therapies to eradicate gastric cancer than the simple technical aspects of noninvasive extirpative surgery.

A large prospective random assignment study from Korea is underway in which 1,415 patients with EGC (pT1-2 N0) are randomly assigned to receive either open or laparoscopic distal gastrectomy.[291] Final results of this expected "definitive" phase 3 study are expected to be available in September 2015. A similar large phase 3 study for stage IA and stage IB gastric cancer was initiated in Japan in March 2010. This study randomizes 920 patients from 33 institutions, with the primary end point of OS.[292] Together, it is anticipated that these two pivotal studies will definitively define the role of laparoscopic-assisted gastrectomy in EGC.

Adjuvant Therapy

Patients with EGCs (e.g., patients with AJCC stage I and some stage II) have a good chance of cure with surgery alone. However, the Japanese S-1 adjuvant study indicates that the prognosis for even stage II tumors can be improved with systemic chemotherapy.

Adjuvant therapy indicates administration of a treatment following a potential curative resection of the primary tumor and regional lymph nodes. Therapy after resections that leave microscopic or gross disease are not adjuvant treatment, but rather therapy for known disease, which is palliative in nature. Neoadjuvant chemotherapy involves the use of systemic treatment before potentially curative surgery.

There are several theoretical reasons for beginning adjuvant therapy soon after operation (perioperative chemotherapy). Studies have shown a rapid increase in cell growth of metastases after a primary tumor has been removed related to a decline in certain circulating factors, which serve to inhibit angiogenesis or other cell-cycle promotors, once the primary tumor is removed. Perioperative or neoadjuvant chemotherapy has been studied because the ability to perform a R0 resection in gastric cancer is difficult. In addition, a substantial number of patients undergoing gastrectomy have prolonged recovery. Neoadjuvant chemotherapy has a dual goal: allowing a higher rate of R0 resections and treatment of micrometastatic disease early in the course of treatment.

Adjuvant Systemic Therapy. The results of selected recent RCTs comparing adjuvant chemotherapy with surgery alone are summarized in Table 38.5. Japanese investigators studied S-1, an oral fluoropyrimidine, in a group of 1,059 patients (stages II to IIIB). S-1 was given for 12 months (4 weeks on/2 weeks off). A total of 529 patients received S-1 plus operation and 530 patients underwent operation only. The 3-year OS was 80.1% and 70.1%, respectively (HR = 0.68).[293]

The 5-year survival update was recently reported and demonstrated a sustained benefit in 5-year OS of 71.7% with adjuvant S-1 versus 61.1% with surgery alone (HR = 0.669; 95% CI = 0.540 to 0.828).[294] In addition, another Asian study from Korea reported the results of adjuvant capecitabine and oxaliplatin.[295] In this study, patients were required to have a D2 resection, and those with stage II-IIIB were then randomly assigned to receive 6 months (eight cycles) of capecitabine/oxaliplatin or observation. This was a large study, in which 520 patients were randomly assigned to receive adjuvant chemotherapy and 515 to surgery alone. The study met its primary endpoint of 3-year DFS (74% [95% CI = 69 to 79] with chemotherapy versus 59% [53% to 64%] with surgery alone; $p < 0.0001$). In contradistinction to the positive results using S-1, and the MAGIC and ACCORD 07 trials described later, Di Costanzo et al.[296] did not find a benefit to the use of cisplatin, epirubicin, leucovorin, and 5-FU as adjuvant therapy.

TABLE 38.5

Adjuvant Therapy for Gastric Cancer: Phase 3 Trials

Study (Ref.)	No. of Patients	Three-y DFS (%)	Overall 5-y Survival (%)	HR
S-1[293]				
Surgery	530	60	70	
Adjuvant	529	72	80	0.38
INT-116[339]				
Surgery	275	31	41	1.35
Adjuvant	281	48	50	
GOIRC[296]				
Surgery	128	42[a]	49	0.90
Adjuvant	130	43[a]	48	
MAGIC[327]				
Surgery	253	25	23	0.75
Neoadjuvant	250	38	36	
ACCORD-07[318]				
Surgery	111	25	21	0.69
Neoadjuvant	113	40	34	

DFS, disease-free survival; HR, hazard ratio; INT, Intergroup Trial; GOIRC, Gruppo Oncologico Italiano di Ricerca Clinica; MAGIC, Medical Research Council Adjuvant Gastric Infusional Chemotherapy; ACCORD, the French Action Clinique Coordonnées en Cancérologie Digestive.
[a] Five-year DFS.

Several meta-analyses of adjuvant chemotherapy in gastric cancer have been reported. Recently, Buyse et al.[297] reported a meta-analysis that included individual patient data; 16 trials involving 3,710 patients were available for analysis. They found an OS benefit in favor of adjuvant chemotherapy (HR = 0.83; 95% CI = 0.76 to 0.91; $p < 0.0001$). The absolute benefit was 6.3% at 5 years. The GASTRIC group conducted a meta-analysis; as of 2010, individual patient data for 17 trials involving 3,838 patients were available for analysis. They found an OS benefit in favor of adjuvant chemotherapy (HR = 0.82; 95% CI = 0.75 to 0.90; $p > 0.001$). The absolute benefit was 5.9% at 5 years.[298] Shown in Table 38.5 are the results of recent trials in which adjuvant chemotherapy plus potentially curative resection was studied. The five most recent trials indicate that adjuvant therapy decreases the risk of recurrence by approximately 10%.[299] The use of systemic therapy plus potentially curative resection is considered a standard of care for patients with locally advanced gastric cancers. The most effective regimen to use, whether or not it is best to give therapy perioperatively, and the role of postoperative radiation *plus* systemic therapy are the focus of ongoing clinical research trials.

Adjuvant Intraperitoneal Chemotherapy.

Peritoneal recurrence is a common pattern of failure for patients with gastric cancer, even after curative resection.[31,298] The median survival time of patients with peritoneal recurrence is 3 to 6 months. The rationale is based on the observation that drug concentrations within the peritoneal cavity are much higher than those achievable by intravenous or oral drug adminsitration. The data are a mixture of retrospective reviews, pilot phase 2 trials, and several small phase 3 trials. No definitive conclusions can yet be drawn regarding the effectiveness of intraperitoneal postoperative chemotherapy in this setting.

There are several modes of administering intraperitoneal chemotherapy: hyperthermic intraoperative peritoneal chemotherapy (HIPEC), normothermic intraoperative chemotherapy (NIIC) given at the conclusion of the operation, early postoperative

intraperitoneal (normothermic) chemotherapy (EPIC), or delayed postoperative intraperitoneal (normothermic) chemotherapy. The theoretical advantage of intraoperative treatment is better drug distribution and the ability to use hyperthermia (HIPEC) to enhance microscopic tumor cytotoxicity. Most trials in gastric cancer have used either 5-FU or floxuridine, mitomycin C, or cisplatin for intraperitoneal chemotherapy.[300–309] Yan et al.[310] performed a meta-analysis of the RCTs reporting on adjuvant intraperitoneal chemotherapy for patients undergoing curative gastric resection; 10 trials involving 1,474 patients were included. A total of 775 patients had resection alone, and 873 patients had resection plus intraperitoneal treatment. A significant improvement in survival was associated with HIPEC (HR = 0.6; 95% CI = 0.43 to 0.83; $p = 0.002$) or HIPEC plus EPIC (HR = 0.45; 95% CI = 0.29 to 0.68; $p = 0.0002$). There was only a trend toward survival benefit with NIIC ($p = 0.06$), but this was not significant with either EPIC alone or delayed postoperative intraperitoneal (normothermic) chemotherapy. The authors concluded that HIPEC with or without EPIC after curative gastric resection is associated with modest improvement in survival and increased complication rate.

Recently, Kang et al.[311] reported on 640 patients with serosal-positive gastric cancer who underwent resection and were then randomized to receive intravenous mitomycin-C (20 mg/m^2) at 3 to 6 weeks after surgery and oral doxifluridine (460 to 600 mg/m^2 per day) starting 4 weeks after the administration of mitomycin-C and continuing for 3 months, or to receive intraperitoneal cisplatin (100 mg), intravenous mitomycin-C (15 mg/m^2) on postoperative day 1, followed by oral doxifluridine for 12 months, and six monthly intravenous cisplatin (60 mg/m^2). Results indicated potential improvement in progression-free survival (PFS) and OS for the intraperitoneal cisplatin therapy arm. Kuramoto et al.[312] reported in a retrospective fashion that extensive intraperitoneal lavage performed with 10 L of normal saline after curative resection and before NIIC is superior to surgery alone or to surgery plus NIIC.

Immunochemotherapy

The use of adjuvant immunostimulants given in combination with cytotoxic chemotherapy (immunchemotherapy) has been studied primarily in Asia. The detailed results of these trials have been discussed in the previous edition of this textbook. Although the data available suggest that immunochemotherapy may be valuable, larger and adequately powered clinical trials are necessary to evaluate the clinical utility and efficacy this approach.

Perioperative and Neoadjuvant Chemotherapy. Perioperative (pre- and postoperative) or neoadjuvant chemotherapy is an attractive concept in gastric cancer because many patients have locally advanced tumors at diagnosis, particularly in Western countries. There are two goals of perioperative treatment: to increase the likelihood of an R0 resection, and treat micrometastatic disease early. After gastric resection, many patients have a prolonged recovery, delaying initiation of adjuvant therapy. Phase 2 trials involving either purely preoperative or perioperative treatment demonstrated that there was no increase in anticipated surgical morbidity or mortality when compared to controls.[313,314] Brenner et al.[314] reported on patients with locally advanced, high-risk gastric cancer who received preoperative CF followed by intraperitoneal chemotherapy after resection. At 43 months of follow-up, 39.5% of patients were still alive. Evaluating efficacy at the primary site is difficult in gastric cancer. Kelsen et al.[313] compared EUS with pathologic stage in assessing objective regression after neoadjuvant chemotherapy. They found that even though EUS was an accurate test in previously untreated patients following administration of chemotherapy, after chemotherapy and prior to surgery, EUS was inaccurate in measuring the depth of invasion (T stage) or lymph node involvement.

FDG-PET scan as a predictive marker of response to preoperative chemotherapy has been studied in patients with gastric cancer. Ott et al.[77] reported on 44 patients with locally advanced gastric cancer who underwent PET scans prior to and after receiving chemotherapy. A decreased SUV was able to differentiate between patients who responded pathologically to treatment and those who did not.[315] These data suggest that functional imaging may eventually prove to be a useful predictive marker for efficacy. Studies in which systemic therapy is changed on the basis of an early PET scan are now under way. As previously noted, for patients with gastric cancer, approximately 20% to 25% of patients will not have an informative PET scan, so this technique cannot be used as a predictive marker for these patients.

FDG-PET and PET/CT scan are being evaluated in Japan as a potentially useful modality for the purpose of gastric cancer. A recently published trial from the National Center for Global Health and Medicine in Tokyo studied over 150,000 asymptomatic patients as part of it FDG-PET screening.[316] With a sensitivity and positive predictive value of 38% and 34%, respectively, the authors appropriately concluded that gastric endoscopy should be included as part of screening programs in order to increase rate of gastric cancer detection.[316]

After phase 2 studies demonstrated safety and suggested efficacy, several perioperative chemotherapy phase 3 trials were conducted (see Table 38.5). English investigators led by Cunningham et al.[317] reported the final results of a well-designed, random assignment study comparing surgery alone with surgery and perioperative chemotherapy in patients with gastroesophageal junction and gastric cancers (the MAGIC trial). All patients had potentially resectable disease prior to entrance into the study. Patients assigned to perioperative chemotherapy were treated with the epirubicin-cisplatin–5-FU (ECF) regimen. Chemotherapy was given both before and after surgery. A total of 503 patients were entered into the study; three-quarters had gastric cancer and one-quarter had gastroesophageal junction or lower esophageal adenocarcinomas. The ECF chemotherapy was well tolerated, with no increase in surgical morbidity or mortality. There was a shift to an earlier stage overall in patients receiving perioperative chemotherapy, as well as an improved R0 resection rate. With a median follow-up of 4 years, there was a significant improvement in both disease-free and OS for patients receiving perioperative chemotherapy: 5-year survival rate was 36% for those receiving perioperative chemotherapy and 23% for those receiving surgery alone (HR = 0.75; 95% CI = 0.6 to 0.9; $p = 0.009$). The authors concluded that ECF perioperative chemotherapy improves outcome for patients with resectable gastric cancer without increasing operative morbidity or mortality. This important trial was a well-designed, adequately powered study demonstrating an advantage of systemic treatment plus surgery when compared with operation alone.

More recently, French investigators reported the results of a similar trial (ACCORD 07-FFCD 9703) using CF prior to surgery versus surgery alone.[318] Approximately half the patients receiving preoperative chemotherapy also received postoperative treatment using the same regimen. The results were similar to those of the MAGIC trial, with 5-year OS being 24% for those undergoing operation alone versus 30% for those who received perioperative chemotherapy. There was a similar improvement in DFS. The results of the ACCORD 07 trial support the results of the MAGIC study.

Summary for Neoadjuvant Chemotherapy.

The results of the MAGIC and ACCORD 07 trials have shown that systemic chemotherapy regimens that are only modestly effective in palliating patients with advanced disease can have a small but clinically meaningful effect on survival when given in the perioperative setting. New and potentially effective cytotoxic agents as well as new biologic agents are now being introduced in the treatment of patients with gastric malignancy. Studies involving perioperative chemotherapy using these agents are now in the advanced planning stage. The results of the perioperative chemotherapy, MAGIC and

ACCORD 07, trials and of postoperative S-1, and Intergroup Trial (INT 0116) chemoradiation studies support the use of systemic therapy as an important component of the treatment plan for patients with locally advanced gastric cancers. The best strategy to pursue—that is, whether to give systemic therapy first followed by operation or to proceed directly to operation followed by systemic treatment plus or minus radiation given after surgery—has yet to be determined.

Given that the role of neoadjuvant chemotherapy in gastric cancer remains controversial, a systematic review and meta-analysis of six RCTs (aggregate $n = 781$) was conducted to gain insights about the potential benefit of neoadjuvant chemotherapy followed by surgery as compared to surgery alone.[319] Outcomes analyzed in this meta-analysis were OS, rate of R0 resection, downstaging effect of neoadjuvant chemotherapy, operative morbidity, and mortality. No significant difference were evident when comparing neoadjuvant chemotherapy and surgery to surgery alone for these outcome variables; odds ratios were as follows for OS 1.16 (0.85 to 1.58; $p = 0.36$), R0 resection 1.24 (0.78 to 1.96; $p = 0.36$), operative morbidity 1.25 (0.75 to 2.09; $p = 0.39$), and mortality 3.60 (0.59 to 22.45; $p = 0.17$).

Adjuvant Radiation and Chemoradiation Therapy.

The recognition of the high rates of local and regional failure following surgery in patterns of failure analyses has served as the basis for clinical trials assessing the value of radiation therapy with and without chemotherapy as an adjuvant treatment in gastric cancer. Although these studies have all addressed the important question of whether clinical outcome is enhanced by adjuvant radiation therapy, there has been marked variability in radiation dose and schedule, sequence with surgery (preoperatively, intraoperatively, or postoperatively), and the use of concurrent and maintenance chemotherapy. These differences in study design may explain in part the conflicting results observed in phase 3 studies.

Two randomized phase 3 trials have studied the use of external beam radiation therapy (EBRT) alone with surgery.[320–322] Although both studies used similar radiation dose and schedule, sequence with surgery differed. In the British Stomach Cancer Group study, 436 patients were randomized to surgery alone, postoperative radiation therapy (45 to 50 Gy in 25 to 28 fractions), or cytotoxic chemotherapy with mitomycin, doxorubicin, and 5-FU.[320,321] The 5-year survival for surgery alone was 20%, for surgery plus radiation therapy 12%, and for surgery plus chemotherapy 19%. In this study, no survival advantage was observed for patients who received postoperative EBRT, although there was an apparent improvement in local control, demonstrating that local disease could be affected by adjuvant radiation therapy. Locoregional failure was documented in only 15 of 153 (10%) in the radiation arm versus 39 of 145 (27%) in the surgery-alone arm, and 26 of 138 (19%) in the mitomycin, doxorubicin, and 5-FU group. Interpretation of these results is complicated by the inclusion of 171 patients undergoing resection with gross or microscopic residual carcinoma. These patients would not be candidates for current gastric surgical adjuvant trials in the United States. In addition, approximately one-third of patients randomized to receive adjuvant treatment did not receive the assigned therapy. Of 153 patients randomized to the postoperative radiation arm, only 104 (68%) received a dose of 40.5 Gy or more, and 36 (24%) received none.

In contrast, the results of a phase 3 study from Beijing demonstrated a survival benefit for patients with gastric cardia carcinoma receiving preoperative radiation and surgery versus surgery alone.[322] In this study, 370 patients with gastric cardia carcinoma were randomized to 40 Gy in 20 fractions over 4 weeks of preoperative irradiation and surgery or surgery alone. The 5-year survival rates of preoperative radiation and surgery and the surgery-alone group were 30% and 20%, respectively (10-year, 20% and 13%, respectively; $p = 0.009$). Further, both local and regional nodal control was improved in patients undergoing preoperative radiation and surgery (61% and 61%, respectively) versus surgery

(48% and 45%, respectively) only. Morbidity and mortality rates were not increased in patients receiving preoperative therapy.[323]

As the price role of adjuvant radiation in resectable gastric cancer remains controversial, an updated systematic review and meta-analysis of 13 RCTs[324] was conducted to gain insights about the potential benefit of adjuvant (including neoadjuvant) radiation and surgery versus surgery alone for resectable gastric cancer.[323] Outcomes analyzed in this meta-analysis were OS, and DFS. Postoperative radiation was associated with a significant improvement in both OS (HR = 0.78; 95% CI = 0.70 to 0.86; $p < 0.001$) and DFS (HR = 0.71; 95% CI = 0.63 to 0.80; $p < 0.001$). Similar improvement in OS (HR = 0.83; 95% CI = 0.67 to 1.03; $p = 0.087$) and DFS (HR = 0.77; 95% CI = 0.91 to 0.65; $p = 0.002$) was observed in five RCTs comparing surgery + adjuvant chemoradiation to surgery + adjuvant chemotherapy for resectable gastric cancer. This meta-analysis suggests that radiation following gastrectomy translates to ~20% DFS and OS benefit.

An alternative approach to postoperative or preoperative radiation is intraoperative radiation therapy (IORT).[325] The advantage of this technique is the ability to deliver a single large fraction (10 to 35 Gy) of radiation to the tumor or tumor bed while excluding or protecting surrounding normal tissue from the high-dose field. This approach permits high-dose radiation with minimal normal tissue treatment. Two randomized trials have examined the efficacy of IORT in combination with surgery for patients with gastric carcinoma.[326,327] Abe et al.[326] from Kyoto University performed a randomized trial of 211 patients with gastric cancer comparing surgery alone with surgery and IORT (28 to 35 Gy). For patients with tumor confined to the gastric wall (stage I), 5-year survival rates were similar for IORT and for resection alone. However, patients with Japanese stages II to IV disease who received IORT in conjunction with resection showed improved survival over patients who underwent resection without radiation. Among patients with stage IV disease (who usually had local residual disease after maximal resection), there were no 5-year survivors who received surgery alone; however, 15% of the patients who received IORT were alive at 5 years. The experience with IORT in gastric cancer at Kyoto University suggested that IORT may be beneficial in the treatment of locally advanced carcinoma of the stomach.

To further evaluate this approach, Sindelar et al.[327] at the National Cancer Institute conducted a prospective RCT comparing surgical resection and IORT with conventional therapy in gastric carcinoma. Patients in the experimental group underwent gastrectomy, and IORT was administered to the gastric bed (20 Gy). Patients in the control group underwent resection and postoperative EBRT to the upper abdomen (50 Gy in 25 fractions) for advanced-stage cancers extending beyond the gastric wall. Of the 100 patients screened for the study, 60 were randomized and underwent exploratory surgery. Nineteen patients were excluded intraoperatively because of unresectability or metastases, leaving 41 patients in the study. The median survival for patients with tumors of all stages was 25 months for the IORT group and 21 months for the control group (p = NS). Locoregional disease relapse occurred in 7 of 16 IORT patients (44%), and in 23 of 25 patients (92%) control patients ($p < 0.001$). Complication rates were similar between IORT and control patients. Although IORT was not associated with a significant advantage over conventional therapy in terms of OS, IORT did significantly improve locoregional disease control. Based on these results, the use of IORT in gastric cancer remains investigational.

Because of the promising results in the early studies of combined-modality therapy for locally advanced (unresectable) or subtotally resected gastric cancer, investigators also have studied this combination of surgery and radiation in resectable gastric carcinoma. A small study from South Africa randomized 66 patients with resected gastric cancer (T (1–3), N (1–2), M0) to low-dose postoperative radiation (20 Gy in eight fractions over 10 days) and 5-FU, or to no further therapy after surgery.[328] No difference in survival was observed between the patients undergoing surgery and adjuvant

therapy and those undergoing surgery alone. Given the subtherapeutic doses of radiation used in this study, it is difficult to draw any definitive conclusions as to the efficacy of adjuvant radiation therapy and 5-FU. In 1984, Moertel et al.[329] reported the results of a prospective randomized trial conducted at the Mayo Clinic with 62 patients with poor prognosis, but completely resected gastric cancers who were randomized to either surgery alone or surgery followed by radiation (37.5 Gy in 24 fractions over 4 to 5 weeks) with concurrent 5-FU. A nonstratified, prerandomization scheme was used with a 2:3 ratio favoring treatment. Ten of the thirty-nine patients refused further therapy and were observed. When analyzed by intent to treat, the adjuvant arm had statistically significant improvement in both relapse-free survival and OS (overall 5-year survival 23% versus 4%; $p < 0.05$). When patient outcome was compared with actual treatment received (29 adjuvant treatment, 33 surgery alone), 5-year survival continued to favor the adjuvant group (20% versus 12%), but the differences were not statistically significant in view of the small patient numbers. The 10 patients who refused assignment to adjuvant treatment had more favorable prognostic findings than the other two groups of patients. When the two groups with equally poor prognostic factors were compared, the 5-year OS was 20% versus 4%, with an advantage to those receiving adjuvant radiation and 5-FU treatment. When analyzed by treatment delivered, locoregional relapse was decreased with adjuvant treatments (54% with surgery alone versus 39% with irradiation and 5-FU).

The Intergroup Trial (INT 0116) randomized patients to receive surgery alone or surgery plus postoperative 5-FU–based chemotherapy and radiation.[330] The trial included patients with stages IB–IVA nonmetastatic adenocarcinoma of the stomach or GEJ. After en bloc resection, 556 patients were randomized to either observation alone or postoperative combined-modality therapy consisting of one monthly 5-day cycle of 5-FU and leucovorin, followed by 45 Gy in 25 fractions plus concurrent 5-FU and leucovorin (4 days in week 1, 3 days in week 5) followed by two monthly 5-day cycles of 5-FU and leucovorin. Nodal metastases were present in 85% of the cases. With 5 years of median follow-up, 3-year relapse-free survival was 48% for adjuvant treatment and 31% for observation ($p = 0.001$); 3-year OS was 50% for treatment and 41% for observation ($p = 0.005$). The median OS in the surgery-only group was 27 months, compared with 36 months in the chemoradiotherapy group; the HR for death was 1.35 (95% CI = 1.09 to 1.66; $p = 0.005$). The hazard ratio for relapse in the surgery-only group as compared with the chemoradiotherapy group was 1.52 (95% CI = 1.23 to 1.86; $p < 0.001$). The median duration of relapse-free survival was 30 months in the chemoradiotherapy group and 19 months in the surgery-only group. Patterns of failure were based on the site of first relapse only and were categorized as local, regional, or distant. Local recurrence occurred in 29% of the patients who relapsed in the surgery-only group and 19% of those who relapsed in the chemoradiotherapy group. Regional relapse, typically abdominal carcinomatosis, was reported in 72% of those who relapsed in the surgery-only group and 65% of those who relapsed in the chemoradiotherapy group. Extra-abdominal distant metastases were diagnosed in 18% of those who relapsed in the surgery-only group and 33% of those who relapsed in the chemoradiotherapy group. Treatment was tolerable, with three (1%) toxic deaths. Grade 3 and 4 toxicity occurred in 41% and 32% of cases, respectively. The results of this large study demonstrate a clear survival advantage for the use of postoperative chemoradiation and strongly support the integration of postoperative chemoradiation into the routine care of patients with curatively resected high-risk carcinoma of the stomach and GEJ.

The US Gastrointestinal Intergroup has recently completed a second randomized prospective trial (Cancer and Leukemia Group B 80101) in patients with completely resected high-risk gastric cancer, comparing two chemotherapy regimens given before and after 5-FU–based chemoradiation. This study examines the use of one cycle of postoperative ECF (epirubicin 50 mg/m², cisplatin 60 mg/m², and continuous infusion 5-FU 200 mg/m² per day for 21 days) followed by radiation therapy with concurrent continuous infusion 5-FU (200 mg/m^2 per day) and two additional cycles of ECF. This is compared with one cycle of postoperative 5-FU and leucovorin followed by concurrent continuous infusion 5-FU (200 mg/m^2 per day) and two additional cycles of 5-FU and leucovorin. This study was recently reported in abstract form and failed to demonstrate a survival advantage of the addition of ECF therapy to standard 5-FU and leucovorin.[331]

To address the important question of the value of postoperative radiation following D2 resection, a Korean phase 3 study comparing postoperative cisplatin/capecitabine (XP) versus postoperative XP with capecitabine and radiation was reported.[332] In this study, 458 patients were enrolled, with 228 randomly assigned to receive adjuvant chemotherapy (XP for six cycles) and 230 patients assigned to receive adjuvant chemoradiation (XPx2 → capecitabine and radiation → XPx2). Although the primary end point of improved 3-year DFS was not met ($p = 0.862$), in the subset of patients with node-positive gastric cancer ($n = 396$), adjuvant chemoradiotherapy was associated with a superior DFS (HR = 0.6865; 95% CI = 0.4735 to 0.9952; $p = 0.471$). Based on these intriguing data, the investigators have initiated a confirmatory study limited to patients with lymph node–positive resected gastric cancer (ARTIST-II).

To address the role of adjuvant chemoradiation in light of the MAGIC trial, the Dutch Colorectal Cancer Group has initiated the CRITICS trial. This study is a phase 3 prospective randomized trial that investigates whether chemoradiotherapy (45 Gy in 5 weeks with daily cisplatin and capecitabine) after preoperative chemotherapy (3 × epirubicin, cisplatin, and capecitabine) and adequate (D1+) gastrectomy leads to improved survival in comparison with postoperative chemotherapy alone (3 × epirubicin, cisplatin, and capecitabine). Further evaluating the role of adjuvant radiation therapy, a Korean phase 3 trial (the ARTIST study) is randomizing patients undergoing D2 gastrectomy to adjuvant cisplatin and capecitabine, with or without radiation therapy.

Although no phase 3 trials have tested the value of preoperative radiation plus chemotherapy for patients with gastric cancer, two phase 2 trials for patients with esophagus cancer have included either lesions of the gastric cardia or the EGJ.[333,334] In both trials, the trimodality study arm demonstrated an improvement in OS when compared with the control arm of surgery alone. The series by Walsh et al.[333] (adenocarcinoma of the esophagus or gastric cardia) demonstrated a median survival of 16 months versus 11 months, and 3-year survival of 32% versus 6% ($p = 0.01$), with the statistically significant advantage to trimodality treatment. The US GI Intergroup phase 3 trial (adenocarcinoma or squamous cell of esophagus or EGJ), which closed prematurely because of low accrual, reported a median survival of 54 months versus 22 months, and 5-year survival of 39% versus 16% ($p = 0.008$), with a significant advantage associated with the trimodality arm.[334] In addition, a recent phase 3 randomized German trial compared preoperative chemotherapy alone (5-FU, leucovorin, and cisplatin) versus the same regimen followed by low-dose radiation therapy (30 Gy) with concurrent cisplatin and etoposide in patients with adenocarcinoma of the lower esophagus or gastric cardia. Although the trial was closed early because of poor accrual (126 patients), patients receiving radiation therapy had significantly higher pathologic complete response rates (2% versus 16%; $p = 0.03$) and trend toward improved survival (3-year survival 47% versus 28%; $p = 0.07$).[335]

Preoperative chemoradiation data for patients with gastric cancer exclusively is limited to phase 2 studies from single institutions and cooperative groups. The MD Anderson Cancer Center has reported a study in which 33 patients completed a preoperative protocol that started with induction chemotherapy of 5-FU, leucovorin, and cisplatin, followed by 45 Gy of radiation therapy in 25 fractions over 5 weeks with concurrent infusional 5-FU. In 28 patients (85%), a gastrectomy was performed and D2 lymph node dissection was attempted. Pathologic complete and partial responses were found in 64% of all operated patients. These patients showed a significant longer median survival of 64 months in comparison with 13 months in patients with tumors that showed no pathologic response to preoperative chemoradiation.[336] In a study from the same institution, 41 patients with operable gastric cancer received two cycles of continuous 5-FU, paclitaxel, and cisplatin followed by 45 Gy of radiation therapy with concurrent 5-FU and paclitaxel. An R0 resection was achieved in 78% of patients; pathologic complete response was seen in 25% and pathologic partial response in 15% of patients. Pathologic response, R0 resection, and postoperative T and N stage correlated with overall and DFS.[337]

The Radiation Therapy Oncology Group (RTOG 9904) reported the results of a phase 2 study of 49 patients undergoing induction 5-FU, leucovorin, and cisplatin followed by concurrent radiation therapy, and infusional 5-FU and paclitaxel. Resection was attempted 5 to 6 weeks after chemoradiation. The pathologic complete response and R0 resection rates were 26% and 77%, respectively. At 1 year, more patients with tumors exhibiting a pathologic complete response (89%) were alive than patients with tumors having less favorable pathologic treatment response (66%). Grade 4 toxicity occurred in 21% of patients. These data appear to support a phase 3 study evaluating preoperative radiation therapy and chemotherapy versus postoperative radiation therapy and chemotherapy.[338]

TECHNICAL TREATMENT-RELATED ISSUES

Surgery

Surgery begins with careful laparoscopic staging and examination. Inspection for the presence of ascites, hepatic metastases, peritoneal seeding, disease in the pelvis (such as a "drop" metastasis), or ovarian involvement should be performed. Once distant metastases have been ruled out, depending on the location of the lesion, a bilateral subcostal incision or a midline abdominal incision can be used to gain adequate exposure to the upper abdomen. The stomach should be inspected to assess the location and extent of the primary tumor. The size and location of the primary tumor dictate the extent of gastric resection. A D2 lymphadenectomy sparing the spleen and pancreas can be done safely, and provides an excellent surgical specimen for pathologic staging, but this procedure should only be performed by or with an experienced surgeon.

The D2 subtotal gastrectomy commences with mobilization of the greater omentum from the transverse colon. After the omentum is mobilized, the anterior peritoneal leaf of the transverse mesocolon is incised along the lower border of the colon, and a plane is developed down to the head of the pancreas. The infrapyloric lymph nodes are dissected and the origin of the right gastroepiploic artery and vein are ligated. With a combination of blunt and sharp dissection, the plane of dissection continues on to the anterior surface of the pancreas, extending to the level of the common hepatic and splenic arteries. This maneuver can be tedious, but it theoretically provides additional protection against serosal spread of tumor to the local peritoneal surface. The right gastric artery is ligated. At this point, the duodenum is divided distal to the pylorus. The stomach and omentum are then reflected cephalad. The gastrohepatic ligament is divided close to the liver up to the gastroesophageal junction. Dissection is then continued along the hepatic artery toward the celiac axis. Once near the celiac axis, the lymph node–bearing tissue is dissected until the left gastric artery is visualized and can be divided at its celiac origin. The proximal peritoneal attachments of the stomach and distal esophagus can then be incised, and the proximal extent of resection is defined. For tumors of the mid- and proximal stomach, dissection of the lymph nodes along the splenic artery and splenic hilum is important. This technique is not indicated for antral tumors, given the low rate of splenic hilar nodal metastases seen with tumors in this anatomical location. The stomach is then divided 5 cm proximal to the tumor, which dictates the extent of gastric resection. Despite the fact that the entire blood supply of the stomach has been interrupted, a cuff of proximal stomach invariably shows good vascularization from the feeding distal esophageal arcade. When feasible, most surgeons prefer to anastomose jejunum to stomach rather than to esophagus because of the technical ease and excellent healing seen with gastrojejunal anastomosis. Reconstruction using a variety of techniques has been described and is a matter of personal choice.

Antibiotics Prophylaxis

One RCT ($n = 501$) tested single-dose cefazolin or ampicillin-sulbactam 30 minutes before surgery versus multiple dose regimen for 3 days postoperatively. There were no differences in surgical site infections or complication.[280,339]

Nasogastric Drainage After Gastrectomy

The Italian Total Gastrectomy Study Group reported on the largest RCT comparing total gastrectomy with Roux-en-Y with and without nasogastric tube ($n = 237$). There were no differences in overall morbidity, leak rate, hospital stay, and time to diet.[340] Other authors confirmed that nasogastric tube is not necessary after gastrectomy.[341–343]

Intraperitoneal Drains After Gastrectomy

As with other pathologies, two RCTs concluded that drains after gastrectomy are generally not indicated, and in certain situations can increase significantly operative morbidity.[344,345]

Reconstruction After Gastrectomy

Iivonen et al.[346] compared Roux-en-Y with and without pouch. They randomized 48 patients and found significantly less dumping syndrome and early satiety but with no differences at 15 months of follow-up. Fein et al.[347] reported on 138 patients randomized in a similar fashion; they found similar QOL at 1 year but significantly improved QOL at 3-, 4-, and 5-year follow-up. It seems that reconstruction with pouch has long-term advantages and may be recommended as the standard reconstruction.[280]

Radiation Treatment

Technique of Radiation Therapy

Idealized portals generated from patterns of failure data should be modified on the basis of the individual patient's initial extent of disease.[348,349] Based on the likely sites of locoregional failure, the gastric/tumor bed, anastomosis and gastric remnant, and regional lymphatics should be included in most patients undergoing postgastrectomy radiation.[350–353] Major nodal chains at risk include the lesser and greater curvature; celiac axis; pancreaticoduodenal, splenic, supra-pancreatic, and porta hepatis groups; and, in some, para-aortic to the level of mid-L3.

The relative risk of nodal metastases at a specific nodal location depends on both the site of origin of the primary tumor, and other factors including width and depth of invasion of the gastric wall.[349] Tumors that originate in the proximal portion of the stomach and the GEJ have a higher propensity of spread to nodes in the mediastinum and pericardial region, but a lower likelihood of involvement of nodes in the region of the gastric antrum, periduodenal area, and porta hepatis. Tumors that originate in the body of the stomach can spread to all nodal sites, but have the highest likelihood of spreading to nodes along the greater and lesser curvature near the location of the primary tumor mass. Tumors that originate in the distal stomach, in the region of the gastric antrum, have a high likelihood of spread to the periduodenal, peripancreatic, and porta hepatis nodes, whereas they have a lower likelihood of spread

to the nodes near the cardia of the stomach, the periesophageal and mediastinal nodes, or to the splenic hilar nodes. Any tumor originating in the stomach has a high propensity of spread to nodes along the greater and lesser curvature, although they are most likely to spread to those sites in close anatomic proximity to the primary tumor mass. Guidelines for defining the clinical target volume for postoperative irradiation fields have been developed based on location and extent of the primary tumor (T stage), and location and extent of known nodal involvement (N stage).[349] In general, for patients with node-positive disease, there should be wide coverage of tumor bed, remaining stomach, resection margins, and nodal drainage regions. For node-negative disease, if there is a good surgical resection with pathologic evaluation of at least 15 nodes, and there are wide surgical margins proximal and distal to the primary tumor (at least 5 cm), treatment of the nodal beds is optional. Treatment of the remaining stomach should depend on a balance of the likely normal tissue morbidity and the perceived risk of local relapse in the residual stomach.

Although parallel-opposed anteroposterior/posteroanterior (AP/PA) fields are a practical arrangement for tumor bed and nodal irradiation, three-dimensional multifield techniques should be used if they can improve long-term tolerance of normal tissues. Tightly contoured fields should be designed to spare as much normal tissue as possible. Over the past decade, a shift has occurred toward more sophisticated treatment techniques that use multiple and often noncoplanar beams including three-dimensional and intensity-modulated radiation therapy. Attention has also been placed on accurate three-dimensional target delineated fields based on CT anatomy rather than only two-dimensional field design. In addition to refinements in radiation therapy target definition based on CT planning, technologic advances including study of and solutions for variability in target and normal organ location during a treatment course (day to day interfraction variability) and actual treatment delivered (intrafraction variability caused by respiration) have been undertaken. Interfraction variability in stomach location can be substantial, particularly among patients treated with neoadjuvant chemoradiation because of daily variations in gastric filling. Because of this, patients should generally be treated with an empty stomach. Intrafraction changes in target shape (deformation) and location are asymmetric and mainly from respiratory motion. Movement, particularly in the cranial-caudad dimension, frequently exceeds 1 to 1.5 cm. Image guidance, four-dimensional treatment planning, and respiratory gating have been developed to address these challenges.

More routine use of multiple field techniques should be considered when preoperative imaging exists to allow accurate reconstruction of target volumes. Single-institution data suggest that multiple field arrangements may produce less toxicity.[354] Although AP/PA fields can be weighted anteriorly to keep the spinal cord dose at acceptable levels using only parallel-opposed techniques, a four-field technique, if feasible, can spare spinal cord radiation exposure, with improved dose homogeneity. Dependent on the posterior extent of the gastric fundus, either oblique or more routine lateral portals can be used to deliver a 10- to 20-Gy component of irradiation to spare the spinal cord or kidney. When lateral fields are used, liver and kidney tolerance limits the use of lateral fields to ≤20 Gy. With the wide availability of three-dimensional treatment-planning systems, it may be possible to target more accurately the high-risk volume, and to use unconventional field arrangements to produce superior dose distributions. To accomplish this without marginal misses, it will be necessary to both carefully define and encompass the various target volumes, given that the use of oblique or noncoplanar beams could potentially exclude target volumes that would be included in AP/PA fields or nonoblique four-field techniques (AP/PA and laterals). In most patients, a portion of both kidneys are within the treatment field, but at least two-thirds to three-fourths of one kidney should be excluded beyond a dose of 20 Gy. For proximal gastric lesions, ≥50% of the left kidney is commonly within the irradiation portal, and the right kidney must be appropriately spared. For distal lesions with narrow or positive duodenal margins, a similar amount of right kidney often is included, and every effort must be taken to spare the left kidney from irradiation in order to maintain function. Late renal sequelae have not been encountered with these techniques, assuming normal renal function bilaterally.[355–357]

With proximal gastric lesions or lesions at the EGJ, a 3- to 5-cm margin of distal esophagus should be included. If the lesion extends through the entire gastric wall, a major portion of the left hemidiaphragm should be included. In these circumstances, blocking can decrease the volume of irradiated heart.

TREATMENT OF ADVANCED DISEASE (STAGE IV)

Treatment of Advanced Gastric Cancer: Palliative Systemic Chemotherapy

Chemotherapy Versus Best Supportive Care

The modest activity and substantial toxicity of cytotoxic chemotherapy has raised the question, Does palliative systemic therapy with available agents have clinical utility? That is, there was controversy as to whether a meaningful advantage is attained by early initiation of systemic therapy as opposed to providing best supportive care. Although this is a difficult hypothesis to test because of patient and physician preferences and biases, several random assignment trials were performed in the 1990s in patients with advanced incurable gastric cancer addressing this issue.

Wagner et al.[358] performed a meta-analysis for the Cochrane collaboration. They included three random assignment trials involving a total of 184 patients in whom the study design was to initiate systemic chemotherapy plus best supportive care or to provide best supportive care alone. Median survival and OS were evaluated (Table 38.6). Patients receiving chemotherapy as part of their treatment had better OS than those receiving best supportive care only, with an overall HR of 0.39 (95% CI = 0.28 to 0.52). The median survival was improved from 4.3 months for best supportive care to approximately 11 months for chemotherapy. Note that

the median survival for patients receiving chemotherapy is consistent with several more recent trials. There was also a modest improvement in time to progression (TTP; 7 months for patients receiving chemotherapy versus 2.5 months for patients receiving best supportive care). Wagner et al.[358] concluded that the evidence supporting initiating chemotherapy for patients with advanced incurable gastric cancer was convincing.

In a fourth trial, QOL was assessed. The average quality-adjusted survival for patients undergoing chemotherapy was superior to patients receiving best supportive care (6 months versus 12 months). Importantly, in those best supportive care trials that reported 2-year survival ($\geq$24 months), only patients undergoing chemotherapy survived for that period of time. The 2-year survival rate was 5% to 14% for patients receiving combination chemotherapy versus 0% for patients receiving best supportive care. More recently, the preliminary results of a small study testing the use of single-agent chemotherapy versus best supportive care in patients who have already received chemotherapy were reported. Previously treated patients were randomly assigned to best supportive care or to single-agent irinotecan plus best supportive care. Although the study was initially powered to require 120 patients, accrual to this type of trial was difficult and a total of only 40 patients were eventually randomized. There was a modest improvement in OS, with median survival for those receiving irinotecan of 123 days, and median survival for those with best supportive care 73 days (HR = 2.85).[359] These results are in concert with the earlier studies in previously untreated patients and indicate that systemic therapy has a modest but real and clinically meaningful effect on outcome. Many cytotoxic agents have been studied in patients with advanced gastric cancer; when used as single agents, modest activity has been identified for drugs from five different classes. More recently, targeted therapy has been tested. The following section summarizes the data for the use of systemic cytotoxic chemotherapy when given with palliative intent. An extensive discussion of older agents can be found in prior editions of this textbook.

Single-Agent Chemotherapy

For most drugs, a variety of doses and schedules have been studied. In the absence of comparative trials using the same agent with different doses and schedules, superiority of one regimen over the other cannot be assessed. Table 38.7 gives a listing of agents that have demonstrated at least modest activity in the treatment of gastric cancer and which are routinely employed as part of standard practice options. Drugs with little or no activity, especially if they were evaluated prior to 2000, are not included in this table.

5-FU is the parent fluorinated pyrimidine that has been the most extensively studied single agent in gastric cancer. An antimetabolite, the drug has been used in a variety of schedules and doses in various epithelial malignancies of gastrointestinal origin. One method involved the use of rapid intravenous injections on a weekly basis, or daily for 5 consecutive days. In gastric cancer, continuous infusion 5-FU has been used more recently. During the 1990s, in several studies, 5-FU was the control arm of a random assignment trial or was studied as a single agent (with leucovorin) in a prospective phase 2 trial. This allowed an assessment using more modern criteria of activity. The studies from the 1990s suggest overall response rates of 10% to 20%, with a median duration of response, or TTP, of approximately 4 months. As is the case in other diseases, the major toxicities reported in gastric cancer for 5-FU are mucositis, diarrhea, or mild myelosuppression. Because continuous intravenous infusion schedules can be cumbersome, oral analogues of 5-FU have been studied in gastric cancer. Three oral drugs of this class have undergone study in gastric cancer. These are tegafur and uracil (UFT), S-1 (tegafur and two modulators, 5-chloro-2,4-dihydroxypyridine and potassium oxonate), and capecitabine (Xeloda, Hoffmann-La Roche, Basel, Switzerland). The data for these agents are also shown in Table 38.7. S-1 has been most extensively studied in Japan. Although a response rate to

---

TABLE 38.6

Chemotherapy for Advanced Gastric Cancer: Treatment Versus Best Supportive Care

Regimen	No. of Patients	Median Survival (mo)	Survival Rate (%) 1y	Survival Rate (%) 2y
FAMTX	30	10	40	6
BSC	10	3	10	0
FEMTX	17	12	—	—
BSC	19	3	—	—
ETOPLF	10	10	—	—
BSC	8	4	—	—
ELF	52	10.2	34.6	9.6
BSC	51	5	7.8	0
Irinotecan	21	123[a]	—	—
BSC	19	73[a]	—	—

F, fluorouracil; A, doxorubicin; MTX, methotrexate; BSC, best supportive care; E, epirubicin; ETOP, etoposide; L, leucovorin.
[a] Median survival in days.
Modified from Wils J. The treatment of advanced gastric cancer. *Semin Oncol* 1996;23:397.

TABLE 38.7

Activity of Selected Single Agents in Advanced Gastric Cancer

Drug	Response Rate (%)
Fluorinated Pyrimidines	
5-Fluorouracil	21
UFT	28
S-1	49
Capecitabine	26
Antibiotics	
Doxorubicin hydrochloride	17
Epirubicin hydrochloride	19
Heavy Metals	
Cisplatin	19
Taxanes	
Paclitaxel	17
Docetaxel	19
Camptothecans	
Irinotecan hydrochloride	23

UFT, tegafur and uracil; S-1, tegafur and two modulators, 5-chloro-2, 4-dihydroxypyridine and potassium oxonate.
From van De Velde CJH, Kelsen D, Minsky B. Gastric cancer: clinical management. In: Kelsen D, Daly JM, Kern SE, et al., eds. *Principles and Practice of Gastrointestinal Oncology*. 2nd ed. Philadelphia: Lippincott Williams & Wilkins; 2008, with permission.

single-agent S-1 of 44% to 54% was reported in Japanese patients, the response rate among European patients was substantially lower. Like capecitabine, S-1 is now undergoing study in combination with other agents, particularly cisplatin. UFT combines tegafur and uracil. In gastric cancer, a response rate of 28% was seen in Japanese patients. In a small European study, Okines et al.[360] reported the results of a European Organisation for Research and Treatment of Cancer (EORTC) study combining UFT and leucovorin. A 16% response rate was seen in a group of 23 patients. Capecitabine has been tested in fewer single-agent studies in gastric cancer. The data available suggest similar activity as seen with other oral fluorinated pyrimidines. Capecitabine has recently been extensively studied in combination with cisplatin or oxaliplatin (see "The REAL-2 Trial").

Platinum compounds are an important part of the treatment of gastric cancer. The parent analogue, cisplatin, was studied in the 1980s. In both previously treated and untreated patients, a response rate of approximately 15% was reported. The major toxicities for cisplatin are nausea and vomiting, peripheral neuropathy, ototoxicity, and nephropathy. The development of efficacious antiemetics has significantly improved control of nausea and vomiting. An analogue of cisplatin, carboplatin, has been less well studied in gastric cancer; it appears to have less activity in this disease, as compared to other epithelial malignancies. Most recently, oxaliplatin, a diamino cyclohexane extensively used in the treatment of colorectal cancer, was included as part of combination chemotherapy for gastric cancer. The data for combination therapy, including oxaliplatin and data from the REAL-2 trial, are shown later.

A third class of cytotoxic agents with activity in gastric cancer is the taxanes. Both paclitaxel and docetaxel have been studied as single agents in gastroesophageal cancers. Docetaxel has been more extensively studied than paclitaxel. De Cosimo et al.[361] reviewed trials in which docetaxel was used as single agent. Patients may have received prior treatment, and 262 patients were evaluable for response. The overall response rate was 19%. The major toxicities were neutropenia, alopecia, and edema. Allergic reactions were seen in about 25% of patients. The most common dosing schedule for docetaxel is 100 mg/m^2 every 3 weeks. When reported, the median TTP while on docetaxel therapy was 6 months. A schedule using lower doses given once weekly has also been studied with similar activity. On the basis of a large randomized study comparing CF to docetaxel-cisplatin–5-FU (DCF), docetaxel was approved by the US Food and Drug Administration for the treatment of advanced gastric cancer. Paclitaxel has also been studied in gastric cancer, although in smaller numbers of patients, and has a similar degree of cytotoxic activity.

A fourth class of active agent is represented by irinotecan. It has been studied both as a single agent and in combination with other cytotoxic agents. When used alone, response rates of 15% to 25% have been reported in both previously treated and untreated patients with advanced gastric cancer. Wagner et al.[358] reviewed the data for combinations, including irinotecan versus multidrug combinations not including irinotecan. They concluded that irinotecan-containing multidrug chemotherapy combinations had a modest survival benefit, which was not statistically significant, when compared with regimens not including irinotecan. The major toxicities of irinotecan are myelosuppression and diarrhea.

Anthracyclines also have activity in gastric cancer. Single-agent data from the 1960s and 1970s show a response rate for doxorubicin of 17%, and for epirubicin a similar response rate of approximately 19%. The anthracyclines have undergone more extensive study in combination chemotherapy for advanced gastric cancer.

Single-Agent Versus Combination Chemotherapy

The potential advantage of giving combination chemotherapy versus single-agent chemotherapy has been evaluated by Wagner et al.[358] in an update of their original Cochrane review. They found that combination chemotherapy had a significant survival advantage when compared to single-agent chemotherapy (HR = 0.82; 95% CI = 0.74 to 0.90). The difference in average median survival, however, was modest: 8.3 months for combination chemotherapy versus 6.7 months for single-agent chemotherapy. In the updated analysis, a test for heterogeneity was not statistically significant; they concluded that this indicated that the results of the different studies were consistent. A secondary analysis for response rate and for TTP also favored combination chemotherapy. Not surprisingly, toxicity is higher when several agents are given together, although this was not statistically significant. Treatment-related mortality was only slightly higher (1.5%) for patients receiving combination chemotherapy versus 1.1% when single-agent chemotherapy was used.

They also evaluated the role of several different combinations of cytotoxic agents, including anthracyclines as part of combination chemotherapy. In this analysis, three studies with a total of 500 patients were included. Wagner et al.[358] found that including anthracyclines in a CF combination had a modest survival advantage over CF alone (HR = 0.77; 95% CI = 0.62 to 0.95). A similar advantage to anthracyclines in combination was found when 5-FU–anthracycline combinations without cisplatin were studied. In contrast to anthracyclines, there was a more modest, albeit not statistically significant, benefit for irinotecan-containing combinations. Once again, there was a modest improvement in OS for docetaxel-containing regimens, but this did not reach statistical significance. The response rate as a secondary objective was 36% for docetaxel-containing regimens versus 31% for nondocetaxel-containing regimens (not statistically significant). Oral fluoropyrimidines when compared to intravenous fluoropyrimidine therapy also showed no significant difference in median OS. The meta-analysis is in concert with the results of the REAL-2 trial, which indicated noninferiority for oral capecitabine when compared to intravenous 5-FU. Similarly, oxaliplatin regimens were compared to cisplatin-containing regimens with modest superiority to oxaliplatin.

In summary, there are five classes of cytotoxic chemotherapy agents in which single agents have modest activity in gastric cancer. The response rates range from 10% to 25%, and the median duration of response is relatively short (4 to 6 months). As a result of the single-agent trials, 5-FU or capecitabine (or other oral fluoropyrimidines), cisplatin or oxaliplatin, docetaxel, and less commonly, paclitaxel, epirubicin, and irinotecan are the major components of conventional combination cytotoxic systemic chemotherapy regimens.

Like other malignancies, multidrug regimens using agents that have single-agent activity have been extensively studied in gastric cancer. This section will focus on phase 3 random assignment trials. For some combinations, only phase 2 data are available. The recent Cochrane review summarizing a comparison of different regimens including three-drug versus two-drug combinations has already been discussed.[358]

Cisplatin-Fluorouracil. One of the most widely used combination chemotherapy regimens in upper gastrointestinal tract malignancies, including gastric cancer, is the two-drug combination of CF. Although this regimen has been used for several decades, with a variety of doses and schedules employed, since 2000, several phase 3 random assignment trials have been performed in which CF was the control arm. This allowed an opportunity for an evaluation of the efficacy of this combination, in patients with advanced incurable gastric cancer, both in terms of response rate, PFS, and OS, using currently accepted criteria for efficacy and toxicity of treatment. Table 38.8 shows the data from six studies in which CF was the control arm.[362] The doses of cisplatin used were 80 to 100 mg/m^2 per course. 5-FU was given as a continuous 24-hour infusion from days 1 through 5 at a dose of 800 to 1,000 mg/m^2 per day. Cycles were usually given on an every-28-day basis. Efficacy outcomes were consistent across these trials. Response rates, PFS, and OS were quite similar. Major objective tumor regression was reported in 20% to 30% of patients; complete clinical remission was very uncommon, however. The median TTP or PFS, depending on the study, ranged from 3.7 months to 4.1 months, with median survival ranging from 7.2 months to 8.6 months. Two-year survival was between 7% and 10%. CF was compared to a variety of other agents in these trials.

Vanhoefer et al.,[363] reporting for EORTC, compared CF to methotrexate, 5-FU, and doxorubicin (FAMTX); a third group of patients received etoposide, leucovorin, and 5-FU combination. There was no significant difference in outcome among the three arms. A Japanese study (JC 09205) also had three systemic therapy arms.[364] 5-FU was compared to CF, and to a third arm of uracil/tegafur plus mitomycin. In this study, there was no advantage for the two-drug combination of CF over 5-FU alone. The final results of the TAX315 trial have recently been published.[365] The details of this study are described later. An advantage was seen for the DCF arm. The CF control arm results were similar to those seen in the earlier trials previously described. The two-drug combination of 5-FU plus irinotecan was compared to CF by Dank et al.[366] CF was equivalent to irinotecan plus 5-FU. Kang et al.[367] reported the results of the RCT comparison between CF versus cisplatin-capecitabine. This study was designed as a noninferiority trial with the hypothesis that capecitabine-cisplatin was not inferior to CF. The end point was PFS. The dose of cisplatin was slightly lower than in the studies described earlier (80 mg/m^2). However, therapy was given on every-3-week basis; 316 patients were treated. The median PFS was 5 months for CF; median survival was 9.3 months. Ajani et al.[368] reported the results of the FLAGS trial, which is described in more detail later. In this study involving 1,029 eligible patients, the control arm of CF had a median OS of 7.9 months.

In summary, the random assignment trials discussed previously indicate consistent data for efficacy (and toxicity) for the two-drug combination CF. The Japanese study raises the question as to whether there is a substantial clinical advantage to CF over

TABLE 38.8

Combination Chemotherapy in Advanced Gastric Cancer: Cisplatin-Fluorouracil-Containing Regimens Used as the Control Arm in Random Assignment Trials

Study (Ref.)	Drug	Dose (mg/ml)	Schedule (d)	No. of Patients	RR (%)	Median TTP/ PFS (mo)	Median Survival (mo)	Two-y Survival (%)
EORTC[363]	C	100	1	127	20	4.1	7.2	~10
	F	1,000	1–5					
JCOG[364]	C	20	1–5	105	36	7.3	3.9	7
	F	800	1–5					
Dank et al.[366]	C	100	1	163	26	4.2	8.7	~10
	F	1,000	1–5					
TAX325[365]	C	100	1	224	25	3.7	8.6	9
	F	1,000	1–5					
FLAGS[368]	C	100	1	508	32	5.5	7.9	~10
	F	1,000	1–5					
Kang et al.[367]	C	80	1	156	32	5.5	9.3	~10
	F	800	1–5					
REAL-2[360,362,374]	E	50	1	289	41	6.2	9.9	~15
	C	60	1					
	F	200	Daily					

RR, recovery rate; TTP, time to progression; PFS, progression-free survival; EORTC, European Organisation for Research and Treatment of Cancer; C, cisplatin; F, fluorouracil; JCOG, Japan Clinical Oncology Group; E, epirubicin; FLAGS, Cisplatin/S-1 With Cisplatin/Infusional Fluorouracil in Advanced Gastric or Gastroesophageal Adenocarcinoma Study; REAL, Randomized Trial of EOC +/− Panitumumab for Advanced and Locally Advanced Esophagogastric Cancer.
Modified from van De Velde CJH, Kelsen D, Minsky B. Gastric cancer: clinical management. In: Kelsen D, Daly JM, Kern SE, et al., eds. *Principles and Practice of Gastrointestinal Oncology*. 2nd ed. Philadelphia: Lippincott Williams & Wilkins; 2008, with permission.

5-FU alone, but the meta-analysis performed by Wagner et al.[358] supports the use of combination over single-agent chemotherapy. Although still commonly used as a conventional standard of practice palliative treatment, the recent demonstration of modest superiority when docetaxel is added to CF (assuming that a more well-tolerated regimen using the three agents can be developed) as well as the noncomparative data using ECF, which is discussed later, suggest that CF may not be the most effective option for therapy in patients with advanced gastric cancer. The slight advantage in longer-term survival (2-year survival) in the TAX325 and in the irinotecan–5-FU–leucovorin (FOLFIRI) studies of 15% to 20%, as compared to 15% to 20% for ECF, suggests that at least some patients may have longer-term survival with newer regimens.

Although type and incidence of treatment-related toxicity is consistent across most CF trials and is generally tolerable, it can be severe on occasion. For example, in the EORTC trial, grade 3 or 4 neutropenia was seen in approximately one-third of patients; one-quarter of patients had grade 3 or 4 nausea or vomiting. Similarly, in the more recent TAX325 trial, overall grade 3 or 4 toxicity was seen in 75% of patients receiving CF; in the FLAGS trial, treatment-related mortality occurred in 4.9% of patients receiving CF. Some toxicity may be ameliorated by improved supportive care. For example, newer antiemetics such as aprepitant should improve control of severe nausea and vomiting. More widespread use of supportive cytokine agents may decrease the incidence of neutropenic fever. Nonetheless, it should be recognized that CF, using the doses and schedules described previously, is associated with substantial toxicity in some patients.

The use of oral fluoropyrimidines in place of intravenous 5-FU has been studied in several phase 3 trials, including that of Kang et al.[367] described earlier, the REAL-2 trial, and the FLAGS trial comparing CF to cisplatin–S-1. In FLAGS trial, 1,029 patients received either cisplatin 100 mg/m^2 and 5-FU 1,000 mg/m^2 as a continuous 5-day infusion or a slightly lower dose of cisplatin plus oral S-1.[368] Median OS was 8.6 months for patients receiving cisplatin plus S-1 versus 7.9 months in the CF arm, with less toxicity for the cisplatin–S-1 combination. These three trials indicate that oral fluoropyrimidine when given with a platinum compound is not inferior to intravenous 5-FU plus cisplatin.

Docetaxel, Cisplatin, and Fluorouracil. Van Cutsem et al.[365] have reported the final results of a large-scale random assignment trial comparing the DCF combination to CF (the TAX325 trial). Previously untreated patients with advanced gastric cancer received either DCF (221 analyzable patients) or CF using the doses and schedules previously described (224 patients). The primary end point of the study was TTP and was powered to detect an increase in median TTP from 4 to 6 months. The two arms of the study were well balanced for prognostic factors, including weight loss, performance status, and extent of disease. The median TTP was 3.7 months for patients receiving CF and 5.6 months for those receiving DCF (HR = 1.47; p = 0.0004). As a secondary end point, survival was also modestly increased from 8.6 months for CF to 9.2 months for DCF. The 2-year survival rate, however, was increased greater than two-fold in the DCF treatment arm (2-year OS: 8.8% for CF and 18.4% for DCF). Another measure of efficacy favoring DCF was tumor response to treatment (37% for DCF and 25% for CF). Although this study indicated an advantage to the three-drug combination of DCF, toxicity was also increased and was very substantial. Eighty-one percent of all patients receiving DCF had at least one grade 3 or 4 nonhematologic toxicity, as well as substantially more hematologic toxicity. Of the patients receiving CF, 14% had neutropenic fever, as did 30% of patients receiving DCF. However, there was no difference in the treatment-related mortality rate for the two arms. This study led to the recent approval of docetaxel by the US Food and Drug Administration for the treatment of gastric cancer when given in association with CF.

Like epirubicin, docetaxel, when added to CF, has a modest improvement in efficacy. The very substantial toxicity seen with the DCF regimen, however, has led to concerns regarding its general use. A number of studies have been performed using modifications of DCF to develop a more tolerable regimen. Several strategies have been pursued, most of which involve using somewhat lower doses of docetaxel and 5-FU, or modifications in the schedule as to duration of 5-FU infusion or timing of the cisplatin dose. The preliminary results of a phase 2 trial comparing one of these modified DCF regimes to the original DCF schedule indicate that modifications of the treatment schedule may decrease toxicity while maintaining treatment efficacy.[369]

Irinotecan Plus Fluorouracil-Leucovorin. A three-drug combination of FOLFIRI has been studied extensively in metastatic colorectal cancer. A random-assignment phase 2 study comparing FOLFIRI with cisplatin-irinotecan indicated a potential advantage for the FOLFIRI-type regimen.[370] Therefore, a definitive phase 3 trial was performed with CF as the control arm.[366] A total of 170 patients received irinotecan–5-FU) and 163 received CF. The primary end point was TTP. The analysis allowed for a noninferiority comparison between the two arms. The study was reasonably well balanced for the usual prognostic indicators; approximately 20% of patients had EGJ tumors. There was no significant difference in the major objective response rate (32% for irinotecan–5-FU and 26% for CF) nor in median TTP (5 months for irinotecan–5-FU and 4.2 months for CF). Overall median survival was also similar between groups (9 months for irinotecan–5-FU and 8.7 months for CF). Time to treatment failure was 4 months versus 3.4 months for irinotecan–5-FU and CF, respectively (p = 0.018). Irinotecan–5-FU was better in terms of toxic deaths (0.6% versus 3%), discontinuation for toxicity (10% versus 22%), neutropenia, thrombocytopenia, and stomatitis but not diarrhea than CF. The investigator's final conclusion was that irinotecan–5-FU was not inferior to CF and was somewhat less toxic.

Epirubicin, Cisplatin, and Fluorouracil. English investigators have extensively studied the three-drug combination ECF. Two random-assignment phase 3 trials have compared the ECF with a noncisplatin-containing combination (FAMTX) or with a mitomycin-cisplatin–5-FU (MCF) combination.[371] In the first study, ECF was more effective than FAMTX both in terms of response rate and median OS (8.7 months versus 6.1 months). Two-year survival was also superior for the ECF combination (14% versus 5%). In the second study, Ross et al.[371] compared ECF with MCF. In this larger study, 574 patients were treated. The primary end point was 1-year survival. The overall objective response rates were similar between the two arms (ECF 50% and MCF 55%). Toxicity was tolerable, although myelosuppression was greater for the experimental MCF arm. There was a slightly improved median duration of survival for ECF (9.4 months versus 8.7 months) and for 1-year survival (40% for ECF and 32% for MCF). There was no significant difference in 2-year survival, which was approximately 15% for both arms. Several studies have demonstrated that a small percentage of patients with advanced unresectable gastric cancer actually survive 2 years. Data for the ECF regimen as the control arm of the REAL-2 trial are discussed later.

Cisplatin Plus Irinotecan. Cisplatin is a commonly used agent in gastric cancer, and irinotecan has been combined with this drug as well as with other agents. In single-arm phase 2 studies, response rates were encouraging and toxicity was tolerable with irinotecan-cisplatin. This observation led to a somewhat larger random-assignment phase 2 trial comparing irinotecan-cisplatin with the irinotecan–5-FU regimen previously described.[370] Sixty-two patients received irinotecan–5-FU and 61 received irinotecan-cisplatin. The dose schedule used for the irinotecan-cisplatin arm was higher than that from earlier irinotecan-cisplatin regimens. In this study, the response rate was higher for irinotecan–5-FU than for irinotecan-cisplatin, as was the TTP. Although irinotecan-cisplatin in the dose and schedule used in the random-assignment phase 2 trial previously described was less effective than irinotecan–5-FU, other investigators have pursued this regimen using different schedules. These studies have been performed in patients with esophageal, gastroesophageal, and gastric cancers. One irinotecan-cisplatin regimen was used with bevacizumab.[372]

Fluorouracil-Leucovorin-Oxaliplatin.

As is the case for irinotecan-containing regimens, oxaliplatin plus 5-FU is a standard practice option for patients with both metastatic and locally advanced colon cancer. In part because of this data, 5-FU–leucovorin-oxaliplatin (FOLFOX) regimens have also been studied in gastric cancer. The toxicity spectrum is similar to that seen in patients with colorectal cancer, with the dose-limiting toxicity of peripheral neuropathy (oxaliplatin). Myelosuppression, mucositis, and diarrhea typical for 5-FU regimens were noted as well. Several FOLFOX phase 2 studies have now been reported in gastric cancer. Overall response rates of approximately 50% were observed, with median TTP of 5 to 6 months and median OS ranging from 10 to 12 months.[373]

The REAL-2 Trial

Partly on the basis of these studies, a phase 3 trial comparing an oxaliplatin-based regimen with cisplatin-containing combinations was performed. Cunningham et al.[374] in the REAL-2 trial studied 1,002 patients who were randomized to one of four treatment groups: a control arm of ECF and three investigational arms. The central question in this study was: Can capecitabine be substituted for 5-FU and/or oxaliplatin substituted for cisplatin. The four arms were ECF, epirubicin-oxaliplatin–5-FU, epirubicin-cisplatin-capecitabine, and epirubicin-oxaliplatin-capecitabine (EOX). The four regimens are shown in Table 38.9. Patients were stratified for performance status and extent of disease. The primary end point was in OS. The study

TABLE 38.9

REAL-2 Regimens

Drug	Dose (mg/m²)	Day(s)	Week(s)[a]
ECF			
Epirubicin	50 mg/m² IV	1	Every 3 wk
Cisplatin	60 mg/m² IV	1	
PVI 5-FU	200 mg/m²/d[b]	1	
EOF			
Epirubicin	50 mg/m² IV	1	Every 3 wk
Oxaliplatin	130 mg/m² IV	1	
PVI 5-FU	200 mg/m²/d[b]	1	
ECX			
Epirubicin	50 mg/m² IV	1	Every 3 wk
Cisplatin	60 mg/m² IV	1	
Capecitabine	625 mg/m²/BID	1	
EOX			
Epirubicin	50 mg/m² IV	1	Every 3 wk
Oxaliplatin	130 mg/m² IV	1	
Capecitabine	625 mg/m²/BID	1	

REAL, Randomized Trial of EOC +/− Panitumumab for Advanced and Locally Advanced Esophagogastric Cancer; ECF, epirubicin-cisplatin-fluorouracil; PVI, protracted venous-infusion; 5-FU, 5-fluorouracil; EOF, epirubicin-oxaliplatin-5-FU; IV, intravenously; ECX, epirubicin-cisplatin-capecitabine; BID, twice a day; EOX, epirubicin-oxaliplatin-capecitabine.
[a] Planned treatment duration 24 weeks (eight cycles).
[b] PVI 5-FU delivered by central venous access catheter.
Modified from Cunningham D, Okines AF, Ashley S, et al. Capecitabine and oxaliplatin for advanced esophagogastric cancer. *N Engl J Med* 2008;358:36.

was powered to show noninferiority for capecitabine compared with 5-FU and oxaliplatin compared with cisplatin. There were approximately 250 patients per arm. The study design was a two-by-two comparison. A total of 40% of patients had primary gastric cancer, and the remainder had either EGJ or esophageal cancers, with 10% of patients having squamous cell cancer of the esophagus. There was no difference in median OS between the arms (ECF 9.9 months, epirubicin-oxaliplatin–5-FU 9.3 months, epirubicin-cisplatin-capecitabine 9.9 months, and EOX 11.2 months). The 1-year OS was also similar and ranged from 38% to 47%, the best outcome evident with EOX and the lowest with the control arm of ECF. The authors concluded the oxaliplatin could be substituted for cisplatin, and capecitabine could be substituted for 5-FU in the palliative setting.

Al-Batran et al.[375] reported the results of a trial comparing a FOLFOX regimen with 5-FU–leucovorin-cisplatin (FLP). A modified FOLFOX-6 schedule was used for the experimental arm. The FLP regimen used slightly lower doses of 5-FU and cisplatin (50 mg/m²) every 2 weeks. The study was powered for superiority of FOLFOX over FLP. A total of 220 patients were randomized between the two arms. There was no significant difference in TTP ($p = 0.08$) and OS (10.7 fluorouracil 2,600 mg/m² via 24-hour infusion, leucovorin 200 mg/m², and oxaliplatin 85 mg/m² [FLO] every 2 weeks versus 8.8 [FLP] months). Although this study did not demonstrate superiority for oxaliplatin-containing regimens, it does support the results of the REAL-2 study for noninferiority comparing oxaliplatin and cisplatin. The FOLFOX regimen was slightly less toxic.

Finally, Kang et al.[367] compared XP with CF. A total of 160 patients received XP and 156 patients received CF. The XP arm was not inferior, with a median PFS of 5.6 months versus 5 months for CF. OS was 10.5 months versus 9.3 months for XP versus CF (HR = 0.85; 95% CI = 0.64 to 1.13; $p = 0.008$ versus noninferiority margin of 1.25). The authors concluded that XP can be considered an effective alternative to CF.

It is of note that FOLFOX, FOLFIRI, and capecitabine-containing regimens are widely used in colorectal cancer. In metastatic colorectal cancer, the median TTP using these regimens is approximately 7 to 8 months and the median survival (even without the use of bevacizumab) is 20 to 24 months. The 1-year survival for patients with stage IV unresectable colon cancer is approximately 70%, and, using these regimens, 2-year survival approaches 40%. As shown earlier, the same regimens used in patients with gastric or EGJ tumors result in substantially shorter times to progression and significantly shorter median survivals. There are more classes of active cytotoxic agents with demonstrated activity in EGJ than there are for colorectal cancer. In upper gastrointestinal tract malignancies, oxaliplatin, cisplatin, 5-FU, irinotecan, capecitabine, taxane, and anthracyclines have at least modest single-agent activity, whereas the taxanes and anthracyclines are not active in colorectal cancer. These differences in efficacy outcomes suggest biologic differences between these malignancies, despite the histologic similarities (e.g., "intestinal-type" gastric cancers).

As is the case for other solid epithelieal malignancies, an important area of investigation is the development of better preclinical models, such as murine models, and the identification of predictive and prognostic biomarkers, which may well be different between gastrointestinal tumors arising in the upper and lower gastrointestinal tract. On the other hand, using targeted therapies, predictive markers may be the same in different cancers; for example, overexpression or amplification of *HER2* is a predictive marker for the use of the monoclonal antibody trastuzumab in both breast and now gastric cancers. It is also possible that the use of another cytotoxic treatment regimen (second-line treatment) after progression of disease on the first treatment regimen in gastroesophageal cancers would lead to a similar outcome as seen in colorectal cancers. For example, in the REAL-2 trial, only 15% of patients received additional therapy at the time of progression of disease. The irinotecan versus best supportive care study described previously suggests that at least some patients will have a modest survival benefit to second-line treatment.

Second-Line Therapy

Despite numerous chemotherapy options, the majority of patients who progress on first-line therapy are currently not treated with second-line chemotherapy in the West. In several series, only 20% to 50% of patients received second-line treatment.[376,377] Patients with gastric cancer often have numerous comorbidities and complications of their malignancy (i.e., failure to thrive with significant protein-calorie losses, peritoneal carcinomatosis with limited bowel function) that preclude the safe administration of second-line therapy. Alternatively, as many as 70% of patients from Japan and other parts of Asia receive second-line therapy. Recently, there have been two random assignment studies that demonstrate the benefits of second-line therapy.[378,379]

In one study, previously treated patients were randomly assigned to best supportive care or to single-agent irinotecan plus best supportive care. Although the study was initially powered to require 120 patients, accrual to this type of trial was difficult and a total of only 40 patients were eventually randomized. Despite the small sample size, the investigators observed a significant improvement in the HR for death (HR = 0.48) with the administration of irinotecan ($p = 0.012$).[359] In a more recent and larger Korean study, 201 patients were randomized to second-line chemotherapy (either irinotecan or docetaxel) after progression on CF therapy. These investigators confirm an improvement in median OS with chemotherapy from 3.8 months with best supportive care alone to 5.1 months with the addition of chemotherapy.[379] Together, these studies definitely establish that patients with metastatic gastric cancer who have maintained their performance status should be considered for second-line palliative chemotherapy as a standard of practice.

A random assignment study was conducted in patients with advanced gastric cancer comparing paclitaxel and irinotecan in the refractory setting.[380] In this study, 223 patients were randomly assigned to either cytotoxic drug, with no difference in OS observed (median OS 9.5 months with paclitaxel and 8.4 months with irinotecan; HR = 1.13; $p = 0.38$).

Targeted Therapy

The Epidermal Growth Factor Receptor Superfamily: Monoclonal Antibodies

Trastuzumab. Overexpression or amplification of *HER2* (*EGFR2*) occurs in approximately 20% of patients with gastric cancer; it varies with the subtype. A phase 3 study of trastuzumab plus chemotherapy versus chemotherapy alone was performed in patients with gastric cancer overexpressing *HER2*. The preliminary results of the ToGA trial have been recently reported.[381] Among 3,807 patients, 594 patients had *HER2*-positive gastric cancer. They were randomized to receive either CF or XP given every 3 weeks for six cycles, or the same chemotherapy plus trastuzumab. The median OS was 13.5 months for patients receiving trastuzumab plus chemotherapy versus 11.1 months for those receiving chemotherapy alone (HR = 0.74; $p = 0.0048$). The response rate was 47% for patients receiving trastuzumab plus chemotherapy versus 35% for those receiving chemotherapy alone. There was no significant difference in toxicity between treatment arms. Trastuzumab has been approved in Europe for *HER2*-positive gastric cancer. The ToGA trial used a *HER2* scoring system similar to that used in breast cancer. *HER2* was more likely to be positive in patients with EGJ tumors than in more distal tumors (33% versus 20%); patients with diffuse gastric cancer were much less likely to have an *HER2*-positive (6%) tumor.[382]

Cetuximab and Panitumumab. Cetuximab is an antibody against epidermal growth factor receptors. In a trial combining cetuximab plus weekly infusions of oxaliplatin and 5-FU, and DL-folinic acid, 46 patients with advanced gastric cancer were treated.

Toxicity was tolerable; the response rate was 56%; however, OS was 9.5 months. K-Ras mutations were rare.[383]

The Epidermal Growth Factor Receptor Superfamily: Tyrosine Kinase Inhibitors

Lapatinib. Lapatinib is the first dual inhibitor of HER1 (EGFR1) and HER2 (EGFR2). Two phase 2 trials have evaluated lapatinib monotherapy in patients with advanced gastric cancer. In one study, 3 of 46 patients had partial responses. In the second study, 21 patients with EGJ adenocarcinomas were treated without objective responses.

Gefitnib and Erlotinib. Both are epidermal growth factor receptor tyrosine kinase inhibitors. In a large study, a 9% response rate was seen for EGJ tumors versus no responses among patients with gastric cancer; other studies have failed to demonstrate activity even in EGJ tumors.

The Vascular Endothelial Growth Factor Superfamily: Monoclonal Antibodies

Bevacizumab. Bevacizumab is a humanized monoclonal antibody that binds the vascular endothelial growth factor ligand (VEGF-A). In gastric cancer, Shah et al.[372] reported on combining cisplatin plus irinotecan with bevacizumab (phase 2). Among 47 patients, the median TTP was 9.9 months. A second phase 2 study evaluating bevacizumab with DCF also showed promising activity, with median PFS of 12 months and median OS of 17 months.[384] This trial demonstrated potential efficacy with acceptable toxicity; follow-up phase 2 trials also demonstrated acceptable toxicity.[385] The AVAGAST multinational phase 3 trial comparing bevacizumab plus CP versus CP alone has now completed accrual.[386,387] Results have been reported.[388]

In this phase 3 study, 774 patients were randomly assigned to XP ($n = 387$) or XP/bevacizumab ($n = 387$). The study did not meet the primary end point of improving OS (12.1 months with XP/bevacizuamb versus 10.1 months with XP; $p = 0.1002$), but did demonstrate improvement in PFS (6.7 months versus 5.3 months; $p = 0.0037$) and overall response rates (46.0% versus 37.4%; $p = 0.0315$) with XP/bevacizumab versus XP alone, respectively.[386,387] In this study, there was distinct geographic variation in which patients enrolled from Asia appeared not to have significant benefit from the addition of bevacizumab. These results support the concept of significant worldwide disease heterogeneity.

A biomarker evaluation was prospectively performed from the AVAGAST study, in which plasma samples were available from 92% of the study population and tissue samples were available from 94% of the study population.[389] In this analysis, baseline plasma VEGF-A levels and tumor neuropilin-1 expression were identified as potential predictors of bevacizumab efficacy. Specifically, patients with high baseline plasma VEGF-A appeared to benefit from bevacizumab therapy (HR = 0.72; 95% CI = 0.57 to 0.93), and similarly, patients with low baseline expression of neuropilin-1 also showed a trend toward improved OS with bevacizumab (HR = 0.75; 95% CI = 0.59 to 0.97). These data, if validated, may provide important insights pertaining to the geographic heterogeneity observed with this international phase 3 study, and importantly, may identify a population of patients for whom bevacizumab would have substantial efficacy when combined with chemotherapy.

The Vascular Endothelial Growth Factor Superfamily: Tyrosine Kinase Inhibitors

Sunitinib. Sunitinib is an oral inhibitor of VEGF receptor [VEGFR]-1, -2, -3, and PDGFR-α, -β, and c-kit. Bang et al.[389] reported on a phase 2 trial of sunitinib as second-line treatment for advanced gastric cancer. Response rate, PFS, and OS were 2 of 72 patients, 11.1 weeks, and 47.7 weeks, respectively. Sorafenib is another multityrosine kinase inhibitor (VEGFR-2, -3; platelet-derived growth factor receptor–β; Flt-3; Raf-1; and c-kit). The ECOG5203, a phase 2 trial investigating docetaxel plus cisplatin plus sorafenib in gastric cancer, suggested clinical efficacy (response rate = 39%; PFS = 5.8 months; OS = 15.9 months).[390]

Recently, a random assignment phase 2 study of apatinib, a tyrosine kinase inhibitor that selectively inhibits VEGFR2, appears to be active in advanced gastric cancer.[391] In this study, 144 patients were randomly assigned to placebo or two different doses of apatinib. Patients assigned to apatinib had a statistically significant improved OS (4.83 and 4.27 months in the apatinib arms versus 2.5 months in the placebo; $p = 0.0017$), with nine patients demonstrating a radiographic partial response.

In addition, a second study has demonstrated efficacy of VEGFR2 inhibition as monotherapy in gastric cancer. Ramucirumab (IMC-1121B) is a fully human IgG1 monoclonal antibody targeting VEGFR-2. The Regard study was a placebo-controlled, double blind, phase 3 international trial conducted in the second-line setting in patients with metastatic gastric or EGJ adenocarcinoma. Median OS was 5.2 months for ramucirumab and 3.8 months for placebo (HR = 0.776; 95% CI = 0.603 to 0.998; $p = 0.0473$). The significance of this study is that it provides a proof-of-principal that antiangiogenic therapy does have activity in gastroesophageal malignancies. The Regard study supports the concept that subtypes of gastric cancer exist and may be differentially sensitive to antiangiogenic therapy.[392]

Inhibition of Mammalian Target of Rapamycin (Protein Kinase)

Everolimus. An oral inhibitor of the mammalian target of rapamycin has shown activity against gastric cancer in preclinical phase 1 studies.[393,394] Doi et al.[394] reported on a phase 2 trial testing everolimus in metastatic gastric cancer. In 53 patients, the disease control rate (complete response rate plus partial response plus stable disease) was 56%, and the median PFS and OS were 2.7 and 10.1 months, respectively. Based on these encouraging results, a phase 3 study was performed comparing everolimus to best supportive care.[395] In this study, 656 patients were randomized in a 2:1 fashion to everolimus versus placebo. Median OS was similar in both arms, 5.4 months versus 3.2 months (HR = 0.9; 95% CI = 0.75 to 1.08; $p = 0.12$).

In summary, new agents targeting dysregulated cancer pathways are now undergoing study in gastric cancer. At the present time, trastuzumab remains the only drug of this type that has demonstrated efficacy, in combination with cytotoxic chemotherapy, in gastric cancer.

Predictive Markers and Early Assessment of Response in Gastric and Gastroesophageal Tumors

The recognition that several different classes of cytotoxic anticancer agents and targeted pathway agents have activity in subgroups of patients suggests the possibility that predictive markers or a gene signature might allow "customized" precision cancer care that will spare patients from unnecessary toxicity from ineffective therapy, such as testing for *HER2* identifies patients who could benefit from trastuzumab. Molecular markers that might indicate resistance or sensitivity to CF are reviewed elsewhere in this book.[396] Ooi et al.[396] and other investigators[397–399] have used gene expression arrays to identify pathways and gene signatures to predicting clinical prognosis. Ott et al.[77] reported that a drop in SUV of 35% after neoadjuvant chemotherapy was associated with significant pathologic response to systemic treatment. Similar findings were reported by Shah et al.[400] and Weber.[401] Overall, PET may allow early identification of patients responding to systemic therapy.

SURGERY IN TREATMENT OF METASTATIC GASTRIC CANCER

Given the recent improvements in systemic therapy for gastric cancer, the question whether resection of limited metastases from gastric cancer can provide survival benefit remains unanswered. To ask this question in a scientific manner, the surgery branch of the National Institutes of Health/National Cancer Institute is currently accruing patients to a prospective RCT comparing gastrectomy, metastasectomy plus systemic therapy, versus systemic therapy alone (the GYMSSA Trial, clinicaltrials.gov no. NCT00941655).[402]

The GYMSSA trial randomized patients with metastatic gastric cancer to gastrectomy, cytoreductive surgery (CRS)/HIPEC plus Folfoxiri (GYMS arm) versus Folfoxiri alone (SA arm) to study OS. All patients underwent comprehensive staging including laparoscopy. To date, the study accrued 16 evaluable patients. Seven of nine patients in the multimodality GYMS arm achieved complete cytoreduction, with median follow-up of 23 months. Median OS was 12 months in the GYMS arm and 10.2 months in the SA arm; 1- and 2-year OS was 44% and 22% versus 0% and 0%, respectively. Two patients in the GYMS arm lived beyond 23 months, and one up to 12 months. No patient in the SA arm lived longer than 12 months.

Kerkar et al.[401,402] reviewed the published data reporting on liver resection for gastric cancer; 19 studies reported on 436 patients. The majority of the patients had synchronous isolated liver gastric metastases. Overall, the 1-, 3-, and 5-year survival rates were 62%, 30%, and 27%, respectively; 13% (48/358) were alive at 5 years, and in studies with >10 years of follow-up, 4% (48/358) survived for >10 years.[402]

Standard of care for patients with pulmonary gastric metastases is chemotherapy with a median survival of 6 months.[403] Kemp et al.[403] reviewed the published data reporting on lung resections for gastric cancer; 21 studies reported on 43 patients. Eighty-two percent of patients (34/43) had a solitary lesion. At a median follow-up of 23 months, 15 of 43 (35%) patients had no evidence of disease. The overall 5-year survival was 33%.

Gastric carcinomatosis occurs in 5% to 50% of patients undergoing surgery with curative intent.[404–410] The median survival for such patients is 1.5 months to 3.1 months.[404,411–413] Overall data are limited; however, several investigators reported on CRS plus HIPEC for gastric carcinomatosis; the median OS ranged from 6 to 21 months, and 5-year survival ranged from 6% to 16% with operative mortality of 2% to 7% mortality. In patients with optimal cytoreduction-CCR-0/1 (no macroscopic or disease <5 mm), the 5-year survival was 16% to 30%. Complete cytoreduction was possible in only 44% to 51% of the patients.[309,414–418] In 2008, the Fifth International Workshop on Peritoneal Surface Malignancy indicated that peritonectomy, intraoperative, and early postoperative HIPEC potentially can be a powerful therapy against gastric cancer peritoneal carcinomatosis.[419–424]

Bidirectional chemotherapy utilizing intraperitoneal and systemic induction chemotherapy prior to CRS and HIPEC has been studied (retrospectively) in patients with peritoneal carcinomatosis of gastric origin undergoing treatment in a specialized peritoneal surface malignancy unit in Japan. A recent study of 194 patients with gastric carcinomatosis treated initially and responsive (response rate 78%) to intraperitoneal docetaxel (20 mg/m^2) and cisplatin (30 mg/m^2) followed by four cycles of oral S-1 (60 mg/m^2), followed by CRS/HIPEC reported median OS of 16 months and 1-, 2-, and 5-year survival of 66%, 32%, and 11%, respectively.[425] Operative morbidity and moratlity were 24% and 4%, respectively. Response to bidirectional intraperitoneal and systemic chemotherapy, low tumor burden (peritoneal cancer index ≤6) and completeness of cytoreduction (CCR0/1) were independently associated with improved OS on multivariate analysis.

Surgery for Palliation

Because survival for patients with advanced gastric cancer is poor, any proposed operation could have a good chance of providing sustained symptomatic relief while minimizing the attendant morbidity and need for prolonged hospitalization. Ekbom and Gleysteen[426] have reviewed the results of palliative resection versus intestinal bypass (gastrojejunostomy) in 75 patients with advanced gastric cancer. The most frequent symptoms for which patients underwent operation included pain, hemorrhage, nausea, dysphasia, or obstruction. Operative mortality was 25% for gastrojejunostomy, 20% for palliative partial or subtotal gastrectomy, and 27% for total or proximal palliative gastrectomy. The most common and often fatal complication was anastomotic leak. After gastrojejunostomy, 80% of patients had relief of symptoms for a mean of 5.9 months compared with palliative resection, which provided relief of symptoms in 88% of patients for a mean of 14.6 months. Although the duration of palliation was significantly longer after resection ($p < 0.01$), the selection criteria for resection versus bypass were not controlled, and some bias against performing a palliative resection in high-risk patients with more advanced disease may have occurred. Meijer et al.[427] also reported on a retrospective analysis of 51 patients undergoing either palliative intestinal bypass or resection. In 20 of 26 patients (77%) undergoing resection, palliation was considered moderate to good with a mean survival of 9.5 months. After gastroenterostomy, some palliation was noted in 8 of 25 patients (30%), and survival was 4.2 months. Butler et al.[428] have presented the results of total gastrectomy for palliation in 27 patients with advanced gastric cancer. Operative mortality was only 4%, whereas morbidity occurred in 48% of patients. Median survival was 15 months, with a survival rate of 38% at 2 years. This substantial survival rate at 2 years reflects that, although all patients were symptomatic before surgery, only half had stage IV disease. Patients with linitis plastica present a very difficult therapeutic challenge. Resection may provide palliation of symptoms; however, survival after total gastrectomy is exceedingly poor, ranging from 3 months to 1 year.

Bozzetti et al.[429,430] have reviewed the outcomes of 246 patients with advanced gastric cancer who underwent simple exploratory laparotomy alone, gastrointestinal bypass, or palliative resection at the National Cancer Institute of Milan. When survival was compared in patients with similar type and extent of disease, a consistent trend was seen for improved median OS with palliative resection in patients with local spread (4 months versus 8 months) and distant spread of disease (3 months versus 8 months). Boddie et al.[431] have reported similar results in 45 patients undergoing palliative resection at the MD Anderson Cancer Center for advanced gastric cancer. Operative mortality for resection was 22%. In 21 patients who had undergone a palliative bypass procedure, OS was significantly shorter than for those undergoing palliative gastric resection ($p < 0.01$).

In select patients with symptomatic advanced gastric cancer, resection of the primary disease appears to provide symptomatic relief with acceptable morbidity and mortality, even in the presence of macroscopic residual disease.

RADIATION FOR PALLIATION

To date, no studies have evaluated the use of radiation therapy in patients with locally recurrent or metastatic carcinoma of the stomach. Its use is likely to be limited to palliation of symptoms such as bleeding or controlling pain secondary to local tumor infiltration. Although minimal data are available, radiation therapy seems to be anecdotally effective in controlling bleeding, as is true in other primary tumor sites. Pain from local tumor invasion can also be palliated with radiation. On rare occasions, a case may arise of a patient with a focal local recurrence without metastases who would be amenable to relatively high-dose radiation therapy in order to try to prolong quality-adjusted survival or in whom radiation therapy would be given as an adjuvant to surgical resection. At present, however, no data support such an approach.

REFERENCES

1. Ferlay JB, Parkin F, Pisani DMP, eds. *Cancer Incidence and Mortality Worldwide*. ISRC Cancer Bases No. 5; 2001, 2000.
2. Jemal A, Bray F, Center MM, et al. Global cancer statistics. *CA Cancer J Clin* 2011;61:69–90.
3. Jemal A, Siegel R, Ward E, et al. Cancer statistics, 2009. *CA Cancer J Clin* 2009;59:225–249.
4. Siegel R, Ma J, Zou Z, et al. Cancer statistics, 2014. *CA Cancer J Clin* 2014;64:9–29.
5. Anderson WF, Fraumeni FJ, Rosenberg PS, et al. Age-specific trends in incidence of noncardia gastric cancer in US adults. *JAMA* 2010;303:1723–1728.
6. Keeney S, Bauer TL. Epidemiology of adenocarcinoma of the esophagogastric junction. *Surg Oncol Clin N Am* 2006;15:687–696.
7. Pacelli F, Cusumano G, Marrelli D, et al. Multivisceral resection for locally advanced gastric cancer: an Italian multicenter observational study. *JAMA Surg* 2013;148:353–360.
8. Lewin JKA. Gastrointestinal tract: stomach. In: Juan R, editor. *Surgical Pathology*. Maryland Heights, MO: Mosby; 2004.
9. Zullo A, Hassan C, Andriani A, et al. Eradication therapy for Helicobacter pylori in patients with gastric MALT lymphoma: a pooled data analysis. *Am J Gastroenterol* 2009;104:1932–1937, quiz 1938.
10. Luminari S, Cesaretti M, Marcheselli L, et al. Decreasing incidence of gastric MALT lymphomas in the era of anti-Helicobacter pylori interventions: results from a population-based study on extranodal marginal zone lymphomas. *Ann Oncol* 2010;21:855–859.
11. Houghton J, Stoicov C, Nomura S, et al. Gastric cancer originating from bone marrow-derived cells. *Science* 2004;306:1568–1571.
12. Stoicov C, Saffari R, Cai X, et al. Molecular biology of gastric cancer: Helicobacter infection and gastric adenocarcinoma: bacterial and host factors responsible for altered growth signaling. *Gene* 2004;341:1–17.
13. Stoicov C, Li H, Carlson J, et al. Bone marrow cells as the origin of stomach cancer. *Future Oncol* 2005;1:851–862.
14. Li HC, Stoicov C, Rogers AB, et al. Stem cells and cancer: evidence for bone marrow stem cells in epithelial cancers. *World J Gastroenterol* 2006;12:363–371.
15. Avital I, Moreira AL, Klimstra DS, et al. Donor-derived human bone marrow cells contribute to solid organ cancers developing after bone marrow transplantation. *Stem Cells* 2007;25:2903–2909.
16. Saikawa Y, Fukuda K, Takahashi T, et al. Gastric carcinogenesis and the cancer stem cell hypothesis. *Gastric Cancer* 2010;13:11–24.
17. Takaishi S, Okumura T, Tu S, et al. Identification of gastric cancer stem cells using the cell surface marker CD44. *Stem Cells* 2009;27:1006–1020.
18. The general rules for The gastric cancer study in surgery. *Jpn J Surg* 1973;3:61–71.
19. Ming SC. The classification and significance of gastric polyps. *Monogr Pathol* 1977;(18):149–175.
20. Bearzi I, Ranaldi R. Early gastric cancer: a morphologic study of 41 cases. *Tumori* 1982;68:223–233.
21. Laurén P. The two histological main types of gastric carcinoma: diffuse and so-called intestinal-type carcinoma: an attempt at a histo-clinical classification. *Acta Pathol Microbiol Scand* 1965;64:31–49.
22. Machado JC, Soares P, Carneiro F, et al. E-cadherin gene mutations provide a genetic basis for the phenotypic divergence of mixed gastric carcinomas. *Lab Invest* 1999;79:459–465.
23. Soga K, Ichikawa D, Yasukawa S, et al. Prognostic impact of the width of subserosal invasion in gastric cancer invading the subserosal layer. *Surgery* 2010;147:197–203.
24. Zinninger MM. Extension of gastric cancer in the intramural lymphatics and its relation to gastrectomy. *Am Surg* 1954;20:920–927.
25. Zinninger MM, Collins WT. Extension of Carcinoma of the Stomach into the Duodenum and Esophagus. *Ann Surg* 1949;130:557–566.
26. Kakeji Y, Tsujitani S, Baba H, et al. Clinicopathological features and prognostic significance of duodenal invasion in patients with distal gastric carcinoma. *Cancer* 1991;68:380–384.
27. Nogueira AM, Silva AC, Paiva EB, et al. [Distal gastric carcinoma with duodenal invasion: histopathologic study and review of the literature]. *Arq Gastroenterol* 2000;37:168–173.
28. Barbour AP, Rizk NP, Gonen M, et al. Adenocarcinoma of the gastroesophageal junction: influence of esophageal resection margin and operative approach on outcome. *Ann Surg* 2007;246:1–8.
29. Miyazaki M, Itoh H, Nakagawa K, et al. Hepatic resection of liver metastases from gastric carcinoma. *Am J Gastroenterol* 1997;92:490–493.
30. Kim JP, Lee JH, Kim SJ, et al. Clinicopathologic characteristics and prognostic factors in 10 783 patients with gastric cancer. *Gastric Cancer* 1998;1:125–133.

31. D'Angelica M, Gonen M, Brennan MF, et al. Patterns of initial recurrence in completely resected gastric adenocarcinoma. *Ann Surg* 2004;240:808–816.

32. Namieno T, Koito K, Higashi T, et al. General pattern of lymph node metastasis in early gastric carcinoma. *World J Surg* 1996;20:996–1000.

33. Maruyama K, Gunvén P, Okabayashi K, et al. Lymph node metastases of gastric cancer. General pattern in 1931 patients. *Ann Surg* 1989;210:596–602.

34. Yoo CH, Noh SH, Shin DW, et al. Recurrence following curative resection for gastric carcinoma. *Br J Surg* 2000;87:236–242.

35. Zacherl J, Zacherl M, Scheuba C, et al. Analysis of hepatic resection of metastasis originating from gastric adenocarcinoma. *J Gastrointest Surg* 2002;6:682–689.

36. Sakamoto Y, Ohyama S, Yamamoto J, et al. Surgical resection of liver metastases of gastric cancer: an analysis of a 17-year experience with 22 patients. *Surgery* 2003;133:507–511.

37. Classic articles in colonic and rectal surgery. George Blumer, M.D.: The rectal shelf. *Dis Colon Rectum* 1980;23(6):445.

38. Kong SH, Park DJ, Lee HJ, et al. Clinicopathologic features of asymptomatic gastric adenocarcinoma patients in Korea. *Jpn J Clin Oncol* 2004;34:1–7.

39. Wanebo HJ, Kennedy BJ, Chmiel J, et al. Cancer of the stomach. A patient care study by the American College of Surgeons. *Ann Surg* 1993;218:583–592.

40. Maconi G, Manes G, Porro GB. Role of symptoms in diagnosis and outcome of gastric cancer. *World J Gastroenterol* 2008;14:1149–1155.

41. Axon A. Symptoms and diagnosis of gastric cancer at early curable stage. *Best Pract Res Clin Gastroenterol* 2006;20:697–708.

42. Dewys WD, Begg C, Lavin PT, et al. Prognostic effect of weight loss prior to chemotherapy in cancer patients. Eastern Cooperative Oncology Group. *Am J Med* 1980;69:491–497.

43. Kahrilas PJ, Kishk SM, Helm JF, et al. Comparison of pseudoachalasia and achalasia. *Am J Med* 1987;82:439–446.

44. Gilliland R, Gill PJ. Incidence and prognosis of Krukenberg tumour in Northern Ireland. *Br J Surg* 1992;79:1364–1366.

45. Morgenstern L. The Virchow-Troisier node: a historical note. *Am J Surg* 1979;138:703.

46. Graham DY, Asaka M. Eradication of gastric cancer and more efficient gastric cancer surveillance in Japan: two peas in a pod. *J Gastroenterol* 2010;45:1–8.

47. Rugge M, Kim JG, Mahachai V, et al. OLGA gastritis staging in young adults and country-specific gastric cancer risk. *Int J Surg Pathol* 2008;16:150–154.

48. Ohata H, Kitauchi S, Yoshimura N, et al. Progression of chronic atrophic gastritis associated with Helicobacter pylori infection increases risk of gastric cancer. *Int J Cancer* 2004;109:138–143.

49. Watabe H, Mitsushima T, Yamaji Y, et al. Predicting the development of gastric cancer from combining Helicobacter pylori antibodies and serum pepsinogen status: a prospective endoscopic cohort study. *Gut* 2005;54:764–768.

50. Yoshihara M, Sumii K, Haruma K, et al. Correlation of ratio of serum pepsinogen I and II with prevalence of gastric cancer and adenoma in Japanese subjects. *Am J Gastroenterol* 1998;93:1090–1096.

51. Talley NJ, Fock KM, Moayyedi P. Gastric Cancer Consensus conference recommends Helicobacter pylori screening and treatment in asymptomatic persons from high-risk populations to prevent gastric cancer. *Am J Gastroenterol* 2008;103:510–514.

52. Leung WK, Wu MS, Kakugawa Y, et al. Screening for gastric cancer in Asia: current evidence and practice. *Lancet Oncol* 2008;9:279–287.

53. Parsonnet J, Harris RA, Hack HM, et al. Modelling cost-effectiveness of Helicobacter pylori screening to prevent gastric cancer: a mandate for clinical trials. *Lancet* 1996;348:150–154.

54. Roderick P, Davies R, Raftery J, et al. Cost-effectiveness of population screening for Helicobacter pylori in preventing gastric cancer and peptic ulcer disease, using simulation. *J Med Screen* 2003;10:148–156.

55. Mason J, Axon AT, Forman D, et al. The cost-effectiveness of population Helicobacter pylori screening and treatment: a Markov model using economic data from a randomized controlled trial. *Aliment Pharmacol Ther* 2002;16:559–568.

56. Marrelli D, Roviello F, De Stefano A, et al. Prognostic significance of CEA, CA 19–9 and CA 72–4 preoperative serum levels in gastric carcinoma. *Oncology* 1999;57:55–62.

57. Nakane Y, Okamura S, Akehira K, et al. Correlation of preoperative carcinoembryonic antigen levels and prognosis of gastric cancer patients. *Cancer* 1994;73:2703–2708.

58. Ychou M, Duffour J, Kramar A, et al. Clinical significance and prognostic value of CA72-4 compared with CEA and CA19-9 in patients with gastric cancer. *Dis Markers* 2000;16:105–110.

59. Pectasides D, Mylonakis A, Kostopoulou M, et al. CEA, CA 19-9, and CA-50 in monitoring gastric carcinoma. *Am J Clin Oncol* 1997;20:348–353.

60. Kodera Y, Yamamura Y, Torii A, et al. The prognostic value of preoperative serum levels of CEA and CA19-9 in patients with gastric cancer. *Am J Gastroenterol* 1996;91:49–53.

61. Kochi M, Fujii M, Kanamori N, et al. Evaluation of serum CEA and CA19–9 levels as prognostic factors in patients with gastric cancer. *Gastric Cancer* 2000;3:177–186.

62. Park SH, Ku KB, Chung HY, et al. Prognostic significance of serum and tissue carcinoembryonic antigen in patients with gastric adenocarcinomas. *Cancer Res Treat* 2008;40:16–21.

63. Liu H, Li YQ, Yu T, et al. Confocal endomicroscopy for in vivo detection of microvascular architecture in normal and malignant lesions of upper gastrointestinal tract. *J Gastroenterol Hepatol* 2008;23:56–61.

64. Hyatt BJ, Paull PE, Wassef W. Gastric oncology: an update. *Curr Opin Gastroenterol* 2009;25:570–578.

65. Kwee RM, Kwee TC. Imaging in local staging of gastric cancer: a systematic review. *J Clin Oncol* 2007;25:2107–2116.

66. Bentrem D, Gerdes H, Tang L, et al. Clinical correlation of endoscopic ultrasonography with pathologic stage and outcome in patients undergoing curative resection for gastric cancer. *Ann Surg Oncol* 2007;14:1853–1859.

67. Hwang SW, Lee DH, Lee SH, et al. Preoperative staging of gastric cancer by endoscopic ultrasonography and multidetector-row computed tomography. *J Gastroenterol Hepatol* 2010;25:512–518.

68. Yan C, Zhu ZG, Yan M, et al. Value of multidetector-row computed tomography in the preoperative T and N staging of gastric carcinoma: a large-scale Chinese study. *J Surg Oncol* 2009;100:205–214.

69. Chen CY, Hsu JS, Wu DC, et al. Gastric cancer: preoperative local staging with 3D multi-detector row CT–correlation with surgical and histopathologic results. *Radiology* 2007;242:472–482.

70. Anzidei M, Napoli A, Zaccagna F, et al. Diagnostic performance of 64-MDCT and 1.5-T MRI with high-resolution sequences in the T staging of gastric cancer: a comparative analysis with histopathology. *Radiol Med* 2009;114:1065–1079.

71. Sohn KM, Lee JM, Lee SY, et al. Comparing MR imaging and CT in the staging of gastric carcinoma. *AJR Am J Roentgenol* 2000;174:1551–1557.

72. Kawamura T, Kusakabe T, Sugino T, et al. Expression of glucose transporter-1 in human gastric carcinoma: association with tumor aggressiveness, metastasis, and patient survival. *Cancer* 2001;92:634–641.

73. Dassen AE, Lips DJ, Hoekstra CJ, et al. FDG-PET has no definite role in preoperative imaging in gastric cancer. *Eur J Surg Oncol* 2009;35:449–455.

74. Chen J, Cheong JH, Yun MJ, et al. Improvement in preoperative staging of gastric adenocarcinoma with positron emission tomography. *Cancer* 2005;103:2383–2390.

75. Yang QM, Kawamura T, Itoh H, et al. Is PET-CT suitable for predicting lymph node status for gastric cancer? *Hepatogastroenterology* 2008;55:782–785.

76. Yun M, Lim JS, Noh SH, et al. Lymph node staging of gastric cancer using (18) F-FDG PET: a comparison study with CT. *J Nucl Med* 2005;46:1582–1588.

77. Ott K, Fink U, Becker K, et al. Prediction of response to preoperative chemotherapy in gastric carcinoma by metabolic imaging: results of a prospective trial. *J Clin Oncol* 2003;21:4604–4610.

78. Lordick F, Ott K, Krause BJ, et al. PET to assess early metabolic response and to guide treatment of adenocarcinoma of the oesophagogastric junction: the MUNICON phase II trial. *Lancet Oncol* 2007;8:797–805.

79. Kwee RM, Kwee TC. Imaging in assessing lymph node status in gastric cancer. *Gastric Cancer* 2009;12:6–22.

80. Kim EY, Lee WJ, Choi D, et al. The value of PET/CT for preoperative staging of advanced gastric cancer: comparison with contrast-enhanced CT. *Eur J Radiol* 2011;79:183–188.

81. Smyth E, Schöder H, Strong VE, et al. A prospective evaluation of the utility of 2-deoxy-2-[(18) F]fluoro-D-glucose positron emission tomography and computed tomography in staging locally advanced gastric cancer. *Cancer* 2012;118:5481–5488.

82. Goldfarb M, Brower S, Schwaitzberg SD. Minimally invasive surgery and cancer: controversies part 1. *Surg Endosc* 2010;24:304–334.

83. Conlon KC. Staging laparoscopy for gastric cancer. *Ann Ital Chir* 2001;72:33–37.

84. Burke EC, Karpeh MS, Conlon KC, et al. Laparoscopy in the management of gastric adenocarcinoma. *Ann Surg* 1997;225:262–267.

85. Sarela AI, Lefkowitz R, Brennan MF, et al. Selection of patients with gastric adenocarcinoma for laparoscopic staging. *Am J Surg* 2006;191:134–138.

86. Tirindelli Danesi D, Cucchiara G, Picconi A, et al. Retrospective analysis of the prognostic significance of DNA ploidy patterns in gastric cancer. *Eur J Histochem* 1997;41:147–148.

87. Muntean V, Mihailov A, Iancu C, et al. Staging laparoscopy in gastric cancer. Accuracy and impact on therapy. *J Gastrointestin Liver Dis* 2009;18:189–195.

88. Lehnert T, Rudek B, Kienle P, et al. Impact of diagnostic laparoscopy on the management of gastric cancer: prospective study of 120 consecutive patients with primary gastric adenocarcinoma. *Br J Surg* 2002;89:471–475.

89. Blackshaw GR, Barry JD, Edwards P, et al. Laparoscopy significantly improves the perceived preoperative stage of gastric cancer. *Gastric Cancer* 2003;6:225–229.

90. Bentrem D, Wilton A, Mazumdar M, et al. The value of peritoneal cytology as a preoperative predictor in patients with gastric carcinoma undergoing a curative resection. *Ann Surg Oncol* 2005;12:347–353.

91. Dalal KM, Woo Y, Kelly K, et al. Detection of micrometastases in peritoneal washings of gastric cancer patients by the reverse transcriptase polymerase chain reaction. *Gastric Cancer* 2008;11:206–213.

92. Wilkiemeyer MB, Bielig SC, Ashfaq R, et al. Laparoscopy alone is superior to peritoneal cytology in staging gastric and esophageal carcinoma. *Surg Endosc* 2004;18:852–856.

93. Nakagawa S, Nashimoto A, Yabusaki H. Role of staging laparoscopy with peritoneal lavage cytology in the treatment of locally advanced gastric cancer. *Gastric Cancer* 2007;10:29–34.

94. Wong J, Schulman A, Kelly K, et al. Detection of free peritoneal cancer cells in gastric cancer using cancer-specific Newcastle disease virus. *J Gastrointest Surg* 2010;14:7–14.

95. Smith A, Finch MD, John TG, et al. Role of laparoscopic ultrasonography in the management of patients with oesophagogastric cancer. *Br J Surg* 1999;86:1083–1087.

96. Lavonius MI, Gullichsen R, Salo S, et al. Staging of gastric cancer: a study with spiral computed tomography, ultrasonography, laparoscopy, and laparoscopic ultrasonography. *Surg Laparosc Endosc Percutan Tech* 2002;12:77–81.

97. Hulscher JB, Nieveen van Dijkum EJ, de Wit LT, et al. Laparoscopy and laparoscopic ultrasonography in staging carcinoma of the gastric cardia. *Eur J Surg* 2000;166:862–865.

98. Edge SB, Compton CC. The American Joint Committee on Cancer: the 7th edition of the AJCC Cancer Staging Manual and the future of TNM. *Ann Surg Oncol* 2010;17:1471–1474.

99. Karpeh MS, Leon L, Klimstra D, et al. Lymph node staging in gastric cancer: is location more important than number? An analysis of 1,038 patients. *Ann Surg* 2000;232:362–371.

100. Smith DD, Schwarz RR, Schwarz RE. Impact of total lymph node count on staging and survival after gastrectomy for gastric cancer: data from a large US-population database. *J Clin Oncol* 2005;23:7114–7124.

101. Ichikura T, Tomimatsu S, Uefuji K, et al. Evaluation of the New American Joint Committee on Cancer/International Union against cancer classification of lymph node metastasis from gastric carcinoma in comparison with the Japanese classification. *Cancer* 1999;86:553–558.

102. Schwarz RE, Smith DD. Clinical impact of lymphadenectomy extent in resectable gastric cancer of advanced stage. *Ann Surg Oncol* 2007;14:317–328.

103. Kattan MW, Karpeh MS, Mazumdar M, et al. Postoperative nomogram for disease-specific survival after an R0 resection for gastric carcinoma. *J Clin Oncol* 2003;21:3647–3650.

104. Ichikura T, Ogawa T, Chochi K, et al. Minimum number of lymph nodes that should be examined for the International Union Against Cancer/American Joint Committee on Cancer TNM classification of gastric carcinoma. *World J Surg* 2003;27:330–333.

105. Aurello P, D'Angelo F, Rossi S, et al. Classification of lymph node metastases from gastric cancer: comparison between N-site and N-number systems. Our experience and review of the literature. *Am Surg* 2007;73:359–366.

106. Hundahl SA, Phillips JL, Menck HR. The National Cancer Data Base Report on poor survival of U.S. gastric carcinoma patients treated with gastrectomy: Fifth Edition American Joint Committee on Cancer staging, proximal disease, and the "different disease" hypothesis. *Cancer* 2000;88:921–932.

107. Bando E, Yonemura Y, Taniguchi K, et al. Outcome of ratio of lymph node metastasis in gastric carcinoma. *Ann Surg Oncol* 2002;9:775–784.

108. Sun Z, Zhu GL, Lu C, et al. The impact of N-ratio in minimizing stage migration phenomenon in gastric cancer patients with insufficient number or level of lymph node retrieved: results from a Chinese mono-institutional study in 2159 patients. *Ann Oncol* 2009;20:897–905.

109. Huang CM, Lin JX, Zheng CH, et al. Prognostic impact of metastatic lymph node ratio on gastric cancer after curative distal gastrectomy. *World J Gastroenterol* 2010;16:2055–2060.

110. Inoue K, Nakane Y, Iiyama H, et al. The superiority of ratio-based lymph node staging in gastric carcinoma. *Ann Surg Oncol* 2002;9:27–34.

111. Xu DZ, Geng QR, Long ZJ, et al. Positive lymph node ratio is an independent prognostic factor in gastric cancer after d2 resection regardless of the examined number of lymph nodes. *Ann Surg Oncol* 2009;16:319–326.

112. Sun Z, Xu Y, Li de M, et al. Log odds of positive lymph nodes: a novel prognostic indicator superior to the number-based and the ratio-based N category for gastric cancer patients with R0 resection. *Cancer* 2010;116:2571–2580.

113. Japanese Gastric Cancer Association. Japanese Classification of Gastric Carcinoma - 2nd English Edition. *Gastric Cancer* 1998;1:10–24.

114. Kurihara M, Aiko T. The new Japanese classification of gastric carcinoma: revised explanation of "response assessment of chemotherapy and radiotherapy for gastric carcinoma." *Gastric Cancer* 2001;4:9–13.

115. Japanese Gastric Cancer Association. Japanese classification of gastric carcinoma–2nd English edition–response assessment of chemotherapy and radiotherapy for gastric carcinoma: clinical criteria. *Gastric Cancer* 2001;4:1–8.

116. Aikou T, Hokita S, Natsugoe S. [Japanese Classification of Gastric Carcinoma (the 13th edition, June 1999): points to be revised]. *Nippon Rinsho* 2001;59:159–165.

117. Sayegh ME, Sano T, Dexter S, et al. TNM and Japanese staging systems for gastric cancer: how do they coexist? *Gastric Cancer* 2004;7:140–148.

118. Aiko T, Sasako M. The new Japanese Classification of Gastric Carcinoma: Points to be revised. *Gastric Cancer* 1998;1:25–30.

119. Zhang M, Zhu G, Ma Y, et al. Comparison of four staging systems of lymph node metastasis in gastric cancer. *World J Surg* 2009;33:2383–2388.

120. Siewert JR, Stein HJ. Classification of adenocarcinoma of the oesophagogastric junction. *Br J Surg* 1998;85:1457–1459.

121. Siewert JR, Feith M, Werner M, et al. Adenocarcinoma of the esophagogastric junction: results of surgical therapy based on anatomical/topographic classification in 1002 consecutive patients. *Ann Surg* 2000;232:353–361.

122. Feith M, Stein HJ, Siewert JR. Adenocarcinoma of the esophagogastric junction: surgical therapy based on 1602 consecutive resected patients. *Surg Oncol Clin N Am* 2006;15:751–764.

123. Hermanek P, Wittekind C. Residual tumor (R) classification and prognosis. *Semin Surg Oncol* 1994;10:12–20.

124. Peeters KC, Kattan MW, Hartgrink HH, et al. Validation of a nomogram for predicting disease-specific survival after an R0 resection for gastric carcinoma. *Cancer* 2005;103:702–707.

125. Novotny AR, Schuhmacher C, Busch R, et al. Predicting individual survival after gastric cancer resection: validation of a U.S.-derived nomogram at a single high-volume center in Europe. *Ann Surg* 2006;243:74–81.

126. Strong VE, Song KY, Park CH, et al. Comparison of gastric cancer survival following R0 resection in the United States and Korea using an internationally validated nomogram. *Ann Surg* 2010;251:640–646.

127. Han MA, Oh MG, Choi IJ, et al. Association of family history with cancer recurrence and survival in patients with gastric cancer. *J Clin Oncol* 2012;31:701–708.

128. Nishi M, Omori Y, Miwa K, eds. *Japanese Research Society for Gastric Cancer. Japanese Classification Of Gastric Carcinoma*. Kanehara, Tokyo: 1995:73.

129. Schlemper RJ, Itabashi M, Kato Y, et al. Differences in diagnostic criteria for gastric carcinoma between Japanese and western pathologists. *Lancet* 1997;349:1725–1729.

130. Gotoda T, Yanagisawa A, Sasako M, et al. Incidence of lymph node metastasis from early gastric cancer: estimation with a large number of cases at two large centers. *Gastric Cancer* 2000;3:219–225.

131. Kwee RM, Kwee TC. Predicting lymph node status in early gastric cancer. *Gastric Cancer* 2008;11:134–148.

132. Haruta H, Hosoya Y, Sakuma K, et al. Clinicopathological study of lymph-node metastasis in 1389 patients with early gastric cancer: assessment of indications for endoscopic resection. *J Dig Dis* 2008;9:213–218.

133. Jeong O, Ryu SY, Park YK. Accuracy of surgical diagnosis in detecting early gastric cancer and lymph node metastasis and its role in determining limited surgery. *J Am Coll Surg* 2009;209:302–307.

134. Li H, Lu P, Lu Y, et al. Predictive factors of lymph node metastasis in undifferentiated early gastric cancers and application of endoscopic mucosal resection. *Surg Oncol* 2010;19:221–226.

135. Park JM, Kim SW, Nam KW, et al. Is it reasonable to treat early gastric cancer with signet ring cell histology by endoscopic resection? Analysis of factors related to lymph-node metastasis. *Eur J Gastroenterol Hepatol* 2009;21:1132–1135.

136. Hirasawa T, Gotoda T, Miyata S, et al. Incidence of lymph node metastasis and the feasibility of endoscopic resection for undifferentiated-type early gastric cancer. *Gastric Cancer* 2009;12:148–152.

137. Holscher AH, Drebber U, Mønig SP, et al. Early gastric cancer: lymph node metastasis starts with deep mucosal infiltration. *Ann Surg* 2009;250:791–797.

138. Matsumoto M, Natsugoe S, Ishigami S, et al. Lymph node micrometastasis and lymphatic mapping determined by reverse transcriptase-polymerase chain reaction in pN0 gastric carcinoma. *Surgery* 2002;131:630–635.

139. Bennett C, Wang Y, Pan T. Endoscopic mucosal resection for early gastric cancer. *Cochrane Database Syst Rev* 2009;(4):CD004276.

140. Jee YS, Hwang SH, Rao J, et al. Safety of extended endoscopic mucosal resection and endoscopic submucosal dissection following the Japanese Gastric Cancer Association treatment guidelines. *Br J Surg* 2009;96:1157–1161.

141. Kojima T, Parra-Blanco A, Takahashi H, et al. Outcome of endoscopic mucosal resection for early gastric cancer: review of the Japanese literature. *Gastrointest Endosc* 1998;48:550–554, discussion 554–555.

142. Giovannini M, Bernardini D, Moutardier V, et al. Endoscopic mucosal resection (EMR): results and prognostic factors in 21 patients. *Endoscopy* 1999;31:698–701.

143. Oda I, Saito D, Tada M, et al. A multicenter retrospective study of endoscopic resection for early gastric cancer. *Gastric Cancer* 2006;9:262–270.

144. Yokoi C, Gotoda T, Hamanaka H, et al. Endoscopic submucosal dissection allows curative resection of locally recurrent early gastric cancer after prior endoscopic mucosal resection. *Gastrointest Endosc* 2006;64:212–218.

145. Ida K, Nakazawa S, Yoshino J, et al. Multicenter collaborative prospective study of endoscopic treatment of early gastric cancer. *Dig Endos* 2004;16:295–302.

146. Nelson DB, Block KP, Bosco JJ, et al. Technology status evaluation report: computerized endoscopic medical record systems: November 1999. *Gastrointest Endosc* 2000;51:793–796.

147. Noda M, Kodama T, Atsumi M, et al. Possibilities and limitations of endoscopic resection for early gastric cancer. *Endoscopy* 1997;29:361–365.

148. Tanabe S, Koizumi W, Kokutou M, et al. Usefulness of endoscopic aspiration mucosectomy as compared with strip biopsy for the treatment of gastric mucosal cancer. *Gastrointest Endosc* 1999;50:819–822.

149. Oizumi H. Endoscopic resection for early gastric cancer. *Stomach & Intestine* 1991;26:289.

150. Watanabe Y, Kato N, Maehata T, et al. Safer endoscopic gastric mucosal resection: preoperative proton pump inhibitor administration. *J Gastroenterol Hepatol* 2006;21:1675–1680.

151. Fukase K, Matsuda T, Suzuki M, et al. Evaluation of the efficacy of endoscopic treatment for gastric cancer considered in terms of long-term prognosis. A comparison with surgical treatment. *Digestive Endoscopy* 1994;6:241–247.

152. Fukase K, Kawata S. Evaluation of the efficacy of endoscopic treatment for early gastric cancer considered in terms of long-term prognosis more than 10 years — a comparison with surgical treatment. *Yamagata Med J* 2004;22:1.

153. Park IS, Lee YC, Kim WH, et al. Clinicopathologic characteristics of early gastric cancer in Korea. *Yonsei Med J* 2000;41:607–614.

154. Kim HS, Lee DK, Baik SK, et al. Endoscopic mucosal resection with a ligation device for early gastric cancer and precancerous lesions: comparison of its therapeutic efficacy with surgical resection. *Yonsei Med J* 2000;41:577–583.

155. Takekoshi T, Baba Y, Ota H, et al. Endoscopic resection of early gastric carcinoma: results of a retrospective analysis of 308 cases. *Endoscopy* 1994;26:352–358.

156. Chonan A, Mochizuki F, Ando M, et al. Endoscopic ultrasonography for the diagnosis of gastric malignant lymphoma. *Endoscopy* 1998;30:A76–A77.

157. Hiki Y, Sakakibara J, Mieno H, et al. Endoscopic treatment of gastric cancer. *Surg Endosc* 1991;5:11–13.

158. Kondo H, Gotoda T, Ono H, et al. Early gastric cancer: endoscopic mucosal resection. *Ann Ital Chir* 2001;72:27–31.

CANCERS OF THE GASTROINTESTINAL TRACT

159. Ono H, Kondo H, Gotoda T, et al. Endoscopic mucosal resection for treatment of early gastric cancer. *Gut* 2001;48:225–229.

160. Tada M, Tokiyama H, Nakamura H, et al. Endoscopic resection for early gastric cancer. *Acta Endoscopica* 1998;28:87–95.

161. Tada M, Matsumoto Y, Murakami A, et al. Problems and their solutions in curative endoscopic resection of early gastric carcinomas. *Endosc Digest* 1993;5:1169–1174.

162. Park JC, Lee SK, Seo JH, et al. Predictive factors for local recurrence after endoscopic resection for early gastric cancer: long-term clinical outcome in a single-center experience. *Surg Endosc* 2010;24:2842–2849.

163. Nakamoto S, Sakai Y, Kasanuki J, et al. Indications for the use of endoscopic mucosal resection for early gastric cancer in Japan: a comparative study with endoscopic submucosal dissection. *Endoscopy* 2009;41:746–750.

164. Tomita R, Fujisak S, Park YJ. Mini-laparotomy with abdominal wall lifting for partial gastrectomy in patients with early gastric mucosal cancer at lesser curvature of the middle stomach. *Hepatogastroenterology* 2009;56:1768–1772.

165. Yamaguchi N, Isomoto H, Fukuda E, et al. Clinical outcomes of endoscopic submucosal dissection for early gastric cancer by indication criteria. *Digestion* 2009;80:173–181.

166. Gouzi JL, Huguier M, Fagniez PL, et al. Total versus subtotal gastrectomy for adenocarcinoma of the gastric antrum. A French prospective controlled study. *Ann Surg* 1989;209:162–166.

167. Robertson CS, Chung SC, Woods SD, et al. A prospective randomized trial comparing R1 subtotal gastrectomy with R3 total gastrectomy for antral cancer. *Ann Surg* 1994;220:176–182.

168. Bozzetti F, Marubini E, Bonfanti G, et al. Subtotal versus total gastrectomy for gastric cancer: five-year survival rates in a multicenter randomized Italian trial. Italian Gastrointestinal Tumor Study Group. *Ann Surg* 1999;230:170–178.

169. Hulscher JB, van Sandick JW, de Boer AG, et al. Extended transthoracic resection compared with limited transhiatal resection for adenocarcinoma of the esophagus. *N Engl J Med* 2002;347:1662–1669.

170. Kitajima M, Kitagawa Y. Surgical treatment of esophageal cancer–the advent of the era of individualization. *N Engl J Med* 2002;347:1705–1709.

171. Hundahl SA. Staging, stage migration, and patterns of spread in gastric cancer. *Semin Radiat Oncol* 2002;12:141–149.

172. Kodera Y, Schwarz RE, Nakao A. Extended lymph node dissection in gastric carcinoma: where do we stand after the Dutch and British randomized trials? *J Am Coll Surg* 2002;195:855–864.

173. Siewert JR, Böttcher K, Stein HJ, et al. Relevant prognostic factors in gastric cancer: ten-year results of the German Gastric Cancer Study. *Ann Surg* 1998; 228:449–461.

174. Cheong O, Kim BS, Yook JH, et al. Modified radical lymphadenectomy without splenectomy in patients with proximal gastric cancer: comparison with standard D2 lymphadenectomy for distal gastric cancer. *J Surg Oncol* 2008;98:500–504.

175. Deng JY, Liang H, Sun D, et al. The most appropriate category of metastatic lymph nodes to evaluate overall survival of gastric cancer following curative resection. *J Surg Oncol* 2008;98:343–348.

176. Woodall CE III, Scoggins CR, McMasters KM, et al. Adequate lymphadenectomy results in accurate nodal staging without an increase in morbidity in patients with gastric adenocarcinoma. *Am J Surg* 2008;196:413–417.

177. Schoenleber SJ, Schnelldorfer T, Wood CM, et al. Factors influencing lymph node recovery from the operative specimen after gastrectomy for gastric adenocarcinoma. *J Gastrointest Surg* 2009;13:1233–1237.

178. Songun I, van de Velde CJ. Optimal surgery for advanced gastric cancer. *Expert Rev Anticancer Ther* 2009;9:1849–1858.

179. Songun I, van de Velde CJ. How does extended lymphadenectomy influence practical care for patients with gastric cancer? *Nat Clin Pract Oncol* 2009;6: 66–67.

180. Ielpo B, Pernaute AS, Elia S, et al. Impact of number and site of lymph node invasion on survival of adenocarcinoma of esophagogastric junction. *Interact Cardiovasc Thorac Surg* 2010;10:704–708.

181. Lim do H, Kim HS, Park YS, et al. Metastatic lymph node in gastric cancer; is it a real distant metastasis? *BMC Cancer* 2010;10:25.

182. Moon YW, Jeung HC, Rha SY, et al. Changing patterns of prognosticators during 15-year follow-up of advanced gastric cancer after radical gastrectomy and adjuvant chemotherapy: a 15-year follow-up study at a single korean institute. *Ann Surg Oncol* 2007;14:2730–2737.

183. Kodera Y, Yamamura Y, Shimizu Y, et al. The number of metastatic lymph nodes: a promising prognostic determinant for gastric carcinoma in the latest edition of the TNM classification. *J Am Coll Surg* 1998;187:597–603.

184. Methasate A, Trakarnsanga A, Akaraviputh T, et al. Lymph node metastasis in gastric cancer: result of D2 dissection. *J Med Assoc Thai* 2010;93:310–317.

185. Qureshi AP, Ottensmeyer CA, Mahar AL, et al. Quality indicators for gastric cancer surgery: a survey of practicing pathologists in Ontario. *Ann Surg Oncol* 2009;16:1883–1889.

186. Printz C. New AJCC cancer staging manual reflects changes in cancer knowledge. *Cancer* 2010;116:2–3.

187. Edge SB, Compton CC. The American Joint Committee on Cancer: the 7th edition of the AJCC cancer staging manual and the future of TNM. *Ann Surg Oncol* 2010;17:1471–1474.

188. Dent DM, Madden MV, Price SK. Randomized comparison of R1 and R2 gastrectomy for gastric carcinoma. *Br J Surg* 1988;75:110–112.

189. Cuschieri A, Weeden S, Fielding J, et al. Patient survival after D1 and D2 resections for gastric cancer: long-term results of the MRC randomized surgical trial. Surgical Co-operative Group. *Br J Cancer* 1999;79:1522–1530.

190. Bonenkamp JJ, Hermans J, Sasako M, et al. Extended lymph-node dissection for gastric cancer. *N Engl J Med* 1999;340:908–914.

191. Degiuli M, Sasako M, Calgaro M, et al. Morbidity and mortality after D1 and D2 gastrectomy for cancer: interim analysis of the Italian Gastric Cancer Study Group (IGCSG) randomised surgical trial. *Eur J Surg Oncol* 2004;30: 303–308.

192. Wu CW, Hsiung CA, Lo SS, et al. Nodal dissection for patients with gastric cancer: a randomised controlled trial. *Lancet Oncol* 2006;7:309–315.

193. Cuschieri A, Fayers P, Fielding J, et al. Postoperative morbidity and mortality after D1 and D2 resections for gastric cancer: preliminary results of the MRC randomised controlled surgical trial. The Surgical Cooperative Group. *Lancet* 1996;347:995–999.

194. Siewert JR, Böttcher K, Roder JD, et al. Prognostic relevance of systematic lymph node dissection in gastric carcinoma. German Gastric Carcinoma Study Group. *Br J Surg* 1993;80:1015–1018.

195. Kajitani T. The general rules for the gastric cancer study in surgery and pathology: art I: clinical classification. *Jpn J Surg* 1981;11:127–139.

196. Songun I, Putter H, Kranenbarg EM, et al. Surgical treatment of gastric cancer: 15-year follow-up results of the randomised nationwide Dutch D1D2 trial. *Lancet Oncol* 2010;11:439–449.

197. Bonenkamp JJ, Hermans J, Sasako M, et al. Quality control of lymph node dissection in the Dutch randomized trial of D1 and D2 lymph node dissection for gastric cancer. *Gastric Cancer* 1998;1:152–159.

198. Bunt TM, Bonenkamp HJ, Hermans J, et al. Factors influencing noncompliance and contamination in a randomized trial of "Western" (r1) versus "Japanese" (r2) type surgery in gastric cancer. *Cancer* 1994;73:1544–1551.

199. Bonenkamp JJ, Songun I, Hermans J, et al. Randomised comparison of morbidity after D1 and D2 dissection for gastric cancer in 996 Dutch patients. *Lancet* 1995;345:745–748.

200. Roggin KK, Posner MC. D3 or not D3. . . that is not the question. *Lancet Oncol* 2006;7:279–280.

201. Chen XZ, Hu JK, Zhou ZG, et al. Meta-analysis of effectiveness and safety of D2 plus para-aortic lymphadenectomy for resectable gastric cancer. *J Am Coll Surg* 2010;210:100–105.

202. Fujimura T, Nakamura K, Oyama K, et al. Selective lymphadenectomy of para-aortic lymph nodes for advanced gastric cancer. *Oncol Rep* 2009;22: 509–514.

203. Brennan MF. Lymph-node dissection for gastric cancer. *N Engl J Med* 1999;340:956–958.

204. Sano T, Sasako M, Yamamoto S, et al. Gastric cancer surgery: morbidity and mortality results from a prospective randomized controlled trial comparing D2 and extended para-aortic lymphadenectomy—Japan Clinical Oncology Group study 9501. *J Clin Oncol* 2004;22:2767–2773.

205. Sasako M, Sano T, Yamamoto S, et al. D2 lymphadenectomy alone or with para-aortic nodal dissection for gastric cancer. *N Engl J Med* 2008;359:453–4662.

206. Yonemura Y, Wu CC, Fukushima N, et al. Randomized clinical trial of D2 and extended paraaortic lymphadenectomy in patients with gastric cancer. *Int J Clin Oncol* 2008;13:132–137.

207. Kulig J, Popiela T, Kolodziejczyk P, et al. Standard D2 versus extended D2 (D2+) lymphadenectomy for gastric cancer: an interim safety analysis of a multicenter, randomized, clinical trial. *Am J Surg* 2007;193:10–15.

208. Cady B. Basic principles in surgical oncology. *Arch Surg* 1997;132:338–346.

209. Degiuli M, Sasako M, Ponti A, et al. Randomized clinical trial comparing survival after D1 or D2 gastrectomy for gastric cancer. *Br J Surg* 2014; 101:23–31.

210. Jiang L, Yang KH, Chen Y, et al. Systematic review and meta-analysis of the effectiveness and safety of extended lymphadenectomy in patients with resectable gastric cancer. *Br J Surg* 2014;101:595–604.

211. Kodera Y, Sasako M, Yamamoto S, et al. Identification of risk factors for the development of complications following extended and superextended lymphadenectomies for gastric cancer. *Br J Surg* 2005;92:1103–1109.

212. Furukawa H, Hiratsuka M, Ishikawa O, et al. Total gastrectomy with dissection of lymph nodes along the splenic artery: a pancreas-preserving method. *Ann Surg Oncol* 2000;7:669–673.

213. Doglietto GB, Pacelli F, Caprino P, et al. Pancreas-preserving total gastrectomy for gastric cancer. *Arch Surg* 2000;135:89–94.

214. Schwarz RE, Zagala-Nevarez K. Gastrectomy circumstances that influence early postoperative outcome. *Hepatogastroenterology* 2002;49:1742–1746.

215. Schwarz RE. Spleen-preserving splenic hilar lymphadenectomy at the time of gastrectomy for cancer: technical feasibility and early results. *J Surg Oncol* 2002;79:73–76.

216. Kimura W, Yano M, Sugawara S, et al. Spleen-preserving distal pancreatectomy with conservation of the splenic artery and vein: techniques and its significance. *J Hepatobiliary Pancreat Surg* 2009;17:813–823.

217. Yao XX, Yan C, Yan JM, et al. [A comparative study on the efficacy of spleen-preserving modified D2 radical gastrectomy and D2 radical gastrectomy with splenectomy]. *Zhonghua Wei Chang Wai Ke Za Zhi* 2010;13:111–114.

218. Oh SJ, Hyung WJ, Li C, et al. The effect of spleen-preserving lymphadenectomy on surgical outcomes of locally advanced proximal gastric cancer. *J Surg Oncol* 2009;99:275–280.

219. Csendes A, Burdiles P, Rojas J, et al. A prospective randomized study comparing D2 total gastrectomy versus D2 total gastrectomy plus splenectomy in 187 patients with gastric carcinoma. *Surgery* 2002;131:401–407.

220. Yu W, Choi GS, Chung HY. Randomized clinical trial of splenectomy versus splenic preservation in patients with proximal gastric cancer. *Br J Surg* 2006;93:559–563.

221. Kunisaki C, Makino H, Suwa H, et al. Impact of splenectomy in patients with gastric adenocarcinoma of the cardia. *J Gastrointest Surg* 2007;11: 1039–1044.

222. Sano T, Yamamoto S, Sasako M. Randomized controlled trial to evaluate splenectomy in total gastrectomy for proximal gastric carcinoma: Japan clinical oncology group study JCOG 0110-MF. *Jpn J Clin Oncol* 2002;32:363–364.

223. Wang W, Li Z, Tang J, et al. Laparoscopic versus open total gastrectomy with D2 dissection for gastric cancer: a meta-analysis. *J Cancer Res Clin Oncol* 2013;139:1721–1734.

224. Coburn N, Seevaratnam R, Paszat L, et al. Optimal management of gastric cancer: results from an international RAND/UCLA expert panel. *Ann Surg* 2014;259:102–108.

225. Kampschoer GH, Maruyama K, van de Velde CJ, et al. Computer analysis in making preoperative decisions: a rational approach to lymph node dissection in gastric cancer patients. *Br J Surg* 1989;76:905–908.

226. Bollschweiler E, Boettcher K, Hoelscher AH, et al. Preoperative assessment of lymph-node metastases in patients with gastric-cancer: evaluation of the Maruyama computer program. *Br J Surg* 1992;79:156–160.

227. Guadagni S, Catarci M, Valenti M, et al. Evaluation of the Maruyama computer program accuracy for preoperative extimation of lymph node metastases from gastric cancer. *World J Surg* 2000;24:1550–1558.

228. Hundahl SA, Macdonald JS, Benedetti J, et al. Surgical treatment variation in a prospective, randomized trial of chemoradiotherapy in gastric cancer: the effect of undertreatment. *Ann Surg Oncol* 2002;9:278–286.

229. Mekicar J, Omejc M. Computer-guided surgery for gastric carcinoma. *Coll Antropol* 2008;32:761–766.

230. Mekicar J, Omejc M. Preoperative prediction of lymph node status in gastric cancer patients with the help of computer analysis. *Dig Surg* 2009;26: 256–261.

231. Yoo MW, Park do J, Ahn HS, et al. Evaluation of the Adequacy of lymph node dissection in pylorus-preserving gastrectomy for early gastric cancer using the maruyama index. *World J Surg* 2010;34:291–295.

232. Catarci M, Guadagni S, Zaraca F, et al. Prospective randomized evaluation of preoperative endoscopic vital staining using CH-40 for lymph node dissection in gastric cancer. *Ann Surg Oncol* 1998;5:580–284.

233. Yanagita S, Natsugoe S, Uenosono Y, et al. Sentinel node micrometastases have high proliferative potential in gastric cancer. *J Surg Res* 2008;145:238–243.

234. Arigami T, Natsugoe S, Uenosono Y, et al. Evaluation of sentinel node concept in gastric cancer based on lymph node micrometastasis determined by reverse transcription-polymerase chain reaction. *Ann Surg* 2006;243:341–347.

235. Higashi H, Natsugoe S, Uenosono Y, et al. Particle size of tin and phytate colloid in sentinel node identification. *J Sur Res* 2004;121:1–4.

236. Aikou T, Higashi H, Natsugoe S, et al. Can sentinel node navigation surgery reduce the extent of lymph node dissection in gastric cancer? *Ann Surg Oncol* 2001;8:90S–93S.

237. Kitagawa Y, Watanabe M, Hasegawa H, et al. Sentinel node mapping for colorectal cancer with radioactive tracer. *Dis Colon Rectum* 2002;45: 1476–1480.

238. Kitagawa Y, Fujii H, Mukai M, et al. Radio-guided sentinel node detection for gastric cancer. *Br J Surg* 2002;89:604–608.

239. Kitagawa Y, Kitajima M. Gastrointestinal cancer and sentinel node navigation surgery. *J Surg Oncol* 2002;79:188–193.

240. Ichikura T, Morita D, Uchida T, et al. Sentinel node concept in gastric carcinoma. *World J Surg* 2002;26:318–322.

241. Miwa K, Kinami S, Taniguchi K, et al. Mapping sentinel nodes in patients with early-stage gastric carcinoma. *Br J Surg* 2003;90:178–182.

242. Miwa K, Kinami S, Taniguchi K, et al. Mapping sentinel nodes in patients with early-stage gastric carcinoma. *Gastroenterology* 2000;118:A263.

243. Hayashi H, Ochiai T, Mori M, et al. Sentinel lymph node mapping for gastric cancer using a dual procedure with dye- and gamma probe-guided techniques. *J Am Coll Surg* 2003;196:68–74

244. Gretschel S, Bembenek A, Hünerbein M, et al. Efficacy of different technical procedures for sentinel lymph node biopsy in gastric cancer staging. *Ann Surg Oncol* 2007;14:2028–2035.

245. Becher RD, Shen P, Stewart JH, et al. Sentinel lymph node mapping for gastric adenocarcinoma. *Am Surg* 2009;75:710–714.

246. Lee JH, Ryu KW, Nam BH, et al. Factors associated with detection failure and false-negative sentinel node biopsy findings in gastric cancer: results of prospective single center trials. *J Surg Oncol* 2009;99:137–142.

247. Lee SE, Lee JH, Ryu KW, et al. Sentinel node mapping and skip metastases in patients with early gastric cancer. *Ann Surg Oncol* 2009;16:603–608.

248. Kitagawa Y, Takeuchi H, Takagi Y, et al. Sentinel node mapping for gastric cancer: a prospective multicenter trial in Japan. *J Clin Oncol* 2013;31:3704–3710.

249. Miyashiro I, Hiratsuka M, Sasako M, et al. High false-negative proportion of intraoperative histological examination as a serious problem for clinical application of sentinel node biopsy for early gastric cancer: final results of the Japan Clinical Oncology Group multicenter trial JCOG0302. *Gastric Cancer* 2014;17:316–323.

250. Birkmeyer JD, Skinner JS, Wennberg DE. Will volume-based referral strategies reduce costs or just save lives? *Health Affairs* 2002;21:234–241.

251. Birkmeyer JD, Finlayson EVA. Volume and outcome - Reply. *N Eng J Med* 2002;347:693–696.

252. Birkmeyer JD, Siewers AE, Finlayson EV, et al. Hospital volume and surgical mortality in the United States. *N Eng J Med* 2002;346:1128–1137.

253. Birkmeyer JD, Stukel TA, Siewers AE, et al. Surgeon volume and operative mortality in the United States. *N Eng J Med* 2003;349:2117–2127.

254. Goodney PP, Stukel TA, Lucas FL, et al. Hospital volume, length of stay, and readmission rates in high-risk surgery. *Ann Surg* 2003;238:161–167.

255. Finlayson EV, Goodney PP, Birkmeyer JD. Hospital volume and operative mortality in cancer surgery: a national study. *Arch Surg* 2003;138:721–725, discussion 726.

256. Goodney PP, Lucas FL, Birkmeyer JD. Should volume standards for cardiovascular surgery focus only on high-risk patients? *Circulation* 2003;107:384–387.

257. Hannan EL, Radzyner M, Rubin D, et al. The influence of hospital and surgeon volume on in-hospital mortality for colectomy, gastrectomy, and lung lobectomy in patients with cancer. *Surgery* 2002;131:6–15.

258. Lin HC, Xirasagar S, Lee HC, et al. Hospital volume and inpatient mortality after cancer-related gastrointestinal resections: the experience of an Asian country. *Ann Surg Oncol* 2006;13:1182–1188.

259. Birkmeyer JD, Sun Y, Goldfaden A, et al. Volume and process of care in high-risk cancer surgery. *Cancer* 2006;106:2476–2481.

260. Hollenbeck BK, Wei YL, Birkmeyer JD. High volume hospitals do not have better long term outcomes following cystectomy for bladder cancer. *J Urol* 2006;175:8.

261. Birkmeyer JD, Dimick JB, Staiger DO. Operative mortality and procedure volume as predictors of subsequent hospital performance. *Ann Surg* 2006; 243:411–417.

262. Callahan MA, Christos PJ, Gold HT, et al. Influence of surgical subspecialty training on in-hospital mortality for gastrectomy and colectomy patients. *Ann Surg* 2003;238:629–636, discussion 636–639.

263. Callahan MA, Christos PJ, Gold HT, et al. Influence of surgical subspecialty training on in-hospital mortality for gastrectomy and colectomy patients. *Ann Surg* 2003;238:629–636, discussion 636–639.

264. Waljee JF, Greenfield LJ, Dimick JB, et al. Surgeon age and operative mortality in the United States. *Ann Surg* 2006;244:353–362.

265. Ritchie WP Jr, Rhodes RS, Biester TW. Work loads and practice patterns of general surgeons in the United States, 1995–1997: a report from the American Board of Surgery. *Ann Surg* 1999;230:533–542, discussion 542–543.

266. Lauren P. The two histological main types of gastric carcinoma: diffuse and so-called intestinal-type carcinoma. An attempt at a histo-clinical classification. *Acta Pathol Microbiol Scand* 1965;64:31–49.

267. Noguchi Y, Yoshikawa T, Tsuburaya A, et al. Is gastric carcinoma different between Japan and the United States? A comparison of patient survival among three institutions. *Cancer* 2000;89:2237–2246.

268. Gill S. Ethnicity-related gastric cancer survival. In reply. *J Clin Oncol* 2003;21:4253.

269. Gill S, Shah A, Le N, et al. Asian ethnicity-related differences in gastric cancer presentation and outcome among patients treated at a Canadian Cancer Center. *J Clin Oncol* 2003;21:2070–2076.

270. Schlemper RJ. Differences in diagnostic criteria for gastric carcinoma between Japanese and western pathologists (Erratum). *Lancet* 1997;350:524.

271. Schlemper RJ, Itabashi M, Kato Y, et al. Differences in diagnostic criteria for gastric carcinoma between Japanese and western pathologists. *Lancet* 1997;349:1725–1729.

272. Schlemper RJ, Itabashi M, Kato Y, et al. Differences in the diagnostic criteria of gastric carcinoma between Japanese and Western pathologists. *Lancet* 1997;349:1725–1729.

273. Lauwers GY, Riddell RH. Gastric epithelial dysplasia. *Gut* 1999;45:784–790.

274. Lauwers GY, Shimizu M, Correa P, et al. Evaluation of gastric biopsies for neoplasia: differences between Japanese and Western pathologists. *Am J Surg Pathol* 1999;23:511–518.

275. Rugge M, Correa P, Dixon MF, et al. Gastric dysplasia: the Padova international classification. *Am J Surg Pathol* 2000;24:167–176.

276. Schlemper RJ, Riddell RH, Kato Y, et al. The Vienna classification of gastrointestinal epithelial neoplasia. *Gut* 2000;47:251–255.

277. Hundahl SA. Staging, stage migration, and patterns of spread in gastric cancer. *Semi Radiat Oncol* 2002;12:141–149.

278. Bunt AM, Hermans J, Smit VT, et al. Surgical/pathologic-stage migration confounds comparisons of gastric cancer survival rates between Japan and Western countries. *J Clin Oncol* 1995;13:19–25.

279. Davis PA, Sano T. The difference in gastric cancer between Japan, USA and Europe: what are the facts? what are the suggestions? *Crit Rev Oncol Hematol* 2001;40:77–94.

280. Mezhir JJ, Pillarisetty VG, Shah MA, et al. Randomized clinical trials in gastric cancer. *Surg Oncol Clin N Am* 2010;19:81–100.

281. Huscher CG, Mingoli A, Sgarzini G, et al. Re: "laparoscopic assisted distal gastrectomy for early gastric cancer: five years' experience." *Surgery* 2005;138:543.

282. Huscher CG, Mingoli A, Sgarzini G, et al. Laparoscopic versus open subtotal gastrectomy for distal gastric cancer: five-year results of a randomized prospective trial. *Ann Surg* 2005;241:232–237.

283. Kitano S, Shiraishi N, Fujii K, et al. A randomized controlled trial comparing open vs laparoscopy-assisted distal gastrectomy for the treatment of early gastric cancer: an interim report. *Surgery* 2002;131:S306–S311.

284. Hayashi H, Ochiai T, Shimada H, et al. Prospective randomized study of open versus laparoscopy-assisted distal gastrectomy with extraperigastric lymph node dissection for early gastric cancer. *Surg Endosc* 2005;19:1172–1176.

285. Kim YW, Baik YH, Yun YH, et al. Improved quality of life outcomes after laparoscopy-assisted distal gastrectomy for early gastric cancer: results of a prospective randomized clinical trial. *Ann Surg* 2008;248:721–727.

286. Kim HH, Han SU, Kim MC, et al. Long-term results of laparoscopic gastrectomy for gastric cancer: a large-scale, case-control and case-matched Korean multicenter study. *J Clin Oncol* 2014:32:627–633.

287. Ohtani H, Tamamori Y, Noguchi K, et al. A meta-analysis of randomized controlled trials that compared laparoscopy-assisted and open distal gastrectomy for early gastric cancer. *J Gastrointest Surg* 2010;14:958–964.

288. Lee JH, Han HS. A prospective randomized study comparing open vs laparoscopy-assisted distal gastrectomy in early gastric cancer: early results. *Surg Endosc* 2005;19:168–173.

289. Jiang L, Yang KH, Guan QL, et al. Laparoscopy-assisted gastrectomy versus open gastrectomy for resectable gastric cancer: an update meta-analysis based on randomized controlled trials. *Surg Endosc* 2013;27:2466–2480.

290. Liang Y, Li G, Chen P, et al. Laparoscopic versus open gastrectomy for early distal gastric cancer: a meta-analysis. *ANZ J Surg* 2011;81:673–680.

291. Kim HH, Han SU, Kim MC, et al. Prospective randomized controlled trial (phase III) to comparing laparoscopic distal gastrectomy with open distal gastrectomy for gastric adenocarcinoma (KLASS 01). *J Korean Surg Soc* 2013;84:123–130.

292. Nakamura K, Katai H, Mizusawa J, et al. A phase III study of laparoscopy-assisted versus open distal gastrectomy with nodal dissection for clinical stage IA/IB gastric Cancer JCOG0912). *Jpn J Clin Oncol* 2013;43:324–327.

293. Sakuramoto S, Sasako M, Yamaguchi T, et al. Adjuvant chemotherapy for gastric cancer with S-1, an oral fluoropyrimidine. *N Engl J Med* 2007;357:1810–1820.

294. Sasako M, Sakuramoto S, Katai H, et al. Five-year outcomes of a randomized phase III trial comparing adjuvant chemotherapy with S-1 versus surgery alone in stage II or III gastric cancer. *J Clin Oncol* 2011;29:4387–4393.

295. Bang YJ, Kim YW, Yang HK, et al. Adjuvant capecitabine and oxaliplatin for gastric cancer after D2 gastrectomy (CLASSIC): a phase 3 open-label, randomised controlled trial. *Lancet* 2012;379:315–321.

296. Di Costanzo F, Gasperoni S, Manzione L, et al. Adjuvant chemotherapy in completely resected gastric cancer: a randomized phase III trial conducted by GOIRC. *J Natl Cancer Inst* 2008;100:388–398.

297. Buyse ME, Pignon J. Meta-analyses of randomized trials assessing the interest of postoperative adjuvant chemotherapy and prognsotic factors in gastric cancer. *J Clin Oncol* 2009;27:4539.

298. Sugarbaker PH, Yu W, Yonemura Y. Gastrectomy, peritonectomy, and perioperative intraperitoneal chemotherapy: the evolution of treatment strategies for advanced gastric cancer. *Semin Surg Oncol* 2003;21:233–248.

299. GASTRIC (Global Advanced/Adjuvant Stomach Tumor Research International Collaboration) Group, Paoletti X, Oba K, et al. Benefit of adjuvant chemotherapy for resectable gastric cancer: a meta-analysis. *JAMA* 2010;303:1729–1737.

300. Hamazoe R, Maeta M, Kaibara N. Intraperitoneal thermochemotherapy for prevention of peritoneal recurrence of gastric cancer. Final results of a randomized controlled study. *Cancer* 1994;73:2048–2052.

301. Takahashi T, Hagiwara A, Shimotsuma M, et al. Prophylaxis and treatment of peritoneal carcinomatosis: intraperitoneal chemotherapy with mitomycin C bound to activated carbon particles. *World J Surg* 1995;19:565–569.

302. Fujimoto S, Takahashi M, Mutou T, et al. Successful intraperitoneal hyperthermic chemoperfusion for the prevention of postoperative peritoneal recurrence in patients with advanced gastric carcinoma. *Cancer* 1999;85:529–534.

303. Yonemura Y, de Aretxabala X, Fujimura T, et al. Intraoperative chemohyperthermic peritoneal perfusion as an adjuvant to gastric cancer: final results of a randomized controlled study. *Hepatogastroenterology* 2001;48:1776–1782.

304. Rosen HR, Jatzko G, Repse S, et al. Adjuvant intraperitoneal chemotherapy with carbon-adsorbed mitomycin in patients with gastric cancer: results of a randomized multicenter trial of the Austrian Working Group for Surgical Oncology. *J Clin Oncol* 1998;16:2733–2738.

305. Yu W, Whang I, Suh I, et al. Prospective randomized trial of early postoperative intraperitoneal chemotherapy as an adjuvant to resectable gastric cancer. *Ann Surg* 1998;228:347–354.

306. Yu W, Whang I, Chung HY, et al. Indications for early postoperative intraperitoneal chemotherapy of advanced gastric cancer: results of a prospective randomized trial. *World J Surg* 2001;25:985–990.

307. Wei G, Fang GE, Bi JW, et al. [Efficacy of intraoperative hypotonic peritoneal chemo-hyperthermia combined with early postoperative intraperitoneal chemotherapy on gastric cancer]. *Ai Zheng* 2005;24:478–482.

308. Sautner T, Hofbauer F, Depisch D, et al. Adjuvant intraperitoneal cisplatin chemotherapy does not improve long-term survival after surgery for advanced gastric cancer. *J Clin Oncol* 1994;12:970–974.

309. Xu DZ, Zhan YQ, Sun XW, et al. Meta-analysis of intraperitoneal chemotherapy for gastric cancer. *World J Gastroenterol* 2004;10:2727–2730.

310. Yan TD, Black D, Sugarbaker PH, et al. A systematic review and meta-analysis of the randomized controlled trials on adjuvant intraperitoneal chemotherapy for resectable gastric cancer. *Ann Surg Oncol* 2007;14:2702–2713.

311. Kang Y, Chang H, Zang D, et al. Postoperative adjuvant chemotherapy for grossly serosa-positive advanced gastric cancer: A randomized phase III trial of intraperitoneal cisplatin and early mitomycin-C plus long-term doxifluridine plus cisplatin (iceMFP) versus mitomycin-C plus short-term doxifluridine (Mf) (AMC 0101) (NCT00296322). *J Clin Oncol* 2008;26:LBA4511.

312. Kuramoto M, Shimada S, Ikeshima S, et al. Extensive intraoperative peritoneal lavage as a standard prophylactic strategy for peritoneal recurrence in patients with gastric carcinoma. *Ann Surg* 2009;250:242–246.

313. Kelsen D, Karpeh M, Schwartz G, et al. Neoadjuvant therapy of high-risk gastric cancer: a phase II trial of preoperative FAMTX and postoperative intraperitoneal fluorouracil-cisplatin plus intravenous fluorouracil. *J Clin Oncol* 1996;14:1818–1828.

314. Brenner B, Shah MA, Karpeh MS, et al. A phase II trial of neoadjuvant cisplatin-fluorouracil followed by postoperative intraperitoneal floxuridine-leucovorin in patients with locally advanced gastric cancer. *Ann Oncol* 2006;17:1404–1411.

315. Downey RJ, Akhurst T, Ilson D, et al. Whole body 18FDG-PET and the response of esophageal cancer to induction therapy: results of a prospective trial. *J Clin Oncol* 2003;21:428–432.

316. Minamimoto R, Senda M, Jinnouchi S, et al. Performance profile of a FDG-PET cancer screening program for detecting gastric cancer: results from a nationwide Japanese survey. *Jpn J Radiol* 2014;32:253–259.

317. Cunningham D, Allum WH, Stenning SP, et al. Perioperative chemotherapy versus surgery alone for resectable gastroesophageal cancer. *N Engl J Med* 2006;355:11–20.

318. Boige V, Pignon J, Saint-Aubert B, et al. Final results of a randomized trial comparing preoperative 5-fluorouracil (F)/cisplatin (P) to surgery alone in adenocarcinoma of stomach and lower esophagus (ASLE): FNLCC ACCORD07-FFCD 9703 trial. *J Clin Oncol* 2007;25:4510.

319. Liao Y, Yang ZL, Peng JS, et al. Neoadjuvant chemotherapy for gastric cancer: a meta-analysis of randomized, controlled trials. *J Gastroenterol Hepatol* 2013;28:777–782.

320. Allum WH, Hallissey MT, Ward LC, et al. A controlled, prospective, randomised trial of adjuvant chemotherapy or radiotherapy in resectable gastric cancer: interim report. British Stomach Cancer Group. *Br J Cancer* 1989;60:739–744.

321. Hallissey MT, Dunn JA, Ward LC, et al. The second British Stomach Cancer Group trial of adjuvant radiotherapy or chemotherapy in resectable gastric cancer: five-year follow-up. *Lancet* 1994;343:1309–1312.

322. Zhang ZX, Gu XZ, Yin WB, et al. Randomized clinical trial on the combination of preoperative irradiation and surgery in the treatment of adenocarcinoma of gastric cardia (AGC)—report on 370 patients. *Int J Radiat Oncol Biol Phys* 1998;42:929–934.

323. Ohri N, Garg MK, Aparo S, et al. Who benefits from adjuvant radiation therapy for gastric cancer? A meta-analysis. *Int J Radiat Oncol Biol Phys* 2013;86:330–335.

324. Liao Y, Yang ZL, Peng JS, et al. Neoadjuvant chemotherapy for gastric cancer: a meta-analysis of randomized, controlled trials. *J Gastroenterol Hepatol* 2013;28:777–782.

325. Gunderson L, Willet G, Harrisson B, et al., eds. *Intraoperative Irradiation: Techniques and Results*. Totowa, NJ: Humana Press; 1999.

326. Abe M, Takahashi M, Ono K, et al. Japan gastric trials in intraoperative radiation therapy. *Int J Radiat Oncol Biol Phys* 1988;15:1431–1433.

327. Sindelar WF, Kinsella TJ, Tepper JE, et al. Randomized trial of intraoperative radiotherapy in carcinoma of the stomach. *Am J Surg* 1993;165:178–186, discussion 186–187.

328. Dent DM, Werner ID, Novis B, et al. Prospective randomized trial of combined oncological therapy for gastric carcinoma. *Cancer* 1979;44:385–391.

329. Moertel CG, Childs DS, O'Fallon JR, et al. Combined 5-fluorouracil and radiation therapy as a surgical adjuvant for poor prognosis gastric carcinoma. *J Clin Oncol* 1984;2:1249–1254.

330. Macdonald JS, Smalley SR, Benedetti J, et al. Chemoradiotherapy after surgery compared with surgery alone for adenocarcinoma of the stomach or gastroesophageal junction. *N Engl J Med* 2001;345:725–730.

331. Fuchs CS, Tepper JE, Niedzwiecki D, et al. Postoperative adjuvant chemoradiation for gastric or gastroesophageal junction (GEJ) adenocarcinoma using epirubicin, cisplatin, and infusional (CI) 5-FU (ECF) before and after CI 5-FU and radiotherapy (CRT) compared with bolus 5-FU/LV before and after CRT: Intergroup trial CALGB 80101. *J Clin Oncol* 2011;29:4003.

332. Lee J, Lim do H, Kim S, et al. Phase III trial comparing capecitabine plus cisplatin versus capecitabine plus cisplatin with concurrent capecitabine radiotherapy in completely resected gastric cancer with D2 lymph node dissection: the ARTIST trial. *J Clin Oncol* 2012;30:268–273.

333. Walsh TN, Noonan N, Hollywood D, et al. A comparison of multimodal therapy and surgery for esophageal adenocarcinoma. *N Engl J Med* 1996;335:462–467.

334. Tepper J, Krasna MJ, Niedzwiecki D, et al. Phase III trial of trimodality therapy with cisplatin, fluorouracil, radiotherapy, and surgery compared with surgery alone for esophageal cancer: CALGB 9781. *J Clin Oncol* 2008;26:1086–1092.

335. Stahl M, Walz MK, Stuschke M, et al. Phase III comparison of preoperative chemotherapy compared with chemoradiotherapy in patients with locally advanced adenocarcinoma of the esophagogastric junction. *J Clin Oncol* 2009;27:851–856.

336. Ajani JA, Mansfield PF, Janjan N, et al. Multi-institutional trial of preoperative chemoradiotherapy in patients with potentially resectable gastric carcinoma. *J Clin Oncol* 2004;22:2774–2780.

337. Ajani JA, Mansfield PF, Crane CH, et al. Paclitaxel-based chemoradiotherapy in localized gastric carcinoma: degree of pathologic response and not clinical parameters dictated patient outcome. *J Clin Oncol* 2005;23:1237–1244.

338. Ajani JA, Winter K, Okawara GS, et al. Phase II trial of preoperative chemoradiation in patients with localized gastric adenocarcinoma (RTOG 9904): quality of combined modality therapy and pathologic response. *J Clin Oncol* 2006;24:3953–3958.

339. Mohri Y, Tonouchi H, Kobayashi M, et al. Randomized clinical trial of single-versus multiple-dose antimicrobial prophylaxis in gastric cancer surgery. *Br J Surg* 2007;94:683–688.

340. Doglietto GB, Papa V, Tortorelli AP, et al. Nasojejunal tube placement after total gastrectomy: a multicenter prospective randomized trial. *Arch Surg* 2004;139:1309–1313, discussion 1313.

341. Yoo CH, Son BH, Han WK, et al. Nasogastric decompression is not necessary in operations for gastric cancer: prospective randomised trial. *Eur J Surg* 2002;168:379–383.

342. Lee JH, Hyung WJ, Noh SH. Comparison of gastric cancer surgery with versus without nasogastric decompression. *Yonsei Med J* 2002;43:451–456.

343. Yang Z, Zheng Q, Wang Z. Meta-analysis of the need for nasogastric or nasojejunal decompression after gastrectomy for gastric cancer. *Br J Surg* 2008;95:809–816.

344. Kim J, Lee J, Hyung WJ, et al. Gastric cancer surgery without drains: a prospective randomized trial. *J Gastrointest Surg* 2004;8:727–732.

345. Alvarez Uslar R, Molina H, Torres O, et al. Total gastrectomy with or without abdominal drains. A prospective randomized trial. *Rev Esp Enferm Dig* 2005; 97:562–569.

346. Iivonen MK, Koskinen MO, Ikonen TJ, et al. Emptying of the jejunal pouch and Roux-en-Y limb after total gastrectomy–a randomised, prospective study. *Eur J Surg* 1999;165:742–747.

347. Fein M, Fuchs KH, Thalheimer A, et al. Long-term benefits of Roux-en-Y pouch reconstruction after total gastrectomy: a randomized trial. *Ann Surg* 2008;247:759–765.

348. Smalley SR, Gunderson L, Tepper J, et al. Gastric surgical adjuvant radiotherapy consensus report: rationale and treatment implementation. *Int J Radiat Oncol Biol Phys* 2002;52:283–293.

349. Tepper JE, Gunderson LL. Radiation treatment parameters in the adjuvant postoperative therapy of gastric cancer. *Semin Radiat Oncol* 2002;12:187–195.

350. Gilbertson V. Results of treatment of stomach cancer. An appraisal of efforts for more extensive surgery and a report of 1938 cases. *Cancer* 1969;23: 1305–1308.

351. Gunderson LL, Sosin H. Adenocarcinoma of the stomach: areas of failure in a re-operation series (second or symptomatic look) clinicopathologic correlation and implications for adjuvant therapy. *Int J Radiat Oncol Biol Phys* 1982;8:1–11.

352. McNeer G, Vandenberg H Jr, Donn FY, et al. A critical evaluation of subtotal gastrectomy for the cure of cancer of the stomach. *Ann Surg* 1951;134:2–7.

353. Stout AP. Pathology of carcinoma of the stomach. *Arch Surg* 1943;46:807–822.

354. Henning GT, Schild SE, Stafford SL, et al. Results of irradiation or chemoirradiation following resection of gastric adenocarcinoma. *Int J Radiat Oncol Biol Phys* 2000;46:589–598.

355. Gunderson LL, Hoskins RB, Cohen AC, et al. Combined modality treatment of gastric cancer. *Int J Radiat Oncol Biol Phys* 1983;9:965–975.

356. Regine WF, Mohiuddin M. Impact of adjuvant therapy on locally advanced adenocarcinoma of the stomach. *Int J Radiat Oncol Biol Phys* 1992;24: 921–927.

357. A comparison of combination chemotherapy and combined modality therapy for locally advanced gastric carcinoma. Gastrointestinal Tumor Study Group. *Cancer* 1982;49:1771–1777.

358. Wagner AD, Unverzagt S, Grothe W, et al. Chemotherapy for advanced cancer. *Cochrane Database Syst Rev* 2010;(3):CD004064.

359. Thuss-Patience PC, Kretzschmar A, Deist T, et al. Irinotecan versus best supportive care as second-line therapy in gastric cancer: a randomized phase III study of the Arbeitsgemeinschaft Internistische Onkologie (AIO). *J Clin Oncol* 2009;27:Abstr 4540.

360. Okines AF, Norman AR, McCloud P, et al. Meta-analysis of the REAL-2 and ML17032 trials: evaluating capecitabine-based combination chemotherapy and infused 5-fluorouracil-based combination chemotherapy for the treatment of advanced oesophago-gastric cancer. *Ann Oncol* 2009;20:1529–1534.

361. Di Cosimo S, Ferretti G, Fazio N, et al. Docetaxel in advanced gastric cancer—review of the main clinical trials. *Acta Oncol* 2003;42:693–700.

362. Cunningham D, Rao S, Starling N, et al. Randomized multicentre phase III study comparing capecitabine with fluorouracil and oxaliplatin with cisplatin in patients with advanced oesophagogastric (OG) cancer: The REAL-2 trial. *J Clin Oncol* 2006;24:LBA4017.

363. Vanhoefer U, Rougier P, Wilke H, et al. Final results of a randomized phase III trial of sequential high-dose methotrexate, fluorouracil, and doxorubicin versus etoposide, leucovorin, and fluorouracil versus infusional fluorouracil and cisplatin in advanced gastric cancer: a trial of the European Organization for Research and Treatment of Cancer Gastrointestinal Tract Cancer Cooperative Group. *J Clin Oncol* 2000;18:2648–2657.

364. Ohtsu A, Shimada Y, Shirao K, et al. Randomized phase III trial of fluorouracil alone versus fluorouracil plus cisplatin versus uracil and tegafur plus mitomycin in patients with unresectable, advanced gastric cancer: the Japan Clinical Oncology Group Study (JCOG9205). *J Clin Oncol* 2003;21:54–59.

365. Van Cutsem E, Moiseyenko VM, Tjulandin S, et al. Phase III study of docetaxel and cisplatin plus fluorouracil compared with cisplatin and fluorouracil as first-line therapy for advanced gastric cancer: a report of the V325 Study Group. *J Clin Oncol* 2006;24:4991–4997.

366. Dank M, Zaluski J, Barone C, et al. Randomized phase III study comparing irinotecan combined with 5-fluorouracil and folinic acid to cisplatin combined with 5-fluorouracil in chemotherapy naive patients with advanced adenocarcinoma of the stomach or esophagogastric junction. *Ann Oncol* 2008;19: 1450–1457.

367. Kang YK, Kang WK, Shin DB, et al. Capecitabine/cisplatin versus 5-fluorouracil/cisplatin as first-line therapy in patients with advanced gastric cancer: a randomised phase III noninferiority trial. *Ann Oncol* 2009;20:666–673.

368. Ajani JA, Rodriguez W, Bodoky G, et al. Multicenter phase III comparison of cisplatin/S-1 with cisplatin/infusional fluorouracil in advanced gastric or gastroesophageal adenocarcinoma study: the FLAGS trial. *J Clin Oncol* 2010;28:1547–1553.

369. Shah MA, Stoller R, Shibata S, et al. Random assignment multicenter phase II study of modified docetaxel, sisplatin, flourouracil (mDCF) versus DCF with growth factor support (GCSF) in metastatic gastroesophageal adenocarcinoma (GE). *J Clin Oncol* 2010;28:Abstr 4014.

370. Pozzo C, Barone C, Szanto J, et al. Irinotecan in combination with 5-fluorouracil and folinic acid or with cisplatin in patients with advanced gastric or esophageal-gastric junction adenocarcinoma: results of a randomized phase II study. *Ann Oncol* 2004;15:1773–1781.

371. Ross P, Nicolson M, Cunningham D, et al. Prospective randomized trial comparing mitomycin, cisplatin, and protracted venous-infusion fluorouracil (PVI 5-FU) with epirubicin, cisplatin, and PVI 5-FU in advanced esophagogastric cancer. *J Clin Oncol* 2002;20:1996–2004.

372. Shah MA, Ramanathan RK, Ilson DH, et al. Multicenter phase II study of irinotecan, cisplatin, and bevacizumab in patients with metastatic gastric or gastroesophageal junction adenocarcinoma. *J Clin Oncol* 2006;24:5201–5206.

373. Nardi M, Azzarello D, Maisano R, et al. FOLFOX-4 regimen as first-line chemotherapy in elderly patients with advanced gastric cancer: a safety study. *J Chemother* 2007;19:85–89.

374. Cunningham D, Okines AF, Ashley S, et al. Capecitabine and oxaliplatin for advanced esophagogastric cancer. *N Engl J Med* 2008;358:36–46.

375. Al-Batran SE, Hartmann JT, Probst S, et al. Phase III trial in metastatic gastroesophageal adenocarcinoma with fluorouracil, leucovorin plus either oxaliplatin or cisplatin: a study of the Arbeitsgemeinschaft Internistische Onkologie. *J Clin Oncol* 2008;26:1435–1442.

376. Catalano V, Graziano F, Santini D, et al. Second-line chemotherapy for patients with advanced gastric cancer: who may benefit? *Br J Cancer* 2008;99:1402–1407.

377. Lee J, Lim T, Uhm JE, et al. Prognostic model to predict survival following first-line chemotherapy in patients with metastatic gastric adenocarcinoma. *Ann Oncol* 2007;18:886–891.

378. Thuss-Patience PC, Kretzschmar A, Bichev D, et al. Survival advantage for irinotecan versus best supportive care as second-line chemotherapy in gastric cancer—a randomised phase III study of the Arbeitsgemeinschaft Internistische Onkologie (AIO). *Eur J Cancer* 2011;47:2306–2314.

379. Park SH, Lim DH, Park K, et al. A multicenter, randomized phase III trial comparing second-line chemotherapy (SLC) plus best supportive care (BSC) with BSC alone for pretreated advanced gastric cancer (AGC). *J Clin Oncol* 2011;29:Abstr 4004.

380. Hironaka S, Ueda S, Yasui H, et al. Randomized, open-label, phase III study comparing irinotecan with paclitaxel in patients with advanced gastric cancer without severe peritoneal metastasis after failure of prior combination chemotherapy using fluoropyrimidine plus platinum: WJOG 4007 trial. *J Clin Oncol* 2013;31:4438–4444.

381. Van Cutsem E, Kang Y, Chung H, et al. Efficacy results from the ToGA trial: a phase III study of trastuzumab added to standard chemotherapy (CT) in first-line human epidermal growth factor receptor 2 (HER2)-positive advanced gastric cancer (GC). *J Clin Oncol* 2009;27:Abstr LBA450.

382. Bang Y, Chung H, Sawaki A, et al. HER2-positivity rates in advanced gastric cancer (GC): results from a large international phase III trial. *J Clin Oncol* 2008;26:Abstr 4526.

383. Lordick F, Luber B, Lorenzen S, et al. Cetuximab plus oxaliplatin/leucovorin/5-fluorouracil in first-line metastatic gastric cancer: a phase II study of the Arbeitsgemeinschaft Internistische Onkologie (AIO). *Br J Cancer* 2010;102:500–505.

384. Kubo T, Kuroda Y, Shimizu H, et al. Resequencing and copy number analysis of the human tyrosine kinase gene family in poorly differentiated gastric cancer. *Carcinogenesis* 2009;30:1857–1864.

385. Kang Y, Ohtsu A, Van Cutsem E, et al. AVAGAST: a randomized, double blind, placebo-controlled, phase III study of first-line capecitabine and cisplatin plus bevacizumab or placebo in patients with advanced gastric cancer. *J Clin Oncol* 2010;28:LBA4007.

386. Shah MA, Ilson D, Kelsen DP. Thromboembolic events in gastric cancer: high incidence in patients receiving irinotecan- and bevacizumab-based therapy. *J Clin Oncol* 2005;23:2574–2576.

387. Ohtsu A, Shah MA, Van Cutsem E, et al. Bevacizumab in combination with chemotherapy as first-line therapy in advanced gastric cancer: a randomized, double-blind, placebo-controlled phase III study. *J Clin Oncol* 2011;29:3968–3976.

388. Van Cutsem E, de Haas S, Kang YK, et al. Bevacizumab in combination with chemotherapy as first-line therapy in advanced gastric cancer: a biomarker evaluation from the AVAGAST randomized phase III trial. *J Clin Oncol* 2102;30:2119–2127.

389. Bang Y, Kang Y, Kang W, et al. Preliminary results from a phase II study of sunitnib as second-line treatment for advanced gastric cancer. *Eur J Cancer* Suppl, 2007;5:272.

390. Li J, Qin S, Xu J, et al. Apatinib for chemotherapy-refractory advanced metastatic gastric cancer: results from a randomized, placebo-controlled, parallel-arm, phase II trial. *J Clin Oncol* 2013;31:3219-3225.

391. Fuchs CS, Tomasek J, Yong CJ, et al. Ramucirumab monotherapy for previously treated advanced gastric or gastro-oesophageal junction adenocarcinoma (REGARD): an internatinoal, randomised, multicenter, placebo-controlled, phase 3 trial. *Lancet* 2014;383:31–39.

392. Okamoto I, Doi T, Ohtsu A, et al. Phase I clinical and pharmacokinetic study of RAD001 (everolimus) administered daily to Japanese patients with advanced solid tumors. *Jpn J Clin Oncol* 2010;40:17–23.

393. Takiuchi H, Doi T, Muro K, et al. Everolimus in patients with previously treated metestatic gastric cancer: Final results of a multicenter Phase II study. *J Clin Oncol* 2010.

394. Doi T, Muro K, Boku N, et al. Multicenter phase II study of everolimus in patients with previously treated metastatic gastric cancer. *J Clin Oncol* 2010;28:1904–1910.

395. Metzger R, Leichman CG, Danenberg KD, et al. ERCC1 mRNA levels complement thymidylate synthase mRNA levels in predicting response and survival for gastric cancer patients receiving combination cisplatin and fluorouracil chemotherapy. *J Clin Oncol* 1998;16:309–316.

396. Ooi CH, Ivanova T, Wu J, et al. Oncogenic pathway combinations predict clinical prognosis in gastric cancer. *PLoS Genet* 2009;5:e1000676.

397. Kim HK, Choi IJ, Kim CG, et al. Gene expression signatures to predict the response of gastric cancer to cisplatin and fluorouracil. *J Clin Oncol* 2009; 27:Abstr 4628.

398. Janjigian Y, Kelsen DP, Ilson D, et al. HER2 status of patients with gastric cancer (GC) in the United States. *J Clin Oncol* 2010;27:Abstr 30.

399. Shah MA, Yeung H, Coit D, et al. A phase II study of preoperative chemotherapy with irinotecan(CPT) and cisplatin(CIS) for gastric cancer(NCI 5917): FDG-PET/CT predicts patient outcome. *J Clin Oncol* 2007;25:4502.

400. Weber WA. Chaperoning drug development with PET. *J Nucl Med* 2006; 47:735–737.

401. Kerkar SP, Kemp CD, Duffy A, et al. The GYMSSA trial: a prospective randomized trial comparing gastrectomy, metastasectomy plus systemic therapy versus systemic therapy alone. *Trials* 2009;10:121.

402. Kerkar SP, Kemp CD, Avital I. Liver resections for metastatic gastric cancer. *HPB (Oxford)* 2010;12:589–596.

403. Kemp CD, Kerkar KM, Ripley TR, et al. Pulmonary resection for metastatic gastric cancer. *J Thorac Oncol* 2010;5:1796–1805.

404. Okajima K, Yamada S. [Surgical treatment of far-advanced gastric cancer]. *Gan No Rinsho* 1986;32:1203–1209.

405. Sugarbaker PH, Yonemura Y. Clinical pathway for the management of resectable gastric cancer with peritoneal seeding: best palliation with a ray of hope for cure. *Oncology* 2000;58:96–107.

406. Boku T, Nakane Y, Minoura T, et al. Prognostic significance of serosal invasion and free intraperitoneal cancer cells in gastric cancer. *Br J Surg* 1990;77: 436–439.

407. Moriguchi S, Maehara Y, Korenaga D, et al. Risk factors which predict pattern of recurrence after curative surgery for patients with advanced gastric cancer. *Surg Oncol* 1992;1:341–346.

408. Roviello F, Marrelli D, de Manzoni G, et al. Prospective study of peritoneal recurrence after curative surgery for gastric cancer. *Br J Surg* 2003;90: 1113–1119.

409. Maehara Y, Hasuda S, Koga T, et al. Postoperative outcome and sites of recurrence in patients following curative resection of gastric cancer. *Br J Surg* 2000;87:353–357.

410. Lee CC, Lo SS, Wu CW, et al. Peritoneal recurrence of gastric adenocarcinoma after curative resection. *Hepatogastroenterology* 2003;50: 1720–1722.

411. Sadeghi B, Arvieux C, Glehen O, et al. Peritoneal carcinomatosis from nongynecologic malignancies: results of the EVOCAPE 1 multicentric prospective study. *Cancer* 2000;88:358–363.

412. Chu DZ, Lang NP, Thompson C, et al. Peritoneal carcinomatosis in nongynecologic malignancy. A prospective study of prognostic factors. *Cancer* 1989;63:364–367.

413. Yamada S, Takeda T, Matsumoto K. Prognostic analysis of malignant pleural and peritoneal effusions. *Cancer* 1983;51:136–140.

414. Glehen O, Gilly FN, Arvieux C, et al. Peritoneal carcinomatosis from gastric cancer: a multi-institutional study of 159 patients treated by cytoreductive surgery combined with perioperative intraperitoneal chemotherapy. *Ann Surg Oncol* 2010;17:2370–2377.

415. Yonemura Y, Kawamura T, Bandou E, et al. Treatment of peritoneal dissemination from gastric cancer by peritonectomy and chemohyperthermic peritoneal perfusion. *Br J Surg* 2005;92:370–375.

416. Hall JJ, Loggie BW, Shen P, et al. Cytoreductive surgery with intraperitoneal hyperthermic chemotherapy for advanced gastric cancer. *J Gastrointest Surg* 2004;8:454–463.

417. Brigand C, Arvieux C, Gilly FN, et al. Treatment of peritoneal carcinomatosis in gastric cancers. *Dig Dis* 2004;22:366–373.

418. Glehen O, Schreiber V, Cotte E, et al. Cytoreductive surgery and intraperitoneal chemohyperthermia for peritoneal carcinomatosis arising from gastric cancer. *Arch Surg* 2004;139:20–26.

419. Ajani JA, Ota DM, Jackson DE. Current strategies in the management of locoregional and metastatic gastric carcinoma. *Cancer* 1991;67:260–265.

420. Kusamura S, Baratti D, Younan R, et al. The Delphi approach to Attain consensus in methodology of local regional therapy for peritoneal surface malignancy. *J Surg Oncol* 2008;98:217–219.

421. Baratti D, Kusamura S, Deraco M. The Fifth International Workshop on Peritoneal Surface Malignancy (Milan, Italy, December 4–6, 2006): methodology of disease-specific consensus. *J Surg Oncol* 2008;98:258–262.

422. Younan R, Kusamura S, Baratti D, et al. Morbidity, toxicity, and mortality classification systems in the local regional treatment of peritoneal surface malignancy. *J Surg Oncol* 2008;98:253–257.

423. Gonzalez-Moreno S, Kusamura S, Baratti D, et al. Postoperative residual disease evaluation in the locoregional treatment of peritoneal surface malignancy. *J Surg Oncol* 2008;98:237–241.

424. Verwaal VJ, Kusamura S, Baratti D, et al. The eligibility for local-regional treatment of peritoneal surface malignancy. *J Surg Oncol* 2008;98:220–223.

425. Canbay E, Mizumoto A, Ichinose M, et al. Outcome data of patients with peritoneal carcinomatosis from gastric origin treated by a strategy of bidirectional chemotherapy prior to cytoreductive surgery and hyperthermic intraperitoneal chemotherapy in a single specialized center in Japan. *Ann Surg Oncol* 2014;21:1147–1152.

426. Ekbom GA, Gleysteen JJ. Gastric malignancy: resection for palliation. *Surgery* 1980;88:476–481.

427. Meijer S, De Bakker OJ, Hoitsma HF. Palliative resection in gastric cancer. *J Surg Oncol* 1983;23:77–80.

428. Butler JA, Dubrow TJ, Trezona T, et al. Total gastrectomy in the treatment of advanced gastric cancer. *Am J Surg* 1989;158:602–604, discussion 604–605.

429. Bozzetti F, Doci P, Bignami P, et al. Patterns of failure following surgical resection of colorectal cancer liver metastases. Rationale for a multimodal approach. *Ann Surg* 1987;205:264–270.

430. Bozzetti F, Bonfanti G, Audisio RA, et al. Prognosis of patients after palliative surgical procedures for carcinoma of the stomach. *Surg Gynecol Obstet* 1987; 164:151–154.

431. Boddie AW Jr, McMurtrey MJ, Giacco GG, et al. Palliative total gastrectomy and esophagogastrectomy: a reevaluation. *Cancer* 1983;51:1195–1200.

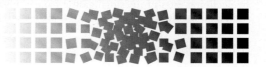

39 Genetic Testing in Stomach Cancer

Nicki Chun and James M. Ford

INTRODUCTION

Gastric cancer encompasses a heterogeneous collection of etiologic and histologic subtypes associated with a variety of known and unknown environmental and genetic factors. It is a global public health concern, accounting for 700,000 annual deaths worldwide, and currently ranks as the fourth leading cause of cancer mortality, with a 5-year survival of only 20%. The incidence and prevalence of gastric cancer vary widely, with Asian/Pacific regions bearing the highest rates of disease.

Recent and rapid advances in molecular genetics have provided an understanding of the cause for many inherited cancer syndromes, offering possibilities for individual genetic testing, family counseling, and preventive approaches. For most cancer syndromes, however, not every individual tested is found to have inherited a germ-line mutation in a candidate gene, suggesting additional uncharacterized alterations in other genes that result in similar outcomes. Nevertheless, the ability to genetically define many individuals and families with inherited cancer syndromes allows for a multidisciplinary approach to their management, often including the consideration of surgical and medical preventive measures. Without question, such complex management and decision making should be centered in the high-risk cancer genetics clinic, where physicians, genetic counselors, and other health professionals jointly consider optimal management for patients and families at high risk for developing cancer.

Approximately 3% to 5% of gastric cancers are associated with a hereditary predisposition, including a variety of Mendelian genetic conditions and complex genetic traits. Identifying those gastric cancers associated with an inherited cancer risk syndrome is the purview of cancer genetics clinics. The keystone to any cancer genetics evaluation is a complete, three-generation family history. Pedigree analyses suggesting an inherited gastric cancer risk include familiar features such as multiple affected relatives tracking along one branch of the family in an autosomal-dominant pattern, young ages at onset, and additional associated malignancies related to an identified syndrome. It is imperative to document the histology of the gastric tumors and other familial cancers because this is the initial node in the decision tree of an inherited gastric cancer syndrome differential. Finally, there are clinical criteria for recognized gastric cancer syndromes published by expert consensus panels that assist genetic practitioners in assessing both the likelihood of identifying an underlying germ-line DNA mutation and guide management in the absence of a molecular confirmation. Herein, we review the literature regarding incidence, recurrence risks, and defined gastric cancer genetic syndromes to assist in providing genetic counseling for families affected by gastric cancer.

HISTOLOGIC DEFINITIONS AND DESCRIPTIONS

Gastric cancer has traditionally been subtyped pathologically according to Lauren's[1] classification published in 1965 and revised by Carneiro et al.[2] in 1995. The four histologic categories include: (1) glandular/intestinal, (2) border foveal hyperplasia, (3) mixed intestinal/diffuse, and (4) solid/undifferentiated.

More clinically relevant, the majority of gastric cancers can be subdivided into intestinal type or diffuse type. Diffuse tumors exhibit isolated cells that typically develop below the mucosal lining and often spread and thicken until the stomach appears hardened into the morphologic designation called *linitis plastica*. Diffuse gastric tumors frequently feature *signet ring cells*, named for the marginalization of the nucleus to the cell periphery due to high mucin content. Intestinal-type gastric tumors more often present as solid masses with atrophic gastritis and intestinal metaplasia at the periphery. The intestinal subtype is seen more commonly in older patients, whereas the diffuse type affects younger patients and has a more aggressive clinical course. The relative proportions of gastric cancer subtypes worldwide are 74% intestinal versus 16% diffuse and 10% other,[3] although diffuse gastric cancer is becoming relatively more common in Western countries. The importance of distinguishing these two main histopathologic types of gastric cancer is highlighted by finding specific genetic changes associated with the different types. For the purposes of genetic counseling, E-cadherin (*CDH1*) mutations are found exclusively in the diffuse type.[4–8] Whereas intestinal-type hereditary gastric cancer families have been identified clinically, no genetic associations have yet been discovered.

As individual molecular profiling of solid tumors becomes more common in the future, we expect classification systems will evolve based on tumor biology more than histology. Advances in deciphering the mechanisms of gene alterations that lead to gastric cancer include gene mutation, amplification, deletion, and epigenetic methylation.[9] For example, two recent studies have performed whole-exome sequencing of human gastric tumors and identified a number of known (e.g., *p53*, *PTEN*, *PIK3CA*), but also previously unreported somatic gene mutations and pathway alterations. Both found *ARID1A* inactivating gene mutations in the majority of microsatellite-instable tumors, a member of the SWI-SNF chromatin remodeling family.[10,11] However, whether any of these somatic gene alterations are found to confer cancer risk when mutated in the germ line remains to be determined.

ETIOLOGY

Analogous to other common cancers, a host of factors are implicated as causes of gastric cancer. Widely diverse geographical disparities suggest both environmental and genetic contributions. Furthermore, a strong association with endemic *Helicobacter pylori* carrier rates implicates infection as a major risk factor. There are likely to be a host of factors contributing to the development of most gastric cancers.

Environmental Risk Factors

Geographic variations in gastric cancer rates have prompted investigations of shared diet and lifestyle variables. Gastric cancer is correlated with the chronic ingestion of pickled vegetables, salted fish, excessive dietary salt, smoked meats, and with smoking.[12–16]

Fruits and vegetables may have a protective effect. The influence of environmental factors as causes of gastric cancer is highlighted by declining rates of intestinal gastric cancer among immigrants from high-incident countries to low-incident countries.

Infectious Risk Factors

H. pylori infection is endemic in the Asian–Pacific basin.[17] Transmission routinely occurs through family contacts in childhood and leads to atrophic gastritis.[18,19] As evidenced by high indigenous infection rates, *H. pylori* is insufficient to singularly cause gastric cancer, suggesting complex interactions between virus and host genetic backgrounds. However, *H. pylori* species are consistently implicated as a major risk factor primarily associated with intestinal-type gastric cancer. Studies in a variety of high- and low-risk populations have found odds ratios ranging from 2.56 to 6 for noncardia gastric cancer.[20]

The Epstein-Barr virus has recently been implicated in about 10% of gastric carcinoma worldwide, or an estimated 80,000 cases annually. Epstein-Barr virus–associated gastric cancer shows some distinct clinicopathologic characteristics, such as male predominance, predisposition to the proximal stomach, and a high proportion in diffuse-type gastric carcinomas. Mechanistically, Epstein-Barr virus gastric tumors display epigenetic promoter methylation of many cancer-related genes, causing downregulation of their expression.[21]

Genetics

Five to 10% of gastric cancer is associated with strong familial clustering and attributable to genetic factors. Shared environmental factors account for the majority of familial clustering of the intestinal type; however, approximately 5% of the total gastric cancer burden is thought to be due to germ-line mutations in genes causing highly penetrant, autosomal-dominant gastric cancer risk of both intestinal and diffuse subtypes. We review the definitions of hereditary gastric cancer families and recognize genetic syndromes associated with increased gastric cancer risk.

EPIDEMIOLOGY OF GASTRIC CANCER

Gastric cancer is now the fourth most common malignancy worldwide, with rates having fallen steadily since 1975 when global statistics were first compared. The incidence and prevalence of gastric cancer vary widely among world populations. High-risk countries (reported incidence × 100,000 per year) include Korea (41.4), China (41.3), Japan (31.1), Portugal (34.4), and Colombia (20.3). Intermediate-risk countries include Malaysia, Singapore, and Taiwan (11 to 19, respectively), whereas low-risk areas include Thailand (8), Northern Europe (5.6), Australia (5.4), India (5.3), and North America (4.3). More than 70% of cases occur in developing countries, and men have roughly twice the risk of women.[22] In 2008, estimates of gastric cancer burden in the United States were 21,500 cases (13,190 men and 8,310 women) and 10,880 deaths.[23] The median age at diagnosis for gastric cancer is 71 years, and 5-year survival is approximately 25%.[24] Only 24% of stomach cancers are localized at the time of diagnosis, 30% have lymph node involvement, and another 30% have metastatic disease. Survival rates are predictably higher for those with localized disease, with corresponding 5-year survival rates of 60%.

The worldwide decline in the incidence of gastric cancer has been attributed to modifications in diet, improved food storage and preservation, and decreased *H. pylori* infection. Fresh fruit and vegetable consumption, refrigeration, decreased urban crowding, and improved living conditions have reduced *H. pylori* exposure and carrier rates. By contrast, the incidence of diffuse-type gastric cancer is stable, and in North America, it may even be increasing.[16,25–27]

TABLE 39.1

Clinical Criteria for CDH1 Testing Defined by the 2010 International Gastric Cancer Linkage Consortium

1. Two gastric cancer cases in the family: one confirmed diffuse type and one diagnosed at the age of <50 y
2. Three confirmed diffuse gastric cancers in first- or second-degree relatives independent of age
3. Diffuse gastric cancer diagnosed at age <40 y (no additional family history needed)
4. Personal or family history (first- or second-degree) of diffuse gastric cancer and lobular breast cancer, one diagnosed at age <50 y

From Fitzgerald RC, Hardwick R, Huntsman D, et al. Hereditary diffuse gastric cancer: Updated consensus guidelines for clinical management and directions for future research. *J Med Genet* 2010;47:436–444.

Familial Gastric Cancer

Shared environmental factors, such as diet and *H. pylori* infection, account for the majority of familial clustering of the intestinal type of gastric cancer, with no known causative germ-line variants. However, few nongenetic risks for diffuse gastric cancer have been identified, supporting a larger role for hereditary factors. Approximately 5% of the total gastric cancer burden is thought to be due to germ-line mutations in genes causing a highly penetrant, autosomal-dominant predisposition. The International Gastric Cancer Linkage Consortium (IGCLC) has redefined genetic classification of familial intestinal gastric cancer to reflect the background incidence rate in a population (Table 39.1).

Thus, countries with high incidence of intestinal-type gastric cancer (China, Korea, Japan, Portugal) use criteria analogous to the Amsterdam criteria invoked for Lynch syndrome:

- At least three relatives with intestinal gastric cancer, one a first-degree relative of the other two
- At least two successive generations affected, and
- Gastric cancer diagnosed before the age of 50 years in at least one individual

In countries with a low incidence of intestinal-type gastric cancer (United States, United Kingdom):

- At least two first-/second-degree relatives affected by intestinal gastric cancer, one diagnosed before the age of 50 years, or
- Three or more relatives with intestinal gastric cancer at any age

Familial intestinal gastric cancer families are similarly prevalent as familial diffuse gastric cancer families, yet a germ-line genetic defect underlying the disease remains to be identified.[28] Hemminki et al.[29] reported Swedish data on all available types of cancer in first-degree relatives by both parent and sibling probands. The relative risks (RR) for gastric cancer were greater than 3 for siblings with any relative with gastric cancer and greater than 5 when a sibling was younger than 50 years. Shin et al.[30] assessed 428 gastric cancer subjects and 368 controls in Korea for the risk of gastric cancer in first-degree relatives and found an RR of 2.85 with one first-degree relative and greater than 5 in a first-degree relative with *H. pylori* and a positive family history. Therefore, in the high-incident countries of Japan and Taiwan, population screening for gastric cancer has greatly enhanced early detection, leading to 5-year survival rates of greater than 90%.[31]

Hereditary Diffuse Gastric Cancer

In 1999, the first IGCLC defined hereditary diffuse gastric cancer (HDGC) as families with (1) two cases diffuse gastric cancer in first-/second-degree relatives with one younger than 50 years, and

(2) three cases diffuse gastric cancer at any age.[32] The first clear evidence for a gastric cancer susceptibility genetic locus was the identification in 1998 of a germ-line inactivating mutation in the gene encoding for E-cadherin (CDH1) in a large, five-generation Maori family from New Zealand with 25 kindred with early-onset diffuse gastric cancer.[33] The age at diagnosis of gastric cancer ranged upward from 14 years, with the majority occurring in individuals younger than 40 years. The pattern of inheritance of gastric cancer was consistent with an autosomal-dominant susceptibility gene with incomplete penetrance. Similar reports of CDH1 mutations in widely diverse HDGC cohorts from Asia, Europe, and North America followed soon thereafter.[34–39] Germ-line CDH1 mutations have been found to be associated with approximately 30% of families with HDGC, with a lifetime risk for gastric cancer of greater than 80%, and up to 60% risk for female carriers developing lobular breast cancer.[40] To date, CDH1 is the only gene implicated in HDGC. Worldwide, about 100 CDH1 mutation–positive families have been reported.[41]

E-cadherin Mutations and Gastric Cancer

The E-cadherin gene coding sequence gives rise to a mature protein consisting of three major domains, a large extracellular domain (exons 4 to 13), smaller transmembranes (exons 13 to 14), and cytoplasmic domains (exons 14 to 16). As in other autosomal-dominant cancer predisposing genes, only one CDH1 allele is mutated in the germ line, and the majority of genetic changes lead to truncation of the protein, with mutations distributed throughout the gene's 2.6 kb of coding sequence and 16 exons without any apparent hotspots. Somatic CDH1 mutations have been identified in about half of sporadic diffuse gastric cancers, but occur rarely in intestinal gastric cancer. CDH1 encodes the calcium-dependent cell-adhesion glycoprotein E-cadherin. E-cadherin is a transmembrane protein that connects to the actin cytoskeleton through a complex with catenin proteins.[5,42] Functionally, E-cadherin impacts the maintenance of normal tissue morphology and cellular differentiation. With regard to HDGC, it is believed that CDH1 acts as a tumor suppressor gene, with the mutation of CDH1 leading to a loss of cell adhesion, proliferation, invasion, and metastasis.[43]

Genetic Testing for HDGC

At the second meeting of the IGCLC in 2010, HDGC guidelines[44] were extended to recommend CDH1 genetic testing to families with the following:

- Cases of gastric cancer in which one case is histopathologically confirmed as diffuse and younger than 50 years
- Families with both lobular breast cancer and diffuse gastric cancer, with one diagnosed younger than 50 years
- Probands diagnosed with diffuse gastric cancer younger than 40 years, with no family history of gastric cancer

Using the initial IGCLC criteria for HDGC, CDH1 mutation testing yielded a detection rate of 30% to 50%.[45] Interestingly, a pattern began to emerge of lower CDH1 mutation rates among HDGC families in high gastric cancer incidence populations and higher rates in low-incident countries.[46,47] Other reports suggest that the rate of CDH1 mutations in isolated cases of diffuse gastric cancer younger than 35 years is similar in both low- and high-risk countries, hovering at around 20%.[48] Approximately 50% to 70% of clinically diagnosed HDGC families have no identifiable genetic mutation. Multiple candidate loci have been investigated without identifying causative mutations that would account for the large number of non-CDH1 HDGC families.[49–51] Huntsman's group has published a report of multiplex ligation-dependent probe amplification-based exon duplication/deletion studies performed on 93 non-CDH1 families

and found 6.5% carried large genomic deletions, bringing the detection rate up to 45.6% in their cohort of 160 families.[52]

As CDH1 mutation families were identified, data on these families provided the foundation for genetic counseling information. Initially, the cumulative risk of gastric cancer by the age of 80 years in HDGC families was initially estimated as 67% for men and 83% for women. The age at onset shows marked variation between and within families. The median age at onset in the 30 Maori CDH1 mutation carriers who developed gastric cancer was 32 years, which was significantly younger than the median age of 43 years in individuals with gastric cancer from other ethnicities.[53] More recent reports of the lifetime risks of diffuse gastric cancer suggest greater than 80% in both men and women by the age of 80 years.[48,54]

The lifetime risk for lobular breast cancer among female CDH1 carriers, originally estimated to be in the range of 20% to 40%, now approaches 60%, with an average age of 53 years at the time of diagnosis.[36,54,55] Of note, CDH1 mutations have been seen in up to 50% of sporadic lobular breast cancer. Pathologic similarities between diffuse gastric and lobular breast carcinomas such as high mucin content with associated signet ring features and loss of E-cadherin on immunohistochemistry hint at a common molecular mechanism.[56,57] To evaluate the CDH1 carrier rate in women with lobular breast cancer without a family history of diffuse gastric cancer, a multicenter study of 318 women with lobular-type breast cancer diagnosed before the age of 45 years and known to be BRCA1/2-negative were sequenced for CDH1 mutations. Only four possibly pathogenic mutations were identified for a rate of 1.3%, suggesting CDH1 is a rare cause of early lobular cancer without associated gastric cancer family history.[58]

Signet ring colon cancer has been reported in two families with germ-line CDH1, but no screening guidelines have been suggested.[45,59] Nonsyndromic cleft lip and/or palate was reported in seven individuals from three families in the Netherlands and in four individuals from two families in France. There is speculation that defects in the cell-adhesion role of E-cadherin may contribute to this developmental anomaly, although no association can be drawn from these scant case reports.[40,60]

Like other familial cancer syndromes with an autosomal-dominant inheritance pattern, high penetrance for heterozygotes, and significant mortality unless diagnosed early, genetic counseling and testing should occur early, and a comprehensive screening plan should be developed, as well as the consideration of prophylactic surgery. Pretest and posttest genetic counseling should be provided to individuals from HDGC kindred who are undergoing genetic testing for germ-line CDH1 mutations. Because cases of gastric cancer in HDGC families have been reported in individuals as young as 14 years, HDGC may be considered one of the sets of hereditary cancer syndromes, such as MEN 2–associated medullary thyroid cancer, Li–Fraumeni syndrome (LFS), and familial adenomatous polyposis (FAP), in which genetic testing is potentially clinically useful in children.

SCREENING AND MANAGEMENT OF CANCER RISK IN HDGC

Diagnosing gastric cancer in its early stages provides the best chance for curative resection but is a difficult task. Symptoms due to gastric cancer are generally nonspecific and do not appear until the disease is more advanced. The survival of early gastric cancer (e.g., not beyond the mucosa or submucosa) is much better than advanced lesions, so identifying these lesions at the earliest of stages is imperative for optimal survival. Endoscopy is generally considered to be the best method to screen for gastric cancer, but diagnosing diffuse gastric carcinoma is most difficult, because these lesions tend not to form a grossly visible exophytic mass, but rather spread submucosally as single cells or clustered islands of cells. Improved chromoendoscopic-aided methods for directed biopsies to diagnose these early diffuse lesions may prove beneficial, but so far all approaches at screening, including computed tomography and positron emission tomography imaging, have proven disappointing.[61]

Given the inadequacy of clinical screening in HDGC, prophylactic total gastrectomy is offered to carriers of germ-line *CDH1* mutations.[62,63] In every published series of this approach, nearly all specimens contain multiple foci of intramucosal diffuse signet ring cell cancer. Currently, there is information available from 96 total gastrectomies in the setting of HDGC,[44] approximately three-quarters of which were performed in asymptomatic *CDH1* carriers following negative screening endoscopy and biopsies. Only three cases did not show evidence for early invasive carcinoma, and in two of these, tiny foci of in situ signet ring cell carcinoma were observed.[44] Although malignant foci are generally localized to the proximal one-third of the stomach,[64] lesions may be distributed throughout the entire stomach, necessitating a total gastrectomy for comprehensive prevention. The optimal timing of prophylactic gastrectomy is unknown but is generally recommended when the unaffected carrier is 5 years younger than the youngest family member who has developed clinical symptoms of HDGC. Clinical management and screening strategies remain uncertain for families who meet criteria for HDGC but are negative for *CDH1* mutations or variants of unknown significance, although a screening endoscopy is often suggested.

The impact and long-term outcomes of prophylactic gastrectomy on carriers' lifestyle and health are significant, particularly because 20% to 30% of carriers may never develop invasive gastric cancer. Certainly, all patients experience some level of morbidity, including diarrhea, weight loss, and difficulty eating. Mortality due to this indication for a gastrectomy has not been reported. Early evidence suggests that women can successfully carry healthy pregnancies after a gastrectomy.[65] Most importantly, to date, there have been no reports of gastric cancer recurrence in a member of an HDGC family after a prophylactic total gastrectomy.

Women with HDGC also exhibit up to 60% lifetime risk for developing breast cancer, primarily of the lobular type, and as more women are prevented from developing diffuse gastric cancer, breast cancer screening is of great relevance. The correct approach to screening for lobular breast cancer in women with HDGC is not known, but is based on approaches used in other hereditary breast cancer susceptibility syndromes. Although prophylactic mastectomies have been shown to effectively prevent the development of breast cancer and result in improved long-term survival in *BRCA1/2* mutation carriers, such an approach remains completely investigational for women in HDGC families. The prognosis of lobular cancers that develop in HDGC patients is currently unknown, and given the relatively late onset compared with breast cancers in *BRCA1/2* carriers, prophylactic mastectomies may not be appropriate. Therefore, standard screening recommendations include annual breast magnetic resonance imaging (MRI) and mammogram starting at the age of 35 years.[66,67] An open question is whether chemoprevention with tamoxifen may benefit women with HDGC, given its role in reducing breast cancer risk in half in women at elevated risk because of age, family history, or history of biopsy-proven lobular carcinoma in situ.[68]

In summary, individuals from HDGC families with inherited germ-line mutations in the *CDH1* gene face up to an 80% likelihood of developing gastric cancer and, for women, an additional 60% chance of developing lobular breast cancer during their lifetime, with significant risk beginning at relatively young ages. Such levels of overall cancer risk are similar to that of developing breast or colon cancer for carriers of *BRCA1* or 2 gene mutations, or mismatch repair gene mutations, respectively. Therefore, rigorous surveillance and the consideration of prophylactic surgery are important for the management of these individuals. At the very least, a regular endoscopic examination with a random biopsy of the stomach should be performed every 6 to 12 months, probably starting 10 years earlier than the youngest affected patient in the

family, or by the age of 25 years. Because mucosal abnormalities tend to occur late in diffuse gastric cancer and delay the endoscopic diagnosis, a prophylactic gastrectomy should be seriously considered as a means of preventing gastric carcinoma, although it clearly comes with high morbidity. It is somewhat less clear as to the correct approach for the screening and prevention of lobular breast cancer in women with HDGC. Adherence to standard recommendations for screening mammographies for breast cancer should be followed. The consideration of investigative approaches to screening with MRI and chemoprevention with tamoxifen or other agents are appropriate. The decision to perform a prophylactic gastrectomy should be balanced with age-based risk, based on age-specific penetrance data, as well as many other personal factors. Therefore, it is essential that patients carrying the gene have the opportunity for extensive counseling, discussion, and reflection with knowledgeable clinicians, geneticists, and counselors before making the decision to proceed.

OTHER HEREDITARY CANCER SUSCEPTIBILITY SYNDROMES WITH INCREASED GASTRIC CANCER RISK

Lynch Syndrome

The seminal report of a family with dominantly inherited colon and gastrointestinal (GI) cancers in 1979 by Lynch and Lynch[69] began decades of defining and refining this hereditary syndrome. Lynch syndrome is caused by a germ-line mutation in a mismatch DNA repair gene (*MLH1, MSH2, MSH6, PMS2,* or *EPCAM*) and is thus associated with tumors exhibiting microsatellite instability (MSI). It is estimated that 2% to 4% of all diagnosed colorectal cancers[70] and 2% to 5% of all diagnosed endometrial cancers[71] are due to Lynch syndrome. With a frequency estimated at 1 in 440 in the United States,[72] it is similar to the BRCA carriage rate. The lifetime risks for Lynch syndrome–associated cancers are highest for colorectal cancer at 52% to 82% (mean age at diagnosis, 44 to 61 years), followed by an endometrial cancer risk of 25% to 60% in women (mean age at diagnosis, 48 to 62 years), a 6% to 13% risk for gastric cancer (mean age at diagnosis, 56 years), and 4% to 12% for ovarian cancer (mean age at diagnosis, 42.5 years).[70–78]

Lynch syndrome–associated gastric cancers predominantly show intestinal histology (more than 90% of the cases). This correlation echoes the strong association between MSI tumor phenotype and intestinal gastric cancer. The International Collaborative Group on hereditary nonpolyposis colorectal cancer (HNPCC) developed the original Amsterdam Criteria in 1991. Revisions followed, with Bethesda criteria outlined in 1997 and revisions in 2004 with the inclusion of extracolonic tumor risks, including gastric cancer.[79,80]

MSI screening by molecular and/or immunohistochemistry for the four common Lynch protein products (MSH2, MSH6, MLH1, and PMS2) should be considered in families who meet the Bethesda criteria. Because 15% of all gastric tumors exhibit MSI histology, the majority of these have acquired this mutator phenotype through sporadic mutations, and further germ-line testing of individuals with MSI-positive tumors is necessary to confirm a molecular diagnosis of Lynch syndrome.

Hereditary Breast Ovarian Cancer Syndrome

Hereditary breast and ovarian cancer due to germ-line *BRCA1* and *BRCA2* mutations is perhaps the most well-defined and recognized inherited cancer syndrome. With a prevalence of 1 in 300 to 400 in most populations and up to 1 in 40 in selected groups with founder mutations (most notably those with Ashkenazi Jewish ancestry), it represents the most common of the hereditary disorders due to high-risk mutations. Carriers face a five- to six-fold increased risk of generally early-onset breast cancer and 10- to 20-fold increased risk for ovarian, fallopian, and primary peritoneal malignancies. Male carriers have a recognized increased risk for prostate cancer and male breast cancer. *BRCA1* and *BRCA2* have been implicated in multiple cellular functions but serve primary roles as tumor suppressor genes recruited to maintain genomic stability through DNA double-strand break repair. Following the cloning of the *BRCA1* and *BRCA2* genes in 1994 and 1995,[81,82] the Breast Cancer Linkage Consortium convened to pool data and generate a body of clinical information to assist in the counseling and management of BRCA carriers, resulting in a seminal publication outlining the spectrum of *BRCA* mutation–associated cancer risks. In 173 breast–ovarian cancer families with *BRCA2* mutations from 20 centers in Europe and North America, the RR of gastric cancer was 2.59 (95% confidence interval [CI], 1.46 to 4.61).[83] Carriers of the 6174 delT *BRCA2* Ashkenazi Jewish founder mutation in Israel found gastric cancer to be the most common malignancy after breast and ovarian. Conversely, 5.7% of patients with gastric cancer in Israel were found to carry this *BRCA2* mutation[84]; 20.7% of a Polish cohort of families with both gastric and breast malignancies were attributable to mutations in *BRCA2*. A *BRCA2* mutation was also found in 23.5% of women with ovarian cancer and a family history of stomach cancer in this population.[85,86]

Several studies have implicated *BRCA1* mutations as a risk factor for gastric cancer. A large Swedish population-based study published in 1999 involving 150 malignant tumors from 1,145 relatives in *BRCA1* found an RR of 5.86 (95% CI, 1.60 to 15.01) and observed that gastric cancer diagnosed before the age of 70 years was twice as common in carrier families compared with the general population. They did not observe the same risk with *BRCA2*.[87,88]

Brose et al.[89] observed the highest RR for gastric cancer (6.9) in 147 families with *BRCA1* mutations in Pennsylvania. Risch et al.[90] also observed an RR of 6.2 in first-degree relatives of 39 *BRCA1* mutation carrier families and, to a lesser extent, in 21 *BRCA2* families in Ontario, Canada.

More recently, a meta-analysis of more than 30 studies of tumor risk in *BRCA1* and *BRCA2* carriers found an RR of 1.69 (95% CI, 1.21 to 2.38) for gastric cancer, the highest risk after breast, ovarian, and prostate, followed closely by pancreatic cancer, with an RR of 1.62 (1.31 to 2.00).[91] No pathology details were included in these studies, and it is unknown if one of the histologic subtypes of gastric cancer predominates in BRCA-associated tumors.

Familial Adenomatous Polyposis

FAP is a rare colon cancer syndrome associated with the striking presentation of early-onset multiple colonic adenomas and, in classic form, a near-complete certainty of early colon cancer without prophylactic surgical intervention. Incidence estimates for FAP range from 1 in 10,000 to 20,000, and almost one-third of those diagnosed carry a de novo mutation, making family history unreliable for ascertainment of many cases. Extracolonic findings include upper GI adenomas, fundic gland polyps, and desmoids tumors. A wide spectrum of extracolonic tumors can occur, including relatively rare cancers such as hepatoblastomas, duodenal adenocarcinomas, and adrenal, pancreatic, thyroid, biliary tract, and brain tumors. Additional diagnostic aids can include the finding of congenital hypertrophy of the retinal pigment epithelium, supernumerary teeth, osteomas, cutaneous lipomas, and cysts.

It is estimated that the lifetime risk for upper GI cancer in FAP is approximately 4% to 12%, of which only 0.5% to 2% are gastric cancers, although this risk has been reported as 7- to 10-fold higher in Asia.[75,92,93] Approximately 50% of individuals with FAP have gastric fundus polyps, and 10% have adenomas of the stomach. Although gastric fundus polyps are unlikely to have malignancy potential, gastric adenomas can occasionally develop into invasive

disease.[94] Prophylactic gastrectomies are even discussed for diffuse fundic gland polyps showing high-grade dysplasia or large polyps.[95] Attenuated FAP is a muted form of classic FAP characterized by fewer than 100 colonic adenoma, a later median age and lower overall risk of colon cancer, and a high proportion of fundic gland polyps, suggesting a measurable risk for gastric cancer.[96–99]

Li–Fraumeni Syndrome

LFS is a devastating cancer syndrome with an extremely high risk for a multitude of tumor types. The most common malignancies are early-onset breast cancers and sarcomas, followed by brain tumors, leukemia, lung cancer, and then gastric cancer.[100] Four families were originally described by Drs. Li and Fraumeni[101] in 1969. The risk of an initial primary cancer is 50% by the age of 30 years and 90% by the age of 70 years,[102] with sex-specific differences in lifetime cancer risk of 73% in males and close to 100% in females primarily accounted for by an excessively high breast cancer risk.[103] There are high risks for multiple primary cancers, with 60% of carriers developing a second tumor and 4% developing a third malignancy.[104] Previously thought to be extraordinarily rare with an incidence of 1 in 50,000 to 100,000, recently relaxed testing criteria suggest the actual carrier rate may be several times higher. Of individuals who meet classic LFS clinical criteria, 70% are found to carry a *TP53* germ-line mutation. The de novo mutation rate is now estimated at 7% to 20%.[105] A negative family history can no longer exclude the consideration of LFS, and clinical criteria have been updated to recommend P53 testing for single cases of adrenal cortical carcinoma, choroid plexus carcinoma, and breast cancer under the age of 30 years.

Although not one of the hallmark tumors of LFS, the International Agency for Research on Cancer database reports that gastric cancer is frequency seen in up to 2.8% of LFS families.[106] Somatic *TP53* alterations are associated with both the intestinal and diffuse forms of gastric cancer in equal frequency. However, *TP53* constitutional mutations are very rarely documented in the overall gastric cancer mutational spectrum. Among 62 TP53 mutant LFS families seen at the Dana-Farber Cancer Institute in Boston and the National Cancer Institute, gastric cancer was diagnosed in 4.9% of affected members.[107] The mean and median ages at gastric cancer diagnosis were 43 and 36 years, respectively (range, 24 to 74 years), compared with the median age of 71 years in the general population based on Surveillance Epidemiology and End Results (SEER) data. Five families (8.1%) reported two or more cases of gastric cancer. A pathology review of the available tumors revealed both intestinal and diffuse histologies. A study of 180 families with LFS in the Netherlands found a concordant rate of gastric cancer among carriers with an RR of 2.6 (95% CI, 0.5 to 7.7).[108]

Peutz–Jeghers Syndrome

Peutz–Jeghers syndrome (PJS) is a rare inherited disorder of GI hamartomas, polyposis, and, most strikingly, early development of pigmented lesions on the lips, oral mucosa, and fingers. Incidence rates are estimated in the range of 1 in 25,000 to 250,000. Initially described by Peutz[109] in 1921 and subsequently by Jeghers et al.[110] in 1949, PJS is characterized by both hamartomatous and adenomatous polyposis throughout the GI tract and a high predisposition to GI malignancies. The clinical diagnosis of PJS is made on the basis of histologically confirmed hamartomatous polyps and two of the following: (1) positive family history, (2) hyperpigmentation of the digits and mucosa of the external genitalia, and (3) small bowel polyposis.[111] The mucocutaneous hyperpigmentation characteristically occurs on the buccal mucosa or near the eyes, nose, mouth, axilla, or fingertips. Typically noticeable by the age of 5 years, they frequently fade by puberty. Classic pigmented lesions in a first-degree relative of a diagnosed individual are sufficient to meet criteria for PJS.

TABLE 39.2

Inherited Cancer Syndromes with Associated Gastric Cancer Risks

Cancer Syndrome	Gene	Frequency	Gastric Cancer Risk (%)	Reference
HDGC	CDH1	Vary rare	>801	Fitzgerald et al.[44]
Hereditary breast/ovarian cancer	BRCA1/2	1/40–1/400	2.6–5.5	Brose et al.[89]
Lynch syndrome	MLH1, MSH2, MSH6, PMS2, Epcam	1/440	6–13	Chen et al.,[72] Watson et al.[77]
Li–Fraumeni syndrome	P53	1/5,000	2.8	Gonzalez et al.[105]
FAP	APC	1/10–20,000	0.5–2.0	Garrean et al.[92]
Juvenile polyposis	SMAD4, BMPR1A	1/16–100,000	21	Howe et al.[121]
PJS	STK11	1/25–250,000	29	Giardiello et al.,[113] van Lier et al.[114]

Chronic GI bleeds, anemia, and recurrent obstruction due to intussusception are frequent complications and often require surgical intervention. Among GI cancers, gastric cancer was found to be the third most frequent tumor in PJS, after small intestine and colorectal carcinoma. The cumulative cancer risk is 47% at the age of 65 years.[112] RRs reported for colon, stomach, and small intestine neoplasms have been as high as 84, 213, and over 500, respectively.[113] Increased risk is also present for other GI cancers (e.g., pancreatic, esophageal), as well as neoplasms outside the GI tract (lung, breast, ovarian, and endometrial). Other tumors associated with PJS are benign ovarian tumors called sex cord tumors with annular tubules, calcifying Sertoli tumors of the testes, and adenoma malignum of the cervix.

A Dutch team reviewed 20 PJS cohort studies and 1 meta-analysis published between 1975 and 2007 with a total of 1,644 patients.[114,115] They found the cumulative lifetime risks of GI cancers of 38% to 66%, and for all cancers, a lifetime risk range of 37% to 93%. Specifically, the gastric cancer risks were 29%, the third most common malignancy after colorectal and breast cancers. Understandably, this prompted a call for screening upper endoscopies every 2 to 5 years starting at the age of 20 years, whereas others suggested initiating endoscopies at the age of 8 years with addition of colonoscopies at the age of 20 years and breast screening at the age of 25 years.

STK11/LKB1 is the only gene identified to cause PJS, and mutations are found in 70% of those who meet clinical criteria.[116] Of affected individuals, 50% have a family history of PJS, and 50% may represent de novo mutations, although the penetrance of PJS has yet to be confirmed. The absence of a mutation in STK11 does not preclude a diagnosis of PJS in individuals meeting the clinical diagnostic criteria.

Juvenile Polyposis Syndrome

Juvenile polyposis syndrome (JPS) is another very rare, hereditary cancer syndrome with a broadly defined incidence rate between 1 in 16,000 and 1 in 100,000.[117–120] The diagnosis is based on the presence of multiple hamartomatous polyps with a distinct morphology termed *juvenile*, although JPS is not restricted to development in childhood. Solitary juvenile polyps occur in 1% to 2% of the general population.

The diagnosis of JPS requires more than five juvenile polyps in the colorectum, multiple juvenile polyps throughout the GI tract, or a number of juvenile polyps in an individual with a known family history of juvenile polyps. There is wide interfamilial and intrafamilial variability in number and distribution of polyps. Juvenile polyps are commonly benign, but the risk of malignant transformation is present. Larger polyps have been noted to contain adenomatous regions, resulting in a high lifetime risk of colorectal cancer approaching 20% by the age of 35 years and 68% by the age of 60 years. Gastric cancer has been found in 21% of JPS patients affected with gastric polyps, and increased incidence of pancreatic and small bowel cancers has also been reported (Table 39.2).[121]

Approximately 75% of JPS cases are familial, and 25% of JPS cases appear to be de novo. Two genes have been implicated as the cause of JPS in 40% of affected individuals: SMAD4 (or MADH4) and BMPR1A, with an approximate equal frequency.[121,122] The majority of JPS cases are due to as yet unidentified gene(s). Mutations in SMAD4 are also associated with hereditary hemorrhagic telangiectasia (HHT), also known as Osler–Weber–Rendu syndrome. HHT is associated with visceral bleeding, telangiectasias, or arteriovenous malformations. Currently, 15% to 22% of SMAD4 mutation carriers are suspected of having combined JPS/HHT.[123]

Surveillance recommendations for screening individuals with JPS include monitoring for rectal bleeding, anemia, and GI symptoms from infancy and additional complete blood counts, upper endoscopies, and colonoscopies at the age of 15 years, or when symptoms are present. An endoscopy is repeated every 1 to 3 years, depending on polyp load. In families with SMAD4 mutations, HHT surveillance begins in early childhood.

CONCLUSIONS

Hereditary gastric cancer is a relatively unusual disease. Given the very poor prognosis for most gastric cancer patients once diagnosed, every effort should be made to identify lesions early when they are still curable. Genetic testing for gastric cancer susceptibility allows for the identification of families with elevated risk for this and other tumors and the development of rational surveillance strategies for early detection. Unfortunately, reliable screening tools for gastric cancer are not available, and prophylactic surgical gastrectomies have proven beneficial in certain autosomal-dominant, high-penetrance genetic syndromes, including HDGC caused by germ-line CDH1 mutations. Genetic testing for other gastric cancer risk genes may also be warranted, as reviewed here. Major goals for clinical cancer genetics include identifying additional risk alleles to explain cancer susceptibility in families without known germ-line variants and to develop more robust tools for clinical screening for gastric cancer in high-risk individuals. Finally, the advent of whole genome sequencing of germ-line DNA and tumor genomes will lead to the rapid identification of novel variants and risk alleles of various penetrance. A challenge for the next generation of cancer genetics professionals will be the interpretation of multiple rare variants found in personal genomes and integration with schemes for the prevention and early detection of gastric cancer.

REFERENCES

1. Lauren P. The two histological main types of gastric carcinoma: diffuse and so-called intestinal-type carcinoma. An attempt at a histo-clinical classification. *Acta Pathol Microbiol Scand* 1965;64:31–49.
2. Carneiro F, Seixas M, Sobrinho-Simoes M. New elements for an updated classification of the carcinomas of the stomach. *Pathol Res Pract* 1995;191:571–584.
3. Wu H, Rusiecki JA, Zhu K, et al. Stomach carcinoma incidence patterns in the United States by histologic type and anatomic site. *Cancer Epidemiol Biomarkers Prev* 2009;18:1945–1952.
4. Machado JC, Soares P, Carneiro F, et al. E-cadherin gene mutations provide a genetic basis for the phenotypic divergence of mixed gastric carcinomas. *Lab Invest* 1999;79:459–465.
5. Becker KF, Atkinson MJ, Reich U, et al. E-cadherin gene mutations provide clues to diffuse type gastric carcinomas. *Cancer Res* 1994;54:3845–3852.
6. Tamura G, Sakata K, Nishizuka S, et al. Inactivation of the E-cadherin gene in primary gastric carcinomas and gastric carcinoma cell lines. *Jpn J Cancer Res* 1996;87:1153–1159.
7. Muta H, Noguchi M, Kanai Y, et al. E-cadherin gene mutations in signet ring cell carcinoma of the stomach. *Jpn J Cancer Res* 1996;87:843–848.
8. Carneiro F, Santos L, David L, et al. T (Thomsen-Friedenreich) antigen and other simple mucin-type carbohydrate antigens in precursor lesions of gastric carcinoma. *Histopathology* 1994;24:105–113.
9. Jang BG, Kim WH. Molecular pathology of gastric carcinoma. *Pathobiology* 2011;78:302–310.
10. Wang K, Kan J, Yuen ST, et al. Exome sequencing identifies frequent mutation of ARID1A in molecular subtypes of gastric cancer. *Nat Genet* 2011;43:1219–1223.
11. Zang ZJ, Cutcutache I, Poon SL, et al. Exome sequencing of gastric adenocarcinoma identifies recurrent somatic mutations in cell adhesion and chromatin remodeling genes. *Nat Genet* 2012;44:570–574.
12. Pedrazzani C, Corso G, Velho S, et al. Evidence of tumor microsatellite instability in gastric cancer with familial aggregation. *Fam Cancer* 2009;8:215–220.
13. Palli D, Russo A, Ottini L, et al. Red meat, family history, and increased risk of gastric cancer with microsatellite instability. *Cancer Res* 2001;61:5415–5419.
14. Buermeyer AB, Deschenes SM, Baker SM, et al. Mammalian DNA mismatch repair. *Annu Rev Genet* 1999;33:533–564.
15. La Torre G, Chiaradia G, Gianfagna F, et al. Smoking status and gastric cancer risk: an updated meta-analysis of case-control studies published in the past ten years. *Tumori* 2009;95:13–22.
16. McMichael AJ, McCall MG, Hartshorne JM, et al. Patterns of gastro-intestinal cancer in European migrants to Australia: The role of dietary change. *Int J Cancer* 1980;25:431–437.
17. Nomura A, Stemmermann GN, Chyou PH, et al. *Helicobacter pylori* infection and gastric carcinoma among Japanese Americans in Hawaii. *N Engl J Med* 1991;325:1132–1136.
18. Parsonnet J, Friedman GD, Vandersteen DP, et al. Helicobacter pylori infection and the risk of gastric cancer. *N Engl J Med* 1991;325:1127–1131.
19. Helicobacter and Cancer Collaborative Group. Gastric cancer and *Helicobacter pylori*: a combined analysis of 12 case control studies nested within prospective cohorts. *Gut* 2001;49:347–353.
20. Cavaleiro-Pinto M, Peleteiro B, Lunet N, et al. Helicobacter pylori infection and gastric cardia cancer: Systematic review and meta-analysis. *Cancer Causes Control* 2011;22:375–387.
21. Chen JN, He D, Tang F, et al. Epstein-Barr virus–associated gastric carcinoma: A newly defined entity. *J Clin Gastroenterol* 2010;46:262–271.
22. Ferlay J, Shin HR, Bray F, et al. Estimates of worldwide burden of cancer in 2008: GLOBOCAN 2008. *Int J Cancer* 2008;127:2893–2917.
23. Jemal A, Siegel R, Ward E, et al. Cancer statistics, 2008. *CA Cancer J Clin* 2008;58:71–96.
24. Correa P. Is gastric cancer preventable? *Gut* 2004;53:1217–1219.
25. Henson DE, Dittus C, Younes M, et al. Differential trends in the intestinal and diffuse types of gastric carcinoma in the United States, 1973–2000: Increase in the signet ring cell type. *Arch Pathol Lab Med* 2004;128:765–770.
26. Roosendaal R, Kuipers EJ, Buitenwerf J, et al. Helicobacter pylori and the birth cohort effect: Evidence of a continuous decrease of infection rates in childhood. *Am J Gastroenterol* 1997;92:1480–1482.
27. Borch K, Jonsson B, Tarpila E, et al. Changing pattern of histological type, location, stage and outcome of surgical treatment of gastric carcinoma. *Br J Surg* 2000;87:618–626.
28. Oliveira C, Seruca R, Carneiro F. Genetics, pathology, and clinics of familial gastric cancer. *Int J Surg Pathol* 2006;14:21–33.
29. Hemminki K, Li X, Czene K. Swedish empiric risks: familial risk of cancer: data for clinical counseling and cancer genetics. *Int J Cancer* 2004;108:109–114.
30. Shin CM, Kim N, Yang HJ, et al. Stomach cancer risk in gastric cancer relatives: Interaction between Helicobacter pylori infection and family history of gastric cancer for the risk of stomach cancer. *J Clin Gastroenterol* 2010;44:e34–e39.
31. Yokota T, Kunii Y, Teshima S, et al. Significant prognostic factors in patients with early gastric cancer. *Int Surg* 2000;85:286–290.
32. Caldas C, Carneiro F, Lynch HT, et al. Familial gastric cancer: Overview and guidelines for management. *J Med Genet* 1999;36:873–880.
33. Guilford P, Hopkins J, Harraway J, et al. E-cadherin germline mutations in familial gastric cancer. *Nature* 1998;392:402–405.
34. Gayther SA, Gorringe KL, Ramus SJ, et al. Identification of germ-line E-cadherin mutations in gastric cancer families of European origin. *Cancer Res* 1998;58:4086–4089.
35. Guilford PJ, Hopkins JB, Grady WM, et al. E-cadherin germline mutations define an inherited cancer syndrome dominated by diffuse gastric cancer. *Hum Mutat* 1999;14:249–255.
36. Keller G, Vogelsang H, Becker I, et al. Diffuse type gastric and lobular breast carcinoma in a familial gastric cancer patient with an E-cadherin germline mutation. *Am J Pathol* 1999;155:337–342.
37. Richards FM, McKee SA, Rajpar MH, et al. Germline E-cadherin gene (CDH1) mutations predispose to familial gastric cancer and colorectal cancer. *Hum Mol Genet* 1999;8:607–610.
38. Shinmura K, Kohno T, Takahashi M, et al. Familial gastric cancer: Clinico-pathological characteristics, RER phenotype and germline p53 and E-cadherin mutations. *Carcinogenesis* 1999;20:1127–1131.
39. Yoon KA, Ku JL, Yang HK, et al. Germline mutations of E-cadherin gene in Korean familial gastric cancer patients. *J Hum Genet* 1999;44:177–180.
40. Kluijt I, Siemerink EJ, Ausems MG, et al. CDH1-related hereditary diffuse gastric cancer syndrome: Clinical variations and implications for counseling. *Int J Cancer* 2012;131:367–376.
41. Guilford P, Humar B, Blair V. Hereditary diffuse gastric cancer: Translation of CDH1 germline mutations into clinical practice. *Gastric Cancer* 2010;13:1–10.
42. Grunwald GB. The structural and functional analysis of cadherin calcium-dependent cell adhesion molecules. *Curr Opin Cell Biol* 1993;5:797–805.
43. Birchmeier W. E-cadherin as a tumor (invasion) suppressor gene. *Bioessays* 1995;17:97–99.
44. Fitzgerald RC, Hardwick R, Huntsman D, et al. Hereditary diffuse gastric cancer: updated consensus guidelines for clinical management and directions for future research. *J Med Genet* 2010;47:436–444.
45. Brooks-Wilson AR, Kaurah P, Suriano G, et al. Germline E-cadherin mutations in hereditary diffuse gastric cancer: assessment of 42 new families and review of genetic screening criteria. *J Med Genet* 2004;41:508–517.
46. Oliveira C, de Bruin J, Nabais S, et al. Intragenic deletion of CDH1 as the inactivating mechanism of the wild-type allele in an HDGC tumour. *Oncogene* 2004;23:2236–2240.
47. Suriano G, Yew S, Ferreira P, et al. Characterization of a recurrent germ line mutation of the E-cadherin gene: Implications for genetic testing and clinical management. *Clin Cancer Res* 2005;11:5401–5409.
48. Oliveira C, Sousa S, Pinheiro H, et al. Quantification of epigenetic and genetic 2nd hits in CDH1 during hereditary diffuse gastric cancer syndrome progression. *Gastroenterology* 2009;136:2137–2148.
49. Keller G, Vogelsang H, Becker I, et al. Germline mutations of the E-cadherin (CDH1) and TP53 genes, rather than of RUNX3 and HPP1, contribute to genetic predisposition in German gastric cancer patients. *J Med Genet* 2004;41:e89.
50. Kim IJ, Park JH, Kang HC, et al. A novel germline mutation in the MET extracellular domain in a Korean patient with the diffuse type of familial gastric cancer. *J Med Genet* 2003;40:e97.
51. Oliveira C, Ferreira P, Nabais S, et al. E-cadherin (CDH1) and p53 rather than SMAD4 and caspase-10 germline mutations contribute to genetic predisposition in Portuguese gastric cancer patients. *Eur J Cancer* 2004;40:1897–1903.
52. Oliveira C, Senz J, Kaurah P, et al. Germline CDH1 deletions in hereditary diffuse gastric cancer families. *Hum Mol Genet* 2009;18:1545–1555.
53. Pharoah PD, Guilford P, Caldas C. Incidence of gastric cancer and breast cancer in CDH1 (E-cadherin) mutation carriers from hereditary diffuse gastric cancer families. *Gastroenterology* 2001;121:1348–1353.
54. Kaurah P, MacMillan A, Boyd N, et al. Founder and recurrent CDH1 mutations in families with hereditary diffuse gastric cancer. *JAMA* 2007;297:2360–2372.
55. Schrader KA, Masciari S, Boyd N, et al. Hereditary diffuse gastric cancer: association with lobular breast cancer. *Fam Cancer* 2008;7:73–82.
56. Berx G, Becker KF, Hofler H, et al. Mutations of the human E-cadherin (CDH1) gene. *Hum Mutat* 1998;12:226–237.
57. Berx G, Cleton-Jansen AM, Strumane K, et al. E-cadherin is inactivated in a majority of invasive human lobular breast cancers by truncation mutations throughout its extracellular domain. *Oncogene* 1996;13:1919–1925.
58. Schrader KA, Masciari S, Boyd N, et al. Germline mutations in CDH1 are infrequent in women with early-onset or familial lobular breast cancers. *J Med Genet* 2011;48:64–68.
59. Oliveira C, Bordin MC, Grehan N, et al. Screening E-cadherin in gastric cancer families reveals germline mutations only in hereditary diffuse gastric cancer kindred. *Hum Mutat* 2002;19:510–517.
60. Frebourg T, Oliveira C, Hochain P, et al. Cleft lip/palate and CDH1/E-cadherin mutations in families with hereditary diffuse gastric cancer. *J Med Genet* 2006;43:138–142.
61. Cisco RM, Ford JM, Norton JA. Hereditary diffuse gastric cancer: Implications of genetic testing for screening and prophylactic surgery. *Cancer* 2008;113:1850–1856.
62. Huntsman DG, Carneiro F, Lewis FR, et al. Early gastric cancer in young, asymptomatic carriers of germ-line E-cadherin mutations. *N Engl J Med* 2001;344:1904–1909.

CANCERS OF THE GASTROINTESTINAL TRACT

63. Norton J, Ham C, Van Dam J, et al. CDH1 truncating mutations in the E-cadherin gene: An indication for total gastrectomy to treat hereditary diffuse gastric cancer. *Ann Surg* 2007;45:873–879.

64. Rogers W, Dobo E, Norton J, et al. Risk-reducing total gastrectomy for germline mutations in E-cadherin (CDH1): pathologic findings with clinical implications. *Am J Surg Pathol* 2008;32:799–809.

65. Kaurah P, Fitzgerald R, Dwerryhouse S, et al. Pregnancy after prophylactic total gastrectomy. *Fam Cancer* 2010;9:331–334.

66. Saslow D, Boetes C, Burke W, et al. American Cancer Society guidelines for breast screening with MRI as an adjunct to mammography. *CA Cancer J Clin* 2007;57:75–89.

67. Daly M, Axilbund J, Buys S, et al. Genetic/familial high-risk assessment: breast and ovarian. *J Natl Compr Cancer Netw* 2010;8:562–594.

68. Wolmark N, Dunn BK. The role of tamoxifen in breast cancer prevention: Issues sparked by the NSABP Breast Cancer Prevention Trial (P-1). *Ann N Y Acad Sci* 2001;949:99–108.

69. Lynch HT, Lynch PM. The cancer-family syndrome: a pragmatic basis for syndrome identification. *Dis Colon Rectum* 1979;22:106–110.

70. Palomaki GE, McClain MR, Melillo S, et al. EGAPP supplementary evidence review: DNA testing strategies aimed at reducing morbidity and mortality from Lynch syndrome. *Genet Med* 2009;11:42–65.

71. Meyer LA, Broaddus RR, Lu KH. Endometrial cancer and Lynch syndrome: clinical and pathologic considerations. *Cancer Control* 2009;16:14–22.

72. Chen S, Wang W, Lee S, et al. Prediction of germline mutations and cancer risk in the Lynch syndrome. *JAMA* 2006;296:1479–1487.

73. Aarnio M, Salovaara R, Aaltonen LA, et al. Features of gastric cancer in hereditary non-polyposis colorectal cancer syndrome. *Int J Cancer* 1997;74:551–555.

74. Aarnio M, Sankila R, Pukkala E, et al. Cancer risk in mutation carriers of DNA-mismatch-repair genes. *Int J Cancer* 1999;81:214–218.

75. Park YJ, Shin KH, Park JG. Risk of gastric cancer in hereditary nonpolyposis colorectal cancer in Korea. *Clin Cancer Res* 2000;6:2994–2998.

76. Vasen HF, Wijnen JT, Menko FH, et al. Cancer risk in families with hereditary nonpolyposis colorectal cancer diagnosed by mutation analysis. *Gastroenterology* 1996;110:1020–1027.

77. Watson P, Vasen HF, Mecklin JP, et al. The risk of extra-colonic, extra-endometrial cancer in the Lynch syndrome. *Int J Cancer* 2008;123:444–449.

78. Gylling A, Abdel-Rahman WM, Juhola M, et al. Is gastric cancer part of the tumour spectrum of hereditary non-polyposis colorectal cancer? A molecular genetic study. *Gut* 2007;56:926–933.

79. Rodriguez-Bigas MA, Boland CR, Hamilton SR, et al. A National Cancer Institute Workshop on hereditary nonpolyposis colorectal cancer syndrome: meeting highlights and Bethesda guidelines. *J Natl Cancer Inst* 1997;89:1758–1762.

80. Umar A, Boland CR, Terdiman JP, et al. Revised Bethesda guidelines for hereditary nonpolyposis colorectal cancer (Lynch syndrome) and microsatellite instability. *J Natl Cancer Inst* 2004;96:261–268.

81. Miki Y, Swensen J, Shattuck-Eidens D, et al. A strong candidate for the breast and ovarian cancer susceptibility gene BRCA1. *Science* 1994;266:66–71.

82. Wooster R, Bignell G, Lancaster J, et al. Identification of the breast cancer susceptibility gene BRCA2. *Nature* 1995;378:789–792.

83. The Breast Cancer Linkage Consortium. Cancer risks in BRCA2 mutation carriers. *J Natl Cancer Inst* 1999;91:1310–1316.

84. Figer A, Irmin L, Geva R, et al. The rate of the 6174delT founder Jewish mutation in BRCA2 in patients with non-colonic gastrointestinal tract tumours in Israel. *Br J Cancer* 2001;84:478–481.

85. Jakubowska A, Nej K, Huzarski T, et al. BRCA2 gene mutations in families with aggregations of breast and stomach cancers. *Br J Cancer* 2002;87:888–891.

86. Jakubowska A, Scott R, Menkiszak J, et al. A high frequency of BRCA2 gene mutations in Polish families with ovarian and stomach cancer. *Eur J Hum Genet* 2003;11:955–958.

87. Johannsson O, Loman N, Moller T, et al. Incidence of malignant tumours in relatives of BRCA1 and BRCA2 germline mutation carriers. *Eur J Cancer* 1999;35:1248–1257.

88. Lorenzo B, Hemminki K. Risk of cancer at sites other than the breast in Swedish families eligible for BRCA1 or BRCA2 mutation testing. *Ann Oncol* 2004;15:1834–1841.

89. Brose MS, Rebbeck TR, Calzone KA, et al. Cancer risk estimates for BRCA1 mutation carriers identified in a risk evaluation program. *J Natl Cancer Inst* 2002;94:1365–1372.

90. Risch H, McLaughlin J, Cole D, et al. Prevalence and penetrance of germline BRCA1 and BRCA2 mutations in a population series of 649 women with ovarian cancer. *Am J Hum Genet* 2001;68:700–710.

91. Friedenson B. BRCA1 and BRCA2 pathways and the risk of cancers other than breast or ovarian. *MedGenMed* 2005;7:60.

92. Garrean S, Hering J, Saied A, et al. Gastric adenocarcinoma arising from fundic gland polyps in a patient with familial adenomatous polyposis syndrome. *Am Surg* 2008;74:79–83.

93. Offerhaus GJ, Giardiello FM, Krush AJ, et al. The risk of upper gastrointestinal cancer in familial adenomatous polyposis. *Gastroenterology* 1992;102:1980–1982.

94. Burt RW. Gastric fundic gland polyps. *Gastroenterology* 2003;125:1462–1469.

95. Lynch HT, Snyder C, Davies JM, et al. FAP, gastric cancer, and genetic counseling featuring children and young adults: A family study and review. *Fam Cancer* 2010;9:581–588.

96. Lynch HT, Smyrk T, McGinn T, et al. Attenuated familial adenomatous polyposis (AFAP). A phenotypically and genotypically distinctive variant of FAP. *Cancer* 1995;76:2427–2433.

97. Abraham SC, Nobukawa B, Giardiello FM, et al. Fundic gland polyps in familial adenomatous polyposis: neoplasms with frequent somatic adenomatous polyposis coli gene alterations. *Am J Pathol* 2000;157:747–754.

98. Bianchi LK, Burke CA, Bennett AE, et al. Fundic gland polyp dysplasia is common in familial adenomatous polyposis. *Clin Gastroenterol Hepatol* 2008;6:180–185.

99. Dunn K, Chey W, Gibbs J. Total gastrectomy for gastric dysplasia in a patient with attenuated familial adenomatous polyposis syndrome. *J Clin Oncol* 2008;26:3641–3642.

100. Olivier M, Goldgar DE, Sodha N, et al. Li-Fraumeni and related syndromes: correlation between tumor type, family structure, and TP53 genotype. *Cancer Res* 2003;63:6643–6650.

101. Li F, Fraumeni JJ. Soft-tissue sarcomas, breast cancer, and other neoplasms. A familial syndrome? *Ann Intern Med* 1969;71:747–752.

102. Malkin D, Li F, Strong L, et al. Germ line p53 mutations in a familial syndrome of breast cancer, sarcomas, and other neoplasms. *Science* 1990;250:1233–1238.

103. Wu CC, Shete S, Amos CI, et al. Joint effects of germ-line p53 mutation and sex on cancer risk in Li-Fraumeni syndrome. *Cancer Res* 2006;66:8287–8292.

104. Hisada M, Garber J, Fung C, et al. Multiple primary cancers in families with Li-Fraumeni syndrome. *J Natl Cancer Inst* 1998;90:606–611.

105. Gonzalez K, Buzin C, Noltner K, et al. High frequency of de novo mutations in Li-Fraumeni syndrome. *J Med Genet* 2009;46:689–693.

106. Corso G, Pedrazzani C, Marrelli D, et al. Familial gastric cancer and Li-Fraumeni syndrome. *Eur J Cancer Care (Engl)* 2010;19:377–381.

107. Masciari S, Dewanwala A, Stoffel EM, et al. Gastric cancer in individuals with Li-Fraumeni syndrome. *Genet Med* 2011;13:651–657.

108. Ruijs MW, Verhoef S, Rookus MA, et al. TP53 germline mutation testing in 180 families suspected of Li-Fraumeni syndrome: Mutation detection rate and relative frequency of cancers in different familial phenotypes. *J Med Genet* 2010;47:421–428.

109. Peutz J. Very remarkable case of familial polyposis of mucous membrane of intestinal tract and nasopharynx accompanied by peculiar pigmentations of skin and mucous membrane. *Nederl Maandschr Geneesk* 1921;10:134–146.

110. Jeghers H, Mc KV, Katz KH. Generalized intestinal polyposis and melanin spots of the oral mucosa, lips and digits; a syndrome of diagnostic significance. *N Engl J Med* 1949;241:1031–1036.

111. Giardiello FM, Welsh SB, Hamilton SR, et al. Increased risk of cancer in the Peutz-Jeghers syndrome. *N Engl J Med* 1987;316:1511–1514.

112. Lim W, Olschwang S, Keller JJ, et al. Relative frequency and morphology of cancers in STK11 mutation carriers. *Gastroenterology* 2004;126:1788–1794.

113. Giardiello F, Brensinger J, Tersmette A, et al. Very high risk of cancer in familial Peutz-Jeghers syndrome. *Gastroenterology* 2000;119:1447–1453.

114. van Lier MG, Wagner A, Mathus-Vliegen EM, et al. High cancer risk in Peutz-Jeghers syndrome: A systematic review and surveillance recommendations. *Am J Gastroenterol* 2010;105:1258–1264.

115. van Lier MG, Westerman AM, Wagner A, et al. High cancer risk and increased mortality in patients with Peutz-Jeghers syndrome. *Gut* 2011;60:141–147.

116. Gruber SB, Entius MM, Petersen GM, et al. Pathogenesis of adenocarcinoma in Peutz-Jeghers syndrome. *Cancer Res* 1998;58:5267–5270.

117. Allen BA, Terdiman JP. Hereditary polyposis syndromes and hereditary non-polyposis colorectal cancer. *Best Pract Res Clin Gastroenterol* 2003;17:237–258.

118. Finan MC, Ray MK. Gastrointestinal polyposis syndromes. *Dermatol Clin* 1989;7:419–434.

119. Lindor NM, Greene MH. The concise handbook of family cancer syndromes. Mayo Familial Cancer Program. *J Natl Cancer Inst* 1998;90:1039–1071.

120. Utsunomiya J, Gocho H, Miyanaga T, et al. Peutz-Jeghers syndrome: its natural course and management. *Johns Hopkins Med J* 1975;136:71–82.

121. Howe JR, Sayed MG, Ahmed AF, et al. The prevalence of MADH4 and BM-PR1A mutations in juvenile polyposis and absence of BMPR2, BMPR1B, and ACVR1 mutations. *J Med Gene* 2004;41:484–491.

122. Sayed MG, Ahmed AF, Ringold JR, et al. Germline SMAD4 or BMPR1A mutations and phenotype of juvenile polyposis. *Ann Surg Oncol* 2002;9:901–906.

123. Gallione C, Richards J, Letteboer T, et al. SMAD4 mutations found in unselected HHT patients. *J Med Genet* 2006;43:793–797.

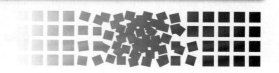

40 Molecular Biology of Pancreas Cancer

Scott E. Kern and Ralph H. Hruban

INTRODUCTION

Pancreatic cancer is a genetic disease. This perspective is supported by reproducible patterns of genetic mutations that accumulate during pancreatic tumorigenesis. These patterns indicate the operation of a selective process favoring the emergence of specific constellations of genetic changes. According to this genetic theory, most pancreatic cancers share a common foundation of genetic mutations disrupting specific cellular regulatory controls. These shared abnormalities are responsible for the processes of cancer growth, invasion, and metastasis in individual patients.

Four categories of mutated genes play a role in the pancreatic tumorigenesis: oncogenes, tumor-suppressor genes, genome-maintenance genes, and tissue-maintenance genes (summarized in Table 40.1). Some of these mutations are germline (i.e., they are transmitted within a family), whereas somatic mutations, acquired during life, contribute to tumorigenesis within a tissue but are not passed to offspring.

The most common cancer type of pancreatic cancer is pancreatic ductal adenocarcinoma (PDA). PDA is the primary focus of clinical and molecular research and is thus highlighted in this chapter. Other clinically and molecularly distinct forms of cancer occur in the pancreas and must be distinguished from PDA; they are discussed here in lesser detail.

In recent years, techniques were developed to sequence all of the genes of individual cancers. Whole-exome sequencing of PDAs revealed an average of 63 somatic mutations per tumor.[1] Most of these mutations undoubtedly are nonfunctional *passenger* mutations, each mutated at a low frequency and not contributing to tumorigenesis. Indeed, most passenger mutations might arise as tissues age before tumorigenesis even begins.[2] Smoking is associated with a doubling of the risk for pancreatic cancer, and remarkably, it is also associated with a 40% increase of the prevalence of low-frequency mutations in the cancers.[3] Only a subset of the mutations in PDA, however, are responsible for *driving* the neoplastic process in the ducts; only they are discussed further here. Modeling of a comprehensive study mapping gene mutations in multiple regions of primary PDAs and their metastases indicated a general timeline of tumorigenesis, invasion, and metastasis. According to this model, about a decade of time passes between the first driver mutation initiating the precursor neoplasm and the emergence of the first cell having the genotype of the invasive cancer; metastatic ability is acquired after another 5 years, and with patient death following about 2 years later.[4]

Telomere abnormalities and manifestations of chromosome instability are the most common alterations in pancreatic neoplasia. Four genes are mutated in most PDAs: the *KRAS*, *p16/CDKN2A*, *TP53*, and *SMAD4/DPC4* genes. Other recurrent genetic abnormalities are seen at a lower frequency, including internal deletions of exons of *FAM190A/CCSER1*; mutations in the genes *BRCA2*, *PALB2*, *FANCC*, *FANCG*, *FBXW7*, *BAX*, and *RB1*, in the transforming growth factor beta (TGF-β) receptors *TGFBR1* and *TGFBR2*, in the activin receptors *ACVR1B* and *ACVR2*, in various chromatin-remodeling genes such as *ARID1A*, in the genes *MKK4*, *STK11*, *MLL3*, *ATM*, *GUCY2F*, *NTRK3*, and *EGFR*, and in cationic trypsinogen; alterations in the mitochondrial genome; amplifications; various chromosomal deletions; inactivation of DNA mismatch-repair genes; and rarely, the maintenance of the Epstein-Barr virus genome as an episome. Irregular sizes and numbers of centrosomes were observed in 85% of pancreatic cancers and some adenomas, but in no tissues of chronic pancreatitis or normal pancreas.[5]

Knowing the genes that are mutated in a cancer can have direct clinical impact. For example, some patients develop pancreatic cancer because of an inherited mutation, and these patients and their families could benefit from genetic counseling.[6–9] A distinct morphologic subtype of pancreatic cancer, the medullary cancer, can suggest such an inherited mutation.[10,11] Another example of clinical impact includes the analysis of the genetic alterations in precursors to invasive pancreatic neoplasia, which indicated that most carcinomas arise by a process of progressive intraductal tumorigenesis, suggesting that these intraductal lesions might be detected and treated before a patient develops an invasive cancer.[12] Epigenetic changes in DNA methylation and in gene expression are also highly specific for the cancerous cells and can serve as markers of disease.

COMMON MOLECULAR CHANGES

Telomere shortening is an early and prevalent genetic change identified in the pancreatic precursor lesions.[13] Telomere shortening experimentally predisposes cells to chromosome fusion (translocations) and the missegregation of genetic material during mitosis.[14] Later in tumorigenesis, the telomerase is often reactivated,[15,16] moderating the telomere erosive process while permitting continued chromosomal instability.[17]

The *KRAS* gene mediates signals from growth factor receptors and other signaling inputs (Fig. 40.1). The mutations present in most pancreatic cancers convert the normal Kras protein (a protooncogene) to an oncogene, causing the protein to become overactive in transmitting growth factor–initiated signals.[18] *KRAS* is mutated in over 90% of conventional pancreatic ductal carcinomas.[19] Among the first genetic changes in the ducts is a *KRAS* gene mutation (see Table 40.1),[20,21] and recent evidence from advanced gene sequencing techniques indicates that their prevalence in early lesions is higher than was previously thought.[22]

As one of the most commonly mutated genes in pancreatic cancer, the Ras protein is an attractive target for the development of gene-specific therapies, and an understanding of the normal biology of the Ras protein should help in the development of these Ras-targeted therapies. Ras proteins require an attachment to the plasma membrane for activity. For many proteins, including Ras, a hydrophobic prenyl group is essential for the attachment. Either farnesyl (15-carbon) or geranylgeranyl (20-carbon) makes a covalent thioether linkage at a cysteine residue located near the C-terminal end of Ras proteins, termed the CAAX motif. Working mostly in artificial legacy models of the *HRAS* oncogene (rather than the more widely available but experimentally less tractable natural *KRAS*-mutant cancer cell lines), the farnesylation reaction

TABLE 40.1

Genetic Profile of Pancreatic Ductal Carcinoma

Gene	Gene Locations	Frequency in Cancers (%)	Timing During Tumorigenesis[a]	Mutation Origin
Oncogenes				
KRAS	12p	95	Early–Mid	Som.
BRAF	7q	4		Som.
AKT2	19q	10–20		Som.
GUCY2F	Xq	3		Som.
NTRK3	15q	1		Som.
EGFR	7p	1		Som.
EBV genome		<1		
Tumor-Suppressors/Genome-Maintenance Genes				
CDKN2A/p16	9p	>90	Mid–Late	Som. > Germ.
TP53	17p	75	Late	Som.
SMAD4	18q	55	Late	Som.
BRCA2 and PALB2	13q/16p	5	Late	Germ. > Som.
FANCC and FANCG	9q/9p	3		Germ. or Som.
CCSER1/FAM10A	4q	4[c]		Som.
MAP2K4	17p	4		Som.
LKB1/STK11	19p	4		Som. > Germ.
ACVR1B	12q	2		Som.
TGFBR1[b]	9q	1		Som.[c]
MSI⁻/TGFBR2[b]	3p	1		Som.[c]
MSI⁺/TGFBR2	3p	4		Som. > Germ.[d]
ACVR2	2q	4		Som. > Germ.[d]
BAX	19q	4		Som. > Germ.[d]
MLH1	3p	4		Som. > Germ.[d]
FBXW7/Cyclin E deregulated	4q	6		Som.[e]
ATM	11q	<1[f]		Germ.
Tissue-Maintenance Genes				
PRSS1	7q	<1[f]	Prior	Germ.

[a] Stage of appearance of the genetic changes during the intraductal precursor phase of the neoplasm, where known. For BRCA2, most mutations are inherited, but the loss of the second allele is reported only in a single advanced pancreatic intraepithelial neoplasia.
[b] Few homozygous deletions of the TGFBR1 gene and the TGFBR2 gene have been identified in non-MSI (microsatellite instability) pancreatic cancers.
[c] The prevalence of exonic transcript deletions is much higher than the prevalence of homozygously deleted exons given here.
[d] In MSI+ tumors, the mismatch repair defect is usually somatic in origin; the TGFBR2, ACVR2, and BAX alterations are somatic.
[e] A single example of homozygous mutation of the FBXW7 gene is reported in a series having a 6% prevalence of cyclin E overexpression. To date, cyclin E amplification is reported only in cell lines.
[f] The prevalence of mutations in severely affected families is higher than the prevalence among unselected cancers given here.
Som., (prevalence of) somatic mutation or methylation; Germ., (prevalence of) germline mutation.

was readily inhibited by various means; in these models, the Ras protein was rendered inactive and was often accompanied by cytotoxicity limited to the mutant cells.

Although many types of compounds capable of blocking the farnesyltransferase enzyme were developed as drugs, they have not been successful anticancer agents. Reasons are many. Although the Hras protein is linked predominantly through farnesyl groups, the Kras protein can be alternately prenylated by geranylgeranyl linkages. The latter is thought to be critical for a wider number of cellular proteins, and for fear of excessive toxicity, geranylgeranyl linkages have not usually been considered as an attractive drug target. The Kras protein may bind more tightly than Hras to the farnesyltransferase enzyme, necessitating higher drug concentrations.[18]

Additionally, the artificial models usually employed the engineered overexpression of the Ras protein, a situation in which the unattached Ras proteins would serve as a dominant-negative inhibitor, binding the essential interacting proteins and sequestering them in the cytoplasm to ensure the inactivation of the many downstream Ras pathways. Such a concentration-driven mechanism would presumably not occur under the normal levels of Ras proteins present in human cancers.[23] Indeed, it is proposed that the limited efficacy of farnesyltransferase inhibitors (FTI) observed in some experimental models and in clinical trials may be attributable to a cellular target not yet identified.[24] Attention has turned to compounds that target the downstream mediators, such as Raf and Mek protein kinase inhibitors.

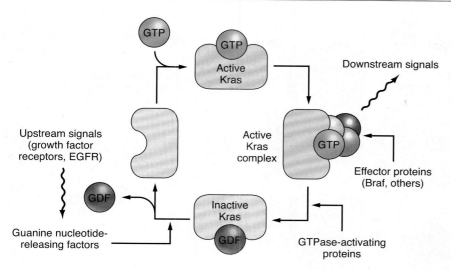

Figure 40.1 The KRAS pathway. KRAS normally integrates and regulates signals arising in the growth factor receptors that are passed to KRAS using the Grb2 and the Sos1 nucleotide exchange factor. The active GTP-bound form of KRAS recruits effector proteins such as Raf1 and Braf, in turn stimulating the downstream mitogen-activated protein kinases, such as MEK and ERK, and activating certain transcription factors. The EGF receptor can be overexpressed and occasionally mutated to provide inappropriately strong upstream signals, and the BRAF protein can be activated by point mutation, but more often in pancreatic cancer, the Kras protein is mutated. These latter mutations impair the GTPase-activating protein (GAP)–stimulated reaction that normally returns KRAS to the inactive state.

The Smad pathway mediates signals initiated upon the binding of the extracellular proteins TGF-β, activin, and bone morphogenic proteins to their receptors (Fig. 40.2). These signals are transmitted to the nucleus by proteins of the Smad family of related genes, including *SMAD4 (DPC4)*.[25] Once in the nucleus, Smad protein complexes bind specific recognition sites on DNA and cause the transcription of certain genes.[26] Mutations in the *SMAD4* gene are found in nearly half of pancreatic carcinomas, including homozygous deletions or intragenic mutations combined with loss of heterozygosity (LOH).[27] Other Smad genes are also occasionally mutated in pancreatic cancer.[1] Also, homozygous deletions and mutation/LOH affecting the TGF-β receptor genes are seen in a few pancreatic cancers.[28] A more common abnormality, in pancreatic as well as in other tumor types, is the underexpression of TGF-β receptors, which may render cells resistant to the normal suppressive effects of the TGF-β ligand.[29]

The *p16/RB1* pathway is a key control of the cell division cycle (Fig. 40.3). The retinoblastoma protein (Rb1) is a transcriptional regulator and regulates the entry of cells into S phase. A complex of cyclin D and a cyclin-dependent kinase (Cdk4 and Cdk6) phosphorylates and thereby regulates Rb1. The p16 protein is a Cdk-inhibitor that binds Cdk4 and Cdk6.[30–32] Virtually all pancreatic carcinomas suffer a loss of *p16* gene function through homozygous deletions, a mutation combined with LOH, or promoter

methylation of the *p16/CDKN2A* gene associated with a lack of gene expression.[33,34] In addition, inherited mutations of the *p16/CDKN2A* gene cause a familial melanoma/pancreatic cancer syndrome known as familial atypical multiple mole melanoma (FAMMM).[35–39] Only rare pancreatic cancers have an inactivating mutation of the *RB1* gene.[40]

The protein product of the *TP53* gene, Tp53, binds to specific sites of DNA and activates the transcription of certain genes that control the cell division cycle and apoptosis.[41,42] The Tp53 protein, normally a short-lived protein, becomes phosphorylated and stabilized after DNA damage and other cellular stresses (Fig. 40.4). In about 75% of pancreatic cancers, the *TP53* gene has point mutations that inhibit the ability of p53 to bind DNA or, occasionally, other types of inactivating mutation.[43–45]

Most human carcinomas have chromosomal instability (CIN), which produces changes in chromosomal copy numbers or aneuploidy.[46] Most pancreatic cancers have complex karyotypes, including deletions of whole chromosomes and subchromosomal regions.[47–49] CIN is the process that causes most of the tumor deletions (i.e., LOH).[50] A few percent of pancreatic carcinomas, however, do not have significant gross or numerical chromosomal changes and instead have a different form of genetic instability; they have defects in DNA mismatch repair, producing high mutation rates at sites of simple repetitive sequences (microsatellites), termed microsatellite instability (MSI).[10,11,51–54] The pattern of

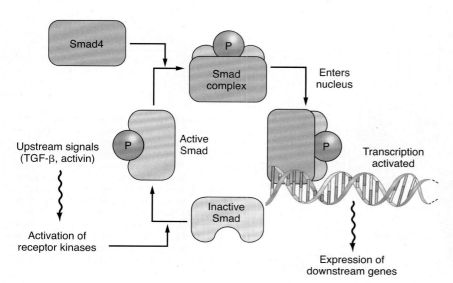

Figure 40.2 The TGF-β/Activin/Smad pathway. Dimeric kinase receptors of the TGF-β superfamily respond to extracellular ligands, causing phosphorylation of one or more of the receptor-associated Smad proteins and leading them to complex with the unphosphorylated common Smad, Smad4. This complex binds to specific DNA sequences and works with other transcription factors to stimulate gene expression. Mutations in pancreatic cancer can inactivate either partner of the dimeric receptors that respond to extracellular TGF-β or activin. More commonly, however, mutations and large deletions in the SMAD4 gene destabilize its protein product or ablate gene expression.

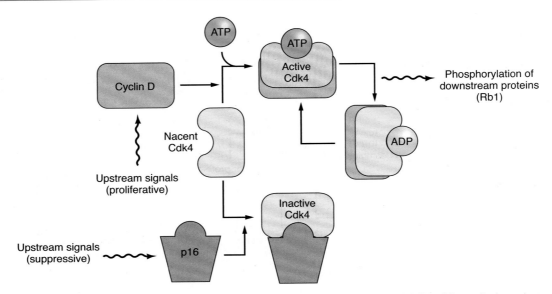

Figure 40.3 The p16/RB1 pathway. p16 binds to, inhibits, and thereby controls the availability of the cyclin-dependent kinases Cdk4 and Cdk6 (not shown). When activated by binding to cyclin D, these kinases phosphorylate and thereby inactivate the Rb1 tumor-suppressor protein. The activity of p16 is controlled in a complex manner, through changes in gene expression and by displacement reactions involving other similar kinase inhibitor proteins. p16 mutations and deletions are nearly ubiquitous in pancreatic cancer, resulting in dysregulation of these cyclin-dependent kinases that regulate the cell division cycle.

genetic damage in these carcinomas differs considerably from the pattern in carcinomas with CIN. The type II TGF-β and activin receptors (*TGFBR2*) and (*ACVR2*), as well as the *BAX* gene, have a repetitive sequence within their protein-coding regions, and biallelic inactivating mutations of these sequences are seen in many MSI pancreatic cancers.[28,54–57]

There are also alterations in pancreatic carcinomas, some probably being important to tumorigenesis, that are not attributed to genetic mutations. These include the expression of telomerase,[15,16] the underexpression of TGF-β receptors,[29] and the overexpression of the growth-stimulating Her-2/neu cell surface receptor[58–61] and growth factor-related proteins.[62] Some of these activities are proposed to be attractive as therapeutic targets, although supportive clinical evidence is not yet available. Pancreatic carcinomas also have reproducible alterations in gene expression, such as overexpression of the proteins mesothelin and prostate stem cell antigen (PSCA), that currently can serve as diagnostic aids in the histopathologic interpretation of biopsies and surgical resections.[57–59]

The epigenetic patterns of gene hypermethylation and various patterns of overexpression of RNA transcripts and proteins in pancreatic cancers are considered promising for developing additional diagnostic markers for the analysis of pancreatic secretions and for noninvasive diagnostic screening.[63]

Genetic patterns are also found among other diagnostic categories of pancreatic neoplasia. The precursor lesions of PDAs, termed pancreatic intraepithelial neoplasia (PanIN), in their most advanced grade closely resemble the genetic patterns of the conventional invasive PDAs. However, the lesions other than the PDAs, including the intraductal papillary mucinous neoplasms (IPMN), the mucinous cyctic neoplasms (MCNs), acinar cell carcinomas, well-differentiated neuroendocrine tumors, pancreatoblastomas, and solid pseudopapillary neoplasms (SPNs), diverge significantly from the patterns of PanINs and typical invasive PDAs. These differences could be used in the future for differential diagnosis of lesions upon biopsy.

Cystic neoplasms such as IPMNs, serous cystadenomas (SCAs), MCNs, and SPNs appear to have relatively few mutant genes in

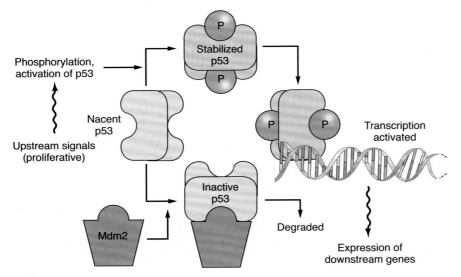

Figure 40.4 The p53 pathway. Many modes of control affect p53 activity, one of which is shown in the diagram. Stresses such as DNA damage result in the phosphorylation of p53, preventing its degradation by an Mdm2-directed pathway. When stabilized, p53 binds to specific DNA sequences and activates the transcription of many genes, including Mdm2 as part of a negative feedback loop. When p53 is mutated, it fails to bind effectively to DNA to activate transcription. Because Mdm2 then lacks its transcriptional stimulus from p53, mutant but inactive p53 proteins are usually expressed at very high levels.

each tumor, yet the genes involved are remarkably distinct.[64–66] Mutations in *GNAS* or *KRAS* were found in 96% of IPMNs; those in *RNF43* were present in many IPMNs and MCNs; those in *CTNNB1* were ubiquitous among the SPNs; and those in *VHL* affected half of the SCAs. *GNAS* mutations were found in collected pancreatic secretions samples of two thirds of familial and sporadic cases of IPMNs, but not in controls, and their presence predicted subsequent emergence or increasing size of detected cysts.[67] *PIK3CA* mutations are present in some IPMNs and the colloid carcinomas that can derive from them.[68] *CTNNB1* (beta-catenin) mutations are present in virtually all solid-pseudopapillary neoplasms[69] and pancreatoblastomas.[70] These genetic data suggested utilities in detection, diagnostic classification, and prognostication when clinically managing pancreatic cysts.

Mutations of *MEN1* and either the *DAXX* or *ATRX* genes are found in most well-differentiated pancreatic neuroendocrine tumors (PanNET).[71,72] Nearly two thirds of these tumors (a subset uniformly harboring *DAXX* or *ATRX* mutations) were found to have abnormal telomeres, indicating an active process termed alternative lengthening of telomeres (ALT). ALT is distinct from the typical activation of telomerase implicated in most types of cancer.[73] The distinguishing patterns of mutations also firmly establish that high-grade small- and large-cell neuroendocrine carcinomas of the pancreas, despite having histologic similarities with well-differentiated PanNETs, arise through different tumorigenic mechanisms.[74]

Lower-Frequency Genetic Changes

The causative genes of *Fanconi anemia* play a role in human tumorigenesis. The *BRCA2* gene represents Fanconi complementation group D1 and is thought to aid DNA strand repair.[75] Because of this function, it is perhaps best to categorize *BRCA2* as a genome-maintenance gene rather than a conventional tumor-suppressor. As many as 7% of apparently *sporadic* pancreatic cancers (more, in instances of familial aggregation) harbor an inactivating intragenic inherited mutation of one copy of the *BRCA2* gene, accompanied by LOH.[1,2,66] The *PALB2* gene represents Fanconi group N, and its protein product functions by binding the Brca2 protein.[76] Three percent of familial pancreatic cancers harbored a germ-line inactivating mutation of *PALB2*, and in a tumor studied in depth, the other copy was inactivated by a somatic mutation.[1,77,78] The *FANCC* and *FANCG* genes have somatic or germ-line mutations in some pancreatic cancer patients, again with loss of the wild-type allele in the cancer.[79] The known hypersensitivity of Fanconi cells to interstrand DNA crosslinking agents, such as cisplatin, melphalan, and mitomycin C, suggested that pancreatic cancers with Fanconi pathway genetic defects would be especially susceptible to treatment with such agents.[80–83] Occasional complete remissions of pancreatic cancer have been reported with therapies that included DNA cross-linkers,[84–88] and there are recent reports of prolonged responses using such agents in patients having *BRCA2* mutations.[89,90] Cells made experimentally deficient for Fanconi genes are also hypersensitive to certain nongenotoxic compounds,[91] and patients that have *BRCA2*-mutant cancers other than pancreatic cancer are reported to respond to therapeutic drug inhibition of the poly (ADP-ribose) polymerase enzyme, which normally becomes activated to facilitate DNA-strand repair.[92] These opportunities are being explored in clinical trials.

A genomic mutational pattern (a *signature*) typical of cancers having *BRCA1* or *BRCA2* inactivation is reported in about 12% of pancreatic cancers.[93] This pattern involves nucleotide substitutions of broad diversity and indicates that the functions of BRCA genes extend to repair mechanisms not yet well explored. Among natural compounds tested, *BRCA2*- and *PALB2*-null cancers seem most hypersensitive to the toxicity of acetaldehyde,[94] a requisite metabolite of alcohol and a natural food constituent. Acetaldehyde

creates deoxynucleotide adducts, but the mutagenic effects of acetaldehyde in carriers of *BRCA2* and *PALB2* mutations are not yet explored with focused epidemiologic studies. Remarkably, *BRCA1* gene mutations were not found in unselected pancreatic cancers or pancreatic cancer families.[95] Nonetheless, pancreatic cancers do occur in carriers of *BRCA1*-inactivating mutations.[96,97] In these persons, the relatively high rate of LOH affecting the other *BRCA1* copy indicates that a loss of *BRCA1* function likely fosters tumorigenesis in these patients.[96]

A hotspot of genomic homozygous deletions affects the *FAM190A* gene, producing deletions of internal exons and typically resulting in in-frame deletions of the protein-coding sequence.[98,99] In addition to these genomic mutations, more than a third of PDAs have similar in-frame deletions affecting the *FAM190A* transcripts and/or defective expression of the Fam190A protein, but yet without an identifiable genomic mutation.[99,100] Fam190a functions in mitosis and in ensuring mononuclear daughter cells after the abscission (separation) phase of cell division.[100] Fam190a abnormalities thus might contribute to chromosomal instability during tumorigenesis.

The *mitochondrial genome* is mutated in a majority of pancreatic cancers.[101–103] These mutations most likely represent genetic drift, and perhaps do not directly contribute to the process of tumorigenesis.[103] Such mutations, however, could potentially serve as a diagnostic target due to the large number of copies of the mitochondrial genome in human carcinoma cells.[102,103]

Genes encoding components of the SWI/SNF chromatin-remodeling complex, including *ARID1A*, *ARID1B*, and *PBRM1*, are each occasionally mutated in PDA, in total affecting nearly a third of these tumors.[104,105]

The *MAP2K4* (*MKK4*) gene participates in a stress-activated protein kinase pathway.[81,82] It is stimulated by various influences, including chemotherapy, and its downstream effects include apoptosis and cellular differentiation. The *MKK4* gene is inactivated by homozygous deletions or mutation coupled with LOH in about 4% of pancreatic cancers.[106,107] The experimental loss of one or both copies of the *MKK4* gene in cancer cells reduced Jun kinase activation and its expression. Such gene dose-dependent effects could rationalize the high rate of loss of chromosomal arm 17p, affecting 90% of pancreatic cancers and more than half of TP53 wild-type cancers.[108]

Germ-line mutations of the *STK11* (*LKB1*) gene, a serine-threonine kinase, are responsible for Peutz-Jeghers syndrome (PJS).[109,110] PJS was anecdotally associated with pancreatic cancer.[111] A follow-up study examined lifetime risk, finding nearly a third of PJS patients to have developed pancreatic cancer.[112] Sporadic pancreatic cancers, independent of PJS, also can lose the gene by homozygous deletion or by somatic mutation/LOH in about 4% of cases.[113]

Kinase oncogenes are mutated at low frequency, including the *GUCY2F*, *EGFR*, and *NTRK3* genes.[91,92] This class of mutations is important in that these mutations can be targeted with antikinase drugs.[93]

Gene amplification also occurs in pancreatic cancer. Amplified regions include the *AKT2* gene within an amplicon on chromosome 19q, which involves about 10% to 20% of cases studied.[94–96] About 6% of pancreatic cancers overexpress the oncogene *CCNE1* (cyclin E). Two mechanisms have been demonstrated, cyclin E gene amplification and the genetic inactivation of the *FBXW7* (*AGO*) gene, which normally serves to degrade cyclin E during the normal phases of the cell division cycle.[1,114]

The patterns of *chromosomal deletion* in pancreatic cancer are complex. In one study, from 1.5% to 32% of all tested loci in the PDAs of different patients had a deletion.[115] For most lost regions, we know of no particular tumor-suppressor genes targeted by the deletions. Conversely, in some regions known to harbor tumor-suppressor genes, the known mutated genes do not justify the high observed prevalence rates of LOH unless gene dose-dependent effects are postulated.[108] Individual homozygous deletions are found at some additional genetic locations, again without a definitive target gene yet identified for most of these events.[98]

Defects in DNA mismatch repair (microsatellite instability, MSI) are seen in a small minority of pancreatic cancers. These cancers typically have a medullary histologic phenotype[10] and mutations of the type II TGF-β (*TGFBR2*) and activin (*ACVR2*) receptor genes.[28,55,56] They can also have mutations of the pro-apoptotic *BAX* gene[54] and of the growth factor pathway mediator *BRAF* gene (affecting the same pathway, presumably, as mutations of the *KRAS* gene).[10,11,54,114] The MSI tumors do not have the propensity for large chromosomal alterations and gross aneuploidy.[17,116] In a study of four cases of pancreatic cancers having MSI, all lacked expression of the Mlh1 protein.[11] Not all cancers with a medullary phenotype have MSI. Yet, medullary pancreatic carcinomas as a whole have a number of clinical and genetic differences as compared to those with conventional histologic appearance; the carcinomas have pushing rather than infiltrative borders, the *KRAS* gene often is wild type, and there is often a family history of malignancy.[5,6,47] A reported case of Epstein-Barr virus (EBV)–associated pancreatic cancer[11] had a medullary phenotype with heavy lymphocytic infiltration. Due to its distinctive features, it is advisable to separately designate the medullary category in the reporting of all clinical, genetic, and pathologic studies of pancreatic cancer.

Inherited or somatic inactivating mutations in the *ATM* gene accompany the loss of the wild-type allele of the cancers, indicating another tumor-suppressor gene for PDAs.[117,118]

Inherited mutations of the *cationic trypsinogen* (*PRSS1*) gene prevent the inactivation of prematurely activated trypsin within the ducts, causing a familial form of severe, early-onset acute pancreatitis.[119] Some affected kindred have a cumulative risk of pancreatic cancer that approaches 40% by the time the affected individuals reach 60 years of age.[120] This cancer diathesis falls in a unique category of cancer susceptibility, in that the predisposition emanates from genetic alterations of a tissue-maintenance gene, one that is not an oncogene, a tumor-suppressor gene, or a genome-maintenance gene.

In summary, pancreatic cancer is fundamentally a genetic disease. An understanding of the genes altered in pancreatic cancer has led to a better understanding of the familial aggregation of pancreatic cancer, which in turn, it is hoped, will lead to effective gene-specific targeted therapies for this deadly form of cancer.

REFERENCES

1. Jones S, Zhang X, Parsons DW, et al. Core signaling pathways in human pancreatic cancers revealed by global genomic analyses. *Science* 2008;321:1801–1806.
2. Shibata DK, Kern SE. Ancestral trees for modeling stem cell lineages genetically rather than functionally: Understanding mutation accumulation and distinguishing the restrictive cancer stem cell propagation theory and the unrestricted cell propagation theory of human tumorigenesis. *Breast Dis* 2008;29:15–25.
3. Blackford A, Parmigiani G, Kensler TW, et al. Genetic mutations associated with cigarette smoking in pancreatic cancer. *Cancer Res* 2009;69:3681–3688.
4. Yachida S, Jones S, Bozic I, et al. Distant metastasis occurs late during the genetic evolution of pancreatic cancer. *Nature* 2010;467:1114–1117.
5. Sato N, Mizumoto K, Nakamura M, et al. Centrosome abnormalities in pancreatic ductal carcinoma. *Clin Cancer Res* 1999;5:963–970.
6. Goggins M, Schutte M, Lu J, et al. Germline BRCA2 gene mutations in patients with apparently sporadic pancreatic carcinomas. *Cancer Res* 1996;56:5360–5364.
7. Ozcelik H, Schmocker B, Di Nicola N, et al. Germline BRCA2 6174delT mutations in Ashkenazi Jewish pancreatic cancer patients. *Nat Genet* 1997;16:17–18.
8. Murphy KM, Brune KA, Griffin C, et al. Evaluation of candidate genes MAP2K4, MADH4, ACVR1B, and BRCA2 in familial pancreatic cancer: deleterious BRCA2 mutations in 17%. *Cancer Res* 2002;62:3789–3793.
9. Hahn SA, Greenhalf B, Ellis I, et al. BRCA2 germline mutations in familial pancreatic carcinoma. *J Natl Cancer Inst* 2003;95:214–221.
10. Goggins M, Offerhaus GJA, Hilgers W, et al. Adenocarcinomas of the pancreas with DNA replication errors (RER+) are associated with wild-type K-ras and characteristic histopathology: poor differentiation, a syncytial growth pattern, and pushing borders suggest RER+. *Am J Pathol* 1998;152:1501–1507.
11. Wilentz RE, Goggins M, Redston M, et al. Genetic, immunohistochemical, and clinical features of medullary carcinomas of the pancreas: a newly described and characterized entity. *Am J Pathol* 2000;156:1641–1651.
12. Hruban RH, Wilentz R, Kern SE. Genetic progression in the pancreatic ducts. *Am J Pathol* 2000;156:1821–1825.
13. van Heek NT, Meeker AK, Kern SE, et al. Telomere shortening is nearly universal in pancreatic intraepithelial neoplasia. *Am J Pathol* 2002;161:1541–1547.
14. Gisselsson D, Jonson T, Petersen A, et al. Telomere dysfunction triggers extensive DNA fragmentation and evolution of complex chromosome abnormalities in human malignant tumors. *Proc Natl Acad Sci U S A* 2001;98:12683–12688.
15. Hiyama E, Kodama T, Shinbara K, et al. Telomerase activity is detected in pancreatic cancer but not in benign tumors. *Cancer Res* 1997;57:326–331.
16. Iwao T, Hiyama E, Yokoyama T, et al. Telomerase activity for the preoperative diagnosis of pancreatic cancer. *J Natl Cancer Inst* 1997;89:1621–1623.
17. Montgomery E, Wilentz RE, Argani P, et al. Analysis of anaphase figures in routine histologic sections distinguishes chromosomally unstable from chromosomally stable malignancies. *Cancer Biol Ther* 2003;2:248–252.
18. Cox AD, Der CJ. Ras family signaling: therapeutic targeting. *Cancer Biol Ther* 2002;1:599–606.
19. Almoguera C, Shibata D, Forrester K, et al. Most human carcinomas of the exocrine pancreas contain mutant c-K-ras genes. *Cell* 1988;53:549–554.
20. Caldas C, Hahn SA, Hruban RH, et al. Detection of K-ras mutations in the stool of patients with pancreatic adenocarcinoma and pancreatic ductal hyperplasia. *Cancer Res* 1994;54:3568–3573.
21. Klimstra DS, Longnecker DS. K-ras mutations in pancreatic ductal proliferative lesions. *Am J Pathol* 1994;145:1547–1550.
22. Kanda M, Matthaei H, Wu J, et al. Presence of somatic mutations in most early-stage pancreatic intraepithelial neoplasia. *Gastroenterology* 2012;142:730–773.e9.
23. Lerner EC, Qian Y, Blaskovich MA, et al. Ras CAAX peptidomimetic FTI-277 selectively blocks oncogenic Ras signaling by inducing cytoplasmic accumulation of inactive Ras-Raf complexes. *J Biol Chem* 1995;270:26802–26806.
24. Cox AD, Der CJ. Farnesyltransferase inhibitors: promises and realities. *Curr Opin Pharmacol* 2002;2:388–393.
25. Riggins GJ, Thiagalingam S, Rozenblum E, et al. Mad-related genes in the human. *Nat Genet* 1996;13:347–349.
26. Zawel L, Dai JL, Buckhaults P, et al. Human Smad3 and Smad4 are sequence-specific transcription activators. *Mol Cell* 1998;1:611–617.
27. Hahn SA, Schutte M, Hoque ATMS, et al. DPC4, a candidate tumor-suppressor gene at 18q21.1. *Science* 1996;271:350–353.
28. Goggins M, Shekher M, Turnacioglu K, et al. Genetic alterations of the TGF beta receptor genes in pancreatic and biliary adenocarcinomas. *Cancer Res* 1998;58:5329–5332.
29. Baldwin RL, Friess H, Yokoyama M, et al. Attenuated ALK5 receptor expression in human pancreatic cancer: correlation with resistance to growth inhibition. *Int J Cancer* 1996;67:283–288.
30. Serrano M, Hannon GJ, Beach D. A new regulatory motif in cell-cycle control causing specific inhibition of cyclin D/CDK4. *Nature* 1993;366:704–707.
31. Russo AA, Tong L, Lee JO, et al. Structural basis for inhibition of the cyclin-dependent kinase Cdk6 by the tumour suppressor p16INK4a. *Nature* 1998;395:237–243.
32. Coleman KG, Wautlet BS, Morrissey D, et al. Identification of CDK4 sequences involved in cyclin D1 and p16 binding. *J Biol Chem* 1997;272:18869–18874.
33. Caldas C, Hahn SA, da Costa LT, et al. Frequent somatic mutations and homozygous deletions of the p16 (MTS1) gene in pancreatic adenocarcinoma. *Nat Genet* 1994;8:27–31.
34. Schutte M, Hruban RH, Geradts J, et al. Abrogation of the Rb/p16 tumor-suppressive pathway in virtually all pancreatic carcinomas. *Cancer Res* 1997;57:3126–3130.
35. Goldstein AM, Fraser MC, Struewing JP, et al. Increased risk of pancreatic cancer in melanoma-prone kindreds with p16INK4 mutations. *N Engl J Med* 1995;333:970–974.
36. Moskaluk CA, Hruban RH, Lietman AS, et al. Novel germline p16INK4A allele (Asp145Cys) in a family with multiple pancreatic carcinomas. *Hum Mutat* 1998;12:70.
37. Whelan AJ, Bartsch D, Goodfellow PJ. Brief report: a familial syndrome of pancreatic cancer and melanoma with a mutation in the CDKN2 tumor-suppressor gene. *N Engl J Med* 1995;333:975–977.
38. Ciotti P, Strigini P, Bianchi-Scarra G. Familial melanoma and pancreatic cancer. *N Engl J Med* 1996;334:469–470.
39. Bartsch DK, Langer P, Habbe N, et al. Clinical and genetic analysis of 18 pancreatic carcinoma/melanoma-prone families. *Clin Genet* 2009;77:333–341.
40. Huang L, Lang D, Geradts J, et al. Molecular and immunochemical analyses of RB1 and cyclin D1 in human ductal pancreatic carcinomas and cell lines. *Mol Carcinog* 1996;15:85–95.

41. Kern SE, Kinzler KW, Bruskin A, et al. Identification of p53 as a sequence-specific DNA-binding protein. *Science* 1991;252:1708–1711.

42. El-Deiry WS, Tokino T, Velculescu VE, et al. WAF1, a potential mediator of p53 tumor suppression. *Cell* 1993;75:817–825.

43. Kern SE, Pietenpol JA, Thiagalingam S, et al. Oncogenic forms of p53 inhibit p53-regulated gene expression. *Science* 1992;256:827–830.

44. Redston MS, Caldas C, Seymour AB, et al. p53 mutations in pancreatic carcinoma and evidence of common involvement of homocopolymer tracts in DNA microdeletions. *Cancer Res* 1994;54:3025–3033.

45. Rozenblum E, Schutte M, Goggins M, et al. Tumor-suppressive pathways in pancreatic carcinoma. *Cancer Res* 1997;57:1731–1744.

46. Lengauer C, Kinzler KW, Vogelstein B. Genetic instabilities in human cancers. *Nature* 1998;396:643–649.

47. Johansson B, Bardi G, Heim S, et al. Nonrandom chromosomal rearrangements in pancreatic carcinomas. *Cancer* 1992;69:1–8.

48. Griffin CA, Hruban RH, Morsberger LA, et al. Consistent chromosome abnormalities in adenocarcinoma of the pancreas. *Cancer Res* 1995;55:2394–2399.

49. Brat DJ, Hahn SA, Griffin CA, et al. The structural basis of molecular genetic deletions: An integration of classical cytogenetic and molecular analyses in pancreatic adenocarcinoma. *Am J Pathol* 1997;150:383–391.

50. Hahn SA, Seymour AB, Hoque ATMS, et al. Allelotype of pancreatic adenocarcinoma using a xenograft model. *Cancer Res* 1995;55:4670–4675.

51. Ionov Y, Peinado MA, Malkhosyan S, et al. Ubiquitous somatic mutations in simple repeated sequences reveal a new mechanism for colonic carcinogenesis. *Nature* 1993;363:558–561.

52. Thibodeau SN, Bren G, Schaid D. Microsatellite instability in cancer of the proximal colon. *Science* 1993;260:816–819.

53. Aaltonen LA, Peltomäki P, Leach FS, et al. Clues to the pathogenesis of familial colorectal cancer. *Science* 1993;260:812–816.

54. Yamamoto H, Itoh F, Nakamura H, et al. Genetic and clinical features of human pancreatic ductal adenocarcinomas with widespread microsatellite instability. *Cancer Res* 2001;61:3139–3144.

55. Markowitz S, Wang J, Myeroff L, et al. Inactivation of the type II TGF-beta receptor in colon cancer cells with microsatellite instability. *Science* 1995;268:1336–1338.

56. Hempen PM, Zhang L, Bansal RK, et al. Evidence of selection for clones having genetic inactivation of the activin A type II receptor (ACVR2) gene in gastrointestinal cancers. *Cancer Res* 2003;63:994–999.

57. Rampino N, Yamamoto H, Ionov Y, et al. Somatic frameshift mutations in the BAX gene in colon cancers of the microsatellite mutator phenotype. *Science* 1997;275:967–969.

58. Day JD, DiGiuseppe JA, Yeo CJ, et al. Immunohistochemical evaluation of Her-2/neu oncogene expression in pancreatic adenocarcinoma and pancreatic intraepithelial neoplasms. *Human Pathol* 1996;27:119–124.

59. Lei S, Appert HE, Nakata B, et al. Overexpression of HER2/neu oncogene in pancreatic cancer correlates with shortened survival. *Int J Pancreatol* 1995;17:15–21.

60. Yamanaka Y, Friess H, Kobrin MS, et al. Overexpression of HER2/neu oncogene in human pancreatic carcinoma. *Hum Pathol* 1993;24:1127–1134.

61. Sakorafas GH, Lazaris A, Tsiotou AG, et al. Oncogenes in cancer of the pancreas. *Eur J Surg Oncol* 1995;21:251–253.

62. Preis M, Korc M. Signaling pathways in pancreatic cancer. *Crit Rev Eukaryot Gene Expr* 2011;21:115–129.

63. Matsubayashi H, Canto M, Sato N, et al. DNA methylation alterations in the pancreatic juice of patients with suspected pancreatic disease. *Cancer Res* 2006;66:1208–1217.

64. Jiang X, Hao HX, Growney JD, et al. Inactivating mutations of RNF43 confer Wnt dependency in pancreatic ductal adenocarcinoma. *Proc Natl Acad Sci U S A* 2013;110:12649–12654.

65. Wu J, Jiao Y, Dal Molin M, et al. Whole-exome sequencing of neoplastic cysts of the pancreas reveals recurrent mutations in components of ubiquitin-dependent pathways. *Proc Natl Acad Sci U S A* 2011;108:21188–21193.

66. Wu J, Matthaei H, Maitra A, et al. Recurrent GNAS mutations define an unexpected pathway for pancreatic cyst development. *Sci Transl Med* 2011;3:92ra66.

67. Kanda M, Knight S, Topazian M, et al. Mutant GNAS detected in duodenal collections of secretin-stimulated pancreatic juice indicates the presence or emergence of pancreatic cysts. *Gut* 2013;62:1024–1033.

68. Schonleben F, Qiu W, Ciau NT, et al. PIK3CA mutations in intraductal papillary mucinous neoplasm/carcinoma of the pancreas. *Clin Cancer Res* 2006;12:3851–3855.

69. Abraham SC, Klimstra DS, Wilentz RE, et al. Solid-pseudopapillary tumors of the pancreas are genetically distinct from pancreatic ductal adenocarcinomas and almost always harbor beta-catenin mutations. *Am J Pathol* 2002;160:1361–1369.

70. Abraham SC, Wu TT, Klimstra DS, et al. Distinctive molecular genetic alterations in sporadic and familial adenomatous polyposis-associated pancreatoblastomas: frequent alterations in the APC/beta-catenin pathway and chromosome 11p. *Am J Pathol* 2001;159:1619–16127.

71. Chung DC, Brown SB, Graeme-Cook F, et al. Localization of putative tumor suppressor loci by genome-wide allelotyping in human pancreatic endocrine tumors. *Cancer Res* 1998;58:3706–3711.

72. Jiao Y, Shi C, Edil BH, et al. DAXX/ATRX, MEN1, and mTOR pathway genes are frequently altered in pancreatic neuroendocrine tumors. *Science* 2011;331:1199–1203.

73. Heaphy CM, de Wilde RF, Jiao Y, et al. Altered telomeres in tumors with ATRX and DAXX mutations. *Science* 2011;333:425.

74. Yachida S, Vakiani E, White CM, et al. Small cell and large cell neuroendocrine carcinomas of the pancreas are genetically similar and distinct from well-differentiated pancreatic neuroendocrine tumors. *Am J Surg Pathol* 2012;36:173–184.

75. Mizuta R, LaSalle JM, Cheng HL, et al. RAB22 and RAB163/mouse BRCA2: proteins that specifically interact with the RAD51 protein. *Proc Natl Acad Sci U S A* 1997;94:6927–6932.

76. Xia B, Sheng Q, Nakanishi K, et al. Control of BRCA2 cellular and clinical functions by a nuclear partner, PALB2. *Mol Cell* 2006;22:719–729.

77. Jones S, Hruban RH, Kamiyama M, et al. Exomic sequencing identifies PALB2 as a pancreatic cancer susceptibility gene. *Science* 2009;324:217.

78. Slater EP, Langer P, Niemczyk E, et al. PALB2 mutations in European familial pancreatic cancer families. *Clin Genet* 2010;78:490–494.

79. van der Heijden MS, Yeo CJ, Hruban RH, et al. Fanconi anemia gene mutations in young-onset pancreatic cancer. *Cancer Res* 2003;63:2585–2588.

80. Kern SE, Hruban RH, Hidalgo M, et al. An introduction to pancreatic carcinoma genetics, pathology, and therapy. *Cancer Biol Ther* 2002;1:607–613.

81. Moynahan ME, Cui TY, Jasin M. Homology-directed DNA repair, mitomycin-c resistance, and chromosome stability is restored with correction of a Brca1 mutation. *Cancer Res* 2001;61:4842–4850.

82. Tutt A, Bertwistle D, Valentine J, et al. Mutation in Brca2 stimulates error-prone homology-directed repair of DNA double-strand breaks occurring between repeated sequences. *Embo J* 2001;20:4704–4716.

83. Gallmeier E, Calhoun ES, Rago C, et al. Targeted disruption of FANCC and FANCG in human cancer provides a preclinical model of specific therapeutic options. *Gastroenterology* 2006;130:2145–2154.

84. Todd KE, Gloor B, Lane JS, et al. Resection of locally advanced pancreatic cancer after downstaging with continuous-infusion 5-fluorouracil, mitomycin-C, leucovorin, and dipyridamole. *J Gastrointest Surg* 1998;2:159–166.

85. Takada T, Nimura Y, Katoh H, et al. Prospective randomized trial of 5-fluorouracil, doxorubicin, and mitomycin C for non-resectable pancreatic and biliary carcinoma: multicenter randomized trial. *Hepatogastroenterology* 1998;45:2020–2026.

86. Sadoff L, Latino F. Complete clinical remission in a patient with advanced pancreatic cancer using mitomycin C-based chemotherapy: the role of adjunctive heparin. *Am J Clin Oncol* 1999;22:187–190.

87. Miura T, Endo Y, Matumoto Y, et al. [Intra-arterial infusion chemotherapy in combination with microwave hyperthermia for cancer of head of pancreas and liver metastasis—a case of 16 years survival]. *Gan To Kagaku Ryoho* 2000;27:1794–1800.

88. Vaughn C, Chapman J, Chinn B, et al. Activity of 5-fluorouracil, mitomycin C, and methyl CCNU in inoperable adenocarcinoma of pancreas. *Am J Clin Oncol* 1989;12:49–52.

89. James E, Waldron-Lynch MG, Saif MW. Prolonged survival in a patient with BRCA2 associated metastatic pancreatic cancer after exposure to camptothecin: a case report and review of literature. *Anticancer Drugs* 2009;20:634–638.

90. Chalasani P, Kurtin S, Dragovich T. Response to a third-line mitomycin C (MMC)-based chemotherapy in a patient with metastatic pancreatic adenocarcinoma carrying germline BRCA2 mutation. *JOP* 2008;9:305–308.

91. Gallmeier E, Kern SE. Targeting Fanconi anemia/BRCA2 pathway defects in cancer: the significance of preclinical pharmacogenomic models. *Clin Cancer Res* 2007;13:4–10.

92. Fong PC, Boss DS, Yap TA, et al. Inhibition of poly(ADP-ribose) polymerase in tumors from BRCA mutation carriers. *N Engl J Med* 2009;361:123–134.

93. Alexandrov LB, Nik-Zainal S, Wedge DC, et al. Signatures of mutational processes in human cancer. *Nature* 2013;500:415–421.

94. Ghosh S, Sur S, Yerram SR, et al. Hypersensitivities for acetaldehyde and other agents among cancer cells null for clinically-relevant Fanconi anemia genes. *Am J Pathol* 2014;184:260–270.

95. Axilbund JE, Argani P, Kamiyama M, et al. Absence of germline BRCA1 mutations in familial pancreatic cancer patients. *Cancer Biol Ther* 2009;8:131–135.

96. Al-Sukhni W, Rothenmund H, Borgida AE, et al. Germline BRCA1 mutations predispose to pancreatic adenocarcinoma. *Hum Genet* 2008;124:271–278.

97. Lal G, Liu G, Schmocker B, et al. Inherited predisposition to pancreatic adenocarcinoma: role of family history and germ-line p16, BRCA1, and BRCA2 mutations. *Cancer Res* 2000;60:409–416.

98. Calhoun ES, Hucl T, Gallmeier E, et al. Identifying allelic loss and homozygous deletions in pancreatic cancer without matched normals using high-density single-nucleotide polymorphism arrays. *Cancer Res* 2006;66:7920–7928.

99. Scrimieri F, Calhoun ES, Patel K, et al. FAM190A rearrangements provide a multitude of individualized tumor signatures and neo-antigens in cancer. *Oncotarget* 2011;2:69–75.

100. Patel K, Scrimieri F, Ghosh S, et al. FAM190A deficiency creates a cell division defect. *Am J Pathol* 2013;183:296–303.

101. Polyak K, Li Y, Zhu H, et al. Somatic mutations of the mitochondrial genome in human colorectal tumours. *Nat Genet* 1998;20:291–293.

102. Fliss MS, Usadel H, Caballero OL, et al. Facile detection of mitochondrial DNA mutations in tumors and bodily fluids. *Science* 2000;287:2017–2019.

103. Jones JB, Song JJ, Hempen PM, et al. Detection of mitochondrial DNA mutations in pancreatic cancer offers a "mass"-ive advantage over detection of nuclear DNA mutations. *Cancer Res* 2001;61:1299–1304.

104. Jones S, Li M, Parsons DW, et al. Somatic mutations in the chromatin remodeling gene ARID1A occur in several tumor types. *Hum Mutat* 2011;33:100–103.

105. Shain AH, Giacomini CP, Matsukuma K, et al. Convergent structural alterations define SWItch/Sucrose NonFermentable (SWI/SNF) chromatin remodeler as a central tumor suppressive complex in pancreatic cancer. *Proc Natl Acad Sci U S A* 2012;109:E252–E259.

106. Su GH, Hilgers W, Shekher M, et al. Alterations in pancreatic, biliary, and breast carcinomas support MKK4 as a genetically targeted tumor-suppressor gene. *Cancer Res* 1998;58:2339–2342.

107. Teng DH-F, Perry III WL, Hogan JK, et al. Human mitogen-activated protein kinase kinase 4 as a candidate tumor suppressor. *Cancer Res* 1997;57:4177–4182.

108. Cunningham SC, Gallmeier E, Hucl T, et al. Theoretical proposal: allele dosage of MAP2K4/MKK4 could rationalize frequent 17p loss in diverse human cancers. *Cell Cycle* 2006;5:1090–1093.

109. Hemminki A, Markie D, Tomlinson I, et al. A serine/threonine kinase gene defective in Peutz-Jeghers syndrome. *Nature* 1998;391:184–187.

110. Jenne DE, Reimann H, Nezu J, et al. Peutz-Jeghers syndrome is caused by mutations in a novel serine threonine kinase. *Nature Genet* 1998;18:38–43.

111. Giardiello FM, Welsh SB, Hamilton SR, et al. Increased risk of cancer in the Peutz-Jeghers syndrome. *N Engl J Med* 1987;316:1511–1514.

112. Giardiello FM, Brensinger JD, Tersmette AC, et al. Very high risk of cancer in familial Peutz-Jeghers syndrome. *Gastroenterology* 2000;119:1447–1453.

113. Su GH, Hruban RH, Bova GS, et al. Germline and somatic mutations of the STK11/LKB1 Peutz-Jeghers gene in pancreatic and biliary cancers. *Am J Pathol* 1999;154:1835–1840.

114. Calhoun ES, Jones JB, Ashfaq R, et al. BRAF and FBXW7 (CDC4, FBW7, AGO, SEL10) mutations in distinct subsets of pancreatic cancer: potential therapeutic targets. *Am J Pathol* 2003;163:1255–1260.

115. Iacobuzio-Donahue CA, van der Heijden MS, Baumgartner MR, et al. Large-scale allelotype of pancreaticobiliary carcinoma provides quantitative estimates of genome-wide allelic loss. *Cancer Res* 2004;64:871–875.

116. Lengauer C, Kinzler KW, Vogelstein B. Genetic instability in colorectal cancers. *Nature* 1997;386:623–627.

117. Roberts NJ, Jiao Y, Yu J, et al. ATM mutations in patients with hereditary pancreatic cancer. *Cancer Discov* 2012;2:41–46.

118. Biankin AV, Waddell N, Kassahn KS, et al. Pancreatic cancer genomes reveal aberrations in axon guidance pathway genes. *Nature* 2012;491:399–405.

119. Whitcomb DC, Gorry MC, Preston RA, et al. Hereditary pancreatitis is caused by a mutation in the cationic trypsinogen gene. *Nature Genet* 1996;14:141–145.

120. Lowenfels AB, Maisonneuve P, DiMagno EP, et al. Hereditary pancreatitis and the risk of pancreatic cancer. International Hereditary Pancreatitis Study Group. *J Natl Cancer Inst* 1997;89:442–446.

Cancer of the Pancreas

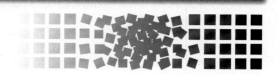

Jordan M. Winter, Jonathan R. Brody, Ross A. Abrams, Nancy L. Lewis, and Charles J. Yeo

INTRODUCTION

Pancreatic ductal adenocarcinoma (PDA) is the 12th most common cancer in the United States, but the 4th most frequent cause of cancer-related death.[1] There are 44,000 new cases of PDA each year in the United States and 38,000 deaths.[2] Although the death rates of most common cancers have declined over the past 80 years, the death rates for PDA have remained flat to slightly increased.[1] Based on demographic, incidence, and survival projections, PDA death rates are expected to eclipse death rates from breast and colon cancer within the next decade, and become the 2nd most deadly cancer. In short, PDA remains a deadly disease and is currently only curable in a minority of patients with localized and resectable disease.

Disease-specific survival has not changed significantly in the past 4 decades, regardless of disease stage. Patients with metastatic disease continue to have a 5-year survival of 2% or less.[1,3,4] A recent single-institution, retrospective analysis of patients with resected PDA revealed similar overall survivals in the 2000s and the 1980s.[5] The similarity in overall survival over time is not at all surprising considering the relatively modest advances in chemotherapy during this time. Although targeted and immunotherapies are now routinely used to treat certain other cancer types, personalized medicines with novel biologic therapies have not yet been successful for PDA.

This chapter provides a comprehensive overview of the pathobiology and management of pancreatic cancer, focusing on PDA. The less common types of pancreatic cancer (e.g., pancreatic neuroendocrine tumors and pancreatic cysts) will be discussed briefly. Current management strategies are placed in an historical context, and the latest understanding of the genetics and molecular biology of pancreatic cancer is reviewed. The management of PDA requires a multidisciplinary approach that involves surgeons, medical oncologists, radiation oncologists, radiologists, gastroenterologists, palliative medicine specialists, nurses, nutritionists, and many others. Herein, the roles of surgery, chemotherapy, and radiation will be emphasized. As much as possible, treatment strategies are framed in the context of the American Joint Committee on Cancer (AJCC) 7th edition staging scheme.[6]

STAGING

Pancreatic cancer is staged according to the AJCC, 7th edition, TNM staging system (Table 41.1).[6] Presented survival data are based on 1998 data.[7] T-stage is defined as follows: Tis is carcinoma in situ (pancreatic intraepithelial neoplasia [PanIN-3]); T1 is 2 cm or less and confined to the pancreas; T2 is greater than 2 cm and confined to the pancreas; T3 extends beyond the pancreas; and T4 invades visceral vessels, rendering the tumor unresectable. N-stage is defined as follows: N0 reflects no regional lymph node metastases; and N1 reflects regional lymph node metastases. M-stage is defined as follows: M0 reflects no distant metastases; and M1 reflects distant metastases.

EPIDEMIOLOGY

Like most cancers, PDA develops as a result of acquired genetic defects over many years, and therefore, most often occurs in the elderly. The median age at onset is 71 years, and nearly 74% of patients are diagnosed between the ages of 55 and 84. Only 12% of patients are diagnosed under 55, and 14% after the age of 84. The age-adjusted incidence rate in the United States is 12 out of 100,000, and the lifetime risk of developing PDA is 1.5%, or 1 in 67. African Americans have a slightly increased risk compared to Caucasians.[8]

Genetic Risk Factors

The greatest risk factor for pancreatic cancer is a strong family history. Approximately 10% of all pancreatic cancers are familial, defined as a family history involving at least two affected first-degree relatives (FDR) (e.g., parents, offspring, and siblings).[9] The lifetime risk is 40% (32-fold) for patients with three or more affected FDRs, 10% for patients with two FDRs (6.4-fold), and 6% for patients with 1 FDR (4.6-fold).[10] Some of the genetic defects underlying familial pancreatic cancer have been discovered, but known genetic defects only account for 10% to 15% of all familial cases.[11] Specific genetic abnormalities are discussed in greater detail in the Pathology and Biology section.

Environmental Risk Factors: Tobacco, Occupational Hazards, and Alcohol Consumption

Many environmental risk factors have been formally evaluated via meta-analyses performed by the Pancreatic Cancer Case Control Consortium (PanC4, http://panc4.org/index.html). Smoking tobacco is the best characterized environmental risk factor for PDA. A large meta-analysis of 83 studies calculated a relative risk increase at 1.74 for active smokers (this is substantially less than having even a single FDR).[12] Importantly, the risk decreases for former smokers, and returns to baseline after 20 years of smoking cessation.[12] These results were confirmed by the PanC4 consortium, which also noted that the number of daily cigarettes is directly proportional to the risk of developing PDA.[13] Not surprising, high-risk individuals with a family history who also smoke carry twice the risk, compared to similar patients who do not smoke.[14,15] Cigars are also associated with an increased risk for PDA, whereas smokeless tobacco is not.[16] The impact of environmental tobacco smoke (i.e., second-hand smoke) on long-term risk is unclear.[17,18] Among the many carcinogens in tobacco products, N-nitrosamines and the polycyclic aromatic hydrocarbons (PAH) are suspected to be the greatest culprits.[19]

With regard to occupational risk hazards, chlorinated hydrocarbons and PAHs have been most consistently found to correlate with PDA, and to increase relative risk by a comparable degree

TABLE 41.1

American Joint Committee on Cancer Staging for Pancreatic Cancer

Stage	T	N	M	Median Survival, All Patients (Months)	Median Survival, Resected Patients (Months)
0	Tis	N0	M0	N/A	N/A
1A	T1	N0	M0	10.0	24.1
1B	T2	N0	M0	9.1	20.6
IIA	T3	N0	M0	8.1	15.4
IIB	T1	N1	M0	9.7	12.7
	T2	N1	M0		
	T3	N1	M0		
III	T4	Any N	M0	7.7	10.6
IV	Any T	Any N	M1	2.5	4.5
Total				4.4	12.6

Modified from Bilimoria KY, Bentrem DJ, Ko CY, et al. Validation of the 6th edition AJCC Pancreatic Cancer Staging System: report from the National Cancer Database. *Cancer* 2007; 110:738–744.

as smoking.[20] The former compound type is associated with dry cleaning and metal work, and, with the latter, exposure occurs with metalwork and aluminum production. According to the PanC4 consortium, mild or moderate alcohol consumption does not predispose one to PDA, whereas heavy alcohol consumption (≥9 drinks per day) is associated with an odds ratio (OR) of 1.6.[21]

Medical Risk Factors: Pancreatitis, Diabetes, and Obesity

Like smoking, chronic pancreatitis is a well-accepted risk factor for PDA, with an OR of 2.7 for patients with over 2 years of disease. The OR skyrockets for patients with less than 2 years of chronic pancreatitis (13.6), in large part because the pancreatitis in these patients represents a presenting symptom of PDA, as oppose to a contributing cause.[22] A preponderance of the evidence from over a dozen studies suggests that obesity is a mild contributing risk factor for PDA (OR 1 to 1.5). Proposed mechanistic links include hormonal (e.g., insulin and insulin-like growth factor 1 [IGF-1]) and inflammatory influences on pancreatic cells, as well as increased carcinogen exposure related to food consumption.[23] Although a link between type II diabetes mellitus (DM) and pancreatic cancer has been extensively studied, a causal association has not been clearly established. Two meta-analyses have been performed that examined more than 30 studies performed over 4 decades. Type II DM is associated with a twofold risk increase for PDA. Patients with long-standing DM (>5 years) have a mildly increased risk compared to patients without DM, suggesting that the disease may indeed contribute to tumorigenesis. Similar to obesity, increased levels of insulin and IGF-1 have been implicated. As with chronic pancreatitis, the highest risk for PDA is clearly in patients with recent onset of DM (<5 years, and particularly within 1 year), suggesting that DM is principally a manifestation of PDA, as opposed to a true risk factor in these patients.[24,25]

PATHOLOGY AND BIOLOGY

The normal pancreas contains two epithelial cell types: exocrine and endocrine cells. Most of the pancreas is comprised of exocrine cells, which line an organized ductal network. Acinar cells line the smallest ducts; they synthesize and secrete digestive enzymes. Larger ducts are lined by intercalated duct cells, and secrete bicarbonate and water. Ultimately, the ducts converge into the main pancreatic duct, which drains into the duodenum. The endocrine component makes up just 1% of the pancreas, and consists of islets of Langerhans. These hormone-producing cell clusters are primarily involved with glucose homeostasis. The principal endocrine cell types include the A (alpha), B (beta), and D (delta) cells, which synthesize glucagon, insulin, and somatostatin, respectively. The different cell types are believed to give rise to the different variants of pancreatic neoplasms.

Pancreatic cancer refers to a heterogeneous group of malignant pathologies that originate in the pancreas, and nearly all are epithelial in origin. They are categorized by their gross appearance (solid or cystic), as well as the predominant cell differentiation pattern (ductal, acinar, or endocrine). Primary pancreatic mesenchymal (e.g., sarcomas) and lymphoid neoplasms are exceptionally rare, and will not be reviewed here. Dozens of different epithelial pancreatic neoplasms have been described, but over 85% are the conventional pancreatic (tubular) ductal adenocarcinomas, and more than 98% of cancers fit into one of the following additional diagnoses: solid types, which include pancreatic endocrine neoplasms, acinar cell carcinomas, and pancreatoblastomas; and cystic types, which include mucinous cystic neoplasms, intraductal papillary mucinous neoplasms, and solid-pseudopapillary neoplasms. These diagnoses are typically made based on microscopic appearance, but a diagnosis may be confirmed with immunolabeling of specific proteins. Uncommon variants of ductal adenocarcinoma that are rarely encountered will not be reviewed. These include adenosquamous carcinoma, colloid noncystic adenocarcinoma, hepatoid carcinoma, signet ring carcinoma, medullary carcinoma, and undifferentiated carcinoma. The classification and nomenclature of pancreatic epithelial neoplasms has been reviewed by Klimstra, Pitman, and Hruban.[26]

EXOCRINE PANCREATIC CANCERS

Pancreatic Ductal Adenocarcinoma

Although the molecular mechanisms that underlie aggressive PDA biology remain poorly understood, there are certain features of PDA that are unique or defining, and will be highlighted in this section on pathobiology as well as in the Future Directions and Challenges section at the end of the chapter. These include molecular heterogeneity, a tendency for perineural invasion, remarkable tolerance to nutrient deprivation, and abundant stroma.

PDA Pathology

PDAs appear as ill-defined, sclerotic, yellow-white masses on gross inspection. The edges are poorly defined and infiltrative. Histologically, they are characterized by perineural invasion in almost all cases (much more frequently than in other common adenocarcinomas like colon and breast). Microscopic vessel and lymphatic invasion are common, and tumor necrosis is frequently present. Even in localized and resected cases, PDAs are rarely encountered at the T1 stage nor are they well differentiated, which drives home the fact that PDA is seldom diagnosed *early* in the life span of the tumor, at a *curable* stage.[27] On light microscopy, the cells typically form infiltrative gland-forming structures, separated from each other by a tenacious desmoplastic reaction. Lymph node spread is present in the majority of resection specimens with localized disease. Immunohistochemical markers typically seen include cytokeratins (e.g., 7, 8, 13, 18, 19), CA19-9, B72.3, CA-125, and DUPAN-2. The nonneoplastic desmoplastic (stromal) component comprises more than 70% of the tumor mass (a higher proportion than other common solid tumors), and is commonly referred to as

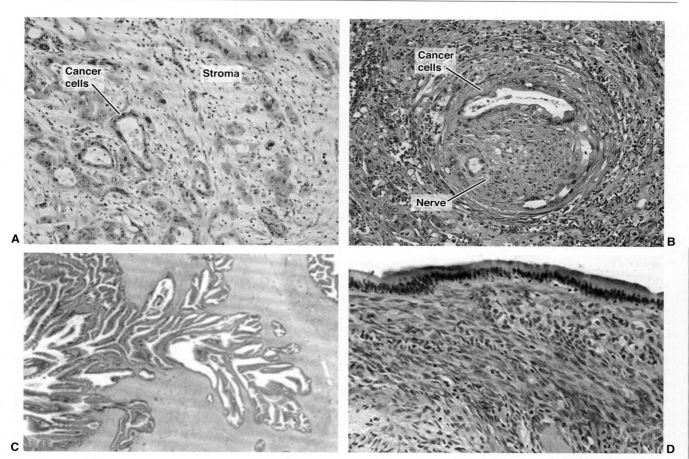

Figure 41.1 High-power photographs of PDA. **(A)** PDA containing dense stroma. **(B)** PDA with perineural invasion. **(C)** Intraductal papillary mucinous neoplasms. **(D)** Mucinous cystic neoplasms.

the tumor microenvironment (TME). The stroma consists of an extracellular matrix and numerous cell types, including inflammatory cells, pancreatic stellate cells, endothelial cells, nerve cells, fibroblasts, and myofibroblasts. The stroma is hypovascular with a low vessel density and high interstitial fluid pressure, resulting in a poorly perfused epithelial compartment, and the characteristic *hypodense* appearance on cross-sectional imaging obtained with intravenous contrast. Classic histologic features of PDA are depicted in Figure 41.1.[28]

The stroma creates a barrier to effective drug delivery[29] and is believed to contribute to the overall virulence of the tumor. Sophisticated mathematical modeling reveals that austere conditions in the TME impose profound selection pressures on cancer cells, leading to the generation and dominance of aggressive cancer subclones.[30] These subclones are chemoresistant and well adapted to survive extreme conditions present in the TME. Not surprisingly, PDA cells are more resistant to nutrient deprivation than most aggressive cancer types.[31] There is now a concerted effort to develop strategies to target the tumor microenvironment in PDA (see Future Directions and Challenges).

PDA development follows an adenoma to carcinoma sequence, similar to previous descriptions for colon cancer.[32] Precursor lesions are referred to as PanIN lesions (pancreatic intraepithelial neoplasia), and are graded from PanIN-1 to PanIn-3. Early PanIN lesions are common (present 20% of individuals at autopsy[33]) and most do not progress to PDA in an individual's lifetime. PanIN-1A lesions are tall columnar cells with abundant mucin; PanIN-1B lesions are similar but have a papillary appearance. PanIN-2 lesions have nuclear abnormalities. PanIN-3 lesions were formerly called carcinoma in situ; they exhibit true cribriforming, budding cells

into lumen, loss of nuclear polarity, and mitoses. PanIN-3 lesions are found in roughly 2% of autopsy specimens from individuals who died from nonpancreatic diseases (Fig. 41.2).[33] The similar lifetime risk of PDA suggests that a high proportion of PanIN-3 lesions develop into clinically significant cancer. Future effective early detection strategies would ideally discover and treat PanIN-3 lesions.[28]

PDA Genetics

Unlike breast and other cancers, PDA cannot be subgrouped by molecular characteristics at the present time to guide therapy or to inform prognosis. However, whole-exome sequencing of numerous PDAs were performed and provided unprecedented insight into the genetics of PDA.[34,35] High throughput sequencing data emphasize the molecular complexity of PDA. Out of 24 PDA genomes, 1,327 different genes (~7% of coding genes) were found to have at least one somatic mutation, and 148 different genes had at least two mutations (0.7%).[35] There were an average of 60 genetic alterations per tumor, and each PDA had a unique genetic fingerprint. Unfortunately, sequencing studies did not identify any novel high frequency mutated *cancer genes* as promising therapeutic targets. A more practical approach to *personalized therapy* is to group the genetically altered genes into 12 core signaling pathways (e.g., apoptosis, DNA damage, and 10 others), as proposed by Jones et al.[35] These pathways are universally dysregulated and therefore may be more realistic therapeutic targets than single genes.[35] A separate study found that axon guidance genes were also mutated at a higher rate than what was expected by chance, although the functional importance of these neuron-related genes in cancer is still unknown.[34]

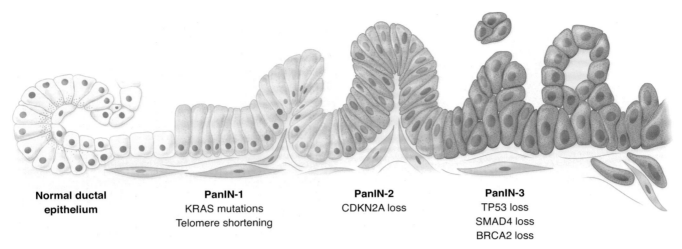

| Normal ductal epithelium | PanIN-1
KRAS mutations
Telomere shortening | PanIN-2
CDKN2A loss | PanIN-3
TP53 loss
SMAD4 loss
BRCA2 loss |

Figure 41.2 PanIN sequence with observed molecular changes. (From Maitra A, Hruban RH. Pancreatic cancer. *Annu Rev Pathol* 2008;3:157–188.)

A genetically altered gene may be categorized as an oncogene (with gain-of-function mutations), a tumor suppressor gene (loss-of-function), or a genome maintenance gene (loss-of-function). For the latter two gene types, both copies of the gene are typically inactivated; one allele is lost by somatic mutation and the other by chromosomal or allelic loss (loss of heterozygosity [LOH]). Oncogenic Kras is altered in more than 90% of PDAs, and is usually an early event in tumorigenesis.[28,35,36] Somatic Kras mutations mostly occur in codon 12, and rarely occur in codons 13 and 61.[37] The sequence alterations inactivate GTPase function, leaving GTP continuously engaged and the oncogene constitutively activated. Activated Kras positively regulates multiple signaling pathways, including the BRAF/mitogen-activated protein kinase (MAPK) pathway (proliferation), phosphatidylinositol 3-kinase (PI3K)/mammalian target of rapamycin (mTOR) (cell growth and survival), and Phospholipase C (PLC)/Protein kinase C (PKC)/Ca^{++} (calcium and second messenger signaling).[38] To date, attempts to pharmacologically inhibit Kras have been unsuccessful.[39] However, because of its early development in nearly all PDAs, the importance of this molecule will continue to preoccupy pancreatic researchers in hopes of finding an effective targeted therapy with a large therapeutic window (see Future Directions section).

The remaining *high frequency* mutated pancreatic cancer genes are tumor suppressor genes. The pattern of frequent allelic loss mutations in PDA due to chromosome instability (losses are more common than gains[40]), promotes a fertile environment of genetic experimentation that favors loss of function mutations. Allelotype mapping reveals that genetic loss ranges from 17% to 80% of the genome in a given PDA.[41] Allelic loss is nonrandom across the PDA genome; LOH *hot spots* (areas where genetic loss most commonly occurs) harbor the most important tumor suppressors genes in PDA: CDKN2A (9p), TP53 (19p), and SMAD4 (18q).

CDKN2A (p16) is inactivated in roughly 95% of PDAs, either through homozygous deletion (deletion of both alleles), somatic mutation combined with LOH (deletion of one allele), or promoter hypermethylation. Inactivation of the gene abrogates the RB1-mediated G1/S checkpoint in the cell cycle (which allows unchecked inhibition of RB1 by CDK4), promoting cell cycle progression and cancer cell proliferation.[42,43] TP53 mutations combined with LOH also occur in the majority of PDAs (~75%).[44] TP53 is a critical component of the DNA damage response. In the face of a cytotoxic stress, TP53 induces cell cycle arrest (at G1 or G2 of the cell cycle), allowing cells to repair their DNA prior to DNA synthesis or mitosis. Thus, TP53 loss contributes to chromosome instability and aneuploidy observed in PDA.[45] TP53 has been targeted experimentally by reactivating the mutant isoform[46] or by targeting the G2/M checkpoint with WEE1 inhibitors

(TP53-deficient tumors are particularly dependent on the G2/M checkpoint).[47] SMAD4/DPC4 is inactivated in roughly half of PDAs through either homozygous deletion or mutation combined with LOH.[48,49] SMAD4 is part of the transforming growth factor β (TGFβ) receptor pathway, and like the other two aforementioned tumor suppressor genes, regulates the cell cycle at the G1/S checkpoint.[28] Interestingly, preservation of SMAD4 protein expression is associated with a local predominant progression pattern in PDA, which could be used to guide patient selection for radiotherapy.[49]

A group of genome maintenance genes (BRCA2, PALB2, FANCC, FANCG) involved in the Fanconi anemia DNA repair pathway (mutated in <10% of PDAs) are particularly intriguing because tumors deficient in this pathway are highly susceptible to DNA damaging agents and poly(ADP-ribose) polymerase (PARP) inhibitor therapy.[28] Mutations in these genes are often present in the germline, and will be discussed further in the section on genetic syndromes associated with pancreatic cancer.

Analyses of laser capture microdissected pancreatic tissues have elucidated the chronologic sequence of major genetic changes in pancreatic tumorigenesis. Telomere shortening and *Kras* mutations are believed to be the earliest events (PanIN-1)[50,51]; *p16* loss occurs at the PanIN-2 stage[52]; and TP53, SMAD4, and BRCA2 inactivation occur later during the PanIN-3 stage (see Fig. 41.2).[53,54] Major chromosome instability, characterized by large-scale allelic copy number changes, is rarely observed in PanIN lesions, and is principally limited to LOH *hot spots*.[55–57]

Iacobuzio-Donahue and colleagues[49] recently launched into pioneering work by extending the molecular progression model of pancreatic cancer to the most advanced stages of disease, through a rapid autopsy program in which primary tumors and paired metastases were sequenced and compared. The investigators distinguished *founder mutations* (those that arise early in tumorigenesis and are present throughout a tumor; about two-thirds of mutations) from *progressor mutations* (mutated in subclonal populations of cells, and absent in the parental clones; about one-third of mutations).[58] Interestingly, progressor mutations that existed throughout a metastatic deposit were also identified in certain microdissected foci in the primary tumor, but not throughout the primary. This finding demonstrated that parent clones giving rise to specific metastases can actually be defined and mapped in the primary tumor. Although previous sequencing studies highlighted intertumoral heterogeneity, this study was the first to identify intratumoral genetic heterogeneity in PDAs, with profound implications on therapy.

Roughly 10% of PDAs are familial, and only 10% of the familial subgroup are associated with a previously defined genetic syndrome.[59] Table 41.2 summarizes those familial syndromes and

TABLE 41.2

Familial Disorders Linked to Prediposition to Pancreatic Ductal Adenocarcinoma

Disease	Gene/Pathway	Lifetime Risk
Inherited pancreatitis	SPINK1/PRSS1	40%
Peutz-Jeghers syndrome	LKB1	30%
Familial atypical multiple mole melanoma (FAMMM)	CDKN2A	15%
Hereditary breast and ovarian cancer	BRCA2	5%
Familial breast cancer	PALB2	?
Ataxia telangiectasia	ATM	?
Familial (>3 FDRs)	Unknown	40%
Familial (2 FDRs)	Unknown	10%
Familial (1 FDRs)	Unknown	6%

FDR, first-degree relative.

genetic defects that have been identified in pancreatic cancer kindreds. Hereditary breast and ovarian cancer is the most common familial syndrome, and the Peutz-Jeghers syndrome confers the highest lifetime risk. Importantly, several of the familial syndromes are associated with defects in DNA repair pathways (BRCA2, PALB2), which likely render tumors particularly susceptible to therapy with DNA damaging agents (e.g., mitomycin C, platinum agents) and PARP inhibitors.[11] Other genetic predisposition alterations, such as single nucleotide polymorphisms (SNP) likely play a role in cancer risk, but remain to be fully characterized. Ongoing whole-exome sequencing efforts in familial patients will almost certainly uncover additional genetic abnormalities that predispose individuals to PDA.

There are currently no universal guidelines or proven strategies for screening high-risk individuals. The Cancer of the Pancreas Screening (CAPS) project has been the principal mechanism to study this patient population and generate recommendations. In one CAPS study, 225 asymptomatic, high-risk individuals were screened with magnetic resonance imaging (MRI), computed tomography (CT) scans, or endoscopic ultrasound (EUS) and the results were interpreted in a blinded fashion. An abnormality was identified in 92 patients (42%), and 5 were recommended to undergo a pancreatectomy (2%). High-grade dysplasia was present in three out of the five specimens.[60] These data highlight that while successes are possible, the general yield of screening programs, even in this high-risk group, is relatively low.

Recently, a 49 member multidisciplinary panel made the following recommendations (with varying degrees of agreement amongst panelists): candidates for screening include FDRs of individuals with familial pancreatic cancer (at least two FDRs); patients with Peutz-Jeghers syndrome; and p16, BRCA2, and HNPCC mutation carriers with one affected FDR. There was also consensus that EUS and MRI were the preferred surveillance strategies. Routine surveillance should be performed annually, and suspicious solid masses should be further evaluated by CT scanning. Screening should begin around 50 years of age.[61]

Other Aspects of PDA Biology

Genetically engineered mouse models (GEMM) of PDA have provided a valuable research tool to study PDA biology.[62] The workhorse of pancreatic cancer research in this area has been the conditional Kras model, where pancreas-specific promoters are exploited to target oncogenic Kras expression exclusively to the pancreas. Kras mutant mice develop pancreatic precursor lesions

(e.g., PanIN lesions). Compound mutant mice with an additional genetic abnormality (e.g., mutant TP53 or CDKN2A) develop invasive and metastatic PDA, simulating human PDA. Similarly, Kras mutant mice with induced pancreatitis also develop invasive PDA. Genetic variations have also been generated that recapitulate pancreatic cystic tumors (SMAD4 loss or TGFα overexpression). The contributions of these models have been immeasurable. For instance, cell lineage tracing experiments in GEMMs reveal that PDA likely originates from acinar or centroacinar cells, as opposed to ductal cells (i.e., acinar-to-ductal metaplasia). GEMMs are enabling the development of molecular and bioimaging assays to detect late PanIN and early invasive lesions. Because GEMMs develop tumors with a robust stroma compartment, therapeutic strategies targeting the stroma can be tested. Early results suggest that this strategy enhances therapeutic efficacy of standard cytotoxic therapy. Finally, these models can be used to test and refine chemoprevention strategies before moving to humans.

Cancer genetics (e.g., mutations) have been prioritized over the last few decades in PDA cancer research, in large part because of the reproducibility of the findings and because the genetic model of tumorigenesis is straightforward and accepted. However, it is now clear that other molecular changes are also paramount for PDA development and maintenance. These include epigenetic abnormalities (methylation and histone modification), transcriptional regulation, and posttranscriptional regulation (microRNAs and RNA binding proteins).[28]

Less Common Pancreatic Cancers

Acinar Cell Carcinoma

Acinar cell carcinomas may have a slightly better prognosis (median survival of 33 months) than conventional PDA. The presentation is similar, except that patients may occasionally develop a paraneoplastic syndrome related to lipase hypersecretion, leading to subcutaneous fat necrosis and polyarthralgia. Microscopically, tumors grow in a trabecular pattern with minimal intervening stroma. Immunohistochemical confirmation is made with positive labeling for pancreatic enzymes (e.g., lipase, trypsin, chymotrypsin, amylase).[63] Cystic variants have been reported as well, and described as acinar cystadenoma or cystadenocarcinoma.[26] Twice the number of somatic mutations per tumor is present (~130 per tumor) compared to PDA, and allelic loss is comparable (27% fractional loss). Whole-exome sequencing did not reveal a consistent genetic pattern; no gene was mutated in more than 30% of cancers, and mutant genes previously identified in diverse pancreatic tumor types (e.g., TP53, SMAD4, RNF43, MEN1, GNAS) and nonpancreatic tumors (e.g., BRAF, PTEN, RB1, APC) were identified. Additionally, some mutant familial genes were identified (e.g., ATM, BRCA2, PALB2), suggesting that this tumor may arise in a familial pattern.[64] Interestingly, no Kras mutations were identified.

Pancreatoblastoma

Pancreatoblastoma is the most common pancreatic malignancy in children and usually occurs in the first 8 years of life. These tumors have been associated with the Beckwith-Wiedmann and familial adenomatous polyposis syndromes. Elevated levels of serum α-fetoprotein and hormones have been described. Cures are often achievable with resection in children, although one-third of patients present with metastatic disease. Cases have been reported in adults as well, with survival after resection that is comparable to conventional PDA.[65] Microscopically, these tumors contain acinar cells, but other cell types (e.g., neuroendocrine, ductal) are often present. Pancreatoblastomas have been whole-exome sequenced in only two adult cases.[64] These tumors acquire relatively few mutations (~15 per tumor), and SMAD4 and CTNNB1 are typical. Kras mutations have not been reported.

Intraductal Papillary Mucinous Neoplasms

Intraductal papillary mucinous neoplasms (IPMN) are mucin-producing cystic neoplasms that arise from (and therefore communicate with) pancreatic ducts.[66] Similar to PanIN lesions, they follow a progression pattern: low-grade dysplasia, moderate-grade dysplasia, high-grade dysplasia, and frank invasive carcinoma. Benign IPMNs are subgrouped according to their papillary appearance on microscopy (see Fig. 41.1), with each type associated with a particular mucin expression pattern: intestinal (MUC5AC, MUC2), gastric-foveolar (MUC5AC, MUC6), pancreatobiliary (MUC5AC, MUC1), and intraductal oncocytic neoplasm (MUC1, MUC6). Clinically, IPMNs are classified as involving the side-branch ducts or the main-pancreatic duct, with some tumors involving both of these. IPMNs are the most common pancreatic cystic neoplasms and with increased usage of high-resolution cross-sectional imaging, are believed to develop in roughly 1% to 5% of the general population.[67] Although all benign IPMNs are technically *premalignant*, there is a wide range of malignant potential amongst encountered cysts. For instance, main duct IPMNs harbor associated cancers 40% of the time, whereas small side-branched IPMNs without any concerning radiographic features have a cancer risk closer to 5% or less.[68] Thus, there has been considerable effort to try to determine which IPMNs harbor invasive cancer or are at highest risk for malignant transformation and warrant resection. The Sendai guidelines recommend resection for IPMNs that are either symptomatic, >3 cm in diameter, contain solid components (e.g., mural nodules), have malignant cells on cytology, or involve the main pancreatic duct.[68] Invasive cancer associated with IPMNs are most commonly either tubular (conventional PDA) or colloid subtypes. The former is typically more aggressive and develops from pancreatobiliary IPMNs, whereas the latter usually develops from intestinal subtypes. Although IPMN-associated cancers have a more favorable prognosis than conventional PDA, this has been attributed to the lower stage at diagnosis; when matched stage for stage, the two pancreatic cancer types are associated with similar outcomes.[69] Moreover, a recent multi-institution analysis of IPMNs with small foci of invasion (all <2 cm invasive component) indicates a significant recurrence risk (~20%) regardless of the size of the invasive component (Jordan M. Winter, MD, unpublished, July 2014).

Whole-exome sequencing of IPMN lesions revealed roughly half the number of mutations (~27 per tumor) compared to PDA. There was a high incidence of RNF43 mutations, which is a tumor suppressor with E3 ubiquitin ligase activity (involved in protein degradation).[70] Additionally, Kras and GNAS mutations occurred with high frequency.

Mucinous Cystic Neoplasms

Mucinous cystic neoplasms (MCN) are typically large cysts lined by tall, columnar epithelium (see Fig. 41.1). Benign MCNs are categorized similar to IPMNs from low- to high-grade dysplasia, and roughly one-third of cases harbor invasive cancer. Additionally, RNF43 and Kras mutations are frequently present (as with IPMNs). Distinguishing features of MCNs (from IPMNs) include a large predominance in woman, the cysts are typically localized on the left side of the pancreas, ovarian stroma underlying the epithelial component is pathognomonic (even in men), there is no communication with the pancreatic duct, and GNAS mutations have not been identified.[26,70]

Solid-Pseudopapillary Neoplasms

Solid-pseudopapillary neoplasms (SPNs) solid and cystic tumors are eponymously referred to as Hamoudi or Franz tumors. They typically occur in young women and may arise throughout the gland. Histologically, they consist of noncohesive polygonal cells that form solid masses, but develop cystic components over time with frequent intracystic hemorrhage. The tumors are considered low-grade malignancies, with a 10% risk of lymph node spread in resected specimens, and a 95% lifetime recurrence-free survival rate after resection.[71] SPNs develop fewer than five somatic mutations per tumor, but virtually all SPNs harbor CTNNB1 (β-catenin) mutations. This molecular abnormality is believed to contribute to the poor cohesion between cells apparent on microscopy (wild type β-catenin interacts with E-cadherin at cell–cell junctions).

ENDOCRINE PANCREATIC CANCERS

The classification of pancreatic neuroendocrine tumors (PNET) has been challenging based on the heterogenous biology of this tumor type. Recent staging systems have been adopted based on size and lymph node metastases, with different versions in the United States (AJCC 7th ed. 2010, same as exocrine pancreatic cancer) and Europe (European Neuroendocrine Tumor Society [ENETS]).[72] The ENETS system also considers biologic parameters and has simplified the World Health Organization classification according to the following scheme: G1 (well differentiated, <2 mitoses per 10 High power field (HPF), <3% KI67 index); G2 (well differentiated, intermediate grade: 2 to 20 mitoses per 10 HPF, 3% to 20% KI67 index); and G3 (high grade or poorly differentiated: >20 mitoses per 10 HPF, >20% KI67 index).[73] Typically, G1 tumors are considered benign and cured with resection, whereas G2 tumors are considered malignant. However, the distinction (benign versus malignant) is not always clear. Older studies observed that half of PNETs were nonfunctional and half were functional due to the presence of measurable hormones in serum.[74] The balance has shifted dramatically toward nonfunctional tumors being more common, in large part due to small, incidentally discovered PNETs identified on cross-sectional imaging obtained for nonpancreatic reasons.

Pancreatic neuroendocrine cancers have an incidence of roughly 0.2 out of 100,000 (versus 12 out of 100,00 for PDAs), yet autopsy studies show that small PNETs are very common (~10% of deceased individuals).[75] They comprise roughly 5% of all resected pancreatic cancers (on par with IPMN associated cancers).[27] PNETs are typically well demarcated and hypervascular. Therefore, they focally enhance on the arterial phase in imaging studies with intravenous contrast. Microscopically, neoplastic cells are arranged in a nested fashion with a high density of intratumoral microvessels (in contrast to PDA). The majority of well-differentiated PNETs have an indolent course and are cured with surgery alone. Even patients with metastatic disease have a 5-year survival around 50%.[72] Insulinomas are the most common functional PNETs (30% to 45%) and symptoms are associated with excessive endogenous insulin production (Whipple triad: documented hypoglycemia, symptoms of hypoglycemia, improved symptoms with correction of hypoglycemia).[76] Gastrinomas comprise roughly 20% of functional PNETs, and cause peptic ulcer disease and diarrhea from hypergastrinemia. Less common functional PNETs include glucagonomas (associated with glucose intolerance and migratory necrolytic erythema), VIPomas (watery diarrhea), and somatostatinomas (steatorrhea, diabetes mellitus, and gallstones). Familial syndromes associated with the development of PNETs include multiple endocrine neoplasia 1 (MEN1 gene), von Hippel-Lindau disease (VHL), neurofibromatosis (NF1), and tuberous sclerosis (TSC1 or TSC2).

The genetic landscape of PNETs has now been defined through whole-exome sequencing.[77] Compared to PDAs, there are fewer somatic mutations per tumor (~16). Kras mutations have not been observed. Commonly mutated genes included MEN1 (44% of PNETs), chromatin remodeling genes (43%: DAXX and ATRX), and mTOR pathway genes (15%: phosphatase and tensin homolog [PTEN], PIK3CA, and TSC2). This latter gene group likely renders many PNETs vulnerable to systemic targeted therapy using mTOR inhibitors. Although surgery is the principal therapy for local disease, treatment options have greatly expanded for advanced disease, and include local liver-directed therapies (radiofrequency ablation), regional liver-directed therapies (bland, chemo, and radioembolization), and systemic therapies (cytotoxic drugs, targeted agents, somatostatin analogs including radio-labeled drugs). The complex management of PNETs is discussed in other reviews on the subject.[78]

STAGE I AND II: LOCALIZED PANCREATIC DUCTAL ADENOCARCINOMA

Anatomy

The evaluation and treatment of localized pancreatic cancer requires a strong understanding of the anatomy of the pancreas and nearby structures. The pancreas is an elongated gland in the retroperitoneum that crosses the midline at the L2 spinal level (Fig. 41.3). It is bounded anteriorly by the stomach and posteriorly by the inferior vena cava, aorta, left adrenal gland, and left kidney. The descriptive anatomy of the gland is grossly separated into four components. The head is the right-most portion, and sits within the duodenal C-loop. It includes parenchyma to the right of the superior mesenteric vessels and contains the uncinate process, which projects inferomedially, extending to the right lateral border of the superior mesenteric artery. The common bile duct runs

within (or rarely just posterior) to the pancreatic head and enters the duodenum at the ampulla of Vater with the main pancreatic duct. Moving leftward, the neck of the pancreas lies anterior to the superior mesenteric vein–portal vein axis. The superior mesenteric vessels run posterior to the pancreatic neck, and course inferiorly across the anterior border of the third portion of the duodenum. The body of the pancreas extends to the left of the superior mesenteric vessels. The gland transitions distally into the pancreatic tail anterior to the left kidney, and courses toward the splenic hilum.

Presentation

The most common presenting symptoms associated with PDA located in the right side of the pancreas (head, neck, or uncinate process) include jaundice (75%), weight loss (50%), abdominal pain (40%), or nausea (10%).[27] Jaundice occurs as a result of obstruction of the common bile duct and is often associated with pruritus. Other symptoms or findings associated with an obstructed bile duct include acholic stools and tea-colored urine. An obstructed pancreatic duct may induce acute pancreatitis and result in exocrine insufficiency associated with steatorrhea. Patients with left-sided PDAs (body or tail) typically experience abdominal pain, back pain, and nausea. New onset DM (within 1 year of diagnosis) occurs in roughly 10% of patients with PDA, based on our own institutional experience and others (unpublished).[79]

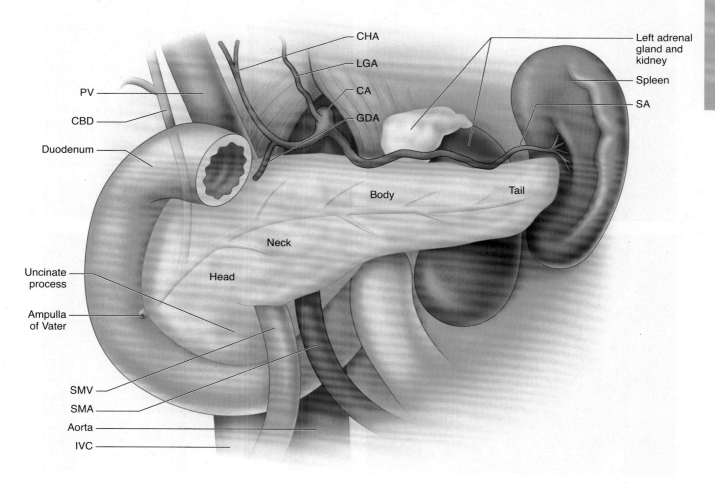

Figure 41.3 Pancreatic and peripancreatic anatomy. CBD, common bile duct; PV, portal vein; CHA, common hepatic artery; LGA, left gastric artery; CA, celiac axis; GDA, gastroduodenal artery; SA, splenic artery; SMV, superior mesenteric vein; SMA, superior mesenteric artery; IVC, inferior vena cava. (Courtesy of Jennifer Brumbaugh, Department of Surgery, Thomas Jefferson University.)

Evaluation and Assessing Resectability

Although periampullary cancer (adenocarcinoma of the pancreas, ampulla of Vater, bile duct, or periampullary duodenum) should be considered in any patient who presents with a conjugated hyperbilirubinemia, the likelihood is highest in older patients (e.g., >55 years). In individuals with an expected pancreatic cancer, a thorough history and physical should be performed, followed by appropriate imaging for staging and to assess resectability. Critical findings on physical exam include scleral icterus, jaundice, and lymphadenopathy (e.g., Sister Mary Joseph or Virchow nodes). A chest x-ray or chest CT scan is performed to assess for pulmonary metastases and as a baseline study. Either a high-quality MRI or CT scan of the abdomen is performed to evaluate the pancreas and measure the extent of disease. We typically prefer CT for its superior resolution and detailed depiction of the relevant vasculature. Water is administered as oral contrast, and nonionic intravenous contrast is rapidly injected. Slices are captured at 1-mm intervals from the diaphragm to the iliac crests at three different times or phases: early arterial, late arterial, and venous. Multiplanar reformatting and three-dimensional (3D) surface rendering is performed during the early arterial and venous phases (Fig. 41.4).[80] Positron-emission tomography (PET)/CT scans do

not add much additional value and are not routinely performed in the initial assessment for resectability.

Resection is attempted if (1) patients are medically fit for a pancreatectomy, (2) there is no evidence of metastases, and (3) patients are believed to have *resectable* disease. Resectability is ultimately decided by the operating surgeon, but general guidelines have been proposed and are based on the likelihood of achieving a complete, margin-negative resection.[81,82] Resectability equates to a high probability of an R_0 resection; borderline resectability equates to a likely result of an R_1 resection (positive microscopic margins); and unresectable (or locally advanced) PDA is likely to result in R_2 resection (residual macroscopic disease). Resectable lesions do not invade the superior mesenteric artery (SMA), celiac axis (CA), common hepatic artery (CHA), or superior mesenteric–portal vein axis (SMV-PV). In contrast, locally advanced lesions encase (i.e., >180° invasion) any of the previously mentioned arteries or occlude the SMV-PV such that no reconstructive options remain. Borderline resectable lesions involve the visceral vessels to a lesser extent; they can abut the visceral arteries (<180° invasion), distort the visceral veins, or even occlude the SMV-PV, but with venous reconstruction still technically feasible (Table 41.3).[83] Most pancreatic surgeons offer patients with resectable lesions an attempt at resection (although some centers advocate neoadjuvant treatment prior to resection even for resectable lesions[84]). Patients with locally advanced lesions are recommended

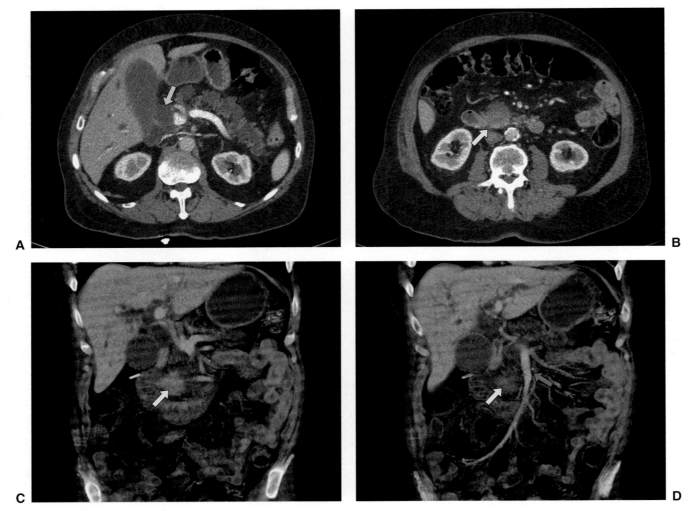

Figure 41.4 Slices from a triphasic CT scan in a patient with resectable pancreatic cancer. **(A)** Late arterial phase. Double duct sign with dilated common bile and pancreatic ducts, and an atrophic pancreatic body. **(B)** Mass. **(C)** Coronal reconstructions, venous phase, with the mass apparent, and **(D)** clearly away from the superior mesenteric–portal vein axis (SMV/PV) axis. *Yellow arrow* = PDA; *green arrow* = common bile duct; *red arrow* = pancreatic duct; and *blue arrow* = SMV. (Courtesy of Jennifer Brumbaugh, Department of Surgery, Thomas Jefferson University.)

TABLE 41.3

Criteria for Resectability

Vessel	Resectable R₀ Resection Likely	Borderline Resectable R₁ Resection Likely	Locally Advanced R₂ Resection Likely
SMA	No abutment	Tumor abutment	Tumor encasement
Celiac axis/ hepatic artery	No abutment	Tumor abutment	Tumor encasement
SMV–PV	Abutment may be present but no vein distortion	Vein Distortion or short-segment occlusion with suitable vessel above and below	Occluded and no technical option for reconstruction

Note: R_0 = gross total resection; histologically <u>negative</u> margins.
R_1 resection = gross total resection; one or more histologically <u>positive</u> margins.
R_2 resection = subtotal resection, visible tumor unresected.
Abutment is ≤180° vessel circumference; encasement is >180° vessel circumference.
SMA, superior mesenteric artery; SMV–PV, superior mesenteric vein–portal vein.
Modified from Varadhachary GR, Tamm EP, Abbruzzese JL, et al. Borderline resectable pancreatic cancer: definitions, management, and role of preoperative therapy. *Ann Surg Oncol* 2006;13:1035–1046.

to undergo palliative treatment without the intent to cure. Considerable debate remains for borderline PDAs; resection may be offered, but increasingly, neoadjuvant treatment is recommended for even abutment or narrowing of the SMV-PV.[81] Neoadjuvant chemotherapy (± radiation) can facilitate resection, and may improve the likelihood of a complete resection with negative margins, even in the absence of a radiographic response.[85]

Obtaining a tissue diagnosis is not essential for all cases. Indications include instances when (1) neoadjuvant treatment is advised or (2) the pretest probability of an alternative diagnosis is considerable (e.g., suspicion for benign causes of pancreatitis, medically managed neoplasms such as lymphoma, or a benign stricture). In these instances, an EUS with fine-needle aspiration (FNA) biopsy is an effective method for obtaining tissue and has an accuracy in excess of 90%.[86] When the diagnosis is clear based on imaging and history, it is appropriate to proceed to attempted resection without a preoperative tissue diagnosis. Similarly, placement of an endoscopic biliary stent is frequently performed in jaundiced patients preoperatively, but is essential in only selected cases. A multicenter prospective and randomized trial compared routine preoperative biliary drainage with delayed resection to early surgery without stenting in jaundiced patients with pancreatic cancer. Serious complications were increased nearly twofold in the routine biliary drainage group (74% versus 39%; p <0.001), suggesting that biliary decompression be reserved for jaundiced patients unable to undergo resection in a short-time frame (1 to 2 weeks).[86] A pancreaticoduodenectomy is safely performed, even when the total bilirubin is markedly elevated. Patients, who are otherwise healthy, with normal renal function and clotting parameters will usually tolerate a safely performed pancreaticoduodenectomy with a total bilirubin as high as 20 mg/dL.

Surgery

Technical aspects of a pancreatectomy are detailed elsewhere and are well beyond the scope of this chapter, hence will only be reviewed briefly here. For right-sided pancreatic cancers, a pancreaticoduodenectomy (PD) is performed. The specimen includes the gallbladder, duodenum, head of the pancreas (the pancreatic transection typically is at the level of the neck), proximal jejunum, and distal common bile duct. The most proximal retained jejunum is brought up into the right upper quadrant, and three anastomoses to the pancreas remnant, common hepatic duct, and proximal duodenum (or stomach) are performed (Fig. 41.5A). A distal pancreatectomy for PDA involves resection of the pancreatic body and tail, with an en bloc splenectomy performed to ensure a proper lymphadenectomy. The transected surface of the

pancreatic remnant is closed with suture (Fig. 41.5B) or staples. A central pancreatectomy or local excision for a PDA is seldom if ever performed for PDA due to inadequate lymph node harvest.

A minimally invasive pancreatectomy using laparoscopy or a robotic-assisted approach may be safely performed. Although a minimally invasive approach is more common for benign and premalignant lesions, a presumed diagnosis of PDA is not a contraindication.[87] A meta-analysis comparing open versus laparoscopic distal pancreatectomies for PDA revealed similar oncologic and pathologic outcomes in the two groups. Patients undergoing laparoscopy had a shorter postoperative stay by 4 days, less blood loss, and fewer surgical site infections.[88] Importantly, studies comparing the two techniques have not been prospective and randomized, and are, therefore, all subject to selection bias, with the more difficult resections falling into the open group. Although most high-volume pancreatic centers offer minimally invasive left-sided resections, laparoscopic PD is more technically challenging, and only a handful of centers have a significant experience.[89] These centers report comparable outcomes with minimally invasive versus open pancreatic surgery in their own experience, although an advantage of laparoscopic PD has not yet been proven in a prospective and randomized study.

International Study Group of Pancreatic Surgery Contributions

Surgically related mortality after PD has improved dramatically over the last 3 decades, and is lower than 5% at most high volume centers.[27] However, morbidity remains high (~40%). The most common complications include pancreatic leak (20%), delayed gastric emptying (15%), and wound infection (10%). Bile and duodenal leaks occur in roughly 3% and 1% of patients, respectively.[27] The greatest limitation to studies focused on pancreatectomy-related complications has been a lack of standard definitions across institutions, making comparisons between institutions' reports difficult. The formation of an International Study Group of Pancreatic Surgery (ISGPS) to address this issue has been a great advance in pancreatic surgery–related outcomes research. The group has published consensus criteria and definitions for complication grading on the following pancreatic-specific morbidities: postoperative pancreatic fistula (leak),[90] delayed gastric emptying,[91] and postpancreatectomy hemorrhage.[92] In addition, the group established concrete guidelines on reporting features and management of the pancreatic remnant/anastomosis (e.g., duct size, gland texture, mobilization distance, type of anastomosis, suture used, use of stent).[93] Definitions of postpancreatectomy-related mortality, bile leak,[94] and wound infection also vary in the literature, and

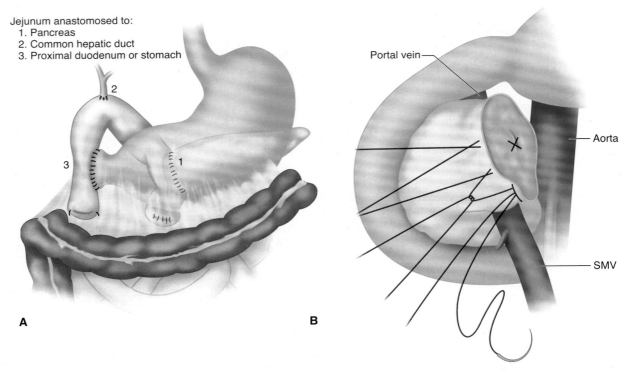

Figure 41.5 **(A)** Standard reconstruction after a pancreaticoduodenectomy, with an end-to-side pancreaticojejunostomy, an end-to-side hepatic jejunostomy, and a retro-colic and end-to-side duodenojejunostomy. **(B)** Suture closure of the pancreatic remnant after distal pancreatectomy.

a strategy to standardize terms and complication grading for these outcomes would enhance the surgical literature.

Surgical Trials

There have been numerous prospective and randomized surgical trials that have shaped the surgical management of PDA. A trial unique to PDA, compared to other common cancers, is a study demonstrating superiority of resection over best nonoperative therapy for the management of resectable disease.[95] A total of 42 patients in Japan with resectable PDA were randomized to either standard pancreatectomy without adjuvant treatment or to chemoradiation alone (50.4 Gy with continuous fluorouracil [5-FU] at 200 mg/m^2 per day) without surgery. Randomization occurred at laparotomy and patients randomized to chemoradiation had only an open biopsy and abdominal closure. The only multivariate predictor of survival in the study was the treatment group (hazard ratio [HR] = 0.4; p = 0.02), with the group undergoing resecting having superior survival (median overall survival (OS), 13 versus 9 months).

Pancreaticoduodenectomy

A comprehensive list of surgical trials in patients undergoing pancreaticoduodenectomy is provided in Table 41.4. Regarding technical aspects of the operation, one of the more studied questions compares pylorus preserving pancreaticoduodenectomy (PPPD) to distal gastrectomy plus pancreaticoduodenectomy (classic PD).[96–102] Karanicolas et al.[97] performed a meta-analysis of six randomized trials including 574 patients. PPPD was associated with a reduced operative time by more than 1 hour (p <0.001), less blood loss (284 mL; p <0.001), and fewer blood transfusions. There was a nonsignificant trend toward improved mortality in the same direction (0.4; p = 0.09). There was not a significant difference in delayed gastric emptying. Multiple randomized studies have also

examined the location of the enteroenterostomy (antecolic versus retrocolic), and no significant differences were observed.[103–107]

A postoperative pancreatic fistula (POPF) remains the most challenging complication after PD. Clinically significant leaks (e.g., requiring treatment intervention) occur in roughly 10% of cases. Risk factors include soft pancreatic texture, a fatty pancreas, a small pancreatic duct, high intraoperative blood loss, and a high postoperative serum amylase level.[108,109] Numerous randomized trials have attempted to reduce the pancreatic leak rate, although few have succeeded. Ineffective interventions include fibrin glue,[110,111] octreotide,[112–119] and internal pancreatic stenting.[27] Mixed results have been reported with pancreaticogastrostomy (versus standard pancreaticojejunostomy).[120–126] The pancreaticojejunostomy *technique* was recently examined, comparing a two-layered invagination technique with interrupted outer stitches and a continuous inner layer, against a duct-to-mucosa technique. The pancreatic leak rate was more than twofold higher with the latter approach (7% grade B/C versus 17%; p = 0.03).[127] A binding pancreaticojejunostomy (versus invagination) is a second technique shown to have a decreased pancreatic leak rate. With this technique, an end-to-end pancreaticojejunostomy is performed; 3 cm of the pancreatic remnant is mobilized and telescoped within the jejunum. No leaks were observed in 106 patients in the latter group, although these data have not yet been replicated.[128] Interestingly, there now have been three randomized trials showing a lower pancreatic leak rate associated with external pancreatic duct stenting (the pancreatic duct stent is brought out through the bowel and skin as a drain),[129–131] whereas a fourth study revealed no benefit.[132] In the past, trials using somatostatin or its analogs have had mixed outcomes in lowering pancreatic leak rates. Recently, a phase III trial using pasireotide (SOM230, a potent somatostatin analog) was completed at Memorial Sloan-Kettering Cancer Center, and revealed a statistically significant lower pancreatic leak rate in patients receiving subcutaneous injections of the study drug

TABLE 41.4

Randomized Surgical Trials with Pancreaticoduodenectomy

Author	Year	Trial	Result
Doi[95]	2008	Surgery vs. chemoradiation for PDA	↑ Survival with surgery
Riall[137]	2005	PD vs. PD with lymphadenectomy	= Survival
Pedrazzoli[136]	1998	PD vs. PD with lymphadenectomy	= Survival
Farnell[135]	2005	PD vs. PD with lymphadenectomy	= Survival
Brennan[138]	1994	Preoperative TPN vs. none	↑ Morbidity with TPN
Ke[133]	2013	Roux-en-Y PJ vs. standard	↓ Grade B POPF with Roux-en-Y
Fischer[281]	2010	Hemodilution vs. standard intraoperative IVF	↑ POPF with hemodilution
Uemura[282]	2008	Ulinastatin vs. placebo	↓ Pancreatitis with ulinastatin
Jo[283]	2006	Glutamine supplement vs. none	= Morbidity
Conlon[139]	2001	Drain vs. no drain	= Complications and mortality
Bassi[284]	2010	Late vs. early drain removal	↑ Complications with late
Van Buren[140]	2013	Drain vs. no drain	↑ Mortality with drain
Van der Gaag[86]	2010	Preoperative biliary drainage vs. none	↑ Morbidity with drainage
Poon[130]	2007	External MPD stent vs. no stent	↓ POPF with external stent
Kuroki[285]	2011	External MPD stent vs. no stent	= POPF
Pessaux[129]	2011	External MPD stent vs. no stent	↓ POPF with external stent
Motoi[131]	2012	External MPD stent vs. no stent	↓ POPF with external stent
Kamoda[286]	2008	External MPD stent vs. internal stent	= POPF
Tani[287]	2010	External MPD stent vs. internal stent	= POPF
Winter[27]	2006	Internal MPD stent vs. no stent	= POPF
Yeo[126]	1995	PG vs. PJ	= POPF
Arnaud[121]	1999	PG vs. PJ	↓ POPF with PG
Takano[125]	2000	PG vs. PJ	↓ POPF with PG
Duffas[123]	2005	PG vs. PJ	= POPF
Bassi[122]	2005	PG vs. PJ	= POPF
Fernandez-Cruz[124]	2008	PG vs. PJ	↓ POPF with PG
Klempa[119]	1991	Octreotide vs. none	= POPF
Beguiristain[113]	1995	Octreotide vs. none	= POPF
Yeo[112]	2000	Octreotide vs. placebo	= POPF
Gouillat[115]	2001	Octreotide vs. placebo	= POPF
Shan[117]	2003	Octreotide vs. none	= POPF
Kollmar[116]	2008	Octreotide vs. placebo	= POPF
Fernandez-Cruz[114]	2013	Octreotide vs. placebo	= POPF
Wang[118]	2013	Octreotide vs. placebo	= POPF
Allen[a]	2013	SOM230 vs. placebo	↓ POPF with SOM230
Reissman[288]	1995	MPD duct ligation vs. PJ	↑ POPF with ligation
Tran[289]	2002	MPD duct ligation vs. PJ	= POPF
Lillemoe[110]	2004	Fibrin glue to PJ vs. none	= POPF
Martin[111]	2013	Fibrin glue to PJ vs. none	= POPF
Bassi[290]	2003	Invagination PJ vs. duct-to-mucosa	= POPF
Berger[127]	2009	Invagination PJ vs. duct-to-mucosa	↓ POPF with invagination
Peng[128]	2007	Binding PJ vs. invagination	↓ POPF with binding PJ
Yeo[291]	1993	Erythromycin vs. placebo	↓ DGE with erythromycin
Tani[107]	2006	Antecolic vs. retrocolic DJ	↓ DGE with antecolic DJ
Gangavatiker[104]	2011	Antecolic vs. retrocolic DJ	= DGE

(continued)

Randomized Surgical Trials with Pancreaticoduodenectomy *(continued)*

Author	Year	Trial	Result
Imamura[103]	2013	Antecolic vs. retrocolic DJ	= DGE
Tamandl[106]	2013	Antecolic vs. retrocolic DJ	= DGE
Eshuis[105]	2014	Antecolic vs. retrocolic DJ	= DGE
Paquet[99]	1998	PPPD vs. classic	= DGE
Bloechle[96]	1999	PPPD vs. classic	= DGE
Wenger[102]	1999	PPPD vs. classic	= Morbidity
Tran[101]	2004	PPPD vs. classic	= DGE
Lin[98]	2005	PPPD vs. classic	↑ DGE with PPPD
Seiler[107]	2005	PPPD vs. classic	= DGE

Note: Shading pattern highlights similar trials.
[a] Personal communication with senior author.
TPN, total parenteral nutrition; PJ, pancreaticojejunostomy; POPF, postoperative pancreatic fistula; IVF, intravenous fluid; MPD, main pancreatic duct; PG, pancreaticogastrostomy; DJ, duodenojejunostomy; DGE, delayed gastric emptying; PPPD, pylorus preserving pancreaticoduodenectomy.

(Peter J. Allen, email communication, January 2014). Roux-en-Y reconstruction performed to isolate the pancreaticojejunostomy (PJ) from the other two anastomoses did not decrease the overall leak rate, but the proportion of clinically significant leaks was substantially reduced (74% versus 29% of all leaks; p = 0.01).[133]

In addition to these important technical trials relevant to the management of right-sided pancreatic neoplasms, other studies have informed the management of patients undergoing PD. A group of studies established that a radical retroperitoneal lymphadenectomy does not confer improved cancer-specific survival (four randomized trials).[134–137] Additionally, routine adjuvant parenteral nutrition has proven to be detrimental.[138] A previous single-institution randomized trial suggested that routine nondrainage after a pancreatic resection is safe,[139] whereas a recent multi-institution and randomized study revealed a much higher mortality rate in patients without drains,[140] leaving this issue unresolved.

Distal Pancreatectomy

A distal pancreatectomy and splenectomy for left-sided PDA is a simpler operation than pancreaticoduodenectomy, yet also carries significant risk. POPF is the principal morbidity associated with distal pancreatectomy. Clinically significant leaks occur in roughly 10% of cases. In 10% to 20% of cases, a leak is appreciable as amylase-rich fluid in surgical drains, but does not add morbidity. There are now roughly a half-dozen randomized clinical trials examining the effect of pancreatic stump management on POPF, ranging from staplers to mattress sutures. In summary, no positive interventions have been discovered. The DISPACT trial was the largest of these trials. This European multi-institution study analyzed 352 patients, and compared stapled and hand-sewn closures. The pancreatic leak rate was roughly 30% in both groups (p = 0.56).[141] Fibrin sealant and falciform ligament patches have also been tested, with no observed benefit.[142, 143] Interestingly, ultrasonic dissection of the pancreas with ligation of all visualized ducts in nonfibrotic glands was associated with improved pancreatic leak rates compared to conventional division and suturing (n = 58, 4% versus 26%, p = 0.02). Roughly 20 4-0 silk ligatures were used per neck transection in the ultrasonic dissection group, and transection took 10 extra minutes, on average.[144]

Palliative Surgery

There have been five randomized trials directly comparing hepaticojejunostomy with endoscopic or percutaneous biliary decompression for patients with malignant periampullary obstruction.[145]

A meta-analysis revealed that OS is the same between the groups, although total hospital days after randomization was twofold more in the stenting group, principally related to recurrent biliary obstruction requiring intervention. The authors recommend that for patients projected to live more than 6 months, a surgical biliary (as well as gastric bypass) be considered. Two separate randomized studies have demonstrated that prophylactic gastrojejunostomy in nonobstructed patients decreased the absolute risk of subsequent gastric outlet obstruction by roughly 20%, but did not affect OS.[146,147] Finally, there is evidence that celiac neurolysis with alcohol injected at laparotomy in patients with unresectable disease improves quality of life and OS.[148]

Operative and Surgical Pathology Reporting

Just as the ISGPS has sought to standardize complication reporting, there have been efforts to standardize operative and pathology reporting to facilitate collaboration between institutions, establish a minimum standard of quality, and provide consistency to the literature. With regard to the operative dictation, a description of the clinical stage (relationship to mesenteric vessels and evidence of metastatic disease) is important. Specific mention of the liver, peritoneum, and small intestines is necessary. Blood loss and the need for transfusion are recorded. The surgical technique used to dissect the uncinate process should be described, as well as the management of the SMA and SMV (e.g., were they skeletonized? resected? the method of visceral vessel repair?). The anastomotic techniques need to be described. The important elements of the pancreaticojejunostomy have been addressed by the ISGPS, as mentioned previously.[93] If a frozen section analysis was performed, the results should be stated. Similarly, any gross residual disease must be reported.[149]

Standards for pathology reporting have been established by the College of American Pathologists, and protocols are available at the Web site (http://www.cap.org/apps/cap.portal). On the pathology review, tumor site (e.g., head, uncinate, body, tail), maximum tumor diameter (in centimeters), histologic type or subtype, and histologic grade (well, moderate, or poor) are provided. Extension into extrapancreatic tissue is described. Margins are assessed (e.g., involvement or distance), including the uncinate, pancreatic neck, common bile duct, and duodenum. The distance to the margin (in millimeters) from the tumor should be stated. The posterior pancreatic surface margin is also reported, although this is not a transected or surgical margin. Microscopic invasion of the lymphatics, small vessels, and nerves are indicated. The TNM stage and the component elements are provided according to the

AJCC 7th edition staging system. A minimum of 12 lymph nodes should be evaluated. Treatment effect is described if the patient has received neoadjuvant therapy.

Assessing Prognosis

Although PDA is widely viewed as an aggressive cancer, like other common cancers, tumors display a wide range of biology. The median survival after resection for PDA is around 18 months in large series[27]; roughly 20% of patients survive more than 5 years, and a comparable number suffer cancer-specific mortality within just 1 year of surgery.[5] There would be substantial value in accurately predicting patients' cancer-specific outcome; at the present time, there are no reliable tests to predict prognosis. The most frequently considered adverse prognostic factors include conventional pathologic features (lymph node metastases, poor differentiation, tumor size >3cm, and positive resection margins). The approximate proportions of resected PDAs that fulfill each criterion are 75%, 40%, 50%, and 40%, respectively.[27] It must be remembered that each of these individual prognostic factors are weak predictors of outcome, with multivariate Cox proportional hazards ratios only around 1.5. Winter et al.,[162] studied 137 patients who underwent resection for PDA and died within 1 year from their disease or survived more than 30 months (patients with intermediate survival were excluded). Adverse pathologic features were frequently present in long-term survivors; for instance, 65% of patients in the long survivor group had lymph node metastases in the resected specimen. Conversely, lymph node metastases were not detected in 17% of the short survivor group, yet they still recurred early after resection and succumbed to their disease.

Perhaps the most robust prognostic marker routinely used in patients with localized and resectable PDA is the *postoperative* CA 19-9 level. CA 19-9 is a high–molecular-weight glycolipid that is a sialylated derivative of the Lewis a antigen (normally expressed by epithelial cells and absorbed onto the surface of erythrocytes). The oligosaccharide epitope is also present on mucins secreted by pancreatic cancer cells and detectable in the serum. A markedly elevated *preoperative* CA 19-9 level has some prognostic value (on par with conventional pathologic features). *Preoperative* CA 19-9 has also been used by some surgeons as a predictor of unresectable disease when the lesion appears resectable on imaging. Roughly 30% of patients with serum values above 300 U/mL were found to have a contraindication to resection on staging laparoscopy.[150] However, preoperative CA 19-9 is particularly limited in patients with biliary obstruction because the antigen is falsely elevated in this setting.[151–153] In addition, the sensitivity suffers because 5% to 10% of the population are unable to express CA 19-9 due to Lewis antigen variability (related to the presence or absence of a fucosyl-transferase).[154–156] As noted previously, CA 19-9 is most informative after resection when biliary obstruction is no longer a confounding variable and there has been macroscopic clearance of the disease. In a landmark ad hoc analysis of the Radiation Therapy Oncology Group (RTOG) 9704 adjuvant trial, an elevated postoperative CA 19-9 level (≥180 U/mL, drawn 1 to 2 months after resection) was associated with a multivariate proportional HR of 3.6.[154] Interestingly, Lewis antigen-negative individuals (who cannot express elevated serum CA 19-9) had the same survival as patients with low CA 19-9 levels for unclear reasons.

Patterns of Failure

Although OS after resection for PDA is roughly 18 months,[27] patients typically recur by 1 year,[159] indicating a short survival time once a recurrence is detected (comparable in survival to patients with metastatic disease). Recurrences have been reported in virtually every organ site, but most commonly occur in the retroperitoneum (57%), liver (51%), peritoneum (35%), and lung (15%). Interestingly, lung recurrences are typically delayed, and rarely

occur early after resection. A study of recurrence patterns out of Memorial Sloan-Kettering revealed that 12% of resected patients developed a local-only recurrence pattern; 33% had metastatic disease only and 46% had both local and metastatic disease (recurrence status was unknown in the remaining patients).[160]

Identifying biomarkers to predict patterns of recurrence could help select the patients who are most likely to benefit from intensive local therapy (radiation). The most intriguing biomarker to date in this area of research has been SMAD4. A study of pancreatic adenocarcinomas from an autopsy series (n = 65) revealed that a local predominant pattern was associated with intact SMAD4 expression (7 of 9 cases), whereas a disseminated pattern was associated with absent SMAD4 expression (16 of 22 cases).[49] This pattern was confirmed in tissue samples of patients from a phase II trial of locally advanced PDA.[161] Out of 15 patients with SMAD4-positive tumors, 11 had progression in a local-predominant pattern. In contrast, 10 of 14 patients with absent SMAD4 had significant distant spread. These studies suggest that patients having tumors with intact SMAD4 are most likely to benefit from radiation, whereas those patients with absent SMAD4 should only receive systemic therapy. However, a study of resected PDA samples revealed that resection alters the natural history of PDA recurrence, such that SMAD4 status is no longer predictive of recurrence pattern in this setting.[160] Other biomarkers[162] were examined as part of that study, and MUC1 expression was associated with a metastatic recurrence pattern. In a multivariate analysis, lymph node spread was the only variable (including the tested biomarkers) associated with pattern of failure. Patients without regional lymph node metastases had an increased risk of a local-only recurrence, typically in a relatively delayed fashion.[160] These data highlight that some patients would likely benefit from intensified local therapy, whereas others are best suited to receive systemic therapy only. Future studies are needed to define a personalized approach.

Adjuvant Therapy

According to the National Comprehensive Cancer Network (NCCN) guidelines, adjuvant chemotherapy is recommended for patients who recover well from pancreatic resection. Acceptable strategies include chemotherapy alone (gemcitabine, 5-FU, or capecitabine monotherapy), or chemoradiation plus chemotherapy (gemcitabine or 5-FU monotherapy, either given before or after chemoradiation).[157] Unfortunately, these regimens all consist of single-agent therapy with minimally effective agents. A meta-analysis of five randomized adjuvant trials including 951 patients concluded that adjuvant therapy provides a 3-month median survival advantage, and a 3% absolute improvement in 5-year survival. To put these findings in perspective, patients typically require a 6-month course of adjuvant treatment to achieve a 3-month survival.[158] Although these figures may appear unappealing to many patients, the reality is more complex; many patients receive no benefit at all, and may even be harmed with treatment, whereas a subset of patients receive a robust and durable survival benefit with these adjuvant treatments. Identifying which patients are most likely to experience a survival benefit is as important as discovering superior treatment regimens.

Adjuvant Trials

There have been eight prospective and randomized adjuvant trials that have shaped current treatment recommendations, including: five European trials, two in the United States, and one in Japan (Table 41.5).[163–170] Out of these eight trials, only four were considered positive with respect to the planned primary end point (one in the United States and three in Europe).[164,165,168,169] The continent where these trials were performed has played an important factor in defining the standard of care adjuvant treatment strategy around the world; chemoradiation is commonly performed in addition to chemotherapy in the United States, whereas chemotherapy

TABLE 41.5

Prospective and Randomized Adjuvant Trials for Pancreatic Cancer

Trial	Year	N	Randomization	OS (Months)	P
GITSG[168]	1985	43	Bolus 5-FU/4,000 cGy vs. observation	**20 vs. 11**	**0.04**
Bakkevold[169a]	1993	61	AMF vs. observation	**23 vs. 11**	**0.04**
EORTC[163a]	1999	218	Continuous 5-FU/4,000 cGy vs. observation	21.6 vs. 19.2	0.5
ESPAC-1[165]	2004	289	Bolus 5-FU vs. observation (2 × 2 design)	**20.1 vs. 15.5**	**0.009**
Japan[167]	2006	89	5-FU/cisplatin vs. observation	12.5 vs. 15.8	0.9
ESPAC-3[166]	2010	1088	Gemcitabine vs. 5-FU	23.6 vs. 23.0	0.4
RTOG 9704[170]	2011	451	Gemcitabine + ChemoXRT vs. 5-FU + ChemoXRT	18.7 vs. 17.3	0.9
CONKO-001[164]	2013	368	Gemcitabine vs. observation	**22.8 vs. 20.2**	**0.01**

Note: Statistically significant findings in bold (p <0.05).
[a] Included all periampullary cancers.
OS, overall survival; AMF, adriamycin, mitomycin C, 5-FU; ChemoXRT, Chemoradiation.

(without radiation) is the standard in Europe. The principal adjuvant trials will briefly be reviewed, emphasizing the strengths and weaknesses of the studies.

The Gastrointestinal Tumor Study Group (GITSG) trial was the first of the adjuvant trials and was a small phase III trial (by today's standards, n = 49 patients treated between 1974 and 1982) performed in the United States. Patients in the experimental arm received 40 Gy (split course with 20 Gy in each course, and a 2-week break in the middle). Bolus 5-FU was administered weekly for 2 years as maintenance therapy (500 mg/m^2), but was given daily for the first 3 days of each radiation course. The treatment arm was compared to an observation only arm, and the chemoradiation group had superior survival (20 versus 11 months; p = 0.04). The study has been criticized for its small sample size. Furthermore, it is not known whether the observed benefit was attributable to chemoradiation, to maintenance chemotherapy, or to both. Nevertheless, this landmark study established a role for adjuvant chemoradiation as an acceptable treatment for resected PDA in the United States.

Two small trials (in Norway[169] and Japan[167]) were performed over the last 15 years that provided equivocal results for chemotherapy alone, compared to surgery only. In the Norwegian trial, authored by Bakkevold et al.,[169] 61 patients with periampullary cancer (only 47 with PDA) were randomized to receive doxorubicin, mitomycin C, and 5-FU (six cycles), or observation. Patients receiving adjuvant chemotherapy had an improved median survival (23 versus 11 months; p = 0.04), but 2-year survival was similar (43% versus 32%; p = 0.1). In the Japanese trial, 89 patients were randomized to just two cycles (separated by 4 to 8 weeks) of 5-FU (500 mg/m^2 as a continuous infusion over 5 days) plus cisplatin (80 mg/m^2 on day 1 of each cycle), versus observation. OS was similar in the two groups (12.5 versus 15.8, respectively; p = 0.9).

The European Organization for Research and Treatment of Cancer (EORTC) trial was Europe's response to the GITSG trial and proved to be the largest adjuvant trial for PDA at that time.[163] A total of 218 patients with either PDA or other periampullary cancer were randomized to chemoradiation or observation. The treatment arm received split-course radiation for 40 Gy (as with GITSG). However, 5-FU was given as a continuous infusion (as opposed to bolus) on days 1 through 5 of each radiation course (for a total of 125 mg/m^2). No maintenance chemotherapy was administered. OS was 21.6 months with treatment and 19.2 months with observation (p = 0.5).

The European Study Group for Pancreatic Cancer (ESPAC-1) was the next large randomized adjuvant trial.[165] A total of 289 patients were randomized to a 2×2 design, with one of the four groups receiving no treatment. Treatment groups included (1) chemoradiation (40 Gy split-course radiation with bolus 5-FU at 500 mg/m^2 on days 1 through 3 of radiation, as with GITSG)

followed by chemotherapy (bolus leucovorin at 20 mg/m^2 and 5-FU at 425 mg/m^2 daily for 5 days, every 28 days for six cycles); (2) adjuvant chemotherapy only (without chemoradiation) as previously defined for group 1; (3) chemoradiation only (without chemotherapy) as previously defined for group 1; and (4) no treatment. The two groups receiving chemotherapy (groups 1 and 2) had superior survival as compared to those who did not (20.1 versus 15.5 months; p = 0.009). When chemoradiation was analyzed separately, the OS were 15.9 months with the two chemoradiation groups (groups 1 and 3) and 17.9 months without chemoradiation (groups 2 and 4; p = 0.05). When patients who received chemotherapy only were excluded from the no chemoradiation group (leaving just patients in the observation group), there was still a strong trend toward improved survival without chemoradiation. The results have been widely questioned because of the complex study design and because patients apparently received suboptimal radiation therapy (split course, no central quality of radiation control, 9% protocol violation, a very high [62%] local failure rate compared to recent trials). Although this study established chemotherapy alone as an acceptable standard of care in Europe and other parts of the world, oncologists in North America remain largely divided on the role of chemoradiation.

The Charité Onkologie (CONKO-001) trial primarily took place in German centers between 1998 and 2004,[159] with updated results recently reported.[164] The trial was an appropriate follow-up to ESPAC-1, which was interpreted in Europe as evidence in favor of adjuvant chemotherapy (without chemoradiation). Moreover, only 5-FU–based adjuvant chemotherapy had been tested up to that point, whereas the superiority of gemcitabine over 5-FU had been established for patients with advanced PDA (discussed in the Stage IV: Metastatic Disease section).[171] A total of 368 patients were randomized to receive six cycles of gemcitabine (4-week cycles) at a weekly dose of 1,000 mg/m^2 every 3 weeks with a 1 week break versus observation alone. Chemoradiation was not included in the treatment arm. The initial report reached its primary end point of disease-free survival (13.4 versus 6.9 months; p <0.001), but OS was not significantly different.[159] However, the updated analysis demonstrated improved OS with gemcitabine (22.8 versus 20.2 months; p = 0.01).[164] The small absolute difference in survival could be explained, in part, by the fact that 38% of patients did not receive the planned dose of gemcitabine and 13% did not receive at least one full cycle. In addition, most patients in the control arm received palliative chemotherapy once a recurrence was detected. Grade 3 through 4 toxicities were extremely rare in the treatment arm (no specific toxicity occurred in more than 3% of patients in the gemcitabine group). Although the median survival advantage is modest, it should be emphasized that the 5-year survival advantage was 10% (20.7% versus 10.2%; p <0.05) and the 10-year survival advantage was 5% (12.2% versus 7.7%).

Overall survival

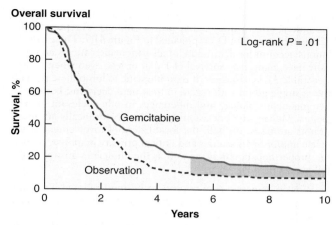

Figure 41.6 Improved long-term survival with gemcitabine monotherapy, in the CONKO-001 trial. The *highlighted area* represents patients who likely had a substantial benefit from gemcitabine monotherapy. (Modified from Oettle H, Neuhaus P, Hochhaus A, et al. Adjuvant chemotherapy with gemcitabine and long-term outcomes among patients with resected pancreatic cancer: the CONKO-001 randomized trial. *JAMA* 2013;310: 1473–1481.)

These data provide very strong evidence that, in a small subset of patients (i.e., 1 in 10), gemcitabine monotherapy is highly effective (Fig. 41.6). The opportunity to achieve long-term survival due to gemcitabine (albeit uncommon) is an important consideration for patients contemplating adjuvant treatment, despite the meager improvement in median survival.

The European ESPAC-3 trial is the largest adjuvant trial to date, and directly compared chemotherapy with gemcitabine (1,000 mg/m^2 over 30 minutes weekly, 3 out of 4 weeks) versus 5-FU (bolus folinic acid at 20 mg/m^2 plus bolus 5-FU at 425 mg/m^2 on days 1 to 5, every 28 days for six cycles as administered in ESPAC-1). As with CONKO-001, no adjuvant chemoradiation was given. Median OS were 23.6 and 23.0 months, respectively (p = 0.4), demonstrating equivalence between the two agents. However, this study did not change the emerging paradigm of frontline gemcitabine monotherapy at most centers, because toxicity was less with gemcitabine (14% serious adverse events with 5-FU versus 7.5% with gemcitabine; p <0.001). The increased toxicity due to 5-FU was primarily related to increased stomatitis and diarrhea.

Finally, RTOG 9704 was the second United States adjuvant trial, completed in 2002[172] and updated in 2011.[170] The trial's treatment arms paralleled the ESPAC-3 study (5-FU versus gemcitabine), except patients in both treatment groups received 5-FU–based chemoradiation in the middle of their adjuvant chemotherapy course. Total treatment duration in both groups was 6 months, and the study question related to chemotherapy (5-FU versus gemcitabine), and not the role of chemoradiation. A total of 451 patients were randomized to chemotherapy with 5-FU at 250 mg/m^2 per day given as a continuous infusion (different from ESPAC-3) or gemcitabine 1,000 mg/m^2 given weekly. Patients received one chemotherapy cycle prior to chemoradiation (3 weeks) and 12 additional weeks afterwards (two cycles of 5-FU consisting of 4 weeks on and 2 weeks off; three cycles of gemcitabine with 3 weeks on and 1 week off). Chemoradiation was given to all study patients as 50.4 Gy with continuous infusion 5-FU (250 mg/m^2 per day), and prospective quality assurance was performed. The primary end points of the study were OS for the whole cohort and for pancreatic head cancers. For all patients, OS was similar in the gemcitabine and 5-FU arms (18.5 versus 16.4 months; p = 0.5). In patients with pancreatic head tumors (86% of the total study population), those receiving gemcitabine had a trend toward superior survival in the multivariate analysis (20.5 versus 17.1 months; p = 0.08). The site of first relapse was recorded in this study, and was distant in roughly

70% of patients, and local–regional in 30% (a low figure relative to the local recurrence rate reported in ESPAC-1). Subsequent sites of recurrence were not reported. The RTOG-9704 study had several additional informative findings. Patients treated at centers that did not meet the quality assurance standards had inferior outcomes.[173] As previously described, postoperative CA 19-9 was identified as an important prognostic variable and should be considered in planning future adjuvant trials.[154] Finally, the inferior outcomes in patients with PDA of the left side of the pancreas raises questions about whether this group should be included in adjuvant trials with chemoradiation.

Future Questions and Ongoing Adjuvant Trials

Based on these trials, 6 months of adjuvant therapy is clearly supported as the standard of care for patients with resected PDA. Whether adjuvant chemoradiation is important remains an unanswered question, and is the subject of an ongoing randomized trial in the United States (RTOG 0848, NCT01013649). The study compares the impact of chemotherapy alone to chemotherapy plus chemoradiation. Patients in the radiation arm will receive 28 fractions of 1.8 Gy (50.4 Gy total, either 3-D conformal or intensity-modulated radiotherapy) and either capecitabine (825 mg/m^2 twice daily) or 5-FU (250 mg/m^2 per day as a continuous infusion for the duration of radiation) as a radiosensitizer. Unlike the RTOG 9704 trial, chemoradiation is administered after five cycles of gemcitabine-based chemotherapy have been completed. This trial design reflects an emerging trend in many centers toward deferring chemoradiation until after chemotherapy is completed in order to maximize systemic control early on and to spare patients who recur early at distant sites the cost and morbidity of radiation. The next ESPAC trial (ESPAC-4, ISRCTN96397434) is evaluating the role of doublet therapy (gemcitabine plus capecitabine versus gemcitabine alone) in the adjuvant setting. It is worth pointing out that this regimen did not improve OS in advanced pancreatic cancer (see the Stage IV: Metastatic Disease section).[174] CONKO-005 (DRKS00000247) is testing the addition of erlotinib to the standard-of-care gemcitabine (versus gemcitabine alone) based on a small, but statistically significant improvement in survival in the metastatic setting.[175,176] As discussed later in detail, two regimens, (1) gemcitabine plus nab-paclitaxel and (2) FOLFIRINOX, were recently shown to be superior to gemcitabine in the metastatic setting.[177,178] In light of these encouraging results, there are plans to test both regimens in the adjuvant setting (NCT01964430 and NCT01526135, respectively), using a similar control arm in both studies (gemcitabine monotherapy). Finally, the role of neoadjuvant chemotherapy in patients with resectable disease is not known. There are selected centers that routinely treat patients with resectable disease with neoadjuvant therapy,[84] and the NCCN guidelines recommend that such an approach be conducted as part of a clinical trial. In one of the largest series, from the M.D. Anderson Cancer Center,[84] outcomes are favorable (34 months) for patients who ultimately make it to pancreatic resection. The median survival of the entire cohort (22.7 months) in an intent-to-treat analysis is similar to historical controls with localized disease (see Table 41.5). Proponents argue that a neoadjuvant approach allows for an objective assessment of treatment response, early treatment of microscopic metastases, and an additional 3 to 6 months to monitor disease biology before committing to an operation with substantial risk. It is likely that as adjuvant treatment improves, more centers will move to a neoadjuvant paradigm, similar to the treatment of other upper gastrointestinal cancers.

Surveillance Postresection

The current NCCN guidelines recommend that patient follow-up after resection should include visits every 3 to 6 months for 2 years, and then annually. Surveillance CT scans and serial tumor markers (CA 19-9 at minimum) should be assessed, along with a history and physical exam. These recommendations are not based on Level 1 evidence, but rather expert consensus.[179] In practice, surveillance patterns range widely from close follow-up with CT imaging and CA 19-9 levels every 3 months, to no routine surveillance at all.[180] Poor outcomes after recurrence (roughly 6 to 12 months in the adjuvant trials discussed previously), and a lack of proven benefit for salvage chemotherapy, argue against close surveillance. However, as the number of second-line agents with activity against PDA increases, so will the opportunity to prolong survival with early detection of recurrence and intervention. It should be noted that a rise in CA 19-9 often precedes radiographic evidence of recurrence by 3 to 12 months.[181] However, initiating chemotherapy based on changes in tumor marker levels alone is not currently recommended (although widely practiced), due to the risk of false positive and false negative results.[153,154]

There are a few reports that support the benefit of close surveillance and early intervention. One study, presented in abstract form, described 139 patients who underwent resection for PDA. All patients were advised to have CT scan and CA 19-9 surveillance every 3 months in the first year, every 6 months in the 2nd year, and annually thereafter. The patients were retrospectively analyzed in three groups: those who followed the recommendations, those who underwent surveillance but with less frequency than recommended, and those who did not follow up. Survivals in the three groups were 16.6, 15.7, and 8.7 months, respectively. The authors concluded that close follow-up is advisable. Notably, the proportions of patients who received adjuvant treatment in each group were not reported.

Selected patients may even benefit from a metastasectomy. Pulmonary metastases (as compared to liver or peritoneal metastases) typically occur in a delayed fashion after surgery.[160] Therefore, the biology and natural history of patients who develop isolated pulmonary metastases may represent a unique subgroup where resection of these lesions is beneficial. The Johns Hopkins group identified 31 patients with isolated lung metastases at a median of 34 months post pancreatectomy. A total of 9 had the lung lesion resected, and these patients survived an additional 19 months (range 5 to 29 months) after the intervention.[182]

STAGE III: LOCALLY ADVANCED DISEASE

AJCC Staging Versus "Intent of Management"–Based Staging

In the current (7th) edition of AJCC staging for pancreatic adenocarcinoma, stage III cancers are T_4, N_{any} M_0 malignancies, with T_4 defined as a "tumor [that] involves the celiac axis or the superior mesenteric artery (unresectable primary tumor)." A representative CT scan of stage III PDA is provided in Figure 41.7. These presentations account for about 30% of all pancreatic cancers and typically have an average survival of 1 year or less, even when treated (see Table 41.1). However, it is problematic to lump these patients into a single group with regard to treatment decisions, because of heterogeneous biology and differences in other relevant clinical factors. Management decisions for patients with locally advanced tumors are based on both the local extent of involvement of the celiac and/or SMA arteries and critical primary branches, such as the proper hepatic artery, as well as the clinician's answer to the following questions:

1. What therapeutic goal appears to be most rational based not only on the tumor staging, but also on performance status, weight loss, and significant comorbid illnesses? Along these lines, is the treatment potentially curative? Is minimal or moderate antineoplastic intensity more appropriate? Or is treatment supportive and purely palliative?
2. What is the level of treatment intensity that this patient would be able to accept and withstand psychologically and emotionally in addition to physiologically?
3. What are the support structures surrounding this patient, and are they up to the challenges that will be incurred by the management selected?

Pragmatically, stage III clinical presentations have been divided into *borderline resectable* and *clearly unresectable* (introduced previously in the section Stage I, II: Localized Disease, Evaluation and Assessing Resectability), with the conceptual distinction being the probability of safely and successfully resecting the tumor without antecedent chemotherapy or chemoradiotherapy.

Basic Management Considerations

The initial evaluation of patients with presumed pancreatic adenocarcinoma will be the same whether the patient ultimately is demonstrated to have a resectable, borderline resectable, or locally unresectable disease at presentation. This component of management has been addressed previously in the chapter (see Stage I, II: Localized Disease, Presentation and Evaluation and Assessing Resectability). For patients treated initially with chemotherapy or chemoradiation, several additional management considerations need to be considered (also relevant for patients with resectable disease who are to receive neoadjuvant treatment).

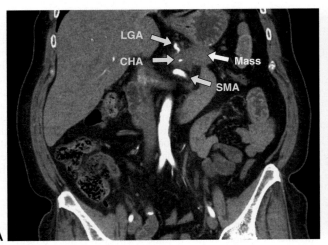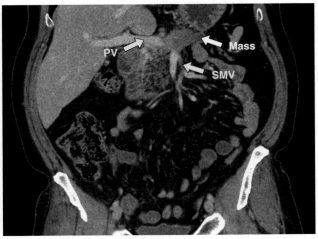

Figure 41.7 CT scans of a locally advanced, stage III PDA in the pancreatic body. Coronal images. **(A)** The arterial phase. Visceral arteries named are left gastric artery (LGA), common hepatic artery (CHA), and superior mesenteric artery (SMA). The CHA is encased. **(B)** The venous phase. The portal splenic confluence is completely occluded.

Patients generally require histologic confirmation of a pancreatic cancer diagnosis prior to treatment. Additionally, relief of obstructive jaundice and duodenal obstruction is necessary when present. These interventions will be concurrent with other basic assessments and interventions such as nutritional optimization, treatment of dehydration and electrolyte abnormalities, pain management, and attention to depression if present. It is important to emphasize that multidisciplinary teams with focused, management experience for gastrointestinal (GI) malignancies of the upper abdomen achieve the best results, and include expertise in pathology, chemotherapeutic, radiotherapeutics, surgical management, interventional radiology, and endoscopy, as mentioned in the opening of the chapter.[183]

Local–Regional Unresectable Disease

Impact of Prognostic Factors in the Management of Locally Unresectable Patients

Patients with locally advanced, or stage III, PDA have an average OS between 7 and 12 months (Table 41.6). Several patient-specific factors have been adversely associated with outcome in this context, including anemia, poor performance status, elevated CA 19-9, and elevated Charlson Comorbidity Score. In addition, use and response to systemic chemotherapy as the initial treatment, prior to chemoradiotherapy, appears to favorably predict (and possibly impact) survival.[184–187]

Evolution of Management for Local–Regional Unresectable Disease

The early, practice defining, randomized experiences have been reviewed in many prior publications and textbooks,[188] and key ones are highlighted in Table 41.6. It is important to remember how dated some studies are with respect to patient selection and evaluation, chemotherapy selection, and radiation planning and delivery (typically delivered as 2-D nonconformal, split course, low-dose therapy). Nevertheless, these papers established proof of principle for treatment feasibility with acceptable toxicity, and the value of 5-FU–based radiosensitization in this context.

From the mid 1990s through the first decade of the current century, there have been a series of important lessons learned in the management of locally advanced pancreatic cancer. Acceptable chemoradiation strategies integrating insights gained from past studies are summarized in Table 41.7. There is a biologic basis for needing both improved local control and improved systemic control to optimize results.

Improved local control in pancreatic cancer has been strongly suggested by the autopsy studies by Iacobuzio-Donahue et al.,[49] previously described (see the Stage I, II: Localized Disease, Adjuvant Therapy section), and validated in patients with locally advanced disease.[161] Investigators observed that patients with tumors having intact SMAD4 expression were more likely to have locally destructive tumors and a lower burden of metastatic disease than patients with tumors showing SMAD4 loss. Recently, Oshima et al.[189] found that abnormal TP53 expression (either absence or

TABLE 41.6

Selected Locally Advanced Pancreatic Ductal Adenocarcinoma Randomized Trials

Year	Study Name	Patient Number	Radiation (Gy)	Chemotherapy	Median Survival (Months)
1980[292]	SWOG	33	60	MeC, 5-FU, SMF	8.8
		29	60	MeC, 5-FU, testolactone	6.9
1981[293]	GITSG	83	60	5-FU	**9.4**
		86	40	5-FU	**9.8**
		25	60	None	5.3
1985[192]	ECOG	37	40	5-FU	8.3
		34	None	5-FU	8.2
1985[294]	GITSG	73	60	5-FU	8.5
		70	40	Doxorubicin	7.6
1988[190]	GITSG	22	54	5-FU, SMF	**9.7**
		21	None	SMF	7.4
1994[295]	Mayo Clinic	44	50–60	5-FU	7.8
		43	50–60	Hycanthone	7.8
2005[296]	ECOG	62	60	None	8.4
		64	60	5-FU, MMC	7.1
2008[191]	FFCD/SFRO	59	60	Gemcitabine	8.6
		60	None	Gemcitabine	**13**
2011[193]	ECOG	34	50	Gemcitabine	**11.1**
		37	None	Gemcitabine	**9.2**
2013[207]	SCALOP	38	50, Gemcitabine	Gemcitabine, Capecitabine	**15.2**
		36	50, Capecitabine	Gemcitabine, Capecitabine	**13.4**

Note: Statistically significant findings are in bold (p <0.05).
MeC, Methyl-CCNU; SMF, streptozotocin, mitomycin C, 5-FU.

TABLE 41.7

Recommended Radiation Treatment Volumes in Commonly Used Chemoradiation Regimens for Localized Pancreatic Cancer

Chemotherapy Choice	Chemotherapy Dose and Schedule	Radiation Dose and Schedule	No Arterial Involvement or Abutment with Likely Resectability (T3 or T4)	Extensive Arterial Involvement with Uncertain Resectability or Arterial Encasement/Unresectable (T4)
Gemcitabine	400–500 mg/m² weekly	50.4 Gy over 5.5 wks (good PS) or 30 Gy over 2 wks (poor PS)	GTV only	GTV only
	1 g/m² weekly	36 Gy over 3 wks	GTV only	GTV only
	40 mg/m² twice weekly	50.4 Gy over 5.5 wks	GTV + ENI	GTV only
Capecitabine	800–825 mg/m² twice per day on days of radiation	50.4 Gy over 5.5 wks (good PS) or 30 Gy over 2 wks (poor PS)	GTV + ENI	GTV only
PVI 5-FU	225 mg/m² daily or 300 mg/m² on days of radiation	50.4 Gy over 5.5 wks (good PS) or 30 Gy over 2 wks (poor PS)	GTV + ENI	GTV only

PS, performance status; GTV, gross tumor volume; ENI, elective nodal irradiation; PVI, protracted venous infusion.
Modified from Royal RE, Wolfe RA, Crane CH. Cancer of the pancreas. In: DeVita VT Jr, Lawrence TS, Rosenberg SA, eds. *DeVita, Hellman, and Rosenberg's Cancer: Principles & Practice of Oncology.* 9th ed. Philadelphia: Lippincott Williams & Wilkins; 2011.

nuclear accumulation) was associated with a local–regional recurrence pattern in patients with resected PDA, whereas CDKN2A loss was associated with widespread metastases.[189] Similar to an aforementioned study by Winter et al.,[160] SMAD4 expression was not associated with pattern of failure in this patient cohort following resection.[189]

Past studies suggest that the controversy of using chemotherapy alone versus chemoradiotherapy should be reframed to acknowledge that there might be potential roles of each. There have been several randomized trials comparing chemotherapy to chemotherapy plus chemoradiation,[190–193] with mixed results (each appear in Table 41.6). An older ECOG study published in 1985 (with the aforementioned limitations) compared weekly 5-FU against the same chemotherapy treatment preceded by 40 Gy radiation (combined with 5-FU) and found no difference in survival. The multiinstitution French Fédération Francophone de Cancérologie Digestive-Société Française de Radiothérapie Oncologie (FFCD/SFRO) study found decreased survival in patients receiving 60 Gy radiation concomitantly with 5-FU and cisplatin, and followed with maintenance gemcitabine, compared to gemcitabine alone (8.6 versus 13 months). The chemoradiation regimen used in this trial has been criticized as being particularly toxic (more on this in the following).[191] The LAP-07 trial with gemcitabine or gemcitabine plus erlotinib for four cycles, followed by either chemoradiotherapy or additional chemotherapy (two cycles), failed to show any difference in survival between the two arms. About one-third of patients had progressed by the time of the second randomization. The trial results, although final, have only been reported in abstract form.[194] However, a GITSG study from 1988 comparing 5-FU and radiation followed by streptozotocin, mitomycin C, and 5-FU chemotherapy to the same chemotherapy alone showed an improved median survival (9.7 versus 7.4 months) with multimodality therapy.[190] Most recently, ECOG 4201 from 2011 suggested that locally advanced patients randomly assigned to receive chemoradiotherapy with gemcitabine followed by five cycles of gemcitabine alone did better than patients receiving gemcitabine without radiotherapy (11.1 versus 9.2 months; p = 0.016).[193] It is noted that this trial was closed, with only 71 patients accrued and analyzed, a potential criticism of the results. Other nonrandomized studies suggesting benefit to using a combination of modalities, rather than one modality, include the recently reported Massachusetts General Hospital experience (improved survival with chemotherapy plus chemoradiation versus chemoradiation alone, HR = 0.46; p <0.001),[184] and a German study in which treatment decisions were assigned from tumor board discussions

(chemoradiotherapy plus chemoradiation, median survival 13.0 months versus 8.0 months without additional chemotherapy).[195] On further analysis, the authors could not find prognostic factor variation between to the two groups to explain this difference.

Gemcitabine has been found to be marginally superior to 5-FU in the metastatic setting.[171] The drug also has marginal efficacy as a single-agent adjuvant therapy after resection for PDA.[164] There is some suggestion that it may be better than 5-FU in the adjuvant setting, when chemoradiation is included,[170] although there is no such trend in a European trial comparing these agents without chemoradiation.[166,170] Thus, there has been interest in exploring gemcitabine as a radiation sensitizer; indeed, the drug is potent in this role based on preclinical and clinical data.[196] Investigators from the M.D. Anderson Cancer Center, the University of Michigan, and other sites explored the use of gemcitabine with radiotherapy in various contexts, with the following observations: Radiotherapy fields designed to cover gross tumor and at risk nodal basins cannot safely be targeted with concurrent gemcitabine unless the gemcitabine dose is reduced from the chemotherapy-only level of 1,000 mg/m² to 300 to 600 mg/m². Additionally, the daily fraction size should not exceed 1.8 Gy when targeting expanded fields with draining lymph nodes. If the desire is to administer full-dose gemcitabine (1,000 mg/m²) weekly with higher radiation doses (e.g., 2.4 Gy fractions), then radiotherapy must be limited to gross tumor only with tight margins, and special attention must be given toward inadvertent targeting organs such as the duodenum, stomach, and small bowel. Subsequent studies have demonstrated that respecting these guidelines allows for acceptable toxicity, especially when combined with appropriate supportive care measures, treatment planning that accounts for target and organ movement with respiration, and intensity modulated planning and delivery aimed at minimizing doses to sensitive critical organs.[196–200]

The work of Ben Joseph et al.[197] at the University of Michigan validates this approach. Investigators conducted a phase I/II dose escalating study of radiotherapy dose over 25 fractions (totaling 50 to 60 Gy) in 50 patients, all deemed to have locally advanced PDA (not borderline resectable). The maximal tolerated dose was 55 Gy (2.2 Gy per fraction) in combination with fixed-dose rate gemcitabine (1,000 mg/m²). Patients had a median survival of 14.8 months and 24% (12 of 50 patients, a very high rate compared to previous studies[161,191,201,202]) underwent resection (10 R0 and 2 R1). Among resected patients, the median survival was 32 months. A meta-analysis of three randomized trials and one comparative retrospective study (including 229 patients) revealed a small but significant survival advantage with gemcitabine-based chemoradiation (at 12 months: HR, 1.5; p = 0.03), over 5-FU–based treatment, although toxicity was higher.[203]

Technologic advances combined with greater understanding of the mechanisms and impact of acute radiation toxicity have improved the safety profile of treatment. Excessive acute toxicity quickly results when the radiation fractional dose increases, the total dose increases, the field sizes are too large for the degree of drug sensitization or intensity, or radiation is delivered without careful consideration of limiting dose volume to the stomach, duodenum, small bowel, or other critical organs. There is increasing consensus that such toxicity can be associated with symptoms, increased costs, and decreased survival.[191,200]

Capecitabine is an appealing alternative to 5-FU or gemcitabine as a radiosensitizer. Capecitabine is a prodrug of 5-FU with near-complete oral bioavailability. It is converted to its active form through a three-step process, with the last step occurring more reliably within tumor cells than in nonmalignant cells, due to higher thymidine phosphorylase levels. Thus, systemic levels of active 5-FU are actually decreased with capecitabine, theoretically widening the therapeutic window of the drug. Aside from hand–foot syndrome associated with capecitabine, clinical trials reproducibly demonstrate an improved safety profile. The efficacy of capecitabine is comparable to 5-FU, at least in studies of other cancer types that directly compare them.[204] Importantly, oral dosing obviates the need for semipermanent venous access and the attendant risks of thrombosis and infection. Nonrandomized data demonstrate that capecitabine (typically administered at a daily dose of around 1,600 mg/m^2) has comparable efficacy to continuous infusion 5-FU, and an improved toxicity profile, as a radiosensitizer in patients with locally advanced PDA receiving intensity-modulated radiation therapy (IMRT).[205,206] Finally, the recently published SCALOP I randomized trial in patients with locally advanced PDA, has suggested mildly increased efficacy (OS 15.2 versus 13.4 months; p = 0.01) and decreased toxicity of capecitabine with irradiation, as compared to gemcitabine. In this study, sensitized radiation was administered after four cycles of gemcitabine and capecitabine chemotherapy (randomization was performed after three cycles).[207] Note that the chemosensitizing dose of gemcitabine (300 mg/m^2) was lower than the fixed-dose rate levels successfully used in the abovementioned Ben Josef study.[197]

A final lesson from previous studies of chemoradiation for locally advanced pancreatic adenocarcinoma demonstrate that induction chemotherapy prior to chemoradiation has advantages. Nevertheless, chemotherapy, chemoradiation, or both have been studied and are acceptable approaches for locally advanced PDA. There are no level 1 data conclusively supporting one approach over the other. However, several studies provide a meaningful rationale for beginning with induction chemotherapy. Roughly two-thirds of patients with locally advanced PDA develop systemic metastases during treatment. Some of these individuals are less likely to benefit from radiation, and the costs and side effects of local radiation therapy may be avoided.[208] An ad hoc analysis of a prospective, nonrandomized study (GERCOR), revealed that patients with locally advanced PDA who received consolidation chemoradiation after induction chemotherapy had improved survival, as compared to those who had chemotherapy alone (15.0 versus 11.7 months; p <0.001).[208] This has been validated by other retrospective data.[209] The SCALOP trial, as previously described, showed that sequenced chemoradiation after chemotherapy achieves very good results with locally advanced PDA.[207] The GERCOR LAP-07, described previously, warrants additional mention here, because no benefit was observed with chemoradiation (50.4 Gy plus capecitabine) after chemotherapy (gemcitabine plus erlotinib of gemcitabine alone), as compared to additional chemotherapy (n = 269; OS, 15.2 versus 16.4 months; p = 0.8).[194]

Along these lines, certain multidrug combinations with higher response rates for advanced PDA than gemcitabine monotherapy (see the Stage IV: Metastatic Disease section) are also promising regimens for locally advanced PDA. FOLFIRINOX (5-FU, oxaliplatin, leucovorin, and irinotecan) has a response rate of 27% in the locally advanced setting,[210] which rivals the best results with multimodality therapy.[197,207] Planned and ongoing trials with FOLFIRINOX, as well as with nab-paclitaxel plus gemcitabine (with or without radiation), will help establish the role of these treatments for locally advanced PDA.

Management of Borderline Resectable Patients

Current NCCN guidelines for borderline resectable patients favor neoadjuvant therapy over directly going to surgery, while acknowledging the validity of both approaches and the absence of phase III data to definitively answer the issue.[157] A meta-analysis of 182 patients from 10 prospective trials of borderline resectable patients included seven studies reporting on the impact of chemoradiation (with or without chemotherapy) and three on chemotherapy alone.[211] At restaging following neoadjuvant therapy, 16% of patients responded to treatment, 69% had stable disease, and 19% showed progression. The median survival for the cohort was 22.0 months, and treatment-related grade 3 to 4 toxicity was observed in 32% of patients. Surgical exploration was performed in 69% of patients, and 80% of surgically explored patients were resected. Moreover, 83% of resected specimens had microscopically negative resection margins. Among resected patients, 61% were alive at 1 year, and 44% were alive at 2 years. The median survival in this highly selected and favorable group was 22.0 months.

Although the survival of patients with borderline PDA after neoadjuvant treatment and resection is comparable to patients with resectable PDA,[27] these data should be interpreted with a few points of caution. First, the study was underpowered and not designed to determine the best neoadjuvant regimen; thus, treatment choice is largely dependent on institutional preferences. Second, resected patients represent 56% of the total cohort, and are enriched for patients with tumors that have favorable biology. In these nonrandomized studies, it is possible that intrinsic biologic factors were more important determinants of survival than neoadjuvant treatment. Notably, nonresected patients with borderline PDA have a survival around 1 year, which is similar to patients with locally advanced disease.[212] Finally, roughly 40% of patients with potentially resectable tumors do not undergo resection when a neoadjuvant approach is used. Whether unresected patients suffered a missed opportunity for resection (and therefore for long-term survival) or were spared ineffective surgery is unknown. Most likely, the answer lies somewhere in the middle.

EMERGING ROLE OF STEREOTACTIC BODY RADIOTHERAPY

SBRT is hypofractionated (one to five fractions) radiotherapy given in doses that, in aggregate, do not exceed 50 to 60 Gy per course. Single fraction courses are usually in the dose range of 20 to 25 Gy. The number of fractions and dose per fraction is determined by tumor size and radiation tolerance of the involved and/or adjacent organs. To be safe, these large-dose fractions are given with extra attention to immobilization, controlling for respiratory movement, image guidance, and dose shaping around critical structures. The risk of severe or lethal normal organ damage is substantial in the absence of proper attention to all required, relevant considerations. In pancreatic applications, the primary dose-limiting structure is the duodenum, followed by the stomach, remaining small bowel, and other adjacent organs/structures. This approach has been applied with and without chemotherapy in a variety of pancreatic contexts, including locally unresectable, borderline resectable, locally recurrent, and as an adjuvant management boost after conventional radiotherapy.[213–215] These studies demonstrated feasibility and acceptable toxicity in experienced hands, although the exact role of this modality remains to be defined.

STAGE IV: METASTATIC DISEASE

Approximately 50% of patients with PDA will be diagnosed with distant metastatic (stage IV) disease at the time of presentation.[1] Prognosis is dismal, with a median OS of less than 6 months and an estimated 2-year survival of only 2%.[3,7] Chemotherapy in this setting improves survival by just a few additional months. Therefore, the goals of therapy in this patient population are to prolong survival, as well as to palliate symptoms.

Gemcitabine as a Gold-Standard Therapy for Metastatic Pancreatic Adenocarcinoma

5-FU was the principal treatment option for metastatic pancreatic cancer through the 1990s, although response rates were under 20% and median survival was just 6 months.[216] Other agents or combinations of drugs failed to show any improvement over 5-FU monotherapy until a landmark study in 1997 by Burris et al.[171] demonstrating the superiority of gemcitabine for advanced PDA. Since that study, gemcitabine has become the single most important pancreatic cancer therapy, and the standard treatment arm in at least 19 phase III studies (Table 41.8).

Gemcitabine (difluorodeoxycytidine [dFdC]) is a nucleoside analog of deoxycytidine, and it is administered as a prodrug. Upon entry into the cell, gemcitabine is phosphorylated by deoxycytidine kinase (DCK) to a monophosphate form (dFdCMP). Similar to the association between thymidine phosphorylase and the prodrug capecitabine, elevated DCK levels in tumor cells (compared to normal tissues)[217] enhance the therapeutic window of gemcitabine. dFdCMP is then phosphorylated into active diphosphate (dFdCDP) and triphosphate (dFdCTP) forms. The active metabolites incorporate into DNA and inhibit chain elongation. Moreover, they deplete nucleotide pools by competitively inhibiting ribonucleotide reductase.[218]

In the 1997 Burris trial, 126 patients with advanced pancreas cancer were randomized to either of two arms: (1) gemcitabine 1,000 mg/m^2 weekly for 7 weeks followed by 1 week of rest, then 3 doses per week every 4 weeks thereafter, or (2) bolus 5-FU 600 mg/m^2 once per week.[171] Patients primarily had metastatic disease, although 26% had locally advanced disease. Treatment in both arms was generally well tolerated. Grade 3 through 4 hematologic toxicities were higher with gemcitabine, including neutropenia (25.9% versus 4.9%), thrombocytopenia (9.7% versus 0%) and anemia (9.7% versus 0%). Grade 3 through 4 nausea was also more frequent in the gemcitabine arm (9.5% versus 4.8%). Clinical benefit, based on pain score, performance status, and weight, was noted in 23.8% of patients in the gemcitabine arm versus only 4.8% in the 5-FU arm (p = 0.0022). The survival advantage with gemcitabine was just over 5 weeks, with median OS of 5.65 and 4.41 months, respectively (p = 0.0025). Survival at 12 months was 18% in the gemcitabine arm versus 2% in the 5-FU arm. Partial tumor responses were observed in 5% of patients in the gemcitabine group, and stable disease was observed in 39%. In contrast, no partial tumor responses were observed with 5-FU, and only 19% of patients experienced stable disease. As a result, gemcitabine was approved by the U.S. Food and Drug Administration (FDA) in 1997 for first-line treatment for locally advanced unresectable or metastatic pancreas cancer.

Two studies have focused on modifying the dosing and infusion rates of gemcitabine in order to increase the concentration of intracellular, activated gemcitabine. Tempero et al.[219] compared two

TABLE 41.8

Phase III Studies of Gemcitabine + Drug "X", Compared to Gemcitabine

Author	Year	N	Drug "X"	Gemcitabine OS (Months)	Combination OS (Months)	P Value
Collucci[223]	2002	107	Cisplatin	5.0	7.5	0.43
Berlin[199]	2002	327	5-FU	5.4	6.7	0.09
Bramhall[229]	2002	239	Marimastat	5.8	5.98	0.95
Rocha Lima[227]	2004	360	Irinotecan	6.6	6.3	0.79
Richards[297]	2004	565	Pemetrexed	6.3	6.2	0.85
Van Cutsem[233]	2004	688	Tipifarnib	6.5	6.9	0.75
Louvet[226]	2005	300	Oxaliplatin	7.1	9.0	0.13
Herrmann[174]	2005	319	Capecitabine	7.3	8.4	0.31
Heinemann[225]	2006	192	Cisplatin	6.0	7.5	0.15
Stathopoulous[228]	2006	130	Irinotecan	6.5	6.4	0.97
Abou-Alfa[221]	2006	349	Exatecan	6.2	6.7	0.52
Moore[175]	2007	569	Erlotinib	6.2	5.9	**0.04**
Poplin[220]	2009	574	Oxaliplatin	4.9	5.7	0.10
Cunningham[224]	2009	533	Capecitabine	6.2	7.1	0.08
Philip[232]	2010	745	Cetuximab	5.9	6.3	0.23
Kindler[231]	2010	602	Bevacizumab	5.9	5.8	0.95
Kindler[230]	2011	632	Axitinib	8.3	8.5	0.54
Conroy[177]	2011	342	FOLFIRINOX[a]	6.8	11.1	**<0.001**
Von Hoff[178]	2013	861	Nab-paclitaxel	6.7	8.5	**<0.001**

Note: Statistically significant findings are in bold (p <0.05).
[a] The experimental arm was FOLFIRINOX alone; all other experimental arms listed in this table include a drugs in combination with gemcitabine.

different dose-intense regimens (compared to the Burris regimen) in a randomized phase II study. A total of 92 patients were randomized to either *standard* 30 minute infusion at a dose of 2,200 mg/m^2 versus 1,500 mg/m^2 over 150 minutes at a fixed-dose rate (FDR) of 10 mg/m^2 per minute.[219] All patients had locally advanced (8%) or metastatic pancreatic cancer (92%). Although there was no difference in the primary end point (i.e., time to treatment failure), patients in the standard arm had a median OS of 5 months, whereas those in the FDR had a median survival of 8 months (p = 0.013). Pharmacokinetic analyses showed a twofold increase in the intracellular (peripheral mononuclear cells) concentration of gemcitabine triphosphate with FDR gemcitabine, even though the total dose given was 30% less. Consistent with these data, grade 3 to 4 hematologic toxicity was also greater with FDR gemcitabine. Subsequently, the Eastern Cooperative Oncology Group (ECOG) conducted a three-arm phase III study (E6201) comparing gemcitabine (1,000 mg/m^2) plus oxaliplatin (100 mg/m^2) every 2 weeks versus a weekly 30-minute infusion of gemcitabine (1,000 mg/m^2) versus weekly FDR gemcitabine (1,500 mg/m^2 as previous).[220] A total of 832 patients were enrolled. The study confirmed an increase in OS for the FDR arm compared to the 30-minute infusion of gemcitabine arm (6.2 months versus 4.9 months; p = 0.04). However, the OS benefit actually did not meet the prespecified criteria for significance (a 33% decrease in survival). In addition, patients experienced greater toxicities with grade 3 to 4 neutropenia and thrombocytopenia in the FDR gemcitabine arm, consistent with the earlier phase II trial. Of note, there was no survival advantage with the combination of gemcitabine and oxaliplatin. Based on these data, the fixed-dose rate of gemcitabine can be considered a reasonable alternative to the standard 30-minute gemcitabine infusion, albeit with greater toxicity.

A Decade of Failed Attempts to Move Beyond Gemcitabine Monotherapy

In addition to oxaliplatin, there have been numerous attempts over the past decade to augment the therapeutic benefit of gemcitabine in patients with advanced disease, using additional therapeutic agents in combination with gemcitabine (see Table 41.8). Conventional cytotoxic agents that have been tested include cisplatin, oxaliplatin, 5-FU, capecitabine, irinotecan, and exatecan. Despite promising phase II data, the aforementioned doublets all failed to show any benefit over gemcitabine monotherapy.[174,220–228] In addition, novel targeted or biologic therapies have been tested in combination with gemcitabine, including marimastat (metalloproteinase inhibitor), tipifarnib (a farnesyltransferase inhibitor, targeting Kras signaling), cetuximab (epidermal growth factor receptor [EGFR] inhibitor), bevacizumab (angiogenesis inhibitor), and axitinib (multitarget tyrosine kinase inhibitor).[229–233] In general, the addition of these agents to gemcitabine failed to markedly change OS.

A few of the biologic agents warrant special mention based on the promise of therapeutic efficacy in other cancer types or in early phase clinical trial data in the treatment of advanced PDA. EGFR is expressed in 60% of PDAs,[162] and amplification or high polysomy at the EGFR locus is identified in half of the affected patients.[234] Moreover, targeting EGFR is effective in certain nonpancreatic cancers (e.g., lung, colorectal, head and neck). Therefore, there is a strong therapeutic rationale for targeting EGFR in the treatment of PDA. Cetuximab is a monoclonal antibody with affinity for EGFR, which was tested in a small phase II study in patients with advanced pancreatic cancer as a combination therapy with gemcitabine.[235] In the 41 patients with EGFR-positive tumors, the median OS was 7.1 months with a 1-year OS of 31.7%, suggesting a potential benefit when compared to historical controls.[171] However, in the large and definitive phase III trial conducted by the Southwest Oncology Group (SWOG S0205),[232] this combination failed to improve the outcome of patients when compared

to gemcitabine alone. A total of 745 patients were accrued, with median survivals of 6.3 (combination) and 5.9 months, respectively (p = 0.23). Objective response rates and progression-free survival were also similar between the two groups.

Angiogenesis has proven to be a worthy target in the solid tumor arena, and prior successes served as the impetus for the Cancer and Leukemia Group B (CALGB 80303) double-blind, placebo-controlled randomized phase III trial comparing gemcitabine plus bevacizumab versus gemcitabine alone.[231] A total of 602 treatment-naïve patients with advanced pancreatic cancer were accrued. The median OS were 5.8 and 5.9 months, respectively (p = 0.95). Again, response rates and progression-free survival were similar. Axitinib is another antiangiogenic factor, and a potent inhibitor of vascular endothelial growth factor receptor (VEGFR)1, 2, and 3. A randomized phase II trial with 103 patients demonstrated a nonsignificant improvement in OS; this prompted a larger phase III trial comparing gemcitabine 1,000 mg/m^2 on days 1, 8, and 15 every 28 days plus axitinib 5 to 10 mg orally daily, or gemcitabine plus placebo.[230] There were 632 patients in the trial, which closed at an interim analysis when the futility boundary was crossed. Median OS was 8.5 months in the gemcitabine/axitinib arm and 8.3 months in the gemcitabine/placebo arm.

Two recently published meta-analyses examined the numerous randomized controlled clinical trials of gemcitabine-based combination therapy in aggregate. These studies included more than 8,000 patients enrolled in over 25 trials.[236,237] Despite the fact that virtually all of these studies were negative independently, both meta-analyses found a small survival benefit (OR >0.9 with p <0.05) with combination therapy, although toxicity was higher. Although these findings do not justify routine use of the examined regimens, they suggest that a small subset of patients (~10% to 20%) do receive a benefit and affirm that further work to identify the best candidates for specific combination therapies is warranted.

Modest Breakthroughs in the Treatment of Advanced Pancreatic Cancer

Two additional treatments have been approved for the treatment of advanced PDA by the FDA: erlotinib and nab-paclitaxel. The former drug is an oral tyrosine kinase inhibitor of the EGFR that was approved in 2005 for use in combination with gemcitabine for locally advanced unresectable or metastatic pancreatic cancer.[175] The National Cancer Institute of Canada Clinical Trials Group (NCIC-CTG) conducted a large international phase III double-blind randomized trial of 569 patients with advanced or metastatic pancreatic adenocarcinoma, comparing gemcitabine intravenous (IV) 1,000 mg/m^2 weekly × 7 weeks followed by 1 week of rest, then weekly × 3 every 4 weeks plus erlotinib 100 mg or 150 mg per day orally versus gemcitabine plus placebo. Toxicities, including diarrhea and the typical acneiform rash associated with EGFR inhibitors, were slightly worse in the erlotinib arm. Nevertheless, these toxicities were mostly grade 1 to 2 and easily manageable. The gemcitabine/erlotinib arm experienced an improved median OS (6.24 months versus 5.91 month), with 1-year OS of 23% and 17%, respectively. Based on this study, combination gemcitabine and erlotinib became a standard of care in the first-line treatment of locally advanced or metastatic pancreas cancer in patients with a reasonably good performance status at many centers. Enthusiasm for the combination has certainly been tempered by the fact that the survival benefit amounted to just 10 days with the combination therapy. Moreover, erlotinib adds roughly $10,000 per month to the cost of treatment.[238] With that said, gemcitabine/erlotinib is clearly a more effective treatment for a subgroup of 5% to 10% of patients than gemcitabine monotherapy, and identifying predictive markers to select these individuals would be a significant advance and a step towards personalized treatment for pancreatic cancer. Notably, individuals who experienced a skin rash had improved disease control (p = 0.05) and improved survival

(Cox regression HR = 0.37; p = 0.04). Kras mutation status was tested based on prior data that wild-type Kras in colorectal cancers is predictive of response to anti-EGR therapy.[239] Unfortunately, no such correlation was found, although the study was underpowered, in large part because nearly all PDAs harbor Kras mutations.[234]

Building on the modest success of the gemcitabine/erlotinib doublet, Van Cutsem et al.[240] evaluated the same combination with or without bevacizumab in a randomized phase III study (published prior to the negative phase III gemcitabine/bevacizumab study).[240] Six hundred and seven patients were randomized to receive gemcitabine 1,000 mg/m^2 per week × 7 weeks over 8 weeks and × 3 every 4 weeks for subsequent cycles plus erlotinib 100 mg per day and bevacizumab 5 mg/kg every 2 weeks, or gemcitabine/erlotinib plus placebo. The median OS were 7.1 months for the bevacizumab arm and 6.0 months for the control arm (p = 0.2). Of note, there was an improvement in progression-free survival with the experimental treatment (4.6 versus 3.6 months; p = 0.0002). Grade 3 through 5 adverse events were comparable. Although the primary end point of OS was not met, there was an apparent favorable trend across all end points, providing a modicum of optimism that the gateway towards improved outcomes was opening, if ever so slightly.

Nab-paclitaxel was approved by the FDA in September 2013 as a second agent indicated for combination therapy with gemcitabine. Paclitaxel binds with high affinity to microtubules, thereby stabilizing tubule polymerization and inhibiting cell mitosis. Nab-Paclitaxel is bound to albumin, resulting in improved pharmokinetic efficiency and higher intratumoral drug levels, compared to the standard solvent-based paclitaxel formulation (standard paclitaxel pharmokinetics is otherwise limited by the hydrophobic nature of the molecule).[241] The exact mechanism of improved nab-paclitaxel delivery is not completely understood, but evidence points to protein–protein interactions between albumin and receptors that mediate transport (e.g., gp60) or that enhance drug targeting in the stroma (secreted protein, acidic, cysteine-rich [SPARC]).[242] Interestingly, a recent study of drug pharmokinetics in a genetically engineered SPARC-null mouse demonstrated that intratumoral nab-paclitaxel levels were not dependent on SPARC expression and that the drug does not target the stroma in this model.[243]

In an early phase I/II study, gemcitabine 1,000 mg/m^2 with nab-paclitaxel 125 mg/m^2 weekly × 3 every 28 days, resulted in tumor shrinkage in 48% of patients (substantially higher than the 5% rate previously seen with gemcitabine alone[171]) and a median OS of 12.2 months (more than twice the survival with gemcitabine).[244] With these promising results, a large international phase III study was conducted, randomizing 861 patients with advanced PDA to receive either gemcitabine/nab-paclitaxel or gemcitabine alone.[178] The MPACT study met its primary end point (Fig. 41.8), with a

Overall survival

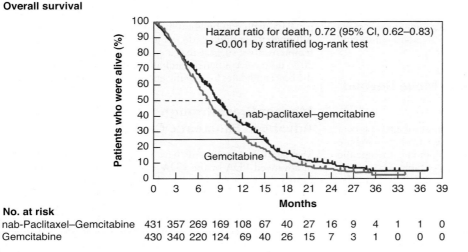

A

Progression-free survival, according to independent review

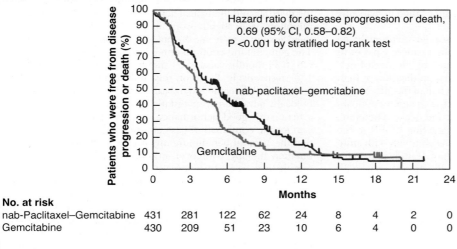

B

Figure 41.8 Kaplan–Meier curves for survival and progression-free survival for nab-paclitaxel versus gemcitabine. CI, confidence interval. (From Von Hoff DD, Ervin T, Arena FP, et al. Increased survival in pancreatic cancer with nab-paclitaxel plus gemcitabine. *N Engl J Med* 2013;369:1691–1703.)

median OS of 8.5 months in the gemcitabine/nab-paclitaxel arm and 6.7 months in the gemcitabine group (p <0.001). Progression-free survivals were 5.5 and 3.7 months, respectively (p <0.001). The 1-year OS were 35% versus 22%, and the 2-year OS were 9% versus 4%, respectively. Patients receiving combination therapy had a higher response rate as well (23% versus 7%; p <0.001). Grade 3 or higher toxicities that were more common in the nab-paclitaxel arm included neutropenia (38% versus 27%), fatigue (17% versus 7%), and neuropathy (17% versus 1%). Given the results of this trial, gemcitabine combined with nab-paclitaxel has eclipsed gemcitabine plus erlotinib as a standard of care in the first-line treatment of advanced, unresectable, or metastatic pancreatic adenocarcinoma. Importantly, the cost of adding nab-paclitaxel is not trivial ($8,000 per month).

Although gemcitabine has served as the principal backbone for pancreatic cancer therapy in most clinical trials, including patients with advanced PDA, studies were also being conducted on a combination of other drugs with proven success in colorectal cancer, including FOLFIRINOX. In 2003, the results of a phase I study were reported, which included 34 evaluable patients in total, and 6 with advanced pancreatic cancer. Two of the patients with pancreatic cancer experienced an objective response, with one complete responder.[245] These observations spawned a single-arm phase II trial in 47 chemotherapy-naïve patients with advanced pancreatic

cancer.[210] In the 46 evaluable patients, the overall response rate was 26%, with a 4% complete response rate. Median time to progression was 8.2 months and the median OS was 10 months. A randomized phase II trial was initiated, comparing the regimen to gemcitabine. Promising results in 88 patients were presented at the American Society of Clinical Oncology (ASCO) 2007 conference (response rate of 38.7% versus 11.7%), and the study continued on as the large, randomized phase III PRODIGE 4/ACCORD 11 study.[246]

The PRODIGE 4/ACCORD 11 study randomized 342 patients with a performance status of ECOG 0-1 to receive FOLFIRI-NOX (oxaliplatin 85 mg/m^2, irinotecan 180 mg/m^2, leucovorin 400 mg/m^2, and 5-FU 400 mg/m^2 IV bolus followed by 5-FU 2,400 mg/m^2 as a 46-hour continuous infusion every 2 weeks) versus gemcitabine 1,000 mg/m^2 weekly × 7 weeks followed by 1 week of rest, then 3 times per weekly × 3 every 4 weeks.[177] The primary end point was overall survival OS (Fig. 41.9). The FOLFIRINOX group had a median OS of 11.1 months compared to 6.8 months in the gemcitabine alone arm (p <0.001). Median progression-free survivals were 6.4 months and 3.3 months (p <0.001), respectively. Objective response rates were 31.6% versus 9.4% (p <0.001), and disease control rates (response + disease stability) were 70.2% and 50.9%, respectively. The FOLFIRINOX regimen resulted in substantially more toxicity, including higher grade 3 and 4 neutropenia (45% versus 21%), febrile neutropenia (5.4%

CANCERS OF THE GASTROINTESTINAL TRACT

Overall survival

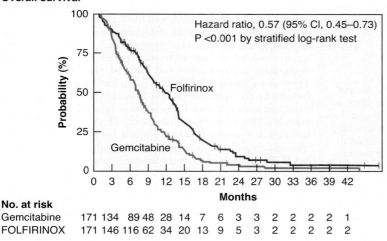

No. at risk

Gemcitabine	171	134	89	48	28	14	7	6	3	3	2	2	2	2	1
FOLFIRINOX	171	146	116	62	34	20	13	9	5	3	2	2	2	2	2

A

Progression-free survival

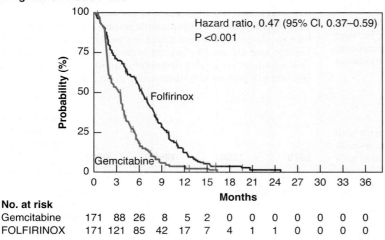

No. at risk

Gemcitabine	171	88	26	8	5	2	0	0	0	0	0	0	0
FOLFIRINOX	171	121	85	42	17	7	4	1	1	0	0	0

B

Figure 41.9 Kaplan–Meier curves for survival and progression-free survival for FOLIRINOX. (From Conroy T, Desseigne F, Ychou M, et al. FOLFIRINOX versus gemcitabine for metastatic pancreatic cancer. *N Engl J Med* 2011;364:1817–1825.)

versus 1.2%), thrombocytopenia (9.1% versus 3.6%), diarrhea (12.7% versus 1.8%), and sensory neuropathy (9% versus 0%). Despite these significant side effects, only 31% of patients in the FOLFIRINOX group had a definitive degradation in quality of life (QoL), as compared to 66% in the gemcitabine group. The time to definitive deterioration (based on the EORTC QoL questionnaire) was also significantly longer for the FOLFIRINOX group in the areas of global health status; physical, cognitive, and social functioning; and multiple symptom domains (e.g., fatigue and pain).[247]

Finally, a recently reported phase III trial in Japan compared gemcitabine alone (standard dosing) versus S-1 alone (80 to 120 mg per day for 28 days every 42 days) versus the combination of gemcitabine (1,000 mg/m^2 × 2 every 21 days) plus S-1 (60 to 100 mg per day for 14 days every 21 days). S-1 is an oral fluoropyrimidine derivative available in Japan with activity against PDA. A total of 832 patients with locally advanced or metastatic PDA were included in the analysis. OS were 8.8, 9.7, and 10.1 months (p = 0.15 for combination therapy compared to gemcitabine alone), respectively. Objective responses were higher with S-1 monotherapy (21%) and combination therapy (29%), than gemcitabine alone (13%). Gemcitabine was associated with more hematologic toxicities compared to S-1, whereas S-1 was associated with more diarrhea.[248] Combination therapy was the most toxic regimen.

Taken together, these trials establish gemcitabine alone, S-1 (in Japan), gemcitabine plus nab-paclitaxel, gemcitabine plus erlotinib, and FOLFIRINOX as the current standard of care treatments for metastatic pancreatic cancer. The latter regimen is recommended for patients with excellent performance status (ECOG 0 or 1), whereas the other regimens are applicable for a broader patient population (ECOG 0–2).

Monitoring Treatment Response

In the current era, with multiple active drugs available to treat PDA, patients increasingly have second-line options after a first-line therapy fails. Therefore, it is important for oncologists to closely monitor patients for signs of progression. Patients typically have weekly laboratory testing, and are seen biweekly or monthly by medical oncologists who assess for signs of treatment toxicity. With regard to treatment response, patients undergo repeat imaging (CT scans or magnetic resonance imaging [MRI]) every 8 weeks and responses are assessed by Response Evaluation Criteria in Solid Tumors (RECIST) criteria. CA 19-9 levels are serially drawn every 8 weeks. A falling CA 19-9 level in response to treatment is associated with improved survival, with the greatest decreases being associated with the best outcomes.[249–253] CEA and CA-125 are not FDA-approved biomarkers for PDA, and have far less accuracy then CA 19-9. Nevertheless, they may be helpful to monitor response to therapy, particularly in patients who do not express CA 19-9 due to Lewis antigen polymorphism variability. In the face of rising tumor markers and tumor progression, oncologists should pay close attention to performance status, because patients with an ECOG status of 2 or greater have an expected survival around 2 months and are not likely to benefit from additional chemotherapy.[231]

Symptom Palliation

Although extending survival is a primary objective in patients with PDA, the palliation of symptoms is equally important. As with other aspects of care, palliative-focused therapy in the patient with PDA requires a multidisciplinary team approach. Treatment recommendations are often based on the etiology of the symptoms, which may be multifactorial. Contributing factors include the metabolic burden of the tumor, treatment toxicity, or mechanical obstruction from the tumor. Optimization of nutritional intake is paramount and could be exacerbated by cancer cachexia and pancreatic insufficiency. Aggressive pain management frequently requires minimally invasive interventions such as celiac plexus neurolysis (endoscopic or percutaneous), in addition to systemic narcotics. Active surveillance and prompt treatment of thromboembolic events, biliary obstruction, and gastric outlet obstruction are critical. Psychosocial issues for the patient and family must be addressed. Often, the extent of symptoms and deterioration in performance status precludes additional antitumor-directed therapy. Even with expert care, there is a 1% to 4% mortality rate related to treatment.[177,178] Therefore, oncologists need to have frank discussions with patients and family members about best supportive care (e.g., no chemotherapy or radiation) when appropriate.

FUTURE DIRECTIONS AND CHALLENGES

The timeline of pancreatic cancer therapy can be summarized as follows (Fig. 41.10): Through the 1970s, no effective therapies existed; between 1980 and 2000, surgical outcomes markedly improved, permitting safe treatment of early stage PDA at high volume centers; between 2000 and the present, modest improvements in chemotherapy and radiation have improved outcomes and the safety profile of these treatments. Over the same time span, there have been dramatic advances in the genetic and molecular understanding of pancreatic cancer development and survival, although this new knowledge has not yet translated into improved patient outcomes. It is becoming more apparent, however, that the field is on the cusp of substantial breakthroughs, similar to those experienced recently in many other cancer types (e.g., breast, colon, melanoma). The next decade will likely produce improved molecular diagnostics (markers for detection, prognosis, and treatment response), targeted therapies (personalized oncology), antistromal agents used in tandem with antineoplastic agents, and immunotherapies (e.g., vaccines and immune checkpoint inhibitors). There is a growing trend toward multi-institutional collaboration fostered by the National Cancer Institute (NCI), private foundations, and industry, as well as scheduled national meetings focused entirely on pancreatic cancer research. This surge in collaboration and communication between thought leaders, coupled with increased national attention (e.g., the Recalcitrant Cancer Research Act of 2012, which identified pancreatic cancer as a high priority), will undoubtedly jolt the field forward in the coming years.

In this closing section, we will broadly discuss some of the most encouraging areas of research, address some of the greatest challenges, and highlight areas that warrant investigative pursuit.

Biomarkers: Diagnostic, Prognostic, and Predictive

Biomarkers can be separated into three categories. *Diagnostic* biomarkers detect the presence of disease. They are relevant for *early detection*, as well as to measure disease burden in response to therapy. *Prognostic* markers gauge disease aggressiveness or tumor biology, and are used to forecast outcome or recurrence pattern. *Predictive* markers predict treatment response, and are the key ingredient to a personalized therapeutic approach.

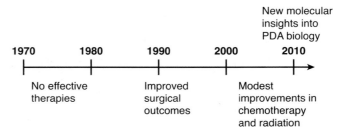

Figure 41.10 Timeline of advances in PDA-related therapy and science.

Effective early detection of PDA could have the greatest impact on PDA-specific outcomes, but may also be the least likely to come to fruition. Such a test would need to identify premalignant lesions that are at very high risk of developing into an invasive lesion (PanIN-3). Genetically engineered mouse data suggest that tumor dissemination can still occur even at the premalignant stage[254]; nevertheless, it is still believed (albeit unproven) that treatment of PanIN-3 lesions would be curative for most patients. Moreover, PanIN-3 (i.e., carcinoma in situ) lesions are likely far enough along in the tumor progression sequence that the risk of overtreatment would not outweigh the potential benefit of treatment (including surgical intervention).[33,255]

There are several challenges associated with early detection research. First, most diagnostic biomarker research to date merely distinguishes invasive PDA (in resected patients) from normal controls. This research largely misses the point, because the index lesions are not *curable* precursor lesions. Most individuals with *localized* invasive cancer already harbor occult metastases. Presently, only 6% of resected PDAs (and <1% of all PDAs) are diagnosed at stage I, and the resection of PanIN-3 disease in the absence of invasive carcinoma is exceedingly rare.[27,256] Second, current CT scanning technology fails to reliably detect PDAs below 2 cm, because PDAs are poorly demarcated and are hypodense compared to normal pancreata.[80] Curable lesions (i.e., PanIN-3 lesions) are likely one-quarter the size of this lower limit.[224] Third, the sensitivity required for effective screening tests is much higher than commonly appreciated. Pannala et al.[79] calculated that an early detection biomarker with 99% sensitivity and specificity would detect all PDAs in the general population, but would also result in a 1% false positive rate due to the relatively low prevalence of PDA (false positives outnumbering true positives by an astounding 25:1). Restricting early detection tests to *high-risk* individuals would improve the positive predictive value, but of course end up missing sporadic PDAs, which comprise the large majority of cases. Finally, serum based tests have a low pretest probability of detecting molecular analytes derived from *noninvasive* lesions that do not have access to the circulatory system. As an illustration of this point, we recently prepared plasma from fresh phlebotomy draws in patients with PDA, and performed a Kras mutation screen using a high-sensitivity commercial mutation detection assay (BEAMing, which detects mutant genes in a background of wild-type DNA at ratios >1:10,000).[257] Mutations were detected at low rates even in patients with high invasive disease burden: two out of nine patients with metastatic disease and zero out of three with localized disease (Jordan M. Winter, unpublished observation). With improved high-throughput instrumentation and bioinformatics strategies available, researchers are now better equipped to interrogate analytes beyond DNA (e.g., metabolome, transcriptome, proteome) in search of a molecular beacon of early PDA. National tissue banking programs, such as the NCI-sponsored Early Detection Research Network, are critical to this pursuit.

There are currently no effective prognostic panels for PDA, akin to the validated Oncotype Dx panels for breast, colon, and prostate cancers. Limitations are primarily due to relatively low tissue availability and to a tighter survival distribution necessitating even higher sample numbers for analyses. Nevertheless, the technology currently exists (e.g., gene expression arrays or Nanostring multiplex gene expression analyses [Seattle, WA]) to develop prognostic panels for PDA. Improved prognostics could identify patients who harbor particularly aggressive tumors that may appear resectable by imaging, yet are best managed with neoadjuvant chemotherapy to treat occult metastases and perhaps avoid ineffective surgery.

There has been some intriguing work in this area. Stratford et al.[258] used fresh frozen tumors from 15 resected PDAs and 15 metastatic PDAs (from autopsies) to identify a gene expression signature using cDNA microarrays associated with metastatic disease. The researchers then tested the derived signature in two separate cohorts of patients with resected disease and found that the panel predicted poor survival. The gene signature has not yet been validated by a separate group.[258] In a separate study, protein expression patterns of 13 putative PDA biomarkers were examined in a large cohort of short- and long-term survivors after resection. The investigators found that MUC1 and mesothelin (MSLN) expression were far more predictive of early cancer-specific death than conventional pathologic features. Again, these findings require validation.[162]

There are no proven predictive markers for standard pancreatic cancer therapies. Data from the phase II gemcitabine/nab-paclitaxel study suggested that stromal SPARC expression is associated with improved outcome.[244] Data from the more recent phase III study are forthcoming. No predictive markers of gemcitabine have been consistently validated in samples from randomized trials. Human equilibrative nucleoside transporter 1 (hENT1) is a nucleoside transporter involved in gemcitabine uptake. Increased expression was associated with improved survival in patients receiving gemcitabine in the RTOG 9704 study,[259] but no association was observed in a randomized study comparing gemcitabine and an hENT1-independent gemcitabine derivative.[260] Brody et al. have identified the RNA binding protein, HuR, as a candidate predictive marker of gemcitabine efficacy in two retrospective institutional cohorts.[261,262] HuR regulates and stabilizes DCK, which phosphorylates and activates gemcitabine. Investigators are currently evaluating samples from the adjuvant ESPAC3 trial (gemcitabine versus 5-FU) to validate this finding. Finally, our group at Thomas Jefferson recently observed that DCK expression was associated with improved survival in patients receiving 5-FU chemotherapy in the RTOG 9704 trial. This finding was recapitulated in cell lines (unpublished).

Targeted Therapy

As a result of whole-exome sequencing, the vast majority of genes mutated in PDA with high frequency are now known. Unfortunately, no novel high frequency *druggable* targets were identified. Many mutated genes can be categorized within core signaling pathway (12 were initially described),[35] and there have growing efforts to try to develop therapies targeting these pathways (as opposed to a specific genetically altered gene). In addition, there has been a redoubling of efforts to target Kras, as a result of the empty genetic search for promising new targets. As stated, Kras is mutated in virtually every PDA, as well as most cells within each PDA. Although attempts to inhibit Kras have eluded researchers thus far, numerous innovative approaches are currently under investigation. These include developing novel compounds to directly bind and inhibit RAS through rational drug design; developing drugs that restore GTP hydrolytic function in mutant RAS; interference with RAS posttranslational modification (e.g., prenylation, proteolytic processing, carboxyl methylation); inhibition of RAS expression (e.g., RNA interference); inhibition of downstream RAS signaling (e.g., Raf-MEK-ERK and PI3K pathways); and identifying pathways that are required for survival in Kras mutant cells (synthetic lethal approach). As evidence of the importance that the NCI has placed on this research, the NCI recently announced an initiative focused on targeting Kras, and plans to divert $10 million annually to support the program (http://frederick.cancer.gov/News/RASCancerGeneticsInitiative.aspx).

Heterogeneity as an Obstacle to Targeted Therapy

PDAs exhibit tremendous molecular heterogeneity, both between and within tumors. The genetic fingerprint of each tumor is unique: each with a different set of mutated genes and chromosome copy number changes.[35,41] Yachida et al.[255] revealed that

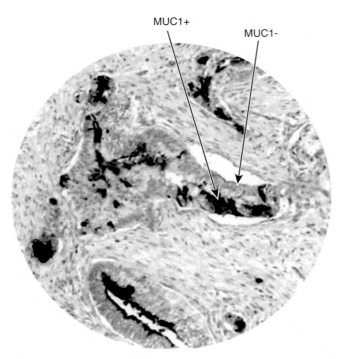

MUC1+

MUC1-

Figure 41.11 MUC1 expression in a pancreatic cancer. A focus of invasive cancer reveals areas of positive (+) and negative (−) MUC1 expression *(arrows).*

genetic abnormalities differ across a given pancreatic tumor, with genetically distinct foci in the primary, that give rise to clonal populations in metastatic deposits. An immunohistochemical survey of pancreatic cancer biomarkers illustrates the diversity in protein expression.[162] For instance, MUC1 is absent in 15% of PDAs, but is diffusely expressed (>75% of neoplastic cells) in 30%. Even a single focus of PDA containing both MUC1-positive and MUC1-negative cells illustrates biologic variation within a given tumor (Fig. 41.11). Keeping with this pattern, metabolic gradients exist in tumors due to the proximity of neoplastic cells to patent blood vessels as well as due to the dynamic nature of the tumor microenvironment. Microecologic niches result,[263] which are reflected in the varied expression patterns of metabolic enzymes across tumor sites (e.g., primary and metastases) in patients with PDA.[264] Basic cell cycle dynamics drive proteomic changes in a single cell over time, even in the most stable circumstances. PDA heterogeneity is, therefore, a certainty, yet has emerged as the unaddressed truth, as the cancer field pursues a *personalized* approach to cancer therapy. Single molecule targeting is likely to fail because of PDA heterogeneity. An example from another cancer type is illustrative. Extreme heterogeneity, based on the expression pattern of the estrogen receptor, was observed in a human ovarian cancer prior to treatment. After treatment, the expression pattern was dramatically altered in the same tumor sample, when only chemoresistant clones survived.[265] A multitargeted approach may be necessary, similar to the standard treatment strategy against HIV. Therapeutic strategies that are significantly more *tunable* than conventional medicinal pharmacology may also be useful, such as nanoparticle-delivered gene therapy.[266]

Targeting the Stroma

Over 70% of a PDA is comprised of stroma, and a worse outcome was observed in patients with tumors exhibiting a higher stromal content.[267] The hypovascular stroma is viewed as an obstacle to drug delivery, and explains why gemcitabine is potent against xenografts (with low stromal content), but ineffective in autochthonous genetically engineered mouse models of PDA.[268] Stromal depletion in KPC mice (mice with conditional and pancreatic-specific expression of mutant Kras and TP53) with a Hedgehog pathway inhibitor improved gemcitabine delivery to tumors and decreased tumor burden. The same effects were observed in a separate study that used a drug targeting the extracellular matrix protein, hyaluronic acid.[269] Thus, targeting the tumor stroma is a promising strategy to improve the efficacy of conventional pancreatic cancer treatments and is a high research priority.

Metabolism

There is a growing appreciation and understanding of the malignant metabolic phenotype, although Otto Warburg first observed fundamental metabolic differences between cancer and normal cells nearly 100 years ago. The proliferative demands of pancreatic cancer cells, along with the adaptive requirements for survival in an austere tumor microenvironment (characterized by an abundant, yet nutrient-deprived stroma), require complex mechanisms to reprogram metabolic pathways.[270] In fact, PDA cells are particularly tolerant to nutrient deprivation compared to other cancers.[31] Recently, mutant Kras was found to alter metabolic pathways, leading to increased glycolysis,[271] altered amino acid metabolism through noncanonical enzyme pathways,[272] and macropinocytosis of protein as an additional fuel source.[273] Metabolic reprogramming through posttranscriptional regulation of metabolic enzymes by a stress response RNA-binding protein was found to be an independent survival mechanism of PDA cells under nutrient deprivation.[274] A better understanding of PDA metabolism will likely expose metabolic dependencies as important therapeutic targets.

Immunotherapy

Immunotherapy was the 2013 Science Breakthrough of the Year,[275] as a result of multiple new therapies for nonpancreatic malignancies (especially melanoma). Many of the treatments work by targeting immunologic checkpoints (i.e., immunosuppressive pathways induced by cancer cells). Inhibition of these molecules with antibodies unleashes the body's immune system against the tumor in some patients.[276,277] T-cell adoptive therapy is another emerging immunotherapy with successes in nonpancreatic cancers, where T cells from patients are genetically engineered ex vivo to target the patient's own tumor.[278] Thus, there is an urgent need to understand how these strategies can be used or modified to treat pancreatic cancer.

There are immunotherapies that have had some preclinical and early clinical trial success against pancreatic cancer. CD40 is a molecule on the surface of tumor-associated macrophages that stimulates T-cell–dependent antitumor immunity. In a recent phase I study, patients with treatment-naïve advanced PDA were treated with gemcitabine and a monoclonal antibody that binds and stimulates CD40. There was a 19% response rate and biologic indicators of a strong immune response (e.g., increased cytokine levels).[279] A pancreatic cancer vaccine (algenpantucel-L, NewLink Genetics Corporation, Ames, IA) has also been developed in which pancreatic cancer cell lines are genetically engineered to express an immunogenic nonhuman epitope. The vaccine is delivered intradermally, and was given to 70 patients as part of a phase II study, along with gemcitabine and chemoradiation (similar to the RTOG 9704 regimen). The 12-month OS of patients who received the vaccine and conventional adjuvant treatment was 86%, which compared favorably with historical controls.[280] Vaccine-related toxicity was minimal. A phase III adjuvant trial was recently completed in North America, and the results are pending.

CONCLUSION

Improvements in pancreatic cancer treatment over the past 2 decades include safer surgical management, safer radiation treatment, and modest but notable improvements in systemic treatments. With modern chemotherapy, roughly half of patients experience temporary disease control. Nevertheless, the disease is still lethal in most patients and survival beyond 2 years is a rare event. For those of us who routinely treat this disease, progress cannot come soon enough. However, advances are imminent, and there is reason for optimism. The Pancreatic Cancer Action Network has publicized its desire to dramatically improve patient outcomes by the year 2020, and the scientific community is rallying to the charge.

REFERENCES

1. Siegel R, Naishadham D, Jemal A. Cancer statistics, 2013. *CA Cancer J Clin* 2013;63:11–30.
2. American Cancer Society. *Cancer Facts & Figures.* Atlanta: American Cancer Society; 2013.
3. Riall TS, Nealon WH, Goodwin JS, et al. Pancreatic cancer in the general population: Improvements in survival over the last decade. *J Gastrointest Surg* 2006;10:1212–1223.
4. Worni M, Guller U, White RR, et al. Modest improvement in overall survival for patients with metastatic pancreatic cancer: a trend analysis using the Surveillance, Epidemiology, and End Results Registry From 1988 to 2008. *Pancreas* 2013;42:1157–1163.
5. Winter JM, Brennan MF, Tang LH, et al. Survival after resection of pancreatic adenocarcinoma: results from a single institution over three decades. *Ann Surg Oncol* 2012;19:169–175.
6. Edge SE, Byrd DR. *AJCC Cancer Staging Manual.* New York: Springer; 2009.
7. Bilimoria KY, Bentrem DJ, Ko CY, et al. Validation of the 6th edition AJCC Pancreatic Cancer Staging System: report from the National Cancer Database. *Cancer* 2007;110:738–744.
8. National Cancer Institute. SEER Stat Fact Sheets: Pancreas Cancer. http://seer.cancer.gov/statfacts/html/pancreas.html.
9. Solomon S, Das S, Brand R, et al. Inherited pancreatic cancer syndromes. *Cancer J* 2012;18:485–491.
10. Klein AP, Brune KA, Petersen GM, et al. Prospective risk of pancreatic cancer in familial pancreatic cancer kindreds. *Cancer Res* 2004;64:2634–2638.
11. Klein AP. Genetic susceptibility to pancreatic cancer. *Mol Carcinog* 2012;51:14–24.
12. Iodice S, Gandini S, Maisonneuve P, et al. Tobacco and the risk of pancreatic cancer: a review and meta-analysis. *Langenbecks Arch Surg* 2008;393:535–545.
13. Bosetti C, Lucenteforte E, Silverman DT, et al. Cigarette smoking and pancreatic cancer: an analysis from the International Pancreatic Cancer Case-Control Consortium (Panc4). *Ann Oncol* 2012;23:1880–1888.
14. Silverman DT, Schiffman M, Everhart J, et al. Diabetes mellitus, other medical conditions and familial history of cancer as risk factors for pancreatic cancer. *Br J Cancer* 1999;80:1830–1837.
15. Schenk M, Schwartz AG, O'Neal E, et al. Familial risk of pancreatic cancer. *J Natl Cancer Inst* 2001;93:640–644.
16. Bertuccio P, La Vecchia C, Silverman DT, et al. Cigar and pipe smoking, smokeless tobacco use and pancreatic cancer: an analysis from the International Pancreatic Cancer Case-Control Consortium (PanC4). *Ann Oncol* 2011;22:1420–1426.
17. Zhou J, Wellenius GA, Michaud DS. Environmental tobacco smoke and the risk of pancreatic cancer among non-smokers: a meta-analysis. *Occup Environ Med* 2012;69:853–857.
18. Chuang SC, Gallo V, Michaud D, et al. Exposure to environmental tobacco smoke in childhood and incidence of cancer in adulthood in never smokers in the European Prospective Investigation into Cancer and Nutrition. *Cancer Causes Control* 2011;22:487–494.
19. Hecht SS. Tobacco carcinogens, their biomarkers and tobacco-induced cancer. *Nat Rev Cancer* 2003;3:733–744.
20. Andreotti G, Silverman DT. Occupational risk factors and pancreatic cancer: a review of recent findings. *Mol Carcinog* 2012;51:98–108.
21. Lucenteforte E, La Vecchia C, Silverman D, et al. Alcohol consumption and pancreatic cancer: a pooled analysis in the International Pancreatic Cancer Case-Control Consortium (PanC4). *Ann Oncol* 2012;23:374–382.
22. Duell EJ, Lucenteforte E, Olson SH, et al. Pancreatitis and pancreatic cancer risk: a pooled analysis in the International Pancreatic Cancer Case-Control Consortium (PanC4). *Ann Oncol* 2012;23:2964–2970.
23. Bracci PM. Obesity and pancreatic cancer: overview of epidemiologic evidence and biologic mechanisms. *Mol Carcinog* 2012;51:53–63.
24. Huxley R, Ansary-Moghaddam A, Berrington de Gonzalez A, et al. Type-II diabetes and pancreatic cancer: a meta-analysis of 36 studies. *Br J Cancer* 2005;92:2076–2083.
25. Ben Q, Xu M, Ning X, et al. Diabetes mellitus and risk of pancreatic cancer: A meta-analysis of cohort studies. *Eur J Cancer* 2011;47:1928–1937.
26. Klimstra DS, Pitman MB, Hruban RH. An algorithmic approach to the diagnosis of pancreatic neoplasms. *Arch Pathol Lab Med* 2009;133:454–464.
27. Winter JM, Cameron JL, Campbell KA, et al. 1423 pancreaticoduodenectomies for pancreatic cancer: A single-institution experience. *J Gastrointest Surg* 2006;10:1199–1210.
28. Winter JM, Maitra A, Yeo CJ. Genetics and pathology of pancreatic cancer. *HPB (Oxford)* 2006;8:324–336.
29. Neesse A, Michl P, Frese KK, et al. Stromal biology and therapy in pancreatic cancer. *Gut* 2011;60:861–868.
30. Anderson AR, Weaver AM, Cummings PT, et al. Tumor morphology and phenotypic evolution driven by selective pressure from the microenvironment. *Cell* 2006;127:905–915.
31. Izuishi K, Kato K, Ogura T, et al. Remarkable tolerance of tumor cells to nutrient deprivation: possible new biochemical target for cancer therapy. *Cancer Res* 2000;60:6201–6207.
32. Cho KR, Vogelstein B. Genetic alterations in the adenoma—carcinoma sequence. *Cancer* 1992;70:1727–1731.
33. Kozuka S, Sassa R, Taki T, et al. Relation of pancreatic duct hyperplasia to carcinoma. *Cancer* 1979;43:1418–1428.
34. Biankin AV, Waddell N, Kassahn KS, et al. Pancreatic cancer genomes reveal aberrations in axon guidance pathway genes. *Nature* 2012;491:399–405.
35. Jones S, Zhang X, Parsons DW, et al. Core signaling pathways in human pancreatic cancers revealed by global genomic analyses. *Science* 2008;321:1801–1806.
36. Caldas C, Kern SE. K-ras mutation and pancreatic adenocarcinoma. *Int J Pancreatol* 1995;18:1–6.
37. Smit VT, Boot AJ, Smits AM, et al. KRAS codon 12 mutations occur very frequently in pancreatic adenocarcinomas. *Nucleic Acids Res* 1988;16:7773–7782.
38. Suda K, Tomizawa K, Mitsudomi T. Biological and clinical significance of KRAS mutations in lung cancer: an oncogenic driver that contrasts with EGFR mutation. *Cancer Metastasis Rev* 2010;29:49–60.
39. Baines AT, Xu D, Der CJ. Inhibition of Ras for cancer treatment: the search continues. *Future Med Chem* 2011;3:1787–1808.
40. Schleger C, Arens N, Zentgraf H, et al. Identification of frequent chromosomal aberrations in ductal adenocarcinoma of the pancreas by comparative genomic hybridization (CGH). *J Pathol* 2000;191:27–32.
41. Calhoun ES, Hucl T, Gallmeier E, et al. Identifying allelic loss and homozygous deletions in pancreatic cancer without matched normals using high-density single-nucleotide polymorphism arrays. *Cancer Res* 2006;66:7920–7928.
42. Caldas C, Hahn SA, da Costa LT, et al. Frequent somatic mutations and homozygous deletions of the p16 (MTS1) gene in pancreatic adenocarcinoma. *Nat Genet* 1994;8:27–32.
43. Schutte M, Hruban RH, Geradts J, et al. Abrogation of the Rb/p16 tumor-suppressive pathway in virtually all pancreatic carcinomas. *Cancer Res* 1997;57:3126–3130.
44. Scarpa A, Capelli P, Mukai K, et al. Pancreatic adenocarcinomas frequently show p53 gene mutations. *Am J Pathol* 1993;142:1534–1543.
45. Schmitt CA, Fridman JS, Yang M, et al. Dissecting p53 tumor suppressor functions in vivo. *Cancer Cell* 2002;1:289–298.
46. Yu X, Vazquez A, Levine AJ, et al. Allele-specific p53 mutant reactivation. *Cancer Cell* 2012;21:614–625.
47. Meng X, Laidler LL, Kosmacek EA, et al. Induction of mitotic cell death by overriding G2/M checkpoint in endometrial cancer cells with non-functional p53. *Gynecol Oncol* 2013;128:461–469.
48. Hahn SA, Schutte M, Hoque AT, et al. DPC4, a candidate tumor suppressor gene at human chromosome 18q21.1. *Science* 1996;271:350–353.
49. Iacobuzio-Donahue CA, Fu B, Yachida S, et al. DPC4 gene status of the primary carcinoma correlates with patterns of failure in patients with pancreatic cancer. *J Clin Oncol* 2009;27:1806–1813.
50. Shi C, Hong SM, Lim P, et al. KRAS2 mutations in human pancreatic acinar-ductal metaplastic lesions are limited to those with PanIN: implications for the human pancreatic cancer cell of origin. *Mol Cancer Res* 2009;7:230–236.
51. van Heek NT, Meeker AK, Kern SE, et al. Telomere shortening is nearly universal in pancreatic intraepithelial neoplasia. *Am J Pathol* 2002;161:1541–1547.
52. Rosty C, Geradts J, Sato N, et al. p16 Inactivation in pancreatic intraepithelial neoplasias (PanINs) arising in patients with chronic pancreatitis. *Am J Surg Pathol* 2003;27:1495–1501.
53. McCarthy DM, Brat DJ, Wilentz RE, et al. Pancreatic intraepithelial neoplasia and infiltrating adenocarcinoma: analysis of progression and recurrence by DPC4 immunohistochemical labeling. *Hum Pathol* 2001;32:638–642.
54. Wilentz RE, Iacobuzio-Donahue CA, Argani P, et al. Loss of expression of Dpc4 in pancreatic intraepithelial neoplasia: evidence that DPC4 inactivation occurs late in neoplastic progression. *Cancer Res* 2000;60:2002–2006.

CANCERS OF THE GASTROINTESTINAL TRACT

55. Baumgart M, Werther M, Bockholt A, et al. Genomic instability at both the base pair level and the chromosomal level is detectable in earliest PanIN lesions in tissues of chronic pancreatitis. *Pancreas* 2010;39:1093–1103.

56. Hong SM, Vincent A, Kanda M, et al. Genome-wide somatic copy number alterations in low-grade PanINs and IPMNs from individuals with a family history of pancreatic cancer. *Clin Cancer Res* 2012;18:4303–4312.

57. Luttges J, Galehdari H, Brocker V, et al. Allelic loss is often the first hit in the biallelic inactivation of the p53 and DPC4 genes during pancreatic carcinogenesis. *Am J Pathol* 2001;158:1677–1683.

58. Yachida S, Iacobuzio-Donahue CA. Evolution and dynamics of pancreatic cancer progression. *Oncogene* 2013;32:5253–5260.

59. Roberts NJ, Jiao Y, Yu J, et al. ATM mutations in patients with hereditary pancreatic cancer. *Cancer Discov* 2012;2:41–46.

60. Canto MI, Hruban RH, Fishman EK, et al. Frequent detection of pancreatic lesions in asymptomatic high-risk individuals. *Gastroenterology* 2012;142:796–804.

61. Canto MI, Harinck F, Hruban RH, et al. International Cancer of the Pancreas Screening (CAPS) Consortium summit on the management of patients with increased risk for familial pancreatic cancer. *Gut* 2013;62:339–347.

62. Perez-Mancera PA, Guerra C, Barbacid M, et al. What we have learned about pancreatic cancer from mouse models. *Gastroenterology* 2012;142:1079–1092.

63. Seth AK, Argani P, Campbell KA, et al. Acinar cell carcinoma of the pancreas: an institutional series of resected patients and review of the current literature. *J Gastrointest Surg* 2008;12:1061–1067.

64. Jiao Y, Yonescu R, Offerhaus GJ, et al. Whole exome sequencing of pancreatic neoplasms with acinar differentiation. *J Pathol* 2014;232:428–435.

65. Salman B, Brat G, Yoon YS, et al. The diagnosis and surgical treatment of pancreatoblastoma in adults: a case series and review of the literature. *J Gastrointest Surg* 2013;17:2153–2161.

66. Shi C, Hruban RH. Intraductal papillary mucinous neoplasm. *Hum Pathol* 2012;43:1–16.

67. Laffan TA, Horton KM, Klein AP, et al. Prevalence of unsuspected pancreatic cysts on MDCT. *AJR Am J Roentgenol* 2008;191:802–807.

68. Tanaka M, Chari S, Adsay V, et al. International consensus guidelines for management of intraductal papillary mucinous neoplasms and mucinous cystic neoplasms of the pancreas. *Pancreatology* 2006;6:17–32.

69. Poultsides GA, Reddy S, Cameron JL, et al. Histopathologic basis for the favorable survival after resection of intraductal papillary mucinous neoplasm-associated invasive adenocarcinoma of the pancreas. *Ann Surg* 2010;251:470–476.

70. Wu J, Jiao Y, Dal Molin M, et al. Whole-exome sequencing of neoplastic cysts of the pancreas reveals recurrent mutations in components of ubiquitin-dependent pathways. *Proc Natl Acad Sci U S A* 2011;108:21188–21193.

71. Reddy S, Cameron JL, Scudiere J, et al. Surgical management of solid-pseudopapillary neoplasms of the pancreas (Franz or Hamoudi tumors): a large single-institutional series. *J Am Coll Surg* 2009;208:950–957.

72. Ellison TA, Wolfgang CL, Shi C, et al. A single institution's 26-year experience with nonfunctional pancreatic neuroendocrine tumors: a validation of current staging systems and a new prognostic nomogram. *Ann Surg* 2014;259:204–212.

73. Klimstra DS, Modlin IR, Coppola D, et al. The pathologic classification of neuroendocrine tumors: a review of nomenclature, grading, and staging systems. *Pancreas* 2010;39:707–712.

74. Phan GQ, Yeo CJ, Hruban RH, et al. Surgical experience with pancreatic and peripancreatic neuroendocrine tumors: review of 125 patients. *J Gastrointest Surg* 1998;2:472–482.

75. Kimura W, Kuroda A, Morioka Y. Clinical pathology of endocrine tumors of the pancreas. Analysis of autopsy cases. *Dig Dis Sci* 1991;36:933–942.

76. Whipple AO. The surgical therapy of hyperinsulinism. *J Int Chir* 1938;3:237–276.

77. Jiao Y, Shi C, Edil BH, et al. DAXX/ATRX, MEN1, and mTOR pathway genes are frequently altered in pancreatic neuroendocrine tumors. *Science* 2011;331:1199–1203.

78. Falconi M, Bartsch DK, Eriksson B, et al. ENETS Consensus Guidelines for the management of patients with digestive neuroendocrine neoplasms of the digestive system: well-differentiated pancreatic non-functioning tumors. *Neuroendocrinology* 2012;95:120–134.

79. Pannala R, Basu A, Petersen GM, et al. New-onset diabetes: a potential clue to the early diagnosis of pancreatic cancer. *Lancet Oncol* 2009;10:88–95.

80. Fong ZV, Tan WP, Lavu H, et al. Preoperative imaging for resectable periampullary cancer: clinicopathologic implications of reported radiographic findings. *J Gastrointest Surg* 2013;17:1098–1106.

81. Callery MP, Chang KJ, Fishman EK, et al. Pretreatment assessment of resectable and borderline resectable pancreatic cancer: expert consensus statement. *Ann Surg Oncol* 2009;16:1727–1733.

82. Evans DB, Erickson BA, Ritch P. Borderline resectable pancreatic cancer: definitions and the importance of multimodality therapy. *Ann Surg Oncol* 2010;17:2803–2805.

83. Varadhachary GR, Tamm EP, Abbruzzese JL, et al. Borderline resectable pancreatic cancer: definitions, management, and role of preoperative therapy. *Ann Surg Oncol* 2006;13:1035–1046.

84. Evans DB, Varadhachary GR, Crane CH, et al. Preoperative gemcitabine-based chemoradiation for patients with resectable adenocarcinoma of the pancreatic head. *J Clin Oncol* 2008;26:3496–3502.

85. Katz MH, Fleming JB, Bhosale P, et al. Response of borderline resectable pancreatic cancer to neoadjuvant therapy is not reflected by radiographic indicators. *Cancer* 2012;118:5749–5756.

86. van der Gaag NA, Rauws EA, van Eijck CH, et al. Preoperative biliary drainage for cancer of the head of the pancreas. *N Engl J Med* 2010;362:129–137.

87. Kooby DA, Hawkins WG, Schmidt CM, et al. A multicenter analysis of distal pancreatectomy for adenocarcinoma: is laparoscopic resection appropriate? *J Am Coll Surg* 2010;210:779–785.

88. Venkat R, Edil BH, Schulick RD, et al. Laparoscopic distal pancreatectomy is associated with significantly less overall morbidity compared to the open technique: a systematic review and meta-analysis. *Ann Surg* 2012;255:1048–1059.

89. Kendrick ML. Laparoscopic and robotic resection for pancreatic cancer. *Cancer J* 2012;18:571–576.

90. Bassi C, Dervenis C, Butturini G, et al. Postoperative pancreatic fistula: an international study group (ISGPF) definition. *Surgery* 2005;138:8–13.

91. Wente MN, Bassi C, Dervenis C, et al. Delayed gastric emptying (DGE) after pancreatic surgery: a suggested definition by the International Study Group of Pancreatic Surgery (ISGPS). *Surgery* 2007;142:761–768.

92. Wente MN, Veit JA, Bassi C, et al. Postpancreatectomy hemorrhage (PPH): an International Study Group of Pancreatic Surgery (ISGPS) definition. *Surgery* 2007;142:20–25.

93. Shukla PJ, Barreto SG, Fingerhut A, et al. Toward improving uniformity and standardization in the reporting of pancreatic anastomoses: a new classification system by the International Study Group of Pancreatic Surgery (ISGPS). *Surgery* 2010;147:144–153.

94. Burkhart RA, Relles D, Pineda DM, et al. Defining treatment and outcomes of hepaticojejunostomy failure following pancreaticoduodenectomy. *J Gastrointest Surg* 2013;17:451–460.

95. Doi R, Imamura M, Hosotani R, et al. Surgery versus radiochemotherapy for resectable locally invasive pancreatic cancer: final results of a randomized multi-institutional trial. *Surg Today* 2008;38:1021–1028.

96. Bloechle C, Broering DC, Latuske C, et al. Prospective randomized study to evaluate quality of life after partial pancreatoduodenectomy according to whipple versus pylorus preserving pancreatoduodenectomy according to longmir-traverso for periampullary carcinoma. *Deutsche Gesellschaft Chir* 1999;Suppl 1:661–664.

97. Karanicolas PJ, Davies E, Kunz R, et al. The pylorus: take it or leave it? Systematic review and meta-analysis of pylorus-preserving versus standard whipple pancreaticoduodenectomy for pancreatic or periampullary cancer. *Ann Surg Oncol* 2007;14:1825–1834.

98. Lin PW, Shan YS, Lin YJ, et al. Pancreaticoduodenectomy for pancreatic head cancer: PPPD versus Whipple procedure. *Hepatogastroenterology* 2005;52:1601–1604.

99. Paquet KJ. Comparison of Whipples pancreaticoduodenectomy with the pylorus-preserving pancreaticoduodenectomy—a prospectively controlled, randomized long-term trial. *Chir Gastroenterol* 1998;14:54–58.

100. Seiler CA, Wagner M, Bachmann T, et al. Randomized clinical trial of pylorus-preserving duodenopancreatectomy versus classical Whipple resection-long term results. *Br J Surg* 2005;92:547–556.

101. Tran KT, Smeenk HG, van Eijck CH, et al. Pylorus preserving pancreaticoduodenectomy versus standard Whipple procedure: a prospective, randomized, multicenter analysis of 170 patients with pancreatic and periampullary tumors. *Ann Surg* 2004;240:738–745.

102. Wenger FA, Jacobi CA, Haubold K, et al. [Gastrointestinal quality of life after duodenopancreatectomy in pancreatic carcinoma. Preliminary results of a prospective randomized study: pancreatoduodenectomy or pylorus-preserving pancreatoduodenectomy]. *Chirurg* 1999;70:1454–1459.

103. Imamura N, Chijiiwa K, Ohuchida J, et al. Prospective randomized clinical trial of a change in gastric emptying and nutritional status after a pylorus-preserving pancreaticoduodenectomy: comparison between an antecolic and a vertical retrocolic duodenojejunostomy. *HPB (Oxford)* 2014;16:382–394.

104. Gangavatiker R, Pal S, Javed A, et al. Effect of antecolic or retrocolic reconstruction of the gastro/duodenojejunostomy on delayed gastric emptying after pancreaticoduodenectomy: a randomized controlled trial. *J Gastrointest Surg* 2011;15:843–852.

105. Eshuis WJ, van Eijck CH, Gerhards MF, et al. Antecolic versus retrocolic route of the gastroenteric anastomosis after pancreatoduodenectomy: a randomized controlled trial. *Ann Surg* 2014;259:45–51.

106. Tamandl D, Sahora K, Prucker J, et al. Impact of the reconstruction method on delayed gastric emptying after pylorus-preserving pancreaticoduodenectomy: a prospective randomized study. *World J Surg* 2014;38:465–475.

107. Tani M, Terasawa H, Kawai M, et al. Improvement of delayed gastric emptying in pylorus-preserving pancreaticoduodenectomy: results of a prospective, randomized, controlled trial. *Ann Surg* 2006;243:316–320.

108. Winter JM, Cameron JL, Yeo CJ, et al. Biochemical markers predict morbidity and mortality after pancreaticoduodenectomy. *J Am Coll Surg* 2007;204:1029–1036.

109. Mathur A, Pitt HA, Marine M, et al. Fatty pancreas: a factor in postoperative pancreatic fistula. *Ann Surg* 2007;246:1058–1064.

110. Lillemoe KD, Cameron JL, Kim MP, et al. Does fibrin glue sealant decrease the rate of pancreatic fistula after pancreaticoduodenectomy? Results of a prospective randomized trial. *J Gastrointest Surg* 2004;8:766–772.

111. Martin I, Au K. Does fibrin glue sealant decrease the rate of anastomotic leak after a pancreaticoduodenectomy? Results of a prospective randomized trial. *HPB (Oxford)* 2013;15:561–566.

112. Yeo CJ, Cameron JL, Lillemoe KD, et al. Does prophylactic octreotide decrease the rates of pancreatic fistula and other complications after pancreaticoduodenectomy? Results of a prospective randomized placebo-controlled trial. *Ann Surg* 2000;232:419–429.

113. Beguiristain A, Espi A, Balen E, et al. [Somatostatin prophylaxis following cephalic duodenopancreatectomy]. *Rev Esp Enferm Dig* 1995;87:221–224.

114. Fernandez-Cruz L, Jimenez Chavarria E, Taura P, et al. Prospective randomized trial of the effect of octreotide on pancreatic juice output after pancreaticoduodenectomy in relation to histological diagnosis, duct size and leakage. *HPB (Oxford)* 2013;15:392–399.

115. Gouillat C, Chipponi J, Baulieux J, et al. Randomized controlled multicentre trial of somatostatin infusion after pancreaticoduodenectomy. *Br J Surg* 2001;88:1456–1462.

116. Kollmar O, Moussavian MR, Richter S, et al. Prophylactic octreotide and delayed gastric emptying after pancreaticoduodenectomy: results of a prospective randomized double-blinded placebo-controlled trial. *Eur J Surg Oncol* 2008;34:868–875.

117. Shan YS, Sy ED, Lin PW. Role of somatostatin in the prevention of pancreatic stump-related morbidity following elective pancreaticoduodenectomy in high-risk patients and elimination of surgeon-related factors: prospective, randomized, controlled trial. *World J Surg* 2003;27:709–714.

118. Wang W, Tian B, Babu SR, et al. Randomized, placebo-controlled study of the efficacy of preoperative somatostatin administration in the prevention of postoperative complications following pancreaticoduodenectomy. *Hepatogastroenterology* 2013;60:400–405.

119. Klempa I, Baca I, Menzel J, et al. [Effect of somatostatin on basal and stimulated exocrine pancreatic secretion after partial duodenopancreatectomy. A clinical experimental study]. *Chirurg* 1991;62:293–299.

120. He T, Zhao Y, Chen Q, et al. Pancreaticojejunostomy versus pancreaticogastrostomy after pancreaticoduodenectomy: a systematic review and meta-analysis. *Dig Surg* 2013;30:56–69.

121. Arnaud JP, Tuech JJ, Cervi C, et al. Pancreaticogastrostomy compared with pancreaticojejunostomy after pancreaticoduodenectomy. *Eur J Surg* 1999;165:357–362.

122. Bassi C, Falconi M, Molinari E, et al. Reconstruction by pancreaticojejunostomy versus pancreaticogastrostomy following pancreatectomy: results of a comparative study. *Ann Surg* 2005;242:767–771.

123. Duffas JP, Suc B, Msika S, et al. A controlled randomized multicenter trial of pancreatogastrostomy or pancreatojejunostomy after pancreatoduodenectomy. *Am J Surg* 2005;189:720–729.

124. Fernandez-Cruz L, Cosa R, Blanco L, et al. Pancreatogastrostomy with gastric partition after pylorus-preserving pancreatoduodenectomy versus conventional pancreatojejunostomy: a prospective randomized study. *Ann Surg* 2008;248:930–938.

125. Takano S, Ito Y, Watanabe Y, et al. Pancreaticojejunostomy versus pancreaticogastrostomy in reconstruction following pancreaticoduodenectomy. *Br J Surg* 2000;87:423–427.

126. Yeo CJ, Cameron JL, Maher MM, et al. A prospective randomized trial of pancreaticogastrostomy versus pancreaticojejunostomy after pancreaticoduodenectomy. *Ann Surg* 1995;222:580–588.

127. Berger AC, Howard TJ, Kennedy EP, et al. Does type of pancreaticojejunostomy after pancreaticoduodenectomy decrease rate of pancreatic fistula? A randomized, prospective, dual-institution trial. *J Am Coll Surg* 2009;208:738–747.

128. Peng SY, Wang JW, Lau WY, et al. Conventional versus binding pancreaticojejunostomy after pancreaticoduodenectomy: a prospective randomized trial. *Ann Surg* 2007;245:692–698.

129. Pessaux P, Sauvanet A, Mariette C, et al. External pancreatic duct stent decreases pancreatic fistula rate after pancreaticoduodenectomy: prospective multicenter randomized trial. *Ann Surg* 2011;253:879–885.

130. Poon RT, Fan ST, Lo CM, et al. External drainage of pancreatic duct with a stent to reduce leakage rate of pancreaticojejunostomy after pancreaticoduodenectomy: a prospective randomized trial. *Ann Surg* 2007;246:425–433.

131. Motoi F, Egawa S, Rikiyama T, et al. Randomized clinical trial of external stent drainage of the pancreatic duct to reduce postoperative pancreatic fistula after pancreaticojejunostomy. *Br J Surg* 2012;99:524–531.

132. Imaizumi H, Harada N, Hatori T, et al. Stenting is unnecessary in duct-to-mucosa pancreaticojejunostomy even in the normal pancreas. *Pancreatology* 2002;2:116–121.

133. Ke S, Ding XM, Gao J, et al. A prospective, randomized trial of Roux-en-Y reconstruction with isolated pancreatic drainage versus conventional loop reconstruction after pancreaticoduodenectomy. *Surgery* 2013;153:743–752.

134. Svoronos C, Tsoulfas G, Katsourakis A, et al. Role of extended lymphadenectomy in the treatment of pancreatic head adenocarcinoma: review and meta-analysis. *ANZ J Surg* 2013 [Epub ahead of print].

135. Farnell MB, Pearson RK, Sarr MG, et al. A prospective randomized trial comparing standard pancreatoduodenectomy with pancreatoduodenectomy with extended lymphadenectomy in resectable pancreatic head adenocarcinoma. *Surgery* 2005;138:618–628.

136. Pedrazzoli S, DiCarlo V, Dionigi R, et al. Standard versus extended lymphadenectomy associated with pancreatoduodenectomy in the surgical treatment of adenocarcinoma of the head of the pancreas: a multicenter, prospective, randomized study. Lymphadenectomy Study Group. *Ann Surg* 1998;228:508–517.

137. Riall TS, Cameron JL, Lillemoe KD, et al. Pancreaticoduodenectomy with or without distal gastrectomy and extended retroperitoneal lymphadenectomy for periampullary adenocarcinoma—part 3: update on 5-year survival. *J Gastrointest Surg* 2005;9:1191–1204.

138. Brennan MF, Pisters PW, Posner M, et al. A prospective randomized trial of total parenteral nutrition after major pancreatic resection for malignancy. *Ann Surg* 1994;220:436–441.

139. Conlon KC, Labow D, Leung D, et al. Prospective randomized clinical trial of the value of intraperitoneal drainage after pancreatic resection. *Ann Surg* 2001;234:487–493.

140. Van Buren G, Bloomston M, Hughes SJ, et al. A randomized prospective multicenter trial of pancreaticoduodenectomy with and without routine intraperitoneal drainage. *Ann Surg* 2014;259:605–612.

141. Diener MK, Seiler CM, Rossion I, et al. Efficacy of stapler versus hand-sewn closure after distal pancreatectomy (DISPACT): a randomised, controlled multicentre trial. *Lancet* 2011;377:1514–1522.

142. Carter TI, Fong ZV, Hyslop T, et al. A dual-institution randomized controlled trial of remnant closure after distal pancreatectomy: does the addition of a falciform patch and fibrin glue improve outcomes? *J Gastrointest Surg* 2013;17:102–109.

143. Montorsi M, Zerbi A, Bassi C, et al. Efficacy of an absorbable fibrin sealant patch (TachoSil) after distal pancreatectomy: a multicenter, randomized, controlled trial. *Ann Surg* 2012;256:853–859.

144. Suzuki Y, Fujino Y, Tanioka Y, et al. Randomized clinical trial of ultrasonic dissector or conventional division in distal pancreatectomy for non-fibrotic pancreas. *Br J Surg* 1999;86:608–611.

145. Glazer ES, Hornbrook MC, Krouse RS. A meta-analysis of randomized trials: immediate stent placement vs. surgical bypass in the palliative management of malignant biliary obstruction. *J Pain Symptom Manage* 2014;47:307–314.

146. Lillemoe KD, Cameron JL, Hardacre JM, et al. Is prophylactic gastrojejunostomy indicated for unresectable periampullary cancer? A prospective randomized trial. *Ann Surg* 1999;230:322–328.

147. Van Heek NT, De Castro SM, van Eijck CH, et al. The need for a prophylactic gastrojejunostomy for unresectable periampullary cancer: a prospective randomized multicenter trial with special focus on assessment of quality of life. *Ann Surg* 2003;238:894–902.

148. Lillemoe KD, Cameron JL, Kaufman HS, et al. Chemical splanchnicectomy in patients with unresectable pancreatic cancer. A prospective randomized trial. *Ann Surg* 1993;217:447–455.

149. Katz MH, Merchant NB, Brower S, et al. Standardization of surgical and pathologic variables is needed in multicenter trials of adjuvant therapy for pancreatic cancer: results from the ACOSOG Z5031 trial. *Ann Surg Oncol* 2011;18:337–344.

150. Maithel SK, Maloney S, Winston C, et al. Preoperative CA 19-9 and the yield of staging laparoscopy in patients with radiographically resectable pancreatic adenocarcinoma. *Ann Surg Oncol* 2008;15:3512–3520.

151. Barton JG, Bois JP, Sarr MG, et al. Predictive and prognostic value of CA 19-9 in resected pancreatic adenocarcinoma. *J Gastrointest Surg* 2009;13:2050–2058.

152. Hartwig W, Hackert T, Hinz U, et al. Pancreatic cancer surgery in the new millennium: better prediction of outcome. *Ann Surg* 2011;254:311–319.

153. Marrelli D, Caruso S, Pedrazzani C, et al. CA19-9 serum levels in obstructive jaundice: clinical value in benign and malignant conditions. *Am J Surg* 2009;198:333–339.

154. Berger AC, Garcia M Jr, Hoffman JP, et al. Postresection CA 19-9 predicts overall survival in patients with pancreatic cancer treated with adjuvant chemoradiation: a prospective validation by RTOG 9704. *J Clin Oncol* 2008;26:5918–5922.

155. Narimatsu H, Iwasaki H, Nakayama F, et al. Lewis and secretor gene dosages affect CA19-9 and DU-PAN-2 serum levels in normal individuals and colorectal cancer patients. *Cancer Res* 1998;58:512–518.

156. Tempero MA, Uchida E, Takasaki H, et al. Relationship of carbohydrate antigen 19-9 and Lewis antigens in pancreatic cancer. *Cancer Res* 1987;47:5501–5503.

157. National Comprehensive Cancer Network. NCCN Guidelines. Pancreatic Adenocarcinoma. http://www.nccn.org/professionals/physician_gls/PDF/pancreatic.pdf.

158. Boeck S, Ankerst DP, Heinemann V. The role of adjuvant chemotherapy for patients with resected pancreatic cancer: systematic review of randomized controlled trials and meta-analysis. *Oncology* 2007;72:314–321.

159. Oettle H, Post S, Neuhaus P, et al. Adjuvant chemotherapy with gemcitabine vs observation in patients undergoing curative-intent resection of pancreatic cancer: a randomized controlled trial. *JAMA* 2007;297:267–277.

160. Winter JM, Tang LH, Klimstra DS, et al. Failure patterns in resected pancreas adenocarcinoma: lack of predicted benefit to smad4 expression. *Ann Surg* 2013;258:331–335.

161. Crane CH, Varadhachary GR, Yordy JS, et al. Phase II trial of cetuximab, gemcitabine, and oxaliplatin followed by chemoradiation with cetuximab for locally advanced (T4) pancreatic adenocarcinoma: correlation of Smad4(Dpc4) immunostaining with pattern of disease progression. *J Clin Oncol* 2011;29:3037–3043.

162. Winter JM, Tang LH, Klimstra DS, et al. A novel survival-based tissue microarray of pancreatic cancer validates MUC1 and mesothelin as biomarkers. *PLoS One* 2012;7:e40157.

163. Smeenk HG, van Eijck CH, Hop WC, et al. Long-term survival and metastatic pattern of pancreatic and periampullary cancer after adjuvant chemoradiation or observation: long-term results of EORTC trial 40891. *Ann Surg* 2007;246:734–740.

164. Oettle H, Neuhaus P, Hochhaus A, et al. Adjuvant chemotherapy with gemcitabine and long-term outcomes among patients with resected pancreatic cancer: the CONKO-001 randomized trial. *JAMA* 2013;310:1473–1481.

165. Neoptolemos JP, Stocken DD, Friess H, et al. A randomized trial of chemoradiotherapy and chemotherapy after resection of pancreatic cancer. *N Engl J Med* 2004;350:1200–1210.

CANCERS OF THE GASTROINTESTINAL TRACT

166. Neoptolemos JP, Stocken DD, Bassi C, et al. Adjuvant chemotherapy with fluorouracil plus folinic acid vs gemcitabine following pancreatic cancer resection: a randomized controlled trial. *JAMA* 2010;304:1073–1081.

167. Kosuge T, Kiuchi T, Mukai K, et al. A multicenter randomized controlled trial to evaluate the effect of adjuvant cisplatin and 5-fluorouracil therapy after curative resection in cases of pancreatic cancer. *Jpn J Clin Oncol* 2006;36:159–165.

168. Kalser MH, Ellenberg SS. Pancreatic cancer. Adjuvant combined radiation and chemotherapy following curative resection. *Arch Surg* 1985;120:899–903.

169. Bakkevold KE, Arnesjo B, Dahl O, et al. Adjuvant combination chemotherapy (AMF) following radical resection of carcinoma of the pancreas and papilla of Vater—results of a controlled, prospective, randomised multicentre study. *Eur J Cancer* 1993;29A:698–703.

170. Regine WF, Winter KA, Abrams R, et al. Fluorouracil-based chemoradiation with either gemcitabine or fluorouracil chemotherapy after resection of pancreatic adenocarcinoma: 5-year analysis of the U.S. Intergroup/RTOG 9704 phase III trial. *Ann Surg Oncol* 2011;18:1319–1326.

171. Burris HA 3rd, Moore MJ, Andersen J, et al. Improvements in survival and clinical benefit with gemcitabine as first-line therapy for patients with advanced pancreas cancer: a randomized trial. *J Clin Oncol* 1997;15:2403–2413.

172. Regine WF, Winter KA, Abrams RA, et al. Fluorouracil vs gemcitabine chemotherapy before and after fluorouracil-based chemoradiation following resection of pancreatic adenocarcinoma: a randomized controlled trial. *JAMA* 2008;299:1019–1026.

173. Abrams RA, Winter KA, Regine WF, et al. Failure to adhere to protocol specified radiation therapy guidelines was associated with decreased survival in RTOG 9704—a phase III trial of adjuvant chemotherapy and chemoradiotherapy for patients with resected adenocarcinoma of the pancreas. *Int J Radiat Oncol Biol Phys* 2012;82:809–816.

174. Herrmann R, Bodoky G, Ruhstaller B, et al. Gemcitabine (G) plus capecitabine (C) versus G alone in locally advanced or metastatic pancreatic cancer. A randomized phase III study of the Swiss Group for Clinical Cancer Research (SAKK) and the Central European Cooperative Oncology Group (CECOG). *J Clin Oncol* 2005;23: LBA4010.

175. Moore MJ, Goldstein D, Hamm J, et al. Erlotinib plus gemcitabine compared with gemcitabine alone in patients with advanced pancreatic cancer: a phase III trial of the National Cancer Institute of Canada Clinical Trials Group. *J Clin Oncol* 2007;25:1960–1966.

176. O'Reilly EM. Evolving panorama of treatment for metastatic pancreas adenocarcinoma. *J Clin Oncol* 2013;31:1621–1623.

177. Conroy T, Desseigne F, Ychou M, et al. FOLFIRINOX versus gemcitabine for metastatic pancreatic cancer. *N Engl J Med* 2011;364:1817–1825.

178. Von Hoff DD, Ervin T, Arena FP, et al. Increased survival in pancreatic cancer with nab-paclitaxel plus gemcitabine. *N Engl J Med* 2013;369:1691–1703.

179. O'Reilly EM, Lowery MA. Postresection surveillance for pancreatic cancer performance status, imaging, and serum markers. *Cancer* 2012;18:609–613.

180. Sheffield KM, Crowell KT, Lin YL, et al. Surveillance of pancreatic cancer patients after surgical resection. *Ann Surg Oncol* 2012;19:1670–1677.

181. Locker GY, Hamilton S, Harris J, et al. ASCO 2006 update of recommendations for the use of tumor markers in gastrointestinal cancer. *J Clin Oncol* 2006;24:5313–5327.

182. Arnaoutakis GJ, Rangachari D, Laheru DA, et al. Pulmonary resection for isolated pancreatic adenocarcinoma metastasis: an analysis of outcomes and survival. *J Gastrointest Surg* 2011;15:1611–1617.

183. Fitzgerald TL, Seymore NM, Kachare SD, et al. Measuring the impact of multidisciplinary care on quality for pancreatic surgery: transition to a focused, very high-volume program. *Am Surg* 2013;79:775–780.

184. Cai S, Hong TS, Goldberg SI, et al. Updated long-term outcomes and prognostic factors for patients with unresectable locally advanced pancreatic cancer treated with intraoperative radiotherapy at the Massachusetts General Hospital, 1978 to 2010. *Cancer* 2013;119:4196–4204.

185. Ikeda M, Okada S, Tokuuye K, et al. Prognostic factors in patients with locally advanced pancreatic carcinoma receiving chemoradiotherapy. *Cancer* 2001;91:490–495.

186. Krishnan S, Rana V, Janjan NA, et al. Prognostic factors in patients with unresectable locally advanced pancreatic adenocarcinoma treated with chemoradiation. *Cancer* 2006;107:2589–2896.

187. Rudra S, Narang AK, Pawlik TM, et al. Evaluation of predictive variables in locally advanced pancreatic adenocarcinoma patients receiving definitive chemoradiation. *Pract Radiat Oncol* 2012;2:77–85.

188. Dickler A, Abrams RA. Radiochemotherapy in the management of pancreatic cancer—part II: use in adjuvant and locally unresectable settings. *Semin Radiat Oncol* 2005;15:235–244.

189. Oshima M, Okano K, Muraki S, et al. Immunohistochemically detected expression of 3 major genes (CDKN2A/p16, TP53, and SMAD4/DPC4) strongly predicts survival in patients with resectable pancreatic cancer. *Ann Surg* 2013;258:336–346.

190. Treatment of locally unresectable carcinoma of the pancreas: comparison of combined-modality therapy (chemotherapy plus radiotherapy) to chemotherapy alone. Gastrointestinal Tumor Study Group. *J Natl Cancer Inst* 1988;80:751–755.

191. Chauffert B, Mornex F, Bonnetain F, et al. Phase III trial comparing intensive induction chemoradiotherapy (60 Gy, infusional 5-FU and intermittent cisplatin) followed by maintenance gemcitabine with gemcitabine alone for locally advanced unresectable pancreatic cancer. Definitive results of the 2000-01 FFCD/SFRO study. *Ann Oncol* 2008;19:1592–1599.

192. Klaassen DJ, MacIntyre JM, Catton GE, et al. Treatment of locally unresectable cancer of the stomach and pancreas: a randomized comparison of 5-fluorouracil alone with radiation plus concurrent and maintenance 5-fluorouracil—an Eastern Cooperative Oncology Group study. *J Clin Oncol* 1985;3:373–378.

193. Loehrer PJ, Sr., Feng Y, Cardenes H, et al. Gemcitabine alone versus gemcitabine plus radiotherapy in patients with locally advanced pancreatic cancer: an Eastern Cooperative Oncology Group trial. *J Clin Oncol* 2011;29:4105–4112.

194. Hammel P, Florence H, Van Lathem J, et al. Comparison of chemoradiotherapy (CRT) and chemotherapy (CT) in patients with a locally advanced pancreatic cancer (LAPC) controlled after 4 months of gemcitabine with or without erlotinib: Final results of the international phase III LAP 07 study. *J Clin Oncol* 2013;31:suppl; abstr LBA4003.

195. Brunner TB, Tinkl D, Grabenbauer GG, et al. Maintenance chemotherapy after chemoradiation improves survival of patients with locally advanced pancreatic carcinoma: a retrospective analysis of prospectively recruited patients. *Strahlenther Onkol* 2006;182:210–215.

196. Crane CH, Wolff RA, Abbruzzese JL, et al. Combining gemcitabine with radiation in pancreatic cancer: understanding important variables influencing the therapeutic index. *Semin Oncol* 2001;28:25–33.

197. Ben-Josef E, Schipper M, Francis IR, et al. A phase I/II trial of intensity modulated radiation (IMRT) dose escalation with concurrent fixed-dose rate gemcitabine (FDR-G) in patients with unresectable pancreatic cancer. *Int J Radiat Oncol Biol Phys* 2012;84:1166–1171.

198. Murphy JD, Adusumilli S, Griffith KA, et al. Full-dose gemcitabine and concurrent radiotherapy for unresectable pancreatic cancer. *Int J Radiat Oncol Biol Phys* 2007;68:801–808.

199. Small W Jr, Berlin J, Freedman GM, et al. Full-dose gemcitabine with concurrent radiation therapy in patients with nonmetastatic pancreatic cancer: a multicenter phase II trial. *J Clin Oncol* 2008;26:942–947.

200. Wolff RA, Evans DB, Gravel DM, et al. Phase I trial of gemcitabine combined with radiation for the treatment of locally advanced pancreatic adenocarcinoma. *Clin Cancer Res* 2001;7:2246–2253.

201. Kim HJ, Czischke K, Brennan MF, et al. Does neoadjuvant chemoradiation downstage locally advanced pancreatic cancer? *J Gastrointest Surg* 2002;6:763–769.

202. Crane CH, Abbruzzese JL, Evans DB, et al. Is the therapeutic index better with gemcitabine-based chemoradiation than with 5-fluorouracil-based chemoradiation in locally advanced pancreatic cancer? *Int J Radiat Oncol Biol Phys* 2002;52:1293–1302.

203. Zhu CP, Shi J, Chen YX, et al. Gemcitabine in the chemoradiotherapy for locally advanced pancreatic cancer: a meta-analysis. *Radiother Oncol* 2011;99:108–113.

204. Van Cutsem E, Hoff PM, Harper P, et al. Oral capecitabine vs intravenous 5-fluorouracil and leucovorin: integrated efficacy data and novel analyses from two large, randomised, phase III trials. *Br J Cancer* 2004;90:1190–1197.

205. Kim YJ, Lee WJ, Woo SM, et al. Comparison of capecitabine and 5-fluorouracil in chemoradiotherapy for locally advanced pancreatic cancer. *Radiat Oncol* 2013;8:160.

206. Jackson AS, Jain P, Watkins GR, et al. Efficacy and tolerability of limited field radiotherapy with concurrent capecitabine in locally advanced pancreatic cancer. *Clin Oncol (R Coll Radiol)* 2010;22:570–577.

207. Mukherjee S, Hurt CN, Bridgewater J, et al. Gemcitabine-based or capecitabine-based chemoradiotherapy for locally advanced pancreatic cancer (SCALOP): a multicentre, randomised, phase 2 trial. *Lancet Oncol* 2013;14:317–326.

208. Huguet F, Andre T, Hammel P, et al. Impact of chemoradiotherapy after disease control with chemotherapy in locally advanced pancreatic adenocarcinoma in GERCOR phase II and III studies. *J Clin Oncol* 2007;25:326–331.

209. Krishnan S, Rana V, Janjan NA, et al. Induction chemotherapy selects patients with locally advanced, unresectable pancreatic cancer for optimal benefit from consolidative chemoradiation therapy. *Cancer* 2007;110:47–55.

210. Conroy T, Paillot B, Francois E, et al. Irinotecan plus oxaliplatin and leucovorin-modulated fluorouracil in advanced pancreatic cancer—a Groupe Tumeurs Digestives of the Federation Nationale des Centres de Lutte Contre le Cancer study. *J Clin Oncol* 2005;23:1228–1236.

211. Festa V, Andriulli A, Valvano MR, et al. Neoadjuvant chemo-radiotherapy for patients with borderline resectable pancreatic cancer: a meta-analytical evaluation of prospective studies. *JOP* 2013;14:618–625.

212. Katz MH, Pisters PW, Evans DB, et al. Borderline resectable pancreatic cancer: the importance of this emerging stage of disease. *J Am Coll Surg* 2008;206:833–846.

213. Seo Y, Kim MS, Yoo S, et al. Stereotactic body radiation therapy boost in locally advanced pancreatic cancer. *Int J Radiat Oncol Biol Phys* 2009;75:1456–1461.

214. Rwigema JC, Parikh SD, Heron DE, et al. Stereotactic body radiotherapy in the treatment of advanced adenocarcinoma of the pancreas. *Am J Clin Oncol* 2011;34:63–69.

215. Mahadevan A, Jain S, Goldstein M, et al. Stereotactic body radiotherapy and gemcitabine for locally advanced pancreatic cancer. *Int J Radiat Oncol Biol Phys* 2010;78:735–742.

216. Hansen R, Quebbeman E, Ritch P, et al. Continuous 5-fluorouracil (5FU) infusion in carcinoma of the pancreas: a phase II study. *Am J Med Sci* 1988;295:91–93.

217. Sebastiani V, Ricci F, Rubio-Viqueira B, et al. Immunohistochemical and genetic evaluation of deoxycytidine kinase in pancreatic cancer: relationship to molecular mechanisms of gemcitabine resistance and survival. *Clin Cancer Res* 2006;12:2492–2497.

218. Mini E, Nobili S, Caciagli B, et al. Cellular pharmacology of gemcitabine. *Ann Oncol* 2006;17 Suppl 5:v7–v12.

219. Tempero M, Plunkett W, Ruiz Van Haperen V, et al. Randomized phase II comparison of dose-intense gemcitabine: thirty-minute infusion and fixed dose rate infusion in patients with pancreatic adenocarcinoma. *J Clin Oncol* 2003;21:3402–3408.

220. Poplin E, Feng Y, Berlin J, et al. Phase III, randomized study of gemcitabine and oxaliplatin versus gemcitabine (fixed-dose rate infusion) compared with gemcitabine (30-minute infusion) in patients with pancreatic carcinoma E6201: a trial of the Eastern Cooperative Oncology Group. *J Clin Oncol* 2009;27:3778–3785.

221. Abou-Alfa GK, Letourneau R, Harker G, et al. Randomized phase III study of exatecan and gemcitabine compared with gemcitabine alone in untreated advanced pancreatic cancer. *J Clin Oncol* 2006;24:4441–4447.

222. Berlin JD, Catalano P, Thomas JP, et al. Phase III study of gemcitabine in combination with fluorouracil versus gemcitabine alone in patients with advanced pancreatic carcinoma: Eastern Cooperative Oncology Group Trial E2297. *J Clin Oncol* 2002;20:3270–3275.

223. Colucci G, Giuliani F, Gebbia V, et al. Gemcitabine alone or with cisplatin for the treatment of patients with locally advanced and/or metastatic pancreatic carcinoma: a prospective, randomized phase III study of the Gruppo Oncologia dell'Italia Meridionale. *Cancer* 2002;94:902–910.

224. Cunningham D, Chau I, Stocken DD, et al. Phase III randomized comparison of gemcitabine versus gemcitabine plus capecitabine in patients with advanced pancreatic cancer. *J Clin Oncol* 2009;27:5513–5518.

225. Heinemann V, Quietzsch D, Gieseler F, et al. Randomized phase III trial of gemcitabine plus cisplatin compared with gemcitabine alone in advanced pancreatic cancer. *J Clin Oncol* 2006;24:3946–3952.

226. Louvet C, Labianca R, Hammel P, et al. Gemcitabine in combination with oxaliplatin compared with gemcitabine alone in locally advanced or metastatic pancreatic cancer: results of a GERCOR and GISCAD phase III trial. *J Clin Oncol* 2005;23:3509–3516.

227. Rocha Lima CM, Green MR, Rotche R, et al. Irinotecan plus gemcitabine results in no survival advantage compared with gemcitabine monotherapy in patients with locally advanced or metastatic pancreatic cancer despite increased tumor response rate. *J Clin Oncol* 2004;22:3776–3783.

228. Stathopoulos GP, Syrigos K, Aravantinos G, et al. A multicenter phase III trial comparing irinotecan-gemcitabine (IG) with gemcitabine (G) monotherapy as first-line treatment in patients with locally advanced or metastatic pancreatic cancer. *Br J Cancer* 2006;95:587–592.

229. Bramhall SR, Schulz J, Nemunaitis J, et al. A double-blind placebo-controlled, randomised study comparing gemcitabine and marimastat with gemcitabine and placebo as first line therapy in patients with advanced pancreatic cancer. *Br J Cancer* 2002;87:161–167.

230. Kindler HL, Ioka T, Richel DJ, et al. Axitinib plus gemcitabine versus placebo plus gemcitabine in patients with advanced pancreatic cancer: a double-blind randomised phase 3 study. *Lancet Oncol* 2011;12:256–262.

231. Kindler HL, Niedzwiecki D, Hollis D, et al. Gemcitabine plus bevacizumab compared with gemcitabine plus placebo in patients with advanced pancreatic cancer: phase III trial of the Cancer and Leukemia Group B (CALGB 80303). *J Clin Oncol* 2010;28:3617–3622.

232. Philip PA, Benedetti J, Corless CL, et al. Phase III study comparing gemcitabine plus cetuximab versus gemcitabine in patients with advanced pancreatic adenocarcinoma: Southwest Oncology Group-directed intergroup trial S0205. *J Clin Oncol* 2010;28:3605–3610.

233. Van Cutsem E, van de Velde H, Karasek P, et al. Phase III trial of gemcitabine plus tipifarnib compared with gemcitabine plus placebo in advanced pancreatic cancer. *J Clin Oncol* 2004;22:1430–1438.

234. da Cunha Santos G, Dhani N, Tu D, et al. Molecular predictors of outcome in a phase 3 study of gemcitabine and erlotinib therapy in patients with advanced pancreatic cancer: National Cancer Institute of Canada Clinical Trials Group Study PA.3. *Cancer* 2010;116:5599–5607.

235. Xiong HQ, Rosenberg A, LoBuglio A, et al. Cetuximab, a monoclonal antibody targeting the epidermal growth factor receptor, in combination with gemcitabine for advanced pancreatic cancer: a multicenter phase II Trial. *J Clin Oncol* 2004;22:2610–2616.

236. Ciliberto D, Botta C, Correale P, et al. Role of gemcitabine-based combination therapy in the management of advanced pancreatic cancer: a meta-analysis of randomised trials. *Eur J Cancer* 2013;49:593–603.

237. Sun C, Ansari D, Andersson R, et al. Does gemcitabine-based combination therapy improve the prognosis of unresectable pancreatic cancer? *World J Gastroenterol* 2012;18:4944–4958.

238. Tam VC, Ko YJ, Mittmann N, et al. Cost-effectiveness of systemic therapies for metastatic pancreatic cancer. *Curr Oncol* 2013;20:e90–e106.

239. Karapetis CS, Khambata-Ford S, Jonker DJ, et al. K-ras mutations and benefit from cetuximab in advanced colorectal cancer. *N Engl J Med* 2008;359:1757–1765.

240. Van Cutsem E, Vervenne WL, Bennouna J, et al. Phase III trial of bevacizumab in combination with gemcitabine and erlotinib in patients with metastatic pancreatic cancer. *J Clin Oncol* 2009;27:2231–2237.

241. Yardley DA. nab-Paclitaxel mechanisms of action and delivery. *J Control Release* 2013;170:365–372.

242. Miele E, Spinelli GP, Tomao F, et al. Albumin-bound formulation of paclitaxel (Abraxane ABI-007) in the treatment of breast cancer. *Int J Nanomedicine* 2009;4:99–105.

243. Neesse A, Frese KK, Chan DS, et al. SPARC independent drug delivery and antitumour effects of nab-paclitaxel in genetically engineered mice. *Gut* 2014;63:974–983.

244. Von Hoff DD, Ramanathan RK, Borad MJ, et al. Gemcitabine plus nab-paclitaxel is an active regimen in patients with advanced pancreatic cancer: a phase I/II trial. *J Clin Oncol* 2011;29:4548–4554.

245. Ychou M, Conroy T, Seitz JF, et al. An open phase I study assessing the feasibility of the triple combination: oxaliplatin plus irinotecan plus leucovorin/5-fluorouracil every 2 weeks in patients with advanced solid tumors. *Ann Oncol* 2003;14:481–489.

246. Ychou M, Desseigne F, Guimbaud R, et al. Randomized phase II trial comparing folfirinox (5FU/leucovorin [LV], irinotecan [I] and oxaliplatin [O]) vs gemcitabine (G) as first-line treatment for metastatic pancreatic adenocarcinoma (MPA). First results of the ACCORD 11 trial. *J Clin Oncol* 2007;25:4516.

247. Gourgou-Bourgade S, Bascoul-Mollevi C, Desseigne F, et al. Impact of FOLFIRINOX compared with gemcitabine on quality of life in patients with metastatic pancreatic cancer: results from the PRODIGE 4/ACCORD 11 randomized trial. *J Clin Oncol* 2013;31:23–29.

248. Ueno H, Ioka T, Ikeda M, et al. Randomized phase III study of gemcitabine plus S-1, S-1 alone, or gemcitabine alone in patients with locally advanced and metastatic pancreatic cancer in Japan and Taiwan: GEST study. *J Clin Oncol* 2013;31:1640–1648.

249. Hammad N, Heilbrun LK, Philip PA, et al. CA19-9 as a predictor of tumor response and survival in patients with advanced pancreatic cancer treated with gemcitabine based chemotherapy. *Asia Pac J Clin Oncol* 2010;6:98–105.

250. Heinemann V, Schermuly MM, Stieber P, et al. CA19-9: a predictor of response in pancreatic cancer treated with gemcitabine and cisplatin. *Anticancer Res* 1999;19:2433–2435.

251. Maisey NR, Norman AR, Hill A, et al. CA19-9 as a prognostic factor in inoperable pancreatic cancer: the implication for clinical trials. *Br J Cancer* 2005;93:740–743.

252. Wong D, Ko AH, Hwang J, et al. Serum CA19-9 decline compared to radiographic response as a surrogate for clinical outcomes in patients with metastatic pancreatic cancer receiving chemotherapy. *Pancreas* 2008;37:269–274.

253. Ziske C, Schlie C, Gorschluter M, et al. Prognostic value of CA 19-9 levels in patients with inoperable adenocarcinoma of the pancreas treated with gemcitabine. *Br J Cancer* 2003;89:1413–1417.

254. Rhim AD, Mirek ET, Aiello NM, et al. EMT and dissemination precede pancreatic tumor formation. *Cell* 2012;148:349–361.

255. Yachida S, Jones S, Bozic I, et al. Distant metastasis occurs late during the genetic evolution of pancreatic cancer. *Nature* 2010;467:1114–1117.

256. Andea A, Sarkar F, Adsay VN. Clinicopathological correlates of pancreatic intraepithelial neoplasia: a comparative analysis of 82 cases with and 152 cases without pancreatic ductal adenocarcinoma. *Mod Pathol* 2003;16:996–1006.

257. Diehl F, Li M, Dressman D, et al. Detection and quantification of mutations in the plasma of patients with colorectal tumors. *Proc Natl Acad Sci U S A* 2005;102:16368–16373.

258. Stratford JK, Bentrem DJ, Anderson JM, et al. A six-gene signature predicts survival of patients with localized pancreatic ductal adenocarcinoma. *PLoS Med* 2010;7:e1000307.

259. Farrell JJ, Elsaleh H, Garcia M, et al. Human equilibrative nucleoside transporter 1 levels predict response to gemcitabine in patients with pancreatic cancer. *Gastroenterology* 2009;136:187–195.

260. Poplin E, Wasan H, Rolfe L, et al. Randomized, multicenter, phase ii study of co-101 versus gemcitabine in patients with metastatic pancreatic ductal adenocarcinoma: including a prospective evaluation of the role of hent1 in gemcitabine or co-101 sensitivity. *J Clin Oncol* 2013;31:4453–4461.

261. Costantino CL, Witkiewicz AK, Kuwano Y, et al. The role of HuR in gemcitabine efficacy in pancreatic cancer: HuR Up-regulates the expression of the gemcitabine metabolizing enzyme deoxycytidine kinase. *Cancer Res* 2009;69:4567–4572.

262. Richards NG, Rittenhouse DW, Freydin B, et al. HuR status is a powerful marker for prognosis and response to gemcitabine-based chemotherapy for resected pancreatic ductal adenocarcinoma patients. *Ann Surg* 2010;252:499–505.

263. Sutherland RM. Cell and environment interactions in tumor microregions: the multicell spheroid model. *Science* 1988;240:177–184.

264. Chaika NV, Yu F, Purohit V, et al. Differential expression of metabolic genes in tumor and stromal components of primary and metastatic loci in pancreatic adenocarcinoma. *PLoS One* 2012;7:e32996.

265. Faratian D, Christiansen J, Gustavson M, et al. Heterogeneity mapping of protein expression in tumors using quantitative immunofluorescence. *J Vis Exp* 2011:e3334.

266. Showalter SL, Huang YH, Witkiewicz A, et al. Nanoparticulate delivery of diphtheria toxin DNA effectively kills Mesothelin expressing pancreatic cancer cells. *Cancer Biol Ther* 2008;7:1584–1590.

267. Erkan M, Hausmann S, Michalski CW, et al. The role of stroma in pancreatic cancer: diagnostic and therapeutic implications. *Nat Rev Gastroenterol Hepatol* 2012;9:454–467.

268. Olive KP, Jacobetz MA, Davidson CJ, et al. Inhibition of Hedgehog signaling enhances delivery of chemotherapy in a mouse model of pancreatic cancer. *Science* 2009;324:1457–1461.

269. Provenzano PP, Cuevas C, Chang AE, et al. Enzymatic targeting of the stroma ablates physical barriers to treatment of pancreatic ductal adenocarcinoma. *Cancer Cell* 2012;21:418–429.

270. Vander Heiden MG, Cantley LC, Thompson CB. Understanding the Warburg effect: the metabolic requirements of cell proliferation. *Science* 2009;324:1029–1033.

CANCERS OF THE GASTROINTESTINAL TRACT

271. Ying H, Kimmelman AC, Lyssiotis CA, et al. Oncogenic Kras maintains pancreatic tumors through regulation of anabolic glucose metabolism. *Cell* 2012;149:656–670.

272. Son J, Lyssiotis CA, Ying H, et al. Glutamine supports pancreatic cancer growth through a KRAS-regulated metabolic pathway. *Nature* 2013;496:101–105.

273. Commisso C, Davidson SM, Soydaner-Azeloglu RG, et al. Macropinocytosis of protein is an amino acid supply route in Ras-transformed cells. *Nature* 2013;497:633–637.

274. Burkhart RA, Pineda DM, Chand SN, et al. HuR is a post-transcriptional regulator of core metabolic enzymes in pancreatic cancer. *RNA Biol* 2013;10:1312–1323.

275. Couzin-Frankel J. Breakthrough of the year 2013. Cancer immunotherapy. *Science* 2013;342:1432–1433.

276. Robert C, Thomas L, Bondarenko I, et al. Ipilimumab plus dacarbazine for previously untreated metastatic melanoma. *N Engl J Med* 2011;364:2517–2526.

277. Topalian SL, Hodi FS, Brahmer JR, et al. Safety, activity, and immune correlates of anti-PD-1 antibody in cancer. *N Engl J Med* 2012;366:2443–2454.

278. Hinrichs CS, Rosenberg SA. Exploiting the curative potential of adoptive T-cell therapy for cancer. *Immunol Rev* 2014;257:56–71.

279. Beatty GL, Torigian DA, Chiorean EG, et al. A phase I study of an agonist CD40 monoclonal antibody (CP-870,893) in combination with gemcitabine in patients with advanced pancreatic ductal adenocarcinoma. *Clin Cancer Res* 2013;19:6286–6295.

280. Hardacre JM, Mulcahy M, Small W, et al. Addition of algenpantucel-L immunotherapy to standard adjuvant therapy for pancreatic cancer: a phase 2 study. *J Gastrointest Surg* 2012;17:94–100.

281. Fischer M, Matsuo K, Gonen M, et al. Relationship between intraoperative fluid administration and perioperative outcome after pancreaticoduodenectomy: results of a prospective randomized trial of acute normovolemic hemodilution compared with standard intraoperative management. *Ann Surg* 2010;252:952–958.

282. Uemura K, Murakami Y, Hayashidani Y, et al. Randomized clinical trial to assess the efficacy of ulinastatin for postoperative pancreatitis following pancreaticoduodenectomy. *J Surg Oncol* 2008;98:309–313.

283. Jo S, Choi SH, Heo JS, et al. Missing effect of glutamine supplementation on the surgical outcome after pancreaticoduodenectomy for periampullary tumors: a prospective, randomized, double-blind, controlled clinical trial. *World J Surg* 2006;30:1974–1982.

284. Bassi C, Molinari E, Malleo G, et al. Early versus late drain removal after standard pancreatic resections: results of a prospective randomized trial. *Ann Surg* 2010;252:207–214.

285. Kuroki T, Tajima Y, Kitasato A, et al. Stenting versus non-stenting in pancreaticojejunostomy: a prospective study limited to a normal pancreas without fibrosis sorted by using dynamic MRI. *Pancreas* 2011;40:25–29.

286. Kamoda Y, Fujino Y, Matsumoto I, et al. Usefulness of performing a pancreaticojejunostomy with an internal stent after a pancreatoduodenectomy. *Surg Today* 2008;38:524–528.

287. Tani M, Onishi H, Kinoshita H, et al. The evaluation of duct-to-mucosal pancreaticojejunostomy in pancreaticoduodenectomy. *World J Surg* 2005;29:76–79.

288. Reissman P, Perry Y, Cuenca A, et al. Pancreaticojejunostomy versus controlled pancreaticocutaneous fistula in pancreaticoduodenectomy for periampullary carcinoma. *Am J Surg* 1995;169:585–588.

289. Tran K, Van Eijck C, Di Carlo V, et al. Occlusion of the pancreatic duct versus pancreaticojejunostomy: a prospective randomized trial. *Ann Surg* 2002;236:422–428.

290. Bassi C, Falconi M, Molinari E, et al. Duct-to-mucosa versus end-to-side pancreaticojejunostomy reconstruction after pancreaticoduodenectomy: results of a prospective randomized trial. *Surgery* 2003;134:766–771.

291. Yeo CJ, Barry MK, Sauter PK, et al. Erythromycin accelerates gastric emptying after pancreaticoduodenectomy. A prospective, randomized, placebo-controlled trial. *Ann Surg* 1993;218:229–237.

292. McCracken JD, Ray P, Heilbrun LK, et al. 5-Fluorouracil, methyl-CCNU, and radiotherapy with or without testolactone for localized adenocarcinoma of the exocrine pancreas: a Southwest Oncology Group Study. *Cancer* 1980;46:1518–1522.

293. Moertel CG, Frytak S, Hahn RG, et al. Therapy of locally unresectable pancreatic carcinoma: a randomized comparison of high dose (6000 rads) radiation alone, moderate dose radiation (4000 rads + 5-fluorouracil), and high dose radiation + 5-fluorouracil: The Gastrointestinal Tumor Study Group. *Cancer* 1981;48:1705–1710.

294. Radiation therapy combined with Adriamycin or 5-fluorouracil for the treatment of locally unresectable pancreatic carcinoma. Gastrointestinal Tumor Study Group. *Cancer* 1985;56:2563–2568.

295. Earle JD, Foley JF, Wieand HS, et al. Evaluation of external-beam radiation therapy plus 5-fluorouracil (5-FU) versus external-beam radiation therapy plus hycanthone (HYC) in confined, unresectable pancreatic cancer. *Int J Radiat Oncol Biol Phys* 1994;28:207–211.

296. Cohen SJ, Dobelbower R, Jr., Lipsitz S, et al. A randomized phase III study of radiotherapy alone or with 5-fluorouracil and mitomycin-C in patients with locally advanced adenocarcinoma of the pancreas: Eastern Cooperative Oncology Group study E8282. *Int J Radiat Oncol Biol Phys* 2005;62:1345–1350.

297. Richards DA, Kindler HL, Oettle H, et al. A randomized phase III study comparing gemcitabine + pemetrexed versus gemcitabine in patients with locally advanced and metastatic pancreas cancer. *J Clin Oncol* 2004;22:4007.

42 Genetic Testing in Pancreatic Cancer

Jennifer E. Axilbund and Elizabeth L. Wiley

CANCERS OF THE GASTROINTESTINAL TRACT

INTRODUCTION

It is estimated that 5% to 10% of pancreatic cancer (adenocarcinoma) is familial,[1,2] and individuals with a family history of pancreatic cancer are at a greater risk of developing pancreatic cancer themselves.[3] Although there is evidence of a major pancreatic cancer susceptibility gene,[4] it remains elusive. Therefore, the majority of families with multiple cases of pancreatic cancer do not have an identifiable causative gene or syndrome, making risk assessment and counseling challenging. However, a subset of pancreatic cancer is attributable to known inherited cancer predisposition syndromes (Table 42.1).

SELECTED GENES THAT MAY CAUSE PANCREATIC CANCER

BRCA2

The *BRCA2* gene is associated with hereditary breast and ovarian cancer syndrome, and often presents as premenopausal breast cancer, ovarian cancer, and/or male breast cancer. The Breast Cancer Linkage Consortium[5] reported a 3.5-fold (95% confidence interval [CI], 1.9 to 6.6) increased risk of pancreatic cancer in *BRCA2* gene mutation carriers. Subsequent studies in the United Kingdom and the Netherlands showed a relative risk of 4.1 and 5.9, respectively.[6,7] In a United States–based study, 10.9% (17 out of 156) of families with a *BRCA2* mutation reported a family history of pancreatic cancer. The median ages at diagnosis for males and females were 67 and 59 years, respectively, which differed statistically from the Surveillance, Epidemiology and End Results (SEER) database (70 years old for males and 74 years old for females; $p = 0.011$).[8] Although genotype–phenotype data remain sparse, the *BRCA2* K3326X variant was found in 5.6% (8 out of 144) of familial pancreatic cancer patients compared with 1.2% (3 out of 250) of those with sporadic pancreatic cancer (odds ratio [OR], 4.84; 95% CI, 1.27 to 18.55; $p <0.01$).[9]

Approximately 17% of pancreatic cancer patients who have at least two additional relatives with pancreatic cancer carry deleterious mutations in the *BRCA2* gene.[10] Estimates for the prevalence of *BRCA2* mutations with two first-degree relatives with pancreatic cancer are 6% to 12%,[11,12] and *BRCA2* mutations also explain a portion of apparently sporadic pancreatic cancers.[13] However, prevalence varies between populations. Out of 145 Ashkenazi Jews with pancreatic cancer, 6 (4.1%) were found to have a deleterious *BRCA2* mutation when compared with cancer-free controls (OR, 3.85; 95% CI, 2.1 to 10.8; $p = 0.007$), although no differences were noted in age at diagnosis or clinical pathologic features.[14] An earlier, smaller study found a deleterious *BRCA2* mutation in 3 (13%) of 23 Ashkenazi Jews with pancreatic cancer, unselected for family history.[15] Among Ashkenazi Jewish probands with breast cancer who reported a family history of pancreatic cancer, 7.6% (16 out of 211) had a *BRCA2* mutation.[16] By comparison, no *BRCA2* mutations were found in studies of pancreatic cancer in Korea or Italy.[17,18]

BRCA1

Similar to *BRCA2*, mutations in *BRCA1* are associated with a markedly increased risk for premenopausal breast cancer and ovarian cancer. The Breast Cancer Linkage Consortium reported a 2.26-fold (95% CI, 1.26 to 4.06) increased risk of pancreatic cancer in families with a *BRCA1* mutation,[19] and Brose et al.[20] estimated a threefold higher lifetime risk. However, more recently, in the United Kingdom, Moran et al.[6] found no elevation in pancreatic cancer risk in 268 families with a known *BRCA1* mutation. A United States–based study reported that 11% (24 out of 219) of their families with a *BRCA1* mutation had at least one individual with pancreatic cancer, with median ages at diagnosis of 59 years for males and 68 years for females. Again, this was significantly younger than reported in the SEER database ($p = 0.0014$).[8] Al-Sukhni et al.[21] molecularly evaluated pancreatic tumors from seven known *BRCA1* mutation carriers and found a loss of heterozygosity of *BRCA1* in five (71%), with confirmed loss of the wild-type allele in three of the five compared with only one (11%) of nine sporadic controls. This suggests that *BRCA1* germ-line mutations do, in fact, predispose some individuals to pancreatic cancers.

Familial breast cancer registries in the United States and Israel have evaluated the mutation status of families that reported pancreatic cancer in addition to breast cancer and ovarian cancer. In the US study of 19 families with breast, ovarian, and pancreatic cancer, 15 carried a deleterious mutation in *BRCA1* and 4 in *BRCA2*,[22] whereas the Israeli study reported an equal number of *BRCA1* and *BRCA2* families.[23]

Another study, specifically of Ashkenazi Jewish families, reported a *BRCA1* mutation in 7% of probands with breast cancer who also had a family history of pancreatic cancer,[16] which was, again, equal to the prevalence of *BRCA2* mutations. Thus, within the Ashkenazi Jewish population, *BRCA1* and *BRCA2* mutations may contribute more equally to risk in families with both breast and pancreatic cancer. However, these studies all examined cohorts of families selected because of clustering of breast and/or ovarian cancer with pancreatic cancer. When families were selected on the basis of familial pancreatic cancer alone, *BRCA1* mutations were less prevalent. None of the sixty-six families with three or more cases of pancreatic cancer had a deleterious *BRCA1* mutation, including those who also reported a family history of breast and/or ovarian cancer.[24] An evaluation of Ashkenazi Jewish patients ascertained on the basis of pancreatic cancer alone showed a 1.3% (2 out of 145) prevalence of *BRCA1* mutations.[14] Therefore, *BRCA1* may explain a small subset of families showing a clustering of pancreatic cancer with breast and/or ovarian cancer, but is unlikely to explain most families with site-specific pancreatic cancer.

PALB2

PALB2 (partner and localizer of *BRCA2*) was recognized as the *FANCN* gene in 2007, and biallelic mutation carriers develop

TABLE 42.1

Inherited Cancer Predisposition Syndromes that Increase the Risk for Pancreatic Cancer

Syndrome	Gene(s)	Risk of Pancreatic Cancer	Predominant Features
Hereditary breast and ovarian cancer	BRCA1	RR, 2.26–3	Malignancies: Breast (particularly premenopausal), ovary, male breast, prostate
	BRCA2	RR, 3.5–5.9	Malignancies: Breast (particularly premenopausal), ovary, male breast, prostate, melanoma (cutaneous and ocular)
Familial atypical multiple mole and melanoma	CDKN2A	RR, 7.4–47.8	Malignancies: Melanoma (often multiple and early onset) Other: Dysplastic nevi
Hereditary pancreatitis	PRSS1	SIR, 57	Other: Chronic pancreatitis
Hereditary nonpolyposis colorectal cancer (Lynch syndrome)	MLH1 MSH2 MSH6 PMS2 EPCAM	SIR, 0–8.6	Malignancies: Colorectum, endometrium, ovary, stomach, small bowel, urinary tract (ureter, renal pelvis), biliary, brain (glioblastoma), skin (sebaceous)
PJS	STK11	SIR, 132	Malignancies: Colorectum, small bowel, stomach, breast, gynecologic Other: Melanin pigmentation (mucocutaneous), small-bowel intussusception

SIR, standardized incidence ratio.

Fanconi anemia.[25,26] Monoallelic mutation carriers were shown to be at an increased risk for breast cancer (relative risk [RR], 2.3; 95% CI, 1.4 to 3.9).[27] The prevalence of *PALB2* mutations among familial breast cancer cases is low across ethnicities; *PALB2* mutations are relatively nonexistent in breast cancers in the Irish and Icelandic populations and are found in approximately 1% of Italians, African Americans, Chinese, and Spanish breast cancer families, and in 2% of young South African breast cancer patients.[28–35] An analysis of 1,144 US familial breast cancer cases found a *PALB2* mutation in 3.4% (33 out of 972) of non-Ashkenazi Jews and none (0 out of 172) of Ashkenazi Jews. The estimated risk for breast cancer was 2.3-fold by the age of 55 years (95% CI, 1.5 to 4.2) and 3.4-fold by the age of 85 years (95% CI, 2.4 to 5.9). There was also a fourfold risk for male breast cancer ($p = 0.0003$) and a sixfold risk for pancreatic cancer ($p = 0.002$).[36] Among French Canadian women with bilateral breast cancer, a *PALB2* mutation was found in 0.9% (5 out of 559) compared with none of the 565 women with unilateral breast cancer ($p = 0.04$), and first-degree relatives of *PALB2* mutation carriers had a 5.3-fold risk for breast cancer (95% CI, 1.8 to 13.2).[37]

PALB2 founder mutations have been identified in several populations, including the c.2323C>T (Q775X) mutation in French Canadians.[38] Another example is the Finnish founder mutation c.1592delT. This mutation was found in 2.7% (3 out of 113) of familial breast and/or breast/ovarian cancer families compared with 0.2% (6 out of 2,501) of controls (OR, 11.3; 95% CI, 1.8 to 57.8; $p = 0.005$).[39] One percent (18 out of 1,918) of breast cancer cases unselected for family history also had this founder mutation. The hazard ratio for breast cancer was estimated at 6.1 (95% CI, 2.2 to 17.2; $p = 0.01$), with a penetrance of 40% by the age of 70 years.[40]

PALB2 has not been shown to be a significant contributor to familial clustering of other cancers, including melanoma, ovarian cancer, and prostate cancer,[41–43] but has been identified in familial pancreatic cancer kindreds. Specifically, Jones et al.[44] identified a *PALB2* mutation in a familial pancreatic

cancer proband, and subsequently found *PALB2* mutations in 3 out of 96 additional families, suggesting that 3% to 4% of familial pancreatic cancer may be attributed to this gene. Other populations have found lower mutation frequencies, ranging from absent in the Dutch (0 out of 31) to 3.7% (3 out of 81) in Germans.[45,46] When ascertained on the basis of co-occurrence of breast and pancreatic cancer in the same individual or family, prevalence varied, again, from absent in the Dutch (0 out of 45) and United States–based studies (0 out of 77) to 4.8% (3 out of 62) in Italians.[42,47,48]

CDKN2A

The p16 transcript of the *CDKN2A* gene is an important cell cycle regulator. Germ-line mutations in the *CDKN2A* gene predispose individuals to multiple early-onset melanomas. Somatic *CDKN2A* mutations are also frequently identified in pancreatic adenocarcinomas and precursor lesions, indicating a role for this gene in pancreatic cancer development and progression.[49–51]

The risk of pancreatic cancer with *CDKN2A* mutations varies based on genotype. In a study of 22 families with the Dutch founder mutation, p16-Leiden, which is a 19–base-pair deletion in exon 2, the relative risk of pancreatic cancer was 47.8 (95% CI, 28.4 to 74.7).[52] The age-related risks have been shown to be less than 1%, 4%, 5%, 12%, and 17% by ages 40, 50, 60, 70, and 75 years, respectively.[53] Regarding other mutations, the Genes, Environment and Melanoma Study assessed relative risks for nonmelanoma cancers in 429 first-degree relatives of 65 melanoma patients with a *CDKN2A* mutation. Five pancreatic cancers were reported compared with 41 pancreatic cancers among 23,452 first-degree relatives of 3,537 noncarriers, for a relative risk of 7.4 (95% CI, 2.3 to 18.7; $p = 0.002$).[54] A United States–based study estimated penetrance to be 58% by the age of 80 years (95% CI, 8% to 86%) and noted a hazard ratio of 25.8 ($p = 2.1 \times 10^{2^{13}}$) in those who ever smoked cigarettes.[55]

Mutation prevalence in pancreatic cancer families varies by population. In an Italian study, 5.7% of 225 consecutive patients with pancreatic cancer had an identified *CDKN2A* mutation.[56] The predominant mutations were the E27X and G101W founder mutations, although others were also represented. Of 16 patients classified as having familial pancreatic cancer, 5 (31%) carried *CDKN2A* mutations, leading the authors to conclude that this gene may account for a sizeable subset of Italian familial pancreatic families. By comparison, no *CDKN2A* mutations were found in 51 Polish pancreatic cancer patients diagnosed at younger than 50 years.[57] Similarly, an analysis of 94 German pancreatic cancer patients who had at least one other first-degree relative with pancreatic cancer revealed no *CDKN2A* mutations.[58] However, two of five families with at least one pancreatic cancer and at least one melanoma had an identified mutation.[59] Similarly, a Canadian study found a *CDKN2A* mutation in 2 of 14 families with both pancreatic cancer and melanoma.[60] Finally, a United States–based study found 9 *CDKN2A* mutations in an unselected series of 1,537 pancreatic cancer cases (0.6%). The prevalence increased to 3.3% and 5.3% for those who reported a first-degree relative with pancreatic cancer or melanoma, respectively.[55] Thus, in the majority of populations, the co-occurrence of melanoma appears to be a significant indicator of an underlying *CDKN2A* mutation.

SELECTED SYNDROMES THAT INCREASE THE RISK OF PANCREATIC CANCER

Hereditary Nonpolyposis Colorectal Cancer

Hereditary nonpolyposis colorectal cancer (HNPCC), also referred to as Lynch syndrome, is the most common form of hereditary colon cancer, and it accounts for 2% to 5% of colorectal cancers. In addition to a high lifetime risk for colorectal cancer, affected individuals are at an increased risk for multiple other cancers. HNPCC results from mutations in mismatch repair (MMR) genes, and colon cancers that arise in Lynch syndrome typically demonstrate microsatellite instability (MSI). Four percent of all pancreatic adenocarcinomas demonstrate MSI.[61] Yamamoto et al.[62] assessed tumor characteristics in three *MLH1* mutation carriers with both colon and pancreatic cancer, and found that both tumor types had similar properties, including high MSI, loss of MLH1 protein expression, wild-type KRAS and p53, and poor differentiation. These findings support an inherited basis for the development of both types of cancer.[62]

Pancreatic cancer has been described in HNPCC kindreds as early as 1985, although data regarding the risk of pancreatic cancer in HNPCC have varied.[63–68] Barrow et al.[64] studied 121 families with known MMR mutations; 2 of 282 extracolonic cancers were pancreatic, leading to a 0.4% cumulative lifetime risk for pancreatic cancer (95% CI, 0% to 0.8%). By comparison, Geary et al.[65] studied 130 families with MMR mutations and found 22 cases of pancreatic cancer, half of which were in confirmed or obligate carriers. Pancreatic cancer in these families was seven times more common than expected, and the familial relative risk was 3.8 ($p = 0.02$). In addition, these tumors were 15 times more common in individuals younger than 60 years, suggesting an earlier average age at diagnosis as compared with the general population.[65] Another United States–based study of HNPCC families found the lifetime risk for pancreatic cancer to be 1.31% by the age of 50 years (95% CI, 0.31% to 2.32%) and 3.68% by the age of 70 years (95% CI, 1.45% to 5.88%). These risks are higher than those from the SEER data of 0.04% and 0.52% at ages 50 and 70 years, respectively.[66]

Regarding the prevalence of HNPCC in pancreatic cancer, Gargiulo et al.[69] assessed 135 pancreatic cancer patients. Nineteen of these patients had a family history that was suggestive of HNPCC, and of the 11 patients whose DNA was available for analysis, only one deleterious MMR mutation was found. Thus, MMR mutations presumably account for only a small proportion of pancreatic cancer patients.

Hereditary Pancreatitis

Hereditary pancreatitis (HP) is a rare form of chronic pancreatitis. Several genes have been linked to chronic pancreatitis, including *SPINK1*, *CTFR*, and *CTRC*, but the *PRSS1* gene on chromosome 7q35 accounts for the majority of hereditary cases. *PRSS1* mutations are inherited in an autosomal-dominant fashion and have an 80% penetrance for pancreatitis. Affected individuals begin experiencing symptoms of pancreatic pain and acute pancreatitis early in life. Several studies have shown an increase in pancreatic cancer risk associated with HP, and cumulative lifetime risk estimates range from 18.8% to 53.5%.[70–72] Lowenfels et al.[71] observed an increased risk associated with paternal inheritance. Tobacco use in patients with HP has been shown to increase the risk for pancreatic cancer twofold (95% CI, 0.7 to 6.1), pancreatic and HP patients who smoke developed cancer 20 years earlier than did their nonsmoking counterparts.[73]

Peutz–Jeghers Syndrome

Peutz–Jeghers syndrome (PJS) is an autosomal-dominant condition characterized by mucocutaneous pigmentation and hamartomatous polyps of the gastrointestinal tract. PJS is caused by mutations on the *STK11* (*LKB1*) gene. The lifetime risk to develop any cancer has been estimated to be as high as 93%,[74] with no sex difference in cancer risk noted.[74,75] Risk for pancreatic cancer in PJS is estimated to be 8% to 36% by the age of 70 years.[74–76] Grützmann et al.[77] analyzed 39 individuals with familial pancreatic cancer, and none were found to carry mutations in *STK11*. In 2011, Schneider et al.[58] confirmed these findings in their study of 94 familial pancreatic cancer kindreds. Therefore, although *STK11* mutations confer a high lifetime risk for pancreatic cancer in individuals with PJS, germ-line *STK11* mutations are not thought to account for hereditary pancreatic cancer.

EMPIRIC RISK COUNSELING AND MANAGEMENT

Having a first-degree relative with apparently sporadic pancreatic cancer has a moderate effect on risk (OR, 1.76; 95% CI, 1.19 to 2.61).[78] In familial pancreatic cancer kindreds (defined as a family with a pair of affected first-degree relatives), the risk of pancreatic cancer increases with the number of affected first-degree relatives (Table 42.2).[3] These findings suggest that high-penetrance genes may be causing the clustering of pancreatic cancer in families with two or three pancreatic cancer cases. Thus, individuals with multiple affected first-degree relatives are at an appreciably increased risk for pancreatic cancer and may be candidates for increased surveillance.

TABLE 42.2

Risk of Pancreatic Cancer in Familial Pancreatic Cancer Kindreds Based on Number of Affected First-Degree Relatives

Number of Affected FDRs	SIR (95% CI)
1	4.5 (0.54–16.3)
2	6.4 (1.8–16.4)
3	32 (10.4–74.7)

FDR, first-degree relatives; SIR, standardized incidence ratio.

Ideally, high-risk patients would be able to undergo noninvasive, inexpensive pancreatic cancer screening; however, to date, a highly sensitive and specific method for pancreas surveillance has not been recognized. Screening of high-risk patients with endoscopic ultrasound, magnetic resonance imaging, and/or magnetic resonance cholangiopancreatogram has been shown to be effective at identifying early neoplasms, both benign and malignant.[79-82] However, it is unknown if these methods actually prevent pancreatic cancer or improve overall survival by detecting presymptomatic disease. In addition, there is great interest in developing a biomarker for premalignant or early-stage disease, although none, including CA19-9, have been proven effective.[83] Thus, whenever possible, it is recommended that high-risk patients undergo pancreatic screening through a research study.

REFERENCES

1. Lynch HT, Smyrk T, Kern SE, et al. Familial pancreatic cancer: A review. *Semin Oncol* 1996;23:251–275.
2. Klein AP, Hruban RH, Brune KA, et al. Familial pancreatic cancer. *Cancer J* 2001;7:266–273.
3. Klein AP, Brune KA, Petersen GM, et al. Prospective risk of pancreatic cancer in familial pancreatic cancer kindreds. *Cancer Res* 2004;64:2634–2638.
4. Klein AP, Beaty TH, Bailey-Wilson JE, et al. Evidence for a major gene influencing risk of pancreatic cancer. *Genet Epidemiol* 2002;23:133–149.
5. The Breast Cancer Linkage Consortium. Cancer risks in BRCA2 mutation carriers. *J Natl Cancer Inst* 1999;91:1310–1316.
6. Moran A, O'Hara C, Khan S, et al. Risk of cancer other than breast or ovarian in individuals with BRCA1 and BRCA2 mutations. *Fam Cancer* 2012;11:235–242.
7. van Asperen CJ, Brohet RM, Meijers-Heijboer EJ, et al. Cancer risks in BRCA2 families: Estimates for sites other than breast and ovary. *J Med Genet* 2005;42:711–719.
8. Kim DH, Crawford B, Ziegler J, et al. Prevalence and characteristics of pancreatic cancer in families with BRCA1 and BRCA2 mutations. *Fam Cancer* 2009;8:153–158.
9. Martin ST, Matsubayashi H, Rogers CD, et al. Increased prevalence of the BRCA2 polymorphic stop codon K3326X among individuals with familial pancreatic cancer. *Oncogene* 2005;24:3652–3656.
10. Murphy KM, Brune KA, Griffin C, et al. Evaluation of candidate genes MAP2K4, MADH4, ACVR1B, and BRCA2 in familial pancreatic cancer: Deleterious BRCA2 mutations in 17%. *Cancer Res* 2002;62:3789–3793.
11. Hahn SA, Greenhalf B, Ellis I, et al. BRCA2 germline mutations in familial pancreatic carcinoma. *J Natl Cancer Inst* 2003;95:214–221.
12. Couch FJ, Johnson MR, Rabe KG, et al. The prevalence of BRCA2 mutations in familial pancreatic cancer. *Cancer Epidemiol Biomarkers Prev* 2007;16:342–346.
13. Goggins M, Schutte M, Lu J, et al. Germline BRCA2 gene mutations in patients with apparently sporadic pancreatic carcinomas. *Cancer Res* 1996;56:5360–5364.
14. Ferrone CR, Levine DA, Tang LH, et al. BRCA germline mutations in Jewish patients with pancreatic adenocarcinoma. *J Clin Oncol* 2009;27:433–438.
15. Figer A, Irmin L, Geva R, et al. The rate of the 6174delT founder Jewish mutation in BRCA2 in patients with non-colonic gastrointestinal tract tumours in Israel. *Br J Cancer* 2001;84:478–481.
16. Stadler ZK, Salo-Mullen E, Patil SM, et al. Prevalence of BRCA1 and BRCA2 mutations in Ashkenazi Jewish families with breast and pancreatic cancer. *Cancer* 2012;118:493–499.
17. Cho JH, Bang S, Park SW, et al. BRCA2 mutations as a universal risk factor for pancreatic cancer has a limited role in Korean ethnic group. *Pancreas* 2008;36:337–340.
18. Ghiorzo P, Pensotti V, Fornarini G, et al. Contribution of germline mutations in the BRCA and PALB2 genes to pancreatic cancer in Italy. *Fam Cancer* 2012;11:41–47.
19. Thompson D, Easton DF. Cancer incidence in BRCA1 mutation carriers. *J Natl Cancer Inst* 2002;94:1358–1365.
20. Brose MS, Rebbeck TR, Calzone KA, et al. Cancer risk estimates for BRCA1 mutation carriers identified in a risk evaluation program. *J Natl Cancer Inst* 2002;94:1365–1372.
21. Al-Sukhni W, Rothenmund H, Borgida AE, et al. Germline BRCA1 mutations predispose to pancreatic adenocarcinoma. *Hum Genet* 2008;124:271–278.
22. Lynch HT, Deters CA, Snyder CL, et al. BRCA1 and pancreatic cancer: pedigree findings and their causal relationships. *Cancer Genet Cytogenet* 2005;158:119–125.
23. Danes BS, Lynch HT. A familial aggregation of pancreatic cancer. An in vitro study. *JAMA* 1982;247:2798–2802.
24. Axilbund JE, Argani P, Kamiyama M, et al. Absence of germline BRCA1 mutations in familial pancreatic cancer patients. *Cancer Biol Ther* 2009;8:131–135.
25. Reid S, Schindler D, Hanenberg H, et al. Biallelic mutations in PALB2 cause Fanconi anemia subtype FA-N and predispose to childhood cancer. *Nat Genet* 2007;39:162–164.
26. Xia B, Dorsman JC, Ameziane N, et al. Fanconi anemia is associated with a defect in the BRCA2 partner PALB2. *Nat Genet* 2007;39:159–161.
27. Rahman N, Seal S, Thompson D, et al. PALB2, which encodes a BRCA2-interacting protein, is a breast cancer susceptibility gene. *Nat Genet* 2007;39:165–167.
28. McInerney NM, Miller N, Rowan A, et al. Evaluation of variants in the CHEK2, BRIP1 and PALB2 genes in an Irish breast cancer cohort. *Breast Cancer Res Treat* 2010;121:203–210.
29. Gunnarsson H, Arason A, Gillanders EM, et al. Evidence against PALB2 involvement in Icelandic breast cancer susceptibility. *J Negat Results Biomed* 2008;7:5.
30. Papi L, Putignano AL, Congregati C, et al. A PALB2 germline mutation associated with hereditary breast cancer in Italy. *Fam Cancer* 2010;9:181–185.
31. Ding YC, Steele L, Chu LH, et al. Germline mutations in PALB2 in African-American breast cancer cases. *Breast Cancer Res Treat* 2011;126:227–230.
32. Zheng Y, Zhang J, Niu Q, et al. Novel germline PALB2 truncating mutations in African American breast cancer patients. *Cancer* 2012;118:1362–1370.
33. Cao AY, Huang J, Hu Z, et al. The prevalence of PALB2 germline mutations in BRCA1/BRCA2 negative Chinese women with early onset breast cancer or affected relatives. *Breast Cancer Res Treat* 2009;114:457–462.
34. Blanco A, de la Hoya M, Balmaña J, et al. Detection of a large rearrangement in PALB2 in Spanish breast cancer families with male breast cancer. *Breast Cancer Res Treat* 2012;132:307–315.
35. Sluiter M, Mew S, van Rensburg EJ. PALB2 sequence variants in young South African breast cancer patients. *Fam Cancer* 2009;8:347–353.
36. Casadei S, Norquist BM, Walsh T, et al. Contribution of inherited mutations in the BRCA2-interacting protein PALB2 to familial breast cancer. *Cancer Res* 2011;71:2222–2229.
37. Tischkowitz M, Capanu M, Sabbaghian N, et al. Rare germline mutations in PALB2 and breast cancer risk: A population-based study. *Hum Mutat* 2012;33:674–680.
38. Foulkes WD, Ghadirian P, Akbari MR, et al. Identification of a novel truncating PALB2 mutation and analysis of its contribution to early-onset breast cancer in French-Canadian women. *Breast Cancer Res* 2007;9:R83.
39. Erkko H, Xia B, Nikkilä J, et al. A recurrent mutation in PALB2 in Finnish cancer families. *Nature* 2007;446:316–319.
40. Erkko H, Dowty JG, Nikkilä J, et al. Penetrance analysis of the PALB2 c.1592delT founder mutation. *Clin Cancer Res* 2008;14:4667–4671.
41. Sabbaghian N, Kyle R, Hao A, et al. Mutation analysis of the PALB2 cancer predisposition gene in familial melanoma. *Fam Cancer* 2011;10:315–317.
42. Adank MA, van Mil SE, Gille JJ, et al. PALB2 analysis in BRCA2-like families. *Breast Cancer Res Treat* 2011;127:357–362.
43. Tischkowitz M, Sabbaghian N, Ray AM, et al. Analysis of the gene coding for the BRCA2-interacting protein PALB2 in hereditary prostate cancer. *Prostate* 2008;68:675–678.
44. Jones S, Hruban RH, Kamiyama M, et al. Exomic sequencing identifies PALB2 as a pancreatic cancer susceptibility gene. *Science* 2009;324:217.
45. Harinck F, Kluijt I, van Mil SE, et al. Routine testing for PALB2 mutations in familial pancreatic cancer families and breast cancer families with pancreatic cancer is not indicated. *Eur J Hum Genet* 2012;20:577–579.
46. Slater EP, Langer P, Niemczyk E, et al. PALB2 mutations in European familial pancreatic cancer families. *Clin Genet* 2010;78:490–494.
47. Stadler ZK, Salo-Mullen E, Sabbaghian N, et al. Germline PALB2 mutation analysis in breast-pancreas cancer families. *J Med Genet* 2011;48:523–525.
48. Peterlongo P, Catucci I, Pasquini G, et al. PALB2 germline mutations in familial breast cancer cases with personal and family history of pancreatic cancer. *Breast Cancer Res Treat* 2011;126:825–828.
49. Kanda M, Matthaei H, Wu J, et al. Presence of somatic mutations in most early-stage pancreatic intraepithelial neoplasia. *Gastroenterology* 2012;142:730–733.
50. Remmers N, Bailey JM, Mohr AM, et al. Molecular pathology of early pancreatic cancer. *Cancer Biomark* 2011;9:421–440.
51. Bartsch D, Shevlin DW, Tung WS, et al. Frequent mutations of CDKN2 in primary pancreatic adenocarcinomas. *Genes Chromosomes Cancer* 1995;14:189–195.
52. de Snoo FA, Bishop DT, Bergman W, et al. Increased risk of cancer other than melanoma in CDKN2A founder mutation (p16-Leiden)-positive melanoma families. *Clin Cancer Res* 2008;14:7151–7157.
53. Vasen HF, Gruis NA, Frants RR, et al. Risk of developing pancreatic cancer in families with familial atypical multiple mole melanoma associated with a specific 19 deletion of p16 (p16-Leiden). *Int J Cancer* 2000;87:809–811.
54. Mukherjee B, Delancey JO, Raskin L, et al. Risk of non-melanoma cancers in first-degree relatives of CDKN2A mutation carriers. *J Natl Cancer Inst* 2012;104:953–956.

55. McWilliams RR, Wieben ED, Rabe KG, et al. Prevalence of CDKN2A mutations in pancreatic cancer patients: Implications for genetic counseling. *Eur J Hum Genet* 2011;19:472–478.

56. Ghiorzo P, Fornarini G, Sciallero S, et al. CDKN2A is the main susceptibility gene in Italian pancreatic cancer families. *J Med Genet* 2012;49:164–170.

57. Debniak T, van de Wetering T, Scott R, et al. Low prevalence of CDKN2A/ARF mutations among early-onset cancers of breast, pancreas and malignant melanoma in Poland. *Eur J Cancer Prev* 2008;17:389–391.

58. Schneider R, Slater EP, Sina M, et al. German national case collection for familial pancreatic cancer (FaPaCa): ten years experience. *Fam Cancer* 2011; 10:323–330.

59. Bartsch DK, Sina-Frey M, Lang S, et al. CDKN2A germline mutations in familial pancreatic cancer. *Ann Surg* 2002;236:730–737.

60. Lal G, Liu L, Hogg D, et al. Patients with both pancreatic adenocarcinoma and melanoma may harbor germline CDKN2A mutations. *Genes Chromosomes Cancer* 2000;27:358–361.

61. Goggins M, Offerhaus GJ, Hilgers W, et al. Pancreatic adenocarcinomas with DNA replication errors (RER⁺) are associated with wild-type K-ras and characteristic histopathology. Poor differentiation, a syncytial growth pattern, and pushing borders suggest RER⁺. *Am J Pathol* 1998;152:1501–1507.

62. Yamamoto H, Itoh F, Nakamura H, et al. Genetic and clinical features of human pancreatic ductal adenocarcinomas with widespread microsatellite instability. *Cancer Res* 2001;61:3136–3144.

63. Lynch HT, Voorhees GJ, Lanspa SJ, et al. Pancreatic carcinoma and hereditary nonpolyposis colorectal cancer: a family study. *Br J Cancer* 1985;52: 271–273.

64. Barrow E, Robinson L, Alduaij W, et al. Cumulative lifetime incidence of extracolonic cancers in Lynch syndrome: A report of 121 families with proven mutations. *Clin Genet* 2009;75:141–149.

65. Geary J, Sasieni P, Houlston R, et al. Gene-related cancer spectrum in families with hereditary non-polyposis colorectal cancer (HNPCC). *Fam Cancer* 2008;7:163–172.

66. Kastrinos F, Mukherjee B, Tayob N, et al. Risk of pancreatic cancer in families with Lynch syndrome. *JAMA* 2009;302:1790–1795.

67. Aarnio M, Sankila R, Pukkala E, et al. Cancer risk in mutation carriers of DNA-mismatch-repair genes. *Int J Cancer* 1999;81:214–218.

68. Vasen HF, Offerhaus GJ, den Hartog Jager FH, et al. The tumor spectrum in hereditary non-polyposis colorectal cancer: a study of 24 kindreds in the Netherlands. *Int J Cancer* 1990;46:31–34.

69. Gargiulo S, Torrini M, Ollila S, et al. Germline MLH1 and MSH2 mutations in Italian pancreatic cancer patients with suspected Lynch syndrome. *Fam Cancer* 2009;8:547–553.

70. Howes N, Lerch MM, Greenhalf W, et al. Clinical and genetic characteristics of hereditary pancreatitis in Europe. *Clin Gastroenterol Hepatol* 2004;2:252–261.

71. Lowenfels AB, Maisonneuve P, Di Magno EP, et al. Hereditary pancreatitis and the risk of pancreatic cancer. International Hereditary Pancreatitis Study Group. *J Natl Cancer Inst* 1997;89:442–446.

72. Rebours V, Boutron-Ruault MC, Schnee MF, et al. Risk of pancreatic adenocarcinoma in patients with hereditary pancreatitis: a national exhaustive series. *Am J Gastroenterol* 2008;103:111–119.

73. Lowenfels AB, Maisonneuve P, Whitcomb DC, et al. Cigarette smoking as a risk factor for pancreatic cancer in patients with hereditary pancreatitis. *JAMA* 2001;286:169–170.

74. Giardiello FM, Brensinger JD, Tersmette AC, et al. Very high risk of cancer in familial Peutz–Jeghers syndrome. *Gastroenterology* 2000;119:1447–1453.

75. Lim W, Olschwang S, Keller JJ, et al. Relative frequency and morphology of cancers in STK11 mutation carriers. *Gastroenterology* 2004;126:1788–1794.

76. Hearle N, Schumacher V, Menko FH, et al. Frequency and spectrum of cancers in the Peutz–Jeghers syndrome. *Clin Cancer Res* 2006;12:3209–3215.

77. Grützmann R, McFaul C, Bartsch DK, et al. No evidence for germline mutations of the LKB1/STK11 gene in familial pancreatic carcinoma. *Cancer Lett* 2004;214:63–68.

78. Jacobs EJ, Chanock SJ, Fuchs CS, et al. Family history of cancer and risk of pancreatic cancer: A pooled analysis from the Pancreatic Cancer Cohort Consortium (PanScan). *Int J Cancer* 2010;127:1421–1428.

79. Canto MI, Hruban RH, Fishman EK, et al. Frequent detection of pancreatic lesions in asymptomatic high-risk individuals. *Gastroenterology* 2012;142:796–804.

80. Ludwig E, Olson SH, Bayuga S, et al. Feasibility and yield of screening in relatives from familial pancreatic cancer families. *Am J Gastroenterol* 2011;106:946–954.

81. Verna EC, Hwang C, Stevens PD, et al. Pancreatic cancer screening in a prospective cohort of high-risk patients: A comprehensive strategy of imaging and genetics. *Clin Cancer Res* 2010;16:5028–5037.

82. Langer P, Kann PH, Fendrich V, et al. Five years of prospective screening of high-risk individuals from families with familial pancreatic cancer. *Gut* 2009;58:1410–1418.

83. Goggins M. Markers of pancreatic cancer: working toward early detection. *Clin Cancer Res* 2011;17:635–637.

43 Molecular Biology of Liver Cancer

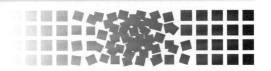

Jens U. Marquardt and Snorri S. Thorgeirsson

INTRODUCTION

Hepatocellular carcinoma (HCC) is the fifth most common cancer in men and the seventh most common cancer in women worldwide, accounting for at least 600,000 deaths annually.[1] Although rates in traditionally high-incidence regions such as southeast Asia and sub-Sahara Africa has stabilized and slowly declined due to generalized vaccination programs, the incidence and mortality rates of HCC have doubled in the United States and Europe in the past 4 decades and are predicted to continue rising.[2] Several confounding factors (e.g., immigration from high-incidence countries) contribute to these high numbers in the western world, and HCC is currently among the fastest growing causes of cancer related deaths in the United States. Small HCCs can be cured by resection and/or liver transplantation. However, at the time of diagnosis, less than 20% of patients are eligible for these treatment options.[3] These observations make it clear that liver cancer is a major health problem in the United States and Europe and highlight the critical need for both improved understanding and treatment options of this deadly disease.

The major etiologic agents responsible for chronic liver disease, cirrhosis, and ultimately, HCC are known and well characterized (e.g., hepatitis B virus [HBV], hepatitis C virus [HCV], ethanol abuse). Other etiologic factors include nonalcoholic fatty liver disease (NAFLD) and other metabolic disorders that have become particularly relevant in Western countries due to a sharp increase in prevalence and a high number of HCCs without underlying cirrhosis.[4]

Over the last decades, molecular mechanisms of liver diseases that are associated with increased risk of HCC as well as several cellular alterations that precede HCC have been identified.[5,6] Research into the molecular pathogenesis of HCC is currently focused on the interrelationship of abnormal genomics, epigenomics, proteomics, and downstream alterations in molecular signaling pathways. The primary goal of this research is to integrate the new data with clinicopathologic features of HCC in order to uncover new diagnostic tools, improve treatment options, and implement effective prevention strategies.[7]

The recent introduction of next-generation whole genomic technologies permits simultaneously detection of the expression of tens of thousands of genes in small samples from normal and diseased tissues.[8] High-throughput microarray-based technologies and the recent advent of next-generation whole genome DNA sequencing offer a unique opportunity to define the descriptive characteristics (i.e., phenotype) of a biologic system in terms of the genomic readout (e.g., gene expression, coding mutations, insertions and deletions in DNA, splicing variants, copy number variations, chromosomal translocations). Integrated analyses and the interpretation of biologic systems has caused a paradigm shift in biologic research, from the classic reductionism to systems biology.[9] Fundamental to the systems approach is the hypothesis that disease processes are driven by aberrant regulatory networks of genes and proteins that differ from the normal counterparts. The application of multiparametric measurements promises to transform current approaches of diagnosis and therapy, providing the foundation for predictive and preventive personalized medicine.[10]

In this chapter we discuss both the molecular hallmarks of hepatocarcinogenesis in the context of next-generation high-throughput genomic technologies, and the implications for clinical and translational efforts.

GENETIC ALTERATIONS IN LIVER CANCER

During the last decade, a detailed map of the structural variation in the human cancer genome has been generated.[11] This map reveals that tumor development is the consequence of intragenic mutations in approximately 140 genes belonging to 12 signaling pathways regulating three core cellular processes—cell fate, cell survival, and genome maintenance—that can promote or "drive" tumorigenesis in the majority of human cancers.[11] Hepatocarcinogenesis can, therefore, be considered a multistep process that is orchestrated by a sequence of epigenetic and genetic alterations leading to disruption in these core processes by the activation or inhibition of key downstream signaling such as p53, WNT, β-catenin, MYC, the ErbB family, as well as chromatin modifications.[11]

Structural variation and chromosomal aberrations in tumors are traditionally regarded as evidence of gene deregulation and genome instability, and may facilitate the identification of crucial genes and regulatory pathways that are perturbed in diseases.[12] Large, genomewide association studies (GWAS) recently identified liver disease–specific susceptibility loci, including in HCC.[13,14] Most of these studies employed powerful high-throughput microarray technology for single nucleotide polymorphism (SNP) genotyping and array-based comparative genomic hybridization (aCGH). These technologies enable a high-throughput analysis of DNA copy number and yield comprehensive information for determining the molecular pathogenesis of human HCC.

A meta-analysis of aCGH studies of chromosome aberrations in human HCC shows that specific chromosomal gains and losses correlate with etiology and histologic grade.[15] In HCC, the most frequent amplifications of genomic material involve 1q (57.1%), 8q (46.6%), 6p (22.3%), and 17q (22.2%), whereas losses are most common in 8p (38%), 16q (35.9%), 4q (34.3%), 17p (32.1%), and 13q (26.2%). Deletions of 4q, 16q, 13q, and 8p correlate with HBV infection and a lack of HCV infection. Chromosomes 13q and 4q are significantly underrepresented in poorly differentiated HCC, and gains of 1q correlate with other high-frequency alterations.[16] Amplifications and deletions often occur on chromosome arms at sites of oncogenes (e.g., MYC on 8q24) and tumor suppressor genes (e.g., RB1 on 13q14), as well as at several loci that contain genes with known and/or suspected oncogenic functions (e.g., FZD3, WISP1, SIAH-1, and AXIN2), all of which modulate the WNT signaling pathway. In these meta-analyses, etiology and poor differentiation of HCC correlated with specific genomic alterations. In preneoplastic dysplastic nodules (DN), amplifications are most frequent in 1q and 8q, whereas deletions occur in 8p, 17p, 5p, 13q, 14q, and 16q.[16] A gain of 1q appears to be an early event that develops in DN, possibly predisposing affected cells to acquire additional chromosomal aberrations.

A comprehensive collection of common aberrations from both human and rodent HCC is provided in the OncoDB.HCC database (http://oncodb.hcc.ibms.sinica.edu.tw).[17] This database provides a useful, validated, and graphic integration of published data derived from loss of heterozygosity (LOH) analyses, aCGH, gene expression microarrays, as well as proteomics, which is publically assessable for the validation of possible molecular targets.

Recently, a systematic strategy to identify potential driver genes by integrating whole genome copy number data with gene expression profiles of HCC patients was introduced.[18] Using regional pattern recognition approaches, the authors discovered the most probable copy number–dependent regions and 50 potential driver genes. At each step of the process, the functional relevance of the selected genes was evaluated by estimating the prognostic significance of the selected genes. Further validation using small interference RNA-mediated knockdown experiments showed proof-of-principle evidence for the potential driver roles of the genes in HCC progression (i.e., NCSTN, SCRIB). In addition, the systemic prediction of drug responses using the Connectivity Map,[19] a compendium of functional connections between drugs and genes, implicated the association of the 50 genes with specific signaling molecules associated with hepatocarcinogenesis (mTOR, AMPK, and EGFR). It was concluded that the application of an unbiased and integrative analysis of multidimensional genomic data sets can effectively screen for potential driver genes and provide novel mechanistic and clinical insight into the pathobiology of HCC.

In a similar approach, a recent study used an integrative approach combining information from high-resolution aCGH and gene expression profiling with clinical data from HCC patients to identify copy-number variations (CNV) in HCC with functional relevance for tumor progression.[20] The investigation was restricted to genes that showed (1) recurrent CNVs, (2) correlation of the CNVs and the transcriptome, and (3) a selective association to patients' outcomes to distinguish "drivers" from passengers. The authors were able to demonstrate significant differences in CNVs between patients with good and poor outcome and generated a 10-gene signature as a molecular predictor of patient survival and validated the signature in several independent cohorts. Both these studies elegantly illustrate the power of multilayer integrative analyses to identify the functional significance of genomic alterations in human HCC.

EPIGENETIC ALTERATIONS IN LIVER CANCER

Epigenetic alterations such as DNA methylation are important factors in tumor development for many cancers.[21] Changes in DNA methylation patterns are believed to be early events in hepatocarcinogenesis, preceding allelic imbalances and ultimately leading to cancer progression, thereby adding considerable complexity to the pathogenesis of liver cancer.[22]

Global hypomethylation and promoter hypermethylation in certain cancer-related genes are known drivers of hepatocarcinogenesis with an association to biologic behavior and prognosis.[23] Methylation patterns can further be used to classify patients according to different etiological factors (e.g. HBV, HCV, alcohol).[24,25] Moreover, in addition to changes in global methylation patterns, distinct methylation patterns strongly correlate with clinical characteristics of HCC patients.[23] Methylation patterns in a 807 cancer-related gene panel could successfully separate primary HCC samples according to their biologic subtype.[26] Consistent with previous studies, patients with progenitor cell origin displayed the worst clinical outcome.[27] The confirmation of a multistep, epigenetic-driven sequence of molecular alteration in hepatocarcinogenesis could further be demonstrated in HBV-related liver cancers. A stepwise hypermethylation of CpG islands of nine well-

described genes was seen from cirrhotic nodules over dysplastic nodules (low and high grade) to early carcinoma (eHCC) and, finally, progressed HCC (pHCC).[28]

More recently, integrative genome-wide methylation analyses have been applied to 71 human HCC patients.[29] The methylation data were combined with those from a microarray analysis of gene reexpression in four hepatoma cell lines following their exposure to DNA methylation inhibitors. A total of 13 candidate tumor suppressor genes were identified using this approach and, subsequently, SMPD3 and NEFH were functionally validated as tumor suppressor genes in HCC. The authors could further show that SMPD3 not only affects tumor aggressiveness, but also that reduced levels are an independent prognostic factor for early recurrence of HCC.

Although genetic changes in chromatin modulators are among the most common alterations in HCC (see the following), the role of epigenetic alterations beyond DNA methylation such as modification of histones (e.g., acetylation, methylation, phosphorylation, ubiquitylation, SUMOylation) are not well studied in HCC.[30] The fact that modifications of both repressing (e.g., H3 lysine 27 and histone H3 Lysine 9) and activating histone marks (e.g., H3 lysines 4) have a significant impact on the expression of critical genes associated with hepatocarcinogenesis highlight the need for whole genomic approaches such as chromatin immunoprecipitation with microarray technology (ChIP-chip) and ChIP sequencing (ChIP-seq) to address the role of these changes in a more global perspective.[31]

MicroRNAs are epigenetically active, small RNAs that are critically involved to regulate protein expression.[32] Distinct MicroRNA expression patterns contribute to the definition of the cellular phenotype, including the regulation of proliferation, cell signaling, and apoptosis. Not surprisingly, the aberrant expression of microRNAs is associated with cancer initiation, propagation, and progression. Several microRNAs are frequently deregulated in HCC and associated with certain clinicopathologic features.[33] Several studies have demonstrated that microRNAs play an essential role in HCC progression by directly contributing to cell proliferation, apoptosis, and metastasis of HCC as well as by targeting a large number of critical protein-coding genes involved in hepatocarciongenesis.[34] The profiling of microRNA expression by microarray revealed subclasses associated with clinicopathologic features as well as mutations in several oncogenic pathways such as β-catenin and HNF1A.[35] Furthermore, microRNA profiling of 89 HCC samples using a ligation-mediated amplification method revealed three distinct clusters HCCs reflecting the clinical behavior of the tumors as well as identifying the microRNAs family mir-517 with increased tumorigenicity of HCC cells.[36]

Ji and colleagues[37] confirmed the therapeutic potential of microRNA-based treatment modalities in HCC. The authors demonstrated that miR-26 levels are associated with a response to adjuvant therapy with interferon α (IFN-α) and, more recently, developed a simple and reliable companion diagnostic (MIR26-DX) to select HCC patients for adjuvant IFN-α therapy as a first step to successfully translate information from large scale analyses into the clinics.[38]

MUTATIONAL LANDSCAPE OF GENETIC ALTERATIONS IN HCC: THE NEXT GENERATION

Sophisticated next-generation sequencing (NGS) technologies are now applied in cancer research for complete and cost-efficient analyses of cancer genomes at a single nucleotide resolution and have advanced into valuable tools in translational medicine.[12] The implementation of NGS to solid tumors like HCC is challenging because the proportion of normal cells or the stromal composition within a given sample contributes to the genomic signature and, therefore, may require additional coverage (i.e., read depth). Also, HCCs often arise in the background of a chronically diseased liver with underlying cirrhosis, fibrosis, or HBV or HCV infection, which may complicate the tumor/normal variant discovery when compared to the peritumoral liver tissue or even blood.[39] Therefore, the number of studies where NGS technologies—in particular, whole exome sequencing—have been applied to investigate HCC is, so far, limited and only conducted on a few patients.[40] However, all the studies revealed that the landscape of molecular alterations in HCC is relatively broad, with the number of mutations found ranging from 5 to 121 mutations per tumor. Thus, due to the genetic heterogeneity, a rather complex interaction of multiple mutations in the development of a singular HCC has to be assumed.[41–44] Although no clear oncogenic addiction has been demonstrated, a high number of mutations in p53 and Wnt/β-catenin signaling were detected (Fig. 43.1). Thus, results from in-depth analyses strengthen existing evidence that p53 and Wnt/β-catenin signaling are among the most common molecular changes involved in HCC development. Another interesting finding is the high frequency of genetic alteration in genes involved in chromatin remodeling. Overall, 16% to 24% of HCCs showed genetic alterations in these pathways, thereby suggesting a causative association with hepatocyte transformation and highlighting recent evidence for the key role of epigenetics in hepatocarcinogenesis.[45]

Two recent studies on whole exome/genome sequencing of 87 and 88 human HCCs as well as matched normal tissue[46,47] con-firmed the previous studies that β-catenin (10% and 15.9%) and TP53 (18% and 35.2%) are the most frequently mutated oncogene and tumor suppressor, respectively, in HCC.[46,47] The study by Kan et al.[47] also detected several drugable mutations, including activating mutations of Janus kinase 1 (9.1%), which might provide an option for novel individualized therapeutic interventions. Interestingly, Nault et al.,[48] using traditional Sanger sequencing, identified somatic mutations activating telomerase reverse transcriptase as both the earliest and the most frequent mutations in human preneoplastic lesions (25%) as well as hepatocellular carcinomas (59%) and is associated with activating CTNNB1 mutations.[48]

Compared to whole-genome sequencing, the application of RNA sequencing in liver cancer is currently limited to three studies. One study investigated the transcriptomes of 10 matched HBV-related HCC cases, identifying a total of 1,378 differentially expressed genes with a specific enrichment of chromosome location on 8q21.3 to 24.3.[49] Another study investigated three paired nontumor and tumor specimens demonstrating that ADAR1-mediated AZIN1 RNA editing is linked to tumor initiation and development in liver cancer.[50]

Sequential molecular alterations during human hepatocarcinogenesis from dysplastic lesions to eHCC and, ultimately, pHCC are not clearly defined. This lack of information represents a major challenge in the clinical management of patients at risk. Although recent results associating MYC activation with early stages of malignant conversion into HCC, detailed molecular sequences that drive premalignant lesions into pHCC still remain

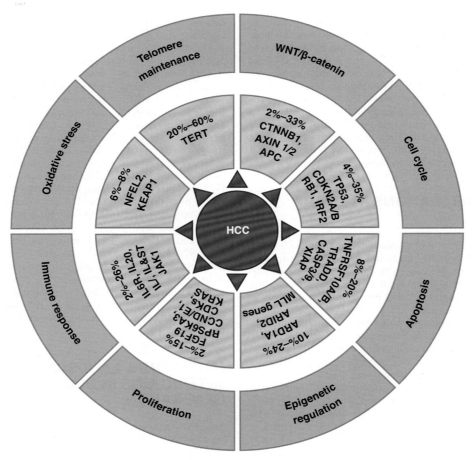

Figure 43.1 Major oncogenic pathways and genetic landscape in hepatocellular carcinoma (HCC). The scheme shows the major disrupted pathways in HCC patients (*outer circle*). The *inner circle* emphasizes the frequency of genetic alterations within the corresponding pathways and their putative contribution to hepatocarcinogenesis. Frequencies are based on results from recent whole genomic studies.[41–44] Representative members of each pathway most frequently altered in HCC are also shown.

to be clarified.[51] In the third study, integrative transcriptome sequencing to the tumor-free surrounding liver (n = 7), low-grade (n = 4) and high-grade dysplastic lesions (n = 9), eHCC (n = 5), and pHCC (n = 3) from eight HCC patients with HBV infections was applied.[52] The results of the study indicate that molecular profiles of dysplastic lesions and eHCC are quite uniform. In contrast, a sharp increase in heterogeneity on both mRNA and DNA levels is observed in progressed HCC. These molecular alterations result in massive deregulation of key oncogenic molecules such as transforming growth factor beta 1 (TGF-β1), MYC, PI3K/AKT, and suggest that activation of prognostically adverse signaling pathways is a late event during hepatocarcinogenesis (Fig. 43.2).

THE MICROENVIRONMENT OF LIVER CANCER

HCC develops on the basis of chronic liver disease and, in more than 80% of the cases, with preexisting liver cirrhosis. For a complete understanding of the molecular mechanisms of hepatocarcinogenesis, the underlying liver disease leading to a chronically altered inflamed liver microenvironment has to be appreciated.[53] Recent research efforts have focused on the identification of key factors that contribute to the disruption of the liver microenvironment and the generation of an adverse niche(s) that promotes he-

patocarcinogenesis. Among the most prominent factors involved in the so called inflammation-fibrosis-cancer axis is the nuclear factor kappa B (NF-κB) pathway.[54] The dominant role of this pathway for hepatocarcinogenesis is well documented.[54] However, the absence of NF-κB by genetic loss of the NF-κB master regulator *NEMO* significantly enhanced liver cancer development in a mouse model, indicating that inhibition of NF-κB may not only exert beneficial effects, but also may negatively impact hepatocyte viability, especially when NF-κB inhibition is pronounced.[55]

The importance of the microenvironment is further highlighted in a recent study demonstrating that transplantation of hepatic progenitor cells gave rise to cancer only when introduced into a liver with chronic damage and compensatory proliferation.[56] Interestingly, similar to observations made in human hepatocarcinogenesis, the cells resembling these progenitor cells quiescently resided within dysplastic lesions for several months before the appearance of HCC. During this time, the progenitor cells acquired autocrine interleukin (IL)-6 signaling that stimulated in vivo growth and malignant progression, which might be a general mechanism of progenitor cell–induced HCC.

However, the microenvironment does not only contribute to tumor initiation. Although gene-expression profiles of tumor tissue failed to yield a significant association with survival, a 186-gene signature generated from the surrounding nontumoral liver tissue was highly correlated with outcomes in a cohort of more than 300

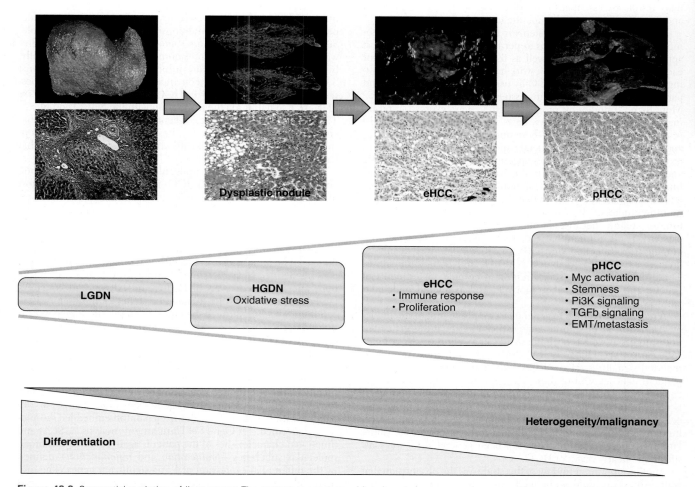

Figure 43.2 Sequential evolution of liver cancer. The current concept considers hepatocarcinogenesis as a multistep process that develops on the basis of a chronically altered microenvironment (i.e., cirrhosis) and progresses from dysplastic nodules (high grade and low grade) over early HCC to progressed HCC *(upper panels)*. On the molecular level, the different stages are characterized by progressive activation of signaling pathways related to oxidative stress, immune response, and proliferation *(middle panel)*. However, the activation of prognostically adverse signaling occurs late during the evolution of liver cancer. During this process, a progressive loss of differentiation with a concomitant acquisition of malignant and invasive properties is observed *(lower panel)*. LGDN, low-grade dysplastic nodule; HGDN, high-grade dysplastic nodule; EMT, epithelial-mesenchymal transition.

HCC patients.[57] Consistently, this poor-prognosis signature contained gene sets associated with inflammation, such as IFN signaling, NF-κB, and tumor necrosis factor α (TNF–α). Further, a gene set enrichment analysis showed that the downstream targets of IL-6 were strongly associated with the poor-prognosis signature, again confirming the importance of this signaling for hepatocarcinogenesis.

Together, these studies demonstrate the complexity of molecular mechanisms influencing the development and progression of liver cancer that are exerted by epigenetic and genetic alterations and a cross-talk between microenvironment and damaged hepatocytes and/or cancer cells, respectively.

CLASSIFICATION AND PROGNOSTIC PREDICTION OF HEPATOCELLULAR CARCINOMA

The application of microarray technologies to characterize tumors on the basis of global gene expression has had a significant impact on both basic and clinical oncology.[10] The goal of tumor microarray studies generally includes the discovery of subsets of tumors (class discovery), which enables diagnostic classification (class comparison), a prediction of clinical outcome (class prediction), and mechanistic analysis. Verification and validation of the primary results are essential for the discovery of oncogenic pathways and the identification of therapeutic targets.[8]

The goal of all staging systems is to separate patients into homogeneous prognostic groups to permit the selection of the most appropriate surveillance as well as to find a specific therapy for each subtype. Although much work has been devoted to establishing prognostic models for HCC by using clinical information and pathologic classification, many issues still remain unresolved.[58] More than 20 studies on prognostic HCC gene expression profiling, as well as several reviews, have appeared during the last 10 years.[4] However, results from these studies are quite heterogeneous and, besides disruption in general cancer-related processes such as proliferation, apoptosis, neoangiogenesis as well as prometastatic and proinflammatory gene sets, the overall similarity was low, thus limiting a successful implementation into clinical practice. A potential explanation is the fact that the interpretation of molecular profiling studies of HCC poses more challenges than other human tumors, mainly because of the complex pathogenesis of this cancer.[59] As already emphasized, HCC arises in diverse settings ranging from infection with HBV or HCV to chronic metabolic diseases as varied as diabetes, NAFLD, and hemochromatosis. These different disease stages represent complex assortments of genetic and epigenetic aberrations as well as altered molecular pathways.[39,60]

A recent study aimed to generate a composite prognostic model by evaluating 22 prognostic gene expression signatures generated from tumors as well as cirrhotic tissues in a cohort of 287 patients with early stage HCC (BCLC 0/A).[61] Overall, most previously reported signatures retained their prognostic ability in this independent data set. Out of these 22 signatures, 17 were able to adequately subclassify patients according to their prognostic trait. It is noteworthy that none of the signatures reflecting a progenitor cell origin (i.e., EpCAM, hepatoblastoma-C2, CK19-rat, CK19-human signature) could be confirmed to be of prognostic value. However, these signatures have not been generated for the classification of early stages of HCC.

Another important finding of this study was the observation that gene expression profiles obtained from paired biopsies from the center and periphery of the same tumor in 15 tumor specimens showed a high (>80%) transcriptomic concordance. Although these observation provide at least some evidence for stability of gene expression signatures in paired biopsies and suggests a low influence of sampling error, more in-depth analyses are needed to better define the intratumoral genetic heterogeneity of HCC that is likely to contribute to the high tumor recurrence and chemoresistance of the disease.[62,63]

Nault et al.[64] aimed to identifying a robust molecular signature to accurately predict the clinical outcome of HCC patients who underwent curative surgical resection. They identified a panel of five genes (TAF9, RAMP3, HN1, KRT19, and RAN) in a training cohort of 314 HCC patients with a strong prognostic relevance and further validated this panel in two independent validation cohorts with different HCC etiologies.[64] The five-genes panel was associated with disease-specific survival both in the training and in the validation cohort, and was found to be significantly more accurate in predicting the patients' prognosis (i.e., survival and recurrence) when compared to known gene expression signatures. Due to the simplicity of the panel and its reproducibility in different technologies (i.e., gene expression microarray and real-time reverse-transcription polymerase chain reaction [qRT-PCR]), the work by Nault et al. has a high potential for implementation into the clinical management of HCC. In particular, the score may be helpful to stratify patients at high risk for relapse and tumor-related death before the decision of liver resection or transplantation is made. However, independent validation of this prognostic algorithm by different groups and independent cohorts is needed before the panel can be used for clinical decision making.

Two independent studies provide evidence that the oncofetal marker SALL4 could be an attractive therapeutic target in HCC with progenitor cell origin.[65,66] High SALL4 expression was significantly associated with overall survival of patients in large independent cohorts. Further, and consistent with its oncofetal role, SALL4 overexpressing tumors shared similar molecular profiles with fetal progenitor cells and stemness-associated HCC. Finally, by using RNAi and a specific inhibitory 12-AA peptide against SALL4, the authors could convincingly show that SALL4 possessed therapeutic potential in HCC by interacting with PTEN/PI3K-AKT signaling via the interaction with the NuRD complex.[67] These studies confirm several recent observations indicating that HCCs harboring phenotypic features of stem/progenitor cells constitute a subclass of therapeutically challenged cancer patients that have a particularly poor prognosis.[27,68,69]

Contrary to HCCs, the molecular pathology of intrahepatic cholangiocellular carcinoma (ICC) is less well investigated. Most of the studies on cholangiocarcinogenesis focused on the investigation of few candidate genes.[70] In a seminal work on both genomic and genetic features of ICC gene expression, profiles of 104 surgically resected cholangiocarcinoma samples were collected and analyzed from patients in Australia, Europe, and the United States.[71] The authors discovered new two prognostic subclasses of patients defined by a 238-gene classifier as well as KRAS mutations and increased levels of EGFR and HER2, and concomitantly validated promising therapeutic strategies in different ICC cell lines, which resembled the different prognostic subtypes. Furthermore, this study also addressed the importance of the stromal component of ICC by laser capture microdissection of epithelial and stromal compartments from 23 tumors. Although the tumor epithelium was defined by deregulation of the HER2 network and frequent overexpression of EGFR, c-MET, pRPS6 as well as proliferation, the stroma was predominantly enriched for inflammatory gene sets. In another study, gene expression analyses of 149 patients with ICC from formalin-fixed paraffin-embedded samples were performed.[72] A Gene Set Enrichment Analysis (GSEA) and functional characteristics of the patients again revealed two broad molecular subclasses—proliferation and inflammation—defined by the differential expression of 1,565 significant genes. The proliferation class was associated with aggressive tumor biology as well as a poor prognosis and was characterized by molecular enrichment of oncogenic pathways (e.g., RAS/RAF/MAPK, VEGF, and PDGF). The inflammation class displayed a better prognosis and enrichment of immune-related signaling, in particular IL-10 and signal transducer and activator of transcription 3 (STAT3) signaling. Furthermore, a subgroup of ICCs in the proliferation class shared features of several previously published prognostic HCC signatures with a possible progenitor cell origin, which supported the hypothesis that these tumors may be derived from a common origin or precursor cell(s). This hypothesis is supported by recent work by Woo et al.,[73] which applied an integrative oncogenomic approach to address the clinical and functional implications of the overlapping phenotype of combined hepatocellular cholangiocarcinoma (CHC), a histopathologic intermediate between HCC and cholangiocellular carcinoma (CC).

CONCLUSION AND PERSPECTIVE

Next-generation technologies, in particular gene expression microarrays and, more recently, next-generation sequencing, have provided an extraordinary opportunity for integrative analyses of the cancer (epi-) genome as well as transcriptome. Array-based gene expression profiling not only has advanced our understanding of cancer biology, but also has begun to influence decision making in clinical oncology, which may ultimately allow for the development of more effective therapies. The power of gene expression profiling of HCC can be further enhanced by cross-comparison analyses of multiple gene expression data sets from human HCC and the rich database of HCC in animal models.[74,75] The success

of these new analytical approaches, comparative and/or integrative functional genomics, suggests that integration of independent data sets will enhance our ability to identify robust predictive markers. Despite the success of these approaches in preclinical translational studies, the clinical application of gene expression profiling is still immature. Although current signatures accurately classify HCCs according to their natural biology, they are unable to predict the response to currently used therapies.[59] Furthermore, HCC with progenitor cell features display a particular aggressive behavior, which might indicate that tumor heterogeneity and resulting chemoresistance might be generated in molecularly plastic cancer stem cells (CSCs).[76] Because CSCs by definition are a rare subpopulation of cells, their molecular profile might be diluted by the bulk of tumor cells, which further hampers therapeutic progress.[77] However, based on the exciting results of recent studies and the advent of NGS technologies that offer unprecedented depths and resolution, it seems reasonable to predict that the genomic technologies will play an increasingly important role in clinical oncology. The immediate focus undoubtedly will be on incorporating these whole-genomic technologies into clinical trials. To achieve this ambitious goal, systematic and standardized collections of tissue specimens from HCC patients (e.g., mandatory biopsies) for subsequent prospective molecular analyses are urgently needed to ultimately improve the diagnosis and treatment of liver cancer patients.

REFERENCES

1. El-Serag HB. Epidemiology of viral hepatitis and hepatocellular carcinoma. *Gastroenterology* 2012;142:1264–1273.e1.
2. El-Serag HB. Hepatocellular carcinoma. *N Engl J Med* 2011;365:1118–1127.
3. Bruix J, Sherman M, American Association for the Study of Liver D. Management of hepatocellular carcinoma: an update. *Hepatology* 2011;53:1020–1022.
4. Marquardt JU, Galle PR, Teufel A. Molecular diagnosis and therapy of hepatocellular carcinoma (HCC): an emerging field for advanced technologies. *J Hepatol* 2012;56:267–275.
5. Bruix J, Boix L, Sala M, et al. Focus on hepatocellular carcinoma. *Cancer Cell* 2004;5:215–219.
6. Thorgeirsson SS, Grisham JW. Molecular pathogenesis of human hepatocellular carcinoma. *Nature Genet* 2002;31:339–346.
7. Zender L, Villanueva A, Tovar V, et al. Cancer gene discovery in hepatocellular carcinoma. *J Hepatol* 2010;52:921–929.
8. Quackenbush J. Microarray analysis and tumor classification. *N Engl J Med* 2006;354:2463–2472.
9. Hood L, Heath JR, Phelps ME, et al. Systems biology and new technologies enable predictive and preventative medicine. *Science* 2004;306:640–643.
10. McDermott U, Downing JR, Stratton MR. Genomics and the continuum of cancer care. *N Engl J Med* 2011;364:340–350.
11. Vogelstein B, Papadopoulos N, Velculescu VE, et al. Cancer genome landscapes. *Science* 2013;339:1546–1558.
12. Meyerson M, Gabriel S, Getz G. Advances in understanding cancer genomes through second-generation sequencing. *Nat Rev Genet* 2010;11:685–696.
13. Krawczyk M, Mullenbach R, Weber SN, et al. Genome-wide association studies and genetic risk assessment of liver diseases. *Nat Rev Gastroenterol Hepatol* 2010;7:669–681.
14. Kumar V, Kato N, Urabe Y, et al. Genome-wide association study identifies a susceptibility locus for HCV-induced hepatocellular carcinoma. *Nat Genet* 2011;43:455–458.
15. Moinzadeh P, Breuhahn K, Stutzer H, et al. Chromosome alterations in human hepatocellular carcinomas correlate with aetiology and histological grade—results of an explorative CGH meta-analysis. *Br J Cancer* 2005;92:935–941.
16. Poon TC, Wong N, Lai PB, et al. A tumor progression model for hepatocellular carcinoma: bioinformatic analysis of genomic data. *Gastroenterology* 2006;131:1262–1270.
17. Su WH, Chao CC, Yeh SH, et al. OncoDB.HCC: an integrated oncogenomic database of hepatocellular carcinoma revealed aberrant cancer target genes and loci. *Nucleic Acids Res* 2007;35:D727–D731.
18. Woo HG, Park ES, Lee JS, et al. Identification of potential driver genes in human liver carcinoma by genomewide screening. *Cancer Res* 2009;69:4059–4066.
19. Lamb J. The Connectivity Map: a new tool for biomedical research. *Nat Rev Cancer* 2007;7:54–60.
20. Roessler S, Long EL, Budhu A, et al. Integrative genomic identification of genes on 8p associated with hepatocellular carcinoma progression and patient survival. *Gastroenterology* 2012;142:957–966.e12.
21. Feinberg AP. Phenotypic plasticity and the epigenetics of human disease. *Nature* 2007;447:433–440.
22. Feinberg AP, Ohlsson R, Henikoff S. The epigenetic progenitor origin of human cancer. *Nat Rev Genet* 2006;7:21–33.
23. Calvisi DF, Ladu S, Gorden A, et al. Mechanistic and prognostic significance of aberrant methylation in the molecular pathogenesis of human hepatocellular carcinoma. *J Clin Invest* 2007;117:2713–2722.
24. Hernandez-Vargas H, Lambert MP, Le Calvez-Kelm F, et al. Hepatocellular carcinoma displays distinct DNA methylation signatures with potential as clinical predictors. *PLoS One* 2010;5:e9749.
25. Lambert MP, Paliwal A, Vaissiere T, et al. Aberrant DNA methylation distinguishes hepatocellular carcinoma associated with HBV and HCV infection and alcohol intake. *J Hepatol* 2011;54:705–715.
26. Andersen JB, Factor VM, Marquardt JU, et al. An integrated genomic and epigenomic approach predicts therapeutic response to zebularine in human liver cancer. *Sci Transl Med* 2010;2:54ra77.
27. Lee JS, Heo J, Libbrecht L, et al. A novel prognostic subtype of human hepatocellular carcinoma derived from hepatic progenitor cells. *Nat Med* 2006;12:410–416.
28. Um TH, Kim H, Oh BK, et al. Aberrant CpG island hypermethylation in dysplastic nodules and early HCC of hepatitis B virus-related human multistep hepatocarcinogenesis. *J Hepatol* 2011;54:939–947.
29. Revill K, Wang T, Lachenmayer A, et al. Genome-wide methylation analysis and epigenetic unmasking identify tumor suppressor genes in hepatocellular carcinoma. *Gastroenterology* 2013;145:1424–1435.e1–25.
30. Esteller M. Epigenetics in cancer. *N Engl J Med* 2008;358:1148–1159.
31. Hoshida Y, Toffanin S, Lachenmayer A, et al. Molecular classification and novel targets in hepatocellular carcinoma: recent advancements. *Semin Liver Dis* 2010;30:35–51.
32. Lujambio A, Lowe SW. The microcosmos of cancer. *Nature* 2012;482:347–355.
33. Coulouarn C, Factor VM, Andersen JB, et al. Loss of miR-122 expression in liver cancer correlates with suppression of the hepatic phenotype and gain of metastatic properties. *Oncogene* 2009;28:3526–3536.
34. Mott JL. MicroRNAs involved in tumor suppressor and oncogene pathways: implications for hepatobiliary neoplasia. *Hepatology* 2009;50:630–637.
35. Ladeiro Y, Couchy G, Balabaud C, et al. MicroRNA profiling in hepatocellular tumors is associated with clinical features and oncogene/tumor suppressor gene mutations. *Hepatology* 2008;47:1955–1963.
36. Toffanin S, Hoshida Y, Lachenmayer A, et al. MicroRNA-based classification of hepatocellular carcinoma and oncogenic role of miR-517a. *Gastroenterology* 2011;140:1618–1628.e16.
37. Ji J, Shi J, Budhu A, et al. MicroRNA expression, survival, and response to interferon in liver cancer. *N Engl J Med* 2009;361:1437–1447.
38. Ji J, Yu L, Yu Z, et al. Development of a miR-26 companion diagnostic test for adjuvant interferon-alpha therapy in hepatocellular carcinoma. *Int J Biol Sci* 2013;9:303–312.
39. Arzumanyan A, Reis HM, Feitelson MA. Pathogenic mechanisms in HBV- and HCV-associated hepatocellular carcinoma. *Nat Rev Cancer* 2013;13:123–135.

40. Teufel A, Marquardt JU, Galle PR. Next generation sequencing of HCC from European and Asian HCC cohorts. Back to p53 and Wnt/beta-catenin. *J Hepatol* 2013;58:622–624.

41. Fujimoto A, Totoki Y, Abe T, et al. Whole-genome sequencing of liver cancers identifies etiological influences on mutation patterns and recurrent mutations in chromatin regulators. *Nat Genet* 2012;44:760–764.

42. Guichard C, Amaddeo G, Imbeaud S, et al. Integrated analysis of somatic mutations and focal copy-number changes identifies key genes and pathways in hepatocellular carcinoma. *Nat Genet* 2012;44:694–698.

43. Li M, Zhao H, Zhang X, et al. Inactivating mutations of the chromatin remodeling gene ARID2 in hepatocellular carcinoma. *Nat Genet* 2011;43:828–829.

44. Totoki Y, Tatsuno K, Yamamoto S, et al. High-resolution characterization of a hepatocellular carcinoma genome. *Nat Genet* 2011;43:464–469.

45. Toffanin S, Cornella H, Harrington A, et al. Next-generation sequencing: path for driver discovery in hepatocellular carcinoma. *Gastroenterology* 2012;143:1391–1393.

46. Cleary SP, Jeck WR, Zhao X, et al. Identification of driver genes in hepatocellular carcinoma by exome sequencing. *Hepatology* 2013;58:1693–1702.

47. Kan Z, Zheng H, Liu X, et al. Whole-genome sequencing identifies recurrent mutations in hepatocellular carcinoma. *Genome Res* 2013;23:1422–1433.

48. Nault JC, Mallet M, Pilati C, et al. High frequency of telomerase reverse-transcriptase promoter somatic mutations in hepatocellular carcinoma and preneoplastic lesions. *Nat Commun* 2013;4:2218.

49. Huang Q, Lin B, Liu H, et al. RNA-Seq analyses generate comprehensive transcriptomic landscape and reveal complex transcript patterns in hepatocellular carcinoma. *PLoS One* 2011;6:e26168.

50. Chen L, Li Y, Lin CH, et al. Recoding RNA editing of AZIN1 predisposes to hepatocellular carcinoma. *Nat Med* 2013;19:209–216.

51. Kaposi-Novak P, Libbrecht L, Woo HG, et al. Central role of c-Myc during malignant conversion in human hepatocarcinogenesis. *Cancer Res* 2009;69:2775–2782.

52. Marquardt JU, Seo D, Andersen JB, et al. Sequential transcriptome analysis of human liver cancer indicates late stage acquisition of malignant traits. *J Hepatol* 2014;60:346–353.

53. Hernandez-Gea V, Toffanin S, Friedman SL, et al. Role of the microenvironment in the pathogenesis and treatment of hepatocellular carcinoma. *Gastroenterology* 2013;144:512–527.

54. Karin M. Nuclear factor-kappaB in cancer development and progression. *Nature* 2006;441:431–436.

55. Luedde T, Schwabe RF. NF-kappaB in the liver—linking injury, fibrosis and hepatocellular carcinoma. *Nat Rev Gastroenterol Hepatol* 2011;8:108–118.

56. He G, Dhar D, Nakagawa H, et al. Identification of liver cancer progenitors whose malignant progression depends on autocrine IL-6 signaling. *Cell* 2013;155:384–396.

57. Hoshida Y, Villanueva A, Kobayashi M, et al. Gene expression in fixed tissues and outcome in hepatocellular carcinoma. *N Engl J Med.* 2008;359:1995–2004.

58. Thorgeirsson SS. Genomic decoding of hepatocellular carcinoma. *Gastroenterology* 2006;131:1344–1346.

59. Schirmacher P, Calvisi DF. Molecular diagnostic algorithms in hepatocellular carcinoma: dead-end street or light at the end of the tunnel? *Gastroenterology* 2013;145:49–53.

60. Farazi PA, DePinho RA. Hepatocellular carcinoma pathogenesis: from genes to environment. *Nat Rev Cancer* 2006;6:674–687.

61. Villanueva A, Hoshida Y, Battiston C, et al. Combining clinical, pathology, and gene expression data to predict recurrence of hepatocellular carcinoma. *Gastroenterology* 2011;140:1501–1512.e2.

62. Gerlinger M, Rowan AJ, Horswell S, et al. Intratumor heterogeneity and branched evolution revealed by multiregion sequencing. *N Engl J Med* 2012;366:883–892.

63. Teufel A, Marquardt JU, Galle PR. Novel insights in the genetics of HCC recurrence and advances in transcriptomic data integration. *J Hepatol* 2012;56:279–281.

64. Nault JC, De Reynies A, Villanueva A, et al. A hepatocellular carcinoma 5-gene score associated with survival of patients after liver resection. *Gastroenterology* 2013;145:176–187.

65. Oikawa T, Kamiya A, Zeniya M, et al. Sal-like protein 4 (SALL4), a stem cell biomarker in liver cancers. *Hepatology* 2013;57:1469–1483.

66. Yong KJ, Gao C, Lim JS, et al. Oncofetal gene SALL4 in aggressive hepatocellular carcinoma. *N Engl J Med* 2013;368:2266–2276.

67. Marquardt JU, Thorgeirsson SS. Sall4 in "stemness"-driven hepatocarcinogenesis. *N Engl J Med* 2013;368:2316–2318.

68. Marquardt JU, Raggi C, Andersen JB, et al. Human hepatic cancer stem cells are characterized by common stemness traits and diverse oncogenic pathways. *Hepatology* 2011;54:1031–1042.

69. Yamashita T, Forgues M, Wang W, et al. EpCAM and alpha-fetoprotein expression defines novel prognostic subtypes of hepatocellular carcinoma. *Cancer Res* 2008;68:1451–1461.

70. Andersen JB, Thorgeirsson SS. Genetic profiling of intrahepatic cholangiocarcinoma. *Curr Opin Gastroenterol* 2012;28:266–272.

71. Andersen JB, Spee B, Blechacz BR, et al. Genomic and genetic characterization of cholangiocarcinoma identifies therapeutic targets for tyrosine kinase inhibitors. *Gastroenterology* 2012;142:1021–1031.e15.

72. Sia D, Hoshida Y, Villanueva A, et al. Integrative molecular analysis of intrahepatic cholangiocarcinoma reveals 2 classes that have different outcomes. *Gastroenterology* 2013;144:829–840.

73. Woo HG, Lee JH, Yoon JH, et al. Identification of a cholangiocarcinoma-like gene expression trait in hepatocellular carcinoma. *Cancer Res* 2010;70:3034–3041.

74. Lee JS, Chu IS, Heo J, et al. Classification and prediction of survival in hepatocellular carcinoma by gene expression profiling. *Hepatology* 2004;40:667–676.

75. Lee JS, Thorgeirsson SS. Comparative and integrative functional genomics of HCC. *Oncogene* 2006;25:3801–3809.

76. Marquardt JU, Thorgeirsson SS. Stem cells in hepatocarcinogenesis: evidence from genomic data. *Semin Liver Dis* 2010;30:26–34.

77. Marquardt JU, Factor VM, Thorgeirsson SS. Epigenetic regulation of cancer stem cells in liver cancer: current concepts and clinical implications. *J Hepatol* 2010;53:568–577.

44 Cancer of the Liver

Yuman Fong, Damian E. Dupuy, Mary Feng, and Ghassan Abou-Alfa

CANCERS OF THE GASTROINTESTINAL TRACT

INTRODUCTION

Primary cancers of the liver represent the fifth most common malignancy worldwide and the second most common cause of death from cancer. This is due the relationship of hepatocellular carcinoma to chronic hepatitis B virus (HBV) and hepatitis C virus (HCV) infections.[1] The prognosis of untreated hepatocellular carcinoma (HCC) has a dismal prognosis, with a 5-year survival rate below 10%.[2] The combination of cancer and chronic liver disease add significant complexity to treatment. The great progress in understanding the natural history, pathogenesis, and tumor biology of HCC has resulted in effective treatment options. For localized HCC, surgical resection and orthotopic liver transplantation (OLT) are the gold standard therapies. Formidable radiologic directed local and regional therapies, radiation therapy, and systemic therapies now round out a full arsenal of treatments even for disseminated disease. There have also been marked advances in therapies for hepatitis[3] and in care of the associated liver parenchymal disease. However, this optimism may be negated by the continued lack of a true breakthrough in screening and early detection, and the continued rising incidence of HCC globally.

EPIDEMIOLOGY

The annual number of worldwide liver cancer cases (748,300) closely resembles the number of deaths (695,900). Long-term survival rates are 3% to 5% in most cancer registries. In the United States, approximately 30,640 new tumors of the liver and intrahepatic bile ducts are diagnosed each year, with 21,670 deaths estimated annually.[1] HCC is 2.3 times more common in men than in women, and this difference is consistent globally. Androgen and androgen receptor (AR) have long been implicated in this male-dominance feature.[4] In the United States, rates of HCC are two times higher in Asians than African Americans, which are two times higher than those in Caucasians. There has been a significant overall increase in the incidence of HCC in the United States during the past 25 years.[5] This parallels the increase in HCV infection, the increase in immigrants from HBV-endemic countries, and an increase in nonalcoholic fatty liver disease. The widespread utilization of HBV vaccination is leading to a decrease in liver cancer in some areas. A dramatic demonstration of this is available from Taiwan, where an HBV vaccine was introduced in 1984, and a reduction of liver cancer was observed in children from 0.54 per 100,000 to 0.2 per 100,000 during a 16-year period.[6]

ETIOLOGIC FACTORS

Viral Hepatitis and Hepatocellular Carcinoma

The variable geographic incidence of liver cancer[7] reflects the variable geographic incidence in HCV and HBV infections, which account for 75% of the world's cases. Both case control studies and cohort studies have shown a strong association between chronic hepatitis B carriage rates and increased incidence of HCC. Beasley et al.[8] followed Taiwanese male postal carriers who were hepatitis B surface antigen (HBsAg)-positive and found an annual HCC incidence of 495 per 100,000. This represented a 98-fold greater risk than observed in HBsAg-negative individuals. By evaluating apparently asymptomatic HBsAg-positive blood donors at American Red Cross centers, a relative risk of 12.7 was noted for liver cancer compared with HBsAg-negative individuals. A multivariate analysis has been used to determine *risk scores* for the development of HCC.[9] Factors predictive of HCC include male gender, advanced age, specific promoter mutations, the presence of cirrhosis, and higher viremia levels. If validated, this may improve patient selection for surveillance.

The exact mechanism by which HBV infection causes HCC is not known.[10,11] Some have postulated that the effect of HBV on hepatic carcinogenesis is indirect, through the process of inflammation, regeneration, and fibrosis associated with chronic hepatitis and cirrhosis. Consistent with this hypothesis, 70% of cases of HBV-related HCC occur in association with cirrhosis. It is well known that cirrhosis of all causes may result in HCC.

There is evidence that the effect may be a direct viral effect. HBV DNA may become integrated within the chromosomes of infected hepatocytes, and in some HCCs, this integration of viral genetic material may occur in a critical location within the cellular genome. For example, integration of HBV DNA has been observed within the retinoic acid receptor alpha gene and within the human cyclin A gene, both of which play crucial roles in cellular growth. However, in most cases, the HBV DNA integration appears to be random. The hepatitis B x gene (*HBx*) product has been implicated in causing HCC because it is a transcriptional activator of various cellular genes associated with growth control. *HBx* has been found to interact with *p53*, interfering with its function as a tumor suppressor.

HCV is an RNA virus without a DNA intermediate form, and therefore, cannot integrate into hepatocyte DNA. In contrast to HBV, HCV is more likely to lead to chronic infection (10% versus 60% to 80%), and cirrhosis (20-fold increase).[12] The typical interval between HCV-associated transfusion and subsequent HCC is only about 30 years (compared with 40 to 50 years for HBV). The state of the liver also differs in that HCV-associated HCC patients tend to have more frequent and more advanced cirrhosis. In HBV-associated HCC, only half the patients have cirrhosis. The risk of developing HCC in a patient with HCV-related cirrhosis is 5% per year versus 0.5% per year for HBV-related cirrhosis.

There have been extensive efforts to establish the molecular pathways involved in the pathogenesis of HCC.[13,14] Some of the abnormalities that are commonly found in HCC include (1) cell-cycle dysregulation associated with somatic mutations or loss of heterozygosity in *TP53*, silencing of *CDKN2A* or *RB1*, or *CCND1* overexpression; (2) increased angiogenesis accompanied by overexpression or amplification of *VEGF*, *PDGF*, and *ANGPT2*; (3) evasion of apoptosis as a result of activation of survival signals such as nuclear factor kappa B (NF-κB); and (4) reactivation of *TERT*.

There is emerging evidence of the importance of microRNAs and epigenetic alterations such as hypermethylation in the pathogenesis of HCC. MicroRNA-155 (miR-155) levels were significantly increased in patients infected with HCV, and overexpression of miR-155 was associated with nuclear accumulation of beta-catenin by increased Wnt signaling, thereby implicating this pathway in HCV-associated hepatocellular carcinogenesis.[15]

Alcohol-Induced Hepatocarcinogenesis

There is a strong association between alcoholic cirrhosis and the development of HCC. By itself, chronic alcohol consumption has carcinogenic effects. Thus, chronic alcohol intake is known to lead to oxidative stress in the liver, inflammation, and cirrhosis. Ethanol is metabolized by alcohol dehydrogenases and cytochrome P-450, producing acetaldehyde and reactive oxygen species. Acetaldehyde binds directly to proteins and DNA. It damages mitochondria, initiating apoptosis. P-450 metabolism leads to reactive oxygen species, which lead to lipid consumption peroxidation, protein oxidation, and DNA adducts.[16] Alcohol leads to monocyte activation and inflammatory cytokine production. Oxidative stress has been demonstrated in alcoholic cirrhosis through increased isoprostane, a marker of lipid peroxidation.[17] Oxidative stress promotes the development of fibrosis and cirrhosis, creating a permissive HCC microenvironment. Oxidative stress may also lead to decreased Signal Transducers and Activators of Transcription 1 (STAT1)-directed activation of interferon gamma (IFNγ) signaling with consequent hepatocyte damage.[18]

Nonalcoholic Fatty Liver Disease

HCC has been linked to nonalcoholic fatty liver disease (NAFLD). NAFLD is present in 30% of the general adult population, in 90% of morbidly obese adults (body mass index [BMI] $\geq$40 kg/m^2), and in close to 74% of those with diabetes.[19–21] The risk of HCC due to NAFLD appears to be less than that of chronic hepatitis C. A recent US study reported a 2.6% yearly cumulative incidence of HCC in NAFLD and 4% in HCV cirrhosis.[22] Similarly, a prospective 5-year study from Japan reported a rate of HCC of 11.3% among patients with NAFLD cirrhosis compared to 30.5% among those with HCV-associated cirrhosis.[23] A recent study from Germany identified nonalcoholic steatohepatitis (NASH) as the most common etiology of HCC (24%), surpassing chronic hepatitis C (23.3%), chronic hepatitis B (19.3%), and alcoholic liver disease (12.7%).[24]

Diabetes and obesity have been established as independent risk factors for HCC, and that association holds true in the setting of NAFLD and associated NASH.[25,26] However, there is also increasing evidence suggesting that NAFLD contributes to noncirrhotic HCC, and that HCC can develop in patients with metabolic syndrome and NAFLD in the absence of NASH and fibrosis.[27]

Other Etiologic Considerations

In addition to alcoholic cirrhosis and viral hepatitis, several underlying conditions have been found to be associated with an increased risk for the development of HCC (Table 44.1). These include autoimmune chronic active hepatitis, cryptogenic cirrhosis, and metabolic diseases. Metabolic diseases include hemochromatosis (iron accumulation), Wilson disease (copper accumulation), α$_1$-antitrypsin deficiency, tyrosinemia, porphyria cutanea tarda, glycogenesis types 1 and 3, citrullinemia, and orotic acid urea. In children, congenital cholestatic syndrome (Alagille syndrome) is associated with a familial type of HCC.

Chemical Carcinogens

Probably the best-studied and most potent ubiquitous natural chemical carcinogen is a product of the *Aspergillus* fungus,

TABLE 44.1

Conditions Associated with Human Hepatocellular Carcinoma

Condition	Risk
Cirrhosis	
Hepatitis B virus	High
Hepatitis C virus	High
Alcohol	High
Autoimmune chronic active hepatitis	High
Cryptogenic cirrhosis	High
Cirrhosis due to nonalcoholic fatty liver disease	High
Primary biliary cirrhosis	Low
Hereditary hemochromatosis	High
α$_1$-Antitrypsin deficiency	High
Wilson disease	Low
Metabolic Diseases (without Cirrhosis)	
Hereditary tyrosinemia	High
α$_1$-Antitrypsin deficiency	Moderate
Ataxia telangiectasia	Moderate
Types 1 and 3 glycogen storage disease	Moderate
Galactosemia	Moderate
Citrullinemia	Moderate
Hereditary hemorrhagic telangiectasia	Moderate
Porphyria cutanea tarda	Moderate
Orotic aciduria	Moderate
Alagille syndrome (congenital cholestatic syndrome)	Moderate
Environmental	
Thorotrast	Moderate
Androgenic steroids	Moderate
Cigarette smoking	Low to moderate
Aflatoxin	Moderate

called aflatoxin B$_1$.[28] *Aspergillus flavus* mold and aflatoxin product can be found in a variety of stored grains, particularly in hot, humid parts of the world, where grains such as rice are stored in unrefrigerated conditions. In the months following the monsoons in Southeast Asia, most village-based grains can be seen to be covered by a white layer of aflatoxin that is consumed with the grain. Data on aflatoxin contamination of foodstuffs correlate well with incidence rates of HCC in Africa and to some extent in China.

There is considerable literature on the hepatocarcinogenicity of anabolic steroids as well as the induction of benign adenomas by estrogens.[29] Although estrogens are capable of causing HCC in rodents, an epidemiologic association in humans has never been clearly shown. In an industrial society, a large number of environmental pollutants, particularly pesticides and insecticides, are known rodent hepatic carcinogens. In a recent case-control study, cumulative lifetime tobacco use of more than 11,000 packs and Asian ethnicity were independent predictors of HCC development amongst a cohort of patients with chronic liver disease, including HCV.[30]

STAGING

Multiple clinical staging systems for hepatic tumors have been described. The most widely used is the American Joint Committee on Cancer/tumor-node-metastasis (AJCC/TNM) (Table 44.2).[31] Adverse prognostic features include large size, multiple tumors, vascular invasion, and lymph node spread. Macroscopic or microscopic vascular invasions, in particular, have profound effects on prognosis. Stage III disease contains a mixture of lymph node–positive and –negative tumors. Stage III patients with positive lymph node or stage IV disease have a poor prognosis, and few patients survive 1 year.

The prognosis in patients with HCC is very much influenced by the presence and severity of underlying liver disease as well. The Child-Pugh scoring system is the most commonly used tool for assessing cirrhosis (see Table 44.2).[32] It encompasses five parameters—bilirubin, albumin, prothrombin time, clinical ascites, and clinical encephalopathy—each of which is scored from one to three depending on severity. The key limitation of the Child-Pugh scoring system is its lack of any parameters pertaining to the cancer itself. Despite that, it remains incorporated into many HCC clinical trials as a tool to measure the extent of liver disease in the study populations, and thus, its use may not fade away any time soon. However, this main limitation of the Child-Pugh scoring system has been overcome by other scoring systems. Among those, the first to be established is the Okuda staging system. The

TABLE 44.2A

Staging for Liver Function and Cancer: American Joint Commission on Cancer Staging for Hepatocellular Cancer

T	TX	Primary tumor cannot be assessed		
	T0	No evidence of primary tumor		
	T1	Solitary tumor without vascular invasion		
	T2	Solitary tumor with vascular invasion, or multiple tumors no more than 5 cm		
	T3a	Multiple tumors more than 5 cm		
	T3b	Tumor involving a major branch of the portal or hepatic vein(s)		
	T4	Tumor(s) with direct invasion of adjacent organs other than the gallbladder or with perforation of visceral peritoneum		
N	NX	Regional lymph nodes cannot be assessed		
	N0	No regional lymph node metastasis		
	N1	Regional lymph node metastasis		
M	MX	Distant metastasis cannot be assessed		
	M0	No distant metastasis		
	M1	Distant metastasis		
Stage Grouping				
I	T1	N0	M0
II	T2	N0	M0
IIIA	T3a	N0	M0
IIIB	T3b	N0	M0
IIIC	T4	N0	M0
IVA	Any T	N1	M0
IVB	Any T	Any N	M1

Edge SB, Byrd DR, Compton CC, et al., eds. *The American Joint Committee on Cancer: AJCC Cancer Staging Manual*, 7th ed. New York:Springer;2010:197.

TABLE 44.2B

Child-Pugh Grading of Cirrhosis[a]

Measurement	1 Point	2 Points	3 Points
Bilirubin (mg/dL)	1–1.9	2–2.9	>2.9
Prolongation of PT	1–3	4–6	>6
Albumin (g/dL)	>3.5	2.8–3.4	<2.8
Ascites	None	Mild	Moderate/severe
Encephalopathy	None	Grade 1 or 2	Grade 3 or 4

[a] Grade A = 5–6 points; grade B = 7–9 points; grade C = 10–15 points. PT, prothrombin time.

Cancer of the Liver Italian Program (CLIP) score was defined and studied prospectively in patients with HCC mainly caused by HCV.[33,34] The CLIP score consists of the Child-Pugh score parameters combined with a subjective assessment of tumor in the liver, the presence or absence of portal vein thrombosis, and the alpha-fetoprotein (AFP) level. The addition of vascular endothelial growth factor levels to the CLIP parameters (V-CLIP) has been shown to provide a significantly more precise prognosis, but has yet to be prospectively validated.[35] The Chinese University Prognostic Index (CUPI) scoring system was developed in patients with mainly HBV-related HCC.[36] The CUPI parameters are bilirubin, ascites, AFP, alkaline phosphatase, the tumor extent (AJCC/TNM 5th edition), and clinical symptoms at presentation. A French system called the Groupe d'Etude et de Traitement du Carcinoma Hepatocellulaire (GETCH) staging system consists of bilirubin, Karnofsky performance score, AFP, alkaline phosphatase, and portal vein thrombosis.[37] Another scoring system that is mainly used in Japan is the Japan Integrated Staging (JIS) score.[38]

Another commonly used scoring system is the Barcelona Clinic Liver Cancer (BCLC) classification system.[39] The BCLC couples prognosis with treatment assignment and has been validated prospectively.[40] However, it has been shown to be less valuable in the setting of more advanced disease, defined as BCLC category C.[41,42] In retrospective analyses of patients with advanced-stage HCC seen by medical oncologists, the CLIP scoring system was noted to be the most informative regarding the outcome of this specific patient population.

DIAGNOSIS

The tests used to diagnose HCC include radiologic studies and pathologic diagnosis with biopsy. Core biopsies are most preferred because of the tissue architecture given by this technique. For patients suspected of having portal vein involvement, a core biopsy of the portal vein may be performed.[43] Morphologic features, such as stromal invasion, help distinguish high-grade dysplastic nodules from HCC.[44]

The American Association for the Study of Liver Diseases (AASLD),[45] and the European Association for the Study of the Liver (EASL)[46] have outlined noninvasive criteria for the diagnosis of HCC. EASL recommends that lesions that are greater than 2 cm with characteristic radiologic features of arterial hyperenhancement on two different imaging modalities, or on one imaging modality alongside with a serum AFP of 400 ng/dL or more, are diagnostic of HCC, and no biopsy is needed. The AASLD added venous washout as a requisite radiologic feature. Detection of a lesion larger than 2 cm that exhibits both arterial hyperenhancement and venous washout in a single imaging modality concomitant with an AFP >200 ng/mL is sufficient to diagnose HCC.[47] Bialecki et al.[48] found a sensitivity and specificity of 89.1% and 100%, respectively, for liver biopsy compared to 64.9% and 62.8%, respectively, for the noninvasive EASL criteria. The fear of biopsy-related hemorrhage is dissuaded by a 0.4% rate, and tumor seeding occurs at a low rate of 1.6%. When seeding does occur, it can be treated by local resection and is seldom a cause of morbidity and mortality.[49,50]

TREATMENT OF HEPATOCELLULAR CARCINOMA

Many treatment options for HCC are available (Table 44.3). Resection and liver transplantation represent the potentially curative options with the longest track record. For small tumors, ablation and radiotherapy (RT) are quite effective and may be curative.

Surgical Resection for Hepatocellular Carcinoma

Patient Selection

Liver resection is the preferred treatment for the noncirrhotic patient with HCC. These patients generally have normal liver function, no portal hypertension, and can tolerate major liver resections with acceptable morbidity and low mortality. The selection of noncirrhotic patients with HCC for resection is as for other malignant lesions. Resection should be considered for patients where a complete resection of tumor is possible while preserving greater than 30% functional liver. If the potential remnant liver volume may be less than 30%, portal vein embolization is now a well-accepted preoperative preparatory method for increasing the potential remnant liver volume and safety of the resection.[51]

For cirrhotic patients, the primary determinant of outcome and selection of therapy is the degree of hepatic dysfunction and portal hypertension. Traditionally, only compensated cirrhotics

---

TABLE 44.3

Treatment Options for Hepatocellular Carcinoma

- Surgery
  - Partial hepatectomy
  - Liver transplantation

- Local ablative therapies
  - Cryosurgery
  - Microwave ablation
  - Ethanol injection
  - Acetic acid injection
  - Radiofrequency ablation

- Regional therapies: hepatic artery transcatheter treatments
  - Transarterial chemotherapy
  - Transarterial embolization
  - Transarterial chemoembolization
  - Transarterial yttrium-90 microspheres
  - Transarterial ^{131}I-lipiodol
  - Proton or carbon ion therapy
  - Conformal radiation therapy
  - Stereotactic radiation therapy
  - Palliative low-dose radiation therapy

- Systemic therapies
  - Chemotherapy
  - Targeted therapy (sorafenib)[a]
  - Immunotherapy
  - Hormonal therapy

- Supportive care

[a] Sorafenib is the only systemic therapy with level 1 evidence, proving a survival benefit.

(Child-Turcotte-Pugh class A) were candidates for hepatic resection, whereas patients with significant hepatic functional dysfunction (Child class B or C) are generally not selected for resection because of poor outcome.[51] Portal hypertension can be indirectly assessed clinically by the presence of splenomegaly, esophagogastric varices, and thrombocytopenia (platelet count <100.000/mm^3) or directly determined by hepatic venous wedge pressures (≥ 10 mmHg). With recent advances in perioperative care, there is growing evidence that liver resection for HCC in well-selected patients with mild portal hypertension is safe and can achieve a comparable outcome as in patients without portal hypertension.[52,53]

The future remnant liver mass is another important factor to be considered in cirrhotic patients before resection. A too small remnant liver volume is associated with an increased risk for postresectional liver failure.[54] There is a general consensus that the critical remnant liver volume in cirrhotic patients is 50%,[55] and portal vein embolization should be considered if the future remnant liver volume is expected to be below 50%.[56–59] Some investigators have even attempted to sequential employ transarterial chemoembolization (TACE) to control the tumor or portal vein embolization (PVE) to increase residual liver volume, followed by definitive surgical resection.[56,57] The sequential use of TACE and PVE results in more efficient hypertrophy of the future remnant liver compared to PVE alone.[51]

In other parts of the world, dynamic liver function tests are also employed for the assessment of suitability for liver resection. These include the indocyanine green (ICG) test and technetium-99m diethylenetriaminepentaacetic acid-galactosyl human serum albumin (technetium-99m galactosyl human serum albumin [99mTc-GSA] scintigraphy).[51,55] An ICG retention rate of less than 14% proved to be a safe indicator for major hepatectomy in cirrhotic patients, whereas retention rates above 20% are considered a contraindication for major hepatectomy.[60–62]

Patient medical comorbidities considered are similar to an assessment for any major surgery. Some studies have reported age and gender to be independent risk factors for poor outcome after resection of HCC.[63] Other studies indicate that advanced age is more a surrogate for medical fitness, and that, with careful patient selection, elderly patients benefit as much from resection as younger patients.[64] Comorbidities as represented by American Society of Anesthesia (ASA) grade have been shown to correlate with survival.[65]

Outcomes of Resection and Prognostic Factors

With improving patient selection and perioperative care, the outcome of hepatic resection for HCC has been continuously improved during the past 2 decades. Many large series of the past 10 years show that resection is associated with a perioperative mortality rate of less than 7%, and patients achieve an overall survival rate of 30% to 50% (Table 44.4).[65–75] Many major centers are recently reporting operative mortalities less than 2%,[68,70,74] even in cirrhotic patients.

Tumor factors most important for outcome are TNM staging at presentation, macro- and microvascular invasion, and the number of tumors. Large HCC has a propensity for vascular invasion and growth of tumor intraluminally. This is associated with intrahepatic satellite metastases via the portal venous system and is frequently associated with small satellite tumors. Intraluminal spread through the hepatic veins leads to pulmonary metastases.

One surgical factor prognostic for outcome is surgical margins. There is no clear margin size that has been universally agreed upon, but there is consensus on importance of an R0 resection.[76] Most surgeons prefer at least a 1-cm margin. In one 225 patient study, a 1-cm margin was associated with a 77% 3-year survival versus 21% for those with less than a 1-cm margin.[72] It must be noted that in a randomized controlled trial, a 2-cm margin was associated with a decrease in recurrence as well as improved survival.[77] Studies have demonstrated improved outcome for anatomic versus nonanatomic resections for HCC.[78] In a series of 210 patients, 5-year survival rates were 66% for anatomic versus 35% in

TABLE 44.4

Results of Surgical Resection for Hepatocellular Carcinoma

First Author	Year Published	Number of Patients	Cirrhosis	Minor Resections[a]	Mortality	5-Year Overall Survival Rate
Zhou[66]	2001	2,366	—	72%	2.7%	50%
Kanematsu[68]	2002	303	55%	76%	1.6%	51%
Belghiti[67]	2002	328	50%	—	6.4%	37%
Wayne[69]	2002	249	73%	73%	6.1%	41%
Ercolani[65]	2003	224	100%	—	—	42%
Wu[70]	2005	426	100%	55%	1.6%	46%–61%[b]
Capussotti[71]	2005	216	100%	24%	8.3%	34%
Hasegawa[72]	2005	210	39%	—	0.0%	35%–66%[b]
Nathan[73]	2009	788	—	—	—	39%
Yang[74]	2009	481	77%	—	1.7%	20%–48%[b]
Wang[75]	2010	438	—	—	7.5%	43%

Note: Selected series with more than 200 patients over the past decade. Areas marked by a dash are not defined.
[a] Minor resections are defined as ≤ segmentectomy.
[b] Range of 5-year overall survival among different subgroups.

nonanatomic resections.[72] For small solitary tumors, anatomic resections seem to be less important.[79] Choice of margin and the anatomic approach for cancer clearance must be weighed against better perioperative outcome for limited parenchymal resection in cirrhotic patients.

Liver Transplantation for Hepatocellular Carcinoma

Patient Selection

Theoretically, liver transplantation is the ideal therapy for HCC in cirrhotic patients because it treats both the cancer as well as the underlying parenchymal disease. However, early experience with transplants produced dismal results. Bismuth et al.[80] was one of the first groups to consider that, in advanced disease, the likelihood of systemic disease was so high that recurrence rates, and therefore long-term outcomes, were unacceptably poor. They demonstrated that patients with limited disease (uninodular or binodular <3 cm tumors) had much better outcomes with transplant than resection (83% 5-year survival versus 18%).[80]

The landmark works of Mazzaferro et al.[81] have defined the most commonly used criteria for the selection of patients with HCC for transplantation. In their paper they defined the Milan criteria for transplantation as a single tumor less than 5 cm or three or fewer tumors all individually less than 3 cm (Fig. 44.1). Using these criteria for selection, patients transplanted had a very favorable outcome, including a 4-year actuarial survival rate of 85% and a recurrence-free survival rate of 92%. The suitability of these criteria for the selection of patients for transplant has been confirmed by numerous studies (Table 44.5).[81–94]

The excellent outcomes of HCC patients within the Milan criteria led many to explore more expansive and inclusive criteria.[90] The most accepted of the expanded criteria is that from the University of California San Francisco (UCSF) group. They reported excellent results after transplant for solitary tumor ≤6.5 cm, three or fewer nodules with the largest ≤4.5 cm, and total tumor diameter ≤8 cm (see Fig. 44.1). The UCSF criteria was associated with a survival of 90% and 75% at 1 and 5 years, respectively.[90,95]

The largest experience to date using transplantation for HCC was reported from the University of California, Los Angeles

(UCLA).[96] In this study of 467 transplants performed for HCC, the overall 1-, 3-, and 5-year survivals were 82%, 65%, and 52%, respectively. Transplanted patients with tumors beyond the UCSF criteria had a survival below 50%.

Living Donor Liver Transplant

Because of the shortage of cadaveric livers, living donor liver transplant (LDLT) has become an increasingly utilized modality for the treatment of patients with decompensated cirrhosis. In many Asian countries, where prevalence of HCC is high, living related transplants are the most common liver transplants performed. Survival

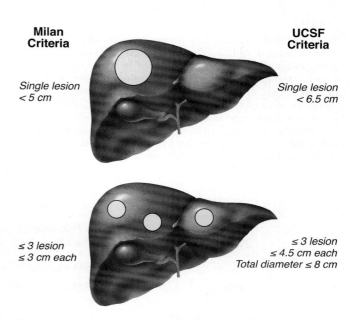

Figure 44.1 Milan (single lesion ≤5 cm, or no more than 3 lesions ≤3 cm) and University of California, San Francisco (UCSF) criteria (single lesion ≤6.5 cm, or no more than 3 lesions ≤4.5 cm and a total diameter of 8 cm) for patients with HCC and who are undergoing liver transplantation.

TABLE 44.5

Results of Liver Transplantation for Early Hepatocellular Carcinoma

Study	Number of Patients	Tumor Number and Size	Neoadjuvant Therapy	Survival (%)[a]
Mazzaferro et al., 2009[81]	444	1 ≤5 cm; 3 ≤3 cm	None	73
	1,112	Beyond Milan criteria	None	54
Pelletier et al., 2009[85]	2,790	1≤5 cm; 3 ≤3 cm	None	61
	346	Beyond Milan criteria	None	32
Herrero et al., 2008[86]	47	1 ≤5 cm; 3 ≤3 cm	None	70
	26	Beyond Milan criteria	None	73
Onaca et al., 2007[87]	631	1 ≤5 cm; 3 ≤3 cm	None	62 (5 y RFS)
	575	Beyond Milan criteria	None	43 (5 y RFS)
Decaens et al., 2006[88]	279	1 ≤5 cm; 3 ≤3 cm	None	60
	44	UCSF criteria	None	46
	145	Beyond UCSF criteria	None	35
Bigourdan et al., 2003[89]	17	1 ≤5 cm; 3 ≤3 cm	TACE	71
Yao et al., 2001[90]	46	1 ≤5 cm; 3 ≤3 cm	TACE/ETOH	72
Tamura et al., 2001[91]	56	<5 cm	± TACE	71
Regalia et al., 2001[92]	122	1 ≤5 cm; 3 ≤3 cm	TACE	80
Jonas et al., 2001[93]	120	1 ≤5 cm; 3 ≤3 cm	None	71
Llovet et al., 1998[94]	58	<5 cm	None	74
Mazzaferro et al., 1996[81]	48	1 ≤5 cm; 3 ≤3 cm	TACE	75 (4 y)

[a] All are 5-year survivals, except where noted.
RFS, recurrence-free survival; ETOH, alcohol.

outcomes for all patients undergoing LDLT are comparable to the results with deceased donors (Table 44.6).[97–102] The disadvantage is clearly the risk to the living donor, with morbidity as high as 40% and a 0.5% mortality. The greatest concern is that LDLT may encourage transplants for patients with unfavorable biology (outside of the established Milan or UCSF criteria) and pose unjustified risk to two lives, including the healthy individual.

Multimodality Management While Awaiting Transplant

To qualify for the wait list, a biopsy or one of the following criteria must be fulfilled: AFP >200 mg/mL, arteriogram confirming the tumor or arterial enhancement followed by portal venous washout on computed tomography (CT) scans or magnetic resonance imaging (MRI), or a history of local–regional treatment. Patients should be assessed radiologically for number and size of tumors, to rule out extrahepatic disease and vascular involvement. Patients with tumors less than 2 cm in size or patients who do not qualify for the Milan criteria can be listed for transplant, but they will receive no additional priority points for the tumor. The tumor should

be assessed every 3 months by CT scans or MRI to rule out progression of disease beyond the established criteria.

To reduce the likelihood of tumor progression while on the wait list, many local treatments are used, including TACE, percutaneous radiofrequency ablation (RFA), or percutaneous ethanol injection (PEI). TACE involves selective embolization of the arterial feeding vessels for the hepatoma with occlusive particles with or without admixed chemotherapeutic agents. TACE limits wait list dropout, decreases posttransplant recurrence, and can downstage HCC that is beyond transplant criteria.[103] A dropout rate of 14% was found in a series of patients treated with TACE as bridge to transplant, which compared very favorably to a dropout rate of 38% for an untreated group of patients reported by the Barcelona Liver Cancer study group.[104,105]

For small, solitary tumor, PEI[106] or RFA can be effective treatment options for use as a bridge to transplant. In a series of 52 patients treated with RFA, the dropout rate was 6% at 12 months due to tumor progression with a 3-year disease-free survival of 76% for the 41 patients eventually transplanted.[107] Mazzaferro et al.[108] reported no dropout for their patients treated with RFA as bridge to transplant, with a 3-year survival of 83%.

TABLE 44.6

Results of Living Donor Liver Transplantation for Hepatocellular Carcinoma with Patient Selection Based on the Milan Criteria

Study	Patients Meeting Milan Criteria		Patients Exceeding Milan Criteria	
	Number	3-Year Survival (%)	Number	3-Year Survival (%)
Todo et al., 2004[99]	137	80	172	60
Hwang et al., 2005[100]	151	91	62	62
Takada et al., 2006[101]	49	68	44	59
Sugawara et al., 2007[102]	68	79	10	60

ADJUVANT AND NEOADJUVANT THERAPY

Adjuvant Therapy

A recent report of a randomized trial of adjuvant IFNα-2b described an improved 5-year survival in patients with stage III/IVA tumor from 24% to 68% ($p = 0.038$).[109] In a separate, larger study, IFNα-2b therapy was not associated with reducing postoperative recurrence in a population at risk for viral hepatitis–induced hepatocellular carcinoma. In this study of 268 patients, the median recurrence-free survival was 42.2 and 48.6 months with observation and IFNα-2b therapy, respectively (p = 0.828).[110]

Another approach that has been evaluated is intrahepatic ^{131}I-lipiodol. In a randomized study of 43 patients, adjuvant ^{131}I-lipiodol administered via the hepatic artery was compared with observation after resection of HCC. There was an improvement in median disease-free survival noted in favor of the ^{131}I-lipiodol arm (57.2 versus 13.6 months; $p = 0.037$).[111] However, a long-term follow-up of this trial at 10 years failed to show the same survival advantage.[112]

The best-studied systemic adjuvant therapy so far is acyclic retinoid, which was evaluated against placebo following surgical resection in 89 patients.[113] Patients who received acyclic retinoid had a recurrence rate of 27% compared with 49% for patients who received placebo ($p = 0.04$) after a median follow-up period of 38 months. The prevention of second primary HCC was more marked after a median follow-up of 62 months ($p = 0.002$, log rank test), but the difference in survival rates did not reach significance until after 6 years, with an estimated 6-year survival of 74% versus 46%, respectively ($p = 0.04$).[114]

Sorafenib, which will be discussed at length in the Systemic Therapy section, was also studied in the adjuvant setting. In a pilot study of 31 patients with HCC who had undergone curative resection and were at high risk of recurrence, sorafenib prolonged the time to recurrence (21.5 versus 13.4 months; $p = 0.006$) and significantly lowered recurrence rate (29.4% versus 70.7%; $p = 0.006$).[115] A currently fully accrued yet not reported phase III trial (STORM) randomized patients to adjuvant sorafenib versus placebo after surgery, radiofrequency ablation, or percutaneous alcohol injection with a primary end point of recurrence-free survival (Clinical Trial: NCT00692770). A phase II randomized, placebo-controlled study evaluating whether adjuvant sorafenib can prevent recurrence of HCC in high-risk orthotopic liver transplant recipients is currently enrolling (Clinical Trial: NCT01624285).

Neoadjuvant Therapy

Two randomized controlled trials and seven nonrandomized trials have evaluated preoperative transarterial chemotherapy. No clear advantage in disease-free or overall survival was found in these studies.[116–118] Postoperative transarterial chemotherapy has been examined in four randomized controlled trials and three nonrandomized controlled trials. A meta-analysis of these trials revealed a significant improvement in disease-free and overall survival.[117] The regimens consisted of Lipiodol and chemotherapy agents, including doxorubicin, mitomycin, and cisplatin. An analysis of postoperative adjuvant systemic chemotherapy trials demonstrated no consistent advantage in terms of disease-free or overall survival.[113,119–122]

A combination regimen of systemic therapy that has been studied extensively in advanced HCC provided input for its potential use in the neoadjuvant setting. PIAF (cisplatin, IFNα-2b, doxorubicin, and 5-fluorouracil) have shown in a phase II study a response rate of 26% with a median survival of approximately 9 months.[123] Of the 13 patients (26%) who had a partial response, 9 underwent surgery and 4 (9%) achieved a complete pathologic response to chemotherapy. These results illustrated that chemotherapy for HCC is effective in selected patients and suggest the possible use of PIAF as neoadjuvant therapy for medically fit patients with good liver function in whom cytoreduction might permit future resectability. The potential for cure would justify the risk of the significant toxicity profile of PIAF.

Choice of Resection, Ablation, or Transplantation

Although liver resection versus liver transplantation as primary therapy for patients with small HCC and adequate hepatic reserve is hotly debated, in most cases resection and OLT are complementary and not competing therapies. A number of studies report comparable overall survival rates for primary resection and primary OLT for transplantable HCC (Table 44.7).[89,124–134]

Patients with limited disease have potentially curative treatment options. There is general consensus that in patients with no underlying liver dysfunction, limited disease should be resected because this gives the best chance of cure without an ongoing need of immunosuppression dictated by transplantation. The outcomes of resection are quite good, with 5-year survivals of 30% to 50% (see Table 44.4).

For patients with end-stage liver disease (ESLD) and limited HCC, OLT is currently the best treatment modality. However, OLT can only be offered only to a small proportion of patients due to donor organ shortage. Therefore, liver resection remains the most important surgical therapy in patients with HCC and well-preserved liver function (Child class A).[51] Using resection as first-line therapy with salvage transplantation saved for recurrence is a common approach, especially for geographic regions with a high incidence of HCC and a low liver donation rate.[135,136] Resection can, therefore, be used as bridge therapy before OLT to control the tumor burden in patients who fulfill the Milan[81] or UCSF[90] criteria. In a study from a large Asian transplant center, the majority of patients (79%) who developed tumor recurrence after resection of small HCC were still eligible for salvage transplantation.[137] Primary resection also allows the opportunity to pathologically assess the tumor and adjacent liver tissue.[136] Pathologic prognostic factors such as micro- or macrovascular invasion, satellitosis, or occult tumors can be used as selection criteria for salvage liver transplantation in the case of recurrent tumor disease.

Patients with large HCC beyond the Milan or UCSF criteria have a less favorable outcome than those with small HCC.[81,90] Patients in the United States outside the accepted criteria can be transplanted based on the physiologic Model for End-Stage Liver Disease (MELD) score but do not receive any exception points for HCC. In an analysis of 94 patients with HCC exceeding the Milan criteria, results of resection was compared to OLT.[138] The overall survival rate was 66% for both groups even though the mean tumor size was 10 cm for the resection group and 6.4 cm for the OLT group. The results suggest that resection and OLT in patients with HCC beyond the Milan criteria have similar outcomes. A proposed algorithm of care from the Barcelona Clinic is shown in Figure 44.2.

Ablative Therapy For Localized Hepatocellular Cancer

Chemical Ablation

Chemicals destroy tumor tissue by direct dehydration of the cytoplasm, protein denaturation, and consequent coagulation necrosis as well as from indirect ischemia from vascular thrombosis from endothelial damage.[139,140] The direct instillation of chemicals such as absolute ethanol or acetic acid has been long studied for the treatment of HCC.[141–143] Chemical ablation is very inexpensive and, therefore, it is more widely used in developing countries with a high incidence of HCC. Intratumoral instillation of acetic acid for the treatment of HCC compares favorably

TABLE 44.7

Recent Studies Comparing Long-Term Outcome of Patients with Hepatocellular Carcinoma Treated Primarily with Resection (and Salvage Transplantation) or Primary Liver Transplantation

First Author	Year Published	Primary Therapy	Sample Size	5-Year Overall Survival Rate (%)	5-Year Disease-Free Survival Rate (%)
Lee[127]	2010	Transplantation	78	68	75[a]
		Resection	130	52	50
Facciuto[128b]	2009	Transplantation	119	62	—
		Resection	60	61	—
Del Gaudio[129]	2008	Transplantation	147	58	54
		Resection	80	66	41
Shah[130]	2007	Transplantation	140	64	78[a]
		Resection	121	56	60
Poon[131]	2007	Transplantation	85	44	—
		Resection	228	60	—
Margarit[126]	2005	Transplantation	36	50	64[a]
		Resection	37	78	39
Bigourdan[89]	2003	Transplantation	17	71	80[a]
		Resection	20	36	40[a]
Adam[132]	2003	Transplantation	195	61[b]	58[a]
		Resection	98	50	18
Belghiti[133]	2003	Transplantation	70	—	59
		Resection	18	—	61
Figueras[134]	2000	Transplantation	85	60	60[a]
		Resection	35	51	31

[a] Significant difference as reported in the original study.
[b] Fourth-year survival rates are reported for patients meeting the Milan criteria.
Adapted from Rahbari NN, Mehrabi A, Mollberg NM, et al. Hepatocellular carcinoma: current management and perspectives for the future. *Ann Surg* 2011;253:453–469, Table 3, with permission from Lippincott Williams & Wilkins.

with that of ethanol treatment.[144,145] Moderate quality evidence supports that RFA is superior to chemical ablation for the treatment of HCC.[146] Chemical ablation requires multiple applications, and thus, thermal ablation has largely replaced chemical ablation in many cases. In certain anatomic locations, such as adjacent to the major biliary tree or gallbladder, the combination of thermal ablation and ethanol ablation has shown some benefit.[147,148]

Radiofrequency Ablation

RFA is currently the most widely used ablative technique for the treatment of liver malignancies. The term *radiofrequency* applies to all electromagnetic energy sources with frequencies less than 30 MHz, although most clinically available devices function in the 375 to 500 kHz range. The technique for thermal ablation in the liver by using RFA was first described in animal liver models in 1990[149,150] and was later reported in a patient in 1995.[151]

In this technique, the RF electrode is placed into the tumor with imaging guidance. The electrode is coupled to an RF generator and is grounded by means of a grounding pad or pads applied to the thighs. The RF generator produces a voltage between the active electrode (applicator) and the reference electrode (grounding pad), establishing electric field lines that oscillate with the alternating current. This oscillating electric field causes electron collisions with the adjacent molecules closest to the applicator, inducing frictional heating.[152] Tissue heating to temperatures greater than 60°C leads to immediate cell death. Thus, for any given RFA procedure, the application of energy from the applicator is maximized to create a zone of tissue necrosis that encompasses the tumor and a margin of normal parenchyma.[153] The volume of ablation achieved is based

on the energy balance between heat conduction of the local RF energy applied and heat convection from the circulating blood and extracellular fluid.

In the United States, there are three commercially available percutaneous RFA systems (Fig. 44.3). Two of the systems (Boston Scientific/RadioTherapeutics and RITA Medical Systems) use a deployable RF array electrode that consists of 4 to 16 small wires (tines) deployed through a 14- to 17-G needle. Because the tines of the Boston Scientific device (LeVeen electrode) curve back toward the handle (see Fig. 44.3), the array is initially deployed in the deep portion of the tumor. In contrast, the RITA electrode tines course forward and laterally so the probe is deployed on the near surface of the tumor. The LeVeen electrode measures impedance only, and treatment time depends on repeated increases in impedance during active heating, which is a measure of tissue desiccation indicative of adequate thermocoagulation. With the RITA system, temperature readings are obtained throughout the ablation cycle from multiple peripheral thermocouples. The RITA system also has perfusion electrodes (see Fig. 44.3) that introduce small amounts of saline into the tissue to enhance the distribution of tissue heating. The third RF system (Cool-tip; Covidien) utilizes a single or triple "cluster" perfusion electrode (three single electrodes spaced 5 mm apart; see Fig. 44.3), the tip of which is positioned in the deepest part of the tumor.

Cold saline or water is pumped internally within the shaft of the electrode to keep its tip cooler than the adjacent heated tissue, thus reducing charring, which in turn helps the thermal conduction to occur at a greater distance from its source. The single or cluster RF electrode contains a thermocouple embedded in its tip, which is used to measure intratumoral temperature. A switching controller can be used with the Covidien system, allowing the placement of up to three separate single electrodes spaced 1.5 to

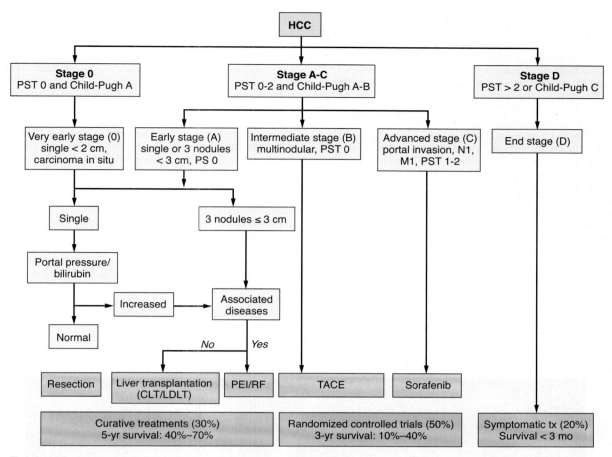

Figure 44.2 Strategy for staging and treatment assignment for patients with HCC according to the BCLC staging system. PST, performance status; CLT, cadaveric liver transplantation; tx, treatment.

2.5 cm apart, thus increasing the duty cycle of the generator to enable the creation of a greater volume of tissue thermocoagulation in a single application, as compared with three separate ablations that might be required with a single electrode. Most of the thermal ablation data regarding the treatment of liver tumors has been reported with RFA.[154–156]

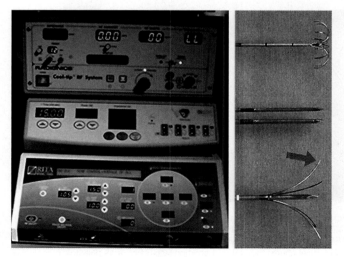

Figure 44.3 Radiofrequency ablation equipment currently available in the United States. The three most popular generators *(left)* and needle designs *(right)* are shown.

Microwave Ablation

Like RFA, microwave ablation (MWA) uses electromagnetic waves to produce heating. Unlike RFA, the MW energy is not an electrical current and is in a much higher frequency range that extends from 300 MHz to 300 GHz. The broader deposition of MW energy creates a much larger zone of active heating. MW applicators available for clinical use generally operate in the 900 to 2,450 MHz range.[157] Microwave tissue heating occurs because of the induction of kinetic energy in surrounding water molecules. Because of their electron configuration, water molecules have highly polar properties and function as small electric dipoles, with the negative charges preferentially localized around the oxygen nucleus. The rapidly alternating electric field of the MW antenna causes water molecules to spin rapidly in an attempt to align with electromagnetic charges of opposite polarity. These spinning water molecules interact with neighboring tissues, transferring a portion of their kinetic energy. Because temperature is merely a proxy measurement of molecular kinetic energy, this energy transfer results in local tissue hyperthermia.

Currently, there are six MWA systems that are commercially available in the United States and Europe.[158] These systems use either a 915-MHz generator (Evident, Covidien; MicrothermX, BSD Medical, Salt Lake City, UT; Avecure, MedWaves, San Diego, CA) or a 2,450-MHz generator (Certus 140, NeuWave Medical, Madison, WI; Amica, Hospital Service, Rome, Italy; Acculis MTA, Microsulis Medical, Hampshire, England) and straight antennae with varying active tips 0.6 to 4.0 cm in length. Perfusion of the antenna shaft is required for five of the six systems, with either room-temperature fluid or carbon dioxide to reduce conductive heating of the nonactive portion of the antenna, thus preventing damage to the skin and tissues proximal to the active tip. A single applicator is used with a single generator in four of the systems. Two have the ability to power up to three antennae with a single generator and treat large tumors (Fig. 44.4). Because most of the microwave systems have only recently received U.S. Food and Drug Administration approval, there are no published data at this time on the differences between systems in clinical safety or effectiveness. Similar safety and efficacy results for the treatment of metastatic colorectal liver metastases have been reported.[159] Perceived advantages of MW over RF energy include a greater heating profile and less severe heat sink effects.[160] Less heat sink effects may reduce local recurrences, and the larger resultant ablative volume when using the synergistic effect of multiple applicators simultaneously will allow a faster treatment time when compared to RFA.[161,162] Large trials evaluating safety show a similar safety profile compared with RF.[163] In Asia, MWA technology has been used for the treatment of liver tumors for a long period of time, and their extensive experience has created the development of appropriate treatment guidelines.[163]

Outcomes of Ablations

To date, the literature is replete with retrospective, single and multicenter cohorts with very few randomized controlled or cooperative group trials evaluating the benefits of liver ablation.

Regardless, many institutions around the world perform liver ablation for primary and metastatic liver tumors given its relative safety, low cost, and low toxicity. Many factors affect the success of thermal ablation treatment for liver malignancies, some of which include: tumor size, proximity to blood vessels, operator experience, the presence of underlying liver disease, extrahepatic disease in patients with secondary liver malignancies, overall patient health, and implementation alongside synergistic therapies in a collegial, multidisciplinary treatment clinic. The ever present argument for surgery as first-line treatment in these patients would be to properly stage the patient because preoperative imaging can underestimate the extent of liver and extrahepatic disease.[164] Of course, not all patients are fit for surgery, and ablation is an attractive minimally invasive option for older and frailer patients. Tumors adjacent to larger (>3 mm) blood vessels may be undertreated due to the thermal sink effect.[165] Proper device selection to effectively eradicate tumors adjacent to vessels should be improved, in theory, with hotter energy sources such as MWA compared to RFA.[166] A novel, largely, nonthermal electrical ablation technology called irreversible electroporation that is purported to be unaffected by thermal sink effects may play a role in treating tumors adjacent to blood vessels and critical structures, but there are no mature data at this time.[167]

With a myriad of thermal ablation devices available to hepatic surgeons, hepatologists, and interventional radiologists, studies

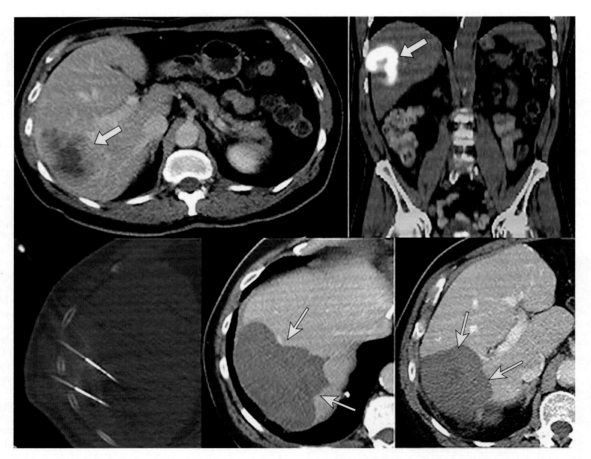

Figure 44.4 A 73-year-old man with previously resected colorectal metastatic disease in the left lobe of the liver who recurred in the right lobe despite 5-flourouracil, oxaliplatin, leukovorin (FOLFOX) chemotherapy. An axial contrast enhanced CT scan and coronal fludeoxyglucose–positron-emission tomography (FDG-PET) CT scan *(top panel)* show a large heterogeneous colorectal cancer (CRC) metastasis in the right lobe. The patient refused additional chemotherapy and ablation was offered as palliative therapy. Given the size of the mass, microwave ablation was performed with multiple antennas under CT guidance *(bottom left)*. The patient responded to the treatment extremely well, and a current 20-month follow-up contrast enhanced CT scan *(bottom right)* shows a large coagulation defect *(small arrows)* without evidence of recurrence in the liver.

have shown that it is incumbent upon these operators to gain experience with a particular device before optimal results can be expected.[164,168] This can be difficult not only in low patient volume ablation practices, but also in general given the rapid technologic changes that occur in this arena whereby a newer technology is perceived to be an improvement over an existing technology prior to rigorous scientific study. The presence of underlying cirrhosis will affect treatment options and outcomes in patients presenting with HCC. In general, HCC patients with Child-Pugh class C cirrhosis who are not on a liver transplant list and do not undergo liver-directed therapies have a median survival of less than 4 months. Therefore, treatment with thermal ablation is unlikely going to affect long-term survival.[169] In patients with Child-Pugh class A cirrhosis, data suggest thermal ablation can rival surgery when tumors are solitary and smaller (<5 cm) and less in number (< three tumors each under 3 cm).[170] However, for patients who are healthier with a normal performance status, surgical resection may provide better long-term survival compared to RFA.[171] It makes clinical sense that in patients with limited extrahepatic disease, liver-directed therapy could improve outcomes, although the outcomes themselves may be as much due to underlying tumor biology and not necessarily the treatment.[154,155] Given the complexity of any given patient with hepatic malignancy, it is important to first and foremost apply any treatment or treatments under the supervision of a team of experts whose primary goal is to provide the most cost-effective, comprehensive treatment based on evidenced-based medicine when available alongside patient centered outcomes.

Liver Resection Versus Ablative Therapy for Hepatocellular Carcinoma

With recent improvements in imaging that allows for the early diagnosis of cancer and facile guidance for interventional therapies, ablative modalities such as RFA are increasingly accepted as effective treatment for small tumors. Ablative techniques are less invasive and have the promise of being better tolerated than resections or transplantation. In retrospective studies, data suggest that for small HCCs (≤2 to 3 cm), RFAs result in similar outcomes as resections.[172–174]

Recently, four randomized trials comparing RFA and hepatic resection have been reported (Table 44.8).[175–178] Two of them, Chen et al. and Huang et al., compared tumors fulfilling the Milan tumor criteria for transplantation. Chen et al.[175] compared resection to RFA for tumors less than 5 cm in size. The 1-, 3- and 4-year survivals were 93%, 73% and 64%, respectively, for resection, and 96%, 71%, and 68%, respectively, for RFA. The authors concluded that RFA was as effective as surgical resection in the treatment of solitary HCCs ≤5 cm in terms of overall and disease-free survival after 4 years with no significant difference in outcome between the two groups on follow-up. Huang et al.[177] concluded that surgical resections have better outcomes than RFAs. This conclusion was based on a recurrence rate at 5 years of 63% in the RFA group and 41% in the resection group. However, it must be pointed out that more patients in the resected group had tumors less than 3 cm in size. In addition, the overall survival was not statistically different between the two treatment groups.

Feng et al.[178] and Liang et al.[176] confirmed the similar efficacy of RFA to resection in tumors <4 cm. Both groups found RFA and resection to have similar overall survival in a follow-up period after 3 years. It appears that for small HCCs, particularly in patients with cirrhosis, RFA can produce similar cancer outcomes with much lower morbidity. Figure 44.5 illustrates a recommended algorithm of care for small HCCs.

Embolic Therapies for Regional Disease

For patients with multifocal liver-predominant disease who are not candidates for resection or transplantation, transcatheter ablative methods have emerged as the most commonly used treatment worldwide. These techniques rely on the dual blood supply of the liver: arterial and portal venous. The portal vein provides over 75% of the blood flow to the hepatic parenchyma, whereas the hepatic artery is the primary nutrient supply of tumors. Selectively delivering agents transarterially targets the tumor while sparing the liver.

There are currently three main categories of percutaneously administered transcatheter intra-arterial therapies: TACE, bland hepatic artery embolization (HAE), and radioembolization (RAE). The usual chemotherapeutic agents used are mitomycin C, doxorubicin, and aclarubicin. The majority of the effects of embolic therapies derive from tumor ischemia produced by occlusion of the arterial vessels. Thus, bland embolizations (without chemotherapy), even with a nonpermanent agent such as Gelfoam, can produce a high likelihood of tumor killing. RAE involves the administration of yttrium-90 (a pure β emitter) that can be loaded in glass or resin microspheres intra-arterially.[179] This is really not an embolization, in that the goal is not occlusion of the arterial inflow, but more brachytherapy. RAE will be further discussed.

Patient Selection

Performance status, underlying liver disease, and degree of portal hypertension are important patient selection criteria. Although minimally invasive, following embolization, patients commonly experience a postembolization syndrome of pain, fever, and nausea that may last for several days to a few weeks. It often takes 4 to 6 weeks to recover to baseline performance status.

Although embolization in patients with normal liver, or well-compensated cirrhosis, has a low risk of liver failure, the risk of further compromising liver function and hastening death in poorly compensated cirrhosis is significant. This is because a basis of TACE is that the portal blood flow will protect the noncancerous liver from the treatment agents and ischemia. Thus, portal vein occlusion is considered a contraindication to both TACE[180] and HAE because of the risk of liver failure. Ascites, which is an indication of severe portal hypertension, or measured reversal of portal blood flow is a relative contraindication.

Results of Treatment

It has always been apparent that embolic therapies can result in a high rate of tumor response (>50%). Excellent results (level IIa evidence) following chemoembolization have also been reported from Japan in 8510 patients treated between 1994 and 2001, with 1-, 3-, and 5-year survival of 82%, 47%, and 26%, respectively.[29] With well-designed trials, there is also now level I evidence of a survival benefit to conventional TACE as demonstrated in randomized trials published by Llovett et al.,[181] Lo et al.,[182] and Becker et al.[183] In the trial by Lo et al.,[182] patients were randomized to TACE (cisplatin + Lipiodol + Gelfoam) versus control (no treatment). The 2-year survival was 31% for TACE versus 11% for controls. In the trial by Llovet et al.,[181] patients randomized to TACE (doxorubicin + Lipiodol + Gelfoam) had a 2-year survival of 63% versus 27% for control. In the study from Becker et al.,[183] TACE (mitomycin C [MMC] + Lipiodol + Gelfoam) + PEI resulted in a 39% 2-year survival compared to 18% for TACE. What seems clear from these data is that arterial embolotherapy is an effective method of treating HCC and can prolong the patient's survival. Comparable, or better, survival results have been demonstrated with bland embolization.[119]

Radiation Therapy for Hepatocellular Carcinoma

Radiation therapy for liver tumors was historically limited by hepatic toxicity but, with improved imaging, treatment planning, and treatment delivery, it now is an excellent option, particularly for patients with unresectable tumors or who are medical inoperable.

TABLE 44.8

Randomized Controlled Trials of Hepatic Resection Versus RF Ablations for HCC Reported After 2000

Author/Year Country	Treatment	Number	Age	Tumor Number	Characteristics Diameter	Disease-Free Survival (%)				Overall Survival (%)				p
						1 Year	3 Years	4 Years	5 Years	1 Year	3 Years	4 Years	5 Years	
Chen (2006)[175]	RES	90	49±11	1	≤5 cm	87	69	46	—	93	73	64	—	NS
	RFA	71	52±11	1	≤5 cm	86	64	52	—	96	71	68	—	
Liang (2008)[176a]	RES	44	49±12	≤3	≤5 cm	—	—	—	—	79	45	31	28	0.8
	RFA	66	55±11	≤3	≤5 cm	—	—	—	—	77	49	40	40	
Huang (2010)[177]	RES	115	56±13	≤3	≤5 cm (77%)	85	61	—	51	98	92	—	76	NS
	RFA	115	57±14	≤3	≤5 cm (73%)	82	46	—	29	87	70	—	55	
Feng (2012)[178]	RES	84	47(18–76)	≤2	≤4 cm	91	61	—	—	96	75	—	—	0.3
	RFA	84	51(24–83)	≤2	≤4 cm	86	50	—	—	93	67	—	—	

[a]Treatments for recurrent disease.

RES, resected patients; OS, overall survival; DFS, disease-free survival; NS, not significant.

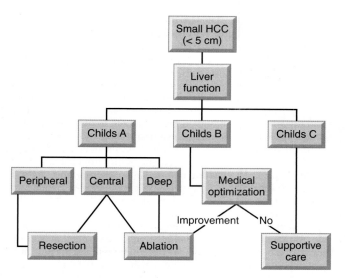

Figure 44.5 The treatment algorithm for a small HCC.

Tumors not likely to be effectively treated by radiofrequency ablation due to size over 3 cm or proximity to the diaphragm, large vessel, or gallbladder are also good candidates for RT. With proper care, tumors near gastrointestinal (GI) structures can also be treated. Side effects are typically minimal, and commonly include mild fatigue, and less commonly include nausea, mild radiation dermatitis, pain associated with tumor edema, or worsening liver dysfunction. Radiation can be delivered using external beam or brachytherapy. Patients with metastases to the bone, brain, adrenals, or other locations can be effectively palliated with RT, as can patients with pain from large primary tumors.[184]

External Beam Radiotherapy

Fractionated Treatment

Because the liver is one of the most radiosensitive organs in the body, treatment planning and delivery must be done carefully to maximize dose to the tumor and to minimize dose to the normal liver. The primary toxicity of concern is radiation-induced liver disease (RILD), which can be categorized as classic and nonclassic. Classic RILD is a constellation of anicteric ascites, hepatomegaly, and elevated liver enzymes (particularly alkaline phosphatase), which typically occurs within 4 months of therapy and is a type of veno-occlusive disease, similar to that which can be seen after high-dose chemotherapy conditioning for bone marrow transplantation.[185] Nonclassic RILD, a recently coined classification, can occur in patients with hepatitis and cirrhosis, and is characterized by jaundice and markedly elevated serum transaminases (>5 times the upper limit of normal) within 3 months of completion of therapy. This is thought to represent direct hepatocyte rather than endothelial injury.[186] RILD is typically self-limited, but can be serious, even leading to mortality. It is managed symptomatically, using diuretics and paracentesis. Even low doses to the whole liver of 25 Gy in 10 fractions or 32 Gy in 1.5 Gy per fraction twice daily are associated with a more than 5% risk of radiation-induced liver disease, particularly for patients with cirrhosis and already compromised liver function. Other toxicities that can occur include gastric or duodenal bleeding,[187] although both of these risks can be minimized using careful treatment planning, image guidance, and treatment delivery. It is important to consider factors including cirrhosis, prior liver-directed therapies, and hepatitis B and C, which add to the dose and volume models for the prediction of RILD. ICG is also used in Asia as a pretreatment assessment for the safety

of RT, similar to its use for the safety of liver resection.[188,189] In the United States, the University of Michigan has pioneered its use to measure individual tolerance to radiation, which can be quite variable. Even some patients with good pretreatment liver function can experience rapid decline, so customizing treatment is crucial.[190]

At the University of Michigan, investigators created the normal-tissue complication probability (NTCP) model that quantitatively described the relationship between radiation dose and liver volumes and the probability of developing RILD.[191] Dose was customized per patient to give an anticipated risk of 5% to 15%. Due to the variety of tumor and liver sizes and geometries, prescribed doses ranged from 40 to 90 Gy. Patients who received 75 Gy or more had a higher median survival of 24 versus 15 months. Progression-free survival was also improved with higher doses.[192–195] A prospective phase II trial from France treated patients to 66 Gy in 2 Gy fractions, with a response rate of 92%.[196] The largest published experiences are from Asia, which has a very high incidence of HCC. In a multicenter retrospective patterns-of-care study among 10 institutions in Korea, 398 patients with HCC were described. Of those, 70% were Child class A, 54% had tumors >5 cm, and 40% had portal vein thrombosis. Nearly all had received prior treatment, mostly TACE. In this series, higher dose (biologic effective dose over 53 Gy) also correlated with better survival.[197] Other groups have combined TACE and RT, with various schedules, although mostly using RT to treat residual disease. In a Korean study of 73 patients with incomplete response to TACE, 38 received RT, whereas the rest received additional TACE. Patients who received radiation had a higher 2-year survival of 37% versus 14% (p = 0.001).[198,199]

Another use for RT is to treat tumor thrombus in the portal vein, with the goals of decreasing portal pressure and allowing the safe delivery of embolic therapies. The largest series from Taiwan reports a 25% response rate. Compared with a dismal 1-year survival of 9% for nonresponders, responders had a better survival of 21% for those still not eligible for definitive therapies, and 29% for those who ultimately had additional therapy.[200]

Other crucial components of a liver RT program not always available for standard RT include adequate imaging with arterial and portal venous phase imaging with CT scans and MRI for tumor delineation, motion assessment, and management tools four-dimensional computed tomography (4D-CT) scan, treatment gating), and precise image guidance (cone beam CT scan) on the treatment machine. Because liver tumors move with respiration, accurate assessment and management of this will aid in proper tumor targeting and normal tissue avoidance. Some common methods include forced breath hold for tumor immobilization and 4D-CT scans to assess and help account for motion.[201,202] Fiducials can also be placed within or near the tumor percutaneously prior to treatment planning, with daily alignment on the treatment machine, because external anatomy is a poor surrogate for internal anatomy and tumor location.

Stereotactic Body Radiotherapy

Stereotactic body radiotherapy (SBRT) is a relatively new method of delivering high-dose, high-precision therapy in just a few treatments, rather than spread out daily over a course of several weeks. With high doses per fraction, the biologic effect is much more than with the same total dose delivered in a standard fractionated course, up to the equivalent to 80 to 150 Gy in 2-Gy fractions (see Fig. 44.5). This technique was pioneered by Blomgren et al.,[203] who treated 20 liver tumors, including 8 HCCs in the 1990s. Since then, the literature has mostly been populated by small retrospective studies. A few prospective studies have been quite informative. Mendez-Romero et al.[204] initially started treating patients with a schedule of 25 Gy in five fractions, but after two patients experienced local failure, the dose was raised to 30 Gy in three fractions for the rest of the study. The 1-year local control was 75%, with all failures in the low-dose group. One Child-Pugh class B patient experienced grade 5 nonclassic RILD, leading the authors to advise others to be very cautious with similar patients.[204] The next and largest studies were a phase I and II trial from Princess Margaret Hospital.[205,206] Of 41 initial patients, 31 had HCC. Patients were treated with a six-fraction course of SBRT delivered over 2 weeks, with the dose individualized based on the University of Michigan NTCP model, escalated from 5% to 20%. The median dose was 36 Gy (range, 24 to 54 Gy) and the median tumor volume was 173 mL (range, 9 to 1,913 mL). Even for these relatively large tumors, approximately 50% had a response to treatment, and 42% had stable disease. Median survival was 12 months. No patients developed classic RILD, although 26% had grade 3 elevation of liver enzymes and 16% had a decline from Child class A to B within 3 months after treatment. Recently, the results from the full 102 patients from both the phase I and II portions of the trial were reported.[206] Of the patients, 93% had underlying liver disease, 52% had received prior therapy, and 55% had tumor vascular thrombosis. The 1-year local control was excellent, at 87%. However, 30% of patients had grade 3 or higher toxicity, some of which possibly contributed to mortality. This illustrates the tenuous balance between treatment safety and efficacy and the need for improved predictive models of safety for individual patients.

Another phase I study reported 100% local control after 36 to 48 Gy in three to five fractions. Similar to what was seen in the Mendez-Romero study, patients with Child-Pugh class B liver failure were prone to liver toxicity.[207] Truly, these patients need extra attention and consideration. Many larger retrospective studies have confirmed these smaller prospective results.[208–210]

Charged particles, including protons and carbon ions, are being investigated for treatment of HCC. These have the advantage of lower entrance and minimal exit dose, due to a difference in dose deposition properties. In a Japanese retrospective review, 162 patients were treated with 72 Gy in 16 fractions using protons with a 5-year local control and survival of 87% and 24%, respectively. There were no grade 3 or higher toxicities.[211] In a phase II proton study, 51 patients received 66 Gy in 10 fractions. The 5-year local control and survival rates were 88% and 39%, respectively. There were no cases of RILD, although 26% had a decline in liver function.[212] Currently, carbon-ion therapy is only available in a few centers worldwide. In Japan, 24 patients were treated on a phase I/II dose-escalation study. Twenty-four patients received from 50 to 80 Gy in 15 fractions, with local control and survival similar to other reports, at 81% and 25%, respectively.[213] Despite the technologic imperative that newer is better, charged particles are not the miracle treatment some may assume. The high-dose treatment region cannot be shaped as conformably as with standard photon radiotherapy (SBRT and intensity modulated radiotherapy [IMRT]), and image guidance is currently rudimentary, therefore, ensuring the accuracy of treatment is difficult. However, because the liver is extremely sensitive to radiation, reducing the moderate and low-dose regions could potentially aid in protecting the normal liver and allowing for escalation of tumor dose. The next few years should yield exciting developments.

Brachytherapy

In contrast to other tumor sites such as prostate, gynecologic, and breast, liver brachytherapy typically involves an injection of a radioisotope for regional therapy, rather than interstitial or intracavitary therapy, although small experiences in interstitial therapy have been reported.[214,215] Radioembolization, like chemoembolization, takes advantage of the liver's dual blood supply and the arterial enhancement of HCC. Rather than chemotherapy and embolic material, radioisotopes linked to either glass (TheraSphere, Nordion, Canada) or resin (SIRTeX Medical, Inc., Lane Cove, New South Wales, Australia) microspheres are injected into the hepatic artery (HA). This outpatient treatment is typically delivered through either the right or the left HA, although with favorable anatomy, it can be delivered more selectively. Whole liver treatment is usually reserved for metastases rather than HCC due to the risk of liver injury. The most common isotope is yttrium-90, a pure beta emitter, with an effective path length of 5 mm and a half-life of 65 hours. Ninety percent of the energy is deposited within 5 mm of the sphere, therefore, side effects are quite localized. The dose to the individual tumors is not well characterized, but is prescribed to 80 to 150 Gy, depending on liver function, to the entire treated portion of the liver, assuming equal distribution and based on pretreatment angiography. Side effects are typically quite tolerable and consist of mild nausea, pain, and fatigue. Rare complications could include hepatobiliary dysfunction, radiation pneumonitis, and GI ulceration. Risk factors associated with early mortality include an infiltrative tumor, a tumor encompassing over 50% to 70% of the liver, albumin <3 g/dL, bilirubin >2 mg/dL, and lung dose >30 Gy.[216] With proper patient selection, this procedure is relatively safe. Although both RAE and chemoembolization can deliver regional therapy, which is particularly useful for multifocal HCC, it is currently unclear which treatment may be preferred for which patients. No randomized trials comparing these two modalities have been completed; however, a retrospective comparison suggests that RAE may have a longer time to progression with reduced toxicity and similar overall survival.[179] In general, response rates are 30% to 50%, with a time to progression of 6 to 16 months depending on stage and portal vein thrombus.[217,218] Treatment may be repeated.[219]

Toxicities

RT is typically very well tolerated. Mild fatigue can be attributed both to the treatment itself and to the travel related to multiple appointments for the treatment. Mild nausea can be prevented by premedicating with an antiemetic. Radiation dermatitis is highly unusual due to the extremely conformal distribution of radiation dose. Occasionally, the treatment of large tumors can cause a pain flare due to local edema. These acute effects typically resolve within a few weeks after treatment. Late effects could include RILD, as discussed previously, in addition to GI ulceration and renal dysfunction, although these risks can be avoided by minimizing the dose to these structures to below acceptable levels.[187]

Systemic Therapy for Hepatocellular Carcinoma

First-Line Single-Agent Therapies

A large number of controlled and uncontrolled clinical studies have been performed with most of the major classes of cancer chemotherapy, given intravenously as single agent or in combination. However, these systemic therapies, and other chemotherapy combinations studied, have had no proven benefits on survival in HCC.[220] Many other nonchemotherapeutic agents have also been tried without definitive success, including luteinizing hormone-releasing hormone agonists, tamoxifen, IFN, Sandostatin, megestrol, vitamin K, thalidomide, interleukin-2, ^{131}I-lipiodol, and ^{131}I-ferritin.

Given the vascular nature of HCC and that vascular endothelial growth factor (VEGF) promotes HCC development and metastasis, antiangiogenic agents have been studied extensively in the setting of advanced HCC. Increased levels of VEGF have been observed and have been associated with inferior survival.[221]

Sorafenib a multi–tyrosine kinase inhibitor with antiangiogenic effects are thought to be mediated by the blockade of VEGFR-2/-3, platelet-derived growth factor receptor (PDGFR)-β, and other receptor tyrosine kinases.[222] The clinical efficacy of sorafenib in HCC was first reported in a multicenter phase II study of 137 patients with systemic treatment-naïve, inoperable HCC and varying hepatic reserve (72% Child-Pugh class A, 28% Child-Pugh class B) received the agent, with a primary end point of evaluating response by World Health Organization (WHO) criteria.[223] Although only

2.2% of the study population achieved a confirmed objective response by WHO criteria, 42% of the study population had extended disease control. There was a median overall survival of 9.2 months, which was encouraging when compared to historical controls. Subsequently, the Sorafenib Hepatocellular Carcinoma Assessment Randomized Protocol (SHARP) trial enrolled 602 patients with advanced HCC, Child-Pugh class A, and who had not received prior systemic therapy.[224] The majority of the study population was recruited from the Western Hemisphere. Patients were randomly assigned to receive sorafenib at 400 mg orally twice a day (N = 299) or best supportive care (N = 303). The coprimary end points of the study were overall survival and time to symptomatic progression. Median overall survival was 10.7 months in the sorafenib arm versus 7.9 months in the placebo arm (hazard ratio [HR] = 0.69; 95% confidence interval [CI], 0.55 to 0.87). A predefined subset analysis indicated that the survival benefit of sorafenib was independent of performance status and disease burden.

Parallel to the SHARP trial, the Asia-Pacific study assessed the efficacy and tolerability of sorafenib in comparison with best supportive care in the patients with advanced HCC geographically localized to Asia.[225] As expected and in contrast to the SHARP trial, the Asia-Pacific study was enriched with patients with HBV-related HCC (73% of the total study population). The trial confirmed that sorafenib, when compared to best supportive care, was tolerable and led to a statistically significant improvement in disease control, time to radiographic progression, and overall survival. However, the magnitude of the overall survival benefit on the Asia-Pacific study was not as substantial as observed on the SHARP study—the median overall survival was only 6.5 and 4.2 months for patients receiving sorafenib and placebo, respectively. The inclusion of patients who were more ill prior to beginning therapy than those patients on the SHARP study might explain this difference. Another postulate is that the observed differential outcomes on the two trials were due to differing treatment patterns between Asia and Western countries. Intense local–regional therapies might be more common in Asia, thus leading to the selection of patients on the Asia-Pacific study who are presenting later in the course of their disease. The inclusion criteria for the Asia-Pacific study, however, do not necessarily support this assertion. Alternatively, specific viral etiologic factors might affect prognosis and influence the responsiveness of liver cancer to sorafenib.

In an unplanned subset analysis of the SHARP study, patients with HBV-related HCC who were treated with sorafenib had a modest prolongation in median overall survival over placebo (9.7 versus 6.1 months).[226] However, HCV-related HCC patients treated with sorafenib appeared to derive a more substantial survival improvement over placebo (14.0 versus 7.4 months). A retrospective analysis of the initial phase II study of sorafenib observed similar etiologic-dependent trends in survival. Patients who were infected with HCV lived longer (N = 13, 12.4 months) than did patients infected with HBV (N = 33, 7.3 months; p = 0.29). The recently reported phase III study of first-line sunitinib indicates that there may in fact be differential outcomes relative to disease cause and ethnic origin, with median overall survival for HCV-associated HCC ranging from 18.3 months for patients with living outside of Asia to 7.9 months for patients living in Asia.[227] Etiologic-dependent genomic differences in HCC might explain improved outcomes to sorafenib in patients with HCV-related HCC. *CTNNB1* mutations are more commonly observed in HCV-related HCC but not in HBV-related HCC and are associated with a specific WNT gene expression profile.[228] Sorafenib can modulate this gene signature, interfere with WNT signaling output, and lead to HCC growth suppression in preclinical models. Etiologic-dependent differences in outcome might also be explained by HCV core protein-induced upregulation of the sorafenib target CRAF, among other kinases.[229] Finally, in vitro data suggest that sorafenib can directly inhibit HCV viral replication, although the clinical importance of this observation is debatable.[230] Although more exploration is certainly required, it should be emphasized that the utility of sorafenib

is not undercut by this observation, and it remains an effective and life prolonging therapy for HCC, irrespective of etiologic factor.

Several other small receptor tyrosine kinase inhibitors have been studied. Thus far, emerging results have been disappointing with the major phase III studies of antiangiogenic therapy failing to improve upon sorafenib in the first-line setting. Sunitinib, an inhibitor of vascular endothelial growth factor receptor (VEGFR)-1/-2 with greater potency than sorafenib, plus an inhibitor of PDGFR-α/β, c-KIT, FLT3, RET, and other kinases, has been studied in three phase II studies with three different dosing schedules of the agent as a treatment for advanced HCC.[231–233] A subsequent randomized phase III study of sunitinib, dosed continuously, versus sorafenib in patients with advanced HCC and Child Pugh class A liver function was initiated and rapidly enrolled 530 patients on the sunitinib arm and 544 on the sorafenib arm.[227] The study, powered to test the dual hypotheses of noninferiority and superiority with regard to overall survival, was halted by an independent data monitoring committee due to futility and safety concerns. The median overall survival for the sunitinib arm was 7.9 versus 10.2 months for the sorafenib arm (HR, 1.30; one-sided p = 0.9990; two-sided p = 0.0014).

Brivanib, a dual inhibitor of VEGFR and fibroblast growth factor receptor (FGFR), demonstrated modest antitumor activity in both treatment-naïve and in those patients who had failed prior antiangiogenic therapy in two separate phase II studies.[234,235] Based on these data, a large randomized phase III study compared brivanib to sorafenib in patients with systemic treatment-naïve, advanced HCC.[236] This noninferiority trial did not meet its primary end point; median overall survival with brivanib treatment was 9.5 months versus 9.9 months with sorafenib (HR, 1.06; 95% CI, 0.93 to 1.22; p = 0.3730).

Linifanib, a selective inhibitor of VEGFR and PDGFR, also failed to improve upon the modest survival advantage of sorafenib despite early encouraging efficacy data.[237] A large multicenter, randomized, phase III study of sorafenib versus linifanib as a first-line therapy for advanced HCC, failed to meet both prespecified end points of superiority and noninferiority. The median overall survival for linifanib was 9.1 months versus 9.8 months for sorafenib (HR = 1.046; 95%, CI 0.896 to 1.221).

Over 20 separate clinical trials have assessed or are assessing bevacizumab, a monoclonal antibody directed against VEGF, in patients with advanced HCC. Evaluated regimens include monotherapy and combination therapy with chemotherapy, targeted agents, and embolization procedures. In general, completed studies have reported higher response rates than those observed with other tyrosine kinase inhibitors; however, adverse events such as arterial/venous thrombotic events and variceal hemorrhage (some fatal) are more common. A phase II study in advanced HCC with extrahepatic disease found a 14% overall response rate with bevacizumab monotherapy.[238] It has not moved to later stage trials due to concerns regarding bleeding.

First-Line Combination Therapies

The addition of cytotoxic chemotherapy or targeted therapy to bevacizumab may augment antitumor activity. Response proportions with various cytotoxic combinations range from 9% to 20%, with disease control rates reportedly as high as 78%.[239–241] Bevacizumab and erlotinib may offer enhanced antitumor activity with a response rate of 24% and favorable patient outcomes with a median overall survival of 13.7 months.[242] A multicenter, randomized phase II trial of bevacizumab combined with erlotinib (Clinical Trial: NCT00881751) versus sorafenib monotherapy is ongoing. Similarly, the SEARCH trial confirmed that the addition of erlotinib to sorafenib provided no benefit in HCC. In this randomized, placebo-controlled, double-blind, phase III study the combination of sorafenib and erlotinib were compared to sorafenib alone in the first-line setting in 720 patients with advanced HCC. There was no statistically significant difference between study arms with regard to the primary end point of overall survival (combination 9.5 months, sorafenib 8.5 months; HR = 0.93; 95%, CI 0.78 to 1.11).

In the attempt to improve upon the modest results observed with sorafenib, investigators have proposed combination strategies with cytotoxic chemotherapy and novel biologic agents. Prior to the approval of sorafenib, doxorubicin was evaluated as monotherapy or in combination with sorafenib in a randomized, double-blind, phase II study.[243] The trial enrolled 96 patients with treatment-naïve advanced HCC and Child-Pugh class A liver function. The primary end point of the study was time to progression. In a planned exploratory analysis, both time to progression, as determined by independent review, and progression-free survival were increased by approximately 4 months, and the median overall survival doubled in favor of combined therapy (13.7 versus 6.5 months; p = 0.006). Cardiac toxicity was notable, with a higher proportion of patients on the combination experiencing left ventricular systolic dysfunction (19% versus 2%). Although the majority of such cases were asymptomatic, the median cumulative doxorubicin dose was limited to 165 mg/m². The dramatic increase in survival over placebo was striking; however, the lack of sorafenib as a comparator arm limits the interpretation of the trial. Doxorubicin may contribute little to outcome. The observed benefit in the doxorubicin–sorafenib group may be due to the effects of sorafenib alone. Alternatively, the combination may be synergistic. Inhibition of the mitogen-activated protein kinase (MAPK) pathway by sorafenib may restore chemosensitivity by enhancing proapoptotic pathways and dampening multidrug resistance (MDR) pathways. Anthracycline-induced cytotoxicity is mediated by the proapoptotic kinase ASK1.[244] Growth factor–induced MAPK activation, via FGF, has been shown to abrogate ASK1 activity. Blockade of the RAF kinases by sorafenib might, therefore, augment the antitumor activity of doxorubicin. Furthermore, MAPK activation leads to the induction of the MDR-1 pump.[245] Sorafenib decreases ATP-binding cassette/MDR protein gene expression, thereby restoring HCC sensitivity to doxorubicin in vitro.[246] A randomized phase III study of sorafenib versus sorafenib and doxorubicin in the first-line setting is currently underway (Clinical Trial: NCT01015833). A phase II study of doxorubicin plus sorafenib in second-line setting after sorafenib failure is currently underway (Clinical Trial: NCT01840592).

Gemcitabine and oxaliplatin (GEMOX) therapy has established efficacy in HCC,[247] and there is reason to believe that addition of sorafenib to gemcitabine might offer synergistic antitumor effects.[246] The GEMOX–sorafenib versus sorafenib was recently tested in a randomized phase II study (GONEXT).[248] The trial enrolled 95 patients with advanced HCC. The primary end point was 4-month progression-free survival of greater than or equal to 50%. The combination of GEMOX plus sorafenib resulted in a 4-month progression-free survival rate of 61% compared to 54% in the sorafenib monotherapy group. The combination was feasible, and efficacy data were encouraging (overall response rate [ORR] 16%, DCR 77%).

Second-Line Therapies

The interest in developing novel agents for advanced HCC and the positive outlook on improved outcome led to a rapidly evolving field studying second-line therapies, with already several phase III clinical trials reported, still on-going, or planned.

Overexpression of c-MET and its ligand hepatocyte growth factor (HGF) occur in up to 80% of human HCC tumors.[249] Transgenic mice that overexpress MET in hepatocytes developed HCC, and inactivation of this transgene leads to tumor regression, mediated by apoptosis and growth suppression.[250] Blocking MET with several different multitargeted tyrosine kinase inhibitors small molecules induce in vitro HCC growth suppression, cell-cycle arrest, and decreased viability as well as growth suppression and survival prolongation in vivo.[251] Based on these data, several MET inhibitors are already being studied in the setting of advanced HCC. Tivantinib, a selective MET receptor tyrosine kinase inhibitor, was

evaluated at two doses in a randomized, placebo-controlled phase II in advanced HCC patients who had progressed after first-line therapy.[252] This study reported a statistically significant difference in outcomes between high-MET expressing tumors in favor of tivantinib. For patients with high MET-expressing tumors (defined as ≥50% 3 to 4+ expression), tivantinib therapy resulted in a median time to progression of 2.7 months in comparisons to 1.4 months for placebo (HR, 0.43; 95% CI, 0.19 to 0.97) and a median overall survival of 7.2 months versus 3.8 months for placebo (HR, 0.38, 0.18 to 0.81). Importantly, no such differences between the agent and placebo were observed in low-MET expression tumors. This strongly suggests that MET expression is a predictive biomarker for MET-directed targeted therapy in HCC. Additionally, in patients on the placebo arm, high tumoral MET expression was associated with an improved overall survival when compared with low tumoral MET expression (3.8 months versus 9 months; HR, 2.94; 95% CI, 1.16 to 7.43). This observation indicates that MET expression may also be prognostic in this disease. Given these data, tivantinib is being compared with placebo in a double-blind, randomized phase III study in patients with advanced HCC and high-MET expressing tumors in the second-line setting (Clinical Trial: NCT01755767). Cabozantinib, an inhibitor of MET and VEGFR-2, has also shown promising efficacy data in a cohort of 41 patients with advanced HCC.[253] In 78% of patients, tumor regression was observed by Response Evaluation Criteria in Solid Tumors (RECIST) with a 5% confirmed partial response rate. Median progression-free survival for the cohort was estimated at 4.2 months, and median overall survival 15.1 months. A phase III study of cabozantinib versus placebo in patients with advanced HCC in the second-line setting is underway (Clinical Trial: NCT01908426). A different view on the biology of met inhibition differs between those two studies, where the tivantinib approach is to treat only patients with met-positive tumors defined as ≥50% 3 to 4+ expression, whereas the cabozantinib study will take all comers, arguing that it is not known yet how much met positivity is needed, if at all, considering the multikinase nature of both drugs.

The mammalian target of rapamycin (mTOR) pathway plays a critical role in hepatocarcinogenesis, and in xenograft mouse models, blockade of this pathway results in HCC growth suppression—but not regression or cellular apoptosis—and in lengthening of survival.[254] These observations, as well as retrospective data indicating enhanced survival among patients receiving sirolimus immunosuppression following liver transplantation for HCC, led to the development of a phase I/II study of everolimus established that 10 mg daily was a safe dose.[255] The phase II portion, a two-stage efficacy design, did not meet its prespecified boundary for expansion to the second stage. Of 25 evaluable patients, 1 (4%) had a partial response and 10 (40%) had stable disease. Median time to progression was 3.9 months and median overall survival was 8.4 months. Nonetheless, everolimus was investigated in the second-line setting after sorafenib failure in the phase III, randomized, placebo-controlled EVOLVE-1 study (Clinical Trial: NCT01035229) that was recently reported as negative.

A randomized phase III study of brivanib after progression of disease on sorafenib versus best supportive care also failed to meet its primary end point of improved overall survival.[256] Among 395 randomized patients, 87% had disease progression while on sorafenib, median overall survival was 9.4 months in the brivanib group versus 8.2 months in the placebo group (HR, 0.89; 95.8% CI, 0.69 to 1.15; p = 0.3307). This study's importance lies in defining what may be the true and current median survival of patients with advanced HCC, preserved liver function, and who have failed at least one prior line of therapy. The median survival of such population seems to be better than anticipated and may be reflective of the involvement of multidisciplines, ensuring better management of patients with advanced HCC. A selection bias, of course, could not be ruled out in the brivanib study as portal invasion and/or thrombosis was noted in 12% of placebo patients versus 25% on the brivanib arm.[256]

Ramucirumab, a monoclonal antibody blocking VEGFR-2, was recently assessed in a phase II study comprised of 43 patients with systemic treatment-naïve advanced HCC.[257] The median progression-free survival was 4 months and the median survival was 12 months. Based on these data, a randomized phase III study of ramucirumab versus best supportive care in the second-line setting is ongoing (Clinical Trial: NCT01140347).

The biosynthesis of the nonessential amino acid arginine occurs as part of the urea cycle and is dependent upon the enzymes argininosuccinate synthetase and argininosuccinate lyase. Messenger RNA encoding argininosuccinate synthetase is not present in subsets of hepatocellular carcinomas; therefore, arginine must be extracted from the circulation.[258] Pegylated arginine deiminase (ADI-PEG 20) is an arginine-degrading enzyme isolated from *Mycoplasma* that is formulated with polyethylene glycol (molecular weight: 20 kDa). In preclinical models, ADI-PEG 20 decreases HCC cell viability at low nanomolar concentrations, reduces serum arginine levels to undetectable levels, and prolongs survival in HCC xenograft mouse models. A phase I/II study demonstrated an excellent safety profile in a patient population comprised with a high burden of disease and impaired hepatic function.[259] The most common events were injection site reactions and isolated lab abnormalities, such as elevated fibrinogen. Of 19 patients evaluable, 2 (10.5%) had a complete response, 7 (36.8%) had a partial response, and 7 (36.8%) had stable disease. The duration of response ranged from 37 to more than 680 days. A subsequent study reported a disease control rate of 63.1%, a 2.6% objective response rate, and a median overall survival of 11.4 months.[260] This exclusively European patient population was composed predominantly of HCV-associated (79%) HCC confined to the liver (84%) with otherwise excellent hepatic function (81%). In contrast, Yang and colleagues[261] tested the agent in a heavily pretreated Asian population with HBV-associated (69%) extrahepatic (58%) hepatocellular carcinoma. In this study, no objective responses were noted and the median overall survival was 7.3 months. Currently, a double-blind placebo-controlled study of ADI-PEG 20 after prior systemic therapy is ongoing (Clinical Trial: NCT01287585).

Systemic Treatments for Patients with Advanced Liver Cirrhosis

Both the SHARP and Asia-Pacific studies were limited to patients with unresectable or metastatic HCC who also had preserved liver function. The benefit of sorafenib in patients with Child-Pugh class B and C has not been established. Sorafenib's safety in patients who are not Child-Pugh class A is of concern. A subgroup analysis of the phase II sorafenib study reported higher rates of hepatic decompensation, represented by worse hyperbilirubinemia, encephalopathy, and ascites in Child-Pugh class B compared to Child-Pugh class A patients.[262] Patients in this subgroup had a shorter treatment duration as well as shorter survival in Child-Pugh class B (3.2 months) versus Child-Pugh class A patients (9.5 months). In a Japanese study, there were no differences in the incidence of adverse events between Child-Pugh class A and B groups, despite a geometric means of area under the curve (AUC_{0-12}) and maximum serum concentration (Cmax) at steady state that were slightly lower in patients with Child-Pugh class B cirrhosis compared with Child-Pugh class A.[263] Similar findings have been reported from the phase IV study of sorafenib known as GIDEON.[264] Child-Pugh class B and C patients were treated for a shorter duration, had a shorter median survival on sorafenib, and were more likely to develop hepatic and serious drug-related adverse events. A phase I study of sorafenib pharmacokinetics in patients with hepatic dysfunction helped establish some guidance on the use of sorafenib among patients with advanced Child-Pugh score.[265] For a serum bilirubin $\leq$1.5 × upper limit of normal (ULN), sorafenib at the full dose of 400 mg twice daily can be given, whereas for a bilirubin 1.6 to 3 × ULN, half that dose should be considered. For albumin <2.5 mg/dL, no more than 200 mg once daily should be given. There was no safe dose identified for patients

with a bilirubin >3 × ULN. Other antiangiogenic therapies have shown to be detrimental in cirrhotics (Fig. 44.6).[237]

TREATMENT OF OTHER PRIMARY LIVER TUMORS

Fibrolamellar Hepatocellular Carcinoma

Fibrolamellar HCC is a rare primary liver cancer that differs significantly from the usual HCC. Fibrolamellar HCC occurs in a much younger age group (peak incidence, 3rd decade), is usually not associated with cirrhosis or viral hepatitis, and affects males and females equally. Additionally, a much higher percentage (>15%) of patients with fibrolamellar HCC presents with positive lymph nodes than normal variant HCC.

Whether the diagnosis of fibrolamellar HCC portends a more favorable outcome after surgical treatment remains controversial.[266–269] Resection is the first-line of therapy. For those patients in whom the tumor is thought to be unresectable, liver transplantation provides an effective alternative. Pinna et al.[269] described 13 patients with fibrolamellar HCC who received transplantation between 1968 and 1995 and reported 1-, 3-, and 5-year patient survival rates of approximately 90%, 75%, and 38%, respectively.[269] Given that most patients transplanted presented as young patients with advanced disease, this is not an unacceptable survival rate. El-Gazzaz et al.[270] reported similar survival rates. Contrary to what was previously reported, in a large 95 patient retrospective analysis, with 50% presented with stage IV disease, median survival was limited to 6.7 years. Factors significantly associated with poor survival were female sex, advanced stage, lymph node metastases, macrovascular invasion, and unresectable disease.[271]

There is a great need for new, effective systemic therapies for advanced fibrolamellar HCC. A study is underway evaluating everolimus plus estrogen deprivation with leuprolide and letrozole for unresectable fibrolamellar HCC (Clinical Trial: NCT01642186).

Hepatoblastoma

Hepatoblastoma is the most common primary cancer of the liver occurring in childhood. The annual incidence of hepatoblastoma ranges from 0.5 to 1.5 cases per million children, with a peak incidence occurring within the first 2 years of life.[272] Hepatoblastoma is highly sensitive to chemotherapy, which often renders unresectable tumors resectable. Surgical resection is considered the first line of therapy. However, for those tumors that cannot be converted to resectable lesions but without distant metastasis, most can be rescued with liver transplantation. Survival rates for these children after liver transplantation is excellent, with 1-, 3-, and 5-year survivals reported at 92%, 92%, and 83%, respectively.[272]

Epithelioid Hemangioendothelioma

Epithelioid hemangioendothelioma is a very rare tumor of vascular origin that can originate in the liver; it occurs predominantly in females. The tumor is often confused with other more aggressive cancers, particularly cholangiocarcinoma, angiosarcoma, and HCC. The clinical course of epithelioid hemangioendothelioma is quite variable. In the review by Makhlouf et al.,[273] 137 cases were described, and survival ranged from 4 months to 28 years. Of interest, one patient who received no treatment survived for 27 years without evidence of metastasis. Surgical resection is considered to be the treatment of choice. However, in multifocal disease, a short observation may be reasonable to help decide between observation, ablation, resection, or transplant as the course of action. The presence of metastatic disease does not seem to influence survival and should not be considered an absolute contraindication to either surgical resection or transplantation.

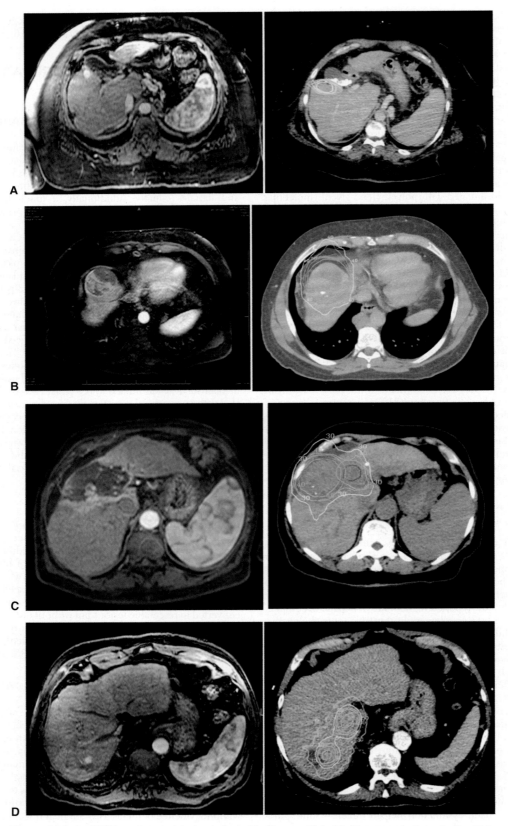

Figure 44.6 An SBRT can be used to treat single **(A, B)** or multiple **(C, D)** tumors in three to five high-dose, highly focused treatments. Planning is typically performed by fusing MRI images **(A, C)** with a planning CT scan **(B, D)** for accurate targeting. Special attention must be given to minimizing radiation dose to the remaining liver, particularly for patients with preexisting liver dysfunction.

REFERENCES

1. Parkin DM, Bray F, Ferlay J, et al. Global cancer statistics, 2002. *CA Cancer J Clin* 2005;55:74–108.
2. Llovet JM, Bustamante J, Castells A, et al. Natural history of untreated nonsurgical hepatocellular carcinoma: rationale for the design and evaluation of therapeutic trials. *Hepatology* 1999;29:62–67.
3. Lawitz E, Poordad FF, Pang PS, et al. Sofosbuvir and ledipasvir fixed-dose combination with and without ribavirin in treatment-naive and previously treated patients with genotype 1 hepatitis C virus infection (LONESTAR): an open-label, randomised, phase 2 trial. *Lancet* 2014;383:515–523.
4. Yu MW, Yang YC, Yang SY, et al. Androgen receptor exon 1 CAG repeat length and risk of hepatocellular carcinoma in women. *Hepatology* 2002; 36:156–163.
5. Kim WR, Gores GJ, Benson JT, et al. Mortality and hospital utilization for hepatocellular carcinoma in the United States. *Gastroenterology* 2005;129: 486–493.
6. Chang MH, Chen TH, Hsu HM, et al. Prevention of hepatocellular carcinoma by universal vaccination against hepatitis B virus: the effect and problems. *Clin Cancer Res* 2005;11:7953–7957.
7. Siegel R, Naishadham D, Jemal A. Cancer statistics, 2013. *CA Cancer J Clin* 2013;63:11–30.
8. Beasley RP, Hwang LY, Lin CC, et al. Hepatocellular carcinoma and hepatitis B virus. A prospective study of 22,707 men in Taiwan. *Lancet* 1981;2: 1129–1133.
9. Yuen MF, Tanaka Y, Fong DY, et al. Independent risk factors and predictive score for the development of hepatocellular carcinoma in chronic hepatitis B. *J Hepatol* 2009;50:80–88.
10. Blum HE, Moradpour D. Viral pathogenesis of hepatocellular carcinoma. *J Gastroenterol Hepatol* 2002;17:S413–S420.
11. Farazi PA, DePinho RA. Hepatocellular carcinoma pathogenesis: from genes to environment. *Nat Rev Cancer* 2006;6:674–687.
12. Rehermann B, Nascimbeni M. Immunology of hepatitis B virus and hepatitis C virus infection. *Nat Rev Immunol* 2005;5:215–229.
13. Hoshida Y, Toffanin S, Lachenmayer A, et al. Molecular classification and novel targets in hepatocellular carcinoma: recent advancements. *Semin Liver Dis* 2010;30:35–51.
14. Villanueva A, Newell P, Chiang DY, et al. Genomics and signaling pathways in hepatocellular carcinoma. *Semin Liver Dis* 2007;27:55–76.
15. Zhang Y, Wei W, Cheng N, et al. Hepatitis C virus-induced up-regulation of microRNA-155 promotes hepatocarcinogenesis by activating Wnt signaling. *Hepatology* 2012;56:1631–1640.
16. Seitz HK, Stickel F. Risk factors and mechanisms of hepatocarcinogenesis with special emphasis on alcohol and oxidative stress. *Biol Chem* 2006;387:349–360.
17. McClain CJ, Hill DB, Song Z, et al. Monocyte activation in alcoholic liver disease. *Alcohol* 2002;27:53–61.
18. Osna NA, Clemens DL, Donohue TM Jr. Ethanol metabolism alters interferon gamma signaling in recombinant HepG2 cells. *Hepatology* 2005;42: 1109–1117.
19. Browning JD, Szczepaniak LS, Dobbins R, et al. Prevalence of hepatic steatosis in an urban population in the United States: impact of ethnicity. *Hepatology* 2004;40:1387–1395.
20. Lazo M, Clark JM. The epidemiology of nonalcoholic fatty liver disease: a global perspective. *Semin Liver Dis* 2008;28:339–350.
21. Williams CD, Stengel J, Asike MI, et al. Prevalence of nonalcoholic fatty liver disease and nonalcoholic steatohepatitis among a largely middle-aged population utilizing ultrasound and liver biopsy: a prospective study. *Gastroenterology* 2011;140:124–131.
22. Ascha MS, Hanouneh IA, Lopez R, et al. The incidence and risk factors of hepatocellular carcinoma in patients with nonalcoholic steatohepatitis. *Hepatology* 2010;51:1972–1978.
23. Yatsuji S, Hashimoto E, Tobari M, et al. Clinical features and outcomes of cirrhosis due to non-alcoholic steatohepatitis compared with cirrhosis caused by chronic hepatitis C. *J Gastroenterol Hepatol* 2009;24:248–254.
24. Ertle J, Dechene A, Sowa JP, et al. Non-alcoholic fatty liver disease progresses to hepatocellular carcinoma in the absence of apparent cirrhosis. *Int J Cancer* 2011;128:2436–2443.
25. Starley BQ, Calcagno CJ, Harrison SA. Nonalcoholic fatty liver disease and hepatocellular carcinoma: a weighty connection. *Hepatology* 2010;51: 1820–1832.
26. Regimbeau JM, Colombat M, Mognol P, et al. Obesity and diabetes as a risk factor for hepatocellular carcinoma. *Liver Transpl* 2004;10:S69–S73.
27. Guzman G, Brunt EM, Petrovic LM, et al. Does nonalcoholic fatty liver disease predispose patients to hepatocellular carcinoma in the absence of cirrhosis? *Arch Pathol Lab Med* 2008;132:1761–1766.
28. Gao J, Xie L, Yang WS, et al. Risk factors of hepatocellular carcinoma—current status and perspectives. *Asian Pac J Cancer Prev* 2012;13:743–752.
29. Henderson BE, Preston-Martin S, Edmondson HA, et al. Hepatocellular carcinoma and oral contraceptives. *Br J Cancer* 1983;48:437–440.
30. Ha NB, Ahmed A, Ayoub W, et al. Risk factors for hepatocellular carcinoma in patients with chronic liver disease: a case-control study. *Cancer Causes Control* 2012;23:455–462.
31. Edge SB, Compton CC. The American Joint Committee on Cancer: the 7th edition of the AJCC cancer staging manual and the future of TNM. *Ann Surg Oncol* 2010;17:1471–1474.
32. Pugh RN, Murray-Lyon IM, Dawson JL, et al. Transection of the oesophagus for bleeding oesophageal varices. *Br J Surg* 1973;60:646–649.
33. A new prognostic system for hepatocellular carcinoma: a retrospective study of 435 patients: the Cancer of the Liver Italian Program (CLIP) investigators. *Hepatology* 1998;28:751–755.
34. Prospective validation of the CLIP score: a new prognostic system for patients with cirrhosis and hepatocellular carcinoma. The Cancer of the Liver Italian Program (CLIP) Investigators. *Hepatology* 2000;31:840–845.
35. Kaseb AO, Hassan MM, Lin E, et al. V-CLIP: Integrating plasma vascular endothelial growth factor into a new scoring system to stratify patients with advanced hepatocellular carcinoma for clinical trials. *Cancer* 2011;117: 2478–2488.
36. Leung TW, Tang AM, Zee B, et al. Construction of the Chinese University Prognostic Index for hepatocellular carcinoma and comparison with the TNM staging system, the Okuda staging system, and the Cancer of the Liver Italian Program staging system: a study based on 926 patients. *Cancer* 2002;94: 1760–1769.
37. Chevret S, Trinchet JC, Mathieu D, et al. A new prognostic classification for predicting survival in patients with hepatocellular carcinoma. Groupe d'Etude et de Traitement du Carcinome Hepatocellulaire. *J Hepatol* 1999; 31:133–141.
38. Kudo M, Chung H, Osaki Y. Prognostic staging system for hepatocellular carcinoma (CLIP score): its value and limitations, and a proposal for a new staging system, the Japan Integrated Staging Score (JIS score). *J Gastroenterol* 2003;38:207–215.
39. Llovet JM, Bru C, Bruix J. Prognosis of hepatocellular carcinoma: the BCLC staging classification. *Semin Liver Dis* 1999;19:329–338.
40. Cillo U, Vitale A, Grigoletto F, et al. Prospective validation of the Barcelona Clinic Liver Cancer staging system. *J Hepatol* 2006;44:723–731.
41. Collette S, Bonnetain F, Paoletti X, et al. Prognosis of advanced hepatocellular carcinoma: comparison of three staging systems in two French clinical trials. *Ann Oncol* 2008;19:1117–1126.
42. Huitzil-Melendez FD, Capanu M, O'Reilly EM, et al. Advanced hepatocellular carcinoma: which staging systems best predict prognosis? *J Clin Oncol* 2010;28:2889–2895.
43. Dusenbery D, Ferris JV, Thaete FL, et al. Percutaneous ultrasound-guided needle biopsy of hepatic mass lesions using a cytohistologic approach. Comparison of two needle types. *Am J Clin Pathol* 1995;104:583–587.
44. Di Tommaso L, Franchi G, Park YN, et al. Diagnostic value of HSP70, glypican 3, and glutamine synthetase in hepatocellular nodules in cirrhosis. *Hepatology* 2007;45:725–734.
45. Bruix J, Sherman M. Management of hepatocellular carcinoma: an update. *Hepatology* 2011;53:1020–1022.
46. Bruix J, Sherman M, Llovet JM, et al. Clinical management of hepatocellular carcinoma. Conclusions of the Barcelona-2000 EASL conference. European Association for the Study of the Liver. *J Hepatol* 2001;35:421–430.
47. Forner A, Vilana R, Ayuso C, et al. Diagnosis of hepatic nodules 20 mm or smaller in cirrhosis: Prospective validation of the noninvasive diagnostic criteria for hepatocellular carcinoma. *Hepatology* 2008;47:97–104.
48. Bialecki ES, Ezenekwe AM, Brunt EM, et al. Comparison of liver biopsy and noninvasive methods for diagnosis of hepatocellular carcinoma. *Clin Gastroenterol Hepatol* 2006;4:361–368.
49. Bret PM, Labadie M, Bretagnolle M, et al. Hepatocellular carcinoma: diagnosis by percutaneous fine needle biopsy. *Gastrointest Radiol* 1988;13:253–255.
50. Durand F, Regimbeau JM, Belghiti J, et al. Assessment of the benefits and risks of percutaneous biopsy before surgical resection of hepatocellular carcinoma. *J Hepatol* 2001;35:254–258.
51. Clavien PA, Petrowsky H, DeOliveira ML, et al. Strategies for safer liver surgery and partial liver transplantation. *N Engl J Med* 2007;356:1545–1559.
52. Capussotti L, Ferrero A, Vigano L, et al. Liver resection for HCC with cirrhosis: surgical perspectives out of EASL/AASLD guidelines. *Eur J Surg Oncol* 2009;35:11–15.
53. Cucchetti A, Ercolani G, Vivarelli M, et al. Is portal hypertension a contraindication to hepatic resection? *Ann Surg* 2009;250:922–928.
54. Shirabe K, Shimada M, Gion T, et al. Postoperative liver failure after major hepatic resection for hepatocellular carcinoma in the modern era with special reference to remnant liver volume. *J Am Coll Surg* 1999;188:304–309.
55. Breitenstein S, Apestegui C, Petrowsky H, et al. "State of the art" in liver resection and living donor liver transplantation: a worldwide survey of 100 liver centers. *World J Surg* 2009;33:797–803.
56. Aoki T, Imamura H, Hasegawa K, et al. Sequential preoperative arterial and portal venous embolizations in patients with hepatocellular carcinoma. *Arch Surg* 2004;139:766–774.
57. Ogata S, Belghiti J, Farges O, et al. Sequential arterial and portal vein embolizations before right hepatectomy in patients with cirrhosis and hepatocellular carcinoma. *Br J Surg* 2006;93:1091–1098.
58. Palavecino M, Chun YS, Madoff DC, et al. Major hepatic resection for hepatocellular carcinoma with or without portal vein embolization: Perioperative outcome and survival. *Surgery* 2009;145:399–405.
59. Seo DD, Lee HC, Jang MK, et al. Preoperative portal vein embolization and surgical resection in patients with hepatocellular carcinoma and small future liver remnant volume: comparison with transarterial chemoembolization. *Ann Surg Oncol* 2007;14:3501–3509.

60. Fan ST, Lo CM, Liu CL, et al. Hepatectomy for hepatocellular carcinoma: toward zero hospital deaths. *Ann Surg* 1999;229:322–330.

61. Poon RT, Fan ST. Assessment of hepatic reserve for indication of hepatic resection: how I do it. *J Hepatobiliary Pancreat Surg* 2005;12:31–37.

62. Yamanaka N, Okamoto E, Toyosaka A, et al. Prognostic factors after hepatectomy for hepatocellular carcinomas. A univariate and multivariate analysis. *Cancer* 1990;65:1104–1110.

63. Liu JH, Chen PW, Asch SM, et al. Surgery for hepatocellular carcinoma: does it improve survival? *Ann Surg Oncol* 2004;11:298–303.

64. Hanazaki K, Kajikawa S, Shimozawa N, et al. Hepatic resection for hepatocellular carcinoma in the elderly. *J Am Coll Surg* 2001;192:38–46.

65. Ercolani G, Grazi GL, Ravaioli M, et al. Liver resection for hepatocellular carcinoma on cirrhosis: univariate and multivariate analysis of risk factors for intrahepatic recurrence. *Ann Surg* 2003;237:536–543.

66. Zhou XD, Tang ZY, Yang BH, et al. Experience of 1000 patients who underwent hepatectomy for small hepatocellular carcinoma. *Cancer* 2001;91:1479–1486.

67. Belghiti J, Regimbeau JM, Durand F, et al. Resection of hepatocellular carcinoma: a European experience on 328 cases. *Hepatogastroenterology* 2002;49:41–46.

68. Kanematsu T, Furui J, Yanaga K, et al. A 16-year experience in performing hepatic resection in 303 patients with hepatocellular carcinoma: 1985–2000. *Surgery* 2002;131:S153–S158.

69. Wayne JD, Lauwers GY, Ikai I, et al. Preoperative predictors of survival after resection of small hepatocellular carcinomas. *Ann Surg* 2002;235:722–730.

70. Wu CC, Cheng SB, Ho WM, et al. Liver resection for hepatocellular carcinoma in patients with cirrhosis. *Br J Surg* 2005;92:348–355.

71. Capussotti L, Muratore A, Amisano M, et al. Liver resection for hepatocellular carcinoma on cirrhosis: analysis of mortality, morbidity and survival—a European single center experience. *Eur J Surg Oncol* 2005;31:986–993.

72. Hasegawa K, Kokudo N, Imamura H, et al. Prognostic impact of anatomic resection for hepatocellular carcinoma. *Ann Surg* 2005;242:252–259.

73. Nathan H, Schulick RD, Choti MA, et al. Predictors of survival after resection of early hepatocellular carcinoma. *Ann Surg* 2009;249:799–805.

74. Yang LY, Fang F, Ou DP, et al. Solitary large hepatocellular carcinoma: a specific subtype of hepatocellular carcinoma with good outcome after hepatic resection. *Ann Surg* 2009;249:118–123.

75. Wang J, Xu LB, Liu C, et al. Prognostic factors and outcome of 438 Chinese patients with hepatocellular carcinoma underwent partial hepatectomy in a single center. *World J Surg* 2010;34:2434–2441.

76. Lise M, Bacchetti S, Da Pian P, et al. Prognostic factors affecting long term outcome after liver resection for hepatocellular carcinoma: results in a series of 100 Italian patients. *Cancer* 1998;82:1028–1036.

77. Shi M, Guo RP, Lin XJ, et al. Partial hepatectomy with wide versus narrow resection margin for solitary hepatocellular carcinoma: a prospective randomized trial. *Ann Surg* 2007;245:36–43.

78. Ikai I, Arii S, Kojiro M, et al. Reevaluation of prognostic factors for survival after liver resection in patients with hepatocellular carcinoma in a Japanese nationwide survey. *Cancer* 2004;101:796–802.

79. Kang CM, Choi GH, Kim DH, et al. Revisiting the role of nonanatomic resection of small (< or = 4 cm) and single hepatocellular carcinoma in patients with well-preserved liver function. *J Surg Res* 2010;160:81–89.

80. Bismuth H, Chiche L, Adam R, et al. Liver resection versus transplantation for hepatocellular carcinoma in cirrhotic patients. *Ann Surg* 1993;218:145–151.

81. Mazzaferro V, Regalia E, Doci R, et al. Liver transplantation for the treatment of small hepatocellular carcinomas in patients with cirrhosis. *N Engl J Med* 1996;334:693–699.

82. Cillo U, Vitale A, Bassanello M, et al. Liver transplantation for the treatment of moderately or well-differentiated hepatocellular carcinoma. *Ann Surg* 2004;239:150–159.

83. Hemming AW, Cattral MS, Reed AI, et al. Liver transplantation for hepatocellular carcinoma. *Ann Surg* 2001;233:652–659.

84. Mazzaferro V, Llovet JM, Miceli R, et al. Predicting survival after liver transplantation in patients with hepatocellular carcinoma beyond the Milan criteria: a retrospective, exploratory analysis. *Lancet Oncol* 2009;10:35–43.

85. Pelletier SJ, Fu S, Thyagarajan V, et al. An intention-to-treat analysis of liver transplantation for hepatocellular carcinoma using organ procurement transplant network data. *Liver Transpl* 2009;15:859–868.

86. Herrero JI, Sangro B, Pardo F, et al. Liver transplantation in patients with hepatocellular carcinoma across Milan criteria. *Liver Transpl* 2008;14:272–278.

87. Onaca N, Davis GL, Goldstein RM, et al. Expanded criteria for liver transplantation in patients with hepatocellular carcinoma: a report from the International Registry of Hepatic Tumors in Liver Transplantation. *Liver Transpl* 2007;13:391–399.

88. Decaens T, Roudot-Thoraval F, Hadni-Bresson S, et al. Impact of UCSF criteria according to pre- and post-OLT tumor features: analysis of 479 patients listed for HCC with a short waiting time. *Liver Transpl* 2006;12:1761–1769.

89. Bigourdan JM, Jaeck D, Meyer N, et al. Small hepatocellular carcinoma in Child A cirrhotic patients: hepatic resection versus transplantation. *Liver Transpl* 2003;9:513–520.

90. Yao FY, Ferrell L, Bass NM, et al. Liver transplantation for hepatocellular carcinoma: expansion of the tumor size limits does not adversely impact survival. *Hepatology* 2001;33:1394–1403.

91. Tamura S, Kato T, Berho M, et al. Impact of histological grade of hepatocellular carcinoma on the outcome of liver transplantation. *Arch Surg* 2001;136:25–30.

92. Regalia E, Coppa J, Pulvirenti A, et al. Liver transplantation for small hepatocellular carcinoma in cirrhosis: analysis of our experience. *Transplant Proc* 2001;33:1442–1444.

93. Jonas S, Herrmann M, Rayes N, et al. Survival after liver transplantation for hepatocellular carcinoma in cirrhosis according to the underlying liver disease. *Transplant Proc* 2001;33:3444–3445.

94. Llovet JM, Bruix J, Fuster J, et al. Liver transplantation for small hepatocellular carcinoma: the tumor-node-metastasis classification does not have prognostic power. *Hepatology* 1998;27:1572–1577.

95. Yao FY, Xiao L, Bass NM, et al. Liver transplantation for hepatocellular carcinoma: validation of the UCSF-expanded criteria based on preoperative imaging. *Am J Transplant* 2007;7:2587–2596.

96. Duffy JP, Vardanian A, Benjamin E, et al. Liver transplantation criteria for hepatocellular carcinoma should be expanded: a 22-year experience with 467 patients at UCLA. *Ann Surg* 2007;246:502–509.

97. Olthoff KM, Merion RM, Ghobrial RM, et al. Outcomes of 385 adult-to-adult living donor liver transplant recipients: a report from the A2ALL Consortium. *Ann Surg* 2005;242:314–323.

98. Sarasin FP, Majno PE, Llovet JM, et al. Living donor liver transplantation for early hepatocellular carcinoma: A life-expectancy and cost-effectiveness perspective. *Hepatology* 2001;33:1073–1079.

99. Todo S, Furukawa H. Living donor liver transplantation for adult patients with hepatocellular carcinoma: experience in Japan. *Ann Surg* 2004;240:451–459.

100. Hwang S, Lee SG, Joh JW, et al. Liver transplantation for adult patients with hepatocellular carcinoma in Korea: comparison between cadaveric donor and living donor liver transplantations. *Liver Transpl* 2005;11:1265–1272.

101. Takada Y, Ueda M, Ito T, et al. Living donor liver transplantation as a second-line therapeutic strategy for patients with hepatocellular carcinoma. *Liver Transpl* 2006;12:912–919.

102. Sugawara Y, Tamura S, Makuuchi M. Living donor liver transplantation for hepatocellular carcinoma: Tokyo University series. *Dig Dis* 2007;25:310–312.

103. Lo CM, Ngan H, Tso WK, et al. Randomized controlled trial of transarterial lipiodol chemoembolization for unresectable hepatocellular carcinoma. *Hepatology* 2002;35:1164–1171.

104. Llovet JM, Fuster J, Bruix J. Intention-to-treat analysis of surgical treatment for early hepatocellular carcinoma: resection versus transplantation. *Hepatology* 1999;30:1434–1440.

105. Maddala YK, Stadheim L, Andrews JC, et al. Drop-out rates of patients with hepatocellular cancer listed for liver transplantation: outcome with chemoembolization. *Liver Transpl* 2004;10:449–455.

106. Vilana R, Bruix J, Bru C, et al. Tumor size determines the efficacy of percutaneous ethanol injection for the treatment of small hepatocellular carcinoma. *Hepatology* 1992;16:353–357.

107. Lu DS, Yu NC, Raman SS, et al. Radiofrequency ablation of hepatocellular carcinoma: treatment success as defined by histologic examination of the explanted liver. *Radiology* 2005;234:954–960.

108. Mazzaferro V, Battiston C, Perrone S, et al. Radiofrequency ablation of small hepatocellular carcinoma in cirrhotic patients awaiting liver transplantation: a prospective study. *Ann Surg* 2004;240:900–909.

109. Lo CM, Liu CL, Chan SC, et al. A randomized, controlled trial of postoperative adjuvant interferon therapy after resection of hepatocellular carcinoma. *Ann Surg* 2007;245:831–842.

110. Chen LT, Chen MF, Li LA, et al. Long-term results of a randomized, observation-controlled, phase III trial of adjuvant interferon Alfa-2b in hepatocellular carcinoma after curative resection. *Ann Surg* 2012;255:8–17.

111. Lau WY, Leung TW, Ho SK, et al. Adjuvant intra-arterial iodine-131-labelled lipiodol for resectable hepatocellular carcinoma: a prospective randomised trial. *Lancet* 1999;353:797–801.

112. Lau WY, Lai EC, Leung TW, et al. Adjuvant intra-arterial iodine-131-labeled lipiodol for resectable hepatocellular carcinoma: a prospective randomized trial-update on 5-year and 10-year survival. *Ann Surg* 2008;247:43–48.

113. Muto Y, Moriwaki H, Ninomiya M, et al. Prevention of second primary tumors by an acyclic retinoid, polyprenoic acid, in patients with hepatocellular carcinoma. Hepatoma Prevention Study Group. *N Engl J Med* 1996;334:1561–1567.

114. Muto Y, Moriwaki H, Saito A. Prevention of second primary tumors by an acyclic retinoid in patients with hepatocellular carcinoma. *N Engl J Med* 1999;340:1046–1047.

115. Wang SN, Chuang SC, Lee KT. Efficacy of sorafenib as adjuvant therapy to prevent early recurrence of hepatocellular carcinoma after curative surgery: a pilot study. *Hepatol Res* 2014;44:523–531.

116. Wu CC, Ho YZ, Ho WL, et al. Preoperative transcatheter arterial chemoembolization for resectable large hepatocellular carcinoma: a reappraisal. *Br J Surg* 1995;82:122–126.

117. Schwartz JD, Schwartz M, Mandeli J, et al. Neoadjuvant and adjuvant therapy for resectable hepatocellular carcinoma: review of the randomised clinical trials. *Lancet Oncol* 2002;3:593–603.

118. Yamasaki S, Hasegawa H, Kinoshita H, et al. A prospective randomized trial of the preventive effect of pre-operative transcatheter arterial embolization against recurrence of hepatocellular carcinoma. *Jpn J Cancer Res* 1996;87:206–211.

119. Shiratori Y, Shiina S, Teratani T, et al. Interferon therapy after tumor ablation improves prognosis in patients with hepatocellular carcinoma associated with hepatitis C virus. *Ann Intern Med* 2003;138:299–306.

120. Takayama T, Sekine T, Makuuchi M, et al. Adoptive immunotherapy to lower postsurgical recurrence rates of hepatocellular carcinoma: a randomised trial. *Lancet* 2000;356:802–807.

121. Mazzaferro V, Romito R, Schiavo M, et al. Prevention of hepatocellular carcinoma recurrence with alpha-interferon after liver resection in HCV cirrhosis. *Hepatology* 2006;44:1543–1554.
122. Breitenstein S, Dimitroulis D, Petrowsky H, et al. Systematic review and meta-analysis of interferon after curative treatment of hepatocellular carcinoma in patients with viral hepatitis. *Br J Surg* 2009;96:975–981.
123. Leung TW, Patt YZ, Lau WY, et al. Complete pathological remission is possible with systemic combination chemotherapy for inoperable hepatocellular carcinoma. *Clin Cancer Res* 1999;5:1676–1681.
124. Cherqui D, Laurent A, Mocellin N, et al. Liver resection for transplantable hepatocellular carcinoma: long-term survival and role of secondary liver transplantation. *Ann Surg* 2009;250:738–746.
125. Chua TC, Saxena A, Chu F, et al. Hepatic resection for transplantable hepatocellular carcinoma for patients within Milan and UCSF Criteria. *Am J Clin Oncol* 2012;35:141–145.
126. Margarit C, Escartin A, Castells L, et al. Resection for hepatocellular carcinoma is a good option in Child-Turcotte-Pugh class A patients with cirrhosis who are eligible for liver transplantation. *Liver Transpl* 2005;11:1242–1251.
127. Lee KK, Kim DG, Moon IS, et al. Liver transplantation versus liver resection for the treatment of hepatocellular carcinoma. *J Surg Oncol* 2010;101:47–53.
128. Facciuto ME, Rochon C, Pandey M, et al. Surgical dilemma: liver resection or liver transplantation for hepatocellular carcinoma and cirrhosis. Intention-to-treat analysis in patients within and outwith Milan criteria. *HPB (Oxford)* 2009;11:398–404.
129. Del Gaudio M, Ercolani G, Ravaioli M, et al. Liver transplantation for recurrent hepatocellular carcinoma on cirrhosis after liver resection: University of Bologna experience. *Am J Transplant* 2008;8:1177–1185.
130. Shah SA, Cleary SP, Tan JC, et al. An analysis of resection vs transplantation for early hepatocellular carcinoma: defining the optimal therapy at a single institution. *Ann Surg Oncol* 2007;14:2608–2614.
131. Poon RT, Fan ST, Lo CM, et al. Difference in tumor invasiveness in cirrhotic patients with hepatocellular carcinoma fulfilling the Milan criteria treated by resection and transplantation: impact on long-term survival. *Ann Surg* 2007;245:51–58.
132. Adam R, Azoulay D, Castaing D, et al. Liver resection as a bridge to transplantation for hepatocellular carcinoma on cirrhosis: a reasonable strategy? *Ann Surg* 2003;238:508–518.
133. Belghiti J, Cortes A, Abdalla EK, et al. Resection prior to liver transplantation for hepatocellular carcinoma. *Ann Surg* 2003;238:885–892.
134. Figueras J, Jaurrieta E, Valls C, et al. Resection or transplantation for hepatocellular carcinoma in cirrhotic patients: outcomes based on indicated treatment strategy. *J Am Coll Surg* 2000;190:580–587.
135. Cucchetti A, Vitale A, Gaudio MD, et al. Harm and benefits of primary liver resection and salvage transplantation for hepatocellular carcinoma. *Am J Transplant* 2010;10:619–627.
136. Belghiti J. Resection and liver transplantation for HCC. *J Gastroenterol* 2009;44:132–135.
137. Poon RT, Fan ST, Lo CM, et al. Long-term survival and pattern of recurrence after resection of small hepatocellular carcinoma in patients with preserved liver function: implications for a strategy of salvage transplantation. *Ann Surg* 2002;235:373–382.
138. Canter RJ, Patel SA, Kennedy T, et al. Comparative analysis of outcome in patients with hepatocellular carcinoma exceeding the Milan criteria treated with liver transplantation versus partial hepatectomy. *Am J Clin Oncol* 2010;34:466–471.
139. Shiina S, Tagawa K, Unuma T, et al. Percutaneous ethanol injection therapy for hepatocellular carcinoma. A histopathologic study. *Cancer* 1991;68:1524–1530.
140. Ohnishi K, Ohyama N, Ito S, et al. Small hepatocellular carcinoma: treatment with US-guided intratumoral injection of acetic acid. *Radiology* 1994;193:747–752.
141. Livraghi T, Giorgio A, Marin G, et al. Hepatocellular carcinoma and cirrhosis in 746 patients: long-term results of percutaneous ethanol injection. *Radiology* 1995;197:101–108.
142. Blendis L. Percutaneous ethanol ablation of small hepatocellular carcinomas: twenty years on. *Gastroenterology* 2006;130:280–282.
143. Mazzanti R, Arena U, Pantaleo P, et al. Survival and prognostic factors in patients with hepatocellular carcinoma treated by percutaneous ethanol injection: a 10-year experience. *Can J Gastroenterol* 2004;18:611–618.
144. Lin SM, Lin CJ, Lin CC, et al. Randomised controlled trial comparing percutaneous radiofrequency thermal ablation, percutaneous ethanol injection, and percutaneous acetic acid injection to treat hepatocellular carcinoma of 3 cm or less. *Gut* 2005;54:1151–1156.
145. Tsai WL, Cheng JS, Lai KH, et al. Clinical trial: percutaneous acetic acid injection vs. percutaneous ethanol injection for small hepatocellular carcinoma—a long-term follow-up study. *Aliment Pharmacol Ther* 2008;28:304–311.
146. Weis S, Franke A, Mossner J, et al. Radiofrequency (thermal) ablation versus no intervention or other interventions for hepatocellular carcinoma. *Cochrane Database Syst Rev* 2013;12:CD003046.
147. Kurokohchi K, Watanabe S, Masaki T, et al. Combination therapy of percutaneous ethanol injection and radiofrequency ablation against hepatocellular carcinomas difficult to treat. *Int J Oncol* 2002;21:611–615.
148. Cha DI, Lee MW, Rhim H, et al. Therapeutic efficacy and safety of percutaneous ethanol injection with or without combined radiofrequency ablation for hepatocellular carcinomas in high risk locations. *Korean J Radiol* 2013;14:240–247.
149. McGahan JP, Browning PD, Brock JM, et al. Hepatic ablation using radiofrequency electrocautery. *Invest Radiol* 1990;25:267–270.
150. Rossi S, Fornari F, Pathies C, et al. Thermal lesions induced by 480 KHz localized current field in guinea pig and pig liver. *Tumori* 1990;76:54–57.
151. Buscarini L, Rossi S, Fornari F, et al. Laparoscopic ablation of liver adenoma by radiofrequency electrocauthery. *Gastrointest Endosc* 1995;41:68–70.
152. Organ LW. Electrophysiologic principles of radiofrequency lesion making. *Appl Neurophysiol* 1976;39:69–76.
153. Nahum Goldberg S, Dupuy DE. Image-guided radiofrequency tumor ablation: challenges and opportunities—part I. *J Vasc Interv Radiol* 2001;12:1021–1032.
154. Siperstein AE, Berber E, Ballem N, et al. Survival after radiofrequency ablation of colorectal liver metastases: 10-year experience. *Ann Surg* 2007;246:559–565.
155. Gillams AR, Lees WR. Five-year survival in 309 patients with colorectal liver metastases treated with radiofrequency ablation. *Eur Radiol* 2009;19:1206–1213.
156. Machi J, Oishi AJ, Sumida K, et al. Long-term outcome of radiofrequency ablation for unresectable liver metastases from colorectal cancer: evaluation of prognostic factors and effectiveness in first- and second-line management. *Cancer J* 2006;12:318–326.
157. Simon CJ, Dupuy DE, Mayo-Smith WW. Microwave ablation: principles and applications. *Radiographics* 2005;25:S69–S83.
158. Ward RC, Healey TT, Dupuy DE. Microwave ablation devices for interventional oncology. *Expert Rev Med Devices* 2013;10:225–238.
159. Pathak S, Jones R, Tang JM, et al. Ablative therapies for colorectal liver metastases: a systematic review. *Colorectal Dis* 2011;13:e252–e265.
160. Dodd GD 3rd, Dodd NA, Lanctot AC, et al. Effect of variation of portal venous blood flow on radiofrequency and microwave ablations in a blood-perfused bovine liver model. *Radiology* 2013;267:129–136.
161. Wright AS, Lee FT Jr, Mahvi DM. Hepatic microwave ablation with multiple antennae results in synergistically larger zones of coagulation necrosis. *Ann Surg Oncol* 2003;10:275–283.
162. Martin RC, Scoggins CR, McMasters KM. Safety and efficacy of microwave ablation of hepatic tumors: a prospective review of a 5-year experience. *Ann Surg Oncol* 2010;17:171–178.
163. Liang P, Yu J, Yu XL, et al. Percutaneous cooled-tip microwave ablation under ultrasound guidance for primary liver cancer: a multicentre analysis of 1363 treatment-naive lesions in 1007 patients in China. *Gut* 2012;61:1100–1101.
164. Mulier S, Ni Y, Jamart J, et al. Local recurrence after hepatic radiofrequency coagulation: multivariate meta-analysis and review of contributing factors. *Ann Surg* 2005;242:158–171.
165. Lu DS, Raman SS, Limanond P, et al. Influence of large peritumoral vessels on outcome of radiofrequency ablation of liver tumors. *J Vasc Interv Radiol* 2003;14:1267–1274.
166. Schramm W, Yang D, Wood BJ, et al. Contribution of direct heating, thermal conduction and perfusion during radiofrequency and microwave ablation. *Open Biomed Eng J* 2007;1:47–52.
167. Kingham TP, Karkar AM, D'Angelica MI, et al. Ablation of perivascular hepatic malignant tumors with irreversible electroporation. *J Am Coll Surg* 2012;215:379–387.
168. Poon RT, Ng KK, Lam CM, et al. Learning curve for radiofrequency ablation of liver tumors: prospective analysis of initial 100 patients in a tertiary institution. *Ann Surg* 2004;239:441–449.
169. Cabibbo G, Maida M, Genco C, et al. Natural history of untreatable hepatocellular carcinoma: A retrospective cohort study. *World J Hepatol* 2012;4:256–261.
170. Ruzzenente A, Guglielmi A, Sandri M, et al. Surgical resection versus local ablation for HCC on cirrhosis: results from a propensity case-matched study. *J Gastrointest Surg* 2012;16:301–311.
171. Hsu CY, Lee YH, Hsia CY, et al. Performance status enhances the selection of treatment for patients with hepatocellular carcinoma within the Milan criteria. *Ann Surg Oncol* 2013;20:2035–2042.
172. Guglielmi A, Ruzzenente A, Valdegamberi A, et al. Radiofrequency ablation versus surgical resection for the treatment of hepatocellular carcinoma in cirrhosis. *J Gastrointest Surg* 2008;12:192–198.
173. Vivarelli M, Guglielmi A, Ruzzenente A, et al. Surgical resection versus percutaneous radiofrequency ablation in the treatment of hepatocellular carcinoma on cirrhotic liver. *Ann Surg* 2004;240:102–107.
174. Wakai T, Shirai Y, Suda T, et al. Long-term outcomes of hepatectomy vs percutaneous ablation for treatment of hepatocellular carcinoma < or =4 cm. *World J Gastroenterol* 2006;12:546–552.
175. Chen MS, Li JQ, Zheng Y, et al. A prospective randomized trial comparing percutaneous local ablative therapy and partial hepatectomy for small hepatocellular carcinoma. *Ann Surg* 2006;243:321–328.
176. Liang HH, Chen MS, Peng ZW, et al. Percutaneous radiofrequency ablation versus repeat hepatectomy for recurrent hepatocellular carcinoma: a retrospective study. *Ann Surg Oncol* 2008;15:3484–3493.
177. Huang J, Yan L, Cheng Z, et al. A randomized trial comparing radiofrequency ablation and surgical resection for HCC conforming to the Milan criteria. *Ann Surg* 2010;252:903–912.
178. Feng K, Yan J, Li X, et al. A randomized controlled trial of radiofrequency ablation and surgical resection in the treatment of small hepatocellular carcinoma. *J Hepatol* 2012;57:794–802.
179. Salem R, Lewandowski RJ, Kulik L, et al. Radioembolization results in longer time-to-progression and reduced toxicity compared with chemoembolization in patients with hepatocellular carcinoma. *Gastroenterology* 2011;140:497–507.

CANCERS OF THE GASTROINTESTINAL TRACT

180. Yamada R, Sato M, Kawabata M, et al. Hepatic artery embolization in 120 patients with unresectable hepatoma. *Radiology* 1983;148:397–401.

181. Llovet JM, Real MI, Montana X, et al. Arterial embolisation or chemoembolisation versus symptomatic treatment in patients with unresectable hepatocellular carcinoma: a randomised controlled trial. *Lancet* 2002;359:1734–1739.

182. Lo CM, Ngan H, Tso WK, et al. Randomized controlled trial of transarterial lipiodol chemoembolization for unresectable hepatocellular carcinoma. *Hepatology* 2002;35:1164–1171.

183. Becker G, Soezgen T, Olschewski M, et al. Combined TACE and PEI for palliative treatment of unresectable hepatocellular carcinoma. *World J Gastroenterol* 2005;11:6104–6109.

184. Soliman H, Ringash J, Jiang H, et al. Phase II trial of palliative radiotherapy for hepatocellular carcinoma and liver metastases. *J Clin Oncol* 2013;31:3980–3986.

185. Lawrence TS, Robertson JM, Anscher MS, et al. Hepatic toxicity resulting from cancer treatment. *Int J Radiat Oncol Biol Phys* 1995;31:1237–1248.

186. Guha C, Kavanagh BD. Hepatic radiation toxicity: avoidance and amelioration. *Semin Radiat Oncol* 2011;21:256–263.

187. Feng M, Normolle D, Pan CC, et al. Dosimetric analysis of radiation-induced gastric bleeding. *Int J Radiat Oncol Biol Phys* 2012;84:e1–e6.

188. Yoon HI, Koom WS, Lee IJ, et al. The significance of ICG-R15 in predicting hepatic toxicity in patients receiving radiotherapy for hepatocellular carcinoma. *Liver Int* 2012;32:1165–1171.

189. Imamura H, Sano K, Sugawara Y, et al. Assessment of hepatic reserve for indication of hepatic resection: decision tree incorporating indocyanine green test. *J Hepatobiliary Pancreat Surg* 2005;12:16–22.

190. Stenmark MH, Cao Y, Wang H, et al. Indocyanine green for individualized assessment of functional liver reserve in patients undergoing liver radiation therapy. *Int J Radiat Oncol Biol Phys* 2013;87:S26–S27.

191. Dawson LA, Normolle D, Balter JM, et al. Analysis of radiation-induced liver disease using the Lyman NTCP model. *Int J Radiat Oncol Biol Phys* 2002;53:810–821.

192. Robertson JM, McGinn CJ, Walker S, et al. A phase I trial of hepatic arterial bromodeoxyuridine and conformal radiation therapy for patients with primary hepatobiliary cancers or colorectal liver metastases. *Int J Radiat Oncol Biol Phys* 1997;39:1087–1092.

193. Ben-Josef E, Normolle D, Ensminger WD, et al. Phase II trial of high-dose conformal radiation therapy with concurrent hepatic artery floxuridine for unresectable intrahepatic malignancies. *J Clin Oncol* 2005;23:8739–8747.

194. Dawson LA, McGinn CJ, Normolle D, et al. Escalated focal liver radiation and concurrent hepatic artery fluorodeoxyuridine for unresectable intrahepatic malignancies. *J Clin Oncol* 2000;18:2210–2218.

195. McGinn CJ, Ten Haken RK, Ensminger WD, et al. Treatment of intrahepatic cancers with radiation doses based on a normal tissue complication probability model. *J Clin Oncol* 1998;16:2246–2252.

196. Mornex F, Girard N, Beziat C, et al. Feasibility and efficacy of high-dose three-dimensional-conformal radiotherapy in cirrhotic patients with small-size hepatocellular carcinoma non-eligible for curative therapies—mature results of the French Phase II RTF-1 trial. *Int J Radiat Oncol Biol Phys* 2006;66:1152–1158.

197. Seong J, Lee IJ, Shim SJ, et al. A multicenter retrospective cohort study of practice patterns and clinical outcome on radiotherapy for hepatocellular carcinoma in Korea. *Liver Int* 2009;29:147–152.

198. Shim SJ, Seong J, Han KH, et al. Local radiotherapy as a complement to incomplete transcatheter arterial chemoembolization in locally advanced hepatocellular carcinoma. *Liver Int* 2005;25:1189–1196.

199. Guo WJ, Yu EX, Liu LM, et al. Comparison between chemoembolization combined with radiotherapy and chemoembolization alone for large hepatocellular carcinoma. *World J Gastroenterol* 2003;9:1697–1701.

200. Huang YJ, Hsu HC, Wang CY, et al. The treatment responses in cases of radiation therapy to portal vein thrombosis in advanced hepatocellular carcinoma. *Int J Radiat Oncol Biol Phys* 2009;73:1155–1163.

201. Balter JM, Brock KK, Litzenberg DW, et al. Daily targeting of intrahepatic tumors for radiotherapy. *Int J Radiat Oncol Biol Phys* 2002;52:266–271.

202. Balter JM, Dawson LA, Kazanjian S, et al. Determination of ventilatory liver movement via radiographic evaluation of diaphragm position. *Int J Radiat Oncol Biol Phys* 2001;51:267–270.

203. Blomgren H, Lax I, Naslund I, et al. Stereotactic high dose fraction radiation therapy of extracranial tumors using an accelerator. Clinical experience of the first thirty-one patients. *Acta Oncol* 1995;34:861–870.

204. Mendez Romero A, Wunderink W, Hussain SM, et al. Stereotactic body radiation therapy for primary and metastatic liver tumors: a single institution phase i-ii study. *Acta Oncol* 2006;45:831–837.

205. Tse RV, Hawkins M, Lockwood G, et al. Phase I study of individualized stereotactic body radiotherapy for hepatocellular carcinoma and intrahepatic cholangiocarcinoma. *J Clin Oncol* 2008;26:657–664.

206. Bujold A, Massey CA, Kim JJ, et al. Sequential phase I and II trials of stereotactic body radiotherapy for locally advanced hepatocellular carcinoma. *J Clin Oncol* 2013;31:1631–1639.

207. Cardenes HR, Price TR, Perkins SM, et al. Phase I feasibility trial of stereotactic body radiation therapy for primary hepatocellular carcinoma. *Clin Transl Oncol* 2010;12:218–225.

208. Liu E, Stenmark MH, Schipper MJ, et al. Stereotactic body radiation therapy for primary and metastatic liver tumors. *Transl Oncol* 2012;6:442–446.

209. Sanuki N, Takeda A, Oku Y, et al. Stereotactic body radiotherapy for small hepatocellular carcinoma: a retrospective outcome analysis in 185 patients. *Acta Oncol* 2014;53:399–404.

210. Bibault JE, Dewas S, Vautravers-Dewas C, et al. Stereotactic body radiation therapy for hepatocellular carcinoma: prognostic factors of local control, overall survival, and toxicity. *PLoS One* 2013;8:e77472.

211. Chiba T, Tokuuye K, Matsuzaki Y, et al. Proton beam therapy for hepatocellular carcinoma: a retrospective review of 162 patients. *Clin Cancer Res* 2005;11:3799–3805.

212. Fukumitsu N, Sugahara S, Nakayama H, et al. A prospective study of hypofractionated proton beam therapy for patients with hepatocellular carcinoma. *Int J Radiat Oncol Biol Phys* 2009;74:831–836.

213. Kato H, Tsujii H, Miyamoto T, et al. Results of the first prospective study of carbon ion radiotherapy for hepatocellular carcinoma with liver cirrhosis. *Int J Radiat Oncol Biol Phys* 2004;59:1468–1476.

214. Goldschmidt RP, Kotzen JA, Giraud RM. Intraductal hepatocellular carcinoma treated by intralumenal brachytherapy. *Clin Oncol (R Coll Radiol)* 1993;5:118–119.

215. Crellin RP, Chan SY. Hepatocellular carcinoma treated by intralumenal brachytherapy. *Clin Oncol (R Coll Radiol)* 1993;5:332.

216. Goin JE, Salem R, Carr BI, et al. Treatment of unresectable hepatocellular carcinoma with intrahepatic yttrium 90 microspheres: factors associated with liver toxicities. *J Vasc Interv Radiol* 2005;16:205–213.

217. Salem R, Lewandowski RJ, Atassi B, et al. Treatment of unresectable hepatocellular carcinoma with use of 90Y microspheres (TheraSphere): safety, tumor response, and survival. *J Vasc Interv Radiol* 2005;16:1627–1639.

218. Sangro B, Salem R, Kennedy A, et al. Radioembolization for hepatocellular carcinoma: a review of the evidence and treatment recommendations. *Am J Clin Oncol* 2011;34:422–431.

219. Young JY, Rhee TK, Atassi B, et al. Radiation dose limits and liver toxicities resulting from multiple yttrium-90 radioembolization treatments for hepatocellular carcinoma. *J Vasc Interv Radiol* 2007;18:1375–1382.

220. Abou-Alfa GK, Venook AP. The impact of new data in the treatment of advanced hepatocellular carcinoma. *Curr Oncol Rep* 2008;10:199–205.

221. Poon RT, Ho JW, Tong CS, et al. Prognostic significance of serum vascular endothelial growth factor and endostatin in patients with hepatocellular carcinoma. *Br J Surg* 2004;91:1354–1360.

222. Wilhelm SM, Carter C, Tang L, et al. BAY 43-9006 exhibits broad spectrum oral antitumor activity and targets the RAF/MEK/ERK pathway and receptor tyrosine kinases involved in tumor progression and angiogenesis. *Cancer Res* 2004;64:7099–7109.

223. Abou-Alfa GK, Schwartz L, Ricci S, et al. Phase II study of sorafenib in patients with advanced hepatocellular carcinoma. *J Clin Oncol* 2006;24:4293–4300.

224. Llovet JM, Ricci S, Mazzaferro V, et al. Sorafenib in advanced hepatocellular carcinoma. *N Engl J Med* 2008;359:378–390.

225. Cheng AL, Kang YK, Chen Z, et al. Efficacy and safety of sorafenib in patients in the Asia-Pacific region with advanced hepatocellular carcinoma: a phase III randomised, double-blind, placebo-controlled trial. *Lancet Oncol* 2009;10:25–34.

226. Bruix J, Raoul JL, Sherman M, et al. Efficacy and safety of sorafenib in patients with advanced hepatocellular carcinoma: subanalyses of a phase III trial. *J Hepatol* 2012;57:821–829.

227. Cheng AL, Kang YK, Lin DY, et al. Sunitinib versus sorafenib in advanced hepatocellular cancer: results of a randomized phase III trial. *J Clin Oncol* 2013;31:4067–4075.

228. Lachenmayer A, Alsinet C, Savic R, et al. Wnt-pathway activation in two molecular classes of hepatocellular carcinoma and experimental modulation by sorafenib. *Clin Cancer Res* 2012;18:4997–5007.

229. Giambartolomei S, Covone F, Levrero M, et al. Sustained activation of the Raf/MEK/Erk pathway in response to EGF in stable cell lines expressing the Hepatitis C Virus (HCV) core protein. *Oncogene* 2001;20:2606–2610.

230. Himmelsbach K, Sauter D, Baumert TF, et al. New aspects of an anti-tumour drug: sorafenib efficiently inhibits HCV replication. *Gut* 2009;58:1644–1653.

231. Zhu AX, Sahani DV, Duda DG, et al. Efficacy, safety, and potential biomarkers of sunitinib monotherapy in advanced hepatocellular carcinoma: a phase II study. *J Clin Oncol* 2009;27:3027–3035.

232. Faivre S, Raymond E, Boucher E, et al. Safety and efficacy of sunitinib in patients with advanced hepatocellular carcinoma: an open-label, multicentre, phase II study. *Lancet Oncol* 2009;10:794–800.

233. Koeberle D, Montemurro M, Samaras P, et al. Continuous Sunitinib treatment in patients with advanced hepatocellular carcinoma: a Swiss Group for Clinical Cancer Research (SAKK) and Swiss Association for the Study of the Liver (SASL) multicenter phase II trial (SAKK 77/06). *Oncologist* 2010;15:285–292.

234. Finn RS, Kang YK, Mulcahy M, et al. Phase II, open-label study of brivanib as second-line therapy in patients with advanced hepatocellular carcinoma. *Clin Cancer Res* 2012;18:2090–2098.

235. Park JW, Finn RS, Kim JS, et al. Phase II, open-label study of brivanib as first-line therapy in patients with advanced hepatocellular carcinoma. *Clin Cancer Res* 2011;17:1973–1983.

236. Johnson PJ, Qin S, Park JW, et al. Brivanib versus sorafenib as first-line therapy in patients with unresectable, advanced hepatocellular carcinoma: results from the randomized phase III BRISK-FL study. *J Clin Oncol* 2013;31:3517–3524.

237. Toh HC, Chen PJ, Carr BI, et al. Phase 2 trial of linifanib (ABT-869) in patients with unresectable or metastatic hepatocellular carcinoma. *Cancer* 2013;119:380–387.

238. Siegel AB, Cohen EI, Ocean A, et al. Phase II trial evaluating the clinical and biologic effects of bevacizumab in unresectable hepatocellular carcinoma. *J Clin Oncol* 2008;26:2992–2998.

239. Zhu AX, Blaszkowsky LS, Ryan DP, et al. Phase II study of gemcitabine and oxaliplatin in combination with bevacizumab in patients with advanced hepatocellular carcinoma. *J Clin Oncol* 2006;24:1898–1903.

240. Hsu CH, Yang TS, Hsu C, et al. Efficacy and tolerability of bevacizumab plus capecitabine as first-line therapy in patients with advanced hepatocellular carcinoma. *Br J Cancer* 2010;102:981–986.

241. Sun W, Sohal D, Haller DG, et al. Phase 2 trial of bevacizumab, capecitabine, and oxaliplatin in treatment of advanced hepatocellular carcinoma. *Cancer* 2011;117:3187–3192.

242. Kaseb AO, Garrett-Mayer E, Morris JS, et al. Efficacy of bevacizumab plus erlotinib for advanced hepatocellular carcinoma and predictors of outcome: final results of a phase II trial. *Oncology* 2012;82:67–74.

243. Abou-Alfa GK, Johnson P, Knox JJ, et al. Doxorubicin plus sorafenib vs doxorubicin alone in patients with advanced hepatocellular carcinoma: a randomized trial. *JAMA* 2010;304:2154–2160.

244. Alavi AS, Acevedo L, Min W, et al. Chemoresistance of endothelial cells induced by basic fibroblast growth factor depends on Raf-1-mediated inhibition of the proapoptotic kinase, ASK1. *Cancer Res* 2007;67:2766–2772.

245. McCubrey JA, Steelman LS, Abrams SL, et al. Roles of the RAF/MEK/ERK and PI3K/PTEN/AKT pathways in malignant transformation and drug resistance. *Adv Enzyme Regul* 2006;46:249–279.

246. Hoffmann K, Franz C, Xiao Z, et al. Sorafenib modulates the gene expression of multi-drug resistance mediating ATP-binding cassette proteins in experimental hepatocellular carcinoma. *Anticancer Res* 2010;30:4503–4508.

247. Zaanan A, Williet N, Hebbar M, et al. Gemcitabine plus oxaliplatin in advanced hepatocellular carcinoma: a large multicenter AGEO study. *J Hepatol* 2013;58:81–88.

248. Assenat E, Boige V, Thézenas S. Sorafenib (S) alone versus S combined with gemcitabine and oxaliplatin (GEMOX) in first-line treatment of advanced hepatocellular carcinoma (HCC): Final analysis of the randomized phase II GONEXT trial (UNICANCER/FFCD PRODIGE 10 trial). Presented at: 2013 ASCO Annual Meeting; 2013; Chicago, IL

249. Chu JS, Ge FJ, Zhang B, et al. Expression and prognostic value of VEGFR-2, PDGFR-beta, and c-Met in advanced hepatocellular carcinoma. *J Exp Clin Cancer Res* 2013;32:16.

250. Wang R, Ferrell LD, Faouzi S, et al. Activation of the Met receptor by cell attachment induces and sustains hepatocellular carcinomas in transgenic mice. *J Cell Biol* 2001;153:1023–1034.

251. Heideman DA, Overmeer RM, van Beusechem VW, et al. Inhibition of angiogenesis and HGF-cMET-elicited malignant processes in human hepatocellular carcinoma cells using adenoviral vector-mediated NK4 gene therapy. *Cancer Gene Ther* 2005;12:954–962.

252. Santoro A, Rimassa L, Borbath I, et al. Tivantinib for second-line treatment of advanced hepatocellular carcinoma: a randomised, placebo-controlled phase 2 study. *Lancet Oncol* 2013;14:55–63.

253. Verslype C, Cohn AL, Kelley RK. Activity of cabozantinib (XL184) in hepatocellular carcinoma: Results from a phase II randomized discontinuation trial (RDT). Presented at: 2012 ASCO Annual Meeting; 2012; Chicago, IL.

254. Villanueva A, Chiang DY, Newell P, et al. Pivotal role of mTOR signaling in hepatocellular carcinoma. *Gastroenterology* 2008;135:1972–1983.

255. Zhu AX, Abrams TA, Miksad R, et al. Phase 1/2 study of everolimus in advanced hepatocellular carcinoma. *Cancer* 2011;117:5094–5102.

256. Llovet JM, Decaens T, Raoul JL, et al. Brivanib in patients with advanced hepatocellular carcinoma who were intolerant to sorafenib or for whom sorafenib failed: results from the randomized phase III BRISK-PS study. *J Clin Oncol* 2013;31:3509–3516.

257. Zhu AX, Finn RS, Mulcahy M, et al. A phase II and biomarker study of ramucirumab, a human monoclonal antibody targeting the VEGF receptor-2, as first-line monotherapy in patients with advanced hepatocellular cancer. *Clin Cancer Res* 2013;19:6614–6623.

258. Ensor CM, Holtsberg FW, Bomalaski JS, et al. Pegylated arginine deiminase (ADI-SS PEG20,000 mw) inhibits human melanomas and hepatocellular carcinomas in vitro and in vivo. *Cancer Res* 2002;62:5443–5450.

259. Izzo F, Marra P, Beneduce G, et al. Pegylated arginine deiminase treatment of patients with unresectable hepatocellular carcinoma: results from phase I/II studies. *J Clin Oncol* 2004;22:1815–1822.

260. Glazer ES, Piccirillo M, Albino V, et al. Phase II study of pegylated arginine deiminase for nonresectable and metastatic hepatocellular carcinoma. *J Clin Oncol* 2010;28:2220–2226.

261. Yang TS, Lu SN, Chao Y, et al. A randomised phase II study of pegylated arginine deiminase (ADI-PEG 20) in Asian advanced hepatocellular carcinoma patients. *Br J Cancer* 2010;103:954–960.

262. Abou-Alfa GK, Amadori D, Santoro A, et al. Safety and efficacy of sorafenib in patients with hepatocellular carcinoma (HCC) and Child-Pugh A versus B cirrhosis. *Gastrointest Cancer Res* 2011;4:40–44.

263. Furuse J, Ishii H, Nakachi K, et al. Phase I study of sorafenib in Japanese patients with hepatocellular carcinoma. *Cancer Sci* 2008;99:159–165.

264. Piperdi B, McGuire B, Parvez M, et al. Second interim analysis of GIDEON (Global Investigation of Therapeutic Decisions in Unresectable HCC and of Its Treatment with Sorafenib): Sorafenib treatment and safety in U.S. patients with Child-Pugh B status. Presented at: 2012 ASCO Annual Meeting; 2012; Chicago, IL.

265. Miller AA, Murry DJ, Owzar K, et al. Phase I and pharmacokinetic study of sorafenib in patients with hepatic or renal dysfunction: CALGB 60301. *J Clin Oncol* 2009;27:1800–1805.

266. Ringe B, Wittekind C, Weimann A, et al. Results of hepatic resection and transplantation for fibrolamellar carcinoma. *Surg Gynecol Obstet* 1992;175:299–305.

267. Soreide O, Czerniak A, Bradpiece H, et al. Characteristics of fibrolamellar hepatocellular carcinoma. A study of nine cases and a review of the literature. *Am J Surg* 1986;151:518–523.

268. Ruffin MT. Fibrolamellar hepatoma. *Am J Gastroenterol* 1990;85:577–581.

269. Pinna AD, Iwatsuki S, Lee RG, et al. Treatment of fibrolamellar hepatoma with subtotal hepatectomy or transplantation. *Hepatology* 1997;26:877–883.

270. El-Gazzaz G, Wong W, El-Hadary MK, et al. Outcome of liver resection and transplantation for fibrolamellar hepatocellular carcinoma. *Transpl Int* 2000;13:S406–S409.

271. Ang CS, Kelley RK, Choti MA, et al. Clinicopathologic characteristics and survival outcomes of patients with fibrolamellar carcinoma: data from the fibrolamellar carcinoma consortium. *Gastrointest Cancer Res* 2013;6:3–9.

272. Cruz RJ Jr, Ranganathan S, Mazariegos G, et al. Analysis of national and single-center incidence and survival after liver transplantation for hepatoblastoma: new trends and future opportunities. *Surgery* 2013;153:150–159.

273. Makhlouf HR, Ishak KG, Goodman ZD. Epithelioid hemangioendothelioma of the liver: a clinicopathologic study of 137 cases. *Cancer* 1999;85:562–582.

CANCERS OF THE GASTROINTESTINAL TRACT

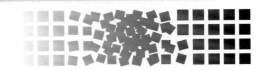

Tushar Patel and Mitesh J. Borad

INTRODUCTION

The biliary tract or the biliary drainage system includes the intra- and extrahepatic bile ducts and the gallbladder. Cancers associated with the biliary tract may be associated with biliary tract epithelia along the entire biliary tract from the intrahepatic ductules to the ampulla of Vater.

Cholangiocarcinomas are cancers of the biliary tract that are associated with the intrahepatic or extrahepatic bile ducts. The term *cholangiocarcinoma* encompasses three distinct tumor types that vary in their risk factors, presentation, natural history, and management.[1,2] Intrahepatic cholangiocarcinomas (iCCA) arise from the intrahepatic biliary tract beyond the second order ducts. Distal extrahepatic cholangiocarcinomas (dCCA) arise from the common hepatic duct extending up to the junction with the cystic duct up to the papilla. Perihilar cholangiocarcinomas (pCCA) arise from the second order ductal division within the liver and the large extracellular ducts up to the confluence with the cystic duct. In addition to cholangiocarcinomas, cancers such as gallbladder cancer and some ampullary cancers also arise from the biliary tract.

The presentation, diagnosis, and management of intrahepatic, perihilar, and distal cholangiocarcinomas and of gallbladder cancer are separately described in this chapter.

Periampullary tumors can arise from biliary as well as pancreatic, duodenal, or ampullary tissues. The presentation, evaluation, and management of periampullary tumors of biliary tract origin are identical to those of any of the other types of periampullary tumors, namely pancreatic, duodenal, or ampullary tumors. In most instances, the distinction between the tissue type of origin is obscure or may only be made on a histopathologic examination. These cancers will not be described in this chapter.

As a group, cancers of the biliary tract are rare. They are often diagnosed at an advanced stage and are associated with a poor prognosis. Management of these patients requires a multidisciplinary approach by a team with experience in their management and which includes hepatobiliary surgeons, hepatologists, gastroenterologists, diagnostic and interventional radiologists, pathologists, medical oncologists, and radiation oncologists. If the relevant and necessary expertise is not available locally, an early referral to experienced centers should be considered.

ANATOMY OF THE BILIARY TRACT

The biliary tract consists of the intrahepatic and extrahepatic bile ducts and is responsible for transporting bile from the liver to the intestine. Development of bile ducts requires complex intercellular interactions and signaling. Notch signaling is a critical determinant of both biliary differentiation and morphogenesis leading to the formation of normal bile ducts. Activation of Notch in liver progenitor cells results in differentiation to biliary ductal cells, whereas activation of Notch signaling in the hepatic lobule promotes ectopic biliary differentiation and duct formation. Experimentally enforced Notch signaling in adult murine hepatocytes causes them to reprogram to a biliary phenotype and can result in cholangiocarcinoma formation.

Within the liver, bile ducts along with branches of the hepatic artery and portal vein constitute the portal triad, which is directed to each lobule of the liver. The adult liver is divided into eight segments delineated by blood supply and venous drainage. These segments delineate and guide the resections of the liver. The main left hepatic duct exits the liver at the base of the umbilical fissure, and the main right hepatic duct exits the liver between segments V and VI. The caudate lobe drains directly into the left main hepatic duct via numerous small branches.

The confluence of the right and left hepatic ducts occurs in the hilum. The porta hepatis consists of the bile duct, the portal vein, and the hepatic artery, from right to left. At the hilum, the portal vein is posterior; the right hepatic artery generally passes between the common bile duct and the portal vein; and the cystic artery passes anterior to the bile duct. The proximity of the portal vein and hepatic artery to the bile duct in the hilum leads to early vessel involvement or occlusion from pCCA, which affects the options for surgical resection. Arterial anomalies are common, and if not recognized, could lead to inadvertent injury during dissection within the porta hepatis.

The cystic duct may enter the common duct near the confluence of the right and left ducts, or distally near the duodenum. It may also enter the right hepatic duct. The distal bile duct travels posterior within the head of the pancreas and then joins the pancreatic duct in a common channel leading to the ampulla of Vater.

The lymph node drainage of the bile ducts involves the superior pancreaticoduodenal, retroportal, or proper hepatic nodes first, then the peripancreatic, celiac, and interaortocaval lymph nodes.[3] Lymph nodes in the porta hepatis may be difficult to remove because of attached venous branches from the portal vein or fixation of tumor-involved lymph nodes to the bile duct, portal vein, hepatic artery, or the head of the pancreas. However, a multi-institutional cohort study reported that the presence of lymph node metastases significantly and adversely affected patient survival (hazard ratio [HR], 2.21; p <0.001), and may explain the survival benefit of a lymphadenectomy for iCCA.

The location of the primary tumor within the gallbladder and the proximity of the portal vein, hepatic artery, and bile duct are all important factors in the surgical management of this tumor. The gallbladder is attached to segments IVb and V of the liver, and these segments may be involved early in tumors of the fundus and body of the gallbladder. The gallbladder has a thin mucosal wall, a narrow lamina propria, and only a single muscle layer. Once this is penetrated, the tumor can access major lymphatic and vascular channels leading to early lymphatic and hematogenous spread. Tumors of the infundibulum or cystic duct can also obstruct the common bile duct and may involve the portal vein.

The lymphatic drainage of the gallbladder first involves cystic and pericholedochal nodes, before extending to nodes posterior to the pancreas, portal vein, and common hepatic artery. Finally, the flow reaches the interaortocaval, celiac, and superior mesenteric artery lymph nodes. Node-bearing adipose tissue posterior to the head of the pancreas and portal vein may be involved early, whereas drainage to the hilum does not occur.[4] Direct connections may exist from the pericholedochal nodes to the interaortocaval nodes, limiting the ability to control disease spread with a regional lymph node dissection.

The upper abdomen contains many organs with relative low tolerance to radiation, such as the spinal cord, kidneys, liver, stomach, duodenum, and small bowel. The tolerance of these at-risk organs poses significant limitations to the dose used in radiation therapy.

CHOLANGIOCARCINOMA

Nomenclature of Cholangiocarcinoma

The nomenclature used for cholangiocarcinomas has evolved over time and has been variably applied. As an example, epidemiological reports have either included perihilar tumors with iCCA or as extrahepatic tumors with dCCA. In addition, iCCA have long been reported along with other primary tumors of the liver. Because of the failure to recognize the different tumor types, the true incidence, prevalence, and natural history are not well established. The relative distribution of tumors within the biliary tract is also unclear. pCCA are the most common type of cholangiocarcinoma (CCA) worldwide. In one study, only 8% of cholangiocarcinomas seen were iCCA.[5] However, these data are not supported by clinical observations in practice and do not accurately reflect disease distribution because they are from a single center series and influenced by referral patterns.[5] The seventh edition of 2010 American Joint Committee on Cancer (AJCC) staging system classifies each of type of cancer of the biliary tract as separate entities with distinct staging and biologic properties.[6]

Classification of all of these diverse cancers as a single group of biliary tract cancers has resulted in a lack of recognition of their distinctive clinical behavior, nature, and management. The individual risk factors and specific molecular pathogenesis of iCCA, pCCA, or dCCA are also not well understood. Likewise, a lack of distinction between these cancers in therapeutic clinical trials has limited progress in identifying useful and optimal therapies for the individual types of cancers. Most clinical studies have included all types of biliary tract cancers, including gallbladder cancer and ampullary cancer, and have reported results in an aggregate fashion. Although specific etiologic and molecular differences are now becoming recognized, an improved understanding will emerge only once these distinctive cancer types are recognized as separate cancers in future population-based reports, patient-based studies, or laboratory investigations.

Etiology of Cholangiocarcinoma

Risk Factors

Although these cancers often occur sporadically without any identifiable risk factors, there are some well-defined risk factors. These include infections, conditions resulting in chronic biliary tract inflammation, drug/toxins, or congenital causes.[1,7–11] Because the individual risk factors for the different types of cholangiocarcinoma have not yet been delineated, we will review common risk factors associated with these cancers in this section. Where tumor specific risk factors are known, they will be discussed in the relevant sections.

Infestation with *Opisthorchis viverrini* and *Clonorchis sinensis* results in chronic inflammation of the bile duct, and are associated with CCAs. These two parasitic liver flukes are classified as group 1 carcinogens by the International Agency for Research on Cancer.[12] These liver flukes are highly prevalent in certain geographic regions such as Southeast Asia and, in particular, in Northeast Thailand. The geographic restriction of liver flukes has resulted in a highly variable disease prevalence in different parts of the world varying from 87 per 100,000 in Thailand to 1 to 2

per 100,000 in the United States.[13] Liver fluke infection with *O. viverrini* or *C. sinensis* species is associated with ingestion of raw fish containing the larva of liver flukes. Infestation is reversible with treatment with praziquantel. The degree of infestation as measured by stool egg count is related to the risk for CCA. Liver fluke infestation is associated with intrahepatic stones as well as with elevated nitrates, and animal and human studies suggest that N-nitroso compounds may be involved in carcinogenesis. The diagnosis of cancer is often difficult and delayed. Once cancer develops, the prognosis is similar to that of CCA in patients that do not have a fluke infestation.

Other infectious diseases that have been associated with CCA include HIV, and chronic hepatitis B virus (HBV) and hepatitis C virus (HCV) infections.[14] A recent meta-analysis of case-control studies reported an increased risk of iCCA in patients with HBV and HCV infection.[15,16] There appear to be regional differences in the risk of chronic hepatitis associated iCCA, although these are not well characterized.

Inflammatory conditions are less common, but their prevalence is more widely distributed. Primary sclerosing cholangitis (PSC) is an autoimmune condition affecting the biliary tract and characterized by inflammation within the biliary tract and subsequent development of diffuse multifocal biliary ductal strictures. CCA can occur in 5% to 10% of patients with PSC[17] and occurs more frequently in patients with chronic ulcerative colitis than in the general population.[18] A high incidence of CCA occurs in patients with coexisting PSC and ulcerative colitis.[19] Up to 50% of patients with PSC with CCA have this diagnosed within a year of their initial diagnosis with PSC.[20] The presence of underlying liver dysfunction resulting from biliary tract disease complicates surgery or chemotherapy.[21]

Chronic calculi of the intrahepatic and extrahepatic bile ducts (hepatolithiasis) outside the gallbladder is rare, but predisposes one to cancer formation. In Southeast Asia, chronic portal bacteremia and portal phlebitis are associated with intrahepatic pigmented stones, and subsequently, increased risk of cholangiocarcinoma. Cancers may develop even after stone removal, potentially related to stasis and cholangitis related to fibrosis induced by stone disease.[22]

An anomalous pancreatic–biliary duct junction may lead to a chronic inflammatory state in the bile duct via reflux of pancreatic juice into the biliary tree. This has been associated with an increased risk of CCA.[23]

Biliary tract cystic diseases are associated with an increased risk of malignancy, which can arise in noncystic portions of the biliary tract. Tumors can occur in patients with untreated choledochal cyst disease.[24,25] A choledochal cyst is a rare condition, manifest by congenital cystic dilatation(s) of the bile ducts. Bile stasis in the cysts leads to chronic inflammation of the duct. Of patients with choledochal cysts, 10% to 20% will develop CCA if left untreated or managed with surgical drainage alone.[26] Early excision of the choledochal cyst has been proposed to reduce the risk of CCA. Caroli disease is a rare variant of choledochal cysts that results in intrahepatic ductal dilatation and an increased risk of developing CCA.[27]

Recent epidemiologic studies indicate that occupational exposure to asbestos or to certain volatile compounds used in the printing industry such as 1,2-dichloropropane may also increase the risk of cancer.[28,29] Exposure to dioxin has also been implicated, although the data are not conclusive. Other potential carcinogens include radionuclides, radon, and nitrosamines.[30] Thorotrast (thorium dioxide) is a vascular contrast agent that is associated with an increased risk of cancer, but has not been used since the 1940s.[31] The risks associated with cigarette smoking are not well quantified.[15,30]

Recently, liver cirrhosis has been identified as a risk factor for iCCA.[15] Consistent with this observation, risk factors for cirrhosis, such as chronic hepatitis C, chronic hepatitis B, and alcohol, are also associated with a higher risk for iCCA.[15,32,33] Because these are also dominant risk factors for hepatocellular cancers, these observations suggest potential common risk mechanisms of tumorigenesis in liver epithelia.

Molecular Pathogenesis of Cholangiocarcinomas

The mechanism and events responsible for neoplastic transformation in the biliary tract are not well understood. It is postulated that chronic inflammation and infection in biliary epithelia and their interactions with other stromal cells' active inflammatory signaling such as those involving interleukin-6 (IL-6), inducible nitric oxide synthase (iNOS), and cyclooxygenase 2 (COX-2).[34] These result in a proliferative stimulus to epithelial cells involving epidermal growth factor receptor (EGFR), RAS/mitogen-activated protein kinase (MAPK), IL-6, or MET signaling. Malignant transformation occurs in the setting of genetic alterations and epigenetic changes on this background, and results in the deregulation of several signaling pathways that can enhance malignant cell growth, apoptosis, and tumor cell behavior. Tumors may arise from malignant transformation of biliary epithelial cells, progenitor cell populations, or transdifferentiation of hepatocytes.

Several genetic and epigenetic alterations and deregulated signaling pathways have been identified.[35] In PSC, inflammation results in the activation of the nuclear factor κB (NF-κB) signaling and increased tumor necrosis factor alpha (TNF-α) and IL-6. IL-6 is an important contributor to cholangiocarcinogenesis and has been associated with several molecular events such as alterations in EGFR, p38, and p42/44 MAPK and altered let-7 microRNAs.[34] Alterations in hepatocyte growth factor/MET signaling and in the EGFR family with overexpression of EGFR and HER-2/neu have been identified. Autocrine growth loops have been identified, involving hepatocellular growth factor (HGF)/MET and IL-6/glycoprotein 130 (gp130).[36] Alterations in the glycosylation of mucins (MUC proteins) and sialosyl-Tn antigen may be relevant, although their contribution in not well defined.[37]

Genetic alterations that have been identified, including activating mutations of KRAS, loss of TP53, mutations in IDH2 and IDH1, and rarely, alterations in BRAF, NRAS, and PI3K.[35,38–40] Tissue-specific activation of the K-ras G12D mutation in genetically engineered mice results in invasive iCCA, which is augmented by the addition of a loss in p53.[41] Mutations of Her-2/neu and c-MET have also been reported.[42] The genetic mutations observed may vary with type of tumor. Thus, IDH1/2 mutations are not seen with pCCA or dCCA, but may occur in up to 25% of iCCA, whereas K-ras mutations are more common in the former.[43,44]

Notch signaling is a complex, evolutionarily conserved pathway that is needed for normal bile duct development. Notch and several of its downstream targets SOX9, sex determining region Y-box 9, and hepatocyte nuclear factor 1β, may be involved in CCA pathogenesis. SOX9 is strongly expressed in intrahepatic bile ducts. Loss of SOX9 in CCA is associated with higher tumor grade and stage, and is an independent adverse prognostic factor for survival.[45] Nuclear colocalization of deltalike ligand 4 (DLL4) with Notch receptor 1 or 3 was associated with nodal metastases, less histologic differentiation, and worse survival of extrahepatic CCA and gallbladder cancer.

In addition to genetic changes, epigenetic changes resulting from alterations in promoter methylation of tumor suppressor genes such as SOCS-3, RASSF1A, p14ARF, and p16[INK4A] as well as changes in some microRNAs such as miR-21 and miR-200c have been described.[35] Genomic studies have started to identify distinct subgroups of iCCA on patterns of gene expression, but these need to be validated and their clinical applications defined.[35,46–48]

Although the specific molecular pathogenesis of pCCA tumors is unknown, it is postulated that tumorigenesis results from a similar sequence of events to that described previously with the additional contribution of cholestasis. The reasons for the predilection

of these tumors to occur in the hilar region are not clear. Morphologically and genetically, pCCA more closely resemble extrahepatic dCCA than iCCA. The pathogenesis of pCCA and dCCA is presumed to be similar to that described for iCCA, with an additional contribution of cholestasis. Some of these tumors may originate from progenitor cell populations in the submucous glands, and in tumors that have maintained differentiation, mucin production may be prominent. A subtype of iCCA may arise from a progenitor cell within the liver that results in tumors with histologic and genetic features of mixed hepatocellular carcinoma–cholangiocellular carcinoma.

A sequence of progression from normal mucosa to adenomatous hyperplasia, dysplasia, carcinoma in situ, and then invasive cancer similar to that described for other mucosal cancers may also occur in the biliary tract. Two precursor lesions are identified: biliary intraepithelial carcinoma neoplasia, which is more common, and intraductal papillary neoplasm of the bile duct.[38]

Pathology of Cholangiocarcinomas

Gross Morphology

The gross morphology can be exophytic, (nodular) mass forming, intraductal, or periductal infiltrating (or sclerosing). Mass-forming and periductal infiltrating (or both combined) are the most common types encountered. iCCAs are more likely to be nodular and mass forming, whereas pCCAs and dCCAs are more likely to be sclerosing, although not exclusively so. The sclerosing type is associated with an intense desmoplastic reaction and often manifest as diffuse thickening of the ducts without a defined mass. The nodular type tends to result in a mass lesion and usually arises within the liver. Intraductal tumors are less common and can encompass a range of lesions from preneoplastic to invasive carcinomas. In some patients, dCCAs may present only as a thickened bile duct wall involved in a dense fibrous scar. Polypoid or papillary cancers have the best prognosis. Papillary cancers represent a low-grade adenocarcinoma that is represented by a polypoid mass filling the lumen of the bile duct, with minimal invasion and no desmoplastic reaction.[49]

Histology

More than 90% of tumors are epithelial adenocarcinomas.[50] Other variants include well-differentiated, pleomorphic, giant cell, adenosquamous, oat cell, and colloid carcinomas. Other types, such as squamous cell carcinomas, sarcomas, small cell cancer, and lymphomas account for less than 5%. Sclerosing tumors are characterized by an extensive fibrous stroma with interspersed tumor cells. Papillary tumors may have papillary fronds with extension into the bile duct lumen, and may produce extracellular mucin. Nodular mass-forming tumors may vary with appearances akin to sclerosing type or with tubular pattern. Satellites are common and may result from spread along the bile ducts or from vascular invasion and intrahepatic metastatic spread. Regional lymph node metastases and perineural invasion are common with pCCAs and dCCAs. Distant metastases can occur, but are unusual.[51]

Intrahepatic Cholangiocarcinoma

Incidence and Etiology

iCCAs are cancers of the biliary tract that arise from intrahepatic bile ducts beyond the second order ductal system within the liver. They are the second most common primary epithelial malignancy of the liver, but are uncommon cancers in the United States. The incidence and mortality from iCCAs have been reported to be increasing in the United States and in many other countries.[52,53] The incidence of these cancers increases with age, with the majority of patients aged 65 years or older. Patients with defined risk factors such as PSC or choledochal cysts tend to develop tumors at a younger age. These tumors are slightly more common in men. There are racial and ethnic variations prevalent, with the highest prevalence among Hispanics in the United States (1.22 per 100,000) and the lowest among African Americans (0.3 per 100,000).[54]

Diagnosis

Patients with iCCAs may be asymptomatic, with the initial presentation being a mass lesion within the liver. When symptoms occur, these may include nonspecific right upper quadrant pain, or weight loss. In contrast to pCCAs or dCCAs where obstructive jaundice occurs early, jaundice occurs late with iCCAs and usually indicates extensive disease.[55] Occasionally, a centrally located iCCA may present with jaundice due to extrinsic compression of the main ducts. Other presentations are rare, and include mucobilia or a tumor embolizing into the extrahepatic bile ducts, resulting in pain, jaundice, or even pancreatitis.[56]

The diagnosis of iCCA involves demonstrating a mass lesion within the liver using abdominal computed tomography (CT) or magnetic resonance imaging (MRI).[57] On CT scan, the lesion is usually of low attenuation with only mild enhancement seen with contrast.[58] On a T1-weighted MRI, iCCAs are usually of low intensity, but may have high intensity on T2-weighted images. Centripetal filling in after gadolinium administration may be observed on MRI. Ductal dilation is often present peripheral to the tumor. Local vascular invasion is often seen by CT scan, MRI, or angiography.[59,60]

The differential diagnosis includes hepatocellular cancer (HCC) or metastatic cancer from other primary tumors. Cirrhosis is a risk factor for both iCCAs and HCCs. Imaging findings are often used to diagnose liver masses as HCCs without obtaining a biopsy. Characteristic imaging features of iCCAs that may be helpful in distinguishing these tumors from HCCs are slow uptake of contrast, particularly in highly desmoplastic tumors, and a peripheral rim of enhancement. A liver biopsy should be considered for a diagnosis if the tumor is inoperable due to extensive spread or if other lesions such as focal nodular hyperplasia are strongly suspected. Otherwise, in potentially resectable cases, further staging studies, including a laparoscopy, would be considered.

Grossly, iCCAs may be well or poorly demarcated, single, or multiple. Mucin production, fibrosis between the acini of tumor tissue, and a more overtly glandular pattern are the main differentiating characteristics from HCC.

Immunohistochemical staining for specific cytokeratins may also be helpful. Unlike HCCs, some cholangiocarcinomas stain positively for CA19-9 or carcinoembryonic antigen (CEA), or $\alpha v\beta 6$ integrin, but not for hepatocyte antigen.[61] It may be difficult to distinguish iCCA from a liver metastasis of extrahepatic origin if a cytological analysis shows adenocarcinoma. Cytokeratin 7 or cytokeratin 20 may be helpful to establish a biliary origin. Cytokeratin 20 expression is focal and rare in iCCAs in contrast to being diffuse and common in colorectal cancer metastases.[62] If a primary site cannot be identified, a diagnosis of iCCA should be presumed.

Staging

The tumor-node-metastasis (TNM) system devised by the AJCC should be used for staging these cancers.[6] The seventh edition (2010) separated the staging of iCCAs from that of hepatocellular cancer, as well as from perihilar or distal CCAs. Table 45.1 shows the staging system for iCCAs.

Management

Most treatment information has been derived from small series gathered over several years, with variable definitions of disease used and, therefore, the best approaches to treatment are not clarified. Consensus guidelines have been proposed for management.[63,64]

TABLE 45.1

American Joint Committee on Cancer TNM Staging for Intrahepatic Cholangiocarcinoma

Primary Tumor (T)

TX	Primary tumor cannot be assessed
T0	No evidence of primary tumor
Tis	Carcinoma in situ (intraductal tumor)
T1	Solitary tumor without vascular invasion
T2a	Solitary tumor with vascular invasion
T2b	Multiple tumors, with or without vascular invasion
T3	Tumor perforating the visceral peritoneum or involving the local extrahepatic structures by direct invasion
T4	Tumor with periductal invasion; the pathologic definition of periductal invasion is the finding of a longitudinal growth pattern along the intrahepatic bile ducts on both gross and microscopic examination

Regional Lymph Nodes (N)

NX	Regional lymph nodes cannot be assessed
N0	No regional lymph node metastasis
N1	Regional lymph node metastasis present

Distant Metastasis (M)

M0	No distant metastasis
M1	Distant metastasis present

Anatomic Stage/Prognostic Groups

Stage 0	Tis	N0	M0
Stage I	T1	N0	M0
Stage II	T2	N0	M0
Stage III	T3	N0	M0
Stage IVA	T4	N0	M0
	Any T	N1	M0
Stage IVB	Any T	Any N	M1

Used with the permission of the American Joint Committee on Cancer (AJCC), Chicago, Illinois. The original source for this material is the *AJCC Cancer Staging Manual*, Seventh Edition (2010) published by Springer Science and Business Media LLC, www.springerlink.com, page 203.

An algorithm for the management of these cancers is shown in Figure 45.1.

Surgery. Indications for resectability are not well described. The goal is to resect the tumor with an adequate margin of normal tissue, and to obtain microscopically free resection margins, while retaining enough liver tissue behind for the patient to have adequate liver function after surgery. The resection may vary from nonanatomic resections to segmental anatomic resections. Intrahepatic metastases tend to occur as multiple satellites, and although their presence impacts prognosis, it should not define resectability. However, for widespread hepatic metastases, curative resection is unlikely, and other forms of therapy should be considered. The presence of underlying advanced cirrhosis with portal hypertension may preclude surgical resection. Extrahepatic spread portends a poor prognosis, and carcinomatosis should be considered a contraindication to resection. A staging laparoscopy can help define respectability prior to a full laparotomy and is recommended.[65]

Outcomes after surgical resection for iCCAs have been reported in small series in the literature. The resectability rate ranges from 32% to 90%. The mortality of resection is slightly higher than se-

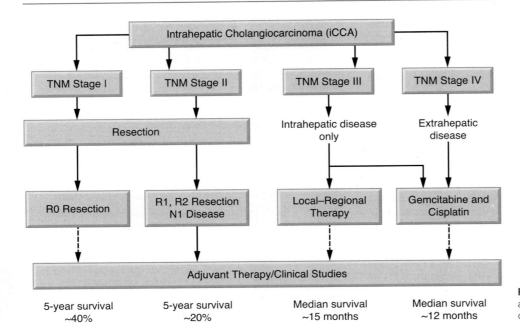

Figure 45.1 Algorithm for the management of intrahepatic cholangiocarcinoma.

ries of hepatic resection for other indications, but is generally less than 10%. Lymph node metastases, positive margin status, and vascular invasion were reported as significant prognostic factors in an analysis of 449 patients.[66] Other prognostic factors include satellite metastases, nodal metastases, tumor size, and a CA19-9 level greater than 1,000. Although rare, intrahepatic intraductal papillary tumors have an excellent prognosis if completely resected.[67,68]

The median survival after surgical resection is ~36 months. The 5-year survival rate with a curative R0 resection is ~60%, but curative resections are possible only in about 30% of patients. There is high risk of tumor recurrence both locally with intrahepatic metastases as well as with extrahepatic disease. However, there are no established guidelines for surveillance and follow-up after surgical resection for iCCAs. As a guide, surveillance could consist of laboratory tests of liver function and CA19-9 and radiologic evaluations every 3 months for the first 2 years after surgery and every 6 months thereafter for the first 5 years could be considered and modified based on the perceived risk. The role and utility of surveillance has not been formally established. Surgery is generally not indicated for recurrent CCAs.

Liver Transplantation. The outcomes from liver transplantation for iCCAs, unlike those for hilar CCAs have been disappointing, with a 5-year survival rate of 29% in data from the European Liver Transplant Registry.[69] As a result of these poor outcomes, liver transplantation is not generally offered for this indication.

Local–Regional Therapies. Local–regional therapy for unresectable iCCAs include transarterial chemoembolization (TACE), transarterial radioembolization (TARE), radiofrequency ablation (RFA), or microwave ablation. They may be used for palliation and local control in persons with a good performance status. A median survival time of 20 months with TACE and 43.7 months with TARE have been reported in case series. For tumors smaller than 3 cm, RFA resulted in a median survival time of 38.5 months. Most tumors present with a large bulky tumor precluding complete ablation, and there is a potential risk of biliary complications arising from bile duct damage.

Chemotherapy. Based on pivotal data from the UK-ABC-02 study, gemcitabine in combination with cisplatin has been

established as the standard of care for patients with biliary cancers.[70] Gemcitabine was dosed at 1000 mg/m^2 in combination with cisplatin at 25 mg/m^2, with both agents given intravenously on days 1 and 8 every 21 days for a maximum of 6 months. The study was conducted using a phase II/III design and enrolled 410 patients across centers in the United Kingdom. Stratification was done based on the extent of disease (locally advanced versus metastatic), primary tumor site (intrahepatic/extrahepatic bile ducts, ampullary, gallbladder), performance status (Eastern Cooperative Oncology Group [ECOG] score 0, 1, or 2), prior therapy (yes/no), and recruiting center. The median overall survival in the gemcitabine/cisplatin group was 11.7 months compared to 8.1 months in the gemcitabine only group (p <0.001; 95% CI, 9.5 to 14.3) with a hazard ratio of 0.64 (95% CI, 0.52 to 0.80). Efficacy was evident across a range of endpoints, including progression-free survival (8 months versus 5 months; HR, 0.63; p <0.001) and response rate (26.1% versus 15.5%). Prespecified subgroups described earlier all derived clinical benefit. Only 17.6% (72 of 410) patients went on to receive second-line therapy. The role of subsequent lines of therapy with regard to survival benefit remains to be defined, but fluoropyrimidine-based regimens have demonstrated preliminary evidence of efficacy in studies with small numbers of patients with cholangiocarcinoma/gallbladder cancer,[71,72] and should be investigated in larger, controlled studies. Of patients, 58.8% (241 of 410) had involvement of the bile ducts in this study; 19.5% (80 of 410) had intrahepatic disease; 17.8% (73 of 410) had intrahepatic involvement; and 13.9% (57 of 410) had hilar disease. Survival benefit was most prominent in the intrahepatic group on a subgroup analysis (HR, 0.57; 95% CI, 0.34 to 0.94). The subgroup analyses were not powered to demonstrate benefit within each subgroup and, as such, should be viewed as hypothesis generating. Response rate was 19% versus 11.7% in the subgroup comprising both biliary and ampullary cancers.

At a conceptual level, there is support for the consideration of combined modality chemoradiation therapy for patients with unresectable disease using gemcitabine- or fluoropyrimidine-based strategies, and efficacy has been observed in small studies.[73,74] However, definitive data through controlled trials remains unavailable and, as such, this remains an area of active investigation, particularly from the standpoint of patient selection and advantages over chemotherapy alone.

The advent of molecular profiling has uncovered putative therapeutic targets, which include aberrations in the Akt–PI3K–mammalian target of rapamycin (mTOR), Fanconi, IDH1/2, ERBB–MEK, and fibroblast growth factor receptor (FGFR) pathways.[43,75,76] Fusions in fused in glioblastoma–repressor of silencing 1 (FIG–ROS1) and various FGFR2 fusions such as FGFR2–BICC and others have been identified, and more such events will be identified with the increasing use of genomic sequencing studies. The pursuit of these targets may lead to an eventual individualized and heterogeneous approach to patients with both refractory and untreated disease in lieu of empiric approaches such as gemcitabine and cisplatin.

Perihilar Cholangiocarcinoma

pCCAs are cancers that arise from the extrahepatic biliary tract from the second order ducts to the origin of the cystic duct. These cancers are amongst the commonest malignancies of the biliary tract encountered in many parts of the world.

pCCAs should be distinguished from nonhilar, distal extracellular tumors because of their distinctive clinical presentations, natural history, staging, and management approaches. Although distinctive molecular and pathologic differences have yet to be determined, and the pathogenesis of these tumors may be similar, dCCAs are far less common than pCCAs and have better treatment outcomes. The reason for the predilection of pCCAs to predominantly arise at the liver hilum is not known.

Tumors that cause ductal obstruction at the hilar region are occasionally referred to as Klatskin tumors. However, the series reported in the classical paper by Klatskin included both intrahepatic and extrahepatic cancers, and was reported in an era in which the biliary tract was inaccessible to noninvasive preoperative imaging.[77] Thus, use of the term Klatskin tumor to describe pCCAs is inaccurate, confusing, and best avoided.

Diagnosis

Patients with early-stage cancers are often asymptomatic. Most patients present with painless jaundice and its clinical sequelae of dark urine, light stool, and pruritus. Nonspecific gastrointestinal symptoms such as anorexia and nausea, as well as mild weight loss and fatigue are not unusual. Most patients will present with painless obstructive jaundice, associated with pruritus, abdominal pain, weight loss (30% to 50%), and fever in about 20%.[78] The clinical presentation of pCCAs are indistinguishable from other malignancies causing large bile ductal obstruction such as dCCAs or pancreatic cancer. Obstruction of the bile duct and biliary stasis may lead to bacterial colonization and cholangitis, particularly in patients with biliary stones. Patients with cholangitis can present with high fever, pain, nausea, vomiting, and rigors.

Serum biochemical tests will reveal the evidence of cholestasis with elevations in bilirubin, alkaline phosphatase, and γ-glutamyltransferase. Serum aminotransferase levels may be normal or mildly elevated in the early stages. Serum CEA and CA19-9 levels are the most commonly elevated serum tumor markers. CA19-9 has limited value because levels can be elevated in benign biliary tract disease, cholangitis, or cholestasis. CA19-9 levels above 100 U/mL were found to be 89% sensitive and 86% specific for the diagnosis of malignancy in patients with PSC.[79,80] CEA levels also have a low predictive value for cancer and are not helpful for a diagnosis.[79,81] Both CA19-9 and CEA levels may be elevated in bile specimens in the presence of cancer.[82] A combined index of CA19-9 and CEA has been proposed, with studies showing mixed results in predicting cancer. The presence of cholangitis or hepatolithiasis can cause elevations of tumor markers, and these tests should be repeated after symptoms have resolved. CA19-9 is a carbohydrate cell–surface antigen related to Lewis blood group antigens. Patients with a negative Lewis blood group antigen (representing 10% of the population) cannot synthesize

CA19-9 and will not manifest an elevation in this marker. Additional potential markers for CCA include CA242, CA72-4, CA50, CA125, RCAS1, and serum MUC5AC. These have all been evaluated with mixed results.[80,83–87] CA19-9 has also been defined as a poor prognostic factor in CCA.[88]

A diagnosis is usually based on history, cholangiography and cytology, or tissue analysis. pCCAs often arise and can progress to obstruction of one of the main bile ducts at the hilum before involving the other main duct. Unilateral obstruction of either the right or left bile duct alone may not lead to jaundice or an elevated bilirubin because of compensation from the normally draining lobe of the liver. However, the alkaline phosphatase and γ-glutamyltransferase may be elevated. Jaundice may occur when the tumor extends down the bile ducts to involve the confluence of the right and left ducts. Unilateral obstruction results in atrophy of the affected side of the liver and hypertrophy of the other side. This atrophy–hypertrophy phenomenon will also occur if the portal vein has also been blocked by the tumor. Because atrophy–hypertrophy results in an axial rotation of structures in the hepatoduodenal ligament, its effects need to be considered when interpreting imaging studies or in planning hepatic resections.[89]

Any patient who has a perihilar stricture, without evidence of ductal disease elsewhere in the biliary tree suggestive of PSC, and who has not had previous biliary surgery that might have resulted in stricture, is considered to have pCCA. The diagnosis and evaluation of these tumors depends on the available diagnostic technologies and expertise. The goals are to (1) ascertain the nature and extent of obstruction, (2) obtain tissue for diagnosis if possible, and (3) stage the tumor to determine spread and metastasis to guide therapy. An abdominal ultrasound will confirm the presence of a biliary obstruction. Additional testing with either a CT or MRI/magnetic resonance cholangiopancreatography (MRCP) is needed to identify the potential and for staging if a malignancy is suspected. The accuracy of CT and MRI/MRCP for the prediction of the extent of ductal involvement ranges from 84% to 91%; for hepatic arterial invasion, it ranges from 83% to 93%; for portal vein invasion, from 86% to 98%, and for lymph node metastasis, from 74% to 84%.[90–92]

Biliary tract imaging (cholangiography) with cytology is used to establish the diagnosis. Tissue biopsies can be obtained under fluoroscopic guidance, or using cholangioscopy during endoscopic retrograde cholangiopancreatography (ERCP). A cholangioscopy may allow for direct visualization, but often provides a lower amount of tissue for analysis.[93–96] In one study, direct visualization for biliary strictures using a miniendoscope identified malignancy in 11 of 20 patients and resulted in modification of diagnosis of biliary stricture in 20 of 29 patients.[97]

Peroral cholangioscopy using the spyglass system may also be associated with a higher rate of cholangitis. Confocal laser endomicroscopy is an emerging technique that may be helpful. Specific criteria (Miami criteria) for the diagnosis of a malignancy within a stricture using this technique have been proposed, but need to be further validated, and the specificity needs to be improved.[98] An endoscopic ultrasound (EUS) with fine-needle aspiration (FNA) may also be helpful for a diagnosis or to predict unresectability by detecting nodal spread. An intraductal ultrasound performed using an ultrasound probe passed into the common bile duct increased the accuracy of ERCP from 58% to 90%.[99]

pCCAs are less accessible than other distal CCAs for sampling. The highly desmoplastic nature of these tumors further limits the amount of cellular material that may be obtained for a cytologic analysis. As a result, establishing a tissue diagnosis of pCCA is extremely difficult. The diagnostic sensitivity of tissue or cytology examination remains poor. Indeed, benign disease has been noted in about 10% of surgical resections performed for presumed pCCAs.[100–102] A positive diagnosis with brush cytology ranges from 44% to 80%,[103–105] with pooled data from over 800 CCA patients reporting a sensitivity of 42%, a specificity of 98%, and a positive predictive value (PPV) of 98% among patients with confirmed cancer.[103] A brush cytology is diagnostic and very useful when positive, but of little value when negative. In a study of 74 patients with pancreaticobiliary strictures, the sensitivity and specificity of brush cytology were 56% and 100%, respectively, and the positive predictive value was 100%.[106] Intraductal tissue biopsies also have a low diagnostic yield with a pooled sensitivity of 56%, a specificity of 97%, and a PPV of 97%. The use of multiple sampling techniques should be considered to improve the diagnostic yield of sampling.

Mucobilia on ERCP is an uncommon finding that is highly suggestive of a papillary CCA. Papillary tumors could be either intrahepatic or extrahepatic. FNA is also useful if a mass can be seen on ultrasound examination or on CT scan.

Staging

Disease staging in pCCA requires an assessment of the extent of ductal involvement as well as the extent of involvement of the liver parenchyma, lymph nodes, and vasculature and distant metastases.[107] The TNM system (Table 45.2) does not help to define surgical resectability and, therefore, may not adequately predict outcome.[51] A classification for hilar tumors was introduced and modified by Bismuth.[108] This classification is based on the level of ductal involvement by the tumor, and provides a guide as to the extent of surgical resection that may be required for tumor eradication. However, it is not a true staging system and has low accuracy.[109] A registry of pCCA has been initiated to collect data that may serve as a resource to guide the development of meaningful future staging classifications.[110]

Management

A suggested approach to the management of pCCA is presented in Figure 45.2. The local extent of the disease along the biliary tree can be determined by direct or imaging-defined cholangiography—either ERCP, magnetic resonance cholangiography MRCP or percutaneous transhepatic cholangiography (PTC). However, the extent of disease may not be appreciated because of tumor spread along the wall of the bile duct without lumenal compromise. PTC or MRCP may be more useful than ERCP in establishing the upper extent of disease. MRCP is less invasive, but may need to be supplemented with direct cholangiography at times. Vascular invasion has been assessed by MRI/MR angiography, angiography, or Doppler ultrasound. An MRI is useful to assess liver invasion or vascular involvement not clearly identified on CT scans. CT scans or MR angiography are replacing the need for an invasive angiography to assess vascular involvement. Color-flow Doppler ultrasound is very dependent on the operator, but can be effective at evaluating portal vein involvement and, in some cases, hepatic artery involvement.[111] Positron-emission tomography (PET)/CT scans, intraductal ultrasound (US), and EUS have all been used for staging. EUS with FNA may also be helpful for a diagnosis by detecting distal lymph node involvement. A staging laparoscopy with or without ultrasound can identify tumor spread beyond that detected on cholangiography, vascular encasement, or lymph node involvement.

Liver Transplantation.
Liver transplantation has emerged as a viable option for the treatment of early stage, unresectable pCCA in highly selected patients.[112] For patients with tumors that are unresectable, a complete hepatectomy with liver transplantation may provide the only chance for a cure. The presence of extrahepatic nodal disease or metastases is a contraindication to transplant. In carefully selected patients, a multimodality approach combining preoperative chemoradiation, staging laparoscopy, and orthotopic liver transplantation has resulted in overall 5-year survival rates of up to 82%. A study of the combined experience of several centers showed an overall survival of 53% on an intention-to-treat analysis, with a 65% recurrence-free survival after 5 years.[112] It should be noted that these data reflect results obtained with a highly selected group of patients.

The availability of adequate organs for transplantation has limited the use of liver transplantation as a treatment modal-

TABLE 45.2

American Joint Committee on Cancer TNM Staging System for Perihilar Cholangiocarcinoma

Primary Tumor (T)

TX	Primary tumor cannot be assessed
T0	No evidence of primary tumor
Tis	Carcinoma in situ
T1	Tumor confined to the bile duct, with extension up to the muscle layer or fibrous tissue
T2a	Tumor invades beyond the wall of the bile duct to surrounding adipose tissue
T2b	Tumor invades adjacent hepatic parenchyma
T3	Tumor invades unilateral branches of the portal vein or hepatic artery
T4	Tumor invades main portal vein or its branches bilaterally, or the common hepatic artery, or the second-order biliary radicals bilaterally, or unilateral second-order biliary radicals with contralateral portal vein or hepatic artery involvement

Regional Lymph Nodes (N)

NX	Regional lymph nodes cannot be assessed
N0	No regional lymph node metastasis
N1	Regional lymph node metastasis (including nodes along the cystic duct, common bile duct, hepatic artery, and portal vein)
N2	Metastasis to periaortic, pericaval, superior mesenteric artery, and/or celiac artery lymph nodes

Distant Metastasis (M)

M0	No distant metastasis
M1	Distant metastasis

Anatomic Stage/Prognostic Groups

Stage 0	Tis	N0	M0
Stage I	T1	N0	M0
Stage II	T2a-b	N0	M0
Stage IIIA	T3	N0	M0
Stage IIIB	T1–3	N1	M0
Stage IVA	T4	N0–1	M0
Stage IVB	Any T	N2	M0
	Any T	Any N	M1

Used with the permission of the American Joint Committee on Cancer (AJCC), Chicago, Illinois. The original source for this material is the *AJCC Cancer Staging Manual*, Seventh Edition (2010) published by Springer Science and Business Media LLC, www.springerlink.com, page 221.

ity for pCCA. The use of living donor liver transplantation may overcome some of the limitations of organ availability for this indication because 5-year survival after living donor living transplantation (LDLT) was 69% compared with 63% after deceased donor transplantation. The outcomes are better in patients with pCCAs arising in the setting of PSC, with a 72% 5-year survival compared with 51% in non-PSC patients. Furthermore, patients with pCCAs undergoing neoadjuvant chemoradiation and liver transplantation have a quality of life that is similar to those for patients undergoing transplantation for other indications.[113] If liver transplantation is being considered as a treatment option, FNA of the hilar lesion by EUS should be avoided because of the risk of tumor seeding.

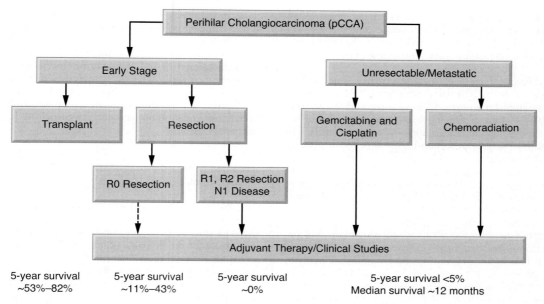

Figure 45.2 Algorithm for the management of perihilar cholangiocarcinoma.

In early reports, EBRT and bolus fluorouracil (5-FU), followed by brachytherapy, 5-FU, and liver transplantation, was used.[114,115] Out of 28 patients, 11 were excluded because of metastatic disease found at the time of exploratory surgery. The rest underwent liver transplantation with an identifiable tumor noted on explant in 10 patients; 2 patients had recurrence after 40 months and 54 months, respectively; and 2 died of non–cancer-related causes. The median duration of follow-up was 41.8 months (range, 2.8 to 105.5 months); the 5-year actuarial survival rate for those transplanted was 87%. A follow-up protocol added a intrabiliary brachytherapy using iridium seeds after external beam radiation therapy (EBRT) and maintenance therapy with capecitabine until transplantation.[115] Out of 56 enrolled patients, 28 received a transplant. The actuarial 1- and 5-year survivals were 88% and 82%, respectively, after transplantation. A similar protocol that combined neoadjuvant brachytherapy and infusional 5-FU followed by transplantation was reported, with 5 of 17 patients (29%) achieving long-term disease-free survival.[93] Other small series have demonstrated 3-year survival rates from 0% to 53%.[116]

Earlier studies of liver transplantation for patients with all types of CCA in unselected patients showed very poor results. Meyer et al.[117] reported the results of liver transplantation for cholangiocarcinoma in 207 patients collected by the Cincinnati Transplant Tumor Registry. Fifty-one percent had recurrence, with a median time of recurrence of 9.7 months, and the median time between recurrence and death being 2 months. In a series of 7 patients undergoing liver-related transplant for CCA, 6 were alive after a median follow-up of 20 months. Recurrences were noted in all patients in this series with iCCA.[118]

Surgery. Surgical resection is complex and associated with mortality and morbidity. The results of surgical resection for pCCA have been reported in many retrospective single-institution surgical series. The goals of surgical resection are to remove the tumor with negative resection margins. An en bloc resection of at least one lobe of the liver, the extrahepatic bile duct, and a complete periportal lymphadenectomy may be required.

The preoperative assessment serves to define the extent of resection that may be required. There is a role for preoperative biliary drainage in some, but not all patients. This could be performed either percutaneously or endoscopically with stenting or placement of a nasobiliary tube. Biliary drainage can alleviate symptoms in patients with severe obstructive jaundice, renal dysfunction, or pruritus.[119] However, preoperative decompression can increase complications during or after surgery.[120–123] Cholangitis may occur following bacterial colonization of bile and stenting may induce fibrosis, making it difficult to delineate the extent of tumor.[120] Five randomized trials and a meta-analysis have not demonstrated a benefit, although retrospective studies suggest a disadvantage to preoperative stenting.[124] It may be appropriate if a hemihepatectomy for CCA is planned in a jaundiced patient or if a pancreaticoduodenectomy is to be done in a patient with long-standing or severe jaundice. Other preoperative preparations include correcting a vitamin K deficiency and bowel preparation. The use of MRCP to guide decision making toward surgical resection may avoid the need for more invasive cholangiography and stenting.

Excision of the bile ducts may be possible up to the first order branches of the right and left bile ducts. If the tumor extends beyond this on one side, a partial hepatectomy may be needed, and a Roux-en-Y reconstruction performed. The contralateral preserved bile duct should be transected at the level of the first segmental branch to maximize the chance of a negative margin. If the resection is extended beyond the first order branches, a main drainage channel may need to be fashioned by suturing the individual segmental or sectoral ducts together. A caudate lobe resection is often routinely performed because invasion of the caudate ducts may occur. Several early branches of the left hepatic duct drain the caudate lobe and can be involved with the tumor involving the left main hepatic duct. Indeed, 46% of pCCAs microscopically involve the caudate lobe.[125,126]

Surgery is indicated in the absence of distant metastases where a preoperative workup suggests that an R0 resection is feasible. Bilateral biliary involvement to the point that all four sectional ducts are involved precludes curative resection.[127] Other indicators of unresectability include bilateral intrahepatic bile duct spread, involvement of the main trunk of the portal vein, involvement of both branches of the portal vein or bilateral involvement of the hepatic artery and portal vein, or a combination of vascular involvement on one side of the liver with extensive bile duct involvement on the other side.[89] With vascular replacement, it may be possible to resect some tumors previously considered unresectable.

A periportal lymphadenopathy is not a contraindication, and resection with microscopic positive margins (R1) determined after resection can provide significant palliation. A lymphadenectomy should include all soft tissue in the porta hepatis, excluding the portal vein and hepatic artery. The common hepatic artery nodes, the celiac artery nodes, the peripancreatic nodes, and the interaortocaval lymph nodes should be assessed because dissection may be indicated. Adequate staging may require sampling of at least seven nodes.[128]

Resectable disease is present in approximately one-third of patients with suspected pCCA. In a series from 2001 to 2008, of 118 patients referred for surgery, 51% were resectable and 41% underwent R0 resection.[129] Operative mortality averaged about 8%[130]; 5-year survival rates after resection have ranged from 10% to 35%. The results of surgical resection highly depend on whether negative resection margins are achieved.[107,131–135] Frozen sections are used to evaluate tumor margins at the time of surgery and to guide the extent of resection. However, the desmoplastic nature of these tumors and fibroinflammatory changes related to the presence of a biliary stent, often restricts an accurate determination of the presence of a tumor in frozen sections.

When negative margins are obtained, median survival of patients with a tumor-free margin is ~3.4 years with a 5-year survival rate from 11% to 43%. However, when margins are positive, median survival is 1 to 1.2 years and 5-year survival is almost zero.[107,132,135,136] With positive microscopic margins, there were no 5-year survivors in one study.[137] Other negative prognostic variables include tumor stage, nodal disease, tumor grade, bilirubin concentration, serum albumin level, postoperative sepsis, and absence of mucobilia.[119,135,136,138,139] Recurrences most commonly occur locally at the resection bed or within the retroperitoneal lymph nodes. Distant metastases occur in one-third of cases, most commonly within the lung, mediastinum, liver, or peritoneum. Improved outcomes seen in more recent series may reflect increasing use of routine liver resections.

There are no established guidelines for surveillance and follow-up after surgical resection. There is high risk of recurrence, with peritoneal spread, hepatic metastases, local extrahepatic recurrence, and distant metastases (most commonly lung). Laboratory and radiologic evaluations every 3 months for the first 2 years after surgery and at longer 6-month intervals thereafter could be considered based on the perceived risk. The role of CA19-9 as a surveillance indicator is not established, but persistently rising levels may precede radiologic evidence of recurrence. The role of CT scans or MRI for surveillance and detection of tumor recurrence has not been evaluated in clinical trials. MRIs may be preferable to CT scans for surveillance because of the ability to concomitantly visualize the biliary tract. In a recent study, PET/CT scans demonstrated a higher positive predictive value compared to CT scans alone (94% versus 78%) for nodal metastases and a higher sensitivity (95% versus 63%) for distant metastases.[140] Surgery is generally not indicated for recurrent CCA. Close surveillance and early diagnosis of recurrences may allow for eligibility for clinical trials.

Adjuvant Therapy. There is a lack of conclusive data regarding the efficacy of adjuvant radiation therapy or chemoradiation therapy for patients who have a gross residual tumor, a tumor involving the resection margins, or regional lymph nodes involved with a tumor after undergoing resection with curative intent. The reported series have been small with the potential for selection bias, and there are no randomized trials that support any particular adjuvant approaches as standard. There is a need to explore and effectively evaluate new regimens for adjuvant therapy in these patients. It is recommended that patients are enrolled in clinical trials to define the role of adjuvant therapy. Similarly, there is a paucity of data upon which to base decisions on the use of adjuvant chemotherapy. In a randomized study, mitomycin C and 5-FU were compared with observation alone in a study of 508 patients with resected pancreaticobiliary cancers that included 139 patients with bile duct cancers.[141] No apparent differences in overall or 5-year disease-free survival were noted. A phase III study comparing adjuvant capecitabine versus observation

alone in surgically resected patients has completed enrollment in the United Kingdom and outcomes data are eagerly awaited (NCT00363584). The primary endpoint of this study is 2-year overall survival. An analogous phase III study using gemcitabine in combination with oxaliplatin versus observation alone is underway in France with disease-free survival as the primary endpoint (NCT01313377). Data from these two pivotal studies will help define the role of adjuvant therapy more definitively. In the interim, the recommendation for patients is to participate in clinical trials whenever feasible.

Palliative Care. For unresectable tumors, palliation may be performed by percutaneous or endoscopic stent placement or by surgical bypass.

Stent Placement. The goal is to drain the most functional lobe of the liver with a stent that traverses the malignant obstruction and allows for internal drainage. Percutaneous biliary drainage is more appropriate for the drainage of intrahepatic ducts and may be required for access to these ducts. Both internal and external biliary drainage are possible. Both plastic or metallic stents may be used, with one study reporting a longer survival and lower complication rates with the latter.[142] Biliary catheters may exit the skin and remain capped. This allows for irrigation and provides easy access for cholangiography and stent changes as needed. However, percutaneous draining catheters may decrease quality of life. An attempt should be made to enable the drainage of greater than 50% of more of the liver volume, irrespective of whether one or more stents are used or one or more segments are drained. Imaging-based volumetric assessments may be useful to determine whether drainage will be adequate. A guided approach using MRCP may be beneficial to routine bilateral stenting. If bilateral stents are placed, they may be used side by side or by contralateral stenting through the mesh of the first stent (stent in stent). Plastic stents typically clog within 2 to 6 months, whereas metal stents last longer, up to 8 to 10 months. Endoscopic metallic stenting should be performed by an experienced biliary endoscopist. Catheter tract recurrence is a rare complication of PTC-placed stents, and was reported in 6 of 441 patients (2.6%) who underwent percutaneous biliary drainage for pCCAs.[143] Patients with catheter tract recurrence had a lower survival than those without recurrence (17.5 months versus 23.0 months; $p = 0.089$).

Surgery. Surgical approaches have not been shown to be superior to percutaneous or endoscopic biliary drainage. A surgical bypass may avoid the need for long-term biliary tube placement, and its associated morbidity, such as cholangitis, occlusion, and need for frequent replacement. The disadvantage of surgical bypass for palliation is the morbidity associated with the procedure when there is limited overall life expectancy. If advanced unresectable disease is encountered at the time of a laparotomy for presumed resectable tumors, a bypass could be performed for palliation to avoid the need for another procedure. A surgical bypass for pCCA involving a bypass to intraparenchymal ducts using a defunctionalized limb of jejunum can be technically challenging but quite effective for palliation. A surgical biliary enteric bypass to segment III (Bismuth–Corlette cholangiojejunostomy), where the bile duct is accessed through the liver parenchyma anteriorly avoids the hilar region that may be involved with the tumor.[144] A bypass to right-sided ducts may be challenging.[145,146] The right lobe could be drained by a bypass to the anterior sectoral bile duct. Surgical implantation of large-bore tubes through the tumor has been used in the past but is rarely employed now.

Photodynamic Therapy. Photodynamic therapy with stenting has shown to improve survival, reduce cholestasis, and improve quality of life compared to stenting alone in a randomized study.[147–149] In a small, multicentered, randomized controlled trial of 39 patients, patients who received photodynamic therapy with biliary stenting survived 493 days compared with 98 days for those treated with stenting alone.[142] In a recently published meta-analysis of 6 studies, 170 patients received photodynamic therapy and were compared with 157 who had biliary stenting alone.[150] There were statistical improvements in patient survival and performance status, and a trend in the decline of serum bilirubin was significantly improved and the risk of biliary sepsis was similar (15%). These data also suggest a possible role for photodynamic therapy in these patients.

Radiation Therapy. There are very few data regarding the efficacy of the use of radiation therapy either alone or in combination with other techniques for advanced stage disease, either unresectable or resected with gross residual tumor. Most of the reported series are small and no randomized comparisons exist. Long-term survivors have been rarely described.

External-beam irradiation was successful in clearing jaundice in 10 of 11 patients in a recent report; no other decompressive measures were used.[151] Brachytherapy has been applied through percutaneous tubes, with a median survival of 23 months.[152] The combination of surgery and radiotherapy was reported to provide a median survival of 14 months in unresectable or recurrent disease.[153] However, other series have reported no benefit with radiation.[154] Stereotactic body radiotherapy (SBRT) may have some efficacy but has the potential for severe toxicity. In a study of 27 patients (26 with pCCA and 1 with iCCA), of whom 18 were treated on a prospective phase II trial and received 45 Gy in three fractions over 5 to 8 days,[155] the median overall survival was 10.6 months and the local control at 1 year was 84% with a median follow-up of 5.4 years. Six patients had severe duodenal or pyloric ulceration, and three patients developed duodenal stenosis. Interestingly, no such toxicity was observed in another group of 13 patients with Klatskin tumors.[156] Eight of these received 48 Gy in four fractions and the others received a range of doses (32 to 56 Gy in 3 to 4 Gy per fraction), and median survival was 33.5 months.

No formal comparative studies have been performed, although the median survival of 1 year observed with radiation therapy appears to be superior to 3 months with chemotherapy or 6 months with best supportive care alone.

Other Approaches. Endobiliary radiofrequency ablation may potentially provide benefits that are similar to the use of photodynamic therapy for palliation of malignant ductal obstruction, but the experience with this has been limited.[157] EUS-guided biliary drainage through a transgastric approach is technically feasible, but has high complication rates, such as bile leakage and peritonitis (20%) even in experienced hands.[158–162]

Systemic Therapy. As described earlier, based on the UK-ABC-02 data, gemcitabine and cisplatin should be regarded as the standard of care for patients with perihilar cholangiocarcinoma with unresectable disease. Although fluoropyrimidine-based therapies have shown evidence of preliminary efficacy, the role of subsequent lines of systemic chemotherapy remains to be definitively defined. Similarly, molecular profiling of these cancers may eventually result in a paradigm shift, allowing for the individualized treatment of patients based on single-agent/combination therapy based on perturbation of aberrant pathways.

Distal Cholangiocarcinoma

dCCAs are cancers arising from the extrahepatic common hepatic duct between the junction of the cystic duct and the papilla, but not involving either the cystic duct or the ampulla of Vater.

There is heterogeneity of cancers that arise from the extrahepatic bile duct. Other cancers that arise from the extrahepatic ducts but are considered separately from dCCAs include tumors at the liver hilum or cystic duct. Cancers arising at the hilum are considered separately as pCCAs, whereas those arising within the cystic duct are considered along with other gallbladder cancers.

Diagnosis

The typical presentation of dCCAs is with obstructive jaundice. In the case of tumors arising below the insertion of the cystic duct, the gallbladder may be palpable. The presentation is similar to that of pCCAs or cancers arising from the head of the pancreas. Patients may present with jaundice associated with pruritus, weight loss, fever, and occasionally, with abdominal pain. Cholangitis may occur, but is rare as a presenting symptom in the absence of prior interventions directed toward the biliary tract such as cannulation or stent placement. Bile is sterile, but can serve as a medium for bacterial growth and can become contaminated with instrumentation. Patients with cholangitis may present with fever, abdominal pain, nausea, vomiting, and rigors. Bacteremia with biliary tract flora such as *Escherichia coli*, Klebsiella, Proteus, *Pseudomonas aeruginosa*, Serratia, Streptococcus, and Enterobacter may be present.

The presence of obstructive jaundice is an indication for further diagnostic testing to evaluate for malignant obstruction resulting from tumors of the bile ducts.

Laboratory tests suggest extrahepatic biliary obstruction with elevations in serum bilirubin, alkaline phosphatase, and γ-glutamyltransferase levels. Transaminase levels may be elevated, but typically to a lesser level.

Tumor markers may not be very helpful. CA19-9 has low accuracy for diagnosis because the levels may be increased in the presence of pancreatic cancer, or in the presence of cholangitis or biliary obstruction from other causes. In patients with PSC, a cutoff of 100 IU has a sensitivity of 89% and specificity of 86% for CCA in PSC.[163] The King's College group index that incorporates both CEA and CA19-9 values has attained similar sensitivities for cancer arising in patients with PSC.[164] Bile CEA levels are reportedly elevated in CCA, but not in benign diseases, other than intrahepatic stones.[138]

Evaluation involves abdominal US, and body imaging with CT scans or MRI, as well as biliary tract imaging with ERCP. US is cheap, noninvasive, and is the best initial test for the detection of biliary stones or for ductal dilation that can occur with long-standing obstruction. Abdominal imaging with either a CT scan or MRI should be obtained for the patient with painless jaundice in whom malignancy is suspected. The advantage of MRI is that an MRCP could also be performed at the same time. Although a CT scan can identify mass lesions, an ERCP or MRCP may be needed to evaluate for the site and nature of biliary obstruction if no mass lesions are noted.

In patients without PSC and with no visible mass lesions, the presence of a single stricture by ERCP indicates a malignancy. In patients with PSC, a malignancy may be associated with the deterioration of clinical status and liver function tests. However, dCCAs may also present in these patients without any change in liver biochemistries. There are no data to determine the efficacy, timing, or effectiveness of screening and surveillance for a malignancy in patients with PSC, although this is often done in clinical practice using CT scans or an MRI/MRCP, with CA19-9.[164] The diagnosis of malignancy in patients who have a biliary tract stricture can be very difficult. Because of the dense associated stroma, well-differentiated cancers with little invasion are difficult to differentiate from the bile duct that has a fibrotic scar or stricture from PSC or other prior biliary injury. The presence of malignant-appearing cells within nerve sheaths (perineural invasion) is an important diagnostic criterion of malignancy that is not present in a benign stricturing disease such as PSC.

The differential diagnosis includes any cause of painless obstructive jaundice such as choledocholithiasis, pCCA, or pancreatic cancer. As with pCCA, dCCAs must be differentiated from benign fibroinflammatory strictures such as from immunoglobulin (Ig) G4 cholangiopathy or sclerosing cholangitis.[165] The former can occur in the extrahepatic and intrahepatic ducts and is diagnosed by an elevated IgG4 in the serum, or by an increased number of IgG4-positive cells in tissue samples. The failure to consider these diagnoses may lead to inappropriate therapies, such as long-term stenting or hepatic resection, and these strictures may respond to corticosteroids.

Cancers of the lower bile ducts may not be readily distinguished from ampullary, duodenal, or pancreatic cancers. Although all of these cancers present in a similar manner to dCCA, establishing a diagnosis is helpful because dCCAs are less likely to metastasize widely and may have a more favorable outcome with aggressive treatment.

Staging

The AJCC's TNM system may be used for staging dCCAs (Table 45.3).[6] Prior TNM staging systems did not consider separate staging systems for extrahepatic bile duct tumors. However, the seventh edition (2010) separated the staging of dCCAs from that of pCCAs. In order to determine resectability of the tumor, staging is necessary to identify the extent of tumor spread and the relationship to portal vein and superior mesenteric artery. EUS with FNA may be useful in determining the extent of tumor spread and involvement of local lymph nodes.[166] Although PET scanning for staging has been proposed, the benefit has not yet been shown.[167] A staging laparoscopy with or without US may enable the direct visualization of the peritoneal surfaces for metastatic implants, as well as detect vascular or nodal invasion, any of which would preclude resection for cure.[127,168,169]

Management

An approach to the evaluation and management of the patient with suspected dCCA is presented in Figure 45.3.

Biliary Decompression. If the distal ducts are dilated and extending into the lower common bile duct, therapeutic decompression by ERCP or percutaneous stenting could be performed at the time of the initial evaluation. We recommend obtaining brushings at ERCP even if no masses have been seen on abdominal imaging studies.

Surgery. Surgical resection can be considered for locally confined dCCA without major vascular involvement or distant metastases. An intraoperative assessment with the help of the pathologist

TABLE 45.3

American Joint Committee on Cancer TNM Staging System for Distal Cholangiocarcinoma

Primary Tumor (T)

TX	Primary tumor cannot be assessed
T0	No evidence of primary tumor
Tis	Carcinoma in situ
T1	Tumor confined to the bile duct histologically
T2	Tumor invades beyond the wall of the bile duct
T3	Tumor invades the gallbladder, pancreas, duodenum, or other adjacent organs without involvement of the celiac axis, or the superior mesenteric artery
T4	Tumor involves the celiac axis, or the superior mesenteric artery

Regional Lymph Nodes (N)

NX	Regional lymph nodes cannot be assessed
N0	No regional lymph node metastasis
N1	Regional lymph node metastasis

Distant Metastasis (M)

M0	No distant metastasis
M1	Distant metastasis

Anatomic Stage/Prognostic Groups

Stage 0	Tis	N0	M0
Stage IA	T1	N0	M0
Stage IB	T2	N0	M0
Stage IIA	T3	N0	M0
Stage IIB	T1	N1	M0
	T2	N1	M0
	T3	N1	M0
Stage III	T4	Any N	M0
Stage IV	Any T	Any N	M1

Used with the permission of the American Joint Committee on Cancer (AJCC), Chicago, Illinois. The original source for this material is the *AJCC Cancer Staging Manual*, Seventh Edition (2010) published by Springer Science and Business Media LLC, www.springerlink.com, page 229.

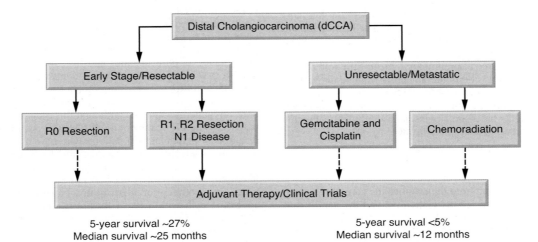

Figure 45.3 Algorithm for the management of distal cholangiocarcinoma.

must dictate the extent of resection. For localized dCCAs, a pancreaticoduodenectomy with resection of the extrahepatic bile duct to the level of the confluence may be required. Although dCCAs often involve the intrapancreatic portion of the common hepatic duct, on rare occasions the tumor may be confined to a small region of the duct and removed by an extrahepatic bile duct resection without a pancreaticoduodenectomy. The peripancreatic and periportal lymph nodes should be removed and examined, along with the interaortocaval lymph nodes, if necessary.

Although the incidence of dCCAs is lower than that of pCCAs, the resectability rate of dCCAs is much higher than that of pCCAs, which may contribute to improved outcomes. A pancreaticoduodenectomy with distal bile duct resection has a reasonable chance of providing a margin-negative resection for dCCAs. There is considerable morbidity and a mortality rate from 2% to 10%. Morbidity can arise from biliary fistulas in about 2% of patients or a fistula from the pancreatic–jejunal anastomosis in 5% to 10% of patients. Although many patients require pancreatic enzyme replacement after this procedure, few develop diabetes. Short-term outcomes and/or quality of life are similar between the pylorus-preserving and standard types of pancreaticoduodenectomy.[170,171] Extensive en bloc–combined hepatic and pancreatic resections could be considered in the rare circumstance that there is extensive involvement of the entire bile duct without any evidence of distant spread. The morbidity of such extensive surgery is very high, and the overall prognosis is poor.[126] The 5-year survival rates after an R0 resection is 27%, with a median survival time of 25 months. The expected 5-year survival is between 23% and 50%. Prognostic factors for poor survival include high p53 expression, nodal metastases, positive margins, pancreatic invasion, and perineural invasion.[172,173]

There are no established guidelines for surveillance and follow-up after surgical resection. Laboratory and radiologic surveillance modalities and intervals will be determined on perceived risk on an individual basis. Tumor recurrence may occur locally within the peritoneum or local nodes or with distant metastases.

Adjuvant Therapy. Postoperative adjuvant radiotherapy can be administered by intraoperative radiotherapy (IORT), EBRT, intrabiliary brachytherapy, or a combination of modalities. EBRT is widely available, noninvasive, and can deliver a homogeneous dose to a large volume. In most series, EBRT has been used to deliver a dose of 40 to 50 Gy (at 1.80 Gy per day) to the tumor bed and draining lymph node basin. In some series, a smaller volume (i.e., a boost) was treated with additional EBRT, intraluminal brachytherapy, or IORT to a total dose of 60 Gy or more. Most commonly, radiotherapy is administered in a continuous course during 5 to 6 weeks. However, the role of radiotherapy from an efficacy standpoint remains to be definitively ascertained. Similarly, as described earlier, the role of chemotherapy remains an area of active investigation in patients with biliary cancers.

Palliative Care. For unresectable dCCA, palliation by stenting for biliary decompression by itself, or in combination with chemotherapy may be considered. Plastic or metal stent placement can be performed at the time of ERCP or PTC, and an internal or external drainage. In general, replaceable plastic stents are used for those with a life expectancy of less than 6 months, and metal stents are used for those with a longer life expectancy, based on results of a randomized controlled trial.[174] Plastic stents need to be replaced every 3 months for best results and to minimize cholangitis. This requires repeated endoscopy procedures. Metal expandable stents remain patent for a longer time and are associated with less cholangitis, but they cannot be readily removed. Tumor advancement may lead to a complete stent occlusion.

A randomized trial of surgical bypass versus endoscopic intubation favored the latter.[175] Unresectability can often be determined preoperatively, but if unresectability is determined only at the time of an open exploration, a palliative bypass for biliary decompression and jejunal bypass may be performed. A surgical bypass to the common bile duct does involve the morbidity associated with laparotomy and bowel anastomosis. A laparoscopic bypass of a distal bile duct obstruction can be performed,[145] usually with a cholecystojejunostomy. This will be unsuccessful if the common bile duct at the level of the cystic duct is involved with the tumor.

The efficacy of radiation therapy for advanced unresectable disease has never been evaluated in prospective randomized trials. Radiation therapy can result in biliary tract and intestinal complications. The available data is based on small retrospective reviews with heterogeneous patient populations that have been treated with a wide variety of modalities and techniques. As described earlier, based on the UK-ABC-02 data, gemcitabine and cisplatin should be regarded as the standard of care for patients with dCCA. Although fluoropyrimidine-based therapies have shown evidence of preliminary efficacy, the role of subsequent lines of systemic chemotherapy remains to be definitively defined. Similarly, molecular profiling of these cancers may eventually result in a paradigm shift, allowing for individualized treatment of patients based on single-agent/combination therapy predicated on the perturbation of aberrant pathways.

GALLBLADDER CANCER

Incidence and Etiology

Gallbladder cancers (GBC) are cancers that arise from the gallbladder mucosa. GBC is the fifth most common malignancy of the gastrointestinal tract. The incidence of GBC correlates with the prevalence of cholelithiasis. Patients who have gallstones for longer than 40 years have a significantly higher incidence of GBC than those who have had gallstones for a shorter time. It has been postulated that 1% of patients aged 65 years or more with gallstones would develop GBC, and this may reflect the duration of stone disease.[176] GBC affects women three to four times more often than men and is more common in Caucasians than in African Americans. The incidence of GBC increases with age, with the greatest incidence in persons aged 65 or more. However, there have been isolated reports of GBC diagnosed in children.[177–179] Mortality trends have been variable. Germany and the Netherlands have relatively high mortality rates from GBC, but have shown declines in most age groups. Sweden, France, and Bulgaria show steady upward trends. In Japan, the incidence increased through the 1980s but has stabilized in recent years.[180] GBC incidence in the United States, Britain, and Canada has stabilized or declined. These changes have occurred coincident with the rise in the number of laparoscopic cholecystectomies.[181]

Geographic Variation

The incidence of GBC varies considerably with geographic location.[224] In the United States, GBC is the most common cancer of the biliary tract, but is a rare cancer with an incidence of 1 to 2 per 100,000. A study based on data from the Surveillance, Epidemiology, and End Results (SEER) program reported an incidence of 1.2 cases per 100,000 population per year in the United States.[182] The highest incidence of GBC occurs in Chileans and Bolivians.[183] Mortality from GBC in Chile is 5.2%, the highest in the world.[184] GBC is the main cause of death from cancer among women in Chile. The incidence of GBC is also high in Native American, Hispanic American, Latin American, Japanese, and Zimbabwean women,[185] and in Americans of Mexican origin.[186] Lower rates of GBC occur among Nigerians, New Zealand Maoris, and Chinese natives and immigrants.[185] Within the United States and the United Kingdom, urban areas show higher incidences than rural regions. It has been suggested that lower socioeconomic status may lead to delayed access to cholecystectomy, which may increase GBC rates.[187]

Ethnicity

There are considerable ethnic differences in the incidence of GBC. In contrast to the general population, the incidence of GBC is much higher in Native Americans in the Southwest United States and in Mexican Americans. In Mexico, the highest incidence of GBC is in *mestizos* (i.e., people of mixed ancestry). The incidence of GBC in Spain, Cuba, and Puerto Rico is low, suggesting that the geographic and ethnic variations noted in GBC incidence in North and South America may be related to Native American rather than Spanish heritage. In Bolivia, differences are related to tribal origin.[185]

Risk Factors

Established risk factors include gallstone disease, bile composition, calcification of the gallbladder wall, congenital biliary cysts or ductal anatomy, some infections, environmental carcinogens, and drugs. Some of the noted geographic differences may reflect genetic differences. Although gallstone disease is associated with GBC, the mechanisms predisposing to this increased risk are not known. Cholecystolithiasis is present in 70% to 90% of patients with GBC, and the incidence of GBC in patients with cholecystolithiasis ranges from 0.5% to 3%.[188] The risk of GBC was increased in a prospective cohort study of patients with gallstones, although the incidence (9 per 10,000 per person-years), and the absolute number of cases of GBC (5 of 2,583 people) in this population was low.[189] The duration of gallstone disease, the patient age, the size of gallstones, and possible carcinogenic effects of gallstones, such as from the chemical composition or bacteria within the stones, may be important; although, in one study patients with cancers did not have larger stones, nor were their stones of higher cholesterol content.[190,191]

Although familial clusters of GBC have been reported, an inherited predisposition has not been found in large series.[192] A recent cohort study from Sweden found an association among first-degree relatives, specifically among parents (relative risk [RR], 5.1; 95% confidence interval [CI], 2.4 to 9.3) or offspring (RR, 4.1; 95% CI, 2.0 to 7.6).[235] Genetic variants in DNA repair pathways may be involved in gallbladder carcinogenesis.[193]

There is a high incidence of GBC in patients with an anomalous pancreatic–biliary duct junction (APBJ), and this risk is independent of the presence of gallstones. Studies from Japan have linked APBJ to other biliary tract cancers as well as GBC.[194] About 2% of Japanese patients examined had APBJ, with about 75% of these cases associated with a choledochal cyst and duct dilation. The rest were noted to have normal caliber bile ducts.[194,195] Patients with APBJ get cancer at a younger age than patients with sporadic GBC. Children with APBJ frequently have epithelial hyperplasia of the gallbladder.[196]

GBC has been associated with partial or complete calcification of the gallbladder wall (porcelain gallbladder). The association is controversial, with some studies reporting an incidence up to 25%, and other studies disputing the association.[197,198]

Salmonella typhi carriage has been associated with GBC. Typhoid carriers may also suffer chronic inflammation of the gallbladder and have a sixfold higher risk of gallbladder cancer.[199] *Helicobacter bilis* and *Helicobacter pylori* have been identified in bile specimens and have been demonstrated to increase the risk of carcinoma by about sixfold.[200,201]

Exposure to toxic environmental factors in the automotive, rubber, textile, and metal industries have been associated with GBC.[183,190,202] Chemicals implicated in gallbladder carcinogenesis include methyldopa, oral contraceptives, isoniazid.[203–205]

An elevated body mass index has been associated with GBC. Although many cohort studies have identified obesity as a risk factor for GBC, this parallels the risk for gallstone disease. Other rare associations with gallbladder cancer include previous gastric surgery, inflammatory bowel disease, and polyposis coli.

Pathology

Sixty percent of GBCs occur in the fundus, 30% occur in the body, and 10% occur in the neck of the gallbladder. Tumors that arise in the neck and the Hartman pouch may infiltrate the cystic and common bile duct, making them clinically and radiographically indistinguishable from pCCAs. They may be isolated tumors or involve the gallbladder through intramural spread analogous to linitis plastica of the stomach. Gallbladder cancer can spread early by direct extension into the liver and other adjacent organs. This cancer also has a propensity to seed and grow in the peritoneal cavity, and along needle biopsy sites and in laparoscopic port sites. At autopsy, GBC patients have a 91% to 94% incidence of lymphatic metastasis, 65% to 82% have an incidence of hematogenous metastasis, and 60% have an incidence of peritoneal spread.[206,207] Hematogenous metastasis tends to be from invasion into small veins that extend directly from the gallbladder into the portal venous system, leading to hepatic metastases in segments IV and V of the liver. There is a high propensity for intra-abdominal recurrence after resection, with distant metastasis occurring late in the course. The only common extra-abdominal site of metastasis is the lung. It is rare, however, to have metastasis to the lung in the absence of advanced local–regional disease.

GBC can be categorized into infiltrative, nodular, and papillary forms. The infiltrative tumors are the most common form and cause thickening and induration of the gallbladder wall, sometimes extending to involve the entire gallbladder. These tumors spread in a subserosal plane. Tumor seeding into the peritoneal cavity can occur if the subserosal plane is violated during and the presence of the tumor is not recognized at the time of cholecystectomy. Advanced tumors can invade the liver and can result in a thick wall of tumor encasing the gallbladder. Nodular or mass-forming GBCs can show early invasion through the gallbladder wall into the liver or neighboring structures. Despite this invasiveness, it may be easier to control surgically than the infiltrative form, where the margins are less defined. Papillary carcinomas exhibit a polypoid or cauliflowerlike appearance and fill the lumen of the gallbladder with only minimal invasion of the gallbladder wall. The prognosis of these tumor is better than other forms of GBC.

Most malignant neoplasms of the gallbladder are adenocarcinomas. Primary malignant mesenchymal tumors of the gallbladder have been described, including embryonal rhabdomyosarcoma, leiomyosarcoma, malignant fibrous histiocytoma, angiosarcoma, and Kaposi sarcoma. Other primary rare tumors of the gallbladder include carcinosarcomas, carcinoids, lymphomas, and melanomas. In addition, the gallbladder can be involved with metastatic cancers from numerous sites. Many tumors exhibit more than one histologic pattern. The only histologic type with clear prognostic significance is the papillary adenocarcinoma, which has a markedly improved survival compared with all other histologic types. There is also evidence to suggest that oat cell carcinomas, adenosquamous tumors, and carcinosarcomas have a poorer survival rate.[208]

Gallstones are found in more than 75% of all patients with GBC. In the presence of gallstones, chronic mucosal irritation predisposes one to malignant transformation. Cholesterol stones are the most common type associated with GBC. Bile from high endemic areas is more mutagenic than that from low endemic areas.[209] Although the chemical composition of stones or bile may be related to the development of cancer, there are no conclusive data linking biliary bile acids to GBC. A potential mechanism of carcinogenesis may involve the excretion of dietary or chemical metabolites within bile, with bile acids acting as cocarcinogens. Experimentally, GBC was induced by the carcinogen dimethylnitrosamine in 68% of hamsters with cholesterol pellets inserted into the gallbladder compared to 6% of controls fed the carcinogen alone.[210] Calcification is the end stage of a long-standing inflammatory process, and calcification of the gallbladder (porcelain gallbladder) is associated with cancer in 10% to 25% of cases. Despite this association, the incidence of GBC in patients with gallstones is only 0.3% to 3%.

Cancers arising from gallbladder mucosa behave similar to other adenocarcinomas of the gastrointestinal tract. Premalignant to invasive malignant changes can be found; metastatic spread occurs by lymphatic and vascular routes; the diagnosis is often delayed; and survival is related to the stage. Interestingly, at the population level, mortality is also inversely related to cholecystectomy rates.[211] GBC originates as mucosal lesions and, as growth progresses, the tumor invades the wall of the gallbladder. The lack of a well-defined muscularis leads to early entry of invasive GBC into the perimuscular connective tissue. Lymphatic, neural, and hematogenous invasions occur earlier with GBC than with other cancers of the gut.

Adenocarcinomas progress from metaplasia–dysplasia to carcinoma in situ to cancer. Chronic inflammation may play a role in the development of premalignant lesions.[212] Two types of metaplasia—intestinal and squamous—have been found in patients with GBC. The relation of intestinal metaplasia to the subsequent development of GBC has not been determined. Squamous metaplasia, in which squamous epithelium replaces the normal gallbladder epithelium, is a rare premalignant lesion associated with squamous cell cancer of the gallbladder. Cholecystitis follicularis, a rare type of inflammation, has been reported in a few cases of GBC, but its premalignant potential is unclear.[212] Progression from dysplasia to carcinoma in situ to invasive cancer in the gallbladder epithelium can take about 15 years.[213] Dysplastic changes are found in adjacent mucosa in most GBCs. Gallbladder adenomas are rarely encountered or associated with dysplasia.

Several mutations have been reported in GBCs. K-ras and p53 mutations are common.[186,214] Mutant *p53* is found in 92% of invasive carcinomas, 86% of carcinoma in situ, and 28% of dysplastic epithelium, but not in adenomas.[215] *K-ras* mutations are identified in 39% of GBCs.[216] Data on the expression of ras and myc are conflicting. In one study, *b-RAF* mutations were evident in 33% of GBCs.[217] The *erbB2* oncoprotein is overexpressed in some patients with GBC, and transgenic mice that express *erbB2* in the gallbladder epithelium develop GBC. Activated *EGFR* and *c-MET* may occur.[218,219] The fragile histidine triad (*FHIT*) gene is a candidate tumor suppressor gene in GBCs.[220] Epigenetic inactivation of *SEMA3B* and *FHIT* occurs in some GBCs.[221]

The malignant potential of APBJ is quite high and this anatomic variant is associated with premalignant histologic changes of epithelial hyperplasia with a papillary or villous appearance. The nonmalignant areas of the gallbladder of patients with APBJ-associated GBC show increased hyperplastic changes in the gallbladder mucosa compared with patients with sporadic GBCs.[222] In a cat model, side-to-side biliary–pancreatic anastomosis produced hyperplastic changes in the gallbladder within 6 months.[223] Although *K-ras* mutations are not commonly observed in lesions associated with gallstones, they are frequently identified in dysplastic lesions associated with APBJ. The differences in presentation, morphology, and molecular changes indicate that there are at least two distinct pathways to gallbladder carcinogenesis associated with either stone disease or with APBJ.[224]

Prevention

The low incidence of GBCs in some countries may be related to the rate of cholecystectomy performed for gallstone disease. However, the prevention of GBCs is not considered as a sole indication to perform cholecystectomy in patients who have asymptomatic gallstones. The incidence of gallbladder cancer is low compared with the incidence of gallstones in the population.

In certain high-risk conditions involving abnormalities within the gallbladder wall, a prophylactic cholecystectomy could be considered. A calcified or *porcelain* gallbladder is an indication

for cholecystectomy in the asymptomatic patient, because up to 25% of cases will be associated with gallbladder cancer. Patients with pancreaticobiliary maljunction and a normal-sized bile duct may benefit from a prophylactic cholecystectomy.[225] A study of northern Indian women reported a benefit of prophylactic cholecystectomy.[226] A serum CA19-9 evaluation and bile cytology may be helpful in making a preoperative diagnosis of cancer. A laparoscopic cholecystectomy could be reserved for those with normal markers and negative cytology. For those highly suspicious of cancer, the laparoscopic approach is not reasonable because of the risk for inadvertent seeding of the peritoneal cavity.

Diagnosis

Patients with gallbladder cancer are often asymptomatic. When symptoms occur, they may be similar to biliary colic or chronic cholecystitis, and are nonspeciifc. In contrast to biliary colic, patients with GBCs may have diffuse abdominal pain of a more constant nature. As a result of the low index of suspicion, patients with gallbladder cancer present with symptoms at an advanced stage of disease, or as incidental findings at the time of imaging or cholecystectomy for unrelated reasons. Recent weight loss and persistent right upper quadrant pain should raise the suspicion of GBCs in elderly patients over 70 years of age.

In early stage disease, symptoms can mimic those of cholelithiasis and cholecystitis or they may be related to associated cholelithiasis. Pain may be dull and aching, colicky, sharp, constant, or intermittent, with radiation to the back and associated with nausea, vomiting, and anorexia. At more advanced stages, jaundice, weight loss, hepatomegaly, a palpable mass, or ascites may develop. Jaundice can result from the obstruction of extrahepatic bile ducts by direct tumor growth or from metastatic disease. Jaundice is a poor prognostic sign, and 85% of patients with jaundice have unresectable tumors.[188] Mirizzi syndrome, in which compression of the common hepatic duct results from an impacted stone in the gallbladder neck, can be a presentation of GBC. Rarely, duodenal or colonic obstruction, cholecystoenteric fistula, or evidence of extraabdominal metastases such as palpable mass, ascites, or paraneoplastic syndromes such as acanthosis nigricans may occur. These indicate an advanced malignancy and unresectable disease.

Tumor spread can involve the liver and the extrahepatic biliary tree by direct spread. Liver metastases without full-thickness invasion of the gallbladder wall occurs in less than 10% of cases. Lymph node metastasis to the cystic, pericholedochal, peripancreatic, and celiac nodes occurs early, and are present at the time of diagnosis in more than half of patients. Direct invasion of the duodenum or colon, intraperitoneal spread, Krukenberg tumors (i.e., ovarian metastases), and hematogenous dissemination can also occur.[3]

Laboratory findings lack specificity and are not diagnostic. Patients may have increased alkaline phosphatase and bilirubin levels as a result of ductal obstruction in advanced cases. Serum CEA or CA19-9 may be elevated, but these tumor markers are not diagnostic. A CA19-9 level above 20 U/mL has a 79% sensitivity and a 79% specificity for the diagnosis of GBCs. A CEA greater than 4 ng/mL is 93% specific for GBCs, but sensitivity is only 50% for detecting cancer. CA125 has also been reported to be a reasonable marker for gallbladder cancer in some small studies.[227]

An ultrasound is the usual initial diagnostic study whenever gall bladder or biliary tract disease is suspected. Findings on ultrasonography of the gallbladder that are suggestive, but not diagnostic, of GBCs include thickening of the wall, a lumenal mass, calcification, or a mass lesion. A comparison between patients with unsuspected GBCs and those with benign gallbladder disease found that a solitary stone or displaced stone, or an intralumenal or invasive mass were more commonly associated with cancer.[228] On ultrasonography, a discontinuous gallbladder mucosa, echogenic mucosa, and submucosal echolucency were significantly more common in GBC than in benign gallbladder disease. A polypoid mass was present in 27% and a gallbladder-replacing or invasive mass was present in 50% of cases of GBC examined.[228]

Mucosal thickening should be viewed with suspicion. US will detect polyps that may represent nonmalignant lesions such as adenomas, papillomas, or cholesterolosis in addition to GBCs. An invasive cancer is more likely in polyps greater than 1 cm in diameter. The accuracy of US for staging disease extent or spread is low (38% in one study).[229] EUS is useful for a further diagnosis of polyps or gallbladder wall thickening. EUS has a higher sensitivity (92% versus 54%) and specificity (88% versus 54%) for GBC than US. It can also enable FNA of any suspicious masses or aspiration of bile for cytology. If a tumor is present, EUS can be useful for staging by assessing tumor wall invasion or distant nodal spread.

Abdominal CT scans or MRI can identify intraluminal polyps, gallbladder wall thickening, mass lesions, hepatic involvement, nodal enlargement, or other distant spread. CT scanning will reveal a mass partially obliterating the gallbladder lumen, a polypoidal mass, or diffuse wall thickening. However, only one-third of pathologically positive nodes are identified preoperatively by CT scan. The use of MRI for the diagnostic workup of GBC can be helpful. MRCP may provide more detailed information than can be provided by US or CT scan.[230] MRI may be helpful in determining vascular invasion and nodal involvement. There is almost no role for cholangiography using ERCP or PTC, although these may occasionally be needed to plan the extent of surgical resection by determining the extent of ductal involvement or spread.[231]

Fluorodeoxyglucose (FDG)-PET scanning has low sensitivity for extrahepatic disease. However, PET scanning may identify a disease that has not been radiologically apparent and resulted in a change in stage and treatment in 17% to 23% of cases with presumed localized resectable disease in one study.[65] For suspicious lesions on US, PET scanning has been reported to have a sensitivity of 0.80 and a specificity of 0.82, a positive predictive value of 0.67, and a negative predictive value of 0.90.[232]

The need for tissue biopsy before definitive exploration and resection of a mass that is suspicious for GBC is controversial because of the risks of the tumor seeding into the peritoneal cavity or abdominal wound. Bile cytology may avoid these and should be performed whenever any patient suspected of having GBC who undergoes ERCP or PTC. The diagnostic accuracy of combined ERCP and bile cytology is 50% for gallbladder cancers. The sensitivity of bile cytology alone for the diagnosis of GBC has been reported between 50% and 73%.[233] If referral for surgical management is being considered, a diagnosis based on bile cytology or percutaneous FNA cytology would be preferable to operative or laparoscopic biopsy.

Percutaneous FNA or core needle biopsy are indicated for unresectable masses. The risk of tumor seeding within the needle tract is greater with the latter. EUS-directed FNA for gallbladder lesions is associated with a 80% sensitivity and 100% specificity.[234] Percutaneous FNA has an 88% accuracy for gallbladder cancers with a negligible false-positive rate.[233] EUS may be useful to distinguish between inflammatory nodes and metastatic disease during an evaluation of periportal and peripancreatic adenopathy. A staging laparoscopy to determine the extent of spread may be helpful for some patients.[127,169]

Survival of patients with GBC is related to stage and histologic type of cancer. Lymph node involvement is rare in stage T1 tumors[235,236]; that is, lymph node involvement almost never occurs until the muscularis has been penetrated. After that, lymph node involvement is common, occurring in about 50% of stage II patients and in 70% to 80% of patients in stage III and IV. There is a close correlation between lymph node involvement and prognosis. Most long-term survivors are patients with well-differentiated tumors that were minimally invasive. These are usually found incidentally at or immediately after cholecystectomy.

GBCs may be identified incidentally at the time of cholecystectomy; the incidence ranges from 0.3% to 1%. If this occurs during a laparoscopic procedure, the potential for port-site implantation should be considered,[237,238] and the gallbladder is extracted in a plastic bag. Implantation can arise due to physical contact between the tumor and port site tissues during extraction, or can be related to positive-pressure pneumoperitoneum.[239] The tissue surrounding the trocar ports is excised because seeding may have occurred. Early reoperation may be necessary if the tumor is discovered on later pathologic examination, or with uncertainty about residual tumor. Stage I gallbladder carcinomas with clear resection margins may not require further surgical treatment.

Gallbladder polyps may be malignant but are rarely so when they are smaller than 1 cm in diameter. In a series of patients with gallbladder polyps, none were malignant if less than 1 cm in diameter, but 23% of polyps larger than 1 cm were malignant.[240] In another series, 88% of polyps larger than 1 cm in diameter were malignant, and polyps larger than 1.8 cm were more likely to contain a more advanced stage of cancer.[241] FNA is an accurate way of distinguishing between polyps due to cholesterolosis and neoplastic polyps,[233] especially for polyps that are larger than 1 cm in diameter[242]; however, it is much less accurate in determining whether a neoplastic polyp is an adenoma or carcinoma.[242] Doppler US imaging of blood flow within a neoplastic polyp may also be useful in distinguishing these lesions from benign polyps.

Staging

Several staging systems have been described for GBC. These systems incorporate clinical and pathologic characteristics with prognostic significance. These include the modified Nevin system, the Japanese Biliary Surgical Society system, and the AJCC TNM staging system.[6,235,243] The use of these different staging systems makes it difficult to compare the treatment results of different series in the literature. The AJCC TNM staging system should be used for the standardization of reporting across studies so as to enable a comparison of treatment results. This staging system is shown in Table 45.4. Stage 1 includes tumors that invade the lamina propria or muscle layer. Tumors can arise in the Rokitansky–Aschoff sinuses and are considered stage I in a subserosal position. Tumors with invasion into the perimuscular connective tissue are considered stage II, and liver invasion is stage III. Extensive nodal metastasis to periaortic, pericaval, superior mesenteric artery, or celiac artery is now considered stage IVA. Patients with distant metastasis are considered stage IVB. GBCs undergo histopathologic grading from G1 (well differentiated) to G4 (undifferentiated). Although the grade does not factor into staging, it has prognostic significance, with high-grade tumors having a worse prognosis.

Management

Most studies of treatment approaches for GBC are from small case series or are heterogenous studies that include other biliary tract cancers. As a result, the optimal approaches to surgery or palliative therapy with chemoradiation are unknown. The stage of the disease determines the treatment approach and prognosis.[235] The diagnosis of GBC usually occurs at advanced stages TNM III or IV, and most patients in advanced stages are not resectable.[244,245] A suggested management scheme is outlined in Figure 45.4.

Surgery. Surgery is the only potentially curative option for GBCs. Absolute contraindications to surgery include distant metastases, vascular involvement, or nodal spread beyond the hepatoduodenal ligament. When GBC is suspected, an open cholecystectomy is preferable to laparoscopic excision to minimize the potential impact of tumor implantation due to gallbladder perforation and bile spillage that are more frequent with the latter. An extraserosal cholecystectomy excises the gallbladder on a deeper plane than a standard cholecystectomy, so that the gallbladder and all connective tissue down to actual liver tissue are removed. The extent of resection will depend on the extent of disease spread. For T1 lesions where the tumor has not penetrated the muscularis mucosa and margins are negative, cholecystectomy is sufficient and can

TABLE 45.4

American Joint Committee on Cancer TNM Staging of Gallbladder Cancer

Primary Tumor (T)

TX	Primary tumor cannot be assessed
T0	No evidence of primary tumor
Tis	Carcinoma in situ
T1	Tumor invades lamina propria or muscular layer
T1a	Tumor invades lamina propria
T1b	Tumor invades muscular layer
T2	Tumor invades perimuscular connective tissue; no extension beyond serosa or into liver
T3	Tumor perforates the serosa (visceral peritoneum) and/or directly invades the liver and/or one other adjacent organ or structure, such as the stomach, duodenum, colon, pancreas, omentum, or extrahepatic bile ducts
T4	Tumor invades main portal vein or hepatic artery or invades two or more extrahepatic organs or structures

Regional Lymph Nodes (N)

NX	Regional lymph nodes cannot be assessed
N0	No regional lymph node metastasis
N1	Metastases to nodes along the cystic duct, common bile duct, hepatic artery, and/or portal vein
N2	Metastases to periaortic, pericaval, superior mesenteric artery, and/or celiac artery lymph nodes

Distant Metastasis (M)

M0	No distant metastasis
M1	Distant metastasis

Anatomic Stage/Prognostic Groups

Stage 0	Tis	N0	M0
Stage I	T1	N0	M0
Stage II	T2	N0	M0
Stage IIIA	T3	N0	M0
Stage IIIB	T1–3	N1	M0
Stage IVA	T4	N0–1	M0
Stage IVB	Any T	N2	M0
	Any T	Any N	M1

Used with the permission of the American Joint Committee on Cancer (AJCC), Chicago, Illinois. The original source for this material is the *AJCC Cancer Staging Manual*, Seventh Edition (2010) published by Springer Science and Business Media LLC, www.springerlink.com, page 213–214.

CANCERS OF THE GASTROINTESTINAL TRACT

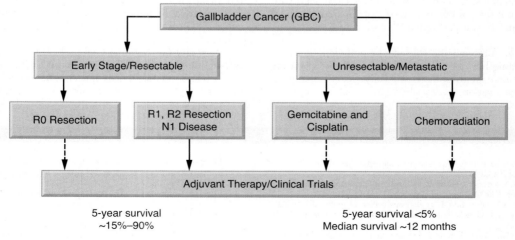

Figure 45.4 Algorithm for the management of gallbladder carcinoma.

be curative. Direct tumor growth into the liver or duodenum or colon is not a contraindication to surgery, but the extent of spread will guide the extent of resection for these T2 to T4 lesions. Thus, wedge resection of the liver, portal lymph node dissection, and extrahepatic bile duct resection, or even a pancreaticoduodenectomy may be needed in addition to a cholecystectomy. If there is obvious penetration to the serosal layer on the deep surface of the gallbladder, or if margins are positive, or the muscularis has been penetrated, resection of at least liver segments IVb and V, and a lymph node dissection are performed. If the cystic duct resection margin is positive, then, in addition, the extrahepatic bile duct is excised to clear margins. A more extensive liver resection may be required if the tumor has penetrated further into the liver. If negative resection margins are achieved, 5-year survival rates range from 90% in stage I disease, 80% in stage II, 40% in stage III, and 15% in stage IV. Lymph node involvement portends a worse prognosis than local hepatic invasion alone.[243,245] A pancreaticoduodenectomy may be considered for T2 to T4 disease, but the results remain poor in advanced stages.[246]

Randomized studies did not show a benefit of preoperative biliary decompression for jaundiced patients.[247–249] However, these studies were performed in an era in which surgical intervention mostly involved palliative bypass of the biliary tree, and the potential benefits of preoperative decompression prior to either pancreaticoduodenectomy or liver resection are not defined.

Adjuvant Therapy.

GBC has a high risk of systemic spread and local–regional failure and adjuvant chemotherapy and radiotherapy are recommended by most cancer centers.

As with other biliary tract cancers, published reports on adjuvant radiotherapy or chemoradiation therapy after a resection for gallbladder cancer consist of retrospective reviews that vary in the type of radiation treatment (e.g., EBRT, brachytherapy, or IORT) and the extent of surgical resection (complete or incomplete). As a result, they cannot provide adequate evidence upon which a standard treatment recommendation could be based.

A median survival of approximately 2 years has been reported for patients receiving adjuvant therapy.

In a study of 21 patients who received postoperative adjunct EBRT with 5-FU, EBRT was applied to a median dose of 54 Gy in fractions of 1.8 to 2.0 Gy per day, with one patient also receiving 15 Gy of IORT after EBRT, the median survival rates were 0.6, 1.4, and 15.1 years, and 2-year local control rates were 0%, 80%, and 88% for patients with gross residual tumor, microscopic residual tumor, and no residual disease, respectively.[250] For six patients who received more than 54 Gy, the 3-year local control rate was 100% compared with 65% for 15 patients who received less than 54 Gy. In a randomized trial comparing mitomycin C and 5-FU with observation alone that enrolled 140 patients with gallbladder cancers, a significantly better 5-year survival was seen with chemotherapy, but these differences were not apparent when an intent-to-treat analysis was performed.[141]

Chemotherapy.

Although the role of chemotherapy given in the adjuvant setting has not been defined definitively, given the poor outcomes for patients with resected disease, it remains an area of active investigation. As described earlier, data from pivotal phase III studies using gemcitabine- or fluoropyrimidine-based regimens is eagerly awaited. New approaches beyond the currently available chemotherapeutic agents are needed for these cancers to achieve any improvements in survival. Understanding the molecular and genomic contributors to this cancer may enable more focused therapy in the future.

Palliative Care.

Advanced GBC has a 1-year survival rate of less than 5%. Although the resection of gross disease may provide palliation and, in some instances, a chance for cure, it may not always be possible. Patients with advanced disease should be considered for clinical trials. The aggressive nature and dismal prognosis of advanced unresectable cancer should be considered when deciding on palliative management. The goals of palliative treatment are to prevent biliary and bowel obstruction and to relieve pain.

Stenting.

If biliary obstruction is present, percutaneous stenting for relief of obstruction can be performed by percutaneous or endoscopic approaches similar to that for other cancers such as dCCAs and pCCAs.

Surgery.

Surgical bypass is not usually warranted because of the poor expected survival. The resection of hematogenous metastasis or of distant nodal disease is not justified.

Chemotherapy.

In the UK-ABC-02 study described earlier, 36.3% (149 of 410) of the patients had advanced gallbladder cancer. The response rate was 37.7% versus 21.4%. Median overall survival and progression-free survival differences were not reported separately, but the survival benefit did demonstrate significance on a subgroup analysis in patients with gallbladder cancer (HR, 0.63; 95% CI, 0.42 to 0.89). As such, the standard of care in patients with advanced GBC is also regarded to be gemcitabine in combination with cisplatin. As described previously, although fluoropyrimidine-based therapies have shown evidence of preliminary efficacy, the role of subsequent lines of systemic chemotherapy remains to be definitively defined. Akin to CCA, therapeutic strategies based on genomic profiling of tumors will also be an area of critical study to best define approaches that can be more individualized in nature.

Regional Therapy.

Regional therapy is possible for gallbladder cancer. In one study, a 48% overall response rate and a prolongation of median survival from 5 to 14 months compared with historical controls was reported with intra-arterial mitomycin C.[251]

Radiation Therapy.

EBRT may be considered for symptomatic patients. The limited data available suggest that tumor control is rarely possible, although some GBCs may be radiosensitive and spread is mainly by local–regional growth.[252,253] However, radiation therapy may be considered for palliation of jaundice in some cases, or used in multimodality approaches combining EBRT with a 5FU-based treatment. The latter approach is supported by consensus guidelines from the European Society of Medical Oncology and the National Comprehensive Cancer Network.[254] Although the benefit of EBRT is minimal, with a median survival of only 6 to 8 months, it does appear to be well tolerated and may improve symptoms and prolong survival in selected patients.

REFERENCES

1. Patel T. Cholangiocarcinoma—controversies and challenges. *Nat Rev Gastroenterol Hepatol* 2011;8:189–200.
2. Razumilava N, Gores GJ. Classification, diagnosis, and management of cholangiocarcinoma. *Clin Gastroenterol Hepatol* 2013;11:13–21.
3. Uesaka K, Yasui K, Morimoto T, et al. Visualization of routes of lymphatic drainage of the gallbladder with a carbon particle suspension. *J Am Coll Surg* 1996;183:345–350.
4. Shirai Y, Yoshida K, Tsukada K, et al. Identification of the regional lymphatic system of the gallbladder by vital staining. *Br J Surg* 1992;79:659–662.
5. DeOliveira ML, Cunningham SC, Cameron JL, et al. Cholangiocarcinoma: thirty-one-year experience with 564 patients at a single institution. *Ann Surg* 2007;245:755–762.
6. Edge SB, Compton CC. The American Joint Committee on Cancer: the 7th edition of the AJCC cancer staging manual and the future of TNM. *Ann Surg Oncol* 2010;17:1471–1474.
7. Patel T. Cholangiocarcinoma. *Nat Clin Pract Gastroenterol Hepatol* 2006;3:33–42.
8. Tyson GL, El-Serag HB. Risk factors for cholangiocarcinoma. *Hepatology* 2011;54:173–184.

9. Ben-Menachem T. Risk factors for cholangiocarcinoma. *Eur J Gastroenterol Hepatol* 2007;19:615–617.

10. Grainge MJ, West J, Solaymani-Dodaran M, et al. The antecedents of biliary cancer: a primary care case-control study in the United Kingdom. *Br J Cancer* 2009;100:178–180.

11. Welzel TM, Graubard BI, El-Serag HB, et al. Risk factors for intrahepatic and extrahepatic cholangiocarcinoma in the United States: a population-based case-control study. *Clin Gastroenterol Hepatol* 2007;5:1221–1228.

12. Shin HR, Oh JK, Masuyer E, et al. Epidemiology of cholangiocarcinoma: an update focusing on risk factors. *Cancer Sci* 2010;101:579–585.

13. Sripa B, Pairojkul C. Cholangiocarcinoma: lessons from Thailand. *Curr Opin Gastroenterol* 2008;24:349–356.

14. Hocqueloux L, Gervais A. Cholangiocarcinoma and AIDS-related sclerosing cholangitis. *Ann Intern Med* 2000;132:1006–1007.

15. Palmer WC, Patel T. Are common factors involved in the pathogenesis of primary liver cancers? A meta-analysis of risk factors for intrahepatic cholangiocarcinoma. *J Hepatol* 2012;57:69–76.

16. Li M, Li J, Li P, et al. Hepatitis B virus infection increases the risk of cholangiocarcinoma: a meta-analysis and systematic review. *J Gastroenterol Hepatol* 2012;27:1561–1568.

17. Broome U, Olsson R, Loof L, et al. Natural history and prognostic factors in 305 Swedish patients with primary sclerosing cholangitis. *Gut* 1996;38:610–615.

18. Ritchie JK, Allan RN, Macartney J, et al. Biliary tract carcinoma associated with ulcerative colitis. *Q J Med* 1974;43:263–279.

19. Ross AP, Braasch JW. Ulcerative colitis and carcinoma of the proximal bile ducts. *Gut* 1973;14:94–97.

20. Razumilava N, Gores GJ, Lindor KD. Cancer surveillance in patients with primary sclerosing cholangitis. *Hepatology* 2011;54:1842–1852.

21. de Groen PC. Cholangiocarcinoma in primary sclerosing cholangitis: who is at risk and how do we screen? *Hepatology* 2000;31:247–248.

22. Jan YY, Chen MF, Wang CS, et al. Surgical treatment of hepatolithiasis: long-term results. *Surgery* 1996;120:509–514.

23. Hasumi A, Matsui H, Sugioka A, et al. Precancerous conditions of biliary tract cancer in patients with pancreaticobiliary maljunction: reappraisal of nationwide survey in Japan. *J Hepatobiliary Pancreat Surg* 2000;7:551–555.

24. Ono J, Sakoda K, Akita H. Surgical aspect of cystic dilatation of the bile duct. An anomalous junction of the pancreaticobiliary tract in adults. *Ann Surg* 1982;195:203–208.

25. Flanigan DP. Biliary carcinoma associated with biliary cysts. *Cancer* 1977;40:880–883.

26. Chapman RW. Risk factors for biliary tract carcinogenesis. *Ann Oncol* 1999;10 Suppl 4:308–311.

27. Taylor AC, Palmer KR. Caroli's disease. *Eur J Gastroenterol Hepatol* 1998;10:105–108.

28. Brandi G, Di Girolamo S, Farioli A, et al. Asbestos: a hidden player behind the cholangiocarcinoma increase? Findings from a case-control analysis. *Cancer Causes Control* 2013;24:911–918.

29. Kumagai S, Kurumatani N, Arimoto A, et al. Cholangiocarcinoma among offset colour proof-printing workers exposed to 1,2-dichloropropane and/or dichloromethane. *Occup Environ Med* 2013;70:508–510.

30. Mitacek EJ, Brunnemann KD, Hoffmann D, et al. Volatile nitrosamines and tobacco-specific nitrosamines in the smoke of Thai cigarettes: a risk factor for lung cancer and a suspected risk factor for liver cancer in Thailand. *Carcinogenesis* 1999;20:133–137.

31. Kato I, Kido C. Increased risk of death in thorotrast-exposed patients during the late follow-up period. *Jpn J Cancer Res* 1987;78:1187–1192.

32. Shaib YH, El-Serag HB, Davila JA, et al. Risk factors of intrahepatic cholangiocarcinoma in the United States: a case-control study. *Gastroenterology* 2005;128:620–626.

33. El-Serag HB, Engels EA, Landgren O, et al. Risk of hepatobiliary and pancreatic cancers after hepatitis C virus infection: A population-based study of U.S. veterans. *Hepatology* 2009;49:116–123.

34. Braconi C, Patel T. Cholangiocarcinoma: new insights into disease pathogenesis and biology. *Infect Dis Clin North Am* 2010;24:871–884.

35. Sia D, Tovar V, Moeini A, et al. Intrahepatic cholangiocarcinoma: pathogenesis and rationale for molecular therapies. *Oncogene* 2013;32:4861–4870.

36. Sugawara H, Yasoshima M, Katayanagi K, et al. Relationship between interleukin-6 and proliferation and differentiation in cholangiocarcinoma. *Histopathology* 1998;33:145–153.

37. Amaya S, Sasaki M, Watanabe Y, et al. Expression of MUC1 and MUC2 and carbohydrate antigen Tn change during malignant transformation of biliary papillomatosis. *Histopathology* 2001;38:550–560.

38. Hezel AF, Deshpande V, Zhu AX. Genetics of biliary tract cancers and emerging targeted therapies. *J Clin Oncol* 2010;28:3531–3540.

39. Hassid VJ, Orlando FA, Awad ZT, et al. Genetic and molecular abnormalities in cholangiocarcinogenesis. *Anticancer Res* 2009;29:1151–1156.

40. Ahrendt SA, Rashid A, Chow JT, et al. p53 overexpression and K-ras gene mutations in primary sclerosing cholangitis-associated biliary tract cancer. *J Hepatobiliary Pancreat Surg* 2000;7:426–431.

41. O'Dell MR, Huang JL, Whitney-Miller CL, et al. Kras(G12D) and p53 mutation cause primary intrahepatic cholangiocarcinoma. *Cancer Res* 2012;72:1557–1567.

42. Aishima SI, Taguchi KI, Sugimachi K, et al. c-erbB-2 and c-MET expression relates to cholangiocarcinogenesis and progression of intrahepatic cholangiocarcinoma. *Histopathology* 2002;40:269–278.

43. Borger DR, Tanabe KK, Fan KC, et al. Frequent mutation of isocitrate dehydrogenase (IDH)1 and IDH2 in cholangiocarcinoma identified through broad-based tumor genotyping. *Oncologist* 2012;17:72–79.

44. Voss JS, Holtegaard LM, Kerr SE, et al. Molecular profiling of cholangiocarcinoma shows potential for targeted therapy treatment decisions. *Hum Pathol* 2013;44:1216–1222.

45. Yoon HA, Noh MH, Kim BG, et al. Clinicopathological significance of altered Notch signaling in extrahepatic cholangiocarcinoma and gallbladder carcinoma. *World J Gastroenterol* 2011;17:4023–4030.

46. Sia D, Hoshida Y, Villanueva A, et al. Integrative molecular analysis of intrahepatic cholangiocarcinoma reveals 2 classes that have different outcomes. *Gastroenterology* 2013;144:829–840.

47. Andersen JB, Spee B, Blechacz BR, et al. Genomic and genetic characterization of cholangiocarcinoma identifies therapeutic targets for tyrosine kinase inhibitors. *Gastroenterology* 2012;142:1021–1031.

48. Andersen JB, Thorgeirsson SS. Genetic profiling of intrahepatic cholangiocarcinoma. *Curr Opin Gastroenterol* 2012;28:266–272.

49. Martin RC, Klimstra DS, Schwartz L, et al. Hepatic intraductal oncocytic papillary carcinoma. *Cancer* 2002;95:2180–2187.

50. Lim JH. Cholangiocarcinoma: morphologic classification according to growth pattern and imaging findings. *AJR Am J Roentgenol* 2003;181:819–827.

51. Burke EC, Jarnagin WR, Hochwald SN, et al. Hilar Cholangiocarcinoma: patterns of spread, the importance of hepatic resection for curative operation, and a presurgical clinical staging system. *Ann Surg* 1998;228:385–394.

52. Patel T. Increasing incidence and mortality of primary intrahepatic cholangiocarcinoma in the United States. *Hepatology* 2001;33:1353–1357.

53. Patel T. Worldwide trends in mortality from biliary tract malignancies. *BMC Cancer* 2002;2:10.

54. McLean L, Patel T. Racial and ethnic variations in the epidemiology of intrahepatic cholangiocarcinoma in the United States. *Liver Int* 2006;26:1047–1053.

55. Chen MF. Peripheral cholangiocarcinoma (cholangiocellular carcinoma): clinical features, diagnosis and treatment. *J Gastroenterol Hepatol* 1999;14:1144–1149.

56. Capizzi PJ, Rosen CB, Nagorney DM. Intermittent jaundice by tumor emboli from intrahepatic cholangiocarcinoma. *Gastroenterology* 1992;103:1669–1673.

57. Choi BI, Han JK, Shin YM, et al. Peripheral cholangiocarcinoma: comparison of MRI with CT. *Abdom Imaging* 1995;20:357–360.

58. Soyer P, Bluemke DA, Hruban RH, et al. Intrahepatic cholangiocarcinoma: findings on spiral CT during arterial portography. *Eur J Radiol* 1994;19:37–42.

59. Soyer P, Bluemke DA, Sibert A, et al. MR imaging of intrahepatic cholangiocarcinoma. *Abdom Imaging* 1995;20:126–130.

60. Gautier AL, Vilgrain V, Flejou JF, et al. [Imaging of peripheral cholangiocarcinoma. Comparison with pathological anatomy]. *Gastroenterol Clin Biol* 1996;20:139–145.

61. Patsenker E, Wilkens L, Banz V, et al. The alphavbeta6 integrin is a highly specific immunohistochemical marker for cholangiocarcinoma. *J Hepatol* 2010;52:362–369.

62. Rullier A, Le Bail B, Fawaz R, et al. Cytokeratin 7 and 20 expression in cholangiocarcinomas varies along the biliary tract but still differs from that in colorectal carcinoma metastasis. *Am J Surg Pathol* 2000;24:870–876.

63. Khan SA, Davidson BR, Goldin R, et al. Guidelines for the diagnosis and treatment of cholangiocarcinoma: consensus document. *Gut* 2002;51:VII–VI9.

64. Khan SA, Davidson BR, Goldin RD, et al. Guidelines for the diagnosis and treatment of cholangiocarcinoma: an update. *Gut* 2012;61:1657–1669.

65. Goere D, Wagholikar GD, Pessaux P, et al. Utility of staging laparoscopy in subsets of biliary cancers: laparoscopy is a powerful diagnostic tool in patients with intrahepatic and gallbladder carcinoma. *Surg Endosc* 2006;20:721–725.

66. Ribero D, Pinna AD, Guglielmi A, et al. Surgical Approach for long-term survival of patients with intrahepatic cholangiocarcinoma: a multi-institutional analysis of 434 patients. *Arch Surg* 2012;147:1107–1113.

67. Nakanuma Y, Sasaki M, Ishikawa A, et al. Biliary papillary neoplasm of the liver. *Histol Histopathol* 2002;17:851–861.

68. Poultsides GA, Zhu AX, Choti MA, et al. Intrahepatic cholangiocarcinoma. *Surg Clin North Am* 2010;90:817–837.

69. Pascher A, Jonas S, Neuhaus P. Intrahepatic cholangiocarcinoma: indication for transplantation. *J Hepatobiliary Pancreat Surg* 2003;10:282–287.

70. Valle J, Wasan H, Palmer DH, et al. Cisplatin plus gemcitabine versus gemcitabine for biliary tract cancer. *N Engl J Med* 2010;362:1273–1281.

71. Lee S, Oh SY, Kim BG, et al. Second-line treatment with a combination of continuous 5-fluorouracil, doxorubicin, and mitomycin-C (conti-FAM) in gemcitabine-pretreated pancreatic and biliary tract cancer. *Am J Clin Oncol* 2009;32:348–352.

72. Moretto R, Raimondo L, De Stefano A, et al. FOLFIRI in patients with locally advanced or metastatic pancreatic or biliary tract carcinoma: a monoinstitutional experience. *Anticancer Drugs* 2013;24:980–985.

73. Nakagawa K, Katayose Y, Unno M. [Efficacy of neoadjuvant chemoradiation therapy for clinical Stage II cholangiocarcinoma as a preoperative diagnosis]. *Gan To Kagaku Ryoho* 2012;39:1945–1947.

74. Katayose Y, Rikiyama T, Motoi F, et al. Phase I trial of neoadjuvant chemoradiation with gemcitabine and surgical resection for cholangiocarcinoma patients (NACRAC study). *Hepatogastroenterology* 2011;58:1866–1872.

75. Arai Y, Totoki Y, Hosoda F, et al. FGFR2 tyrosine kinase fusions define a unique molecular subtype of cholangiocarcinoma. *Hepatology* 2014;59:1427–1434.

76. Wu YM, Su F, Kalyana-Sundaram S, et al. Identification of targetable FGFR gene fusions in diverse cancers. *Cancer Discov* 2013;3:636–647.

77. Klatskin G. Adenocarcinoma of the hepatic duct at its bifurcation within the porta hepatis. An unusual tumor with distinctive clinical and pathological features. *Am J Med* 1965;38:241–256.

78. Lee CC, Wu CY, Chen JT, et al. Comparing combined hepatocellular-cholangiocarcinoma and cholangiocarcinoma: a clinicopathological study. *Hepatogastroenterology* 2002;49:1487–1490.

79. Siqueira E, Schoen RE, Silverman W, et al. Detecting cholangiocarcinoma in patients with primary sclerosing cholangitis. *Gastrointest Endosc* 2002;56:40–47.

80. Hultcrantz R, Olsson R, Danielsson A, et al. A 3-year prospective study on serum tumor markers used for detecting cholangiocarcinoma in patients with primary sclerosing cholangitis. *J Hepatol* 1999;30:669–673.

81. Bjornsson E, Kilander A, Olsson R. CA 19-9 and CEA are unreliable markers for cholangiocarcinoma in patients with primary sclerosing cholangitis. *Liver* 1999;19:501–508.

82. Chen CY, Shiesh SC, Tsao HC, et al. The assessment of biliary CA 125, CA 19-9 and CEA in diagnosing cholangiocarcinoma—the influence of sampling time and hepatolithiasis. *Hepatogastroenterology* 2002;49:616–620.

83. Ozkan H, Kaya M, Cengiz A. Comparison of tumor marker CA 242 with CA 19-9 and carcinoembryonic antigen (CEA) in pancreatic cancer. *Hepatogastroenterology* 2003;50:1669–1674.

84. Carpelan-Holmstrom M, Louhimo J, Stenman UH, et al. CEA, CA 19-9 and CA 72-4 improve the diagnostic accuracy in gastrointestinal cancers. *Anticancer Res* 2002;22:2311–2316.

85. Nehls O, Gregor M, Klump B. Serum and bile markers for cholangiocarcinoma. *Semin Liver Dis* 2004;24:139–154.

86. Enjoji M, Nakashima M, Yamaguchi K, et al. Significance of RCAS1 antigen in hepatocellular, cholangiocellular and pancreatic carcinomas. *J Gastroenterol Hepatol* 2005;20:1143–1148.

87. Wongkham S, Sheehan JK, Boonla C, et al. Serum MUC5AC mucin as a potential marker for cholangiocarcinoma. *Cancer Lett* 2003;195:93–99.

88. Hatzaras I, Schmidt C, Muscarella P, et al. Elevated CA 19-9 portends poor prognosis in patients undergoing resection of biliary malignancies. *HPB (Oxford)* 2010;12:134–138.

89. Blumgart LH, Stain SC. Surgical treatment of cholangiocarcinoma. *Cancer Treat Res* 1994;69:75–96.

90. Masselli G, Gualdi G. Hilar cholangiocarcinoma: MRI/MRCP in staging and treatment planning. *Abdom Imaging* 2008;33:444–451.

91. Masselli G, Manfredi R, Vecchioli A, et al. MR imaging and MR cholangiopancreatography in the preoperative evaluation of hilar cholangiocarcinoma: correlation with surgical and pathologic findings. *Eur Radiol* 2008;18:2213–2221.

92. Lee MG, Park KB, Shin YM, et al. Preoperative evaluation of hilar cholangiocarcinoma with contrast-enhanced three-dimensional fast imaging with steady-state precession magnetic resonance angiography: comparison with intraarterial digital subtraction angiography. *World J Surg* 2003;27:278–283.

93. Chen YK, Parsi MA, Binmoeller KF, et al. Single-operator cholangioscopy in patients requiring evaluation of bile duct disease or therapy of biliary stones (with videos). *Gastrointest Endosc* 2011;74:805–814.

94. Fukuda Y, Tsuyuguchi T, Sakai Y, et al. Diagnostic utility of peroral cholangioscopy for various bile-duct lesions. *Gastrointest Endosc* 2005;62:374–382.

95. Shah RJ, Langer DA, Antillon MR, et al. Cholangioscopy and cholangioscopic forceps biopsy in patients with indeterminate pancreaticobiliary pathology. *Clin Gastroenterol Hepatol* 2006;4:219–225.

96. Itoi T, Osanai M, Igarashi Y, et al. Diagnostic peroral video cholangioscopy is an accurate diagnostic tool for patients with bile duct lesions. *Clin Gastroenterol Hepatol* 2010;8:934–938.

97. Fishman DS, Tarnasky PR, Patel SN, et al. Management of pancreaticobiliary disease using a new intra-ductal endoscope: the Texas experience. *World J Gastroenterol* 2009;15:1353–1358.

98. Meining A, Chen YK, Pleskow D, et al. Direct visualization of indeterminate pancreaticobiliary strictures with probe-based confocal laser endomicroscopy: a multicenter experience. *Gastrointest Endosc* 2011;74:961–968.

99. Stavropoulos S, Larghi A, Verna E, et al. Intraductal ultrasound for the evaluation of patients with biliary strictures and no abdominal mass on computed tomography. *Endoscopy* 2005;37:715–721.

100. Verbeek PC, van Leeuwen DJ, de Wit LT, et al. Benign fibrosing disease at the hepatic confluence mimicking Klatskin tumors. *Surgery* 1992;112:866–871.

101. Juntermanns B, Kaiser GM, Reis H, et al. Klatskin-mimicking lesions: still a diagnostical and therapeutical dilemma? *Hepatogastroenterology* 2011;58:265–269.

102. Wetter LA, Ring EJ, Pellegrini CA, Way LW. Differential diagnosis of sclerosing cholangiocarcinomas of the common hepatic duct (Klatskin tumors). *Am J Surg* 1991;161:57–62.

103. de Bellis M, Sherman S, Fogel EL, et al. Tissue sampling at ERCP in suspected malignant biliary strictures (Part 2). *Gastrointest Endosc* 2002;56:720–730.

104. De Bellis M, Sherman S, Fogel EL, et al. Tissue sampling at ERCP in suspected malignant biliary strictures (Part 1). *Gastrointest Endosc* 2002;56:552–561.

105. Fogel EL, deBellis M, McHenry L, et al. Effectiveness of a new long cytology brush in the evaluation of malignant biliary obstruction: a prospective study. *Gastrointest Endosc* 2006;63:71–77.

106. Ferrari Junior AP, Lichtenstein DR, Slivka A, et al. Brush cytology during ERCP for the diagnosis of biliary and pancreatic malignancies. *Gastrointest Endosc* 1994;40:140–145.

107. Jarnagin WR, Fong Y, DeMatteo RP, et al. Staging, resectability, and outcome in 225 patients with hilar cholangiocarcinoma. *Ann Surg* 2001;234:507–517.

108. Bismuth H, Nakache R, Diamond T. Management strategies in resection for hilar cholangiocarcinoma. *Ann Surg* 1992;215:31–38.

109. Paul A, Kaiser GM, Molmenti EP, et al. Klatskin tumors and the accuracy of the Bismuth-Corlette classification. *Am Surg* 2011;77:1695–1699.

110. Deoliveira ML, Schulick RD, Nimura Y, et al. New staging system and a registry for perihilar cholangiocarcinoma. *Hepatology* 2011;53:1363–1371.

111. Neumaier CE, Bertolotto M, Perrone R, et al. Staging of hilar cholangiocarcinoma with ultrasound. *J Clin Ultrasound* 1995;23:173–178.

112. Darwish Murad S, Kim WR, Harnois DM, et al. Efficacy of neoadjuvant chemoradiation, Followed by liver transplantation, for perihilar cholangiocarcinoma at 12 US centers. *Gastroenterology* 2012;143:88–98.

113. Murad SD, Heimbach JK, Gores GJ, et al. Excellent quality of life after liver transplantation for patients with perihilar cholangiocarcinoma who have undergone neoadjuvant chemoradiation. *Liver Transpl* 2013;19:521–528.

114. Hassoun Z, Gores GJ, Rosen CB. Preliminary experience with liver transplantation in selected patients with unresectable hilar cholangiocarcinoma. *Surg Oncol Clin N Am* 2002;11:909–921.

115. Heimbach JK, Haddock MG, Alberts SR, et al. Transplantation for hilar cholangiocarcinoma. *Liver Transpl* 2004;10:S65–S68.

116. Shimoda M, Farmer DG, Colquhoun SD, et al. Liver transplantation for cholangiocellular carcinoma: analysis of a single-center experience and review of the literature. *Liver Transpl* 2001;7:1023–1033.

117. Meyer CG, Penn I, James L. Liver transplantation for cholangiocarcinoma: results in 207 patients. *Transplantation* 2000;69:1633–1637.

118. Jonas S, Mittler J, Pascher A, et al. Extended indications in living-donor liver transplantation: bile duct cancer. *Transplantation* 2005;80:S101–S104.

119. Lillemoe KD, Cameron JL. Surgery for hilar cholangiocarcinoma: the Johns Hopkins approach. *J Hepatobiliary Pancreat Surg* 2000;7:115–121.

120. Hochwald SN, Burke EC, Jarnagin WR, et al. Association of preoperative biliary stenting with increased postoperative infectious complications in proximal cholangiocarcinoma. *Arch Surg* 1999;134:261–266.

121. Sakata J, Shirai Y, Wakai T, et al. Catheter tract implantation metastases associated with percutaneous biliary drainage for extrahepatic cholangiocarcinoma. *World J Gastroenterol* 2005;11:7024–7027.

122. Ferrero A, Lo Tesoriere R, Vigano L, et al. Preoperative biliary drainage increases infectious complications after hepatectomy for proximal bile duct tumor obstruction. *World J Surg* 2009;33:318–325.

123. Liu F, Li Y, Wei Y, et al. Preoperative biliary drainage before resection for hilar cholangiocarcinoma: whether or not? A systematic review. *Dig Dis Sci* 2011;56:663–672.

124. Sewnath ME, Karsten TM, Prins MH, et al. A meta-analysis on the efficacy of preoperative biliary drainage for tumors causing obstructive jaundice. *Ann Surg* 2002;236:17–27.

125. Tabata M, Kawarada Y, Yokoi H, et al. Surgical treatment for hilar cholangiocarcinoma. *J Hepatobiliary Pancreat Surg* 2000;7:148–154.

126. Nimura Y, Kamiya J, Kondo S, et al. Aggressive preoperative management and extended surgery for hilar cholangiocarcinoma: Nagoya experience. *J Hepatobiliary Pancreat Surg* 2000;7:155–162.

127. Callery MP, Strasberg SM, Doherty GM, et al. Staging laparoscopy with laparoscopic ultrasonography: optimizing resectability in hepatobiliary and pancreatic malignancy. *J Am Coll Surg* 1997;185:33–39.

128. Ito K, Ito H, Allen PJ, et al. Adequate lymph node assessment for extrahepatic bile duct adenocarcinoma. *Ann Surg* 2010;251:675–681.

129. Rocha FG, Matsuo K, Blumgart LH, et al. Hilar cholangiocarcinoma: the Memorial Sloan-Kettering Cancer Center experience. *J Hepatobiliary Pancreat Sci* 2010;17:490–496.

130. Nagino M, Kamiya J, Uesaka K, et al. Complications of hepatectomy for hilar cholangiocarcinoma. *World J Surg* 2001;25:1277–1283.

131. Bengmark S, Ekberg H, Evander A, et al. Major liver resection for hilar cholangiocarcinoma. *Ann Surg* 1988;207:120–125.

132. Washburn WK, Lewis WD, Jenkins RL. Aggressive surgical resection for cholangiocarcinoma. *Arch Surg* 1995;130:270–276.

133. Pinson CW, Rossi RL. Extended right hepatic lobectomy, left hepatic lobectomy, and skeletonization resection for proximal bile duct cancer. *World J Surg* 1988;12:52–59.

134. Iwasaki Y, Okamura T, Ozaki A, et al. Surgical treatment for carcinoma at the confluence of the major hepatic ducts. *Surg Gynecol Obstet* 1986;162:457–464.

135. Su CH, Tsay SH, Wu CC, et al. Factors influencing postoperative morbidity, mortality, and survival after resection for hilar cholangiocarcinoma. *Ann Surg* 1996;223:384–394.

136. Nagorney DM, Donohue JH, Farnell MB, et al. Outcomes after curative resections of cholangiocarcinoma. *Arch Surg* 1993;128:871–877.

137. Otani K, Chijiiwa K, Kai M, et al. Outcome of surgical treatment of hilar cholangiocarcinoma. *J Gastrointest Surg* 2008;12:1033–1040.

138. Nakeeb A, Pitt HA, Sohn TA, et al. Cholangiocarcinoma. A spectrum of intrahepatic, perihilar, and distal tumors. *Ann Surg* 1996;224:463–473.

139. Klempnauer J, Ridder GJ, von Wasielewski R, et al. Resectional surgery of hilar cholangiocarcinoma: a multivariate analysis of prognostic factors. *J Clin Oncol* 1997;15:947–954.

140. Lee SW, Kim HJ, Park JH, et al. Clinical usefulness of 18F-FDG PET-CT for patients with gallbladder cancer and cholangiocarcinoma. *J Gastroenterol* 2010;45:560–566.

141. Takada T, Amano H, Yasuda H, et al. Is postoperative adjuvant chemotherapy useful for gallbladder carcinoma? A phase III multicenter prospective randomized controlled trial in patients with resected pancreaticobiliary carcinoma. *Cancer* 2002;95:1685–1695.

142. Hii MW, Gibson RN, Speer AG, et al. Role of radiology in the treatment of malignant hilar biliary strictures 2: 10 years of single-institution experience with percutaneous treatment. *Australas Radiol* 2003;47:393–403.

143. Kang MJ, Choi YS, Jang JY, et al. Catheter tract recurrence after percutaneous biliary drainage for hilar cholangiocarcinoma. *World J Surg* 2013;37: 437–442.

144. Jarnagin WR, Burke E, Powers C, et al. Intrahepatic biliary enteric bypass provides effective palliation in selected patients with malignant obstruction at the hepatic duct confluence. *Am J Surg* 1998;175:453–460.

145. Witzigmann H, Lang H, Lauer H. Guidelines for palliative surgery of cholangiocarcinoma. *HPB (Oxford)* 2008;10:154–160.

146. Zhang BH, Cheng QB, Luo XJ, et al. Surgical therapy for hiliar cholangiocarcinoma: analysis of 198 cases. *Hepatobiliary Pancreat Dis Int* 2006;5: 278–282.

147. Ortner ME, Caca K, Berr F, et al. Successful photodynamic therapy for nonresectable cholangiocarcinoma: a randomized prospective study. *Gastroenterology* 2003;125:1355–1363.

148. Zoepf T, Jakobs R, Arnold JC, et al. Palliation of nonresectable bile duct cancer: improved survival after photodynamic therapy. *Am J Gastroenterol* 2005;100:2426–2430.

149. Cheon YK, Cho YD, Baek SH, et al. [Comparison of survival of advanced hilar cholangiocarcinoma after biliary drainage alone versus photodynamic therapy with external drainage]. *Korean J Gastroenterol* 2004;44:280–287.

150. Leggett CL, Gorospe EC, Murad MH, et al. Photodynamic therapy for unresectable cholangiocarcinoma: a comparative effectiveness systematic review and meta-analysis. *Photodiagnosis Photodyn Ther* 2012;9:189–195.

151. Ohnishi H, Asada M, Shichijo Y, et al. External radiotherapy for biliary decompression of hilar cholangiocarcinoma. *Hepatogastroenterology* 1995;42: 265–268.

152. Leung J, Guiney M, Das R. Intraluminal brachytherapy in bile duct carcinomas. *Aust N Z J Surg* 1996;66:74–77.

153. Kuvshinoff BW, Armstrong JG, Fong Y, et al. Palliation of irresectable hilar cholangiocarcinoma with biliary drainage and radiotherapy. *Br J Surg* 1995;82: 1522–1525.

154. Pitt HA, Nakeeb A, Abrams RA, et al. Perihilar cholangiocarcinoma. Postoperative radiotherapy does not improve survival. *Ann Surg* 1995;221:788–797.

155. Kopek N, Holt MI, Hansen AT, et al. Stereotactic body radiotherapy for unresectable cholangiocarcinoma. *Radiother Oncol* 2010;94:47–52.

156. Momm F, Schubert E, Henne K, et al. Stereotactic fractionated radiotherapy for Klatskin tumours. *Radiother Oncol* 2010;95:99–102.

157. Steel AW, Postgate AJ, Khorsandi S, et al. Endoscopically applied radiofrequency ablation appears to be safe in the treatment of malignant biliary obstruction. *Gastrointest Endosc* 2011;73:149–153.

158. Yamao K, Hara K, Mizuno N, et al. EUS-guided biliary drainage. *Gut Liver* 2010;4 Suppl 1:S67–S75.

159. Yamao K, Bhatia V, Mizuno N, et al. EUS-guided choledochoduodenostomy for palliative biliary drainage in patients with malignant biliary obstruction: results of long-term follow-up. *Endoscopy* 2008;40:340–342.

160. Park do H, Koo JE, Oh J, et al. EUS-guided biliary drainage with one-step placement of a fully covered metal stent for malignant biliary obstruction: a prospective feasibility study. *Am J Gastroenterol* 2009;104:2168–2174.

161. Kahaleh M, Hernandez AJ, Tokar J, et al. EUS-guided pancreaticogastrostomy: analysis of its efficacy to drain inaccessible pancreatic ducts. *Gastrointest Endosc* 2007;65:224–230.

162. Maranki J, Hernandez AJ, Arslan B, et al. Interventional endoscopic ultrasound-guided cholangiography: long-term experience of an emerging alternative to percutaneous transhepatic cholangiography. *Endoscopy* 2009;41: 532–538.

163. Nichols JC, Gores GJ, LaRusso NF, et al. Diagnostic role of serum CA 19-9 for cholangiocarcinoma in patients with primary sclerosing cholangitis. *Mayo Clin Proc* 1993;68:874–879.

164. Ramage JK, Donaghy A, Farrant JM, et al. Serum tumor markers for the diagnosis of cholangiocarcinoma in primary sclerosing cholangitis. *Gastroenterology* 1995;108:865–869.

165. Stamatakis JD, Howard ER, Williams R. Benign inflammatory tumour of the common bile duct. *Br J Surg* 1979;66:257–258.

166. Tio TL, Cheng J, Wijers OB, et al. Endosonographic TNM staging of extrahepatic bile duct cancer: comparison with pathological staging. *Gastroenterology* 1991;100:1351–1361.

167. Kluge R, Schmidt F, Caca K, et al. Positron emission tomography with [(18)F]fluoro-2-deoxy-D-glucose for diagnosis and staging of bile duct cancer. *Hepatology* 2001;33:1029–1035.

168. Warshaw AL, Tepper JE, Shipley WU. Laparoscopy in the staging and planning of therapy for pancreatic cancer. *Am J Surg* 1986;151:76–80.

169. John TG, Greig JD, Crosbie JL, et al. Superior staging of liver tumors with laparoscopy and laparoscopic ultrasound. *Ann Surg* 1994;220:711–719.

170. McLeod RS, Taylor BR, O'Connor BI, et al. Quality of life, nutritional status, and gastrointestinal hormone profile following the Whipple procedure. *Am J Surg* 1995;169:179–185.

171. Strasberg SM, Drebin JA, Soper NJ. Evolution and current status of the Whipple procedure: an update for gastroenterologists. *Gastroenterology* 1997; 113:983–994.

172. Cheng Q, Luo X, Zhang B, et al. Distal bile duct carcinoma: prognostic factors after curative surgery. A series of 112 cases. *Ann Surg Oncol* 2007;14: 1212–1219.

173. Murakami Y, Uemura K, Hayashidani Y, et al. Pancreatoduodenectomy for distal cholangiocarcinoma: prognostic impact of lymph node metastasis. *World J Surg* 2007;31:337–342.

174. Prat F, Chapat O, Ducot B, et al. A randomized trial of endoscopic drainage methods for inoperable malignant strictures of the common bile duct. *Gastrointest Endosc* 1998;47:1–7.

175. Smith AC, Dowsett JF, Russell RC, et al. Randomised trial of endoscopic stenting versus surgical bypass in malignant low bileduct obstruction. *Lancet* 1994;344:1655–1660.

176. Glenn F, Hays DM. The scope of radical surgery in the treatment of malignant tumors of the extrahepatic biliary tract. *Surg Gynecol Obstet* 1954;99: 529–541.

177. Rudolph R, Cohen JJ. Cancer of the gallbladder in an 11-yr-old Navajo girl. *J Pediatric Surg* 1972;7:66–67.

178. De Aretxabala X, Roa I, Araya JC, et al. Gallbladder cancer in patients less than 40 years old. *Br J Surg* 1994;81:111.

179. de Aretxabala XA, Roa IS, Burgos LA, et al. Curative resection in potentially resectable tumours of the gallbladder. *Eur J Surg* 1997;163:419–426.

180. Randi G, Franceschi S, La Vecchia C. Gallbladder cancer worldwide: geographical distribution and risk factors. *Int J Cancer* 2006;118:1591–1602.

181. Saika K, Matsuda T. Comparison of time trends in gallbladder cancer mortality (1990-2006) between countries based using the WHO mortality database. *Jpn J Clin Oncol* 2010;40:374–375.

182. Carriaga MT, Henson DE. Liver, gallbladder, extrahepatic bile ducts, and pancreas. *Cancer* 1995;75:171–190.

183. Strom BL, Soloway RD, Rios-Dalenz JL, et al. Risk factors for gallbladder cancer. An international collaborative case-control study. *Cancer* 1995;76: 1747–1756.

184. Nervi F, Duarte I, Gomez G, et al. Frequency of gallbladder cancer in Chile, a high-risk area. *Int J Cancer* 1988;41:657–660.

185. Strom BL, Nelson WL, Henson DE, et al. Carcinoma of the gallbladder. In: Cohen S, Soloway RD, eds. *Gallstones.* New York: Churchill Livingstone; 1985: 275.

186. Lazcano-Ponce EC, Miquel JF, Munoz N, et al. Epidemiology and molecular pathology of gallbladder cancer. *CA Cancer J Clin* 2001;51:349–364.

187. Serra I, Calvo A, Baez S, et al. Risk factors for gallbladder cancer. An international collaborative case-control study. *Cancer* 1996;78:1515–1517.

188. Piehler JM, Crichlow RW. Primary carcinoma of the gallbladder. *Surg Gynecol Obstet* 1978;147:929–942.

189. Maringhini A, Moreau JA, Melton LJ 3rd, et al. Gallstones, gallbladder cancer, and other gastrointestinal malignancies. An epidemiologic study in Rochester, Minnesota. *Ann Intern Med* 1987;107:30–35.

190. Strom BL, Soloway RD, Rios-Dalenz J, et al. Biochemical epidemiology of gallbladder cancer. *Hepatology* 1996;23:1402–1411.

191. Diehl AK. Gallstone size and the risk of gallbladder cancer. *JAMA* 1983;250: 2323–2326.

192. Fernandez E, La Vecchia C, D'Avanzo B, et al. Family history and the risk of liver, gallbladder, and pancreatic cancer. *Cancer Epidemiol Biomarkers Prev* 1994;3:209–212.

193. Srivastava K, Srivastava A, Mittal B. Polymorphisms in ERCC2, MSH2, and OGG1 DNA repair genes and gallbladder cancer risk in a population of Northern India. *Cancer* 2010;116:3160–3169.

194. Chijiiwa K, Kimura H, Tanaka M. Malignant potential of the gallbladder in patients with anomalous pancreaticobiliary ductal junction. The difference in risk between patients with and without choledochal cyst. *Int Surg* 1995;80: 61–64.

195. Todani T, Toki A. [Cancer arising in choledochal cyst and management]. *Nihon Geka Gakkai zasshi* 1996;97:594–598.

196. Tokiwa K, Iwai N. Early mucosal changes of the gallbladder in patients with anomalous arrangement of the pancreaticobiliary duct. *Gastroenterology* 1996; 110:1614–1618.

197. Stephen AE, Berger DL. Carcinoma in the porcelain gallbladder: a relationship revisited. *Surgery* 2001;129:699–703.

198. Towfigh S, McFadden DW, Cortina GR, et al. Porcelain gallbladder is not associated with gallbladder carcinoma. *Am Surg* 2001;67:7–10.

199. Welton JC, Marr JS, Friedman SM. Association between hepatobiliary cancer and typhoid carrier state. *Lancet* 1979;1:791–794.

200. Matsukura N, Yokomuro S, Yamada S, et al. Association between Helicobacter bilis in bile and biliary tract malignancies: H. bilis in bile from Japanese and Thai patients with benign and malignant diseases in the biliary tract. *Jpn J Cancer Res* 2002;93:842–847.

201. Mishra RR, Tewari M, Shukla HS. Helicobacter species and pathogenesis of gallbladder cancer. *Hepatobiliary Pancreat Dis Int* 2010;9:129–134.

202. Neugut AI, Wylie P, Brandt-Rauf PW. Occupational cancers of the gastrointestinal tract. II. Pancreas, liver, and biliary tract. *Occup Med* 1987;2:137–153.

203. Broden G, Bengtsson L. Biliary carcinoma associated with methyldopa therapy. *Acta Chir Scand Suppl* 1980;500:7–12.

204. Lowenfels AB, Norman J. Isoniazid and bile duct cancer. *JAMA* 1978;240: 434–435.

205. Ellis EF, Gordon PR, Gottlieb LS. Oral contraceptives and cholangiocarcinoma. *Lancet* 1978;1:207.

206. Kimura W, Nagai H, Kuroda A, et al. Clinicopathologic study of asymptomatic gallbladder carcinoma found at autopsy. *Cancer* 1989;64:98–103.

207. Perpetuo MD, Valdivieso M, Heilbrun LK, et al. Natural history study of gall-bladder cancer: a review of 36 years experience at M. D. Anderson Hospital and Tumor Institute. *Cancer* 1978;42:330–335.

208. Okabayashi T, Sun ZL, Montgomey RA, et al. Surgical outcome of car-cinosarcoma of the gall bladder: a review. *World J Gastroenterol* 2009;15:4877–4882.

209. Mano H, Roa I, Araya JC, et al. Comparison of mutagenic activity of bile be-tween Chilean and Japanese female patients having cholelithiasis. *Mutat Res* 1996;371:73–77.

210. Kowalewski K, Todd EF. Carcinoma of the gallbladder induced in hamsters by insertion of cholesterol pellets and feeding dimethylnitrosamine. *Proc Soc Exp Biol Med* 1971;136:482–486.

211. Diehl AK, Beral V. Cholecystectomy and changing mortality from gallbladder cancer. *Lancet* 1981;2:187–189.

212. Albores-Saavedra J, Henson DE. *Atlas of Tumor Pathology, 2nd Series, Fascicle 22: Tumors of the Gallbladder and Extrahepatic Bile Ducts.* Washington DC: Armed Forces Institute of Pathology; 1986.

213. Roa I, Araya JC, Villaseca M, et al. Preneoplastic lesions and gallbladder cancer: an estimate of the period required for progression. *Gastroenterology* 1996;111:232–236.

214. Itoi T, Watanabe H, Ajioka Y, et al. APC, K-ras codon 12 mutations and p53 gene expression in carcinoma and adenoma of the gall-bladder suggest two genetic pathways in gall-bladder carcinogenesis. *Pathol Int* 1996;46:333–340.

215. Wistuba II, Albores-Saavedra J. Genetic abnormalities involved in the pathogenesis of gallbladder carcinoma. *J Hepatobiliary Pancreat Surg* 1999;6:237–244.

216. Imai M, Hoshi T, Ogawa K. K-ras codon 12 mutations in biliary tract tumors detected by polymerase chain reaction denaturing gradient gel electrophoresis. *Cancer* 1994;73:2727–2733.

217. Saetta AA, Papanastasiou P, Michalopoulos NV, et al. Mutational analysis of BRAF in gallbladder carcinomas in association with K-ras and p53 mutations and microsatellite instability. *Virchows Arch* 2004;445:179–182.

218. Leone F, Cavalloni G, Pignochino Y, et al. Somatic mutations of epidermal growth factor receptor in bile duct and gallbladder carcinoma. *Clinical Cancer Research* 2006;12:1680–1685.

219. Nakazawa K, Dobashi Y, Suzuki S, et al. Amplification and overexpression of c-erbB-2, epidermal growth factor receptor, and c-MET in biliary tract cancers. *J Pathol* 2005;206:356–365.

220. Koda M, Yashima K, Kawaguchi K, et al. Expression of Fhit, Mlh1, and P53 protein in human gallbladder carcinoma. *Cancer Lett* 2003;199:131–138.

221. Riquelme E, Tang M, Baez S, et al. Frequent epigenetic inactivation of chro-mosome 3p candidate tumor suppressor genes in gallbladder carcinoma. *Cancer Lett* 2007;250:100–106.

222. Hanada K, Itoh M, Fujii K, et al. K-ras and p53 mutations in stage I gallbladder carcinoma with an anomalous junction of the pancreaticobiliary duct. *Cancer* 1996;77:452–458.

223. Kaneko T, Ando H, Umeda T, et al. A new model for pancreaticobiliary maljunction without bile duct dilatation: demonstration of cell proliferation in the gallbladder epithelium. *J Surg Res* 1996;60:115–121.

224. Wistuba II, Gazdar AF. Gallbladder cancer: lessons from a rare tumour. Nature reviews. *Cancer* 2004;4:695–706.

225. Kamisawa T, Tu Y, Kuwata G, et al. Biliary carcinoma risk in patients with pan-creaticobiliary maljunction and the degree of extrahepatic bile duct dilatation. *Hepatogastroenterology* 2006;53:816–818.

226. Mohandas KM, Patil PS. Cholecystectomy for asymptomatic gallstones can reduce gall bladder cancer mortality in northern Indian women. *Indian J Gas-troenterol* 2006;25:147–151.

227. Shukla VK, Gurubachan, Sharma D, et al. Diagnostic value of serum CA242, CA 19-9, CA 15-3 and CA 125 in patients with carcinoma of the gallbladder. *Trop Gastroenterol* 2006;27:160–165.

228. Wibbenmeyer LA, Sharafuddin MJ, Wolverson MK, et al. Sonographic diag-nosis of unsuspected gallbladder cancer: imaging findings in comparison with benign gallbladder conditions. *AJR Am J Roentgenol* 1995;165:1169–1174.

229. Pandey M, Sood BP, Shukla RC, et al. Carcinoma of the gallbladder: role of sonography in diagnosis and staging. *J Clin Ultrasound* 2000;28:227–232.

230. Schwartz LH, Coakley FV, Sun Y, et al. Neoplastic pancreaticobiliary duct obstruction: evaluation with breath-hold MR cholangiopancreatography. *AJR Am J Roentgenol* 1998;170:1491–1495.

231. Ohtani T, Shirai Y, Tsukada K, et al. Spread of gallbladder carcinoma: CT eval-uation with pathologic correlation. *Abdom Imaging* 1996;21:195–201.

232. Rodriguez-Fernandez A, Gomez-Rio M, Medina-Benitez A, et al. Application of modern imaging methods in diagnosis of gallbladder cancer. *J Surg Oncol* 2006;93:650–664.

233. Akosa AB, Barker F, Desa L, et al. Cytologic diagnosis in the management of gallbladder carcinoma. *Acta Cytologica* 1995;39:494–498.

234. Meara RS, Jhala D, Eloubeidi MA, et al. Endoscopic ultrasound-guided FNA biopsy of bile duct and gallbladder: analysis of 53 cases. *Cytopathology* 2006;17:42–49.

235. Nevin JE, Moran TJ, Kay S, et al. Carcinoma of the gallbladder: staging, treat-ment, and prognosis. *Cancer* 1976;37:141–148.

236. Tsukada K, Hatakeyama K, Kurosaki I, et al. Outcome of radical surgery for carcinoma of the gallbladder according to the TNM stage. *Surgery* 1996;120:816–821.

237. Johnstone PA, Rohde DC, Swartz SE, et al. Port site recurrences after laparo-scopic and thoracoscopic procedures in malignancy. *J Clin Oncol* 1996;14:1950–1956.

238. Copher JC, Rogers JJ, Dalton ML. Trocar-site metastasis following laparoscop-ic cholecystectomy for unsuspected carcinoma of the gallbladder. Case report and review of the literature. *Surg Endosc* 1995;9:348–350.

239. Doudle M, King G, Thomas WM, et al. The movement of mucosal cells of the gallbladder within the peritoneal cavity during laparoscopic cholecystectomy. *Surg Endosc* 1996;10:1092–1094.

240. Toda K, Souda S, Yoshikawa Y, et al. Significance of laparoscopic excisional biop-sy for polypoid lesions of the gallbladder. *Surg Laparosc Endosc* 1995;5:267–271.

241. Kubota K, Bandai Y, Noie T, et al. How should polypoid lesions of the gallbladder be treated in the era of laparoscopic cholecystectomy? *Surgery* 1995;117:481–487.

242. Wu SS, Lin KC, Soon MS, et al. Ultrasound-guided percutaneous transhepatic fine needle aspiration cytology study of gallbladder polypoid lesions. *Am J Gas-troenterol* 1996;91:1591–1594.

243. Onoyama H, Yamamoto M, Tseng A, et al. Extended cholecystectomy for car-cinoma of the gallbladder. *World J Surg* 1995;19:758–763.

244. Chao TC, Wang CS, Jeng LB, et al. Primary carcinoma of the gallbladder in Taiwan. *J Surg Oncol* 1996;61:49–55.

245. Ruckert JC, Ruckert RI, Gellert K, et al. Surgery for carcinoma of the gallblad-der. *Hepatogastroenterology* 1996;43:527–533.

246. Miyazaki M, Itoh H, Ambiru S, et al. Radical surgery for advanced gallbladder carcinoma. *Br J Surg* 1996;83:478–481.

247. Hatfield AR, Tobias R, Terblanche J, et al. Preoperative external biliary drain-age in obstructive jaundice. A prospective controlled clinical trial. *Lancet* 1982;2:896–899.

248. McPherson GA, Benjamin IS, Hodgson HJ, et al. Pre-operative percutane-ous transhepatic biliary drainage: the results of a controlled trial. *Br J Surg* 1984;71:371–375.

249. Pitt HA, Gomes AS, Lois JF, et al. Does preoperative percutaneous biliary drain-age reduce operative risk or increase hospital cost? *Ann Surg* 1985;201:545–553.

250. Kresl JJ, Schild SE, Henning GT, et al. Adjuvant external beam radiation therapy with concurrent chemotherapy in the management of gallbladder car-cinoma. *Int J Radiat Encol Biol Phys* 2002;52:167–175.

251. Makela JT, Kairaluoma MI. Superselective intra-arterial chemotherapy with mitomycin for gallbladder cancer. *Br J Surg* 1993;80:912–915.

252. Uno T, Itami J, Aruga M, et al. Primary carcinoma of the gallbladder: role of external beam radiation therapy in patients with locally advanced tumor. *Strahlenther Onkol* 1996;172:496–500.

253. Todoroki T, Iwasaki Y, Orii K, et al. Resection combined with intraoperative radiation therapy (IORT) for stage IV (TNM) gallbladder carcinoma. *World J Surg* 1991;15:357–366.

254. Eckel F, Brunner T, Jelic S, Grp EGW. Biliary cancer: ESMO Clinical Prac-tice Guidelines for diagnosis, treatment and follow-up. *Ann Oncol* 2011;22:vi40–vi44.

46 Cancer of the Small Bowel

Ronald S. Chamberlain, Krishnaraj Mahendraraj, and Syed Ammer Shah

SMALL BOWEL CANCER

Although the small intestine comprises 75% of the length and 90% of the total absorptive surface of the gastrointestinal tract, less than 3% of gastrointestinal malignancies occur in the small bowel.[1] Small bowel cancers (SBC) are 40- to 60-times less common than colorectal cancer. The rarity of SBCs makes them difficult to diagnose, especially considering their varied clinical presentation. With an increasing incidence and advanced stage at diagnosis, it has become even more important to understand the pathology of these rare but deadly cancers.

Epidemiology

SBC accounts for ~3% of all the gastrointestinal cancers with an equal male to female ratio and a median age of 66 years. The American Cancer Society estimates there will be 9,160 new cases of SBCs in 2014, with 1,210 deaths.[2,3] This number represents a steady increase in the incidence of SBCs from ~6,100 new cases per year in the 1980s based on information derived from the Surveillance, Epidemiology, and End Results (SEER) database registries.[1–5,8]

There are more than 40 SBC histologic subtypes, with 93% of them comprised of four major types: carcinoid (37.4%), adenocarcinoma (36.9%), lymphoma (17.3%), and gastrointestinal stromal tumors (8.4%).[6] Historically, adenocarcinoma had a higher incidence than carcinoid tumors, but this has changed over the past decade.[5–8] In terms of the location, ≠50% of SBC occur in the duodenum, where adenocarcinoma predominates, followed by the jejunum (30%) and ileum, where lymphoma is more common proximally, and carcinoid tumors distally. There is an increased incidence of SBC among colon cancer patients and the reverse is true also, suggesting a similar causal mechanism rather than a surveillance bias or the carcinogenic effects treating the index primary.[6,9,10]

Pathogenesis and Risk Factors

Proposed risk factors for the predisposition to small bowel neoplasms are varied, although it is notable that 64% of small bowel tumors are malignant. Proposed factors that have been associated with SBC include:

1. Advanced age: SBCs occur predominantly in the elderly with a mean age of ≠66 years.
2. Specific inheritable syndromes predisposing to SBC[11–32]:

   - *Familial adenomatosis polyposis (FAP) syndromes.* FAP is an autosomal-dominant disorder attributable to a mutation in the adenomatosis polyposis coli (*APC*) gene and characterized by the development of hundreds or thousands of polyps throughout the gastrointestinal tract, but predominately in the large bowel. FAP patients have a 100% lifetime risk of developing colorectal cancer, and this has led to a clearly defined role for total colectomy or proctocolectomy to prevent cancer development. FAP patients also inherit a 4% to 12% lifetime risk of developing adenocarcinoma of the duodenum or periampullary region, which is 300 times that of the general population, necessitating screening esophagogastroduodenoscopy (EGD) as part of the work-up.[11–18]
   - *Hereditary nonpolyposis colon cancer (HNPCC).* HNPCC, also known as Lynch syndrome, is a hereditary condition that results from a germ-line mutation in DNA mismatch repair genes, primarily *MSH2* and *MLH1*. This mutation predisposes one not only to an 80% lifetime risk of colorectal cancer, but also to an increased risk of endometrial, gastric, ovarian, urinary, small bowel, biliary, and skin cancers.[19,20] HNPCC patients have a SBC lifetime risk of 1% to 4%, or a 100-fold greater risk than the general population, which also tends to present 10 to 20 years earlier.[20] SBC may be the initial presentation of HNPCC in a small cohort of patients, and some clinicians recommend small bowel surveillance for this group.[20–25]
   - *Peutz-Jeghers syndrome* (PJS). PJS is an autosomal-dominant disorder characterized by benign hamartomatous polyps in the intestine along with melanocytic macules on the lips and oral mucosa. PJS is due to a mutation in the *STK11* (*LKB1*) tumor suppressor gene, which results in a significant increased inherited risk for multiple cancer types, with the highest risk involving the gastrointestinal tract. By the age of 70 years, the cumulative gastrointestinal (GI) cancer risk is approximately 57% (colon cancer followed by SBC), which represents a 15-fold increased risk compared to the general population.[27,28]
   - *MUTYH-associated polyposis (MAP).* First described in 2002, the *MUTYH* gene encodes for DNA glycosylase, which is involved in oxidative DNA damage repair and belongs to the family of DNA mismatch repair genes. Mutations in this gene result in heritable predisposition to GI cancers, including SBC in an autosomal-recessive fashion. Mutations of this gene results in G to T transversions, usually involving the *APC* and *KRAS* gene, thus predisposing individuals to cancer development.[29,30]
   - *Cystic fibrosis.* A marginally increased risk of SBC has been documented in cystic fibrosis patients.[31]

3. *Inflammatory bowel disease.* Although only 2% of Crohn disease (CD) patients will develop a small bowel malignancy (typically an adenocarcinoma associated with >10 years of disease and involving the distal small bowel), this represents a 10- to 60-times higher risk than the general population.[33–35] Specifically, SBCs in CD occur more commonly in men, in the distal ileal location, are more common in small bowel bypass loops and in strictures, and in patients with exposure to asbestos or other carcinogens such as halogenated aromatic compounds.[36] A meta-analysis identified a 33.2 relative risk (95% confidence interval [CI], 15.9 to 60.9) of developing small bowel cancer among CD patients.[37–39]

4. *Celiac disease or sprue (CS).* CS is an autoimmune disorder characterized by villous atrophy, crypt hyperplasia, and increased intraepithelial lymphocytes caused by a reaction to the wheat protein gliadin in the presence of specific pairs of allelic variants in two HLA *DQ2/DQ8* genes. CS is associated with an increased risk of *enteropathy-associated T-cell lymphoma* (EATL), which can occur in up to 39% of patients with severe or refractory CS (RCS). The overall prevalence of RCS is low (0.6% to 1.5%). RCS can be subclassified into RCS type 1, which is characterized by increased but nonclonal expansion of intraepithelial lymphocytes (IEL), or RCS type 2, which displays clonal expansion of IELs that evolve into EATL in 60% to 80% of such patients within 5 years.[40–42]

5. *Immunosuppression.* Iatrogenic (therapeutic) or posttransplant immunosuppression is a generalized dysregulator of homeostasis and predisposes certain patients to both lymphomas and sarcomas. Small bowel lymphomas that develop in these patients are predominantly B-cell as opposed to T-cell lymphomas. Posttransplant lymphoproliferative disorders (PTLD) that occur develop primarily post–Epstein Barr viral infection and are typically B-cell lymphomas.

6. *Other malignancies.* The patient with other primary malignancies may also be at increased risk for SBCs. This includes patients with prior colorectal, pancreas, periampullary, uterine, ovarian, prostate, thyroid, skin, and soft tissue tumors.[9,10,43] In fact, 30% to 40% of patients with SBCs have a synchronous malignancy, which may be associated with the primary pathologic entity or may reflect shared genetic or environmental risk factors.

7. *Modifiable risk factors.* Modifiable risk factors implicated in SBCs include alcohol use and obesity. In a recent large Asian study involving over 500,000 patients with a 10.6-year follow-up, a higher body mass index (>27.5 kg/m^2) and alcohol use (>400 g of ethanol per week) were associated with increased SBC risk. Notably, smoking is not associated with an increased risk of developing SBC.[44–46] Abstinence, weight loss, and dietary modifications (including adhering to a gluten-free diet in those with celiac disease) have been suggested to reduce the risk of SBCs.

Clinical Features

SBC presents in a variety of ways and is more likely to be symptomatic early in the disease course compared to benign tumors.[47,48] The most common presenting symptoms are abdominal pain (45% to 76%), nausea and vomiting (16% to 52%), weight loss (28% to 45%), fatigue and anemia (15% to 30%), and gastrointestinal bleeding (7% to 23%).[49–52] The most common clinical sign of pallor is seen in ~40% of patients. Up to 77% of SBCs present acutely with either small bowel obstruction or perforation, particularly adenocarcinomas.[47] Patients with familial or genetic predisposition to SBCs present, on average, 10 years earlier compared to sporadic cases.[52–56]

In comparing different SBC histologies, adenocarcinoma is most often associated with abdominal pain and obstruction, whereas sarcomas and lymphomas are more often associated with bleeding and perforation, respectively. Adenocarcinomas are frequently found in the duodenum, carcinoid tumors affect the ileum and sarcomas, and lymphomas are found throughout the entire small bowel.

Diagnosis

The diagnosis of SBC is often delayed as a result of its rarity and nonspecific presentation. The mean duration of symptoms prior to an accurate SBC diagnosis ranges from 8 to 12 months.[48–51] A high index of clinical suspicion is imperative if the diagnosis is to be made early. In many instances, a preoperative diagnosis is not established because patients present emergently with hemorrhage, perforation, or obstruction. No single diagnostic test has sufficient sensitivity or specificity to be considered a gold standard.[141–167]

Conventional abdominal radiographs have a limited, nonspecific role in the diagnosis of SBCs. Plain abdominal radiographs are helpful when an obstruction exists, but even then accuracy is only 50% to 60%. A single or double contrast small bowel follow through (SBFT) is well suited for examination of luminal abnormalities and mucosal abnormalities, but is time consuming and associated with an accuracy ranging from 33% to 60%.[78–82] Small bowel enteroclysis may improve this accuracy to 90%.[57] A major limitation of both SBFT and enteroclysis is their inability to evaluate extraluminal pathology, which is circumvented by cross-sectional imaging, such as computed tomography (CT) scans and magnetic resonance imaging (MRI). CT- and MRI-based enteroclysis has improved the sensitivity and specificity of small bowel tumor detection compared to conventional enteroclysis.[58–60]

In clinical practice, a CT scan of the abdomen with oral and intravenous contrast is the most common diagnostic test utilized in the acute and chronic setting. Pathognomonic CT signs that differentiate between types of small bowel lesions have been well described. Adenocarcinoma appears as a discrete tumor mass with annular narrowing, abrupt concentric or irregular "overhanging edges," or as an ulcerative lesion. Lesions in the duodenum are typically intraluminal polyps, whereas more distal polypoid lesions present with intussusception and a characteristic "target sign" (Figs. 46.1 and 46.2).[61]

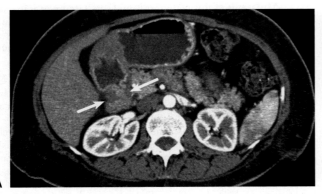
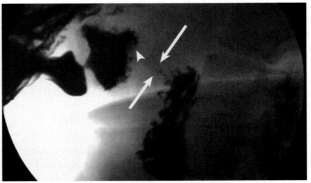

Figure 46.1 Moderately differentiated primary small bowel adenocarcinoma. **(A)** The contrast-enhanced axial computed tomography image shows an annular soft tissue lesion (*arrows*) in the duodenum, resulting in circumferential luminal narrowing and wall thickening. **(B)** A lateral image from subsequent upper gastrointestinal series shows the annular "apple-core" lesion, resulting in advanced narrowing of the duodenal lumen (*arrows*). Note the compressed, overhanging edges (*arrowhead*) of the small bowel at the margin of the mass.

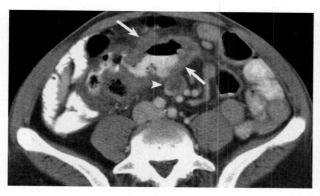
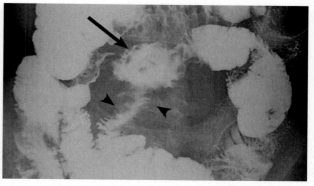

Figure 46.2 A small bowel intussusception due to primary small bowel adenocarcinoma. **(A)** A contrast-enhanced axial computed tomography image shows a small bowel target sign consistent with intussusception; the intussusceptum (*arrowhead*) telescopes into the intussuscipiens (*arrow*). The lead point for the intussusceptions was a primary small bowel carcinoma. **(B)** An image from small bowel follow through shows the "coiled spring" appearance of the intussusceptum (arrowhead) as it telescopes into the intussuscipiens (*arrow*).

Carcinoid tumors appear as hyperintense luminal masses due to increased vascularity. The tumors typically have intense desmoplastic reaction in response to biochemical products produced by the tumor that results in puckering of the adjacent mesentery, giving a characteristic stellate pattern on the CT scan not necessarily reflecting mesenteric invasion (Fig. 46.3).

Small bowel lymphomas present as circumferential mural thickening with low homogeneous attenuation and a characteristic aneurysmal dilatation in which the involved segment shows cavitary dilatation with a nodular, irregular luminal contour and peripheral bowel wall thickening (Fig. 46.4).[62] Sarcomas appear as homogeneous, well-circumscribed, hypervascular masses on CT (Fig. 46.5).[63–65]

The MRI has a defined niche in the assessment of early small bowel lesions given its improved soft tissue delineation and it may be pivotal in detecting early small bowel pathology (Table 46.1).[66–70] Somatostatin receptor scans (octreoscan) and metaiodobenzylguanidine (MIBG) scans may be helpful in localizing and diagnosing of small bowel carcinoid tumors. Octreoscan employs a ^{111}In-diethylenetriaminepentaacetic acid analog that targets somatostatin receptors. Over 90% of carcinoid tumors express somatostatin receptors, and this test has a sensitivity of 80% to 100%. Octreoscans may also provide a functional map of the tumor for anticipated radiolabelled immunotherapy-targeted therapy depending on the stage of the disease.[71]

Positron emission tomography (PET)/CT scans are useful in the initial diagnosis and in disease staging for small bowel adenocarcinomas (SBA), lymphomas, and gastrointestinal stromal tumor (GIST).[72,74] Fludeoxyglucose ([18]FDG)-PET has a limited role in the diagnosis and staging of carcinoid tumors because they are not [18]FDG avid; however, it may play important role in ascertaining treatment response and detecting disease recurrence.[72–74]

Two notable advances are double-balloon enteroscopy, or push enteroscopy, and video capsule endoscopy (VCE), which were both introduced in 2001. Double-balloon enteroscopy is a technically challenging procedure that permits the evaluation of the entire small bowel and tissue sampling, which is not possible with VCE. Double-balloon enteroscopy most commonly detects symptomatic lesions, including areas of ulceration, stenosis, and GI bleeds, with a sensitivity of 74% to 81%.[75–83] VCE is effective at identifying 50% of new SBC lesions and 87% of all lesions, with a relatively low miss rate of 10%.[84–93]

ADENOCARCINOMA

Adenocarcinoma of the small bowel is the second most common histologic SBC subtype, comprising 36.9% of cases.[94] The annual incidence is estimated at 7.3 case per million worldwide. In the United States, 3,050 new cases of SBA are anticipated in 2013.[94,95] Patients with SBA usually present between the 6th and 8th decade of life, with earlier presentations in patients with genetic, autoimmune, or inflammatory conditions (Table 46.2).

SBAs display a slight predominance for men, with age-adjusted incidence rates highest among African Americans (14.1 per 10[6]) followed by Caucasians (7.7 per 10[6]), Hispanics (6.2 per 10[6]), and

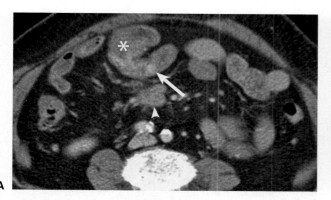
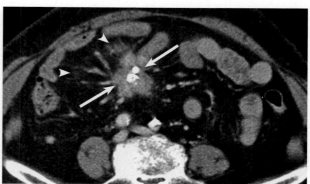

Figure 46.3 Primary ileal carcinoid. **(A)** A contrast-enhanced computed tomography (CT) shows a tethered and thickened segment of ileum (*asterisk*) containing a small submucosal enhancing lesion (*arrow*), consistent with primary carcinoid. Note partially imaged metastasis (*arrowhead*) in the adjacent mesentery. **(B)** A more inferior CT image shows a stellate mesenteric carcinoid metastasis (*arrows*) with central calcification and desmoplastic reaction (*arrowheads*) in the adjacent fat.

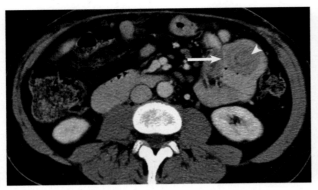
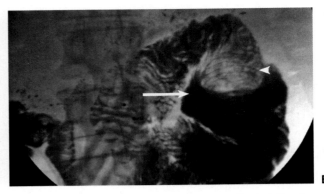

Figure 46.4 Primary small bowel lymphoma. **(A)** A contrast-enhanced computed tomography (CT) image shows aneurysmal luminal dilatation and extensive wall thickening of a segment of small bowel (*arrows*). Note enlarged adjacent mesenteric node (*arrowhead*). **(B)** A radiograph from the small bowel follow through shows a small bowel segment with luminal dilatation (*arrow*) and extensive mural thickening and irregularity (*arrowheads*) corresponding to the diseased segment on the CT.

Asian/Pacific Islanders (5.5 per 10^6). Adenocarcinoma incidence decreases distally in the small bowel, with the highest incidence in the duodenum (50% to 5%), followed by the jejunum (16%) and ileum (13%). Most SBA patients present at an advanced stage (American Joint Committee on Cancer [AJCC] stage III or greater) resulting in a poor overall 5-year disease-free survival (of about 30%) and mean survival (20 months).[50] Outcomes are worse for duodenal tumors (28% 5-year survival) compared to jejunal and ileal lesions (38% 5-year survival).

Etiology

SBA shares several etiologic features with colorectal cancers (CRC), leading to the adoption of similar treatment strategies, although they are biologically distinct diseases. The most obvious similarity between SBA and CRC is a common etiopathogenic pathways because both cancers are more common in patients with FAP, HNPCC, and inflammatory bowel disease. Available data imply a similar adenoma to carcinoma sequence in both SBA and CRC. As with CRC, the risk of progression is associated with the size of the adenoma (8.3% for lesions <1 cm and 30% for lesions >1 cm) and histology (14.3 % for tubular, 23.1% for tubulovillous, and 36% for villous).[96–99] A number of molecular similarities and dissimilarities between these two cancers have also been reported. In a recent genomic hybridization study looking at GI cancers, SBA was more similar to CRC than to stomach cancer.[100] In addition, *HER2* oncogene amplification is low in SBA similar to CRC in contrast to gastric cancer.[97,98,101,102] Microsatellite instability (MSI) and loss of mismatch repair proteins is present in 18% to

35% of SBAs versus 15% of CRCs.[77–79] Approximately 50% of the SBA cases reflect sporadic methylation of the *MLH1* gene with a relatively high incidence of MSI and MLH1 methylation in CD associated SBA (67% to 73%).[106–117]

Staging and Prognosis

The AJCC staging system for SBA is depicted in Table 46.3. Given the nonspecific initial presentation of SBAs, 32% of patients present with stage IV disease, 27% present with stage III, 30% present with stage II, and 10% present with stage I.[102] Less than 50% of SBA patients are curative surgical candidates. Survival by stage is 63% for stage I, 48% for stage II, 32% for stage III, and about 4% for stage IV.[102] Multivariate regression analyses identified age over 55 years, males, African Americans, T4 tumor, lymph node involvement and ratio, duodenal followed by ileal primary, poor differentiation, metastatic disease, and positive margins as associated with a poor prognosis.[94,102,120–122] Recent investigations into molecular determinants have also identified the CpG island methylator phenotype (CIMP) status, E-cadherin loss, and aberrant β-catenin expression as also associated with a worse prognosis.[106,118]

Management

The site of the disease, the stage at presentation, the available expertise, patient comorbidities, and patient performance status are all important considerations in determining the optimal management for individual SBA patients.

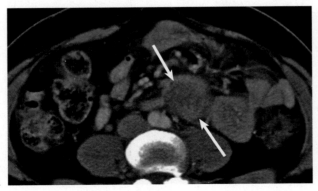
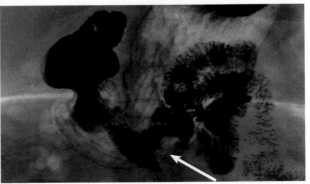

Figure 46.5 A gastrointestinal stromal tumor of the small bowel. **(A)** A contrast-enhanced computed tomography image shows a solid, heterogeneously enhancing mass (*arrows*) arising from the submucosa of the third portion of the duodenum. **(B)** An image from upper gastrointestinal series shows a filling defect (*arrow*) in the third portion of the duodenum due to the submucosal gastrointestinal stromal tumor.

TABLE 46.1

Risk Factors and Predisposing Conditions in the Development of Small Bowel Cancer

Risk Factor	Lifetime Risk	Small Bowel Cancer Type
Genetic		
FAP (2%–5%)	2%–5%	Periampullary adenocarcinoma, duodenal/jejunal adenocarcinoma,
HNPCC	1%–4%	adenocarcinoma, Gardner syndrome, desmoid duodenal adenocarcinoma,
Peutz-Jeghers syndrome	15-fold	gastrointestinal cancers
MUTYH-associated polyposis	4%	
Cystic fibrosis		
Autoimmune/Inflammatory		
Crohn disease	(>10 yr) 2%	Ileal adenocarcinoma, jejunal lymphoma/ adenocarcinoma, celiac disease immunosuppressive lymphoma, posttransplant lymphoproliferative disorder, neurofibromatosis, paragangliomas

Malignant Conditions
Colorectal, prostate, pancreas, uterine, skin and soft tissue tumors

Benign Conditions
Cholecystectomy, peptic ulcer disease

Other Conditions
Male gender, African American, advanced age, high-fat diet, obesity, alcohol

TABLE 46.2

Magnetic Resonance Findings of Common Small Bowel Neoplasms

Tumor Type	Growth Pattern	Margins	Secondary Intestinal Findings	Type of Lymphatic and Mesenteric Spread	MRI Findings
Adenocarcinoma	Short annular lesion with intraluminal growth, predominantly in duodenum	Irregular margins	Stenotic lesion with proximal obstruction	Local–regional metastases	Isointense to muscle on T1, heterogeneous signal on T2, hypovascular after Gd
Lymphoma	Long segmental infiltrating lesion	Smooth regular contours with preservation of the perivisceral fat plane	Aneurysmal dilatation without obstruction	Bulky retroperitoneal metastases	Isointense to muscle on T1, heterogeneous signal on T2, moderate enhancement after Gd
GIST	Intramural submucosal mass with extraserosal extension	Smooth lobulated contours	Aneurysmal dilatation, stenosis or obstruction usually absent	Peritoneal metastatic nodules, adenopathy rare	Inhomogeneous lesions, isointense on T1, mildly hyperintense on T2, peripheral enhancement in large lesions
Carcinoid	Focal asymmetric predominantly in ileum	Irregular margins; mesenteric stranding and kinking of the involved segment	Intermittent obstruction possible proximal to the kinked loop	Hypervascular mesenteric metastases with spiculated margins and local adenopathy with calcification	Isointense to muscle on T1, heterogeneous hyperintense on T2, hypervascular on Gd

Gd, gadolinium.
Adapted from Crusco F, Giovagnoni A, et al. Malignant small bowel neoplasms: spectrum of disease on MR imaging. *Radiol Med* 2010;115:1279–1291.

TABLE 46.3

American Joint Committee on Cancer Staging of Small Intestinal Cancer

Primary Tumor

Tx	Primary tumor cannot be assessed
T0	No evidence of primary tumor
Tis	*Carcinoma in situ*
T1a	Tumor invades lamina propria
T1b	Tumor invades submucosa[a]
T2	Tumor invades muscularis propria
T3	Tumor invades through the muscularis propria into the subserosa or into the nonperitonealized perimuscular tissue (mesentery or retroperitoneum) with extension ≤2 cm[a]
T4	Tumor perforates the visceral peritoneum or directly invades other organs or structures (includes other loops of small intestine, mesentery, or retroperitoneum >2 cm, and abdominal wall by way of serosa; for duodenum only, invasion of pancreas or bile duct)

Regional Lymph Nodes

Nx	Regional lymph nodes cannot be assessed
N0	No regional lymph node metastasis
N1	Metastasis in 1–3 regional lymph nodes
N2	Metastases in ≥4 regional lymph nodes

Distant Metastasis

M0	No distant metastasis
M1	Distant metastasis

Anatomic Stage/Prognostic Group

Stage	T	N	M
0	Tis	N0	M0
I	T1	N0	M0
	T2	N0	M0
IIA	T3	N0	M0
IIB	T4	N0	M0
IIIA	Any T	N1	M0
IIIB	Any T	N2	M0
IV	Any T	Any N	Any M

[a] The nonperitonealized perimuscular tissue is, for the jejunum and ileum, part of the mesentery. For the duodenum in areas where serosa is lacking, it is part of the interface with the pancreas.

Used with the permission of the American Joint Committee on Cancer (AJCC), Chicago, Illinois. The original source for this material is the *AJCC Cancer Staging Manual*, Seventh Edition (2010) published by Springer Science and Business Media LLC, www.springerlink.com, page 129.

Surgery for Local–Regional Disease

Surgery is the treatment for local–regional confined SBAs.[50] The 5-year survival of resected versus unresected patients is 54% versus 0%.[122] The optimal surgical treatment depends on the location of the primary tumor, with duodenal adenocarcinomas managed by either a pancreaticoduodenectomy or segmental resection. Both procedures are equivalent with regard to long-term survival, with segmental resection associated with less postoperative morbidity and length of hospitalization.[122–125] Jejunal and ileal adenocarcinomas

are treated with oncologic-appropriate segmental resection. A right hemicolectomy is the appropriate oncologic approach to tumors near the ileocecal valve.

Adjuvant Therapy

Recurrence in SBAs is predominantly distant and rarely local–regional (86% versus 18%, respectively).[50] Although duodenal SBAs have a higher incidence of local failure, distant recurrence still predominates (59% versus 19%, respectively, and combined, 22%).[94,126,127] Most treatment strategies are based on fluorouracil (5-FU) or, more recently, 5-FU/oxaliplatin–based regimens. Overman et al.[129] reported adjuvant therapy improved disease-free survival (hazard ration [HR], 0.23, 95% CI, 0.06 to 0.89, p = 0.03), but not overall survival (HR, 0.48, 95% CI, 0.13 to 1.74, p = 0.26) in patients receiving adjuvant chemotherapy (5-FU or platinum based).[129] Multiple retrospective studies have demonstrated a mixed response for adjuvant chemotherapy in SBAs.[49,50,128–130]

The role of hyperthermic intraperitoneal chemotherapy (HIPEC) in the treatment of SBCs has been investigated in four small trials involving a total of 30 patients with peritoneal carcinomatosis. These patients underwent HIPEC followed by adjuvant chemotherapy, with a reported mean overall survival of 22.2 months compared to 12 months on conventional treatment strategies. The results are encouraging, but the numbers are too small to draw any robust conclusions.[140]

Treatment for Metastatic Disease

Limited randomized controlled trials defining a role for chemotherapy versus best supportive care (BSC) in patients with advanced SBAs have been performed. Multiple retrospective studies have demonstrated a small survival advantage for palliative chemotherapy approaches compared to BSC alone (Table 46.4).[49,50,131–136]

Although there are *no* randomized trials comparing different regimens, a number of SBA clinical trials are currently accruing in an effort to more precisely define the role of chemotherapy in advanced SBA. The role of surgery for all advanced/metastatic SBC is purely palliative. Specific patients might benefit from an intestinal bypass to maintain an enteral means of nutrition and an improved quality of life.[120,137–139]

CARCINOID TUMORS

Carcinoid tumors are slow growing neoplasms that arise from the neuroendocrine cells of Kulchitsky. Of these cells, 75% occur in the gastrointestinal tract (44.7% in the small bowel and 19.6% in the rectum), followed by the lung, bronchus, and rarely the liver, pancreas, or gonads. Given the fourfold increase in the incidence of carcinoids that has occurred over the past 2 decades, carcinoids are now the most common SBC (36.9%) according to the National Cancer Database.[167,168]

Clinical Presentation and Prognosis

Of small bowel carcinoids, 44.7% occur in the small bowel, and over 50% of these are found in the ileum.[168] Carcinoid tumors are most common in the 7th decade of life (mean age, 66 years), in males (52.4%), and in Caucasians (80.4%). Most carcinoids present in an advanced stage (75%) as a result of a significant delay and difficulty in diagnosis. Despite the advanced stage, most carcinoids follow an indolent course, with an overall 5-year survival ranging from 52% to 77%.[170–174] Tumors over 10 mm and those with a transmural depth of invasion are the primary risk factors for local–regional progression and metastasis.[175]

TABLE 46.4

Current Clinical Trials for Advanced Small Bowel Adenocarcinoma

Identifier	Phase	Tumor Type	N	Therapy Line	Agent
NCT00354887	II	Small bowel adenocarcinoma and ampullary	30	1st	CAPOX + bevacizumab
NCT00433550	II	Small bowel adenocarcinoma	33	1st	CAPOX + irinotecan
NCT01202409	II	Small bowel adenocarcinoma and ampullary	20	1st	CAPOX + panitumumab (KRAS wild type)
NCT00987766	1b	Duodenal + ampullary	22	1st	GEMOX + erlotinib
NCT01730586	II	Small bowel adenocarcinoma	10	>2nd	Nab-paclitaxel

CAPOX, capecitabine + oxaliplatin, GEMOX, gemcitabine + oxaliplatin, Nab-paclitaxel, nano-article albumin-bound paclitaxel.
Adapted from Raghav K, Overman MJ. Small bowel adenocarcinoma—existing evidence and evolving paradigms. *Nat Rev Clin Oncol* 2013;10:534–544.

Carcinoid Syndrome

Carcinoid syndrome is an array of symptoms that occurs in patients with carcinoid tumors of the bronchus or metastatic to the liver. Symptoms of carcinoid syndrome include diarrhea, cutaneous flushing, and wheezing. These symptoms are precipitated by stress, alcohol intake, and certain physical activities, and are secondary to the systemic release of several tumor-derived factors, including serotonin, dopamine, tachykinins, histamine, and prostaglandins, all of which are metabolized by the liver. Up to 80% of patients with small bowel carcinoids develop carcinoid syndrome, and it is the presenting complaint in 10% to 17% of patients. The mainstay of treatment for carcinoid syndrome is somatostatin, which prevents the secretion of hormones by binding to a specific receptor on the tumor surface.[192,193] Although octreotide is effective in most patients, interferon α (IFN-α) may benefit patients who do not respond to octreotide alone.[187] The antihistamine cyproheptadine has also been used successfully for refractory carcinoid symptoms.[188]

Management

Surgery for Local–Regional Disease

An oncologic segmental resection of the tumor is the preferred treatment for localized small bowel carcinoids.[176] Five-year survival after resection of localized disease ranges between 50% and 85%. Of small bowel carcinoids, 29% are associated with other noncarcinoid neoplasms, necessitating a thorough inspection of the entire bowel at surgery. Appendiceal carcinoids smaller than 2 cm can be treated with a simple appendectomy, whereas larger tumors require a right hemicolectomy. Pretreatment with octreotide prior to anesthetic induction is recommended because surgical intervention/manipulation can precipitate a carcinoid crisis.[177–180]

Surgery for Metastatic Disease

The liver is the most common site of carcinoid metastasis. Liver resection along with primary tumor resection is recommended for resectable metastatic disease. More radical surgical debulking or cytoreductive surgery has been used for patients with extensive bilobar liver disease, liver failure, or extensive metastatic disease to provide prolonged disease-free survival. Several studies have shown that liver resection can improve the 5-year survival rate from 36% to 61% compared to historic controls.[181–183] Although long-term data are lacking, percutaneous or laparoscopic local ablative techniques such as radiofrequency, microwave, or cryoablation represent alternative cytoreductive modalities for the treatment of metastatic carcinoid tumors. Cytoreductive strategies not only prolong survival, but are also associated with a decrease in octreotide doses required to control carcinoid symptoms. A number of retrospective series have demonstrated that surgical resection is superior to systemic therapy with regard to both overall survival and symptom management.[184]

Hepatic Artery Embolization

Transcatheter hepatic arterial embolization (HAE) with or without chemotherapy has been utilized extensively for both symptom control and as a definitive treatment for unresectable carcinoid liver metastasis.[185] HAE may be performed with gel foam, polyvinyl alcohol, or microspheres. The addition of chemotherapy allows for the delivery of much higher intratumoral concentrations than can be achieved with systemic therapy. Known complications include transient or fulminant liver failure, liver abscesses, and postembolization syndrome (fever, abdominal pain, leukocytosis, elevations in liver function tests).[185]

Systemic Chemotherapy

Several chemotherapeutics have been studied extensively in the management of carcinoid metastases, including 5-FU, streptozotocin, and doxorubicin. All have yielded modest response rates of ~20%. In addition, IFN-α has been purported to achieve tumor stabilization in 20% to 40% of cases, and octreotide has been shown to prevent the progression of metastatic carcinoids in several small case series.[186–190] Tyrosine–kinase inhibitors like imatinib or sunitinib can induce a delay in tumor cell growth in preclinical studies and disease stability in 83% of patients treated over a 1-year period. In a recent phase II study, bevacizumab, a monoclonal antibody that targets vascular endothelial growth factor (VEGF), was shown to stabilize disease in 95% of patients when combined with octreotide compared to 68% stabilization when octreotide was combined with IFN-α.[191,218,219]

Palliative Surgery

The decision to perform palliative resection for disseminated carcinoid tumors should carefully balance the surgical risks and perceived patient benefits. Orthotopic liver transplantation for patients with unresectable liver-only disease remains investigational and is currently performed by only a small number of transplant centers.

SMALL BOWEL LYMPHOMA

Lymphoma is the third most common SBC, comprising 10% to 20% of cases. Of such cases, 20% to 40% are extranodal lymphomas, which arise within a solid organ, and ~50% of extranodal lymphomas are GI lymphomas.[194–198] Of GI lymphomas, 75% are located in the stomach, followed by the small bowel, colon, and other organs such as the pancreas and the liver. GI lymphomas have a peak incidence in the 7th decade of life, with a male to female ratio of 1.5:1. The incidence of small bowel lymphomas has increased in the United States over the last 2 decades, correlating with an increase in lymphomas among immunocompromised patients. Increased immigration from the Middle East—where primary intestinal lymphoma constitutes the most common primary extranodal disease—may also account for some of the increase in small bowel lymphomas. Additional risk factors include Crohn disease and prior radiation exposure.

Staging and Prognosis

The most important prognostic indicator for intestinal lymphoma is tumor spread. Most GI lymphomas are of the non-Hodgkin type and are staged based on the Ann Arbor staging system: stage I disease is limited to a single site; stage II tumors are confined to below the diaphragm and are separated into two subgroups, namely stage II with regional (stage II 1E) and distant (stage II 2E) lymph node involvement; stage III has involvement of organs on both sides of the diaphragm; and stage IV represents widespread dissemination, including the liver and the spleen. Primary intestinal lymphomas can be differentiated from secondary lymphomas by the absence of superficial and mediastinal lymphadenopathies on work-up, if there is no evidence of disease on both peripheral blood smears and bone marrow biopsies, if the disease is localized to a specific small bowel segment and regional draining mesenteric lymph nodes only, and if there is no evidence of hepatic or splenic involvement (except via direct extension from the primary tumor).

Variants

Mucosal-Associated Lymphoid Tissue Lymphoma

Marginal zone B-cell lymphomas (MALT) are the most common primary gastrointestinal lymphomas. They occur more commonly in the stomach, followed by the small bowel (most commonly, the ileocecal region), the colon, and the esophagus. MALTs occur predominately in men and peak in the 6th decade of life. They present as unifocal, ulcerated overhanging lesions, characterized by cellular heterogeneity and bearing close resemblance to normal gut-associated lymphoid tissue (Peyer patch and mesenteric nodal tissue). Nonneoplastic reactive lymphoid follicles surrounded by centrocytes are characteristic, with the neoplastic focus occupying the marginal zone or intrafollicular region. These tumor cells express elevated levels of immunoglobulin (Ig)M and B-cell–associated antigens (including CD19, CD20, CD22, and CD79a). Most tumors are CD5, CD10, and CD23 negative and CD43 variable. MALT lymphomas are not associated with *Bcl-2* or *Bcl-1* rearrangements.

MALT lymphomas may be associated with chronic inflammatory conditions, including autoimmune disorders such as Sjögren syndrome and Hashimoto thyroiditis. The majority of patients present with stage I or II disease. Therapy is multimodal and includes surgical resection and/or chemoradiation therapy, with small bowel lymphomas having a better prognosis than gastric tumors. Some studies suggest that MALT tumors may be antigen driven, especially by *Campylobacter jejuni* and *Helicobacter pylori*. Regression has been reported with eradication of *H. pylori* infection using antibiotics.[194]

Diffuse Large B-Cell Lymphoma

The second most common small bowel lymphoma is diffuse large B-cell lymphoma (DLBCL), also known as large cell immunoblastic, large-cleaved follicular center cell, centroblastic D immunoblastic cell, or diffuse mixed lymphocytic and histiocytic cell. DLBCL occurs more frequently in men, with a median age of 54 to 61 years, and primarily involves the ileocecal region. DLBCLs present as unifocal ulcerated lesions, composed of diffuse large B cells with large nuclei that are twice the size of a normal lympho-

cyte. Tumor cells are CD19, CD20, CD22, and CD79a positive. *Bcl-2 gene* mutation is present in approximately 30% of the cases. Immunosuppression is an important risk factor for DLBCL. Surgery is the mainstay of treatment for localized disease, followed by adjuvant radiation or chemotherapy.[195] Overall 5-year survival is between 50% and 70% with multimodality therapy.[196]

Burkitt Lymphoma

Burkitt lymphoma of the small bowel accounts for <5% of all small bowel lymphomas. It can occur endemically or sporadically and is highly aggressive. The endemic subtype is seen predominantly in Central Africa; it affects children with a peak incidence at 8 years of age, is associated with Epstein-Barr virus (EBV) infection, and involves the GI tract in only 20% to 30% of cases. Conversely, sporadic Burkitt lymphoma occurs more commonly in Westernized countries, affects a broader age group, is not associated with EBV infections and commonly affects the GI tract (ileocecal region). Clinically, they can mimic appendicitis by presenting as large masses. Microscopically, cells are monomorphic medium-sized cells with round nuclei and an abundant basophilic cytoplasm. It is a rapidly growing tumor with short doubling time; the high rate of proliferation gives it a *starry sky* pattern due to the numerous macrophages that have ingested apoptotic tumor cells. Treatment primarily consists of chemotherapy, usually vincristine, cyclophosphamide, doxorubicin, and methotrexate.[197]

Mantle Cell Lymphoma

Mantle cell lymphoma (MCL) is a rare primary GI lymphoma that follows either an indolent or very aggressive course. MCL commonly affects men (ratio, 4:1) in their 6th or 7th decades of life and has a predilection for the small bowel and colon. Macroscopically, MCLs appear as multiple, whitish polypoid lesions that share morphologic features with nodal lymphomas. CD5+ B cells are located within the mantle zone that surrounds the germinal centers. Four histologic subtypes have been described: nodular, diffuse, mantle zone, and blastic. The blastic type has the worst prognosis, whereas the nodular and diffuse types have the best prognosis. MCLs have been associated with t(11;14) (q13; q32) chromosomal translocation, causing overexpression of cyclin D1. The vast majority of MCLs present in stage IV disease.

T-Cell Lymphoma

T-cell lymphomas (TCL) of the small bowel are less common than their B-cell counterparts, accounting for approximately 15% of all small bowel lymphomas. TCLs affect men and women equally and most commonly arise in the jejunum or the proximal ileum. TCLs may remain localized; however, dissemination is common. They typically present as large circumferential ulcers, in the absence of large masses, with associated mesenteric lymphadenopathy. As with other types of lymphomas, obstruction and perforation are common presentations. Microscopically, transmural replacement of the intestinal wall by highly pleomorphic lymphoid cells may be seen. A large number of surrounding intraepithelial lymphocytes may also show cellular atypia. Tumor cells stain positive for CD3, CD7, CD8, and CD103 and negative for CD4. Small bowel TCLs are known as EATLs due to their association with long-standing enteropathies, primarily celiac disease. EATL is described in approximately 5% to 10% of all patients with celiac disease, and the relative risk of developing a lymphoma in this setting is 25- to 100-fold higher than normal patients. Prognosis is generally poor, with a 5-year survival rate of 10%.[198]

GASTROINTESTINAL STROMAL TUMORS

GIST tumors arise from the intestinal cells of Cajal and are characterized by the presence of a gain-of-function c-kit (CD117) mutation. The c-kit protein codes for a tyrosine–kinase receptor involved in cellular proliferation, apoptosis, and differentiation.

Epidemiology and Genetics

GISTS are the most common mesenchymal tumor of the small bowel, despite comprising only 0.5% to 1% of all GI tumors. There are between 4,500 to 6,000 GISTs per year in the United States, with the stomach being the most common site.[199–204] Incidence rates are equal in both genders and peak between 50 and 60 years of age. Small bowel GISTs are most commonly found in the jejunum, followed by the ileum, and the duodenum and typically present with pain, intussusception, or bleeding. Approximately 80% to 90% of all GIST tumors contain a c-kit mutation (CD117), whereas the remainder have a mutation in another tyrosine–kinase receptor gene or platelet-derived growth factor (PDGF) receptor alpha. It is now recognized that a vast majority of tumors previously identified as leiomyomas and leiomyosarcomas were actually CD117+ GIST. The molecular discoveries have allowed for the development of the specific c-kit tyrosine–kinase inhibitor imatinib (Gleevec), a drug initially designed to treat chronic myelogenous leukemia.

Prognosis and Behavior

All GISTs have the potential for malignancy, and approximately 50% of resected patients will have disease recurrence within 5 years. Of GISTs, 30% to 50% are clinically malignant. Most GISTs have a c-kit gain-of-function mutation, allowing for the prediction of clinical behavior and recurrence risk stratification.[205–208] Tumors larger than 2 cm have a higher risk of recurrence and metastasis. This risk increases significantly for tumors larger than 3 cm to 5 cm. The mitotic rate has also been studied, and GISTs with five or more mitoses per 50 high-powered field (HPF) have a worse prognosis, whereas mitotic rates higher than 10 per 50 HPF predicts high recurrence and metastatic rates regardless of tumor size or location, with 5-year survival rates ~25%. The tumor site also plays an important role in prognosis, with jejunal and ileal GISTs displaying more malignant behavior compared to duodenal, rectal, or gastric GISTs.

Management

Surgery

R0 surgical resection is the mainstay therapy for all GISTs. Extensive resection of the surrounding uninvolved tissue has not been shown to improve outcomes. A routine lymphadenectomy is not indicated because GISTs rarely metastasize to regional lymph nodes. Intraoperative tumor rupture and spillage has been linked to carcinomatosis, necessitating a meticulous surgical technique. The peritoneum and liver are the main sites of metastasis and recurrence, and both should be inspected during surgical exploration.[209–212]

Adjuvant Therapy

Adjuvant imatinib therapy improves recurrence-free survival after complete surgical resection of localized disease. The ACOSOG Z9001 trial was a randomized phase III double-blinded, placebo-controlled multicenter trial where 713 patients were assigned to receive either 400 mg of imatinib or placebo daily for 1 year after complete resection of a c-kit–positive, 3 cm (or more) GIST. One-year progression-free survival was 98% in the imatinib arm and 83% in the placebo arm.[213]

Similar results were found in the Z9000 trial, a phase II, intergroup trial led by the American College of Surgeons Oncology Group, in which 106 patients who had undergone complete surgical resection of GIST were prescribed imatinib 400 mg per day for 1 year followed by serial radiologic evaluation. At 7.7 years of follow-up, the patients receiving imatinib had 1-, 3-, and 5-year overall survival rates of 99%, 97%, and 83%, respectively,

compared to a 5-year overall survival rate of 35% for historic controls. Progression-free survival for 1, 3, and 5 years was 96%, 60%, and 40%, respectively.[214]

In patients in whom the initial complete surgical resection is not possible, the use of imatinib therapy has resulted in a significant prolongation of survival, with 80% of patients achieving a 5-year overall survival versus 9 months' survival with no therapy.[215] Neoadjuvant imatinib is also effective at reducing large tumor burdens and may facilitate margin-negative, organ-sparing resections.[216,217] Regorafenib is another novel multitargeted kinase inhibitor being used in GIST management that inhibits the Ras/Raf/Mek pathways as well as VEGF receptor 2 (VEGFR2) signaling.[219]

OTHER MESENCHYMAL TUMORS

Leiomyomas and Leiomyosarcomas

Small bowel leiomyomas and leiomyosarcomas arise from the muscularis propria and muscularis mucosa. They have a varied presentation, primarily involving tumor ulceration and bleeding as the tumor enlarges. Because tumor growth is initially localized and primarily extraluminal, obstruction does not occur until very late in the disease course.[223] Leiomyosarcomas stain positive for desmin and actin and are negative for CD117 (c-kit and CD34). Metastasis is via hematologic routes and is mainly to the liver and peritoneum. About one third of patients have metastasis at the time of diagnosis, and prognosis is very poor.[228–231]

Desmoid Tumors

Frequently confused with GISTs, these spindle cell tumors originate from musculoaponeurotic structures throughout the body and are histologically defined by fibroblastic proliferation and the formation of bundles of spindle cells around blood vessels in a dense hypocellular fibrous stroma. Desmoids occur with higher frequency in patients with FAP and Gardner syndrome.[234] Few mitotic figures are seen, and necrosis is usually absent. Desmoids stain for vimentin, smooth muscle actin, and nuclear beta catenin. Although desmoids tumors are benign with no potential for metastasis, they tend to be locally aggressive and recur even after complete resection.[238] Treatment is surgical resection with a wide margin to ensure negative microscopic margins; however, this may be difficult due to the anatomic location and the involvement of vital structures. Other treatment modalities include chemotherapy (methotrexate and vinblastine, doxorubicin), radiation therapy, nonsteroidal anti-inflammatory agents, and antiestrogens (tamoxifen).[235–237]

Inflammatory Fibroid Polyps

These benign lesions are uncommonly seen in the small bowel. They are typically submucosal and consist of a mixture of small granulation tissue–like vessels, spindle cells, and inflammatory cells. They can stain positively for CD34; however, they do not stain for CD117 with the exception of very small areas of stroma within these tumors.[232,233]

Schwannomas

Although relatively rare in the small bowel, schwannomas of the GI tract are often found in the stomach, colon, and esophagus. They are benign lesions, and present as rubbery yellowish trabeculated tumors characterized by lymph node aggregates around their periphery with nuclear palisading Verocay bodies and hyalinized vessels similar to schwannomas found elsewhere in the body. Schwannomas stain strongly for S100 and glial fibrillary acidic protein, but are CD117, CD 34, and smooth muscle actin negative.[224,225]

Inflammatory and Myofibroblastic Tumors

Inflammatory mesenchymal tumors typically present as solid white masses with infiltrative margins. Although their precise etiology is uncertain, several authors have suggested that they are benign reactions to infectious processes, although local recurrence has been reported. These tumors rarely behave in a malignant fashion and are histologically composed of spindle cells admixed with lymphocytes and plasma cells. Unlike GIST, they stain negatively for CD117 and CD 34, but positive for desmin, muscle-specific actin, and cytokeratin.[226,227]

METASTATIC CANCER TO THE SMALL BOWEL

Metastatic tumors to the small intestine are 2.5 times more common than are primary SBCs. Metastatic spread to the small intestine from distant primary sites is more frequent than to any other site in the GI tract. The main routes by which secondary neoplasms reach the small bowel is primary dependent and includes direct extension (for colonic, pancreatic, and gastric cancers), intraperitoneal spread (ovarian cancer), and lympho- or hematogenous embolization (melanoma, and lung and breast cancers).

Epidemiology

Melanoma is the most common cancer to metastasize to the small bowel, with up to 4.4% of all melanoma patients demonstrating small bowel metastases. Malignant melanoma is the primary tumor in 50% to 70% of all small bowel metastases, with the terminal ileum being the most often affected site.[220–223] Primary melanomas of the intestine are extremely rare, with few case reports found in the literature.[239]

Clinically, small bowel metastases can present with obstruction, perforation, intussusception, malabsorption, and/or GI bleeding. Obstruction is commonly seen in association with metastatic lobular breast carcinoma. A wide array of nonspecific symptoms may also be present, including abdominal discomfort, distension, and diarrhea. Typical features of intestinal metastases include intestinal wall thickening, submucosal spread, and ulcers. Melanomas and sarcomas may appear as nodules or polyps. Metastases are typically located deep within the submucosa or the muscularis propria of the small bowel, with little involvement of the mucosa.[221–223]

Intestinal metastases usually represent at a late stage of the disease, during which other sites of hematogenous metastases are also frequently found. However, the prognosis for patients with small bowel metastasis varies widely according to the primary tumor type and patient-specific factors. Metastatic melanomas or renal carcinomas with isolated metastasis to the small bowel may be associated with prolonged survival after resection. Other more common primary tumors that metastasize to the small bowel are uterus, cervix, colon, lung, and breast tumors.

Management

The management of small bowel metastatic disease is defined by the primary tumor of origin. Isolated small bowel metastasis warrants segmental resection to prevent bowel obstruction, to maintain nutrition, or as part of a debulking procedure (e.g., ovarian, appendiceal). Most often, systemic therapy is the modality of choice for advanced/diffuse small bowel involvement. A diffuse disease may rarely warrant debulking or treatment with HIPEC on established protocols.

REFERENCES

1. Zollinger RM Jr. Primary neoplasms of the small intestine. *Am J Surg* 1986;151:654–658.
2. Siegel R, Ma J, Zou Z, et al. Cancer statistics, 2014. *CA Cancer J Clin* 2014;64:9–29.
3. DiSario JA, Burt RW, Vargas H, et al. Small bowel cancer: epidemiological and clinical characteristics from a population-based registry. *Am J Gastroenterol* 1994;89:699–701.
4. Hatzaras I, Palesty JA, Abir F, et al. Small-bowel tumors: epidemiologic and clinical characteristics of 1260 cases from the connecticut tumor registry. *Arch Surg* 2007;142:229–235.
5. Haselkorn T, Whittemore AS, Lilienfeld DE. Incidence of small bowel cancer in the United States and worldwide: geographic, temporal, and racial differences. *Cancer Causes Control* 2005;16:781–787.
6. Jemal A, Siegel R, Ward E, et al. Cancer statistics, 2008. *CA Cancer J Clin* 2008;58:71–96.
7. Talamonti MS, Goetz LH, Rao S, et al. Primary cancers of the small bowel: analysis of prognostic factors and results of surgical management. *Arch Surg* 2002;137:564–570.
8. Chow JS, Chen CC, Ahsan H, et al. A population-based study of the incidence of malignant small bowel tumours: SEER, 1973-1990. *Int J Epidemiol* 1996;25:722–728.
9. Neugut AI, Santos J. The association between cancers of the small and large bowel. *Cancer Epidemiol Biomarkers Prev* 1993;2:551–553.
10. Scelo G, Boffetta P, Anderson A, et al. Associations between small intestine cancer and other primary cancers: an international population-based study. *Int J Cancer* 2006;118:189–196.
11. Schiessling S, Kihm M, Ganschow P, et al. Desmoid tumour biology in patients with familial adenomatous polyposis coli. *Br J Surg* 2013;100:694–703.
12. Ghoshal UC, Sengar V, Srivastava D. Colonic transit study technique and interpretation: can there be uniform globally in different populations with non-uniform colon transit time? *J Neurogastroenterol Motil* 2012;18:227–228.
13. Kim SK. Small intestine transit time in the normal small bowel study. *Am J Roentgenol Radium Ther Nucl Med* 1968;104:522–524.
14. Belchetz LA, Berk T, Bapat BV, et al. Changing causes of mortality in patients with familial adenomatous polyposis. *Dis Colon Rectum* 1996;39:384–387.
15. Bjork J, Akerbrant H, Iselius L, et al. Periampullary adenomas and adenocarcinomas in familial adenomatous polyposis: cumulative risks and APC gene mutations. *Gastroenterology* 2001;121:1127–1135.
16. Burke CA, Beck GJ, Church JM, et al. The natural history of untreated duodenal and ampullary adenomas in patients with familial adenomatous polyposis followed in an endoscopic surveillance program. *Gastrointest Endosc* 1999;49:358–364.
17. Kadmon M, Tandara A, Herfarth C. Duodenal adenomatosis in familial adenomatous polyposis coli. A review of the literature and results from the Heidelberg Polyposis Register. *Int J Colorectal Dis* 2001;16:63–75.
18. Watson P, Lynch HT. Extracolonic cancer in hereditary nonpolyposis colorectal cancer. *Cancer* 1993;71:677–685.
19. Boland CR. Evolution of the nomenclature for the hereditary colorectal cancer syndromes. *Fam Cancer* 2005;4:211–218.
20. Lynch HT, Lynch PM, Lanspa SJ, et al. Review of the Lynch syndrome: history, molecular genetics screening, differential diagnosis, and medicolegal ramifications. *Clin Genet* 2009;76:1–18.
21. Morpurgo E, Vitale GC, Galandiuk S, et al. Clinical characteristics of familial adenomatous polyposis and management of duodenal adenomas. *J Gastrointest Surg* 2004;8:559–564.
22. Nugent KP, Spigelman AD, Phillips RK. Life expectancy after colectomy and ileorectal anastomosis for familial adenomatous polyposis. *Dis Colon Rectum* 1993;36:1059–1062.
23. Schulmann K, Brasch FE, Kunstmann E, et al. HNPCC-associated small bowel cancer: clinical and molecular characteristics. *Gastroenterology* 2005;128:590–599.
24. Park JG, Kim DW, Hong CW, et al. Germ line mutations of mismatch repair genes in hereditary nonpolyposis colorectal cancer patients with small bowel cancer: International Society for Gastrointestinal Hereditary Tumours Collaborative Study. *Clin Cancer Res* 2006;12:3389–3393.
25. Watson P, Lynch HT. Cancer risk in mismatch repair gene mutation carriers. *Fam Cancer* 2001;1:57–60.
26. Koornstra JJ, Kleibeuker JH, Vasen HF. Small-bowel cancer in Lynch syndrome: is it time for surveillance? *Lancet Oncol* 2008;9:901–905.
27. Hearle N, Schumacher V, Menko FH, et al. Frequency and spectrum of cancers in the Peutz-Jeghers syndrome. *Clin Cancer Res* 2006;12:3209–3215.
28. Hemminki A. The molecular basis and clinical aspects of Peutz-Jeghers syndrome. *Cell Mol Life Sci* 1999;55:735–750.
29. Yamaguchi S, Ogata H, Katsumata D, et al. MUTYH-associated colorectal cancer and adenomatous polyposis. *Surg Today* 2014;44:593–600.
30. Al-Tassan N, Chmiel NH, Maynard J, et al. Inherited variants of MYH associated with somatic G:C—>T:A mutations in colorectal tumors. *Nat Genet* 2002;30:227–232.

31. Maisonneuve P, Marshall BC, Knapp EA, et al. Cancer risk in cystic fibrosis: a 20-year nationwide study from the United States. *J Natl Cancer Inst* 2013;105:122–129.

32. Agaimy A, Vassos N, Croner RS. Gastrointestinal manifestations of neurofibromatosis type 1 (Recklinghausen's disease): clinicopathological spectrum with pathogenetic considerations. *Int J Clin Exp Pathol* 2012;5:852–862.

33. von Roon AC, Reese G, Teare J, et al. The risk of cancer in patients with Crohn's disease. *Dis Colon Rectum* 2007;50:839–855.

34. Sigel JE, Petras RE, Lashner BA, et al. Intestinal adenocarcinoma in Crohn's disease: a report of 30 cases with a focus on coexisting dysplasia. *Am J Surg Pathol* 1999;23:651–655.

35. Lashner BA. Risk factors for small bowel cancer in Crohn's disease. *Dig Dis Sci* 1992;37:1179–1184.

36. Pan SY, Morrison H. Epidemiology of cancer of the small intestine. *World J Gastrointest Oncol* 2011;3:33–42.

37. Canavan C, Abrams KR, Mayberry J. Meta-analysis: colorectal and small bowel cancer risk in patients with Crohn's disease. *Aliment Pharmacol Ther* 2006;23:1097–1104.

38. Hemminki K, Li X, Sundquist J, et al. Cancer risks in ulcerative colitis patients. *Int J Cancer* 2008;123:1417–1421.

39. Bernstein CN, Blanchard JF, Kliewer E, et al. Cancer risk in patients with inflammatory bowel disease: a population-based study. *Cancer* 2001;91:854–862.

40. Di Sabatino A, Biagi F, Gobbi PG, et al. How I treat enteropathy-associated T-cell lymphoma. *Blood* 2012;119:2458–2468.

41. Malamut G, Afchain P, Verkarre V, et al. Presentation and long-term follow-up of refractory celiac disease: comparison of type I with type II. *Gastroenterology* 2009;136:81–90.

42. Silano M, Volta U, Mecchia AM, et al. Delayed diagnosis of coeliac disease increases cancer risk. *BMC Gastroenterology* 2007;7:8.

43. Ripley D, Weinerman BH. Increased incidence of second malignancies associated with small bowel adenocarcinoma. *Can J Gastroenterol* 1997;11:65–68.

44. Mohandas KM, Desai DC. Epidemiology of digestive tract cancers in India. V. Large and small bowel. *Indian J Gastroenterol* 1998;18:118–121.

45. Chen CC, Neugut AI, Rotterdam H. Risk factors for adenocarcinomas and malignant carcinoids of the small intestine: preliminary findings. *Cancer Epidemiol Biomarkers Prev* 1994;3:205–207.

46. Boffetta P, Hazelton WD, Chen Y, et al. Body mass, tobacco smoking, alcohol drinking and risk of cancer of the small intestine—a pooled analysis of over 500,000 subjects in the Asia Cohort Consortium. *Ann Oncol* 2012;23:1894–1898.

47. Neugut AI, Jacobson JS, Suh S, et al. The epidemiology of cancer of the small bowel. *Cancer Epidemiol Biomarkers Prev* 1998;7:243–251.

48. Ciresi DL, Scholten DJ. The continuing clinical dilemma of primary tumors of the small intestine. *Am J Surg* 1995;61:698–702.

49. Halfdanarson TR, McWilliams RR, Donohue JH, et al. A single-institution experience with 491 cases of small bowel adenocarcinoma. *Am J Surg* 2010;199:797–803.

50. Dabaja BS, Suki D, Pro B, et al. Adenocarcinoma of the small bowel: presentation, prognostic factors, and outcome of 217 patients. *Cancer* 2004;101:518–526.

51. Talamonti MS, Goetz LH, Rao S, et al. Primary cancers of the small bowel: analysis of prognostic factors and results of surgical management. *Arch Surg* 2002;137:564–570.

52. Rodriguez-Bigas MA, Vasen HF, Lynch HT, et al. Characteristics of small bowel carcinoma in hereditary nonpolyposis colorectal carcinoma. International Collaborative Group on HNPCC. *Cancer* 1998;83:240–244.

53. Giardiello FM, Brensinger JD, Tersmette AC, et al. Very high risk of cancer in familial Peutz-Jeghers syndrome. *Gastroenterology* 2000;119:1447–1453.

54. Negri E, Bosetti C, Vecchia C, et al. Risk factors for adenocarcinoma of the small intestine. *Int J Cancer* 1999;82:171–174.

55. Green PH, Cellier C. Celiac disease. *N Engl J Med* 2007;357:1731–1743.

56. Jess T, Winther KV, Munkholm P, et al. Intestinal and extra-intestinal cancer in Crohn's disease: follow-up of a population-based cohort in Copenhagen County, Denmark. *Aliment Pharmacol Ther* 2004;19:287–293.

57. Bessette JR, Maglinte DD, Kelvin FM, et al. Primary malignant tumors in the small bowel: a comparison of the small-bowel enema and conventional follow-through examination. *AJR Am J Roentgenol* 1989;153:741–744.

58. Pilleul F, Penigaud M, Milot L, et al. Possible small-bowel neoplasms: contrast-enhanced and water-enhanced multidetector CT enteroclysis. *Radiology* 2006;241:796–801.

59. Van Weyenberg SJ, Meijerink MR, Jacobs MA, et al. MR enteroclysis in the diagnosis of small-bowel neoplasms. *Radiology* 2010;254:765–773.

60. Minordi LM, Vecchioli A, Mirk P, et al. CT enterography with polyethylene glycol solution vs CT enteroclysis in small bowel disease. *Br J Radiol* 2011;84:112–119.

61. Gore RM, Mehta UK, Newmark GM, et al. Diagnosis and staging of small bowel tumours. *Cancer Imaging* 2006;6:209–212.

62. Balthazar EJ, Noordhoorn M, Megibow AJ, et al. CT of small-bowel lymphoma in immunocompetent patients and patients with AIDS: comparison of findings. *AJR Am J Roentgenol* 1997;168:675–680.

63. Levy AD, Remotti HE, Thompson WM, et al. Gastrointestinal stromal tumors: radiologic features with pathologic correlation. *Radiographics* 2003;23:283–304.

64. Burkill GJ, Badran M, Al-Muderis O, et al. Malignant gastrointestinal stromal tumor: distribution, imaging features, and pattern of metastatic spread. *Radiology* 2003;226:527–532.

65. Hong X, Choi H, Chusilp C, et al. Gastrointestinal stromal tumor: role of CT in diagnosis and in response evaluation and surveillance after treatment with imatinib. *Radiographics* 2006;26:481–495.

66. Albert JG, Martiny F, Krummenerl A, et al. Diagnosis of small bowel Crohn's disease: a prospective comparison of capsule endoscopy with magnetic resonance imaging and fluoro- scopic enteroclysis. *Gut* 2005;54:1721–1727.

67. Masselli G, Gualdi G. MR Imaging of small bowel. *Radiology* 2012;264:333–348.

68. Albert JG, Martiny F, Krummenerl A, et al. Diagnosis of small bowel Crohn's disease: a prospective comparison of capsule endoscopy with magnetic resonance imaging and fluoroscopic enteroclysis. *Gut* 2005;54:1721–1727.

69. Van Weyenberg SJ, Van Waesberghe JH, Ell C, et al. Enteroscopy and its relationship to radiological small bowel imaging. *Gastrointest Endosc Clin N Am* 2009;19:389–407.

70. Crusco F, Maselli PA, Pelliccia G, et al. Malignant small bowel neoplasms: spectrum of disease on MR imaging. *Radiol Med* 2010;115:1279–1291.

71. Khan MU, Morse M, Coleman RE. Radioiodinated metaiodobenzylguanidine in the diagnosis and therapy of carcinoid tumors. *Q J Nucl Med Mol Imaging* 2008;52:441–454

72. Cronin CG, Swords R, Truong MT, et al. Clinical utility of PET/CT in lymphoma. *AJR Am J Roentgenol* 2010;194:W91–W103.

73. Ullerich H, Franzius CH, Domagk D, et al. 18F-Fluorodeoxyglucose PET in a patient with primary small bowel lymphoma: the only sensitive method of imaging. *Am J Gastroenterol* 2001;96:2497–2499.

74. Cronin CG, Scott J, McDermott R, et al. Utility of PET/CT in the evaluation of small bowel pathology. *Br J Radiol* 2012;85:1211–1221.

75. Mensink PB, Haringsma J, Kucharzik T, et al. Complications of double balloon enteroscopy: a multicenter survey. *Endoscopy* 2007;39:613–615.

76. Kita H, Yamamoto H, Yano T, et al. Double balloon endoscopy in two hundred fifty cases for the diagnosis and treatment of small intestinal disorders. *Inflammopharmacology* 2007;15:74–77.

77. Zhong J, Ma T, Zhang C, et al. A retrospective study of the application on double-balloon enteroscopy in 378 patients with suspected small-bowel diseases. *Endoscopy* 2007;39:208–215.

78. Yamamoto H, Sekine Y, Sato Y, et al. Total enteroscopy with a nonsurgical steerable double-balloon method. *Gastrointest Endosc* 2001;53:216–220.

79. May A, Nachbar L, Wardak A, et al. Double-balloon enteroscopy: preliminary experience in patients with obscure gastrointestinal bleeding or chronic abdominal pain. *Endoscopy* 2003;35:985–991.

80. Cazzato IA, Cammarota G, Nista EC, et al. Diagnostic and therapeutic impact of double-balloon enteroscopy (DBE) in a series of 100 patients with suspected small bowel diseases. *Dig Liver Dis* 2007;39:483–487.

81. May A, Nachbar L, Pohl J, et al. Endoscopic interventions in the small bowel using double balloon enteroscopy: feasibility and limitations. *Am J Gastroenterol* 2007;102:527–535.

82. Suzuki T, Matsushima M, Okita I, et al. Clinical utility of double-balloon enteroscopy for small intestinal bleeding. *Dig Dis Sci* 2007;52:1914–1918.

83. Imaoka H, Higaki N, Kumagi T, et al. Characteristics of small bowel tumors detected by double balloon endoscopy. *Dig Dis Sci* 2011;556:2366–2371.

84. Liao Z, Gao R, Xu C, et al. Indications and detection, completion, and retention rates of small-bowel endoscopy: a systematic review. *Gastrointest Endosc* 2009;71:280–286.

85. Bailey AA, Debinski HS, Appleyard MN, et al. Diagnosis and outcome of small bowel tumors found by capsule endoscopy: a three-center Australian experience. *Am J Gastroenterol* 2006;101:2237–2243.

86. Schwartz GD, Barkin JS. Small-bowel tumors detected by wireless capsule endoscopy. *Dig Dis Sci* 2007;52:1026–1030.

87. Bailey AA, Debinski HS, Appleyard MN, et al. Diagnosis and outcome of small bowel tumors found by capsule endoscopy: a three-center Australian experience. *Am J Gastroenterol* 2006;101:2237–2243.

88. Lewis BS, Eisen GM, Friedman S. A pooled analysis to evaluate results of capsule endoscopy trials. *Endoscopy* 2005;37:960–965.

89. Lewis BS, Eisen GM, Freidman S. A pooled analysis to evaluate to evaluate results of capsule endoscopy trials. *Endoscopy* 2005;37:960–965.

90. DeLeusse A, Vahedi K, Jian R, et al. Capsule endoscopy or push enteroscopy for first-line exploration of obscure gastrointestinal bleeding? *Gastroenterology* 2007;132:855–862.

91. Morgan D, Upchurch B, Chiorean M, et al. Spiral enteroscopy: prospective US multicenter study in patients with small bowel disorders. *Gastrointest Endosc* 2010;72:992–998.

92. Triester SL, Leighton JA, Leontiadias GI, et al. A meta-analysis of yield of the yield of capsule endoscopy compared to other diagnostic modalities in patients with obscure gastrointestinal bleeding. *Am J Gastroenterol* 2005;100:2407–2418.

93. Akerman PA, Agrawal D, Cantero D, et al. Spiral enteroscopy with the new DSB overtube: a novel technique for deep peroral small-bowel intubation. *Endoscopy* 2008;40:974–978.

94. Bilimoria KY, Bentrem DJ, Wayne DJ, et al. Small bowel cancer in United States: changes in epidemiology, treatment and survival over the last 20 years. *Ann Surg* 2009;249:63–71.

95. American Cancer Society. Small Intestine Cancer. http://www.cancer.org/acs/groups/cid/documents/webcontent/003140-pdf.pdf. Accessed December 13, 2013.

96. Zouhairi ME, Venner A, Charabaty A, et al. Small bowel adenocarcinoma. *Curr Treat Options Oncol* 2008;9:388–399.

97. Pan SY, Morrison H. Epidemiology of cancer of the small intestine. *World J Gastrointest Oncol* 2011;3:33–42.

CANCERS OF THE GASTROINTESTINAL TRACT

98. Raghav K, Overman MJ. Small bowel adenocarcinomas-existing evidence and evolving paradigms. *Nat Rev Clin Oncol* 2013;10:534–544.

99. Sellner F. Investigations on the significance of the adenoma carcinoma sequence in the small bowel. *Cancer* 1990;66:702–715.

100. Haan JC, Buffart TE, Eijk PP, et al. Small bowel adenocarcinoma copy number profiles are more closely related to colorectal cancer than to gastric cancers. *Ann Oncol* 2012;23:367–374.

101. Chan OT, Chen ZM, Chung F, et al. Lack of HER2 overexpression and amplification in small intestinal adenocarcinoma. *Am J Clin Pathol* 2010;134:880–885.

102. Overman MJ, Hu CY, Kopetz S, et al. A population-based comparison of adenocarcinoma of large and small intestine: insights into a rare disease. *Ann Surg Oncol* 2012;19:1439–1445.

103. Jess T, Winther KV, Binder V, et al. Intestinal and extraintestinal cancer in Crohn's disease: follow-up of a population-based cohort in Copenhagen county, Denmark. *Ailment Pharmacol Ther* 2004;19:287–293.

104. Jess T, Gamborg M, Matzen P, et al. Increased risk of intestinal cancer in Crohn's disease: a meta-analysis of a population based cohort. *Am J Gastroentrol* 2005;100:2724–2729.

105. Green PH, Fleischauer AT, Bhagat G, et al. Risk of malignancy in patients with Celiac disease. *Am J Med* 2003;115:191–195.

106. Lee HJ, Lee OJ, Jang KT, et al. Combined loss of E-cadherin and aberrant β-catenin protein expression correlates with poor prognosis for small intestinal adenocarcinomas. *Am J Clin Pathol* 2013;139:167–176.

107. Murata M, Iwao K, Miyoshi Y, et al. Molecular and biological analysis of carcinoma of small intestine: beta-catenin gene mutation by interstitial deletion involving exon 3 and replication error phenotype. *Am J Gastroentrol* 2000;95:1576–1580.

108. Breuhahan K, Singh S, Blaker H. Large scale N-terminal deletions but not point mutations stabilize beta-catenin in small bowel carcinomas, suggesting divergent molecular pathways of small and large intestinal carcinogenesis. *J Pathol* 2008;215:300–307.

109. Ilyas M, Tomlinson IP, Bodmer WF. Beta-catenin mutations in the cell lines established from human colorectal cancers. *Proc Natl Acad Sci U S A* 1997;94:10330–10334.

110. Bläker H, von Herbay A, Penzel R, et al. Genetics of adenocarcinoma of small intestine: frequent deletions at chromosome 18q and mutations of SMAD4 gene. *Oncogene* 2002;21:158–164.

111. Bläker H, Aulmann S, Helmchen B, et al. Loss of SMAD4 function in small intestinal adenocarcinoma: comparison of genetic and immunohistochemical findings. *Pathol Res Pract* 2004;200:1–7.

112. Rashid A, Hamilton SR. Genetic alterations in sporadic and Crohn's associated adenocarcinomas of small intestine. *Gastroenterology* 1997;113:127–135.

113. Nishiyama K, Yao T, Yonemasu H, et al. Overexpression of p53 protein and point mutation of K-ras genes in primary carcinoma of small intestine. *Oncol Rep* 2002;9:293–300.

114. Boland CR, Thibodeau SN, Hamilton SR, et al. A National Cancer Institute Workshop on Microsatellite instability for cancer detection and familial predisposition: development of international criteria for the determination of microsatellite instability in colorectal cancer. *Cancer Res* 1998;58:5248–5257.

115. Overman MJ, Pozadzides J, Kopetz S, et al. Immunophenotype and molecular characterization of adenocarcinoma of small intestine. *Br J Cancer* 2010;102:144–150.

116. Plank M, Ericson K, Piotrowska Z, et al. Microsatellite instability and expression of MLH1 and MSH2 in carcinomas of small intestine. *Cancer* 2003;97:1551–1557.

117. Diosdado B, Buffart TW, Watkins R, et al. High-resolution array comparative genomic hybridization in sporadic and celiac disease-related small bowel adenocarcinomas. *Clin Cancer Res* 2010;16:1391–1401.

118. Fu T, Pappou EP, Guzzetta AA, et al. CpG island methylator phenotype-positive tumours in the absence of MLH1 methylation constitute a distinct subset of duodenal adenocarcinomas and are associated with poor prognosis. *Clin Cancer Res* 2012;18:4743–4752.

119. Potter DD, Murray JA, Donohue JH, et al. The role of defective mismatch repair in small bowel adenocarcinoma in celiac disease. *Cancer Res* 2004;64:7073–7077.

120. Howe JR, Karnell LH, Menck HR, et al. American College of Surgeons Commission on Cancer and the American Cancer Society. Adenocarcinoma of the small bowel: review of national cancer database 1985-1995. *Cancer* 1999;86:2693–2706.

121. Overman MJ, Hu CY, Wolff RA, et al. Prognostic value of lymph node evaluation in small bowel adenocarcinoma: analysis of the surveillance, epidemiology, and end results database. *Cancer* 2010;116:5374–5382.

122. Barnes G Jr, Romero L, Hess KR, et al. Primary adenocarcinoma of the duodenum: management and survival in 67 patients. *Ann Surg Oncol* 1994;1:73–78.

123. Bakaeen FG, Murr MM, Sarr MG, et al. What prognostic factors are important in duodenal adenocarcinoma? *Arch Surg* 2000;135:635–641.

124. Kaklamanos IG, Bathe OF, Franceschi D, et al. Extent of resection in the management of duodenal adenocarcinoma. *Am J Surg* 2000;179:37–41.

125. Joesting DR, Beart RW Jr, van Heerden JA, et al. Improving survival in adenocarcinoma of the duodenum. *Am J Surg* 1981;141:228–231.

126. Poultsides GA, Huang LC, Camerson JL, et al. Duodenal adenocarcinoma: clinicopathologic analysis and implications for treatment. *Ann Surg Oncol* 2012;19:1928–1935.

127. Lepage C, Bouvier AM, Manfredi S, et al. Incidence and management of primary malignant small bowel cancers: a well-defined French population study. *Am J Gastroenterol* 2006;101:2826–2832.

128. Sohn TA, Lillemoe KD, Cameron JL, et al. Adenocarcinoma of the duodenum: factors influencing long-term survival. *J Gastrointest Surg* 1998;2:79–87.

129. Overman MJ, Kopetz S, Lin E, et al. Is there a role for adjuvant therapy in resected adenocarcinoma of the small intestine. *Acta Oncol* 2010;49:474–479.

130. Kelsey CR, Nelson JW, Willett CG, et al. Duodenal adenocarcinoma: patterns of failure after resection and the role of chemoradiotherapy. *Int J Radiat Oncol Biol Phys* 2007;69:1436–1441.

131. Fishman PN, Pond GR, Moore MJ, et al. Natural history and chemotherapy effectiveness for advanced adenocarcinoma of the small bowel: a retrospective review of 113 cases. *Am J Clin Oncol* 2006;29:225–231.

132. Koo DH, Yun SC, Hong YS, et al. Systemic chemotherapy for treatment of advanced small bowel adenocarcinoma with prognostic factor analysis: retrospective study. *BMC Cancer* 2011;11:205.

133. Czaykowski P, Hui D. Chemotherapy in small bowel adenocarcinoma: 10-year experience of the British Columbia Cancer Agency. *Clin Oncol (R Coll Radiol)* 2007;19:143–149.

134. Ouriel K, Adams JT. Adenocarcinoma of the small intestine. *Am J Surg* 1984;147:66–71.

135. Locher C, Malka D, Boige V, et al. Combination chemotherapy in advanced small bowel adenocarcinoma. *Oncology* 2005;69:290–294.

136. Zaanan A, Gauthier M, Malka D, et al. Second-line chemotherapy with fluorouracil, leucovorin, and irinotecan (FOLFIRI regimen) in patients with advanced small bowel adenocarcinoma after failure of first-line platinum-based chemotherapy: a multicentre AGEO study. *Cancer* 2011;117:1422–1428.

137. Jeurnink SM, van Eijck CH, Steyerberg EW, et al. Stent versus gastrojejunostomy for the palliation of gastric outlet obstruction: a systematic review. *BMC Gastroenterol* 2007;7:18.

138. Ercolani G, Grazi GL, Ravaioli M, et al. The role of liver resections for noncolorectal, nonneuroendocrine metastases: experience with 142 observed cases. *Ann Surg Oncol* 2005;12:459–466.

139. Adam R, Chiche L, Aloia T, et al. Hepatic resection for noncolorectal nonendocrine liver metastases: analysis of 1,452 patients and development of a prognostic model. *Ann Surg* 2006;244:524–535.

140. Yankai S, Stewart J, Levine E. Cytoreductive surgery and hyperthermic intraperitoneal chemotherapy for peritoneal carcinomatosis from small bowel adenocarcinoma. *Am Surg* 2013;79:644–648.

141. Bessette JR, Maglinte DD, Kelvin FM, et al. Primary malignant tumors in the small bowel: a comparison of the small-bowel enema and conventional follow-through examination. *AJR Am J Roentgenol* 1989;153:741–744.

142. Gourtsoyiannis N, Makó E. Imaging of primary small intestinal tumours by enteroclysis and CT with pathological correlation. *Eur Radiol* 1997;7:625–642.

143. Buckley JA, Fishman EK. CT evaluation of small bowel neoplasms: spectrum of disease. *Radiographics* 1998;18:379–392.

144. Buckley JA, Siegelman SS, Jones B, et al. The accuracy of CT staging of small bowel adenocarcinoma: CT/pathologic correlation. *J Comput Assist Tomogr* 1997;21:986–991.

145. Buckley JA, Jones B, Fishman EK. Small bowel cancer. Imaging features and staging. *Radiol Clin North Am* 1997;35:381–402.

146. Laurent F, Drouillard J, Lecesne R, et al. CT of small-bowel neoplasms. *Semin Ultrasound CT MR* 1995;16:102–111.

147. Maglinte DT, Reyes BL. Small bowel cancer. Radiologic diagnosis. *Radiol Clin North Am* 1997;35:361–380.

148. Horton KM, Juluru K, Montgomery E, et al. Computed tomography imaging of gastrointestinal stromal tumors with pathology correlation. *J Comput Assist Tomogr* 2004;28:811–817.

149. Horton KM, Fishman EK. The current status of multidetector row CT and three-dimensional imaging of the small bowel. *Radiol Clin North Am* 2003;41:199–212.

150. Dudiak KM, Johnson CD, Stephens DH. Primary tumors of the small intestine: CT evaluation. *AJR Am J Roentgenol* 1989;152:995–998.

151. Horton KM, Fishman EK. Multidetector-row computed tomography and 3-dimensional computed tomography imaging of small bowel neoplasms: current concept in diagnosis. *J Comput Assist Tomogr* 2004;28:106–116.

152. Ramachandran I, Sinha R, Rajesh A, et al. Multidetector row CT of small bowel tumours. *Clin Radiol* 2007;62(7):607.

153. Maglinte DD, Sandrasegaran K, Lappas JC. CT enteroclysis: techniques and applications. *Radiol Clin North Am* 2007;45:289–301.

154. Pilleul F, Penigaud M, Milot L, et al. Possible small-bowel neoplasms: contrast-enhanced and water-enhanced multidetector CT enteroclysis. *Radiology* 2006;241:796–801.

155. Bender GN, Timmons JH, Williard WC, et al. Computed tomographic enteroclysis: one methodology. *Invest Radiol* 1996;31:43–49.

156. Yamamoto H, Sekine Y, Sato Y, et al. Total enteroscopy with a nonsurgical steerable double-balloon method. *Gastrointest Endosc* 2001;53:216–220.

157. May A, Nachbar L, Wardak A, et al. Double-balloon enteroscopy: preliminary experience in patients with obscure gastrointestinal bleeding or chronic abdominal pain. *Endoscopy* 2003;35:985–991.

158. Mensink PB, Haringsma J, Kucharzik T, et al. Complications of double balloon enteroscopy: a multicenter survey. *Endoscopy* 2007;39:613–615.

159. Kita H, Yamamoto H, Yano T, et al. Double balloon endoscopy in two hundred fifty cases for the diagnosis and treatment of small intestinal disorders. *Inflammopharmacology* 2007;15:74–77.

160. Suzuki T, Matsushima M, Okita I, et al. Clinical utility of double-balloon enteroscopy for small intestinal bleeding. *Dig Dis Sci* 2007;52:1914–1918.

161. Zhong J, Ma T, Zhang C, et al. A retrospective study of the application on double-balloon enteroscopy in 378 patients with suspected small-bowel diseases. *Endoscopy* 2007;39:208–215.

162. Cazzato IA, Cammarota G, Nista EC, et al. Diagnostic and therapeutic impact of double-balloon enteroscopy (DBE) in a series of 100 patients with suspected small bowel diseases. *Dig Liver Dis* 2007;39:483–487.

163. May A, Nachbar L, Pohl J, et al. Endoscopic interventions in the small bowel using double balloon enteroscopy: feasibility and limitations. *Am J Gastroenterol* 2007;102:527–535.

164. Triester SL, Leighton JA, Leontiadis GI, et al. A meta-analysis of the yield of capsule endoscopy compared to other diagnostic modalities in patients with obscure gastrointestinal bleeding. *Am J Gastroenterol* 2005;100: 2407–2418.

165. Liao Z, Gao R, Xu C, et al. Indications and detection, completion, and retention rates of small-bowel endoscopy: a systematic review. *Gastrointest Endosc* 2009;71:280–286.

166. Schwartz GD, Barkin JS. Small-bowel tumors detected by wireless capsule endoscopy. *Dig Dis Sci* 2007;52:1026–1030.

167. Mazzarolo S, Brady P. Small bowel capsule endoscopy: a systematic review. *South Med J* 2007;100:274–280.

168. Modlin IM, Lye KD, Kidd M. A 5-decade analysis of 13,715 carcinoid tumors. *Cancer* 2003;97:934–959.

169. Maggard MA, O'Connell JB, Ko CY. Updated population-based review of carcinoid tumors. *Ann Surg* 2004;240:117–122.

170. Stinner B, Kisker O, Zielke A, et al. Surgical management for carcinoid tumors of small bowel, appendix, colon, and rectum. *World J Surg* 1996;20: 183–188.

171. Akerström G, Makridis C, Johansson H. Abdominal surgery in patients with midgut carcinoid tumors. *Acta Oncol* 1991;30:547–553.

172. Makridis C, Oberg K, Juhlin C, et al. Surgical treatment of mid-gut carcinoid tumors. *World J Surg* 1990;14:377–383.

173. Shebani KO, Souba WW, Finkelstein DM, et al. Prognosis and survival in patients with gastrointestinal tract carcinoid tumors. *Ann Surg* 1999;229: 815–821.

174. Soga J. Early-stage carcinoids of the gastrointestinal tract: an analysis of 1914 reported cases. *Cancer* 2005;103:1587–1595.

175. Soga J. Carcinoids of the small intestine: a statistical evaluation of 1102 cases collected from the literature. *J Exp Clin Cancer Res* 1997;16:353–363.

176. Akerström G, Hellman P. Surgery on neuroendocrine tumours. *Best Pract Res Clin Endocrinol Metab* 2007;21:87–109.

177. Hellman P, Lundstrom T, Ohrvall U, et al. Effect of surgery on the outcome of midgut carcinoid disease with lymph node and liver metastases. *World J Surg* 2002;26:991–997.

178. Givi B, Pommier SJ, Thompson AK, et al. Operative resection of primary carcinoid neoplasms in patients with liver metastases yields significantly better survival. *Surgery* 2006;140:891–897.

179. Söreide JA, van Heerden JA, Thompson GB, et al. Gastrointestinal carcinoid tumors: long-term prognosis for surgically treated patients. *World J Surg* 2000;24:1431–1436.

180. Gronbech JE, Soreide O, Bergan A. The role of resective surgery in the treatment of the carcinoid syndrome. *Scand J Gastroenterol* 1992;27:433–437.

181. McEntee GP, Nagorney DM, Kvols LK. Cytoreductive hepatic surgery for neuroendocrine tumors. *Surgery* 1990;108:1091–1096.

182. Sarmiento JM, Heywood G, Rubin J, et al. Surgical treatment of neuroendocrine metastases to the liver: a plea for resection to increase survival. *J Am Coll Surg* 2003;197:29–37.

183. Sarmiento JM, Que FG. Hepatic surgery for metastases from neuroendocrine tumors. *Surg Oncol Clin North Am* 2003;12:231–242.

184. Osborne DA, Zervos EE, Strosberg J, et al. Improved outcome with cytoreduction versus embolization for symptomatic hepatic metastases of carcinoid and neuroendocrine tumors. *Ann Surg Oncol* 2006;13:572–581.

185. Gupta S, Yao JC, Ahrar K, et al. Hepatic artery embolization and chemoembolization for treatment of patients with metastatic carcinoid tumors: the M.D. Anderson experience. *Cancer J* 2003;9:261–267.

186. Kulke M. Advances in the treatment of neuroendocrine tumors. *Curr Treat Options Oncol* 2005;6:397–409.

187. Tiensuu Janson EM, Ahlström H, Andersson T, et al. Octreotide and interferon alfa: a new combination for the treatment of malignant carcinoid tumours. *Eur J Cancer* 1992;28:1647–1650.

188. Moertel CG, Kvols LK, Rubin J. A study of cyproheptadine in the treatment of metastatic carcinoid tumor and the malignant carcinoid syndrome. *Cancer* 1991;67:33–36.

189. Virgolini I, Patri P, Novotny C, et al. Comparative somatostatin receptor scintigraphy using in-111-DOTA-lanreotide and in-111-DOTA-Tyr3-octreotide versus F-18-FDG-PET for evaluation of somatostatin receptor-mediated radionuclide therapy. *Ann Oncol* 2001;12:S41–S45.

190. Kwekkeboom DJ, Teunissen JJ, Kam BL, et al. Treatment of patients who have endocrine gastroenteropancreatic tumors with radiolabeled somatostatin analogues. *Hematol Oncol Clin North Am* 2007;21:561–573.

191. Yao JC, Hoff PM. Molecular targeted therapy for neuroendocrine tumors. *Hematol Oncol Clin North Am* 2007;21:575–581.

192. Kvols LK, Moertel CG, O'Connell MJ, et al. Treatment of the malignant carcinoid syndrome: evaluation of a long-acting somatostatin analogue. *N Engl J Med* 1986;315:663–666.

193. Kvols LK, Moertel CG, Schutt AJ, et al. Treatment of the malignant carcinoid syndrome with a long acting somatostatin analogue (SMS 201–995): preliminary evidence that more is not better. *Proc Am Soc Clin Oncol* 1987;6:95.

194. Suarez F, Lortholary O, Hermine O, et al. Infection-associated lymphomas derived from marginal zone B cells: a model of antigen-driven lymphoproliferation. *Blood* 2006;107:3034–3044.

195. Fischbach W, Dragosics B, Kolve-Goebeler ME, et al. Primary gastric B-cell lymphoma: results of a prospective multicenter study. The German-Austrian Gastrointestinal Lymphoma Study Group. *Gastroenterology* 2000;119: 1191–1202.

196. Koniaris LG, Drugas G, Katzman PJ, et al. Management of gastrointestinal lymphoma. *J Am Coll Surg* 2003;197:127–141.

197. Blum KA, Lozanski G, Byrd JC. Adult Burkitt leukemia and lymphoma. *Blood* 2004;104:3009–3020.

198. Al-Toma A, Verbeek WH, Hadithi M, et al. Survival in refractory coeliac disease and enteropathy associated T cell lymphoma: retrospective evaluation of single centre experience. *Gut* 2007;56:1373–1378.

199. Miettinen M, Lasota J. Gastrointestinal stromal tumors: review on morphology, molecular pathology, prognosis, and differential diagnosis. *Arch Pathol Lab Med* 2006;130:1466–1478.

200. Blanke C, Eisenberg BL, Heinrich M. Epidemiology of GIST. *Am J Gastroenterol* 2005;100:2366.

201. Perez EA, Livingstone AS, Franceschi D, et al. Current incidence and outcomes of gastrointestinal mesenchymal tumors including gastrointestinal stromal tumors. *J Am Coll Surg* 2006;202:623–629.

202. Nilsson B, Bumming P, Meis-Kindblom JM, et al. Gastrointestinal stromal tumors: the incidence, prevalence, clinical course, and prognostication in the pre-imatinib mesylate era—a population-based study in western Sweden. *Cancer* 2005;103:821–829.

203. Tryggvason G, Kristmundsson T, Orvar K, et al. Clinical study on gastrointestinal stromal tumors (GIST) in Iceland, 1990–2003. *Dig Dis Sci* 2007;52: 2249–2253.

204. Tryggvason G, Gislason HG, Magnusson MK, et al. Gastrointestinal stromal tumors in Iceland, 1990–2003: the Icelandic GIST study, a population-based incidence and pathologic risk stratification study. *Int J Cancer* 2005; 117:289–293.

205. Miettinen M, Lasota J. Gastrointestinal stromal tumors: pathology and prognosis at different sites. *Semin Diagn Pathol* 2006;23:70–83.

206. Miettinen M, Sobin LH, Sarlomo-Rikala M. Immunohistochemical spectrum of GISTs at different sites and their differential diagnosis with a reference to CD117 (KIT). *Mod Pathol* 2000;13:1134–1142.

207. Fletcher CD, Berman JJ, Corless C, et al. Diagnosis of gastrointestinal stromal tumors: a consensus approach. *Hum Pathol* 2002;33:459–465.

208. Fletcher CD, Berman JJ, Corless C, et al. Diagnosis of gastrointestinal stromal tumors: a consensus approach. *Int J Surg Pathol* 2002;10:81–89.

209. Pitsinis V, Khan AZ, Cranshaw I, et al. Single center experience of laparoscopic vs. open resection for gastrointestinal stromal tumors of the stomach. *Hepatogastroenterology* 2007;54:606–608.

210. Feliu X, Besora P, Claveria R, et al. Laparoscopic treatment of gastric tumors. *J Laparoendosc Adv Surg Tech A* 2007;17:147–152.

211. Novitsky YW, Kercher KW, Sing RF, et al. Long-term outcomes of laparoscopic resection of gastric gastrointestinal stromal tumors. *Ann Surg* 2006;243: 738–745.

212. Nguyen SQ, Divino CM, Wang JL, et al. Laparoscopic management of gastrointestinal stromal tumors. *Surg Endosc* 2006;20:713–716.

213. Dematteo RP, Ballman KV, Antonescu CR, et al. Adjuvant imatinib mesylate after resection of localised, primary gastrointestinal stromal tumour: a randomised, double-blind, placebo-controlled trial. *Lancet* 2009;373:1097–1104.

214. DeMatteo RP, Ballman KV, Antonescu CR, et al. Long-term results of adjuvant imatinib mesylate in localized, high-risk, primary gastrointestinal stromal tumor: ACOSOG Z9000 (Alliance) Intergroup phase 2 trial. *Ann Surg* 2013;258:422–429.

215. Blanke CD, Demetri GD, von Mehren M, et al. Long-term results from a randomized phase II trial of standard- versus higher-dose imatinib mesylate for patients with unresectable or metastatic gastrointestinal stromal tumors expressing KIT. *J Clin Oncol* 2008;26:620–625.

216. Hohenberger P, Oladeji O, Licht T, et al. Neoadjuvant imatinib and organ preservation in locally advanced gastrointestinal stromal tumors (GIST). *J Clin Oncol* 2009;27:abst 10550.

217. Cassier PA, Blesius AA, Perol D, et al. Neoadjuvant imatinib in patients with locally advanced GIST in the prospective BFR14 trial. *J Clin Oncol* 2009;27:abst 10551.

218. Yao JC, Shah MH, Ito T, et al. Everolimus for advanced pancreatic neuroendocrine tumors. *N Engl J Med* 2011;364:514–523.

219. Raymond E, Dahan L, Raoul JL, et al. Sunitinib malate for the treatment of pancreatic neuroendocrine tumors. *N Engl J Med* 2011;364:501–513.

220. Demetri GD, Reichardt P, Kang YK, et al. Efficacy and safety of regorafenib for advanced gastrointestinal stromal tumours after failure of imatinib and sunitinib (GRID): an international, multicentre, randomised, placebo-controlled, phase 3 trial. *Lancet* 2013;381:295–302.

221. Bender GN, Maglinte DD, McLarney JH, et al. Malignant melanoma: patterns of metastasis to the small bowel, reliability of imaging studies, and clinical relevance. *Am J Gastroenterol* 2001;96:2392–2400.

CANCERS OF THE GASTROINTESTINAL TRACT

222. Berger A, Cellier C, Daniel C, et al. Small bowel metastases from primary carcinoma of the lung: clinical findings and outcome. *Am J Gastroenterol* 1999;94:1884–1887.

223. Buckley JA, Fishman EK. CT evaluation of small bowel neoplasms: spectrum of disease. *Radiographics* 1998;18:379–392.

224. Eskelinen M, Pasanen P, Kosma VM, Alhava E. Primary malignant schwannoma of the small bowel. *Ann Chir Gynaecol* 1991;81:326–328.

225. Levy AD, Quiles AM, Miettinen M, et al. Gastrointestinal schwannomas: CT features with clinicopathologic correlation. *Am J Roentgenol* 2005;184:797–802.

226. Kovach SJ, Fischer AC, Katzman PJ, et al. Inflammatory myofibroblastic tumors. *J Surg Oncol* 2006;94:385–391.

227. Day DL, Sane S, Dehner LP. Inflammatory pseudotumor of the mesentery and small intestine. *Pediatr Radiol* 1986;16:210–215.

228. Arts R, Bosscha K, Ranschaert E, et al. Small bowel leiomyosarcoma: a case report and literature review. *Turk J Gastroenterol* 2012;23:381–384.

229. Deck KB, Silberman H. Leiomyosarcomas of the small intestine. *Cancer* 1979;44:323–325.

230. Akwari OE, Dozois RR, Weiland LH, et al. Leiomyosarcoma of the small and large bowel. *Cancer* 1978;42:1375–1384.

231. Ashley SW, Wells SA Jr. Tumors of the small intestine. *Semin Oncol* 1988;15:116–128.

232. Shimer GR, Helwig EB. Inflammatory fibroid polyps of the intestine. *Am J Clin Pathol* 1984;81:708–714.

233. Harned RK, Buck JL, Shekitka KM. Inflammatory fibroid polyps of the gastrointestinal tract: radiologic evaluation. *Radiology* 1992;182:863–866.

234. Jones IT, Jagelman DG, Fazio VW, et al. Desmoid tumors in familial polyposis coli. *Ann Surg* 1986;204:94–97.

235. Dickson PV, Pollock R. Surgical management of desmoid tumors. In: Litchman C, ed. *Desmoid Tumors*. Netherlands: Springer; 2012:77–90.

236. Alman B. Desmoid tumors: are they benign or malignant? In: Litchman C, ed. *Desmoid Tumors*. Netherlands: Springer; 2012:195–203.

237. de Camargo VP, Keohan ML, D'Adamo DR, et al. Clinical outcomes of systemic therapy for patients with deep fibromatosis (desmoid tumor). *Cancer* 2010;116:2258–2265.

238. Reitamo JJ, Schelnin TM, Häyry P. The desmoid syndrome: new aspects in the cause, pathogenesis and treatment of the desmoid tumor. *Am J Surg* 1986;151:230–237.

239. Sachs DL, Lowe L, Chang AE, et al. Do primary small intestinal melanomas exist? Report of a case. *J Am Acad Dermatol* 1999;41:1042–1044.

47 Gastrointestinal Stromal Tumor

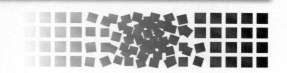

Paolo G. Casali, Angelo Paolo Dei Tos, and Alessandro Gronchi

INTRODUCTION

Gastrointestinal stromal tumors (GIST) are mesenchymal neo-plasms of the gastrointestinal tract, whose tumor cell's normal counterpart is the interstitial cell of Cajal. This serves as a *pacemaker* of gastrointestinal motility, providing an interface between autonomic nerve stimulation and the muscle layer of the gastro-intestinal wall.[1] GISTs are rare cancers, which were defined as a distinct disease in the 1990s, having been classified within smooth muscle neoplasms for decades from their first description in the 1960s.[2,3] Coincidentally, in 2000, they became targetable by new tyrosine-kinase inhibitors (TKI), given the role played by KIT and platelet-derived growth factor receptor alpha (PDGFRA) in their pathogenesis.[4–7] As of today, GISTs serve as an advanced model displaying both potentials and limits of currently available molecularly targeted agents in medical oncology of solid cancers.

From the clinical point of view, surgery is the mainstay treatment when GISTs are localized, and adjuvant therapy is used depending on their risk of relapse. Apparently, adjuvant therapy with TKIs is mainly able to delay relapse, if due to occur, rather than to avoid it. In the advanced disease, TKIs have substantially improved the prognosis of KIT-mutated GISTs and have become standard treatment. They face the major limiting factor of secondary resistance, which affects most patients and is marked by genetic het-erogeneity. A minority of GISTs do not harbor mutations to either KIT or PDGFRA genes and, therefore, are called *wild type* (WT). They are less amenable to available TKIs, although their natural history tends to be less aggressive. Their variegated nature adds to the complexity of GISTs as a whole.

In brief, GISTs are more complex than initially believed, whereas targeted therapy has substantially improved their progno-sis but is challenged by its apparent inability to eradicate the disease (even minimum residual disease), and by the heterogeneity of the secondary resistance it often gives rise to in the advanced setting. Intense translational and clinical research is underway. All this and the rarity of the disease strongly suggest to refer GIST patients to institutions or networks specializing in their treatment and study.

INCIDENCE AND ETIOLOGY

GISTs are rare cancers. Their crude incidence is suggested to be approximately 1.5 out of 100,000 per year (roughly 5,000 new cases in the United States yearly), with the limitations deriving from the fact that only recently were they identified as a clinicopathologic entity.[8,9] However, there are a number of small GISTs that are clini-cally meaningless and generally go undetected. In addition, micro-scopic GISTs (micro-GIST) might be found incidentally in as many as 10% to 25% of stomachs.[10,11] The reasons why the vast majority do not give rise to clinically overt diseases are not known, especially considering the fact that most of them harbor the same mutations to KIT and PDGFRA of fully developed diseases, which implies that alterations of these proto-oncogenes are not solely the pathogenetic drivers of GISTs.[12] Thus, the incidence of histologic GISTs may be much higher than that of clinical cases, which remains low. Preva-lence is low as well, although roughly half of clinical GISTs are cured by surgery, and the median survival of advanced GISTs has improved with the use of TKIs and is likely still improving.

GISTs can occur at any age, with a median occurrence at 60 to 65 years. A small minority of GISTs affect children and adoles-cents: most of them are WT for KIT and PDGFRA and may take place within selected syndromes. In general, GISTs are slightly more incident in males than females. Succinate dehydrogenase (SDH)-deficient WT GISTs typically occur in young females.

No specific causes are known, although the pathogenesis of KIT- and PDGFRA-mutated GISTs has been elucidated in es-sence. There are some predisposing conditions for WT GISTs, which include the Carney triad (marked by GIST, pulmonary chondromas, and extra-adrenal paragangliomas), the hereditary Carney-Stratakis syndrome (marked by GIST and familial para-gangliomas), and type 1 neurofibromatosis (NF-1).[13–15] Hereditary syndromes driven by germ-line mutations to KIT or PDGFRA are very rare but well recognized.[16,17]

ANATOMY AND PATHOLOGY

More than half of GIST cases arise from the stomach, one-fourth from the small bowel, roughly 5% from the rectum, and a small minority from the esophagus.[7] Some GISTs have been labeled as *extragastrointestinal*, apparently arising from the mesentery, omen-tum, and retroperitoneum; however, it remains unknown whether these are lesions detached from their gastrointestinal origin and/or are metastases from an unknown primary tumor.

Morphologically, GISTs can be made up of spindle cells (in more than two-thirds of cases), epithelioid cells, or both (Fig. 47.1 A,B).[18] Epithelioid-cell GISTs are more common in the stomach and include those that are PDGFRA mutated. Aside from this, there are no major clinical implications in the microscopic aspect of lesions. Importantly, there are no pathologic clues to make a distinction between malignant GISTs and others whose clinical behavior is actually benign. Thus, many GISTs behave as benign diseases as a matter of fact, but this cannot be forecast histologi-cally or molecularly. It follows that all GISTs are currently con-sidered malignant neoplasms, although with a highly variable risk of distant relapse, which is negligible in a significant proportion of them. This is the reason why risk classification systems are gener-ally used in the clinic as prognosticators, being based today on a pathologic factor (i.e., the mitotic count) and two clinical variables (tumor size and tumor site).[19–24]

Immunohistochemically, the hallmark of most GISTs is their positivity for KIT (CD117) and DOG-1 (Fig. 47.2 A,B).[25–27] A low proportion of GISTs are CD117 negative, which is typical of PDG-FRA-mutated GISTs, but immunohistochemical status does not reflect the mutational status with regard to KIT and PDGFRA, per se, so that it has no concrete predictive value for sensitivity to TKIs. Thus, CD117 has only a meaning in the pathologic differential diagnosis. Given their morphology, GISTs must be differentiated

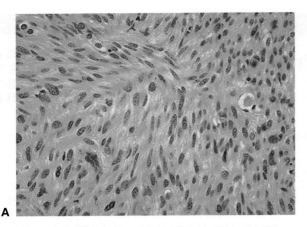
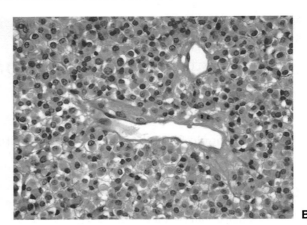

Figure 47.1 (A) Spindle-cell GIST. **(B)** Epithelioid-cell GIST.

from other soft tissue tumors of the gastrointestinal wall, including those of smooth muscle and neural origin and desmoid-type fibromatosis, endocrine tumors, melanocytic tumors, lymphomas, etc. Desmin is rarely positive, as opposed to vimentin and CD34. A negative stain for SDHB identifies the subgroup of SDH-deficient WT GISTs.[28,29]

Molecularly, GIST have become a relatively heterogeneous and complex group of lesions.[30] Gain-of-function mutations of the oncogenes located on chromosome 4 (4q12) coding for the type III receptor tyrosine kinases KIT and PDGFRA can be found in approximately 80% of GISTs.[5,6,31] Pathogenetically, they are the drivers of the disease and, therapeutically, underlie the efficacy of currently used TKIs. They are mutually exclusive and result in the constitutive activation of either KIT or PDGFRA, which normally are autoinhibited, being activated by the binding of their respective ligands (i.e., stem-cell factor [Steel factor] and platelet-derived growth factor A). The activation of the receptor binds two molecules of KIT or PDGFRA (dimerization), giving rise to downstream oncogenic signaling, which for both KIT and PDGFRA involves the RAS/MAPK and the PI3K/AKT/mammalian target of rapamycin (mTOR) pathways (Fig. 47.3). Mutations can be deletions, insertions, and missense mutations. They affect: exon 11 of the KIT oncogene, encoding for the juxtamembrane domain of the KIT receptor, in slightly less than 70% of GISTs; exon 9 of KIT, encoding for the extracellular domain of the receptor, in less than 10%; exon 13 and 17 of KIT, encoding for the intracellular ATP-binding pocket and activation loop domains, respectively, in a small minority of GISTs. Approximately 10% of GIST have mutations homologous to these, which affect PDGFRA (i.e., exon 12, 14, and 18 of the oncogene, with 70% being represented by the

exon 18 D842V mutation). The latter is known for its wide lack of sensitivity to available TKIs, along with a few other rare exon 18 mutations, whereas the deletion of codons 842 to 845 is sensitive. Possibly because of their similarity with different kinds of normal interstitial cell of Cajal, some tumor cell mutations correlate with elective primary sites of origin. In particular, exon 9 mutations of KIT are preferably found in the small bowel, and PDGFRA mutations are found in the stomach.

Approximately 10% to 15% of GISTs are WT for KIT and PDGFRA. They make up a family of tumor subsets with different pathogenetic backgrounds and, to some extent, different natural histories (see Fig. 47.3). Their classification is evolving.[5,6,31] In essence, as of today, one may identify: (1) SDH-deficient GISTs; (2) neurofibromatosis (NF)-1–related GISTs; or (3) others, including those with the BRAF V600E mutation. In fact, half of WT GISTs are marked by alterations involving the SDH complex, which is crucial for the Krebs cycle and mitochondrial respiratory cell function. Immunohistochemically, these GIST are negative to SDHB staining. A group of them includes *pediatric* GISTs and can be associated with the Carney triad.[13] In fact, these GISTs tend to arise in children and young adults of the female sex, are gastric and multifocal, can metastasize to lymph nodes, have a rather indolent evolution. When the Carney triad is fully expressed, it includes GISTs, pulmonary chondromas, and paragangliomas. Given the absence of mutations to the SDH complex, a posttranscriptional defect leading to dysfunctions of the SDH complex may be in place. These GISTs are SDHA positive. On the other hand, a group of SDH-deficient GISTs carries germ-line mutations of the SDHA, SDHB, or SDHC units of the SDH complex[32,33] and may be related to the Carney-Stratakis syndrome.[14] This is marked by

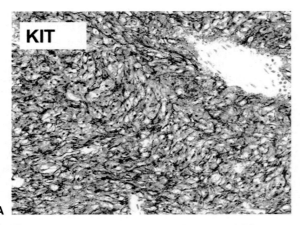
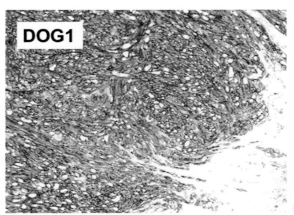

Figure 47.2 Immunostaining for KIT (CD117) and DOG1.

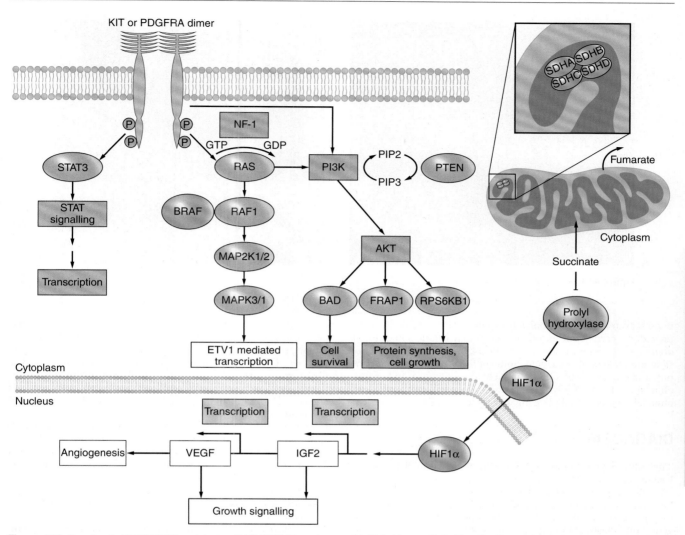

Figure 47.3 Signaling in KIT/PDGFRA-mutated and WT GIST. (From Joensuu H, Hohenberger P, Corless CL. Gastrointestinal stromal tumour. *Lancet* 2013;382:973–983.)

GIST and paragangliomas. Immunohistochemically, GISTs with SDHA mutations are negative to SDHA staining. The median age of these patients is somewhat higher and the female to male predominance is lower, but the course of disease is indolent as well. Then, WT SDHB-positive GISTs can occur in the context of NF-1, and their pathogenetic mechanism is supposed to be the absence of neurofibromin (i.e., the product of the NF-1 gene), which is mutated.[34,35] This may lead to increased activity of the RAS pathway. GISTs related to NF-1 are typically multicentric as well, and have a rather indolent course, but arise from the small bowel. Of course, NF-1 may coexist with a non–NF-1-related GISTs. Finally, the remaining SDHB-positive GISTs are probably a basket of different conditions: some were reported to have the V600E mutation of BRAF[36,37] or, more rarely, HRAS, NRAS, and PIK3 mutations.[5] All this makes the so-called WT GISTs a variegated family of tumors, which can now be identified not only through a negative definition (i.e., by the lack of KIT and PDGFRA mutations), but through immunohistochemical or cytogenetic markers, pointing to specific subsets with different natural histories.

A very rare subset of familial GISTs does exist, being marked by mutations of KIT or PDGFRA affecting the germ line.[16,17] They parallel mutations found in sporadic GISTs and lead to the multicentric and multifocal occurrence of GISTs. The behavior of these GISTs is variable (i.e., it is often indolent but some lesions turn out to become aggressive). Hyperplasia of interstitial cells of Cajal can be found, which may entail altered motility of the gastrointestinal tract. Urticaria pigmentosa and other alterations of skin pigmentation may complete the syndrome.

It is then clear how important genotyping has become for GIST patients. In fact, genotyping has an obvious predictive value, which is crucial for all patients who are candidates for medical therapy, whether in the advanced or in the adjuvant setting. In addition, genotyping has prognostic implications, at least given the peculiar natural history of WT GISTs. Finally, genotyping confirms the pathologic diagnosis in KIT/PDGFRA-mutated GIST, or leads to further pathologic and molecular assessments in WT GISTs. Thus, although there are subsets of GISTs with such a low risk of relapse as not to make them candidates for any medical therapy, a mutational analysis is currently felt as a companion to virtually any pathologic diagnosis of GISTs.

SCREENING

GISTs are rare cancers. Therefore, population-based screening policies are unforeseeable. As for all rare cancers, the clinical aim should be a timely diagnosis in the individual patient with symptoms and/or signs of disease. A difficulty thereof is the anatomical tendency of GIST lesions to grow outwards from the gastrointestinal wall, so that they may go undetected for long

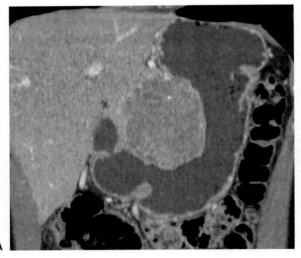
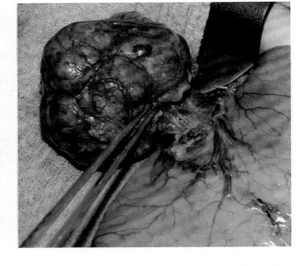

Figure 47.4 GIST growing outward of the gastric wall.

periods even when endoscopically explored. However, endoscopic procedures carried out for other reasons may lead to some risk of *overdiagnosis*, even in such a rare disease, when small gastric lesions are incidentally detected. Some of them will be benign entities, and others will be GISTs unlikely to ever grow as to become clinically relevant. Only a minority of them will turn out to be clinically aggressive GISTs caught in their making.

DIAGNOSIS

The outward growth of many GISTs (Fig. 47.4) within the gastrointestinal wall is one of the reasons why several are diagnosed relatively late, either as major abdominal masses or as causes of gastrointestinal bleeding, hemoperitoneum, perforations (Fig. 47.5). Therefore, as many as one-fourth of GISTs are diagnosed in a clinical emergency, often leading to surgical explorations resulting in the unexpected finding of the disease. One-fourth of GISTs are discovered incidentally during diagnostic assessments (whether an endoscopic procedure, ultrasound, or computed tomography [CT] scan) done for other reasons. The remaining are diagnosed because of symptoms of compression from an abdominal mass, or chronic anemia, fatigue, and the like. Therefore, GISTs should be included in the differential diagnosis of abdominal masses. When their pertinence

to the gastrointestinal wall is clear, the possibility of a GIST may be obvious, with a differential diagnosis mainly against epithelial tumors, small bowel endocrine tumors, lymphomas, paragangliomas, etc. Otherwise, retroperitoneal sarcomas and desmoid-type fibromatosis, germ cell tumors, and lymphomas are the main alternatives. Notably, when this is the clinical presentation, surgery is of choice only for some of the possible alternatives within the clinical differential diagnosis. In addition, preoperative treatments may be resorted to even in some of the surgical indications. On top of this, an intraoperative pathologic differential diagnosis is prohibitive. In principle, therefore, a diagnostic core needle biopsy is suggested by many, allowing pathologic diagnosis and, in the case of GIST, a mutational analysis, prior to any surgical exploration. In the case of gastric or rectal lesions, a biopsy can be carried out by means of endoscopic ultrasound, although, for gastric tumors, the risk of perforation should be factored in depending on the presentation. A CT/ultrasound-guided percutaneous biopsy is the other option, apparently with a negligible risk of dissemination if done at a center of expertise, again factoring in the clinical presentation.[38] There may remain some cases in which the difficulty of an endoscopic or percutaneous biopsy and the easiness of a surgical exploration would suggest the latter. In general, however, a biopsy prior to any therapeutic planning can minimize the number of abdominal masses undergoing futile surgery.

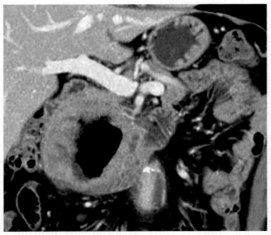
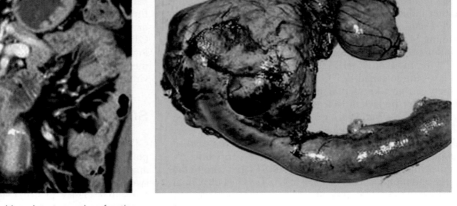

Figure 47.5 Duodenal GIST with an intratumoral perforation.

Follow-ups after potentially eradicating surgery is aimed at picking up relapses at an early stage. Local relapses are infrequent and tend to develop outwards from the gastrointestinal wall: therefore, an endoscopy is generally not used as a routine follow-up procedure. A CT scan is the most sensitive exam to pick up peritoneal and liver metastases and is recommended. It can be replaced by magnetic resonance imaging (MRI), while ultrasound is much less sensitive on the peritoneum. The maximum risk interval averages 2 to 3 years after surgery or, if an adjuvant therapy was done, after its completion. Long-term relapses are unlikely, although they are occasionally observed, especially in GISTs with a low mitotic rates. All this helps drive rational follow-up policies for potentially cured patients, though there is a lack of any empirical evidence of their effectiveness.[39]

STAGING

Conventional stage classification is seldom used.[40] Clinicians mainly distinguish localized from metastatic disease and, if the disease is localized and amenable to complete surgery, quantify the risk of relapse.[20,22,24]

Current risk classification systems are based on the combination of mitotic count, tumor size, and site of origin. Indeed, the mitotic count is the main prognostic factor, proportionally correlating to the risk of relapse. Its downside has turned out to be its possibly low reproducibility rate, but clearly this can be higher if the pathologist is aware of its importance in driving treatment choices. Tumor size is the next prognostic factor. On one side, it singles out very small gastric lesions (<2 cm), which may undergo watchful surveillance if incidentally discovered endoscopically. On the other, it highlights lesions in excess of 5 to 10 cm, which have a worse prognosis. With regard to the primary site, gastric lesions have a better prognosis than small bowel and rectal GISTs. Thus, the combination of these three factors allows one to forecast a risk of relapse by using tools such as the Armed Forces Institute of Pathology (AFIP) risk classification, the Memorial Sloan Kettering Cancer Center (MSKCC) nomogram, or the contour maps. The contour maps have the advantage of treating both the mitotic rate and tumor size as continuous variables as they are, so that the accuracy is increased especially for intermediate-risk cases (Fig. 47.6). Also, reproducibility issues become less crucial by factoring mitotic count as a continuous variable. In addition, contour maps segregate the prognosis

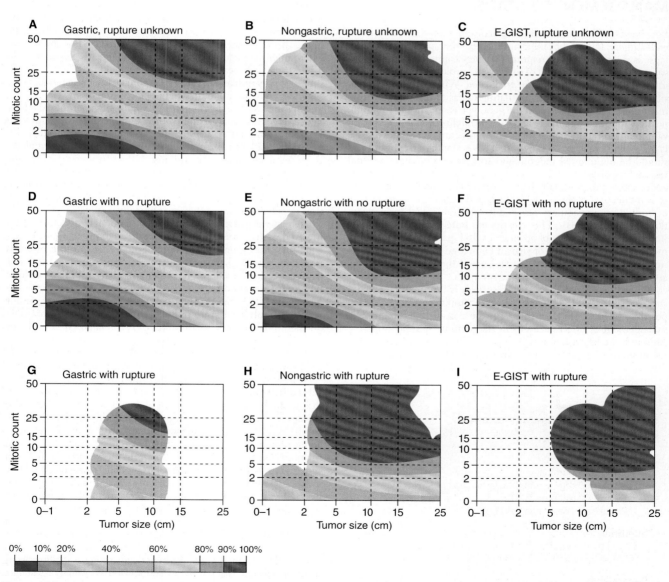

Figure 47.6 Contour prognostic maps in localized GISTs. (From Joensuu H, Vehtari A, Riihimäki J, et al. Risk of gastrointestinal stromal tumour recurrence after surgery: an analysis of pooled population-based cohorts. *Lancet Oncol* 2012;13:265–274.)

CANCERS OF THE GASTROINTESTINAL TRACT

of lesions that underwent tumor rupture, which is a highly adverse prognostic factor in diseases anatomically facing the peritoneum.[41]

The natural history of advanced GISTs is marked by their potential extension to the peritoneum and/or the liver. Thus, a CT scan is the staging procedure of choice to rule out metastatic disease. Lung metastases are rare, with the possible exception of rectal GISTs, although a chest CT scan is generally used to extend a staging workup to lungs and the mediastinum. Bone metastases are possible, but they are usually confined to the very advanced stages of disease, so that the skeleton is not routinely assessed in the lack of symptoms.[42] Other sites of distant metastases are exceedingly rare. Lymph node regional metastases are not typical of GISTs, as for mesenchymal tumors in general, with the remarkable exception of WT GISTs occurring in children and/or within syndromes. In addition, all *syndromic* GISTs may be multifocal and multicentric.[43,44] This is not tantamount to metastatic spread, being rather a marker of their inherent natural history. All these features of the natural history of GISTs drive staging procedures, in addition to the potential for other syndromic correlates, depending on the presentation.

MANAGEMENT BY STAGE

Localized GISTs with no evidence of distant metastases are treated with surgery, followed by adjuvant medical therapy if the risk of relapse is significant. This treatment strategy capitalizes on the consolidated curative potential of surgery and prolongs the relapse-free interval of patients who are not eradicated. When surgery is unfeasible or could be made less mutilating or easier through downsizing, medical therapy is used if the genotype is sensitive to imatinib, possibly followed by surgery and the completion of a medical adjuvant treatment if the risk of relapse is significant. When the disease is metastatic, medical therapy with TKIs is standard treatment and should be maintained indefinitely. Surgery of metastatic residual responding disease can be used when reasonably feasible, but its added value prognostically is unproven. When imatinib fails and/or is ineffective, other available TKIs and judicious use of surgery of limited progression are resorted to (see Table 47.1 for conventionally used agents). This treatment strategy has substantially improved the prognosis of advanced GIST patients by increasing median survival in terms of years if compared to any historical series, with a proportion of patients, limited though it may be, becoming long-term progression-free survivors.

When the disease is localized, surgery is the treatment mainstay. Indeed, all GISTs ≥2 cm in size should be resected when possible, because none of them can be considered *benign*. The management of GISTs <2 cm in size is more questionable.[45–47] Although the low risk of progression of GISTs <2 cm leads to the recommendation of a conservative approach, a reliable mitotic

index cannot be determined by biopsy or fine-needle aspiration (FNA), thus preventing the identification of those at higher risk. Therefore, both observation and resection for GISTs 1 to 2 cm can be considered, and the risks and benefits of one versus the other should be discussed with the patient. The endoscopic resection of small gastric GISTs could be an option in these presentations. Risks of perforation may be low, although the decision is made on a case-by-case basis. Regardless of their size, any small GIST that is symptomatic (e.g., bleeding from erosions through the mucosa) or increases in size on serial follow-up should be resected.

A laparotomic or laparoscopic/laparoscopy-assisted resection of primary GISTs should be performed following standard oncologic principles. On laparotomy/laparoscopy, the abdomen should be thoroughly explored to identify and remove any previously undetected peritoneal metastatic deposits.[48–51] Although primary GISTs may demonstrate inflammatory adhesions to surrounding organs, true invasion is not frequent. The goal of surgery is R0 excision. A macroscopically complete resection with negative or positive microscopic margins (R0 or R1 resection, respectively) is associated with a better prognosis than a macroscopically incomplete excision (R2 excision).[52,53] Available series have not clearly shown that R1 surgery is associated with a definitely higher risk of local failure, so that the decision whether to reexcise a lesion already operated on with microscopically positive margins is doubtful, aside from the fact that sometimes a reexcision may not be technically foreseeable in the gastrointestinal tract. An exception are GIST of the rectum, where microscopically positive margins are clearly associated with a higher risk of local failure.[54] In general, local relapse after R0 surgery is very unlikely in GISTs. Of course, the margins of a big lesion toward the peritoneum will not be covered by any clean tissue, and this may well be the main reason for the high peritoneal relapse rate of large tumors even after complete surgery. Tumor rupture or violation of the tumor capsule during surgery are associated with a very high risk of recurrence, and therefore should be avoided.[41] Some clinicians approach ruptured GISTs as already metastatic, although there may be different kinds of *rupture*, possibly leading to different risk levels. A lymphadenectomy is not routinely required, because lymph nodes are rarely involved (in adult patients) and are thus resected only when they are clinically suspect.

In general, surgery is a wedge or segmental resection of the involved gastric or intestinal tract, with margins that can be less wide than for an adenocarcinoma. Sometimes, a more extensive resection (e.g., total gastrectomy for a large proximal gastric GIST, pancreaticoduodenectomy for a periampullary GIST, or abdominoperineal resection for a low rectal GIST) is needed. In the rare syndromic GIST (either SDH deficient or NF-1 related), tumors are often multifocal and confined either to the stomach (SDH-deficient GIST) or the small bowel (NF-1–related GIST). The extent of surgery should be decided on a case-by-case basis, taking into account the risk of recurrence, the lack of benefit from currently available TKIs, and the actual behavior of the underlying disease.[55]

Adjuvant medical therapy with imatinib was demonstrated to substantially improve relapse-free intervals, although with a trend to lose the benefit in a time span of 1 to 3 years from the end of therapy.[56–58] This was shown through randomized trials that compared 1 and 2 years of adjuvant therapy with imatinib versus no adjuvant therapy, and 3 years versus 1 year of adjuvant therapy with imatinib. As of today, the suggestion from these studies is that adjuvant therapy with TKIs can delay, but probably not avoid, a relapse, if this is due to occur. This correlated with a survival improvement in one trial[57] and with a trend to improvement of a potential surrogate for survival in another,[58] where the surrogate was survival free from changing the original tyrosine kinase inhibitor (TKI)—in practice, survival without secondary resistance. In fact, secondary resistance is the limiting factor of TKIs in the advanced setting, so that an adjuvant therapy will be beneficial as long as it either avoids recurrences or at least prolongs freedom from secondary resistance, but by no means shortens it. Thus, the risk of any detrimental effect was ruled out for adjuvant therapy durations up to 3 years. In this

---

TABLE 47.1

Standard Medical Agents Currently Used in GIST

Imatinib
- 400 mg by mouth daily
- Possibly 800 mg by mouth daily, in case of:
  - Exon 9 KIT-mutated GIST
  - Progression on imatinib 400 mg

Sunitinib
- 50 mg by mouth daily for 4 wks every 6 wks
- 37.5 mg by mouth daily continuously

Regorafenib
- 160 mg by mouth daily for 3 wks every 4 wks

sense, going beyond 3 years would seem logical, given the tendency to lose the benefit after 1 to 3 years from stopping adjuvant therapy, but such a policy should be validated by clinical trials ruling out any adverse effect on secondary resistance. Results from clinical studies on longer durations of adjuvant therapy are therefore expected. Currently, adjuvant therapy is recommended for 3 years and is reserved for patients with a significant risk of relapse, as long as the benefit in absolute terms will be higher as the risk increases, as is the case with all adjuvant therapies. In a sense, the lack of a tangible impact on the long-term relapse rate encourages one to exclude relatively low-risk patients, which is, to some extent, at odds with what is done with adjuvant cytotoxic chemotherapy in some solid cancers. This said, the magnitude of risk that is worth an adjuvant therapy with imatinib for 3 years may well be subject to a shared decision making with the individual patient, and, as a matter of fact, is generally placed above 30% to 50%. Logically, a benefit can be expected for patients whose genotype is potentially sensitive to imatinib.[59] In practice, this leads to the selection of all patients with a KIT-mutated GIST or a PDGFRA-mutated sensitive GIST (with the exception of the D842V exon 18 mutation and the few others which are insensitive in vitro and in vivo to imatinib). Given the benefit shown with the use of a double dose of imatinib (800 mg daily) for advanced GIST patients with an exon 9 KIT-mutated GIST,[60] such a dosage can be selected for them, although there is a lack of any formal demonstration in the adjuvant setting. WT GISTs are much less sensitive to imatinib, and adjuvant studies

are lacking with other TKIs, which may be potentially more active. Even more importantly, the natural history of WT GISTs is often less aggressive. These are the reasons why many clinicians currently do not select WT GISTs patients for any adjuvant treatment.

Given the extensive use of adjuvant therapy with imatinib in the high-risk populations and the activity of the drug, several recent multi-institutional retrospective series have questioned the need for extensive resections such as pancreaticoduodenectomy, abdominal perineal resection, or total/proximal gastrectomy, when tumor downsizing can be likely achieved with a preoperative medical treatment. In practice, preoperative imatinib can shrink gastric, periampullary, or rectal GISTs to such an extent as to allow more limited excisions (wedge gastrectomy, excision of periampullary lesions, transanal/perineal resection of rectal GISTs, respectively), and imatinib can then be continued postoperatively to complete the *adjuvant* treatment (Fig. 47.7). Thus, if extensive surgery is required for complete tumor removal, preoperative imatinib should be considered.[61–64] In addition to this, there are some big abdominal masses that may be felt by the surgeon as implying a significant risk of tumor rupture during surgery, which can be treated with preoperative imatinib. Because downsizing is the clinical end point in these cases, the duration of pre-operative medical therapy is generally 6 to 12 months, which corresponds to the time interval when the maximum degree of tumor shrinkage was shown to occur in studies on advanced GISTs.[65] In addition, mutational status is important in order to select patients likely to respond to imatinib,

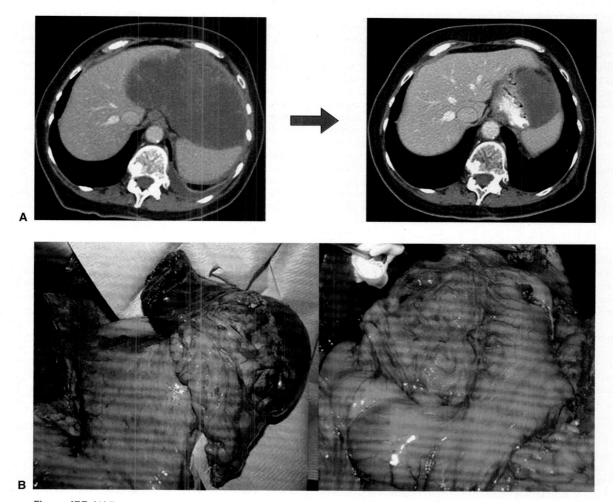

Figure 47.7 (A) Tumor shrinkage of a gastric primary GIST after 12 months of preoperative imatinib, **(B)** allowing for a sleeve gastrectomy plus splenectomy and liver resection with preservation of most of the stomach after resection.

and tumor response should be monitored closely. Positron-emission tomography (PET) scans are a resource, because they can demonstrate tumor responsiveness in a matter of weeks.

Syndromic GISTs can present with multifocal and/or multicentric disease, which may imply delicate surgical decisions. Thus, in WT GISTs, such as those occurring in children and young adults or in NF-1 patients, one should take into account the indolent behavior of many lesions and the possible presence of hyperplasia of the interstitial cells of Cajal on one side, and the possibility that single lesions may be aggressive on the other. Surgery should judiciously factor in all this. In addition, the relative lack of sensitivity of WT GISTs to available TKIs may suggest to resort to surgery more liberally than is currently done with KIT-mutated GISTs.

With regard to the highly rare syndromes of familial GISTs from germ-line mutations of KIT or PDGFRA, treatment is challenging and may involve resorting to surgery and/or TKIs depending on the behavior and extent of clinically relevant lesions.

When the disease is metastatic or locally advanced, medical therapy is the best choice and is currently based on imatinib continued indefinitely.[66–69] However, given the limiting factor of secondary resistance, some clinicians prefer to surgically resect some highly localized first distant relapses, thus delaying the start of imatinib to a subsequent relapse. It is unproven whether this approach may delay progression, its rationale being to delay the onset of time to secondary resistance by delaying the onset of any use of TKIs. Theoretically, the downside may be starting medical therapy with a higher tumor burden, which was shown to be related to a shorter time to secondary resistance to imatinib.

In fact, initial tumor burden is virtually the only prognostic factor in the metastatic GIST patient starting imatinib.[70] On the other hand, although above 80% overall, the probability of response is strictly correlated with the mutational status, which is, therefore, the main predictive factor.[71–73] KIT-mutated GIST are responsive in most cases, including the most frequent genotype, marked by mutations of exon 11. This applies also to patients who underwent adjuvant imatinib and who did not experience tumor relapse during the adjuvant period, so that these patients are currently approached the same way as those who have not been already exposed to imatinib. The standard daily dosage of imatinib is 400 mg. However, there are data derived from retrospective subgroup analyses that suggest progression-free survival is better with doses higher than 400 mg (i.e., 800 mg daily) for exon 9 KIT-mutated GIST patients.[60] Thus, many institutions treat these patients with 800 mg. PDGFRA-mutated GIST patients can be sensitive to imatinib as well, with the remarkable exception of the D842V mutation, which is the most frequent amongst PDGFRA mutations, and a few others. WT GISTs are less sensitive to imatinib, which may, however, be active in some patients. Sunitinib is an alternative option, because it was shown to have some activity in WT GISTs.[74] Generally, the clinical decision in WT GISTs, and of course PDGFRA D842–mutated patients, takes into account the natural history of these subtypes, which is often less aggressive than in KIT-mutated GISTs. Thus, surgical options, including ablations, may be resorted to when the relapse is limited. However, in sensitive genotypes medical therapy is an option even when surgery is feasible, and any decision on surgery is usually delayed to when the tumor response has been established. This allows for the possibility of being certain about a patient's responsiveness to a medical therapy that will need to be prolonged indefinitely because the disease is metastatic.

In fact, a discontinuation trial showed that stopping therapy after 1, 3, or 5 years is followed by progression in a matter of months.[75] It is true that reestablishing therapy generally leads to a new response, but its quality may be inferior to the previous one.[76] In any case, intervals to progression would be remarkably short, and an untenable *stop-and-go* treatment policy would be the result.

Imatinib is generally well tolerated, with fatigue, edema, mild diarrhea, and anemia as frequent complaints, along with less frequent toxicities, such as neutropenia, skin rash, and others.[67–69]

Clinical wisdom needs to be exercised in order to maintain dose intensity vis-à-vis side effects.[77] The number of patients truly intolerant to imatinib should be exceedingly low.

Secondary resistance is the limiting factor of imatinib, with a median time to the event averaging 2 years in the frontline advanced setting. One cannot rule out that current patients, who are generally put on therapy with lower tumor burdens, may show improved progression-free survival intervals over the earliest series. More importantly, the range of time to secondary resistance is wide, with a limited proportion of patients, averaging 10%, who become long-term progression-free survivors. Currently, there are no known prognostic factors for long-term progression-free survivorship, excluding the mutational status, which affects tumor response to imatinib, and tumor burden at the onset of imatinib therapy, which affects the duration of response. The group of long-term progression-free survivors may thus represent either just the "tail" of a curve driven by the stochastic mechanisms of secondary resistance, or the result of specific genomic profiles, still to be elucidated.

In an attempt to download tumor burden, thus potentially prolonging time to secondary resistance, surgery of residual responding disease has been resorted to in many institutions, and its results were retrospectively, but not prospectively, evaluated, with the exception of an underpowered randomized prospective study in patients who had only peritoneal disease.[78–83] These case series analyses showed a better prognosis for patients undergoing surgery, but a selection bias may well explain the results. Prospective trials have not been successful; therefore, the decision whether to surgically excise metastatic lesions responding to imatinib is currently left to a shared decision making with the patient in conditions of uncertainty. Of course, clinical presentations are manifold, and sometimes the easiness of the surgical resection is the main factor leading to the decision, and vice versa. In general, many institutions currently avoid resorting to major surgery for responding metastases. In any case, only patients amenable to complete resection of all lesions should be candidates for this kind of surgery. In this sense, surgery may be less often indicated in peritoneal compared to liver metastases, because the former are frequently underestimated by available imaging modalities and the selection of completely clearable tumors is less feasible. However, the clinician must be aware that imatinib needs to be continued after surgery, even if surgery was complete. In fact, some patients enrolled in the discontinuation trial of imatinib had had a complete excision of their metastatic lesions.[74] In addition, surgery of metastatic GISTs was never proved to be eradicating in the pre-imatinib era.[84]

Progression during therapy with imatinib is often due to secondary resistance, which essentially is marked by the occurrence of new mutations to the same primarily mutated oncogene, or, less frequently, oncogene amplifications or alterations of alternative pathways.[5] It is left to elucidate whether these secondary mutations should be biologically viewed as developing de novo. Secondary mutations entail such consequences as to lower the binding capacity of the KIT or PDGFRA receptor for imatinib and/or to circumvent its inhibiting action by escape mechanisms.[85] It was demonstrated that secondary resistance can be heterogeneous, so that more mutations can be detected in different lesions, or even within the same lesion.[86,87] Of course, this is a major limiting factor for second-line agents targeting KIT or PDGFRA. Secondary mutations in KIT-mutated GISTs are relatively limited in number, affecting exons 13 and 14, which encode the ATP-binding pocket, or exons 17 and 18, which encode the activation loop. Many resistant PDGFRA-mutated GISTs acquire the D842V mutation, which encodes for the activation loop of the receptor.

Clinically, the progression may be *limited* in a substantial proportion of cases. This means that progression is radiologically evident only in one or a few lesions, with the others still progressing. A typical clinical pattern is the *nodule within the nodule* (i.e., a small hyperdensity within a responding hypodense lesion on CT scan).[88] Given the scope of activity of further-line therapies, many clinicians now tend to treat limited progression conservatively from the medical point of view, resorting to selected surgical or ablative procedures to get rid of the progressing component of the disease, while continuing imatinib for the remaining. This might delay the moment when the first TKI is switched to a second-line one. Though this policy is not based on prospective clinical studies, it makes sense in the economy of advanced GISTs following the introduction of TKIs. Clearly this does not apply to *generalized* progressions.

Radiologic progression should be confirmed, taking into account the peculiarities of tumor response patterns in GISTs undergoing TKIs. Furthermore, before attributing progression on frontline imatinib to molecular secondary resistance, one should rule out any lack of patient compliance with therapy, which may often go unnoticed and even be underappreciated by the patient. Another mechanism leading to resistance can lie in changes of the pharmacokinetics of the drug. There is evidence that pharmacokinetics can undergo variations with time, in addition to being variable across individuals.[89] This has led to the evaluation of the importance of maintaining target plasma levels of imatinib.[90] There are limitations to the standardization of such assessments, and available data pointing to a correlation with progression-free survival are retrospective in nature. Thus, at the moment, we lack any convincing formal demonstration that pharmacokinetics is a factor able to personalize medical therapy (i.e., to drive changes in drug dosages in the lack of evident progression). However, available evidence also suggests that it can well be a variable with many orally administered targeted agents. At least, plasma levels may be assessed in the single patient: in case of clinical progression, to rule out that a major pharmacokinetic issue does exist at that stage; in case of unexpected side effects; and in case of comedications potentially able to interfere with the drug metabolism.

In the case of clinical progression with imatinib 400 mg daily, an option widely used is to increase the dose to 800 mg daily. This proved temporarily successful in a limited proportion of patients crossing over to the higher dose in randomized trials that compared 400 mg with 800 mg as frontline therapy for advanced GISTs.[91] When valuing this benefit, one should probably discount patients who had an exon 9 mutation and who started with 400 mg, and possibly some patients failing to comply with therapy, whereas other patients may have benefited due to the correction of pharmacokinetics problems.

Standard second-line therapy is sunitinib, which is a TKI inhibiting KIT and PDGFRA but also displaying antiangiogenic activity by the inhibition of vascular endothelial growth factor receptor (VEGFR)1, 2, and 3. It was shown to be effective at increasing progression-free survival by 5 months in a randomized trial versus placebo in patients failing (or intolerant) to imatinib.[92] Its molecular profile is such as to include activity on exon 9 KIT mutations as well as on secondary mutations of regions coding for the ATP-binding pocket, thus potentially covering mutations which are, respectively, less affected or not affected by imatinib.[93] What limits the potential of molecular prediction in further-line therapies of GISTs is basically the heterogeneity that often underlies secondary resistance, so that the presence of a secondary mutation is unlikely to be alone, although potentially sensitive to available agents. However, the activity of sunitinib against some secondary mutations and probably its antiangiogenic activity underlie its clinical efficacy after failing to imatinib. Its tolerability profile is less favorable, with fatigue and hand–foot syndrome as its main side effects, variable though they may be across patients. Although the clinical trial evaluated a regimen of sunitinib given 50 mg daily for 4 weeks, with a 2-week rest, a continuous regimen with a daily dose of 37.5 mg can be used as well.[94]

Regorafenib, another TKI with activity on KIT and PDGFRA as well as VEGFR1, 2, and 3, and thus with antiangiogenic properties, is standard third-line therapy for advanced GIST patients. In fact, it was shown to be effective as a third-line therapy in patients failing both imatinib and sunitinib, by providing a median advantage of 4 months of progression-free survival over placebo in a randomized clinical trial.[95] Its tolerability profile is close to sunitinib,

with hand–foot syndrome, hypertension, fatigue, and diarrhea as main side effects.[96]

An observation made in this trial was the persistence of some activity when therapy was carried on beyond progression.[97] In other words, a subset of patients, although arbitrarily selected by investigators on clinical grounds, went on with therapy beyond their first progression, achieving a second progression-free interval that approximated the previous one. This would suggest that a subset of progressing patients have a disease that might be slowed down by continuing the TKI in spite of the progression. This observation likely applies to all TKIs, at least in selected patients, and is worth testing prospectively by developing criteria to single out those patients who are more likely to benefit. In general, this parallels the clinical feeling that stopping any kind of TKI may accelerate tumor progression, even when resistance to that TKI has been established. Indeed, a criticism that was made to placebo-controlled trials on new TKIs in GIST is the lack of any tyrosine kinase inhibition in the control group, possibly worsening its outcome in comparison to what could happen by continuing the TKI already in use or by rechallenging the disease with a TKI used earlier.

In fact, in anecdotal cases and also in a small randomized clinical trial, it was shown that rechallenging a progressing GIST patient with TKIs used at an earlier stage can be beneficial, at least temporarily.[98] In other words, reestablishing imatinib in patients who underwent the drug as frontline therapy and then switched to others results in a benefit in terms of progression-free survival that is not far from what is achievable with further-line agents. One may speculate that there is a process of reexpansion of tumor clones that were sensitive to imatinib and might have been narrowed by the selective pressure of the drug, as long as resistant clones were emerging.

Following third-line therapy, there is no standard option at the moment, aside from rechallenge, and clearly patients are eligible for clinical studies on new agents. New drugs investigated in currently ongoing trials include other TKIs targeting KIT and PDGFRA; agents targeting downstream pathways (e.g., PI3K/AKT); agents targeting heat shock proteins, given their chaperone function for KIT and PDGFRA; among others. Clearly, agents with a mechanism of action other than imatinib, sunitinib, and regorafenib try to address the limiting factor of the heterogeneous nature of secondary resistance. Combinations of agents with different mechanisms of action are tried as well, although their added toxicity may be prohibitive even when they are reasonably well tolerated as single drugs. Future directions might try to exploit molecular diagnostics such as the *liquid biopsy* (i.e., the assessment of secondary mutations on circulating DNA shed by tumor cells). The sensitivity of this technique for primary and secondary mutations of GISTs has been demonstrated.[99] Thus, it looks promising for the future, to allow a degree of molecular personalization of therapy, whether following secondary resistance or before it establishes clinically, as a means to avoid or delay its occurrence. Combinations or rotations of TKIs might be tested, rationally driven by liquid biopsies. This could exploit the peculiarities of resistance seen with TKIs in GISTs. In fact, the efficacy of treatment beyond progression and of rechallenge suggests that sensitive and resistant clones may fluctuate within the tumor load, depending on the selective pressure they are exposed to. This would be consistent with the model of a *liquid resistance*, which, clinically, could be exploited by employing new strategies as from the upfront approach with TKIs.

A methodologic issue in the medical therapy of GISTs with all TKIs lies in the peculiar patterns displayed by tumor response as compared to those observed with standard cytotoxic chemotherapy of solid cancers and lymphomas.[100,101] These patterns of tumor response are marked by the possible lack of tumor shrinkage in the face of substantial changes in tumor tissue and tumor metabolic activity. Although most observations derive from imatinib in frontline therapy, in essence, they regard all TKIs, the main difference being possibly the weakness of tumor response to further-line therapies, so that some of these aspects may look less clear cut in the further-line therapy setting as opposed to the frontline. Under these patterns of tumor response, first of all, in the presence of symptoms, a subjective response may take place very early. In a matter of days, if not hours, after starting an effective TKI, a symptomatic patient may well feel a clear degree of subjective improvement. As far as imaging is concerned, this is paralleled by metabolic response as assessed through a fludeoxyglucose (FDG)-PET scan.[102] A positive PET scan may turn negative in a few days. Of course, this does not correspond to the disappearance of the tumor lesion, but rather be the consequence of the metabolic *switch off* that the tumor undergoes when an effective TKI targets its cells. The reverse is true as well, so that any stop of therapy rapidly entails a *switch on* of functional imaging. Again, this does not correspond to clinical progression, which would follow only for longer interruptions of therapy. This should be taken into account when assessing functional tumor response, because, for instance, any lack of compliance with therapy in the days the exam is made might affect metabolic response as detected through PET scanning. For example, metabolic switch on was observed by PET scans performed during the 2 weeks off of therapy with sunitinib. In principle, this adds to the feeling that TKIs need to be maintained in order to preserve tumor response, in the context of a *clinically cytostatic* effect. It goes without saying that when a PET scan has become negative, the tumor lesion will not be visible to functional imaging, so that a CT scan, MRI, or ultrasounds need to be used in order to appreciate the evolution of tumor lesions. The radiologic response, as assessed through CT scans and MRI, is marked by tumor shrinkage and/or changes in tumor tissue. Tumor shrinkage may well appear very early, but, in some cases, it is lacking in the early phases of treatment, or even later on, so that tumor lesions look unchanged dimensionally. Sometimes tumor size may even increase. In these cases, however, if a response is in place, the radiologic aspect will show substantial changes to the tumor tissue. On a CT scan, this means a decrease in density of responding lesions, with decreased contrast enhancement. On an MRI, it entails an hypointense signaling on T1-weighted images and hyperintense on T2-weighted images, and decreased contrast enhancement. These changes are substantial in GIST patients undergoing frontline therapy with imatinib, so that recording tumor response is generally unchallenging for the clinician, provided tumor shrinkage is not the only criterion. Signs of nondimensional response may prove less obvious when the tumor response is less clear cut, as with further-line therapy with TKIs. Functional imaging may help, although it is exposed to the same limitations as well if the response is less striking. However, when the response is overt, the main shortfalls of nondimensional tumor response assessments lie in the difficulty to standardize reproducible (i.e., reliable) instruments, as is needed in clinical trials. In this sense, Response Evaluation Criteria in Solid Tumors (RECIST) criteria for tumor response assessment are based on the measurement on one diameter of selected target lesions and, thus, have a good record of reproducibility.[103] However, their *validity* is, by definition, unsatisfactory in the presence of a nondimensional response. Choi criteria were worked out in GISTs to accommodate these patterns of response, by factoring tumor hypodensity on CT scans in addition to a decrease in size.[104] Their validity in predicting progression-free survival was demonstrated and compared favorably with RECIST criteria, while paralleling functional imaging with PET scanning. Then, aside from the need to use easily reproducible instruments in the research setting, for the clinician the message coming from the GIST model is simple, inasmuch as it points to the existence of nondimensional patterns of tumor response, which can be easily highlighted through CT scans and MRI on one side and through functional imaging with PET scan on the other. One should be aware that the meaning of a radiologic response through CT scans or MRI is deeply different from metabolic response assessed through a PET scan. In fact, a PET

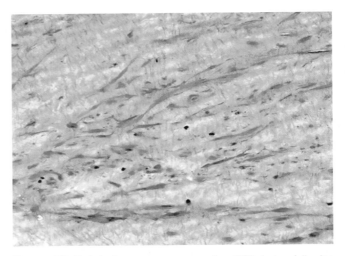

Figure 47.8 Pathologic tumor response of a GIST lesion following therapy with imatinib.

scan measures the biological effect of a TKI on the tumor cells very early, but does not necessarily imply any anatomical change in the tumor. On the contrary, CT scans and MRI detect actual changes in the tumor tissue, which correspond to pathologic signs of tumor response. These were found to take shape in terms of a myxoid degeneration widely affecting responding tumor lesions, with signs of apoptosis (Fig. 47.8). A variable proportion of vital cells may be detected, especially to the periphery of lesions (pointing in principle to the prospects of regrowth in case of discontinuation of the TKI). In this sense, a nondimensional tumor response does not mean just *absence of progression*; indeed, it is all about an actual pathologic response, with major changes to the tumor tissue. Of course, all tumor changes one can see when a tumor response is in place have their counterparts when the tumor progresses. Thus, increased tumor density and contrast enhancement on a CT scan will mark tumor progression, with or without an increase in tumor size. This may well affect just a portion of the tumor lesions, such as its periphery or a small part (as is the case with the *nodule within the nodule*). In brief, the quality of the tumor tissue should be observed, in addition to its size, in order to detect both response and progression in GISTs undergoing a TKI. Whatever the response pattern, whether dimensional or not, a tumor response on a CT scan or MRI says that the tumor is undergoing pathologic changes that clearly correlate with the prognosis. In fact, both dimensional and nondimensional tumor responses have clearly correlated with improved outcome in clinical trials, as opposed to progression. Only secondary resistance, or treatment interruption, will terminate a dimensional or nondimensional tumor response, with radiological signs that, as said, will be dimensional or nondimensional as well.

PALLIATIVE CARE

The natural history of GISTs that are not cured by initial surgery is dominated by abdominal spread involving the liver and the peritoneum. Liver failure as well as intestinal and urinary obstructions are thus the main palliative challenges. This may well carry the need of palliative surgery in selected patients. Extra-abdominal metastases are occasionally seen, mainly to the bone, and can require palliative irradiation. A systemic sign such as fatigue may add to asthenia induced by anemia as well as directly by TKIs. In fact, the existence of three lines of standard medical therapy, the potentials of rechallenge, and the availability of many agents of interest, either within clinical studies or among TKIs developed for other diseases, lead to treating many GIST patients with molecularly targeted therapy even in the very advanced stages of disease. In this sense, the usual palliative challenges of abdominal malignancies meet the new palliative challenges posed by the use of TKIs, which revolutionized the field of the disease.

Indeed, all phases of treatment of GIST are currently a model for the medical oncology of new molecularly targeted agents. The model continues to shed light on their potentials in solid cancers as well as on their current limitations. It also demonstrates how clinical methodology is deeply affected by these agents, not only for medical oncologists, but for all members of the multidisciplinary cancer team, from surgeons to palliative physicians. Interestingly, the model of GISTs shows how a multidisciplinary approach remains crucial in solid cancers, in all phases of disease, and in the era of molecularly targeted therapies, too.

REFERENCES

1. Kindblom L-G, Remotti HE, Aldenborg F, et al. Gastrointestinal pacemaker cell tumor (GIPACT): gastrointestinal stromal tumors show phenotypic characteristics of the interstitial cell of Cajal. *Am J Pathol* 1998;152:1259–1269.
2. Martin JF, Bazin P, Feroldi J, et al. Tumeurs myoides intra-murales de l'estomac. Considérations microscopiques à propos de 6 cas. *Ann Anat Pathol* 1960;5:484–497.
3. Stout AP. Bizarre smooth muscle tumors of the stomach. *Cancer* 1967;15:400–409.
4. Hirota S, Isozaki K, Moriyama Y, et al. Gain of function mutations of c.kit in human gastrointestinal stroma tumors. *Science* 1998;279:577–580.
5. Corless CL. Gastrointestinal stromal tumors: what do we know now? *Mod Pathol* 2014;27:S1–S16.
6. Barnett CM, Corless CL, Heinrich MC. Gastrointestinal stromal tumors: molecular markers and genetic subtypes. *Hematol Oncol Clin North Am* 2013;27:871–888.
7. Joensuu H, Hohenberger P, Corless CL. Gastrointestinal stromal tumour. *Lancet* 2013;382:973–983.
8. Nilsson B, Bumming P, Meis-Kindblom JM, et al. Gastrointestinal stromal tumors: the incidence, prevalence clinical course, and prognostication in the pre-imatinib mesylate era – a populationbased study in western Sweden. *Cancer* 2005;103:821–829.
9. Goettsch WG, Bos SD, Breekveldts-Postma N, et al. Incidence of gastrointestinal stromal tumours is underestimated: result of a nation-wide study. *Eur J Cancer* 2005;41:2868–2872.
10. Agaimy A, Wunsch PH, Hofstaedter F, et al. Minute gastric sclerosing stromal tumors (GIST tumorlet) are common in adults and frequently show c-kit mutations. *Am J Surg Pathol* 2007;31:113–120.
11. Kawanowa K, Sakuma Y, Sakurai S, et al. High incidence of microscopic gastrointestinal stromal tumors in the stomach. *Hum Pathol* 2006;37:1527–1535.
12. Rossi S, Gasparotto D, Toffolatti L, et al. Molecular and clinicopathologic characterization of gastrointestinal stromal tumors (GISTs) of small size. *Am J Surg Pathol* 2010;34:1480–1491.
13. Carney JA. Gastric stromal sarcoma, pulmonary chondroma, and extraadrenal paraganglioma (Carney Triad): natural history, adrenocortical component, and possible familial occurrence. *Mayo Clin Proc* 1999;74:543–552.
14. Stratakis CA, Carney JA. The triad of paragangliomas, gastric stromal tumors and pulmonary chondromas (Carney triad) and the dyad of paragangliomas and gastric stromal sarcomas (Carney–Stratakis syndrome): molecular genetics and clinical implications. *J Intern Med* 2009;266:43–52.
15. Fuller CE, Williams GT. Gastrointestinal manifestations of type 1 neurofibromatosis (von Recklinghausen's disease). *Histopathology* 1991;19:1–11.
16. Li FP, Fletcher JA, Heinrich MC, et al. Familial gastrointestinal stromal tumor syndrome: phenotypic and molecular features in a kindred. *J Clin Oncol* 2005;23:2735–2743.
17. Postow MA, Robson ME. Inherited gastrointestinal stromal tumor syndromes: mutations, clinical features, and therapeutic implications. *Clin Sarcoma Res* 2012;2:16.
18. Miettinen MM, Corless CL, Debiec-Rychter M, et al. Gastrointestinal stromal tumors. In: Fletcher CDM, Bridge JA, Hogendoorn PCW, Mertens F, eds. Lyon, France: IARC; 2013: 164–167.
19. Fletcher CDM, Bermann JJ, Corless C, et al. Diagnosis of gastrointestinal stromal tumor: a consensus approach. *Hum Pathol* 2002;33:459–465.
20. Miettinen M, Lasota J. Gastrointestinal stromal tumors: pathology and prognosis at different sites. *Semin Diagn Pathol* 2006;23:70–83.
21. Joensuu H. Risk stratification of patients diagnosed with gastrointestinal stromal tumors. *Hum Pathol* 2008;39:1411–1419.
22. Gold JS, Gonen M, Gutierrez A, et al. Development and validation of a prgnostic nomongram for recurrence-free survival after complete surgical resection of localized primary gastrointestinal stromal tumour: a retrospective analysis. *Lancet Oncol* 2009;10:1045–1052.
23. Rossi S, Miceli R, Messerini L, et al. Natural history of imatinib-naive GISTs: a retrospective analysis of 929 cases with long-term follow-up and development of a survival nomogram based on mitotic index and size as continuous variables. *Am J Surg Pathol* 2011;35:1646–1656.
24. Joensuu H, Vehtari A, Riihimäki J, et al. Risk of gastrointestinal stromal tumour recurrence after surgery: an analysis of pooled population-based cohorts. *Lancet Oncol* 2012;13:265–274.
25. Sarlomo-Rikala M, Kovatich AJ, Barusevicius A, et al. CD117: a sensitive marker for gastrointestinal stromal tumors that is more specific than CD34. *Mod Pathol* 1998;11:728–734.
26. West RB, Corless CL, Chen X, et al. The novel marker, *DOG1*, is expressed ubiquitously in gastrointestinal stromal tumors irrespective of *KIT* or *PDGFRA* mutational status. *Am J Pathol* 2004;165:107–113.
27. Novelli M, Rossi S, Rodriguez-Justo M, et al. DOG1 and CD117 are the antibodies of choice in the diagnosis of gastrointestinal stromal tumours. *Histopathology* 2010;57:259–270.
28. Doyle LA, Nelson D, Heinrich MC, et al. Loss of succinate dehydrogenase subunit B (SDHB) expression is limited to a distinctive subset of gastric wild-type gastrointestinal stromal tumours: a comprehensive genotype-phenotype correlation study. *Histopathology* 2012;61:801–809.
29. Wagner AJ, Remillard SP, Zhang YX, et al. Loss of expression of SDHA predicts SDHA mutations in gastrointestinal stromal tumors. *Mod Pathol* 2013;26:289–294.
30. Ricci R, Dei Tos AP, Rindi G. GISTogram: a graphic presentation of the growing GIST complexity. *Virchows Arch* 2013;463:481–487.
31. Nannini M, Biasco G, Astolfi A, et al. An overview on molecular biology of KIT/PDGFRA wild type (WT) gastrointestinal stromal tumours (GIST). *J Med Genet* 2013;50:653–661.
32. Janeway KA, Kim SY, Lodish M, et al. Defects in succinate dehydrogenase in gastrointestinal stromal tumors lacking KIT and PDGFRA mutations. *Proc Natl Acad Sci U S A* 2011;108:314–318.
33. Miettinen M, Killian JK, Wang ZF, et al. Immunohistochemical loss of succinate dehydrogenase subunit A (SDHA) in gastrointestinal stromal tumors (GISTs) signals SDHA germline mutation. *Am J Surg Pathol* 2013;37:234–240.
34. Kinoshita K, Hirota S, Isozaki K, et al. Absence of c-kit gene mutations in gastrointestinal stromal tumours from neurofibromatosis type 1 patients. *J Pathol* 2004;202:80–85.
35. Maertens O, Prenen H, Debiec-Rychter M, et al. Molecular pathogenesis of multiple gastrointestinal stromal tumors in NF1 patients. *Hum Mol Genet* 2006;15:1015–1023.
36. Agaram NP, Wong GC, Guo T, et al. Novel V600E BRAF mutations in imatinib-naive and imatinib-resistant gastrointestinal stromal tumors. *Genes Chromosomes Cancer* 2008;47:853–859.
37. Hostein I, Faur N, Primois C, et al. BRAF mutation status in gastrointestinal stromal tumors. *Am J Clin Pathol* 2010;133:141–148.
38. Eriksson M, Reichardt P, Sundby Hall K, et al. Needle biopsy through the abdominal wall for the diagnosis of GIST – Does it pose any risk for tumor cell seeding and recurrence? Presented at: 2012 Connective Tissue Oncology Society Meeting; November 17, 2012; Prague.
39. Plumb AA, Kochhar R, Leahy M, et al. Patterns of recurrence of gastrointestinal stromal tumour (GIST) following complete resection: implications for follow-up. *Clin Radiol* 2013;68:770–775.
40. Edge S, Byrd DR, Compton CC, eds. *AJCC Cancer Staging Manual*. 7th ed. New York: Springer; 2010.
41. Hohenberger P, Ronellenfitsch U, Oladeji O, et al. Pattern of recurrence in patients with ruptured primary gastrointestinal stromal tumour. *Br J Surg* 2010;97:1854–1859.
42. Jati A, Tatlı S, Morgan JA, et al. Imaging features of bone metastases in patients with gastrointestinal stromal tumors. *Diagn Interv Radiol* 2012;18:391–396.
43. Kaemmer DA, Otto J, Lassay L, et al. The Gist of literature on pediatric GIST: review of clinical presentation. *J Pediatr Hematol Oncol* 2009;31:108–112.
44. Kim SY, Janeway K, Pappo A. Pediatric and wild-type gastrointestinal stromal tumor: new therapeutic approaches. *Curr Opin Oncol* 2010;22:347–350.
45. Bruno M, Carucci P, Repici A, et al. The natural history of gastrointestinal subepithelial tumors arising from muscularis propria: an endoscopic ultrasound survey. *J Clin Gastroenterol* 2009;43:821–825.
46. Gill KR, Camellini L, Conigliaro R, et al. The natural history of upper gastrointestinal subepithelial tumors: a multicenter endoscopic ultrasound survey. *J Clin Gastroenterol* 2009;43:723–726.
47. Lim YJ, Son HJ, Lee JS, et al. Clinical course of subepithelial lesions detected on upper gastrointestinal endoscopy. *World J Gastroenterol* 2010;16:439–444.
48. Karakousis GC, Singer S, Zheng J, et al. Laparoscopic versus open gastric resections for primary gastrointestinal stromal tumors (GISTs): a size-matched comparison. *Ann Surg Oncol* 2011;18:1599–1605.
49. Catena F, Di Battista M, Fusaroli P, et al. Laparoscopic treatment of gastric GIST: report of 21 cases and literature's review. *J Gastrointest Surg* 2008;12:561–568.
50. Ohtani H, Maeda K, Noda E, et al. Meta-analysis of laparoscopic and open surgery for gastric gastrointestinal stromal tumor. *Anticancer Res* 2013;33:5031–5041.
51. Frankel TL, Chang AE, Wong SL. Surgical options for localized and advanced gastrointestinal stromal tumors. *J Surg Oncol* 2011;104:882–887.

52. DeMatteo RP, Lewis JJ, Leung D, et al. Two hundred gastrointestinal stromal tumors: recurrence patterns and prognostic factors for survival. *Ann Surg* 2000;231:51–58.

53. McCarter MD, Antonescu CR, Ballman KV, et al. Microscopically positive margins for primary gastrointestinal stromal tumors: analysis of risk factors and tumor recurrence. *J Am Coll Surg* 2012;215:53–59.

54. Jakob J, Mussi C, Ronellenfitsch U, et al. Gastrointestinal stromal tumor of the rectum: results of surgical and multimodality therapy in the era of imatinib. *Ann Surg Oncol* 2013;20:586–592.

55. Mussi C, Schildhaus HU, Gronchi A, et al. Therapeutic consequences from molecular biology for gastrointestinal stromal tumor patients affected by neurofibromatosis type 1. *Clin Cancer Res* 2008;14:4550–4555.

56. Dematteo RP, Ballman KV, Antonescu CR, et al. Adjuvant imatinib mesylate after resection of localised, primary gastrointestinal stromal tumour: a randomised, double-blind, placebo-controlled trial. *Lancet* 2009;373:1097–1104.

57. Joensuu H, Eriksson M, Sundby Hall K, et al. One vs three years of adjuvant imatinib for operable gastrointestinal stromal tumor: a randomized trial. *JAMA* 2012a;307:1265–1272.

58. Casali PG, Le Cesne A, Poveda Velasco A, et al. Imatinib failure-free survival (IFS) in patients with localized gastrointestinal stromal tumors (GIST) treated with adjuvant imatinib (IM): The EORTC/AGITG/FSG/GEIS/ISG randomized controlled phase III trial. *J Clin Oncol* 2013;31:abstr 10500.

59. Casali PG, Fumagalli E, Gronchi A. Adjuvant therapy of gastrointestinal stromal tumors (GIST). *Curr Treat Options Oncol* 2012;13:277–284.

60. Gastrointestinal Stromal Tumor Meta-Analysis Group (MetaGIST). Comparison of two doses of imatinib for the treatment of unresectable or metastatic gastrointestinal stromal tumors: a meta-analysis of 1,640 patients. *J Clin Oncol* 2010;28:1247–1253.

61. Fiore M, Palassini E, Fumagalli E, et al. Preoperative imatinib mesylate for unresectable or locally advanced primary gastrointestinal stromal tumors (GIST). *Eur J Surg Oncol* 2009;35:739–745.

62. Rutkowski P, Gronchi A, Hohenberger P, et al. Neoadjuvant imatinib in locally advanced gastrointestinal stromal tumors (GIST): the EORTC STBSG experience. *Ann Surg Oncol* 2013;20:2937–2943.

63. Koontz MZ, Visser BM, Kunz PL. Neoadjuvant imatinib for borderline resectable GIST. *J Natl Compr Canc Netw* 2012;10:1477–1482.

64. Wang D, Zhang Q, Blanke CD, et al. Phase II trial of neoadjuvant/adjuvant imatinib mesylate for advanced primary and metastatic/recurrent operable gastrointestinal stromal tumors: long-term follow-up results of Radiation Therapy Oncology Group 0132. *Ann Surg Oncol* 2012;19:1074–1080.

65. Tirumani SH, Shinagare AB, Jagannathan JP, et al. Radiologic assessment of earliest, best, and plateau response of gastrointestinal stromal tumors to neoadjuvant imatinib prior to successful surgical resection. *Eur J Surg Oncol* 2014;40:420–428.

66. Joensuu H, Roberts PJ, Sarlomo-Rikala M, et al. Effect of the tyrosine kinase inhibitor STI571 in a patient with a metastatic gastrointestinal stromal tumor. *N Engl J Med* 2001;344:1052–1056.

67. Blanke CD, Demetri GD, von Mehren M, et al. Long-term results from a randomized phase II trial of standard- versus higher-dose imatinib mesylate for patients with unresectable or metastatic gastrointestinal stromal tumors expressing KIT. *J Clin Oncol* 2008;26:620–625.

68. Verweij J, Casali PG, Zalcberg J, et al. Progression-free survival in gastrointestinal stromal tumours with high-dose imatinib: randomised trial. *Lancet* 2004;364:1127–1134.

69. Blanke CD, Rankin C, Demetri GD et al. Phase III randomized, intergroup trial assessing imatinib mesylate at two dose levels in patients with unresectable or metastatic gastrointestinal stromal tumors expressing the kit receptor tyrosine kinase: S0033. *J Clin Oncol* 2008;26:626–632.

70. Van Glabbeke M, Verweij J, Casali PG, et al. Initial and late resistance to imatinib in advanced gastrointestinal stromal tumors are predicted by different prognostic factors: a European Organisation for Research and Treatment of Cancer-Italian Sarcoma Group-Australasian Gastrointestinal Trials Group study. *J Clin Oncol* 2005;23:5795–5804.

71. Heinrich MC, Owzar K, Corless CL, et al. Correlation of kinase genotype and clinical outcome in the North American Intergroup Phase III Trial of imatinib mesylate for treatment of advanced gastrointestinal stromal tumor: CALGB 150105 Study by Cancer and Leukemia Group B and Southwest Oncology Group. *J Clin Oncol* 2008;26:5360–5367.

72. Heinrich MC, Corless CL, Blanke CD, et al. Molecular correlates of imatinib resistance in gastrointestinal stromal tumors. *J Clin Oncol* 2006;24:4764–4774.

73. Barnett CM, Corless CL, Heinrich MC. Gastrointestinal stromal tumors: molecular markers and genetic subtypes. *Hematol Oncol Clin North Am* 2013;27:871–888.

74. Janeway KA, Albritton KH, Van Den Abbeele AD, et al. Sunitinib treatment in pediatric patients with advanced GIST following failure of imatinib. *Pediatr Blood Cancer* 2009;52:767–771.

75. Le Cesne A, Ray-Coquard I, Bui BN, et al. French Sarcoma Group. Discontinuation of imatinib in patients with advanced gastrointestinal stromal tumours after 3 years of treatment: an open-label multicentre randomised phase 3 trial. *Lancet Oncol* 2010;11:942–949.

76. Patrikidou A, Chabaud S, Ray-Coquard I, et al. Influence of imatinib interruption and rechallenge on the residual disease in patients with advanced GIST: results of the BFR14 prospective French Sarcoma Group randomised, phase III trial. *Ann Oncol* 2013;24:1087–1093.

77. Joensuu H, Trent JC, Reichardt P. Practical management of tyrosine kinase inhibitor-associated side effects in GIST. *Cancer Treat Rev* 2011;37:75–88.

78. DeMatteo RP, Maki RG, Singer S, et al. Results of tyrosine kinase inhibitor therapy followed by surgical resection for metastatic gastrointestinal stromal tumor. *Ann Surg* 2007;245:347–352.

79. Sym SJ, Ryu MH, Lee JL, et al. Surgical intervention following imatinib treatment in patients with advanced gastrointestinal stromal tumors (GISTs). *J Surg Oncol* 2008;98:27–33.

80. Raut CP, Wang Q, Manola J, et al. Cytoreductive surgery in patients with metastatic gastrointestinal stromal tumor treated with sunitinib malate. *Ann Surg Oncol* 2010;17:407–415.

81. Mussi C, Ronellenfitsch U, Jakob J, et al. Post-imatinib surgery in advanced/metastatic GIST: is it worthwhile in all patients? *Ann Oncol* 2010;21:403–408.

82. Wang D, Zhang Q, Blanke CD, et al. Phase II trial of neoadjuvant/adjuvant imatinib mesylate for advanced primary and metastatic/recurrent operable gastrointestinal stromal tumors: long-term follow-up results of Radiation Therapy Oncology Group 0132. *Ann Surg Oncol* 2012;19:1074–1080.

83. Wang YP, Jie ZG, He YL, et al. Is there a role of surgery in patients with recurrent or metastatic gastrointestinal stromal tumours responding to imatinib: a prospective randomised trial in China. *Eur J Cancer* 2014;50:1772–1778.

84. Bamboat ZM, DeMatteo RP. Metastasectomy for gastrointestinal stromal tumors. *J Surg Oncol* 2014;109:23–27.

85. Wang WL, Conley A, Reynoso D, et al. Mechanisms of resistance to imatinib and sunitinib in gastrointestinal stromal tumor. *Cancer Chemother Pharmacol* 2011;67:S15–S24.

86. Liegl B, Kepten I, Le C, et al. Heterogeneity of kinase inhibitor resistance mechanisms in GIST. *J Pathol* 2008;216:64–74.

87. Wardelmann E, Merkelbach-Bruse S, Pauls K, et al. Polyclonal evolution of multiple secondary KIT mutations in gastrointestinal stromal tumors under treatment with imatinib mesylate. *Clin Cancer Res* 2006;12:1743–1749.

88. Shankar S, vanSonnenberg E, Desai J, et al. Gastrointestinal stromal tumor: new nodule-within-a-mass pattern of recurrence after partial response to imatinib mesylate. *Radiology* 2005;235:892–898.

89. Judson I, Ma P, Peng B, et al. Imatinib pharmacokinetics in patients with gastrointestinal stromal tumour: a retrospective population pharmacokinetic study over time. EORTC Soft Tissue and Bone Sarcoma Group. *Cancer Chemother Pharmacol* 2005;55:379–386.

90. Demetri GD, Wang Y, Wehrle E, et al. Imatinib plasma levels are correlated with clinical benefit in patients with unresectable/metastatic gastrointestinal stromal tumors. *J Clin Oncol* 2009;27:3141–3147.

91. Zalcberg JR, Verweij J, Casali PG, et al. EORTC Soft Tissue and Bone Sarcoma Group, the Italian Sarcoma Group; Australasian Gastrointestinal Trials Group. Outcome of patients with advanced gastro-intestinal stromal tumours crossing over to a daily imatinib dose of 800 mg after progression on 400 mg. *Eur J Cancer* 2005;41:1751–1757.

92. Demetri GD, van Oosterom AT, Garrett CR, et al. Efficacy and safety of sunitinib in patients with advanced gastrointestinal stromal tumour after failure of imatinib: a randomised controlled trial. *Lancet* 2006;368:1329–1338.

93. Heinrich MC, Maki RG, Corless CL, et al. Primary and secondary kinase genotypes correlate with the biological and clinical activity of sunitinib in imatinib-resistant gastrointestinal stromal tumor. *J Clin Oncol* 2008;26:5352–5359.

94. George S, Blay JY, Casali PG, et al. Clinical evaluation of continuous daily dosing of sunitinib malate in patients with advanced gastrointestinal stromal tumour after imatinib failure. *Eur J Cancer* 2009;45:1959–1968.

95. Demetri GD, Reichardt P, Kang YK, et al. Efficacy and safety of regorafenib for advanced gastrointestinal stromal tumours after failure of imatinib and sunitinib (GRID): an international, multicentre, randomised, placebo-controlled, phase 3 trial. *Lancet* 2013;381:295–302.

96. De Wit M, Boers-Doets CB, Saettini A, et al. Prevention and management of adverse events related to regorafenib. *Support Care Cancer* 2014;22:837–846

97. Casali PG, Reichardt P, Kang Y, et al. Clinical benefit with regorafenib across subgroups and post-progression in patients with advanced gastrointestinal stromal tumor (GIST) after progression on imatinib (IM) and sunitinib (SU): phase 3 GRID trial update. *Ann Oncol* 2012;23:ix478.

98. Kang YK, Ryu MH, Yoo C, et al. Resumption of imatinib to control metastatic or unresectable gastrointestinal stromal tumours after failure of imatinib and sunitinib (RIGHT): a randomised, placebo-controlled, phase 3 trial. *Lancet Oncol* 2013;14:1175–1182.

99. Demetri GD, Jeffers M, Reichardt P, et al. Mutational analysis of plasma DNA from patients (pts) in the phase III GRID study of regorafenib (REG) versus placebo (PL) in tyrosine kinase inhibitor (TKI)-refractory GIST: correlating genotype with clinical outcomes. *J Clin Oncol* 2013;31:abstr 10503.

100. Benjamin RS, Debiec-Rychter M, Le Cesne A, et al. Gastrointestinal stromal tumors II: medical oncology and tumor response assessment. *Semin Oncol* 2009;36:302–311.

101. Tirumani SH, Jagannathan JP, Krajewski KM, et al. Imatinib and beyond in gastrointestinal stromal tumors: A radiologist's perspective. *AJR Am J Roentgenol* 2013;201:801–810.

102. Van den Abbeele AD. The lessons of GIST—PET and PET/CT: a new paradigm for imaging. *Oncologist* 2008;13:8–13.

103. Eisenhauer EA, Therasse P, Bogaerts J, et al. New response evaluation criteria in solid tumours: revised RECIST guideline (version 1.1). *Eur J Cancer* 2009;45:228–247.

104. Choi H, Charnsangavej C, Faria SC, et al. Correlation of computed tomography and positron emission tomography in patients with metastatic gastrointestinal stromal tumor treated at a single institution with imatinib mesylate: proposal of new computed tomography response criteria. *J Clin Oncol* 2007;25:1753–1759.

48 Molecular Biology of Colorectal Cancer

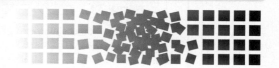

Ramesh A. Shivdasani

INTRODUCTION

The cumulative lifetime risk of developing colorectal cancer (CRC) in the United States is about 6% (www.cancer.gov/statistics) and increases about fourfold in persons with a family history of CRC. Fewer than 5% of cases, however, occur in patients with inherited predisposition syndromes. Most CRCs are therefore considered sporadic, although 20% to 30% of cases might have a familial basis despite the absence of a known germ-line defect, and genomewide association (GWA) studies reveal at least 20 alleles that elevate the risk of developing CRCs. Characteristic somatic mutations, DNA repair defects, chromosomal instability, and epigenetic alterations promote the disease. Predisposing conditions and somatic mutations profoundly inform the molecular understanding of CRCs and serve as a paradigm for the genetic basis of cancer.

MULTISTEP MODELS OF COLORECTAL TUMORIGENESIS

The genetic basis of CRC is best appreciated in light of the adenoma–carcinoma sequence. CRCs invariably arise within benign precursor polyps that show epithelial overgrowth, dysplasia, abnormal differentiation, and, sometimes, foci of tissue invasion. Pedunculated polyps are the most significant precursor lesions, with those larger than 1 cm harboring about a 15% risk of progressing to carcinoma over 10 years; endoscopic removal of these adenomas reduces CRC incidence and mortality.[1] The prevalence of polyps in the United States, estimated at up to 50% by age 70,[2] dwarfs the 6% lifetime risk of CRCs because few adenomas progress to invasive cancer and the successive aberrations that promote invasion and malignancy take 1 to 3 decades to accumulate.[3]

Nonclassical adenomas, such as hyperplastic polyps, were previously thought to have little potential to spawn invasive CRCs, but two serrated precursor lesion forms are now recognized.[4] Serrated adenomas with cytologic dysplasia occasionally evolve into common CRCs with chromosomal instability and *KRAS* mutation, whereas sessile serrated adenomas that lack dysplasia can spawn CRCs with microsatellite instability (MSI-hi), *BRAF* mutation, and abundant CpG island methylation.[5,6] About 8% of sporadic CRCs originate in such lesions, retain a serrated epithelium with characteristic nuclear morphology, and carry a relatively poor prognosis.

Although cancer progression has both genetic (somatic mutations) and epigenetic (unrelated to altered DNA sequence) underpinnings, we presently know more about the former than the latter. Alterations in several classes of genes drive tumors: oncogenes; tumor suppressors, including genes that repair damaged DNA; and those that help control other genes (epigenetic modifiers). Selected mutations appear at high frequencies in different tumor types and stages, allowing for the assignment of typical sequences (Fig. 48.1), although mutational order can vary and most tumors do not carry every alteration. These mutations support the idea of cancer as a multifaceted disease that breaches natural checks on cell survival, growth, and invasion.[7] Few specific mutations correlate strongly with particular histologic features or patient survival and most affect multiple cellular functions. Particular genotypes do, however, define CRC subtypes and response to certain therapies. MSI-hi tumors typically arise in the ascending colon and carry a good prognosis; adjuvant 5-fluorouracil provides little benefit in stage II cases of this variety. *KRAS* or *BRAF* mutations, together accounting for about half of all cases, limit response to epidermal growth factor receptor (EGFR) antibodies[8,9] and are contraindications for this treatment. The prognostic and predictive value of other molecular features will become clearer as new therapies enter the clinic. Meanwhile, specific mutations reveal normal controls on colonic cells, possibly guiding future prevention strategies and key signaling pathways for rational drug development.

Global Events in Colorectal Cancer

CRCs acquire genetic instability in stereotypic ways that favor the accumulation of hundreds to thousands of somatic aberrations (see Fig. 48.1). About 80% of tumors display widespread chromosomal gains, losses, and translocations—phenomena that lead to gene amplifications, rearrangements, and deletions.[10] These tumors carry, on average, below 100 somatic nonsynonymous point mutations. Chromosomal segregation defects may account for chromosomal instability (CIN), as the segregation factor *Bub1* illustrates in mice,[11] but few specific gene defects are implicated confidently. Beyond weak associations with structural changes on chromosomes 8 and 18,[12] specific cytogenetic features barely influence disease patterns or patient outcomes.

About 15% of CRCs appear globally euploid but carry thousands of point mutations and small deletions or insertions near nucleotide repeat tracts—the defect designated as MSI-hi.[13] Features and the molecular determinants of disease progression in MSI-hi adenomas differ from those associated with CIN; for example, *BRAF* V600E mutations are more common in MSI+ precursor adenomas than in other types.[14] Because hypermutability, whether associated with CIN or MSI, results in many changes that are inconsequential or even detrimental to tumors, the mere presence of a mutation does not signify a pathogenic role. Therefore, two features are used to distinguish *driver* from *passenger* mutations: appearance in a high fraction of tumor specimens, and ideally, the experimental demonstration of its contribution to a malignant property.

Epigenetic mechanisms may be as significant as mutations in cancer but are less well understood. Various covalent histone modifications and methylation of cytosine residues in DNA represent prominent modes of gene regulation,[15] the latter being far better characterized in CRCs than the former. 5′-CpG-3′ dinucleotide pairs are particular targets for methylation in localized areas of high CpG content in promoters, where methylation silences adjacent genes. CRCs show 8% to 15% lower total DNA methylation than normal tissue,[16] even in colorectal adenomas.[17] Reduced pericentromeric methylation might decrease the fidelity of chromosomal segregation and altered methylation or loss of imprinting at the *IGF2* locus increase CRC risk,[18] suggesting broad effects of global hypomethylation on cell growth. However,

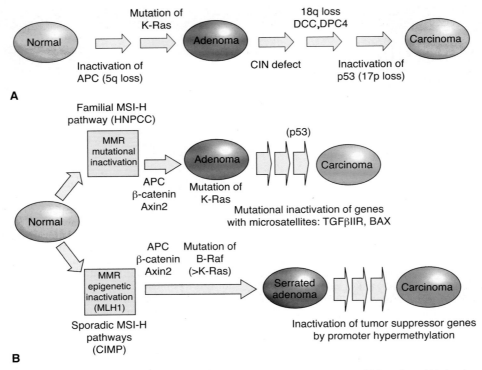

Figure 48.1 Genetic pathways to colorectal carcinoma. All colorectal cancers (CRCs) arise within benign adenomatous precursors, fueled by mutations that serially enhance malignant behavior. Mutations that activate the Wnt signaling pathway seem to be necessary initiating events, after which two possible courses contribute to the accumulation of additional mutations. **(A)** Chromosomal instability is a feature of up to 80% of CRCs and is commonly associated with activating KRAS point mutations and loss of regions that encompass *P53* and other tumor suppressors on 18q and 17p, often but not necessarily in that order. **(B)** About 20% of CRCs are euploid but defective in DNA mismatch repair (MMR), resulting in high microsatellite instability (MSI-hi). MMR defects may develop sporadically, associated with CpG island methylation (CIMP), or as a result of familial predisposition in hereditary nonpolyposis colorectal cancer (HNPCC). Mutations accumulate in the *KRAS* or *BRAF* oncogenes, *p53* tumor suppressor, and in microsatellite-containing genes vulnerable to MMR defects, such as *TGFβIIR*. Epigenetic inactivation of the MMR gene *MLH1* and activating *BRAF* point mutations are especially common in serrated adenomas, which progress, in part, through the silencing of tumor suppressor genes by promoter hypermethylation. Progression from adenoma to CRC takes years to decades, a process that accelerates in the presence of MMR defects. CIN, chromosomal instability.

its precise significance is unclear because some animals show increased tumor susceptibility with global hypomethylation,[19] whereas *Apc*Min mice lacking or overexpressing the de novo DNA methyltransferase DNMT3B show reduced or accelerated progression of small adenomas, respectively.[20,21]

Against a backdrop of genomewide *hypo*methylation, a distinct subset of CRCs shows coordinate *hyper*methylation of many CpG-rich promoters, conferring the CpG island methylator phenotype (CIMP), with transcriptional attenuation of tumor suppressor genes such as *HIC1* and Wnt-inhibiting *SFRPs*.[22,23] Whole-genome methylation analyses have confirmed the existence of this once controversial entity[24] and features that distinguish it from *KRAS*-mutant CIN disease—origin in sessile serrated adenomas; strong association with *BRAF*-mutant, right-sided MSI-hi tumors with *MLH1* gene methylation;[25] and distinctive gene expression patterns.[26]

Although the features cited previously, especially MMR and CIMP, overlap to some degree, CRCs seem to fall into three general categories: (1) traditional, (2) alternative, and (3) serrated, which are characterized by CIN, DNA mismatch repair, and CIMP, respectively (see Fig. 48.1). The Cancer Genome Atlas (TCGA) Network classified CRCs into nonhypermutated (generally CIN+) and hypermutated (encompassing MMR and CIMP) categories.[26] Other variations on the classical adenoma–carcinoma sequence are also recognized. A 10-fold elevated risk of CRC in patients with long-standing ulcerative colitis (UC)[27] likely reflects

heightened mutation in a setting of ongoing mucosal injury and repair. UC-associated CRCs often arise within flat adenomatous plaques and nonadenomatous areas of dysplasia. Compared to sporadic cases, *TP53* mutations occur earlier in the cancer sequence,[28] *APC* inactivation is less frequent, and methylation of the *p16*INK4a tumor suppressor gene is more common.[29]

INHERITED SYNDROMES OF INCREASED CANCER RISK HIGHLIGHT EARLY EVENTS AND CRITICAL PATHWAYS IN COLORECTAL TUMORIGENESIS

Two uncommon but highly penetrant Mendelian syndromes, familial adenomatous polyposis (FAP) and hereditary nonpolyposis colorectal cancer (HNPCC), together account for almost 5% of cases. *MYH*-associated polyposis (MAP), polymerase proofreading-associated polyposis (PPAP), familial juvenile polyposis (FJP), Peutz-Jeghers syndrome (PJS), and Cowden disease, each occurring in fewer than 1 in 200,000 births, also elevate the risk of CRCs (Table 48.1). Knowledge about the genes responsible for these inherited disorders allows for accurate molecular diagnosis, risk assessment, and targeted prevention in affected families. It also profoundly informs understanding of the considerably larger proportion of sporadic cases.

TABLE 48.1

Genetics of Inherited Colorectal Tumor Syndromes

Syndrome	Features Commonly Seen in Affected Individuals	Gene Defect
Syndromes with Adenomatous Polyps		
Familial adenomatous polyposis (FAP)	Multiple adenomas (>100) and colorectal carcinomas; duodenal polyps and carcinomas; gastric fundus polyps; congenital hypertrophy of retinal epithelium	*APC* (>90%)
– Gardner syndrome	Same as FAP, with desmoid tumors and mandibular osteomas	*APC*
– Turcot syndrome	Polyposis and CRC with brain tumors (medulloblastoma, glioblastoma)	*APC, MLH1*
Attenuated adenomatous polyposis coli (AAPC)	Less than 100 polyps, although marked variation in polyp number (from ~5 to >1,000 polyps) seen in mutation carriers within a single family	*APC* (5' mutations)
Hereditary nonpolyposis colorectal cancer (HNPCC)	CRC with modest polyposis; high risk of endometrial cancer; some risk of ovarian, gastric, urothelial, hepatobiliary, and brain cancers	*MSH2, MLH1, MSH6* (together >90%), *PMS2* (about 5%)
MYH-associated polyposis (MAP)	Multiple gastrointestinal polyps, autosomal recessive	*MYH*
Polymerase proofreading-associated polyposis (PPAP)	Large adenomas, early-onset CRC, elevated risk of endometrial cancer only	*POLE* or *POLD1*
Syndromes with Atypical Polyps		
Peutz-Jeghers syndrome (PJS)	Hamartomatous polyps throughout the gastrointestinal (GI) tract; mucocutaneous pigmentation; estimated 9- to 13-fold increased risk of GI and non-GI cancers	*STK11* (30%–70%)
Cowden disease	Multiple hamartomas involving breast, thyroid, skin, brain, and GI tract; increased risk of breast, uterus, thyroid, and some GI cancers	*PTEN* (85%)
Juvenile polyposis syndrome	Multiple hamartomas in youth, predominantly in colon and stomach; variable increase in colorectal and stomach cancer risk; facial changes	*BMPR1A* (25%), *SMAD4* (15%), *ENG*
Hereditary mixed polyposis (HMPS)	Polyps of highly heterogeneous form and size, a few of which progress to CRC; confined to rare Ashkenazi Jewish kindreds; only CRC risk is elevated	*GREM1* (imputed)

Familial Adenomatous Polyposis and the Central Importance of Wnt Signaling

FAP is an autosomal-dominant monogenic disorder that underlies about 0.5% of all CRCs. Individuals develop hundreds to thousands of colonic polyps by their early 20s, and the lifetime risk of CRC approaches 100% at a median age of 39. Extraintestinal manifestations include (1) duodenal and gastric adenomas; (2) congenital hypertrophy of the retinal pigmented epithelium; (3) osteomas and mesenteric desmoid tumors in the Gardner syndrome variant[30]; (4) brain tumors in the Turcot syndrome variant[31]; and rarely, (5) cutaneous cysts, thyroid tumors, or adrenal adenomas. Although most of these extraintestinal features are benign, rare patients develop hepatoblastoma or thyroid cancer. Reflecting similar homeostatic mechanisms in the small and large bowel epithelia, a 5% to 10% risk of periampullary adenocarcinoma mandates endoscopic monitoring of the duodenum after prophylactic colectomy.[32]

The gene responsible for FAP, *adenomatous polyposis coli* (*APC*), encodes a 300 kDa protein. Germ-line mutations occur throughout the locus, clustering in the 5' half and exon 15,[33] mostly introducing premature truncations. A few mutations correlate with phenotypic severity or specific extraintestinal manifestations, but identical mutations can produce different features. Mutations clustered in the extreme 5' or 3' ends of *APC* exons lead to the variant attenuated APC, with few polyps or CRCs developing late in life.[34] The *I1307K* allele, present in Ashkenazi Jews,

barely doubles the lifetime risk of CRC over the background and does not affect APC protein function but replaces an $(A)_3T(A)_4$ coding sequence with an $(A)_8$ tract that is occasionally targeted for nearby truncating mutations.[35] The identification of specific *APC* mutations in probands allows for a reliable testing of family members. Minimal recommendations for carriers include screening colonoscopy annually after age 10, gastroduodenoscopy after age 25, and treatment with nonsteroidal anti-inflammatory drugs to reduce CRC risk.[36] A prophylactic colectomy is highly recommended, with continued vigilance over the rectal stump and other at-risk tissues.

The larger significance of the *APC* gene derives from its somatic inactivation in about 80% of sporadic CRCs and adenomas,[37] including tiny polyps without dysplasia. APC inactivation is a rate-limiting step in the development of most polyps, and knowledge of its cellular functions supports this gatekeeper role. Attesting to the tumor suppressor function, CRCs that arise sporadically or in FAP show loss of heterozygosity and biallelic APC inactivation, with one copy usually lost by deletion. Because *APC* encodes several functional domains, truncated mutant proteins might interfere with various cellular activities. Disruption of its role in chromosome segregation might, for example, contribute to CIN.[38] However, attention on *APC* rightly centers on its control of the Wnt signaling pathway. About half the sporadic CRCs with intact *APC* function carry activating point mutations in *CTNNB1*,[39,40] which encodes β-catenin, a transcriptional effector of Wnt signaling; many of the rest carry fusions of genes that encode R-spondin cofactors.[41] Moreover, acute APC loss in mice produces intestinal defects identical to those observed upon Wnt pathway activation.[42] APC mutations are uncommon in sporadic cancers outside the intestine.

Wnts are secreted glycoprotein morphogens with diverse developmental and homeostatic functions, and, especially in the intestine, their role is intimately tied to that of R-spondins.[43,44] In the absence of Wnt ligands, cells use a complex containing APC, AXIN2, and other cytosolic proteins to promote casein kinase I- and glycogen synthase kinase (GSK)-3β-mediated phosphorylation of conserved serine and threonine residues at the N-terminus of β-catenin; this phosphorylation targets β-catenin for ubiquitin-mediated proteasomal degradation. The binding of Wnt ligands to a surface complex containing a FRIZZLED protein and the obligate coreceptor LRP5/6 inhibits the APC-AXIN2 destruction complex and stabilizes a pool of cytosolic β-catenin (Fig. 48.2), distinct from the abundant cellular stores that attach to E-cadherin on the inner cell surface. Accumulated β-catenin translocates to the cell nucleus, where it coactivates genes bound by sequence-specific transcription factors of the T-cell factor (TCF) family. Of the four proteins in this family, TCF4 is especially important in normal bowel epithelium and CRCs[39,45] and nuclear β-catenin is necessary to activate target genes.[46]

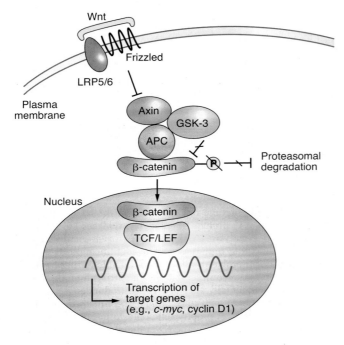

Figure 48.2 Outline of Wnt signaling, the key driver pathway in colorectal cancer. Members of the Wnt family of glycoprotein morphogens bind the cell surface coreceptors Frizzled and LRP5/6. In the absence of Wnt binding, normal cells use a complex containing APC, Axin, and other cytoplasmic proteins to promote GSK-3β–mediated phosphorylation of the β-catenin N-terminus, which targets β-catenin for proteasomal degradation (from Clevers H. Wnt/β-catenin signaling in development and disease. *Cell* 2006;127:469). Binding of a Wnt ligand to Frizzled and its obligate coreceptor LRP5/6 antagonizes the APC/Axin destruction complex, stabilizing β-catenin (CTNNB1), which moves into the nucleus and coactivates genes through T-cell factor/lymphoid enhancer factor (TCF/LEF) transcription factors. Either of the two principal gatekeeper events in colorectal cancer, inactivating APC or activating CTNNB1 mutations, results in constitutive, Wnt-independent stabilization of β-catenin and unregulated activation of the cognate transcriptional program. Wnt signaling in the intestine is normally confined to crypt progenitors, and its aberrant activation by APC or CTNNB1 mutations confers a permanent cryptlike state that favors cell replication.

CTNNB1 mutations in CRC invariably target residues for N-terminal phosphorylation and the mutant protein hence, resists degradation. Thus, both alternative gatekeeper lesions in CRC, inactivating APC or activating CTNNB1 mutations, result in constitutive, Wnt ligand-independent stabilization of β-catenin. R-SPONDIN genes are translocated in up to 10% of cases, all with wild-type APC and CTNNB1,[41] and the gene fusions are probably pathogenic because they potentiate Wnt signaling. TCF4 (also known as TCF7L2) mutations are surprisingly common,[26] but their roles and effects are unclear, as is the functional significance of rare AXIN2 mutations in MSI[+] cases[47] and of TCF3 or TCF4 gene fusions in microsatellite stability (MSS) cases.[48]

Normal intestinal crypt stem and progenitor cells require Wnt signaling to proliferate, and APC or CTNNB1 mutation-induced loss of this ligand dependence liberates cells from a potent regulatory restraint. Accordingly, the Wnt-dependent transcriptional program in CRC cell lines overlaps significantly with that in intestinal crypts.[49] Cycling crypt base cells that express the surface marker LGR5 are especially vulnerable to Wnt-induced transformation in mice, suggesting that CRC arises from stem cells and not from mature descendants.[50] Laboratory evidence suggests that even advanced CRCs remain dependent on constitutive Wnt pathway activity.[49] The TCF4–β-catenin complex controls hundreds of candidate genes,[49,51] but the individual significance of most target genes is unclear. Apc mutant mice lacking CD44 and selected other Wnt-pathway targets develop fewer adenomas,[52] but MYC seems especially vital because its absence in mouse intestines completely abrogates effects of acute APC loss.[53,54]

Hereditary Nonpolyposis Colorectal Cancer and the Role of DNA Mismatch Repair

HNPCC, or Lynch syndrome, an autosomal-dominant disorder that confers about 70% lifetime risk of developing CRCs, usually before age 50, is estimated to account for 2% to 4% of all cases. Affected individuals do not lack colonic polyps (nearly all CRCs, syndromic or sporadic, arise within benign precursors), but develop many fewer polyps than patients with FAP, a condition that must be excluded to satisfy diagnostic criteria for HNPCC (Table 48.2).[55] Cancers tend to develop in the ascending colon and patients are also predisposed to develop tumors of the endometrium (35% to 50% lifetime risk), ovary and upper urothelium (7% to 8% risk), stomach, small intestine, biliary tract, and brain—a spectrum reflected in the revised Amsterdam II criteria (see Table 48.2).[56] Cancers in HNPCC show pronounced variation in the lengths of microsatellite DNA sequences, and MSI at two or more among a panel of five mono- and dinucleotide tracts (BAT26, BAT25, D5S346, D2S123, and D17S250) confers the MSI-hi designation. CRCs harboring CIN represent a distinct class and show MSS or, in a small fraction, instability of unclear significance at just one of the five test regions (MSI-lo).

HNPCC results from germ-line mutations in any of several genes that enable DNA mismatch repair (MMR), a proofreading process that corrects base-pair mismatches and short insertions and deletions in the normal course of DNA replication. MMR in mammalian cells is mediated by homologs of bacterial and yeast repair proteins, MutS homologs (MSH) 1 through 6, MutL homologs (MLH) 1 through 3, PMS1, and PMS2. Both MLH1 and PMS2 are recruited to sites of DNA mismatch as a MutLα complex and in turn recruit MSH2-MSH6 (MutSβ) or MSH2-MSH3 (MutSβ) heterodimers to sites of 1-bp or 2- to 4-bp errors, respectively. These proteins efficiently excise the strand that carries the mismatch and resynthesize and ligate the repaired DNA. Germ-line mutations in MSH2, MLH1, MSH6, and PMS2 together explain about 95% of kindreds,[57–59] including a subset with germ-line loss of the stop codon of TACSTD1, which results in silencing of its 3' neighbor MSH2 by hypermethylation.[60,61]

TABLE 48.2

Criteria for Clinical Diagnosis of Hereditary Nonpolyposis Colorectal Cancer

A. Revised Amsterdam Criteria (Clinical Diagnosis)
1. Three or more family members with histologically verified HNPCC-related cancers, one of whom is a first-degree relative of the other two
2. Two successive affected generations
3. One or more of the HNPCC-related cancers (see C, which follows) diagnosed before age 50
4. Exclusion of familial adenomatous polyposis (FAP)

B. Revised Bethesda Guidelines (Criteria to Prompt Microsatellite Instability Testing of Tumors)
1. Diagnosis of CRC before age 50
2. Synchronous or metachronous presence of CRC or other HNPCC-associated cancer
3. CRC diagnosed before age 60 with histopathologic features associated with MSI-hi
4. CRC in at least one first-degree relative with an HNPCC-related tumor, with one of the cancers diagnosed before age 50
5. CRC in two or more first-degree relatives with HNPCC-related tumors, regardless of age

C. Spectrum of Sites for HNPCC-related Cancers
Colon and rectum, endometrium, stomach, ovary, pancreas, ureter and renal pelvis, biliary tract, small intestine, brain, sebaceous gland adenomas, and keratoacanthomas

MSI-hi colon cancers typically show exophytic growth, lymphoid infiltrates, mucinous signet-ring differentiation, and a medullary growth pattern; Bethesda guidelines (see Table 48.2) combine clinical and phenotypic features to facilitate a diagnosis of HNPCC.[62] When these criteria are met, tumor DNA should be tested either for MSI in a simple, polymerase chain reaction (PCR)-based assay or by immunohistochemistry for the absence of the commonly implicated MLH1, MSH2, and MSH6 proteins.[63] Because Bethesda guidelines might miss up to a quarter of cases, experts now recommend testing all colon cancers arising in patients under 70 years.[64,65] Coupled with thorough personal and family histories, positive results should prompt DNA testing for MLH1, MSH2, MSH6, or PMS2 mutations.[66] The identification of mutant alleles and carriers allows for the targeting of cost-effective screening and interventions that are proven to reduce mortality[65] (e.g., preventive colonoscopy screening every 1 to 2 years, starting around 30 years of age; family counseling; aspirin therapy). Carriers should consider prophylactic subtotal colectomy, hysterectomy, and oophorectomy; females should at least have an annual endometrial evaluation soon after age 30.

In incipient cancers, random events first disrupt function of the wild-type allele of a mutant MMR gene and the resulting *mutator phenotype* promotes DNA replication errors at rates 10^2 to 10^3 times higher than the background.[13,57] Consequently, adenomas progress into carcinomas over 3 to 5 years instead of 2 or more decades.[67] Paradoxically, the prognosis for patients with MSI-hi CRCs is better than for those with sporadic MSS disease, perhaps because many resulting somatic mutations place tumors at a disadvantage. Both of the most commonly inactivated genes, ACVR2A and TGFBR2, encode receptors for specific ligands of the transforming growth factor beta (TGF-β) family and contain vulnerable mononucleotide tracts in their coding sequences.[26,68] TGF-β inhibits the proliferation of intestinal epithelial cells, and biallelic TGFBR2 inactivation is detected in over 90% of MSI-hi and 15% of MSS, sporadic CRCs.[69] Other genes mutated in familial MSI-hi colon tumors encode the proapoptotic genes

CASP5 and BAX[70]; transcription factor genes, including TCF4[71]; and the epidermal growth factor receptor (EGFR)[72]; but KRAS and, especially, BRAF mutations are rare. CRC pathogenesis requires deregulated APC–β-catenin gatekeeper function irrespective of MMR status.[73]

MSI-hi is observed in 12% to 15% of sporadic cases of CRC,[74] often in older patients with early-stage disease. Such tumors seem to arise from sessile serrated adenomas in the ascending colon and do not reflect unrecognized germ-line mutation or somatic disruption of a known MMR gene.[75] Rather, most but not all cases reflect MLH1 gene inactivation by biallelic promoter hypermethylation and show activating BRAF mutations and CIMP.[76–78]

MYH-Associated Polyposis and Polymerase Proofreading-Associated Polyposis

Germ-line mutations in MYH, a homolog of the *Escherichia coli* base excision-repair gene MutY cause MAP, a recessively inherited syndrome of multiple adenomas and CRC.[79] CRC develops later in life than in FAP, polyp numbers vary widely, and extracolonic tumors are less frequent than in HNPCC (see Table 48.1). Because MYH is a DNA glycosylase that helps repair oxidative DNA damage, tumors are not associated with MSI but with somatic G:C to T:A mutations, including in the APC gene. Two alleles, Y165C and G382D, account for most cases, and CRCs develop in homozygotes or compound heterozygotes, with no risk elevation in monoallelic carriers.[80] Surveillance recommendations are the same as in HNPCC.

Rare kindreds with a dominantly inherited high risk of CRC carry particular germ-line defects in POLE and POLD1, which encode the proofreading exonuclease activities of the leading- and lagging-strand DNA polymerases ε and δ, respectively.[81] Clinical findings of large adenomas and early-onset CRCs resemble those in HNPCC or MAP, including elevated endometrial cancer risk in women with mutant POLD1. Tumors carry thousands of mutations, but stable microsatellite tracts reveal a third familial *mutator* mechanism in CRCs. Hypermutation in the absence of MSI accounts for about 3% of sporadic CRCs, nearly all of which have a somatic POLE exonuclease domain and also APC mutations.[26] POLE and POLD1 are nonclassical tumor suppressors because, instead of deletion or truncation, specific missense mutations affect proofreading function, and the wild-type allele is usually retained. Until further characterization of PPAP leads to formal surveillance recommendations, it is prudent to adopt those developed for HNPCC.

Familial Juvenile Polyposis and the Peutz-Jeghers, Hereditary Mixed Polyposis, and Cowden Syndromes

Patients with FJP develop premalignant hamartomatous polyps in the stomach or the small or large intestine by adolescence[82,83] and may give a revealing family history, although a significant minority represent the first case in their families. Germ-line mutations in genes encoding the bone morphogenetic protein (BMP) receptor BMPR1A, the accessory TGF-β receptor endoglin, ENG, or the SMAD4 signal transducer emphasize the role of TGF-β signaling in disease pathogenesis (see Table 48.1).[84,85] Indeed, sporadic CRCs are often insensitive to the growth inhibitory effects of TGF-β and loss of BMP function in mice expands stem and progenitor cells, leading to polyposis or ectopic crypts.[86–88] Not all patients carry these mutations, indicating that additional genes remain undiscovered. Notably, a conditional *Smad4* deletion from mouse intestinal cells does not affect growth, whereas selective loss in T lymphocytes causes intestinal mucosal thickening and polyps.[89] These findings confound simple interpretations of TGF-β function and implicate stromal inflammation in intestinal tumorigenesis.

Patients with PJS also develop benign tumors that contain differentiated but disorganized cells (hamartomas), mainly in the small intestine but also in the colon or stomach, sometimes leading to hemorrhage or intussusception. PJS shows autosomal-dominant inheritance and is associated with macular lesions on the skin and buccal mucosa; bladder and bronchial polyps; and a propensity to develop a range of cancers, including those of the lung, breast, and female reproductive organs (see Table 48.1). The lifetime risk for all cancers exceeds 90%, the incidence of small intestine, stomach, and pancreas cancers is 50 to 500 times higher than the general population, and CRC risk is elevated nearly 100-fold.[90] *Serine–threonine kinase 11 (STK11,* also known as *LKB1),* the implicated tumor suppressor gene,[91] acts at the nexus of diverse cellular pathways and functions. Its principal activity, exerted through the adenosine monophosphate (AMP)-activated protein kinase AMPK, seems to be in linking nutrient and energy utilization to controls over cellular structure, particularly cell polarity.[92] STK11 also modulates the Rheb-GDP:Rheb-GTP cycle and downstream activities of the tuberous sclerosis gene *TSC2* and the mammalian target of rapamycin (mTOR),[93] key regulators of protein synthesis and cell growth. The roles of STK11 in cell polarity and metabolism are busy areas of research, likely to hold vital clues into CRC pathogenesis and rational therapy.

Confined to rare Ashkenazi Jewish kindreds descended from a single founder, patients with HMPS develop polyps of several diverse morphologies and CRCs but no other cancers.[94] A 40-kb duplication upstream of *GREM1* seems to activate a distant enhancer of this BMP antagonist gene, driving ectopic and high expression in the colonic epithelium.[95] The resulting increased crypt cell turnover likely accelerates the accumulation of oncogenic mutations. *GREM1* is also the locus of a CRC risk allele identified at 15q13.3 in a GWA study.[96]

Cowden disease encompasses diverse mucosal lesions, specific cutaneous lesions (facial trichilemmomas and acral verrucous papules), and breast fibroadenomas, neurofibromas, lipomas, and meningiomas.[97] The syndrome results from germ-line mutations in *PTEN,* a tumor suppressor gene encoding the phosphatase and tensin homolog deleted on chromosome 10,[98] and the second most frequently mutated gene in cancers after *TP53.* The lipid phosphatase PTEN dephosphorylates key phosphoinositide (PI) signaling molecules[99] and accordingly regulates intracellular growth signaling negatively through PI-3 kinase and its downstream effectors AKT and mTOR. The CRC risk in Cowden syndrome is modest, and *PTEN* mutations are rare in sporadic cases, but protein immunostaining is lost in about 40% of CRCs, often as a result of promoter hypermethylation,[100] thus highlighting its tumor suppressor role.

Significance of Inherited Syndromes of Elevated Colorectal Cancer Risk

Following a clinical diagnosis of the previous Mendelian syndromes, patients and family members should be tested for pertinent germ-line mutations, receive genetic counseling, and enter programs for cancer prevention and screening. The corresponding molecular defects profoundly inform an understanding of sporadic CRCs, in particular, revealing the seminal role of Wnt signaling and early, rate-limiting effects of *APC* inactivation or *CTNNB1* activation. Similarly, *STK11* and *PTEN* loss in inherited and sporadic CRCs shed light on crucial molecular pathways, whereas HNPCC and PPAP help classify the disease and reveal the significance of features such as MSI, which is present in 12% to 15% of sporadic cases. Even in the absence of a recognized predisposition syndrome, individuals with a history of CRC in a first-degree relative are up to 4 times more likely to develop CRC than those without a family history. Specific environmental factors that compound the risk of developing CRCs are complex and insufficiently characterized, but include obesity, excessive consumption of red meat, physical inactivity, and vitamin D deficiency.[101] Because many of these factors converge on insulin signaling, some experts propose that insulin and insulinlike growth factors play a seminal role in CRCs.[102] However, three of every four CRCs arise in individuals lacking a well-defined risk factor, and it is unknown to what extent particular genotypes confer sensitivity to environmental variables.

The cancer spectrum in HNPCC or PPAP and the particular predilection for CRC remain unexplained. Colonic, endometrial, and selected other epithelia may be especially sensitive to the kind of mutations that occur in the setting of defective DNA mismatch and base-excision repair, loss of wild-type tumor suppressor alleles may occur more readily in these tissues, or they may lack repair safeguards that protect other cell types.

Insights from Genomewide Association Studies

The quarter or more of sporadic CRC cases with a familial component[103,104] probably have diverse molecular etiologies, with low risk conferred by some common genetic variants and interaction of individual risk alleles with other genes and with environmental factors. Large multinational GWA studies have interrogated thousands of genomes and, to date, have uncovered statistical association of CRC risk with at least 20 distinct loci, including those linked to single nucleotide polymorphisms (SNPs) rs6983267 at 8q24.21, rs4939827 on 18q21, and rs3802842 at 11q23 (Table 48.3). The frequency of risk alleles ranges from less than 10% to half or more of the human population and each one elevates CRC risk no more than 7% to 25% above the background in persons with the nonrisk allele.[105,106] Even if homozygosity at some loci and additive effects compound this risk, allele frequencies are such that the cumulative risk rises no more than 50% to 250% over the background. As a result, the total effect of all identified risk variants explains, at most, 5% to 7% of cases with a family history; it is not presently feasible to predict an individual's precise risk or modify screening recommendations on the basis of known genotypes. Nevertheless, the identification of risk loci is a crucial advance for an eventually thorough understanding of disease determinants.

The specific causal significance of most of these DNA sequence variants is unclear and many localize far from coding genes, with growing evidence that they correspond to regulatory regions for control of nearby genes. This implies that an altered expression of the linked genes either transforms normal colonocytes at low frequency or, more likely, influences the oncogenic potential of other events. Particularly strong association occurs with the SNP rs6983267 at 8q24.21, which lies in a gene desert near low-risk susceptibility alleles for breast and prostate cancers. Molecular studies indicate that each culpable region acts as a tissue-specific enhancer controlling the nearest gene, *CMYC,*[107–109] thereby modulating disease risk.[110] Attesting to the role of TGF-β signaling in colonic epithelial homeostasis, risk alleles on chromosomes 18q21 and 14q22 are linked to *SMAD7* and *BMP4,* respectively.[111,112] Some genes near risk variants are not expressed in the colonic mucosa, suggesting a role for extraepithelial genetic effects from stromal or immune cells. In summary, at least 20 common polymorphisms elevate CRC risk modestly and with sufficiently low penetrance that effect detection requires large population-based analyses. The pathophysiologic functions of these loci will likely inform future prevention and screening strategies and help determine how risk alleles interact with environmental factors.

ONCOGENE AND TUMOR SUPPRESSOR GENE MUTATIONS IN COLORECTAL CANCER PROGRESSION

Building on the foundation of lost gatekeeper functions in Wnt signaling, somatic mutations in oncogenes and tumor suppressor

TABLE 48.3

Single Nucleotide Polymorphisms Conferring Increased Risk of Colorectal Cancer

Chromosomal Location	Imputed SNP (Risk Allele)	Nearest Gene	Risk Allele Frequency in Controls	Odds Ratio, 95% CI	P Value
18q21.1	rs4939827 (T)	SMAD7	0.53	1.16–1.24	8×10^{-28}
8q23.3	rs16892766 (C)	EIF3H	0.07	1.20–1.34	3×10^{-18}
8q24.21	rs6983267 (G)	MYC	0.49	1.16–1.39	1×10^{-14}
10p14	rs10795668 (A)		0.48	1.10–1.16	3×10^{-13}
6p21	rs1321311 (A)	CDKN1A	0.25	1.07–1.13	1×10^{-10}
20p12.3	rs961253 (A)		0.36	1.08–1.16	2×10^{-10}
11q13.4	rs3824999 (C)	POLD3	0.51	1.05–1.10	4×10^{-10}
11q23.1	rs3802842 (C)	C11orf93	0.29	1.08–1.15	6×10^{-10}
Xp22.2	rs5934683 (T)	SHROOM2	0.38	1.04–1.10	7×10^{-10}
14q22.2	rs4444235 (C)	BMP4	0.46	1.08–1.15	8×10^{-10}
19q13.11	rs10411210 (C)	RHPN2	0.90	1.10–1.20	5×10^{-9}
16q22.1	rs9929218 (G)	CDH1	0.29	1.06–1.12	1×10^{-8}
15q13.3	rs4779584 (T)	GREM1	0.19	1.14–1.34	5×10^{-7}
1q41	rs6691170 (T)		0.35	1.13	
20q13.33	rs4925386 (C)	LAMA5	0.68	1.11	
12q13.3	rs11169552 (C)		0.72	1.12	
3q26.2	rs10936599 (C)	MYNN	0.76	1.07	

CI, confidence interval.

genes cumulatively confer malignant properties. The particular spectrum of recurring mutations in CRC provides a framework to decipher the oncogenic signaling circuits and develop rational targeted drugs (Table 48.4). The high collective frequency of recurrent *KRAS*, *BRAF*, and *PIK3CA* mutations places EGFR and downstream extracellular signal-regulated kinase (ERK, also known as mitogen-activated protein kinase [MAPK]) signaling at the center of research and therapeutic efforts.

The *KRAS*, *BRAF*, and *PIK3CA* Oncogenes

Ras-family G-proteins transduce growth factor signals and are aberrantly activated in a wide variety of cancers. *KRAS* is mutated in about 40% of CRCs[113] and *NRAS* in another 5% to 8% of cases. Mutations in both genes cluster in codons 12 or 13, and less frequently at codon 61. *KRAS* mutations appear even in lesions of low malignant potential, such as aberrant crypt foci lacking dysplasia,[114] and certainly in small polyps, although their frequency increases with lesion size.[115] A *KRAS* mutation is not required to initiate adenomas, but contributes to disease progression when combined with other genetic alterations, and specific interference with mutant *KRAS* in CRC cells and xenografts impedes cell growth.[116,117] Among the many different growth factor receptor signals that KRAS transduces in diverse cells, its activity in the colonic epithelium and CRC is particularly related to EGFR signaling, which is important for two reasons. First, inasmuch as Wnt and EGFR signaling drive normal gut epithelial turnover, CRC appears to subvert tissue-specific homeostatic circuits. Second, because a *KRAS* mutation introduces intracellular defects that lock EGFR signaling in the "on" state, EGFR antibodies are ineffective in this subset of CRCs[8] and targeted therapies will need to interfere further downstream in the signaling pathway.

Because KRAS acts early in transducing signals from EGFR and other receptor tyrosine kinases, *KRAS* mutations can potentially deregulate several effector pathways for cell survival, proliferation, invasion, and metastasis (Fig. 48.3). Constitutive phosphorylation of ERKs accompanies *KRAS* mutation, reflecting the activation of the ERK/MAPK pathway.[118] KRAS-mediated growth factor signaling recruits RAF kinases to the plasma membrane and triggers MEK1 and MEK2 kinases to activate ERK1 and ERK2, which in turn phosphorylate proteins that control the G_1–S cell cycle transition, among other substrates.[119] Although other, non–KRAS-mediated growth factor pathways also activate the MAPK cascade, signaling in CRC is most often deregulated through activating mutations in *KRAS* or *BRAF*. *BRAF* is mutated in about 10% of CRCs, especially those associated with MSI and CIMP.[120,121] The most common *BRAF* mutation in CRCs, melanoma, and selected other cancers, *V600E*, affects a residue within the activation loop of the kinase domain and constitutively activates kinase function, probably by several hundred-fold and acting as a phosphomimetic.[122] Like mutant KRAS, activated BRAF also phosphorylates ERKs, lifting intrinsic restraints on cell growth. Indeed, *KRAS*, *NRAS*, and *BRAF* mutations are mutually exclusive in CRCs,[26,120] highlighting their actions in a common cellular pathway and reflecting alternative routes to the same end.

Several features of *BRAF*-mutant CRCs are noteworthy. First, the defect confers a worse prognosis than *KRAS* mutations in advanced disease,[9,123] which indicates distinctive molecular or cellular features. Second, the *BRAF* mutation is a hallmark of nonfamilial MSI-hi CRC and occurs early in the natural history of sessile serrated adenomas.[121] Third, whereas forced *Kras* activation in the mouse intestine has a modest independent consequence,[124,125] *Braf*V600E expression rapidly induces persistent generalized hyperplasia with a high penetrance of crypt dysplasia, serrated morphology, and MSI-hi invasive cancers that show Wnt pathway activation.[126] Fourth, tumors mutant for either KRAS or BRAF intrinsically resist treatment with EGFR antibodies.[9,123] Fifth, *BRAF*V600E mutant melanomas initially respond to selective,

CANCERS OF THE GASTROINTESTINAL TRACT

Recurrent Somatic Gene Mutations in Human Colorectal Cancers

Gene	Frequency	CRC Class	Known Cellular or Oncogenic Function
Oncogenes			
KRAS	35%–40%	CIN	RTK signaling
PIK3CA	18%–20%	Mostly CIN	RTK signaling
BRAF	7%–15%	MSI-hi, CIMP	RTK signaling
NRAS	9%	CIN	RTK signaling
ERBB3	~8%	CIN	RTK signaling
CTNNB1	~5%	All	Wnt pathway activation
Tumor Suppressor Genes			
APC	85%	All	Wnt pathway inactivation
TP53	50%	CIN predominant	Stress, hypoxia response; DNA replication
SMAD4	10%	CIN	
FBXW7	10%	CIN	
SOX9	5%	CIN	Wnt-dependent ISC function
ACVR2A		MSI-hi	Wnt pathway activity
TGFBR2		MSI-hi	TGF-β signaling
MSH3		MSI-hi	DNA mismatch repair
MSH6		MSI-hi	DNA mismatch repair
POLE		Hypermutated (non-MSI)	DNA polymerase ε
Epigenetic Modifier Genes (Roles Are Emerging)			
ARID1A		MSI-hi	Chromatin remodeling
SIN3A			Transcriptional repression
SMARCA5			Chromatin remodeling
NCOR1			Transcriptional repression
JARID2			Histone modification
TET1, 2, 3			DNA demethylation

RTK, receptor tyrosine kinase; ISC, intestinal stem cell.

ATP-competitive BRAF inhibitors such as vemurafenib and take months to manifest secondary resistance,[127] whereas *BRAFV600E* mutant CRCs are intrinsically resistant and barely respond to the same agents. This is because BRAF inhibition in CRC quickly induces feedback EGFR signaling through KRAS and CRAF, restoring stimuli for cell replication (melanoma cells hardly express EGFR and therefore avoid this feedback activation).[128,129] Because BRAF inhibition renders cells newly sensitive to direct antagonism of EGFR, a combined antagonism of BRAF and EGFR signaling may be beneficial.

KRAS signals are transduced not only through ERKs, but also through phosphatidylinositol (PI) 3-kinase (PI3K),[118,130] which phosphorylates the intracellular lipid PI-4,5-bisphosphate at the three position, triggering a cascade that promotes cell survival and growth.[131] Up to 20% of CRCs carry activating mutations in *PIK3CA*, the gene encoding the catalytic p110 subunit of PI3K. Mutations cluster in exons 9 and 20 and seem to arise late in the adenoma–carcinoma sequence, possibly coincident with invasion[132]; many fewer CRCs carry related *PIK3R1* mutations. Cellular PI3K activity is countered by the product of the *PTEN* gene, which is inactivated (usually by deletion) in another 10% of cases. Although both PI3K and BRAF act downstream of KRAS, only *BRAF* and *KRAS* mutations are mutually exclusive; up to one-fifth of *KRAS*-mutant CRCs also have *PIK3CA* mutations, implying that these oncogenes are not trivially redundant. One reason could

be that mutant KRAS activates PI3K signaling inefficiently.[133] More likely, oncogenic signaling pathways are less strictly linear than is convenient to depict. Indeed, seemingly parallel streams of KRAS signaling through RAF–MEK and PI3K (see Fig. 48.3) interact extensively with one another and both streams feed into the mTOR, which coordinates cell growth with nutrient responses.[134] Lastly, insulinlike growth factor 2 (IGF2) is overexpressed in at least 15% of CRCs as a result of focal gene amplifications, loss of imprinting, and other mechanisms.[26] Overexpression of *IGF2* and its downstream effector IRS2 is mutually exclusive with *PIK3CA* mutations and *PTEN* deletions, strongly implying that the underlying genetic aberrations represent alternative means to disrupt the same signaling circuit.

MYC, CDK8, and Control of Cell Growth and Metabolism

Although the *MYC* and *CDK8* oncogenes are rarely mutated in CRC, considerable gene amplification is seen in at least 10% of cases, with moderate increases in copy number and expression in up to 25% of cases.[26,135] Aberrant *MYC* gene regulation likely explains the significant GWA studies risk allele rs6983267 and MYC expression is not only a prominent outcome of Wnt signaling,[49] but may account for the bulk of the tumor effect in *Apc*-mutant

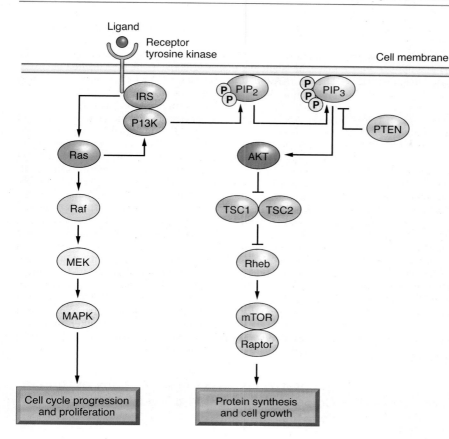

Figure 48.3 Signaling pathways, oncogenic mutations, and therapeutic opportunities in CRC. It is instructive to consider common genetic alterations in CRC in light of a common canonical outline of signaling through receptor tyrosine kinases, among which the EGFR is a prime example. *KRAS*, the oncogene mutated in up to 40% of CRCs, signals receptor activation through RAF proteins (including BRAF, which is mutated in 5% to 8% of CRCs) and phosphatidylinositol 3-kinase (PI3K), whose catalytic PIK3CA subunit is mutated in 15% to 20% of CRCs. These transducers in turn activate the intracellular mitogen-activated protein kinase and AKT or mTOR pathways, respectively. Hence, common mutations confer growth factor independence on cells, resulting in dysregulated proliferation, protein synthesis, and metabolism. They also represent promising targets for therapeutic interference with aberrantly activated signaling cascades.

mouse intestines.[54] CDK8, a cyclin-dependent kinase component of the Mediator complex, couples transcription factors to the basal transcriptional machinery and hence resembles MYC in regulating thousands of genes, including those necessary for cellular metabolism, proliferation, and self-renewal. CDK8 activity in CRC is particularly associated with β-catenin.[135] Indeed, although *APC*, *CTNNB1*, and probably *RSPO* mutations kick start colonic adenomas, additional genetic events in CRC potentiate Wnt activity. Disrupting this seminally important pathway and/or its downstream effector MYC may therefore be imperative in CRC therapy, but poses formidable challenges, in part because that requires interfering with protein–protein interactions downstream of conventional druggable nodes.[136]

TP53 and Other Tumor Suppressors

The allelic loss of chromosome 17p is observed in three of every four CRCs but <10% of adenomatous polyps.[115] The remaining *TP53* allele is inactivated in most tumors with 17p loss of heterozygosity (LOH), most often at codons 175, 245, 248, 273, or 282.[137] *TP53* mutations, found in half of all CRCs and LOH of 17p thus appear to arise late in the transition from adenoma to carcinoma, possibly facilitating progression. Cells with an intact *TP53* function undergo cell cycle arrest and apoptosis when faced with stress from DNA damage, hypoxia, reduced nutrient access, or aneuploidy. *TP53* loss may allow cells to overcome these barriers to tumor survival and progression, but confers no specific disease features in CRCs.

LOH of chromosome 18q, which is rare in small to midsize adenomas, is observed in >60% of CRCs and nearly all liver metastases from MSS tumors.[138] This sequence implicates loss of resident genes in disease progression, but 18q LOH does not by itself confer a poor prognosis.[139] The minimal common region of LOH contains two candidate tumor suppressor genes[140]: *SMAD4* (*DPC4*) in about one-third of cases and *DCC* (deleted in

colorectal cancer, a receptor for Netrin axonal guidance proteins) in the rest. *SMAD4/DPC4* and *SMAD2* are positive and negative regulators of TGF-β signaling, respectively, and closely linked on 18q. Somatic *SMAD4* mutations are present in 10% to 15% of CRCs with LOH, and germ-line mutations are noted in some FJP kindreds[141]; *SMAD2* and *DCC* are rarely mutated in CRC,[142] but *DCC* mRNA and protein are lost in >50% of cases.[143] Together, these findings suggest a complex, multifactorial basis for the selection of 18q LOH in CRC.

FBXW7 (F-box and WD40 repeat domain containing 7), another gene frequently inactivated in CRCs, encodes a receptor subunit of Skp, Cullin, F-box-containing (SCF)-E3 ubiquitin ligase complexes, which target multiple regulators of cell growth, such as MYC and JUN transcription factors, for degradation. Monoallelic missense mutations tend to cluster in arginine residues within a β-propeller domain that recognizes specific substrates, including NOTCH, JUN, DEK, and TGIF1 in intestinal cells.[144,145]

THE MUTATIONAL LANDSCAPE OF COLORECTAL CANCER

Early analyses of protein-coding genes in a few CRCs produced average estimates of 81 mutations per tumor and spawned the useful idea that the mutational landscape of CRC contains few mountains (genes such as *APC*, *KRAS*, *TP53*, and *PIK3CA*, with frequent mutations) or hills (less frequent but functional mutations [e.g., *BRAF*^{V600E}]).[146] Although many additional events are individually infrequent and may contribute to neoplasia sporadically or represent *passenger* mutations, they tend to congregate in genes that control cell adhesion, signaling, DNA topology, and the cell cycle.[147] In general, CRCs show a genomewide bias toward C:G to T:A transitions at 5′-CpG-3′ sites and a lower frequency of mutations in 5′-TpC-3′ dinucleotides than observed, for example, in breast cancer.[146] Such findings may eventually link specific environmental factors to characteristic mutational spectra. Moreover, an average of 17 genes are deleted or amplified to 12 or more copies per CRC cell,[148] and the oncogenes *ERBB2, MYC, KRAS, MYB, IGF2, CCND1,* and *CDK8* are in aggregate amplified or overexpressed in most cases, usually together with neighboring genes. Nearly half the copy number alterations—28 amplifications and 22 deletions, including 15 recurrent changes encompassing <12 genes—identified in one study[149] also appear in other cancers. CRCs thus reflect the perturbation of selected pathways of replicative and tissue homeostasis, some in common with most cancers and others restricted to CRCs.

Detailed data from two genome-scale studies of nearly 300 CRCs and matched normal tissue corroborate these general observations and provide reliable catalogs of genetic alterations.[26,41] These comprehensive efforts revealed *RSPO* gene fusions and up to 10% incidence of monoallelic missense mutations in *SOX9*, a transcription factor target of Wnt signaling that is highly expressed and active in intestinal crypt stem and progenitor cells.[150] Additionally, MSI-hi tumors showed frequent mutations in the *ARID1A* chromatin remodeling factor gene, which may affect a broad swath of other genes. An updated, partial list of recurrent genetic alterations in CRC (see Table 48.4) indicates that few new mutations fall in genes that appeal to the pharmaceutical industry, such as tyrosine or serine/threonine kinases.

Prognostic and Predictive Value of Molecular Properties and Tumor Genotypes

These specific genetic alterations might confer particular clinical behaviors, prognoses, or drug responses. Mutational, chromosome structural, and gene expression profiles are virtually identical in colonic and rectal adenocarcinomas. Aneuploidy and tetraploidy confer a worse prognosis than MSI-hi status in early-stage disease,[151] and the benefits of adjuvant 5-fluorouracil therapy may be restricted to patients with MSS tumors.[152,153] Because nearly all CRCs have a constitutive Wnt pathway activity, this element alone has limited prognostic value and outcomes seem unaffected by whether *APC* or *CTNNB1* mutations stimulate the pathway. The presence of *KRAS* or *BRAF* mutations and possibly also *PIK3CA* mutation or loss of PTEN expression predicts a lack of response to EGFR monoclonal antibodies.[8,154] These are important observations because they direct treatment decisions and because, unlike leukemias or breast cancer, CRCs had previously resisted subgrouping on the basis of specific gene alterations. For example, mutations in the two most frequently affected oncogenes, *KRAS* or *PIK3CA*, seem not to impact survival in stage III or stage IV disease treated with chemotherapy,[9,155] although they will likely predict responses to new agents that target MEK or PI3 kinase signaling, respectively. Patients with metastatic *BRAF*-mutant CRC have especially low survival and respond poorly to current chemotherapy regimens, including adjuvant fluoropyrimidines in stage III disease.[9,156]

AN INTEGRATED MODEL FOR COLORECTAL CANCER INITIATION AND PROGRESSION

Intensive molecular investigation has informed our understanding of CRC for more than 2 decades, with crucial independent contributions from delineation of the adenoma–carcinoma sequence, uncommon familial syndromes, the Wnt–Rspo–β-catenin pathway, and EGFR signaling through the KRAS–BRAF–ERK and PIK3CA–AKT–mTOR pathways. Together with whole-genome analyses of CRC and refined investigation of intestinal crypt biology in animals, a large corpus of knowledge now permits a coherent model of disease initiation and advance.

Animal Models of Colorectal Cancer Genetics

Similar intestinal cell properties and genetics in humans and mice make the laboratory mouse valuable in the investigation of CRCs. The *multiple intestinal neoplasia* (*Min*) strain has a truncating mutation in *Apc* and phenocopies human FAP with respect to intestinal adenomas,[157] although tumors form mainly in the small bowel. *Apc*[Min] mice are a cornerstone for the genetic analysis of intestinal polyps and deregulated Wnt signaling, but other *Apc* mutants also have value. A *D716* allele increases the number of adenomas, all with loss of the wild-type copy,[158] whereas a larger fraction of *Apc*[1638N] adenomas appear in the colon[159]; *Apc*[Pirc] rats carry a stop codon at position 1137 and more than half the tumors arise in the colon.[160] Deletion of the N-terminal degradation domain of murine β-catenin also stabilizes the protein and induces widespread intestinal polyposis.[161] Expression of activated *Kras* alleles in the intestinal epithelium of otherwise intact mice barely affects cell signaling or proliferation, but similar to human CRCs, expression on *Apc* mutant backgrounds expands progenitor cell numbers and hastens adenoma progression.[124,125] In contrast, activated *Braf* induces crypt hyperplasia, followed by invasive cancers with deregulated Wnt and ERK signaling.[126] The inactivation of murine genes for DNA MMR[162] leads to more lymphomas than intestinal tumors, with some mutants showing neither but revealing roles in meiosis; MMR is nevertheless necessary for protecting cells from mutation and malignancy.

Integrated Insights from the Study of Human Colorectal Cancers and Mouse Intestinal Crypts

Animal studies strongly suggest that CRCs originate in resident intestinal epithelial stem cells.[50] These cells, characterized mainly in the mouse small bowel, replicate frequently and neutral drift ensures that each normal crypt contains a monoclonal population of five to eight functional stem cells.[163,164] Gatekeeper mutations in *APC* or *CTNNB1* in one such cell induce constitutive Wnt pathway activity; the attendant growth advantage allows this mutant stem cell to dominate that crypt and eventually take hold as a monoclonal population. Notably, the outcome of this stochastic process is not inevitable: Neutral drift permits either wild-type or *APC*-mutant cells to replace each other quite rapidly, but a selective advantage in the latter gives them a demonstrable edge over their wild-type siblings.[165] Once a mutant stem cell clone is established, with no competing wild-type cells remaining in that crypt, it can flourish indefinitely and accumulate mutations as they occur, by chance or by virtue of a hypermutable state, so long as a mutation is not lethal or severely detrimental. Again, the outcome is not inevitable: Few polyps advance into carcinomas and others may even regress. Eventually, various combinations of mutations that co-opt existing signaling circuits confer invasive properties on a fraction of adenomas. Indeed, the bulk of observed mutations represent alternative means to dysregulate the same few pathways—Wnt, EGFR, TGF-β, IGF2, and PI3K—that control normal colonic cell turnover. Therefore, although specific genes, such as *BRAF* and *PIK3CA*, represent obvious targets for molecular therapy, it may be more useful in the long run to consider CRCs with broad respect to the pathways in which commonly mutated genes operate.

SUMMARY

The adenoma–carcinoma sequence represents the overt pathologic manifestation of sequential genetic alterations that promote cell growth, survival, and invasion. Molecular genetic studies have revealed crucial underlying mutations and the contribution of specific defects toward CRC pathogenesis. Colonic adenomas begin with deregulated Wnt signaling and this pathway's functions in intestinal crypt homeostasis lead us to interpret cancer in relation to pools of normal tissue stem cells. MSI-hi distinguishes CRCs that arise in the setting of HNPCC and about 15% of sporadic cases from the larger fraction of cases with CIN, leading to a molecular classification into at least three disease subgroups with distinctive features, natural histories, and treatment considerations. Somatic mutations associated with tumor progression involve a small selection of signaling and homeostatic pathways, revealing candidate therapeutic targets. Further work on the biologic functions of inherited and somatic mutations will help design novel, rational, and targeted therapies. Much also remains unknown about how environmental factors impinge on the implicated key pathways to modulate CRC risk and about specific interventions to prevent a cancer whose incidence and lethality in developed countries is second only to lung cancer.

REFERENCES

1. Levin B, Lieberman DA, McFarland B, et al. Screening and surveillance for the early detection of colorectal cancer and adenomatous polyps, 2008: a joint guideline from the American Cancer Society, the US Multi-Society Task Force on Colorectal Cancer, and the American College of Radiology. *Gastroenterology* 2008;134:1570–1595.
2. Winawer SJ, Zauber AG, O'Brien MJ, et al. The National Polyp Study. Design, methods, and characteristics of patients with newly diagnosed polyps. The National Polyp Study Workgroup. *Cancer* 1992;70:1236–1245.
3. Jones S, Chen WD, Parmigiani G, et al. Comparative lesion sequencing provides insights into tumor evolution. *Proc Natl Acad Sci USA* 2008;105:4283–4288.
4. East JE, Saunders BP, Jass JR. Sporadic and syndromic hyperplastic polyps and serrated adenomas of the colon: classification, molecular genetics, natural history, and clinical management. *Gastroenterol Clin North Am* 2008;37:25–46.
5. Noffsinger AE. Serrated polyps and colorectal cancer: new pathway to malignancy. *Annu Rev Pathol* 2009;4:343–364.
6. Leggett B, Whitehall V. Role of the serrated pathway in colorectal cancer pathogenesis. *Gastroenterology* 2010;138:2088–2100.
7. Hanahan D, Weinberg RA. Hallmarks of cancer: the next generation. *Cell* 2011;144:646–674.
8. Van Cutsem E, Köhne CH, Hitre E, et al. Cetuximab and chemotherapy as initial treatment for metastatic colorectal cancer. *N Engl J Med* 2009;360:1408–1417.
9. Souglakos J, Philips J, Wang R, et al. Prognostic and predictive value of common mutations for treatment response and survival in patients with metastatic colorectal cancer. *Br J Cancer* 2009;101:465–472.
10. Pino MS, Chung DC. The chromosomal instability pathway in colon cancer. *Gastroenterology* 2010;138:2059–2072.
11. Baker DJ, Jin F, Jeganathan KB, et al. Whole chromosome instability caused by Bub1 insufficiency drives tumorigenesis through tumor suppressor gene loss of heterozygosity. *Cancer Cell* 2009;16:475–486.
12. Bardi G, Fenger C, Johansson B, et al. Tumor karyotype predicts clinical outcome in colorectal cancer patients. *J Clin Oncol* 2004;22:2623–2634.
13. Ionov Y, Peinado MA, Malkhosyan S, et al. Ubiquitous somatic mutations in simple repeated sequences reveal a new mechanism for colonic carcinogenesis. *Nature* 1993;363:558–561.
14. Spring KJ, Zhao ZZ, Karamatic R, et al. High prevalence of sessile serrated adenomas with BRAF mutations: a prospective study of patients undergoing colonoscopy. *Gastroenterology* 2006;131:1400–1407.
15. Plass C, Pfister SM, Lindroth AM, et al. Mutations in regulators of the epigenome and their connections to global chromatin patterns in cancer. *Nat Rev Genet* 2013;14:765–780.
16. Goelz SE, Vogelstein B, Hamilton SR, et al. Hypomethylation of DNA from benign and malignant human colon neoplasms. *Science* 1985;228:187–190.
17. Feinberg AP, Gehrke CW, Kuo KC, et al. Reduced genomic 5-methylcytosine content in human colonic neoplasia. *Cancer Res* 1988;48:1159–1161.
18. Cui H, Cruz-Correa M, Giardiello FM, et al. Loss of IGF2 imprinting: a potential marker of colorectal cancer risk. *Science* 2003;299:1753–1755.
19. Eden A, Gaudet F, Waghmare A, et al. Chromosomal instability and tumors promoted by DNA hypomethylation. *Science* 2003;300:455.
20. Lin H, Yamada Y, Nguyen S, et al. Suppression of intestinal neoplasia by deletion of Dnmt3b. *Mol Cell Biol* 2006;26:2976–2983.
21. Linhart HG, Lin H, Yamada Y, et al. Dnmt3b promotes tumorigenesis in vivo by gene-specific de novo methylation and transcriptional silencing. *Genes Dev* 2007;21:3110–3122.
22. Toyota M, Ahuja N, Ohe-Toyota M, et al. CpG island methylator phenotype in colorectal cancer. *Proc Natl Acad Sci U S A* 1999;96:8681–8686.
23. Suzuki H, Watkins DN, Jair KW, et al. Epigenetic inactivation of SFRP genes allows constitutive WNT signaling in colorectal cancer. *Nat Genet* 2004;36:417–422.
24. Xu Y, Hu B, Choi AJ, et al. Unique DNA methylome profiles in CpG island methylator phenotype colon cancers. *Genome Res* 2012;22:283–291.
25. Hinoue T, Weisenberger DJ, Lange CP, et al. Genome-scale analysis of aberrant DNA methylation in colorectal cancer. *Genome Res* 2012;22:271–282.
26. Cancer Genome Atlas Network. Comprehensive molecular characterization of human colon and rectal cancer. *Nature* 2012;487:330–337.
27. Jess T, Loftus EV Jr, Velayos FS, et al. Risk of intestinal cancer in inflammatory bowel disease: a population-based study from olmsted county, Minnesota. *Gastroenterology* 2006;130:1039–1046.
28. Hussain SP, Amstad P, Raja K, et al. Increased p53 mutation load in noncancerous colon tissue from ulcerative colitis: a cancer-prone chronic inflammatory disease. *Cancer Res* 2000;60:3333–3337.
29. Hsieh CJ, Klump B, Holzmann K, et al. Hypermethylation of the p16INK4a promoter in colectomy specimens of patients with long-standing and extensive ulcerative colitis. *Cancer Res* 1998;58:3942–3945.
30. Gardner EJ. A genetic and clinical study of intestinal polyposis, a predisposing factor for carcinoma of the colon and rectum. *Am J Hum Genet* 1951;3:167–176.
31. Hamilton SR, Liu B, Parsons RE, et al. The molecular basis of Turcot's syndrome. *N Engl J Med* 1995;332:839–847.
32. Parc Y, Piquard A, Dozois RR, et al. Long-term outcome of familial adenomatous polyposis patients after restorative coloproctectomy. *Ann Surg* 2004;239:378–382.
33. Miyoshi Y, Nagase H, Ando H, et al. Somatic mutations of the APC gene in colorectal tumors: mutation cluster region in the APC gene. *Hum Mol Genet* 1992;1:229–233.
34. Spirio L, Olschwang S, Groden J, et al. Alleles of the APC gene: an attenuated form of familial polyposis. *Cell* 1993;75:951–957.
35. Laken SJ, Petersen GM, Gruber SB, et al. Familial colorectal cancer in Ashkenazim due to a hypermutable tract in APC. *Nat Genet* 1997;17:79–83.
36. Smalley WE, DuBois RN. Colorectal cancer and nonsteroidal anti-inflammatory drugs. *Adv Pharmacol* 1997;39:1–20.
37. Powell SM, Zilz N, Beazer-Barclay Y, et al. APC mutations occur early during colorectal tumorigenesis. *Nature* 1992;359:235–237.
38. Hadjihannas MV, Brückner M, Jerchow B, et al. Aberrant Wnt/beta-catenin signaling can induce chromosomal instability in colon cancer. *Proc Natl Acad Sci U S A* 2006;103:10747–10752.
39. Morin PJ, Sparks AB, Korinek V, et al. Activation of beta-catenin-Tcf signaling in colon cancer by mutations in beta-catenin or APC. *Science* 1997;275:1787–1790.
40. Sparks AB, Morin PJ, Vogelstein B, et al. Mutational analysis of the APC/beta-catenin/Tcf pathway in colorectal cancer. *Cancer Res* 1998;58:1130–1134.
41. Seshagiri S, Stawiski EW, Durinck S, et al. Recurrent R-spondin fusions in colon cancer. *Nature* 2012;488:660–664.
42. Sansom OJ, Reed KR, Hayes AJ, et al. Loss of Apc in vivo immediately perturbs Wnt signaling, differentiation, and migration. *Genes Dev* 2004;18:1385–1390.
43. Carmon KS, Gong X, Lin Q, et al. R-spondins function as ligands of the orphan receptors LGR4 and LGR5 to regulate Wnt/beta-catenin signaling. *Proc Natl Acad Sci U S A* 2011;108:11452–11457.
44. de Lau W, Barker N, Low TY, et al. Lgr5 homologues associate with Wnt receptors and mediate R-spondin signalling. *Nature* 2011;476:293–297.
45. Korinek V, Barker N, Moerer P, et al. Depletion of epithelial stem-cell compartments in the small intestine of mice lacking Tcf-4. *Nat Genet* 1998;19:379–383.
46. Roose J, Clevers H. TCF transcription factors: molecular switches in carcinogenesis. *Biochim Biophys Acta* 1999;1424:M23–M37.
47. Liu W, Dong X, Mai M, et al. Mutations in AXIN2 cause colorectal cancer with defective mismatch repair by activating beta-catenin/TCF signalling. *Nat Genet* 2000;26:146–147.
48. Bass AJ, Lawrence MS, Brace LE, et al. Genomic sequencing of colorectal adenocarcinomas identifies a recurrent VTI1A-TCF7L2 fusion. *Nat Genet* 2011;43:964–968.
49. van de Wetering M, Sancho E, Verweij C, et al. The beta-catenin/TCF-4 complex imposes a crypt progenitor phenotype on colorectal cancer cells. *Cell* 2002;111:241–250.
50. Barker N, Ridgway RA, van Es JH, et al. Crypt stem cells as the cells-of-origin of intestinal cancer. *Nature* 2009;457:608–611.
51. van der Flier LG, van Gijn ME, Hatzis P, et al. Transcription factor achaete scute-like 2 controls intestinal stem cell fate. *Cell* 2009;136:903–912.
52. Zeilstra J, Joosten SP, Dokter M, et al. Deletion of the WNT target and cancer stem cell marker CD44 in Apc(Min/+) mice attenuates intestinal tumorigenesis. *Cancer Res* 2008;68:3655–3661.
53. He TC, Sparks AB, Rago C, et al. Identification of c-MYC as a target of the APC pathway. *Science* 1998;281:1509–1512.
54. Sansom OJ, Meniel VS, Muncan V, et al. Myc deletion rescues Apc deficiency in the small intestine. *Nature* 2007;446:676–679.
55. Vasen HF, Watson P, Mecklin JP, et al. New clinical criteria for hereditary nonpolyposis colorectal cancer (HNPCC, Lynch syndrome) proposed by the International Collaborative group on HNPCC. *Gastroenterology* 1999;116:1453–1456.

CANCERS OF THE GASTROINTESTINAL TRACT

56. Watson P, Vasen HF, Mecklin JP, et al. The risk of extra-colonic, extra-endometrial cancer in the Lynch syndrome. *Int J Cancer* 2008;123:444–449.

57. Fishel R, Kolodner RD. Identification of mismatch repair genes and their role in the development of cancer. *Curr Opin Genet Dev* 1995;5:382–395.

58. Vasen HF, Boland CR. Progress in genetic testing, classification, and identification of Lynch syndrome. *JAMA* 2005;293:2028–2030.

59. Liu T, Yan H, Kuismanen S, et al. The role of hPMS1 and hPMS2 in predisposing to colorectal cancer. *Cancer Res* 2001;61:7798–7802.

60. Ligtenberg MJ, Kuiper RP, Chan TL, et al. Heritable somatic methylation and inactivation of MSH2 in families with Lynch syndrome due to deletion of the 3' exons of TACSTD1. *Nat Genet* 2009;41:112–117.

61. Kovacs ME, Papp J, Szentirmay Z, et al. Deletions removing the last exon of TACSTD1 constitute a distinct class of mutations predisposing to Lynch syndrome. *Hum Mutat* 2009;30:197–203.

62. Umar A, Boland CR, Terdiman JP, et al. Revised Bethesda Guidelines for hereditary nonpolyposis colorectal cancer (Lynch syndrome) and microsatellite instability. *J Natl Cancer Inst* 2004;96:261–268.

63. Pinol V, Castells A, Andreu M, et al. Accuracy of revised Bethesda guidelines, microsatellite instability, and immunohistochemistry for the identification of patients with hereditary nonpolyposis colorectal cancer. *JAMA* 2005; 293:1986–1994.

64. Hampel H, Frankel WL, Martin E, et al. Screening for the Lynch syndrome (hereditary nonpolyposis colorectal cancer). *N Engl J Med* 2005;352: 1851–1860.

65. Vasen HF, Blanco I, Aktan-Collan K, et al. Revised guidelines for the clinical management of Lynch syndrome (HNPCC): recommendations by a group of European experts. *Gut* 2013;62:812–823.

66. Balmana J, Stockwell DH, Steyerberg EW, et al. Prediction of MLH1 and MSH2 mutations in Lynch syndrome. *J Am Med Assoc* 2006;296: 1469–1478.

67. Dove-Edwin I, de Jong AE, Adams J, et al. Prospective results of surveillance colonoscopy in dominant familial colorectal cancer with and without Lynch syndrome. *Gastroenterology* 2006;130:1995–2000.

68. Markowitz S, Wang J, Myeroff L, et al. Inactivation of the type II TGF-beta receptor in colon cancer cells with microsatellite instability. *Science* 1995;268:1336–1338.

69. Grady WM, Myeroff LL, Swinler SE, et al. Mutational inactivation of transforming growth factor beta receptor type II in microsatellite stable colon cancers. *Cancer Res* 1999;59:320–324.

70. Rampino N, Yamamoto H, Ionov Y, et al. Somatic frameshift mutations in the BAX gene in colon cancers of the microsatellite mutator phenotype. *Science* 1997;275:967–969.

71. Duval A, Gayet J, Zhou XP, et al. Frequent frameshift mutations of the TCF-4 gene in colorectal cancers with microsatellite instability. *Cancer Res* 1999;59:4213–4215.

72. Yuan Z, Shin J, Wilson A, et al. An A13 repeat within the 3'-untranslated region of epidermal growth factor receptor (EGFR) is frequently mutated in microsatellite instability colon cancers and is associated with increased EGFR expression. *Cancer Res* 2009;69:7811–7818.

73. Huang J, Papadopoulos N, McKinley AJ, et al. APC mutations in colorectal tumors with mismatch repair deficiency. *Proc Natl Acad Sci U S A* 1996;93: 9049–9054.

74. Thibodeau SN, French AJ, Cunningham JM, et al. Microsatellite instability in colorectal cancer: different mutator phenotypes and the principal involvement of hMLH1. *Cancer Res* 1998;58:1713–1718.

75. Liu B, Nicolaides NC, Markowitz S, et al. Mismatch repair gene defects in sporadic colorectal cancers with microsatellite instability. *Nat Genet* 1995;9: 48–55.

76. Cunningham JM, Christensen ER, Tester DJ, et al. Hypermethylation of the hMLH1 promoter in colon cancer with microsatellite instability. *Cancer Res* 1998;58:3455–3460.

77. Kambara T, Simms LA, Whitehall VL, et al. BRAF mutation is associated with DNA methylation in serrated polyps and cancers of the colorectum. *Gut* 2004;53:1137–1144.

78. Weisenberger DJ, Siegmund KD, Campan M, et al. CpG island methylator phenotype underlies sporadic microsatellite instability and is tightly associated with BRAF mutation in colorectal cancer. *Nat Genet* 2006;38:787–793.

79. Sieber OM, Lipton L, Crabtree M, et al. Multiple colorectal adenomas, classic adenomatous polyposis, and germ-line mutations in MYH. *N Engl J Med* 2003;348:791–799.

80. Balaguer F, Castellvi-Bel S, Castells A, et al. Identification of MYH mutation carriers in colorectal cancer: a multicenter, case-control, population-based study. *Clin Gastroenterol Hepatol* 2007;5:379–387.

81. Palles C, Cazier JB, Howarth KM, et al. Germline mutations affecting the proofreading domains of POLE and POLD1 predispose to colorectal adenomas and carcinomas. *Nat Genet* 2013;45:136–144.

82. Giardiello FM, Hamilton SR, Kern SE, et al. Colorectal neoplasia in juvenile polyposis or juvenile polyps. *Arch Dis Child* 1991;66:971–975.

83. Jass JR, Williams CB, Bussey HJ, et al. Juvenile polyposis—a precancerous condition. *Histopathology* 1988;13:619–630.

84. Howe JR, Sayed MG, Ahmed AF, et al. The prevalence of MADH4 and BMPR1A mutations in juvenile polyposis and absence of BMPR2, BMPR1B, and ACVR1 mutations. *J Med Genet* 2004;41:484–491.

85. Sweet K, Willis J, Zhou XP, et al. Molecular classification of patients with unexplained hamartomatous and hyperplastic polyposis. *J Am Med Assoc* 2005;294:2465–2473.

86. Haramis AP, Begthel H, van den Born M, et al. De novo crypt formation and juvenile polyposis on BMP inhibition in mouse intestine. *Science* 2004;303:1684–1686.

87. He XC, Zhang J, Tong WG, et al. BMP signaling inhibits intestinal stem cell self-renewal through suppression of Wnt-beta-catenin signaling. *Nat Genet* 2004;36:1117–1121.

88. Batts LE, Polk DB, Dubois RN, et al. Bmp signaling is required for intestinal growth and morphogenesis. *Dev Dyn* 2006;235:1563–1570.

89. Kim BG, Li C, Qiao W, et al. Smad4 signalling in T cells is required for suppression of gastrointestinal cancer. *Nature* 2006;441:1015–1019.

90. Giardiello FM, Brensinger JD, Tersmette AC, et al. Very high risk of cancer in familial Peutz-Jeghers syndrome. *Gastroenterology* 2000;119:1447–1453.

91. Hemminki A, Markie D, Tomlinson I, et al. A serine/threonine kinase gene defective in Peutz-Jeghers syndrome. *Nature* 1998;391:184–187.

92. Hezel AF, Bardeesy N. LKB1; linking cell structure and tumor suppression. *Oncogene* 2008;27:6908–6919.

93. Shaw RJ, Bardeesy N, Manning BD, et al. The LKB1 tumor suppressor negatively regulates mTOR signaling. *Cancer Cell* 2004;6:91–99.

94. Whitelaw SC, Murday VA, Tomlinson IP, et al. Clinical and molecular features of the hereditary mixed polyposis syndrome. *Gastroenterology* 1997; 112:327–334.

95. Jaeger E, Leedham S, Lewis A, et al. Hereditary mixed polyposis syndrome is caused by a 40-kb upstream duplication that leads to increased and ectopic expression of the BMP antagonist GREM1. *Nat Genet* 2012;44:699–703.

96. Jaeger E, Webb E, Howarth K, et al. Common genetic variants at the CRAC1 (HMPS) locus on chromosome 15q13.3 influence colorectal cancer risk. *Nat Genet* 2008;40:26–28.

97. Rustgi AK. The genetics of hereditary colon cancer. *Genes Dev* 2007;21: 2525–2538.

98. Liaw D, Marsh DJ, Li J, et al. Germline mutations of the PTEN gene in Cowden disease, an inherited breast and thyroid cancer syndrome. *Nat Genet* 1997;16:64–67.

99. Maehama T, Dixon JE. The tumor suppressor, PTEN/MMAC1, dephosphorylates the lipid second messenger, phosphatidylinositol 3,4,5-trisphosphate. *J Biol Chem* 1998;273:13375–13378.

100. Goel A, Arnold CN, Niedzwiecki D, et al. Frequent inactivation of PTEN by promoter hypermethylation in microsatellite instability-high sporadic colorectal cancers. *Cancer Res* 2004;64:3014–3021.

101. Kim YS, Milner JA. Dietary modulation of colon cancer risk. *J Nutr* 2007; 137:2576S–2579S.

102. Slattery ML, Fitzpatrick FA. Convergence of hormones, inflammation, and energy-related factors: a novel pathway of cancer etiology. *Cancer Prev Res* 2009;2:922–930.

103. Cannon-Albright LA, Skolnick MH, Bishop DT, et al. Common inheritance of susceptibility to colonic adenomatous polyps and associated colorectal cancers. *N Engl J Med* 1988;319:533–537.

104. Johns LE, Houlston RS. A systematic review and meta-analysis of familial colorectal cancer risk. *Am J Gastroenterol* 2001;96:2992–3003.

105. Tomlinson I, Webb E, Carvajal-Carmona L, et al. A genome-wide association scan of tag SNPs identifies a susceptibility variant for colorectal cancer at 8q24.21. *Nat Genet* 2007;39:984–988.

106. Tenesa A, Farrington SM, Prendergast JG, et al. Genome-wide association scan identifies a colorectal cancer susceptibility locus on 11q23 and replicates risk loci at 8q24 and 18q21. *Nat Genet* 2008;40:631–637.

107. Pomerantz MM, Ahmadiyeh N, Jia L, et al. The 8q24 cancer risk variant rs6983267 shows long-range interaction with MYC in colorectal cancer. *Nat Genet* 2009;41:882–884.

108. Tuupanen S, Turunen M, Lehtonen R, et al. The common colorectal cancer predisposition SNP rs6983267 at chromosome 8q24 confers potential to enhanced Wnt signaling. *Nat Genet* 2009;41:885–890.

109. Ahmadiyeh N, Pomerantz MM, Grisanzio C, et al. 8q24 prostate, breast, and colon cancer risk loci show tissue-specific long-range interaction with MYC. *Proc Natl Acad Sci U S A* 2010;107:9742–9746.

110. Sur IK, Hallikas O, Vähärautio A, et al. Mice lacking a Myc enhancer that includes human SNP rs6983267 are resistant to intestinal tumors. *Science* 2012;338:1360–1363.

111. Broderick P, Carvajal-Carmona L, Pittman AM, et al. A genome-wide association study shows that common alleles of SMAD7 influence colorectal cancer risk. *Nat Genet* 2007;39:1315–1317.

112. Houlston RS, Webb E, Broderick P, et al. Meta-analysis of genome-wide association data identifies four new susceptibility loci for colorectal cancer. *Nat Genet* 2008;40:1426–1435.

113. Bos JL, Fearon ER, Hamilton SR, et al. Prevalence of ras gene mutations in human colorectal cancers. *Nature* 1987;327:293–297.

114. Pretlow TP. Aberrant crypt foci and K-ras mutations: earliest recognized players or innocent bystanders in colon carcinogenesis? *Gastroenterology* 1995;108:600–603.

115. Vogelstein B, Fearon ER, Hamilton SR, et al. Genetic alterations during colorectal-tumor development. *N Engl J Med* 1988;319:525–532.

116. Shirasawa S, Furuse M, Yokoyama N, et al. Altered growth of human colon cancer cell lines disrupted at activated Ki-ras. *Science* 1993;260:85–88.

117. Barbie DA, Tamayo P, Boehm JS, et al. Systematic RNA interference reveals that oncogenic KRAS-driven cancers require TBK1. *Nature* 2009;462:108–112.

118. Ebi H, Corcoran RB, Singh A, et al. Receptor tyrosine kinases exert dominant control over PI3K signaling in human KRAS mutant colorectal cancers. *J Clin Invest* 2011;121:4311–4321.

119. Downward J. Targeting RAS signalling pathways in cancer therapy. *Nat Rev Cancer* 2003;3:11–22.

120. Rajagopalan H, Bardelli A, Lengauer C, et al. Tumorigenesis: RAF/RAS oncogenes and mismatch-repair status. *Nature* 2002;418:934.

121. Tanaka H, Deng G, Matsuzaki K, et al. BRAF mutation, CpG island methylator phenotype and microsatellite instability occur more frequently and concordantly in mucinous than non-mucinous colorectal cancer. *Int J Cancer* 2006;118:2765–2771.

122. Davies H, Bignell GR, Cox C, et al. Mutations of the BRAF gene in human cancer. *Nature* 2002;417:949–954.

123. Di Nicolantonio F, Martini M, Molinari F, et al. Wild-type BRAF is required for response to panitumumab or cetuximab in metastatic colorectal cancer. *J Clin Oncol* 2008;26:5705–5712.

124. Sansom OJ, Meniel V, Wilkins JA, et al. Loss of Apc allows phenotypic manifestation of the transforming properties of an endogenous K-ras oncogene in vivo. *Proc Natl Acad Sci U S A* 2006;103:14122–14127.

125. Feng Y, Bommer GT, Zhao J, et al. Mutant KRAS promotes hyperplasia and alters differentiation in the colon epithelium but does not expand the presumptive stem cell pool. *Gastroenterology* 2011;141:1003–1013.e1–10.

126. Rad R, Cadinanos J, Rad L, et al. A genetic progression model of Braf(V600E)-induced intestinal tumorigenesis reveals targets for therapeutic intervention. *Cancer Cell* 2013;24:15–29.

127. Flaherty KT, Puzanov I, Kim KB, et al. Inhibition of mutated, activated BRAF in metastatic melanoma. *N Engl J Med* 2010;363:809–819.

128. Corcoran RB, Ebi H, Turke AB, et al. EGFR-mediated re-activation of MAPK signaling contributes to insensitivity of BRAF mutant colorectal cancers to RAF inhibition with vemurafenib. *Cancer Discov* 2012;2:227–235.

129. Prahallad A, Sun C, Huang S, et al. Unresponsiveness of colon cancer to BRAF(V600E) inhibition through feedback activation of EGFR. *Nature* 2012;483:100–103.

130. Gupta S, Ramjaun AR, Haiko P, et al. Binding of ras to phosphoinositide 3-kinase p110alpha is required for ras-driven tumorigenesis in mice. *Cell* 2007;129:957–968.

131. Cantley LC. The phosphoinositide 3-kinase pathway. *Science* 2002;296:1655–1657.

132. Samuels Y, Wang Z, Bardelli A, et al. High frequency of mutations of the PIK-3CA gene in human cancers. *Science* 2004;304:554.

133. Li W, Zhu T, Guan KL. Transformation potential of Ras isoforms correlates with activation of phosphatidylinositol 3-kinase but not ERK. *J Biol Chem* 2004;279:37398–37406.

134. Shaw RJ, Cantley LC. Ras, PI(3)K and mTOR signalling controls tumour cell growth. *Nature* 2006;441:424–430.

135. Firestein R, Bass AJ, Kim SY, et al. CDK8 is a colorectal cancer oncogene that regulates beta-catenin activity. *Nature* 2008;455:547–551.

136. Lepourcelet M, Chen YN, France DS, et al. Small-molecule antagonists of the oncogenic Tcf/beta-catenin protein complex. *Cancer Cell* 2004;5:91–102.

137. Baker SJ, Fearon ER, Nigro JM, et al. Chromosome 17 deletions and p53 gene mutations in colorectal carcinomas. *Science* 1989;244:217–221.

138. Vogelstein B, Fearon ER, Kern SE, et al. Allelotype of colorectal carcinomas. *Science* 1989;244:207–211.

139. Ogino S, Nosho K, Irahara N, et al. Prognostic significance and molecular associations of 18q loss of heterozygosity: a cohort study of microsatellite stable colorectal cancers. *J Clin Oncol* 2009;27:4591–4598.

140. Thiagalingam S, Lengauer C, Leach FS, et al. Evaluation of candidate tumour suppressor genes on chromosome 18 in colorectal cancers. *Nat Genet* 1996;13:343–346.

141. Howe JR, Roth S, Ringold JC, et al. Mutations in the SMAD4/DPC4 gene in juvenile polyposis. *Science* 1998;280:1086–1088.

142. Riggins GJ, Kinzler KW, Vogelstein B, Thiagalingam S. Frequency of Smad gene mutations in human cancers. *Cancer Res* 1997;57:2578–2580.

143. Mehlen P, Fearon ER. Role of the dependence receptor DCC in colorectal cancer pathogenesis. *J Clin Oncol* 2004;22:3420–3428.

144. Sancho R, Jandke A, Davis H, et al. F-box and WD repeat domain-containing 7 regulates intestinal cell lineage commitment and is a haploinsufficient tumor suppressor. *Gastroenterology* 2010;139:929–941.

145. Babaei-Jadidi R, Li N, Saadeddin A, et al. FBXW7 influences murine intestinal homeostasis and cancer, targeting Notch, Jun, and DEK for degradation. *J Exp Med* 2011;208:295–312.

146. Sjoblom T, Jones S, Wood LS, et al. The consensus coding sequences of human breast and colorectal cancers. *Science* 2006;314:268–274.

147. Vogelstein B, Papadopoulos N, Velculescu VE, et al. Cancer genome landscapes. *Science* 2013;339:1546–1558.

148. Leary RJ, Lin JC, Cummins J, et al. Integrated analysis of homozygous deletions, focal amplifications, and sequence alterations in breast and colorectal cancers. *Proc Natl Acad Sci U S A* 2008;105:16224–16229.

149. Martin ES, Tonon G, Sinha R, et al. Common and distinct genomic events in sporadic colorectal cancer and diverse cancer types. *Cancer Res* 2007;67:10736–10743.

150. Blache P, van de Wetering M, Duluc I, et al. SOX9 is an intestine crypt transcription factor, is regulated by the Wnt pathway, and represses the CDX2 and MUC2 genes. *J Cell Biol* 2004;166:37–47.

151. Sinicrope FA, Rego RL, Halling KC, et al. Prognostic impact of microsatellite instability and DNA ploidy in human colon carcinoma patients. *Gastroenterology* 2006;131:729–737.

152. Ribic CM, Sargent DJ, Moore MJ, et al. Tumor microsatellite-instability status as a predictor of benefit from fluorouracil-based adjuvant chemotherapy for colon cancer. *N Engl J Med* 2003;349:247–257.

153. Popat S, Hubner R, Houlston RS. Systematic review of microsatellite instability and colorectal cancer prognosis. *J Clin Oncol* 2005;23:609–618.

154. Sartore-Bianchi A, Di Nicolantonio F, Nichelatti M, et al. Multi-determinants analysis of molecular alterations for predicting clinical benefit to EGFR-targeted monoclonal antibodies in colorectal cancer. *PLoS One* 2009;4:e7287.

155. Ogino S, Meyerhardt JA, Irahara N, et al. KRAS mutation in stage III colon cancer and clinical outcome following intergroup trial CALGB 89803. *Clin Cancer Res* 2009;15:7322–7329.

156. Ogino S, Shima K, Meyerhardt JA, et al. Predictive and prognostic roles of BRAF mutation in stage III colon cancer: results from intergroup trial CALGB 89803. *Clin Cancer Res* 2012;18:890–900.

157. Moser AR, Pitot HC, Dove WF. A dominant mutation that predisposes to multiple intestinal neoplasia in the mouse. *Science* 1990;247:322–324.

158. Oshima M, Oshima H, Kitagawa K, et al. Loss of Apc heterozygosity and abnormal tissue building in nascent intestinal polyps in mice carrying a truncated Apc gene. *Proc Natl Acad Sci U S A* 1995;92:4482–4486.

159. Yang K, Edelmann W, Fan K, et al. A mouse model of human familial adenomatous polyposis. *J Exp Zool* 1997;277:245–254.

160. Amos-Landgraf JM, Kwong LN, Kendziorski CM, et al. A target-selected Apc-mutant rat kindred enhances the modeling of familial human colon cancer. *Proc Natl Acad Sci U S A* 2007;104:4036–4041.

161. Harada N, Tamai Y, Ishikawa T, et al. Intestinal polyposis in mice with a dominant sf mutation of the beta-catenin gene. *EMBO J* 1999;18:5931–5942.

162. Wei K, Kucherlapati R, Edelmann W. Mouse models for human DNA mismatch-repair gene defects. *Trends Mol Med* 2002;8:346–353.

163. Lopez-Garcia C, Klein AM, Simons BD, et al. Intestinal stem cell replacement follows a pattern of neutral drift. *Science* 2010;330:822–825.

164. Snippert HJ, van der Flier LG, Sato T, et al. Intestinal crypt homeostasis results from neutral competition between symmetrically dividing Lgr5 stem cells. *Cell* 2010;143:134–144.

165. Vermeulen L, Morrissey E, van der Heijden M, et al. Defining stem cell dynamics in models of intestinal tumor initiation. *Science* 2013;342:995–998.

CANCERS OF THE GASTROINTESTINAL TRACT

49 Cancer of the Colon

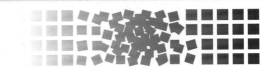

Steven K. Libutti, Leonard B. Saltz, Christopher G. Willett,
and Rebecca A. Levine

INTRODUCTION

A more thorough understanding of the molecular basis for this disease, coupled with the development of new therapeutic approaches, has dramatically altered the way in which patients with colorectal cancer (CRC) are managed. This chapter and the one that follows will provide an up-to-date description of the current state of the science and outline a multidisciplinary approach to the patient with colon or rectal cancer.

EPIDEMIOLOGY

Incidence and Mortality

Globally, nearly 1,200,000 new CRC cases are believed to occur, which accounts for approximately 10% of all incident cancers, and mortality from CRC is estimated at nearly 609,000.[1] In 2010, there were an estimated 141,570 new cases of CRC and 51,370 deaths in the United States.[2] As such, CRC accounts for nearly 10% of cancer mortality in the United States. Prevalence estimates reveal that in unscreened individuals age 50 years or older, there is a 0.5% to 2.0% chance of harboring an invasive CRC, a 1.0% to 1.6% chance of an in situ carcinoma, a 7% to 10% chance of a large (≥1 cm) adenoma, and a 25% to 40% chance of an adenoma of any size.[3]

Age impacts CRC incidence greater than any other demographic factor. To that end, sporadic CRC increases dramatically above the age of 45 to 50 years for all groups. In almost all countries, age-standardized incidence rates are less for women than for men. Although CRC incidence has been steadily decreasing in the United States and Canada, the incidence is rapidly increasing in Japan, Korea, and China.[1] In the United States from 2002 to 2006, the age-standardized incidence rates per 100,000 population were 59.0 for men and 43.6 for women when combined for all races.[2] Recognizing that decreases in age-standardized CRC incidence and mortality rates are apparent in the United States over the past 10 to 15 years, such trends may be counterbalanced by prolonged longevity.

While the incidence of CRC in the United States has decreased overall, presumably due to aggressive screening of the population over age 50, there has been a dramatic increase in younger patients. A new study using data from the Surveillance Epidemiology and End Results (SEER) program found a rising incidence of CRC over the last 20 years in patients aged 20 to 49. The most pronounced growth was in the age group 40 to 44 where colon and rectal cancer increased 56% and 94%, respectively. Based on these findings and the fact that CRC in younger patients tends to be more advanced, the authors recommend lowering the age for average risk screening by 10 years.[4,5]

Geographic Variation

The incidence rate for Alaskan Natives exceeds 70 per 100,000,[6] while that for Gambia and Algeria is <2 per 100,000.[7] Generally speaking, CRC incidence and mortality rates are the greatest in developed Western nations.[1,7] The reader is referred to the most recent detailed incidence and mortality rates in different countries over time according to gender, ethnicity, and anatomic site as established by the National Cancer Institute on their website.

As mentioned, there appears to be a recent decrease in age-standardized CRC incidence and mortality rates within the United States. From 1999 to 2006, CRC incidence and mortality both decreased.[2] Furthermore, 5-year survival improved. These trends are apparent regardless of gender, race, or ethnic group, except for Native Americans. Although at an initial glance one might invoke alterations in dietary and lifestyle factors, or the utilization of chemopreventive agents, it is clear that enhanced use of colonoscopy with polypectomy represents a significant reason for the improvements in trends in some areas.[8]

Emigration Patterns in Population Groups

Seminal studies have revealed that migrants from low-incident areas to high-incident areas assume the incidence of the host country within one generation.[9–12] For example, for Chinese who immigrate to the United States, higher CRC rates have been ascribed to greater meat consumption and diminished physical activity in contrast to controls within their original country.[10] These and other studies underscore the importance of environmental exposure in CRC incidence and provide a platform for attention to dietary and lifestyle modification as preventive measures.

Race and Ethnicity

Although dietary and lifestyle factors are of paramount importance in low-incident regions of the world, especially Asia and Africa, nonetheless there are certain trends along racial or ethnic lines. For example, an inherited adenomatosis polyposis coli (APC) gene mutation, I1307K, confers a higher risk of CRC within certain Ashkenazi Jewish families that is not apparent in other ethnic groups.[13,14] Inherited mutations in the DNA mismatch repair genes may be more common among African Americans,[15] in part accounting for anatomic variation in colon cancers among races in the United States,[16,17] an area that is receiving much attention in epidemiology- and biology-based research.

One recent study extracted data from the Adjuvant Colon Cancer ENdpoinTs (ACCENT) collaborative group database to analyze time-to-event end points for black and white patients participating in 12 randomized controlled adjuvant phase 3 trials of resected stage II and III colon cancer. In this cohort of 14,611 patients—controlling for sex, stage, age, and treatment type—both overall 5-year survival rates and 3-year recurrence-free survival rates were significantly worse for black patients (68.2% versus 72.8% and 68.4% versus 72.1%, respectively). However, recurrence-free interval was similar, arguing against a differential response to the adjuvant therapy itself. The authors concluded that poorer outcomes were more likely related to confounding factors not measured such as toxicity, comorbid conditions, and racial disparities in care for recurrent disease.[18]

Socioeconomic Factors

Generally, cancer incidence and mortality rates have been higher in economically advantaged countries.[19,20] This may be related to consumption of a high fat and high red meat diet, lack of physical activity with resulting obesity, and variations in mortality causes over a longitudinal period of time.

Anatomic Shift

Classically, colon cancer was believed to be a disease of the left or distal colon. However, the incidence of right-sided or proximal colon cancer has been increasing in North America[17,21] and Europe.[22] Similar trends have been observed in Asian countries.[23] This anatomic shift is likely multifactorial: (1) due to increased longevity; (2) as a response to luminal procarcinogens and carcinogens, which can vary between different sites of the colon and rectum; and (3) because of genetic factors, which can preferentially involve defects in mismatch repair genes with resulting microsatellite instability (MSI) in proximal colon cancers and chromosomal instability pathway predominant in left-sided colon and rectal cancers. These developments in anatomic variation will necessarily impact considerably on screening procedures, response to chemoprevention, response to chemotherapy, and, ultimately, disease-specific survival.[24–26]

ETIOLOGY: GENETIC AND ENVIRONMENTAL RISK FACTORS

Inherited Predisposition

Family history confers an increased lifetime risk of CRC, but that enhanced risk varies depending on the nature of the family history (Table 49.1). Familial factors contribute importantly to the risk of sporadic CRC, depending upon the involvement of first- or second-degree relatives and the age of onset of CRC. Involvement of at least one first-degree relative with CRC serves to double the risk of CRC.[27] There is further enhancement of the risk if a case is affected prior to the age of 60. Similarly, the likelihood of harboring premalignant adenomas or CRC is increased in first-degree

TABLE 49.1

Etiology of Colon Cancer: Environmental Factors

Increased Incidence	Decreased Incidence
High-caloric diet	High-fiber diet??
High red meat consumption	Antioxidant vitamins
Overcooked red meat??	Fresh fruit/vegetables
High saturated fats	Nonsteroidal anti-inflammatories
Excess alcohol consumption	Coffee
Cigarette smoking	High calcium
Sedentary lifestyle	High Magnesium
Obesity	Bisphosphonates
Diabetes	

relatives of persons with CRC.[28,29] The National Polyp Study reveals compelling data; the relative risk (RR) for parents and siblings of patients with adenomas compared to spousal controls was 1.8, which increased to 2.6 if the proband was younger than age 60 at adenoma detection.[30]

Provocative assessments of population groups suggest a dominantly inherited susceptibility to colorectal adenomas and cancer, which may account for the majority of sporadic CRC, but this may have variable inheritance based on the degree of exposure to environmental factors.[31] What are these susceptibility factors? The answer has yet to emerge. Nonetheless, genetic polymorphisms may be of paramount importance, such as in glutathione-s-transferase,[32] ethylene tetrahydrofolate reductase,[33,34] and N-acetyltransferases, especially NAT1 and NAT2.[35] In fact, genetic polymorphisms can vary among different racial and ethnic groups, which may provide clues to the geographic variation of CRC as well.

Environmental Factors

Seminal studies have underscored the importance of environmental factors as contributing to the pathogenesis of CRC. One has to take population-based studies into the context of methodologies employed, lead-time bias, time-lag issues, definition of surrogate and true end points, and the role of susceptibility factors.

One such population-based study recently evaluated risk factors for CRC from the Women's Health Initiative, a comprehensive prospectively collected database of 150,912 postmenopausal women, in which 1,210 developed colon cancer and 282 developed rectal cancer. Eleven risk factors were independently associated with colon cancer, some which have little or no previous support in the literature (age, waist girth, use of hormone therapy at baseline [protective], years smoked, arthritis [protective presumably due to medications used], relatives with CRC, lower hematocrit levels, fatigue, diabetes, less use of sleep medication, and cholecystectomy). Three of these factors were also significantly associated with an increased risk of rectal cancer (age, waist girth, and not taking hormone therapy).[36]

Diet

Total Calories

Obesity and total caloric intake are independent risk factors for CRC as revealed by cohort and case-control studies.[37,38] Increased body mass may result in a two-fold increase in CRC risk, with a strong association in men with colon but not rectal cancer. Weight gains during early to middle adulthood have also recently been linked with increased risk of colon but not rectal cancer. This relationship too seems more prominent in men than women in a large prospective study.[39]

Meat, Fat, and Protein

Ingestion of red meat but not white meat is associated with an increased CRC risk,[40,41] and as such, per capita consumption of red meat is a potent independent risk factor. Whether the total abstinence from red meat leads to a decreased CRC incidence has not been clarified, as there are studies with opposing results.[42] Also unclear is whether the type of red meat or the degree of processing or cooking method make any difference. While Probst-Hensch et al.[43] found fried, barbecued, and processed meats to be associated with CRC risk, especially for rectal cancer, with odds ratio (OR) of 6, follow-up reports do not consistently support these claims. In the population-based Norwegian Women and Cancer cohort including 84,538 participants, highly processed meat intake (especially sausage) was associated with increased CRC risk but meat cooking methods and total meat intake were not.[44]

A second study of 53,988 participants reported no difference with processed meat intake either. The authors did find that cancer risk was associated with different meat subtypes (i.e., animal of origin) which varied by tumor location—specifically, colon cancer risk was significantly elevated in the setting of high lamb intake (incidence rate ratio = 1.07) and rectal cancer risk was affected by pork (incidence rate ratio = 1.18).[45] However, McCullough et al.[46] recently reported a positive association in patients with non-metastatic CRC between red and processed meat consumption before cancer diagnosis with higher risk of death after definitive surgery.

Coffee

Coffee contains numerous bioactive compounds that may modulate cancer risk but previous epidemiologic studies investigating its role in CRC have yielded ambiguous results. In a recent meta-analysis of 41 studies (25,965 patients), Li et al.[47] found a significant inverse association from case-control data for CRC (OR = 0.85) and colon cancer (OR = 0.79), but not rectal cancer. This was particularly true among females and in Europe.[47] Stronger evidence comes from the National Institutes of Health–AARP Diet and Health Study, a large prospective US cohort including 489,706 members. In this report, both caffeinated and decaffeinated coffee drinkers had a decreased risk of colon cancer, particularly of proximal tumors (hazard ratio [HR] for more than six cups a day = 0.62), and decaffeinated coffee drinkers also had a decreased risk of rectal cancer. While known confounders such as smoking and red meat consumption were adjusted for, further investigation is warranted to confirm and clarify this association.[48]

Fiber

Classically, a high-fiber diet was associated with a low incidence of CRC in Africa,[49] with numerous studies substantiating this premise.[50] Protection was believed to be afforded from wheat bran, fruit, and vegetables.[41] A high-fiber diet was believed to dilute fecal carcinogens, decrease colon transit time, and generate a favorable luminal environment. The European Prospective Investigation into Cancer and Nutrition is an ongoing multicenter prospective cohort study, which was one of the largest and most influential studies to initially report an inverse association between dietary fiber and CRC. More long-term data, with a mean follow-up of 11 years and a near three-fold increase in CRC cases, further supports this claim while providing a more precise estimation by fiber food source as well. After multivariable adjustments, total dietary fiber was found to be inversely associated with both colon and rectal cancers (HR per 10 g/day increased in fiber = 0.87), and this did not differ by age, sex, lifestyle, or other dietary factors.[51] However, other large, well-controlled studies show no inverse relationship between CRC and fiber intake.[52] In a study of nearly 90,000 women from ages 34 to 59 who were followed for 16 years, no protective effect was noted between fiber and incidence of either adenomatous polyp or CRC.[52] This was further corroborated by two large randomized controlled trials that evaluated high-fiber diets for moderate duration and discovered a lack of effect on the number, size, and histology of polyps found on colonoscopy.[53,54] At this point, therefore, it is unclear whether dietary fiber plays any substantial role in the risk of developing CRC.

Vegetables and Fruit

A protective effect of vegetables and fruits against CRC is generally believed to be true.[40] This has been observed with raw, green, and cruciferous vegetables. Whether certain agents such as antioxidant vitamins (E, C, and A), folate, thioethers, terpenes, and plant phenols may translate into effective chemopreventive strategies requires further investigation, although the data for folate intake are sound.[55]

Taking this nutritional data a step further, Bamia et al.[56] recently evaluated the impact of the Mediterranean diet on CRC risk in a large European cohort. This diet, introduced in the 1960s as "health-protecting," includes a high intake of vegetables, fruits, nuts, fish, cereals, and legumes with moderate alcohol consumption and low consumption of dairy and meat. The authors found an 8% to 11% decreased CRC risk when comparing patients with the highest to lowest diet adherence rates (HR = 0.89). The association was strongest for women and colon tumors.[56]

Other dietary factors under recent investigation include calcium, magnesium, and vitamin D. Calcium has been historically implicated as having a protective effect, perhaps due to its ability to bind injurious bile acids with reduction of colonic epithelial proliferation.[57] This is supported through cell culture models. However, population-based studies are not definitive.

A recent meta-analysis evaluating the influence of magnesium intake demonstrated a modest risk reduction, with pooled RRs of 0.81 for colon cancer and 0.94 for rectal cancer. This association persisted even after results were adjusted for calcium intake in six of the analyzed studies.[58]

Vitamin D has been shown to inhibit cell proliferation and increase apoptosis in vitro, and its deficiency is considered an important risk factor for many types of solid cancers. In a meta-analysis of 18 prospective studies, vitamin D intake and blood 25 (OH)D levels were found to be inversely associated with the risk of CRC as well (RR = 0.79 and 0.62 for colon cancer, respectively; RR = 0.78 and 0.61 for rectal cancer, respectively). While this report offers only preliminary observational data, larger randomized trials for vitamin D supplementation are warranted[59] and would be needed before routine vitamin D supplementation could be recommended for the purpose of CRC prevention. It is noteworthy that the Institute of Medicine, while supporting vitamn D supplementation to maintain bone health, found the evidence insufficient to support vitamin D as being protective against colorectal or any other cancer.[60]

Lifestyle

Physical inactivity has been associated with CRC risk, for colon more than rectal cancer. A sedentary lifestyle may account for an increased CRC risk, although the mechanism is unclear. Data suggest that physical activity after the diagnosis of stages I to III colon cancer may reduce the risk of cancer-related and overall mortality, and that the amount of aerobic exercise correlates with a reduced risk of recurrence following resection of stage III colon cancer.[61] More recently, positive associations have been established between increased amounts of recreational physical activity before and after CRC diagnosis and lower mortality.[62]

Most studies of alcohol have demonstrated at most a minimally positive effect. Associations are strongest between alcohol consumption in men and risk of rectal cancer. Perhaps interference with folate metabolism through acetaldehyde is responsible.[63]

Prolonged cigarette smoking is associated with the risk of CRC.[40] Cigarette smoking for >20 pack-years was associated with large adenoma risk and >35 pack-years with cancer risk. To examine the impact of smoking cessation on the attenuation of this risk, Gong et al.[64] conducted a pooled analysis of eight studies, including 6,796 CRC cases and 7,770 controls. The authors found that former smokers also remained at increased risk for up to 25 years after quitting. However, this varied substantially by cancer subsite with risk declining immediately for proximal colon and rectal cases but not until 20 years after smoking cessation for distal colon tumors.[64]

Diabetes

Type 2 diabetes has previously been implicated in the development of CRC, but it has been difficult to separate this association from other confounding lifestyle factors such as smoking and obesity.

Two recent meta-analyses provide further evidence that this condition is in fact a significant indepent risk factor. Yuhara et al.[65] identified 14 studies, most of which controlled for smoking, obesity, and physical exercise, and demonstrated that diabetes was associated with increased risk of both colon and rectal cancer (RR = 1.38 and RR = 1.20, respectively).[65] A second report, analyzing 24 studies, found a similar association (RR = 1.26) with even higher risk for those patients on insulin therapy (RR = 1.61).[66]

Drugs

Nonsteroidal Anti-Inflammatory Drugs

Population-based studies strongly support inverse associations between use of aspirin and other nonsteroidal anti-inflammatory drugs (NSAID) and the incidences of both CRC and adenomas.[67–69] As a result, NSAIDs and selective cyclooxygenase 2 (COX-2) inhibitors have been investigated intensively in hereditary and sporadic CRC.

Long-term results have just been reported from the CAPP2 study, the first double-blind randomized controlled trial of aspirin chemoprevention with cancer as the primary end point. In this study, 861 carriers of Lynch syndrome were randomly assigned to aspirin or placebo. With a mean follow-up of 55.7 months, the authors report a significantly decreased incidence of CRC in the treatment group as well as a trend toward reduction in extracolonic Lynch syndrome–associated cancers. Importantly, there was no significant difference in adverse events such as gastrointestinal (GI) bleeding, ulcers, or anemia during the intervention period. These data provide strong rationale for the routine use of aspirin chemoprevention in Lynch syndrome and establish a foundation for further study in sporadic neoplasia. In a combined analysis of four large randomized trials of lower-dose aspirin (75 to 300 mg/day) involving 14,033 patients, aspirin taken for 5 years or more was associated with a reduced 20-year incidence and mortality due to CRC (absolute reduction = 1.76%; 95% confidence interval [CI] = 0.61 to 2.91; p = 0.001). Reduction was largely confined to right-sided tumors.[70] In addition to generalized chemoprevention, the question of aspirn and other NSAIDs in patients with a diagnosis of CRC has been addressed. Liao et al.[71] have reported evidence that suggests that aspirin therapy after CRC diagnosis may be beneficial to those patients whose tumors have a PIK3CA mutation, but not in those with wild-type PIK3CA.[71] However, PIK3CA mutation status had no impact on the influence of the COX-2 inhibitor rofecoxib on cancer recurrence.[72]

Bisphosphonates

In addition to being one of the most commonly used medications for osteoporosis, bisphosphonates have been shown to have various antiproliferative, antiangiogenic, proapoptotic, and antiadhesive effects in preclinical studies. Practical impact on malignant disease, however, has been inconsistent. Singh et al.[73] performed a recent meta-analysis demonstrating a statistically significant 17% reduction in CRC incidence with bisphosphonate use. This finding was observed independently for both proximal and distal colon cancers as well as rectal cancers, highlighting another potential pathway for chemoprevention.[73]

Biomarkers

In an effort to improve screening protocols and advance understanding of colorectal carcinogenesis, investigators are focusing on a variety of biomarkers for increased risk as well.

Toriola et al.[74] evaluated the role of C-reactive protein and serum amyloid A, two common inflammatory mediators, in the Women's Health Initiative Observational Study. With over 900 case-control pairs for each marker, the authors found that elevated concentrations of both C-reactive protein and serum amyloid A conferred significantly increased risk of colon cancer (OR = 1.50, p = 0.006). This is not surprising given the role inflammation plays in colorectal carcinogenesis as well as the new promising data surrounding NSAID chemoprevention.[74]

Leptin, a peptide hormone produced by adipocytes, is also thought to contribute to CRC pathogenesis. A recent prospective analysis found that soluble leptin receptor levels, which may regulate leptin function, was strongly inversely associated with both CRC and colon cancer risk (RR = 0.55 and RR = 0.42, respectively). This finding was independent of leptin levels and other circulating biomarkers.[75] Chi et al.[76] performed a similar investigation of insulin-like growth factor peptides, also implicated in CRC carcinogenesis, and found that high levels of insulin-like growth factor I and insulin-like growth factor II significantly increased cancer risk (OR = 1.25 and OR = 1.52, respectively).[76] Along these lines, high circulating levels of C-peptide, a direct marker of hyperinsulinemia, may also be a predictive factor for increased CRC risk, as indicated in a recent meta-analysis.[77]

Human Papillomavirus

While human papillomavirus is well-established as the critical pathogenic force behind cervical and anogenital cancer, its role in colorectal malignancy is less clear. An association between the two was first reported in 1990 and since then, a growing number of studies have detected the virus in colon adenocarcinoma specimens. In the first meta-analysis to address this topic (including 16 articles and 1,436 patients), Damin, Ziegelmann, and Damin[78] not only reported a high prevalence of human papillomavirus (31.9%) in affected patients, but also found a strong correlation between human papillomavirus positivity and increased CRC risk (OR = 10.04; 95% CI = 3.7 to 27.5). These results may indicate an alternative pathway of colorectal carcinogenesis that could have vast implications for treatment and prevention.[78]

FAMILIAL COLORECTAL CANCER

Familial Adenomatous Polyposis

Familial adenomatous polyposis (FAP) constitutes 1% of all CRC incidence (Table 49.2). Hallmark features include hundreds to thousands of colonic polyps that develop in patients in their teens to 30s, and if the colon is not surgically removed, 100% of patients progress to CRC. Extracolonic manifestations include benign conditions—congenital hypertrophy of the retinal pigment epithelium, mandibular osteomas, supernumerary teeth, epidermal cysts, adrenal cortical adenomas, desmoid tumors (although these tumors may lead to obstruction)—and malignant conditions—thyroid tumors, gastric small intestinal polyps with a 5% to 10% risk of duodenal or ampullary adenocarcinoma, and brain tumors.[79] The brain tumors may be of two types—glioblastoma multiforme or medulloblastoma—and the particular association of brain tumors and colonic polyposis is called Turcot syndrome.[80] The colonic polyps in Turcot syndrome are fewer and larger than in classic FAP. An attenuated form of FAP harbors up to 100 colonic polyps and has a predisposition to colorectal cancer in patients when they are in their 50s or 60s.[81]

FAP is an autosomally dominant disorder with nearly 100% penetrance. However, about 30% of patients have de novo mutations and are without an ostensible family history. Based on karyotypic analysis that reveals an interstitial deletion on human chromosome 5q and subsequent genetic linkage analysis to 5q21, the gene responsible for FAP was identified as APC. Patients with FAP inherit a mutated copy of the APC gene, thereby predisposing them to early onset polyposis. During life, patients with FAP acquire inactivation of the remaining APC gene copy, which accelerates the progression to CRC. Interesting genotypic-phenotypic

TABLE 49.2

Familial and Nonfamilial Causes of Colorectal Cancer

Syndromes with Adenomatous Polyps

APC gene mutations (1%):
- Familial adenomatous polyposis
- Attenuated APC
- Turcot syndrome (two-thirds of families)

MMR gene mutations (3%):
- Hereditary nonpolyposis colorectal cancer types I and II
- Muir-Torre syndrome
- Turcot syndrome (one-third of families)

Syndromes with hamartomatous polyps (<1%)

Peutz-Jeghers (*LKB1*)

Juvenile polyposis (*SMAD4, PTEN*)

Cowden (*PTEN*)

Bannayan-Ruvalcaba-Riley

Mixed polyposis

Other Familial Causes (up to 20%–25%)

Family history of adenomatous polyps (*MYH*)

Family history of colon cancer:
- Risk more than three times greater if two first-degree relatives or one first-degree relative <50 y with colon cancer
- Risk two times greater if second-degree relative affected

Familial colon-breast cancer

Nonfamilial Causes

Personal history of adenomatous polyps

Personal history of colorectal cancer

Inflammatory bowel disease (ulcerative colitis, Crohn's colitis)
- Radiation colitis
- Ureterosigmoidostomy
- Acromegaly
- Cronkhite-Canada syndrome

TABLE 49.3

Criteria for Identifying At-Risk Individuals for Mismatch Repair Deficiency (High Microsatellite Instability)

Amsterdam I Criteria

At least three relatives with colorectal cancer

One relative should be a first-degree relative of the other two

At least two successive generations should be affected

At least one colorectal cancer case before age 50

FAP should be excluded

Tumors should be verified histopathologically

Amsterdam II Criteria

At least three relatives with HNPCC-associated cancer (colorectal, endometrial, small bowel, ureter, or renal pelvis)

At least two successive generations should be affected

At least one case before age 50

FAP should be excluded

Tumors should be verified histopathologically

Bethesda Criteria (for Identification of Patients with Colorectal Tumor who Should Undergo Testing for MSI)

Cancer in families that meet Amsterdam criteria

Two HNPCC-related cancers, including colorectal or extracolonic

Colorectal cancer and a first degree relative with colorectal cancer and/or HNPCC-related extracolonic cancer and/or colorectal adenoma: one cancer before age 45 and adenoma before age 40

Colorectal cancer or endometrial cancer before age 45

Right-sided colorectal cancer with an undifferentiated pattern on histopathology before age 45

Signet-ring cell type colorectal cancer before age 45

Adenoma before age 40

FAP, familial adenomatous polyposis; HNPCC, hereditary nonpolyposis colorectal cancer; MSI, microsatellite instability.

associations exist between the location of the *APC* gene mutation and certain clinical manifestations, such as congenital hypertrophy of the retinal pigment epithelium, desmoid tumors, and classic FAP versus attenuated FAP.

The *APC* gene comprises 15 exons and encodes a protein of nearly 2,850 amino acids (310 kDa). Nearly all germline mutations in the *APC* gene lead to a truncated protein, which can be detected through molecular diagnostic assays that can be integrated into genetic counseling and genetic testing of affected patients and at-risk family members.[82,83] The functions of the APC protein and the interrelated pathways and regulatory molecules will be discussed later.

Hereditary Nonpolyposis Colorectal Cancer

Hereditary nonpolyposis CRC (HNPCC) accounts for about 3% of all CRCs. Salient features include up to 100 colonic polyps (hence the term nonpolyposis), preferentially, albeit not exclusively, in the right or proximal colon.[84] There is an accelerated rate of progression to CRC in these diminutive, at times flat, polyps with mean age of onset of CRC being 43 years. This is designated HNPCC type I. HNPCC type II is distinguished by extracolonic tumors that originate in the stomach, small bowel, bile duct, renal pelvis, ureter, bladder, uterus and ovary, skin, and perhaps the pancreas.

The lifetime risk of CRC in HNPCC is 80%, up to 50% to 60% for endometrial cancer, and 1% to 13% for all other cancers.[84,85] Of note, a variant of HNPCC involves skin tumors and is designated as Muir-Torre syndrome. HNPCC is defined classically by the modified Amsterdam criteria (Table 49.3).

HNPCC is an autosomally dominant disorder with about 80% penetrance. Genetic and biochemical approaches led to the discovery of the involvement of human DNA mismatch repair genes in HNPCC. Recognized as the human orthologues of mismatch repair genes described in bacteria and yeast, human mismatch repair genes encode enzymes that repair errors during DNA replication that may occur spontaneously or upon exposure to an exogenous agent (e.g., ultraviolet light, chemical carcinogen). Mutations in one of these mismatch repair genes results in MSI, which creates a milieu of somatic mutations of target genes—TGF-β2 receptor, *bax, IGF* type I receptor, among others—in HNPCC-associated tumors.[86] About 60% of germline mutations in HNPCC are found in either the *hMLH1* gene or the *hMSH2* gene, but mutations in other members of this family—*hMSH6, hPMS1, hPMS2*—are rare, thereby indicating that other genes are involved but have yet to be discovered. Genetic testing is not facile for HNPCC as it is for FAP, but it involves sequencing both the *hMLH1* and *hMSH2* genes (Table 49.4). If a germline mutation is found, then the remaining at-risk family members can be genetically screened.

TABLE 49.4

Genetic Testing in Inherited Colorectal Cancer

FAP	APC protein truncating testing (preferred). If APC mutation found, screen for mutation in family. Less desirable alternatives: gene sequencing, linkage testing.
HNPCC	MSI testing in tumor.[a] If MSI present, proceed to sequencing of both *hMLH1* and *hMSH2* genes. If mutation found, screen for mutation in family.

FAP, familial adenomatous polyposis; APC, adenomatosis polyposis coli; HNPCC, hereditary nonpolyposis colorectal cancer; MSI, microsatellite instability.
[a] Immunohistochemistry may be an option.

MSI testing and hMLH1/hMSH2 immunohistochemistry (IHC) can be performed on tumor specimens as a possible prelude to genetic testing.

Hamartomatous Polyposis Syndromes

Hamartomatous polyposis syndromes are rare syndromes, mostly affecting the pediatric and adolescent population, and represent <1% of CRCs annually. Peutz-Jeghers syndrome involves large but few colonic and small bowel polyps that can manifest by GI bleeding or obstruction and an increased risk of CRC. The polyps are distinguished by a smooth muscle band in the submucosa. Hallmark clinical features on physical examination include freckles on the hands, around the lips, in the buccal mucosa, and periorbitally. Associated characteristics include sinus, bronchial, and bladder polyps, and about 5% to 10% of patients have sex cord tumors. Patients can also develop lung and pancreatic adenocarcinomas. The gene responsible for this syndrome is *LKB1*, a serine threonine kinase.

Juvenile polyposis have overlapping clinical manifestations with Peutz-Jeghers, but the polyps tend to be confined to the colon, although cases of gastric and small bowel polyps have been described and there is an increased risk of CRC. Extracolonic manifestations are not prevalent. This is a polygenic disease, involving germline mutations in *PTEN*, *SMAD4*, *BMPR1*, or other genes yet to be identified.

Cowden syndrome harbors hamartomatous polyps anywhere in the GI tract, and surprisingly, there is no increased risk of CRC. However, about 10% of patients will have thyroid tumors and nearly 50% of patients have breast tumors. Germline *PTEN* mutations have been reported.

It is estimated that about 20% to 30% of CRCs are compatible with an inherited predisposition, independent of known syndromes.[87] The identification of other responsible genes will have great clinical impact. Intensive approaches are being pursued through sibling-pair studies and other familial studies. As previously mentioned, patients may be predisposed to an increased risk of adenomatous polyps as well in the context of a family history of sporadic adenomatous polyps.

ANATOMY OF THE COLON

The colon and rectum make up the segment of the digestive system commonly referred to as the large bowel. Defined as the portion of intestine from the ileocecal valve to the anus, the large bowel is approximately 150 cm in length. It is divided into five segments defined by its vascular supply and by its extraperitoneal or retroperitoneal location: the cecum (with appendix) and ascending colon, the transverse colon, the descending colon, the sigmoid colon, and the rectum. The anatomy of the rectum will be discussed in detail in the chapter on rectal cancer. The large bowel has a muscular wall and can be distinguished from the small intestine by its increased diameter, the presence of haustra, appendices epiploicae, and tenia coli. The tenia consist of condensations of longitudinal muscle fibers starting near the base of the appendix and continuing throughout the abdominal colon to form a continuous longitudinal muscle coat in the upper rectum. Haustra are outpouchings of bowel wall separated by folds that give a classic appearance on radiography or barium enema.

The right colon is made up of the cecum (with appendix) and ascending colon. It is anterior to the right kidney and the duodenum. Its vascular supply is from branches of the superior mesenteric artery (SMA). The SMA divides into the middle colic artery and the trunk of the SMA. The middle colic artery immediately forms two to three large arcades in the transverse mesocolon. The SMA ileocolic arterial branches then extend from the SMA. The right colic artery arises as a separate branch from the SMA in 10.7% of cases.[88] The ileocolic artery gives off a right colic artery to the upper ascending colon and forms an anastomosis with branches from the middle colic artery. The ileal branch of the ileocolic artery gives off branches to the distal small bowel and cecum, whereas the colic branch supplies the ascending colon. An anastomosis occurs between the distal SMA and the ileal branch of the ileocolic artery at the junction of the terminal ileum and cecum. The right colon is a retroperitoneal structure.

The transverse colon is supplied by branches of the middle colic artery. It is the first portion of the colon considered to be intraperitoneal, and its length can vary. Its boundaries are defined by the hepatic flexure on the right and the splenic flexure on the left. Both of these points are fixed. The hepatic flexure abuts the gallbladder fossa, while the splenic flexure lies anterior to the splenic hilum and the tail of the pancreas. The descending colon is where the colon once again becomes a retroperitoneal structure, and it is defined as the segment of colon from the splenic flexure to the sigmoid colon. The descending colon is the first segment of the left side of the colon and receives its blood supply from the inferior mesenteric artery. The inferior mesenteric artery arises from the aorta and gives off the left colic artery. It also gives off three to four sigmoidal arteries, which supply the intraperitoneal sigmoid colon. The anastomosis between the vessels of the middle colic artery and those of the left colic artery and right colic artery is known as the marginal artery of Drummond. The arcade, which effectively connects the left and right circulations, is known as the arc of Riolan. The arterial supply to the colon is depicted in Fig. 49.1.

The venous and lymphatic drainage of the colon parallels the arterial supply, and all three vessels course and divide within the colonic mesocolon (Fig. 49.2). The mesocolon therefore contains the regional lymph nodes (LN) for the segment of colon it supplies and drains. The efferent lymphatic channels pass from the submucosa to the intramuscular and subserosal plexus of the bowel to the first tier of LNs lying adjacent to the large intestine and known as *epicolic nodes*.[89] *Paracolic nodes* lie on the marginal vessels along the mesenteric side of the colon and are frequently involved in metastases. *Intermediate nodes* are found along the major arterial branches of the SMA and inferior mesenteric artery in the mesocolon. The *principal nodes* are found around the origin of these vessels from the aorta, and they drain into retroperitoneal nodes. The drainage of the superior and inferior mesenteric veins, which drain the ascending, transverse, descending, and sigmoid colon, is to the portal vein. The rectum is drained by rectal tributaries to the vena cava.

The extent of resection of the colon is defined by the vascular supply and by the need to take the regional draining LNs.[90,91] A careful understanding of the colonic anatomy, structure, location, and vascular supply is therefore critical in order to perform a safe and effective cancer operation. The segmental resections important for removal of lesions in various locations within the colon will be described in greater detail in later sections.

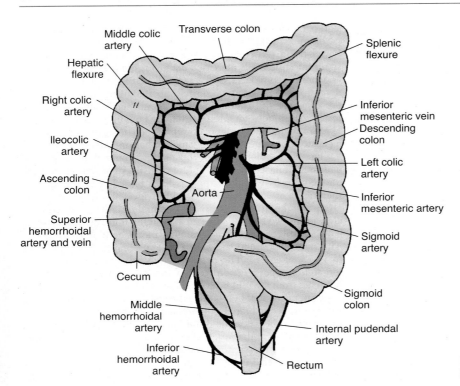

Figure 49.1 The anatomy of the colon with particular emphasis on the vascular supply.

DIAGNOSIS OF COLORECTAL CANCER

Symptoms associated with CRC include lower GI bleeding, change in bowel habits, abdominal pain, weight loss, change in appetite, and weakness, and in particular, obstructive symptoms

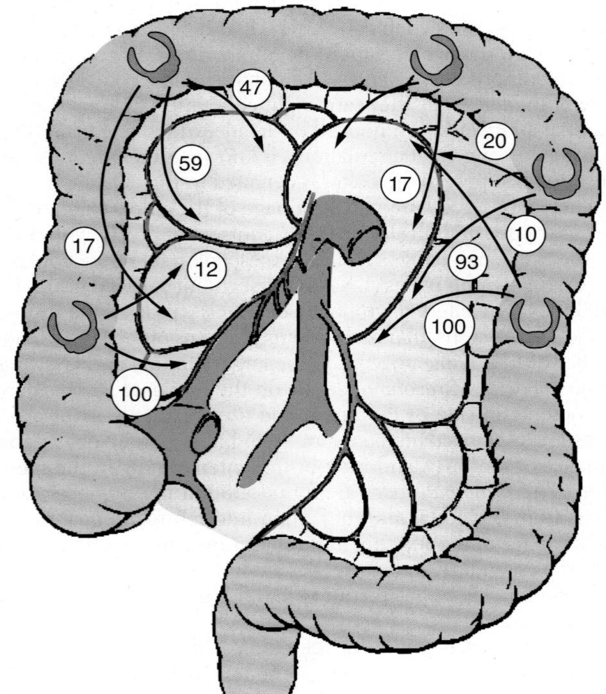

Figure 49.2 The lymphatic drainage of lesions in various anatomic locations throughout the colon.

are alarming.[92] However, apart from obstructive symptoms, other symptoms do not necessarily correlate with stage of disease or portend a particular diagnosis.[93]

Physical examination may reveal a palpable mass, bright blood per rectum (usually left-sided colon cancers or rectal cancer) or melena (right-sided colon cancers), or lesser degrees of bleeding (hemoccult-positive stool). Adenopathy, hepatomegaly, jaundice, or even pulmonary signs may be present with metastatic disease. Obstruction by colon cancer is usually in the sigmoid or left colon, with resulting abdominal distention and constipation, whereas right-sided colon cancers may be more insidious in nature. Complications of CRC include acute GI bleeding, acute obstruction, perforation, and metastasis with impairment of distant organ function.

Laboratory values may reflect iron-deficiency anemia, electrolyte derangements, and liver function abnormalities. The carcinoembryonic antigen (CEA) may be elevated and is most helpful to monitor postoperatively, if reduced to normal as a result of surgery.[94]

Evaluation should include complete history, family history, physical examination, laboratory tests, colonoscopy, and pan-body computed tomography (CT) scan.[95] For rectal cancer, additional imaging techniques, such as magnetic resonance imaging or endoscopic ultrasound, are utilized to further characterize the primary tumor prior to therapy (see Chapter 52). Upon completion of diagnosis and staging for both colon and rectal tumors, it is essential to incorporate the expertise from medical, radiation, and surgical oncologists in order to formulate and implement an optimal treatment plan.

With the advent of molecular biologic techniques, attention has been drawn to stool-based tools and new blood-based tests. Technology now exists to extract genomic DNA or protein from stool and assay for evidence of genetic alterations.[96,97] Large-scale validation studies are in progress, one of which has just been published, describing an automated multitarget sDNA assay (fecal immunochemical testing) with a 90% specificity and 98% sensitivity for the detection of CRC, as well 83% sensitivity for advanced adenoma with high-grade dysplasia.[98] In addition, Epi proColon (Epigenomics AG, Berlin, Germany), a blood-based test, was shown to be noninferior to fecal immunochemical testing in preliminary results from a multicenter double blind comparative study (press release from Epigenomics AG, December 4, 2012). One particularly attractive pathway for stool-based diagnostics would be able to stratify patients as high, moderate, or low risk for CRC and thus influence screening modalities and frequency of screening. In a complementary fashion, functional genomics are being applied to pair-wise comparisons of normal colon and CRCs to sample the entire human genome of nearly 30,000 genes to discover those genes, known and novel, that may be upregulated or downregulated and possibly linked to detection, prognosis, and therapy.

SCREENING FOR COLORECTAL CANCER

Debate is vigorous as to the best approaches for screening, and multiple factors influence that decision: simplicity and rapidity so as to enhance patient compliance, benefit to risk ratio, sensitivity, specificity, cost-effectiveness, and other economic factors. To that end, currently, optical colonoscopy likely offers the most effective approach when one considers all of these factors.

The average-risk patient is defined as a man or woman above the age of 50 without personal or family history of adenomatous polyps or CRC and absence of any occult or acute GI bleeding. Screening recommendations or guidelines for average-risk and high-risk individuals are presented in Table 49.5.

Optical colonoscopy is currently the most sensitive method for screening. Advantages include direct visualization, with the ability to remove polyps (with rate-limiting factors of size and anatomic location) and to obtain biopsies. Disadvantages involve the preparation, invasive nature of the procedure, and potential side effects that include perforation (although this is <1%).

The digital rectal examination should be part of the general physical examination. Anorectal masses may be palpated. Flexible sigmoidoscopy does not require conscious sedation and hemodynamic monitoring, and will typically allow visualization of the rectum, sigmoid colon, and descending colon to the splenic flexure. Flexible sigmoidoscopy should not be considered as a single screening measure but requires coupling with barium enema. Barium enema allows visualization of the entire colon, and experience is necessary to ensure proper visualization of the rectum. Barium enema affords advantages of ease of preparation, lack of conscious sedation and hemodynamic monitoring, and ability to visualize polyps and masses. However, small polyps may be missed. Furthermore, if a luminal polyp or mass is identified, then colonoscopy will be necessary for polypectomy or biopsies.

New noninvasive technologies, such as CT and magnetic resonance colonography, are receiving increased attention in clinical studies, which demonstrate overall feasibility, as well as some advantages.[99]

Two meta-analyses published in 2011 provide strong support for the implementation of CT colonography as a viable alternative to optical colonoscopy in both average and high-risk populations.

CANCERS OF THE GASTROINTESTINAL TRACT

TABLE 49.5

Recommendations for Colorectal Cancer Screening in Average-Risk and Increased-Risk Patients from the Gastrointestinal Consortium Panel

Average-Risk Patient (Different Options)
1. FOBT: Offer yearly screening with FOBT using a guaiac-based test with dietary restriction or an immunochemical test without dietary restriction. Two samples from each of three consecutive stools should be examined without rehydration. Patients with a positive test on any specimen should be followed up with colonoscopy.
2. Flexible sigmoidoscopy: Offer flexible sigmoidoscopy every 5 y.
3. FOBT plus flexible sigmoidoscopy: Offer screening with FOBT every year combined with flexible sigmoidoscopy every 5 y. When both tests are performed, the FOBT should be done first.
4. Colonoscopy: Offer every 10 y.
5. DCBE: Offer every 5 y.

Increased Risk for Colorectal Cancer
1. Family history of colorectal cancer or polyps. People with a first-degree relative (parent, sibling, or child) with colon cancer or adenomatous polyp diagnosed at age <60 y or two first-degree relatives diagnosed with colorectal cancer at any age should be advised to have screening colonoscopy starting at age 40 y or 10 y younger than the earliest diagnosis in the family, whichever comes first, and repeated every 5 y.
2. FAP: Flexible sigmoidoscopy to start at ages 10 to 12 y. Genetic testing (for FAP, upper endoscopy with side-viewing scope) should be done every 1 to 3 y.
3. HNPCC: Colonoscopy every 1 to 2 y starting at ages 20 to 25 y or 10 y younger than the earliest case in the family, whichever comes first. Genetic testing (for HNPCC, consideration should be given to screening for uterine and ovarian cancer with hysteroscopy and transvaginal ultrasound, the frequency of which varies within centers).
4. Personal history of adenomatous polyps
   A. If one or more polyps that are malignant or large and sessile or colonoscopy is incomplete, then follow-up colonoscopy should be in the short term.
   B. If three of more polyps, follow-up colonoscopy in 3 y.
   C. If one or two polyps (<1 cm), follow-up colonoscopy in 5 y (or more).
5. Personal history of colorectal cancer
   A. Colonoscopy is incomplete at time of diagnosis of colorectal cancer due to obstruction, then repeat colonoscopy 6 mo after surgical resection.
   B. Colonoscopy is complete at time of diagnosis of colorectal cancer, then repeat colonoscopy in 3 y, and if that is normal, then repeat every 5 y.
6. Inflammatory bowel disease (ulcerative colitis, Crohn's colitis). Surveillance colonoscopy is recommended.

FOBT, fecal occult blood testing; DCBE, double-contrast barium enema; FAP, familial adenomatous polyposis; HNPCC, hereditary nonpolyposis colorectal cancer. From Rex DK, Johnson DA, Lieberman DA, et al. Colorectal cancer prevention 2000: screening recommendations of the American College of Gastroenterology. American College of Gastroenterology. *Am J Gastroenterol* 2000;95:868–877; Winawer S, Fletcher R, Rex D, et al. Colorectal cancer screening and surveillance: clinical guidelines and rationale-Update based on new evidence. *Gastroenterology* 2003;124:544–560.

In a review of 4,086 asymptomatic patients, de Haan et al.,[100] estimates sensitivities of 82.9% and 87.9% and specificities of 91.4% and 97.6% for adenomas ≥6 mm and ≥10mm, respectively.

In a complementary analysis looking exclusively at cancer detection, Pickhardt et al.[101] concludes that CT colonography is not only clinically equivalent to colonoscopy but perhaps even more suitable for initial investigation given consistently high sensitivity (96.1%) without heterogeneity across 49 studies, and 11,151 patients, despite wide variation in technique.

Other reports suggest advantages in long-term costs and patient compliance, although these issues remain controversial.[102,103]

Lastly, CT colonography may also offer improvements in preoperative staging as one study found this technique to be highly predictive of T3-4 tumors. Whether this information will prove as clinically relevant in colon cancer as it is for the rectum remains to be seen.[104]

STAGING AND PROGNOSIS OF COLORECTAL CANCER

This discussion will focus primarily on those prognostic and predictive indicators that are best supported by available data and are appropriate for use and consideration in current practice. The reader should remain aware of the potential for rapid changes and advances in this area, however.

Staging

Although many factors have been identified that have an impact on recurrence and survival, none exceeds stage in terms of prognostic significance.[105] Staging of CRC should be done using the current TNM (tumor, node, metastasis) classification of the American Joint Committee on Cancer (AJCC)/International Union Against Cancer (UICC) staging system (Table 49.6).[106] Other systems should be regarded as of historical significance only and must be comprehended solely for the purposes of understanding the studies that were performed and reported in the past using these older classifications.

TABLE 49.6

Tumor (T) Node (N) Metastasis (M) Classification of Colorectal Cancer

Stage	T	N	M
0	Tis	N0	M0
I	T1	N0	M0
	T2	N0	M0
IIA	T3	N0	M0
IIB	T4a	N0	M0
IIC	T4b	N0	M0
IIIA	T1-T2	N1-N2a	M0
IIIB	T3-T4a	N1	M0
	T2-T3	N2a	M0
	T1-T2	N2b	M0
IIIC	T4a	N2a	M0
	T3-T4a	N2b	M0
	T4b	N1-N2	M0
IVA	T any	N any	M1a
IVB	T any	N any	M1b

Used with the permission of the American Joint Committee on Cancer (AJCC), Chicago, Illinois. The original source for this material is the *AJCC Cancer Staging Manual*, Seventh Edition (2010) published by Springer Science and Business Media LLC, www.springer.com, page 144.

The Dukes Classification and Its Modifications

In the 1930s, Cuthbert Dukes, a Scottish pathologist working predominantly on a classification scheme for rectal cancer, developed the classification system that bears his name. The system, and the several modifications to it made by Dukes and others, is at this time of historical interest only, and the reader is referred to chapters in earlier editions of this book for further details.

Tumor, Node, Metastasis Classification

The current AJCC/UICC staging system for CRC is now the only classification system that should be used.[106] The TNM system classifies colorectal tumors on the basis of the invasiveness (not size) of the primary (T stage), the number (not size or location) of local-regional LNs containing metastatic cancer (N stage), and the presence or absence of distant metastatic disease (M stage) (see Table 49.6).

T Stage. A designation of Tx refers to the inability to describe the extent of tumor invasion due to incomplete information. In situ adenocarcinoma (Tis) includes cancers confined to the glandular basement membrane or lamina propria. The terms *high-grade dysplasia* and *severe dysplasia* are synonymous with in situ carcinoma and are also classified as Tis. T1 tumors invade into but not through the submucosa. T2 tumors invade into but not through the muscularis propria, and T3 tumors invade through the muscularis propria into the subserosa or into nonperitonealized pericolic or perirectal tissue. T4 tumors perforate the visceral peritoneum (T4a) or invade other named organs or structures (T4b). Tumors invading other colorectal segments by way of the serosa (i.e., carcinoma of the cecum invading the sigmoid) are classified as T4b. A tumor that is adherent to other structures or organs macroscopically is classified clinically as T4b; however, if the microscopic examination of the adhesions is negative, then the pathologic classification is pT3. The V and L substaging should be used to identify the presence or absence of vascular or lymphatic invasion. The "p" prefix denotes pathologic (rather than clinical) assessment, and the "y" prefix is attached to those tumors that are being reported after neoadjuvant (presurgical) treatment. For example, the pathologic T stage of a tumor showing only penetration into the submucosa after preoperative therapy would be ypT1. Recurrent tumors are reported with an "r" prefix (rpT3).

N Stage. Because of the prognostic significance associated with increased numbers of LNs inspected (see the following discussion), the current TNM classification scheme calls for at least 12 LNs to be analyzed, and both the number of nodes that are positive for tumor and the total number of nodes inspected should be reported. The term Nx is applied if no description of LN involvement is possible because of incomplete information. A pN0 designation may be made even if fewer than the recommended number of nodes are present; however, the prognostic significance of this pN0 designation is weaker. N0 denotes that all nodes examined are negative. N1a includes tumors with metastasis in one regional LN. N1b refers to involvement of two or three nearby LNs. N1c defines the presence of cancer cells found in areas of fat near LNs, but not in the LNs themselves. N2a indicates metastasis in four to six regional LNs. N2b denotes involvement of greater than seven nodes. Metastatic nodules or foci found in the pericolic, perirectal, or adjacent mesentery without evidence of residual LN tissue are regarded as being equivalent to a regional node metastasis and are counted accordingly.

Stage I disease is defined as T1-2N0 in a patient without distant metastases (M0). Stage II disease is defined as T3-4N0M0. The T-stage carries prognostic significance for stage II, and therefore T3N0 is classified as IIA, and T4a-bN0 is classified as IIB and IIC, respectively.

Node positivity in the absence of M1 disease defines stage III CRC. Recently, the prognostic significance of tumor invasiveness (T stage) has been reincorporated into the assessment of risk in stage III patients. In an exhaustive review of over 50,000 patients, Greene et al.[107] demonstrated the prognostic significance of T stage within node-positive patients. Within the N1 category T stage was found to be highly prognostic, with T1-2 patients fairing significantly better than T3-4. Within the N2 population, the prognosis was worse than either subgroup of N1 patients, with T stage no longer carrying prognostic significance. Thus T stage is prognostic in patients with N0 and N1 but not N2 disease. The current TNM staging system takes these findings into account and now stratifies stage III patients into IIIA (T1-2N1), IIIB (T3-4N1), and IIIC (T any, N2). Stages IIIA, B, and C are highly prognostic for survival.

M Stage. Patients are designated M0 if no evidence of distant metastases is present. Identification of distant metastases denotes a classification of M1. Involvement of the external iliac, common iliac, para-aortic, supraclavicular, or other nonregional LNs is classified as distant metastatic (M1) disease. The M1 category is subdivided into M1a, defined as spread of tumor to one distant organ or set of distant LNs, and M1b, where spread has occurred to more than one distant organ or sets of LNs or spread has occurred to the peritoneum. Although the TNM staging system is regarded as the most comprehensive tool for prognostic and predictive purposes, a major criticism of the last two revisions is that survival of stage IIIA patients continues to be superior to stage IIB. This disparity, which is actually more pronounced in the seventh edition of AJCC manual, has been attributed to inadequate LN assessment and understaging. However, a recent review of SEER data showed this problem persists even in a subset analysis of patients with >12 LNs, highlighting the need for additional refinement and perhaps the incorporation of nonanatomic prognostic factors.[108]

Residual Tumor (R Stage) at Margins of Resection. Tumors that are completely resected with histologically negative margins are classified as R0. Tumors with a complete gross resection but with microscopically positive margins are classified as R1, the positive margin indicating that at least microscopic tumor remains in the patient. Patients who have incomplete resections with grossly positive margins are classified as having had an R2 resection. The R0, R1, and R2 designations carry strong prognostic implications.

Identification of the proximal and distal margins of resection is relatively straightforward, and definitions of these margins are well understood. A more complex and often misunderstood (as well as underreported) margin of resection is the circumferential radial margin (CRM). All three margins (proximal, distal, and CRM) should be specifically commented upon in the pathology report, as all three have prognostic significance.

The CRM is, by definition, a surgically dissected surface. It is defined as the cut retroperitoneal or perineal soft tissue margin closest to the deepest penetration of tumor. It is considered positive if tumor is present microscopically (R1) or macroscopically (R2) on a *cut* radial or lateral aspect of the surgical specimen. For the ascending colon, descending colon, and upper rectum, which are incompletely encased by peritoneum, the CRM is created by dissection of the retroperitoneal aspect of the bowel. In the case of the lower rectum, which is not encased by peritoneum, the CRM is created by sharp dissection of the mesorectum.

A tumor simply penetrating into pericolonic or perirectal fat does not necessarily constitute a positive CRM, but rather is simply a description of a T3 primary. A tumor that involves a peritonealized surface of the bowel and not a surgically cut surface does not constitute a positive CRM, but rather constitutes a T4a primary. If, however, the cut surface at the deepest penetration of the tumor is positive, then the CRM is positive and the resection is staged R1 (microscopic) or R2 (macroscopic). A positive CRM is highly predictive of local recurrence and should prompt consideration of adjuvant treatment.

Prognosis

Histologic Grade

Although histologic grade has been shown to have prognostic significance, there is significant subjectivity involved in scoring of this variable, and no one set of criteria for determination of grade are universally accepted.[105] The majority of staging systems divide tumors into grade 1 (well differentiated), grade 2 (moderately differentiated), grade 3 (poorly differentiated), and grade 4 (undifferentiated). Many studies collapse this into low grade (well to moderately differentiated) and high grade (poorly differentiated or undifferentiated). Greene et al.[107] demonstrated that this two-tiered split has important prognostic significance.

College of American Pathologists Consensus Statement. The College of American Pathologists (CAP) has published an expert panel consensus statement outlining their interpretation of the validity and usefulness of a large number of putatively prognostic and predictive factors in CRC.[109] Variables were categorized as belonging to categories I through IV. Category I was defined as those factors proven to be of prognostic import based on evidence from multiple, statistically robust, published trials and generally used in patient management. Category IIA included factors intensively studied biologically or clinically and repeatedly shown to have prognostic value for outcome or predictive value for therapy that is of sufficient import to be included in the pathology report, but that remains to be validated in statistically robust studies. Category IIB included factors shown to be promising in multiple studies but lacking sufficient data for inclusion in category I or IIA. Category III included factors felt to be not yet sufficiently studied to determine their prognostic value, and category IV included those factors that are adequately studied to have convincingly shown no prognostic significance. A number of these factors are discussed in further detail in the following.

The T, N, and M categories of the current AJCC/UICC staging system were all classified as category I. Other category I inclusions were blood or lymphatic vessel invasion and residual tumor following surgery with curative intent (the R category). Although not assessed pathologically, an elevation of the preoperative CEA level was also felt to merit category I inclusion. Factors in category IIA included tumor grade, radial margin status (for resection of specimens with nonperitonealized surfaces), and residual tumor in the resection specimen following neoadjuvant therapy. Factors in category IIB (many of which are discussed in further detail in the following) included histologic type, histologic features associated with MSI (i.e., host lymphoid response to tumor and medullary or mucinous histologic type), high degree of MSI (MSI-H), loss of heterozygosity (LOH) of 18q (*DCC* [deleted in colon cancer] gene loss), and tumor border configuration (infiltrating versus pushing border). Factors grouped in category III included DNA content, all other molecular markers except for LOH of 18q/DCC and MSI-H, perineural invasion, microvessel density, tumor cell–associated proteins or carbohydrates, peritumoral fibrosis, peritumoral inflammatory response, focal neuroendocrine differentiation, nuclear organizing regions, and proliferation. Those factors in category IV (proven to be of no significance) included tumor size and gross tumor configuration.

Total Number of Lymph Nodes

It has been well established that an adequate number of LNs must be sampled before a patient can be considered node negative, and careful pathologic technique has been demonstrated to be crucial to adequate nodal interpretation. Failure to adequately dissect and display the mesentery will lead to underreporting and understaging.[110,111] It should be noted that an insufficient number of LNs reported could be due to a suboptimal nodal dissection at operation, a less than thorough search for nodes by the pathologist, or some combination of the two. Additional patient- and tumor-related factors may also affect LN count independent of pathologist or surgeon. Belt et al.[112] found a significant association between MSI phenotype and high LN yield in both stage II and III colon cancers, with the strongest effect in the latter group. The authors postulate that this may be due to a more prominent lymphocytic antitumor response known to be exhibited by MSI-H cancers.[112] Another report suggests that low body mass index is associated with increased LN yield, although it did not affect relapse-free or overall survival in stage III cancers. Proximal tumor location, well- or moderately differentiated histology, and stage IIIC cancer were also significant variables for adequate LN recovery.[113] Finally, a multivariate analysis of two large prospective US cohort databases (121,701 women and 51,529 men) demonstrated that specimen length, tumor size, ascending tumor location, T3N0M0 stage, and year of diagnosis were positively associated with negative node count ($p <0.002$). Mutation of KRAS was borderline significant and requires further study. The authors recommend that these variables be taken into account when judging adequacy of LN harvest and devising individualized treatment plans in the future.[114] An analysis was reported on outcome versus nodal sampling in the patients who participated in an Intergroup trial (INT-0089), a large four-arm trial of different 5-fluorouracil (5-FU)–based adjuvant chemotherapies in patients with colon cancer. Multivariate analyses were performed on the node-positive (2,768 patients) and node-negative (648 patients) groups separately. The median number of LNs reported in the assessable patients on this trial was 11 (range, 1 to 87). Survival (overall, cancer-specific, and disease-free [DFS]) was found to decrease with an increasing number of involved LNs ($p = 0.0001$ for all three survival end points). However, after controlling for the number of involved nodes, survival increased with the total number of nodes (positive plus negative) reported ($p = 0.0001$ for overall survival, cancer-specific survival, and DFS). Even in patients who were node negative, overall survival ($p = 0.0005$) and cancer-specific survival ($p = 0.007$) were significantly increased as the number of reported LNs increased.

In a different secondary analysis of the Intergroup trial (INT-0089), a mathematical model was created to estimate the probability of a true node-negative result on the basis of the number of LNs examined in a subset of patients who had at least 10 LNs reported in their resection specimen.[115] A total of 1,585 patients with stage III or high-risk stage II colon cancer were evaluated. This model concluded that when 18 nodes are examined, there is a <25% probability of true node negativity in T1 and T2 tumors. However, examination of <10 LNs was needed in T3 and T4 tumors to achieve the same probability. The overall conclusions of this analysis were that a very significant proportion of patients are understaged, and that such understaging could have important implications for decisions regarding adjuvant therapy and for overall prognosis.

The CAP consensus statement suggests that a minimum of 12 to 15 LNs should be examined in order to determine node negativity.[109] Availability of fewer nodes should therefore be regarded as a relative high-risk factor in terms of prognosis and should be factored into decisions regarding adjuvant therapy. Further support for this recommendation comes from a newly published Danish cohort study that indicates that the advantage of larger LN harvest extends beyond more accurate staging. In addition to improved outcomes for node-negative patients, the authors found a significant increase in overall survival for stage III patients with >12 LNs removed as well (58.6% versus 45.2% for <12 LNs), despite a higher prevalence of N2 disease in this group. This may be related to better surgical technique or an underlying benefit of wider lymphadenectomy in general. LN ratio was also shown to be an important independent prognostic indicator and, in fact, superior to N-stage in predicting survival for stage III patients. This finding is consistent with a number of previous reports, many of which have advocated for incorporation of this parameter into the AJCC staging system.[116–120]

Microscopic Nodal Metastases

The advent of improved pathologic techniques and sensitive methods such as IHC or polymerase chain reaction may have an impact on the number of positive LNs detected and may have important prognostic significance.[121,122] However, the prognostic value of these positive LNs, which otherwise would not be detected, remains controversial. In a recent review of 16 studies with survival data, Sirop et al.[123] found only 8 papers that reported definitely poorer outcomes, whereas the remainder were either equivocal in their conclusions or demonstrated no influence on outcome at all. Jeffers et al.[124] evaluated LNs from 77 patients who were found to have negative LNs by routine examination with immunocytochemical staining for cytokeratin AE1:AE3. Nineteen patients (25%) were found to have immunohistochemical evidence of micrometastases; however, there was no difference in survival between the microscopically positive and negative patients. A larger trial by Faerden et al.,[125] on the other hand, did demonstrate adverse prognostic impact. In this study, 39 of 126 patients with stage I/II colon cancer were noted to have micrometastases or isolated tumor cells (MM/ITC+) on IHC staining. Prospective median 5-year follow-up of MM/ITC+ compared to MM/ITC− patients revealed recurrence rates of 23% versus 7% ($p = 0.010$) and 5-year DFS of 75% versus 93% ($p = 0.012$), respectively.[125] If micrometastases are reported, the methodology by which they are detected should be specified, as it is likely that differences in reliability and reproducibility of different techniques will emerge. Although the actual TNM staging is not altered by the presence of micrometastases, many clinicians choose to regard the presence of such a finding as a poor prognostic variable in their consideration of adjuvant treatment.

Sentinel Node Analysis

Sentinel node analysis is an approach that has received attention in the management of cutaneous melanoma and breast cancer.[126,127] This technique has been proposed as a means of increasing the yield and the diagnostic information for colon cancer.[91,92] The technique for sentinel node mapping and biopsy for colon cancer has been described by Saha et al.[128] Unlike sentinel node approaches for melanoma and breast, where the goal is to potentially limit the extent of an unnecessary formal dissection of a node basin, the goal of the sentinel node in colon cancer is to focus the pathologic analysis on fewer nodes so a more extensive study can be performed. The same extent of node dissection is performed regardless of the sentinel node procedure. The initial studies of sentinel node biopsy demonstrated it was technically feasible, with accuracy rates >80% and upstaging in 15.4% of patients according to a recent prospective trial.[129–131] In addition, Saha et al.[132] suggest that sentinel LN mapping may not just improve staging accuracy but influence the extent of nodal dissection as well. In this study, sentinel LN mapping detected aberrant lymphatic drainage in 22%, which in turn led to a change in operation (i.e., more extensive resection). In two patients, the aberrant sentinel nodes were the only positive nodes identified.[132] However, not all subsequent studies have shown positive results. False-negative rates as high as 60% have been reported, and some studies have failed to demonstrate any change in the stage determination of the lesion.[133] Based on the available data, two conclusions can be reached. First, from a technical standpoint, sentinel node dissection at the time of a colon resection can be performed and the sentinel node accurately identified. Second, the utility of this technique has not yet been established and further large-scale trials are required to establish its role in the staging of patients with CRC.

Blood or Lymphatic Vessel Invasion

Although there have been conflicting reports in the literature, the CAP consensus statement gave blood and lymphatic vessel invasion category I status, indicating that the preponderance of evidence strongly supports the reliability of these findings as indicators of poorer prognosis.[109] Unfortunately, considerable heterogeneity exists in the methodology for examining and reporting of vessel involvement. The finding of vessel involvement increases with the number of sections examined, and differentiation of postcapillary venules from lymphatics is often not possible. These aspects can make interpretation of some older data on this topic potentially problematic. Current recommendations are that at least three blocks of tumor (optimally five or more) each have a single section examined using hematoxylin and eosin stain to look for tumor invasion of vessels. Vessels not definitively interpreted as venules or lymphatics should be reported as angiolymphatic vessels.

Histologic Type

Several histologic types of CRC carry specific independent prognostic significance. Signet ring carcinomas are characterized by >50% of cells demonstrating the "signet ring" morphology in which intracellular mucin accumulation displaces the nuclei and cytoplasm toward the cellular periphery. This histology carries an adverse prognosis.[134,135] The prognostic significance of the finding of mucinous (>50% mucinous) carcinoma remains controversial. Although some reports list mucinous type as an adverse histology, this has not been consistently demonstrated. Most findings of adverse prognosis with mucinous histology are based on univariate analyses. The one finding in a multivariate analysis of a poor prognostic outcome with mucinous tumors was based on a study of tumors presenting with obstruction, a presentation that is in itself high risk. Some reports have lumped mucinous and signet cell tumors together and found this to be a negative prognostic factor; however, this may simply reflect the negative impact of the signet cell tumors, and its meaning regarding the risk of a mucinous histology is unclear. Small cell (extrapulmonary oat cell) tumors are high-grade neuroendocrine tumors with clearly adverse prognostic features. The prognostic significance of focal neuroendocrine differentiation is, however, unclear (CAP category III). Most data indicate that extensive neuroendocrine differentiation is associated with a poorer prognosis.[136] Medullary carcinoma is a subtype characterized by an absence of glands and distinctive growth pattern that previously would have been classified as undifferentiated. It is typically infiltrated with lymphocytes. This histologic subtype is tightly associated with MSI-H and carries a more favorable prognosis.[137] Histologic types other than signet ring, small cell, and medullary carcinomas are routinely designated in the pathology report; however, the majority of these other histologic types carry no established independent prognostic significance.

Microsatellite Instability

As discussed earlier in this chapter, there are two distinct mutational pathways that can give rise to CRC: the MSI pathway or the chromosomal instability pathway. Microsatellites are sections of DNA in which a short sequence of nucleotides (most commonly a dinucleotide) is repeated multiple times.[138] MSI is a situation in which a microsatellite has gained or lost repeat units and so has undergone a change in length, resulting in frame shift mutations or base-pair substitutions. Approximately 15% of CRCs display these mutations. This form of genetic destabilization is typically associated with defective DNA mismatch repair function. Studies of HNPCC tumor specimens demonstrated mutations in mismatch repair genes such as *MLH1* and *MSH2*. These genes encode proteins that repair nucleotide mismatches. The phenotype of tumors with this defect is termed the MSI-H–instability phenotype.

The majority (approximately 85%) of patients with CRC have cancers characteristic of the chromosomal instability pathway, typically having genetic alterations involving LOH, chromosomal amplifications, and chromosomal translocations. These are known as the microsatellite-stable (MSS) tumors. MSI-H tumors have a number of different features relative to low MSI (MSI-L)

or MSS colorectal tumors.[139,140] MSI-L and MSS tumors tend to behave and present similarly. MSI-H tumors are more frequently right-sided, high grade, and mucinous type.[24,141] They are characteristically associated with increased peritumoral lymphocytic infiltration and are characteristically diploid, whereas MSS tumors are more likely to be aneuploid.[142,143] MSI-H CRCs are more likely to have a larger primary at the time of diagnosis but are more likely to be node negative. Patients with MSI-H CRCs have a better long-term prognosis than stage-matched patients with cancers exhibiting MSS.[144]

Watanabe et al.[145] evaluated MSI status as well as allelic loss from chromosomes 18q, 17b, and 8p, as well as cellular levels of p53 and p21$^{wafl/clpl}$ proteins as potential prognostic markers. Tumors were analyzed from 460 stage III and high-risk stage II patients who had been treated with 5-FU–based adjuvant therapy. A total of 62 of 298 tumors evaluated for MSI status (21%) were found to be MSI-H. Of the MSI-H tumors, 38 (61%) had a mutation of the gene for type II receptor of transforming growth factor (TGF)-β1. In this analysis, MSI-H was a favorable prognostic indicator for 5-year DFS ($p = 0.02$) and trended toward being a favorable independent prognostic indicator, but did not reach statistical significance for overall survival ($p = 0.20$). However, the 5-year survival among patients with MSI-H was 74% in the presence of a mutated gene for the type II receptor of TGF-β1 and 46% in patients whose tumors lacked this mutation (RR = 2.90; 95% CI = 1.14 to 7.34; $p = 0.04$). MSI-H cells are relatively resistant to 5-FU in vitro.[146] All of the patients in Watanabe et al.'s[145] analysis received 5-FU–based chemotherapy. The TGF-β1 pathway inhibits tumor proliferation by causing a late G_1 cell cycle arrest. Therefore, a mutated and presumably nonfunctional *TGF-β1* gene could favor increased proliferation, which would be anticipated to confer increased susceptibility to cytotoxic chemotherapy. A recent evaluation of the prognostic significance of MSI in the N0147 adjuvant trial[147] demonstrated a more nuanced result. When looking at the colon overall, MSI was not found to be predictive. However, when divided by side, MSI was found to carry a favorable prognosis for right-sided colon lesions, but was a negative prognostic factor in left-sided colon lesions. The reasons for this difference is not clear; however, the different embryologic origins of the left and right colon may play a role in these observations.

BRAF

BRAF mutation, present in 10% to 20% of CRCs, is linked to a subset of MSI-H tumors that are sporadic and generally have poorer prognosis. Ogino et al.[148] confirmed this relationship in comparative analysis of 506 stage III patients enrolled in the Cancer and Leukemia Group B (CALGB) 89803 trial. BRAF-mutated patients had significantly worse overall survival (HR = 1.66) compared to wild-type, a finding that was most pronounced in the setting of MSS.[148] In a follow-up study, Lochhead et al.[149] also identified combined BRAF/MSI status as a powerful prognosticator and recommends stratification of all patients into poor (MSS/BRAF mutant), intermediate (MSS/BRAF wild-type), and favorable (MSI-H/BRAF wild-type) groups in order better inform treatment strategies. Douillard et al.[150] confirmed BRAF mutation to be a poor prognostic factor in patients with stage IV disease as well.

Allelic Loss of 18q (*DCC* Gene Loss)

Allelic LOH that involves chromosome 18q occurs in half or more of all CRCs. Allelic loss of 18q typically involves the *DCC* gene; however, other genes in this region, such as Smad2 and Smad4, may also be relevant to CRC development. DCC expression is greatly reduced or absent in many colorectal carcinomas, and loss of DCC is associated with metastasis and an adverse prognosis.[151] The specific product of the DCC gene has been shown to be the netrin-1 receptor. In the nonpathologic state, this receptor guides the migration of neuronal axons. DCC induces apoptosis in the absence of netrin-1 binding. DCC is cleaved by caspase, and mutation of the site at

TABLE 49.7

Loss of Heterozygosity (Allelic Loss) at 18q and Prognosis in Patients with Stage III Colon Cancer

Allelic Status of 18q	No. of Patients	Five-Y Survival (%)	P Value
No loss	112	69	0.005
Loss	109	50	

From Watanabe T, Wu TT, Catalano PJ, et al. Molecular predictors of survival after adjuvant chemotherapy for colon cancer. *N Engl J Med* 2001;344: 1196–1206.

which caspase 3 cleaves DCC suppresses the proapoptotic effect of DCC completely. Binding of netrin-1 to DCC blocks apoptosis.[152] Loss of DCC as a result of allelic loss in 18q could therefore be anticipated to impair apoptosis, thereby resulting in greater resistance to chemotherapy. This hypothesized mechanism of action of 18q LOH is attractive; however, it should be emphasized that it is not at all clear to what extent DCC is the active moiety in the setting of 18q allelic loss. Watanabe et al.[145] evaluated allelic loss from chromosome 18q as a potential prognostic indicator in archived specimens of tumors from patients who were treated in one of two national Intergroup adjuvant trials (INT 0035 or INT 0089). MSI status was also evaluated, as were 17p, 8p, and cellular levels of p53 and p21[wafl/clp1] proteins. Tumors were analyzed from 460 stage III and high-risk stage II patients who had been treated with 5-FU–based adjuvant therapy. Allelic loss of 18q was present in 155 of 319 cancers (49%). Allelic loss in 18q was highly prognostically significant in this analysis (Table 49.7). In the stage III patients with allelic loss of 18q, 5-year overall survival was 50%, while in those with retained 18q alleles, 5-year survival was 69% ($p = 0.005$). Other markers evaluated in this analysis were not shown to be prognostically significant.

Host Lymphoid Response

Lymphocytic infiltration has been identified as a favorable prognostic indicator. Whether this is a truly independent predictor of outcome is not clear, however, as this finding is tightly associated with MSI-H, a favorable prognostic factor. Along these lines, the prognostic value of neutrophil-to-lymphocyte ratio has also been recently evaluated. Chiang et al.[153] found that elevated preoperative neutrophil-to-lymphocyte ratio (>3) was associated with significantly worse DFS in stage I to III colon but not rectal cancers on multivariate analysis. In another study, neutrophil-to-lymphocyte ratio (>5) was also found to be an independent risk factor for recurrence. While the direct impact of this parameter is difficult to explain, the authors of the first study postulate that it may represent a measure of innate-to-adaptive immunity under stress with relative lymphopenia, as a marker of depressed cell-mediated immunity, conferring survival disadvantage.[153,154]

Tumor Border Configuration

The configuration of the tumor border (infiltrating versus pushing border) has been shown to have independent prognostic significance. An infiltrating border, characterized by an irregular, infiltrating pattern at the tumor edge (also known as focal dedifferentiation or tumor budding), has been shown in multivariate analyses to portend a poorer prognosis than tumors with smooth, pushing borders.

Carcinoembryonic Antigen

An elevated preoperative CEA is a poor prognostic factor for cancer recurrence. Although there is variability in the available data regarding the level that denotes a prognostic cutoff, a preoperative CEA level >5 ng/ml is considered a category I poor prognostic indicator

by the CAP consensus panel.[109] Patients in whom the elevated CEA fails to normalize after a potentially curative operation are at particularly high risk. Several authors have presented evidence that indicates that CEA is an independent prognostic factor. In a report of 572 patients who underwent curative resection for node-negative colon cancer, the preoperative CEA level and the stage of disease predicted survival by both univariate and multivariate analyses.[155] Given the prognostic significance of the preoperative CEA, it is reasonable to recommend that all patients who undergo operation for CRC have a serum CEA drawn prior to operation.

No other serum markers have been demonstrated to be reliably prognostic or predictive in CRC. Cancer antigen (CA) 19-9, a factor that has become widely used for pancreas cancer, has no role at this time in the routine management of CRC.

Obstruction and Perforation

Carcinoma of the colon that is complicated by obstruction or perforation has been recognized as having a poorer prognosis. Data obtained from 1,021 patients with Dukes stage B and C CRC, who were entered into randomized clinical trials of the National Surgical Adjuvant Breast and Bowel Project (NSABP) showed that the presence of bowel obstruction strongly influenced the outcome. The effect of bowel obstruction was more pronounced when the obstruction was located in the right colon. The larger-sized tumor needed to block the ascending colon completely might allow a longer time for these tumors to grow and spread when compared with tumors located in the descending colon.

A review of the Massachusetts General Hospital records compared patients who presented with obstruction or perforation with a control group who underwent curative resection. The actuarial 5-year survival rate seen in patients who presented with obstruction was 31%, in contrast to 59% in historical controls. For patients with localized perforation, the 5-year actuarial survival rate was 44%. The Gastrointestinal Tumor Study Group (GITSG) multivariate analysis concluded that obstruction was an important indicator of prognosis, independent of Dukes stage. Bowel perforation was a poor prognostic factor only for DFS.

Category III Factors

Multiple factors, while of investigational interest, are at this time not appropriate for routine clinical use and have so been designated as category III (defined as not sufficiently studied to prove their prognostic value) by the CAP consensus panel. These include DNA content, or ploidy, and proliferation indices. Also included in category III are all molecular markers other than MSI and 18q deletions, such as thymidylate synthase (TS), dihydropyrimidine dehydrogenase (DPD), and p53 mutational status. Perineural invasion, microvessel density, tumor cell–associated proteins or carbohydrates, peritumoral fibrosis, peritumoral inflammatory response, and focal neuroendocrine differentiation are also category III. The area of molecular prognostic markers is one of particular activity, however, and it is anticipated that clinical trials that are now ongoing will shed light on these important areas.

Perineural Invasion

The ability of CRCs to invade perineural spaces as far as 10 cm from the primary tumor has long been described. Early reports suggest an increased disease recurrence rate and worse 5-year survival. Multivariate analyses have failed to show the prognostic significance of this finding. The CAP consensus panel classified perineural invasion as category III (insufficient evidence of determine prognostic significance).

Tumor Size and Configuration

Studies have consistently shown that both the size and configuration of the primary tumor in CRC do not carry prognostic significance (CAP category IV). In a review of 391 patients, the mean diameter of Dukes stage B2 tumors was actually greater than the mean diameter of stage C2 tumors ($p < 0.001$) and D tumors ($p < 0.05$). The size of the primary tumor showed no relationship to 5-year adjusted survival. These results were confirmed by the NSABP experience.[156] Tumor configuration is described as exophytic (fungating), endophytic (ulcerative), diffusely infiltrative (linitis plastica), or annular. The vast majority of studies have failed to show any of these configurations to have consistent independent prognostic significance. Linitis plastica has been related to a poor prognosis; however, this may be due to the signet cell and other high-grade features of the tumors that are typically associated with this morphology.

Hemorrhage or Rectal Bleeding

It has been speculated that tumors that present with bleeding might be found earlier and therefore might be associated with a better prognosis. This has not been confirmed by data. In the GITSG multivariate analysis, the presence of melena or rectal bleeding showed a trend as a prognostic factor for prolonged survival but failed to reach statistical significance ($p = 0.08$). One large study found bleeding to be a favorable prognostic indicator on univariate analysis; however, this finding disappeared on multivariate analysis. Bleeding at presentation does not appear to carry any significance.

Primary Tumor Location

Large retrospective reviews of data from the NSABP suggest that right-sided colon cancers carry a worse prognosis than left-sided ones. However, poorer prognosis for patients with disease in the left colon has also been reported. Several investigators report no difference based on the location of the primary tumor. The large GITSG colon cancer experience showed that tumor location (left, right, and rectosigmoid or sigmoid) was of low prognostic value. A recent analysis of SEER-Medicare data by Weiss et al.[157] provides additionally ambiguous results. Of 53,801 patients, 67% had right-sided colon cancer and were more likely to be older, women, and diagnosed with more advanced stage and with more poorly differentiated tumors. However, on multivariate analysis, there was no significant difference in mortality for all stages combined or for stage I. Compared to left-sided lesions, right-sided cancers were associated with a lower mortality within the stage II subgroup (HR = 0.92; $p = 0.001$) but higher mortality within stage III (HR = 1.12; $p = 0.001$). Critics of this report point out that a less aggressive treatment approach was likely employed in this older study population, as at least 40% of stage III cases did not receive adjuvant therapy and nearly half underwent inadequate LN harvest. Regardless, these results further dispel the notion of a straightforward relationship between tumor location and mortality.[157]

Body Mass Index

While obesity is known to be a risk factor for the development of colon cancer, the prognostic impact of body mass index on long-term outcomes is controversial. In a cohort study conducted within a large randomized trial of 3,759 patients with high-risk stage II or III colon cancer (INT-0089), obese women had significantly worse overall mortality (HR = 1.34; 95% CI = 1.07 to 1.67); however, this finding was not apparent in men.[158] Sinicrope et al.[159] found the opposite gender correlation using the ACCENT database, a pooled resource of 25,291 participants in national and international adjuvant chemotherapy trials. On multivariate analysis, with a median follow-up of 7.8 years, obese and underweight men, but not women, had significantly poorer survival compared to overweight and normal weight patients.[159] And in another prospective cohort of 913 patients with stage II and III colon cancer, Alipour et al.[160] found no association between obesity (as measured by either body mass index or body surface area) and oncologic outcomes. Evidently, this topic warrants further study before any conclusions can be drawn.[160]

Diabetes Mellitus

The influence of diabetes mellitus on outcome is also unclear. In the INT-0089 cohort, diabetes conferred a strong disadvantage with affected patients experiencing a significantly worse DFS (48% versus 59%; $p < 0.0001$), overall survival (57% versus 66%; $p < 0.0001$), and recurrence-free survival (56% versus 64%; $p = 0.012$) at 5 years. Median survival for diabetics was 6 years, whereas for nondiabetics it was 11.3 years.[158] Other reports, however, have generated less consistent results. Among 2,278 subjects from the Cancer Prevention Study-II Nutrition Cohort, patients with CRC and type 2 diabetes were at higher risk of all-cause mortality (ACM; RR = 1.53), but only those without insulin use were at higher risk for CRC-specific mortality. These results are in line with previous evidence that hyperinsulinemia (as in poorly controlled diabetes) plays an important role in tumorigenesis and metastasis of CRC.[161] Another population-based study did not find any such an association in 6,974 patients with colon cancer. Disease-specific mortality was only significantly increased for patients with rectal cancer ($n = 3,888$, 10% of whom were diabetic; HR = 1.30). While hyperinsulinemia is again implicated, the authors call for additional study to clarify specific pathways responsible for these rectum-specific findings.[162]

Gender

Female sex has generally been considered a favorable prognostic factor, but data is limited and inconclusive. In the first study to examine the impact of gender in the era of oxaliplatin-based therapy, Cheung et al.[163] performed a prospectively planned, pooled analysis of 33,345 patients participating in the ACCENT database of randomized trials. The authors found a significant but very modest survival advantage for women with early stage disease that persisted across all ages, stages, and types of adjuvant therapy. Sex was not a predictive factor for treatment efficacy, however, suggesting that chemotherapy regimens should be not be altered based on this parameter.[163]

Smoking

As discussed earlier, prolonged cigarette smoking appears to be a moderate risk factor for CRC with continued effect even after smoking cessation. Increasing evidence indicates that this association differs not just by tumor site but also by molecular features, such as the presence of MSI-H and BRAF mutations, which cumulatively seem to confer the strongest risk. Impact on survival has now also been reported in a recent study analyzing data from a large multicenter randomized adjuvant chemotherapy trial (N0147). The authors found that smokers experienced significantly shorter 3-year DFS (74% versus 70%; HR = 1.21) that was most evident in BRAF wild-type and KRAS-mutated tumors.[164]

Blood Transfusions

Considerable controversy has surrounded the question of an association between perioperative blood transfusions and the recurrence rate of CRC. Some investigators have reported worse DFS in patients who require transfusions. By multivariate analysis in a large prospective study, however, no negative influence of transfusion on survival could be detected, and it does not appear that perioperative blood transfusions carry negative prognostic value. A retrospective analysis evaluating 1,051 patients treated with curative surgery for stage II or III colorectal adenocarcinoma at the Mayo Clinic demonstrated that the use of blood components probably had no impact on disease recurrence, and the documented adverse impact of transfusions is more likely due to other variables or to the underlying illness necessitating the transfusion.[165]

Oncogenes and Molecular Markers

Oncogenes and molecular markers are discussed extensively in another chapter. At present, none of the markers under investigation has achieved adequate validity to permit routine clinical use. However, the study of molecular markers continues to progress and continues to advance the understanding of the development and treatment of CRC. TS continues to be a major area of investigation. Data are conflicting on its prognostic significance; however, preliminary studies suggest that high TS levels may be predictive for resistance to 5-FU–based therapies.[166] At present, there is no role for TS determinations in routine clinical practice. The *p53* gene located on chromosome 17p is a well-known tumor suppressor gene. The abnormal *p53* appears to be a late phenomenon in colorectal carcinogenesis. This mutation may allow the growing tumor with multiple genetic alterations to evade cell cycle arrest and apoptosis. In a retrospective review of 141 patients with resected stage II and III colon carcinoma, a *p53* mutation increased the risk of death by 2.82 times in patients with stage II disease and by 2.39 times in patients with stage III colon carcinoma. The Southwest Oncology Group assessed the prognostic value of p53 in 66 patients with stage II and 163 stage III colon cancer. *p53* expression was found in 63% of cancers and was associated with favorable survival in stage III but not stage II disease. Seven-year survival with stage III disease was 56% with *p53* expression versus 43% with no*p53* expression ($p = 0.012$).[167] Overall, the data are conflicting on the utility of *p53* as a prognostic variable, and it does not have a use at this time in standard practice.

Epidermal growth factor receptor (EGFR) is an important molecular target for antibody-based therapy in various cancer types and is ubiquitous in colonic tissue. The prognostic impact of this biomarker was recently addressed in a meta-analysis demonstrating worse postoperative survival in patients with high compared to low EGFR expression (HR = 2.34).[168]

Genetic Polymorphisms

Extensive preliminary work is indicating that genetic polymorphisms can potentially have important predictive implications in terms of both efficacy and toxicity with chemotherapy. For example, the UGT1A1 polymorphism has been correlated with CPT-11 toxicity, and TS and XRCC1 polymorphisms may predict efficacy for oxaliplatin or 5-FU combinations.[169] Although a commercial assay is currently available for measurement of UGT1A1 polymorphisms, it is not, at this time, clear how, or if, this assay should be used in routine practice. Currently, there are no specific guidelines for dose modifications on the basis of UGT1A1polymorphism, and the 7/7 mutation, associated with higher toxicity, has also been associated with greater antitumor activity. These approaches will require considerable more validation and exploration before they can be considered for standard management.[170]

APPROACHES TO SURGICAL RESECTION OF COLON CANCER

The management of colon cancer is best understood as a multimodality approach tailored to the stage of disease. However, there are certain basic tenets of surgical management for the resection of the primary lesion that can be applied across various pathologic stages. Therefore, in order to provide a clear description of these techniques, they will first be described based on the type of surgical resection. These procedures will then be referred to throughout the discussion of stage-specific treatment.

Colonoscopic Resection of Polyps

Many lesions of the colon are first detected during endoscopic procedures. These lesions can range from small hyperplastic polyps to large fungating invasive carcinomas. The appearance of these lesions often indicates their relative potential for malignancy. However, the only definitive way to make a diagnosis is through a pathologic examination of the tissue. Therefore, the goal of a colonoscopic biopsy or resection is to, whenever feasible, remove the lesion in its entirety and preserve a tissue architecture in order to achieve both a therapeutic resection and an accurate pathologic diagnosis. Various techniques can be employed for the removal of lesions in the colon depending on their size and location. Biopsy forceps and snares are the two most commonly employed instruments used during a colonoscopy. These devices are fashioned from flexible coated wires that can conform to the shape of the colonoscope and can also conduct electrical current in order to achieve coagulation and hemostasis.

Bleeding and perforation, while uncommon, are seen at an increased frequency during a therapeutic as opposed to a diagnostic colonoscopy.[171,172] Small polypoid lesions (up to 5 to 8 mm) that are found during the course of a colonoscopic examination can often be removed in their entirety along with a small amount of normal mucosa using a biopsy forceps. Bleeding is usually minimal but can be controlled by electrocautery if persistent. Larger well-pedunculated polyps can often be removed using a technique employing a snare and electrocautery. The snare is placed over the polypoid lesion and cinched down at the base of the polyp. Once tightened, an electrical current is applied and the polyp is resected. If the lesions are too large to be retrieved through the working port of the colonoscope, they can be held in place with a snare just beyond the tip of the colonoscope where they can be kept in view and withdrawn with the scope from the patient. It is important, when sending these specimens to pathology, to properly orient the polyp so as to indicate the base where the resection took place as well as the other positions of the lesion. This will allow the pathologist to provide important information as to the margin status for the resection. Carcinoma in situ as well as stage I invasive carcinomas found in a well-pedunculated polyp can be treated with colonoscopic resection, as described previously, and no further surgical management is needed as long as there is a negative margin >2 mm and the tumor is well-differentiated without lymphovascular invasion or extension of malignant cells beyond the stalk (Haggitt levels 1 to 3).[173] If these criteria are not met, further therapy is required. It is for this reason that it is often helpful to mark the site of the polyp resection with an agent that will leave a "tattoo" to guide additional intervention.

Larger lesions with a broad base or sessile lesions are best biopsied to make a diagnosis rather than resected using the colonoscope. The risk of perforation or inadequate resection margins is greatly increased with broad-based and sessile lesions. Multiple biopsies should be taken in order to determine whether the lesion harbors an invasive cancer, and further resection decisions are made based on the pathologic findings. In cases where there is low suspicion for malignancy, an endoscopic mucosal or submucosal resection may be attempted, usually by a gastroenterologist with advanced interventional endoscopic expertise. However, if such a lesion is left behind, it is of critical importance to note the position of the lesion in order that it might be more easily found if a subsequent procedure is required. In addition to determining the depth of insertion of the scope, which can be highly inaccurate with flexible instruments, other landmarks including the appendiceal orifice or ileocecal valve in the cecum and the liver/splenic shadows at the flexures should be noted. The most important step however is to properly mark the polyp site with 1 ml of tattoo injected submucosally in each of four quadrants for definitive intra- and extraluminal recognition at a later date.[174]

For lesions that cannot be resected through the scope or are found to be invasive carcinomas that are sessile or broad based, a variety of surgical resections can be employed depending on the position of the lesion and its T stage. It is important to keep in mind, however, that the formal staging of the lesion does not occur until after the resection is completed; therefore, if there is any suspicion of an invasive carcinoma being present, a definitive oncologic resection should be performed.[175]

Bowel Preparation

An important part of the preoperative regimen for a colon resection is the proper cleansing of the bowel in order to reduce the risk of postoperative complications as well as to allow for easier visualization during the procedure, particularly with the laparascopic approach. A variety of regimens have been described, and there are many that have demonstrated efficacy.[176,177] Although there are several choices described in the literature, the basic components of a bowel preparation are a mechanical cleansing of the bowel using a cathartic or volume-displacing agent and appropriate antibiotic prophylaxis.[178,179] Recently, some studies have suggested that mechanical bowel preparation may be unnecessary; however, this remains controversial.[180,181]

For rectal and low sigmoid tumors, a number of surgeons also perform distal rectal washout prior to resection, with the professed intention of eliminating exfoliated intraluminal cancer cells that may increase local recurrence risk. There has been little evidence to support this theory, and washout has not been routinely recommended as standard practice. However, a recent meta-analysis of nine studies and 5,395 patients is the first to demonstrate a significant benefit to this maneuver with a nearly two-fold reduction in local recurrence rates (5.79% versus 10.05%; $p < 0.00001$). While the lack of randomized controlled trials limits the strength of this data, the authors conclude that distal washout should be reconsidered in all patients given the minimal cost, time, and risk it entails.[182]

Anatomic Resection

For invasive carcinomas of the colon, stages I through III, the surgical approach will be dictated by the size and location of lesions in the colon.[183,184] The location will determine what region of bowel is removed, and the extent of its resection is dictated by its vascular and lymphatic supply.

Resection of the Right Colon

Lesions in the cecum and ascending colon are managed with a right hemicolectomy (Fig. 49.3A,B). The right colon is mobilized from the retroperitoneum by incising its retroperitoneal attachments, taking care to avoid injury to the ureter, inferior vena cava, duodenum, and gonadal vessels. The colon is mobilized from the ileum to the transverse colon, taking care at the hepatic flexure not to injure the gallbladder or duodenum. The ileocolic, right colic, and right branch of middle colic vessels are then ligated and divided. A proximal ligation in order to allow for the removal of colonic mesentery along with LNs is performed for staging purposes. Once the vascular supply is divided and the intervening mesenteric tissue ligated and divided, attention can be addressed to the resection of the colonic tissue.

There are a variety of techniques for dividing the colon. This can be done between clamps using scalpel or using a variety of stapling devices. One method would be to use a linear GI anastigmatic stapler. After making a small hole just below the colonic wall though the mesentery at the point chosen for resection, the stapler can be positioned across the colon and fired, thus dividing the tissue. This is then repeated across the ileum just proximal to the ileocecal valve. Once divided, all remaining mesenteric tissue is carefully ligated and divided, and the colonic specimen can be removed. Although a no-touch "technique" has been advocated in the past, studies have demonstrated that this has no influence on recurrence or seeding of distant disease.[185] Once the right colon has been removed, intestinal continuity can be re-established by creating an anastomosis between the terminal ileum and the remaining transverse colon using either a hand-sewn or stapled technique.

Resection of the Transverse Colon

For lesions located in the transverse colon, a variety of approaches can be undertaken. Those lesions that are proximal and

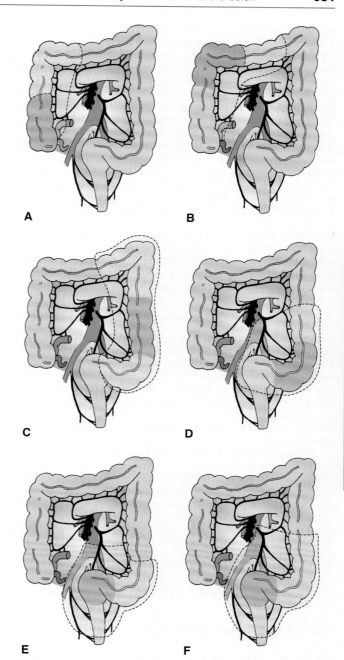

Figure 49.3 **(A)** Surgical resection for a cecal or ascending colon cancer. **(B)** Surgical resection for a cancer at the hepatic flexure. **(C)** Surgical resection for a descending colon cancer. **(D)** Preferred surgical procedure for cancer of the middle and proximal sigmoid colon. In poor-risk patients, the inferior mesenteric artery and the left colic artery may be preserved. **(E)** Surgical resection for cancer of the rectosigmoid. **(F)** A more radical surgical resection for cancer of the rectosigmoid.

near the hepatic flexure can be resected with an extended right hemicolectomy. This extension should encompass up to and include the middle colic vessel. The advantage of such a resection over a true transverse colectomy is that the anastomosis performed to restore intestinal continuity involves an anastomosis between the ileum and the remaining colon. Due to the improved blood supply delivered by the small bowel mesentery, there is a decreased risk of an anastomotic leak in an ileocolic as opposed to a colocolic anastomosis.[175] Likewise, a lesion in the distal transverse colon can be resected with an extended left hemicolectomy, which will be described in more detail in the following section. For those lesions that are in the midportion of the transverse colon, however, a transverse colectomy can be performed. This procedure requires mobilization of the right colon in order to allow this tissue to be brought over for an anastomosis following the resection.

The omentum is divided from the greater curvature of the stomach up to and including its attachments at the splenic helium. The omentum can often be a source of micrometastatic disease and therefore its resection at the time a transverse colectomy is indicated. After dividing the omentum and mobilizing the right and transverse colon up to and including the splenic flexure, the middle colic artery is ligated at its trunk and smaller vessels from the right and left colic artery branches can be ligated and divided as required. A linear stapler can once again be used to divide the colonic tissue, and then the mobilized right colon can be anastomosed to the descending colon in an end-to-end fashion using a hand-sewn anastomosis or using a side-to-side stapled technique. Depending on the size of the transverse colon, however, it is often safer and easier to resect the right and transverse colon and connect the ileum to the descending colon. This allows enough colonic reserve for water absorption and normal bowel movements.

Resection of the Descending and Sigmoid Colon

For lesions in the proximal descending colon, the splenic flexure is mobilized and the left colic artery can be ligated and divided with the portion of colon removed by mobilizing the splenic flexure and dividing the omentum (Fig. 49.3C,D). The transverse colon can be brought over to the region of the sigmoid colon for anastomosis. For lesions in the midportion of the descending colon, a left hemicolectomy can be performed, taking care to ligate the left colic vessel along with some sigmoidal branches and taking an adequate portion of mesentery for staging purposes.

For lesions that involve the sigmoid colon, a sigmoid colectomy can be performed with margins of resection on either side of the lesion. The descending colon is mobilized (together with the splenic flexure as needed) and connected to the rectum using either a hand-sewn anastomosis or stapling device. The mesentery can be divided either at the level of the sigmoidal branches with preservation of the left colic artery or at the origin of the inferior mesenteric pedicle (Fig. 49.3E,F). While the latter approach is preferred by some to achieve greater mobilization and higher lymph node counts, neither this nor a more extensive left hemicolectomy has resulted in improved survival.

The approaches to the resection of lesions below the peritoneal reflection will be discussed in the chapter on rectal cancer.

Total Abdominal Colectomy

For patients with ulcerative colitis or familial polyposis syndrome who either have evidence of invasive carcinoma or are at significant risk for the development of invasive carcinoma, a total abdominal colectomy may be required. This can be performed by mobilization of the right colon, transverse colon along the omentum, taking the omentum as part of the resection, the hepatic and splenic flexures, as well as the complete mobilization of the descending colon down to the peritoneal reflection. Ligation of the ileocolic, right colic, middle colic, left colic, and sigmoid branches will allow for removal of the colon down to the peritoneal reflection. For ulcerative colitis and familial polyposis syndromes without evidence of carcinoma below the peritoneal reflection, the operation can be terminated at this point with ileorectal anastomoses and careful surveillance of the remaining rectum via proctoscopy. However, in order to remove all tissue at risk for further lesions, a total protocolectomy is often advocated.[186,187] Although this procedure can be performed as an abdominal perineal resection with a permanent end ileostomy, most surgeons now advocate one of many continent pull-through procedures in order to preserve fecal continence in a patient population that is often very young. Such

procedures provide very good control of continence and a relatively normal lifestyle.[188]

SURGICAL MANAGEMENT OF COMPLICATIONS FROM PRIMARY COLON CANCER

Patients with primary lesions of the colon can present with obstruction, bleeding, and perforation. The surgical management of these patients can be complex, requiring intraoperative decisions tailored to the situation encountered. Blood per rectum can be one of the most frightening experiences for patient and physician alike. Bleeding from a CRC can occur anywhere from the cecum to the distal rectum. Although bleeding can be temporized with endoscopic fulguration and the patient supported with transfusion, definitive management of the lesion with either surgery or radiation therapy will ultimately be required. Other maneuvers such as angiographic embolization may provide only a temporary solution. Fortunately, life-threatening hemorrhage due to a colon cancer primary is a rare occurrence. More often, these lesions lead to a chronic blood loss, resulting in anemia.

Colonic obstruction due to a primary tumor is not uncommon. Obstructing colon lesions present several important issues. First, the acute obstruction must be managed. Ideally, an exploration with resection of the tumor and primary anastomosis with or without a diversion is ideal. However, given the fact that the operation will be performed on unprepared bowel and the patient's physical condition may be less than optimal, resection without an anastomosis and an end colostomy should be considered. In some instances, the obstructing lesion may present significant technical hurdles for resection in the setting of an acutely dehydrated and ill patient. In these circumstances, a decompression maneuver that can be performed rapidly and with minimal morbidity such as a transverse loop colostomy or a colostomy and mucous fistula can be performed to temporize the situation and allow the patient to be prepared and resuscitated adequately for a definitive resection at a second exploration.

Bypass operations should be reserved only for the most extreme circumstances as complications following these procedures due to repeat obstructions and leakage with abdominal sepsis are not insignificant.

Another option is to place an endoscopic stent either for temporary decompression or for definitive palliation of unresectable lesions. Multiple studies over the past 10 years have demonstrated the feasibility and safety of this maneuver in selected patients.[189–194] As a bridge to surgery, stenting can provide a minimally invasive means for converting an emergency situation into an elective one, allowing time for resuscitation, bowel prep, and adjuvant therapies. In a small randomized, controlled trial from 2009, Cheung et al.[195] reported additional advantages including significantly reduced rates of perioperative morbidity and stoma creation.

While short-term data seem to support the use of self-expanding metallic stents (SEMS) as a bridge to surgery, other reports as well long-term results from a recent comparative trial do not.[196,197] Sabbagh et al.[198] performed a head-to-head, intention-to-treat analysis of 87 patients undergoing either stenting or emergency surgery, using a propensity score to correct for selection bias. Overall survival at 3 and 5 years was significantly better in the surgery group (66% versus 44%, $p = 0.015$, and 62% versus 25%, $p = 0.0003$, respectively) and remained superior even when patients with perforation and metastatic disease were excluded (74% versus 51%, $p = 0.02$, and 67% versus 30%, $p = 0.001$, respectively). Five-year cancer-specific mortality was significantly higher in the SEMS group (48% versus 21%, $p = 0.02$) and there were trends toward worse 5-year DFS and increased recurrence as well as mean time to recurrence. Based on these findings, the authors have markedly changed their management of left-sided malignant obstruction, now reserving SEMS strictly for palliative indications and patients with high postoperative mortality risk.[198]

Laparoscopic Colon Resection

Since its introduction to the field of general surgery for gallbladder resection, the use of laparoscopic surgery has found increasing applications.[199] Laparoscopic surgery has become a particularly important addition to the armamentarium of the surgical oncologist. The use of laparoscopy for the staging of the extent of disease for peritoneal malignancies, pancreatic cancer, colon cancer, and gastric cancer is now widely accepted.[200–202] Laparoscopic resection has also found a niche for the removal of adrenal tumors, the spleen, and distal pancreas.[203,204] The use of laparoscopic approaches for the resection of malignant lesions in the colon is now becoming more common.

With the increasing application of laparoscopic techniques to colon cancer surgery, concerns ranging from inadequacy of resection margins, inadequacy of LN sampling, and the potential seeding of port sites with malignant cells have been raised.[205–207] Although these concerns are important, there are several potential advantages for laparoscopic approaches to the surgical management of colon cancer. Issues regarding length of incision, patient recovery time, and return to bowel function are often cited as justification for a laparoscopic approach. However, just as important are the technical advantages of surgery utilizing laparoscopic systems. The improved visualization due to magnification provided by video laparoscopy allows much more intricate and careful dissections in the deep pelvis, which could potentially reduce postoperative morbidity from low anterior resections that utilize a mesorectal excision technique. The ability to carefully trace vessels in the mesentery under magnification could improve the ability to perform high ligations in order to retrieve a greater number of LNs for sampling.

The technical difficulties faced during laparoscopic resection of the colon relate, in general, to the size of the specimen being removed and the need to perform an anastomosis. Each of these can be overcome through careful placement of incisions for specimen removal as well as a judicious use of stapling devices in order to perform both intracorporeal as well as a combination of intracorporeal and extracorporeal anastomotic techniques. A number of studies have examined the relative risks and benefits of the laparoscopic resection of colon cancer.[205,208–210] A prospective random assignment trial conducted by Clinical Outcomes of Surgical Therapy Study Group examined both the oncologic outcomes with respect to DFS and overall survival as well as the impact of laparoscopic versus open surgery on patient recovery, pain management, and time to return of bowel function. An initial report on quality of life showed only a modest short-term benefit for laparoscopic resection versus a conventional open procedure,[211] but the overall results of the trial with respect to oncologic outcomes demonstrated equivalence between the laparoscopic and open approach.[212]

Long-term follow-up from the corresponding UK randomized study (CLASICC Trial Group), which was similarly designed to compare laparoscopic to conventional surgery for colon and rectal cancer, and that initially reported noninferiority results in 2007, lends further support to the laparoscopic approach. With a median follow-up of 62.9 (range, 22.9 to 92.8) months, the authors found no statistically significant differences in overall survival (82.7% versus 78.3%), DFS (77% versus 89.5%), or local recurrence.[213,214]

Over a period of 10 years, the group from the Colon and Rectal Clinic of Orlando, Florida, performed a prospective nonrandomized study comparing laparoscopic to open resection for colorectal carcinoma. Laparoscopic resection was offered selectively in the absence of a large mass, invasion into the abdominal wall or adjacent organs, or if the patient did not have multiple prior operations.[205] All laparoscopic resections were performed with curative intent, and 20% of the patients whose procedures were converted to open resection were included in the laparoscopic resection group based

on an intention-to-treat model. The study measured oncologic outcomes and compared them with a computerized case-matched open resection group, using case-matching variables consisting of age, gender, site of primary tumor (colon versus rectum), and TNM stage. The group who received laparoscopic resection was followed prospectively and the data were updated on a regular basis. Follow-up of these patients consisted of a combination of office visits, telephone calls, and a review of the US Social Security Death Index Database. There were 172 patients in each group, and the groups were well matched for age, TMM stage, prior chemo- or radiation therapy, and site of the primary tumor (colon versus rectum).

Thirty-day mortality was 1.2% in the laparoscopic resection group and 2.4% in the open resection group; however, this difference was not statistically significant. The local recurrence rate of the laparoscopic group was 3.5% compared to a local recurrence rate in the open group of 2.9%. The stage-for-stage overall 5-year survival rate between the two groups was similar, and the conclusion of the authors, while acknowledging drawbacks based on the nonrandomized nature of the study, was that there was no significant difference in outcomes between using laparoscopic approaches versus an open approach in the management of primary colon and rectal tumors. There was, however, no formal cost analysis in this study, and, therefore, although oncologic outcomes were no different between the two groups, it is impossible to determine whether one group was superior to the other with respect to other outcomes.

A case-matched comparison of clinical and financial outcomes following laparoscopic and open colorectal surgery has been performed.[206] The group at the Cleveland Clinic studied patients from a prospective database who had undergone laparoscopic or open colectomy and were matched for age, gender, and disease-related groupings. A group of 150 patients undergoing laparoscopic colectomy was compared to a matched group of patients undergoing open colectomy. There was no difference found between the two groups for diagnosis, complications, or 30-day readmission rate. Although operating room costs were significantly higher after laparoscopic colectomy, this was offset by a decrease in the length of hospital stay with an overall significant reduction in total costs. This is attributed mainly to a lower cost for pharmacy, laboratory, and ward nursing expenses.

The ultimate role of laparoscopic resection in the management of CRC has yet to be determined. The studies discussed have shed some light on the relative risks and benefits as well as costs of these two procedures. The questions will remain, however, if the procedures are equivalent and whether deviating from the accepted gold standard of open resection for the management of CRC will be warranted. Longer follow-up will hopefully assist in this assessment.

In the meantime, exploration of other minimally invasive approaches to resection is ongoing. Early studies report the feasibility and safety of single port surgery, or "SILC" (single-incision laparoscopic colectomy), as well as equivalent oncologic outcomes at 2 years, and robotic colectomy has also been performed although its greatest potential is thought to lie with rectal dissection.[215–221] Natural orifice surgery is another area of interest with data accumulating on transvaginal specimen extraction as well as a pure transrectal approach.[222–224] Whether any of these novel modalities will offer real advantages (other than cosmesis) to offset the significant drawbacks of increased technical difficulty, operating time, and cost remains to be seen.

POLYPS AND STAGE I COLON CANCER

The management of polyps and stage I colon cancer is through surgical resection. Most cancer in polyps is not diagnosed until after the polypectomy is performed. Therefore, with respect to pedunculated lesions, care should be taken to resect the stalk completely, down to its base. Invasive early stage I cancers found in a polyp managed by polypectomy do not require further resection if there is a negative margin >2 mm and the tumor is well-differentiated without lymphovascular invasion or extension of malignant cells beyond the stalk (Haggitt levels 1 to 3).[173,225] Sessile lesions that are biopsied and shown to harbor an invasive cancer should be managed with a segmental colon resection. Large polypoid lesions may also require a segmental resection.

Because the stage of the lesion will not be determined until after the resection, all colon cancer lesions managed with a segmental resection should be approached the same way. The type of resection will be dictated by the location of the lesion, as has been described. Following a complete resection of a stage I lesion, no further adjuvant therapy is required. Patients managed in this way can expect a 5-year survival of over 95%.[225] Those that recur are most likely improperly classified stage II or III lesions.

STAGE II AND STAGE III COLON CANCER

Adjuvant Chemotherapy Considerations

The earliest clinical trials of adjuvant chemotherapy in colon cancer were conducted in the 1950s, utilizing the limited arsenal of anticancer agents that were available at that time. Many of these agents are now known to have no meaningful activity in metastatic CRC, and thus would not be studied in the adjuvant setting today.

The adjuvant trials of the 1950s through the mid-1980s tended to be small by current standards. Based perhaps on an unrealistically optimistic expectation of what magnitude of benefit might be achieved from the use of available chemotherapies, the size of the trials did not allow evaluation of more modest clinical benefits. A large meta-analysis of controlled randomized trials of adjuvant therapy published through 1986 indicated a nonsignificant trend toward an overall survival benefit, with a mortality OR of 0.83 in favor of therapy (95% CI = 0.70 to 0.98).[226] This sobering analysis suggested that substantially larger trials would be needed to detect the modest advantages that available chemotherapies might afford.

Large-Scale Randomized Trials

The large-scale 5-FU trials have been well summarized previously, and the reader who is interested in the details is referred to subject-relevant chapters in the previous edition of this book.[227] The outcome of numerous trials performed largely in the 1990s can be briefly summarized as follows. Trials comparing 5-FU–based therapy to surgery only demonstrated a clear benefit in terms of 5-year DFS (essentially, an increased cure rate) for stage III patients who received chemotherapy.[228,229] Six months of chemotherapy was sufficient, and no further benefit was provided by extending treatment to either nine or twelve months. Levamisole, an agent initially thought to be active, was, in fact inactive, and high-dose leucovorin did not confer superior efficacy over low-dose leucovorin, so comparisons of various 5-FU/leucovorin schedules did not demonstrate clear superiority of one schedule over the other in terms of efficacy. However, the Mayo Clinic daily times five schedule was substantially more toxic than either weekly bolus of biweekly infusion schedules. Alfa interferon conferred substantial toxicity and provided no benefit.[230–234]

Oral Fluoropyrimidine Therapies

Oral administration of 5-FU proved to be problematic secondary to erratic bioavailability. This was likely due in large part to variable effects of DPD, the rate-limiting enzyme in catabolism of 5-FU, on the first pass clearance of oral 5-FU by the liver. Two oral 5-FU prodrugs, capecitabine and uracil/tegafur (UFT), have demonstrated efficacy in metastatic disease that is comparable to the Mayo Clinic schedule of parenteral 5-FU/leucovorin. Both of

these agents have now been studied in the adjuvant setting in comparison to the now defunct Mayo Clinic 5-FU schedule. In a study designed to assess for noninferiority in 3-year DFS, Twelves et al.[235] randomly assigned 1,987 patients with resected stage III colon cancer to receive either oral capecitabine (1,004 patients) or Mayo Clinic bolus 5-FU plus leucovorin (983 patients). Each treatment was planned for 24 weeks. DFS in the capecitabine group was at least equivalent to that in the 5-FU/leucovorin group (in the intention-to-treat analysis [p <0.001] for the comparison of the upper limit of the HR with the noninferiority margin of 1.20), and capecitabine resulted in significantly fewer adverse events than Mayo Clinic bolus 5-FU/leucovorin (p <0.001). Overall, this trial demonstrates that capecitabine is a reasonable alternative to intravenous 5-FU/leucovorin in the adjuvant treatment of colon cancer in reliable, motivated patients who are able to comply with a complex schedule of oral medication. However, as discussed in the following, while possibly appropriate for some stage II patients, 5-FU/leucovorin alone is no longer the standard postsurgical adjuvant treatment for stage III colon cancer. As such, the role of single-agent capecitabine in the adjuvant management of resected colon cancer remains limited at this time. Data supporting its use with concurrent intravenous oxaliplatin are discussed subsequently.

The NSABP C-06 trial assessed the use of oral UFT plus oral leucovorin in the treatment of stage II and III colon cancer.[236] A total of 1,608 patients with stage II (47%) and stage III (53%) colon cancer were randomly assigned to receive either oral UFT with leucovorin or intravenous 5-FU with leucovorin. With a median follow-up of 62.3 months, there were no significant differences in DFS or overall survival between the treatment groups. Toxicity and primary quality of life end points were similar in the two groups. As such, similar to the situation with capecitabine, the combination of oral UFT with leucovorin is an acceptable alternative to parenteral 5-FU/leucovorin; however, use of fluoropyrimidine plus leucovorin alone is no longer routine standard practice (see the following) in the adjuvant treatment of at least stage III disease. Furthermore, UFT is not commercially available in the United States.

Combination Adjuvant Therapies

Clinical trials in the metastatic setting have established the antitumor activity of combinations of agents, including irinotecan, oxaliplatin, bevacizumab, cetuximab, and panitumumab (see discussion of treatment of metastatic disease for more details). Although it had been assumed that activity in the metastatic setting would translate into an increased cure rate in the adjuvant setting, this assumption has turned out to be overly simplistic and often untrue. Of the agents listed previously, only the addition of oxaliplatin to fluoropyrimidines has resulted in benefit in the adjuvant setting.

Oxaliplatin

Oxaliplatin plus biweekly infusional 5-FU/leucovorin was first evaluated in the adjuvant setting in the Multicenter International Study of Oxaliplatin/5-Fluorouracil/Leucovorin in the Adjuvant Treatment of Colon Cancer (MOSAIC) trial.[237] The results of this trial are summarized in Table 49.8. A total of 2,246 stage II and III patients were randomized to the LV5FU2 regimen, a biweekly infusional and bolus 5-FU/leucovorin regimen that has been demonstrated to have comparable efficacy to the Mayo Clinic daily times five bolus schedule in the adjuvant setting, or to the FOLFOX-4 regimen, which is LV5FU2 plus oxaliplatin on day 1.[230] For the combined stage II and III study population, the 5-year DFS rates were 73.3% and 67.4% in the FOLFOX-4 and LV5FU2 groups, respectively (HR = 0.80; 95% CI = 0.68 to 0.93; p = 0.003).[237] Six-year overall survival rates were statistically significantly improved by 2.5% (78.5% versus 76.0% in the FOLFOX-4

TABLE 49.8

Results of The Mosaic Trial: Biweekly Infusional Fluorouracil/Leucovorin Versus 5-Fluorouracil/Leucovorin Plus Oxaliplatin in Patients with Stage II and III Colon Cancer

	FOLFOX (%)	5FULV2 (%)	*P* Value
Five-y disease-free survival (stage II+III)	73.3	67.4	0.003
Six-y overall survival (stage II+III)	78.5	76.0	0.046
Six-y overall survival (stage III only)	72.9	68.7	0.023
Six-y overall survival (stage II only)	85	83.3	0.65
Grade 3–4 neutropenia	41	5	
Grade 3–4 diarrhea	11	7	
Grade 3 neuropathy	12	0	
Grade 2 neuropathy	32	0	

FOLFOX, fluorouracil/leucovorin plus oxaliplatin; 5FULV2, fluorouracil/leucovorin.

and LV5FU2 groups, respectively; HR = 0.84; 95% CI = 0.71 to 1.00; p = 0.046). For the stage III population, the 6-year overall survival rates were improved by 4.2% (72.9% versus 68.7%, respectively; HR = 0.80; 95% CI = 0.65 to 0.97; p = 0.023), whereas for the stage II population, the addition of oxaliplatin conferred no survival benefit (6-year survival 85.0% and 83.3%, respectively; p = 0.65). A more recent update showed that even amongst the stage II patients with high-risk factors, an improved outcome with the addition of oxaliplatin was not evident. While toxicity was regarded as manageable, the FOLFOX-4 regimen resulted in 41% grade 3 or 4 neutropenia versus 5% in the control arm, and 11% grade 3 or 4 diarrhea versus 7%. All-cause mortality in the first 60 days was 0.5% in each arm. Peripheral sensory neuropathy, a toxicity not present in the LV5FU2 control arm, was a frequent occurrence on the FOLFOX-4 arm. Grade 2 neuropathy was reported in 32% of the patients, and grade 3 occurred in 12%. In some cases, the duration of the neuropathy was substantial. One year after completion of therapy, 30% of patients still experienced some grade of neuropathy (0.8% grade 2 and 1.3% grade 3). Four years after completion of therapy, 15.4% still had some degree of neuropathy, and 0.7% still had grade 3 neuropathy. It is reasonable to assume that the toxicity still present at 4 years out from the last treatment is essentially permanent.

Oxaliplatin has also been combined with a weekly bolus 5-FU regimen in an adjuvant trial. The NSABP C-07 trial studied the FLOX regimen of oxaliplatin given on weeks 1, 3, and 5 plus weekly bolus 5-FU/leucovorin on weeks 1 through 6, repeated at 8-week cycles, versus the standard weekly Roswell Park regimen of 5-FU/leucovorin.[238] A total of 2,409 patients were randomized to FLOX or to 5-FU/leucovorin. A total of 29% of patients had stage II disease and 71% had stage III. With a median follow-up of 8 years, FLOX showed a superior DFS, with 69.4% versus 64.2% alive and free of disease at five years (HR = 0.82; 95% CI = 0.72 to 0.93; p = 0.002). However, the overall survival difference was not statistically significantly different between the two arms. Treatment-related deaths were 1.3% versus 1.1% in the FLOX and 5-FU/leucovorin arms, respectively. Grade 2 or higher neurotoxicity was reported in 30.4% of patients on the FLOX arm versus 3.6% on 5-FU/leucovorin. Grade 3 diarrhea was 38.1% and 32.4% in the two arms, respectively, reflecting the higher incidence of serious diarrhea with the weekly bolus 5-FU regimen. Kidwell et al.[239] published long-term data regarding the persistent neurotoxic side effects of oxaliplatin beyond 4 years from this same NSABP C-07 trial, and found that there was a statistically but not clinically significant increase in total neurotoxicity for those who received the agent, with initial differences between the two groups dissipating by 7 years. However specific symptoms of numbness and tingling in the hands and feet did remain substantially elevated over time.[239]

Another recent study examined the effect of diabetes and other comorbidities on oxaliplatin-induced neuropathy. With symptoms identified in 65% of patients, hypertension, smoking, and diabetes were associated with higher trends although not statistically significant differences in severe neuropathy. Additionally, patients with diabetes developed oxaliplatin-induced neuropathy at a significantly lower cumulative dose, highlighting the importance of tailoring patient-specific regimens to minimize toxicity.[240]

In an exploratory analysis, however, the authors noted significant age-related differences in response to oxaliplatin, finding statistically improved overall survival in patients <70 years old, whereas older patients actually fared worse with increased grade 4-5 toxicity (OR = 1.59) and a 4.7% decrease in 5-year overall survival.

This age-treatment interaction has also been supported by a 2012 pooled analysis of 5,489 patients >75 years old from four large data sets that demonstrated minimal benefit of oxaliplatin in this group.[241] Moreover, post hoc analysis of MOSAIC data as well as revised findings from the ACCENT study (which initially showed no age-related difference) further indicate the limited clinical utility of this agent in older patients.[241,242] Taking all this into account, the 2013 National Comprehensive Cancer Network (NCCN) guidelines now recommend individualizing the decision to add oxaliplatin to adjuvant regimens in the elderly.[243]

More recently, a 1,866-patient study comparing capecitabine plus oxaliplatin (Cape/Ox) with bolus 5-FU/leucovorin in the adjuvant treatment of stage III colon cancer has been reported.[244] The Cape/Ox regimen had a statistically significant DFS advantage over 5-FU/leucovorin, with 66.1% of patients alive and disease-free at 5 years with Cape/Ox versus 59.8% with 5-FU/leucovorin. The difference between arms in overall survival at 5 years favored the Cape/Ox arm by 3.4%; however, this difference did not reach statistical significance at the time of this analysis (p = 0.15). The efficacy results of the FOLFOX and Cape/Ox studies appear more similar than different at this point in time and appear to justify interchangeability of these regimens in the adjuvant setting. Data for FLOX regimens appear to show higher rates of serious or life-threatening diarrhea, and the lack of a statistically significant survival benefit at 6 years is notable. The higher degree of severe and life-threatening diarrhea seen with FLOX would appear to be a potential reason for favoring FOLFOX or Cape/Ox over FLOX, although in the absence of a head-to-head comparison, the relative safety and efficacy when comparing one or these regimens to the other is impossible to know with certainty. The Cape/Ox regimen is a reasonable consideration only in highly reliable, motivated patients who can be expected to comply with taking multiple pills of capecitabine orally (typically three to five pills, twice daily) for 2 weeks on, 1 week off, in the setting of concurrent emetogenic intravenous chemotherapy.

Irinotecan

Based on improved overall survival in the first- and second-line metastatic settings, it was widely assumed that irinotecan would be beneficial to patients in the adjuvant setting.[245–247] This assumption has turned out to be incorrect, however, and the results of the adjuvant trials with this agent underscore the importance of both performing trials in the adjuvant setting and waiting for the results of those trials before adopting changes in practice.

The CALGB studied the weekly schedule of irinotecan plus bolus 5-FU and leucovorin (IFL). Early safety analysis of this trial identified an alarming elevation in early mortality for the experimental arm on this trial, with 18 deaths within the first 4 months of treatment on the IFL arm versus 6 deaths within the same time period on the control arm ($p = 0.008$).[248] At a median follow-up of 2.1 years in each arm, futility boundaries for both DFS and overall survival had been crossed; thus, the final result of this trial is that the addition of irinotecan provided no benefit, while increasing toxicity, including lethal toxicity.[249]

Results of adding irinotecan to biweekly infusional 5-FU/leucovorin (LV5FU2 versus FOLFIRI) were also negative. In the ACCORD 02 trial, 400 patients with high-risk stage III disease (defined as four or more positive nodes or perforated or obstructed primary tumors) were randomly assigned to LV5FU2 versus FOLFIRI. In this high-risk population, there was no benefit seen in the FOLFIRI group, and in fact the study trended insignificantly in favor of the nonirinotecan-containing arm (3-year DFS 60% for LV5FU2 versus 51% for FOLFIRI).[250]

A second, larger trial of LV5FU2 versus FOLFIRI was conducted by the PETACC-3 investigators.[251] The prespecified primary efficacy analysis of this trial was based on 2,094 patients with stage III disease. At a median follow-up of 6.5 years, there was no statistically significant difference in the 5-year DFS (56.7% versus 54.3% for FOLFIRI versus LV5FU2, respectively; $p = 0.1$) or in 5-year overall survival (73.6% versus 71.3%, respectively; $p = 0.94$). FOLFIRI was associated with an increased incidence of grade 3 or 4 GI events and neutropenia.

Taken together, the results of these three trials to evaluate irinotecan in the adjuvant setting clearly establish that despite having substantial activity in the metastatic setting, irinotecan has no meaningful activity, and no role, in the adjuvant treatment of colon cancer. Of interest, an analysis from the CALGB trial suggested that patients with MSI-H showed a benefit from inclusion of irinotecan in their adjuvant treatment; however, a similar, substantially larger analysis from the PETACC-3 trial contradicted this and showed no benefit from adding irinotecan in patients with MSI-H.[252,253]

Bevacizumab

As detailed subsequently, bevacizumab has demonstrated the ability to favorably augment standard chemotherapy for metastatic disease and has become a part of standard management in that arena. This led to evaluation of this agent in the adjuvant setting. In the NSABP C-08 trial, 2,672 patients, 25% with stage II and 755 with stage III colon cancer, were randomized to receive modified FOLFOX-6, either alone or with bevacizumab.[254] A design imbalance that could have been problematic had this been a positive trial, the FOLFOX was given for 6 months in each arm, while the bevacizumab was given both with the FOLFOX and then for an additional 6 months, for a total of 1 year of bevacizumab. This was, however, a fully negative trial, so the issues regarding the design of the trial are moot. With a median follow-up of 5 years, the addition of bevacizumab to FOLFOX did not improve either the DFS or the overall survival. DFS was 77.9% versus 75.1% ($p = 0.35$) for the study overall, and DFS was 73.5% versus 71.7% ($p = 0.55$) for the

stage III patients. Five-year overall survival was 82.5% versus 80.7% ($p = 0.56$) for the entire study, and 78.7% versus 77.6% for the stage III patients. There was a separation between the curves at the 1-year mark; however, this began to diminish a few months later and was all but absent by year 3. This finding suggests that bevacizumab did delay progression of micrometastases in some patients, but only for as long as it was continued. Bevacizumab did not contribute to the eradication of micrometastases and thus did not improve the cure rate in the adjuvant setting. Although some might choose to interpret these data to suggest that if bevacizumab were continued indefinitely, an improved survival *might* be seen, the long-term consequences of lifelong suppression of vascular endothelial growth factor (VEGF), as well as the psychological, social, and economic considerations involved, render such an approach inappropriate, especially considering that only a very small percentage of patients so treated would actually have the potential to benefit, if there is a benefit. Another trial, termed the AVANT trial, also explored the use of bevacizumab in the adjuvant treatment of stage III colon cancer, and also found no benefit.[255] This study randomized 3,451 patients, 2,876 of whom had stage III disease, to FOLFOX4, FOLFOX4 plus bevacizumab, or Cape/Ox plus bevacizumab. The bevacizumab-containing arms did not achieve a statistically significant improvement in DFS. After a minimum of 60 months follow-up, overall survival data suggested a possible detriment with the addition of bevacizumab, as the survival in the two bevacizumab-containing arms trended toward inferior to the FOLFOX-alone control arm; however, these differences did not reach statistical significance.

Thus, the available evidence suggests that bevacizumab is not beneficial in the treatment of colon cancer in the adjuvant setting, and might, in fact, be harmful. Until and unless data to the contrary emerge, bevacizumab should not be used in the adjuvant treatment of stage II and III colon cancer.

Cetuximab

As outlined in detail in the following, cetuximab has demonstrated clinical activity in metastatic CRC, prompting investigation of its usefulness in the adjuvant setting. Intergroup trial N0147 randomized patients with stage III colon cancer to modified FOLFOX-6 with or without cetuximab.[256] Once investigators became aware that the study included only patients whose tumors lacked mutations in the KRAS gene (see the following), the study was modified to obtain KRAS genotyping on all patients and to only enroll those with wild-type KRAS. Despite this selection, this large, adequately powered, randomized phase 3 trial showed no benefit for the addition of cetuximab to FOLFOX in the adjuvant treatment of patients with KRAS–wild-type stage III colon cancer. DFS and overall survival curves trended insignificantly in favor of the FOLFOX-alone control arm, and the addition of cetuximab was overtly harmful in patients >70 years of age. Cetuximab should therefore not be used in the treatment of stage III colon cancer.

Panitumumab

Panitumumab, like cetuximab, is a monoclonal antibody that blocks ligand binding to the EGFR. Although no investigations have been reported to evaluate panitumumab in the adjuvant setting, results in the metastatic setting suggest that panitumumab and cetuximab are extremely similar in terms of target, mechanism of action, mechanisms of resistance, and clinical activity. It is therefore extremely unlikely that these agents would differ in the adjuvant setting, and statements regarding cetuximab in this setting may be reasonably applied to panitumumab.

TREATMENT OF STAGE II PATIENTS

The optimal management of patients with stage II colon cancer remains undefined. Although the role of adjuvant therapy in patients with stage II colon cancer has not been firmly established, it is interesting to see what practice patterns have been emerging. Using the SEER-Medicare linked database, Schrag et al.[257] identified 3,151 patients age 65 to 75 with resected stage II colon cancer and no adverse prognostic features. Using Medicare billing records, they identified those patients who did or did not receive chemotherapy within 3 months of operation. Their review identified that 27% of patients received chemotherapy during the 3-month postoperative period. Younger age, white race, unfavorable tumor grade, and low comorbidity were associated with a greater likelihood of receiving treatment. The 5-year survival was 75% for untreated patients and 78% for those patients who received therapy in this nonrandomized comparison. After adjusting for known between-group differences, the HR for survival associated with adjuvant treatment was 0.91 (95% CI = 0.77 to 1.09). Thus, despite the lack of proven benefit, a substantial percentage of Medicare beneficiaries have received adjuvant chemotherapy for stage II disease.

Because stage II patients as a group have a relatively favorable prognosis, benefits from treatment could only be expected if either a highly efficacious therapy were used or if extremely large trials were done to detect very subtle differences. The International Multicentre Pooled Analysis of B2 Colon Cancer Trials meta-analysis provides one of the largest samples of stage II patients.[258] A total of 1,016 stage II patients were randomized between 5-FU/leucovorin and surgery alone. The surgery-only arm had a long-term overall survival rate of 81% versus 83% for those stage II patients who received adjuvant 5-FU/leucovorin. This absolute difference of 2% closely approached, but did not reach, statistical significance.

More recently, published studies have not generated any consensus on this topic. In a large retrospective, population-based analysis of 3,716 patients undergoing surgery for stage II disease with or without adjuvant chemotherapy, there was a statistically significant survival advantage for the adjuvant group (12 years versus 9.2 years). However, this is not a randomized trial, and patients receiving chemotherapy were more likely to be younger, with left-sided lesions and a higher LN yield, all of which are now known to be favorable prognostic factors. As such, it is difficult to draw conclusions from this study.[259] Another study that evaluated data from 24,847 patients, 75% of whom had one or more prognostic features, found no survival benefit from an adjuvant regimen.[260] Finally, Wu et al.[261] performed a systematic review of 12 randomized controlled trials including both colon and rectal cancers that suggested some improvement in 5-year overall survival and DFS for both tumor sites as well as a significant reduction in recurrence risk for stage II colon cancers. While the review has substantial flaws that limit interpretation of these results, it does indicate that larger, higher-quality trials are warranted.[261] One such study underway is the SACURA trial, a multicenter, randomized phase 3 study designed to evaluate the superiority of a 1-year adjuvant regimen compared to observation in stage II colon cancer. Investigators will seek to identify "high-risk factors of recurrence/death" as well as predictors of efficacy and toxicity in the adjuvant arm. End points include DFS, overall survival, and recurrence-free survival as well as the incidence and severity of adverse events. Results from this trial will hopefully facilitate a definitive therapeutic strategy for stage II colon cancers moving forward.[262]

Several prognostic indicators have been identified that correlate with a higher risk for subsequent failure in stage II patients. These include obstruction or perforation of the bowel wall as well as other less-established risk factors, such as elevated preoperative or postoperative CEA, poorly differentiated histology, and tumors not demonstrating high levels of MSI, or an 18q deletion in colorectal tumors, which may correlate with a poor prognosis.[145,263–265] Additionally cited poor prognostic factors include macroscopically infiltrating-type tumors, high serum CA 19-9 levels, extensive venous invasion, male gender, age >50 years old, and <12 dissected LNs.[266] It appears that stage II patients with one or more of these risk factors have a poorer prognosis, one closer to patients with stage III disease. Whether adjuvant chemotherapy can provide similar benefits in these patients as it does in stage III

patients remains a matter of conjecture, and in the absence of definitive data, definitive recommendations on this topic cannot be made at this time. In fully informed high-risk stage II patients, it is reasonable to consider adjuvant treatment. All reports form the MOSAIC trial have shown no benefit for the addition of oxaliplatin to 5-FU/leucovorin in terms of overall survival of stage II patients. Uniquivocally, stage II patients lacking high-risk factors have not been shown to benefit from oxliplatin, and considering the short- and long-term toxicities of this agent, oxaliplatin should not be used in the management of good-risk stage II patients. A recent update of the outcomes for stage II patients on the MOSAIC trial demonstrates no benefit to use of oxaliplatin, even in patients on the trial with one or more high-risk factors.[242] Whereas patients with exceptionally poor risk stage II tumors may still seem reasonable for consideration of oxaliplatin-containing regimens, these negative data suggest that routine use of oxaliplatin in most patients with stage II colon cancer is unlikely to be appropriate.

Impact of Microsatellite Instability on Treatment in Stage II and III Colon Cancer

Ribic et al.[267] investigated the usefulness of MSI status as a predictor of benefit from 5-FU–based adjuvant chemotherapy in 570 stage II and III patients from five randomized trials in which no treatment control arm was used. MSI-H was exhibited in 95 patients (16.7%), MSI-L in 60 patients (10.5%), and MSS in 415 patients (72.8%). In the 287 patients who did not receive adjuvant chemotherapy, those with tumors exhibiting MSI-H had superior 5-year survival compared to patients with MSI-L or MSS tumors (HR = 0.31; $p = 0.004$). In the population of patients who received adjuvant chemotherapy, there was no difference in survival between the patients with MSI-H and patients without MSI-H ($p = 0.8$). In the patients with MSI-L or MSS tumors, chemotherapy resulted in improved survival versus no chemotherapy (HR = 0.72; $p = 0.04$). However, 5-FU/leuvocorin did not improve survival in the patients with MSI-H tumors (Table 49.9).

5-FU/leuvocorin was associated with improved outcome in both stage II and III patients with MSS or MSI-L, with an HR of 0.67 (95% CI = 0.39 to 1.15) in stage II patients and 0.69 (95% CI = 0.47 to 1.01) in patients with stage III cancer. In contrast, in patients with MSI-H tumors, treatment did not improve survival,

TABLE 49.9

Microsatellite Instability Versus Outcome with 5-Fluorouracil-Based Adjuvant Chemotherapy

	No. of Patients	Five-Y Disease-Free Survival (%)	P Value
All Patients			
Adjuvant chemotherapy	285	70	0.06
No adjuvant chemotherapy	287	62	
Patients with MSI-L/MSS			
Adjuvant chemotherapy	230	70	0.01
No adjuvant chemotherapy	245	59	
Patients with MSI-H			
Adjuvant chemotherapy	53	69	0.11
No adjuvant chemotherapy	42	83	

MSI-L, low level of microsatellite instability; MSS, microsatellite stable; MSI-H, high level of microsatellite instability.
From Ribic CM, Sargent DJ, Moore MJ, et al. Tumor microsatellite-instability status as a predictor of benefit from fluorouracil-based adjuvant chemotherapy for colon cancer. *N Engl J Med* 2003;349:247–257.

and in fact was associated with a trend toward worse outcome for both stage II (HR for death = 3.28; 95% CI = 0.86 to 12.48) and stage III cancers (HR = 1.42; 95% CI = 0.36 to 5.56). Of note, an analysis of MSI status from the NSABP failed to corroborate the results of the Ribic et al.[267] study, and the authors concluded that in their trial there was no interaction between MSI status and treatment effect, and that their data do not support the use of MSI-H as a predictive marker for chemotherapy benefit.[268] However, an updated expansion on the data from the Ribic et al.[267] report appears to corroborate the original findings, leading the authors of that study to suggest that MSI determinations should be performed on all stage II patients, and that stage II patients with MSI-H should not be treated with fluoropyrimidines alone.[269] The Eastern Cooperative Oncology Group I is leading a trial (ECOG 5202) in which patients with MSI-H and absence of LOH in chromosome 18q are being selected for observation, on the hypothesis that these patients will have a highly favorable prognosis with observation alone, whereas others are being assigned to FOLFOX chemotherapy and randomized to with or without bevacizumab. This trial has accrued and data are pending at the time of this writing.

An analysis of data indicate that patients with MSI-H stage III tumors, while having a more favorable prognosis than MSS tumors, do nevertheless achieve benefit from, and in the absence of contraindications, should receive, 5-FU–based adjuvant therapy.[270] This recommendation is further supported when considering oxaliplatin-based chemotherapy in stage III disease. This would be reasonable to expect, as platinum-DNA adducts are not removed by the mismatch repair enzymes that are deficient in MSI tumors. A more recent analysis of MSI impact in stage III disease in the N0147 trial suggested a more complex and nuanced impact, with MSI-H tumors having a favorable prognostic impact when arising in the right side of the colon, but actually having a negative prognostic impact when occurring in the left colon.[147] The reasons for this difference remain unclear; however, the different embryologic origins of the left and right colon, and the resultant different venous drainages, may contribute to this.

The incidence of MSI has more recently been shown to vary with stage of disease presentation, with 22% of stage II patients, 12% of stage III, and only 3.5% of stage IV patients found to exhibit MSI, consistent with the data that MSI-H is a favorable *prognostic* factor. Data from the PETACC-3 trial suggest that it is a strong prognostic factor in stage II disease; however, it was less so in stage III.[271–273]

Other Molecular Markers

As the majority of stage II, and even stage III, patients do not benefit from adjuvant therapy, it would be highly desirable to be able to identify those patients who are both at risk for recurrent disease (i.e., harbor micrometastases) and those whose micrometastases are sensitive to, and will be eradicated by, a particular chemotherapy. At present there are no such validated markers, with the possible exception of MSI, as discussed previously. KRAS mutations have no prognostic value in the adjuvant setting, and as there is no role for use of anti-EGFR agents in the adjuvant setting, the expense of genotyping patients with less than stage IV disease is difficult to justify.[273,274] BRAF mutations appear to be prognostic of poorer overall survival in stage II disease that is not MSI-H; however, this appears to be regardless of therapy, and so again it provides no information to inform treatment decision making.[275] At present, no molecular test has been validated as useful for making adjuvant treatment decisions, and none should be utilized outside of a clinical trial. More recently, a genetic profiling assay utilizing 21-gene signature analysis has become available.[271] This assay has been shown to provide risk stratification with stage II patients who are classified as having from 8% to 22% chance of recurrence. However, there was no interaction with treatment, meaning that the test is prognostic, identifying relatively lower or higher risk

individuals, but it provided no guidance on whom to treat. Thus, despite the interesting data outlined in the following, it would appear to be of little value in decision making at this time.

Despite this limitation, research efforts have been increasingly focused on developing and refining such gene signatures over the past few years, with three that stand out presently, promising to improve and possibly replace current risk stratification models.[275] Unfortunately, none of these approaches are able to predict who will or will not benefit from adjuvant chemotherapy. While these prognostic scores may be of scientific interest, at present they are not recommended for routine clinical use in NCCN guidelines, as they appear to offer little if any guidance in terms of treatment decisions.

The Oncotype DX Recurrence Score, which is the only externally validated assay available for commercial use, is based on a 12-gene signature that separates 3-year recurrence risk into low, intermediate, and high (12%, 18%, 22%, respectively), independent of clinicopathologic features, and with enhanced accuracy. It has been shown to be highly prognostic in stage II and III patients receiving 5-FU/leucovorin, and enables better discrimination of absolute oxaliplatin benefit as a function of risk. A recent analysis of long-term costs and outcomes in "average-risk" stage II colon cancers (T3, MSS) concluded that this signature, when applied appropriately, could potentially reduce adjuvant chemotherapy use by 17% with increased quality-adjusted life expectancy of 0.035 years and cost-savings of $2,971 per patient.[276]

Another interesting signature, ColoPrint (Agendia Inc. USA, Irvine, CA), is an 18-gene prognostic classifier developed on fresh-frozen tumor tissue to identify 5-year metastasis-free survival. Separating patients into two risk categories, this assay is particularly precise in identifying low-risk stage II cases that be managed without chemotherapy irrespective of MSI status. It also appears to better classify high-risk patients than clinicopathologic factors alone. While the signature has been validated twice in retrospective trials, it is not yet available for commercial use. A large prospective clinical validation study is under way (PARSC: Prospective Analysis of Risk Stratification by ColoPrint) that may better clarify the role of ColoPrint specifically in the management of stage II disease.[277]

Colorectal Cancer DSA (Almac Diagnostics, Craigavon, Unite Kingdom) is the most recently reported signature, based on 634 genes, developed to identify stage II patients at higher risk of recurrence (HR = 2.53) and cancer-related death (HR = 2.21) at 5 years. It has been shown to perform independently of known prognostic factors. While this assay is also not available for commercial use at the time of this writing, a prospective validation trial in stage II patients is being planned.[278]

The lack of clear direction on the matter of treatment of good-risk stage II patients is reflected in a current consensus statement, which, while not recommending therapy for all stage II patients, does recommend a medical oncology consultation for the purpose of discussing the pros and cons of chemotherapy for all stage II patients.[279]

TREATMENT OPTIONS FOR STAGE III PATIENTS

It is clear that in the absence of medical or psychiatric contraindications, patients with node-positive colon cancer should receive postoperative chemotherapy. At the very least, a 5-FU–based regimen would appear to be appropriate, and approximately 6 months of therapy would be supported by the majority of trials. The daily times five Mayo Clinic schedule or a variant has been shown to be more toxic than other 5-FU/leucovorin schedules; therefore, daily times five schedules should not be used. Oral capecitabine or oral UFT/leucovorin are acceptable alternatives if a fluoropyrimidine-only approach is selected. At this time, the data for incorporation of oxaliplatin into the routine adjuvant treatment of colon cancer appears compelling, and the FOLFOX schedule is now the most widely used adjuvant therapy. FLOX is an acceptable alternative; however, nonrandomized comparisons suggest that FLOX may carry a higher risk of serious diarrhea than FOLFOX. Cape/Ox is also an acceptable alternative in appropriately motivated and reliable patients. Although the pivotal adjuvant study was done with FOLFOX-4, in practice this regimen is rarely used, and the modified FOLFOX-6 regimen, which has been the basis for all FOLFOX-based National Cancer Institute Intergroup adjuvant and metastatic trials, is routinely used due to its greater convenience. The risk of peripheral neuropathy and the possibility of long-term neuropathy must be considered in the selection of therapy. At the time of this writing, FOLFOX or Cape/Ox are the regimens of choice in treatment of all patients with stage III colon cancer in the absense of specific contraindications. The long-term morbidity of oxaliplatin treatment has become more appreciated; however, it is anticipated that risk stratification strategies may become available in the near future to identify those patients who are likely to benefit from oxaliplatin treatment.

Irinotecan-based regimens should not be used in the adjuvant setting, as randomized data have shown increased toxicity and no long-term benefit. Bevacizumab, cetuximab, and panitumumab should also not be used in the adjuvant setting, as they add toxicity and expense, and do not add benefit.

Timing of Treatment

Traditionally, adjuvant chemotherapy is commenced within 8 weeks of surgery. However, this time frame is somewhat arbitrary, based largely on what has been mandated in clinical trials. A 2010 meta-analysis pooled data from 13,158 patients with stage II or III disease and concluded that delaying treatment beyond this interval was associated with interior survival (RR = 1.20).[280] However, these data are retrospective, nonrandomized, and fail to adequately consider the collateral implications of whatever medical and surgical conditions might have contributed to the delay in start of therapy. As such, these findings should be regarded as hypothesis-generating only, and certainly not definitive. Another study that included only stage III cancers found no such clear correlation. Secondary analysis did demonstrate a trend toward poorer outcomes after 8 weeks, particularly in younger patients (<66 years) as well as significantly inferior survival for patients beginning chemotherapy after 9 and 10 weeks (HR of death = 1.68 and 1.67, respectively).[281]

Investigational Adjuvant Approaches

Portal Vein Infusion

The NSABP C-02 trial randomized 1,158 patients with Dukes A, B, or C colon cancers to either a 7-day portal vein infusion of 5-FU (600 mg/m^2 per day) or to surgery alone.[282] A modest, albeit statistically significant, advantage in DFS (74% versus 64% at 4 years) was demonstrated for the group who received intraportal chemotherapy; however, no difference was seen in the incidence of hepatic recurrences.

Similar findings were reported from a 533 patient trial performed by the Swiss Group for Clinical Cancer Research.[283,284] In this trial, intraportal chemotherapy included 10 mg/m^2 mitomycin C by 2-hour infusion followed by a 7-day infusion of 5-FU at a dose of 500 mg/m^2 per day. The 5-year DFS and overall survival were modestly improved in the intraportal treatment versus surgery-only groups (57% versus 48%, and 66% versus 55%, respectively).

Subsequently, a large meta-analysis of intraportal chemotherapy trials involving over 4,000 patients in 10 randomized studies revealed only a 4% improvement in 5-year overall survival for the patients who received portal infusion. At present, intraportal adjuvant chemotherapy has not been accepted as routine practice and remains limited to clinical investigations.

Intraperitoneal Chemotherapy

A small, single-arm study explored the feasibility of immediate postoperative intraperitoneal floxuridine and leucovorin plus systemic 5-FU and levamisole.[285] A randomized trial of 241 stage II and III patients compared intraperitoneal plus systemic 5-FU/leucovorin to systemic 5-FU/levamisole.[286] With 4 years' median follow-up, no benefit was seen for the stage II patients. Among the 196 eligible patients with stage III disease, however, a 43% reduction in mortality was seen. This small trial is encouraging but would require further corroboration before being accepted into standard practice.

Hyperthermic intraperitoneal chemotherapy has been explored as a possible means of providing a benefit in patients at high risk for developing peritoneal metastases. Sammartino et al.[287] explored this hypothesis in a small case control study of patients with T3/4 lesions and mucinous or signet ring cell histology who underwent either standard resection or extended surgery (including omentectomy, bilateral adnexectomy, hepatic round ligament resection, and appendectomy) followed by hyperthermic intraperitoneal chemotherapy. The experimental group experienced statistically significantly decreased rates of peritoneal recurrence (4% versus 22%) as well as improved DFS (36.8 months versus 21.9 months; p <0.01). Large randomized trials would be necessary, however, before nonresearch use of this highly aggressive and potentially toxic treatment strategy could be considered.[287]

Vaccines

Vaccination strategies endeavor to stimulate the patient's immune system to recognize and eradicate the patient's tumor cells. An ideal immunologic target molecule would be a highly antigenic epitope that is always expressed on the tumor and never expressed on normal tissue. Such an ideal target has yet to be identified; however, a number of approaches have been explored.

CEA is a commonly expressed antigen in colorectal carcinomas. Unfortunately, CEA does not appear to be particularly immunogenic. Several approaches have been pursued in an attempt to increase immune recognition of CEA. Thus, a number of avenues of investigation are being pursued; however, at this time the use of vaccine therapy for treatment of resected colon cancer remains highly investigational.

One tumor-associated antigen that may be a more promising candidate is the MUC1 glycoprotein, which is abnormally expressed on neoplastic cells in a hypoglycosylated form that induces humoral and cellular response. A vaccine based on this antigen was found to be highly immunogenic in the premalignant setting, inducing long-term memory responses and no significant toxicity when administered to patients with advanced colonic adenomas. Subsequent studies will determine whether these results translate into meaningful clinical outcomes.[288]

Active Specific Immunotherapy

Irradiated cancer cells maintain their immunogenicity; however, they are unable to proliferate. Active specific immunotherapy is a maneuver in which patients are immunized with a preparation of their own irradiated tumor cells plus an immunostimulant such as bacillus Calmette-Guérin. This technique has been explored for some time now as a potential adjuvant immunotherapy for CRC. Overall, trials have failed to show a benefit for the use of active specific immunotherapy in the management of colon cancer, and its use should remain limited to investigational settings.

Preoperative Chemotherapy

Investigators are currently exploring the role of preoperative chemotherapy in the management of nonmetastatic disease. A pilot phase of the first randomized trial to address this topic (FOx-TROT) has recently been completed, demonstrating the feasibility and safety of this approach in locally advanced, operable colon cancer. The 150 patients who underwent meticulous radiologic staging were randomly assigned to receive 6 weeks of preoperative oxaliplatin/5-FU/l-folinic acid followed by surgery and 18 weeks of postoperative chemotherapy or upfront resection followed by

24 weeks of treatment. There were no significant differences in postoperative morbidity between the two groups. While a small proportion of the patients receiving preoperative therapy had apparent progression during the time between staging and surgery, there were no tumor-related complications during this interval. Overall, preoperative therapy resulted in significant downstaging, including reductions in apical node involvement and incomplete resections as well as two pathologic complete responses. Whether these results will translate into improved survival and potentially change the accepted pathway for management of nonmetastatic disease remains to be seen. A larger phase 3 trial now under way will hopefully shed light on this issue in the near future.[289]

FOLLOW-UP AFTER MANAGEMENT OF COLON CANCER WITH CURATIVE INTENT

Follow-up after definitive management has two primary goals. First, patients with a history of CRC are at higher risk than the general population for a second colon cancer primary.[290,291] A colonoscopic screening may benefit in the early detection of a second primary malignancy or detection of a benign polyp, which can then be resected, potentially preventing the development of an invasive cancer.

Second, surveillance may increase the chance of identifying local regional or distant recurrence that is potentially curable by surgery. It should be noted that it is this detection of potentially curable recurrent or second primary disease that justifies routine postoperative surveillance. To date, there are no compelling data that indicate that early detection of unresectable asymptomatic metastatic disease is of benefit to the patient. In other words, if recurrent disease is unresectable and therefore incurable, there is no urgency to identify it; there is no compelling evidence that the early initiation of palliative chemotherapy is of benefit in the asymptomatic, incurable patient. Although the choice of follow-up routine and which studies to include in that follow-up have been the subject of much debate in the colon cancer literature,[292–295] subsequent analyses have shown that most interventions that have been considered are not value-added and not appropriate for routine use. The American Society of Clinical Oncology (ASCO) has recently updated its guidelines for postsurgical follow-up.[296] These recommendations are for physical examination and blood CEA monitoring every 3 to 6 months for the first 3 years, and every 6 months for years 4 and 5. CT scans of the chest and abdomen are recommended once a year for the first 3 years. Positron emission tomography (PET) scans are specifically not recommended for routine screening and surveillance. NCCN guidelines differ only slightly in that they recommend annual CT scanning for up to 5 years and include CT scans of the pelvis. Colonoscopy is recommended at 1 year after resection (or 3 to 6 months after resection if a complete colonoscopy was not performed prior to surgery) and then 3 years later, and then every 5 years. CT scans

and CEA monitoring should not be continued beyond 5 years. Of note, older studies advocating routine monitoring of complete blood count, liver function studies, lactate dehydrogenase, chest X-rays, and fecal occult blood monitoring have not been supported by subsequent data, and none of these are recommended for routine monitoring of patients at this time. The role of CEA measurement in patients following definitive management of CRC has been controversial.[94,297,298] ASCO carefully reviewed its utility in an additional panel guided in 1996.[299] Their recommendation for CEA monitoring then, which was confirmed in the surveillance guideline panel review, was postoperative serum CEA testing to be performed every 3 months in patients with stage II or III disease for up to 3 years after diagnosis. An elevated CEA level, if confirmed by retesting, warranted further evaluation for metastatic disease.

This further workup of an elevated CEA typically consists of a colonoscopy and a CT scan of the chest, abdomen, and pelvis. If these studies are negative, the clinician is faced with a dilemma. The question of what to do in the face of a rising serum CEA level in the absence of imageable disease by conventional imaging modalities is one that has been addressed in clinical trials.[300–305] Strategies to image CEA expression might improve upon the detection capability of standard imaging studies. Several studies were performed using immunoscintigraphy with an antibody directed against CEA or Tag72, a CEA-like glycoprotein (CEA scan and OncoScint [Cytogen Corp, Lonza Biologics, Princeton, NJ] scan, respectively).[306–308] The results of these studies using antibody-directed immunoscintigraphy were variable, and at this time, CEA scintigraphy is no longer considered in standard care. In an older study, in order to more directly address this clinical dilemma, a prospective study was performed comparing CEA immunoscintigraphy to PET using 18-fluorodeoxyglucose (FDG) and blind "second look" laparotomy.[303]

In this study patients with a rising CEA level without imageable disease by CT scan of the chest, abdomen, and pelvis as well as colonoscopy and abdominal ultrasound were enrolled along with patients with a single site of otherwise resectable disease. All patients had a CEA scan performed as well as a PET scan with FDG. All patients who failed to demonstrate evidence of disease outside of the abdominal cavity went on to have an exploratory laparotomy by a surgeon who had no knowledge of the CEA or the FDG scan results. A second surgeon participated in the remainder of the exploration after thoroughly reviewing all studies including the nuclear medicine scans. Twenty-eight patients were studied in this fashion, and the trial demonstrated that PET scan with FDG was far superior to CEA scans in detecting recurrence; roughly 30% of the patients on the study potentially benefited by having recurrent disease treated at the time of surgery (Fig. 49.4).

Based on these findings, it appears that serum CEA surveillance following definitive management of a primary CRC is a reasonable surveillance technique. If the CEA level is elevated on repeat testing, imaging studies should be performed consisting of CT scans and a through evaluation of the colon with colonoscopy

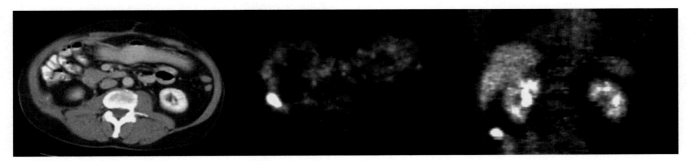

Figure 49.4 From left to right, the *first panel* depicts a contrast-enhanced computed tomography scan image of a patient with a rising carcinoembryonic antigen following a definitive resection of a right colon cancer. The *middle and far panels* show the same region imaged with fluorodeoxyglucose position emission tomography. (From Libutti SK, Alexander HR Jr, Choyke P, et al. A prospective study of 2-[18F] fluoro-2-deoxy-D-glucose/positron emission tomography scan, 99mTc-labeled arcitumomab [CEA-scan], and blind second-look laparotomy for detecting colon cancer recurrence in patients with increasing carcinoembryonic antigen levels. *Ann Surg Oncol* 2001;8:779.)

performed as well. If no recurrence or second primary is detected, watchful waiting and repeat of CT imaging at approximately 3-month intervals versus a PET scan with FDG can be considered. If disease is discovered, it should be managed as indicated. If no disease is detected, then continued surveillance is warranted with repeat CEA levels and CT or magnetic resonance imaging at intervals.[303,309]

The role of physical examination has also been evaluated.[310] The ASCO panel noted that no formal examination of the contribution of physician's history and physical examination to help outcomes of CRC has been performed. However, data from the larger studies of surveillance showed that 80% of recurrences were found by CEA testing, whereas only 20% were found by routine history and physical examination done at the same time.[311] This has been confirmed by other studies.[312,313] Although no direct effects were shown on history or physical examination about the impact and detection or outcome in the surveillance period, a physician–patient encounter provides a vital link for other studies that may influence outcome. Therefore, while not in itself substantiated by the data in the literature, it is felt that routine postresection visits be performed every 3 to 6 months for the first 3 years following resection and every 6 months during years 4 and 5.

The role of liver function tests as a means for detecting colorectal recurrence has also been carefully evaluated. No studies that were reviewed by the ASCO panel demonstrated any benefit for the routine use of liver function test measurements in the postsurveillance period.[310,314] In fact, studies suggest that other routine blood tests such as CEA detected recurrence far earlier than liver function test abnormalities.[94] Therefore, the 2005 ASCO consensus panel did not recommend the routine use of liver function test measurements in the postresection surveillance period.

Routine fecal occult blood testing, routine complete blood counts, and routine chest X-rays were all not thought to be of benefit in postoperative surveillance. Although the panel was not in uniform agreement with respect to chest X-ray, it was thought that all three of these modalities should be reserved for the evaluation of the patient with evidence of recurrence such as a rising CEA level or a positive endoscopy. Each of these modalities in and of itself was not found to be useful.

The panel recommended that annual CT of the chest and abdomen (with pelvis for rectal cancer) be performed for 3 years in those patients at higher risk for recurrence who could be candidates for curative-intent surgery of a recurrence. With respect to colonoscopy and flexible proctosigmoidoscopy, the panel, after reviewing the literature, recommended that all patients have a colonoscopy for the pre- or perioperative documentation of the cancer and to ascertain that the remainder of the colon is free from polyps. Further, the panel agreed that the data were sufficient to recommend colonoscopy at 3 years to detect new cancers and polyps and then every 5 years if normal. However, they did not recommend routine annual colonoscopy as follow-up following definitive management of patients with CRC. Further, the panel concluded that colonoscopy was superior to flexible proctosigmoidoscopy and therefore should be performed as previously discussed for patients following both colon and rectal cancer surgery. Other studies have also supported the routine use of colonoscopic examination following definitive management of CRC.[315,316]

A meta-analysis and systematic review of randomized trials to address the impact of close postoperative surveillance on overall survival following definitive management of CRC was also performed by Renehan et al.[317] A total of five randomized trials that met their inclusion criteria were reviewed, representing 1,342 patients. For four of the studies, intensive follow-up consisted of blood work including serum CEA, colonoscopy, physical examination, abdominal ultrasound, and CT scans. In one study, no CEA measurements or CT scans were performed. Follow-up in the intensive arm was performed every 3 months for 2 years and then every 6 months thereafter up to 5 years, with yearly CT scans and endoscopy. All five studies had a control arm subjected to a less aggressive follow-up regimen, which varied from study to study

ranging from no specific follow-up to interval laboratory tests and plain X-rays or ultrasound. They found that there was an absolute reduction in mortality of 9% to 13% by employing an aggressive follow-up regimen, consisting of serum CEA measurements and CT scans. Two studies in particular showed the greatest impact on survival.

In summary, a rational postoperative surveillance program would include CEA measurements every 3 to 6 months and a yearly CT scan of the chest, abdomen, and pelvis (for rectal cancer) for the first 3 years. Colonoscopy can be performed every 3 to 5 years following the resection. At the time of CEA measurements, a physician encounter should be scheduled where a discussion of patient symptoms and a physical examination can be performed. If a rising serum CEA is detected on two consecutive measurements in the absence of imageable disease by CT scan, a PET scan with FDG can be considered. Lesions found on colonoscopy should be managed appropriately either with colonoscopic resection or surgical management. These surveillance guidelines should allow for the early detection of either resectable recurrence or second primary lesions and therefore the potential to impact patient outcome.

SURGICAL MANAGEMENT OF STAGE IV DISEASE

For a select group of patients with metastatic CRC, complete surgical resection of stage IV disease (discussed in detail in Chapter 52) may be an option and may provide a long-term survival advantage. This is especially true with respect to metastatic sites in the liver and lung. Resection of locoregional recurrence can also benefit the patient with respect to local control and overall outcome. Numerous regional approaches have also been explored for the treatment of stage IV colon cancer depending on the organ or body cavity involved. Organ-specific infusional therapy, isolated or continuous perfusion therapy, radiofrequency ablation or cryotherapy, surgical debulking, and radiation are all technical approaches that have been performed. Many of these regional strategies as well as surgical metastasectomy will be discussed in separate chapters and therefore will not be specifically addressed here.

MANAGEMENT OF UNRESECTABLE METASTATIC DISEASE

Unresectable metastatic CRC is generally not curable with current technology. Management centers around palliation and control of symptoms, control of tumor growth, and attempts to lengthen progression-free and overall survival. Given the palliative nature of such treatments, extreme care must be taken to adequately assess each individual's potential for both benefit and harm from chemotherapy. Care must also be taken with surgical interventions as well. Quality-of-life issues must be frankly and objectively discussed with patients and their caregivers so that informed decisions can be made and expectations can be contained within a realistic framework. The issue of whether patients presenting with unresectable stage IV disease should have their primary tumors resected has been the matter of some debate. Although such resections had been routinely performed in the past, more recent data suggest that such interventions are not required, and may in fact be counterproductive. Temple et al.[318] reviewed the linked SEER-Medicare databases and found that of 9,011 elderly patients presenting with synchronous stage IV disease, that 72% had undergone resection of the primary, and that the 30-day mortality for these resections was 10%. In a retrospective review, Poultsides et al.[319] demonstrated that 93% of 233 patients never required surgical intervention on their primary tumors. More recently, the NSABP C-10 trial prospectively addressed this question, treating

90 patients with unresectable stage IV disease and intact, asymptomatic primary tumors with initial medical management with FOLFOX-6 plus bevacizumab. Twelve patients (14%) experienced major morbidity due to the intact primary tumor. This study met its prespecified end points for acceptability of intial nonoperative management, and the investigators concluded that good performance status patients with asymptomatic primaries can be spared initial noncurative resection of their primaries.[320]

Surgical intervention can be a very effective method of palliation and is often indicated in cases of impending obstruction, perforation, bleeding, or pain. However, it can also be associated with high postoperative morbidity and mortality. Stillwell et al.[321] identifies several adverse prognostic factors that can guide clinicians considering surgical palliation versus other less aggressive maneuvers. In a retrospective analysis of 379 patients who underwent palliative resection, elderly (≥70 years) patients with advanced local disease or extrahepatic metastases were at greatest risk for postoperative mortality. Other independently associated factors included emergency operation and medical complications. Advanced nodal disease (N2) and poor tumor differentiation were significant predictors of decreased long-term survival.[321]

The chemotherapy options available and the developmental work that supports their utility are outlined subsequently. It is of paramount importance to keep in mind that virtually all of the clinical trials done in patients with metastatic disease were performed by design on patients who were in good overall general medical condition. Entry criteria for most trials require a favorable performance status and acceptable bone marrow, renal, and hepatic function, and they often specify evidence of reasonable nutritional intake.

It is not reasonable to extrapolate the results of these trials to patients who do not conform to these entry criteria. The likelihood of benefit in a poor performance status patient is substantially diminished, and the likelihood of a serious adverse event is greatly increased. Patients with hepatic or renal dysfunction may be particularly prone to additional toxicity if the drug is cleared or metabolized by these organs. Patients with marginal nutritional intake may have their nutritional deficiencies further exacerbated by drugs that produce nausea or anorexia, and patients with partial or complete bowel obstruction or other causes of prolonged GI transit time may have increased toxicity from those drugs that undergo an enterohepatic recirculation.

Thus, chemotherapy for patients with incurable metastatic disease should be approached with appropriate caution. Good performance status in well-motivated patients with good bone marrow reserve and good organ function portend a significant potential for substantial benefits from chemotherapy and should be strongly considered for aggressive therapy. Patients with poor performance status and significant comorbidities should be considered for either less aggressive therapies or for supportive care only.

Fluorouracil

Virtually the entire history of chemotherapy for CRC has revolved around the use of 5-FU. Developed by Heidelberger et al.[322] and patented in 1957, it is a source of frustration and humility for investigators working to move beyond it that over 50 years later this agent remains at the very core of most chemotherapeutic approaches to CRC.

5-FU must be metabolized before it can exert cytotoxic activity. The details of 5-FU metabolism are covered in a separate chapter. The history of investigations of 5-FU in CRC treatment has been well summarized in previous editions of this book.[227] 5-FU remained the only drug available to treat CRC for almost four decades, during which time numerous agents were studied for their ability to "biomodulate" 5-FU. Of these, only leucovorin remains in use today, and it is debatable whether this reduced folate truly contributes to the efficacy of 5-FU. Most studies that evaluate the same dose of 5-FU with or without leucovorin find that both activity and toxicity are increased in the leucovorin arm, whereas studies that evaluate single-agent 5-FU versus an equitoxic schedule of a lower dose of 5-FU plus leucovorin find equivalent activity. Nevertheless, use of leucovorin persists in most standard regimens today. Data comparing bolus versus infusional schedules of 5-FU show a slight benefit for infusions. These infusional schedules achieved widespread acceptance in Europe sooner than in the United States. It was not until the advent of combination schedules of 5-FU plus other active agents that the benefits of infusional schedules, especially in terms of improved toxicity, asserted themselves in North American practice. A selection of commonly used 5-FU regimens is outlined in Table 49.10.[323–325]

TABLE 49.10

Commonly Used 5-Fluorouracil Regimens[a]

Name of Regimen	Author (Ref.)	Schedule (All Agents Administered Intravenously)
Roswell Park	Haller et al., 1998[231]	LV 500 mg/m² over 2 hr; 5-FU 500 mg/m² by bolus 1 hr into LV infusion. Treatments given weekly for 6 consecutive wk, repeated every 8 wk.
Low-dose weekly LV	Jager et al., 1996[323]	LV 20 mg/m² over 5–15 min, followed by bolus 5-FU 500 mg/m²; treatments given weekly for 6 consecutive wk, repeated every 8 wk.
Protracted venous infusion	Lokich et al., 1989[324]	5-FU 300 mg/m²/d by continuous infusion.
AIO (weekly 24-hr infusion)	Kohne et al., 1998[325]	LV 500 mg/m² over 2 hr, followed by 5-FU 2,600 mg/m² over 24 hr, repeated weekly.
LV5FU2	de Gramont et al., 1997[341]	LV 200 mg/m² over 2 hr days 1 and 2, followed by bolus 5-FU 400 mg/m²/day 1 and 2, followed by 5-FU 600 mg/m² over 22 hr days 1 and 2; cycle repeated every 14 d.
Simplified LV5FU2	Adapted from Andre et al., 1999[333]	LV 400 mg/m² over 2 hr, followed by bolus 5-FU 400 mg/m², followed by 5-FU 1,200 mg/m²/d times 2 d (2,400 mg/m² over 46–48 hr); cycles repeated every 14 d.

LV, leucovorin; 5-FU, 5-fluorouracil; AIO, Arbeitsgemeinschaft Internistische Onkologie (Oncology Working Group, Germany).
[a] Doses listed are recommended starting doses for good performance status patients with normal renal, hepatic, and bone marrow function. Individual dose adjustments may be required.

Capecitabine

Capecitabine is a 5-FU precursor that is administered orally. It is absorbed intact through the gut and then activated by a series of enzymatic alterations. Some data suggest that thymidine phosphorylase levels are higher in tumor than in normal tissue. This could, in theory, provide a degree of preferential intratumoral activation; however, clinical trials do not appear to support a substantially better therapeutic index than 5-FU.[326] Phase 2 studies demonstrate that this agent has substantial activity in CRC, with an acceptable toxicity profile.[327] Because the addition of leucovorin did not appear to show any benefit, clinical development went forward without additional biomodulation. Phase 3 randomized clinical trials, performed both in the United States and Europe, have now shown that this orally administered agent is at least as effective as intravenous 5-FU/leucovorin, and the side effect profile of capecitabine is superior to the daily times five Mayo Clinic schedule of 5-FU/leucovorin.[328,329] However, as this bolus daily times five schedule is now known to be unacceptably toxic and is not used anymore, the relevance of the toxicity comparison is questionable. Head-to-head studies of modern infusional 5-FU/leucovorin regimens versus capecitabine have never been done; however, a reasonable extrapolation from available data would suggest that these two approaches are extremely similar in efficacy and tolerability. The dose used in these pivotal trials was 1,250 mg/m^2 given twice daily for 14 days followed by a 7-day rest. The major side effects of capecitabine appear to be palmar-plantar erythrodysesthesia, commonly called hand-foot syndrome, and to a lesser extent diarrhea. The hand-foot toxicity is frequently a dose-limiting side effect, and although the approved starting dose is 1,250 mg/m^2 twice daily, this dose is based on trials conducted mainly in Europe. For unclear reasons, possibly related to higher serum folate levels, American patients tolerate capecitabine less well than European patients, and clinicians in the United States often choose to initiate therapy at a lower dose and escalate if little or no toxicity is seen.

Irinotecan

Irinotecan (CPT-11) is a semisynthetic derivative of camptothecin, a plant alkaloid extracted from the wood of the Asian tree *Camptotheca acuminate*.[330] CPT-11 possesses a bulky dipiperidino side chain linked to the camptothecin molecule via a carboxyl-ester bond. This side chain provides solubility but greatly decreases anticancer activity. Carboxylesterase, a ubiquitous enzyme with primary activity in the liver and gut, cleaves the carboxyl-ester bond to form the more active metabolite 7-ethyl-10-hydroxycamptothecin (SN-38).[331] SN-38 is as much as 1,000-fold more potent in inhibiting topoisomerase I than irinotecan and is thus the predominant active form of the drug. CPT-11 is often considered to be a prodrug for SN-38; however, this concept may be a bit too simplistic, as achieved CPT-11 concentrations may be several logs higher than those of SN-38.

Camptothecin, CPT-11, and SN-38 function as inhibitors of topoisomerase I (topo I). Topo I is a nuclear enzyme that aids in DNA uncoiling for replication and transcription. When topo I binds to DNA, it causes a reversible single-stranded break in the DNA, allowing the intact strand to pass through the break to relieve torsional stress on the coiled helix, and then reseals the break. CPT-11 and SN-38 stabilize these single-stranded breaks. Although the stabilized breaks do not cause irreversible damage, the collision of replication forks with open single-stranded breaks results in double-stranded breaks, leading to lethal DNA fragmentation. The early development of irinotecan and its single-agent schedules have been well documented in earlier editions of this textbook.[227]

CPT-11 in First-Line Combination Regimens

Numerous phase 1 combinations of 5-FU, usually with leucovorin, plus CPT-11, were tried. Saltz et al.[332] reported a phase 1 trial built on the weekly CPT-11 schedule that had been selected for phase 1 development in North America. A low dose of weekly leucovorin was utilized in order to reduce the potential for 5-FU/leucovorin–induced diarrhea. The phase 1 trial showed that the full single-agent dose of 125 mg/m^2 of CPT-11 could be given with 500 mg/m^2 of 5-FU and 20 mg/m^2 leucovorin, with all drugs given weekly for 4 consecutive weeks followed by a 2-week break. This and other CPT-11/5-FU/leucovorin regimens are summarized in Table 49.11. This combination of IFL was compared to the Mayo Clinic schedule of 5-FU/leucovorin in a multicenter, multinational phase 3 trial.[247] For regulatory reasons, a single-agent CPT-11 arm was included as well. The IFL arm was found to be superior to Mayo Clinic 5-FU/leucovorin in terms of response rate, time to tumor progression, and overall survival. The CPT-11–alone arm appeared to be comparable in efficacy to the 5-FU/leucovorin arm. The overall incidence of severe toxicity was similar in all arms of this trial. More serious diarrhea and vomiting were seen with IFL, while more neutropenia, neutropenic fever, and stomatitis were seen with 5-FU/leucovorin. Treatment-related deaths occurred in 1% of patients in each arm of this trial. Although this IFL schedule represented a step forward over the Mayo Clinic 5-FU/leucovorin schedule, neither of these are recommended for current use. As outlined in the following, the infusional 5-FU schedules have a superior safety and efficacy profile and are preferred for use, especially in combination regimens.

TABLE 49.11

Commonly Used Irinotecan/5-Fluorouracil Combination Regimens[a]

Name of Regimen	Author (Ref.)	Schedule (All Agents Administered Intravenously)
FOLFIRI	Douillard et al., 2000[246]	Irinotecan 180 mg/m^2 over 2 hr; LV 200 mg/m^2 concurrently with irinotecan (can be given in same line through "Y" connector); followed by 5-FU bolus 400 mg/m^2, followed by 5-FU 600 mg/m^2 infusion over 22 hr. Irinotecan given day 1 only. All other meds given days 1 and 2. Cycle repeated every 14 d.
FOLFIRI (simplified)	Andre et al., 1999[333]	Irinotecan 180 mg/m^2 over 90 min; LV 400 mg/m^2 concurrently with irinotecan (can be given in same line through "Y" connector); followed by 5-FU bolus 400 mg/m^2, followed by 5-FU 1,200 mg/m^2/d times 2 d (2,400 mg/m^2 infusion over 46–48 hr). Cycle repeated every 14 d.
FUFIRI	Douillard et al., 2000[246]	Irinotecan 80 mg/m^2, then LV 500 mg/m^2, followed by 5-FU 2,300 mg/m^2; all drugs given weekly for 6 wk, repeated every 7 wk.

FOLFIRI, irinotecan, 5-FU, LV; LV, leucovorin; 5-FU, 5-fluorouracil; FUFIRI, 5-FU, LV.
[a] Doses listed are recommended starting doses for good performance status patients with normal renal, hepatic, and bone marrow function. Individual dose adjustments may be required.

In Europe, a parallel study to investigate the benefit of adding irinotecan to a 5-FU–based schedule was undertaken.[246] Two high-dose intermittent infusional schedules were developed. In France, a biweekly treatment for 2 consecutive days was explored, while German investigators, building on their experience with weekly 24-hour high-dose infusions of 5-FU, combined CPT-11 with this schedule. A randomized phase 3 trial was performed in which a participating center chose which of these two schedules would be used, and then the patients were randomized to that 5-FU/leucovorin schedule plus or minus CPT-11. Again, response rate, progression-free survival, and overall survival were superior in the CPT-11–containing arm of the trial. Of note, only the cohort treated with the biweekly schedule demonstrated a statistically superior survival over the 5-FU/leucovorin control arm, and the biweekly combination schedule is the only one registered for use in the United States.

More recently, the biweekly schedule of LV5FU2 plus irinotecan has been studied with a simplified LV5FU2 infusion schedule.[333] This schedule, known as FOLFIRI (FOL for folinic acid, F for 5-FU, and IRI for irinotecan), was initially studied as a salvage regimen; however, this has now gained widespread acceptance as a first-line treatment option, based on the data discussed subsequently.

The BICC-C (Bolus, Infusional, or Capecitabine with Camptosar-Celecoxib) trial is the only trial to directly compare weekly bolus IFL to FOLFIRI.[334] This trial utilized a modified bolus IFL schedule, giving treatment on days 1 and 8, repeated on a 3-week cycle. This modified IFL was compared to FOLFIRI as well as to capecitabine/irinotecan. The first phase of this trial (430 patients) confirmed the superior safety and efficacy of FOLFIRI over IFL (median progression-free survival 7.6 months for FOLFIRI versus 5.8 months; $p = 0.007$) and over capecitabine/irinotecan (progression-free survival 5.7 months; $p = 0.003$). The trial was halted when bevacizumab (see the following) became commercially available, and a second phase randomized 117 patients to modified IFL plus bevacizumab versus FOLFIRI plus bevacizumab (capecitabine/irinotecan was dropped from the second phase of this trial). This second phase showed a significant overall survival advantage for FOLFIRI/bevacizumab over modified IFL/bevacizumab ($p = 0.002$). The BICC-C trial also had a second randomization of all patients to celecoxib versus placebo. Celecoxib was found to provide no benefit in terms of either safety or efficacy and does not appear to have a role as part of standard chemotherapy of this disease.

Oxaliplatin

Oxaliplatin (1,2-diaminocyclohexane (trans-l) oxalatoplatinum) is a third-generation platinum compound of the diaminocyclohexane family. Initial single-agent phase 1 studies established that oxaliplatin could be safely administered, with evidence of clinical activity.[335,336] No significant nephrotoxicity was seen. Nausea and vomiting, minimal leucopenia, and rare thrombocytopenia were observed. Extra et al.[335] were the first to describe in detail the most notable toxicity encountered with oxaliplatin: neurotoxicity. This neurotoxicity manifested as paresthesias and dysesthesias of the hands, feet, perioral region, and throat. Pharyngolaryngeal dysesthesia, a sensation of choking without overt airway blockage, was described as well. These neurologic toxicities were induced or worsened by exposure to cold. Early single-agent explorations with oxaliplatin have been well outlined in the prior edition of this textbook.[337]

Oxaliplatin/5-Fluorouracil/Leucovorin Combination Trials

Based on a series of phase 2 trials by Levi et al., Giachetti et al.[338] from the same group reported a phase 3 trial of chronomodulated

5-FU/leucovorin alone or with oxaliplatin.[338–340] Two hundred patients were randomly assigned to receive a 5-day course every 3 weeks of chronomodulated 5-FU and leucovorin (700 and 300 mg/m^2 per day, respectively; peak delivery rate at 4 a.m.) with or without oxaliplatin on the first day of each course (125 mg/m^2, as a 6-hour infusion). The group who received oxaliplatin had a superior response rate (53% versus 16%; $p < 0.001$). Progression-free survival was also superior, just reaching statistical significance (8.7 months versus 7.4 months; $p = 0.048$). There were no differences in median overall survival (19.4 months and 19.9 months, respectively). Survival outcomes in this trial are somewhat difficult to interpret as extensive use of resection of metastatic disease was applied in both arms.

Most of the combination 5-FU/leucovorin/oxaliplatin trials have used flat (nonchronomodulated) administration of agents and have centered on variants of the FOLFOX regimen. The acronym FOLFOX (FOL for folinic acid [leucovorin], F for fluorouracil, OX for oxaliplatin) refers to a series of combinations of these agents. These are biweekly (every other week) regimens using 2 days of infusional 5-FU on a 14-day cycle (LV5FU2).[341] The FOLFOX-1, -2, and -3 regimens employed various alterations in dosing of each oxaliplatin, 5-FU, and leucovorin.[342,343] They are of historical interest, but were never evaluated in randomized trials. FOLFOX-3 and FOLFOX-4 were reported in a combined series to have a response rate of 21% in a population of patients who had progressed on the same 5-FU/leucovorin schedule without oxaliplatin.[342] The FOLFOX-4 regimen had a modestly higher response rate and lower toxicity than FOLFOX-3 (which used higher doses of 5-FU and leucovorin), and FOLFOX-4 appeared to be better tolerated. The more commonly used oxaliplatin/5-FU/leucovorin combinations are outlined in Table 49.12.[344,345]

A randomized phase 3 trial was undertaken to evaluate FOLFOX-4 versus the LV5FU2 schedule in patients with previously untreated metastatic CRC (essentially a trial of LV5FU2 with or without oxaliplatin).[346] Patients treated with FOLFOX-4 had a statistically significantly superior outcome in terms of response rate (51% versus 22%; $p = 0.001$) and progression-free survival (9 months versus 6.2 months; $p = 0.0003$). The FOLFOX arm had a 1.5-month improvement in median overall survival; however, this did not reach statistical significance (16.2 months versus 14.7 months; $p = 0.12$). The number of patients experiencing grade 3 or 4 neutropenia was increased with FOLFOX-4 over 340 (42% versus 5% of patients). Grade 3 or 4 diarrhea (12% versus 5%) was also increased in the FOLFOX arm. Neurotoxicity, virtually absent in the LV5FU2 arm, was frequent in the FOLFOX arm, with 18% of patients experiencing grade 3 neurosensory toxicity.

The FOLFOX-4 regimen has also been evaluated in a multicenter randomized trial in second-line therapy following failure of first-line IFL chemotherapy.[347] Patients were randomly assigned to one of three arms: FOLFOX-4, LV5FU2, or single-agent oxaliplatin. Response rates were 10% for FOLFOX, 0% for LV5FU2, and 1% for oxaliplatin alone ($p < 0.0001$ for FOLFOX versus LV5FU2). Time to tumor progression was also superior for FOLFOX-4 (4.6 months) versus LV5FU2 (2.7 months) and oxaliplatin alone (1.6 months). These data confirm initial clinical impressions that oxaliplatin/5-FU combinations have superior activity to single-agent oxaliplatin, even in 5-FU–refractory disease. FOLFOX-4 has activity in IFL-refractory disease; however, single-agent oxaliplatin essentially does not.

Further modifications have been made to the FOLFOX schedule. FOLFOX-5 was designed with an increased dose of oxaliplatin to 100 mg/m^2 every 14 days; however, this regimen was never tested in clinical trials. FOLFOX-6 utilized this 100 mg/m^2 oxaliplatin dose with a simplified 5-FU/leucovorin schedule.[348] Oxaliplatin 100 mg/m^2 is given over 2 hours, with leucovorin 400 mg/m^2 given concurrently via a "T" connector. These are then followed by a 400 mg/m^2 bolus of 5-FU, and then a 46-hour infusion of 5-FU at 2,400 to 3,000 mg/m^2. More recently, the FOLFOX-7 regimen has been reported, utilizing a 130 mg/m^2 dose of oxaliplatin

TABLE 49.12

Selected Commonly Used Oxaliplatin/5-Fluorouracil Combination Regimens[a]

Name of Regimen	Author (Ref.)	Schedule (All Agents Administered Intravenously)
FOLFOX-4	de Gramont et al., 2000[346]	Oxaliplatin 85 mg/m^2 over 2 hr; LV 200 mg/m^2 concurrently with oxaliplatin (can be given in same line through "Y" connector); followed by 5-FU bolus 400 mg/m^2, followed by 5-FU 600 mg/m^2 infusion over 22 hr. Oxaliplatin given day 1 only. All other meds given days 1 and 2. Cycle repeated every 14 d.
FOLFOX-6	Tournigand et al., 2004[349]	Oxaliplatin 100 mg/m^2 over 2 hr; LV 400 mg/m^2 concurrently with oxaliplatin (can be given in same line through "Y" connector); followed by 5-FU bolus 400 mg/m^2, followed by 5-FU 1,200 mg/m^2/d times 2 d (2,400 mg/m^2 infusion over 46–48 hr). Cycle repeated every 14 d.
Modified FOLFOX-6	Widely used in current phase 3 trials, Wolmark et al. 2009[344]	Oxaliplatin 85 mg/m^2 over 2 hr; LV 400 mg/m^2 concurrently with oxaliplatin (can be given in same line through "Y" connector); followed by 5-FU bolus 400 mg/m^2, followed by 5-FU 1,200 mg/m^2/d times 2 d (2,400 mg/m^2 infusion over 46–48 hr). Cycle repeated every 14 d.
FUFOX	Grothey et al., 2002[345]	Oxaliplatin 50 mg/m^2 over 2 hr, followed by LV 500 mg/m^2, followed by 5-FU 2,000 mg/m^2 over 24 hr, weekly for 5 wk, repeated every 6 wk.

FOLFOX, folinic acid, 5-FU, oxaliplatin; LV, leucovorin; 5-FU, 5-fluorouracil; FUFOX, 5-FU, folinic acid.
[a] Doses listed are recommended starting doses for good performance status patients with normal renal, hepatic, and bone marrow function. Individual dose adjustments may be required.

every 14 days. The simplified leucovorin/5-FU administration of FOLFOX-6 is maintained, with deletion of the bolus 5-FU. Oxaliplatin is discontinued after 3 months, with planned reintroduction after 12 weeks or sooner if clinical progression occurs.[349] This rationale appears promising, both for treatment of metastatic disease and for potential use in the adjuvant setting. Given the similar response rates after 12 weeks, it would appear that the increased dose of oxaliplatin in FOLFOX-7 is unnecessary. A reasonable approach to standard use of FOLFOX in the metastatic setting is to use a modified FOLFOX-6, with 85 mg/m^2 of oxaliplatin and simplified LV5FU2 at a dose of 2,400 mg/m^2 over 46 to 48 hours (1,200 mg/m^2 per day for 2 consecutive days). As discussed in the following, the OPTIMOX trial data support cessation of oxaliplatin after 12 weeks and reintroduction of the oxaliplatin at a later date upon disease progression. It had been previously hypothesized that administration of high doses of calcium and magnesium with oxaliplatin would be protective against neurotoxicity, but a definitive trial has now demonstrated that this is not the case.[350]

Comparisons of Oxaliplatin- and Irinotecan-Based Combinations

With both oxaliplatin- and irinotecan-based regimens showing encouraging activity, the question of which agent to use first was addressed by a number of investigators. Tournigand et al.[349] reported a phase 3 trial of FOLFOX-6 versus FOLFIRI. This trial utilized identical simplified LV5FU2 schedules, with the only variable being oxaliplatin or irinotecan. All patients were planned to crossover to the other regimen at time of progression, and the primary end point was time to tumor progression after *both* chemotherapy regimens. Results are shown in Table 49.13. Although the study is somewhat underpowered at a total of 226 patients, the

TABLE 49.13

Comparison of First-Line Use of Irinotecan Versus Oxaliplatin in Conjunction with the Same Simplified Biweekly Infusional 5-Fluorouracil/Leucovorin Schedule

	FOLFIRI (n = 109 Patients Treated)	FOLFOX-6 (n = 111 Patients Treated)	P Value
Major objective response rate (partial plus complete responses)	56%	54%	0.68
Time to tumor progression (on first-line regimen)	8.5 mo	8.1 mo	0.65
Time to tumor progression (after first- and second-line regimen)	14.4 mo	11.5 mo	0.65
Overall survival (from initial randomization)	20.4 mo	21.5 mo	0.9
Two-yr overall survival	41%	45%	
Grade 3–4 neutropenia	25%	44%	
Neutropenic fever	6%	1%	
Grade 3–4 diarrhea	14%	11%	
Neuropathy (grade 3)	0%	34%	
Alopecia (grade 2)	24%	9%	

FOLFIRI, irinotecan, 5-fluorouracil, leucovorin; FOLFOX, folinic acid, 5-fluorouracil, oxaliplatin.
From Tournigand C, Andre T, Achille E, et al. FOLFIRI followed by FOLFOX6 or the reverse sequence in advanced colorectal cancer: a randomized GERCOR study. *J Clin Oncol* 2004;22:229–237.

results show a striking consistency between regimens, suggesting that use of either FOLFOX-6 or FOLFIRI in first-line treatment is acceptable. A somewhat larger trial of 360 patients randomized to FOLFOX-4 versus the equivalent FOLFIRI schedule, utilizing the same LV5FU2 dose and schedule in each arm, again shows comparable efficacy data, with differing and predictable toxicity profiles.[351]

The North Central Cancer Treatment Group–led US Intergroup study N9741, a complex and important trial that underwent many iterations before its completion, initially opened as a four-arm trial comparing the Mayo Clinic 5-FU/leucovorin control arm to three different CPT-11/5-FU/leucovorin regimens: weekly bolus IFL as reported by Saltz et al.,[247] a "Mayo II" schedule of CPT-11 on day 1 and bolus 5-FU/low-dose leucovorin on days 2 to 5, or the biweekly infusional schedule of LV5FU2 plus CPT-11 as reported by Douillard et al.[246] and Goldberg.[352] After accruing a small number of patients, the trial was closed to incorporate three oxaliplatin-containing arms: FOLFOX-4, IROX (a once every 3 weeks combination of irinotecan and oxaliplatin, without 5-FU), and a modified Mayo Clinic schedule of bolus 5-FU plus low-dose leucovorin days 1 through 5, with oxaliplatin given on day 1. The infusional LV5FU2 plus CPT-11 arm was dropped. This created a six-arm trial. In March 2000, the trial was again halted, based on presentation of evidence that the combination of CPT-11/5-FU/ leucovorin, using either bolus or infusional schedules, was superior to 5-FU/leucovorin. The Mayo Clinic control arm of N9741 was now dropped, and weekly bolus IFL became the control arm. At the same time, ongoing real-time monitoring of fatal toxicities identified unacceptably high rates of treatment-related mortality in the oxaliplatin plus Mayo Clinic 5-FU/leucovorin and in the CPT-11 plus 5-FU/leucovorin arms. These schedules were also dropped from the trial and from further development, leaving a three-arm trial of CPT-11 plus bolus 5-FU/leucovorin (IFL), oxaliplatin plus infusional LV5FU2 (FOLFOX-4), and oxaliplatin plus CPT-11 (IROX).

The trial was stopped a third time in April 2001, when monitoring of the trial indicated what appeared to be a higher than expected early mortality in the IFL control arm.[248] This observation, however, was based on utilization of a new metric, the 60-day ACM. This metric records death from *any* cause within 60 days of initial therapy. The 60-day ACM of the IFL arm was initially noted to be 4.5%. Because this was a new metric, however, there were no readily available historical controls; no one had ready access to data to say what the 60-day ACM had been in previous trials, either with IFL or with 5-FU/leucovorin regimens. The 4.5% ACM was therefore compared to the previously reported death rate for the IFL regimen, which was 0.9%. However, the previously reported death rate was the treatment-related death rate, the percentage of deaths judged by the investigators to have been caused by treatment, not all deaths within 60 days of starting therapy. Of further concern to the safety monitoring committee, however, the experimental arms (FOLFOX-4 and IROX) each showed 60-day ACMs of 1.8% (compared to 4.5% for the IFL control arm). This information was difficult to put into context, however, because the efficacy of the two experimental arms had not yet been established.

In fact, the 60-day ACM on the original phase 3 trial of IFL (subsequently calculated after N9741 was halted) was 6.7%, and the 60-day ACM for the Mayo Clinic control arm of that trial was found to be 7.3%. Although the 7.3% 60-day ACM appeared subjectively to be unusually high, no historical baseline data on 60-day ACM in 5-FU–based regimens were readily available. To help interpret these data, an analysis was undertaken to determine the 60-day ACM in multiple large-scale randomized trials that had used 5-FU/leucovorin schedules over the prior decade. This analysis confirmed that 60-day ACM regularly was encountered at a rate of 5% to 8% in the treatment of metastatic CRC.[353] Thus the 60-day ACM for the IFL regimen was actually *lower* on N9741 than in previous trials and was *lower* than what had been seen consistently with 5-FU/leucovorin regimens alone. In the final analysis of N9741, the 60-day ACM seen in the IFL, FOLFOX-4, and IROX arms were 4.5%, 2.6%, and 2.7%, respectively, and these differences were not statistically significant.

The efficacy results of N9741, however, were statistically significant and showed superior outcome for the patients randomized to FOLFOX-4, as compared to those randomized to either IFL or IROX, in terms of response rate, time to tumor progression, and overall survival (Table 49.14).[354] Toxicity for FOLFOX-4 was also superior for virtually all parameters, except of course neurotoxicity. The results of the IROX arm did not statistically significantly differ from those of the IFL arm in terms of toxicity, response, or time to tumor progression; however, survival was borderline statistically significantly better in the IROX arm than the IFL arm ($p = 0.04$).

TABLE 49.14

Results of Intergroup Trial N9741: Irinitecan Plus Bolus 5-Fluorouracil/Leucovorin, Oxaliplatin Plus Infusional 5-Fluorouracil/Leucovorin, and Irinotecan Plus Oxaliplatin in First-Line Treatment of Patients with Metastatic Colorectal Cancer

	IFL (*n* = 264)	FOLFOX-4 (*n* = 267)	IROX (*n* = 264)	*P* Value (IFL vs. FOLFOX)
Major objective response rate (partial plus complete responses)	31%	45%	35%	0.03
Time to tumor progression	6.9 mo	8.7 mo	6.5 mo	0.001
Overall survival	15.0 mo	19.5 mo	17.4 mo	0.0001
Received second-line therapy with active drug not included in first-line regimen	24% (oxaliplatin)	60% (irinotecan)	50% (fluorouracil)	Not given
Grade 3–4 neutropenia	40%	50%	36%	0.35
Neutropenic fever	15%	4%	11%	0.001
Grade 3–4 diarrhea	28%	12%	24%	0.001
Grade 3–4 nausea	16%	6%	19%	0.001
Grade 3 neuropathy	3%	18%	7%	0.001
60-d all cause mortality	4.5%	2.6%	2.7%	Not significant

IFL, 5-fluorouracil, leucovorin; FOLFOX4, oxaliplatin plus infusional 5-fluorouracil/leucovorin; IROX, irinotecan plus oxaliplatin
From Goldberg RM, Sargent DJ, Morton RF, et al. A randomized controlled trial of fluorouracil plus leucovorin, irinotecan, and oxaliplatin combinations in patients with previously untreated metastatic colorectal cancer. *J Clin Oncol* 2004;22:23–30.

Taken together, where do these trials leave us in terms of first-line use of oxaliplatin- and irinotecan-based regimens? Data from trial N9741 indicate that FOLFOX-4 is superior to IFL in both response rate and time to tumor progression. Overall survival was superior in the FOLFOX-4 arm versus IFL as well; however, interpretation of the survival results of N9741 is somewhat complicated due to imbalances between arms in availability of effective second-line therapy. Second-line CPT-11 was available to all patients who had received FOLFOX-4. Oxaliplatin, however, was not commercially available in the United States during the course of N9741. To what degree this imbalance in second-line therapy may have influenced the survival result is unknown. Also, as IFL contains bolus 5-FU, while FOLFOX-4 contains infusional leucovorin/5-FU2, it is difficult to isolate the irinotecan versus oxaliplatin component from the 5-FU bolus versus 5-FU infusion component.

Two other trials indicate that the FOLFOX and FOLFIRI regimens have similar safety and efficacy, with differing toxicity profiles.[349,351] Thus, FOLFOX has comparable efficacy to FOLFIRI, whereas FOLFOX has a superior response rate, time to tumor progression, and possibly some degree of survival benefit over IFL. Toxicity with irinotecan-based regimens shows a higher degree of alopecia. Diarrhea and neutropenia are increased on the bolus 5-FU schedule but are similar between FOLFOX and FOLFIRI. Oxaliplatin-based regimens, however, have neurotoxicity, absent from the irinotecan-based regimens, which can be problematic in some patients. It would therefore seem reasonable at this time to favor the use of a high-dose intermittent infusional 5-FU/leucovorin schedule plus either oxaliplatin (i.e., FOLFOX) or CPT-11 (i.e., FOLFIRI). Data do not support continued routine use of the bolus IFL schedule, nor are there randomized data to support the routine use of a bolus 5-FU/leucovorin schedule with oxaliplatin in the metastatic setting. Routine use of IROX is also not supported by the currently available body of data.

Whether to use an irinotecan-based or oxaliplatin-based combination in first-line treatment of good performance status patients can be considered a matter of patient preference, and discussion of the differing toxicity profiles is appropriate to help individuals decide. It is hoped that in the near-term future molecular prognostic indicators and pharmacogenomics will provide useful guidance for the individualization of therapies, but such approaches remain investigational at this time.

The only oxaliplatin schedule registered for use in the United States is FOLFOX-4; however, the modified FOLFOX-6 would appear at this time to be a very reasonable schedule for routine clinical use when the decision is made to use an oxaliplatin/5-FU combination.

The recognition of neurotoxicity as a major limitation of the FOLFOX regimens led to the investigation of optimization of oxaliplatin (the OPTIMOX study).[355] In this trial, patients were randomly assigned to receive either standard FOLFOX-4 until progression or 12 weeks of FOLFOX-7, followed by planned cessation of oxaliplatin and continuation of the LV5FU2. As designed, the study called for a reintroduction of oxaliplatin after 6 months of LV5FU2, although this actually occurred in the minority of patients and outcomes were superior in those patients in whom reintroduction of oxaliplatin occurred.[356] The primary end point was duration of disease control, the time from initiation of treatment until either progression through all agents (including failure after reintroduction of oxaliplatin if this was done), or death. Duration of disease control as well as progression-free survival and overall survival were not statistically significantly different between the two arms. As anticipated, toxicity, including neurotoxicity, was substantially reduced in the OPTIMOX arm. This OPTIMOX strategy of planned interruption of oxaliplatin can be considered a standard care option in metastatic disease. It is important to discuss plans for such planned interruptions with patients at the beginning of therapy so that they will not be surprised or alarmed at the removal of one of the drugs.

Although a regimen of oxaliplatin, weekly bolus 5-FU, and low-dose weekly leucovorin (bFOL) appeared promising in an initial phase 2 trial, two sequential randomized phase 2 trials, known as TREE-1 and TREE-2, suggest modestly inferior activity for the bFOL schedule compared with FOLFOX or Cape/Ox.[357,358] Thus, in the metastatic setting, oxaliplatin with bolus 5-FU schedules is therefore not recommended for routine use.

Use of planned sequential administration of FOLFOX and FOLFIRI has also been proposed, both in terms of pretreatment for potentially resectable patients with liver metastases and in terms of adjuvant treatment of earlier stage disease. Several groups are also exploring the use of "triple therapy" with oxaliplatin, CPT-11, and 5-FU/leucovorin (FOLFOXIRI). A randomized phase 3 trial conducted in Italy reported that FOLFOXIRI is tolerable and offers a modest survival benefit over FOLFIRI. These trials utilized higher doses of 5-FU than are likely to be tolerable by American patients, and use of this combination has not gained widespread acceptance.[359]

As discussed previously, a trial comparing FOLFIRI to capecitabine/irinotecan suggested inferior outcome for the capecitabine-containing regimen.[334] However, a large randomized trial has now compared Cape/Ox versus FOLFOX. The study also had a two-by-two randomization to with or without bevacizumab (discussed subsequently). This trial demonstrated the Cape/Ox regimen to be noninferior to FOLFOX, and each had acceptable toxicity, indicating that Cape/Ox is an acceptable alternative to FOLFOX.[360] It should be noted that the Cape/Ox regimen requires a motivated, reliable patient who will be able to take multiple pills of oral medication on a complex schedule, even in the setting of potentially emetogenic oxaliplatin.

Duration of Therapy

Controversy continues to exist regarding the optimal duration of chemotherapy for palliation of metastatic disease. Traditional practice for many years had been to continue chemotherapy until either unacceptable toxicity, clinical deterioration, or disease progression. When efficacy of treatment was more limited, with the duration of therapy typically limited to a small number of months, the issue of treatment breaks did not seem relevant. Now, with patients typically living multiple years with metastatic CRC and with some treatments maintaining control for more extended periods of time, the need for patients to have breaks (often referred to as "treatment holidays" or "chemotherapy-free intervals" [CFI]) is greater, and there is considerable interest in using these approaches. Both physically and psychologically, many patients appear to both need and derive benefit from these treatment interruptions.

The concept of noncontinuous chemotherapy has been investigated for some time now. Maughan et al.[361] conducted a randomized trial of continuous versus interrupted treatment in 354 patients who were responding or who had stable disease after receiving 12 weeks of either 5-FU– or raltitrexed-based chemotherapy. Patients were randomized to either continue chemotherapy until progression or to stop chemotherapy after the first 12 weeks, followed by a planned restarting on the same chemotherapy at the time of progression. At randomization, 41% of patients had achieved a major objective response and 59% had stable disease. There was no evidence of a difference in overall survival, the primary end point, between the two groups, with an HR of 0.87 ($p = 0.23$, favoring the intermittent arm).

More recently, the idea of planned early cessation of all chemotherapy was investigated in the OPTIMOX-2 trial.[362] A total of 202 patients with previously untreated metastatic CRC were treated. All patients received six cycles of modified FOLFOX-7 followed by either continued LV5FU2 until progression, or a complete cessation of all chemotherapy (a CFI). Patients on both arms were planned to receive retreatment with FOLFOX following tumor progression. The results of this study did not support the use of this planned, early interruption in therapy, as the median duration of disease control, progression-free survival, and overall survival were all inferior in the arm with the early planned CFI. This should not be misconstrued as evidence that CFIs are contraindicated, but rather that early planned CFIs for all patients is not an appropriate strategy. The authors suggest that this study indicates there are no pretreatment parameters that can identify a priori those patients who can successfully benefit from a CFI. Thus, specific decisions regarding use and timing of CFIs cannot be made in advance of starting treatment; rather, clinical judgment must be exercised in deciding on treatment interruptions for CFIs in responding patients after a favorable response. In a retrospective review of 822 patients in the two OPTIMOX studies, after excluding those patients who had early progression within the first 3 months of treatment as well as those who underwent complete gross resection of metastatic disease within 3 months of stopping chemotherapy, Perez-Staub et al.[363] noted that there was no indication of a detriment in survival when comparing those patients who took a CFI versus those who did not. In fact, in this retrospective, nonrandomized analysis, the median survival was 37.5 months in patients who had a CFI versus 21.2 months in matched patients who did not have a CFI. Of note, median overall survival of patients who stopped chemotherapy earlier than 3 months was 24 months, whereas it was 42 months when a CFI was taken between 3 and 9 months into therapy, and 44 months when a CFI was taken later than 9 months into chemotherapy. These studies were accomplished prior to the use of bevacizumab. Some clinicians have advocated the continuation of bevacizumab during CFIs. Such an approach is not supported by data, and given the absence of activity of single-agent bevacizumab in CRC, use of single-agent bevacizumab during otherwise CFIs is not recommended at this time.

Other investigators specifically addressed the question of whether rechallenge with 5-FU after a planned treatment interruption could produce a response. A pooled analysis was conducted on 613 patients involved in three randomized trials of first-line 5-FU–based therapy.[364] All patients had a planned maximum treatment period of 6 months. Patients with responding or stable disease at the end of that period were observed off treatment with a plan for retreatment at the time of disease progression. Median time to rechallenge was 11.7 months. Seventeen percent of patients had an objective response to rechallenging. Median survival for the group was 14.8 months. These nonrandomized data indicate that patients have a meaningful response rate at time of reinstitution of chemotherapy.

A similar approach was explored in patients who received second-line irinotecan therapy.[365] A total of 333 patients entered into a trial to receive 24 weeks of irinotecan. Patients who remained in the study at the end of that time were to be randomized to either continue treatment or to stop therapy. Of the 333 patients, most came off the study due to progression or toxicity before reaching the 24-week mark. Fifty-five patients with responding or stable disease agreed to randomization. Although the numbers available for comparison were small, there were no differences between the

arms in progression-free survival or overall survival, nor were there differences in quality-of-life scores.

Overall, there appears to be no compelling evidence that continuation of chemotherapy indefinitely is necessary for optimal control of metastatic disease. The option of discontinuation of therapy after a reasonable period of time appears to be an appropriate consideration in standard practice.

Combination versus Single-Agent Chemotherapy

Given that combination regimens are invariably associated with more toxicity than single agents, the question of the need for universal upfront use of these combinations was investigated. The CAIRO (CApecitabine, IRinotecan, Oxaliplatin) trial randomized 820 patients to sequential versus concurrent therapies (Table 49.15).[366] In the sequential arm, first-line therapy was single-agent capecitabine. Upon failure, single-agent irinotecan was used, and then third-line therapy was Cape/Ox (since single-agent oxaliplatin is essentially inactive in 5-FU–refractory CRC). The combination arm used Cape/Ox as first-line therapy and capecitabine and irinotecan as second-line therapy. The primary end point, median overall survival, was not statistically significantly different between the two arms (17.4 months for combination versus 16.3 months for the sequential arm; $p = 0.33$). Dose-limiting toxicity (grade 3 or 4) was not significantly different between the two groups; in fact, grade 3 hand-foot syndrome was somewhat more common in the sequential arm (13% versus 7%; $p = 0.004$).

Similar findings were reported in the FOCUS study.[367] In this trial, a total of 2,135 patients were randomized to one of three arms. Arm A was sequential therapy, with initial treatment given with 5-FU on the leucovorin/5-FU2 (biweekly infusional) schedule until progression, at which point second-line therapy was given with single-agent irinotecan. Arm B also gave biweekly LV5FU2 until failure, and then LV5FU2 was continued with the addition of either oxaliplatin or irinotecan (this was a second randomization within this arm). Thus, second-line therapy was a change from biweekly LV5FU2 to either FOLFOX or FOLFIRI in this arm. In arm C, patients began with combination chemotherapy, and within this arm were randomized to either FOLFOX or FOLFIRI. The primary end point, median overall survival, for arm A was 13.9 months. For arm B, survival was 15.0 months for irinotecan and 15.2 months for oxaliplatin. Arm C had a median overall survival of 16.7 months for the FOLFIRI patients and 15.4 months for those treated with FOLFOX. Only the difference between arm A and the irinotecan arm of arm C reached statistical significance ($p = 0.01$). Arm B (initial LV5FU2 followed by FOLFOX or FOLIRI) was noninferior to arm C (initial FOLFOX or FOLIRI) (HR = 1.06; 90% CI = 0.97 to 1.17).

Taken together, the CAIRO and FOCUS trials provide a strong argument that not all patients with unresectable metastatic disease require exposure to the toxicity of combination therapy, and

TABLE 49.15

Sequential Versus Combination Chemotherapy with Capecitabine, Irinotecan, and Oxaliplatin in Advanced Colorectal Cancer: Efficacy End Points

	Overall Survival	One-Yr Survival	Progression-Free Survival (First Line)	Response Rate
Sequential Cape, then Iri, then Cape/Ox ($n = 401$)	16.3 mo	64%	5.8 m	20%
Combination Cape/Iri, then Cape/Ox ($n = 402$)	17.4 mo	67%	7.8 m	41%
P value	0.33	0.38	0.0002	0.0001

Cape, capecitabine; Iri, irinotecan; Ox, oxaliplatin.
From Koopman M, Antonini NF, Douma J, et al. Sequential versus combination chemotherapy with capecitabine, irinotecan, and oxaliplatin in advanced colorectal cancer (CAIRO): a phase III randomised controlled trial. *Lancet* 2007;370:135–142.

TABLE 49.16A

Efficacy Outcomes, First-Line Treatment of Metastatic Colorectal Cancer: Irinotecan Plus Bolus 5-Fluorouracil/Leucovorin Plus Placebo Versus 5-Fluorouracil/Leucovorin Plus Bevacizumab

Regimen	No. of Patients	Response Rate	Progression-Free Survival	Overall Survival
IFL + placebo	411	34.8%	6.2 mo	15.6 mo
IFL + bevacizumab	402	44.8% $p = 0.004$	10.6 mo $p < 0.001$	20.3 mo $p < 0.001$

IFL, 5-fluorouracil, leucovorin.

that initial use of fluorinated pyrimidine alone in patients with previously untreated metastatic CRC is a treatment alternative that needs to be carefully considered.

Bevacizumab

Bevacizumab is a humanized monoclonal antibody that binds to VEGF, thereby substantially reducing the amount of circulating ligand and thus preventing receptor activation.[368,369] The first trial of bevacizumab in CRC was a modest-sized, three-arm, randomized phase 2 trial in which a total of 104 patients were randomly assigned to either one of two different doses levels of bevacizumab (5 mg/kg or 10 mg/kg) plus weekly 5-FU/leucovorin or to 5-FU/leucovorin alone.[370] The response rate, time to tumor progression, and overall survival were superior in the 5-FU/leucovorin with 5 mg/kg bevacizumab arm. Despite the small size and limited statistical power of this study, this result would served as the basis for design of the pivotal phase 3 trial of bevacizumab in CRC.

The initial design of the phase 3 pivotal trial was a comparison between 5-FU/leucovorin plus placebo to 5-FU/leucovorin plus 5 mg/kg of bevacizumab. However, as the randomized phase 2 trial, discussed previously, was nearing completion, the randomized phase 3 trial was reported, which demonstrated a modest but statistically significant survival advantage for the IFL regimen (irinotecan plus weekly bolus 5-FU/leucovorin) compared with 5-FU/leucovorin alone.[247] As a result of this trial, the IFL regimen was then felt to be the appropriate control arm for subsequent phase 3 trials. There were no safety data at the time, however, on the combination of bevacizumab plus IFL. As a result of this, a three-arm trial was designed that contained (1) 5-FU/leucovorin/bevacizumab, (2) IFL/bevacizumab, and (3) IFL/placebo (the control arm).[371] The design included a preplanned analysis of safety on all arms when enrollment reached 100 patients per arm, with a further plan to close the 5-FU/leucovorin/bevacizumab arm at that time if the safety data indicated acceptable tolerability and safety of the IFL/bevacizumab arm.

In the final efficacy analysis, the IFL/bevacizumab cohort experienced superior outcome compared to the IFL/placebo group in response rate (45% versus 35%; $p < 0.003$), progression-free survival (10.6 months versus 6.2 months; $p < 0.00001$), and overall survival (20.3 months versus 15.6 months; $p = 0.00003$) (Table 49.16A).

It should be noted that no crossover to second-line bevacizumab in the IFL/placebo control arm was allowed in this trial.

In order to better understand the effects of bevacizumab in conjunction with 5-FU/leucovorin, Kabbinavar et al.[372] combined the data from three separate modest-sized trials to create a more robust data set. In this combined analysis of 5-FU/leucovorin with or without bevacizumab, there was a statistically significant survival advantage for the patients who received bevacizumab. Given the favorable aspects of the biweekly infusional LV5FU2 schedule used in the FOCUS trial, the LV5FU2 schedule would seem most appropriate for combination with bevacizumab.[373] At the same time as the pivotal front-line study was accruing, the Eastern Cooperative Oncology Group (ECOG) also performed a trial (ECOG-3200) to evaluate the use of bevacizumab in the second-line setting.[374] This trial randomized patients who had failed irinotecan and 5-FU but were naive to bevacizumab, to one of three arms: bevacizumab/FOLFOX, FOLFOX alone, or bevacizumab. The investigators chose to investigate a 10 mg/kg bevacizumab dose. Overall, a modest but statistically significant improvement in median overall survival was demonstrated for FOLFOX-4 with bevacizumab versus FOLFOX-4 alone (12.5 months versus 10.7 months; $p = 0.0024$), and grade 3 or 4 toxicities were not increased. The bevacizumab-alone arm had substantially inferior progression-free survival and an investigator-adjudicated response rate of 3%, suggesting that single-agent bevacizumab does not have meaningful activity in CRC and should not be used. It is important to note that this trial was performed *exclusively* in patients who had *not* received bevacizumab in the first-line setting. This trial provides no data on whether use of bevacizumab with a second-line regimen after progression on a first-line bevacizumab-containing regimen is efficacious.

Although it was performed in second-line patients, the ECOG-3200 trial was the first trial to provide safety data for the combination of bevacizumab plus FOLFOX. As a result of this, even before front-line data were available, bevacizumab plus FOLFOX had become widely accepted as a front-line option in the United States for metastatic CRC. More recently, the NO16966 trial directly addressed the question of front-line bevacizumab plus oxaliplatin-based therapy (Table 49.16B).[375] In this trial, 1,400 patients with previously untreated CRC were randomly assigned to

TABLE 49.16B

Efficacy Outcomes, First-Line Treatment of Metastatic Colorectal Cancer: Capeox/Folfox Plus Placebo Versus Capeox/Folfox Plus Bevacizumab

Regimen	No. of Patients	Response Rate	Progression-Free Survival	Overall Survival
CapeOx/FOLFOX + placebo	701	49%	8.0 mo	19.9 mo
CapeOx/FOLFOX + bevacizumab	699	47% $p = 0.31$	9.4 mo $p = 0.0023$	21.3 mo $p = 0.078$

CapeOx, capecitabine, oxaliplatin; FOLFOX, fluorouracil, leucovorin, oxaliplatin.
From Saltz LB, Clarke S, Diaz-Rubio E, et al. Bevacizumab in combination with oxaliplatin-based chemotherapy as first-line therapy in metastatic colorectal cancer: a randomized phase III study. *J Clin Oncol* 2008;26:2013–2019.

either FOLFOX-4 or Cape/Ox and then to either placebo or bevacizumab, in a two-by-two randomization. Although the study did show a statistically significant progression-free survival advantage for the addition of bevacizumab (9.4 months versus 8.0 months for chemotherapy with bevacizumab versus chemotherapy with placebo, respectively; HR = 0.83; p = 0.003), this difference was more modest than the 4.4-month progression-free survival difference seen in the initial bevacizumab with IFL front-line trial. Overall survival improvement with bevacizumab approached, but did not reach, statistical significance (21.3 months versus 19.9 months; HR = 0.89; p = 0.077) Also, in the NO16966 trial, the addition of bevacizumab to front-line oxaliplatin-based chemotherapy did not confer any response benefit. It is noteworthy that the majority of patients on this trial discontinued treatment, presumably due to nonbevacizumab-related toxicity issues, before progression. This may have diminished the impact of bevacizumab on survival and progression-free survival but would not have impacted the response rate.

Toxicity

In terms of toxicity, grade 3 hypertension was higher in the bevacizumab/IFL arm than in the placebo/IFL arm (11% versus 2%) in the IFL/bevacizumab study.[371] Hypertension is now widely recognized as a common side effect of bevacizumab, and monitoring for and treatment of hypertension with antihypertensive medications is a routine part of bevacizumab management. Incidences of overall thromboembolic events and proteinuria were not statistically different between the two arms. However, two rare but extremely serious toxicities were encountered with increased frequency in the bevacizumab-containing arm: GI perforations and arterial thrombotic events.

The GI perforations were a group of events that included a perforated gastric ulcer, small bowel perforations, and free air under the diaphragm without identified sources. Although these were somewhat heterogeneous in nature, it was noted that six such events occurred on the bevacizumab-containing arm (one fatal) compared with none on the chemotherapy-alone arm. No clear risk factors for these perforations could be identified from this trial. Interestingly, GI perforations were not frequent occurrences in large cooperative group trials in patients with lung cancer or breast cancer; however, an unusually high GI perforation rate has recently halted accrual on a trial of bevacizumab in patients with ovarian cancer. These ovarian observations illustrate an important aspect about GI perforations in association with bevacizumab: there is not an association between the presence of an intact primary tumor in the colon and a GI perforation. Concerns have been expressed by some clinicians about the possibility of needing to remove an asymptomatic primary colorectal tumor in a patient with synchronous stage IV disease before using bevacizumab out of an unsubstantiated fear that the primary will put the patient at risk for perforation. At present, there are no data to support this assumption, and surgery for an asymptomatic primary tumor in a stage IV patient is not routinely indicated, regardless of whether there are plans to use a bevacizumab-containing chemotherapy regimen.[319]

The other rare but very serious identified increased risk with bevacizumab-containing treatment was that of arterial thrombotic events. Initially, no clear indication of this risk was detected in the pivotal phase 3 trial. However, in a combined analysis of several trials, an important observation was made. Here again, multiple events were combined into one metric. Thus, cerebral vascular accidents, myocardial infarctions, transient ischemic attacks, and angina were combined to create the metric of arterial thrombotic events. The observed incidence of these events was 2.5% in the nonbevacizumab-containing control arms versus 5.0% in the bevacizumab-containing experimental arms. It was noted that patients who had histories of cardiovascular or atherosclerotic disease appeared to be at greater risk for increased bevacizumab-related arterial thrombotic complications. In addition, a further

analysis of these events suggested that the risk was essentially linear over time, indicating that the risk of a new arterial thrombotic event was the same in earlier versus later months of exposure.[376]

Another complication of bevacizumab that has been rarely described in the literature is fistula formation. Ganapathi et al.[377] reports a 4.1% incidence of this problem in a review of 222 patients with metastatic CRC. Two-thirds were perineal or anal with the remainder colovesicular, occuring an average of 3.9 months after initiation of treatment. Cessation of bevacizumab led to fistula healing in nearly all cases; however, three patients required fecal diversion. The authors suggest that this complication has been underreported thus far and stress the importance of early recognition.[377]

Bevacizumab Beyond Progression

Prior studies had demonstrated the activity of bevacizumab when added to first-line chemotherapy, and the ECOG 3200 trial had shown that bevacizumab added to second-line chemotherapy in bevacizumab-naïve patients. Until recently, however, data were lacking regarding the question of continuation of bevacizumab with second-line therapy after progression of disease through a first-line, bevacizumab-containing regimen. This question has now been addressed by the TML trial.[378] In this trial, 820 patients who had progressed through a first-line, bevacizumab-containing regimen were assigned to a noncross-resistant chemotherapy regimen (irinotecan plus fluoropirymidine if previously treated with oxliplatin or oxaliplatin-fluoropyrimidine if previously treated with irinotecan) and then randomized to receive bevacizumab with this second-line chemotherapy or not. The arm receiving bevacizumab showed a modest but statistically significant survival benefit of 1.4 months (overall survival of 11.2 months versus 9.8 months; HR = 0.81; 95% CI = 0.69 to 0.94; p = 0.0062). Grade 3 to 5 bleeding or hemorrhage (8 [2%] versus 1 [1%]), GI perforation (7 [2%] versus 3 [1%]), and venous thromboembolisms (19 [5%] versus 12 [3%]) were more common in the bevacizumab plus chemotherapy group than in the chemotherapy-alone group.

Aflibercept

Aflibercept is a fusion molecule containing the binding domains of VEGF receptors 1 and 2 bound to the human immunoglobulin (Ig) G Fc fragment, forming a VEGF trap molecule. Aflibercept binds all human VEGF A isoforms, VEGF B, and placental growth factor with greater affinity than the native receptors for these ligands. Aflibercept has been evaluated in the large scale phase 3 VELOUR trial, in which 1,226 patients who had progressed on a first-line oxaliplatin-containing regimen were randomized to receive second-line FOLFIRI plus aflibercept 4 mg/kg versus FOLFIRI plus placebo. All treatments were given every 2 weeks. Thirty percent of patients had received prior bevacizumab with their first-line treatment regimen, while the remainder were naïve to anti-VEGF therapy. The group receiving aflibercept achieved a modest, but statistically significant overall survival benefit of 1.4 months (13.50 months versus 12.06 months; HR = 0.817; 95% CI = 0.713 to 0.937; p = 0.0032).[379] PFS was also statistically significantly improved from 4.67 months to 6.9 months with the addition of aflibercept (p <0.0001). Reponse rate was improved from 11.1% to 19.8%.

The findings of the VELOUR and TML trials show striking similarities to one another. Each utilized an anti-VEGF strategy in second-line treatment in conjunction with active chemotherapy, and each shows a 1.4-month survival benefit. Given these findings, use of either with second-line FOLFIRI (if second-line FOLFIRI is deemed appropriate) would seem reasonable. Aflibercept has not demonstrated benefit in conjunction with oxaliplatin-based regimens at the time of this writing, and so use of aflibercept with oxaliplatin-based chemotherapy is not recommended. Furthermore, a change from FOLFIRI-aflibercept to

FOLFIRI-bevacizumab (or vice versa) is not supported by current data, nor is use of either aflibercept or bevacizumab as a single agent. As such, aflibercept presents an option for second-line therapy in conjunction with FOLFIRI, but does not create a new line of therapy in the continuum of treatment.

Regorafenib

Regorafenib is a small molecule multitargeted tyrosine kinase inhibitor. It is closely related to its parent compound, sorafenib, and differs only by the addition of a fluorine atom. After phase 1 trials identified preliminary evidence of activity in patients with refractory CRC, a large phase 3 trial of regorafenib versus placebo was undertaken.[380] A total of 760 patients, all with ECOG grade 0 or 1 performance status, who had progressed through all standard therapies, were randomized 2:1 to received regorafenib 160 mg orally daily versus placebo. The regorafenib group achieved a modest but statistically significant overall survival benefit of 1.4 months (6.4 months versus 5.0 months; HR = 0.77; 95% CI = 0.64 to 0.94; p = 0.0052). Response was essentially nonevident, with a response rate of 1% in the regorafenib arm. Grade 3 hand-foot syndrome (17%) and grade 3 fatigue (10%) were the most common toxicities encountered on the regorafenib arm. Regorafenib monotherapy can be considered as a standard care option for good performance status patients who have progressed through standard therapies. Studies assessing the use of regorafenib in earlier lines of therapy and in combination with cytotoxic agents are in progress at the time of this writing.

Cetuximab and Panitumumab

The EGFR, also called HER-1, is a transmembrane glycoprotein receptor. When the external binding domain of the EGFR binds specific ligands, such as epidermal growth factor or TGF-α, receptor dimerization occurs (either homodimerization with another EGFR or heterodimerization with another member of the EGFR family). This in turn stimulates phosphorylation of the tyrosine kinases on the intracellular domain of the receptor, which initiates a signaling cascade, which ultimately regulates cell proliferation, migration, adhesion, differentiation, and survival.[381–383] Cetuximab (c-mab), is a chimeric IgG$_1$ monoclonal antibody that recognizes and binds to the extracellular domain of the EGFR. Panitumumab (p-mab) is a fully human IgG$_2$ monoclonal antibody that also targets the EGFR. Binding of either c-mab or p-mab to this receptor does not cause receptor activation, but rather results in a steric interference with the ligand binding site.[384]

Preclinical models of cetuximab, or its murine precursor, demonstrated more substantial activity when given in combination with cytotoxic chemotherapy. Based on these observations, and on a single anecdotal report of a major response to cetuximab plus irinotecan in a young woman with irinotecan-refractory CRC, a multicenter phase 2 trial was initiated. This trial, reported in abstract form only, was conducted in patients who were determined by their treating investigator to have progressed on irinotecan.[385] Patients were treated with cetuximab at a dose of 400 mg/m^2 loading dose week 1 over 2 hours, followed by weekly 250 mg/m^2 over 1 hour. Irinotecan was given on the same dose and schedule as had previously failed. Irinotecan dose reductions made previously, prior to study entry, were maintained upon initiation of the study treatment.

One hundred twenty patients with irinotecan-refractory CRC were identified and enrolled. In addition, in a parallel portion of the trial, 28 patients with clinically and radiographically stable disease after receiving a minimum of 3 months of irinotecan therapy were also enrolled and treated by the addition of cetuximab to their ongoing irinotecan therapy. The response outcome of this "stable disease cohort" was not reported; only those patients who were felt to be irinotecan refractory were included in the initial report. As reported by an independent response assessment committee, 22.5% of irinotecan-refractory patients achieved a major objective response. The irinotecan-related toxicity was relatively mild in this population, at least in part because many patients had already had irinotecan dose modifications made prior to starting on this trial. Of the side effects specifically attributable to cetuximab, 3% of patients developed an allergic, anaphylactoid reaction requiring discontinuation of cetuximab therapy, and 75% of patients experienced a skin rash (12% grade 3), a rash now recognized to be characteristic of all EGFR inhibitors. This rash superficially resembles acne, leading to its initial description as an acneiform rash. However, microscopically this is not acne, and topical acne medications are ineffective in its management. An interesting observation from this trial, which has since been corroborated in multiple trials, is that the presence and severity of the rash appeared to be associated with response in this study.

The results seen in the phase 2 cetuximab plus irinotecan combination trial raised the question, both from a scientific and from a regulatory perspective, of the activity of single-agent cetuximab in irinotecan-refractory CRC. A small phase 2 trial was therefore quickly designed and accrued. In this trial, 5 of 57 patients (9%) achieved a partial response confirmed by an independent radiologic review.[386]

Based on the preliminary results of the initial phase 2 cetuximab plus irinotecan study, described previously, a subsequent larger trial, ultimately reported by Cunningham et al.,[245] was designed to provide confirmatory evidence of the activity of cetuximab in CRC (Table 49.17). This large, randomized phase 2 trial in patients with irinotecan-refractory CRC, which has become known as the BOND trial, compared cetuximab plus irinotecan to cetuximab monotherapy in a two-to-one schema. A total of 329 patients were randomized in a two-to-one schema. The response rates of 22.9% for cetuximab plus irinotecan and 10.8% for cetuximab alone were virtually identical to the response rates that had been reported previously in the two US phase 2 trials, confirming the activity of this agent in CRC. Time to tumor progression in the Cunningham et al.[245] study was

TABLE 49.17

Efficacy Outcomes: Cetuximab Plus Irinotecan Versus Cetuximab Alone in Irinotecan-Refractory Colorectal Cancer

	No. of Patients	Response Rate (95% CI)	Disease Control (95% CI)	Median TTP (mo)	Median OS (mo) (95% CI)
Cetuximab	111	11% (6%–18%)	32% (24%–42%)	1.5	6.9 (5.6–9.1)
Cetuximab + irinotecan	218	23% (18%–29)[a]	56% (49%–62%)[b]	4.1[c]	8.6 (7.6–9.6)

CI, confidence interval; TTP, time to progression; OS, overall survival.
[a] p = 0.0074.
[b] p = 0.0001.
[c] p < 0.0001.
From Cunningham D, Humblet Y, Siena S, et al. Cetuximab monotherapy and cetuximab plus irinotecan in irinotecan-refractory metastatic colorectal cancer. *N Engl J Med* 2004;351:337–345.

4.1 months for the combination versus 1.5 months for single-agent cetuximab. Survival in the two arms was not significantly different; however, the study was neither designed nor powered to address the issue of a survival advantage for cetuximab, and cetuximab was given to all patients on both arms of the study.

A National Cancer Institute Canada phase 3 trial compared cetuximab plus best supportive care to best supportive care alone in 572 patients who had exhausted standard treatment options.[387] The median overall survival was improved by 1.5 months (from 4.6 months to 6.1 months) in the cetuximab group compared to supportive care alone. Partial responses occurred in 23 patients (8.0%) in the cetuximab group versus none in the supportive care group (p <0.001).

Similar results were reported with panitumumab. As seen with single-agent cetuximab, phase 2 evaluations of panitumumab in patients with CRC indicate approximately a 10% response rate, with over 90% of patients experiencing some degree of acneiform-like rash.[388,389] The fully human nature of this antibody appears to reduce the likelihood of anaphylactoid infusion reactions, with only 1 of the 148 patients treated after experiencing a dose-limiting allergic reaction. A randomized trial of panitumumab versus best supportive care in the salvage setting demonstrated a modest (8 weeks versus 7.3 weeks) but highly statistically significant improvement in median progression-free survival for single-agent panitumumab over best supportive care (HR = 0.54; p <0.000000001). Response rate to p-mab was 10%. There was no difference in overall survival; however, there was extensive postprogression crossover, which obscures this end point.[390]

KRAS and Other Determinants of Anti–Epidermal Growth Factor Receptor Resistance

Perhaps the most important development in the use of anti-EGFR agents over the past several years has been the recognition that these agents only have the potential to be beneficial to patients whose tumors have nonmutated, or wild-type, KRAS gene. KRAS is a signal transduction protein that is a critical intermediate in transmission of growth and survival signals from the EGFR to the nucleus. Mutations in exon 2 of the gene that encodes for the KRAS protein lead to constitutive activation of this signaling pathway, which renders blocking of the EGFR-binding site on the surface useless. Several small retrospective series identified KRAS mutations as being incompatible with responses to cetuximab.[391,392] Subsequently, Amado et al.[393] demonstrated that the activity of panitumumab in the registration study referenced previously was limited to those patients with wild-type KRAS. In this trial, 92% of patients had tissue available for KRAS genotyping, and 43% of tumors were found to harbor a mutation in codons 12 or 13 in exon 2 of KRAS. The objective response rate to single-agent panitumumab was 17% in KRAS wild-type tumors and 0% in those tumors that had a KRAS

mutation. The progression-free survival in the patients with KRAS wild-type tumor who received panitumumab was 12.3 weeks versus 7.3 weeks for best supportive care. In patients with KRAS-mutated tumors, there was no difference in progression-free survival with panitumumab versus best supportive care. Again, overall survival in this trial could not be interpreted due to extensive postprogression crossover.

Similarly, analysis of the National Cancer Institute Canada study, discussed previously, demonstrated that activity of cetuximab as a single agent in chemotherapy-refractory disease was limited to the KRAS wild-type patients only (Table 49.18).[394] Approximately 70% of patients in this trial had tissue available for KRAS genotyping, and 42% were found to have mutated KRAS. Those with mutated KRAS showed no evidence of clinical benefit from cetuximab, while patients whose tumors had wild-type K-ras showed a 4.7-month improvement in median overall survival with cetuximab versus best supportive care (9.5 months versus 4.8 months; HR for death = 0.55; 95% CI = 0.41 to 0.74; p <0.001). In the control group who received best supportive care, KRAS mutation status had no impact on median overall survival (p = 0.97). Although some data have suggested that tumors with KRAS exon 2, codon 13 mutatuions might still garner some benefit from first-line treatment with cetuximab or panitumumab,[395] subsequent data have refuted this, and any KRAS exon 2 mutation remains a firm contraindication to treatment with an EGFR inhibitor. (More recently, a retrospective analysis suggested that in addition to exon 2 KRAS mutations, tumors with mutated BRAF, NRAS, or PIK3CA were significantly associated with a low response rate to cetuximab or panitumumab.[396]) The question of the impact of other KRAS mutations outside of exon 2 has been further addressed, as has the impact of NRAS mutations. Data strongly suggest that the presence of any KRAS or NRAS mutation confers resistance to cetuximab and panitumumab, and that these agents should not be used in patients whose tumors harbor any of these mutations.[150] The role of BRAF genotyping remains less definitive. While an unpreplanned retrospective subset analysis of a combination of two first-line trials suggests some possible contribution of cetuximab in patients with BRAF-mutated tumors, most published datasets of patients treated in the nonfirst-line setting show essentially no activity for cetuximab or panaitumumab in patients with BRAF-mutated tumors.

Genotyping for KRAS mutation status should now be regarded as standard practice in all patients with stage IV disease, and cetuximab and panitumumab should only be considered in patients with nonmutated KRAS.[397] Importantly, using a matched set of resected metastases and primary tumors from 84 patients, Vakiani et al.[398] demonstrated near-complete concordance between primary and metastasis for RAS, BRAF, and PIK3CA. Therefore, genotyping of the primary tumor is sufficient and patients do not need to be subjected to a biopsy of a metastatic site for the purposes of tissue genotyping.

It is prudent to obtain KRAS genotyping at the time that stage IV disease is diagnosed, not necessarily because the information is needed for first-line therapy, as only a minority of patients will be

TABLE 49.18

Cetuximab Versus Best Supportive Care in Metastatic Chemotherapy-Refractory Colorectal Cancer

	Overall Survival		Progression-Free Survival		Response Rate	
	KRAS Wt	KRAS Mut	KRAS Wt	KRAS Mut	KRAS Wt	KRAS Mut
Cetux	9.5 mo	4.5 mo	3.7 mo	1.8 mo	12.8%	1.2%
BSC	4.8 mo	4.6 mo	1.9 mo	1.8 mo	0%	0%
P value	0.001	0.89	0.001	0.96	NR	NR

Wt, wild type; Mut, mutant; Cetux, cetuximab; BSC, best supportive care; NR, not reported.
From Karapetis CS, Khambata-Ford S, Jonker DJ, et al. K-ras mutations and benefit from cetuximab in advanced colorectal cancer. *N Engl J Med* 2008;359:1757–1765.

appropriate for first-line anti-EGFR therapy, but because whether a patient can consider the use of cetuximab or panitumumab in the course of multiple lines of therapy is easier to both determine and to deal with early on when there are multiple options, rather than waiting until all other options are exhausted. At present, there is no role for determining KRAS status in stage I, II, or III disease, as there is no basis for use of EGFR agents in other than stage IV.

Preliminary data suggests that KRAS status might play a role in oxaliplatin sensitivity as well. In vitro analysis, published by Lin et al.[399] demonstrated that this mutation caused downregulation of ERCC1 (excision repair cross-complementation group 1), which led to enhanced oxaliplatin sensitivity. Overexpression of ERCC1 has been shown previously to be associated with resistance to platinum-based therapy in a number of cancers. Improved understanding of this pathway may prove critical toward defining new targets for KRAS-mutant CRC treatment.[399]

Cetuximab or Panitumumab in First-Line Therapy

A 1,200-patient study of FOLFIRI with or without cetuximab, known at the CRYSTAL trial, has been reported.[400] The primary end point of the trial, progression-free survival, was statistically significantly improved with the addition of cetuximab, albeit by only 0.9 month, or 27 days. When the study was analyzed in terms of KRAS genotype, those patients with mutated KRAS showed no benefit, while those with wild-type KRAS showed a progression-free survival improvement of 1.2 months, or 37 days, but also a median overall survival improvement from 20.0 months to 23.5 months (HR = 0.796; p = 0.0093).[401] Response rates were also statistically significantly higher (57.3% versus 39.7%) in the cetuximab arm for the KRAS wild-type tumors. Skin rash and diarrhea were increased in the cetuximab arm. As has been noted in virtually all trials of anti-EGFR agents, there is a strong correlation between severity of skin rash and clinical benefit, with progression-free survival advantage being limited to those patients with grade 2 or 3 skin rash. BRAF was confirmed as a poor prognostic factor but was not predictive of response to cetuximab in this trial. The numbers of BRAF-mutated tumors limit the power to detect a predictive role of BRAF in this trial, however.

FOLFOX with or without cetuximab had been initially investigated in a randomized phase 2 trial in which the primary end point was response rate.[402] A total of 337 patients were treated. The overall response rate was improved by the addition of cetuximab from 36% to 46%, a result that did not achieve statistical significance (p = 0.64). For the KRAS wild-type patients, however, the result was more robust, with an improvement from 37% to 61% (p = 0.011). Progression-free survival was very modestly, albeit statistically significantly improved in the KRAS wild-type patients by a median of 15 days; however, progression-free survival was statistically significantly worse in the cetuximab arm in those patients whose tumors had mutated KRAS.

However, several larger phase 3 trials have cast considerable doubt on the role of cetuximab in conjunction with oxaliplatin-based therapy. In the Medical Research Council COIN trial, 1,603 patients with previously untreated metastatic CRC were treated with oxaliplatin plus a fluoropyrimidine (either the FOLFOX or Cape/Ox regimen) and randomized to receive cetuximab in addition or not. In the patients with KRAS wild-type tumors (367 with cetuximab plus oxaliplatin-containing chemotherapy and 362 with oxaliplatin-containing chemotherapy alone), there was no improvement in overall survival (17.9 months versus 17 months; HR = 1.04; p = 0.67) or in progression-free survival (8.6 months versus 8.6 months in the two arms). Overall response rate increased from 57% to 64% with the addition of cetuximab (p = 0.049). The data from this trial do not support use of cetuximab with front-line oxaliplatin-based chemotherapy. Outcomes were worse with the addition of cetuximab to capecitabine plus oxaliplatin, and the use of that combination is specifically not recommended.[403] In addition, the Nordic VII trial investigated the addition of cetuximab to the Nordic FLOX regimen of oxaliplatin, bolus 5-FU and leucovorin in a 571-patient phase 3 trial.[404]

Patients were randomized to one of three arms: Nordic FLOX given continuously, cetuximab plus Nordic FLOX given continuously, or cetuximab plus Nordic FLOX given intermittently. There were no statistically significant differences in the median progression-free survival between the three arms (7.9 months, 8.3 months, and 7.3 months, respectively). Overall survival also showed no difference between the three arms (20.4 months, 19.7 months, and 20.3 months, respectively). Even in patients with KRAS wild-type tumors, cetuximab did not provide demonstrable benefit.

Taken in the aggregate, the data do not lend substantial support to the use of cetuximab with oxaliplatin-based chemotherapy. Curiously, however, the results with panitumumab are somewhat different. In a phase 3 trial of FOLFOX with or without panitumumab (6 mg/kg every 14 days), 1,183 patients were randomized, of whom 60% had wild-type KRAS.[405] Progression-free survival was modestly but statistically significantly improved with panitumumab in the KRAS wild-type patients (9.6 months versus 8 months; p = 0.02), and response rate was increased from 48% to 55%. However, as was seen with cetuximab, in the patients with KRAS-mutated tumors, the addition of panitumumab resulted in a statistically significant worsening of median progression-free survival from 8.8 months in the control arm to 7.3 months in the panitumumab-containing arm. In an updated analysis focusing on KRAS wild-type patients only, as statistically significant survival benefit was seen with the addition of panitumumab in this cohort.[150] The addition of panitumumab resulted in increased skin rash, diarrhea, and hypomagnesemia.

Also reported in abstract form is a phase 3 trial of second-line FOLFIRI with or without panitumumab.[406] Despite this being a second-line study, patients had an excellent performance status (ECOG 0 or 1 in 94% of patients). KRAS mutations were present in 45% of patients. For the patients with KRAS wild-type tumors, the progression-free survival was statistically significantly improved in the panitumumab-containing arm (5.9 months versus 3.9 months; p = 0.004), and response rate was improved as well (35% versus 10%). Overall survival differences in favor of the panitumumab arm (14.5 months versus 12.5 months) did not reach statistical significance (p = 0.1). There were no differences in efficacy outcomes with the addition of panitumumab in the patients with KRAS-mutated tumors. Again, skin rash, diarrhea, and hypomagnesemia were increased in the panitumumab arm.

More recently the long-awaited initial results of the NCI cooperative group 80405 study have been reported in abstract form. In this trial, patients with previously untreated metastatic colorectal cancer with wild-type KRAS were enrolled. Patients were assigned to receive either FOLFOX or FOLFIRI per physician preference, and then randomized to receive either cetuximab or bevacizumab. There was no difference in overall survival, the primary study endpoint, between the cetuximab and bevacizumab arms (29.0 months vs 29.9 months, p = 0.34).[407]

Toxicities of Anti–Epidermal Growth Factor Receptor Monoclonal Antibodies

The primary toxicity of cetuximab and panitumumab is an acne-like rash, which is seen to some degree in from 75% to 100% of patients treated. This rash is not acne, and it is accompanied by skin dryness and paronychial cracking. Other than moisturizers, which are recommended, no topical agents have been shown to be of benefit in the treatment of this rash. Drying agents and retinoids, such as are used in the treatment of acne, are contraindicated. Anecdotal reports of benefit for topical steroids or antibiotics do not have supportive randomized data, and as the natural history of the rash is to wax and wane, interpretation of these anecdotal reports is problematic. There are data suggesting that prophylactic use of oral antibiotics may somewhat mitigate the severity of the rash.[408] Importantly, it has been well established that there is a clear correlation between severity of skin rash and favorable outcome with

EGFR agents.[409] The mechanism of this correlation has not yet been determined; however, it is clear that benefit from these agents is virtually confined to those patients who experience a grade 2 or 3 skin rash. A severe rash does not guarantee a response or clinical benefit; however, absence of a rash after the first month of therapy is virtually incompatible with clinical benefit from these agents. This is an important point to consider, especially in consideration of front-line use; only those patients with a very substantial rash stand a chance of benefit.

Hypersensitivity reactions, which are anaphylactoid in nature and are completely separate and distinct from the skin rash toxicity discussed previously, occur in approximately 3% of patients with cetuximab and <1% of patients with panitumumab. Almost all of these reactions are first-dose events. Dramatic regional differences in the frequency of these reactions have been noted, with serious hypersensitivity reactions to cetuximab noted in up to 20% of patients in North Carolina and Tennessee, while the serious hypersensitivity reaction rate in the northeastern United States is <1%.[410] Subsequently, it has been demonstrated that there is a high prevalence of cetuximab-specific IgE in Tennessee, suggesting cross-reactivity with an environmental allergen.[411] Panitumumab does not appear to exhibit this marked regional variation in incidence of hypersensitivity reaction, and would be the clearly preferred agent over cetuximab in these areas of high incidence of cetuximab hypersensitivity.

It should be noted that the incidence of skin rash appears to be quite similar between cetuximab and panitumumab, as does the degree of clinical activity. Thus, outside of the areas that see high frequency of cetuximab hypersensitivity reactions, there appears to be little reason to favor one agent over the other. Case reports and anecdotal evidence suggest that patients who experience hypersensitivity to cetuximab do typically tolerate panitumumab. There is no basis, however, for using one of these agents after clinical failure on the other.

Another more recently recognized toxicity of anti-EGFR therapy is hypomagnesemia.[412] This result is due to hypermagnesemia, presumably promoted by EGFR antagonism in the loop of Henle. Regular monitoring of serum magnesium levels, and intravenous magnesium supplementation, when indicated, should be practiced routinely with anti-EGFR therapies. Oral magnesium is unlikely to provide adequate supplementation, as diarrhea from this is often dose-limiting.

Cetuximab and Panitumumab in Epidermal Growth Factor Receptor–Negative Patients

From the outset of clinical development, the assumption was made that quantitative EGFR expression would be predictive of the activity, or lack thereof, of an anti-EGFR antibody, and that an absence of demonstrable EGFR expression would therefore preclude clinical activity of cetuximab or panitumumab. For this reason, all early trials with these agents required that the patient's tumor shows EGFR positivity by IHC as a criterion for study eligibility. This assumption, that EGFR expression would be predictive, has never been supported by clinical or preclinical data and has been refuted by all clinical data that have addressed the issue. All of the reported cetuximab trials to date, the earlier ones of which excluded EGFR-negative patients altogether, have demonstrated absolutely no correlation between the intensity of the EGFR expression and clinical response.[245,385] Additionally, the results of a small cohort of nine patients who were EGFR-negative and treated with cetuximab were reported in abstract form.[413] Two major objective responses were reported by the investigators, one of which was confirmed as a major response by third-party review and one of which was not.

On the basis of the lack of correlation between EGFR staining intensity and response, as well as the small data set outlined previously, a decision was made at Memorial Sloan Kettering Cancer Center in New York that patients with EGFR-negative CRC would not be excluded from standard off-protocol treatment with cetuximab simply on the basis of EGFR status. Subsequently, a retrospective review was conducted using the computerized pharmacy records to identify all patients who had received non-research cetuximab-based therapy at Memorial Sloan Kettering Cancer Center in the first 3 months of cetuximab's commercial availability. This review identified 16 patients with irinotecan-refractory, EGFR-negative CRC who had been treated. Fourteen of these patients had received cetuximab in combination with irinotecan and two had received cetuximab alone. Of the 16, four patients experienced major objective (response rate = 25%; 95% CI = 4% to 46%), demonstrating that the hypothesis that a negative EGFR stain would preclude the possibility of response to cetuximab is false.[414] A similar lack of correlation of EGFR staining and activity with panitumumab has also more recently been reported.[415]

Because current EGFR IHC techniques have no predictive value, these techniques have no role in current management of CRC. The exclusion of a patient from cetuximab-based or panitumumab-based therapy solely on the basis of EGFR IHC is not appropriate. Likewise, no patient, with CRC or otherwise, should be given an anti-EGFR treatment solely on the basis of a high EGFR IHC expression.

Bevacizumab Plus Anti–Epidermal Growth Factor Receptor Agents

Given the reported activity of both bevacizumab and cetuximab, investigators logically became interested in the idea of concurrent use of these agents. Both some limited preclinical data, as well as mechanistic understandings of potential interaction between anti-EGFR and anti-VEGF pathways, supported the concept. As will be discussed subsequently, this concept serves as yet another example of perfectly logical, well-thought out assumptions supported by preliminary clinical evidence that turned out to be incorrect when subjected to the appropriately rigorous test of an adequately powered clinical trial.

The first study to attempt to administer bevacizumab and cetuximab concurrently was a small randomized phase 2 study of bevacizumab added to cetuximab alone or to cetuximab plus irinotecan in patients with irinotecan-refractory CRC.[416] This was a feasibility trial to assess the safety of concurrent administration of these agents and to look for preliminary evidence of efficacy. The study concluded that coadministration of these two monoclonal antibodies together was feasible, and that the preliminary data were encouraging. It should be noted, however, that this was a small feasibility trial with 41 and 40 patients, respectively, reported in each arm. Furthermore, this study was conducted in patients who were naive to both cetuximab and bevacizumab. As most patients now receive bevacizumab with their first-line regimen, the results in the bevacizumab-naive population might not necessarily have a bearing on current practice today. A small follow-up trial in patients with prior progression on a front-line bevacizumab-containing regimen showed far less activity, with 3 of 33 patients (9%) achieving a partial response and a median time to tumor progression of 3.9 months.[417] These small trials were designed to serve as the safety pilots for large-scale front-line studies that combined bevacizumab plus cetuximab with front-line chemotherapy. Two such studies have now been reported, with alarming results, which highlights the dangers of jumping to conclusions prior to the availability of mature, definitive data.

The CAIRO-2 study randomized 755 patients with previously untreated metastatic CRC to Cape/Ox-bevacizumab with or without concurrent cetuximab (Table 49.19A).[418] Not only was there not a benefit to the addition of cetuximab, but the group receiving cetuximab actually had a worse median progression-free survival of 9.4 months, compared to 10.7 months in the Cape/Ox-bevacizumab–alone arm ($p = 0.01$). Response rates were identical

TABLE 49.19A

Capecitabine, Oxaliplatin, and Bevacizumab with or without Cetuximab in Metastatic Colorectal Cancer

Overall	Median Progression-Free Survival	Median Response	Objective Survival Rates
COB (n = 332)	20.3 mo	10.7 mo	50%
COB plus cetux (n = 317)	19.4 mo	9.4 mo	52.7%
P value	0.16	0.01	0.49

COB, capecitabine, oxaliplatin, bevacizumab; cetux, cetuximab.
From Tol J, Koopman M, Cats A, et al. Chemotherapy, bevacizumab, and cetuximab in metastatic colorectal cancer. *N Engl J Med* 2009;360:563–572.

(44%) in the two arms. Furthermore, quality-of-life scores were lower in the cetuximab-containing arm. Overall survival was not statistically significantly different between the two groups. Even for the wild-type KRAS patients, there was no benefit in progression-free survival with the addition of cetuximab. As might now be anticipated (Table 49.19B), within the cetuximab-containing arm, patients whose tumors had mutated KRAS had statistically significantly decreased progression-free survival compared to those with wild-type KRAS tumors (8.1 months versus 10.5 months; $p = 0.04$). However, for the patients with KRAS mutations, those who received cetuximab also had a worse outcome than those on the noncetuximab-containing control arm (progression-free survival 8.1 months versus 12.5 months, $p = 0.003$; overall survival 17.2 months versus 24.9 months, $p = 0.03$).

Another study that investigated the use of combined bevacizumab plus anti-EGFR monoclonal antibody was the Panitumumab in Advanced Colon Cancer Evaluation (PACCE) trial.[419] This trial used FOLFOX-bevacizumab (823 patients) or FOLFIRI-bevacizumab (230 patients) and randomized them with or without concurrent panitumumab. Again, the result of adding the anti-EGFR to chemotherapy plus bevacizumab was not only not beneficial, but was actually detrimental. The median progression-free survival for the overall study was 10.0 months versus 11.4 months for the panitumumab-containing versus chemotherapy-bevacizumab–alone arm. The median overall survival was decreased by 5.1 months, from 24.5 months in the control arm to 19.4 months in the panitumumab arm. Toxicity, including not only skin rash but also diarrhea, infections, and pulmonary embolisms, was more frequent in the panitumumab-containing arm, and worse outcomes were seen in the panitumumab-containing arm regardless of KRAS mutation status.

Clearly, the concurrent use of anti-EGFR monoclonal antibodies, bevacizumab, and cytotoxic chemotherapy, despite supportive encouraging preliminary data, is not an acceptable treatment strategy. The reasons for this unanticipated negative interaction remain unknown at this time.

Oral Epidermal Growth Factor Receptor, Vascular Endothelial Growth Factor, and Cyclooxygenase-2 Inhibitors

The limited experiences with the oral EGFR tyrosine kinase inhibitors gefitinib (ZD1839) and erlotinib (OSI-774) in CRC have been essentially negative, and at present there is no role for these agents in this disease.[420,421] This is consistent with the findings that the activating mutation seen in lung cancer required for anti-EGFR tyrosine kinase activity does not appear to occur in CRC.

Oral VEGF tyrosine kinase inhibitors, with the exception of regorafenib noted previously, have been similarly disappointing. Sunitinib showed essentially no activity as a single agent in chemotherapy-refractory disease, and front-line trials of chemotherapy with or without sunitinib, as well as chemotherapy with or without sorafenib, have now been closed early by their respective data monitoring committees for futility.[422] Two large, randomized trials of FOLFOX with or without the investigational VEGF tyrosine kinase inhibitor PTK-787 have also been reported as negative trials.

Cyclooxygenase-2 Inhibitors. Cyclooxygenase-2 (COX-2) catalyzes the synthesis of prostaglandins in the inflammatory response process. COX-2 has been frequently shown to be upregulated in malignant and premalignant tissues. COX-2 expression has been correlated with increased invasiveness, resistance to apoptosis, and increased angiogenesis.[423] The science behind COX-2 inhibition appeared so compelling that many clinicians had chosen to add drugs such as celecoxib or rofecoxib (now withdrawn from the market for safety reasons) in the absence of efficacy data with the assumption that "it couldn't hurt." Evidence that use of either NSAIDs or selective COX-2 inhibitors has a beneficial role in the treatment of CRC is lacking. The large randomized BICC-C trial showed no benefit whatsoever for the use of celecoxib in terms of either safety or efficacy.[334] In the absence of any emerging data to the contrary, routine use of COX-2 inhibitors with chemotherapy is not recommended.

The role of aspirin as an adjuvant agent is also of particular interest, especially after a recent case-control study suggested that

TABLE 49.19B

Impact of KRAS Mutation Status on Addition of Cetuximab to Capecitabine, Oxaliplatin, and Bevacizumab

	Overall Survival COB + COB cetux	Progression-Free Survival COB + COB cetux
KRAS wild-type	22.4 mo 21.8 mo (p = 0.64)	10.6 mo 10.5 mo (p = 0.30)
KRAS mutated	24.9 mo 17.2 mo (p = 0.03)	12.5 mo 8.1 mo (p = 0.003)

COB, capecitabine, oxaliplatin-bevacizumab; cetux, cetuximab.
From Tol J, Koopman M, Cats A, et al. Chemotherapy, bevacizumab, and cetuximab in metastatic colorectal cancer. *N Engl J Med* 2009;360:563–572.

initiation of this medication after diagnosis reduced overall CRC specific mortality (HR = 0.53; 95% CI = 0.33 to 0.86).[424] The ASCOLT study is the first randomized, placebo-controlled trial designed to investigate this question in patients with stage III-IV and high-risk stage II disease. End points will include DFS and overall survival with anticipated follow-up of 5 years.[425]

In the meantime, a large observational study of 4,481 patients lends further support to the potential therapeutic benefits of aspirin in CRC. The authors report a 23% decrease in disease-specific mortality for patients who took aspirin for any length of time after diagnosis compared to nonaspirin users as well as a 30% lower disease-specific mortality for those who took aspirin for 9 months after diagnosis. A survival benefit was also found for prediagnosis users, although this was less pronounced at 12%.[426]

Other Novel Agents

The number of agents that are undergoing early evaluation in CRC is too large to allow a complete discussion of these in this chapter. Many are variations on the currently available agents and are unlikely to substantially move the field if successful in gaining approval. At present, no new agent with a unique mechanism of action has been identified as having meaningful activity in CRC. Furthermore, all of these at this point are of research interest only and do not have a role in standard treatment of CRC at this time.

MOLECULAR PREDICTIVE MARKERS

With the availability now of a number of active agents, the ability to prospectively select a particular drug or drug combination that would have an increased likelihood of efficacy or a decreased likelihood of toxicity would be clinically useful. Such means of rational selection do not yet exist.

One avenue of investigation has been the elucidation of markers of resistance to 5-FU based on knowledge of its metabolic pathways. Studies have indicated that high levels of either TS, DPD,[427] or thymidine phosphorylase, as measured in a tumor specimen by reverse transcription–polymerase chain reaction, predict for failure to respond to an infusional 5-FU regimen.[166,428,429] These observations are intriguing but are insufficient to exclude the use of 5-FU in a particular patient, and they need to be validated in large-scale prospective trials before being applied to routine practice. There is, at this time, no role for the use of these markers in standard practice. Others have investigated genomic analysis as an indicator of response or toxicity.[170,430] Although these approaches appear promising, they are not yet validated and should not be considered as part of standard care.

A recently reported mechanism of resistance thought to be independent of other mutations or MSI involves the tumor suppressor gene TFAP2E (transcription factor AP-2 epsilon) and its downstream target DKK4(dickkopf homolog 4 protein). In an analysis of 220 patients with CRC, Ebert et al.[431] found that hypermethylation of TFAP2E led to decreased protein expression and was significantly associated with nonresponse to 5-FU–based chemotherapy, whereas hypomethylation yielded a six-fold higher likelihood of response. Moreover, TFAP2E hypermethylation in vitro led to overexpression of DKK4, which was in turn associated with increased chemoresistance to 5-FU but not irinotecan and oxaliplatin. The authors suggest that future studies focus on specific targeting of DKK4 to overcome this pathway of chemoresistance.[431]

REFERENCES

1. Jemal A, Center MM, DeSantis C, et al. Global patterns of cancer incidence and mortality rates and trends. *Cancer Epidemiol Biomarkers Prev* 2010;19:1893–1907.
2. Jemal A, Siegel R, Xu J, et al. Cancer statistics, 2010. *CA Cancer J Clin* 2010;60:277–300.
3. Lieberman DA, Weiss DG, Bond JH, et al. Use of colonoscopy to screen asymptomatic adults for colorectal cancer. Veterans Affairs Cooperative Study Group 380. *N Engl J Med* 2000;343:162–168.
4. Davis DM, Marcet JE, Frattini JC, et al. Is it time to lower the recommended screening age for colorectal cancer? *J Am Coll Surg* 2011;213:352–361.
5. Lee PY, Fletcher WS, Sullivan ES, et al. Colorectal cancer in young patients: characteristics and outcome. *Am Surg* 1994;60:607–612.
6. Brown MO, Lanier AP, Becker TM. Colorectal cancer incidence and survival among Alaska Natives, 1969-1993. *Int J Epidemiol* 1998;27:388–396.
7. Parkin DM, Pisani P, Ferlay J. Global cancer statistics. *CA Cancer J Clin* 1999;49:33–64, 1.
8. Nelson RL, Persky V, Turyk M. Determination of factors responsible for the declining incidence of colorectal cancer. *Dis Colon Rectum* 1999;42:741–752.
9. Staszewski J, Haenszel W. Cancer mortality among the Polish-born in the United States. *J Natl Cancer Inst* 1965;35:291–297.
10. Whittemore AS, Wu-Williams AH, Lee M, et al. Diet, physical activity, and colorectal cancer among Chinese in North America and China. *J Natl Cancer Inst* 1990;82:915–926.
11. McMichael AJ, Giles GG. Cancer in migrants to Australia: extending the descriptive epidemiological data. *Cancer Res* 1988;48:751–756.
12. Kune S, Kune GA, Watson L. The Melbourne colorectal cancer study: incidence findings by age, sex, site, migrants and religion. *Int J Epidemiol* 1986;15:483–493.
13. Laken SJ, Petersen GM, Gruber SB, et al. Familial colorectal cancer in Ashkenazim due to a hypermutable tract in APC. *Nat Genet* 1997;17:79–83.
14. Rozen P, Shomrat R, Strul H, et al. Prevalence of the I1307K APC gene variant in Israeli Jews of differing ethnic origin and risk for colorectal cancer. *Gastroenterology* 1999;116:54–57.
15. Weber TK, Chin HM, Rodriguez-Bigas M, et al. Novel hMLH1 and hMSH2 germline mutations in African Americans with colorectal cancer. *JAMA* 1999;281:2316–2320.
16. Nelson RL, Persky V, Turyk M. Time trends in distal colorectal cancer subsite location related to age and how it affects choice of screening modality. *J Surg Oncol* 1998;69:235–238.
17. Nelson RL, Dollear T, Freels S, et al. The relation of age, race, and gender to the subsite location of colorectal carcinoma. *Cancer* 1997;80:193–197.
18. Yothers G, Sargent DJ, Wolmark N, et al. Outcomes among black patients with stage II and III colon cancer receiving chemotherapy: an analysis of ACCENT adjuvant trials. *J Natl Cancer Inst* 2011;103:1498–1506.
19. Landis SH, Murray T, Bolden S, et al. Cancer statistics, 1998. *CA Cancer J Clin* 1998;48:6–29.
20. Wilmink AB. Overview of the epidemiology of colorectal cancer. *Dis Colon Rectum* 1997;40:483–493.
21. Obrand DI, Gordon PH. Continued change in the distribution of colorectal carcinoma. *Br J Surg* 1998;85:246–248.
22. Kemppainen M, Raiha I, Sourander L. A marked increase in the incidence of colorectal cancer over two decades in southwest Finland. *J Clin Epidemiol* 1997;50:147–151.
23. Ji BT, Devesa SS, Chow WH, et al. Colorectal cancer incidence trends by subsite in urban Shanghai, 1972-1994. *Cancer Epidemiol Biomarkers Prev* 1998;7:661–666.
24. Thibodeau SN, French AJ, Cunningham JM, et al. Microsatellite instability in colorectal cancer: different mutator phenotypes and the principal involvement of hMLH1. *Cancer Res* 1998;58:1713–1718.
25. Fink D, Nebel S, Norris PS, et al. The effect of different chemotherapeutic agents on the enrichment of DNA mismatch repair-deficient tumour cells. *Br J Cancer* 1998;77:703–708.
26. Karnes WE Jr, Shattuck-Brandt R, Burgart LJ, et al. Reduced COX-2 protein in colorectal cancer with defective mismatch repair. *Cancer Res* 1998;58:5473–5477.
27. Fuchs CS, Giovannucci EL, Colditz GA, et al. A prospective study of family history and the risk of colorectal cancer. *N Engl J Med* 1994;331:1669–1674.
28. Pariente A, Milan C, Lafon J, et al. Colonoscopic screening in first-degree relatives of patients with 'sporadic' colorectal cancer: a case-control study. The Association Nationale des Gastroenterologues des Hopitaux and Registre Bourguignon des Cancers Digestifs (INSERM CRI 9505). *Gastroenterology* 1998;115:7–12.
29. Guillem JG, Forde KA, Treat MR, et al. Colonoscopic screening for neoplasms in asymptomatic first-degree relatives of colon cancer patients. A controlled, prospective study. *Dis Colon Rectum* 1992;35:523–529.
30. Winawer SJ, Zauber AG, Gerdes H, et al. Risk of colorectal cancer in the families of patients with adenomatous polyps. National Polyp Study Workgroup. *N Engl J Med* 1996;334:82–87.
31. Ponz de Leon M, Scapoli C, Zanghieri G, et al. Genetic transmission of colorectal cancer: exploratory data analysis from a population based registry. *J Med Genet* 1992;29:531–538.

32. Harris MJ, Coggan M, Langton L, et al. Polymorphism of the Pi class glutathione S-transferase in normal populations and cancer patients. *Pharmacogenetics* 1998;8:27–31.

33. Welfare M, Monesola Adeokun A, Bassendine MF, et al. Polymorphisms in GSTP1, GSTM1, and GSTT1 and susceptibility to colorectal cancer. *Cancer Epidemiol Biomarkers Prev* 1999;8:289–292.

34. Chen J, Giovannucci E, Hankinson SE, et al. A methylenetetrahydrofolate reductase polymorphism and the risk of colorectal cancer. *Cancer Res* 1996;56:4862–4864.

35. Butler LM, Millikan RC, Sinha R, et al. Modification by N-acetyltransferase 1 genotype on the association between dietary heterocyclic amines and colon cancer in a multiethnic study. *Mutat Res* 2008;638:162–174.

36. Hartz A, He T, Ross JJ. Risk factors for colon cancer in 150,912 postmenopausal women. *Cancer Causes Control* 2012;23:1599–1605.

37. Singh PN, Fraser GE. Dietary risk factors for colon cancer in a low-risk population. *Am J Epidemiol* 1998;148:761–774.

38. Slattery ML, Potter J, Caan B, et al. Energy balance and colon cancer—beyond physical activity. *Cancer Res* 1997;57:75–80.

39. Renehan AG, Flood A, Adams KF, et al. Body mass index at different adult ages, weight change, and colorectal cancer risk in the National Institutes of Health-AARP Cohort. *Am J Epidemiol* 2012;176:1130–1140.

40. Potter JD. Colorectal cancer: molecules and populations. *J Natl Cancer Inst* 1999;91:916–932.

41. Willett WC, Stampfer MJ, Colditz GA, et al. Relation of meat, fat, and fiber intake to the risk of colon cancer in a prospective study among women. *N Engl J Med* 1990;323:1664–1672.

42. Key TJ, Fraser GE, Thorogood M, et al. Mortality in vegetarians and nonvegetarians: detailed findings from a collaborative analysis of 5 prospective studies. *Am J Clin Nutr* 1999;70:516S–524S.

43. Probst-Hensch NM, Sinha R, Longnecker MP, et al. Meat preparation and colorectal adenomas in a large sigmoidoscopy-based case-control study in California (United States). *Cancer Causes Control* 1997;8:175–183.

44. Parr CL, Hjartaker A, Lund E, et al. Meat intake, cooking methods and risk of proximal colon, distal colon and rectal cancer: the Norwegian Women and Cancer (NOWAC) cohort study. *Int J Cancer* 2013;133:1153–1163.

45. Egeberg R, Olsen A, Christensen J, et al. Associations between red meat and risks for colon and rectal cancer depend on the type of red meat consumed. *J Nutr* 2013;143:464–472.

46. McCullough ML, Gapstur SM, Shah R, et al. Association between red and processed meat intake and mortality among colorectal cancer survivors. *J Clin Oncol* 2013;31:2773–2782.

47. Li G, Ma D, Zhang Y, et al. Coffee consumption and risk of colorectal cancer: a meta-analysis of observational studies. *Public Health Nutr* 2013; 16:346–357.

48. Sinha R, Cross AJ, Daniel CR, et al. Caffeinated and decaffeinated coffee and tea intakes and risk of colorectal cancer in a large prospective study. *Am J Clin Nutr* 2012;96:374–381.

49. Burkitt DP. Epidemiology of cancer of the colon and rectum. 1971. *Dis Colon Rectum* 1993;36:1071–1082.

50. Howe GR, Benito E, Castelleto R, et al. Dietary intake of fiber and decreased risk of cancers of the colon and rectum: evidence from the combined analysis of 13 case-control studies. *J Natl Cancer Inst* 1992;84:1887–1896.

51. Murphy N, Norat T, Ferrari P, et al. Dietary fibre intake and risks of cancers of the colon and rectum in the European prospective investigation into cancer and nutrition (EPIC). *PLoS One* 2012;7:e39361.

52. Fuchs CS, Giovannucci EL, Colditz GA, et al. Dietary fiber and the risk of colorectal cancer and adenoma in women. *N Engl J Med* 1999;340: 169–176.

53. Schatzkin A, Lanza E, Corle D, et al. Lack of effect of a low-fat, high-fiber diet on the recurrence of colorectal adenomas. Polyp Prevention Trial Study Group. *N Engl J Med* 2000;342:1149–1155.

54. Alberts DS, Martinez ME, Roe DJ, et al. Lack of effect of a high-fiber cereal supplement on the recurrence of colorectal adenomas. Phoenix Colon Cancer Prevention Physicians' Network. *N Engl J Med* 2000;342:1156–1162.

55. Wargovich MJ. New dietary anticarcinogens and prevention of gastrointestinal cancer. *Dis Colon Rectum* 1988;31:72–75.

56. Bamia C, Lajiou P, Buckland G, et al. Mediterranean diet and colorectal cancer risk: results from a European cohort. *Eur J Epidemiol* 2013;28:317–328.

57. Bostick RM, Fosdick L, Wood JR, et al. Calcium and colorectal epithelial cell proliferation in sporadic adenoma patients: a randomized, double-blinded, placebo-controlled clinical trial. *J Natl Cancer Inst* 1995;87:1307–1315.

58. Chen GC, Pang Z, Liu QF. Magnesium intake and risk of colorectal cancer: a meta-analysis of prospective studies. *Eur J Clin Nutr* 2012;66:1182–1186.

59. Ma Y, Zhang P, Wang F, et al. Association between vitamin D and risk of colorectal cancer: a systematic review of prospective studies. *J Clin Oncol* 2011;29:3775–3782.

60. Institute of Medicine. *Dietary Reference Intakes for Calcium and Vitamin D.* Washington, DC: National Academies Press; 2011.

61. Meyerhardt JA, Giovannucci EL, Holmes MD, et al. Physical activity and survival after colorectal cancer diagnosis. *J Clin Oncol* 2006;24:3527–3534.

62. Campbell PT, Patel AV, Newton CC, et al. Associations of recreational physical activity and leisure time spent sitting with colorectal cancer survival. *J Clin Oncol* 2013;31:876–885.

63. Seitz HK, Simanowski UA, Garzon FT, et al. Possible role of acetaldehyde in ethanol-related rectal cocarcinogenesis in the rat. *Gastroenterology* 1990;98:406–413.

64. Gong J, Hutter C, Baron JA, et al. A pooled analysis of smoking and colorectal cancer: timing of exposure and interactions with environmental factors. *Cancer Epidemiol Biomarkers Prev* 2012;21:1974–1985.

65. Yuhara H, Steinmaus C, Cohen SE, et al. Is diabetes mellitus an independent risk factor for colon cancer and rectal cancer? *Am J Gastroenterol* 2011;106:1911–1921, quiz 1922.

66. Deng L, Gui Z, Zhao L, et al. Diabetes mellitus and the incidence of colorectal cancer: an updated systematic review and meta-analysis. *Dig Dis Sci* 2012;57:1576–1585.

67. Giovannucci E, Egan KM, Hunter DJ, et al. Aspirin and the risk of colorectal cancer in women. *N Engl J Med* 1995;333:609–614.

68. Thun MJ, Namboodiri MM, Heath CW Jr. Aspirin use and reduced risk of fatal colon cancer. *N Engl J Med* 1991;325:1593–1596.

69. Rosenberg L, Louik C, Shapiro S. Nonsteroidal antiinflammatory drug use and reduced risk of large bowel carcinoma. *Cancer* 1998;82:2326–2333.

70. Rothwell PM, Wilson M, Elwin CE, et al. Long-term effect of aspirin on colorectal cancer incidence and mortality: 20-year follow-up of five randomised trials. *Lancet* 2010;376:1741–1750.

71. Liao X, Lochhead P, Nishihara R, et al. Aspirin use, tumor PIK3CA mutation, and colorectal-cancer survival. *N Engl J Med* 2012;367:1596–1606.

72. Domingo E, Church DN, Sieber O, et al. Evaluation of PIK3CA mutation as a predictor of benefit from nonsteroidal anti-inflammatory drug therapy in colorectal cancer. *J Clin Oncol* 2013;31:4297–4305.

73. Singh S, Singh AG, Murad MH, et al. Bisphosphonates are associated with reduced risk of colorectal cancer: a systematic review and meta-analysis. *Clin Gastroenterol Hepatol* 2013;11:232–239.e1.

74. Toriola AT, Cheng TY, Neuhouser ML, et al. Biomarkers of inflammation are associated with colorectal cancer risk in women but are not suitable as early detection markers. *Int J Cancer* 2013;132:2648–2658.

75. Aleksandrova K, Boeing H, Jenab M, et al. Leptin and soluble leptin receptor in risk of colorectal cancer in the European Prospective Investigation into Cancer and Nutrition cohort. *Cancer Res* 2012;72:5328–5337.

76. Chi F, Wu R, Zeng YC, et al. Circulation insulin-like growth factor peptides and colorectal cancer risk: an updated systematic review and meta-analysis. *Mol Biol Rep* 2013;40:3583–3590.

77. Chen L, Li L, Wang Y, et al. Circulating C-peptide level is a predictive factor for colorectal neoplasia: evidence from the meta-analysis of prospective studies. *Cancer Causes Control* 2013;24:1837–1847.

78. Damin DC, Ziegelmann PK, Damin AP. Human papillomavirus infection and colorectal cancer risk: a meta-analysis. *Colorectal Dis* 2013;15:e420–e428.

79. Rustgi AK. Hereditary gastrointestinal polyposis and nonpolyposis syndromes. *N Engl J Med* 1994;331:1694–1702.

80. Hamilton SR, Liu B, Parsons RE, et al. The molecular basis of Turcot's syndrome. *N Engl J Med* 1995;332:839–847.

81. Spirio L, Olschwang S, Groden J, et al. Alleles of the APC gene: an attenuated form of familial polyposis. *Cell* 1993;75:951–957.

82. Powell SM, Petersen GM, Krush AJ. Molecular diagnosis of familial adenomatous polyposis. *N Engl J Med* 1993;329:1982–1987.

83. Geller G, Botkin JR, Green MJ, et al. Genetic testing for susceptibility to adult-onset cancer. The process and content of informed consent. *JAMA* 1997;277:1467–1474.

84. Chung DC, Rustgi AK. The hereditary nonpolyposis colorectal cancer syndrome: genetics and clinical implications. *Ann Intern Med* 2003;138:560–570.

85. Marra G, Boland CR. Hereditary nonpolyposis colorectal cancer: the syndrome, the genes, and historical perspectives. *J Natl Cancer Inst* 1995;87:1114–1125.

86. Weber TK, Conlon W, Petrelli NJ, et al. Genomic DNA-based hMSH2 and hMLH1 mutation screening in 32 Eastern United States hereditary nonpolyposis colorectal cancer pedigrees. *Cancer Res* 1997;57:3798–3803.

87. Burt RW. Familial risk and colorectal cancer. *Gastroenterol Clin North Am* 1996;25:793–803.

88. Garcia-Ruiz A, Milsom JW, Ludwig KA, et al. Right colonic arterial anatomy. Implications for laparoscopic surgery. *Dis Colon Rectum* 1996;39:906–911.

89. Chen Y, Liu ZY, Li RX, et al. Structural studies of initial lymphatics adjacent to gastric and colonic malignant neoplasms. *Lymphology* 1999;32:70–74.

90. Colquhoun PH, Wexner SD. Surgical management of colon cancer. *Curr Gastroenterol Rep* 2002;4:414–419.

91. Shatari T, Fujita M, Nozawa K, et al. Vascular anatomy for right colon lymphadenectomy. *Surg Radiol Anat* 2003;25:86–88.

92. Stein W, Farina A, Gaffney K, et al. Characteristics of colon cancer at time of presentation. *Fam Pract Res J* 1993;13:355–363.

93. Majumdar SR, Fletcher RH, Evans AT. How does colorectal cancer present? Symptoms, duration, and clues to location. *Am J Gastroenterol* 1999; 94:3039–3045.

94. Rocklin MS, Senagore AJ, Talbott TM. Role of carcinoembryonic antigen and liver function tests in the detection of recurrent colorectal carcinoma. *Dis Colon Rectum* 1991;34:794–797.

95. Stotland BR, Siegelman ES, Morris JB, et al. Preoperative and postoperative imaging for colorectal cancer. *Hematol Oncol Clin North Am* 1997;11:635–654.

96. Nollau P, Moser C, Weinland G, et al. Detection of K-ras mutations in stools of patients with colorectal cancer by mutant-enriched PCR. *Int J Cancer* 1996;66:332–336.

97. Eguchi S, Kohara N, Komuta K, et al. Mutations of the p53 gene in the stool of patients with resectable colorectal cancer. *Cancer* 1996;77:1707–1710.

98. Lidgard GP, Domanico MJ, Bruinsma JJ, et al. Clinical performance of an automated stool DNA assay for detection of colorectal neoplasia. *Clin Gastroenterol Hepatol* 2013;11:1313–1318.

99. Pickhardt PJ, Choi JR, Hwang I, et al. Computed tomographic virtual colonoscopy to screen for colorectal neoplasia in asymptomatic adults. *N Engl J Med* 2003;349:2191–2200.

100. de Haan MC, van Gelder RE, Graser A, et al. Diagnostic value of CT-colonography as compared to colonoscopy in an asymptomatic screening population: a meta-analysis. *Eur Radiol* 2011;21:1747–1763.

101. Pickhardt PJ, Hassan C, Halligan S, et al. Colorectal cancer: CT colonography and colonoscopy for detection—systematic review and meta-analysis. *Radiology* 2011;259:393–405.

102. Sweet A, Lee D, Gairy K, et al. The impact of CT colonography for colorectal cancer screening on the UK NHS: costs, healthcare resources and health outcomes. *Appl Health Econ Health Policy* 2011;9:51–64.

103. Boone D, Halligan S, Taylor SA. Evidence review and status update on computed tomography colonography. *Curr Gastroenterol Rep* 2011;13:486–494.

104. Flor N, Mezzanzanica M, Rigamonti P, et al. Contrast-enhanced computed tomography colonography in preoperative distinction between T1-T2 and T3-T4 staging of colon cancer. *Acad Radiol* 2013;20:590–595.

105. Compton CC. Surgical pathology of colorectal cancer. In Saltz LB, ed. *Colorectal Cancer: Multimodality Management.* Totowa, NJ: Humana Press; 2002: 247–265.

106. Edge SB, Byrd DR, Compton CC, et al., eds. *AJCC Cancer Staging Manual.* 7th ed. Berlin: Springer; 2010.

107. Greene FL, Stewart AK, Norton HJ. A new TNM staging strategy for node-positive (stage III) rectal cancer: An analysis of 5,988 patients. In: American Society of Clinical Oncology. *Thirty-Ninth Annual Meeting of the ASCO.* Chicago, IL: American Society of Clinical Oncology; 2003.

108. Hari DM, Leung AM, Lee JH, et al. AJCC Cancer Staging Manual 7th edition criteria for colon cancer: do the complex modifications improve prognostic assessment? *J Am Coll Surg* 2013;217:181–190.

109. Compton CC, Fielding LP, Burgart LJ, et al. Prognostic factors in colorectal cancer. College of American Pathologists Consensus Statement 1999. *Arch Pathol Lab Med* 2000;124:979–994.

110. Ratto C, Sofo L, Ippoliti M, et al. Accurate lymph-node detection in colorectal specimens resected for cancer is of prognostic significance. *Dis Colon Rectum* 1999;42:143–154, discussion 154–158.

111. Wong JH, Severino R, Honnebier MB, et al. Number of nodes examined and staging accuracy in colorectal carcinoma. *J Clin Oncol* 1999;17:2896–2900.

112. Belt EJ, te Velde EA, Krijgsman O, et al. High lymph node yield is related to microsatellite instability in colon cancer. *Ann Surg Oncol* 2012;19:1222–1230.

113. Kuo YH, Lee KF, Chin CC, et al. Does body mass index impact the number of LNs harvested and influence long-term survival rate in patients with stage III colon cancer? *Int J Colorectal Dis* 2012;27:1625–1635.

114. Morikawa T, Tanaka N, Kuchiba A, et al. Predictors of lymph node count in colorectal cancer resections: data from US nationwide prospective cohort studies. *Arch Surg* 2012;147:715–723.

115. Joseph NE, Sigurdson ER, Hanson AL, et al. Accuracy of determining nodal negativity in colorectal cancer on the basis of the number of nodes retrieved on resection. *Ann Surg Oncol* 2003;10:213–218.

116. Lykke J, Roikjaer O, Jess P, et al. The relation between lymph node status and survival in Stage I-III colon cancer: results from a prospective nationwide cohort study. *Colorectal Dis* 2013;15:559–565.

117. Greenberg R, Itah R, Ghinea R, et al. Metastatic lymph node ratio (LNR) as a prognostic variable in colorectal cancer patients undergoing laparoscopic resection. *Tech Coloproctol* 2011;15:273–279.

118. Moug SJ, McColl G, Lloyd SM, et al. Comparison of positive lymph node ratio with an inflammation-based prognostic score in colorectal cancer. *Br J Surg* 2011;98:282–286.

119. Hong KD, Lee SI, Moon HY. Lymph node ratio as determined by the 7th edition of the American Joint Committee on Cancer staging system predicts survival in stage III colon cancer. *J Surg Oncol* 2011;103:406–410.

120. Gao P, Song YX, Wang ZN, et al. Integrated ratio of metastatic to examined lymph nodes and number of metastatic lymph nodes into the AJCC staging system for colon cancer. *PLoS One* 2012;7:e35021.

121. Liefers GJ, Cleton-Jansen AM, van de Velde CJ, et al. Micrometastases and survival in stage II colorectal cancer. *N Engl J Med* 1998;339:223–228.

122. Liefers GJ, Tollenaar RA, Cleton-Jansen AM. Molecular detection of minimal residual disease in colorectal and breast cancer. *Histopathology* 1999; 34:385–390.

123. Sirop S, Kanaan M, Korant A, et al. Detection and prognostic impact of micrometastasis in colorectal cancer. *J Surg Oncol* 2011;103:534–537.

124. Jeffers MD, O'Dowd GM, Mulcahy H, et al. The prognostic significance of immunohistochemically detected lymph node micrometastases in colorectal carcinoma. *J Pathol* 1994;172:183–187.

125. Faerden AE, Sjo OH, Bukholm IR, et al. Lymph node micrometastases and isolated tumor cells influence survival in stage I and II colon cancer. *Dis Colon Rectum* 2011;54:200–206.

126. Morton DL, Wen DR, Wong JH, et al. Technical details of intraoperative lymphatic mapping for early stage melanoma. *Arch Surg* 1992;127:392–399.

127. Canavese G, Gipponi M, Catturich A, et al. Sentinel lymph node mapping in early-stage breast cancer: technical issues and results with vital blue dye mapping and radioguided surgery. *J Surg Oncol* 2000;74:61–68.

128. Saha S, Wiese D, Badin J, et al. Technical details of sentinel lymph node mapping in colorectal cancer and its impact on staging. *Ann Surg Oncol* 2000;7:120–124.

129. Paramo JC, Summerall J, Poppiti R, et al. Validation of sentinel node mapping in patients with colon cancer. *Ann Surg Oncol* 2002;9:550–554.

130. Turner RR, Nora DT, Trocha SD, et al. Colorectal carcinoma nodal staging. Frequency and nature of cytokeratin-positive cells in sentinel and nonsentinel lymph nodes. *Arch Pathol Lab Med* 2003;127:673–679.

131. Viehl CT, Guller U, Cecini R, et al. Sentinel lymph node procedure leads to upstaging of patients with resectable colon cancer: results of the Swiss prospective, multicenter study sentinel lymph node procedure in colon cancer. *Ann Surg Oncol* 2012;19:1959–1965.

132. Saha S, Johnston J, Korant A, et al. Aberrant drainage of sentinel lymph nodes in colon cancer and its impact on staging and extent of operation. *Am J Surg* 2013;205:302–305, discussion 305–306.

133. Warner EE, Evans SR. The sentinel node biopsy and colon cancer revisited. *Cancer J* 2002;8:435–437.

134. Cusack JC, Giacco GG, Cleary K, et al. Survival factors in 186 patients younger than 40 years old with colorectal adenocarcinoma. *J Am Coll Surg* 1996;183:105–112.

135. Messerini L, Palomba A, Zampi G. Primary signet-ring cell carcinoma of the colon and rectum. *Dis Colon Rectum* 1995;38:1189–1192.

136. de Bruine AP, Wiggers T, Beek C, et al. Endocrine cells in colorectal adenocarcinomas: incidence, hormone profile and prognostic relevance. *Int J Cancer* 1993;54:765–771.

137. Jessurun J, Romero-Guadarrama M, Manivel JC. Medullary adenocarcinoma of the colon: clinicopathologic study of 11 cases. *Hum Pathol* 1999;30:843–848.

138. de la Chapelle A. Microsatellite instability. *N Engl J Med* 2003;349:209–210.

139. Boland CR, Thibodeau SN, Hamilton SR, et al. A National Cancer Institute Workshop on Microsatellite Instability for cancer detection and familial predisposition: development of international criteria for the determination of microsatellite instability in colorectal cancer. *Cancer Res* 1998;58: 5248–5257.

140. Boland CR, Sato J, Saito K, et al. Genetic instability and chromosomal aberrations in colorectal cancer: a review of the current models. *Cancer Detect Prev* 1998;22:377–382.

141. Thibodeau SN, Bren G, Schaid D. Microsatellite instability in cancer of the proximal colon. *Science* 1993;260:816–819.

142. Jass JR, Do KA, Simms LA, et al. Morphology of sporadic colorectal cancer with DNA replication errors. *Gut* 1998;42:673–679.

143. Jass JR. Diagnosis of hereditary non-polyposis colorectal cancer. *Histopathology* 1998;32:491–497.

144. Gryfe R, Kim H, Hsieh ET, et al. Tumor microsatellite instability and clinical outcome in young patients with colorectal cancer. *N Engl J Med* 2000;342:69–77.

145. Watanabe T, Wu TT, Catalano PJ, et al. Molecular predictors of survival after adjuvant chemotherapy for colon cancer. *N Engl J Med* 2001;344:1196–1206.

146. Carethers JM, Chauhan DP, Fink D, et al. Mismatch repair proficiency and in vitro response to 5-fluorouracil. *Gastroenterology* 1999;117:123–131.

147. Sinicrope FA, Mahoney MR, Smyrk TC, et al. Prognostic impact of deficient DNA mismatch repair in patients with stage III colon cancer from a randomized trial of FOLFOX-based adjuvant chemotherapy. *J Clin Oncol* 2013;31:3664–3672.

148. Ogino S, Shima K, Meyerhardt JA, et al. Predictive and prognostic roles of BRAF mutation in stage III colon cancer: results from intergroup trial CALGB 89803. *Clin Cancer Res* 2012;18:890–900.

149. Lochhead P, Kuchiba A, Imamura Y, et al. Microsatellite instability and BRAF mutation testing in colorectal cancer prognostication. *J Natl Cancer Inst* 2013;105:1151–1156.

150. Douillard JY, Oliner KS, Siena S, et al. Panitumumab–FOLFOX4 treatment and RAS mutations in colorectal cancer. *N Engl J Med* 2013;369: 1023–1034.

151. Fearon E, Cho KR, Nigro JM, et al. Identification of a chromosome 18q gene that is altered in colorectal cancers. *Science* 1990;247:49–56.

152. Mehlen P, Rabizadeh S, Snipas SJ, et al. The DCC gene product induces apoptosis by a mechanism requiring receptor proteolysis. *Nature* 1998;395:801–804.

153. Chiang SF, Hung HY, Tang R, et al. Can neutrophil-to-lymphocyte ratio predict the survival of colorectal cancer patients who have received curative surgery electively? *Int J Colorectal Dis* 2012;27:1347–1357.

154. Mallappa S, Sinha A, Gupta S, et al. Preoperative neutrophil to lymphocyte ratio >5 is a prognostic factor for recurrent colorectal cancer. *Colorectal Dis* 2013;15:323–328.

155. Harrison LE, Guillem JG, Paty P, et al. Preoperative carcinoembryonic antigen predicts outcomes in node-negative colon cancer patients: a multivariate analysis of 572 patients. *J Am Coll Surg* 1997;185:55–59.

156. Wolmark N, Fisher B, Wieand HS. The prognostic value of the modifications of the Dukes' C class of colorectal cancer. An analysis of the NSABP clinical trials. *Ann Surg* 1986;203:115–122.

157. Weiss JM, Pfau PR, O'Connor ES, et al. Mortality by stage for right- versus left-sided colon cancer: analysis of surveillance, epidemiology, and end results—Medicare data. *J Clin Oncol* 2011;29:4401–4409.

158. Meyerhardt JA, Catalano PJ, Haller DG, et al. Impact of diabetes mellitus on outcomes in patients with colon cancer. *J Clin Oncol* 2003;21:433–440.

159. Sinicrope FA, Foster NR, Yothers G, et al. Body mass index at diagnosis and survival among colon cancer patients enrolled in clinical trials of adjuvant chemotherapy. *Cancer* 2013;119:1528–1536.

160. Alipour S, Kennecke HF, Woods R, et al. Body mass index and body surface area and their associations with outcomes in stage II and III colon cancer. *J Gastrointest Cancer* 2013;44:203–210.

161. Dehal AN, Newton CC, Jacobs EJ, et al. Impact of diabetes mellitus and insulin use on survival after colorectal cancer diagnosis: the Cancer Prevention Study-II Nutrition Cohort. *J Clin Oncol* 2012;30:53–59.

162. van de Poll-Franse LV, Haak HR, Coebergh JW, et al. Disease-specific mortality among stage I-III colorectal cancer patients with diabetes: a large population-based analysis. *Diabetologia* 2012;55:2163–2172.

163. Cheung WY, Shi Q, O'Connell M, et al. The predictive and prognostic value of sex in early-stage colon cancer: a pooled analysis of 33,345 patients from the ACCENT database. *Clin Colorectal Cancer* 2013;12:179–187.

164. Phipps AI, Shi Q, Newcomb PA, et al. Associations between cigarette smoking status and colon cancer prognosis among participants in North Central Cancer Treatment Group Phase III Trial N0147. *J Clin Oncol* 2013;31:2016–2023.

165. Donohue J, Williams S, Cha S, et al. Perioperative blood transfusions do not affect disease recurrence of patients undergoing curative resection of colorectal carcinoma: a Mayo/North Central Cancer Treatment Group study. *J Clin Oncol* 1995;13:1671–1678.

166. Leichman CG, Lens HJ, Leichman L, et al. Quantitation of intratumoral thymidylate synthase expression predicts for disseminated colorectal cancer response and resistance to protracted-infusion fluorouracil and weekly leucovorin. *J Clin Oncol* 1997;15:3223–3229.

167. Ahnen DJ, Feigl P, Quan G, et al. Ki-ras mutation and p53 overexpression predict the clinical behavior of colorectal cancer: a Southwest Oncology Group study. *Cancer Res* 1998;58:1149–1158.

168. Hong L, Han Y, Zhang H, et al. High expression of epidermal growth factor receptor might predict poor survival in patients with colon cancer: a meta-analysis. *Genet Test Mol Biomarkers* 2013;17:348–351.

169. Innocenti F, Undevia SD, Iver L, et al. Genetic variants in the UDP-glucuronosyltransferase 1A1 gene predict the risk of severe neutropenia of irinotecan. *J Clin Oncol* 2004;22:1382–1388.

170. McLeod HL. Individualized cancer therapy: molecular approaches to the prediction of tumor response. *Expert Rev Anticancer Ther* 2002;2:113–119.

171. Winawer SJ. Follow-up after polypectomy. *World J Surg* 1991;15:25–28.

172. Lee MG, Hanchard B. Management of colonic polyps by colonoscopic polypectomy. *West Indian Med J* 1991;40:81–85.

173. National Comprehensive Cancer Network Guidelines for Colon Cancer, Version 3.2011, www.nccn.org.

174. Huang EH, Forde KA. Surgical implications of colonoscopy. *Semin Laparosc Surg* 2003;10:13–18.

175. Libutti SK, Forde KA. Surgical considerations III: bowel anastomosis. In Cohen A, Winawer S, eds. *Cancer of the Colon, Rectum and Anus.* New York McGraw Hill; 1995: 445–456.

176. Guenaga KF, Matos D, Willie Jorgensen P, et al. Mechanical bowel preparation for elective colorectal surgery. *Cochrane Database Syst Rev* 2011;(2):CD001544.

177. Makino M, Hisamitsu K, Sugamura K, et al. Randomized comparison of two preoperative methods for preparation of the colon: oral administration of a solution of polyethylene glycol plus electrolytes and total parenteral nutrition. *Hepatogastroenterology* 1998;45:90–94.

178. Chen CF, Lin JK, Leu SY, et al. Evaluation of rapid colon preparation with Golytely. *Zhonghua Yi Xue Za Zhi (Taipei)* 1989;44:45–56.

179. Lewis RT, Goodall RG, Marien B, et al. Is neomycin necessary for bowel preparation in surgery of the colon? Oral neomycin plus erythromycin versus erythromycin-metronidazole. *Can J Surg* 1989;32:265–270.

180. Ram E, Sherman Y, Weil R, et al. Is mechanical bowel preparation mandatory for elective colon surgery? A prospective randomized study. *Arch Surg* 2005;140:285–288.

181. Jung B, Lannerstad O, Pahlman L, et al. Preoperative mechanical preparation of the colon: the patient's experience. *BMC Surg* 2007;7:5.

182. Matsuda A, Kishi T, Musso G, et al. The effect of intraoperative rectal washout on local recurrence after rectal cancer surgery: a meta-analysis. *Ann Surg Oncol* 2013;20:856–863.

183. Benson AB 3rd, Choti MA, Cohen AM, et al. NCCN Practice Guidelines for Colorectal Cancer. *Oncology (Williston Park)* 2000;14:203–212.

184. McGinnis LS. Surgical treatment options for colorectal cancer. *Cancer* 1994;74:2147–2150.

185. Garcia-Olmo D, Ontanon J, Garcia-Olmo DC, et al. Experimental evidence does not support use of the "no-touch" isolation technique in colorectal cancer. *Dis Colon Rectum* 1999;42:1449–1456, discussion 1454–1456.

186. Regimbeau JM, Panis Y, Pocard M, et al. Handsewn ileal pouch-anal anastomosis on the dentate line after total proctectomy: technique to avoid incomplete mucosectomy and the need for long-term follow-up of the anal transition zone. *Dis Colon Rectum* 2001;44:43–50, discussion 50–51.

187. Young CJ, Solomon MJ, Eyers AA, et al. Evolution of the pelvic pouch procedure at one institution: the first 100 cases. *Aust N Z J Surg* 1999;69:438–442.

188. Poppen B, Svenberg T, Bark T, et al. Colectomy-proctomucosectomy with S-pouch: operative procedures, complications, and functional outcome in 69 consecutive patients. *Dis Colon Rectum* 1992;35:40–47.

189. Khot UP, Lang AW, Murali K, et al. Systematic review of the efficacy and safety of colorectal stents. *Br J Surg* 2002;89:1096–1102.

190. Sebastian S, Johnston S, Geoghegan T, et al. Pooled analysis of the efficacy and safety of self-expanding metal stenting in malignant colorectal obstruction. *Am J Gastroenterol* 2004;99:2051–2057.

191. Inaba Y, Arai Y, Yamaura H, et al. Phase II clinical study on stent therapy for unresectable malignant colorectal obstruction (JIVROSG-0206). *Am J Clin Oncol* 2012;35:73–76.

192. Lee HJ, Hong SP, Cheon JH, et al. Long-term outcome of palliative therapy for malignant colorectal obstruction in patients with unresectable metastatic colorectal cancers: endoscopic stenting versus surgery. *Gastrointest Endosc* 2011;73:535–542.

193. Branger F, Thibaudeau E, Mucci-Hennekinne S, et al. Management of acute malignant large-bowel obstruction with self-expanding metal stent. *Int J Colorectal Dis* 2010;25:1481–1485.

194. White SI, Abdool SI, Frenkiel B, et al. Management of malignant left-sided large bowel obstruction: a comparison between colonic stents and surgery. *ANZ J Surg* 2011;81:257–260.

195. Cheung HY, Chung CC, Tsang WW, et al. Endolaparoscopic approach vs conventional open surgery in the treatment of obstructing left-sided colon cancer: a randomized controlled trial. *Arch Surg* 2009;144:1127–1132.

196. Pirlet IA, Slim K, Kwiatkowski F, et al. Emergency preoperative stenting versus surgery for acute left-sided malignant colonic obstruction: a multicenter randomized controlled trial. *Surg Endosc* 2011;25:1814–1821.

197. van Hooft JE, Bemelman WA, Oldenburg B, et al. Colonic stenting versus emergency surgery for acute left-sided malignant colonic obstruction: a multicentre randomised trial. *Lancet Oncol* 2011;12:344–352.

198. Sabbagh C, Brower F, Diouf M, et al. Is stenting as "a bridge to surgery" an oncologically safe strategy for the management of acute, left-sided, malignant, colonic obstruction? A comparative study with a propensity score analysis. *Ann Surg* 2013;258:107–115.

199. Lichten JB, Reid JJ, Zahalsky MP, et al. Laparoscopic cholecystectomy in the new millennium. *Surg Endosc* 2001;15:867–872.

200. Theodoridis TD, Bontis JN. Laparoscopy and oncology: where do we stand today? *Ann N Y Acad Sci* 2003;997:282–291.

201. Hartley JE, Monson JR. The role of laparoscopy in the multimodality treatment of colorectal cancer. *Surg Clin North Am* 2002;82:1019–1033.

202. Mori T, Abe N, Sugiyama M, et al. Laparoscopic hepatobiliary and pancreatic surgery: an overview. *J Hepatobiliary Pancreat Surg* 2002;9:710–722.

203. Grover AC, Skarulis M, Alexander HR, et al. A prospective evaluation of laparoscopic exploration with intraoperative ultrasound as a technique for localizing sporadic insulinomas. *Surgery* 2005;138:1003–1008, discussion 1008.

204. Goletti O, Celona G, Monzani F, et al. Laparoscopic treatment of pancreatic insulinoma. *Surg Endosc* 2003;17:1499.

205. Patankar SK, Larach SW, Ferrara A, et al. Prospective comparison of laparoscopic vs. open resections for colorectal adenocarcinoma over a ten-year period. *Dis Colon Rectum* 2003;46:601–611.

206. Delaney CP, Kiran RP, Senagore AJ, et al. Case-matched comparison of clinical and financial outcome after laparoscopic or open colorectal surgery. *Ann Surg* 2003;238:67–72.

207. Feliciotti F, Paganini AM, Guerrieri M, et al. Results of laparoscopic vs open resections for colon cancer in patients with a minimum follow-up of 3 years. *Surg Endosc* 2002;16:1158–1161.

208. Lezoche E, Feliciotti F, Paganini AM, et al. Results of laparoscopic versus open resections for non-early rectal cancer in patients with a minimum follow-up of four years. *Hepatogastroenterology* 2002;49:1185–1190.

209. Cobb WS, Lokey JS, Schwab DP, et al. Hand-assisted laparoscopic colectomy: a single-institution experience. *Am Surg* 2003;69:578–580.

210. Lauter DM, Lau ST, Lanzafame K. Combined laparoscopic-assisted right hemicolectomy and low anterior resection for synchronous colorectal carcinomas. *Surg Endosc* 2003;17:1498.

211. Weeks JC, Nelson H, Gelber S, et al. Short-term quality-of-life outcomes following laparoscopic-assisted colectomy vs open colectomy for colon cancer: a randomized trial. *JAMA* 2002;287:321–328.

212. Clinical Outcomes of Surgical Therapy Study Group. A comparison of laparoscopically assisted and open colectomy for colon cancer. *N Engl J Med* 2004;350:2050–2059.

213. Jayne DG, Guillou PJ, Thorpe H, et al. Randomized trial of laparoscopic-assisted resection of colorectal carcinoma: 3-year results of the UK MRC CLASICC Trial Group. *J Clin Oncol* 2007;25:3061–3068.

214. Green BL, Marshall HC, Collinson F, et al. Long-term follow-up of the Medical Research Council CLASICC trial of conventional versus laparoscopically assisted resection in colorectal cancer. *Br J Surg* 2013;100:75–82.

215. McNally ME, Todd Moore B, Brown KM. Single-incision laparoscopic colectomy for malignant disease. *Surg Endosc* 2011;25:3559–3565.

216. Gash KJ, Goede AC, Chambers W, et al. Laparoendoscopic single-site surgery is feasible in complex colorectal resections and could enable day case colectomy. *Surg Endosc* 2011;25:835–840.

217. Katsuno G, Fukunaga M, Nagakari K, et al. Single-incision laparoscopic colectomy for colon cancer: early experience with 31 cases. *Dis Colon Rectum* 2011;54:705–710.

218. Chen WT, Chang SC, Chiang HC, et al. Single-incision laparoscopic versus conventional laparoscopic right hemicolectomy: a comparison of short-term surgical results. *Surg Endosc* 2011;25:1887–1892.

219. Yun JA, Yun SH, Park YA, et al. Single-incision laparoscopic right colectomy compared with conventional laparoscopy for malignancy: assessment of perioperative and short-term oncologic outcomes. *Surg Endosc* 2013;27:2122–2130.

220. deSouza AL, Prasad LM, Park JJ, et al. Robotic assistance in right hemicolectomy: is there a role? *Dis Colon Rectum* 2010;53:1000–1006.

221. Luca F, Ghezzi TL, Valvo M, et al. Surgical and pathological outcomes after right hemicolectomy: case-matched study comparing robotic and open surgery. *Int J Med Robot* 2011 [ePub ahead of print].

222. Diana M, Perretta S, Wall J, et al. Transvaginal specimen extraction in colorectal surgery: current state of the art. *Colorectal Dis* 2011;13:e104–e111.

223. Park JS, Choi GS, Kim HJ, et al. Natural orifice specimen extraction versus conventional laparoscopically assisted right hemicolectomy. *Br J Surg* 2011;98:710–715.

224. Rieder E, Spaun GO, Khajanchee YS, et al. A natural orifice transrectal approach for oncologic resection of the rectosigmoid: an experimental study and comparison with conventional laparoscopy. *Surg Endosc* 2011;25: 3357–3363.

225. Nivatvongs S. Surgical management of early colorectal cancer. *World J Surg* 2000;24:1052–1055.

226. Buyse M, Zeleniuch-Jacquotte A, Chalmers TC. Adjuvant therapy of colorectal cancer. Why we still don't know. *JAMA* 1988;259:3571–3578.

227. Libutti S, Saltz L, Tepper J. Cancer of the colon. In: DeVita VT, Hellman S, Rosenberg SA, eds. *Principles and Practice of Oncology*. 8th ed. Philadelphia, PA: Lippincott Williams, & Wilkins; 2008:1261–1264.

228. Efficacy of adjuvant fluorouracil and folinic acid in colon cancer. International Multicentre Pooled Analysis of Colon Cancer Trials (IMPACT) investigators. *Lancet* 1995;345:939–944.

229. Wolmark N, Fisher B, Rockette H, et al. Postoperative adjuvant chemotherapy or BCG for colon cancer: results from NSABP protocol C0-1. *J Natl Cancer Inst* 1988;80:30–36.

230. Andre T, Colin P, Louvet C, et al. Semimonthly versus monthly regimen of fluorouracil and leucovorin administered for 24 or 36 weeks as adjuvant therapy in stage II and III colon cancer: results of a randomized trial. *J Clin Oncol* 2003;21:2896–2903.

231. Haller DG, Catalano PJ, Macdonald JS, et al. Phase III study of fluorouracil, leucovorin, and levamisole in high-risk stage II and III colon cancer: final report of Intergroup 0089. *J Clin Oncol* 2005;23:8671–8678.

232. Kerr DJ, Gray R, McConkey C, et al. Adjuvant chemotherapy with 5-fluorouracil, L-folinic acid and levamisole for patients with colorectal cancer: non-randomised comparison of weekly versus four-weekly schedules—less pain, same gain. QUASAR Colorectal Cancer Study Group. *Ann Oncol* 2000;11:947–955.

233. Comparison of flourouracil with additional levamisole, higher-dose folinic acid, or both, as adjuvant chemotherapy for colorectal cancer: a randomised trial. QUASAR Collaborative Group. *Lancet* 2000;355:1588–1596.

234. O'Connell MJ, Laurie JA, Kahn M, et al. Prospectively randomized trial of postoperative adjuvant chemotherapy in patients with high-risk colon cancer. *J Clin Oncol* 1998;16:295–300.

235. Twelves C, Wong A, Nowacki MP, et al. Capecitabine as adjuvant treatment for stage III colon cancer. *N Engl J Med* 2005;352:2696–2704.

236. Lembersky BC, Wieand HS, Petrelli NJ, et al. Oral uracil and tegafur plus leucovorin compared with intravenous fluorouracil and leucovorin in stage II and III carcinoma of the colon: results from National Surgical Adjuvant Breast and Bowel Project Protocol C-06. *J Clin Oncol* 2006;24: 2059–2064.

237. Andre T, Boni C, Navarro M, et al. Improved overall survival with oxaliplatin, fluorouracil, and leucovorin as adjuvant treatment in stage II or III colon cancer in the MOSAIC trial. *J Clin Oncol* 2009;27:3109–3116.

238. Yothers G, O'Connell MJ, Allegra CJ, et al. Oxaliplatin as adjuvant therapy for colon cancer: updated results of NSABP C-07 trial, including survival and subset analyses. *J Clin Oncol* 2011;29:3768–3774.

239. Kidwell KM, Yothers G, Ganz PA, et al. Long-term neurotoxicity effects of oxaliplatin added to fluorouracil and leucovorin as adjuvant therapy for colon cancer: results from National Surgical Adjuvant Breast and Bowel Project trials C-07 and LTS-01. *Cancer* 2012;118:5614–5622.

240. Uwah AN, Ackier J, Leighton JC Jr, et al. The effect of diabetes on oxaliplatin-induced peripheral neuropathy. *Clin Colorectal Cancer* 2012;11: 275–279.

241. McCleary NJ, Meyerhardt JA, Green E, et al. Impact of age on the efficacy of newer adjuvant therapies in patients with stage II/III colon cancer: findings from the ACCENT database. *J Clin Oncol* 2013;31:2600–2606.

242. Tournigand C, Andre T, Bonnetain F, et al. Adjuvant therapy with fluorouracil and oxaliplatin in stage II and elderly patients (between ages 70 and 75 years) with colon cancer: subgroup analyses of the Multicenter International Study of Oxaliplatin, Fluorouracil, and Leucovorin in the Adjuvant Treatment of Colon Cancer trial. *J Clin Oncol* 2012;30:3353–3360.

243. Benson AB 3rd, Bekali-Saab T, Chan E, et al. Localized colon cancer, version 3.2013: featured updates to the NCCN Guidelines. *J Natl Compr Canc Netw* 2013;11:519–528.

244. Haller DG, Tabernero J, Maroun J, et al. Capecitabine plus oxaliplatin compared with fluorouracil and folinic acid as adjuvant therapy for stage III colon cancer. *J Clin Oncol* 2011;29:1465–1471.

245. Cunningham D, Humblet Y, Siena S, et al. Cetuximab monotherapy and cetuximab plus irinotecan in irinotecan-refractory metastatic colorectal cancer. *N Engl J Med* 2004;351:337–345.

246. Douillard JY, Cunningham D, Roth AD, et al. Irinotecan combined with fluorouracil compared with fluorouracil alone as first-line treatment for metastatic colorectal cancer: a multicentre randomised trial. *Lancet* 2000;355:1041–1047.

247. Saltz LB, Cox JV, Blanke C, et al. Irinotecan plus fluorouracil and leucovorin for metastatic colorectal cancer. Irinotecan Study Group. *N Engl J Med* 2000;343:905–914.

248. Sargent DJ, Niedzwiecki D, O'Connell MJ, et al. Recommendation for caution with irinotecan, fluorouracil, and leucovorin for colorectal cancer. *N Engl J Med* 2001;345:144–145, author reply 146.

249. Saltz LB, Niedzwiecki D, Hollis D, et al. Irinotecan fluorouracil plus leucovorin is not superior to fluorouracil plus leucovorin alone as adjuvant

250. Ychou M, Raoul JL, Douillard JY, et al. A phase III randomised trial of LV5FU2 + irinotecan versus LV5FU2 alone in adjuvant high-risk colon cancer (FNCLCC Accord02/FFCD9802). *Ann Oncol* 2009;20:674–680.

251. Van Cutsem E, Labianca R, Bodoky G, et al. Randomized phase III trial comparing biweekly infusional fluorouracil/leucovorin alone or with irinotecan in the adjuvant treatment of stage III colon cancer: PETACC-3. *J Clin Oncol* 2009;27:3117–3125.

252. Tejpar S, Bosman F, Delorenzi M, et al. Microsatellite instability (MSI) in stage II and III colon cancer treated with 5FU-LV or 5FU-LV and irinotecan (PETACC 3-EORTC 40993-SAKK 60/00 trial). *J Clin Oncol* 2009;27: Abstr 4001.

253. Bertagnolli MM, Niedzwiecki D, Compton CC, et al. Microsatellite instability predicts improved response to adjuvant therapy with irinotecan, fluorouracil, and leucovorin in stage III colon cancer: Cancer and Leukemia Group B Protocol 89803. *J Clin Oncol* 2009;27:1814–1821.

254. Allegra CJ, Yothers G, O'Connell MJ, et al. Bevacizumab in stage II-III colon cancer: 5-year update of the National Surgical Adjuvant Breast and Bowel Project C-08 trial. *J Clin Oncol* 2013;31:359–364.

255. de Gramont A, Van Cutsem E, Schmoll HJ, et al. Bevacizumab plus oxaliplatin-based chemotherapy as adjuvant treatment for colon cancer (AVANT): a phase 3 randomised controlled trial. *Lancet Oncol* 2012;13:1225–1233.

256. Alberts SR, Sargent DJ, Nair S, et al. Effect of oxaliplatin, fluorouracil, and leucovorin with or without cetuximab on survival among patients with resected stage iii colon cancer: a randomized trial. *JAMA* 2012;307: 1383–1393.

257. Schrag D, Rifas-Shiman S, Saltz L, et al. Adjuvant chemotherapy use for Medicare beneficiaries with stage II colon cancer. *J Clin Oncol* 2002;20: 3999–4005.

258. Efficacy of adjuvant fluorouracil and folinic acid in B2 colon cancer. International Multicentre Pooled Analysis of B2 Colon Cancer Trials (IMPACT B2) Investigators. *J Clin Oncol* 1999;17:1356–1363.

259. McKenzie S, Nelson R, Mailey B, et al. Adjuvant chemotherapy improves survival in patients with American Joint Committee on Cancer stage II colon cancer. *Cancer* 2011;117:5493–5499.

260. O'Connor ES, Greenblatt DY, LoConte NK, et al. Adjuvant chemotherapy for stage II colon cancer with poor prognostic features. *J Clin Oncol* 2011;29:3381–3388.

261. Wu X, Zhang J, He X, et al. Postoperative adjuvant chemotherapy for stage II colorectal cancer: a systematic review of 12 randomized controlled trials. *J Gastrointest Surg* 2012;16:646–655.

262. Ishiguro M, Mochizuki H, Tomita N, et al. Study protocol of the SACURA trial: a randomized phase III trial of efficacy and safety of UFT as adjuvant chemotherapy for stage II colon cancer. *BMC Cancer* 2012;12:281.

263. Jen J, Kim H, Piantadosi S, et al. Allelic loss of chromosome 18q and prognosis in colorectal cancer. *N Engl J Med* 1994;331:213–221.

264. Elsaleh H, Iacopetta B. Microsatellite instability is a predictive marker for survival benefit from adjuvant chemotherapy in a population-based series of stage III colorectal carcinoma. *Clin Colorectal Cancer* 2001;1:104–109.

265. Willet CG, Tepper JE, Cohen AM. Obstructive and perforative colonic carcinoma: patterns of failure. *J Clin Oncol* 1985;3:379–384.

266. Sato H, Maeda K, Sugihara K, et al. High-risk stage II colon cancer after curative resection. *J Surg Oncol* 2011;104:45–52.

267. Ribic CM, Sargent DJ, Moore MJ, et al. Tumor microsatellite-instability status as a predictor of benefit from fluorouracil-based adjuvant chemotherapy for colon cancer. *N Engl J Med* 2003;349:247–257.

268. Kim GP, Colangelo H, Wieand HS, et al. Prognostic and predictive roles of high-degree microsatellite instability in colon cancer: a National Cancer Institute-National Surgical Adjuvant Breast and Bowel Project Collaborative Study. *J Clin Oncol* 2007;25:767–772.

269. Sargent DJ, Marsoni S, Thibodeau SN, et al. Confirmation of deficient mismatch repair (dMMR) as a predictive marker for lack of benefit from 5-FU based chemotherapy in stage II and III colon cancer (CC): A pooled molecular reanalysis of randomized chemotherapy trials. *J Clin Oncol* 2008;26:4008.

270. Sinicrope FA, Foster NR, Thibodeau SN, et al. DNA mismatch repair status and colon cancer recurrence and survival in clinical trials of 5-fluorouracil-based adjuvant therapy. *J Natl Cancer Inst* 2011;103:863–875.

271. Kerr D, Gray R, Quirke P, et al. A quantitative multigene RT-PCR assay for prediction of recurrence in stage II colon cancer: Selection of the genes in four large studies and results of the independent, prospectively designed QUASAR validation study. *J Clin Oncol* 2009;27:Abstr 4000.

272. Koopman M, Kortman GA, Mekenkamp L, et al. Deficient mismatch repair system in patients with sporadic advanced colorectal cancer. *Br J Cancer* 2009;100:266–273.

273. Roth AD, Tejpar S, Delorenzi M, et al. Prognostic role of KRAS and BRAF in stage II and III resected colon cancer: results of the translational study on the PETACC-3, EORTC 40993, SAKK 60-00 trial. *J Clin Oncol* 2010;28: 466–474.

274. Ogino S, Nosho K, Irahara N, et al. Prognostic significance and molecular associations of 18q loss of heterozygosity: a cohort study of microsatellite stable colorectal cancers. *J Clin Oncol* 2009;27:4591–4598.

275. Sharif S, O'Connell MJ. Gene signatures in stage II colon cancer: a clinical review. *Curr Colorectal Cancer Rep* 2012;8:225–231.

276. Hornberger J, Lyman GH, Chien R, et al. A multigene prognostic assay for selection of adjuvant chemotherapy in patients with T3, stage II colon

cancer: impact on quality-adjusted life expectancy and costs. *Value Health* 2012;15:1014–1021.

277. Maak M, Simon I, Nitsche U, et al. Independent validation of a prognostic genomic signature (ColoPrint) for patients with stage II colon cancer. *Ann Surg* 2013;257:1053–1058.

278. Kennedy RD, Bylesjo M, Kerr P, et al. Development and independent validation of a prognostic assay for stage II colon cancer using formalin-fixed paraffin-embedded tissue. *J Clin Oncol* 2011;29:4620–4626.

279. Benson AB 3rd, Schrag D, Somerfield MR, et al. American Society of Clinical Oncology recommendations on adjuvant chemotherapy for stage II colon cancer. *J Clin Oncol* 2004;22:3408–3419.

280. Des Guetz G, Nicolas P, Perret GY, et al. Does delaying adjuvant chemotherapy after curative surgery for colorectal cancer impair survival? A meta-analysis. *Eur J Cancer* 2010;46:1049–1055.

281. Czaykowski PM, Gill S, Kennecke HF, et al. Adjuvant chemotherapy for stage III colon cancer: does timing matter? *Dis Colon Rectum* 2011;54:1082–1089.

282. Wolmark N, Rockette H, Wickerham DL, et al. Adjuvant therapy of Dukes' A, B, and C adenocarcinoma of the colon with portal vein fluorouracil hepatic infusion: preliminary results of National Surgical Adjuvant Breast and Bowel Project Protocol C-02. *J Clin Oncol* 1990;8:1466–1475.

283. Long term results of single course of adjuvant intraportal chemotherapy for colorectal cancer. Swiss Group for Clinical Cancer Research (SAKK). *Lancet* 1995;345:349–352.

284. Weber W, Laffer U, Metzger U. Adjuvant portal liver infusion with 5-fluorouracil and mitomycin in colorectal cancer. *Anticancer Res* 1993;13: 1839–1840.

285. Kelsen DP, Saltz L, Cohen AM, et al. A phase I trial of immediate postoperative intraperitoneal floxuridine and leucovorin plus systemic 5-fluorouracil and levamisole after resection of high risk colon cancer. *Cancer* 1994;74: 2224–2233.

286. Scheithauer W, Kornek GV, Marczell A, et al. Combined intravenous and intraperitoneal chemotherapy with fluorouracil + leucovorin vs fluorouracil + levamisole for adjuvant therapy of resected colon carcinoma. *Br J Cancer* 1998;77:1349–1354.

287. Sammartino P, Sibio S, Biacchi D, et al. Prevention of Peritoneal Metastases from Colon Cancer in High-Risk Patients: Preliminary Results of Surgery plus Prophylactic HIPEC. *Gastroenterol Res Pract* 2012;2012:141585.

288. Kimura T, McKolanis JR, Dzubinski LA, et al. MUC1 vaccine for individuals with advanced adenoma of the colon: a cancer immunoprevention feasibility study. *Cancer Prev Res (Phila)* 2013;6:18–26.

289. Foxtrot Collaborative Group. Feasibility of preoperative chemotherapy for locally advanced, operable colon cancer: the pilot phase of a randomised controlled trial. *Lancet Oncol* 2012;13:1152–1160.

290. Muller AD, Sonnenberg A. Prevention of colorectal cancer by flexible endoscopy and polypectomy. A case-control study of 32,702 veterans. *Ann Intern Med* 1995;123:904–910.

291. Burt RW. Colon cancer screening. *Gastroenterology* 2000;119:837–853.

292. Mandel JS, Bond JH, Church TR, et al. Reducing mortality from colorectal cancer by screening for fecal occult blood. Minnesota Colon Cancer Control Study. *N Engl J Med* 1993;328:1365–1371.

293. Graham RA, Wang S, Catalano PJ, et al. Postsurgical surveillance of colon cancer: preliminary cost analysis of physician examination, carcinoembryonic antigen testing, chest x-ray, and colonoscopy. *Ann Surg* 1998;228:59–63.

294. Burke W, Petersen G, Lynch P, et al. Recommendations for follow-up care of individuals with an inherited predisposition to cancer. I. Hereditary nonpolyposis colon cancer. Cancer Genetics Studies Consortium. *JAMA* 1997;277:915–919.

295. Atkin WS, Morson BC, Cuzick J. Long-term risk of colorectal cancer after excision of rectosigmoid adenomas. *N Engl J Med* 1992;326:658–662.

296. Meyerhardt JA, Mangu PB, Flynn PJ, et al. Follow-up care, surveillance protocol, and secondary prevention measures for survivors of colorectal cancer: American Society of Clinical Oncology clinical practice guideline endorsement. *J Clin Oncol* 2013;31:4465–4470.

297. Bruinvels DJ, Stiggelbout AM, Lievit J, et al. Follow-up of patients with colorectal cancer. A meta-analysis. *Ann Surg* 1994;219:174–182.

298. Zeng Z, Cohen AM, Urmacher C. Usefulness of carcinoembryonic antigen monitoring despite normal preoperative values in node-positive colon cancer patients. *Dis Colon Rectum* 1993;36:1063–1068.

299. Clinical practice guidelines for the use of tumor markers in breast and colorectal cancer. Adopted on May 17, 1996 by the American Society of Clinical Oncology. *J Clin Oncol* 1996;14:2843–2877.

300. Martin EW Jr, Minton JP, Carey LC. CEA-directed second-look surgery in the asymptomatic patient after primary resection of colorectal carcinoma. *Ann Surg* 1985;202:310–317.

301. Balz JB, Martin EW, Minton JP. CEA as an early indicator for second-look procedure in colorectal carcinoma. *Rev Surg* 1977;34:1–4.

302. Bruinvels DJ, de Brauw LM, Lievit J, et al. Attitudes towards detection and management of hepatic metastases of colorectal origin: a second look. *HPB Surg* 1994;8:115–122.

303. Libutti SK, Alexander HR Jr, Choyke P, et al. A prospective study of 2-[18F] fluoro-2-deoxy-D-glucose/positron emission tomography scan, 99mTc-labeled arcitumomab (CEA-scan), and blind second-look laparotomy for detecting colon cancer recurrence in patients with increasing carcinoembryonic antigen levels. *Ann Surg Oncol* 2001;8:779–786.

304. Gunderson LL, Sosin H. Areas of failure found at reoperation (second or symptomatic look) following "curative surgery" for adenocarcinoma of the rectum. *Cancer* 1974;34:1278–1292.

305. Ito K, Hibi K, Ando H, et al. Usefulness of analytical CEA doubling time and half-life time for overlooked synchronous metastases in colorectal carcinoma. *Jpn J Clin Oncol* 2002;32:54–58.

306. Takenoshita S, Hashizume T, Asao T, et al. Immunoscintigraphy using 99mTc-labeled anti-CEA monoclonal antibody for patients with colorectal cancer. *Anticancer Res* 1995;15:471–475.

307. Moffat FL Jr, Pinsky CM, Hammershaimb L, et al. Clinical utility of external immunoscintigraphy with the IMMU-4 technetium-99m Fab' antibody fragment in patients undergoing surgery for carcinoma of the colon and rectum: results of a pivotal, phase III trial. The Immunomedics Study Group. *J Clin Oncol* 1996;14:2295–2305.

308. Beatty JD, Hyams DM, Morton BA, et al. Impact of radiolabeled antibody imaging on management of colon cancer. *Am J Surg* 1989;157:13–19.

309. Swanson RS. Is an FDG-PET scan the new imaging standard for colon cancer? *Ann Surg Oncol* 2001;8:752–753.

310. Desch CE, Benson AB 3rd, Somerfield MR, et al. Colorectal cancer surveillance: 2005 update of an American Society of Clinical Oncology practice guideline. *J Clin Oncol* 2005;23:8512–8519.

311. Schoemaker D, Black R, Giles L, et al. Yearly colonoscopy, liver CT, and chest radiography do not influence 5-year survival of colorectal cancer patients. *Gastroenterology* 1998;114:7–14.

312. Makela J, Laitinen S, Kairaluoma MI. Early results of follow-up after radical resection for colorectal cancer. Preliminary results of a prospective randomized trial. *Surg Oncol* 1992;1:157–161.

313. Ohlsson B, Breland U, Ekberg H, et al. Follow-up after curative surgery for colorectal carcinoma. Randomized comparison with no follow-up. *Dis Colon Rectum* 1995;38:619–626.

314. Benson AB 3rd, Desch CE, Flynn PJ, et al. 2000 update of American Society of Clinical Oncology colorectal cancer surveillance guidelines. *J Clin Oncol* 2000;18:3586–3588.

315. Inadomi JM, Sonnenberg A. The impact of colorectal cancer screening on life expectancy. *Gastrointest Endosc* 2000;51:517–523.

316. Fornasarig M, Valentini M, Poletti M, et al. Evaluation of the risk for metachronous colorectal neoplasms following intestinal polypectomy: a clinical, endoscopic and pathological study. *Hepatogastroenterology* 1998;45:1565–1572.

317. Renehan AG, Egger M, Saunders MP, et al. Impact on survival of intensive follow up after curative resection for colorectal cancer: systematic review and meta-analysis of randomised trials. *BMJ* 2002;324:813.

318. Temple LK, Hsieh L, Wong WD, et al. Use of surgery among elderly patients with stage IV colorectal cancer. *J Clin Oncol* 2004;22:3475–3484.

319. Poultsides GA, Servais EL, Saltz LB, et al. Outcome of primary tumor in patients with synchronous stage IV colorectal cancer receiving combination chemotherapy without surgery as initial treatment. *J Clin Oncol* 2009;27:3379–3384.

320. McCahill LE, Yothers G, Sharif S, et al. Primary mFOLFOX6 plus bevacizumab without resection of the primary tumor for patients presenting with surgically unresectable metastatic colon cancer and an intact asymptomatic colon cancer: definitive analysis of NSABP trial C-10. *J Clin Oncol* 2012;30:3223–3228.

321. Stillwell AP, Buettner PG, Siu SK, et al. Predictors of postoperative mortality, morbidity, and long-term survival after palliative resection in patients with colorectal cancer. *Dis Colon Rectum* 2011;54:535–544.

322. Heidelberger C, Chaudhuri NK, Danneberg P, et al. Fluorinated pyrimidines, a new class of tumor inhibitory compounds. *Nature* 1957;179: 663–666.

323. Jager E, Heike M, Bernhard H, et al. Weekly high-dose leucovorin versus low-dose leucovorin combined with fluorouracil in advanced colorectal cancer: results of a randomized mulitcenter trial. *J Clin Oncol* 1996;14: 2274–2279.

324. Lokich JJ, Ahlgren JD, Gullo JJ, et al. A prospective randomized comparison of continuous infusion fluorouracil with a conventional bolus schedule in metastatic colorectal carcinoma: a Mid-Atlantic Oncology Program Study. *J Clin Oncol* 1989;7:425–432.

325. Kohne CH, Schoffski P, Wilke H, et al. Effective biomodulation by leucovorin of high-dose infusion fluorouracil given as a weekly 24-hour infusion: results of a randomized trial in patients with advanced colorectal cancer. *J Clin Oncol* 1998;16:418–426.

326. Schuller J, Cassidy J, Dumont E, et al. Preferential activation of capecitabine in tumor following oral administration to colorectal cancer patients. *Cancer Chemother Pharmacol* 2000;45:291–297.

327. Van Cutsem E, Findlay M, Osterwalder B, et al. Capecitabine, an oral fluoropyrimidine carbamate with substantial activity in advanced colorectal cancer: results of a randomized phase II study. *J Clin Oncol* 2000;18:1337–1345.

328. Hoff PM, Ansari R, Batist G, et al. Comparison of oral capecitabine versus intravenous fluorouracil plus leucovorin as first-line treatment in 605 patients with metastatic colorectal cancer: results of a randomized phase III study. *J Clin Oncol* 2001;19:2282–2292.

329. Van Cutsem E, Twelves C, Cassidy J, et al. Oral capecitabine compared with intravenous fluorouracil plus leucovorin in patients with metastatic colorectal cancer: results of a large phase III study. *J Clin Oncol* 2001;19: 4097–4106.

330. Pizzolato JF, Saltz LB. The camptothecins. *Lancet* 2003;361:2235–2242.

331. Kawato Y, Aonuma M, Hirota Y, et al. Intracellular roles of SN-38, a metabolite of the camptothecin derivative CPT-11, in the antitumor effect of CPT-11. *Cancer Res* 1991;51:4187–4191.

332. Saltz L, Kanowitz J, Kemeny NE, et al. A phase I clinical and pharmacologic trial of irinotecan, 5-fluorouracil, and leucovorin in pateints with advanced solid tumors. *J Clin Oncol* 1996;14:2959–2967.

333. Andre T, Louvet C, Maindrault-Goebel F, et al. CPT-11 (irinotecan) addition to bimonthly, high-dose leucovorin and bolus and continuous-infusion 5-fluorouracil (FOLFIRI) for pretreated metastatic colorectal cancer. GERCOR. *Eur J Cancer* 1999;35:1343–1347.

334. Fuchs CS, Marshall J, Mitchell E, et al. Randomized, controlled trial of irinotecan plus infusional, bolus, or oral fluoropyrimidines in first-line treatment of metastatic colorectal cancer: results from the BICC-C Study. *J Clin Oncol* 2007;25:4779–4786.

335. Extra JM, Espie M, Calvo F, et al. Phase I study of oxaliplatin in patients with advanced cancer. *Cancer Chemother Pharmacol* 1990;25:299–303.

336. Raymond E, Chaney SG, Taamma A, et al. Oxaliplatin: a review of preclinical and clinical studies. *Ann Oncol* 1998;9:1053–1071.

337. Libutti S, Saltz L, Tepper J. Cancer of the colon. In: DeVita VT, Hellman S, Rosenberg SA, eds. *Principles and Practice of Oncology.* 9th ed. Philadelphia, PA: Lippincott Williams, & Wilkins; 2011:1266–1268.

338. Giacchetti S, Perpoint B, Zidani R, et al. Phase III multicenter randomized trial of oxaliplatin added to chronomodulated fluorouracil-leucovorin as first-line treatment of metastatic colorectal cancer. *J Clin Oncol* 2000;18:136–147.

339. Bertheault-Cvitkovic F, Jami A, Ithzaki M, et al. Biweekly intensified ambulatory chronomodulated chemotherapy with oxaliplatin, fluorouracil, and leucovorin in patients with metastatic colorectal cancer. *J Clin Oncol* 1996;14:2950–2958.

340. Levi F, Zidani R, Misset JL. Randomised multicentre trial of chronotherapy with oxaliplatin, fluorouracil, and folinic acid in metastatic colorectal cancer. International Organization for Cancer Chronotherapy. *Lancet* 1997;350:681–686.

341. de Gramont A, Bosset JF, Milan C, et al. Randomized trial comparing monthly low-dose leucovorin and fluorouracil bolus with bimonthly high-dose leucovorin and fluorouracil bolus plus continuous infusion for advanced colorectal cancer: a French Intergroup study. *J Clin Oncol* 1997;15:808–815.

342. Andre T, Bensmaine MA, Louvet C, et al. Multicenter phase II study of bimonthly high-dose leucovorin, fluorouracil infusion, and oxaliplatin for metastatic colorectal cancer resistant to the same leucovorin and fluorouracil regimen. *J Clin Oncol* 1999;17:3560–3568.

343. de Gramont A, Vignoud J, Tournigand C, et al. Oxaliplatin with high-dose leucovorin and 5-fluorouracil 48-hour continuous infusion in pretreated metastatic colorectal cancer. *Eur J Cancer* 1997;33:214–219.

344. Wolmark N, Yothers G, O'Connell MJ, et al. A phase III trial comparing mFOLFOX6 to mFOLFOX6 plus bevacizumab in stage II or III carcinoma of the colon: Results of NSABP Protocol C-08. *J Clin Oncol* 2009;27: Abstr LBA4.

345. Moehler M, Hoffman T, Hildner K, et al. Weekly oxaliplatin, high-dose folinic acid and 24h-5-fluorouracil (FUFOX) as salvage therapy in metastatic colorectal cancer patients pretreated with irinotecan and folinic acid/5 fluorouracil regimens. *Z Gastroenterol* 2002;40:957–964.

346. de Gramont A, Figer A, Seymour M, et al. Leucovorin and fluorouracil with or without oxaliplatin as first-line treatment in advanced colorectal cancer. *J Clin Oncol* 2000;18:2938–2947.

347. Rothenberg ML, Oza AM, Bigelow RH, et al. Superiority of oxaliplatin and fluorouracil-leucovorin compared with either therapy alone in patients with progressive colorectal cancer after irinotecan and fluorouracil-leucovorin: interim results of a phase III trial. *J Clin Oncol* 2003;21:2059–2069.

348. Maindrault-Goebel F, Louvet C, Andre T, et al. Oxaliplatin added to the simplified bimonthly leucovorin and 5- fluorouracil regimen as second-line therapy for metastatic colorectal cancer (FOLFOX6). GERCOR. *Eur J Cancer* 1999;35:1338–1342.

349. Tournigand C, Andre T, Achille E, et al. FOLFIRI followed by FOLFOX6 or the reverse sequence in advanced colorectal cancer: a randomized GERCOR study. *J Clin Oncol* 2004;22:229–237.

350. Loprinzi CL, Qin R, Dakhil SR, et al. Phase III randomized, placebo (PL)-controlled, double-blind study of intravenous calcium/magnesium (CaMg) to prevent oxaliplatin-induced sensory neurotoxicity (sNT), N08CB: An alliance for clinical trials in oncology study. *J Clin Oncol* 2013;31:Abstr 3501.

351. Colucci G, Gebbia V, Paoletti G, et al. Phase III randomized trial of FOLFIRI vs FOLFOX4 in the treatment of advanced colorectal cancer: a multicenter study of the Grupo Oncologico Italia Meridionale. *J Clin Oncol* 2005;23:4866–4875.

352. Goldberg RM. N9741: a phase III study comparing irinotecan to oxaliplatin-containing regimens in advanced colorectal cancer. *Clin Colorectal Cancer* 2002;2:81.

353. Miller L, Emanuel D, Elfring G, et al. 60-day, all-cause mortality with first-line irinotecan/ fluorouracil/leucovorin (IFL) or fluorouracil/leucovorin (FL) for metastatic colorectal cancer (MCRC). *Proc Am Soc Clin Oncol* 2002;21:129a.

354. Goldberg RM, Sargent DJ, Morton RF, et al. A randomized controlled trial of fluorouracil plus leucovorin, irinotecan, and oxaliplatin combinations in patients with previously untreated metastatic colorectal cancer. *J Clin Oncol* 2004;22:23–30.

355. Tournigand C, Cervantes A, Figer A, et al. OPTIMOX1: a randomized study of FOLFOX4 or FOLFOX7 with oxaliplatin in a stop-and-Go fashion in advanced colorectal cancer—a GERCOR study. *J Clin Oncol* 2006;24:394–400.

356. de Gramont A, Buyse M, Abrahantes JC, et al. Reintroduction of oxaliplatin is associated with improved survival in advanced colorectal cancer. *J Clin Oncol* 2007;25:3224–3229.

357. Hochster HS, Hart LL, Ramanathan RK, et al. Safety and efficacy of oxaliplatin/ fluoropyrimidine regimens with or without bevacizumab as first-line treatment of metastatic colorectal cancer (mCRC): final analysis of the TREE-Study. *J Clin Oncol* 2006;24:Abstr 3510.

358. Hochster H, Chachoua A, Speyer J, et al. Oxaliplatin with weekly bolus fluorouracil and low-dose leucovorin as first-line therapy for patients with colorectal cancer. *J Clin Oncol* 2003;21:2703–2707.

359. Falcone A, Ricci S, Brunetti I, et al. Phase III trial of infusional fluorouracil, leucovorin, oxaliplatin, and irinotecan (FOLFOXIRI) compared with infusional fluorouracil, leucovorin, and irinotecan (FOLFIRI) as first-line treatment for metastatic colorectal cancer: the Gruppo Oncologico Nord Ovest. *J Clin Oncol* 2007;25:1670–1676.

360. Cassidy J, Clarke S, Diaz-Rubio E, et al. Randomized phase III study of capecitabine plus oxaliplatin compared with fluorouracil/folinic acid plus oxaliplatin as first-line therapy for metastatic colorectal cancer. *J Clin Oncol* 2008;26:2006–2012.

361. Maughan TS, James RD, Kerr DJ, et al. Comparison of intermittent and continuous palliative chemotherapy for advanced colorectal cancer: a multicentre randomised trial. *Lancet* 2003;361:457–464.

362. Chibaudel B, Maindrault-Goebel F, Lledo G, et al. Can chemotherapy be discontinued in unresectable metastatic colorectal cancer? The GERCOR OPTIMOX2 Study. *J Clin Oncol* 2009;27:5727–5733.

363. Perez-Staub N, Chibaudel B, Figer A, et al. Who can benefit from chemotherapy holidays after first-line therapy for advanced colorectal cancer? A GERCOR study. *J Clin Oncol* 2008;26:Abstr 4037.

364. Yeoh C, Chau I, Cunningham D, et al. Impact of 5-fluorouracil rechallenge on subsequent response and survival in advanced colorectal cancer: pooled analysis from three consecutive randomized controlled trials. *Clin Colorectal Cancer* 2003;3:102–107.

365. Lal KR, et al. A phase II, randomized, multicentre, trial of irinotecan until disease progression (PD) versus 8 cycles, in advanced colorectal cancer (CRC) resistant to fluoropyrimidines. In: *American Society of Clinical Oncology Annual Meeting.* Chicago, IL: American Society of Clinical Oncology; 2003.

366. Koopman M, Antonini NF, Douma J, et al. Sequential versus combination chemotherapy with capecitabine, irinotecan, and oxaliplatin in advanced colorectal cancer (CAIRO): a phase III randomised controlled trial. *Lancet* 2007;370:135–142.

367. Seymour MT, Maughan TS, Ledermann JA, et al. Different strategies of sequential and combination chemotherapy for patients with poor prognosis advanced colorectal cancer (MRC FOCUS): a randomised controlled trial. *Lancet* 2007;370:143–152.

368. Ferrara N, Hillan KJ, Gerber HP, et al. Discovery and development of bevacizumab, an anti-VEGF antibody for treating cancer. *Nat Rev Drug Discov* 2004;3:391–400.

369. Ferrara N. Vascular endothelial growth factor: basic science and clinical progress. *Endocr Rev* 2004;25:581–611.

370. Kabbinavar F, Hurwitz HI, Fehrenbacher L, et al. Phase II, randomized trial comparing bevacizumab plus fluorouracil (FU)/leucovorin (LV) with FU/LV alone in patients with metastatic colorectal cancer. *J Clin Oncol* 2003;21:60–65.

371. Hurwitz H, Fehrenbacher L, Novotny W, et al. Bevacizumab plus irinotecan, fluorouracil, and leucovorin for metastatic colorectal cancer. *N Engl J Med* 2004;350:2335–2342.

372. Kabbinavar FF, Hambleton J, Mass RD, et al. Combined analysis of efficacy: the addition of bevacizumab to fluorouracil/leucovorin improves survival for patients with metastatic colorectal cancer. *J Clin Oncol* 2005;23:3706–3712.

373. Seymour MT. Fluorouracil, oxaliplatin and CPT-11 (irinotecan), use and sequencing (MRC FOCUS): a 2135-patient randomized trial in advanced colorectal cancer (ACRC). *Proc Am Soc Clin Oncol* 2005;23:Abstr 3518. http://www.asco.org/ac/1,1003,_12-002511-00_18-0034-00_19-001999,00.asp.

374. Giantonio BJ, Catalano PJ, Meropol NJ, et al. Bevacizumab in combination with oxaliplatin, fluorouracil, and leucovorin (FOLFOX4) for previously treated metastatic colorectal cancer: results from the Eastern Cooperative Oncology Group Study E3200. *J Clin Oncol* 2007;25:1539–1544.

375. Saltz LB, Clarke S, Diaz-Rubio E, et al. Bevacizumab in combination with oxaliplatin-based chemotherapy as first-line therapy in metastatic colorectal cancer: a randomized phase III study. *J Clin Oncol* 2008;26:2013–2019.

376. Skillings JA, Johnson DH, Miller K, et al. Arterial thromboembolic events (ATEs) in a pooled analysis of 5 randomized, controlled trials (RCTs) of bevacizumab (BV) with chemotherapy. *J Clin Oncol* 2005;23:3019.

377. Ganapathi AM, Westmoreland T, Tyler D, et al. Bevacizumab-associated fistula formation in postoperative colorectal cancer patients. *J Am Coll Surg* 2012;214:582–588, discussion 588–590.

378. Bennouna J, Sastre J, Arnold D, et al. Continuation of bevacizumab after first progression in metastatic colorectal cancer (ML18147): a randomised phase 3 trial. *Lancet Oncol* 2013;14:29–37.

379. Van Cutsem E, Tabernero J, Lakomy R, et al. Addition of aflibercept to fluorouracil, leucovorin, and irinotecan improves survival in a phase III randomized trial in patients with metastatic colorectal cancer previously treated with an oxaliplatin-based regimen. *J Clin Oncol* 2012;30:3499–3506.

380. Grothey A, Van Cutsem E, Sobrero A, et al. Regorafenib monotherapy for previously treated metastatic colorectal cancer (CORRECT): an international, multicentre, randomised, placebo-controlled, phase 3 trial. *Lancet* 2013;381:303–312.

381. Ciardiello F, Tortora G. A novel approach in the treatment of cancer: targeting the epidermal growth factor receptor. *Clin Cancer Res* 2001;7:2958–2970.

382. Real FX, Rettig WJ, Chesa PG, et al. Expression of epidermal growth factor receptor in human cultured cells and tissues: relationship to cell lineage and stage of differentiation. *Cancer Res* 1986;46:4726–4731.

383. Carpenter G, Cohen S. Epidermal growth factor. *J Biol Chem* 1990;265:7709–7712.

384. Thomas SM, Grandis JR. Pharmacokinetic and pharmacodynamic properties of EGFR inhibitors under clinical investigation. *Cancer Treat Rev* 2004;30:255–268.

385. Saltz L, Rubin M, Hochster H, et al. Cetuximab (IMC-C225) plus irinotecan (CPT-11) is active in CPT-11-refractory colorectal cancer (CRC) that expresses epidermal growth factor receptor (EGFR). *J Clin Oncol* 2001;20:Abstr 7.

386. Saltz LB, Meropol NJ, Poehrer PJ Sr, et al. Phase II trial of cetuximab in patients with refractory colorectal cancer that expresses the epidermal growth factor receptor. *J Clin Oncol* 2004;22:1201–1208.

387. Jonker DJ, O'Callaghan CJ, Karapetis CS, et al. Cetuximab for the treatment of colorectal cancer. *N Engl J Med* 2007;357:2040–2048.

388. Van Cutsem E, Siena S, Humblet Y, et al. An open-label, single-arm study assessing safety and efficacy of panitumumab in patients with metastatic colorectal cancer refractory to standard chemotherapy. *Ann Oncol* 2008;19:92–98.

389. Hecht JR, Patnaik A, Berlin J, et al. Panitumumab monotherapy in patients with previously treated metastatic colorectal cancer. *Cancer* 2007;110:980–988.

390. Van Cutsem E, Peeters M, Siena S, et al. Open-label phase III trial of panitumumab plus best supportive care compared with best supportive care alone in patients with chemotherapy-refractory metastatic colorectal cancer. *J Clin Oncol* 2007;25:1658–1664.

391. Lievre A, Bachet JB, Boige V, et al. KRAS mutations as an independent prognostic factor in patients with advanced colorectal cancer treated with cetuximab. *J Clin Oncol* 2008;26:374–379.

392. Khambata-Ford S, Garrett CR, Meropol NJ, et al. Expression of epiregulin and amphiregulin and K-ras mutation status predict disease control in metastatic colorectal cancer patients treated with cetuximab. *J Clin Oncol* 2007;25:3230–3237.

393. Amado RG, Wolf M, Peeters M, et al. Wild-type KRAS is required for panitumumab efficacy in patients with metastatic colorectal cancer. *J Clin Oncol* 2008;26:1626–1634.

394. Karapetis CS, Khambata-Ford S, Jonker DJ, et al. K-ras mutations and benefit from cetuximab in advanced colorectal cancer. *N Engl J Med* 2008;359:1757–1765.

395. Tejpar S, Celik I, Schlichting M, et al. Association of KRAS G13D tumor mutations with outcome in patients with metastatic colorectal cancer treated with first-line chemotherapy with or without cetuximab. *J Clin Oncol* 2012;30:3570–3577.

396. De Roock W, Claes B, Bernasconi D, et al. Effects of KRAS, BRAF, NRAS, and PIK3CA mutations on the efficacy of cetuximab plus chemotherapy in chemotherapy-refractory metastatic colorectal cancer: a retrospective consortium analysis. *Lancet Oncol* 2010;11:753–762.

397. Allegra CJ, Jessup JM, Somerfield MR, et al. American Society of Clinical Oncology provisional clinical opinion: testing for KRAS gene mutations in patients with metastatic colorectal carcinoma to predict response to anti-epidermal growth factor receptor monoclonal antibody therapy. *J Clin Oncol* 2009;27:2091–2096.

398. Vakiani E, Janakiraman M, Shen R, et al. Comparative genomic analysis of primary versus metastatic colorectal carcinomas. *J Clin Oncol* 2012;30:2956–2962.

399. Lin YL, Liau JY, Yu SC, et al. KRAS mutation is a predictor of oxaliplatin sensitivity in colon cancer cells. *PLoS One* 2012;7:e50701.

400. Van Cutsem E, Kohne CH, Hitre E, et al. Cetuximab and chemotherapy as initial treatment for metastatic colorectal cancer. *N Engl J Med* 2009;360:1408–1417.

401. Van Cutsem E, Kohne CH, Lang I, et al. Cetuximab plus irinotecan, fluorouracil, and leucovorin as first-line treatment for metastatic colorectal cancer: updated analysis of overall survival according to tumor KRAS and BRAF mutation status. *J Clin Oncol* 2011;29:2011–2019.

402. Bokemeyer C, Bondarenko I, Makhson A, et al. Fluorouracil, leucovorin, and oxaliplatin with and without cetuximab in the first-line treatment of metastatic colorectal cancer. *J Clin Oncol* 2009;27:663–671.

403. Maughan TS, Adams RA, Smith CG, et al. Addition of cetuximab to oxaliplatin-based first-line combination chemotherapy for treatment of advanced colorectal cancer: results of the randomised phase 3 MRC COIN trial. *Lancet* 2011;377:2103–2114.

404. Tveit KM, Guren T, Glimelius B, et al. Phase III trial of cetuximab with continuous or intermittent fluorouracil, leucovorin, and oxaliplatin (Nordic FLOX) versus FLOX alone in first-line treatment of metastatic colorectal cancer: the NORDIC-VII study. *J Clin Oncol* 2012;30:1755–1762.

405. Douillard JY, Siena S, Cassidy J, et al. Randomized, phase III trial of panitumumab with infusional fluorouracil, leucovorin, and oxaliplatin (FOLFOX4) versus FOLFOX4 alone as first-line treatment in patients with previously untreated metastatic colorectal cancer: the PRIME study. *J Clin Oncol* 2010;28:4697–4705.

406. Peeters M, Price T, Hotko Y, et al. 14LBA Randomized phase 3 study of panitumumab with FOLFIRI vs FOLFIRI alone as second-line treatment (tx) in patients (pts) with metastatic colorectal cancer (mCRC). *EJC Supplements* 2009;7:10.

407. Venook AP, Niedzwiecki D, Heinz-Josef L, et al. CALGB/SWOG 80405: Phase III trial of irinotecan/5-FU/leucovorin (FOLFIRI) or oxaliplatin/5-FU/leucovorin (mFOLFOX6) with bevacizumab (BV) or cetuximab (CET) for patients (pts) with KRAS wild-type (wt) untreated metastatic adenocarcinoma of the colon or rectum (MCRC). *J Clin Oncol* 2014;35:(suppl; abstr LBA3):5s.

408. Scope A, Agero AL, Dusza SW, et al. Randomized double-blind trial of prophylactic oral minocycline and topical tazarotene for cetuximab-associated acne-like eruption. *J Clin Oncol* 2007;25:5390–5396.

409. Perez-Soler R, Saltz L. Cutaneous adverse effects with HER1/EGFR-targeted agents: is there a silver lining? *J Clin Oncol* 2005;23:5235–5246.

410. O'Neil BH, Allen R, Spigel DR, et al. High incidence of cetuximab-related infusion reactions in Tennessee and North Carolina and the association with atopic history. *J Clin Oncol* 2007;25:3644–3648.

411. Chung CH, Mirakhur B, Chan E, et al. Cetuximab-induced anaphylaxis and IgE specific for galactose-alpha-1,3-galactose. *N Engl J Med* 2008;358:1109–1117.

412. Schrag D, Chung KY, Flombaum C, et al. Cetuximab therapy and symptomatic hypomagnesemia. *J Natl Cancer Inst* 2005;97:1221–1224.

413. Lenz HJ, Mayer RJ, Gold PJ, et al. Activity of cetuximab in patients with colorectal cancer refractory to both irinotecan and oxaliplatin. *J Clin Oncol* 2004;22:3510.

414. Chung KY, Shia J, Kemeny NE, et al. Cetuximab shows activity in colorectal cancer patients with tumors that do not express the epidermal growth factor receptor by immunohistochemistry. *J Clin Oncol* 2005;23:1803–1810.

415. Hecht JR, Mitchell E, Neubauer MA, et al. Lack of correlation between epidermal growth factor receptor status and response to Panitumumab monotherapy in metastatic colorectal cancer. *Clin Cancer Res* 2010;16:2205–2213.

416. Saltz LB, Lenz HJ, Kindler HL, et al. Randomized phase II trial of cetuximab, bevacizumab, and irinotecan compared with cetuximab and bevacizumab alone in irinotecan-refractory colorectal cancer: the BOND-2 study. *J Clin Oncol* 2007;25:4557–4561.

417. Segal NH, Reidy-Lagunes D, Capanu M, et al. Phase II study of bevacizumab in combination with cetuximab plus irinotecan in irinotecan-refractory colorectal cancer (CRC) patients who have progressed on a bevacizumab-containing regimen (The BOND 2.5 Study). *J Clin Oncol* 2009;27:Abstr 4087.

418. Tol J, Koopman M, Cats A, et al. Chemotherapy, bevacizumab, and cetuximab in metastatic colorectal cancer. *N Engl J Med* 2009;360:563–572.

419. Hecht JR, Mitchell E, Chidiac T, et al. A randomized phase IIIB trial of chemotherapy, bevacizumab, and panitumumab compared with chemotherapy and bevacizumab alone for metastatic colorectal cancer. *J Clin Oncol* 2009;27:672–680.

420. Oza A, Townsley C, Siu L, et al. Phase II study of erlotinib (OSI-774) in patients with metastatic colorectal cancer. *Proc Am Soc Clin Oncol* 2003;785:50.

421. Dorligschaw O, et al. ZD 1839 (Iressa)-based treatment as last-line therapy in patients with advanced colorectal cancer (ACRC). *Proc Am Soc Clin Oncol* 2003;22.

422. Saltz LB, Rosen LS, Marshall JL, et al. Phase II trial of sunitinib in patients with metastatic colorectal cancer after failure of standard therapy. *J Clin Oncol* 2007;25:4793–4799.

423. Blanke CD. Celecoxib with chemotherapy in colorectal cancer. *Oncology (Huntingt)* 2002;16:17–21.

424. Chan AT, Ogino S, Fuchs CS. Aspirin use and survival after diagnosis of colorectal cancer. *JAMA* 2009;302:649–658.

425. Ali R, Toh HC, Chia WK, et al. The utility of Aspirin in Dukes C and High Risk Dukes B Colorectal cancer—the ASCOLT study: study protocol for a randomized controlled trial. *Trials* 2011;12:261.

426. Bastiaannet E, Sampieri K, Dekkers OM, et al. Use of aspirin postdiagnosis improves survival for colon cancer patients. *Br J Cancer* 2012;106:1564–1570.

427. Schrag D, Garewal HS, Burstein HJ, et al. American Society of Clinical Oncology Technology Assessment: chemotherapy sensitivity and resistance assays. *J Clin Oncol* 2004;22:3631–3638.

428. Metzger R, Danenberg K, Leichman CG, et al. High basal level gene expression of thymidine phosphorylase (platelet-derived endothelial cell growth factor) in colorectal tumors is associated with nonresponse to 5-fluorouracil. *Clin Cancer Res* 1998;4:2371–2376.

429. Salonga D, Danenberg KD, Johnson M, et al. Colorectal tumors responding to 5-fluorouracil have low gene expression levels of dihydropyrimidine dehydrogenase, thymidylate synthase, and thymidine phosphorylase. *Clin Cancer Res* 2000;6:1322–1327.

430. Iqbal S, Lenz HJ. Targeted therapy and pharmacogenomic programs. *Cancer* 2003;97:2076–2082.

431. Ebert MP, Tanzer M, Balluff B, et al. TFAP2E-DKK4 and chemoresistance in colorectal cancer. *N Engl J Med* 2012;366:44–53.

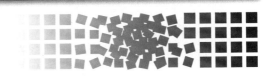

50 Genetic Testing in Colon Cancer (Polyposis Syndromes)

Kory W. Jasperson

INTRODUCTION

Hereditary colonic polyposis conditions account for less than 1% of all colorectal cancers (CRC). Accurate classification of these conditions is imperative, given their distinct cancer risks, management strategies, and consequent risk to relatives. However, overlapping features and atypical or attenuated presentations make diagnosis difficult in some cases. Determining the histologic types of colorectal polyps identified is especially useful in guiding diagnostic strategies. Adenomatous polyps are the predominant lesion in familial adenomatous polyposis (FAP), attenuated FAP (AFAP), and *MUTYH* (MutY human homolog)–associated polyposis (MAP), whereas hamartomatous polyps are the primary gastrointestinal lesion in Peutz–Jeghers syndrome (PJS), juvenile polyposis syndrome (JPS), and Cowden syndrome (CS). Extracolonic features, which are highlighted for each syndrome in Tables 50.1 to 50.3 are also important clues in the diagnostic workup. Genetic testing is now available for these conditions and, in most cases, allows for a precise diagnosis.

ADENOMATOUS POLYPOSIS

Familial Adenomatous Polyposis and Attenuated Familial Adenomatous Polyposis

Of all of the colonic polyposis conditions, FAP is both the most common and the best characterized. FAP is caused by germ-line mutations in the adenomatous polyposis coli (APC) gene and is estimated to occur in about 1 in 10,000 individuals. With the classic presentation of FAP, hundreds to thousands of adenomatous polyps occur by the age of 20 to 40 years.[1] The attenuated or less severe colonic phenotype associated with AFAP may mimic sporadic colon polyps and cancer, or other known syndromes, such as MAP. This creates diagnostic difficulties when evaluating an individual with moderate adenomatous polyposis. Other conditions linked to germ-line APC mutations include Gardner syndrome (with association of colonic polyposis and osteomas, epidermoid cysts, fibromas, and/or desmoid tumors) and Turcot syndrome (with association of colonic polyposis and medulloblastomas).[2] However, it is now believed that the features associated with Gardner syndrome and Turcot syndrome are the result of variable expressivity of APC mutations as opposed to being distinct clinical entities.

Colon Phenotype

Although adenomatous polyps associated with FAP have a similar malignancy rate as those that develop in the general population, the sheer number of polyps present in FAP results in nearly a 100% lifetime risk of CRC in untreated individuals. In FAP, colorectal polyps begin to develop on average around the age of 16 years.[1] The mean age at CRC onset is 39 years, with 7% developing CRC by 21 years and 95% before the age of 50 years.[3]

In AFAP, the lifetime risk of CRC is approximately 70% with an average age at onset in the 50s.[4] The colonic phenotype of AFAP is quite variable, even within the same family. Colonoscopies in 120 mutation-positive individuals within the same family revealed that 37% had less than 10 adenomatous colon polyps (average age, 36 years; range, 16 to 67 years), 28% had 10 to 50 polyps (average age, 39 years; range, 21 to 76 years), and 35% had greater than 50 polyps (average age, 48 years; range, 27 to 49 years).[4] In addition, the total number of polyps per individual ranged from zero to 470.[4]

Extracolonic Features

The most common extracolonic finding in individuals with FAP and AFAP is upper gastrointestinal tract polyps. Although the colonic phenotype in AFAP is less severe than in FAP, the upper gastrointestinal phenotype is comparable. Adenomatous polyps of the duodenum (20% to 100%) and the periampullary region (at least 50%) are common.[5,6] The relative risk of duodenal or periampullary carcinoma in FAP is estimated to be 100 to 330 times greater than the general population, although the absolute risk is only around 5%.[5] The majority of FAP- and AFAP-associated small-bowel carcinomas arise in the duodenum.

Fundic gland polyps are found in most cases of FAP/AFAP and often number in the hundreds.[7] Unlike polyps in the colon or small bowel, fundic gland polyps are a type of hamartoma. They are typically small (1 to 5 mm), sessile, and usually asymptomatic and are located in the fundus and body of the stomach.[7] Adenomatous polyps of the stomach are occasionally found in FAP and AFAP.[8] Gastric cancers arising from fundic gland polyps have been reported in FAP, although most are believed to arise from adenomatous polyps.[8] Individuals with FAP have an 800-fold increased risk for desmoid tumors (aggressive fibromatoses), with a lifetime risk of 10% to 30%.[9–11] Risk factors for desmoid tumors in FAP include a family history of desmoid tumors, APC mutations 3ý to codon 1,399 (genotype–phenotype correlation), female sex, and previous abdominal surgery.[10] Although desmoid tumors do not metastasize, they can be locally invasive, aggressive, and difficult to treat, resulting in significant morbidity and the second leading cause of mortality in FAP.[12]

The phenotypic spectrum of germ-line APC mutations also includes other benign findings such as osteomas, epidermoid cysts, fibromas, dental abnormalities, and congenital hypertrophy of the retinal pigment epithelium (CHRPE). In addition, there are increased risks for other cancers, including those of the pancreas, thyroid, bile duct, brain (typically medulloblastoma), and liver (specifically hepatoblastoma).[6]

Management

Without treatment, CRC is inevitable in FAP. However, with early screening and polypectomies, in addition to prophylactic colectomies after polyps become too difficult to manage endoscopically, most CRCs can be prevented in AFAP and FAP. In FAP, annual

TABLE 50.1

Characteristic Features and Recommendations: Adenomatous Polyposis Conditions

Lifetime Cancer Risks	Management Recommendations	Nonmalignant Features
FAP (*APC*)		
Colorectum (100%)	Annual colonoscopy/sigmoidoscopy by 10–15 y until colectomy or proctocolectomy	100–1,000s of colorectal adenomas
Duodenum (5%)	Upper endoscopy every 1–4 y by 25–30 y	Duodenal polyposis
Stomach (≤1%)	Examine stomach at time of duodenoscopy	Fundic gland polyposis
Thyroid (1%–2%)	Annual physical examination	
Pancreas (1%–2%)		
Hepatoblastoma (1%–2%)		
Medulloblastoma (<1%)		
		CHRPE, epidermoid cysts, osteomas, dental abnormalities, desmoid tumors
AFAP (*APC*)		
Colorectum (70%)	Colonoscopy every 2–3 y by 18–20 y until colectomy	10–100 colonic adenomas (range, 0–100s)
Duodenum (5%)	Upper endoscopy every 1–4 y by 25–30 y	Duodenal polyposis
Stomach (≤1%)		Fundic gland polyposis
Thyroid (1%–2%)	Annual physical examination	
Pancreas (1%–2%)		
MAP (biallelic *MUTYH*)		
Colorectum (80%)	Colonoscopy every 2–3 y by 25–30 y until colectomy	10–100 colonic adenomas (range, 0–100s); Multiple hyperplastic and sessile serrated polyps possible
Duodenum (4%)	Upper endoscopy every 1–4 y by 30–35 y	Duodenal adenomatous polyposis

Adapted with permission from the NCCN Clinical Practice Guidelines in Oncology (NCCN Guidelines®) for Genetic/Familial High-Risk Assessment: Colorectal V.2.2015. © 2015 National Comprehensive Cancer Network, Inc. All rights reserved. The NCCN Guidelines® and illustrations herein may not be reproduced in any form for any purpose without the express written permission of the NCCN. To view the most recent and complete version of the NCCN Guidelines, go online to NCCN.org. NATIONAL COMPREHENSIVE CANCER NETWORK®, NCCN®, NCCN GUIDELINES®, and all other NCCN Content are trademarks owned by the National Comprehensive Cancer Network, Inc.

colonoscopies or flexible sigmoidoscopies are recommended starting around the age of 10 years.[13] In AFAP, screening begins in the late teenage years, and colonoscopies, rather than sigmoidoscopies, are necessary because of proximally located polyps.[13] Colectomies can sometimes be avoided in AFAP, which is not the case for individuals with FAP. After polyps become too numerous (usually >20 to 30 polyps) to manage endoscopically or when adenomas with advanced histology are identified, a prophylactic colectomy is advised.[13] A proctocolectomy with an ileal pouch anal anastomosis is the standard surgery in FAP, whereas a total colectomy with ileorectal anastomosis is often the preferred approach with AFAP or in FAP cases with limited rectal involvement.[13,14] Continued screening of the remaining rectum or ileal pouch is still necessary.[13]

Recently, it has been shown that duodenal cancer detected through surveillance improves survival compared with individuals presenting because of symptoms.[15] The NCCN currently recommends the consideration of an esophagogastroduodenoscopy (EGD) with a side-viewing examination beginning around the age of 25 years for duodenal cancer surveillance.[13] The extent of duodenal polyps, as defined by the Spigelman staging criteria, is used to determine the EGD follow-up interval.[13] Additional considerations for the management in individuals with germ-line APC mutations are outlined and updated annually by the NCCN (www.nccn.org).

Genetic Testing and Counseling

A clinical diagnosis of FAP is considered when at least 100 colorectal adenomatous polyps are detected by the 2nd or 3rd decade of life.[6] Genetic testing of APC is still recommended to clarify extracolonic cancer risks and to help determine FAP status in relatives. Genetic testing has

also been shown to be cost-effective,[16] although it is unlikely to change colon management for cases with extensive adenomatous polyposis.

Given the phenotypic variability, a consensus as to what constitutes a diagnosis of AFAP has not been reached. The National Comprehensive Cancer Network® (NCCN®) currently recommends that individuals with greater than 10 cumulative colorectal adenomas be referred for genetic counseling and the consideration of genetic testing.[13] The identification of an APC mutation in these less severe polyp cases confirms a diagnosis of AFAP. It is also noteworthy that individuals with 100 or more adenomatous polyps may have AFAP if polyp development occurs at a later age (typically after 40 years).

Differentiating among FAP, AFAP, and other colonic polyposis conditions is not always straightforward. Family history, which is consistent with an autosomal-dominant mode of inheritance, is suggestive of FAP/AFAP and increases the likelihood of finding an APC mutation.[6] However, 10% to 30% of probands with germ-line APC mutations are de novo (new mutation) cases, and consequently, their parents are unaffected.[6,17] In addition, it is not uncommon for individuals with AFAP to have less than 10 cumulative adenomatous polyps.[4] In patients with fewer polyps, it is not clear whether genetic testing should be performed.[13] However, it is important that these individuals be closely followed up, and if multiple adenomas continue to develop, genetic testing should be reconsidered.

Unlike what is found in some of the other conditions described in this review, hyperplastic or hamartomatous colon polyps are not known to be associated with FAP/AFAP. Therefore, if multiple hyperplastic or hamartomatous colon polyps are found in an individual, a genetic testing of APC is unlikely to be informative. Other features associated with APC mutations that may assist with making a diagnosis of AFAP or FAP include fundic gland polyposis, duodenal adenomatous polyps, osteomas, CHRPE, desmoid tumors, and hepatoblastoma.[6]

CANCERS OF THE GASTROINTESTINAL TRACT

MUTYH-Associated Polyposis

As the name implies, MAP is a colonic polyposis condition caused by germ-line mutations in the *MUTYH* gene. Contrary to the other conditions described in this review, MAP is inherited in an autosomal-recessive pattern. In 2002, Al-Tassan et al.[18] were the first to describe a family with biallelic (homozygous or compound heterozygous) mutations in *MUTYH*, which is part of the base excision repair system. In this family, three siblings had CRC and/or multiple colorectal adenomas, but no detectable mutations in APC.[18] All three of the affected siblings were found to have compound heterozygous mutations in *MUTYH*, whereas the other four unaffected siblings did not.[18]

It is now widely accepted that MAP is associated with a significant increased risk for multiple colorectal adenomas and cancer. Whether monoallelic *MUTYH* carriers have a modest increase in risk of CRC is debatable.[19] Monoallelic mutations in *MUTYH* are found in 1% to 2% of the general population, whereas biallelic mutations account for less than 1% of all CRCs.[20]

Colonic Phenotype

There are a number of similarities between the colonic phenotype of MAP and AFAP, including the average number, proximal distribution, and young age at onset of adenomas and cancers.[4,19] *MUTYH*-associated polyposis is associated with a 28-fold increased risk of CRC, with a penetrance of 19% by the age of 50 years, 43% by 60 years, and 80% by 70 years.[19,21] Although the risk of CRC has been reported to be as high as 100%,[22] the actual penetrance is likely to be incomplete and similar to that of AFAP. The total number of polyps in MAP is also highly variable, with some individuals developing CRC without polyps, whereas others have more than 500 colorectal polyps.[23] Typically, affected individuals have between 10 and 100 polyps.[23]

Adenomas are the predominant polyp type seen not only in AFAP and FAP, but also in MAP. Unlike individuals with germ-line APC mutations, serrated polyps are common in MAP. Serrated polyps include hyperplastic polyps, sessile serrated polyps (also referred to as sessile serrated adenomas), and traditional serrated adenomas.[24] Boparai et al.[25] evaluated 17 individuals with MAP and found that almost one-half (47%) had hyperplastic and/or sessile serrated polyps. In addition, three met the criteria for hyperplastic polyposis, now known as serrated polyposis. The World Health Organization diagnostic criteria for serrated polyposis include an individual with any of the following: (1) at least five serrated polyps proximal to the sigmoid colon with at least two larger than 10 mm; (2) greater than 20 serrated polyps of any size, but distributed through the colon; and (3) any number of serrated polyps proximal to the sigmoid colon in an individual with a first-degree relative with serrated polyposis.[24] Interestingly, Chow et al.[26] also identified biallelic *MUTYH* mutations in 1 (~3%) of 38 cases meeting hyperplastic polyposis/serrated polyposis criteria. Another family involving three brothers with biallelic *MUTYH* mutations has recently been reported, further highlighting this variability in phenotype. Their history included one with CRC at the age of 48 years but had no additional polyps, another was 38 years old and reportedly met criteria for serrated polyposis but had only two confirmed adenomas, and the other brother was 46 years old and had four hyperplastic polyps removed.[27] Currently, the etiology of serrated polyposis is largely unknown; however, there is growing evidence that the base excision repair pathway may be involved in a minority of these cases.

Boparai et al.[25] also compared the frequency of *KRAS* mutations and G:C to T:A transversions in hyperplastic or sessile serrated polyps in individuals with MAP to controls. In MAP, 51 (70%) of 73 serrated polyps had *KRAS* mutations, and 48 (94%) of these 51 had G:C to T:A transversions, whereas in the control group, only 7 (17%) of 41 serrated polyps had *KRAS* mutations, and 2 (29%) of 7 had G:C to T:A transversions.[25] These findings support an association between MAP and serrated polyps.

Extracolonic Features

A number of extracolonic findings have been reported in individuals with MAP.[23] However, it is still unclear whether most of these manifestations are chance occurrences or due to an underlying defective *MUTYH*. In a study of 276 individuals with MAP, only two developed duodenal cancer.[22] However, compared with the general population, the risk of duodenal cancer was significantly elevated, with a standard incidence ratio of 129 and an estimated lifetime risk of 4%.[22] Although the lifetime risk of duodenal cancer is similar between MAP and FAP/AFAP (4% and 5%), gastric and duodenal polyps are far less common in MAP. Of 150 individuals with MAP who underwent an EGD, 11% had gastric polyps, whereas 17% had duodenal polyps.[22]

Extraintestinal malignancies have also been reported in MAP,[22] although the data supporting an association are conflicting.[28,29] Desmoid tumors, thyroid and brain cancer, CHRPE, osteomas, and epidermoid cysts are rarely seen in MAP.[23]

Genetic Counseling and Testing

Since the first reported family with biallelic *MUTYH* mutations was described in 2002, more than 500 individuals with MAP have been confirmed.[23] As was the case with this first MAP family, genetic testing strategies to evaluate for *MUTYH* are typically targeted toward individuals with multiple colorectal adenomas. However, there are many other factors that can influence genetic testing approaches for *MUTYH* and APC mutations. Family history; age at polyp onset; types, location, and total number of polyps; CRC history (including age at onset and location); ethnicity; and extracolonic features are just some of the factors that influence genetic testing strategies and detection rates. The purpose of this review was not to present every scenario and strategy for *MUTYH* and APC genetic testing, but instead to outline some key concepts and considerations when multiple adenomas are detected.

Given the inheritance pattern of MAP, it is uncommon for more than one generation to be affected; however, a family history of CRC in more than one generation does not exclude MAP. Consanguinity (sharing a common ancestor) is seen in some MAP families and is an important element to evaluate for when taking a history. Siblings of affected individuals have a one in four chance (25%) of having MAP, whereas parents and children are obligate carriers. Therefore, when there is clear evidence of recessive inheritance in a family (more than one sibling affected in a family, but no one else), genetic testing should start with *MUTYH*. APC should still be evaluated in these families if no *MUTYH* mutations are identified, because germ-line mosaicism can result in more than one affected sibling with FAP and unaffected parents.[30] To clarify risk to offspring, spouses of individuals with MAP should also be offered *MUTYH* genetic testing. This strategy has been shown to be cost-effective.[31]

Generally, germ-line APC mutations are more common than biallelic *MUTYH* mutations; therefore, unless there is clear evidence for recessive inheritance in a family, APC genetic testing typically precedes *MUTYH* analysis. There are two common mutations in *MUTYH* that are found in the majority of affected individuals: Y179C and G396D (previously known as Y165C and G382D). These hotspot mutations were found in the original MAP family.[18] According to Nielsen et al.,[23] a review up to 2009 revealed more than 100 distinct *MUTYH* mutations. In individuals with Northern European ancestry and MAP, at least one of the two hotspot mutations are found in 90% of cases.[23,32] Testing specifically for the hotspot mutations, followed by full *MUTYH* sequencing only if one of these mutations is found, is often performed. In other populations, the scope of *MUTYH* mutations is less well understood, and therefore, full gene sequencing of *MUTYH* is often performed in individuals of non–Northern European ancestry. Similar to APC, genetic testing of *MUTYH* is considered when greater than 10 adenomas are documented.[13,23] The detection rates of biallelic *MUTYH* mutations in individuals with 10 to 100 and 100 to 1,000 polyps are 28% and 14%, respectively.[23] Given the growing evidence that hyperplastic and sessile serrated polyps are associated with MAP, these polyps should also be included in the total polyp count when considering when to test someone for *MUTYH* mutations. Individuals with FAP/AFAP are not known to develop numerous serrated polyps; therefore, genetic testing of *APC* in someone with multiple serrated polyps is unlikely to be informative. The NCCN Clinical Practice Guidelines In Oncology (NCCN Guidelines®) Guidelines do not currently recommend genetic testing of *MUTYH* in individuals with multiple serrated polyps and no adenomas.[13]

It is not unusual for individuals with MAP or AFAP to present with early-onset CRC and few to no polyps.[4,33] However, a consensus as to whether genetic testing of *APC* or *MUTYH* should be performed in these cases has not yet been reached.[13,23]

Management

Colonoscopy screening starting at around the age of 25 years is recommended for individuals with MAP.[13] The frequency of screening depends on polyp burden. As is the case with AFAP and FAP, colectomy is advised when polyps become endoscopically uncontrollable. EGDs should be considered in the 30s and, if duodenal adenomas are found, managed the same as in AFAP and FAP.[13] Currently, the evidence does not support increased CRC screening in monoallelic *MUTYH* carriers.

HAMARTOMATOUS POLYPOSIS

Peutz–Jeghers Syndrome

PJS is an autosomal dominant condition caused by mutations in the *STK11/LKB1* gene. It is estimated to occur in 1 in 50,000 to 200,000 births.[34] The two most characteristic manifestations of PJS are the distinct gastrointestinal-type hamartomas, called Peutz–Jeghers polyps, and the mucocutaneous melanin pigmentation. Both of these features are included in the diagnostic criteria for PJS (Table 50.2). Although it is not 100% penetrant and can fade with time, mucocutaneous hyperpigmentation in PJS typically presents in childhood. By the age of 20 years, 50% of individuals present with small-bowel obstruction, intussusception, and/or bleeding due to small-bowel polyps.[35] The polyps in PJS can also number in the hundreds and are most often found in the small intestine, followed by the colon and the stomach.[34]

The cancer risks associated with PJS are more significant after the age of 30 years, although earlier-onset malignancies do occur. In the largest study to date of 419 individuals with PJS, the risk of developing any cancer was 2% by the age of 20 years, 5% by 30 years, 17% by 40 years, 31% by 50 years, 60% by 60 years, and 85% by 70 years.[36] Gastrointestinal tract cancers had the highest cumulative risk. The specific cancer risks associated with PJS are outlined in Table 50.3.

Juvenile Polyposis Syndrome

JPS is an autosomal-dominant condition caused by germ-line mutations in *SMAD4* or *BMPR1A* genes, with an incidence of 0.6 to 1 in 100,000 and a de novo rate of 25% to 50%.[37,38] Juvenile polyps are the hallmark lesion in JPS.[38] They are most commonly found in the colorectum and can number in the hundreds, although the carpeting of polyps is not usually seen in JPS like it is in FAP.[38] Of note, solitary juvenile polyps can occur in children without JPS (see Table 50.2). Hematochezia is the most common presenting symptom and, similar to PJS, intussusception and obstruction are common. The highest risk of cancer (see Table 50.3) in JPS is CRC. Gastric cancers typically occur only in the setting of gastric polyposis, which is more commonly present in individuals with

TABLE 50.2

Testing and Diagnostic Criteria for Peutz–Jeghers Syndrome, Juvenile Polyposis Syndrome, and Cowden Syndrome

PJS

A clinical diagnosis of PJS can be made when an individual has two or more of the following features:
(1) Two or more Peutz-Jeghers-type hamartomatous polyps of the small intestine
(2) Mucocutaneous hyperpigmentation of the mouth, lips, nose, eyes, genitalia, or fingers
(3) Family history of PJS

JPS

A clinical diagnosis of JPS is considered when any of the following are met:
(1) 3–5 juvenile polyps of the colorectum
(2) Juvenile polyps throughout the gastrointestinal tract
(3) ≥1 juvenile polyp in an individual with a family history of JPS

CS[a]

Genetic testing for CS is considered in individuals meeting any of the following criteria:
(1) Adult onset Lhermitte–Duclos disease
(2) Autism spectrum disorder and macrocephaly
(3) ≥2 major criteria (one must be macrocephaly)
(4) ≥3 major criteria without macrocephaly
(5) Bannayan–Riley–Ruvalcaba syndrome
(6) One major and ≥3 minor criteria
(7) ≥2 biopsy-proven trichilemmomas
(8) ≥4 minor criteria

Major Criteria	Minor Criteria
Multiple gastrointestinal (GI) hamartomas/ganglioneuromas	A single GI hamartoma/ ganglioneuroma
Nonmedullary thyroid cancer	Thyroid adenoma or multinodular goiter
Breast cancer	Fibrocystic disease of the breast
Endometrial cancer	Mental retardation (i.e., IQ ≤75)
Mucocutaneous lesions	Autism spectrum disorder
One biopsy proven trichilemmoma	Fibromas
Multiple palmoplantar keratoses	Renal cell carcinoma
Multiple cutaneous facial papules	Uterine fibroids
Macular pigmentation of glans penis	Lipomas
Multifocal/extensive oral mucosal papillomatosis	
Macrocephaly (megalocephaly) (at least 97th percentile)	

IQ, intelligence quotient.
[a] Adapted with permission from the NCCN Clinical Practice Guidelines in Oncology (NCCN Guidelines®) for Genetic/Familial High-Risk Assessment: Colorectal V.2.2015. © 2015 National Comprehensive Cancer Network, Inc. All rights reserved. The NCCN Guidelines® and illustrations herein may not be reproduced in any form for any purpose without the express written permission of the NCCN. To view the most recent and complete version of the NCCN Guidelines, go online to NCCN.org. NATIONAL COMPREHENSIVE CANCER NETWORK®, NCCN®, NCCN GUIDELINES®, and all other NCCN Content are trademarks owned by the National Comprehensive Cancer Network, Inc. Adapted with permission from the NCCN Clinical Practice Guidelines in Oncology (NCCN Guidelines®) for Genetic/Familial High-Risk Assessment: Breast and Ovarian V.1.2016. © 2016 National Comprehensive Cancer Network, Inc. All rights reserved. The NCCN Guidelines® and illustrations herein may not be reproduced in any form for any purpose without the express written permission of the NCCN. To view the most recent and complete version of the NCCN Guidelines, go online to NCCN.org. NATIONAL COMPREHENSIVE CANCER NETWORK®, NCCN®, NCCN GUIDELINES®, and all other NCCN Content are trademarks owned by the National Comprehensive Cancer Network, Inc.

Characteristic Features and Recommendations: Peutz–Jeghers Syndrome and Juvenile Polyposis Syndrome

Lifetime Cancer Risks	Management Recommendations	Nonmalignant Features
PJS (*STK11*)		
Breast (54%)	Annual mammogram and breast magnetic resonance imaging by age 25 y	Mucocutaneous pigmentation
Colon (39%)	Colonoscopy every 2–3 y by late teens	
Pancreas (11%–36%)	Magnetic resonance cholangiopancreatography or endoscopic ultrasound every 1–2 y	Peutz–Jeghers polyps
Stomach (29%)	Upper endoscopy by 2–3 y starting in late teens; consider small-bowel visualization (computed tomography [CT] enterography, small-bowel enteroclysis) by 8–10 y	
Small bowel (13%)	Small bowel visualization (CT or MRI enterography baseline at 8–10 y with follow-up interval based on findings but at least by age 18, then every 2–3 y, though this may be individualized, or with symptoms)	
Ovary[a] (21%) Uterine/cervix[b] (11%)	Annual pelvic examination and Pap smear; Consider transvaginal ultrasound	
Lung (15%)	No specific recommendations	
Testicle[c] (<1%)	Annual testicular examination	
JPS (*SMAD4* and *BMPR1A*)		
Colon (40%–50%)	Colonoscopy by age 15 y repeating annually if polyps are present and every 2–3 y if no polyps	Juvenile polyps Features of hereditary hemorrhagic telangiectasia
Stomach (21% if gastric polyps are present)	Upper endoscopy by age 15 y repeating annually if polyps are present and every 2–3 y if no polyps	Congenital defects

[a] Sex cord tumor with annular tubules.
[b] Adenoma malignum.
[c] Sertoli cell tumor.

mutations in *SMAD4* than in *BMPR1A*.[37] JPS occurring in infancy (also known as juvenile polyposis of infancy) is often fatal, but rare. Hereditary hemorrhagic telangiectasia symptoms, such as arteriovenous malformations, telangiectasia, and epistaxis, occur in some individuals with mutations in *SMAD4*, but not *BMPR1A*.[37]

Cowden Syndrome

CS, which is part of the phosphatase and tensin homolog (PTEN) hamartoma tumor syndrome, occurs in about 1 in 200,000 to 1 in 250,000 individuals and is caused by germ-line mutations in the *PTEN* gene.[39] It is a multisystem disorder associated with characteristic mucocutaneous features, macrocephaly, and a variety of cancers and gastrointestinal manifestations.[39] Although other malignancies may be seen in CS, the primary cancers associated with CS include breast (25% to 50%), nonmedullary thyroid (3% to 10%), and endometrial (5% to 10%).[39] A recent study estimated that the lifetime risk for these cancers in *PTEN* mutation carriers was 85%, 35%, and 28%, respectively.[40] However, these risks are likely overestimates, because Tan et al.[40] failed to accurately account for ascertainment bias in their study.

Gastrointestinal polyps are one of the most common features in CS.[41] Polyps develop throughout the gastrointestinal tract, from the esophagus to the rectum, and numerous polyps or diffuse polyposis can be seen.[41] Multiple, white flat plaques in the esophagus, called glycogenic acanthosis, also occur in the setting of CS. In a large study of 127 individuals with *PTEN* mutations, 39 underwent at least 1 EGD, and 8 (~23%) had glycogenic acanthosis, 26 (~67%) had duodenal and/or gastric polyps, and only 2 (5%) had fundic gland polyps.[41] Of the 67 individuals who underwent

at least 1 colonoscopy, 62 (~93%) had colonic polyps, and 16 met criteria for hyperplastic polyposis.[41] Although hamartomas predominate, a variety of other colon polyps also develop, including adenomatous, hyperplastic, sessile serrated, ganglioneuromatous, inflammatory, lymphoid, and lipomatous. Of all of the mutation carriers in this large study, nine (7%) were diagnosed with CRC.[41]

Peutz–Jeghers Syndrome, Juvenile Polyposis Syndrome, and Cowden Syndrome: Genetic Counseling and Testing

Hamartomatous polyps consist of an overgrowth of cells native to the tissue in which they occur. They are rare, account for a minority of all colon polyps, and can be a red flag for an underlying cancer predisposition syndrome. When hamartomatous polyps are found in an individual, the differential diagnosis depends, in part, on the histologic type, total number, and age at onset of the polyps. Hamartomas can often be misdiagnosed as other polyp types, and therefore, review by a gastrointestinal pathologist should be considered.[42] When hamartomatous colonic polyps are identified, EGD and a thorough physical examination may identify extracolonic manifestations leading to a precise diagnosis. A detailed family history is also imperative. Diagnostic criteria for JPS and PJS are summarized in Table 50.2. Guidelines for genetic testing of CS, which are quite extensive and include a number of extraintestinal features, are also included in Table 50.2. Given the complexity of genetic testing for CS, the NCCN updates their guidelines annually.[13] Management considerations are reviewed for PJS and JPS in Table 50.3 and are also updated annually by the NCCN.[13]

CONCLUSIONS

There are numerous presentations that may warrant genetic testing for hereditary colonic polyposis conditions. Simplified guidelines for referral for genetic counseling include individuals with any of the following: (1) greater than 10 colonic adenomas, (2) three or more hamartomatous polyps, or (3) at least one Peutz–Jeghers polyp. Other manifestations in these individuals may help target genetic testing to a specific condition. Once the genetic cause has been identified in an affected individual, predictive testing in at-risk relatives is critical. Family members who test negative can be spared the increased surveillance and risk-reducing procedures that are warranted for family members who test positive. It is important that health-care providers involved in the care of patients with hereditary colonic polyposis conditions stay updated with management guidelines because recommendations are constantly evolving.

REFERENCES

1. Petersen GM, Slack J, Nakamura Y. Screening guidelines and premorbid diagnosis of familial adenomatous polyposis using linkage. *Gastroenterology* 1991;100:1658–1664.
2. Foulkes WD. A tale of four syndromes: familial adenomatous polyposis, Gardner syndrome, attenuated APC and Turcot syndrome. *QJM* 1995;88:853–863.
3. Jasperson KW, Tuohy TM, Neklason DW, et al. Hereditary and familial colon cancer. *Gastroenterology* 2010;138:2044–2058.
4. Burt RW, Leppert MF, Slattery ML, et al. Genetic testing and phenotype in a large kindred with attenuated familial adenomatous polyposis. *Gastroenterology* 2004;127:444–451.
5. Gallagher MC, Phillips RK, Bulow S. Surveillance and management of upper gastrointestinal disease in familial adenomatous polyposis. *Fam Cancer* 2006;5:263–273.
6. Jasperson KW, Burt RW. APC-associated polyposis conditions. In: Pagon RA, Bird TD, Dolan CR, et al., eds. *Gene Reviews.* Seattle: University of Washington; 1993.
7. Burt RW. Gastric fundic gland polyps. *Gastroenterology* 2003;125:1462–1469.
8. Garrean S, Hering J, Saied A, et al. Gastric adenocarcinoma arising from fundic gland polyps in a patient with familial adenomatous polyposis syndrome. *Am Surg* 2008;74:79–83.
9. Nieuwenhuis MH, Casparie M, Mathus-Vliegen LM, et al. A nation-wide study comparing sporadic and familial adenomatous polyposis-related desmoid-type fibromatoses. *Int J Cancer* 2011;129:256–261.
10. Nieuwenhuis MH, Lefevre JH, Bulow S, et al. Family history, surgery, and APC mutation are risk factors for desmoid tumors in familial adenomatous polyposis: an international cohort study. *Dis Colon Rectum* 2011;54:1229–1234.
11. Sinha A, Tekkis PP, Gibbons DC, et al. Risk factors predicting desmoid occurrence in patients with familial adenomatous polyposis: a meta-analysis. *Colorectal Dis* 2011;13:1222–1229.
12. Nieuwenhuis MH, Mathus-Vliegen EM, Baeten CG, et al. Evaluation of management of desmoid tumours associated with familial adenomatous polyposis in Dutch patients. *Br J Cancer* 2011;104:37–42.
13. Provenzale D, et al. NCCN Clinical Practice Guidelines in Oncology (NCCN Guidelines®) Genetic/Familial High-Risk Assessment: Colorectal Version 2.2015. © 2015 National Comprehensive Cancer Network, Inc. Available at NCCN.org. Accessed: February 1, 2016.
14. Guillem JG, Wood WC, Moley JF, et al. ASCO/SSO review of current role of risk-reducing surgery in common hereditary cancer syndromes. *J Clin Oncol* 2006;24:4642–4660.
15. Bulow S, Christensen IJ, Hojen H, et al. Duodenal surveillance improves the prognosis after duodenal cancer in familial adenomatous polyposis. *Colorectal Dis* 2011;14:947–952.
16. Cromwell DM, Moore RD, Brensinger JD, et al. Cost analysis of alternative approaches to colorectal screening in familial adenomatous polyposis. *Gastroenterology* 1998;114:893–901.
17. Hes FJ, Nielsen M, Bik EC, et al. Somatic APC mosaicism: An underestimated cause of polyposis coli. *Gut* 2008;57:71–76.
18. Al-Tassan N, Chmiel NH, Maynard J, et al. Inherited variants of MYH associated with somatic G:C–>T:A mutations in colorectal tumors. *Nat Genet* 2002;30:227–232.
19. Lubbe SJ, Di Bernardo MC, Chandler IP, et al. Clinical implications of the colorectal cancer risk associated with MUTYH mutation. *J Clin Oncol* 2009;27:3975–3980.
20. Cleary SP, Cotterchio M, Jenkins MA, et al. Germline MutY human homologue mutations and colorectal cancer: a multisite case-control study. *Gastroenterology* 2009;136:1251–1260.
21. Jenkins MA, Croitoru ME, Monga N, et al. Risk of colorectal cancer in monoallelic and biallelic carriers of MYH mutations: a population-based case-family study. *Cancer Epidemiol Biomarkers Prev* 2006;15:312–314.
22. Vogt S, Jones N, Christian D, et al. Expanded extracolonic tumor spectrum in MUTYH-associated polyposis. *Gastroenterology* 2009;137:1976–1985, e1–e10.
23. Nielsen M, Morreau H, Vasen HF, et al. MUTYH-associated polyposis (MAP). *Crit Rev Oncol Hematol* 2011;79:1–16.
24. Snover DC, Ahnen DJ, Burt RW, et al. Serrated polyps of the colon and rectum and serrated polyposis. In: Bosman FT, Carneiro F, Hruban RH, et al., eds. *WHO Classification of Tumours of the Digestive System.* 4th ed. Lyon, France: IARC; 2010:160–165.
25. Boparai KS, Dekker E, Van Eeden S, et al. Hyperplastic polyps and sessile serrated adenomas as a phenotypic expression of MYH-associated polyposis. *Gastroenterology* 2008;135:2014–2018.
26. Chow E, Lipton L, Lynch E, et al. Hyperplastic polyposis syndrome: Phenotypic presentations and the role of MBD4 and MYH. *Gastroenterology* 2006;131:30–39.
27. Zorcolo L, Fantola G, Balestrino L, et al. MUTYH-associated colon disease: Adenomatous polyposis is only one of the possible phenotypes. A family report and literature review. *Tumori* 2011;97:676–680.
28. Out AA, Wasielewski M, Huijts PE, et al. MUTYH gene variants and breast cancer in a Dutch case-control study. *Breast Cancer Res Treat* 2012;134:219–227.
29. Santonocito C, Paradisi A, Capizzi R, et al. Common genetic variants of MUTYH are not associated with cutaneous malignant melanoma: Application of molecular screening by means of high-resolution melting technique in a pilot case-control study. *Int J Biol Markers* 2011;26:37–42.
30. Schwab AL, Tuohy TM, Condie M, et al. Gonadal mosaicism and familial adenomatous polyposis. *Fam Cancer* 2008;7:173–177.
31. Nielsen M, Hes FJ, Vasen HF, et al. Cost-utility analysis of genetic screening in families of patients with germline MUTYH mutations. *BMC Med Genet* 2007;8:42.
32. Goodenberger M, Lindor NM. Lynch syndrome and MYH-associated polyposis: Review and testing strategy. *J Clin Gastroenterol* 2011;45:488–500.
33. Wang L, Baudhuin LM, Boardman LA, et al. MYH mutations in patients with attenuated and classic polyposis and with young-onset colorectal cancer without polyps. *Gastroenterology* 2004; 127:9–16.
34. Offerhaus GJA, Billaud M, Gruber SB. Peutz–Jeghers syndrome. In: Bosman FT, Carneiro F, Hruban RH, et al., eds. *WHO Classification of Tumours of the Digestive System.* 4th ed. Lyon, France: IARC; 2010:168–170.
35. Latchford AR, Phillips RK. Gastrointestinal polyps and cancer in Peutz–Jeghers syndrome: clinical aspects. *Fam Cancer* 2011;10:455–461.
36. Hearle N, Schumacher V, Menko FH, et al. Frequency and spectrum of cancers in the Peutz–Jeghers syndrome. *Clin Cancer Res* 2006;12:3209–3215.
37. Gammon A, Jasperson K, Kohlmann W, et al. Hamartomatous polyposis syndromes. *Best Pract Res Clin Gastroenterol* 2009;23:219–231.
38. Offerhaus GJ, Howe JR. Juvenile polyposis. In: Bosman FT, Carneiro F, Hruban RH, et al., eds. *WHO Classification of Tumours of the Digestive System.* 4th ed. Lyon, France: IARC; 2010:166–167.
39. Pilarski R. Cowden syndrome: a critical review of the clinical literature. *J Genet Couns* 2009;18:13–27.
40. Tan MH, Mester JL, Ngeow J, et al. Lifetime cancer risks in individuals with germline PTEN mutations. *Clin Cancer Res* 2012;18:400–407.
41. Heald B, Mester J, Rybicki L, et al. Frequent gastrointestinal polyps and colorectal adenocarcinomas in a prospective series of PTEN mutation carriers. *Gastroenterology* 2010;139:1927–1933.
42. Sweet K, Willis J, Zhou XP, et al. Molecular classification of patients with unexplained hamartomatous and hyperplastic polyposis. *JAMA* 2005;294:2465–2473.

51 Genetic Testing in Colon Cancer (Nonpolyposis Syndromes)

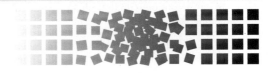

Leigha Senter-Jamieson

INTRODUCTION

Approximately 5% to 10% of colorectal cancers (CRC) are hereditary and are often categorized by the presence or absence of polyposis as a predominant feature. Lynch syndrome (LS), also sometimes referred to as hereditary nonpolyposis CRC, is the most common form of hereditary CRC, accounting for approximately 2.2%[1] of population-based CRCs diagnosed in the United States. LS also accounts for 2.3%[2] of all newly diagnosed endometrial cancers (EC), and individuals with LS also have an increased risk of developing other cancers, including cancers of the ovary, stomach, small bowel, urothelium, and biliary tract.[3] Given these increased cancer risks, cancer screening recommendations for individuals with LS differ significantly from general population screening recommendations with a goal of reducing the cancer risk and burden to the extent possible.

Mutations in one of four mismatch repair genes (*MLH1*, *MSH2*, *MSH6*, and *PMS2*) cause LS, and clinical genetic testing is available for all of them. Unlike most other hereditary cancer syndromes, however, clinical testing for LS typically begins with microsatellite instability (MSI) testing and/or immunohistochemical (IHC) staining of tumor tissue before germ-line genetic testing. This difference in testing approach, although not always possible, allows for targeted genetic analysis and, in most cases, reduced cost. Here, we review key considerations in genetic counseling for LS.

Cancer Risks

CRCs and ECs are the two most common LS-associated malignancies, and there have been several calculations of lifetime cancer risks reported in the literature. Differences in ascertainment and testing approaches have led not only to a wealth of data, but also to a wide range of risk estimates for consideration by clinicians and patients. Consistently, studies have found that the lifetime CRC risk for men with LS is higher than the risk for women with LS. The lifetime CRC risk for males is 27% to 92%, whereas the risk for females is 22% to 68%.[4,5] The most recent large study of carriers of *MLH1*, *MSH2*, and *MSH6* mutations estimated lifetime CRC risks for males and females to be 38% and 31%, respectively.[6] The average age at CRC diagnosis tends to be younger in LS (estimated 45 to 59 years) than that in the general population.[6,7] The lifetime risk of EC for women with LS based on recent data is estimated to be 33% to 39%.[6,8] Individuals with LS who have already been diagnosed with CRC also have an increased risk (10-year risk of 16%) of developing a second primary CRC.[9]

In addition to sex differences in LS-associated cancer risks, there appear to be some differences in gene-specific–associated cancer risks, as well. *MLH1* and *MSH2* seem to be associated with a higher overall cancer risk than risks associated with *MSH6* or *PMS2*.[10,11] A variable expression of phenotype both within and among families with LS is common. Therefore, as a general rule, management of families with LS (discussed later) should always take into account the family history.

Malignancies of the ovary, stomach, small bowel, urothelium, and biliary tract are also seen with greater frequency in individuals with LS when compared with the general population. Although cumulative risk estimates of these less common tumor types have been published, they are usually based on fewer cases than studies focused on CRCs and ECs, and have typically shown a lifetime cancer risk of less than 10%.[3] There have also been reports of LS-associated pancreatic and breast cancers, but the data have been inconsistent. A recent prospective study showed an increased risk of developing both tumor types when comparing carriers of *MMR* gene mutations to their unaffected relatives.[12] Additional data are necessary, however, to determine whether screening recommendations should change based on these reported risks. Some individuals with LS also have a predisposition to developing sebaceous lesions and keratoacanthomas of the skin. When an individual has one of these lesions in addition to a visceral organ malignancy, they have a variant of LS called Muir–Torre syndrome.[13] Some recent studies suggest that these skin lesions are more common in LS than originally thought and that sebaceous tumors of the skin should be considered part of the typical LS spectrum.[14] Another variant of LS characterized by the presence of glioblastomas is called Turcot syndrome. Turcot syndrome is more commonly caused by mutations in the *APC* gene but has been described in individuals with mismatch repair (MMR) deficiency, as well.[15]

CLINICAL CLASSIFICATION: AMSTERDAM CRITERIA AND BETHESDA GUIDELINES

In 1991, the International Collaborative Group on Hereditary Non-Polyposis CRC wrote the Amsterdam I criteria[16] and revised them in 1999 (Amsterdam II criteria)[17] to clinically classify families as having LS (Table 51.1). The Amsterdam criteria rely heavily on extensive family history and do not take into account the full spectrum of possible LS-associated tumors. The less stringent Bethesda guidelines (written in 1997 and revised in 2004)[18,19] (Table 51.2) were written to include these less common LS-associated tumors as well as pathologic features that are common in LS-associated CRCs. Unlike the Amsterdam criteria, which were meant to diagnose LS based on familial criteria, the Bethesda guidelines were meant to determine who should have tumor screenings for LS and relied less on family history. It has been repeatedly shown, however, that these clinical classification systems do not reliably predict LS in all patient populations, particularly for those populations outside the cancer genetics clinics dedicated to high-risk patients.[1,20]

TUMOR SCREENING

Microsatellites are pieces of DNA sequence where a single nucleotide or group of nucleotides is repeated multiple times. In general, the number of repeated nucleotide sequences should remain the same within a person's cells, but when this number of repeats

TABLE 51.1

Revised Amsterdam Criteria

≥3 relatives with colorectal, endometrial, small bowel, ureter, and/or renal pelvis cancer AND

One of these relatives is a first-degree relative[a] of the other two AND

≥2 successive generations are affected AND

At least one diagnosis is at the age of <50 y

Familial adenomatous polyposis is excluded

Tumors should be verified pathologically/histologically

[a] First-degree relative: parent, sibling, or child.
From Vasen HF, Watson P, Mecklin JP, et al. New clinical criteria for hereditary nonpolyposis colorectal cancer (HNPCC, Lynch syndrome) proposed by the International Collaborative group on HNPCC. *Gastroenterology* 1999;116:1453–1456.

TABLE 51.3

Genetic Testing Strategies Based on IHC Pattern

Absence MLH1 and PMS2	*MLH1* methylation and/or *BRAF* testing[a] OR *MLH1* germ-line testing[b] ■ If negative, consider *PMS2* germ-line testing[20]
Absence PMS2 only	*PMS2* germ-line testing ■ If negative consider *MLH1* germ-line testing[21]
Absence MSH2 and MSH6	*MSH2* germ-line testing ■ If negative, *TACSTD1* deletion testing ■ If negative, *MSH6* germline testing
Absence MSH6 only	*MSH6* germ-line testing ■ If negative, consider *MSH2* germ-line testing

[a] If personal/family history highly suggestive of LS, it is appropriate to forgo *MLH1* methylation/*BRAF* testing.
[b] Unless otherwise noted, "germ-line testing" here refers to sequencing/large rearrangement testing.

differs in one or two alleles, MSI is present.[21] In the case of LS, five microsatellite markers are used as the standard with which to measure MSI, and a tumor is considered to have a high level of MSI (MSI-H) if at least 40% of the markers are unstable.[22] Nearly all LS-associated tumors display MSI, but the presence of MSI is not diagnostic of LS, given that approximately 10% to 15% of all CRCs, in general, also display MSI.[23,24] MSI testing, however, can be used as a screening tool to help identify individuals for whom germ-line genetic testing for mutations in *MLH1*, *MSH2*, *MSH6*, and/or *PMS2* is indicated. A clinical diagnosis of LS can be made if a person has an MSI-H CRC and meets the Amsterdam II criteria (see Table 51.1).

Immunohistochemistry can be used to determine the presence or absence of MMR proteins in a tumor specimen and is another available screening test for LS. The absence of one or more MMR proteins in tumor tissue indicates dysfunction of the corresponding *MMR* gene, but additional analyses are required to determine if the dysfunction is germ line or somatic in nature. The benefit of performing IHC staining over MSI testing is that results from IHC staining can direct the approach to genetic testing. For instance, if a patient has CRC that demonstrates an absence of MSH2 and MSH6 proteins, testing for MSH2 with procession to testing for MSH6 if the MSH2 test results are negative is recommended. In

TABLE 51.2

Revised Bethesda Guidelines

Individuals with CRC should be tested for MSI if they have any of the following:
■ CRC at the age of <50 y
■ Synchronous CRC (>1 CRC at the same time) or metachronous CRC (>1 CRC diagnosed at different times) or other LS-associated tumors[a]
■ CRC with MSI-H histology (tumor-infiltrating lymphocytes, Crohnlike lymphocytic reaction, mucinous or signet-ring differentiation, medullary growth pattern) in a patient aged <60 y
■ CRC or LS-associated tumor[a] diagnosed at the age of <50 y in FDR
■ CRC or LS-associated tumor[a] in 2 FDR and/or SDR at any age

[a] CRC, EC, stomach, small bowel, ovary, pancreas, ureter and renal pelvis, biliary tract, brain tumor, sebaceous adenomas, keratoacanthomas.
FDR, first-degree relative (parent, sibling, child); SDR, second-degree relative (grandparent, aunt, uncle, grandchild).
From Umar A, Boland CR, Terdiman JP, et al. Revised Bethesda guidelines for hereditary nonpolyposis colorectal cancer (Lynch syndrome) and microsatellite instability. *J Natl Cancer Inst* 2004;96:261–268.

the context of this IHC result, it is generally not necessary to test for mutations in *MLH1* and/or *PMS2*. Strategies for genetic testing based on IHC results are included in Table 51.3.[25,26] In comparing tumor screening strategies, using MSI and IHC staining together will identify the majority of LS cases. Because the sensitivity of either test is not 100%, using either test alone will leave 5% to 10% of LS cases undetected.[27,28]

Epigenetic events unrelated to LS can cause a tumor to demonstrate MSI and an absence of MLH1 and PMS2 proteins upon IHC staining. These results can often be attributed to hypermethylation of the *MLH1* promoter and/or a somatic *BRAF* mutation (V600E). Several studies have shown that the V600E *BRAF* mutations are not associated with LS, and there have been very few exceptions.[11,29] Both of these tests can be performed on CRC tissue to help determine whether germ-line genetic testing should be pursued, further streamlining the genetic testing process, but this should be interpreted in the context of clinical familial presentation because sensitivities and specificities for these tests are not 100%. It is important to note that it is possible but rare to have inherited *MLH1* promoter hypermethylation.[30]

Similar approaches to screening EC with MSI and/or IHC staining are appropriate. However, because somatic *BRAF* mutations are uncommon in ECs, *BRAF* testing is not an appropriate test for ECs that are MSI-H and/or MLH1- and PMS2-protein deficient.[31] There are less data to support MSI and/or IHC testing using other LS-associated tumor tissue, but many reports suggest that it is at least feasible in the absence of additional testing options.[32]

In 2009, the Evaluation of Genomic Application in Practice and Prevention Working Group recommended that individuals with newly diagnosed CRCs be offered genetic testing for LS. Although the Evaluation of Genomic Application in Practice and Prevention Working Group did not specify the best approach for genetic testing, performing a tumor analysis with IHC staining allows for more targeted genetic testing and was considered to be an acceptable strategy.[33] In addition, multiple reports have shown that tumor screening with IHC staining is a cost-effective strategy for identifying LS in the CRC patient population.[34,35] Ladabaum et al.[35] compared the differences among multiple testing strategies with regard to effect of life-years, cancer morbidity and mortality, and cost. They concluded that IHC staining with inclusion of *BRAF* gene testing if the MLH1 protein was absent was the preferred method of identifying LS among CRC patients.[35] The effectiveness of screening for LS in these reports has been dependent on the ability to test family members of the initially diagnosed

LS patient; therefore, genetic counseling and dissemination of information to relatives of probands are crucial for an effective diagnosis and the prevention of cancer.

GENETIC TESTING

In many situations, as mentioned previously, tumor screening tests are performed before germ-line genetic testing, but there are situations where this is not possible or desired (e.g., sufficient tumor tissue is unavailable, all individuals affected with cancer in a family are deceased). In the absence of IHC results to direct genetic testing, germ-line testing is typically done in a stepwise fashion beginning with *MLH1* and *MSH2*, which account for 32% and 38% of mutations, respectively.[9] If no mutations are identified, testing for mutations in *MSH6* and *PMS2* is indicated. Mutations in these two genes are less common and account for 14% and 15% of LS, respectively.[9] It is important for testing to include sequencing as well as an analysis of deletions and duplications because all mutation types have been reported in the *MMR* genes.

Recently, deletions in *TACSTD1* (also known as *EPCAM*), which is not an *MMR* gene, have been reported to cause an inactivation of *MSH2* and a lack of expression of the MSH2 protein when IHC staining is performed. Therefore, testing for deletions in *TACSTD1* is indicated when the MSH2 protein is absent on IHC staining, but no germ-line *MSHS2* mutation has been identified.[36]

GENETIC COUNSELING FOR LYNCH SYNDROME

Inherited in an autosomal dominant manner, first-degree relatives of individuals with LS have a 50% chance of having inherited the syndrome as well, making the communication of these risks to family members of patients with LS very important. Data have shown that compliance with the screening recommendations, as follows, is effective at reducing the risk of dying of cancer in individuals with LS, and this should be communicated to at-risk families. A large study of *MMR* mutation carriers in Finland found that despite the increased risks of CRCs and ECs, cancer mortality was not increased when individuals followed the intensive screening protocol and/or opted to have prophylactic surgery.[37]

MANAGEMENT OF LYNCH SYNDROME

Individuals with LS require personalized management planning with the goal of reducing their cancer risks. Although many groups have put forth screening recommendations in the literature, the LS surveillance and screening recommendations from the National Comprehensive Cancer Network, which are updated annually, are commonly used in clinical practice. Based on these current recommendations, individuals with LS should have colonoscopy every 1 to 2 years beginning at the age of 20 to 25 years or 2 to 5 years earlier than the youngest CRC in the family if diagnosed before the age of 25 years. (A colonoscopy may be recommended to start at the age of 30 years in families with *MSH6* and *PMS2* mutations if the CRC age at onset in the family is not younger than the age of 30 years given the reduced penetrance with these genes.) Given that there is no clear evidence to support screening for endometrial and/or ovarian cancers, women with LS are recommended to consider a prophylactic hysterectomy and a bilateral salpingo-oophorectomy upon completion of childbearing. Some clinicians may find endometrial sampling, transvaginal ultrasound, and CA-125 serum screening to be helpful; however, these tools should be used at their discretion. To screen for gastric and small-bowel cancers, individuals with LS should consider an esophagogastroduodenoscopy with an extended duodenoscopy and a capsule endoscopy every 2 to 3 years beginning at the age of 30 to 35 years. An annual urinalysis beginning at the age of 25 to 30 years can be used to screen for urothelial cancers, and an annual physical examination to assess for symptoms of central nervous system tumors is reasonable.[38]

A 2011 study by Burn et al.[39] showed through a randomized trial with postintervention double-blind follow-up that daily use of 600 mg of aspirin for a minimum of 25 months reduced the risk of CRCs by almost 60% in individuals with LS. Like other studies of aspirin use on cancer risk, cumulative use seemed to make a difference in the study because a reduced risk became evident over time. The optimum dose and duration of use of aspirin in individuals with LS still need to be established, but based on this evidence, many clinicians are considering aspirin therapy as chemoprevention in this population.

ACKNOWLEDGMENT

The author thanks Kory Jasperson for his review of the manuscript.

REFERENCES

1. Hampel H, Frankel WL, Martin E, et al. Screening for the Lynch syndrome (hereditary nonpolyposis colorectal cancer). *N Engl J Med* 2005;352: 1851–1860.
2. Hampel H, Panescu J, Lockman J, et al. Comment on: Screening for Lynch syndrome (hereditary nonpolyposis colorectal cancer) among endometrial cancer patients. *Cancer Res* 2007;67:9603.
3. Barrow E, Robinson L, Alduaij W, et al. Cumulative lifetime incidence of extracolonic cancers in Lynch syndrome: a report of 121 families with proven mutations. *Clin Genet* 2009;75:141–149.
4. Vasen HF, Wijnen JT, Menko FH, et al. Cancer risk in families with hereditary nonpolyposis colorectal cancer diagnosed by mutation analysis. *Gastroenterology* 1996;110:1020–1027.
5. Quehenberger F, Vasen HF, van Houwelingen HC. Risk of colorectal and endometrial cancer for carriers of mutations of the hMLH1 and hMSH2 gene: correction for ascertainment. *J Med Genet* 2005;42:491–496.
6. Bonadona V, Bonaiti B, Olschwang S, et al. Cancer risks associated with germline mutations in MLH1, MSH2, and MSH6 genes in Lynch syndrome. *JAMA* 2011;305:2304–2310.
7. Hampel H, Stephens JA, Pukkala E, et al. Cancer risk in hereditary nonpolyposis colorectal cancer syndrome: Later age of onset. *Gastroenterology* 2005;129:415–421.
8. Stoffel E, Mukherjee B, Raymond VM, et al. Calculation of risk of colorectal and endometrial cancer among patients with Lynch syndrome. *Gastroenterology* 2009;137:1621–1627.
9. Palomaki GE, McClain MR, Melillo S, et al. EGAPP supplementary evidence review: DNA testing strategies aimed at reducing morbidity and mortality from Lynch syndrome. *Genet Med* 2009;11:42–65.
10. Baglietto L, Lindor NM, Dowty JG, et al. Risks of Lynch syndrome cancers for MSH6 mutation carriers. *J Natl Cancer Inst* 2010;102:193–201.
11. Senter L, Clendenning M, Sotamaa K, et al. The clinical phenotype of Lynch syndrome due to germ-line PMS2 mutations. *Gastroenterology* 2008; 135:419–428.
12. Win AK, Young JP, Lindor NM, et al. Colorectal and other cancer risks for carriers and noncarriers from families with a DNA mismatch repair gene mutation: A prospective cohort study. *J Clin Oncol* 2012;30:958–964.
13. Lynch HT, Lynch PM, Pester J, et al. The cancer family syndrome. Rare cutaneous phenotypic linkage of Torre's syndrome. *Arch Intern Med* 1981;141:607–611.
14. South CD, Hampel H, Comeras I, et al. The frequency of Muir-Torre syndrome among Lynch syndrome families. *J Natl Cancer Inst* 2008;100:277–281.
15. Hamilton SR, Liu B, Parsons RE, et al. The molecular basis of Turcot's syndrome. *N Engl J Med* 1995;332:839–847.
16. Vasen HF, Mecklin JP, Khan PM, et al. The International Collaborative Group on Hereditary Non-Polyposis Colorectal Cancer (ICG-HNPCC). *Dis Colon Rectum* 1991;34:424–425.
17. Vasen HF, Watson P, Mecklin JP, et al. New clinical criteria for hereditary nonpolyposis colorectal cancer (HNPCC, Lynch syndrome) proposed by the International Collaborative group on HNPCC. *Gastroenterology* 1999;116: 1453–1456.

18. Rodriguez-Bigas MA, Boland CR, Hamilton SR, et al. A National Cancer Institute workshop on hereditary nonpolyposis colorectal cancer syndrome: meeting highlights and Bethesda guidelines. *J Natl Cancer Inst* 1997; 89:1758–1762.

19. Umar A, Boland CR, Terdiman JP, et al. Revised Bethesda guidelines for hereditary nonpolyposis colorectal cancer (Lynch syndrome) and microsatellite instability. *J Natl Cancer Inst* 2004;96:261–268.

20. Morrison J, Bronner M, Leach BH, et al. Lynch syndrome screening in newly diagnosed colorectal cancer in general pathology practice: from the revised Bethesda guidelines to a universal approach. *Scand J Gastroenterol* 2012;46:1340–1348.

21. de la Chapelle A, Hampel H. Clinical relevance of microsatellite instability in colorectal cancer. *J Clin Oncol* 2010;28:3380–3387.

22. Boland CR, Thibodeau SN, Hamilton SR, et al. A National Cancer Institute Workshop on Microsatellite Instability for cancer detection and familial predisposition: development of international criteria for the determination of microsatellite instability in colorectal cancer. *Cancer Res* 1998;58: 5248–5257.

23. Hampel H, Frankel WL, Martin E, et al. Feasibility of screening for Lynch syndrome among patients with colorectal cancer. *J Clin Oncol* 2008;26: 5783–5788.

24. Samowitz WS, Curtin K, Lin HH, et al. The colon cancer burden of genetically defined hereditary nonpolyposis colon cancer. *Gastroenterology* 2001;121: 830–838.

25. Niessen RC, Kleibeuker JH, Westers H, et al. PMS2 involvement in patients suspected of Lynch syndrome. *Genes Chromosomes Cancer* 2009;48: 322–329.

26. Zighelboim I, Powell MA, Babb SA, et al. Epitope-positive truncating MLH1 mutation and loss of PMS2: Implications for IHC-directed genetic testing for Lynch syndrome. *Fam Cancer* 2009;8:501–504.

27. Lindor NM, Burgart LJ, Leontovich O, et al. Immunohistochemistry versus microsatellite instability testing in phenotyping colorectal tumors. *J Clin Oncol* 2002;20:1043–1048.

28. Ruszkiewicz A, Bennett G, Moore J, et al. Correlation of mismatch repair genes immunohistochemistry and microsatellite instability status in HNPCC-associated tumours. *Pathology* 2002;34:541–547.

29. Loughrey MB, Waring PM, Tan A, et al. Incorporation of somatic BRAF mutation testing into an algorithm for the investigation of hereditary non-polyposis colorectal cancer. *Fam Cancer* 2007;6:301–310.

30. Hitchins MP, Ward RL. Constitutional (germline) MLH1 epimutation as an aetiological mechanism for hereditary non-polyposis colorectal cancer. *J Med Genet* 2009;46:793–802.

31. Mutch DG, Powell MA, Mallon MA, et al. RAS/RAF mutation and defective DNA mismatch repair in endometrial cancers. *Am J Obstet Gynecol* 2004;190:935–942.

32. Weissman SM, Bellcross C, Bittner CC, et al. Genetic counseling considerations in the evaluation of families for Lynch syndrome—a review. *J Genet Couns* 2011;20:5–19.

33. Evaluation of Genomic Applications in Practice and Prevention (EGAPP) Working Group. Recommendations from the EGAPP Working Group: Genetic testing strategies in newly diagnosed individuals with colorectal cancer aimed at reducing morbidity and mortality from Lynch syndrome in relatives. *Genet Med* 2009;11:35–41.

34. Mvundura M, Grosse SD, Hampel H, et al. The cost-effectiveness of genetic testing strategies for Lynch syndrome among newly diagnosed patients with colorectal cancer. *Genet Med* 2010;12:93–104.

35. Ladabaum U, Wang G, Terdiman J, et al. Strategies to identify the Lynch syndrome among patients with colorectal cancer: A cost-effectiveness analysis. *Ann Intern Med* 2011;155:69–79.

36. Niessen RC, Hofstra RM, Westers H, et al. Germline hypermethylation of MLH1 and EPCAM deletions are a frequent cause of Lynch syndrome. *Genes Chromosomes Cancer* 2009;48:737–744.

37. Jarvinen HJ, Renkonen-Sinisalo L, Aktan-Collan K, et al. Ten years after mutation testing for Lynch syndrome: cancer incidence and outcome in mutation-positive and mutation-negative family members. *J Clin Oncol* 2009;27:4793–4797.

38. National Comprehensive Cancer Network. NCCN Guidelines & Clinical Resources. NCCN Guidelines for Detection, Prevention, and Risk Reduction [v.1.2012]. 2012. http://www.nccn.org/professionals/physician_gls/recently_updated.asp

39. Burn J, Gerdes AM, Macrae F, et al. Long-term effect of aspirin on cancer risk in carriers of hereditary colorectal cancer: an analysis from the CAPP2 randomised controlled trial. *Lancet* 2011;378:2081–2087.

CANCERS OF THE GASTROINTESTINAL TRACT

52 Cancer of the Rectum

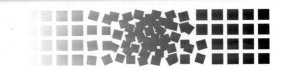

Steven K. Libutti, Christopher G. Willett, Leonard B. Saltz,
and Rebecca A. Levine

INTRODUCTION

Information concerning epidemiology and systemic approaches to
the management of both colon and rectal cancer was given in another chapter in this book. This chapter will focus on issues unique
to rectal cancer with an emphasis on radiation, combined modality therapy, and sphincter-preserving surgery.

ANATOMY

The anatomy of the rectum can be very confusing as there are differing definitions of the relevant landmarks. In the upper portion
of the rectum, there are changes both in the musculature of the
large bowel and in the relationship to the peritoneal covering that
roughly coincide. In the lower portion of the rectum, the mucosal
changes occur at roughly the same location as the anal sphincter.

The anatomy of the rectum is usually divided into three portions (Fig. 52.1). The lower rectum is the area approximately from
3 to 6 cm from the anal verge. The midrectum goes from 5 to 6,
to 8 to 10 cm, and the upper rectum extends approximately from
8 to 10, to 12 to 15 cm from the anal verge, although the retroperitoneal portion of the large bowel often reaches its upper limit
approximately 12 cm from the anal verge. In some patients, especially elderly women, the peritonealized portion of the large bowel
can be located much lower than these definitions. The determination of the location of the boundary between rectum and sigmoid
colon is important in defining adjuvant therapy, with the rectum
usually being operationally defined as that area of the large bowel
that is at least partially retroperitoneal.

Externally, the upper extent of the rectum can be identified
where the tenia spread to form a longitudinal coat of muscle. The
upper third of the rectum is surrounded by peritoneum on its anterior and lateral surfaces but is retroperitoneal posteriorly without
any serosal covering. At the rectovesical or rectouterine pouch, the
rectum becomes completely extra-/retroperitoneal. The rectum
follows the curve of the sacrum in its lower two-thirds. It enters the
anal canal at the level of the levator ani. The anorectal ring is at
the level of the puborectalis sling portion of the levator muscles.

The location of a rectal tumor is most commonly indicated by
the distance between the anal verge, dentate (pectinate or mucocutaneous) line, or anorectal ring and the lower edge of the tumor.
These points of reference are all different for different individuals. Also, these measurements differ depending on the method of
measurement. This can be important clinically, as the measurement from a flexible endoscopy can substantially overestimate
the distance to the tumor from the anal verge or other landmark.
The distance from the anal sphincter musculature is clinically of
more importance than the distance from the anal verge, as it has
implications for the ability to perform sphincter-sparing surgery.
The lack of a peritoneal covering over most of the rectum is a
major reason for the higher risk of local failure after primary surgical management of rectal cancer compared to colon cancer. The
mesorectum is usually used as the structure to define the extent
of a total mesorectal excision (TME), with most of the perirectal
fatty tissue and perirectal lymph nodes (LN) contained within its
boundaries.

Lymphatic Drainage

The lymphatic drainage of the upper rectum follows the course of
the superior hemorrhoidal artery toward the inferior mesenteric
artery. Lymph nodes that are above the midrectum and therefore
drain along the superior hemorrhoidal artery are often part of the
mesentery that is removed during resections of the intraperitoneal
portion of the colon. Lesions that arise in the rectum below approximately 6 cm are in a region of the rectum that is drained
by lymphatics that follow the middle hemorrhoidal artery. Nodes
involved from a cancer in this region can include the internal iliac
nodes and the nodes of the obturator fossa. These regions deserve
particular attention during the resection and irradiation of lesions
in this location. When lesions occur below the dentate line, the
lymphatic drainage is via the inguinal nodes and external iliac
chain, which has major therapeutic implications, especially for
the radiation fields. The corollary of this high risk of inguinal node
involvement for the very low-lying tumors is that tumors located
above the dentate line are at low risk of inguinal node involvement, and these nodes as well as the external iliacs do not need
to be treated.

Bowel Function

Fecal continence is maintained through the function of both the
sphincter mechanism and the preservation of the normal pelvic
floor musculature, which creates a neorectal angle or rectal sling.
The pelvic floor is composed of the levator ani muscles, which
separate the pelvis from the perineum and ischiorectal fossa. The
urethra, vagina, and anus pass through the levator muscles.

Preservation of fecal continence during surgery for rectal
cancer is therefore dependent on a thorough understanding of the
anatomic relationships of the musculature and the sphincter
mechanism. Maintenance of the sphincter apparatus without
preservation of the muscular angles will not have the desired result. These anatomic constraints, especially with respect to lateral
margins, make the use of adjuvant chemotherapy and radiation
therapy critical to a successful surgical outcome. This is true from
both an oncologic as well as a bowel function perspective.

Autonomic Nerves

The preservation of both bladder and sexual function depends on
the surgeon's understanding of the autonomic nerve supply to the
pelvic organs.[1,2] The hypogastric plexus is formed from the sympathetic trunks as they converge over the sacral promontory. These
sympathetic nerves are found beneath the pelvic peritoneum

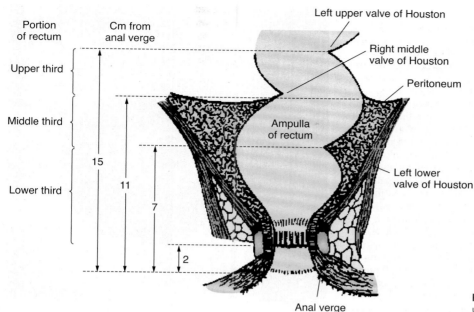

Portion of rectum | Cm from anal verge

Left upper valve of Houston

Right middle valve of Houston

Peritoneum

Upper third

Middle third

Ampulla of rectum

Lower third

15

11

7

Left lower valve of Houston

2

Anal verge

Figure 52.1 Division of the rectum into upper, middle, and lower thirds.

CANCERS OF THE GASTROINTESTINAL TRACT

along the lateral pelvic sidewalls lateral to the mesorectum. The second, third, and fourth sacral nerve roots give rise to parasympathetic fibers to the pelvic viscera. The parasympathetic fibers proceed laterally as the nervi erigentes to join the sympathetic fibers at the site of the pelvic plexus that is just lateral and somewhat anterior to the tips of the seminal vesicle in men.[1,2] In order to preserve these structures and, therefore, sexual and bladder function, a sharp rather than a blunt technique should be used to dissect the mesorectum.[3–6]

STAGING

Standard clinicopathologic staging is the best indicator of prognosis for patients with rectal cancer. For rectal cancer, it is increasingly common to use clinical staging as the basis for the decision to initiate neoadjuvant chemoradiation therapy. Therefore, the accuracy of that initial staging is critically important, both for management and for prognosis. There have been a large number of studies that have evaluated other prognostic markers, including pathologic, socioeconomic, and molecular, as described more fully in Chapter 49. However, even though many of these appear to have prognostic value, there are none that are commonly used to define management. This is related to the large number of tests that could be used, the lack of standardization of these tests, as well as the lack of knowledge as to how to incorporate them into the patient management scheme. The molecular marker that has engendered the most interest is the deletion of 18q.[7] These markers have been fully reviewed elsewhere.[8,9]

The staging system that should be used in the evaluation of patients with rectal cancer is the American Joint Committee on Cancer/International Union Against Cancer TNM (tumor, node, metastases) staging system (fully described in Chapter 49), which has been recently revised to subcategorize patients with stage III (node-positive) tumors. The Dukes staging system or its multiple modifications has been used for many years, but provides less information than the TNM system and should not be used. There have been gradual changes in the TNM system that primarily reflect the stage grouping rather than the system itself. The other systems should be acknowledged for their historical interest and for initially defining many of the high-risk factors for this disease.

Patients now often have both a clinical (preoperative) stage, which may define the need for neoadjuvant therapy, and a

pathologic (postoperative) stage. Initial therapy with chemoradiation can produce substantial downstaging (approximately 15% of patients will have a pathologic complete response, and as many as 40% in those with more favorable tumors). While some believe that the degree of response to neoadjuvant therapy should alter subsequent treatment, and this is in fact an area of active investigation (see later discussion), the current standard of care dictates that all surgical planning and adjuvant therapy be determined based on the initial clinical stage regardless of tumor response. This guideline is based in part on the idea that a good tumor response locally to chemoradiation does not translate into reduced risk of having micrometastatic disease, and thus does not lessen the need for adjuvant postoperative chemotherapy. Whether this will continue to be true in the face of newer data and more aggressive neoadjuvant regimens remains to be seen. Numerous studies have indicated that tumor response to neoadjuvant therapy is an important predictor of multiple oncologic end points for patients completing the full course of multimodal therapy. Patients with pathologic complete response in particular demonstrate excellent long-term results, with local recurrence rates as low as 0.7%, and significantly improved disease-free survival (DFS) and overall survival (OS) compared to nonresponders at 5 years (odds ratio [OR] = 3.28 and OR = 4.33, respectively).[10–12] It is unclear at this time whether such a favorable outcome can be maintained should the course of treatment be altered based on postneoadjuvant reassessment.

Although it is not standard practice to alter treatment based on local response to neoadjuvant therapy, preoperative restaging prior to surgery may still be valuable not only as a prognostic predictor but also for detecting interval metastatic progression. Multiple studies recommend repeating serum carcinoembryonic antigen (CEA) levels, for example, between chemoradiation and surgery as this value as well as the pre- to posttreatment ratio may be more important in predicting survival than the initial measurement.[13–15] In addition, Ayez et al.[16] advocate restaging with chest and abdominal computed tomography (CT), as this changed management in 12% of their patients, and spared 8% from undergoing noncurative rectal surgery, due to new findings of progressive metastatic disease.[16]

The major change that has occurred in the newest version of the staging system is the acknowledgment that both the T stage and the N stage have independent prognostic importance for local control, DFS, and OS.[17,18] Thus, for patients with N0 and N1 tumors viewed separately, the extent of the primary tumor in the rectum is of additional prognostic importance. Patients with T1-2N1 tumors have a relatively favorable prognosis and an outcome superior to that of other stage III patients. In fact, patients with T3N0M0 disease (stage II) have outcomes slightly inferior to those with T1-2N1M0, demonstrating the independent prognostic importance of T stage. These distinctions may allow future decisions to be more individualized as to the adjuvant therapy required.

Although at one level staging is very straightforward, the actuality of proper staging is much more difficult as it relies on multiple quality control issues that can mislead the clinician regarding proper therapy. For instance, it has been well demonstrated that for patients with colon and rectal cancer who are pathologically staged as N0, the prognosis is markedly improved for those in whom more than 12 to 14 nodes were identified by the pathologist compared with those in whom fewer nodes were identified.[19] This could be a surgical issue (fewer nodes were removed) or a pathologist issue (fewer nodes were identified), but it suggests that many patients were inappropriately understaged, which could result in inappropriate therapy. Others have shown that staging accuracy continues to improve as the pathologist recovers more nodes, with accuracy leveling off at approximately 12 to 20 nodes recovered.[20,21] (See discussion in Chapter 49). In rectal cancer, however, N staging presents a particular challenge as there are often fewer LNs in the specimen and preoperative radiotherapy is thought to reduce that number even further.[22–24] In fact, one recent report suggests that LN harvests <12 in pretreated specimens may be a marker of high tumor response and improved rather than compromised oncologic outcome. In this study of 237 patients, local recurrence rates were significantly higher in the LN >12 group as compared to those with "inadequate" LN retrieval (11% versus 0%; $p = 0.004$).[25] As with colon cancer, the percentage of positive nodes is likely of greater prognostic importance than total LN number (M. Meyers, 2007, personal communication).[26–28] The same issue relates to T-stage determination. If the pathologist does not look carefully for evidence of extension of tumor through the muscularis propria, the patient can be understaged, resulting in inappropriate treatment. Close or positive circumferential margins are a poor prognostic factor, which can only be found if the pathologist assiduously evaluates the radial margins.[29,30]

The standard staging procedure for rectal cancer entails a history, physical examination, complete blood cell count, liver and renal function studies, as well as CEA evaluation. The routine laboratory studies are quite insensitive to the presence of metastatic disease, but they are usually ordered as a screen of organ function prior to surgery or chemoradiation therapy. High CEA levels are associated with poorer survival (see Chapter 49) and give an indication as to whether follow-up CEA determinations are likely to be useful. A careful rectal examination by an experienced examiner is an essential part of the pretherapy evaluation in determining distance of the tumor from the anal verge or from the dentate line, involvement of the anal sphincter, amount of circumferential involvement, clinical fixation, sphincter tone, and so forth, and has not been replaced by imaging studies or endoscopy. Colonoscopy or barium enema to evaluate the remainder of the large bowel is essential (if the patient is not obstructed) to rule out synchronous tumors or the presence of polyposis syndromes.

Local staging is completed with one of two imaging modalities, endorectal ultrasound (EUS) or pelvic magnetic resonance imaging (MRI). Each provides similar overall accuracy in T and N determination, and each has its advantages as well as drawbacks. The decision of which to use generally depends on local institutional expertise and resource availability.

EUS defines five interface layers of the rectal wall: mucosa, muscularis mucosa, submucosa, muscularis propria, and perirectal fat, as shown in Figure 52.2. Rectal tumors are generally hypoechoic and disrupt the interfaces depending on the level of tumor extension. The accuracy of EUS depends heavily on the experience and skill of the operator. In experienced hands, EUS has an overall accuracy rate for T stage of 75% to 95% with an

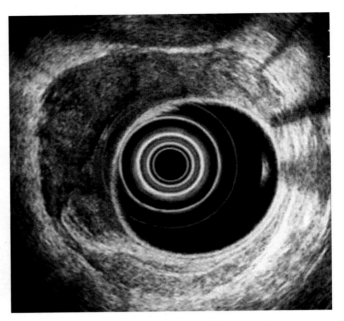

Figure 52.2 Endorectal ultrasound of a T3 tumor of the rectum, extension through the muscularis propria, and into perirectal fat.

overstaging of approximately 10% to 20% in T2 disease because of an inability to distinguish a desmoplastic response and postbiopsy changes from local tumor invasion, and approximately a 10% rate of understaging because of an inability to detect microscopic tumor extension.[31–33]

EUS is less accurate in determining N stage than for T stage, with an overall accuracy rate of 62% to 83%.[31,32] Understaging occurs because many nodal metastases from rectal cancer are small, even micrometastatic, and not easily detected by EUS. In addition, some nodes are located beyond the range of the ultrasound transducer and thus cannot be seen during the procedure. Overstaging is often related to an inflammatory response, perhaps secondary to previous biopsy or manipulation. EUS is not accurate for determining tumor regression after preoperative radiation and chemotherapy, as inflammatory changes and scarring can persist in the rectal wall or in perirectal soft tissue and may not reflect persisting tumor. Newer ultrasound techniques, such as three-dimensional ultrasound, are being explored but have not yet made it into standard practice.

Endorectal coil MRI allows discernment of the layers of the bowel wall and is similar in accuracy to EUS. Thin-section pelvic MRI with a surface coil also allows one to visualize the mesorectal fascia and thus to predict the likely distance of the surgical resection margin when performing a TME. The MERCURY Study Group confirmed this key advantage of MRI in their landmark 2005 multicenter trial, where specificity for predicting clear margins in 408 patients with varying stages of rectal cancer was 92%.[34] Although there has been great interest in this technique since then, follow-up studies still show a disappointing overall accuracy for T and N staging, which fails to surpass EUS in experienced hands. In one study of 96 patients who had MRI followed by TME, of 22 patients classified as having T2 disease on MRI, 3 had T1 and 6 had T3 tumors. Of 61 patients classified as having T3 disease on MRI, 8 had T2 tumors and 2 had T4. Thus, 6 of 22 (27%) patients who might have benefited from preoperative therapy for T3 disease would not have received that therapy. Eight of sixty-one patients (13%) would have received preoperative treatment inappropriately based on the MRI T stage.[35] For nodal status, 8 of 33 MRI-positive nodes were clinically negative, and 7 of 57 MRI-negative nodes were pathologically positive.[36] The presence of nodal disease identified by

MRI is also primarily determined by size, so the accuracy is similar to that of CT (<80%), although defining node positivity based on irregular border or mixed signal intensity could help improve sensitivity and specificity.[35]

While the accuracy of MRI in determining T and N stage is imperfect, newer studies have focused on other radiographic features that may prove more relevant to prognosis and treatment planning than the traditional American Joint Committee on Cancer classification. In addition to defining the circumferential resection margin (CRM) of a low rectal cancer, high-resolution MRI can be used to predict tumor regression grade (TRG) after neoadjuvant therapy. TRG in the surgical specimen is a measure of response to preoperative chemoradiation and has been shown to correlate strongly with OS and DFS. In the first prospective study to address MRI-predicted TRG, Shihab et al.[37] found this too was significantly associated with long-term outcomes. A prognostic role was also demonstrated for pretreatment MRI, specifically in the characterization of tumor invasion into the pelvic floor muscles. Based on these results, the authors postulate that MRI-defined factors may be extraordinarily useful for modifying treatment in both the pre- and postneoadjuvant settings.[37] Patel et al.[38] offer a similar conclusion in their subgroup analysis from the original MERCURY study, which likewise found MRI-predicted TRG and CRM to be significant prognostic markers.

Two studies have taken this issue a step further by investigating exactly how MRI parameters can and should alter therapy. In another extension of the MERCURY trial, Taylor et al.[39] identified patients with "good prognosis" MRI (as defined by predicted negative CRM, absence of extramural venous invasion, and T2/T3a/T3b regardless of N stage) and referred them directly for TME resection without chemoradiation. Survival and recurrence outcomes were highly favorable, suggesting that early MRI can improve patient stratification for more selective and appropriate targeting of preoperative therapy.[39] In the postneoadjuvant setting, MRI can be used to identify poor responders who may require alternative treatments or more radical resection such as the extralevator abdominoperineal approach described by Shihab et al.[40]

Finally, pelvic MRI may also help predict which patients are at increased risk for distant synchronous metastases and would therefore benefit from more extensive pretreatment imaging such as positron emission tomography (PET)/CT or liver MRI. Hunter et al.[41] found that adverse features demonstrated on pelvic MRI (extramural venous invasion, extramural spread of >5 mm or T4, involved CRM or intersphincteric plane for low tumors) were significantly associated with a higher incidence of distant metastases (OR = 6.0; p <0.001). The authors recommend using MRI-based risk stratification to identify patients who may benefit not only from more meticulous staging but also from more aggressive treatment regimens.[41]

M staging for rectal cancer is determined in the same way as colon cancer: with a baseline CT scan to evaluate the chest, abdomen, and pelvis.[42] There has been much debate about the relative value of CT versus MRI or PET, particularly in assessing the liver, without any clear resolution. This decision depends heavily on the institutional expertise and the equipment available.

CT has an overall sensitivity of 70% to 85%, which might be improved with multidetector-improved CT technology, although the data do not yet prove that contention.[43] MRI is superior in characterizing liver lesions and distinguishing cysts and hemangiomas from tumor, especially with the use of enhancement with gadolinium or other agents.[44] PET with [18F]fluorodeoxyglucose shows promise as the most sensitive study for the detection of metastatic disease in the liver and especially in abdominal LNs for which CT and MRI are relatively insensitive. In addition, a meta-analysis of whole-body PET showed a sensitivity of 97% and a specificity of 76% in evaluating for recurrent colorectal cancer.[45] However, PET is not standardly used in preoperative staging, or recommended by National Comprehensive Cancer Network guidelines, and the incremental gain from routine PET scan appears to be small.[46]

A 2013 study has re-emphasized this point, reporting that preoperative PET/CT had no impact on disease management in 96.8% of enrolled patients and advocating against its routine use for primary staging.[47] PET is probably most valuable in restaging patients with recurrence or suspected recurrence to detect additional metastatic sites prior to attempted resection of metastatic disease.

SURGERY

The surgical management of primary rectal cancer presents unique problems for the surgeon based in large part on the anatomic constraints of the pelvis. The primary goal of achieving a complete oncologic resection must be balanced with the desire for optimal nerve and sphincter preservation, which can be quite challenging in such a confined space.

Stage I

The treatment of early-stage rectal cancer can be confusing as there are many approaches that can be used, and patient selection is critical to outcome. In addition, the risk of nerve injury and damage to the anal sphincter is substantial for low-lying tumors and must be taken into consideration, along with the desire not to have a permanent colostomy for early-stage disease. Thus, the options for these patients are primarily those of local therapies without abdominal surgery, abdominal resection of the rectum with anastomosis and retention of the anal sphincter, and abdominal-perineal resection. The last two options are discussed in detail in "Stages II and III Rectal Cancer."

Small early-stage lesions of the rectum that are diagnosed on physical examination or by colonoscopy/proctoscopy can often be managed with local resection. Local resection can be performed colonoscopically (as described in the Chapter 49), or lesions can be removed via a transanal excision with the patient positioned in a prone or lithotomy position. Appropriate retractors can provide visualization, and resection should extend into the perirectal fat with a surrounding margin of normal tissue.[48] For selected T1 and T2 lesions without evidence of nodal disease, transanal excision often provides an adequate resection of the primary tumor mass and can spare the patient the morbidity of a more extensive rectal resection. However, it does not stage the nodal drainage areas and therefore cannot provide as complete staging and management of the tumor as a definitive resection. In the effort to minimize the risk of locoregional failure, criteria for local excision have been established: the tumor must be within 8 to 10 cm of the anal verge, be well or moderately well differentiated, encompass <40% of the circumference of the bowel wall, and contain no evidence of lymphovascular invasion on biopsy. For T2 lesions, local resection should be followed by adjuvant chemoradiation. While these criteria are not strongly evidence-based (and are evolving along with surgical technology), a growing body of literature supports this approach particularly for T1 lesions. In a review of 677 T1 and T2 cancers after TME, Saraste et al.[49] identified three significant risk factors for LN invasion (and hence relative contraindications for local excision): T2 stage (OR = 2.0), poor differentiation (OR = 6.5), and vascular infiltration (OR = 3.4) with likelihood of LN positivity ranging from 6% to 78% depending on how many were found. Further support for these criteria comes from a study of 25 high-risk T1 rectal cancers, half of which were treated by transanal excision only (due to comorbidities or patient refusal to undergo resection) and the remainder with immediate conventional reoperation after local excision. Local recurrence was significantly higher in patients undergoing local excision only (50% versus 7.7%, mean follow-up 62 months), and there was a trend toward decreased 5-year survival (63% versus 89%). There were no differences in age, gender, or tumor characteristics between the two groups.[50] On the other hand, for low-risk T1 lesions in the prospective phase 2 Cancer and Leukemia Group B study, local excision alone was associated with low recurrence and good survival rates that remained durable with long-term follow-up. For T2 lesions, however, even with adjuvant therapy, the role of local excision is less clear, as Saraste et al.[49] would predict, these were associated with higher recurrence rates.[51] Whether the addition of neoadjuvant therapy might be helpful is a focus of multiple investigations. The American College of Surgeons Oncology Group has published preliminary results from its recently completed phase 2 trial of neoadjuvant capecitabine, oxaliplatin, and radiation therapy followed by local excision for ultrasound T2 tumors (ACOSOG Protocol Z6041).[52] The authors report that 49 of 77 patients were downstaged and 44% achieved a complete pathologic response (pCR). There was one positive margin and one patient with a positive node. Rates of treatment-related toxicity and perioperative complications were high, however, requiring dose reduction and potentially compromising response. Follow-up trials are planned to improve upon the therapeutic ratio of this approach and better evaluate long-term efficacy.[53] More long-term results are reported from another prospective trial that supports the role of local excision following neoadjuvant therapy in selected T2N0 lesions with favorable features. Lezoche et al.[54] randomized 100 patients to either endoluminal resection or to laparoscopic or open TME, following neoadjuvant chemoradiation. Downstaging and pCR rates were similar in both groups, occurring in 51% and 28% of patients, respectively. With a mean follow-up of 9.6 years, oncologic outcomes were also essentially equivalent—with similar local recurrence rates and incidence of distant metastases (8% versus 6% and 4% versus 4%, respectively) and no difference in DFS.[54]

Performing a good transanal excision requires substantial technical expertise as the surgeon must retain control over the primary tumor and obtain adequate mucosal margins as well as deep resection into the perirectal fat. Once removed, the tumor must be well laid out for the pathologist so that all relevant margins can be properly evaluated. There is some experience using preoperative radiation therapy and chemotherapy for small lesions, but care must be taken to have the site of the primary tumor well marked with a tattoo if this approach is taken, as excellent regression could make identification of the primary site difficult.

Newer techniques for transanal excision, including transanal endoscopic microsurgery (TEMS) and transanal minimally invasive surgery, have recently gained popularity based on improved visualization of the lesion. TEMS makes use of a standard laparoscopic light source and monitoring system combined with specialized instruments and scopes. The technique allows for videoscopic magnification and the placement of instruments through an operating sigmoidoscope. TEMS and its counterpart transanal minimally invasive surgery, which uses the more basic single port laparoscopic technology, may be applied, in general, to the same patients who are candidates for traditional transanal resection. However, these methods are most useful for excising more proximal lesions that are beyond the reach of standard surgical instruments and too large for removal through a colonoscope. Preliminary data supports the role of TEMS in both benign and early-stage malignant lesions with improved margin negativity and DFS compared to transanal resection for T1 and T2 lesions in a recent report.[55] Another meta-analysis found significant reductions in morbidity and mortality compared to conventional surgery and equivalent 5-year survival rates for T1 tumors.[56] Studies that include T2 lesions and selective use of adjuvant therapy have demonstrated 5-year OS and cancer-specific survivals over 90%, with recurrence rates between 4% to 9%.[57,58] Moreover, the TEMS procedure fairs quite favorably with respect to long-term quality of life and functional outcome as most defecatory parameters return to baseline by 5 years, according to prospective data.[59] Other reports are less encouraging with recurrence rates following TEMS resection as high as 30%,[60] and therefore close endoscopic surveillance is recommended.

Stages II and III Rectal Cancer

The primary treatment of patients with stages II and III rectal cancer (T3-4 and/or node-positive) is surgical. However, in contrast to the treatment of patients with stage I disease, there is a strong body of information to suggest that combined modality therapy with radiation therapy and chemotherapy should be used in conjunction with surgical resection. This conclusion is based on both patterns of failure data, which demonstrate a substantial incidence of local, regional, as well as distant disease failure, and the fact that this incidence of tumor recurrence at all sites is decreased with the use of trimodality therapy.

The desire when performing a resection for rectal cancer is to preserve intestinal continuity and the sphincter mechanism whenever possible while still maximizing tumor control. Therefore, careful preoperative screening is crucial in the determination of the location of the lesion and its depth of invasion. As previously described, it is convenient to think of the rectum as divided into thirds for the purposes of the evaluation and preoperative determination of the surgical approach for resection. The upper third of the rectum is often considered the region of large intestine from the sacral prominence to the peritoneal reflection. These lesions are in almost all cases managed with a low anterior resection in much the same way as a sigmoid colon cancer (see Chapter 49). An adequate 1- to 2-cm distal mucosal margin can be achieved for these lesions well above the sphincter mechanism, and intestinal continuity can be restored using either a hand-sewn technique or a circular stapling device inserted through the rectum.[61,62]

Tumors in the middle and lower thirds of the rectum can be considered as lying entirely below the peritoneal reflection. The resection of these tumors can be challenging because of the confines of the pelvic skeletal structure, and the ability to perform a resection with an adequate distal margin is significantly influenced by the size of the lesion. Nevertheless, tumors of the middle third of the rectum in most cases can be safely resected with a low anterior resection, with restoration of intestinal continuity and preservation of a continent sphincter apparatus.

Lesions in the distal third of the rectum, defined as those within 6 cm of the anal verge, can present the greatest challenge to the surgeon with respect to sphincter preservation. This is often influenced by the extent of lateral invasion of the lesion into the muscles of the sphincter apparatus and how close distally the tumor is to the musculature of the anal canal. The abdominal perineal resection (APR) has historically been considered the standard treatment for patients with rectal cancers located within 6 cm of the anal verge. This procedure requires a transabdominal as well as a transperineal approach with removal of the entire rectum and sphincter complex. A permanent end colostomy is created and the perineal wound either closed primarily or left to granulate in after closure of the musculature.

Although an APR is associated with a relatively low rate of local recurrence, it is not without the obvious problems of the need for a permanent colostomy and loss of intestinal continuity and sphincter function. Therefore, intense interest has been focused on developing approaches to the resection of tumors in the distal third of the rectum that would both avoid local regional recurrence and preserve intestinal continuity and sphincter continence.

Traditionally, tumors within 1 to 2 cm of the dentate line—that is, those that can be removed with at least a 1-cm distal margin—have been considered candidates for sphincter preservation and restoration of intestinal continuity via a coloanal anastomosis, which is commonly protected by a diverting loop ileostomy that can be reversed in 6 to 12 weeks.[63,64] Newer data suggest that when TME and preoperative radiotherapy are routinely employed, even smaller margins are acceptable without oncologic compromise, as long as they are microscopically negative.[65] In fact, one of the advantages of neoadjuvant therapy is thought to be an increase in sphincter-sparing procedures due to reduction in tumor bulk, which would normally preclude identification of this slight but critical margin.[63,66] A recent systematic literature review identified seven studies addressing this topic, most of which implemented pre- or postoperative radiotherapy, and three of which reported results related to a margin of <5 mm. There were no statistically significant differences in local recurrence rates regardless of margin status. This data contributes to the growing evidence that a 1 cm (or even 5 mm) margin may be unnecessary and, more importantly, that strategies employed solely to achieve this margin (such as an APR or intersphincteric resection [ISR] for distal T1 lesions) may in fact be unnecessary as well.[67]

While controversial in the United States, ISR has been described extensively abroad as a method involving at least partial resection of the internal sphincter designed to improve margin status without sacrificing sphincter function.[68] Recently, a large systematic review addressed the efficacy of this approach, identifying 14 (mostly retrospective) studies with 1,289 patients who underwent both open and laparoscopic ISR. Median follow-up was 56 (range, 1 to 227) months. Overall oncologic outcomes did not appear to be compromised with R0 resection achieved in 97% and a mean local recurrence rate of 6.7% (range, 0% to 23%). In addition, mean 5-year OS and DFS rates were 86.3% and 78.6%, respectively. Functional outcomes, however, were widely variable with only 51.2% of patients reporting "perfect continence," while an average of 29.1% experienced fecal soiling, 23.8% incontinence to flatus, and 18.6% complained of urgency.[69]

It has been postulated that neoadjuvant chemoradiation, while improving locoregional control and rates of margin-negative resection, has a deleterious effect on long-term functional outcomes, particularly after surgery for ultralow tumors. However, a recent multivariate analysis did not support this in ISR cases, finding the only significant predictors of continence were distance of the tumor from the anal ring and distance of the anastomosis from the anal verge. There was also no difference with age or extent of internal sphincter resection.[70] Another report did find significant functional differences when comparing partial ISR (resection above the dentate line), subtotal ISR (resection at the dentate line), and total ISR (resection from the intersphincteric groove). Patients with more extensive sphincter resection had higher fecal incontinence scores, more frequent nocturnal leakage, and more problems with discrimination. In addition, manometric studies at 12 months showed greater reductions in mean resting pressure. Overall though, quality of life was maintained in the majority of patients and function improved over time in both studies.[71]

Chemoradiation should be used preoperatively when performing sphincter-preserving resections for T3 or T4 rectal lesions or for any node-positive disease stages II or III. There is some evidence that preoperative radiation results in less morbidity than postoperative radiation therapy when a coloanal anastomosis is planned. In a study of 109 patients treated with a low anterior resection and a straight coloanal anastomosis, those receiving preoperative radiation therapy had a lower incidence of adverse effects on anal function than those receiving postoperative radiation.[72] The authors attributed this to sparing of the neorectum from these effects. Relative benefits and outcomes for preoperative chemoradiation versus postoperative chemoradiation will be discussed in detail in following sections.

Total Mesorectal Resection

The goal of the resection of rectal tumors is the removal of the tumor with an adequate margin as well as removal of draining LNs and lymphatics to properly stage the tumor and to reduce the risk of recurrence and spread. For lesions in the intraperitoneal colon, the lymphatics and vascular supply are found in the mesentery associated with that region of bowel.

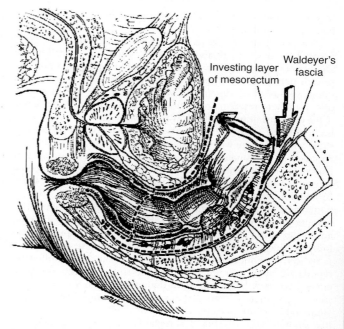

Investing layer of mesorectum

Waldeyer's fascia

Figure 52.3 Total mesorectal excision.

In the rectum, the mesorectum is the structure that contains the blood supply and lymphatics for the upper, middle, and lower rectum. Most involved LNs for rectal cancers are found within the mesorectum, with T1 lesions associated with positive LNs in 5.7% of cases, T2 lesions having positive LNs in 20% of cases, and T3 and T4 lesions having positive LNs in 65% and 78% of cases, respectively.[73]

The anatomy and approach to mesorectal excision is depicted in Figure 52.3. This operation involves a sharp dissection occurring in an avascular plane between the fascia propria of the rectum and the presacral membrane, beyond the region where most of the nodes are located. After a TME, the specimen is typically shiny and bilobed in contrast to the irregular and rough surface after a blunt dissection, where much of the mesorectal fat is left behind. TME attempts not only to clear involved LNs but also to adequately manage the radial margins of the rectal tumor. These radial margins have been shown to be more important with respect to the risk of local regional recurrence than the distal mucosal margin.[66,74] Distal mucosal margins of ≥1 cm are adequate for local control; however, the margin on the mesorectum should extend beyond the distal mucosal margin in order to ensure a successful surgical outcome.[64,66] Numerous studies have demonstrated the benefit of TME, and it is now considered the standard of care for the surgical management of middle and lower third rectal cancers.[5,75–77] Although some studies have suggested that an adequate TME might in and of itself be sufficient management for T2 and T3 rectal cancers, the majority of the literature still supports the use of adjuvant chemoradiation for stages II and III disease even when combined with TME.

Large studies of proctectomy with TME have demonstrated a reduction in the overall incidence of local recurrence to <10%.[4] The consequences of TME can be impairment in erectile and bladder function because of disruption of parasympathetic nerves that are located in proximity to the mesorectum. Several authors have stressed the importance of the experience of the surgeon performing the procedure, and some have suggested specific techniques for monitoring modalities that can be used during this procedure to minimize morbidity.[5,6] A careful understanding of the anatomy and adequate visualization during sharp dissection will help in minimizing injury to the parasympathetic nerves and the consequent morbidity.[3,4]

Adequate visualization in the deep pelvis can often be a challenge. This may be a situation where the visual magnification and ability to enter tight spaces that are unique to the laparoscopic approach may be an advantage. Several groups have demonstrated the feasibility of laparoscopic TME for low rectal cancer as part of a sphincter-preserving operation.[78–80] Some of the larger series, while demonstrating that TME using laparoscopic techniques can be performed safely, do not have adequate follow-up to demonstrate whether there were any oncologic disadvantages to such an approach. Unfortunately, the prospective random assignment trial conducted in the United States to evaluate the role of laparoscopic surgery for colon cancer excluded patients with low rectal lesions. In addition, subgroup analysis from the UK CLASICC trial reported a 34% conversion rate and double the frequency of positive margins compared to open cases (12% versus 6%), prompting the authors to advise against routine practice of laparoscopic proctectomy outside of the research setting.[81] While these results have raised serious concerns regarding oncologic outcomes, follow-up reports are more encouraging. Multiple single-institution experiences have now been published demonstrating not only similar surgical parameters (margin status, LN harvest numbers) but also comparable recurrence and 5-year survival data.[82–86] Furthermore, in a study based on National Surgical Quality Improvement Program data from 5,420 patients, Greenblatt et al.[87] reported significant short-term advantages to laparoscopy, including decreased length of stay (5 days versus 7 days; $p <0.0001$) and 30-day morbidity (20.5% versus 28.8%; $p <0.0001$). Smaller randomized trials as well as two recent large meta-analyses of randomized controlled trials also support the oncologic equivalence of the two approaches, although short-term benefits are mixed.[88–90] In 10-year follow-up data from a pooled analysis of three randomized controlled trials (including 136 laparoscopic and 142 open cases), continued long-term oncologic safety of the laparoscopic approach was demonstrated with no significant differences compared to open in terms of locoregional recurrence (5.5% versus 9.3%), cancer-specific survival (82.5% versus 77.6%), or OS (63% versus 61.1%). Additionally, there was a trend toward lower recurrence among stage III patients in the laparoscopic group (17.7% versus 25.3%), though this did not reach statistical significance.[91] Lujan et al.[92] also reported similar rates of local recurrence and OS in a prospective cohort of 4,405 patients but found decreased complication rates (38.3% versus 45.6%) and improved oncologic parameters with laparoscopy, including decreased margin involvement and more complete TME. Finally, in a smaller study by Westerholm et al.,[93] laparoscopic surgery was found to be an independent predictor of DFS on multivariate analysis with 5-year DFS rates of 50.3% compared to 71.0% after open resection. Definitive recommendations await the results of three ongoing multicenter phase 3 randomized trials: the European COLOR II, the Japanese JCOG 0404, and the ACOSOG Z6051 from the United States.[94]

While laparoscopic TME may be technically feasible, it requires a high level of expertise and can be particularly challenging to perform within the confines of a deep and narrow pelvis. More recently, robotic technology has been applied to rectal dissection, overcoming many of the limitations associated with conventional laparoscopy including limited dexterity, inadequate visualization, and tremor. Robotic surgery offers the advantages of a stable, three-dimensional image, enhanced ergonomics and articulating instruments with seven degrees of freedom, in addition to operator-controlled camera and retraction.[95] Embraced by urologists and gynecologists over the past decade, this technology is ideally suited to pelvic procedures and has the potential to yield enhanced oncologic and functional outcomes in rectal cancer surgery as well. Limited studies so far have demonstrated feasibility and acceptable short-term outcomes.[95–99] In a case-control analysis of 118 patients undergoing laparoscopic versus robotic resection, Kwak et al.[100] reported no differences in surgical oncologic

parameters, postoperative complications, or recurrence rates at a median of 15 months follow-up. When compared to open TME in another case-matched study, the robotic approach was superior in terms of LN harvest, distal margin length, blood loss, and length of stay.[101] Other potential benefits include decreased conversion rates in three large meta-analyses as well as a trend toward reduced anastomotic leaks and CRM positivity with complete autonomic preservation in a recent systematic review of 1,549 patients.[102–105] Whether this data will translate into meaningful long-term advantages that justify the significantly higher cost of this approach remains to be seen.

The Robotic versus Laparoscopic Resection for Rectal Cancer (ROLARR) trial is a prospective, randomized, controlled, multicenter superiority trial that began enrollment in 2010, with a target recruitment of 400 patients. It will evaluate differences in conversion rates; CRM positivity, 3-year local recurrence, DFS and OS, as well as operative morbidity and mortality, quality of life, and cost-effectiveness. Investigators also wish to explore the purported clinical benefits of robotics including preservation of normal bladder and sexual function. Results from this ambitious trial are anxiously awaited.[106]

Resection of Contiguous Organs and Total Pelvic Exenteration

Although aggressive surgical approaches to rectal cancer have resulted in improvement in locoregional recurrence rates, these rates can still be as high as 33%. Not infrequently, large rectal lesions will invade through the wall of the rectum into contiguous structures such as the bladder, prostate, vagina, and uterus. Carefully selected patients with recurrent or locally advanced rectal cancers may benefit from an aggressive approach such as a total pelvic exenteration. Local recurrences remain localized to the pelvis in a significant number of patients, with autopsy studies demonstrating the incidence of pelvic recurrence to be as high as 50%.[107]

Recurrences in the pelvis can result in significant morbidity such as tenesmus, pain, bowel obstruction, and fistula. Although some of these can be ameliorated with radiation, these problems are best managed by preventing their occurrence. Although the impact of total pelvic exenteration on survival has been debated, the potential benefits on controlling locoregional disease and preventing morbidity keeps this technique as one of the tools in the surgeon's armamentarium when approaching large rectal lesions.

Existing literature on multivisceral resection of both primary and recurrent tumors has been recently evaluated in a systematic review of 22 studies comprising 1,575 patients. The authors reported a 4.2% perioperative mortality rate with morbidity of 42.5%. The overall 5-year survival rate was 50.3% with, not surprisingly, worse outcomes in patients with recurrent compared to primary disease (19.5% versus 52.8%). R0 resection was achieved in 79.5% of cases and, also not surprisingly, was the strongest factor associated with long-term survival.[108] Another review focusing only on locally recurrent tumors, reported R0 resection rates from 30% to 45% and 5-year global survival ranging from 30% to 40%, with authors stressing the importance of careful patient selection.[109] To this end, a panel of 36 colorectal surgeons were recently recruited to establish a scoring system for determining patient suitability for pelvic exenteration. A comprehensive list of clinicopathologic and radiographic criteria were considered and ranked by importance and utility in predicting negative resection margin. The authors hope to apply this quantitatively toward improving outcomes for this highly invasive and morbid intervention.[110]

For symptomatic tumors that are not resectable, other palliative options to consider include debulking and ablation. Ripley et al.[111] reported some benefit associated with sequential open radiofrequency ablation and surgical debulking in 16 patients, achieving a median survival of 12 months, with OS 24% at 36 months, and 3 patients remaining with no evidence of disease at 9,

48, and 84 months. There were four cases of significant postoperative morbidity, however, and variable levels of symptom relief.[111] Pusceddu et al.[112] reported far better palliation with CT-guided radiofrequency ablation in 12 patients with painful pelvic recurrence. At the end of follow-up (23±23 months), 92% of patients were symptom free, with a 16% treatment-related morbidity (one rectovesical fistula and one rectal abscess).[112] Finally, transrectal high-intensity focused ultrasonography has now been described in the palliative treatment of rectal cancer. As the only completely noninvasive thermal therapy, it can be delivered by either an intracavitary or extracorporeal device, causing focal ablation via coagulative necrosis. In the first case report, it was well-tolerated and led to immediate symptom relief.[113]

Combined Modality Therapy (Stage II and III)

The use of adjuvant radiation therapy is based on the substantial incidence of locoregional failure with surgical therapy alone. Older studies demonstrate local failure rates of up to 50% in patients with T3-4 or node-positive disease (Table 52.1).[114–120] The locoregional recurrence rates in these studies are in the range of 25% to 50% for patients with T3-4 and/or node-positive disease and is a dominant pattern of failure, although distant recurrence is also of great importance. Local failure is related not just to the stage of the disease, but also the location of the tumor in the rectum (tumors located low in the rectum have a higher incidence of local failure) and the experience and ability of the surgeon. However, the relevance of these older local recurrence data has been brought into question with the advent of the use of TME, as previously described. It is important to realize that the data on local recurrence after primary surgical resection come from selected series with operations performed by experienced surgeons who have been specially trained in TME and may not be relevant to the operations performed by general surgeons who perform the operation only occasionally and who are not specially trained.

Although initial studies reported locoregional failure rates of <5% after TME without the use of any adjuvant therapy,[75,77,121–123] there was concern that these excellent results could not be replicated in larger population-based studies. A number of European countries or regions have shown that the overall locoregional

recurrence risks could be decreased by limiting the surgeons who were authorized to perform rectal surgery to those who were trained and certified in the procedure, and by having educational sessions for those who were performing the surgery.[5] This raised the question of what is the true rate of local failure after TME to help define which patients really require adjuvant therapy.

The most important analysis on local recurrence rates with TME are the data from the Dutch TME study in which patients were randomized to receive either TME alone or a short course of preoperative radiation therapy followed by TME.[77] All patients with rectal cancer were eligible, including those with early-stage disease. Special attempts were made to have good surgical and pathology quality control. The early results (2 years) relating to local tumor recurrence have been reported and are summarized in Table 52.2. The study demonstrates that there are subsets of

TABLE 52.1

Results of Dutch Total Mesorectal Excision Trial

Technique	Preoperative Radiotherapy (5 Gy × 5) + Total Mesorectal Excision	Total Mesorectal Excision Alone
Percentage of Patients		
Stage 0 or I		30
Local failure (2 y)	2.4	8.2
Local failure (4 y)	3	10
Local Failure (Distance from Anal Verge)		
0–5 cm	5.8	10
5–10 cm	1	10.1
10–15 cm	1.3	3.8
Stage III (4-y estimate)		20

From Kapiteijn E, Marijnen CA, Nagtegall ID, et al, Preoperative radiotherapy combined with total mesorectal excision for resectable rectal cancer. *N Eng J Med* 2001;345:638–646, with permission.

TABLE 52.2

Local Failure of Rectal Cancer Surgery Alone (Local Failure Rate Percentage/Number of Patients in Cohort)

Analysis	Gunderson and Sosin[117] Reoperation (Crude)	Rich et al.[119] Clinical Exam + Surgery (Crude)	Minsky et al.[211] First Failure— Clinical Exam + Surgery (5-y Actuarial)	Martling et al.[120] Total Local Recurrence	Mendenhall, Million, and Pfaff[114] Total Local Recurrence— 5-y Follow-up Clinical	Pilipshen et al.[116] First Failure— Clinical	Bonadeo et al.[228] Total Local Recurrence— Clinical[a]
T1N0		8%/39	11%/11	9%/78	0/6	0%/5	3%/103
T2N0			3%/36		38%/16	14%/128	
T3N0	67%/6	24%/42	23%/60	34%/80	40%/30	30%/111	4%/181
T4N0		53%/15	11%/9				
T1-2N+	24%/17	50%/4	14%/11	37%/93	71%/17	22%/49	24%/133
T3N+	83%/40	47%/34	25%/31		65%/17	49%/89	
T4N+		67%/6	22%/10				
Total	64%/75	30%/142	15%/168	27%/251	46%/90		

[a] Local recurrence highly dependent on site in rectum—18% overall for tumors ≤7 cm from anal verge.

TABLE 52.3

Local Control and Survival with and without Radiotherapy—Preoperatively, Postoperatively, and with or without Chemotherapy

Study/Institution[a] (Ref.)	No. of Patients	Local Failure (%)	Disease-Free Survival (%)	Survival (5 y) (%)
NSABP RO-1[129] Surg/Surg + RT (postoperative RT)	184/187	25/16	No difference	No difference
NSABP RO-2[130] Surg + chemo/Surg + chemo + RT (postoperative RT)	348/346	13/8		
GITSG[127] Surg/Surg + RT/Surg + chemo + RT (postoperative RT)	58/50/46	25/20/10	44/50/65	26/33/45
Swedish[215] Surg/Surg + RT (preoperative RT)		27/11		48/58
Stockholm II[120] Surg/Surg + RT (preoperative RT)		34/16 Stage II 37/21 Stage II		
MRC[132] Surg/Surg + RT (postoperative RT)	235/234	34/21		38/41

NSABP, National Surgical Adjuvant Breast and Bowel Project; Surg, surgery; RT, radiotherapy; chemo, chemotherapy; GITSG, Gastrointestinal Study Group; MRC, Medical Research Council.
[a] Randomized studies in either all patients or patients with stage II and III disease.

patients in whom TME alone is likely sufficient for obtaining good pelvic control, including patients with high rectal tumors (some of these may have been sigmoid cancers, rather than rectal) and low-stage tumors (T1-2, N0). On the other hand, low-lying rectal tumors that are moderately advanced (T3-4 and/or node-positive) had a higher incidence of locoregional failure. Local failure after TME alone was 15% in node-positive patients at 2 years, not corrected for site of the primary, and longer-term follow-up will undoubtedly demonstrate higher local failure rates. In addition, as these results were obtained in a controlled setting, one would likely not obtain similarly good results when surgery is done with less careful quality control. There was a consistent decrease in local failure rate by the addition of preoperative radiation therapy, but the absolute magnitude of the effect varied by the tumor characteristics previously discussed. Long-term results from the Dutch TME study have now been published demonstrating a stable, persistent >50% reduction in recurrence risk for the radiotherapy group after a median follow-up of 12 years. For patients with a negative circumferential margin, the benefit was even greater, with the 10-year cumulative incidence of local recurrence 3% after radiotherapy versus 9% after surgery alone ($p <0.0001$) and the incidence of distant recurrence 19% versus 24% ($p = 0.06$). In addition, the incidence of cancer-specific death at 10 years was 17% for the irradiated group versus 22% for surgery alone ($p = 0.04$). OS rates, however, were equivalent.[124]

A trial similar to the Dutch TME study was recently reported. This phase 3 trial randomized 1,350 patients with operable adenocarcinoma of the rectum to short-course preoperative radiotherapy (25 Gy in five fractions; $n = 674$) or to initial surgery with selective postoperative chemoradiotherapy (CRT; 45 Gy in 25 fractions with concurrent 5-fluorouracil [5-FU]) restricted to patients CRM involvement ($n = 676$). The primary outcome measure was local recurrence. At the time of analysis, 330 patients had died (157 preoperative radiotherapy group versus 173 selective postoperative CRT), and median follow-up of surviving patients was 4 years. A total of 99 patients developed local recurrence (27 preoperative radiotherapy versus 72 selective postoperative CRT). A reduction was noted of 61% in the relative risk of local recurrence for patients receiving preoperative radiotherapy (hazard ratio [HR] = 0.39; 95% confidence

interval [CI] = 0.27 to 0.58; $p <0.0001$) and an absolute difference at 3 years of 6.2% (4.4% preoperative radiotherapy versus 10.6% selective postoperative CRT; 95% CI = 5.3–7.1). A relative improvement in DFS of 24% for patients receiving preoperative radiotherapy (HR = 0.76; 95% CI = 0.62 to 0.94; $p = 0.013$), and an absolute difference at 3 years of 6.0% (77.5% versus 71.5%; 95% CI = 5.3 to 6.8) was observed. OS did not differ between the groups (HR = 0.91; 95% CI = 0.73 to 1.13; $p = 0.40$). These findings provide further evidence that short-course preoperative radiotherapy is an effective treatment for patients with operable rectal cancer.[125]

The data are excellent that radiation therapy, especially when combined with chemotherapy, can decrease the local failure rate. This is shown by a Swedish study of preoperative radiation therapy compared with surgery,[126] the Dutch TME trial in the preoperative setting,[76] and by multiple studies in the postoperative setting.[127–132] There are also excellent data to show that locoregional failure is decreased by the use of radiation therapy and is further decreased by the use of concurrent 5-FU–based chemotherapy (Table 52.3).[127,128,133] Most studies have demonstrated that local failure decreases by about 50% with the use of adjuvant radiation therapy, with a greater effect when concurrent 5-FU is used with irradiation. This appears to provide a strong justification for the use of adjuvant radiation therapy. What is less clear is whether trimodality therapy with radiation therapy improves survival, if radiochemotherapy should be given preoperatively or postoperatively, and precisely which patients should be irradiated. To that effect, Schrag et al.[134] investigated the use of a neoadjuvant chemotherapy utilizing a 5-FU–leucovorin-oxaliplatin (FOLFOX)-based regimen, with selective use of chemoradiation therapy only in those patients who had failed to demonstrate tumor improvement on neoadjuvant chemotherapy. Of the 30 patients treated without radiation therapy in this small pilot trial, none experienced local recurrence with a minimum follow-up of 4 years.[134] Three patients experienced distant failure, all in the lungs. This interesting pilot trial has led to the current phase 3 cooperative group trial comparing this approach of neoadjuvant chemotherapy plus selective use of radiation versus standard neoadjuvant chemoradiation therapy. Pending any new information from this randomized trial, neoadjuvant chemoradiation therapy remains appropriate standard practice.

TABLE 52.4

Results of Meta-Analysis, Preoperative Radiotherapy Versus Surgery Alone

Result	Preoperative Radiotherapy vs. Surgery
Overall 5-y mortality	OR = 0.84 (p = 0.03)
5-y cancer mortality	OR = 0.71 (p <0.001)
5-y local recurrence	OR = 0.49 (p <0.001)
5-y distant metastases	OR = 0.93 (p = 0.54)

OR, overall recovery.
From Camma C, Giunta M, Fiorica F, et al. Preoperative radiotherapy for resectable rectal cancer: A meta-analysis. *JAMA* 2000;284:1008–1015, with permission.

DOES ADJUVANT RADIATION THERAPY IMPACT SURVIVAL?

Although there have been multiple randomized trials addressing the use of adjuvant radiation therapy or chemoradiation therapy, and although they consistently show an improvement in local control with adjuvant radiation therapy, the survival outcome data have been mixed. In the past, there have been two meta-analyses performed.[135,136] Table 52.4 shows the results of a meta-analysis by Camma et al.[136] showing a decreased local recurrence rate, cancer mortality rate, and overall mortality rate with the use of preoperative radiation therapy, although without a decrease in distant metastasis rate. The Colorectal Cancer Collaborative Group study (Table 52.5) demonstrates no improvement in the likelihood of curative surgery with preoperative therapy or of OS with all types of radiation therapy combined.[135] Preoperative radiation therapy, however, was shown to improve local control, DFS, and OS compared with surgery alone, although deaths within the first year after surgery were higher after radiation therapy. Local recurrence with preoperative radiation therapy was 46% lower than surgery alone, and cancer deaths were decreased from 50% to 45%. Postoperative radiation therapy was shown to improve local control (although less than preoperative therapy), but did not impact long-term survival. Lending substantial strength to the conclusion that there was a true advantage to radiation therapy is the fact that there was a dose response demonstrated for the radiation effect on local control (i.e., better control was obtained with higher radiation dose). This observation strengthens the conclusion, as it demonstrates a direct correlation between the amount of therapy and outcome. The data from this analysis are heavily influenced by the results of a single Swedish study that showed a long-term survival advantage to the use of preoperative radiation therapy compared with surgery alone.[126] Thus, these data show that improving local control

TABLE 52.5

Colorectal Cancer Collaborative Group 2001 Adjuvant Radiation Therapy in Rectal Cancer

	Preoperative RT vs. Surgery	Postoperative RT vs. Surgery
Yearly risk of local recurrence	46% decrease with RT	37% decrease with RT
Death rate	5% less than with surgery	No difference from surgery

RT, radiotherapy.
From Colorectal Cancer Collaborative Group. Adjuvant radiotherapy for rectal cancer: a systematic overview of 8507 patients from 22 randomised trials. *Lancet* 2001;358:1291–1304, with permission.

with the use of radiation therapy (and presumably with concurrent chemoradiation therapy) is beneficial, and that trimodality therapy, especially when chemoradiation therapy is used preoperatively, can improve survival.

PREOPERATIVE RADIATION THERAPY

The second issue of importance is whether adjuvant therapy should be given preoperatively or postoperatively and the exact timing of the chemotherapy. Current data clearly favor the preoperative approach.

Perhaps the most important study addressing the issue of pre- versus postoperative adjuvant therapy is a German trial of preoperative versus postoperative chemoradiation with radiation therapy given at 1.8 Gy per fraction and using continuous-infusion 5-FU chemotherapy as a 120-hour infusion, for which results have been reported by Sauer et al.[137] This study demonstrates an advantage in sphincter preservation with the use of preoperative therapy. Of the patients thought to need an APR at initial assessment, only 19% had a sphincter-preserving surgery when operation was done immediately versus 39% after preoperative radiation therapy, although there was no difference in the overall sphincter preservation rate. There was a statistically significant decrease in local failure with preoperative radiation therapy compared to postoperative treatment (6% versus 13%; p = 0.006). The relative risk of local failure in the pre- versus postoperative treatment group was 0.46. The 5-year DFS showed a small advantage to preoperative therapy (68% versus 65%; p = 0.32), which was not statistically significant. There was a decrease in late anastomotic strictures with preoperative therapy, and acute toxicity was also decreased by the use of preoperative radiation and chemotherapy, both statistically significant. This provides strong evidence of the superiority of preoperative adjuvant treatment in patients in whom it is determined that adjuvant therapy is needed. Eleven-year follow-up data for this study have just been published, demonstrating a persistently significant improvement in local control for pre- versus postoperative chemoradiation (local relapse rates 7.1% versus 10.1%; p = 0.48). However, there was still no effect on OS or distant metastases, highlighting the need for more effective systemic therapy than just 5-FU–based regimens.[138]

As multimodality treatment regimens are intensified to achieve even better outcomes, it is important to identify subgroups of patients at higher risk for severe toxicity and treatment interruption, both through investigation of predictive markers as well as attention to basic clinical parameters. In an unplanned analysis of the German trial data, Wolff et al.[139] found female gender to be significantly associated with CRT-induced acute toxicity but also associated with improved 10-year OS (62.7% versus 58.4%; p = 0.066). Men with no acute organ toxicities had much poorer OS compared to the rest, leading the authors to conclude that acute toxicity was a significant prognostic parameter and possibly a surrogate for treatment response. Future efforts will need to focus on mitigating this toxicity in susceptible patients without compromising treatment intensity.[139]

Similar to the goals of the German trial, the National Surgical Adjuvant Breast and Bowel Project (NSABP) R-03 trial compared neoadjuvant versus adjuvant CRT in the treatment of locally advanced rectal carcinoma. Patients with clinical T3 or T4 or node-positive rectal cancer were randomly assigned to preoperative or postoperative CRT. Chemotherapy consisted of 5-FU and leucovorin with 45 Gy in 25 fractions with a 5.40-Gy boost within the original margins of treatment. In the preoperative group, surgery was performed within 8 weeks after completion of radiotherapy. In the postoperative group, chemotherapy began after recovery from surgery but no later than 4 weeks after surgery. The primary end points were DFS and OS. A total of 267 patients were randomly assigned to NSABP R-03. The intended sample size was 900 patients. Excluding 11 ineligible and 2 eligible patients without follow-up data, the analysis used data on 123 patients randomly assigned to preoperative and 131 to postoperative CRT. Surviving patients were observed for a median of 8.4 years. The 5-year DFS for preoperative patients was 64.7% versus 53.4% for postoperative patients ($p = 0.011$). The 5-year OS for preoperative patients was 74.5% versus 65.6% for postoperative patients ($p = 0.065$). A pCR was achieved in 15% of preoperative patients. No preoperative patient with a pCR has had a recurrence. The investigators concluded that preoperative CRT, compared with postoperative CRT, significantly improved DFS and showed a trend toward improved OS.[140]

In addition to improving survival, another reason for using preoperative chemoradiation therapy is to increase the chance for sphincter preservation for patients with low-lying tumors of the rectum, where an abdominoperineal resection would be conventionally used. The NSABP R-03 trial was able to obtain worthwhile information regarding this issue. When a patient was first seen, the surgeon was asked (for both preoperative and postoperative patients) what operation was needed. In the patients randomized to postoperative radiation therapy (i.e., immediate surgery), the determination in the office corresponded extremely well to the operation actually performed. However, in the patients who received preoperative radiation therapy, sphincter-preserving surgery was done in 50% of patients compared with 33% of those who had initial surgery.[141] However, the data have been inconsistent overall in demonstrating an advantage to preoperative therapy in terms of sphincter preservation. The analyses are complicated because the decision as to whether sphincter-preserving surgery should be done is heavily dependent on the biases of the surgeon. If the surgeon believes that the same operation should be done regardless of tumor regression, then clearly the same surgery will be done. There are some surgeons who will do sphincter-preserving operations after preoperative irradiation, when they would not have done so if the surgery had been done first.

If one is using preoperative radiotherapy to try to improve the likelihood of sphincter preservation, the radiation must be given in such a way as to maximize the likelihood of this occurring. Specifically, a "standard" long course of irradiation to a dose of approximately 50 Gy at 18 to 20 Gy per fraction over 5 to 5.5 weeks (as given in the German trial mentioned previously) has been thought by most US investigators to be optimal. The short-course therapy with immediate surgery (typically 50 Gy for five fractions given over 1 week), as often used in Europe, followed by immediate surgery is not likely to produce enough tumor shrinkage to allow for sphincter preservation in patients with very low-lying tumors. Bujko et al.[142] have published data that suggest that the short course is as effective in producing local control as the longer course of therapy. A total of 312 patients were randomized to either 25 Gy in 5 fractions followed by surgery within 1 week, or 50.4 Gy in 28 fractions with concurrent bolus 5-FU and leucovorin and surgery 4 to 6 weeks later. DFS was respectively (short- versus long-course therapy) 58.4% versus 55.6%; local recurrence, 9% versus 14.2%; severe late toxicity, 10.1% versus 7.1%; and acute toxicity, 3.2% versus 18.2%. There was no improvement in sphincter preservation with long-course treatment. Although this was a relatively small study, it provides important evidence to support the value of short-course preoperative therapy. A second randomized trial from the Australian Intergroup randomized 326 patients with T3 rectal cancer within 12 cm of the anal verge to short-course radiotherapy (25 Gy in five fractions) or CRT (50.4 Gy with continuous infusion 5-FU). Both arms received adjuvant chemotherapy. The primary end point, locoregional recurrence at 3 years, was not significantly different at 7.5% for short-course radiotherapy and 4.4% for CRT with no difference in distant recurrence rates or OS. At median follow-up of 6 years, there were no differences in late toxicity rates.[143]

Both the Polish and Australian Intergroup trials were relatively small and not powered to show equivalence of long-course CRT and short-course radiotherapy. Both trials have relatively short follow-up and, as indicated by other randomized trials, locoregional recurrence continues to increase with time. In addition, late toxicities may manifest many years following treatment.

Another question is whether the time interval between radiation and surgery is more important than the duration of the preoperative treatment itself. Pettersson et al.[144] evaluated 112 patients who underwent short-course radiotherapy (25 Gy over 5 to 7 days) with delayed surgery >4 weeks and found a significant downstaging effect not previously seen with immediate resection.[144] Another study in which 154 patients receiving short-course radiation were prospectively randomized to immediate surgery (7-day to 10-day interval) versus delayed (4 weeks to 5 weeks) also demonstrated a higher downstaging rate in the latter group (13% versus 44.2%; $p = 0.0001$). In addition, there was reduced systemic recurrence (2.8% versus 12.3%; $p = 0.035$) and a trend toward improved 5-year survival (73% versus 63%). Interestingly, however, delayed surgery was not associated with superior locoregional control or increased rates of sphincter-saving procedures and curative resections.[145] Further trials are necessary to determine the ideal schedule of radiotherapy and surgery that optimizes both downstaging and overall oncologic outcomes. Some clinicians are advocating even more extended intervals between radiation and surgery. In a review of 1,593 patients, the median interval from the start of radiotherapy was 14 weeks (range, 6 weeks to 85 weeks; interquartile range, 12 weeks to 16 weeks) with the highest pCR rate found in patients undergoing resection at 15 weeks to 16 weeks (18%; $p = 0.013$).[146]

There are theoretical reasons to believe that radiation therapy delivered preoperatively would decrease the toxicity of therapy. With postoperative radiation therapy, the soft tissues of the perineum are at risk for involvement after an APR because of surgical manipulation and, therefore, need to be irradiated with its attendant acute skin toxicity. This is not needed with preoperative therapy. With postoperative radiation therapy, normal bowel is moved into the pelvis for the anastomosis after a low anterior resection and therefore is irradiated and at risk for late toxicity. In the preoperative setting, much of the irradiated bowel is removed with the surgical specimen and therefore is not at risk for producing late bowel injury. There is also likely to be a higher risk of having small bowel fixed in the pelvis after surgery secondary to adhesions, which could also lead to late toxicity. On the other hand, many studies have demonstrated that acute surgical morbidity and mortality are not substantially increased with the use of preoperative irradiation, although many surgeons routinely perform a temporary diverting colostomy in order to avoid the problems associated with an anastomotic leak. Except for the German trial previously mentioned, which shows decreased acute and late toxicity, data on late toxicity are not available to directly compare the two techniques when used with concurrent chemotherapy and the commonly used dose/fractionation schedules.

To better evaluate the impact of preoperative chemoradiation on long-term functional outcome, Loos et al.[147] performed a systematic review and meta-analysis of 25 studies and 6,548 patients, including six randomized controlled trials and previously published data from the Dutch TME trial. Although there was substantial heterogeneity of the included trials and low methodologic quality, the authors suggest that preoperative treatment has a largely negative impact on long-term anorectal function but does not significantly affect sexual or urinary performance compared to surgery alone. Without better designed trials, however, that include standardized pre- and postoperative assessment of these parameters as well as direct comparison to postoperative treatment, no definitive conclusions can be drawn.[147]

As the retrospective meta-analyses have generally shown better tumor control locally and better evidence of a survival advantage secondary to preoperative irradiation, many gastrointestinal oncologists prefer preoperative CRT for the patient who clearly requires adjuvant radiation therapy. A reasonable strategy at present is to use preoperative CRT for patients in whom there is little doubt about the advisability of adjuvant therapy (T3 node-positive or T4 disease) or patients with low-lying tumors in whom an APR may still be avoided, but to use initial surgery for other patient cohorts, with postoperative CRT used based on the operative and pathologic findings.

Another issue of importance is the timing of chemotherapy. It has been assumed by many investigators that concurrent preoperative chemotherapy and postoperative adjuvant chemotherapy is the proper way of delivering treatment. A study by the European Organization for Research and Treatment of Cancer, however, questions these assumptions.[148] Patients were randomized to receive either preoperative radiation therapy alone, preoperative CRT, preoperative radiation therapy and postoperative chemotherapy, or preoperative CRT and postoperative chemotherapy. Chemotherapy was bolus 5-FU (350 mg/m^2 per day for 5 days) and leucovorin (20 mg/m^2 for 5 days) with two cycles given with radiation therapy and four cycles postoperatively for the appropriate groups. Local recurrence rates were roughly similar for all patients receiving chemotherapy regardless of timing (7% to 9%) and significantly improved compared with those patients not receiving any chemotherapy (17%). There was no difference in survival outcomes based on the timing of chemotherapy. The 5-year DFS rates were 52.2% and 58.2% in the no adjuvant treatment groups and the adjuvant treatment groups, respectively ($p = 0.13$).

Two recent Cochrane reviews have addressed the role of adding chemotherapy to preoperative radiation regimens. The first included six randomized controlled trials, with a total of 247 patients, comparing preoperative CRT to radiation alone in the treatment of stage III cancers. Thirty-day mortality, sphincter preservation rates, and late toxicity events were similar between groups. A significant increase in acute grade 3/4 toxicity was seen in patients who received CRT versus radiation alone. While there was no difference in OS, CRT was associated with significantly less local recurrence (OR = 0.56; p <0.0001).[149] A second meta-analysis, including five randomized controlled trials, addressed similar questions in stage II-III disease and reported similar findings. The addition of chemotherapy increased grade 3/4 toxicity with no impact on postoperative mortality, anastomotic leak rate, or sphincter preservation. There was also a significant reduction in 5-year local recurrence rate (OR = 0.39 to 0.72; p <0.001) as well as an increase in pCR (OR = 2.12 to 5.84; p <0.00001) in the CRT group, but again no differences in survival. Additional studies with longer follow-up are needed to determine the full benefit of preoperative chemotherapy as well its impact on functional outcome and quality of life.[150]

WHICH PATIENTS SHOULD RECEIVE ADJUVANT THERAPY?

For either pre- or postoperative therapy, the physician needs to address the issue of precisely which patients need to receive adjuvant radiation therapy and chemotherapy. At the present time, these two modalities have been completely linked in US clinical trials, so it is not possible to determine if there are subsets of patients who might benefit from one modality and not the other. In addition, recent US trials have all used chemotherapy concurrent with the radiation therapy in addition to postradiation chemotherapy, so it is not possible to determine the relative importance of each modality.

Based on the historical patterns of failure data, which demonstrated high local failure rates with surgery alone for patients with T3 and/or node-positive disease, virtually all US studies have evaluated this entire patient population. However, many of these studies predate the routine use of now-standard TME surgery, and more detailed analyses have allowed us to define characteristics that help define relatively low-risk and relatively high-risk patient subsets. As mentioned earlier, among the patients conventionally treated with adjuvant CRT, a number of relatively lower risk categories have been identified. Those include patients with T3N0 or

T1-2N1 disease,[17,18,151] those with primary tumors located high in the rectum, those with wide circumferential margins on the final pathology specimen,[29,30] those with node-negative disease after multiple (12 to 14 or more) nodes have been evaluated,[19-21,152] and those in whom TME surgery had been performed by an experienced colorectal oncologic surgeon.[153,154] In the preoperative setting, only some of this information will be available at the time a therapeutic decision must be made, but some information will be available (including knowledge of the surgeon). In addition, one must consider the known inaccuracy of transrectal ultrasound in staging and the experience of the ultrasonographer.[33,60] However, if most of these conditions are met, it is possible that routine adjuvant radiation therapy, and perhaps chemotherapy, is not required for the lower-stage tumors.

Another question is which patients are unlikely to respond to chemoradiation at all and would only be disadvantaged by the toxicities and delay in surgical treatment. Numerous biomarkers and tumor-related features are under investigation as potential predictive factors of response, and this will have important implications for preoperative patient selection as well.[155-165] Among these biomarkers, KRAS has received quite a lot of attention, but results are conflicting. Previous reports suggest that mutated tumors are less likely to develop a pCR compared to wild-type. Duldulao et al.[166] has recently published follow-up data that support this (13% versus 33% pCR in KRAS mutant versus wild-type; $p = 0.006$).[166] However, a larger meta-analysis of eight series and 696 patients showed no association between KRAS status and pCR, tumor downstaging, or cancer-related mortality. Although limited by the heterogeneity of its included studies, this report highlights the need for caution when considering biomarkers in the context of clinical decision making.[167] Another newly described method for predicting response to neoadjuvant therapy involves measuring histologic changes in the tumor soon after the initiation of treatment. Suzuki et al.[168] evaluated biopsies obtained 7 days into the CRT course, comparing expression levels of various apoptotic markers and cellular changes to pretreatment findings as well as to the final surgical specimen. Markers and cellular features of apoptosis at 7 days were strongly correlated with pCR and tumor regression. This study offers another potential strategy for identifying patients who might benefit from early alternative interventions.[168] At the present time, most patients treated outside clinical trials that have T3-4 and/or node-positive disease should probably receive neoadjuvant CRT if there are no extenuating circumstances. However, for patients who meet the previously mentioned favorable criteria, especially those with high rectal T3 N0 tumors, avoiding neoadjuvant radiation therapy and perhaps chemotherapy can be considered. Clinical trials will need to be performed to help resolve which subsets of patients do not require routine adjuvant radiation therapy. New data suggests that for the subset of patients who are confirmed to be node-negative after neoadjuvant chemoradiation and curative surgery, little benefit may be derived from additional postoperative treatment. In two studies, long-term survival and recurrence outcomes were compared between patients with ypN0 rectal cancer who did and did not receive adjuvant chemotherapy. Overall, there was minimal difference between the two groups with prognosis primarily determined by pathologic stage.[169,170] However, these nonrandomized data should be regarded as preliminary and hypothesis-generating; postoperative chemotherapy should be the default position in these patients, and deviations from this plan should only be made on an individual basis after a detailed review of the patient's comorbidities, relative risks, and benefits, and a detailed discussion of this with the patient.

Another important area of investigation is whether patients who have a complete clinical response to neoadjuvant therapy can be safely managed with a nonoperative, "watch and wait" approach. In other words, can the organ-preserving multidisciplinary algorithm, which is now the standard of care for anal cancer, be adopted for rectal malignancy as well? This "wait and see" approach was first seriously addressed in a seminal study by Habr-Gama et al.,[171] which compared the outcomes of 71 clinically complete responders who were observed without surgery to a well-matched group of patients with pCR who were resected. After a mean follow-up of 57 months, there were no cancer-related deaths in the observation group and recurrence rates were extremely low regardless of treatment strategy.[171] Another more recently published study from a different group reported similar results. In this report, 21 patients who achieved a clinical complete response were followed without surgery for a mean of 25 ± 19 months and compared to 20 patients who underwent resection with pCR.[172] There was one local recurrence in the observed group, treated with local excision, and two deaths in the control group. In addition (not surprisingly) functional outcome was significantly better in the patients who did not undergo surgery. Despite the small sample size and short follow-up, these results lend further credibility to the "wait and see" approach in carefully selected patients with rectal cancer. A similar report from yet a third group noted that in 32 patients carefully selected over a 5-year period, with a median follow-up of 28 months, 6 patients experienced local recurrence (3 of whom also had distant recurrence), and all 6 patients were able to undergo resection of the recurrent primary to achieve local control. When compared in an exploratory analysis to a control group of patient treated in the same institution who had undergone resection and had been found to have a pCR, 2-year distant DFS and OS appeared to be similar. Of course, these numbers are small and nonrandomized, and follow-up is short; however, the experience further supports the investigation of selective nonoperative management in patients who achieve a clinical complete response.[173]

Given continued improvements in adjuvant therapies as well as the increasingly sophisticated imaging modalities available for follow-up, a new organ-sparing algorithm for treatment warrants further consideration. At present such an approach outside a clinical trial represents a clear departure from standard practice, and should only be considered in a fully informed patient who is willing and able to comprehend and accept the inherent risks. Logically, this approach seems most appropriate for consideration in those patients with distal tumors, in whom either an APR or a low anastomosis with poor functional outcome would be required. As noted previously, PET scans have insufficient sensitivity and specificity to be relied on in terms of determining the presence or absence of a complete clinical response, and should not be used for this purpose.

One aspect of combined modality therapy, which is undergoing reconsideration at some centers, is the order of administration of modalities of therapy. As noted in detail previously, preoperative chemoradiation followed by surgery followed by postoperative chemotherapy is the most commonly used approach. The role of administering all therapy, both chemotherapy and CRT prior to surgery has become of increasing interest, however. Chau et al.[174] were the first to publish an experience using induction capecitabine plus oxaliplatin (Cape/Ox) for 3 months prior to radiation plus capecitabine in 77 patients with poor-risk rectal cancer.[174] The response rate to Cape/Ox chemotherapy alone was 88%, with 86% of patients achieving symptomatic relieve within a median of 32 days of starting therapy. Fernandez-Martos et al.[175] published a small randomized phase 2 trial in which a total of 108 patients with rectal cancer were randomly assigned to either standard order chemoradiation followed by surgery followed by Cape/Ox chemotherapy, or to Cape/Ox chemotherapy first, followed by surgery. As might be anticipated from the small size of this trial, there were no differences between the arms in terms of efficacy, with pCR rates and R0 resection rates being essentially the same; however, greater dose intensity of both oxaliplatin and capecitabine was achieved in the group receiving preoperative chemotherapy, and higher grades 3 and 4 adverse events were seen during postoperative versus preoperative chemotherapy. The toxicities and dose intensities during the combined CRT were essentially the same in the two arms. Subsequently, several other single-institution experiences with this total neoadjuvant approach

have been reported. Cercek et al.[176] reported a retrospective series of 61 patients who received some or all of their planned chemotherapy as initial treatment for rectal cancer. Of these 61, 19 (31%) had either a pCR (14 patients) or had a complete clinical response and elected to pursue nonoperative management (5 patients). Perez et al.[177] reported preliminary results of a prospective trial of this approach in 36 patients and concluded that a larger proportion of patients were able to complete all planned FOLFOX chemotherapy than would have been expected from postoperative administration. Given the expense of a large-scale trial of initial versus postoperative chemotherapy, it is clear that an adequately powered trial comparing these two approaches will never be done. The potential benefits of initial chemotherapy are several. Firstly, it allows for administration of full-dose chemotherapy earlier in the course of treatment and appears to permit greater dose intensity, which may improve treatment of distant micrometastases and so improve long-term outcome. It also allows for patients requiring temporary ostomies after resection to have those ostomies closed after only 2 months and to not have to tolerate chemotherapy during the time they have an ostomy. In addition, the approach of delivering all planned chemotherapy and radiation therapy preoperatively allows for a favorable platform from which to consider nonoperative management in carefully selected patients.

A critical component of the "wait and see" approach is the ability to accurately identify pathologic complete responders in the preoperative setting. While many strategies have been utilized toward this end, including endoscopic evaluation, imaging, and tissue biopsy, there is no consensus on the optimal method and each has significant limitations. Endoscopic evaluation and close surveillance have long been considered important tools for detecting residual or recurrent malignancy. A recent expert consensus article described the cardinal signs of incomplete tumor response: deep ulceration with or without necrosis, superficial ulceration or mucosal irregularity, a palpable nodule despite mucosal integrity, or significant stenosis.[178] Using these criteria, Smith et al.[179] reported that an endoscopic, or "clinically complete," response was 90% predictive of pCR. Sensitivity of this assessment was low, however, with 61% of the pathologic complete responders demonstrating ultimately false signs of incomplete clinical response.[179]

A variety of imaging modalities have been applied to evaluate tumor burden after neoadjuvant therapy as well. Most are limited by the inability to differentiate postradiation fibrosis from residual cancer cells. Guillem et al.[180] found PET and CT equally inadequate in distinguishing complete from partial pathologic responders in a prospective analysis of 121 patients. Among the 26 patients with a complete response, only 54% and 19% were correctly classified by PET and CT scans, respectively. And of the 95 patients with an incomplete response, 66% and 95% were appropriately recognized by these techniques.[180] Perez et al.[181] also found PET/CT lacking in its ability to definitively identify pCR. In a series of 99 patients, imaging yielded 5 false-negative and 10 false-positive results, giving PET/CT a 93% sensitivity, 53% specificity, 73% negative predictive value, and 87% positive predictive value for the detection of residual cancer. Accuracy of PET/CT was 85%, which was inferior to that of clinical assessment alone at 91%.[181] Much attention has focused on the role of MRI in evaluating tumor burden at all stages of rectal cancer management. Diffusion-weighted MRI has been particularly useful for predicting tumor response in multiple sites and has the advantage of providing a quantitative measurement (apparent diffusion coefficient), which can be tracked longitudinally and compared to pretreatment values. However, this modality is also limited in its ability to distinguish residual solitary tumor cells from a complete response.[182]

Endoscopic biopsies seem to be the most unreliable measure of tumor response, with one study reporting a negative predictive value of 11% (only 3 of the 28 negative biopsies were associated an actual tumor-free specimen after definitive resection).[183] These disappointing results might be explained by the fact that residual tumor cells do not necessarily reside in the most superficial layers of the bowel wall. In fact, Duldulao et al.[184] reports that, in analysis of 94 patients with yPT2-4 tumors, only 13% had cancer cells remaining in the mucosa and only 56% in the submucosa. The majority of tumor burden after neoadjuvant therapy appears to be located at the invasive front, or deepest layer of the bowel wall, suggesting that only a full-thickness or excisional biopsy could accurately detect residual malignancy.[184] The question then becomes where to perform this biopsy. In a recent study, Hayden et al.[185] found that a significant amount of "tumor scatter" occurs after neoadjuvant therapy, with 49.1% of cancer cells located outside the visible ulcer or deep to normal-appearing mucosa. Moreover, the mean distance of distal scatter was 1.0 cm from the visible edge to a maximum of 3 cm, indicating that neither gross ulceration nor the traditional 2 cm margin can be used to adequately guide biopsy or excision of the potential residual tumor.[185] Additionally, even if complete full-thickness excision of the tumor site and all remaining potential cancer cells within the bowel wall were accomplished, a sterile specimen does not guarantee complete nodal response. While the rate of LN involvement in patients with a ypT0 lesion is small, it is not zero (7.7% and 9.1% in recent reports), and therefore there is ultimately no conclusive method for determining a pCR short of total mesenteric excision.[186,187]

CONCURRENT CHEMOTHERAPY

The use of adjuvant chemotherapy has centered on the use of 5-FU chemotherapy, although this drug has been in use for over 50 years and is not very effective for colon or rectal cancer. The initial trials of trimodality therapy in rectal cancer used bolus 5-FU at a dose of 500 mg/m² per day for 3 days during weeks 1 and 5 of the radiation therapy. This was the approach routinely used until the results of the North Central Cancer Treatment Group study testing the use of long-term continuous infusion 5-FU with postoperative radiation therapy (bolus 5-FU was used both before and after the radiation therapy) were reported.[133] This study demonstrated an advantage to continuous infusion 5-FU (only during radiation therapy) compared with bolus 5-FU in terms of local control, DFS, and OS. Because of this result and the encouraging results found with more aggressive therapy in colon cancer, it was logical to think that further intensification of chemotherapy would be of value both for local and systemic control.

Unfortunately, this expectation has not been borne out. Two large US Gastrointestinal Intergroup trials have been run testing intensification with either more aggressive 5-FU and leucovorin, additional continuous infusion 5-FU, and other combinations, with data demonstrating no advantage.[188,189] Thus, we are left with evidence that continuous infusion 5-FU during radiation therapy is of value in improving local control, distant metastases, and survival, but no evidence that anything other than simple 5-FU or 5-FU plus leucovorin should be used during the chemotherapy portion of the therapy. As will be discussed in the following, at present we do not have compelling evidence that addition of other agents, such as oxaliplatin, irinotecan, bevacizumab, cetuximab, or panitumumab, should be included with fluoropyrimidines concurrently with radiation therapy.

In practice, most gastrointestinal oncologists now use capecitabine or continuous infusion 5-FU during radiation therapy. The 1,608-patient phase 3 randomized NSABP R-04 trial has definitively established that capecitabine is noninferior to infusional 5-FU when used concurrently with preoperative radiation therapy in patents with rectal cancer.[190] There were no statistically significant differences in pCR rates, rate of sphincter-sparing surgery, surgical downstaging, or treatment-related toxicities. This study also was a 2 × 2 randomization to include concurrent oxaliplatin with radiation therapy of not. This large

trial showed no benefit for the inclusion of oxaliplatin, with substantially increased toxicity in the oxaliplatin-containing arm. A large trial of capecitabine versus bolus 5-FU confirmed that capecitabine is noninferior to 5-FU in this setting. Final results from this trial are now published, demonstrating superior 5-year OS (76% versus 67%; $p = 0.05$) and 3-year DFS (75% versus 67%; $p = 0.07$) for patients who received capecitabine in both adjuvant and neoadjuvant cohorts. There were similar rates of local recurrence in each group (6% versus 7%), but fewer patients receiving capecitabine developed distant metastases (19% versus 28%; $p = 0.04$).[191] These findings suggest greater systemic efficacy of capecitabine compared to bolus 5-FU and mirror the conclusions drawn from the most recent X-ACT trial data for stage III colon cancer. Long-term follow-up from this study over a median of 6.9 years demonstrated that capecitabine significantly improved both DFS and OS with a better overall safety profile than 5-FU/folinic acid in the adjuvant setting.[192]

There has been greater interest in the use of oxaliplatin added to 5-FU and radiation therapy, although thus far the results have been disappointing. A phase 1/2 study performed by the Cancer and Leukemia Group B demonstrated the feasibility of concurrent oxaliplatin, 5-FU, and radiation therapy,[193] as did a German multicenter phase 2 trial,[194] and the previously mentioned Radiation Therapy Oncology Group randomized phase 2 trial.[195] The NSABP, as part of their R-04 trial, is doing a second randomization to the use of weekly oxaliplatin (50 mg/m² per day) with an evaluation of pCR and local control as end points. However, phase 3 results have begun to emerge, and they are not as encouraging as had been hoped.[196] The French ACCORD cooperative group reported a trial in which 598 patients with locally advanced rectal cancer were randomly assigned to preoperative treatment with 5 weeks of radiation therapy (45 Gy in 25 fractions) with concurrent capecitabine 800 mg/m² twice daily 5 days per week or the same regimen plus oxaliplatin 50 mg/m² once weekly.[197] There was not a statistically significant difference in the primary end point of the trial, the pCR rate, which was 13.9% without and 19.2% with oxaliplatin ($p = 0.09$). More preoperative grade 3–4 toxicity occurred in the oxaliplatin group (25% versus 1%; $p < 0.001$). There were no statistically significant differences between groups in the rate of sphincter-preserving operations (75%), and no differences in terms of rates of serious medical or surgical complications or postoperative deaths at 60 days (0.3%). The authors concluded that the trial did not support the addition of oxaliplatin to this regimen, and that oxaliplatin should not be used with concurrent irradiation in standard practice. They did not detect an improvement in the frequency of clear circumferential radial margins, and they speculated that further investigations are warranted in selected populations. Secondary end point data from this trial have just been published demonstrating no advantage in clinical outcomes with the addition of oxaliplatin either. At 3 years follow-up, there were no significant differences in local recurrence, OS, or DFS.[198]

A large Italian cooperative group phase 3 trial reached a similar result.[199] A total of 747 patients were randomly assigned to either 5-FU infusion (225 mg/m² per day) concomitant with external beam pelvic radiation (50.4 Gy in 28 daily fractions) or the same regimen plus weekly oxaliplatin (60 mg/m² × 6). The primary end point was OS. Data are not yet mature for this end point; however, a secondary end point of primary tumor response to preoperative treatment, as well as toxicity data, have been reported. Overall grade 3–4 toxicity rates on treated patients (mainly diarrhea) were 8% without oxaliplatin and 24% in the oxaliplatin-containing arm ($p < 0.001$). Eighty-two percent of patients receiving oxaliplatin got five or more doses of this drug. pCR rates were 15% and 16% in the 5-FU only and 5-FU–oxaliplatin arms, respectively. The authors concluded that the addition of weekly oxaliplatin to standard 5-FU–based preoperative CRT significantly increases toxicity without affecting local tumor response. Survival data requires further maturation.

As a follow-up to the seminal publication by Sauer et al.,[137] another German trial has been initiated to better evaluate the integration of oxaliplatin into neoadjuvant and adjuvant regimens for rectal cancer. This randomized phase 3 study, entitled CAO/ARO/AIO-04, hopes to achieve an impact on DFS not seen in previous reports. Only preliminary data has been published thus far supporting the feasibility of an oxaliplatin-based regimen, with good compliance and acceptable toxicity and surgical morbidity. Interestingly, in an unplanned analysis, the pCR rate was found to be significantly higher in the oxaliplatin group compared to 5-FU alone (17% versus 13%; $p = 0.038$). Longer follow-up is needed to address the primary end point of DFS, and the finding must be considered in the context of the multiple negative trials regarding concurrent use of oxaliplatin and radiation therapy previously noted.[200]

Postresection use of adjuvant chemotherapy based on the results in colon cancer has become a widespread practice, with oncologists using primarily FOLFOX (biweekly oxaliplatin, 5-FU, and leucovorin; see Chapter 49) as the postradiation chemotherapy. This is based on the reasonable, albeit unproven, extrapolation from data showing that the addition of oxaliplatin to 5-FU/leucovorin improves DFS and OS in the postoperative management of patients with colon cancer (see Chapter 49). In addition to studies that have substituted fluoropyrimidines, there is also substantial interest in the use of other agents added to fluoropyrimidines with concurrent radiation therapy. There have been studies with the addition of irinotecan,[201] but because of the overlapping toxicity of diarrhea with radiation therapy and 5-FU, plus the demonstrated lack of efficacy of irinotecan in the adjuvant treatment of colon cancer, use of irinotecan in the combined mode has not been, and most likely ought not be, heavily pursued. A small randomized phase 3 study showed no benefit to the addition of irinotecan to 5-FU/leucovorin in the nonradiation portion of the treatment.[202] The Radiation Therapy Oncology Group completed a small randomized phase 2 trial of concurrent capecitabine, irinotecan, and radiation therapy versus concurrent oxaliplatin, capecitabine, and radiation therapy.[195] Both on the basis of a lack of data supporting adjuvant irinotecan and a superior pCR rate in the oxaliplatin-containing arm, no further development of the irinotecan-containing schedule is planned.

As biologic agents have a substantial appeal when used in combination with conventional cytotoxics, they also have a large appeal in combination with radiation therapy. There is evidence for a beneficial effect of both cetuximab and bevacizumab when combined with cytotoxics in patients with metastatic colon and rectal cancer (see Chapter 49). There are good laboratory data demonstrating radiation sensitization when these (and similar) agents are used in vitro, and a substantial improvement has been shown in survival in patients with head and neck cancer when cetuximab is added to radiation therapy.[203] Only preliminary studies have been done,[204] but given the lack of encouraging complete responses and the negative results with cetuximab in adjuvant colon cancer (see Chapter 49), it is unlikely that there will be substantial further investigations in this area, and neither cetuximab nor panitumumab should be used in standard practice with radiation therapy for rectal cancer. Similarly, bevacizumab has failed to demonstrate a benefit in adjuvant colon cancer, and should not be used in the routine management of locally advanced rectal cancer.

The literature on this topic continues to grow with a number of new phase 2 trials reporting on the feasibility, safety, and even potential superiority of neoadjuvant regimens that incorporate these agents. Kim et al.[205] found that adding cetuximab to preoperative radiotherapy with irinotecan and capeceitabine was well tolerated in 39 patients and achieved a much higher pCR rate of 23.1%, compared to 10% to 15% with conventional 5-FU regimens. Pinto et al.[206] reported a similarly improved pCR rate of 21.1% in the StarPan/STAR-02 Study, which evaluated panitumumab, oxaliplatin, and 5-FU with concurrent radiotherapy. While this did not reach their anticipated goal, it was a substantial improvement over both 5-FU–only regimens and 5-FU/oxaliplatin combinations from previous reports. The high incidence of grade 3-4 diarrhea with one toxic death, however, mandates modification of this regimen in future trials.[206]

Most recently, in a study evaluating pre- and postoperative Cape/Ox regimens with and without weekly cetuximab, the addition of cetuximab significantly improved radiologic response as well as OS (HR = 0.27; $p = 0.34$).[207] These results are tempered by the negative phase 2 trial of cetuximab in the adjuvant treatment of KRAS wild-type stage III colon cancer. Outside of a clinical trial, neither cetuximab nor panitumumab should be used in the adjuvant or neoadjuvant treatment of locally advanced rectal cancer.

The role of bevacizumab in neoadjuvant therapy is also promising, although dosing schedules, appropriate use of synergistic medications, and patient selection have yet to be defined. When combined with 5-FU ± oxaliplatin in the most recent studies, toxicity levels were manageable and pCR rates ranged from 13% to 36%. In addition, Spigel et al.[208] reported an 85% 1-year DFS.[209,210] However, the negative outcomes of bevacizumab trials in colon cancer adjuvant therapy have greatly dampened enthusiasm for pursuing this approach. Outside of a clinical trial, the use of bevacizumab in the adjuvant treatment of rectal cancer is not recommended.

SYNCHRONOUS RECTAL PRIMARY AND METASTASES

The use of pelvic radiotherapy in patients with synchronous presentation of primary and metastatic disease is controversial. Primary combination chemotherapy can provide substantial palliation and can be considered as initial therapy in many patients with rectal cancer and metastatic disease.[211] Endoscopically placed expandable metal stents can be considered for palliation or protection from impending obstruction. Control of disease in the pelvis can have important implications for patient quality of life; therefore, combined modality therapy, including radiation, chemotherapy, and in some cases palliative surgery, can be appropriate, especially when extrapelvic metastatic disease is small volume and the patient's prognosis is favorable enough that pelvic complications could be anticipated as a long-term problem. No firm guidelines can be made in the management of these complex patients, and treatment decisions must be made on an individual basis.

MANAGEMENT OF UNRESECTABLE PRIMARY AND LOCALLY ADVANCED DISEASE (T4)

Although the majority of patients who present with stage II and III disease have primary tumors that are technically easily resectable, there are a group of patients who have T4 tumors with deep local invasion into adjacent structures, which makes primary resection for cure difficult, if not impossible. Some T4 tumors invade into the vagina, which is easily resectable, but others invade into pelvic sidewall or sacrum, where a complete surgical resection may be impossible (the coccyx and distal sacrum can be resected, if appropriate), and others invade into bladder or prostate, where a more extensive surgical resection can be done, but often at the expense of major morbidity or functional loss. Although there are few randomized trials to define optimal therapy in this group of patients, there are data suggesting that it is appropriate to treat these patients with preoperative radiation therapy combined with chemotherapy, in a manner similar to that described for T3 disease, generally with concurrent 5-FU–based chemotherapy. This will often result in a good clinical response that will allow for a potentially curative resection to be performed. It is preferable to treat a patient preoperatively to try to avoid leaving residual disease rather than attempting to salvage a patient after a clearly inadequate operation.

The use of adjuvant radiation therapy in this clinical situation also allows for treatment of the lymphatics draining the locally invaded organ, such as the internal or external iliacs, that are not typically resected in a low anterior resection or APR, but which may be at substantial risk of secondary involvement from an invaded organ, such as the bladder. Although the definition of "unresectable" is very subjective, a number of studies have shown that preoperative radiation therapy can convert a substantial number of these patients to having resectable disease with substantial cure rates.[212–215]

In a randomized phase 3 trial of 207 patients with locally nonresectable T4 primary rectal carcinoma or local recurrence from rectal cancer, patients received chemotherapy (5-FU/leucovorin) administered concurrently with radiotherapy (50 Gy) and adjuvant for 16 weeks after surgery (98 patients) or radiation therapy (50 Gy) alone (109 patients). The two groups were well balanced according to pretreatment characteristics. An R0 resection was performed in 82 patients (84%) in the CRT group and in 74 patients (68%) in the radiation therapy group ($p = 0.009$). Local control (82% versus 67% at 5 years; log-rank $p = 0.03$), time to treatment failure (63% versus 44%; $p = 0.003$), cancer-specific survival (72% versus 55%; $p = 0.02$), and OS (66% versus 53%; $p = 0.09$) all favored the CRT group. There was no difference in late toxicity.[216] Although the use of preoperative radiation therapy with concurrent 5-FU–based chemotherapy, as described earlier, appears of value in patients with locally advanced disease, there is still a substantial incidence of local failure. Therefore, a number of investigators have explored ways to increase the radiation dose to the highest risk region to try to improve local tumor control. Three main techniques have been used: supplemental postoperative external beam radiation boost, intraoperative electron beam radiation therapy boost, and intraoperative brachytherapy boost.

There are relatively few data on the use of postoperative external beam as a boost, largely because of concerns of normal tissue tolerance after the use of the relatively large fields delivered preoperatively, extensive surgical resection, and the prolonged delay between initial external beam therapy and the final boost after recovery from surgery. The two intraoperative techniques are philosophically the same, although the technique of radiation delivery is different. After a high dose (50 Gy) of preoperative CRT and then a 4- to 6-week break, surgical resection is performed, the extent of which depends on the location and extent of tumor. Areas considered at high risk for residual tumor are determined both by the surgical findings and frozen section pathologic evaluation. For electron beam intraoperative radiotherapy, a treatment cylinder is placed over the high-risk region, often on a pelvic sidewall or the sacrum, and the cylinder is then aligned to the radiation machine, which is either in the operating room or in the radiation therapy department. The cylinder acts both to hold normal tissues outside the radiation beam and to confine the electron beam. The use of electrons allows the radiation oncologist to adjust the depth of penetration of the beam to conform to the local tumor extent. When using brachytherapy, carriers for the radioactive sources are placed over the high-risk region, and the radiation is then given either during the surgery (high-dose rate) or the radioactive sources are inserted approximately 5 days after surgery and left in place for 1 or 2 days (low-dose rate). In all situations, the radiation dose is in the range of 10 to 20 (most commonly 15) Gy when used as a boost to conventional therapy. In both approaches, care must be taken to ensure that normal tissues such as small bowel are out of the irradiated volume.

Techniques similar to this have been used for a number of years and have shown encouraging results, although formal randomized trials have not been performed. Data suggest fairly good levels of local control and long-term survival if a gross total resection can be accomplished, with poorer results if there is gross residual (Table 52.6).[217–220] Use of intraoperative radiotherapy boosts often requires specialized radiation facilities and expertise as well as an experienced team of radiation oncologists, surgical oncologists, urologists, and plastic surgeons. Similar types of surgical and radiation therapy approaches can produce surprisingly good results. For patients who still cannot have a surgical resection performed, either because of the tumor extent or because of coexisting medical problems, attempts should be made to maximize palliation and perhaps local control. Boost doses of radiation are appropriately delivered to the residual tumor to doses of >60 Gy if sensitive normal tissues (primarily small bowel) can be removed from the radiation fields. Only a small percentage (5%) of patients with these advanced tumors will be locally controlled and cured by such an approach, but a substantial percentage will obtain good palliation.[221–223]

RADIATION THERAPY TECHNIQUE

There have been primarily two dosing schemes for radiation therapy that have been used in the treatment of rectal cancer. In the preoperative setting, many European centers have favored a rapid short-course treatment of doses of approximately 25 Gy in five fractions followed by immediate surgery, whereas US centers have generally favored doses of 50.4 Gy given at 1.8 Gy per fraction

CANCERS OF THE GASTROINTESTINAL TRACT

TABLE 52.6

Intraoperative Radiation Therapy for Locally Advanced Rectal Cancer[a]

Resection	Mayo Clinic			Massachusetts General Hospital		
	No. of Patients	Local Failure (%)	Overall Survival (5 y) (%)	No. of Patients	Local Failure (%)	Disease-Specific Survival (%)
Complete resection	18[b]	7	69	40	9	63
Partial resection	35	~20	~40	24	37	35
No resection	1	—	0	—	—	—
Total	56	16	46	64	—	—
Recurrent locally advanced tumor	42	40	19	—	—	—

[a] External beam radiotherapy + resection + intraoperative radiotherapy, no prior radiation therapy.
[b] Two additional patients with no tumor in specimen—both without any tumor recurrence. These are included in the totals.

with a delay of 4 to 8 weeks until surgery. As previously mentioned, an advantage of the long-course therapy is that it provides time to have tumor regression, which appears to facilitate sphincter preservation, although it is more expensive and time-consuming for the patient. In addition, there was substantial late toxicity from the short-course treatment in earlier series, although this was most evident when the radiation therapy techniques were less sophisticated and simple anteroposterior/posteroanterior fields alone were used, which were at times quite large[224]; those techniques are not used at present.

Although major late toxicity is relatively uncommon, functional gastrointestinal disturbances are relatively common. These relate to both surgical effects on bowel with lack of a good reservoir function and possible nerve dysfunction, as well as long-term radiation effects on bowel compliance and neural functioning.[225,226] Many patients continue to have some rectal urgency and food intolerance (especially to roughage), but symptoms tend to improve over time and most patients can live a relatively normal life regarding their gastrointestinal tract. Detailed discussions with the patient about the type of foods likely to cause worsening bowel symptoms, attention to the superimposed problems that can occur from other difficulties such as lactose intolerance, and use of agents such as loperamide all can help the patient deal with bowel problems.

Small bowel–related complications are directly proportional to the volume of small bowel in the radiation field and the radiation dose. In patients receiving combined modality therapy, the volume of irradiated small bowel limits the ability to escalate the dose of 5-FU. A number of simple radiotherapeutic techniques are available to decrease radiation-related small bowel toxicity. First, small bowel contrast or CT scanning during treatment planning allows identification of the location of the small bowel so that fields can be designed to minimize its treatment. Multiple-field techniques (preferably a three- or four-field technique) are now standard to minimize normal tissue irradiation. The use of lateral fields for the boost as well as positioning the patient in the prone position can further decrease the volume of small bowel in the lateral radiation fields.

The treatment should be designed with the use of computerized radiation dosimetry and be delivered by high-energy linear accelerators that deliver a higher dose to the target volume while relatively sparing surrounding normal structures. The advantage of combining a multiple-field technique, high-energy photons, and computerized dosimetry produces a homogenous dose distribution throughout the target volume and minimizes the dose to the small bowel. Although not well studied to date, newer developments in intensity-modulated radiation therapy may allow more conformal radiation dose distributions and a decrease in the irradiation of small bowel. To date, intensity-modulated radiation therapy has not been shown to be of additional value in the adjuvant treatment of rectal cancer.

After pelvic surgery, the small bowel commonly fills the pelvis. Adhesions can form, resulting in fixed loops of small bowel in the radiation fields. In this situation, despite treatment of the patient in the prone position, the use of multiple-field techniques may be of limited value. In contrast, when radiation therapy is delivered preoperatively to a patient who has not undergone prior pelvic surgery, the small bowel is usually mobile. When no small bowel fixation is present, treatment in the prone position can exclude much of the small bowel from the posteroanterior field and completely from the lateral fields.

Various physical maneuvers to exclude small bowel from the pelvis have been examined. Gallagher et al.[227] determined the volume, distribution, and mobility of small bowel in the pelvis after a variety of maneuvers. Regardless of the prior surgical history, a significant decrease was seen in the average small bowel volume when the patients were treated in the prone position with abdominal wall compression and bladder distention compared with the supine position. Treatment in the prone position without abdominal wall compression was not consistently effective in displacing

small bowel and, in some patients (most commonly, obese), the volume of small bowel increased.

Radiation Fields

The precise radiation fields that are used should depend on the individual clinical situation, although the principles of the radiation treatment remain the same. The locoregional failures in rectal cancer occur both because of residual disease in the soft tissues of the pelvis as well as from residual pelvic nodal disease. The nodal disease can be in the internal iliac chain for very low-lying lesions, but only involves the external iliac nodes if the anal canal or sphincter is involved or if an organ is involved that drains into the external iliac system. The internal iliac nodes are not usually dissected by the surgeon, so it is important to treat these for low rectal cancers, but the external iliacs should not be routinely irradiated. The proximal extent of nodal radiation is arbitrary, but the primary drainage of all rectal cancers is along the mesenteric system, and those nodes should primarily be treated surgically. Extending radiation fields to cover para-aortic nodes is not indicated unless there is evidence of disease in those chains.

Because many of the local recurrences occur in the soft tissues of the pelvis, the radiation oncologist must be sure to treat the regions that are least well treated by the surgeon. These include extension to the pelvic sidewall and presacral space, and to the prostate in men and vagina in women. The proximal extent of the radiation field should generally extend to the sacral promontory, as that is the level at which there is an attachment of the posterior peritoneum and where the retroperitoneal rectum becomes the intraperitoneal colon. Above this level, there is little risk of pelvic soft tissue invasion for standard rectal cancer.

The lower extent of the radiation field is more complex. Often, the surgeon will rely on the radiation oncologist to sterilize the most distal extent of the primary tumor in order to perform a sphincter-preserving operation, so the distal margins should be at least a couple of centimeters below the primary tumor mass. Although rectal tumors tend to have only a minimal amount of longitudinal spread along the mucosal margin, they can spread further distally in the perirectal fat and in the LNs in the mesorectum. In fact, this is part of the rationale for a TME. Attempts should thus be made for treatment to at least the level of the dentate line for most low-lying rectal cancers, although this is likely not necessary for rectal cancers in the proximal third. However, it is also likely true that a substantial part of the late toxicity from pelvic radiation therapy is related to dysfunction of the anal sphincter. Thus, it is important to try to minimize the amount of sphincter that is irradiated. Although many textbooks define the lower edge of the radiation field relative to the bones of the pelvis, this is not the proper way to think about irradiating such tumors. The locations of bony anatomic landmarks such as the ischial tuberosity have no consistent relationship to the anal sphincter, anal verge, dentate line, or the rectal cancer. The radiation oncologist must identify the location of these structures as best as possible using radiopaque markers and rectal contrast, and then determine the balance between adequate distal coverage of the tumor as well as minimizing irradiation of the anal sphincter and the perineum (acute toxicity). For anteroposterior or posteroanterior fields, the lateral borders should extend to treat the pelvic sidewall, a possible region for soft tissue extension. The lateral fields should have a similar superior and inferior margin. The posterior border should include all of the presacral soft tissue so the posterior extent of the field should cover the anterior border of the sacrum with at least a 1.5-cm margin for patient motion and dosimetric variation. The anterior border of the lateral fields should cover at least the posterior border of the vagina or the prostate, the anterior extent of the primary rectal tumor, and the anterior edge of the sacral promontory. Examples of typical radiation fields as depicted by a CT simulation are shown in Figure 52.4.

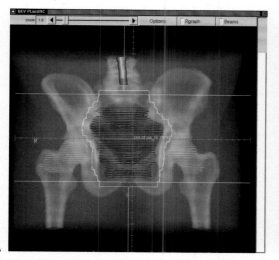
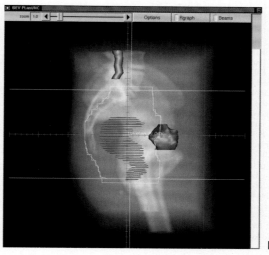
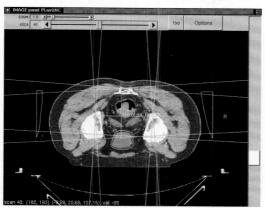

Figure 52.4 Posteroanterior **(A)** and lateral digitally **(B)** reconstructed radiograph of the radiation fields for preoperative radiation therapy of a T3N1 rectal adenocarcinoma. The clinical target volume and rectum are *outlined*. There is a marker at the anal verge to help avoid irradiating the entire anal canal. The field treats the mesorectum and the lymph nodes to the level of the sacral promontory. **(C)** Transverse cut at the middle of the radiation field.

REFERENCES

1. Havenga K, Enker WE, McDermott K, et al. Male and female sexual and urinary function after total mesorectal excision with autonomic nerve preservation for carcinoma of the rectum. *J Am Coll Surg* 1996;182:495–502.
2. Havenga K, DeRuiter MC, Enker WE, et al. Anatomical basis of autonomic nerve-preserving total mesorectal excision for rectal cancer. *Br J Surg* 1996;83:384–388.
3. Mancini R, Cosimelli M, Filippini A, et al. Nerve-sparing surgery in rectal cancer: feasibility and functional results. *J Exp Clin Cancer Res* 2000;19: 35–40.
4. McNamara DA, Parc R. Methods and results of sphincter-preserving surgery for rectal cancer. *Cancer Control* 2003;10:212–218.
5. Wibe A, Eriksen MT, Syse A, et al. Total mesorectal excision for rectal cancer—what can be achieved by a national audit? *Colorectal Dis* 2003;5: 471–477.
6. Hanna NN, Guillem J, Dosoretz A, et al. Intraoperative parasympathetic nerve stimulation with tumescence monitoring during total mesorectal excision for rectal cancer. *J Am Coll Surg* 2002;195:506–512.
7. Watanabe T, Wu TT, Catalamo PJ, et al. Molecular predictors of survival after adjuvant chemotherapy for colon cancer. *N Engl J Med* 2001;344: 1196–1206.
8. Compton CC. Surgical pathology of colorectal cancer. In Saltz LB, ed. *Colorectal Cancer: Multimodality Management.* Totowa, NJ: Humana Press; 2002:247–265.
9. Compton CC, Fielding LP, Burgart LJ, et al. Prognostic factors in colorectal cancer. College of American Pathologists Consensus Statement 1999. *Arch Pathol Lab Med* 2000;124:979–994.
10. Topova L, Hellmich G, Puffer E, et al. Prognostic value of tumor response to neoadjuvant therapy in rectal carcinoma. *Dis Colon Rectum* 2011;54: 401–411.
11. de Campos-Lobato LF, Stochhi L, da Luz Moreira A, et al. Pathologic complete response after neoadjuvant treatment for rectal cancer decreases distant recurrence and could eradicate local recurrence. *Ann Surg Oncol* 2011;18: 1590–1598.
12. Martin ST, Heneghan HM, Winter DC. Systematic review and meta-analysis of outcomes following pathological complete response to neoadjuvant chemoradiotherapy for rectal cancer. *Br J Surg* 2012;99:918–928.
13. Jang NY, Kang SB, Kim DW, et al. The role of carcinoembryonic antigen after neoadjuvant chemoradiotherapy in patients with rectal cancer. *Dis Colon Rectum* 2011;54:245–252.
14. Kim CW, Yu CS, Yang SS, et al. Clinical significance of pre- to post-chemoradiotherapy s-CEA reduction ratio in rectal cancer patients treated with preoperative chemoradiotherapy and curative resection. *Ann Surg Oncol* 2011;18:3271–3277.
15. Song S, Hong JC, McDonnell SE, et al. Combined modality therapy for rectal cancer: the relative value of posttreatment versus pretreatment CEA as a prognostic marker for disease recurrence. *Ann Surg Oncol* 2012;19: 2471–2476.
16. Ayez N, Alberda WJ, Burger JW, et al. Is restaging with chest and abdominal CT scan after neoadjuvant chemoradiotherapy for locally advanced rectal cancer necessary? *Ann Surg Oncol* 2013;20:155–160.
17. Gunderson LL, Sargent DJ, Tepper JE, et al. Impact of T and N substage on survival and disease relapse in adjuvant rectal cancer: a pooled analysis. *Int J Radiat Oncol Biol Phys* 2002;54:386–396.
18. Greene FL, Stewart AK, Norton HJ. New tumor-node-metastasis staging strategy for node-positive (stage III) rectal cancer: an analysis. *J Clin Oncol* 2004;22:1778–1784.
19. Tepper JE, O'Connell MJ, Niedzwiecki D, et al. Impact of number of nodes retrieved on outcome in patients with rectal cancer. *J Clin Oncol* 2001;19: 157–163.
20. Goldstein NS, Sanford W, Coffey M, et al. Lymph node recovery from colorectal resection specimens removed for adenocarcinoma. Trends over time and a recommendation for a minimum number of lymph nodes to be recovered. *Am J Clin Pathol* 1996;106:209–216.
21. Wong JH, Severino R, Honnebier MB, et al. Number of nodes examined and staging accuracy in colorectal carcinoma. *J Clin Oncol* 1999;17: 2896–2900.

22. Doll D, Gertler R, Maak M, et al. Reduced lymph node yield in rectal carcinoma specimen after neoadjuvant radiochemotherapy has no prognostic relevance. *World J Surg* 2009;33:340–347.

23. Rullier A, Laurent C, Capdepont M, et al. Lymph nodes after preoperative chemoradiotherapy for rectal carcinoma: number, status, and impact on survival. *Am J Surg Pathol* 2008;32:45–50.

24. Wang H, Safar B, Wexner S, et al. Lymph node harvest after proctectomy for invasive rectal adenocarcinoma following neoadjuvant therapy: does the same standard apply? *Dis Colon Rectum* 2009;52:549–557.

25. de Campos-Lobato LF, Stocchi L, de Sousa JB, et al. Less than 12 nodes in the surgical specimen after total mesorectal excision following neoadjuvant chemoradiation: it means more than you think! *Ann Surg Oncol* 2013;20:3398–3406.

26. Klos CL, Bordeianou LG, Sylla P, et al. The prognostic value of lymph node ratio after neoadjuvant chemoradiation and rectal cancer surgery. *Dis Colon Rectum* 2011;54:171–175.

27. Kobayashi H, Mochizuki H, Kato T, et al. Lymph node ratio is a powerful prognostic index in patients with stage III distal rectal cancer: a Japanese multicenter study. *Int J Colorectal Dis* 2011;26:891–896.

28. Kang J, Hur H, Min BS, et al. Prognostic impact of the lymph node ratio in rectal cancer patients who underwent preoperative chemoradiation. *J Surg Oncol* 2011;104:53–58.

29. Quirke P, Durdey P, Dixon MF, et al. Local recurrence of rectal adenocarcinoma due to inadequate surgical resection: histopathological study of lateral tumour spread and surgical excision. *Lancet* 1986;2:996–999.

30. Adam IJ, Mohamdee MO, Martin IG, et al. Role of circumferential margin involvement in the local recurrence of rectal cancer. *Lancet* 1994;344:707–711.

31. Kim NK, Kim MJ, Yun SH, et al. Comparative study of transrectal ultrasonography, pelvic computerized tomography, and magnetic resonance imaging in preoperative staging of rectal cancer. *Dis Colon Rectum* 1999;42:770–775.

32. Beynon J. An evaluation of the role of rectal endosonography in rectal cancer. *Ann R Coll Surg Engl* 1989;71:131–139.

33. Garcia-Aguilar J, Pollack J, Lee SH, et al. Accuracy of endorectal ultrasonography in preoperative staging of rectal tumors. *Dis Colon Rectum* 2002;45:10–15.

34. MERCURY Study Group. Diagnostic accuracy of preoperative magnetic resonance imaging in predicting curative resection of rectal cancer: prospective observational study. *BMJ* 2006;333:779.

35. Brown G, Richards CJ, Bourne MW, et al. Morphologic predictors of lymph node status in rectal cancer with use of high-spatial-resolution MR imaging with histopathologic comparison. *Radiology* 2003;227:371–377.

36. Brown G, Richards CJ, Newcombe RG, et al. Rectal carcinoma: thin-section MR imaging for staging in 28 patients. *Radiology* 1999;211:215–222.

37. Shihab OC, Taylor F, Salerno G, et al. MRI predictive factors for long-term outcomes of low rectal tumours. *Ann Surg Oncol* 2011;18:3278–3284.

38. Patel UB, Taylor F, Blomqvist L, et al. Magnetic resonance imaging-detected tumor response for locally advanced rectal cancer predicts survival outcomes: MERCURY experience. *J Clin Oncol* 2011;29:3753–3760.

39. Taylor FG, Quirke P, Heald RJ, et al. Preoperative high-resolution magnetic resonance imaging can identify good prognosis stage I, II, and III rectal cancer best managed by surgery alone: a prospective, multicenter, European study. *Ann Surg* 2011;253:711–719.

40. Shihab OC, How P, West N, et al. Can a novel MRI staging system for low rectal cancer aid surgical planning? *Dis Colon Rectum* 2011;54:1260–1264.

41. Hunter CJ, Garant A, Vuong T, et al. Adverse features on rectal MRI identify a high-risk group that may benefit from more intensive preoperative staging and treatment. *Ann Surg Oncol* 2012;19:1199–1205.

42. National Comprehensive Cancer Network Guidelines for Rectal Cancer, Version 3.2011. www.nccn.org.

43. Haider MA, Amitai MM, Rappaport DC, et al. Multi-detector row helical CT in preoperative assessment of small (< or = 1.5 cm) liver metastases: is thinner collimation better? *Radiology* 2002;225:137–142.

44. Semelka RC, Schlund JF, Molina PL, et al. Malignant liver lesions: comparison of spiral CT arterial portography and MR imaging for diagnostic accuracy, cost, and effect on patient management. *J Magn Reson Imaging* 1996;6:39–43.

45. Huebner RH, Park KC, Shepherd JE, et al. A meta-analysis of the literature for whole-body FDG PET detection of recurrent colorectal cancer. *J Nucl Med* 2000;41:1177–1189.

46. Abdel-Nabi H, Doerr RJ, Lamonica DM, et al. Staging of primary colorectal carcinomas with fluorine-18 fluorodeoxyglucose whole-body PET: correlation with histopathologic and CT findings. *Radiology* 1998;206:755–760.

47. Cipe G, Ergul N, Hasbahceci M, et al. Routine use of positron-emission tomography/computed tomography for staging of primary colorectal cancer: does it affect clinical management? *World J Surg Oncol* 2013;11:49.

48. Canter RJ, Williams NN. Surgical treatment of colon and rectal cancer. *Hematol Oncol Clin North Am* 2002;16:907–926.

49. Saraste D, Gunnarsson U, Janson M. Predicting lymph node metastases in early rectal cancer. *Eur J Cancer* 2013;49:1104–1108.

50. Wu ZY, Zhao G, Chen Z, et al. Oncological outcomes of transanal local excision for high risk T(1) rectal cancers. *World J Gastrointest Oncol* 2012;4:84–88.

51. Greenberg JA, Shibata D, Herndon JE 2nd, et al. Local excision of distal rectal cancer: an update of cancer and leukemia group B 8984. *Dis Colon Rectum* 2008;51:1185–1191, discussion 1191–1194.

52. Ota DM, Nelson H, ACOSOG Group Co-Chairs. Local excision of rectal cancer revisited: ACOSOG protocol Z6041. *Ann Surg Oncol* 2007;14:271.

53. Garcia-Aguilar J, Shi Q, Thomas CR Jr, et al. A phase II trial of neoadjuvant chemoradiation and local excision for T2N0 rectal cancer: preliminary results of the ACOSOG Z6041 trial. *Ann Surg Oncol* 2012;19:384–391.

54. Lezoche E, Baldarelli M, Lezoche G, et al. Randomized clinical trial of endoluminal locoregional resection versus laparoscopic total mesorectal excision for T2 rectal cancer after neoadjuvant therapy. *Br J Surg* 2012;99:1211–1218.

55. Sgourakis G, Lanitis S, Gockel I, et al. Transanal endoscopic microsurgery for T1 and T2 rectal cancers: a meta-analysis and meta-regression analysis of outcomes. *Am Surg* 2011;77:761–772.

56. Wu Y, Wu YY, Li S, et al. TEM and conventional rectal surgery for T1 rectal cancer: a meta-analysis. *Hepatogastroenterology* 2011;58:364–368.

57. Lezoche G, Guerrieri M, Baldarelli M, et al. Transanal endoscopic microsurgery for 135 patients with small nonadvanced low rectal cancer (iT1-iT2, iN0): short- and long-term results. *Surg Endosc* 2011;25:1222–1229.

58. Ramirez JM, Aquilella V, Valencia J, et al. Transanal endoscopic microsurgery for rectal cancer. Long-term oncologic results. *Int J Colorectal Dis* 2011;26:437–443.

59. Allaix ME, Rebecchi F, Giaccone C, et al. Long-term functional results and quality of life after transanal endoscopic microsurgery. *Br J Surg* 2011;98:1635–1643.

60. Ganai S, Kanumuri P, Rao RS, et al. Local recurrence after transanal endoscopic microsurgery for rectal polyps and early cancers. *Ann Surg Oncol* 2006;13:547–556.

61. Herzog U, von Flue M, Tondelli P, et al. How accurate is endorectal ultrasound in the preoperative staging of rectal cancer? *Dis Colon Rectum* 1993;36:127–134.

62. Libutti SK, Forde KA. Surgical considerations III: bowel anastomosis. In Cohen A, Weaver S, eds. *Cancer of the Colon, Rectum and Anus*. New York, NY: McGraw Hill; 1995:445–456.

63. Ota DM, Jacobs L, Kuvshinoff B. Rectal cancer: the sphincter-sparing approach. *Surg Clin North Am* 2002;82:983–993.

64. Moore HG, Riedel E, Minsky BD, et al. Adequacy of 1-cm distal margin after restorative rectal cancer resection with sharp mesorectal excision and preoperative combined-modality therapy. *Ann Surg Oncol* 2003;10:80–85.

65. Fitzgerald TL, Brinkley J, Zervos EE. Pushing the envelope beyond a centimeter in rectal cancer: oncologic implications of close, but negative margins. *J Am Coll Surg* 2011;213:589–595.

66. Kuvshinoff B, Maghfoor I, Miedema B, et al. Distal margin requirements after preoperative chemoradiotherapy for distal rectal carcinomas: are < or = 1 cm distal margins sufficient? *Ann Surg Oncol* 2001;8:163–169.

67. Pahlman L, Bujko K, Rutkowski A, et al. Altering the therapeutic paradigm towards a distal bowel margin of < 1 cm in patients with low-lying rectal cancer: a systematic review and commentary. *Colorectal Dis* 2013;15:e166–e174.

68. Tiret E, Poupardin B, McNamara D, et al. Ultralow anterior resection with intersphincteric dissection—what is the limit of safe sphincter preservation? *Colorectal Dis* 2003;5:454–457.

69. Martin ST, Heneghan HM, Winter DC. Systematic review of outcomes after intersphincteric resection for low rectal cancer. *Br J Surg* 2012;99:603–612.

70. Denost Q, Laurent C, Capdepont M, et al. Risk factors for fecal incontinence after intersphincteric resection for rectal cancer. *Dis Colon Rectum* 2011;54:963–968.

71. Barisic G, Markovic V, Popovic M, et al. Function after intersphincteric resection for low rectal cancer and its influence on quality of life. *Colorectal Dis* 2011;13:638–643.

72. Nathanson DR, Espat NJ, Nash GM, et al. Evaluation of preoperative and postoperative radiotherapy on long-term functional results of straight coloanal anastomosis. *Dis Colon Rectum* 2003;46:888–894.

73. Sitzler PJ, Seow-Choen F, Ho YH, et al. Lymph node involvement and tumor depth in rectal cancers: an analysis of 805 patients. *Dis Colon Rectum* 1997;40:1472–1476.

74. Willett CG. Sphincter preservation in rectal cancer. *Curr Treat Options Oncol* 2000;1:399–405.

75. Enker WE, Thaler HT, Cranor ML, et al. Total mesorectal excision in the operative treatment of carcinoma of the rectum. *J Am Coll Surg* 1995;181:335–346.

76. Kapiteijn E, Marijnen CA, Nagtegall ID, et al. Preoperative radiotherapy combined with total mesorectal excision for resectable rectal cancer. *N Eng J Med* 2001;345:638–646.

77. Tocchi A, Mazzoni G, Lepre L, et al. Total mesorectal excision and low rectal anastomosis for the treatment of rectal cancer and prevention of pelvic recurrences. *Arch Surg* 2001;136:216–220.

78. Zhou ZG, Wang Z, Yu YY, et al. Laparoscopic total mesorectal excision of low rectal cancer with preservation of anal sphincter: a report of 82 cases. *World J Gastroenterol* 2003;9:1477–1481.

79. Tsang WW, Chung CC, Li MK. Prospective evaluation of laparoscopic total mesorectal excision with colonic J-pouch reconstruction for mid and low rectal cancers. *Br J Surg* 2003;90:867–871.

80. Morino M, Parini U, Giraudo G, et al. Laparoscopic total mesorectal excision: a consecutive series of 100 patients. *Ann Surg* 2003;237:335–342.

81. Guillou PJ, Quirke P, Thorpe H, et al. Short-term endpoints of conventional versus laparoscopic-assisted surgery in patients with colorectal cancer (MRC CLASICC trial): multicentre, randomised controlled trial. *Lancet* 2005;365:1718–1726.

82. Cheung HY, Ng KH, Leung AL, et al. Laparoscopic sphincter-preserving total mesorectal excision: 10-year report. *Colorectal Dis* 2011;13:627–631.

83. Lam HD, Stefano M, Tran-Ba T, et al. Laparoscopic versus open techniques in rectal cancer surgery: a retrospective analysis of 121 sphincter-saving procedures in a single institution. *Surg Endosc* 2011;25:454–462.

84. Sartori CA, Dal Pozzo A, Franzato B, et al. Laparoscopic total mesorectal excision for rectal cancer: experience of a single center with a series of 174 patients. *Surg Endosc* 2011;25:508–514.

85. Cone MM, Lu KC, Herzig DO, et al. Laparoscopic proctectomy after neoadjuvant therapy: safety and long-term follow-up. *Surg Endosc* 2011;25:1902–1906.

86. Li S, Chi P, Lin H, et al. Long-term outcomes of laparoscopic surgery versus open resection for middle and lower rectal cancer: an NTCLES study. *Surg Endosc* 2011;25:3175–3182.

87. Greenblatt DY, Rajamanickam V, Pugely AJ, et al. Short-term outcomes after laparoscopic-assisted proctectomy for rectal cancer: results from the ACS NSQIP. *J Am Coll Surg* 2011;212:844–854.

88. Liang X, Hou S, Liu H, et al. Effectiveness and safety of laparoscopic resection versus open surgery in patients with rectal cancer: a randomized, controlled trial from China. *J Laparoendosc Adv Surg Tech A* 2011;21:381–385.

89. Huang MJ, Liang JL, Wang H, et al. Laparoscopic-assisted versus open surgery for rectal cancer: a meta-analysis of randomized controlled trials on oncologic adequacy of resection and long-term oncologic outcomes. *Int J Colorectal Dis* 2011;26:415–421.

90. Ohtani H, Tamamori Y, Azuma T, et al. A meta-analysis of the short- and long-term results of randomized controlled trials that compared laparoscopy-assisted and conventional open surgery for rectal cancer. *J Gastrointest Surg* 2011;15:1375–1385.

91. Ng SS, Lee JF, Yiu RY, et al. Long-term oncologic outcomes of laparoscopic versus open surgery for rectal cancer: a pooled analysis of 3 randomized controlled trials. *Ann Surg* 2014;259:139–147.

92. Lujan J, Valero G, Biondo S, et al. Laparoscopic versus open surgery for rectal cancer: results of a prospective multicentre analysis of 4,970 patients. *Surg Endosc* 2013;27:295–302.

93. Westerholm J, Garcia-Osogobio S, Farrokhysr F, et al. Midterm outcomes of laparoscopic surgery for rectal cancer. *Surg Innov* 2012;19:81–88.

94. Soop M, Nelson H. Laparoscopic-assisted proctectomy for rectal cancer: on trial. *Ann Surg Oncol* 2008;15:2357–2359.

95. deSouza AL, Prasad LM, Marecik SJ, et al. Total mesorectal excision for rectal cancer: the potential advantage of robotic assistance. *Dis Colon Rectum* 2010;53:1611–1617.

96. Koh DC, Tsang CB, Kim SH. A new application of the four-arm standard da Vinci(R) surgical system: totally robotic-assisted left-sided colon or rectal resection. *Surg Endosc* 2011;25:1945–1952.

97. Leong QM, Son DN, Cho JS, et al. Robot-assisted intersphincteric resection for low rectal cancer: technique and short-term outcome for 29 consecutive patients. *Surg Endosc* 2011;25:2987–2992.

98. Bertani E, Chiappa A, Biffi R, et al. Assessing appropriateness for elective colorectal cancer surgery: clinical, oncological, and quality-of-life short-term outcomes employing different treatment approaches. *Int J Colorectal Dis* 2011;26:1317–1327.

99. Baek JH, Pastor C, Pigazzi A. Robotic and laparoscopic total mesorectal excision for rectal cancer: a case-matched study. *Surg Endosc* 2011;25:521–525.

100. Kwak JM, Kim SH, Kim J, et al. Robotic vs laparoscopic resection of rectal cancer: short-term outcomes of a case-control study. *Dis Colon Rectum* 2011;54:151–156.

101. Biffi R, Luca F, Pozzi S, et al. Operative blood loss and use of blood products after full robotic and conventional low anterior resection with total mesorectal excision for treatment of rectal cancer. *J Robot Surg* 2011;5:101–107.

102. Yang Y, Wang F, Zhang P, et al. Robot-assisted versus conventional laparoscopic surgery for colorectal disease, focusing on rectal cancer: a meta-analysis. *Ann Surg Oncol* 2012;19:3727–3731.

103. Trastulli S, Farinella E, Cirocchi R, et al. Robotic resection compared with laparoscopic rectal resection for cancer: systematic review and meta-analysis of short-term outcome. *Colorectal Dis* 2012;14:e134–e156.

104. Memon S, Heriot AG, Murphy DG, et al. Robotic versus laparoscopic proctectomy for rectal cancer: a meta-analysis. *Ann Surg Oncol* 2012;19:2095–2101.

105. Scarpinata R, Aly EH. Does robotic rectal cancer surgery offer improved early postoperative outcomes? *Dis Colon Rectum* 2013;56:253–262.

106. Collinson FJ, Jayne DG, Pigazzi A, et al. An international, multicentre, prospective, randomised, controlled, unblinded, parallel-group trial of robotic-assisted versus standard laparoscopic surgery for the curative treatment of rectal cancer. *Int J Colorectal Dis* 2012;27:233–241.

107. Mukherjee A. Total pelvic exenteration for advanced rectal cancer. *S D J Med* 1999;52:153–156.

108. Mohan HM, Evans MD, Larkin JO, et al. Multivisceral resection in colorectal cancer: a systematic review. *Ann Surg Oncol* 2013;20:2929–2936.

109. Pereira P, Ghouti L, Blanche J. Surgical treatment of extraluminal pelvic recurrence from rectal cancer: oncological management and resection techniques. *J Visc Surg* 2013;150:97–107.

110. Chew MH, Brown WE, Masya L, et al. Clinical, MRI, and PET-CT criteria used by surgeons to determine suitability for pelvic exenteration surgery for recurrent rectal cancers: a Delphi study. *Dis Colon Rectum* 2013;56:717–725.

111. Ripley RT, Gajdos C, Reppert AE, et al. Sequential radiofrequency ablation and surgical debulking for unresectable colorectal carcinoma: thermo-surgical ablation. *J Surg Oncol* 2013;107:144–147.

112. Pusceddu C, Sotgia B, Melis L, et al. Painful pelvic recurrence of rectal cancer: percutaneous radiofrequency ablation treatment. *Abdom Imaging* 2013;38:1225–1233.

113. Monzon L, Wasan H, Leen E, et al. Transrectal high-intensity focused ultrasonography is feasible as a new therapeutic option for advanced recurrent rectal cancer: report on the first case worldwide. *Ann R Coll Surg Engl* 2011;93:e119–121.

114. Mendenhall MW, Million RR, Pfaff PW. Patterns of recurrence in adenocarcinoma of the rectum and rectosigmoid treated with surgery alone: implications in treatment planning with adjuvant radiation therapy. *Int J Radiat Oncol Biol Phys* 1983;9:877–985.

115. Walz B, Lindstrom ER, Butcher HR Jr, et al. Natural history of patients after abdominal-perineal resection implications for radiation therapy. *Cancer* 1977;39:2437–2442.

116. Pilipshen SJ, Heilweil M, Quan SH, et al. Patterns of pelvic recurrence following definitive resections of rectal cancer. *Cancer* 1984;53:1354–1362.

117. Gunderson LL, Sosin H. Areas of failure found at reoperation (second or symptomatic look) following "curative surgery" for adenocarcinoma of the rectum. *Cancer* 1974;34:1278–1292.

118. Stockholm Rectal Cancer Study Group. Preoperative short-term radiation therapy in operable rectal carcinoma. *Cancer* 1990;66:49–55.

119. Rich T, Gunderson LL, Lew R, et al. Patterns of recurrence of rectal cancer after potentially curative surgery. *Cancer* 1983;52:1317–1329.

120. Martling A, Holm T, Johansson H, et al. The Stockholm II trial on preoperative radiotherapy in rectal carcinoma: long-term follow-up of a population-based study. *Cancer* 2001;92:896–902.

121. Heald RJ. The "Holy Plane" of rectal surgery. *J Royal Soc Med* 1988;81:503–508.

122. Heald RJ, Moran BJ, Ryall RD, et al. Rectal cancer: the Basingstoke experience of total mesorecal excision, 1978-1997. *Arch Surg* 1998;133:894–899.

123. Arbman G, Nilsson E, Hallbook O, et al. Local reccurence following total mesorectal excision for rectal cancer. *Br J Surg* 1996;83:375–379.

124. van Gijn W, Marijnen CA, Nagtegaal ID, et al. Preoperative radiotherapy combined with total mesorectal excision for resectable rectal cancer: 12-year follow-up of the multicentre, randomised controlled TME trial. *Lancet Oncol* 2011;12:575–582.

125. Sebag-Montefiore D, Stephens RJ, Steele R, et al. Preoperative radiotherapy versus selective postoperative chemoradiotherapy in patients with rectal cancer (MRC CR07 and NCIC-CTG C016): a multicentre, randomised trial. *Lancet* 2009;373:811–820.

126. Swedish Rectal Cancer Trial. Improved survival with preoperative radiotherapy in resectable rectal cancer. *N Engl J Med* 1997;336:980–987.

127. Prolongation of the disease-free interval in surgically treated rectal carcinoma. Gastrointestinal Tumor Study Group. *N Engl J Med* 1985;312:1465–1472.

128. Krook JE, Moertel CG, Gunderson LL, et al. Effective surgical adjuvant therapy for high-risk rectal carcinoma. *N Engl J Med* 1991;324:709–715.

129. Fisher B, Wolmark N, Rockette H, et al. Postoperative adjuvant chemotherapy or radiation therapy for rectal cancer: results from NSABP protocol R-01. *J Nat Cancer Inst* 1988;80:21–29.

130. Wolmark N, Wieand HS, Hyams DM, et al. Randomized trial of postoperative adjuvant chemotherapy with or without radiotherapy for carcinoma of the rectum: National Surgical Adjuvant Breast and Bowel Project Protocol R-02. *J Natl Cancer Inst* 2000;92:388–396.

131. Balslev IB, Pedersen M, Teglbjaerg PS, et al. Postoperative radiotherapy in Dukes' B and C carcinoma of the rectum and rectosigmoid. A randomized multicenter study. *Cancer* 1986;58:22–28.

132. Medical Research Council Rectal Cancer Working Party. Randomised trial of surgery alone versus surgery followed by radiotherapy for mobile cancer of the rectum. *Lancet* 1996;348:1610–1614.

133. O'Connell MJ, Martenson JA, Wieand HS, et al. Improving adjuvant therapy for rectal cancer by combining protracted-infusion fluorouracil with radiation therapy after curative surgery. *N Engl J Med* 1994;331:502–507.

134. Schrag D, Weiser M, Goodman K, et al. Neoadjuvant chemotherapy without routine use of radiation therapy for patients with locally advanced rectal cancer: a pilot trial. *J Clin Oncol* 2014;32:513–518.

135. Colorectal Cancer Collaborative Group. Adjuvant radiotherapy for rectal cancer: a systematic overview of 8507 patients from 22 randomised trials. *Lancet* 2001;358:1291–1304.

136. Camma C, Giunta M, Fiorica F, et al. Preoperative radiotherapy for resectable rectal cancer: A meta-analysis. *JAMA* 2000;284:1008–1015.

137. Sauer R, Liersch T, Merkel S, et al. Preoperative versus postoperative chemoradiotherapy for rectal cancer. *N Engl J Med* 2004;351:1731–1740.

138. Sauer R, Liersch T, Merkel S, et al. Preoperative versus postoperative chemoradiotherapy for locally advanced rectal cancer: results of the German CAO/ARO/AIO-94 randomized phase III trial after a median follow-up of 11 years. *J Clin Oncol* 2012;30:1926–1933.

139. Wolff HA, Conradi LC, Beissbarth T, et al. Gender affects acute organ toxicity during radiochemotherapy for rectal cancer: long-term results of the German CAO/ARO/AIO-94 phase III trial. *Radiother Oncol* 2013;108:48–54.

140. Roh MS, Colangelo LH, O'Connell MJ, et al. Preoperative multimodality therapy improves disease-free survival in patients with carcinoma of the rectum: NSABP R-03. *J Clin Oncol* 2009;27:5124–5130.

141. Hyams D, Mamounas EP, Petrelli N, et al. A clinical trial to evaluate the worth of preoperative multimodality therapy in patients with operable carcinoma of the rectum: a progress report of National Surgical Breast and Bowel Project Protocol R-03. *Dis Colon Rectum* 1997;40:131–139.

142. Bujko K, Nowacki MP, Nasierowska-Guttmejer A, et al. Long-term results of a randomized trial comparing preoperative short-course radiotherapy with preoperative conventionally fractionated chemoradiation for rectal cancer. *Br J Surg* 2006;93:1215–1223.

143. Ngan SY, Burmeister B, Fisher RJ, et al. Randomized trial of short-course radiotherapy versus long-course chemoradiation comparing rates of local recurrence in patients with T3 rectal cancer: Trans-Tasman Radiation Oncology Group trial 01.04. *J Clin Oncol* 2012;30:3827–3833.

144. Pettersson D, Holm T, Iversen H, et al. Preoperative short-course radiotherapy with delayed surgery in primary rectal cancer. *Br J Surg* 2012;99:577–583.

145. Pach R, Kulig J, Richter P, et al. Randomized clinical trial on preoperative radiotherapy 25 Gy in rectal cancer—treatment results at 5-year follow-up. *Langenbecks Arch Surg* 2012;397:801–807.

146. Sloothaak DA, Geijsen DE, van Leersum NJ, et al. Optimal time interval between neoadjuvant chemoradiotherapy and surgery for rectal cancer. *Br J Surg* 2013;100:933–939.

147. Loos M, Quentmeier P, Schuster T, et al. Effect of preoperative radio(chemo)therapy on long-term functional outcome in rectal cancer patients: a systematic review and meta-analysis. *Ann Surg Oncol* 2013;20:1816–1828.

148. Bosset JF, Collette L, Calais G, et al. Chemotherapy with preoperative radiotherapy in rectal cancer. *N Engl J Med* 2006;355:1114–1123.

149. McCarthy K, Pearson K, Fulton R, et al. Pre-operative chemoradiation for non-metastatic locally advanced rectal cancer. *Cochrane Database Syst Rev* 2012;12:CD008368.

150. De Caluwe L, Van Nieuwenhove Y, Ceelen WP. Preoperative chemoradiation versus radiation alone for stage II and III resectable rectal cancer. *Cochrane Database Syst Rev* 2013;2:CD006041.

151. Willett CG, Badizadegan K, Ancukeiewicz M, et al. Prognostic factors in stage T3N0 rectal cancer: do all patients require postoperative pelvic irradiation and chemotherapy? *Dis Colon Rectum* 1999;42:167–173.

152. Hernanz F, Revuelta S, Redondo C, et al. Colorectal adenocarcinoma: quality of the assessment of lymph node metastases. *Dis Colon Rectum* 1994;37:373–377.

153. Stocchi L, Nelson H, Sargent DJ, et al. Impact of surgical and pathologic variables in rectal cancer: a United States community and cooperative group report. *J Clin Oncol* 2001;19:3895–3902.

154. Martling AL, Holm T, Rutqvist LE, et al. Effect of a surgical training programme on outcome of rectal cancer in the Country of Stockholm. *Lancet* 2000;356:93–96.

155. Kitayama J, Yasuda K, Kawai K, et al. Circulating lymphocyte is an important determinant of the effectiveness of preoperative radiotherapy in advanced rectal cancer. *BMC Cancer* 2011;11:64.

156. Qiu HZ, Wu B, Xiao Y, et al. Combination of differentiation and T stage can predict unresponsiveness to neoadjuvant therapy for rectal cancer. *Colorectal Dis* 2011;13:1353–1360.

157. Nishioka M, Shimada M, Kurita N, et al. Gene expression profile can predict pathological response to preoperative chemoradiotherapy in rectal cancer. *Cancer Genomics Proteomics* 2011;8:87–92.

158. Guedj N, Bretagnol F, Rautou PE, et al. Predictors of tumor response after preoperative chemoradiotherapy for rectal adenocarcinomas. *Hum Pathol* 2011;42:1702–1709.

159. Grimminger PP, Danenberg P, Dellas K, et al. Biomarkers for cetuximab-based neoadjuvant radiochemotherapy in locally advanced rectal cancer. *Clin Cancer Res* 2011;17:3469–3477.

160. Yasuda K, Nirei T, Sunami E, et al. Density of CD4(+) and CD8(+) T lymphocytes in biopsy samples can be a predictor of pathological response to chemoradiotherapy (CRT) for rectal cancer. *Radiat Oncol* 2011;6:49.

161. Moureau-Zabotto L, Farnault B, de Chaisemartin C, et al. Predictive factors of tumor response after neoadjuvant chemoradiation for locally advanced rectal cancer. *Int J Radiat Oncol Biol Phys* 2011;80:483–491.

162. Edden Y, Wexner SD, Berho M. The use of molecular markers as a method to predict the response to neoadjuvant therapy for advanced stage rectal adenocarcinoma. *Colorectal Dis* 2012;14:555–561.

163. Casado E, Garcia VM, Sanchez JJ, et al. A combined strategy of SAGE and quantitative PCR Provides a 13-gene signature that predicts preoperative chemoradiotherapy response and outcome in rectal cancer. *Clin Cancer Res* 2011;17:4145–4154.

164. Shin US, Yu CS, Kim JH, et al. Mucinous rectal cancer: effectiveness of preoperative chemoradiotherapy and prognosis. *Ann Surg Oncol* 2011;18:2232–2239.

165. Chen Z, Liu Z, Li W, et al. Chromosomal copy number alterations are associated with tumor response to chemoradiation in locally advanced rectal cancer. *Genes Chromosomes Cancer* 2011;50:689–699.

166. Duldulao MP, Lee W, Nelson RA, et al. Mutations in specific codons of the KRAS oncogene are associated with variable resistance to neoadjuvant chemoradiation therapy in patients with rectal adenocarcinoma. *Ann Surg Oncol* 2013;20:2166–2171.

167. Clancy C, Burke JP, Coffey JC. KRAS mutation does not predict the efficacy of neo-adjuvant chemoradiotherapy in rectal cancer: a systematic review and meta-analysis. *Surg Oncol* 2013;22:105–111.

168. Suzuki T, Sadahiro S, Tanaka A, et al. Biopsy specimens obtained 7 days after starting chemoradiotherapy (CRT) provide reliable predictors of response to CRT for rectal cancer. *Int J Radiat Oncol Biol Phys* 2013;85:1232–1238.

169. Govindarajan A, Reidy D, Weiser MR, et al. Recurrence rates and prognostic factors in ypN0 rectal cancer after neoadjuvant chemoradiation and total mesorectal excision. *Ann Surg Oncol* 2011;18:3666–3672.

170. Kiran RP, Kirat HT, Burgess AN, et al. Is adjuvant chemotherapy really needed after curative surgery for rectal cancer patients who are node-negative after neoadjuvant chemoradiotherapy? *Ann Surg Oncol* 2012;19:1206–1212.

171. Habr-Gama A, Perez RO, Nadalin W, et al. Operative versus nonoperative treatment for stage 0 distal rectal cancer following chemoradiation therapy: long-term results. *Ann Surg* 2004;240:711–717, discussion 717–718.

172. Maas M, Beets-Tan RG, Lambregts DM, et al. Wait-and-see policy for clinical complete responders after chemoradiation for rectal cancer. *J Clin Oncol* 2011;29:4633–4640.

173. Smith JD, Ruby JA, Goodman KA, et al. Nonoperative management of rectal cancer with complete clinical response after neoadjuvant therapy. *Ann Surg* 2012;256:965–972.

174. Chau I, Brown G, Cunningham D, et al. Neoadjuvant capecitabine and oxaliplatin followed by synchronous chemoradiation and total mesorectal excision in magnetic resonance imaging–defined poor-risk rectal cancer. *J Clin Oncol* 2006;24:668–674.

175. Fernández-Martos C, Pericay C, Aparicio J, et al. Phase II, randomized study of concomitant chemoradiotherapy followed by surgery and adjuvant capecitabine plus oxiplatin (CAPOX) compared with induction CAPOX followed by concomitant chemoradiotherapy and surgery in magnetic resonance imaging-defined, locally advanced rectal cancer: Grupo cancer de recto 3 study. *J Clin Oncol* 2010;28:859–865.

176. Cercek A, Goodman KA, Hajj C, et al. Chemotherapy first, followed by chemoradiation and then surgery, in the management of locally advanced rectal cancer. *J Natl Compr Canc Netw* 2014;12:513–519.

177. Perez K, Pricolo V, Vrees M, et al. A phase II study of complete neoadjuvant therapy in rectal cancer (CONTRE): The Brown University Oncology Group. *ASCO Meeting Abstracts* 2013;31:Abstr 335.

178. Habr-Gama A, Perez RO, Wynn G, et al. Complete clinical response after neoadjuvant chemoradiation therapy for distal rectal cancer: characterization of clinical and endoscopic findings for standardization. *Dis Colon Rectum* 2010;53:1692–1698.

179. Smith FM, Chang KH, Sheahan K, et al. The surgical significance of residual mucosal abnormalities in rectal cancer following neoadjuvant chemoradiotherapy. *Br J Surg* 2012;99:993–1001.

180. Guillem JG, Ruby JA, Leibold T, et al. Neither FDG-PET Nor CT can distinguish between a pathological complete response and an incomplete response after neoadjuvant chemoradiation in locally advanced rectal cancer: a prospective study. *Ann Surg* 2013;258:289–295.

181. Perez RO, Habr-Gama A, Gama-Rodrigues J, et al. Accuracy of positron emission tomography/computed tomography and clinical assessment in the detection of complete rectal tumor regression after neoadjuvant chemoradiation: long-term results of a prospective trial (National Clinical Trial 00254683). *Cancer* 2012;118:3501–3511.

182. Intven M, Reerink O, Philippens ME. Diffusion-weighted MRI in locally advanced rectal cancer : pathological response prediction after neo-adjuvant radiochemotherapy. *Strahlenther Onkol* 2013;189:117–122.

183. Perez RO, Habr-Gama A, Pereira GV, et al. Role of biopsies in patients with residual rectal cancer following neoadjuvant chemoradiation after downsizing: can they rule out persisting cancer? *Colorectal Dis* 2012;14:714–720.

184. Duldulao MP, Lee W, Streja L, et al. Distribution of residual cancer cells in the bowel wall after neoadjuvant chemoradiation in patients with rectal cancer. *Dis Colon Rectum* 2013;56:142–149.

185. Hayden DM, Jakate S, Pinzon MC, et al. Tumor scatter after neoadjuvant therapy for rectal cancer: are we dealing with an invisible margin? *Dis Colon Rectum* 2012;55:1206–1212.

186. Tranchart H, Lefevre JH, Syrcek M, et al. What is the incidence of metastatic lymph node involvement after significant pathologic response of primary tumor following neoadjuvant treatment for locally advanced rectal cancer? *Ann Surg Oncol* 2013;20:1551–1559.

187. Park IJ, You YN, Skibber JM, et al. Comparative analysis of lymph node metastases in patients with ypT0-2 rectal cancers after neoadjuvant chemoradiotherapy. *Dis Colon Rectum* 2013;56:135–141.

188. Tepper JE, O'Connell MJ, Niedzwiecki D, et al. Final report of INT 0114-Aduvant therapy in rectal cancer: analysis by treatment, stage and gender. *Proceedings of the American Society of Clinical Oncology* 2001;20:123a.

189. Smalley S. Intergroup 0144–Phase III trial of 5-FU based chemotherapy regimens plus radiotherapy (XRT) in postoperative adjuvant rectal cancer. Bolus 5-FU vs prolonged venous infusion (PVI) before and after XRT vs bolus-5-FU + leucovorin (LV) + levamisole (LEV) beforeand after XRT + bolus 5-FU + LV. *Proceedings of the American Society of Clinical Oncology* 2003;22:251.

190. Roh MS, Yothers GA, O'Connell MJ, et al. The impact of capecitabine and oxaliplatin in the preoperative multimodality treatment in patients with carcinoma of the rectum: NSABP R-04. *J Clin Oncol* 2011;29:Abstr 3503.

191. Hofheinz RD, Wenz F, Post S, et al. Chemoradiotherapy with capecitabine versus fluorouracil for locally advanced rectal cancer: a randomised, multicentre, non-inferiority, phase 3 trial. *Lancet Oncol* 2012;13:579–588.

192. Twelves C, Scheithauer W, McKendrick J, et al. Capecitabine versus 5-fluorouracil/folinic acid as adjuvant therapy for stage III colon cancer: final results from the X-ACT trial with analysis by age and preliminary evidence of a pharmacodynamic marker of efficacy. *Ann Oncol* 2012;23:1190–1197.

193. Cancer and Leukemia Group B 89901, Ryan DP, Niedzwiecki D, et al. Phase I/II study of preoperative oxaliplatin, fluorouracil, and external-beam radiation therapy in patients with locally advanced rectal cancer: Cancer and Leukemia Group B 89901. *J Clin Oncol* 2006;24:2557–2562.

194. Rodel C, Liersch T, Hermann RM, et al. Multicenter phase II trial of chemoradiation with oxaliplatin for rectal cancer. *J Clin Oncol* 2007;25:110–117.

195. Wong SJ, Winter K, Meropol NJ, et al. RTOG 0247: a randomized phase II study of neoadjuvant capecitabine and irinotecan versus capecitabine and oxaliplatin with concurrent radiation therapy for locally advanced rectal cancer. *J Clin Oncol* 2008;26:Abstr 4021.

196. O'Connell MJ, Colangelo LH, Beart RW, et al. Capecitabine and oxaliplatin in the preoperative multimodality treatment of rectal cancer: surgical end points from National Surgical Adjuvant Breast and Bowel Project trial R-04. *J Clin Oncol* 2014;32:1927–1934.

197. Gerard JP, Azria D, Gourgou-Bourgade S, et al. Comparison of two neoadjuvant chemoradiotherapy regimens for locally advanced rectal cancer: results of the phase III trial ACCORD 12/0405-Prodige 2. *J Clin Oncol* 2010;28:1638–1644.

198. Gerard JP, Azria D, Gourgou-Bourgade S, et al. Clinical outcome of the ACCORD 12/0405 PRODIGE 2 randomized trial in rectal cancer. *J Clin Oncol* 2012;30:4558–4565.

199. Aschele C, Pinto C, Cordio S, et al. Preoperative fluorouracil (FU)-based chemoradiation with and without weekly oxaliplatin in locally advanced rectal cancer: pathologic response analysis of the Studio Terapia Adiuvante Retto (STAR)-01 randomized phase III trial. *J Clin Oncol* 2009;27:Abstr CRA4008.

200. Rodel C, Liersch T, Becker H, et al. Preoperative chemoradiotherapy and postoperative chemotherapy with fluorouracil and oxaliplatin versus fluorouracil alone in locally advanced rectal cancer: initial results of the German CAO/ARO/AIO-04 randomised phase 3 trial. *Lancet Oncol* 2012;13:679–687.

201. Mitchell EP. Irinotecan in preoperative combined-modality therapy for locally advanced rectal cancer. *Oncology (Williston Park)* 2000;14:56–59.

202. Kalofonos HP, Bamias A, Koutras A, et al. A randomised phase III trial of adjuvant radio-chemotherapy comparing Irinotecan, 5FU and Leucovorin to 5FU and Leucovorin in patients with rectal cancer: a Hellenic Cooperative Oncology Group Study. *Eur J Cancer* 2008;44:1693–1700.

203. Bonner JA, Harari PM, Giralt J, et al. Radiotherapy plus cetuximab for squamous-cell carcinoma of the head and neck. *N Engl J Med* 2006;354:567–578.

204. Willett CG, Boucher Y, di Tomaso E, et al. Direct evidence that the VEGF-specific antibody bevacizumab has antivascular effects in human rectal cancer. *Nat Med* 2004;10:145–147.

205. Kim SY, Hong YS, Kim DY, et al. Preoperative chemoradiation with cetuximab, irinotecan, and capecitabine in patients with locally advanced resectable rectal cancer: a multicenter Phase II study. *Int J Radiat Oncol Biol Phys* 2011;81:677–683.

206. Pinto C, Di Fabio F, Maiello E, et al. Phase II study of panitumumab, oxaliplatin, 5-fluorouracil, and concurrent radiotherapy as preoperative treatment in high-risk locally advanced rectal cancer patients (StarPan/STAR-02 Study). *Ann Oncol* 2011;22:2424–2430.

207. Dewdney A, Cunningham D, Tabernero J, et al. Multicenter randomized phase II clinical trial comparing neoadjuvant oxaliplatin, capecitabine, and preoperative radiotherapy with or without cetuximab followed by total mesorectal excision in patients with high-risk rectal cancer (EXPERT-C). *J Clin Oncol* 2012;30:1620–1627.

208. Spigel DR, Bendell JC, McCleod M, et al. Phase II study of bevacizumab and chemoradiation in the preoperative or adjuvant treatment of patients with stage II/III rectal cancer. *Clin Colorectal Cancer* 2012;11:45–52.

209. Nogue M, Salud A, Vicente P, et al. Addition of bevacizumab to XELOX induction therapy plus concomitant capecitabine-based chemoradiotherapy in magnetic resonance imaging-defined poor-prognosis locally advanced rectal cancer: the AVACROSS study. *Oncologist* 2011;16:614–620.

210. Velenik V, Ocvirk J, Music M, et al. Neoadjuvant capecitabine, radiotherapy, and bevacizumab (CRAB) in locally advanced rectal cancer: results of an open-label phase II study. *Radiat Oncol* 2011;6:105.

211. Saltz L, Raben D, Minsky BD, et al. Rectal cancer: presentation with metastatic and locally advanced disease. American College of Radiology. ACR Appropriateness Criteria. *Radiology* 2000;215:1491–1499.

212. Minsky B, Cohen AM, Kemeny N, et al. Pre-operative combined 5-FU, low dose leucovorin, and sequential radiation therapy for unresectable rectal cancer. *Int J Radiat Oncol Biol Phys* 1993;25:821–827.

213. Dosoretz DE, Gunderson LL, Hedberg S, et al. Preoperative irradiation for unresectable rectal and rectosigmoid carcinomas. *Cancer* 1983;52:814–818.

214. Emami B, Pilepich M, Willett C, et al. Effect of preoperative irradiation on resectability of colorectal carcinomas. *Int J Radiat Oncol Biol Phys* 1982;8:1295–1299.

215. Marsh R, Chu NM, Vauthey JN, et al. Preoperative treatment of patients with locally advanced unresectable rectal adenocarcinoma utilizing continuous chronobiologically shaped 5-fluorouracil infusion and radiation therapy. *Cancer* 1996;78:215–225.

216. Braendengen M, Tveit KM, Berglund A, et al. Randomized phase III study comparing preoperative radiotherapy with chemoradiotherapy in nonresectable rectal cancer. *J Clin Oncol* 2008;26:3687–3694.

217. Gunderson LL, Nelson H, Martenson JA, et al. Locally advanced primary colorectal cancer: intraoperative electron and external beam irradiation +/− 5-FU. *Int J Radiat Oncol Biol Phys* 1997;37:601–614.

218. Nakfoor BM, Willett CG, Shellito PC, et al. The impact of 5-fluorouracil and intraoperative electron beam radiation therapy on the outcome of patients with locally advanced primary rectal and rectosigmoid cancer. *Ann Surg* 1998;228:194–200.

219. Tepper JE, Wood WC, Cohen AM. Treatment of locally advanced rectal cancer with external beam radiation, surgical resection, and intraoperative radiation therapy. *Int J Radiat Oncol Biol Phys* 1989;16:1437–1444.

220. Harrison LB, Minsky BD, Enker WE, et al. High dose rate intraoperative radiation therapy (HDR-IORT) as part of the management strategy for locally advanced primary and recurrent rectal cancer. *Int J Radiat Oncol Biol Phys* 1998;42:325–330.

221. Wang C, Schulz M. The role of radiation therapy in the management of carcinoma of the sigmoid, rectosigmoid and rectum. *Radiology* 1962;79:1–5.

222. Overgaard M, Overgaard J. Dose-response relationship for radiation therapy of recurrent, residual, and primarily inoperable colorectal cancer. *Radiother Oncol* 1984;1:217–225.

223. Brierley JD, Cummings BJ, Wong CS, et al. Adenocarcinoma of the rectum treated by radical external radiation therapy. *Int J Radiat Oncol Biol Phys* 1995;31:255–259.

224. Frykholm GJ, Isacsson U, Nygard K, et al. Preoperative radiotherapy in rectal cancer—aspects of acute adverse effects and radiation technique. *Int J Radiat Oncol Biol Phys* 1996;35:1039–1048.

225. Frykholm GJ, Glimelius B, Pahlman L. Preoperative or postoperative irradiation in adenocarcinoma of the rectum: final treatment results of a randomized trial and an evaluation of late secondary effects. *Dis Colon Rectum* 1993;36:564–572.

226. Ooi BS, Tjandra JJ, Green MD. Morbidities of adjuvant chemotherapy and radiotherapy for resectable rectal cancer. *Dis Colon and Rectum* 1999;42:403–418.

227. Gallagher MJ, Brereton HD, Rostock RA, et al. A prospective study of treatment techniques to minimize the volume of pelvic small bowel and reduction of acute and late effects associated with pelvic irradiation. *Int J Radiat Oncol Biol Phys* 1986;12:1565–1573.

228. Bonadeo FA, Vaccaro CA, Benati ML, et al. Rectal cancer: local recurrence after surgery without radiotherapy. *Dis Colon Rectum* 2001;44:374–379.

CANCERS OF THE GASTROINTESTINAL TRACT

53 Cancer of the Anal Region

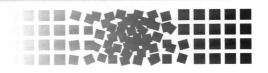

Brian G. Czito, Shahab Ahmed, Matthew Kalady, and Cathy Eng

INTRODUCTION

Carcinoma of the anal canal is a rare malignancy, although its incidence is steadily increasing. The development of anal cancer is a multifocal process largely associated with the human papillomavirus (HPV). The treatment approach to this disease has evolved significantly over recent decades and serves as a model for organ-preserving therapy, transitioning from radical surgery by abdominal perineal resection (APR, entailing permanent colostomy placement with associated high pelvic recurrence rates) to a nonsurgical approach of definitive chemoradiotherapy with 5-fluorouracil (5-FU) and mitomycin C (MMC), leading to successful preservation of anorectal function in the majority of patients. Anal cancer is relatively unique amongst gastrointestinal malignancies in that it has a low propensity for metastatic spread, making local–regional control a paramount endpoint in the approach to this disease. Over the past 2 decades, published randomized trials have demonstrated the superiority of chemoradiotherapy with 5-FU and MMC over radiation therapy alone, radiation with concurrent 5-FU, as well as induction cisplatin/5-FU alone followed by concurrent radiotherapy using the same regimen. Additionally, randomized trials have failed to demonstrate a definitive benefit for radiation dose escalation nor superiority when substituting cisplatin for MMC. Treatment with chemoradiotherapy is associated with significant acute and chronic toxicity rates, and improvement in radiation therapy techniques has been shown to decrease such. Current investigations include the use of novel cytotoxic and inhibitor targeted agents, including epidermal growth factor receptor, in efforts to improve outcomes in patients with more advanced disease, as well as further understanding the molecular etiology and resistance of this disease. This chapter provides an overview of the background, epidemiology, diagnosis, multidisciplinary treatment, and outcomes of tumors arising in the anal canal and perianal skin, as well as anal canal adenocarcinoma and melanoma.

EPIDEMIOLOGY AND ETIOLOGY

Anal cancer is the least prevalent among all gastrointestinal (GI) cancers. It has been reported that anal cancers account for 1% to 2% of all large bowel malignancies. According to the 2014 American Cancer Society statistics, about 7,210 men and women (37% men and 63% women, a ratio of almost 1:2 for men to women) will be diagnosed with anal cancer, and it is estimated that 950 (or 13%) of those diagnosed with anal cancers will die from their disease.[1]

The median age at diagnosis for anal, anal canal, and anorectal cancers was 60 years during 2006 to 2010. This data showed that among all races, Caucasian females experienced the highest incidence rate (2.1 out of 100,000), whereas Asian males had the lowest incidence rate (0.5 out of 100,000) during that time frame (Fig. 53.1). The median age at death was 64 years during this period. It was estimated that African American males

and Caucasian females had the highest mortality rate (0.3 out of 100,000 each) among all races, whereas at the same time, both male and female Asians had the lowest mortality rate (0.1 out of 100,000 each) (see Fig. 53.1).

The incidence of anal cancer has been increasing over the last 30 years in the United States as well as globally.[2,3] This is likely related to the increase in infections by the sexually transmitted HPV and HIV, which may have a significant impact on anal cancer incidence. In one large case-control series, an increasing number of sexual partners was associated with the development of anal cancer in both men and women (odds ratio of 4.5 for women and 2.5 for men with ≥10 sexual partners). This study also demonstrated that a history of anal warts was associated with a higher risk of developing anal cancer, as was receptive anal intercourse in women.[3]

Human Papillomavirus Infection

High-risk HPV type-16 has been detected in almost 90% of cases of squamous cell carcinoma of the anus.[4] A recent meta-analysis suggests that HPV-16 is found more frequently (75%) and HPV-18 less frequently (10%) in anal carcinomas than in cervical carcinomas. Moreover, approximately 80% of anal cancers demonstrated more than one HPV genotype.[5] Anal cancer, now considered to be a predominantly HPV-related cancer, has an incidence 15 times higher in homosexual men than in heterosexual men.[6] In most cases, anal infection with HPV is sexually transmitted, and the risk for cancer is increased in patients with a history of receptive anal intercourse in women and homosexual activity in men.[7] It is also been shown that women with high-grade cervical or vulvar dysplasia are more susceptible to develop anal cancer, as cervical or vulvar HPV infection escalates anal HPV infection risk.[8]

HIV Infection

The incidence of anal cancer in patients who are infected with HIV is estimated to be twice that of HIV-negative patients. Highly active antiretroviral therapy (HAART) has resulted in patients with HIV living longer and the development of related malignancies. In contrast to other HIV-associated malignancies, the incidence of anal cancer has actually risen following implementation of HAART.[9–11] According to the National Cancer Institute (NCI), the rise in anal cancer incidence rates during 1980 to 2005 was predominantly seen in male patients with HIV, relative to their female counterparts.[12] Although HIV has been considered to be a major factor in anal cancer incidence, it is also suggested that HIV may have an impact on the survival of patients with anal cancer, with one report demonstrating that HIV-positive patients with anal cancer tended to develop earlier recurrences than HIV-negative patients by 20 months, although the median survival for HIV-positive patients (34 months) and HIV-negative patients (39 months) were similar (non-significant) (discussed as follows).[13]

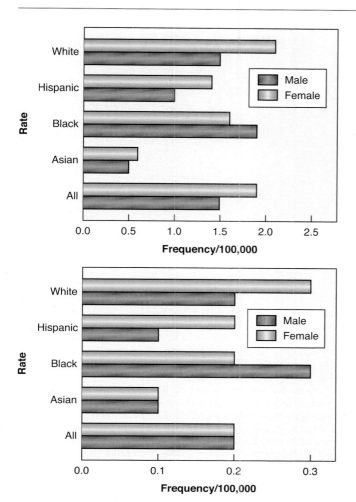

Figure 53.1 Anal cancer distribution among different races. *(Top)* Incidence rate. *(Bottom)* Death rate.

Other Risk Factors

According to the American Society of Colon and Rectal Surgeons (ASCRS), risk factors other than HIV and HPV infections include:

- Age: 67% >55 years.
- Smoking: There are reports demonstrating that that smoking is a risk factor for anal cancer development. According to one study, the relationship between smoking and anal cancer persists for both gender types (adjusted odds ratio for women = 3.8, 95% confidence interval [CI], 2.3 to 6.2; adjusted odds ratio for men = 3.9, 95% CI, 1.9 to 8.0). Similarly, the risk of anal cancer appears to be related to the pack-year history of smoking, with more extensive histories associated with a higher risk.[14]
- Immunosuppression: Solid organ transplant recipients with chronic immunosuppressive therapy have a six times higher risk to develop anal cancer relative to the general population.[15]

Benign anal lesions are no longer thought to contribute to the development of this disease, although anal cancers are frequently misdiagnosed as these conditions.

SCREENING AND PREVENTION

Anal squamous intraepithelial lesions (SIL) or anal intraepithelial neoplasia (AIN) have been recognized as precursors that can progress to anal squamous cell carcinoma (SCC).[16] Although there are no published guidelines that recommend screening of

the general population for anal cancer, there are high-risk groups that may benefit from such, most prominently patients infected with HIV. Although the natural history of SIL is still being unraveled, studies show increased rates of progression in HIV-positive patients with a relative risk of 2.4 and increasing to 3.1 for those with CD4 counts below 200.[17,18] The rationale for screening for SIL is based on the following: there is a high incidence of the anal cancer within the proposed screening population (i.e., HIV-positive patients), available screening tests are effective and cost-efficient, and early detection can change the outcome of the disease. The initial recommended screening test is an "anal Pap smear" that evaluates cells in the anal canal for abnormal cytology through swabbing. Patients with abnormal cytology should then be evaluated by high-resolution anoscopy, which facilitates the visualization of abnormal lesions, allowing biopsy and/or removal.[19,20] Algorithms for the management of low-grade and high-grade SILs remain controversial as more data are needed to determine the effectiveness of intervention on decreasing long-term rates of anal SCC.

Treatment options of high-grade AIN include ablation with electrocautery, topical trichloroacetic acid, topical 5-FU, or imiquimod,[21–23] with estimated lesion control rates ranging from 60% to 80%. A 2012 Cochrane Review highlights the dearth of evidence addressing the efficacy of available interventions for SIL. This review resulted in one randomized trial being identified. This trial evaluated the medication imiquimod versus placebo. Although underpowered, results showed no statistically significant benefit for treatment. The authors concluded that, given the rising incidence of AIN and anal cancer, well-designed randomized controlled trials are urgently needed to address this topic, with emphasis on AIN resolution, downstaging, recurrence, and progression to invasive disease in both HIV-positive and -negative populations.[24]

A promising strategy for the prevention of anal dysplasia and malignancy is HPV vaccination. Two vaccines (Cervarix and Gardasil) are now approved by the U.S. Food and Drug Administration and have been shown to protect against cervical cancer in women.[25,26] The quadrivalent HPV vaccine Gardasil has demonstrated efficacy for prevention of HPV 6-, 11-, 16-, and 18-related genital warts and has been shown to protect against cancers of the anus, vagina, and vulva.[27] In a large, double blind study, 602 healthy men who have sex with men were randomized to receive the quadrivalent HPV vaccine versus placebo. With a 36-month median follow-up for the development of AIN and/or high-risk HPV infection, significantly reduced rates of high-grade anal dysplasia and high-risk HPV infection were demonstrated in the vaccinated group.[28] No cases of anal cancer or vaccine-related serious events were noted. In the context of limited availability and suboptimal outcomes of AIN screening programs, vaccination may reflect the best long-term approach for reducing anal cancer risk and is recommended for girls and boys at age 11 or 12 years and girls 13 to 26 years of age who have not been previously vaccinated.

PATHOLOGY

A variety of malignancies can arise in the anal canal and perianal skin. The typical gross appearance of SCC of the anal canal consists of a lesion with rolled edges, often with central ulceration, with a minority consisting of polypoid lesions (Fig. 53.2). On a practical level, these can be divided into squamous and nonsquamous histologies. The vast majority of anal canal tumors are classified as SCC, which encompasses tumors previously described as basaloid, cloacogenic, transitional, mucoepidermoid, and verrucous mucoepidermoid varieties (Fig. 53.3). These subtypes generally referred to tumors arising in the anal transitional zone, where the anal squamous histology transitions into the glandular epithelium seen in the colorectum. From a treatment standpoint, these are all approached as SCC. The current World Health Organization (WHO)[29] classification does not include these subtypes. The majority of these are

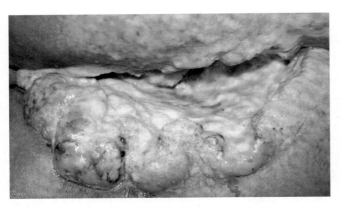

Figure 53.2 A 60-year-old male with advanced squamous cell carcinoma of the anal verge, exhibiting rolled edges with central ulceration.

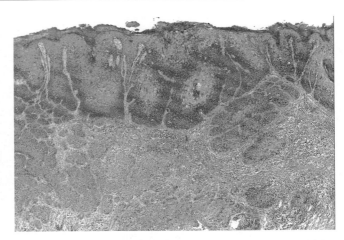

Figure 53.3 A microscopic image of a biopsy revealing nonkeratinizing squamous cell carcinoma.

nonkeratinizing, although tumors arising below the dentate line often display keratinizing properties. Most squamous lesions are moderately to poorly differentiated and display koilocytic changes consistent with HPV infection.

It is believed that most anal cancers arise from precancerous changes (i.e., AIN) of the anal canal and perianal skin epithelium. AIN is a multifocal process associated with HPV, analogous to cervical dysplasia. There is a progression from normal epithelium to condyloma and grade I AIN (associated with mild dysplasia), later progressing to grade II AIN (with moderate dysplasia), and ultimately grade III AIN with severe dysplasia, as well as in situ disease. Once disease has reached grade III AIN, it rarely regresses. It has been estimated that approximately 5% of AIN III patients progress to invasive malignancy, often occurring over a multiyear period. This incidence of progression of AIN III is substantially increased in patients who are immunocompromised.[17,30] The prevalence of AIN among HIV-negative homosexual men is high (>36%), and almost universal among HIV-positive men who have

sexual intercourse with men.[31] The incidence of AIN is believed to be much greater in patients with HIV as exemplified by a French study analyzing 8,153 routine hemorrhoidectomy specimens, finding that only 3 cases of AIN (0.04%) were seen,[32] as compared to 20 cases out of a 103 (19.4%) in specimens from HIV-positive men (Fig. 53.4).[33]

Additional nonsquamous cell histologies arising in the anal canal include adenocarcinoma, small cell carcinoma/neuroendocrine tumors, as well as undifferentiated carcinomas, melanomas, and rarely, lymphomas and sarcomas. Neuroendocrine tumors are thought to arise from endocrine cells in the transitional zone and, like neuroendocrine tumors arising from other sites, tend to disseminate widely. A suspected anal adenocarcinoma may actually reflect an extension from a distal rectal adenocarcinoma in some situations. Mucinous adenocarcinoma is generally thought to arise

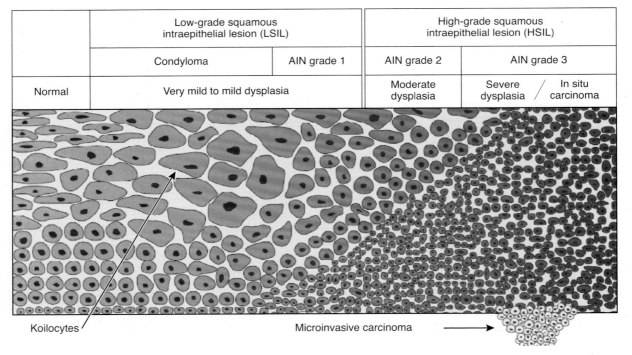

	Low-grade squamous intraepithelial lesion (LSIL)		High-grade squamous intraepithelial lesion (HSIL)	
	Condyloma	AIN grade 1	AIN grade 2	AIN grade 3
Normal	Very mild to mild dysplasia		Moderate dysplasia	Severe dysplasia / In situ carcinoma

Koilocytes

Microinvasive carcinoma →

Figure 53.4 A schematic representation of an anal intraepithelial neoplasia progression. Note that the increasing severity as a proportion of epithelium is replaced by progressive increase in immature-appearing cells, ultimately leading to invasive disease with violation of the basement membrane. (Goldstone SE. Diagnosis and treatment of HPV related squamous intraepithelial neoplasia in men who have sex with men. *PRN Notebook* 2005;10:11–16.)

in the anal glands and ducts and is uncommon. It should be noted that histology is generally more important than location within the anal canal and usually dictates overall patient management.

Tumors of the perianal skin are similar to that seen in the anal canal, primarily comprised of SCC. These tumors are generally well differentiated and keratinizing. Verrucous carcinoma—also sometimes known as a giant condyloma or Buschke-Lowenstein tumor—was initially described in 1925. These tumors are sometimes mistakenly considered to be benign and misdiagnosed as condylomata acuminata, with a subsequent histologic analysis revealing invasion. These are often locally destructive and HPV related. They are often slow growing and can be present for many years before coming to medical attention. Local recurrence rates following excision are high and malignant transformation can be seen in up to 50%.[34] Additional precursor lesions seen in the perianal skin include Bowen disease, which consist of a slow growing intraepidermal SCC that may mimic perianal dermatitis, as well as Paget disease, which is similar to the entity seen associated with breast cancer, with an eczematous appearance. Approximately half of Paget disease patients will harbor an underlying adenocarcinoma, notably in the colorectum.

CLINICAL PRESENTATION AND STAGING

Symptoms of anal cancer can be diverse and include bleeding, pain, sensation of a mass, itching, anal discharge, tenesmus, and a sense of fullness or a lump in the anal canal. The most common presentation is bleeding from the anus. More extensive lesions may present with more ominous symptoms such as incontinence, passage of gas or stool from the vagina, or significant change in bowel habits. Less frequently, an enlarged inguinal lymph node is reported, and 20% of patients are initially asymptomatic. Symptoms may often be dismissed as hemorrhoids or other benign causes, and it is crucial to further evaluate by a physical examination and anoscopy. Any mass should be biopsied for a diagnosis.

Clinical staging is performed by a combination of clinical, endoscopic, and radiographic examinations (Table 53.1). History should include an assessment of anal sphincter function as well as HIV risk factors. Digital rectal examination can identify fixation to the sphincter complex or adjacent organs such as the vagina and prostate. Proctoscopy provides information about the extent of mucosal spread, including the relationship to the dentate line, and facilitates biopsy. It may be necessary to examine patients under anesthesia secondary to pain and sphincter muscle spasms. Female patients should undergo a gynecologic examination to determine vaginal involvement and to exclude other HPV-associated cancers, including evaluation of the cervix. Imaging is used to better delineate the local extent of disease and regional adenopathy, and to determine the presence of distant metastases. An endoanal

ultrasound or pelvic magnetic resonance imaging (MRI) can be considered to assess tumor size and involvement with local structures such as the anal sphincters and vagina or prostate. Computed tomography (CT) scans of the chest, abdomen, and pelvis are commonly employed to evaluate distant disease and adenopathy, particularly in the inguinal regions. Of all patients presenting with palpable inguinal lymph nodes, only 50% are malignant; therefore, fine-needle aspiration is often recommended in suspected cases, and a positive result may guide radiation field design and dose. Some oncologists have suggested a routine sentinel lymph node (SLN) evaluation as a staging technique. A systematic review of 16 published series evaluating the outcome of SLN biopsy of inguinal nodes included 323 patients, and the success in identifying the SLN was 86%. However, the exact role of SNL in the pretreatment evaluation remains undetermined.[35]

A number of recent studies have investigated the role of positron-emission tomography (PET)-CT scans for staging anal cancer. One review described outcomes of patients undergoing conventional staging with ultrasound as well as PET-CT scans. Of 95 patients, the authors found that PET-CT scans were particularly valuable in detecting more extensive nodal and metastatic disease as well as the detection of synchronous malignancies. Upstaging was noted in 14% of patients, and 23% had a change in treatment plan relative to ultrasound staging.[36] Another study comparing the use of conventional imaging with CT scans and MRI found that the addition of PET-CT scans upstaged patients in 20%, downstaged 25%, and altered management in 37%. These authors concluded that PET-CT scans should be a routine part of initial staging of all anal cancers. A lesser impact was seen in patients evaluated in follow-up where PET-CT scans upstaged 11% and downstaged in 6% of cases; however, these changes also led to an altered management in 17%, indicating a potential role for selected PET-CT scan use when there is a question of recurrence or salvage surgery is planned.[37] A study by Vercellino and colleagues[38] similarly found that PET-CT scans were useful in the avoidance of unnecessary biopsies and surgery, with a negative predictive value of 94%, ultimately impacting on treatment plans in 22% of follow-up cases. Finally, PET-CT scans may have prognostic value as well, with one study demonstrating a significant correlation between metabolic response posttreatment and progression-free as well as overall survival.[39] National Comprehensive Cancer Network (NCCN) treatment guidelines include the use of FDG-PET scans with CT scans as part of the staging evaluation, notably for patients with T2-4N0 disease or those with involved lymph nodes.[40] After the previously mentioned evaluation, staging is assigned according to the American Joint Committee on Cancer 2010 (AJCC) (Table 53.2).

PROGNOSTIC FACTORS

Clinical

T and N stages are the most important prognostic factors for anal cancer. According to the AJCC, the 5-year observed overall survival (OS) rates of anal cancer for stage I, II, IIIA, IIIB, and IV are 69.5%, 68.1%, 45.6%, 39.6%, and 15.3%, respectively. It has also been demonstrated that the 5-year OS rates for T1, T2, T3, T4, N0, and node-positive anal cancer are 86%, 86%, 60%, 45%, 76%, and 54%.[41]

There are relatively few studies available that analyze prognostic factors for anal cancer. According to the Radiation Therapy Oncology Group (RTOG) 98-11 study, tumor size (>5 cm), involved lymph nodes (N+), and male sex were associated with worse 5-year disease-free survival (DFS) and OS.[42] Results from European Organisation for Research and Treatment of Cancer (EORTC) 22861 study indicated that skin ulceration, lymph node involvement, and male sex were independent variables associated with local–regional failure (LRF) and OS in multivariate analysis.[43] A secondary analysis of the UK Coordinating Committee on

---

TABLE 53.1

Recommended Diagnostic Evaluation in Newly Diagnosed Anal Cancer

- Digital rectal examination with tumor characterization (location, fixation, extent)
- Examination of inguinal lymph nodes; consideration of biopsy if deemed suspicious
- Endoscopy/proctoscopy
- Gynecologic examination in females to rule out vaginal invasion as well as exclude gynecologic primary
- Positron-emission tomography/computed tomography (PET-CT) scan
- Complete blood count with serum chemistries as well as HIV testing/CD4 levels in the presence of risk factors

TABLE 53.2

TNM Anus Staging According to the American Joint Committee on Cancer

Primary Tumor (T)

TX	Primary tumor cannot be assessed
T0	No evidence of primary tumor
Tis	Carcinoma in situ (Bowen disease, high-grade squamous intraepithelial lesion [HISL], anal intraepithelial neoplasia [AIN] II–III)
T1	Tumor 2 cm or less in greatest dimension
T2	Tumor more than 2 cm but not more than 5 cm in greatest dimension
T3	Tumor more than 5 cm in greatest dimension
T4	Tumor of any size invades adjacent organ(s) (e.g., vagina, urethra, bladder) (direct invasion of rectal wall, perirectal skin, subcutaneous tissue or sphincter muscle is not classified as T4)

Regional Lymph Nodes (N)

NX	Regional lymph nodes cannot be assessed
N0	No regional lymph node metastasis
N1	Metastasis in perirectal lymph nodes(s)
N2	Metastasis in unilateral internal iliac and/or unilateral inguinal lymph node(s)
N3	Metastasis in perirectal and inguinal lymph nodes and/or bilateral internal iliac and/or inguinal lymph nodes

Distant Metastases (M)

M0	No distant metastasis
M1	Distant metastasis

Anatomic Stage/Prognostic Group

Stage 0	Tis	N0	M0
Stage I	T1	N0	M0
Stage II	T2	N0	M0
	T3	N0	M0
Stage IIIA	T1, T2, T3	N1	M0
	T4	N0	M0
Stage IIIB	T4	N1	M0
	Any T	N2, N3	M0
Stage IV	Any T	Any N	M1

From Edge SB, Byrd DB, Compton CC, et al., eds. *AJCC Cancer Staging Manual*, 7th ed. New York: Springer-Verlag; 2010: 171.

Cancer Research (CCCR) Anal Cancer Trial (ACT) 1 trial indicated that palpable lymph nodes as well as male sex portended a poor prognosis, similar to previous studies. In addition, after adjusting for these factors, these investigators also reported that lower hemoglobin and higher white blood cell counts were also prognostic in terms of anal cancer death and worsened overall survival, respectively. Tumor site, T classification, and platelet levels had no influence on outcomes.[44] However, not all studies have confirmed gender as an independent prognostic factor in terms of local control, metastasis, or overall survival.[45,46]

Although well-differentiated histologies have been shown to portend more favorable outcomes in other cancers, the histologic subtypes of anal cancer have not yet been demonstrated as substantial prognostic factors.[47] According to a study by Schlienger and colleagues,[48] there was no significant difference found in survival analysis among cloacogenic, well-differentiated, and moderately or poorly differentiated anal carcinomas.

Molecular

Prognostic biomarkers provide information on patient outcomes regardless of therapy, whereas predictive biomarkers provide information about the effect of specific therapeutic intervention.[49] The ultimate goal of determining prognostic factors is to improve patient survival. Disease processes and progression result from molecular and pathologic pathways, and by targeting altered pathways, potential avenues for therapeutic interventions that could facilitate improvements in survival may emerge. Similarly, molecular analyses of anal cancer to predict treatment response and survival outcomes are essential. Lampejo and colleagues[50] performed a systematic review on anal cancer prognostic biomarkers after reviewing 29 studies for final analysis. The authors found that 13 biomarkers were associated with anal cancer outcomes in only one study, whereas the tumor suppressor genes p53 and p21 as prognostic markers were established by more than one study.

The p53 gene is located in the short arm of chromosome 17 (17p13.1), which encodes a protein (393-amino acid nuclear phosphoprotein) that regulates the cell cycle and is responsible for cell apoptosis.[51,52] Accumulation of nuclear proteins was seen by immunohistochemistry in the cases of muted p53 genes in some studies.[53–55] These studies found that in anal carcinoma, p53 was overexpressed with a range of 34% to 100%. Wong et al.[52] described that increased p53 expression was associated with worse local–regional control ($p = 0.02$) and DFS ($p = 0.01$). Another study of 64 patients suggested that mutant p53 was responsible for inferior LRF rates relative to wild type, although nonsignificant (48 versus 27%, $p = 0.14$).[56] Allal and colleagues[57] reported that anal cancer patients with p53-positive lesions had a lower local–regional control rate (relative risk [RR], 0.38; $p = 0.03$) and shorter DFS (RR, 0.29; $p = 0.003$).

The p21 gene protein, a cyclin-dependent kinase (CDK) inhibitor, is considered to be a mediator of the p53 gene function.[58] Some studies have indicated that the lack of p21 expression is associated with poor prognosis in patients with squamous cell carcinoma of the anal canal (SCCA).[59] Holm et al.[59] reported that a lack of p21 expression was associated with reduced OS ($p = 0.013$), whereas Nilsson and colleagues[60] reported that absence of the same p21 expression was also responsible for an increased LRF rate ($p < 0.05$).

Ajani and colleagues[55] reported epidermal growth factor receptor (EGFR) expression was observed in 86% of patients with anal cancer, but the study was unable to determine the significant correlation between degree of staining and DFS. The same study's multivariate models suggested that Ki67 (negatively, coefficient: -0.04), nuclear factor kappa B (NF-κB) (positively, coefficient: 0.07), Sonic Hedgehog (SHH) (positively, coefficient: 0.05), and Gli-1 (positively, coefficient: 0.03) were associated with DFS ($p = 0.005$, 0.002, 0.02, and 0.02, respectively). Further investigation into the molecular prognostic factors of anal carcinoma is needed.[50]

TREATMENT OF LOCALIZED SQUAMOUS CELL CARCINOMA

Surgery

As with any disease, treatment decisions in anal cancer are made following a consideration of the risks and benefits. Wide local excision may be considered in a highly select subset of patients of anal cancer patients. This approach should generally be reserved for small, well-differentiated, superficial lesions confined to the anal margin, not involving the internal sphincter, and without nodal involvement.[61] For lesions that have residual microscopic disease or have close surgical margins less than 1 mm, further local excision, if technically possible, may be pursued, or adjuvant chemoradiation should be considered.[40]

Prior to the mid 1970s, the standard surgical approach to anal cancer was abdominal perineal resection (APR), which required a permanent colostomy following the removal of the rectum, ischiorectal fat, levator sling, perirectal and superior hemorrhoidal nodes, as well as a wide area of perianal skin, with associated long-term sequelae of sexual and urinary dysfunction. Collectively, long-term DFS results with a surgery alone approach were approximately 50%. A review at the Mayo Clinic of 118 anal cancers treated with APR reported an OS rate of 70% and overall recurrence rate of 40%. Of these, greater than 80% established recurrence sites had either local recurrence alone or some component of such.[62] Similarly, other surgical series using surgery alone results suggested high rates of regional recurrence (up to 60%) following local excision or APR alone across a variety of stages.[63]

Definitive Chemoradiotherapy

Given the relatively poor outcomes obtained with APR alone, Nigro et al., from Wayne State University pioneered incorporating concurrent pelvic radiation therapy and chemotherapy (5-FU and MMC) prior to surgical resection, resulting in high rates of pathologic complete response and survival, later verified by other investigators.[64–69] This led to significant interest in a *definitive* chemoradiotherapy approach.

Initially, the UK CCCR conducted the ACT I study. In this study, 585 patients with SCC of the anal canal or perianal skin were randomized to receive radiation therapy alone (45 Gy in 20 or 25 fractions), followed by additional radiation dose in patients achieving at least a 50% response (delivering an additional 15 to 25 Gy using either external beam radiation therapy or brachytherapy following a 6-week break) versus a similar radiation approach delivered concurrently with infusional 5-FU (750 mg/m^2 or 1,000 mg/m^2 for 5 days given during the first and last weeks of radiation therapy) along with MMC (12 mg/m^2 delivered on day 1 of treatment). Note that ACT I local failure rates captured several events, including persistence of primary disease following combined modality therapy, the requirement for surgery or colostomy because of treatment failure, as well as ongoing requirement for colostomy at 6 months following the completion of treatment. On the initial report, following a median follow-up of 42 months, the 3-year local failure rate was significantly lower in patients receiving chemoradiotherapy (39% versus 61%; p <0.0001), although at the expense of increased treatment-related morbidity. In particular, hematologic, skin, GI, and genitourinary toxicities were higher with the addition of chemotherapy, with six (2%) treatment-related deaths in the chemoradiation arm versus two (0.7%) for the radiation-alone arm. Although no statistically significant advantage was seen in terms of OS (3-year OS 72% versus 65%; p = 0.17), with the addition of chemotherapy, anal cancer-related mortality was significantly improved (28% versus 39%; p = 0.02), leading the authors to conclude that patients with SCC of the anal canal could be treated with definitive chemoradiotherapy with surgery reserved for salvage. In a report of long-term follow-up of this trial, no significant differences were seen in terms of long-term morbidity, although an excess in non–anal cancer deaths was seen in the combined modality group in the first 10 years following treatment (cardiovascular, treatment related, pulmonary disease, and second malignancy), but not beyond. LRF rates remained significantly higher in patients treated with radiation therapy alone (25% absolute difference at 12 years), with a corresponding improvement in relapse-free survival (12% absolute at 12 years) through the addition of chemotherapy, with no significant difference reported between the

two groups in terms of late morbidity.[70,71] Although not statistically significant, an absolute improvement in 12-year survival of 5.6% was seen.

A similar but smaller trial conducted by the EORTC randomized 103 patients with T3-4N0-3 or T1-2N1-3 anal cancer to radiation therapy (45 Gy, with a boost dose of 15 to 20 Gy following a 6-week break, based on disease response), with or without concurrent chemotherapy using infusional 5-FU (750 mg/m^2 per day, days 1 through 5 and days 29 through 33) with MMC (given on day 1 at 15 mg/m^2). Surgery was reserved for patients with less than a partial response. Outcomes from this study revealed that patients treated with concurrent chemotherapy had a higher complete response rate (80% versus 54%) with significant improvement in local–regional control (68 versus 50%), colostomy-free (72% versus 40%) and event-free survival with the addition of chemotherapy at 5 years. Similarly, OS was improved in patients receiving chemotherapy (3 year: 72% versus 65%), although this did not reach statistical significance. Rates of high-grade toxicity were deemed similar between the two groups, although rates of late anal ulceration were higher with the use of concurrent chemotherapy.[43]

The results from these two trials demonstrated that the addition of chemotherapy to definitive radiation therapy significantly improves LRF rates as well as relapse-free and colostomy-free survival rates, although at the expense of increased toxicity.

The Role of Mitomycin in the Combined Modality Therapy Approach of Anal Cancer

Although MMC was delivered concurrently with 5-FU in the aforementioned trials, it's necessity was questioned given the association with significant toxicities, including significant myelosuppression, dermatitis, as well as less common side effects of pulmonary fibrosis, hemolytic-uremic syndrome and therapy-related myelodysplastic syndrome. Given this, a randomized trial conducted by the RTOG and ECOG attempted to deintensify therapy by omitting MMC in efforts to preserve oncologic efficacy while eliminating MMC-related toxicity. In this study, patients with anal cancer of any T or N stage were randomized to radiation therapy (45 to 50.4 Gy, with an additional 9 Gy to patients with biopsy-proven persistence of disease 4 to 6 weeks following the completion of initial therapy) with infusional 5-FU (1,000 mg/m^2 per day on days 1 to 4 and days 29 to 32), with patients randomized to MMC (10 mg/m^2 days 1 and 29) versus not. Note that in patients with a positive biopsy following the first 4- to 6-week treatment, an additional cycle of cisplatin and 5-FU with radiotherapy was delivered. A second biopsy was later obtained and, if positive for residual tumor, patients proceeded to APR. This study enrolled 310 patients, of which 291 were analyzable. Colostomy-free and disease-free survival rates were significantly higher in patients receiving MMC (71% versus 59% and 73% versus 51%, respectively) with significantly lower colostomy (9% versus 22%) and local failure rates (16% versus 34%). OS was not improved, although as in the previously described randomized studies, was numerically superior (76% versus 67%). Also of note is that all grade 4 and 5 toxicities were considerably higher in patients receiving MMC.[47] Table 53.3 summarizes the results of randomized phase III clinical trials evaluating combined modality therapy with radiation, 5-FU, and mitomycin versus radiation therapy alone or radiation therapy with 5-FU.

The Role of Cisplatin Concurrent with Radiation Therapy in Anal Cancer

Given the aforementioned toxicities associated with MMC, there has been interest in substituting with a platinum-based chemotherapy when delivered concurrently with radiation therapy. Initial results using this approach from a Cancer and Leukemia Group B (CALGB) pilot study demonstrated that the use of induction 5-FU with cisplatin for advanced anal cancers (T3 to 4, or

TABLE 53.3

Summary of Randomized Phase III Clinical Trials Evaluating Combined Modality Treatment with Mitomycin-C/5-FU Versus Radiation Therapy Alone Or Radiation Therapy/5-FU for Anal Cancer

Study (Reference)	Treatment Arms[a]	Local–Regional Failure	Relapse-Free Survival	Colostomy-Free Survival	Overall Survival	Acute Toxicity
UKCCR/ ACT I[70,71]	(1) Radiation	(1) 59.1%	(1) 17.7%	(1) 20.1%	(1) 27.5%	(1) "Severe" skin toxicity = 39%; "severe" GI toxicity = 5%
	(2) Radiation + 5-FU + MMC	(2) 33.8% (at 12 years)	(2) 29.7% (at 12 years)	(2) 29.6% (at 12 years)	(2) 33.1% (at 12 years) p = NS	(2) "Severe" skin toxicity = 50%; "severe" GI toxicity = 14%
EORTC[43]	(1) Radiation	18% improvement in arm 2	N/A	32% improvement in arm 2	7% improvement in arm 2 p = NS	(1) Grade 3–4 diarrhea = 8%; grade 3–4 Dermatologic = 50%
	(2) Radiation + 5-FU + MMC					(2) Grade 3–4 diarrhea = 20%; grade 3–4 dermatologic = 57%
RTOG/ ECOG[47]	(1) Radiation + 5-FU	(1) 34%	(1) 51%	(1) 59%	(1) 67%	(1) Grade 4–5 heme = 3%; grade 4–5 nonheme = 4%
	(2) Radiation + 5-FU + MMC	(2) 16%	(2) 73% (disease-free survival at 4 years)	(2) 73% (at 4 years)	(2) 76% (at 4 years) p = NS	(2) Grade 4–5 heme = 18%; grade 4–5 nonheme = 7%

NS, not stated.
Note: + P values significant for comparisons unless otherwise noted.
[a] Details of treatment arms noted in text.

node positive) followed by definitive chemoradiotherapy (45 Gy, with or without a 9 Gy boost) with 5-FU and MMC resulted in an 80% complete response rates with 56% and colostomy-free survival.[72] These and other data led to increasing interest in substituting cisplatin for MMC. The RTOG subsequently conducted a phase III trial (RTOG 98-11), which randomized 644 patients to (1) a standard arm of concurrent chemoradiotherapy (45 to 59 Gy) with continuous infusional 5-FU ($1,000 mg/m^2$ per day) and bolus MMC ($10 mg/m^2$) weeks 1 and 5 versus (2) an experimental arm of two cycles of induction continuous 5-FU ($1,000 mg/m^2$ per day) and bolus cisplatin ($75 mg/m^2$) alone on weeks 1 and 5, followed by concurrent chemoradiotherapy with two cycles of continuous 5-FU ($1,000 mg/m^2$ per day) and bolus cisplatin ($75 mg/m^2$) on weeks 9 and 13. The trial primary endpoint was DFS and secondary endpoint included toxicity analysis. On the initial report, no significant difference was seen in 5-year DFS (60% versus 54%; p = 0.17), OS (75% versus 70%; p = 0.10), or local–regional relapse (25% versus 33%; p = 0.07). However, the 5-year colostomy rate was 10% in the mitomycin group versus 19% in the cisplatin-containing arm (p = 0.02).[73] An update of this trial demonstrated a significant improvement in 5-year DFS (68% versus 58%; p = 0.005), OS (78% versus 71%; p = 0.02), and borderline colostomy-free survival (72% versus 65%; p = 0.05) in the MMC-containing arm, albeit at the expense of increased grade 3 and higher hematologic toxicities (61% versus 42%; p < 0.001). However, nonhematologic toxicity rates were equivalent in both arms, with similar rates of late toxicity.[74] Critics of this study have pointed out that the prolonged the overall treatment duration associated with the use of induction chemotherapy with cisplatin may have allowed for accelerated tumoral repopulation prior to radiation therapy initiation.

A follow-up study from the UK CCCR (the ACT II trial) performed a more direct comparison of the use of cisplatin in conjunction with radiation therapy compared to MMC. In this largest of anal cancer randomized trials, 950 patients with anal or perianal skin cancer were randomized using a 2 × 2 factorial design, with patients randomized to receive infusional 5-FU ($1,000 mg/m^2$ per day, on days 1 to 4 and days 29 to 32) with

pelvic radiation therapy (50.4 Gy) plus MMC ($12 mg/m^2$ on day 1) versus cisplatin ($60 mg/m^2$ on day 1 and 29) with the same 5-FU–radiation regimen. A second randomization was performed following completion of the combined treatment course to no further therapy versus two additional cycles of cisplatin and 5-FU. Grade 3 to 4 acute nonhematologic toxicity rates were similar between the regimens (60% versus 65%; p = 0.17). Not unexpectantly, grade 3 and higher hematologic toxicity rates were greater in the mitomycin group (25% versus 13%; p < 0.001), although no toxic deaths were reported in the trial. In terms of the trial primary endpoint of complete clinical response at 6 months, there was no significant difference between the two groups, and at a median follow-up of 5.1 years, clinical complete response at 26 weeks was 91% in the MMC group compared to 90% in the cisplatin group. Additionally, the 3-year colostomy rate was similar between the two groups (14% mitomycin versus 11% cisplatin). The use of maintenance therapy in this trial showed no obvious benefit, with 3-year recurrence-free survival of 75% in both arms, similar OS rates between the maintenance versus no maintenance groups (85% versus 84%), with 3-year PFS rates of 74% in the maintenance group versus 73% in the nonmaintenance group. The authors concluded that MMC given concurrently with 5-FU and radiation therapy should remain the standard in the treatment of anal cancer, given the following: (1) the high grade hematologic toxicity seen with MMC did not significantly increase sepsis rates; (2) the MMC course was delivered over approximately 10 minutes compared to two courses of either all day or overnight intravenous (IV) hydration with cisplatin, with similar efficacy and overall toxicities between the regimens; (3) fewer chemotherapy cycles were required; (4) there was requirement for fewer nonchemotherapy drugs; (5) there was lesser expense; and (6) there was no risk of neuropathy.[75]

Another phase III trial conducted by the French Federation Nationale des Centres de Lutte Contre La Cancer ACCORD (the ACCORD-03 trial) randomized patients with stage II to III anal cancer to one of four treatment arms: (1) neoadjuvant 5-FU + cisplatin alone followed by 5-FU cisplatin radiation therapy (45 Gy) with a radiation therapy boost (15 Gy) using either external beam or brachytherapy techniques; (2) same as the first arm, except utilizing a higher dose radiation boost (20 to 25 Gy); (3) same as the first arm, but no neoadjuvant chemotherapy; and (4) same as the second arm, but no neoadjuvant chemotherapy. Of note is that a 3-week break was mandated following the completion of the initial 45 Gy, prior to boost treatments. Following a median 50-month follow-up, there was no significant difference in 5-year colostomy-free survival rates (70% to 82%). Similarly, no significant differences were seen between the arms in terms of LRF, cause-specific survival, and OS. The most intensified treatment arm of induction chemotherapy with high-dose radiation boost demonstrated a numerically improved local control (88% versus 72% to 83% on the additional arms). The trial authors indicated that induction chemotherapy does not improve outcomes, with the role of radiation dose escalation in this disease remaining uncertain, but felt that that the combination of induction chemotherapy and radiation dose escalation should be explored further.[76] The results of randomized trials evaluating cisplatin are shown in Table 53.4.

Novel Biologic Radiosensitizing Agents

To date, no biologic agent has been granted U.S. Food and Drug Administration (FDA) approval as an effective radiosensitizer in anal cancer. Early reports have described outcomes of combined treatment modality with EGFR inhibitors, with varying degrees of response and toxicity.[79,80] These and other studies are warranted to assess the role of treatment intensification, particularly in more advanced disease where outcomes are less favorable.

Traditional Radiation and Intensity Modulated Radiation Therapy

The use of combined modality therapy in the definitive treatment of anal cancer results in significant acute as well as late toxicities. All the previously mentioned randomized trials used radiation therapy planned and delivered using either conventional 2-dimensional or 3-dimensional radiation planning techniques. This approach frequently entails treating large volumes of nontarget tissues (bowel, bladder, bone, genitalia), leading to the aforementioned morbidities. Although 3-dimensional planning results in potentially improved normal tissue sparing through the use of axial CT images to define the target volume as well as normal tissue structures, results remain suboptimal. Intensity-modulated radiation therapy is an advanced form of 3-dimensional conformal radiation therapy that implements multiple beams using a nonuniform dose delivery. This can be accomplished in a variety of ways, all of which entail the use of collimating leafs that sweep across the beam path during treatment delivery. Through inverse computer planning techniques, the radiation dose can be more tightly conformed to target tissues with dose reductions to adjacent, nontarget organs. With this technique, there is a significant potential to reduce both acute and long-term morbidity associated with anal cancer treatments. Multiple institutional studies have indicated that, compared to patients treated with non–intensity-modulated radiation therapy (IMRT) techniques, a significant reduction of treatment-related toxicity can be accomplished.[81,82] Additionally, with corresponding reductions in acute toxicity, there may be a reduction in the need for treatment breaks, with the potential to further influence disease-related outcomes.[83] A prospective trial evaluating IMRT for anal cancer was conducted through the RTOG (0529 study). In this phase II trial, patients received concurrent 5-FU with MMC. Radiation therapy was delivered through a *dose-painting* technique, whereby differing target volumes received differing doses of radiation therapy during any one treatment as defined by the study. The primary endpoint of this study included an assessment of grade 2 or higher GI and genitourinary toxicities as compared to the previously described RTOG 98-11 trial (MMC-containing arm). In 52 analyzable patients (out of 63 accrued), rates of grade 3 or higher dermatologic toxicity

were improved in the IMRT study (20% versus 47%; p < 0.001) as were rates of grade 3 or higher GI and genitourinary toxicity (22% versus 36%; p = 0.014). Additionally, median radiation duration was 42.5 days in the IMRT study compared to 49 days in 98-11, with similar 2-year disease-related outcomes when compared to RTOG 98-11.[84,85] An important caveat to this trial was that a central reviewer performed pretreatment quality assurance on all patients. Of initially submitted plans, 81% required planning revisions, with 46% of plans requiring two or more revisions. Although this trial did not formally meet its primary endpoints in reduction and acute toxicities, it does suggest that the use of IMRT can significantly reduce high-grade GI, genitourinary, and skin toxicities without compromising treatment-related outcomes, and that there is also a significant learning curve for the use of IMRT in the treatment of anal cancer. Figure 53.5 demonstrates an example of an anal cancer plan implementing IMRT.

Follow-Up Management

Given that SCC of the anus can regress slowly following treatment completion (up to 12 months), it is generally recommended that patients who have regressive disease do not undergo repeat biopsies given this may lead to nonhealing ulceration and chronic wound infection in previously irradiated tissues.[45,86] Exemplifying this phenomena, in a preliminary report from the ACT II trial, 72% of patients who had not achieved a clinical complete response at 11 weeks ultimately achieved such at 26 weeks from treatment initiation,[87] indicating that premature biopsy following definitive chemoradiotherapy may result in the aforementioned complications as well as premature *salvage* surgery in some cases. Of the 265 patients in the ACT II trial not in complete response at week 11, only 83 ultimately had progression/persistent disease.

Approximately 20% to 25% of patients with SCC treated by chemoradiation will either fail to completely respond or relapse within the first 3 years after treatment. Posttreatment evaluation is critical to assess the effectiveness of therapy and to detect a persistent or recurrent tumor.[86] The first evaluation typically is between 8 to 12 weeks after the completion of chemoradiation. The physical examination should include a visual inspection, a digital rectal exam, an anoscopy, and palpation of the inguinal nodal regions. Ongoing clinical evaluation typically occurs every 3 to 6 months for the first 2 years, then every 6 to 12 months until 5 years following completion of chemoradiation. It may be appropriate to conduct less intense follow-ups following 3 years, given that only 7% of relapses occur beyond this time point.[88] Lesions persisting beyond 3 months following treatment are more concerning for residual disease; however, as stated previously, it is important to assess changes over time. If a tumor continues to shrink, then close clinical surveillance is advised. Chronically persistent or recurrent tumors should be biopsied for confirmation of SCC.[61] Discretion regarding the size and depth of biopsies is needed because extensive biopsies may result in nonhealing ulcers and chronic wound infection.[45] As an adjunct to physical examination, imaging studies for posttreatment surveillance should be considered.[61] Current NCCN guidelines recommend a CT scan of the chest, abdomen, and pelvis annually for 3 years for patients who had T3 or T4 disease or positive inguinal nodes.

Treatment for HIV Population

Unfortunately, the majority of pivotal phase III trials did not allow the inclusion of HIV-positive patients. There are studies suggesting that anal cancer patients with HIV comorbidities have comparable rates of response to HIV-negative patients while being treated with chemoradiation.[89–91] Earlier studies suggested that there was a potential for HIV-positive patients to experience higher toxicities and inferior treatment compliance, which could ultimately alter their outcomes.[92,93] Most studies addressing the application

TABLE 53.4

Phase III Randomized Trials Evaluating the Role of Cisplatin in Anal Cancer

Study (Reference)	Primary site	N	Stage	Treatments	Colostomy-Free Survival (%)[a]	Overall Survival (%)[a]	Grade 3 or 4 Hematological Toxic Effects (%; n/N)[b]	Grade 3 or 4 Nonhematological Toxic Effects (%; n/N)[b]	Late Toxic Effects (%; n/N)[b]
RTOG 98-11[77,78]	Anal canal	682	T2 to T4, N0 to N3	Group 1: EBRT (45–59 Gy) + fluorouracil and mitomycin Group 2: fluorouracil and cisplatin→ EBRT (45–59 Gy) + fluorouracil and cisplatin	Group 1: 71.9% Group 2: 65.0%	Group 1: 78.3% Group 2: 70.7%	Group 1: 61% (199/324) Group 2: 42% (134/320)	Group 1: 74% (240/324) Group 2: 74% (239/320)	Grade 4 small or large bowel: 1% (6/625)
ACCORD[76]	Anal canal	307	≥4cm, <4cm plus N1 to N3	Group 1: fluorouracil and cisplatin →EBRT (45 Gy) + fluorouracil and cisplatin→rest→15 Gy Group 2: fluorouracil and cisplatin →EBRT (45 Gy) + fluorouracil and cisplatin→rest→20–25Gy Group 3: EBRT (45 Gy) + fluorouracil and cisplatin →rest→15 Gy Group 4: EBRT (45 Gy) + fluorouracil and cisplatin →rest→20–25 Gy	Group 1: 69.6% Group 2: 82.4% Group 3: 77.1% Group 4: 72.7%	Group 1 + Group 2: 75% Group 3 + Group 4: 71% Group 1 + Group 3: 71% Group 2 + Group 4: 74%	Group 1 + Group 2: 19% (29/150) Group 3 + Group 4: 12% (19/157)	Group 1 + Group 2 diarrhea: 9% (14/150) Group 3 + Group 4 diarrhea: 12% (18/157)	Grade 4 colostomy: 3% (9/307)
ACTII[75]	Anal canal or anal margin	940	T1 to T4, N– or N+	Group1: EBRT (50.4 Gy) + fluorouracil and cisplatin Group 2: EBRT (50.4 Gy) + fluorouracil and mitomycin Group 3: EBRT (50.4 Gy) + fluorouracil and cisplatin→fluorouracil and cisplatin Group 4: EBRT (50.4 Gy) + fluorouracil and mitomycin→fluorouracil and cisplatin	Group 1: 72% Group 2: 75% Group 3: 75% Group 4: 73%	Group 1: 84% Group 2: 86% Group 3: 83% Group 4: 82%	Mitomycin: 26% (124/472) Cisplatin: 16% (73/468)	Mitomycin: 62% (294/472) Cisplatin: 68% (316/468)	Colostomy: 2% (14/844)

[a] At 5 years in RTOG 98-11 and ACCORD3; at 3 years in ACT II.
[b] (n/N) = affected population/total population.

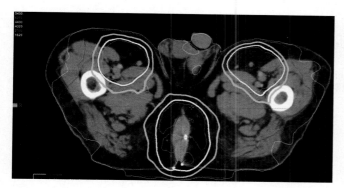

Figure 53.5 An axial CT slice of an intensity-modulated radiation therapy plan of a 56-year-old male with clinical T3N3 squamous cell carcinoma of the anal canal treated with definitive chemoradiotherapy. Note relative organ sparing and *bending* of isodose curves around normal structures including anteriorly based (genitalia) and femora bilaterally while still encompassing the primary target volume of his gross tumor *(red)* as well as local–regional lymph nodes basins (perirectal and inguinal). Note that *colored lines* (isodose curves) represent varying radiation doses.

and outcomes of standard combined regimens for the treatment of anal cancer with HIV-positive patients describe small sample sizes. There are several studies where investigators endeavored to describe the outcomes of treatment modalities for anal carcinomas based on CD4 cell count.[94,95] According to Hoffman et al.,[94] patients with CD4 count ≥200/mm³ tolerated combined therapy (5-FU/MMC/radiation) better (decreased likelihood of toxicity) compared with patients who had CD4 counts <200/mm³. In the Cook County Hospital AIDS Malignancy Project (CHAMP) study, median survival in the HIV-positive versus HIV-negative patients was 34 versus 39 months (p > 0.5). In the HIV-negative population, 22% survived 120 months, whereas no HIV patient survived over 90 months, and time to local recurrence was 20 months shorter in the HIV-positive arm (p < 0.5), with the authors speculating this may imply more aggressive disease. OS based on CD4 count did not differ.[13]

Preliminary safety and efficacy results were presented on the administration of two doses of cetuximab, cisplatin, 5-FU and with radiation therapy (45 to 54 Gy) in immunocompetent (ECOG 3205, n = 28) and HIV-positive (AMC045, n = 45) patients with non-metastatic (stage I to III) squamous cell carcinoma of anal canal.[96] These results showed that the PFS and OS rates in the subsequent 2 years were 80% and 89% for HIV-positive patients with anal cancer, compared to 92% and 93%, respectively for HIV-negative patients. The authors concluded that combined cetuximab, cisplatin, 5FU and radiation combination therapy in HIV positive patients with anal cancer yielded favorable outcomes based on feasibility, safety and efficacy. Further data on these two companion studies are indicated and evaluation within a randomized clinical trial would be required to determine whether patients with anal cancer benefit from an EGFR-targeted therapeutic agent.

HAART is important for bolstering CD4 cell counts in patients with HIV. To analyze the impact of HAART on patients with anal cancer receiving combined modality therapy (CMT), Place and colleagues[95] completed a small study in which patients were divided into two groups: one group received CMT before HAART implementation, and the other group received CMT following HAART therapy. The authors concluded that the patients who received CMT after the advent of HAART had better outcomes, although it was speculated interpretation could be hampered by the fact HAART alone might have altered the immune status of the patients.[95] In a French study, clinical outcomes of anal cancer patients with HIV treated with HAART and chemoradiation were similar to immunocompetent (HIV

negative) controls.[97] More recently, however, a single institution French study[98] reported significantly poorer outcomes for their HIV-positive compared to HIV-negative patients. Local control was achieved in 50% versus 77%, with corresponding 5-year OS rates of 30% versus 84% and DFS rates of 37% versus 75%, respectively. In addition, HIV-infected patients were more likely to be younger and male, although no significant differences were seen in terms of stage or other tumor characteristics. These investigators postulated that the worsened outcomes may have resulted from a higher frequency of advanced disease in their population relative to other studies and a reflection of lack of routine and local screening programs. However, a follow-up study at Case Western University showed that both HIV-positive and HIV-negative patients treated with HAART had comparable treatment efficacy and toxicity rates.[99] Finally, a pooled analysis of 121 patients with anal cancer treated in the HAART era revealed similar complete response and OS rates among HIV-positive and HIV-negative patients, although HIV-positive patients were much more likely to experience local failure (5-year 62% versus 13%; p = 0.008) along with increased acute dermatologic and hematologic toxicities with treatment.[100]

There is a general concern that cancer patients receiving chemotherapy are predisposed to develop immunosuppression, particularly in the setting of an immunodeficiency disease such as HIV, thus complicating the treatment choice and follow-up plan. There is also a potentially greater chance of experiencing adverse treatment reactions that can hinder treatment compliance. Although it is usually not necessary to alter standard management recommendations, HIV-infected patients, especially those with a CD4 count less than 200/μL, should be monitored for an increased risk of toxicity when treated with chemoradiation. Given the previously described ACT I and EORTC trial results, chemotherapy omission is generally not recommended. Thus, factors including pretreatment CD4 cell count, HAART compliance, posttreatment CD4 cell count, and performance status, must come into account in order to formulate a favorable combined treatment modality for anal cancer patients on a personalized, case-by-case basis.

Salvage Therapy for Local Recurrence

APR is recommended for patients who have chronically persistent disease or who develop recurrence. Restaging is performed to evaluate the extent of the disease and determine the presence of extrapelvic metastases. Curative surgery must attain negative margins for oncologic success, and tumor invasion into adjacent organs warrants en bloc resection. Invasion of local structures, including the vagina or prostate, should be approached with an intent of resecting with negative margins. This may involve a multivisceral resection. In instances where there may be close or involved margins at resection, the use of intraoperative radiotherapy or brachytherapy may enhance local control rates. In highly selected cases, there may be a role for low-dose reirradiation with concurrent chemotherapy followed by resection and intraoperative radiotherapy. The majority of published series describing outcomes with salvage surgery have small patient numbers given the relative rarity of such. Five-year survival following resection generally ranges between 30% to 70%, with DFS rates ranging from 30% to 40% (Table 53.5). The most important prognostic factor of survival after resection is margin status, and patients with negative margins (R0) have up to a 75% 5-year OS.[101] Further predictors of a poor OS outcome following surgery include inguinal lymph node involvement, tumor size greater than 5 cm, adjacent organ involvement, male gender, and comorbidities.[102,103] In one of the largest series describing salvage surgery in anal cancer, Correa et al.[104] proposed a scoring system predicting postoperative survival. The three factors included were lymph

TABLE 53.5

Results of Salvage Surgery for Residual or Recurrent Anal Cancer

Study	Patient Number	Negative Margin After Surgery (R0)	5-Year Survival Based on Margin Status	Overall 5-Year Survival
Akbari et al., 2004[102]	62	85%	R0 = 38% R½ = 0%	33%
Nilsson et al., 2002[105]	35	91%	NS	52%
Ghouti et al., 2005[106]	36	NS	NS	69.4% (DFS, 31.1%)
Renehan et al., 2005[107]	73	75%	R0 = 61.4% R½ = 0%	40%
Schiller et al., 2007[103]	40	83%	NS	39% (DFS, 30%)
Ferenschild et al., 2005[109]	18	78%	NS	30%
Sunesen et al., 2009[101]	45	78%	R0 = 75% R1 = 40% R2 = 0%	61%
Eeson et al., 2011[110]	51	63%	R0 = 42% R½ = 0%	29%
Lefevre et al., 2012[111]	105	82%	R0 = 69% R1 = 0%	61%

R0, clear margin; R1, microscopic positive margin; R2, grossly positive margin; NS, not stated.

node involvement, involved surgical margins, and perineural and/or lymphovascular invasion.[104] Patients who had none of these factors (i.e., a score of 0), had an estimated 5-year survival of 55%; however, those with scores of 1 to 3 did much worse, with 5-year survival of 0.03% in patients with all of the factors. The utility of such a system is to define a subgroup that would potentially benefit from additional postoperative treatments. The majority of reported series describing salvage surgery indicate that persistence of disease (as opposed to recurrence) following combined modality therapy was the primary reason for such an approach. In patients undergoing salvage surgery, even with R0 resection, patients with disease persistence tend to have worse outcomes, with 5-year overall survival rates ranging from 31% to 33% as compared to 51% to 82% for truly recurrent patients.[102,105] It is been hypothesized that persistent tumors may harbor a more aggressive tumor biology resistant to chemoradiotherapy, leading to worse outcomes. Overall, length of time to recurrence following resection varies from 1 to 50 months.[101,103,106,107]

Salvage resection is associated with significant morbidity in up to 72% of patients, including side effects of delayed perineal wound healing, pelvic abscesses, perineal wound hernia, urinary retention, as well as the development of impotence. Perineal wound healing difficulties are a result of both the large soft tissue defect created in fully excising these tumors as well as potentially impacted by prior radiation therapy. Closure of the wound by primary intention produces suboptimal results if not combined with flap placement. In one series of 22 patients undergoing salvage APR with primary closure, 59% experience perineal wound break down, with 1 requiring reconstructive operation.[107] Commonly used tissue flaps include an omental pedicle flap, a gracilis muscle flap, and the vertical rectus abdominis myocutaneous flap (VRAM). In one series of 95 patients undergoing salvage APR, patients undergoing an omental pedicle flap, as compared to a VRAM flap, had more perineal wound complications and slower healing.[108] In another smaller series, the perineal wound break-down rate with the use of omental flap reconstruction was 36% versus 0% with a VRAM flap following APR.[110] Finally, a series

of 48 patients who underwent salvage APR reported no delays in wound healing or infectious complications when a VRAM flap was used.[101]

Management of Metastatic Disease

Randomized studies have demonstrated that patients treated with chemoradiation can develop metastatic disease in 10% to 17% of cases.[43,70] Currently, systemic chemotherapy is the treatment of choice for metastatic anal cancer. However, there is little published data in the setting of metastatic disease. Much of the treatment has been extrapolated from more common squamous cell cancers such as head and neck cancer, cervical cancer, etc. A 5-FU/cisplatin combination is recommended by the NCCN[40] guidelines as the first-line regimen to treat metastatic anal SCC.

There are a few small studies that report the benefit of administration of the previous mentioned regimen in patients with metastatic SCCA.[86,112–115] Most notably, according to Faivre et al.,[112] survival at 1 and 5 years were 62.2% and 32.2%, respectively, whereas the median survival was 34.5 months.

MMC and 5-FU may also be considered for first-line therapy[116] for metastatic SCCA. One study showed that patients treated with this regimen ultimately achieved better response that included tumor size shrinkage, pain management, and performance improvement. There are additional combination chemotherapy trials and single agent case reports available that are described briefly in Table 53.6.[117]

Cetuximab has shown favorable outcomes for the treatment of SCC of the head and neck while delivered concurrently with radiation therapy.[125] However, the data supporting the administration of cetuximab in metastatic SCCA is scant. According to a few small studies and case reports, the maximum clinical response achieved was a partial response, with varying ranges of PFS with cetuximab/irinotecan combination therapy.[126–128] Due to the very small sample sizes of these studies, a further evaluation is warranted.

TABLE 53.6

Studies Demonstrating Survival and Response Data on Metastatic Anal Cancer

Study Type (Reference)	Patient Number	Agent(s)	Response Rate or Clinical Response	Progression-Free Survival in Months
Combination[118]	15	Vincristine/bleomycin/methotrexate	25%	2
Combination[119]	**7 (anal only)**	Paclitaxel/carboplatin/5-FU	65%	26
Combination[120]	20	Mitomycin-C/Adriamycin/cisplatin/bleomycin	60%	8
Combination[121]	77	5-FU/cisplatin versus Carboplatin/paclitaxel		8 versus 4
Single-agent case report[122]		Carboplatin	Partial	9
Single-agent case report[123]		Semustine	Partial	15
Single-agent case report[124]		Irinotecan	Partial	Not reported

Like other GI cancers, the liver is the primary site of metastasis from anal cancer. Data on the resection of an isolated hepatic lesion are sparse, and currently, a definitive surgical treatment protocol remains largely undefined in the metastatic setting. That said, surgical resection of metastatic disease can be considered when appropriate, based on the extent of disease and performance status. According to Eng et al.,[121] the median PFS and OS of 33 out of 77 patients with metastatic anal SCCA who received curative surgical treatment for their metastatic disease were 16 (95% CI, 9.2 to 22.8) and 53 months (95% CI, 28.3 to 77.6), respectively. Previously, a multicenter study[129] comprising of 52 patients also suggested that a subset of patients might benefit from surgical resection. According to the study, among 27 metastatic squamous cell anal carcinoma patients pretreated with systemic therapy, the median PFS and OS were 9.6 and 22.3 months, respectively, although definitive selection criteria for surgical resection were lacking.

Outcome, benefit, and toxicity analysis on chemoradiation for metastatic anal cancer is limited. A small study[130] (n = 6) from the M.D. Anderson Cancer Center of patients with para-aortic nodal involvement was reported. In this study, all the patients were treated with IMRT with concurrent infusional 5-FU and cisplatin. The results showed that 3-year actuarial local–regional control, distant control, and survival rates were 100%, 56%, and 63%, respectively. In another study, a short course of chemoradiation comprised of 30 Gy with concurrent 5-FU demonstrated good local–regional control (73% at the median follow-up of 16 months) in elderly patients (median age 81 years).[131] Combined chemoradiation may also be used to palliate symptoms related to metastatic disease.

The International Rare Cancer Initiative (IRCI) in collaboration with the NCI has expressed interest specifically focusing on establishing guidelines for metastatic anal cancer squamous carcinoma patients, including diagnostic imaging, staging, surveillance, and survivorship. The first initiative is an international collaboration with the United Kingdom, EORTC, and ECOG/ACRIN on a randomized phase II trial of 5-FU/cisplatin versus carboplatin/paclitaxel in treatment-naïve patients (InterAACT).

TREATMENT OF OTHER SITES AND PATHOLOGIES

Squamous Cell Carcinoma of the Anal Margin

The definition of anal margin tumors has varied over time, ranging from perianal skin to the distal aspect of the anal canal.

A generally accepted, contemporary definition includes the area extending from the anal verge radially 5 cm outward on the perianal skin. The onset of this disease is frequently seen in the 7th and 8th decades of life, with a slight female predominance.[116,132,133] The majority of these tumors are well differentiated, indicating a slow growing nature with the development of distant metastases rare.[116,134,135] The primary drainage is to the inguinal region and regional nodal metastases directly related to tumoral size. Once series[136] describes that tumors less than 2 cm rarely exhibit lymph node metastases, 2 to 5 cm tumors associated with an approximately 23% node positive rate, and in tumors larger than 5 cm, rates as high as 67%. Therefore, it is important that these tumors be approached on an individual basis based on size, location, and histologic characteristics. Tumors whose epicenter is distal to the anal verge may be managed as skin tumors. Potential treatment options for these patients include local excision with or without adjuvant radiation therapy, or radiation with or without chemotherapy. Treatment considerations in these patients must take into account expected morbidity with such approaches. For smaller tumors, wide local excision with a 1-cm margin is often sufficient. However, surgery for larger tumors may require more aggressive removal, which may entail APR; combined modality therapy may be an appropriate alternative in such cases, particularly where the risk of lymph node involvement is high. Therefore, surgery is often reserved for tumors <2 cm in greatest dimension without adverse histologic features and no involvement of the anal sphincter. APR should generally be reserved for patients with recurrent disease following radiation/chemoradiation or recurrence not amenable to local excision. Chapet and colleagues[137] reviewed an experience of 26 patients with tumors of the perianal skin, 5 with involvement of the anal canal. Most were ≤5 cm in diameter. Fourteen received definitive radiation therapy, with or without chemotherapy, and 12 received radiation therapy following initial local excision. Actuarial local control rate was 61%, and with salvage surgical treatment, this increased to 81%, with a 5-year cause-specific survival of 88%. Khanfir et al.[138] reported similar results in a series of 45 patients. Twenty-nine patients underwent local excision prior to radiation therapy. Five-year local–regional control was 78% with 5-year DFS of 86%. Balmucki et al.[139] updated at University of Florida experience with definitive radiotherapy and chemoradiotherapy in 26 patients with SCC of the perianal skin. Two patients developed local recurrence and two developed regional nodal recurrence, resulting in a 10-year cause-specific survival of 92%. Of note, two patients who had clinically node-negative disease who did not receive prophylactic inguinal nodal radiation developed inguinal recurrences.

Anal Canal Adenocarcinoma

Primary adenocarcinoma of the anal canal is an uncommon tumor. In many situations, this will represent growth of a distal rectal adenocarcinoma into the anal canal and is managed as such. In some instances, this disease is believed to arise from glandular epithelium in the anal canal, accounting for less than 5% of all anal malignancies.[140] Occasionally, adenocarcinoma may occur in patients with ulcerative colitis or Crohn's disease who have ileal pouch–anal anastomosis.[141–143] A study from the Rare Cancer Network registry of 82 patients diagnosed with anal adenocarcinoma was analyzed based on the treatment approach. The actuarial local–regional relapse rate at 5 years was 37%, 36%, and 20%, respectively, in the radiation/surgery, combined chemoradiation therapy alone, and APR alone groups. The 5-year OS rate was 29%, 58%, and 21% and 5-year DFS rate 25%, 54%, and 22%, respectively. A multivariate analysis revealed four independent prognostic factors for survival: T stage, N stage, histologic grade, and treatment modality (chemoradiotherapy). The authors concluded that they observed better survival rates after combined chemoradiotherapy and recommended using APR only for salvage treatment.[144] In contrast, a Surveillance, Epidemiology, and End Results (SEER) study evaluated 165 patients with nonmetastatic adenocarcinoma of the anal canal. Of these, 30 patients were treated with an APR only, 42 patients with an APR and radiation, and 93 patients with radiation alone. The 5-year survival for APR only, APR and radiation, and radiation alone was 58%, 50%, and 30%, respectively (p = 0.04). A multivariate analysis confirmed factors accounting for the survival differences included age, nodal stage, and treatment groups. The authors concluded definitive surgical treatment in the form of an APR with or without radiation is associated with improved survival in these patients.[145] An institutional report from the M. D. Anderson Cancer Center analyzed 16 patients with anal adenocarcinoma and compared outcomes with definitive chemoradiotherapy to similarly treated patients with squamous cell tumors.[146] At 5-years, local failure rate was 54% in the adenocarcinoma group compared to 18% for patients with SCC, with corresponding 5-year DFS of 19% versus 77%, respectively, and OS rates of 64% versus 85%. Given this, patients with primary anal adenocarcinoma are generally treated as if they had rectal adenocarcinomas of similar stage, with surgery remaining as a cornerstone therapy and neoadjuvant radiation therapy or combined modality therapy generally implemented in patients with high-risk features (T3 or T4 and/or nodal involvement).

Anal Paget disease is an intraepithelial adenocarcinoma arising from the dermal apocrine sweat glands, most commonly found in females and in older patients.[34] Although progression from perianal Paget disease to invasive disease is seen in approximately 5% of cases, invasive cancers have been reported up to 40% of patients with untreated Paget disease. Association with tubo-ovarian adenocarcinoma was seen in 7% to 24% and GI cancers in 12% to 14% of cases.[34] Therefore, appropriate imaging and fiber-optic endoscopy studies are recommended to rule out synchronous underlying malignancies.

Melanoma of the Anorectal Region

Anorectal melanoma is a rare disease that accounts for approximately 1% of all malignant melanomas and 0.5% of tumors of anorectal area.[147–149] Symptoms are rather nondescript, with bleeding manifesting as the most common complaint.[150] The gross appearance varies from a small, pigmented lesion to an ulcerated mass. Anal canal melanomas are usually pigmented lesions, but can be amelanotic in as many as 29% of cases.[151] A SEER database review reported a 5-year OS of 2.5%,[152] although some series report up to a 20% survival.[149,150,153] Surgery is the cornerstone of treatment with debate regarding the optimal approach. Traditionally, surgeons adopted a more radical approach utilizing APR with a radical lymph node dissection. However, this approach was associated with significant morbidity without improving OS. Kiran et al.[154] reviewed 109 patients with anorectal melanoma from the SEER database between 1982 and 2002 and reported no significant difference between patients treated by APR or local resection. A retrospective review of 251 patients from the Swedish National Cancer Registry between 1960 and 1999 demonstrated similar findings.[155] A recent systematic review comparing APR to wide local excision in anal melanoma patients reported similar median survivals regardless of treatment approach (21 months for APR, N = 369; 20 months for local excision, N = 324). Similarly, the treatment approach did not significantly impact 5-year survival (14% for APRs, 15% for local excision).[156]

There are some centers that advocate more aggressive treatment for localized disease, arguing for better oncologic outcomes in select subsets. In an older Memorial Sloan Kettering experience, factors associated with long-term survival following APR included female gender, negative lymph nodes, and tumor size less than 2.5 cm, concluding APR may be considered in the subset of patients with these features.[150] A Japanese study that included 79 patients with anorectal melanoma reported 3- and 5-year survival rates of 34.8% and 28.8%, respectively (median survival 22 months), for patients treated by APR.[157] Therefore, the authors of that study recommended local excision for patients with stage 0 melanoma, whereas those with stage 1 cancers or T1 tumors should undergo an APR with lymph node dissection. Ballo et al.[158] reported on 23 patients treated at the M. D. Anderson Cancer Center with sphincter sparing excision and adjuvant radiation therapy using a hypofractionated regimen of 30 Gy delivered in five fractions. Nine patients received systemic therapy. Five-year actuarial overall, disease-free, distant metastases-free, local, and regional nodal control rates were 31%, 37%, 35%, 74%, and 84%, respectively, comparing favorably to varying reports using local excision alone.

REFERENCES

1. Siegel R, Ma J, Zou Z, et al. Cancer statistics, 2014. *CA Cancer J Clin* 2014;64:9–29.
2. Johnson LG, Madeleine MM, Newcomer LM, et al. Anal cancer incidence and survival: the surveillance, epidemiology, and end results experience, 1973-2000. *Cancer* 2004;101:281–288.
3. Frisch M, Melbye M, Moller H. Trends in incidence of anal cancer in Denmark. *BMJ* 1993;306:419–422.
4. Grulich AE, Poynten IM, Machalek DA, et al. The epidemiology of anal cancer. *Sex Health* 2012;9:504–508.
5. Machalek DA, Poynten M, Jin F, et al. Anal human papillomavirus infection and associated neoplastic lesions in men who have sex with men: a systematic review and meta-analysis. *Lancet Oncol* 2012;13:487–500.
6. Lawton MD, Nathan M, Asboe D. HPV vaccination to prevent anal cancer in men who have sex with men. *Sex Transm Infect* 2013;89:342–343.
7. Frisch M, Glimelius B, van den Brule AJ, et al. Sexually transmitted infection as a cause of anal cancer. *N Engl J Med* 1997;337:1350–1358.
8. Goodman MT, Shvetsov YB, McDuffie K, et al. Sequential acquisition of human papillomavirus (HPV) infection of the anus and cervix: the Hawaii HPV Cohort Study. *J Infect Dis* 2010;201:1331–1339.
9. Diamond C, Taylor TH, Aboumrad T, et al. Increased incidence of squamous cell anal cancer among men with AIDS in the era of highly active antiretroviral therapy. *Sex Transm Dis* 2005;32:314–320.
10. Crum-Cianflone NF, Hullsiek KH, Marconi VC, et al. Anal cancers among HIV-infected persons: HAART is not slowing rising incidence. *AIDS* 2010; 24:535–543.
11. Shiels MS, Pfeiffer RM, Gail MH, et al. Cancer burden in the HIV-infected population in the United States. *J Natl Cancer Inst* 2011;103: 753–762.

12. Shiels MS, Pfeiffer RM, Chaturvedi AK, et al. Impact of the HIV epidemic on the incidence rates of anal cancer in the United States. *J Natl Cancer Inst* 2012;104:1591–1598.

13. Rubinstein P, Sreenivasappa S, Gupta S, et al. Concurrent chemoradiotherapy with 5-fluorouracil and mitomycin-C for invasive anal carcinoma in HIV positive patients receiving highly active anti-retroviral therapy versus non-HIV patients. (ASCO 2012). *J Clin Oncol* 2012;30 (supplement).

14. Daling JR, Madeleine MM, Johnson LG, et al. Human papillomavirus, smoking, and sexual practices in the etiology of anal cancer. *Cancer* 2004; 101:270–280.

15. Grulich AE, van Leeuwen MT, Falster MO, et al. Incidence of cancers in people with HIV/AIDS compared with immunosuppressed transplant recipients: a meta-analysis. *Lancet* 2007;370:59–67.

16. Berry JM, Jay N, Cranston RD, et al. Progression of anal high-grade squamous intraepithelial lesions to invasive anal cancer among HIV-infected men who have sex with men. *Int J Cancer* 2014;134:1147–1155.

17. Palefsky JM, Holly EA, Hogeboom CJ, et al. Virologic, immunologic, and clinical parameters in the incidence and progression of anal squamous intraepithelial lesions in HIV-positive and HIV-negative homosexual men. *J Acquir Immune Defic Syndr Hum Retrovirol* 1998;17:314–319.

18. Kreuter A, Potthoff A, Brockmeyer NH, et al. Anal carcinoma in human immunodeficiency virus-positive men: results of a prospective study from Germany. *Br J Dermatol* 2010;162:1269–1277.

19. Jay N, Berry JM, Hogeboom CJ, et al. Colposcopic appearance of anal squamous intraepithelial lesions: relationship to histopathology. *Dis Colon Rectum* 1997;40:919–928.

20. Gimenez F, Costa-e-Silva IT, Daumas A, et al. The value of high-resolution anoscopy in the diagnosis of anal cancer precursor lesions in HIV-positive patients. *Arq Gastroenterol* 2011;48:136–145.

21. Fox PA, Nathan M, Francis N, et al. A double-blind, randomized controlled trial of the use of imiquimod cream for the treatment of anal canal high-grade anal intraepithelial neoplasia in HIV-positive MSM on HAART, with long-term follow-up data including the use of open-label imiquimod. *AIDS* 2010;24:2331–2335.

22. Richel O, Wieland U, de Vries HJ, et al. Topical 5-fluorouracil treatment of anal intraepithelial neoplasia in human immunodeficiency virus-positive men. *Br J Dermatol* 2010;163:1301–1307.

23. Singh JC, Kuohung V, Palefsky JM. Efficacy of trichloroacetic acid in the treatment of anal intraepithelial neoplasia in HIV-positive and HIV-negative men who have sex with men. *J Acquir Immune Defic Syndr* 2009;52:474–479.

24. Macaya A, Munoz-Santos C, Balaguer A, et al. Interventions for anal canal intraepithelial neoplasia. *Cochrane Database Syst Rev* 2012;12:CD009244.

25. FUTURE II Study Group. Quadrivalent vaccine against human papillomavirus to prevent high-grade cervical lesions. *N Engl J Med* 2007;356:1915–1927.

26. Paavonen J, Jenkins D, Bosch FX, et al. Efficacy of a prophylactic adjuvanted bivalent L1 virus-like-particle vaccine against infection with human papillomavirus types 16 and 18 in young women: an interim analysis of a phase III double-blind, randomised controlled trial. *Lancet* 2007;369:2161–2170.

27. Villa LL, Costa RL, Petta CA, et al. High sustained efficacy of a prophylactic quadrivalent human papillomavirus types 6/11/16/18 L1 virus-like particle vaccine through 5 years of follow-up. *Br J Cancer* 2006;95:1459–1466.

28. Palefsky JM, Giuliano AR, Goldstone S, et al. HPV vaccine against anal HPV infection and anal intraepithelial neoplasia. *N Engl J Med* 2011;365: 1576–1585.

29. Fenger C, Frisch M, Marti MC, et al. Tumors of the anal canal. In: Hamilton SR, Aaltonen LA, eds. *World Health Organization Classification of Tumors. Pathology and Genetics of Tumors of the Digestive System.* Lyon, France: IARC Press, 2000:145–155.

30. Scholefield JH, Castle MT, Watson NF. Malignant transformation of high-grade anal intraepithelial neoplasia. *Br J Surg* 2005;92:1133–1136.

31. Glynne-Jones R, Renehan A. Current treatment of anal squamous cell carcinoma. *Hematol Oncol Clin North Am* 2012;26:1315–1350.

32. Lemarchand N, Tanne F, Aubert M, et al. Is routine pathologic evaluation of hemorrhoidectomy specimens necessary? *Gastroenterol Clin Biol* 2004;28:659–661.

33. Kreuter A, Brockmeyer NH, Hochdorfer B, et al. Clinical spectrum and virologic characteristics of anal intraepithelial neoplasia in HIV infection. *J Am Acad Dermatol* 2005;52:603–608.

34. Wietfeldt ED, Thiele J. Malignancies of the anal margin and perianal skin. *Clin Colon Rectal Surg* 2009;22:127–135.

35. Tehranian S, Treglia G, Krag DN, et al. Sentinel node mapping in anal canal cancer: systematic review and meta-analysis. *J Gastrointestin Liver Dis* 2013;22:321–328.

36. Sveistrup J, Loft A, Berthelsen AK, et al. Positron emission tomography/computed tomography in the staging and treatment of anal cancer. *Int J Radiat Oncol Biol Phys* 2012;83:134–141.

37. Wells IT, Fox BM. PET/CT in anal cancer—is it worth doing? *Clin Radiol* 2012;67:535–540.

38. Vercellino L, Montravers F, de Parades V, et al. Impact of FDG PET/CT in the staging and the follow-up of anal carcinoma. *Int J Colorectal Dis* 2011;26: 201–210.

39. Day FL, Link E, Ngan S, et al. FDG-PET metabolic response predicts outcomes in anal cancer managed with chemoradiotherapy. *Br J Cancer* 2011;105:498–504.

40. National Comprehensive Cancer Network (NCCN). NCCN Clinical Practice Guidelines in Oncology - Anal Carcinoma (Version 2.2014). http://www.nccn.org/professionals/physician_gls/pdf/anal.pdf. Accessed June 20, 2014.

41. Touboul E, Schlienger M, Buffat L, et al. Epidermoid carcinoma of the anal canal. Results of curative-intent radiation therapy in a series of 270 patients. *Cancer* 1994;73:1569–1579.

42. Ajani JA, Winter KA, Gunderson LL, et al. Prognostic factors derived from a prospective database dictate clinical biology of anal cancer: the intergroup trial (RTOG 98-11). *Cancer* 2010;116:4007–4013.

43. Bartelink H, Roelofsen F, Eschwege F, et al. Concomitant radiotherapy and chemotherapy is superior to radiotherapy alone in the treatment of locally advanced anal cancer: results of a phase III randomized trial of the European Organization for Research and Treatment of Cancer Radiotherapy and Gastrointestinal Cooperative Groups. *J Clin Oncol* 1997;15:2040–2049.

44. Glynne-Jones R, Sebag-Montefiore D, Adams R, et al. Prognostic factors for recurrence and survival in anal cancer: generating hypotheses from the mature outcomes of the first United Kingdom Coordinating Committee on Cancer Research Anal Cancer Trial (ACT I). *Cancer* 2013;119:748–755.

45. Cummings BJ, Keane TJ, O'Sullivan B, et al. Epidermoid anal cancer: treatment by radiation alone or by radiation and 5-fluorouracil with and without mitomycin C. *Int J Radiat Oncol Biol Phys* 1991;21:1115–1125.

46. Das P, Bhatia S, Eng C, et al. Predictors and patterns of recurrence after definitive chemoradiation for anal cancer. *Int J Radiat Oncol Biol Phys* 2007;68:794–800.

47. Flam M, John M, Pajak TF, et al. Role of mitomycin in combination with fluorouracil and radiotherapy, and of salvage chemoradiation in the definitive nonsurgical treatment of epidermoid carcinoma of the anal canal: results of a phase III randomized intergroup study. *J Clin Oncol* 1996;14:2527–2539.

48. Schlienger M, Krzisch C, Pene F, et al. Epidermoid carcinoma of the anal canal treatment results and prognostic variables in a series of 242 cases. *Int J Radiat Oncol Biol Phys* 1989;17:1141–1151.

49. Oldenhuis CN, Oosting SF, Gietema JA, et al. Prognostic versus predictive value of biomarkers in oncology. *Eur J Cancer* 2008;44:946–953.

50. Lampejo T, Kavanagh D, Clark J, et al. Prognostic biomarkers in squamous cell carcinoma of the anus: a systematic review. *Br J Cancer* 2010;103:1858–1869.

51. Kastan MB, Canman CE, Leonard CJ. P53, cell cycle control and apoptosis: implications for cancer. *Cancer Metastasis Rev* 1995;14:3–15.

52. Wong CS, Tsao MS, Sharma V, et al. Prognostic role of p53 protein expression in epidermoid carcinoma of the anal canal. *Int J Radiat Oncol Biol Phys* 1999;45:309–314.

53. Tanum G, Holm R. Anal carcinoma: a clinical approach to p53 and RB gene proteins. *Oncology* 1996;53:369–373.

54. Indinnimeo M, Cicchini C, Stazi A, et al. Human papillomavirus infection and p53 nuclear overexpression in anal canal carcinoma. *J Exp Clin Cancer Res* 1999;18:47–52.

55. Ajani JA, Wang X, Izzo JG, et al. Molecular biomarkers correlate with disease-free survival in patients with anal canal carcinoma treated with chemoradiation. *Dig Dis Sci* 2010;55:1098–1105.

56. Bonin SR, Pajak TF, Russell AH, et al. Overexpression of p53 protein and outcome of patients treated with chemoradiation for carcinoma of the anal canal: a report of randomized trial RTOG 87-04. Radiation Therapy Oncology Group. *Cancer* 1999;85:1226–1233.

57. Allal AS, Waelchli L, Brundler MA. Prognostic value of apoptosis-regulating protein expression in anal squamous cell carcinoma. *Clin Cancer Res* 2003;9:6489–6496.

58. el-Deiry WS, Tokino T, Velculescu VE, et al. WAF1, a potential mediator of p53 tumor suppression. *Cell* 1993;75:817–825.

59. Holm R, Skovlund E, Skomedal H, et al. Reduced expression of p21WAF1 is an indicator of malignant behaviour in anal carcinomas. *Histopathology* 2001;39:43–49.

60. Nilsson PJ, Lenander C, Rubio C, et al. Prognostic significance of Cyclin A in epidermoid anal cancer. *Oncol Rep* 2006;16:443–449.

61. Steele SR, Varma MG, Melton GB, et al. Practice parameters for anal squamous neoplasms. *Dis Colon Rectum* 2012;55:735–749.

62. Boman BM, Moertel CG, O'Connell MJ, et al. Carcinoma of the anal canal. A clinical and pathologic study of 188 cases. *Cancer* 1984;54:114–125.

63. Singh R, Nime F, Mittelman A. Malignant epithelial tumors of the anal canal. *Cancer* 1981;48:411–415.

64. Nigro ND, Vaitkevicius VK, Considine B Jr. Combined therapy for cancer of the anal canal: a preliminary report. *Dis Colon Rectum* 1974;17:354–356.

65. Nigro ND, Vaitkevicius VK, Buroker T, et al. Combined therapy for cancer of the anal canal. *Dis Colon Rectum* 1981;24:73–75.

66. Nigro ND, Seydel HG, Considine B, et al. Combined preoperative radiation and chemotherapy for squamous cell carcinoma of the anal canal. *Cancer* 1983;51:1826–1829.

67. Leichman L, Nigro N, Vaitkevicius VK, et al. Cancer of the anal canal. Model for preoperative adjuvant combined modality therapy. *Am J Med* 1985;78:211–215.

68. Meeker WR Jr, Sickle-Santanello BJ, Philpott G, et al. Combined chemotherapy, radiation, and surgery for epithelial cancer of the anal canal. *Cancer* 1986;57:525–529.

69. Michaelson RA, Magill GB, Quan SH, et al. Preoperative chemotherapy and radiation therapy in the management of anal epidermoid carcinoma. *Cancer* 1983;51:390–395.

70. Epidermoid anal cancer: results from the UKCCCR randomised trial of radiotherapy alone versus radiotherapy, 5-fluorouracil, and mitomycin. UKCCCR Anal Cancer Trial Working Party. UK Co-ordinating Committee on Cancer Research. *Lancet* 1996;348:1049–1054.

71. Northover J, Glynne-Jones R, Sebag-Montefiore D, et al. Chemoradiation for the treatment of epidermoid anal cancer: 13-year follow-up of the first randomised UKCCCR Anal Cancer Trial (ACT I). *Br J Cancer* 2010;102:1123–1128.

CANCERS OF THE GASTROINTESTINAL TRACT

72. Meropol NJ, Niedzwiecki D, Shank B, et al. Induction therapy for poor-prognosis anal canal carcinoma: a phase II study of the cancer and Leukemia Group B (CALGB 9281). *J Clin Oncol* 2008;26:3229–3234.

73. Ajani JA, Winter KA, Gunderson LL, et al. Fluorouracil, mitomycin, and radiotherapy vs fluorouracil, cisplatin, and radiotherapy for carcinoma of the anal canal: a randomized controlled trial. *JAMA* 2008;299:1914–1921.

74. Gunderson LL, Winter KA, Ajani JA, et al. Long-term update of US GI intergroup RTOG 98-11 phase III trial for anal carcinoma: survival, relapse, and colostomy failure with concurrent chemoradiation involving fluorouracil/mitomycin versus fluorouracil/cisplatin. *J Clin Oncol* 2012;30:4344–4351.

75. James RD, Glynne-Jones R, Meadows HM, et al. Mitomycin or cisplatin chemoradiation with or without maintenance chemotherapy for treatment of squamous-cell carcinoma of the anus (ACT II): a randomised, phase 3, open-label, 2 × 2 factorial trial. *Lancet Oncol* 2013;14:516–524.

76. Peiffert D, Tournier-Rangeard L, Gerard JP, et al. Induction chemotherapy and dose intensification of the radiation boost in locally advanced anal canal carcinoma: final analysis of the randomized UNICANCER ACCORD 03 trial. *J Clin Oncol* 2012;30:1941–1948.

77. Ajani JA, Winter KA, Gunderson LL, et al. Intergroup RTOG 98-11: a phase III randomized study of 5-fluorouracil (5-FU), mitomycin, and radiotherapy versus 5-fluorouracil, cisplatin and radiotherapy in carcinoma of the anal canal. *J Clin Oncol* 2006;24:180s.

78. Gunderson LL, Winter KA, Ajani JA, et al. Intergroup RTOG 9811 phase III comparison of chemoradiation with 5-FU and mitomycin vs 5-FU and cisplatin for anal canal carcinoma: impact of disease-free, overall and colostomy-free survival (abstract). *Int J Radiat Oncol Biol Phys* 2006;66:S24.

79. Garg M, Lee JY, Kachnic L, et al. Phase II trials of cetuximab (CX) plus cisplatin (CDDP), 5-fluorouracil (5-FU) and radiation (RT) in immunocompetent (ECOG 3205) and HIV positive (AMCO45) patients with squamous cell carcinoma of the anal canal (SCAC): Safety and preliminary efficacy results. *J Clin Oncol* 2012;30:abstr 4030.

80. Deutsch E, Lemanski C, Paris E, et al. Cetuximab plus radiochemotherapy in locally advanced anal cancer: Interim results of the French multicenter phase II trial ACCORD16. *J Clin Oncol* 2011;29:abstr 4098.

81. Salama JK, Mell LK, Schomas DA, et al. Concurrent chemotherapy and intensity-modulated radiation therapy for anal canal cancer patients: a multicenter experience. *J Clin Oncol* 2007;25:4581–4586.

82. Pepek JM, Willett CG, Wu QJ, et al. Intensity-modulated radiation therapy for anal malignancies: a preliminary toxicity and disease outcomes analysis. *Int J Radiat Oncol Biol Phys* 2010;78:1413–1419.

83. Ben-Josef E, Moughan J, Ajani JA, et al. Impact of overall treatment time on survival and local control in patients with anal cancer: a pooled data analysis of Radiation Therapy Oncology Group trials 87-04 and 98-11. *J Clin Oncol* 2010;28:5061–5066.

84. Kachnic LA, Tsai HK, Coen JJ, et al. Dose-painted intensity-modulated radiation therapy for anal cancer: a multi-institutional report of acute toxicity and response to therapy. *Int J Radiat Oncol Biol Phys* 2012;82:153–158.

85. Kachnic LA, Winter K, Myerson RJ, et al. RTOG 0529: a phase 2 evaluation of dose-painted intensity modulated radiation therapy in combination with 5-fluorouracil and mitomycin-C for the reduction of acute morbidity in carcinoma of the anal canal. *Int J Radiat Oncol Biol Phys* 2013;86:27–33.

86. Tanum G. Treatment of relapsing anal carcinoma. *Acta Oncol* 1993;32:33–35.

87. Glynne-Jones R, James R, Meadows H, et al, eds. Optimum time to assess complete clinical response (CR) following chemoradiation (CRT) using mitomycin (MMC) or cisplatin (CisP), with or without maintenance CisP/5FU in squamous cell carcinoma of the anus: Results of ACT II. Paper presented at: 2012 ASCO Annual Meeting; 2012; Chicago, IL.

88. Sebag-Montefiore D, James R, Meadows H, et al. The pattern and timing of disease recurrence in cancer of the anus: mature results from the NCRI ACT II trial. J Clin Oncol. 2012;30. 2012 ASCO Annual Meeting.

89. Edelman S, Johnstone PA. Combined modality therapy for HIV-infected patients with squamous cell carcinoma of the anus: outcomes and toxicities. *Int J Radiat Oncol Biol Phys* 2006;66:206–211.

90. Cleator S, Fife K, Nelson M, et al. Treatment of HIV-associated invasive anal cancer with combined chemoradiation. *Eur J Cancer* 2000;36:754–758.

91. Peddada AV, Smith DE, Rao AR, et al. Chemotherapy and low-dose radiotherapy in the treatment of HIV-infected patients with carcinoma of the anal canal. *Int J Radiat Oncol Biol Phys* 1997;37:1101–1105.

92. Oehler-Janne C, Seifert B, Lutolf UM, et al. Local tumor control and toxicity in HIV-associated anal carcinoma treated with radiotherapy in the era of antiretroviral therapy. *Radiat Oncol* 2006;1:29.

93. Kauh J, Koshy M, Gunthel C, et al. Management of anal cancer in the HIV-positive population. *Oncology (Williston Park)* 2005;19:1634–1638.

94. Hoffman R, Welton ML, Klencke B, et al. The significance of pretreatment CD4 count on the outcome and treatment tolerance of HIV-positive patients with anal cancer. *Int J Radiat Oncol Biol Phys* 1999;44:127–131.

95. Place RJ, Gregorcyk SG, Huber PJ, et al. Outcome analysis of HIV-positive patients with anal squamous cell carcinoma. *Dis Colon Rectum* 2001;44:506–512.

96. Garg M, Lee JY, Kachnic L, et al. Phase II trials of cetuximab (CX) plus cisplatin (CDDP), 5-fluorouracil (5-FU) and radiation (RT) in immunocompetent (ECOG 3205) and HIV-positive (AMC045) patients with squamous cell carcinoma of the anal canal (SCAC): Safety and preliminary efficacy results. 2012 ASCO Annual Meeting.

97. Blazy A, Hennequin C, Gornet JM, et al. Anal carcinomas in HIV-positive patients: high-dose chemoradiotherapy is feasible in the era of highly active antiretroviral therapy. *Dis Colon Rectum* 2005;48:1176–1181.

98. Munoz-Bongrand N, Poghosyan T, Zohar S, et al. Anal carcinoma in HIV-infected patients in the era of antiretroviral therapy: a comparative study. *Dis Colon Rectum* 2011;54:729–735.

99. Seo Y, Kinsella MT, Reynolds HL, et al. Outcomes of chemoradiotherapy with 5-Fluorouracil and mitomycin C for anal cancer in immunocompetent versus immunodeficient patients. *Int J Radiat Oncol Biol Phys* 2009;75:143–149.

100. Oehler-Janne C, Huguet F, Provencher S, et al. HIV-specific differences in outcome of squamous cell carcinoma of the anal canal: a multicentric cohort study of HIV-positive patients receiving highly active antiretroviral therapy. *J Clin Oncol* 2008;26:2550–2557.

101. Sunesen KG, Buntzen S, Tei T, et al. Perineal healing and survival after anal cancer salvage surgery: 10-year experience with primary perineal reconstruction using the vertical rectus abdominis myocutaneous (VRAM) flap. *Ann Surg Oncol* 2009;16:68–77.

102. Akbari RP, Paty PB, Guillem JG, et al. Oncologic outcomes of salvage surgery for epidermoid carcinoma of the anus initially managed with combined modality therapy. *Dis Colon Rectum* 2004;47:1136–1144.

103. Schiller DE, Cummings BJ, Rai S, et al. Outcomes of salvage surgery for squamous cell carcinoma of the anal canal. *Ann Surg Oncol* 2007;14:2780–2789.

104. Correa JH, Castro LS, Kesley R, et al. Salvage abdominoperineal resection for anal cancer following chemoradiation: a proposed scoring system for predicting postoperative survival. *J Surg Oncol* 2013;107:486–492.

105. Nilsson PJ, Svensson C, Goldman S, et al. Salvage abdominoperineal resection in anal epidermoid cancer. *Br J Surg* 2002;89:1425–1429.

106. Ghouti L, Houvenaeghel G, Moutardier V, et al. Salvage abdominoperineal resection after failure of conservative treatment in anal epidermoid cancer. *Dis Colon Rectum* 2005;48:16–22.

107. Renehan AG, Saunders MP, Schofield PF, et al. Patterns of local disease failure and outcome after salvage surgery in patients with anal cancer. *Br J Surg* 2005;92:605–614.

108. Lefevre JH, Parc Y, Kerneis S, et al. Abdomino-perineal resection for anal cancer: impact of a vertical rectus abdominis myocutaneous flap on survival, recurrence, morbidity, and wound healing. *Ann Surg* 2009;250:707–711.

109. Ferenschild FT, Vermaas M, Hofer SO, et al. Salvage abdominoperineal resection and perineal wound healing in local recurrent or persistent anal cancer. *World J Surg* 2005;29:1452–1457.

110. Eeson G, Foo M, Harrow S, et al. Outcomes of salvage surgery for epidermoid carcinoma of the anus following failed combined modality treatment. *Am J Surg* 2011;201:628–633.

111. Lefevre JH, Corte H, Tiret E, et al. Abdominoperineal resection for squamous cell anal carcinoma: survival and risk factors for recurrence. *Ann Surg Oncol* 2012;19:4186–4192.

112. Faivre C, Rougier P, Ducreux M, et al. [5-fluorouracile and cisplatinum combination chemotherapy for metastatic squamous-cell anal cancer]. *Bull Cancer* 1999;86:861–865.

113. Jaiyesimi IA, Pazdur R. Cisplatin and 5-fluorouracil as salvage therapy for recurrent metastatic squamous cell carcinoma of the anal canal. *Am J Clin Oncol* 1993;16:536–540.

114. Khater R, Frenay M, Bourry J, et al. Cisplatin plus 5-fluorouracil in the treatment of metastatic anal squamous cell carcinoma: a report of two cases. *Cancer Treat Rep* 1986;70:1345–1346.

115. Ajani JA, Carrasco CH, Jackson DE, et al. Combination of cisplatin plus fluoropyrimidine chemotherapy effective against liver metastases from carcinoma of the anal canal. *Am J Med* 1989;87:221–224.

116. Greenall MJ, Quan SH, Stearns MW, et al. Epidermoid cancer of the anal margin. Pathologic features, treatment, and clinical results. *Am J Surg* 1985;149:95–101.

117. Dewdney A, Rao S. Metastatic squamous cell carcinoma of the anus: time for a shift in the treatment paradigm? *ISRN Oncol* 2012;2012:756591.

118. Wilking N, Petrelli N, Herrera L, et al. Phase II study of combination bleomycin, vincristine and high-dose methotrexate (BOM) with leucovorin rescue in advanced squamous cell carcinoma of the anal canal. *Cancer Chemother Pharmacol* 1985;15:300–302.

119. Hainsworth JD, Burris HA 3rd, Meluch AA, et al. Paclitaxel, carboplatin, and long-term continuous infusion of 5-fluorouracil in the treatment of advanced squamous and other selected carcinomas: results of a Phase II trial. *Cancer* 2001;92:642–649.

120. Jhawer M, Mani S, Lefkopoulou M, et al. Phase II study of mitomycin-C, adriamycin, cisplatin (MAP) and Bleomycin-CCNU in patients with advanced cancer of the anal canal: An eastern cooperative oncology group study E7282. *Invest New Drugs* 2006;24:447–454.

121. Eng C, Rogers J, Chang GJ, et al. Choice of chemotherapy in the treatment of metastatic squamous cell carcinoma of the anal canal. *J Clin Oncol* 2012;30:abstr 4060.

122. Evans TR, Mansi JL, Glees JP. Response of metastatic anal carcinoma to single agent carboplatin. *Clin Oncol (R Coll Radiol)* 1993;5:57–58.

123. Zimm S, Wampler GL. Response of metastatic cloacogenic carcinoma to treatment with semustine. *Cancer* 1981;48:2575–2576.

124. Grifaichi F, Padovani A, Romeo F, et al. Response of metastatic epidermoid anal cancer to single agent irinotecan: a case report. *Tumori* 2001;87:58–59.

125. Bonner JA, Harari PM, Giralt J, et al. Radiotherapy plus cetuximab for squamous-cell carcinoma of the head and neck. *N Engl J Med* 2006;354:567–578.

126. De Dosso S, Martin V, Zanellato E, et al. Molecular characterization and response to cetuximab in a patient with refractory squamous cell anal carcinoma. *Tumori* 2010;96:627–628.

127. Lukan N, Strobel P, Willer A, et al. Cetuximab-based treatment of metastatic anal cancer: correlation of response with KRAS mutational status. *Oncology* 2009;77:293–299.

128. Phan LK, Hoff PM. Evidence of clinical activity for cetuximab combined with irinotecan in a patient with refractory anal canal squamous-cell carcinoma: report of a case. *Dis Colon Rectum* 2007;50:395–398.

129. Pawlik TM, Gleisner AL, Bauer TW, et al. Liver-directed surgery for metastatic squamous cell carcinoma to the liver: results of a multi-center analysis. *Ann Surg Oncol* 2007;14:2807–2816.

130. Hodges JC, Das P, Eng C, et al. Intensity-modulated radiation therapy for the treatment of squamous cell anal cancer with para-aortic nodal involvement. *Int J Radiat Oncol Biol Phys* 2009;75:791–794.

131. Charnley N, Choudhury A, Chesser P, et al. Effective treatment of anal cancer in the elderly with low-dose chemoradiotherapy. *Br J Cancer* 2005;92:1221–1225.

132. Cutuli B, Fenton J, Labib A, et al. Anal margin carcinoma: 21 cases treated at the Institut Curie by exclusive conservative radiotherapy. *Radiother Oncol* 1988;11:1–6.

133. Peiffert D, Bey P, Pernot M, et al. Conservative treatment by irradiation of epidermoid carcinomas of the anal margin. *Int J Radiat Oncol Biol Phys* 1997;39:57–66.

134. Chawla AK, Willett CG. Squamous cell carcinoma of the anal canal and anal margin. *Hematol Oncol Clin North Am* 2001;15:321–344.

135. Morson B. The pathology and results of treatment of squamous cell carcinoma of the anal canal and anal margin. *J R Soc Med* 1960:53.

136. Papillon J, Chassard JL. Respective roles of radiotherapy and surgery in the management of epidermoid carcinoma of the anal margin. Series of 57 patients. *Dis Colon Rectum* 1992;35:422–429.

137. Chapet O, Gerard JP, Mornex F, et al. Prognostic factors of squamous cell carcinoma of the anal margin treated by radiotherapy: the Lyon experience. *Int J Colorectal Dis* 2007;22:191–199.

138. Khanfir K, Ozsahin M, Bieri S, et al. Patterns of failure and outcome in patients with carcinoma of the anal margin. *Ann Surg Oncol* 2008;15:1092–1098.

139. Balamucki CJ, Zlotecki RA, Rout WR, et al. Squamous cell carcinoma of the anal margin: the university of Florida experience. *Am J Clin Oncol* 2011;34:406–410.

140. Deans GT, McAleer JJ, Spence RA. Malignant anal tumours. *Br J Surg* 1994;81:500–508.

141. Chia CS, Chew MH, Chau YP, et al. Adenocarcinoma of the anal transitional zone after double stapled ileal pouch-anal anastomosis for ulcerative colitis. *Colorectal Dis* 2008;10:621–623.

142. Ota H, Yamazaki K, Endoh W, et al. Adenocarcinoma arising below an ileoanal anastomosis after restorative proctocolectomy for ulcerative colitis: report of a case. *Surg Today* 2007;37:596–599.

143. Wong NA, Shirazi T, Hamer-Hodges DW, et al. Adenocarcinoma arising within a Crohn's-related anorectal fistula: a form of anal gland carcinoma? *Histopathology* 2002;40:302–304.

144. Belkacemi Y, Berger C, Poortmans P, et al. Management of primary anal canal adenocarcinoma: a large retrospective study from the Rare Cancer Network. *Int J Radiat Oncol Biol Phys* 2003;56:1274–1283.

145. Kounalakis N, Artinyan A, Smith D, et al. Abdominal perineal resection improves survival for nonmetastatic adenocarcinoma of the anal canal. *Ann Surg Oncol* 2009;16:1310–1315.

146. Papagikos M, Crane CH, Skibber J, et al. Chemoradiation for adenocarcinoma of the anus. *Int J Radiat Oncol Biol Phys* 2003;55:669–678.

147. Weinstock MA. Epidemiology and prognosis of anorectal melanoma. *Gastroenterology* 1993;104:174–178.

148. Iversen K, Robins RE. Mucosal malignant melanomas. *Am J Surg* 1980;139:660–664.

149. Wanebo HJ, Woodruff JM, Farr GH, et al. Anorectal melanoma. *Cancer* 1981;47:1891–1900.

150. Brady MS, Kavolius JP, Quan SH. Anorectal melanoma. A 64-year experience at Memorial Sloan-Kettering Cancer Center. *Dis Colon Rectum* 1995;38:146–151.

151. Quan SH, White JE, Deddish MR. Malignant melanoma of the anorectum. *Dis Colon Rectum* 1959;2:275–283.

152. Metildi C, McLemore EC, Tran T, et al. Incidence and survival patterns of rare anal canal neoplasms using the surveillance epidemiology and end results registry. *Am Surg* 2013;79:1068–1074.

153. Slingluff CL Jr, Seigler HF. Anorectal melanoma: clinical characteristics and the role of abdominoperineal resection. *Ann Plast Surg* 1992;28:85–88.

154. Kiran R, Rottoli M, Pokala N, et al. Long-term outcomes after local excision and radical surgery for anal melanoma: data from a population database. *Dis Colon Rectum* 2010;53:402.

155. Nilsson PJ, Ragnarsson-Olding BK. Importance of clear resection margins in anorectal malignant melanoma. *Br J Surg* 2010;97:98–103.

156. Kanaan Z, Mulhall A, Mahid S, et al. A systematic review of prognosis and therapy of anal malignant melanoma: a plea for more precise reporting of location and thickness. *Am Surg* 2012;78:28–35.

157. Ishizone S, Koide N, Karasawa F, et al. Surgical treatment for anorectal malignant melanoma: report of five cases and review of 79 Japanese cases. *Int J Colorectal Dis* 2008;23:1257–1262.

158. Ballo MT, Gershenwald JE, Zagars GK, et al. Sphincter-sparing local excision and adjuvant radiation for anal-rectal melanoma. *J Clin Oncol* 2002;20:4555–4558.

INDEX

Note: page locators followed by *f* and *t* indicate figure and table, respectively.